APPLIED THERAPEUTICS
The Clinical Use of Drugs

Third Edition ———————————————

Applied Therapeutics

The Clinical Use of Drugs

Edited by

Brian S. Katcher, Pharm.D.
Lecturer in Pharmacy
School of Pharmacy
University of California
San Francisco

Lloyd Y. Young, Pharm.D.
Associate Professor of Clinical Pharmacy
College of Pharmacy
Washington State University
Pullman

Mary Anne Koda-Kimble, Pharm.D.
Associate Clinical Professor of Pharmacy
Vice-Chairwoman, Division of Clinical Pharmacy
School of Pharmacy
University of California
San Francisco

Applied Therapeutics, Inc.
Spokane

Book Design and Layout: Michael Fong
Typesetting: Vera Allen Composition
Printing and Binding: Edwards Brothers

Other publications by Applied Therapeutics, Inc:

DRUG INTERACTIONS NEWSLETTER: A Clinical Perspective and
Analysis of Current Developments, Edited by Philip D. Hansten

Basic Clinical Pharmacokinetics by Michael E. Winter

Applied Pharmacokinetics: Principles of Therapeutic Drug Monitoring, Edited by William E. Evans, Jerome J. Schentag, and William
J. Jusko

Applied Therapeutics, Inc.
P.O. Box 1903
Spokane, WA 99210-1903

Library of Congress Catalog Card Number 82-073291
ISBN 0-915486-05-9

Third Printing—September 1983
Fourth Printing—February 1984
Fifth Printing—July 1984
Sixth Printing—September 1985

Contents

Respiratory Disorders

Gastrointestinal Disorders
John Russo, Jr., Section Editor

Hepatic Disorders

Renal Disorders

Disorders of Metabolism and Nutrition

Infectious Disease
B. Joseph Guglielmo and Steven L. Barriere, Section Editors

Hematopoietic Disorders

Neoplasms

Psychiatric Disorders

Drug Abuse

Neurologic Disorders

Rex S. Lott, Section Editor

Skin Disorders

Eye Disorders

Contraception

Endocrine Disorders

Joint and Connective Tissue Disorders

Special Age Groups

Poisonings

Contributors

Steven R. Abel, Pharm.D.
Assistant Director of Pharmacy, Clinical and Educational Services, Department of Pharmacy, Indiana University Hospitals, Indianapolis.

R. Jon Auricchio, Pharm.D.
Assistant Director, Internal Medicine Spokane; Assistant Professor of Clinical Pharmacy, College of Pharmacy, Washington State University, Pullman.

Steven L. Barriere, Pharm.D.
Associate Clinical Professor of Pharmacy, Division of Clinical Pharmacy, School of Pharmacy; Lecturer in Pharmacology, Pharmacology Department, School of Medicine, University of California, San Francisco.

C.A. Bond, Pharm.D.
Assistant Dean for Professional and Student Affairs, Clinical Associate Professor, School of Pharmacy, University of Wisconsin, Madison.

John A. Bosso, Pharm.D.
Associate Professor of Clinical Pharmacy, Department of Pharmacy Practice, College of Pharmacy; Adjunct Associate Professor of Pediatrics, Department of Pediatrics, School of Medicine, University of Utah, Salt Lake City.

Thomas J. Cali, Pharm.D.
Assistant Professor of Clinical Pharmacy, Department of Clinical Pharmacy, University of Maryland Hospital, University of Maryland, Baltimore.

Moses S. Chow, Pharm.D.
Associate Clinical Professor, School of Pharmacy, University of Connecticut, Storrs; Director of Drug Information Service and Assistant Director of Pharmacy Services, Hartford Hospital, Hartford, Connecticut.

James H. Coleman, Pharm.D.
Clinical Specialist-Psychiatry, Veterans Administration Medical Center, Memphis, Tennessee; Assistant Professor of Clinical Pharmacy in Psychiatry, Department of Psychiatry; Associate Professor, Department of Pharmacy Practice,

University of Tennessee Center for the Health Sciences, Memphis.

Gary C. Cupit, Pharm.D.
Clinical Associate Professor of Pharmacy, Philadelphia College of Pharmacy and Science; Adjunct Assistant Professor of Pharmacy in Pediatrics, School of Medicine, University of Pennsylvania, Philadelphia; Executive Director, Delaware Valley Regional Poison Control Center.

Stephen L. Dahl, Pharm.D.
Clinical Assistant Professor Pharmacy Practice, College of Pharmacy; Adjunct Instructor, Department of Medicine, Division of Rheumatology, University of Utah, Salt Lake City.

Charles C. Depew, Pharm.D.
Pharmacist, Medical/Surgical Intensive Care Unit, Department of Pharmacy, Stanford University Medical Center, Stanford, California.

Richard F. de Leon, Pharm.D.
Associate Professor of Pharmacy, Associate Dean for Clinical Sciences, School of Pharmacy; Director of Pharmacy Services, University Hospitals, University of Michigan, Ann Arbor.

Betty J. Dong, Pharm.D.
Associate Clinical Professor of Pharmacy, Division of Clinical Pharmacy, School of Pharmacy; Associate Clinical Professor, Division of Family and Community Medicine, School of Medicine, University of California, San Francisco.

James E. DuBe, Pharm.D.
Associate Director, Pharmaceutical Services, University of Nebraska Hospitals; Assistant Professor, Department of Pharmacy Practice, College of Pharmacy, University of Nebraska, Omaha.

George E. Dukes, Jr., Pharm.D.
Assistant Professor of Clinical Pharmacy, Department of Pharmacy Practice, College of Pharmacy, University of Utah, Salt Lake City.

Cynthia B. Dunham, M.S.
Instructor of Clinical Pharmacy, Division of Pharmacy Practice, School of Pharmacy, Univer-

sity of North Carolina, Chapel Hill; Clinical Pharmacist, Nephrology Service, North Carolina Memorial Hospital, Chapel Hill.

Thomas W. Dunphy, Pharm.D.
Community Pharmacist; Associate Clinical Professor, Division of Clinical Pharmacy, School of Pharmacy, University of California, San Francisco.

Julia K. Elenbaas, Pharm.D.
Associate Professor of Clinical Pharmacy, Director of Drug Information Service, Division of Professional Practice, University of Missouri, Kansas City.

James C. Eoff, III, Pharm.D.
Associate Professor of Pharmacy Practice, Department of Pharmacy Practice, College of Pharmacy, University of Tennessee, Memphis.

Larry Ereshefsky, Pharm.D.
Associate Professor of Pharmacy, Assistant Professor of Psychiatry and Pharmacology, Clinical Pharmacy Program, Department of Pharmacology, University of Texas Health Science Center, San Antonio, and University of Texas, Austin.

William E. Evans, Pharm.D.
Director, Clinical Pharmacokinetics and Pharmacodynamics Section, St. Jude Children's Research Hospital, Memphis, Tennessee; Associate Professor of Pharmaceutics and Clinical Pharmacy, University of Tennessee, Memphis.

Ronald P. Evens, Pharm.D.
Associate Professor and Chairman (Acting), Department of Pharmacy Practice, College of Pharmacy, University of Tennessee Center for the Health Sciences, Memphis.

Kermit J. Fendler, Pharm.D.
Assistant Professor of Clinical Pharmacy, Division of Pharmacy Practice, School of Pharmacy, University of Missouri, Kansas City.

John G. Gambertoglio, Pharm.D.
Adjunct Associate Professor of Pharmacy, Division of Clinical Pharmacy, School of Pharmacy, University of California, San Francisco.

Joseph P. Gee, Pharm.D.
Assistant Professor of Pharmacy, College of Pharmacy, University of Michigan, Ann Arbor.

Mark A. Gill, Pharm.D.
Assistant Professor of Clinical Pharmacy, School of Pharmacy, University of Southern California, Los Angeles.

Dick R. Gourley, Pharm.D.
Professor and Chairman, Department of Pharmacy Practice, College of Pharmacy, University of Nebraska Medical Center, Omaha.

Barbara L. Greenberg, Pharm.D.
Coordinator of Education and Training, Adjunct Assistant Professor of Clinical Pharmacy, Cincinnati General Division, Department of Pharmacy, University of Cincinnati Hospitals, Cincinnati, Ohio.

B. Joseph Guglielmo, Pharm.D.
Assistant Clinical Professor of Pharmacy, Division of Clinical Pharmacy, School of Pharmacy; Clinical Pharmacist, Cardiothoracic and Vascular Services and Intensive Care Unit, University of California, San Francisco.

Lawrence J. Hak, Pharm.D.
Associate Professor of Clinical Pharmacy, Clinical Assistant Professor of Medicine, University of North Carolina, Chapel Hill.

Linda L. Hart, Pharm.D.
Associate Clinical Professor of Pharmacy, Director, Drug Information Analysis Service, Division of Clinical Pharmacy, School of Pharmacy, University of California, San Francisco.

Robert J. Ignoffo, Pharm.D.
Associate Clinical Professor, Division of Clinical Pharmacy, School of Pharmacy; Clinical Pharmacist, Cancer Research Institute, University of California, San Francisco.

Darryl S. Inaba, Pharm.D.
Director, Haight-Ashbury Free Medical Clinics Drug Detoxification, Rehabilitation and After Care Project; Assistant Clinical Professor of Pharmacy, Division of Clinical Pharmacy, School of Pharmacy, University of California, San Francisco.

Lucia K. Jim, Pharm.D.
Assistant Professor of Pharmacy, College of Pharmacy, University of Michigan, Ann Arbor.

Martin J. Jinks, Pharm.D.
Associate Professor of Clinical Pharmacy, College of Pharmacy, Washington State University, Pullman.

Joseph A. Johnston, Pharm.D.
Clinical Pharmacist, Veterans Administration Hospital, Memphis, Tennessee; Assistant Professor of Clinical Pharmacy, University of Tennessee Center for the Health Sciences, Memphis, Associate Professor of Nursing, Memphis State University.

Philip E. Johnston, Pharm.D.
Associate Professor of Pharmacy Practice and Director of Ambulatory Care Programs, Department of Pharmacy Practice, University of Tennessee Center for the Health Sciences, Memphis.

Brian S. Katcher, Pharm.D.
Lecturer in Pharmacy, School of Pharmacy, University of California, San Francisco.

Steven R. Kayser, Pharm.D.
Associate Clinical Professor of Pharmacy, Division of Clinical Pharmacy, School of Pharmacy; Clinical Pharmacist, Cardiac Care Unit and Cardiac-Anticoagulant Clinic, University of California, San Francisco.

H. William Kelly, Pharm.D.
Associate Professor of Pharmacy and Assistant Professor of Pediatrics, Department of Clinical Pharmacy, College of Pharmacy, University of New Mexico Medical Center, Albuquerque.

Mary Anne Koda-Kimble, Pharm.D.
Associate Clinical Professor of Pharmacy; Vice-Chairwoman, Division of Clinical Pharmacy, School of Pharmacy; Clinical Pharmacist, Diabetic Clinic, University of California, San Francisco.

Donald T. Kishi, Pharm.D.
Clinical Professor of Pharmacy, Vice-Chairman, Division of Clinical Pharmacy, School of Pharmacy, University of California, San Francisco.

Nancy E. Ryti Korman, Pharm.D.
Supervisor, Clinical Pharmacy Section, Veterans Administration Medical Center, San Francisco, California; Associate Clinical Professor, School of Pharmacy, University of California, San Francisco.

Wayne A. Kradjan, Pharm.D.
Associate Professor of Pharmacy Practice, Department of Pharmacy Practice, School of Pharmacy, University of Washington, Seattle.

Kent E. Lieginger, Pharm.D.
Assistant Clinical Professor, Department of Family Practice, School of Medicine; Clinical Pharmacist, Davis Medical Center, University of California, Davis.

Louis C. Littlefield, Pharm.D.
Associate Professor of Pharmacy, Clinical Pharmacy Program, College of Pharmacy, University of Texas, Austin; Associate Professor of Pediatrics and Pharmacology, Clinical Pharmacy Program, Departments of Pharmacology and Pediatrics, University of Texas Health Science Center, San Antonio.

Rex S. Lott, Pharm.D.
Clinical Pharmacist, Minnesota Department of Public Welfare and Anoka State Hospital; Clinical Assistant Professor, College of Pharmacy, University of Minnesota, Minneapolis.

Richard J. Mangini, Pharm.D.
Research Associate, Mediphor/Minerva Project, Division of Clinical Pharmacology, Department of Medicine, Stanford University Medical Center, Stanford, California.

Anthony S. Manoguerra, Pharm.D.
Associate Clinical Professor, Division of Clinical Pharmacy (San Diego program), School of Pharmacy, University of California, San Francisco; Director for Professional Services, Regional Poison Center, University of California, San Diego.

Gail W. McSweeney, Pharm.D.
Assistant Clinical Professor of Pharmacy, Division of Clinical Pharmacy, School of Pharmacy, University of California, San Francisco.

Robert J. Michocki, Pharm.D.
Assistant Professor of Clinical Pharmacy, School of Pharmacy, University of Maryland, Baltimore; Clinical Pharmacy Consultant, Adult Emergency Room, University of Maryland Hospital, Baltimore.

Donald M. Moran, Pharm.D.
Associate Research Instructor, Burroughs Wellcome Postdoctoral Fellowship in Clinical Pharmacy, College of Pharmacy, University of Utah, Salt Lake City.

Kelly D. Mutchie, Pharm.D.
Assistant Professor of Clinical Pharmacy, Department of Pharmacy Practice, College of Phar-

macy; Adjunct Assistant Professor of Pediatrics, Primary Children's Medical Center, University of Utah, Salt Lake City.

Garry M. Oderda, Pharm.D., M.P.H.
Director, Maryland Poison Center; Associate Professor, Department of Clinical Pharmacy, School of Pharmacy, University of Maryland, Baltimore.

Ralph H. Raasch, Pharm.D.
Assistant Professor of Clinical Pharmacy, Division of Pharmacy Practice, School of Pharmacy; Clinical Assistant Professor of Medicine, School of Medicine, University of North Carolina, Chapel Hill.

Juan R. Robayo, Pharm.D.
Associate Professor and Head, Pharmacy Practice Division, College of Pharmacy, Health Sciences Center, University of Oklahoma, Oklahoma City.

Daniel C. Robinson, Pharm.D.
Assistant Professor of Clinical Pharmacy, School of Pharmacy, University of Southern California, Los Angeles.

John C. Rotschafer, Pharm.D.
Section of Clinical Pharmacology, St. Paul Ramsey Medical Center, St. Paul; Assistant Professor, College of Pharmacy, University of Minnesota, Minneapolis.

Michael D. Rotblatt, Pharm.D.
Drug Information Consultant, San Francisco.

John Russo, Jr., Pharm.D.
Associate Editor, ADIS Press (USA) Inc., New York, New York.

Mary E. Russo, Pharm.D.
Assistant Professor of Clinical Pharmacy, Department of Pharmacy Practice, College of Pharmacy; Adjunct Assistant Professor of Medicine, Department of Medicine, School of Medicine, University of Utah, Salt Lake City.

Michael L. Ryan, Pharm.D.
Clinical Assistant Professor of Pharmacy, College of Pharmacy, University of Michigan, Ann Arbor.

Victoria A. Serrano, Pharm.D.
Supervisor, Pediatric Practice Area, Department of Pharmaceutical Services, UCLA Hospital and Clinics, Los Angeles.

Sam K. Shimomura, Pharm.D.
Associate Clinical Professor of Pharmacy, Vice-Chairman, Division of Clinical Pharmacy (Irvine program), School of Pharmacy, University of California, San Francisco.

Gary D. Smith, Pharm.D.
Clinical Assistant Professor of Pharmacy, College of Pharmacy; Clinical Pharmacist, Pediatric Allergy and Pulmonary Division, University of Iowa, Iowa City.

Gary H. Smith, Pharm.D.
Associate Professor of Pharmacy Practice, Assistant Department Head and Director of Drug Information Center, College of Pharmacy, University of Arizona, Tucson.

Catherine A. Sohn, Pharm.D.
Assistant Professor of Clinical Pharmacy, Department of Pharmacy Practice, Philadelphia College of Pharmacy and Science, Philadelphia.

Glen L. Stimmel, Pharm.D.
Associate Professor Clinical Pharmacy, Psychiatry and the Behaviorial Sciences, Schools of Pharmacy and Medicine, University of Southern California, Los Angeles.

Donald L. Uden, Pharm.D.
Associate Director of Pharmacy, Minneapolis Children's Health Center, Minneapolis; Assistant Professor of Clinical Pharmacy, College of Pharmacy, University of Minnesota, Minneapolis.

Earl S. Ward, Jr., Pharm.D.
Assistant Professor of Clinical Pharmacy, School of Pharmacy, Mercer University, Atlanta; Clinical Pharmacist, Pulmonary Rehabilitation Team, Georgia Baptist Medical Center, Atlanta.

William A. Watson, Pharm.D.
Assistant Director, Drug Information Service, Division of Clinical Pharmacy, Department of Pharmacology, University of Texas Health Science Center, San Antonio.

Michael E. Winter, Pharm.D.
Associate Clinical Professor, Director of Clinical Pharmacokinetics Consulting Service, Division of Clinical Pharmacy, School of Pharmacy, University of California, San Francisco.

Thomas H. Wiser, Pharm.D.
Associate Professor, School of Pharmacy; Associate Director, Primary Care, School of Medicine, University of Maryland, Baltimore.

Lana G. Witt, Pharm.D.
Pharmacist, Stanford University Hospital, Stanford, California; Assistant Clinical Professor, School of Pharmacy, University of California, San Francisco.

Lawrence D. Witt, Pharm.D.
Pharmacist, Stanford University Hospital, Stanford, California.

Gary C. Yee, Pharm.D.
Associate in Medical Oncology, Fred Hutchinson Cancer Research Center, Seattle, Washington; Clinical Instructor, Department of Pharmacy Practice, School of Pharmacy, University of Washington, Seattle.

Lloyd Yee Young, Pharm.D.
Associate Professor of Clinical Pharmacy, College of Pharmacy, Washington State University, Pullman.

Preface to the Third Edition

More than a decade ago, when we had to select a title for the first edition of this book, the terms "therapeutics," "applied," "drug therapy," and "clinical pharmacy" all figured prominently in our discussions, and we settled on *Applied Therapeutics for Clinical Pharmacists,* a name that seemed to cover all the bases. However, with this third edition we have given the book a new title to reflect its growing utilization among physicians, medical students, interns and residents, and among nurse practitioners and physicians' assistants. The objectives for this book remain the same as stated in the preface to the first edition. *Applied Therapeutics: The Clinical Use of Drugs* is still designed to illustrate the appropriate clinical application of pharmacology and pharmacokinetics to specific patient problems. We still feel that this objective is best accomplished through the use of case history presentations, pertinent questions, and well-referenced responses, an approach which brings into focus the nature of the decision making process. In this much expanded edition, the format has undergone considerable refinement. The questions and responses are more sharply focused on the cases, and the case presentations are better organized to show the logical flow of data gathering and decision making required for optimal drug therapy. In addition, borrowing from a more traditional approach, we have utilized an extensive system of headings and subheadings within the text to allow the reader to more easily locate specific information. All of the chapters have been completely rewritten and many new ones have been added.

Brian S. Katcher
Lloyd Yee Young
Mary Anne Koda-Kimble

Preface to the First Edition

In the past decade, new roles for the pharmacist have emerged. More and more frequently the pharmacist is placed in increasingly responsible positions within the health care delivery system. In this capacity (s)he is able to have a significant influence on the quality of health care delivered to the patient. M. Silverman and P. Lee have skillfully assessed the current and future role of the pharmacist in *Pills, Profits and Politics.*[1]

". . . It is the pharmacist who can play a vital role in assisting physicians to prescribe rationally, who can help see to it that the right drug is ordered for the right patient at the right time, in the right amounts and with due consideration of costs and that the patient knows how, when and why to use both prescription and non-prescription products.

"It is the pharmacist who has been most highly trained as an expert on drug products, who has the best opportunity to keep up-to-date on developments in this field and who can serve both physician and patient as a knowledgeable adviser. It is the pharmacist who can take a key part in preventing drug misuse, drug abuse and irrational prescribing."

Many schools of pharmacy have made substantial curriculum changes to prepare their graduates for these responsibilities. Although traditional pharmacy courses have imparted factual information about drugs, they have not enabled the student to apply these facts to the drug therapy of patients. Similarly, traditional pharmacology and medical textbooks do not provide the professional with sufficient information to make a judgment regarding the selection and dosing of a particular product for a specific patient. To arrive at this decision, the clinician must consider a number of patient factors including age, renal and hepatic function, concurrent disease states and medications and allergies. (S)he

must also consider drug product factors including bioavailability, pharmacokinetics, efficacy, toxicity, risk to benefit ratio, and cost.

We have found that students have most difficulty in **integrating** and **applying** the multiple components of their education to formulate the safest, most rational drug regimen for a given patient. We have also observed that although the student is able to enumerate the adverse effects of a drug, (s)he is unable to **recognize** or monitor for these effects should they occur in his/her patient.

This text is an outgrowth of the clinical pharmacy courses taught at the University of California and at Washington State University. The major objective of these courses is to enable the student to practice effectively in the clinical setting. Lectures on the pathophysiology and medical management of disease states are supplemented with conferences where students are challenged with drug therapy questions frequently asked by physicians and by case histories which require drug therapy assessment and the selection of appropriate alternatives. The objective of these conferences and this text is to enable the student to identify relevant factors in drug treatment such as the probability of whether or not a specific drug is responsible for a patient's symptoms; the clinical significance of a drug interaction; why a specific drug is not achieving therapeutic blood levels; the dose for a patient with multiple disease states.

The success of the conference portion of our courses was a major determinant of the format used for this text: case histories which simulate the actual practice situation and frequently asked therapeutic questions are followed by well-referenced responses.

The authors have drawn much information from their own clinical experiences. **It remains the responsibility of every practitioner to evaluate the appropriateness of a particular opinion in the context of the actual clinical situation and with due consideration of any new developments in the field.** Although the

[1] Silverman, M. and Lee, P.R.: *Pills, Profits and Politics,* University of California Press, Berkeley, 1974, p. 192.

authors have been careful to recommend dosages that are in agreement with current standards and responsible literature, we suggest the student or practitioner consult several appropriate infor- mation sources when dealing with new and un- familiar drugs.

Mary Anne Koda-Kimble
Lloyd Y. Young
Brian S. Katcher

Acknowledgments

We are indebted to our contributing authors for meeting the many demands required for publication of this book; our many colleagues who wrote extensive critiques of chapters from the previous edition; Linda Young, who skillfully coordinated our editorial offices, and Katy Hilmer and Anne Roorda, who assisted her; Cheryl Case, who assisted with the final stages of manuscript preparation; Todd Dankmyer and Keith Haglund, editors of The New Physician, for their helpful comments on portions of the book which appeared in The New Physician; the American Medical Writers Association, for their kind and encouraging recognition of the previous edition; Michael Fong and the entire staff at Vera Allen Composition who expertly carried out the typesetting of this edition; our students who never let us forget there is more to learn; Sid Riegelman, whose envisionary ideas catalyzed the inception of this text; and to Betty, Linda, Don, and our children who have endured, understood and sustained us throughout the preparation of this third edition.

APPLIED THERAPEUTICS
The Clinical Use of Drugs

Chapter 1

Clinical Pharmacokinetics

Michael E. Winter

BASIC PRINCIPLES

The use of plasma drug concentrations as a means of monitoring drug therapy is increasing. The clinical application of pharmacokinetics allows the clinician to select dosage regimens that are likely to produce therapeutic concentrations. Pharmacokinetic calculations also provide a basis for the modification of dosage regimens in light of laboratory evaluations of plasma drug concentrations.

A complete presentation of this topic is beyond the scope of this chapter. A basic introduction to key pharmacokinetic principles and illustration of their clinical application is presented in *Basic Clinical Pharmacokinetics* (1) and several other pharmacokinetics texts (2–4). This chapter will briefly review pharmacokinetic parameters and then provide examples of some typical situations which demonstrate their clinical application. Other examples of the clinical use of pharmacokinetics appear in various chapters of this book.

Reported or calculated plasma levels are useful in the evaluation of therapy; however, they should only be considered as a *guide* to treatment, not the sole criterion for determination of dosage regimens. A drug level which is reported from the laboratory may be in error or may be the result of a blood sample that was drawn at an inappropriate time. If a calculated regimen appears unreasonable, there is always the possibility that there has been a mathematical error, or that the formula being used is inappropriate for the situation at hand. In some cases, the pharmacokinetic parameters utilized in the calculations may be incorrect for the patient in question. This last point is an important one. Because many of the pharmacokinetic parameters available in the literature are based on a relatively small number of patients or normal volunteers (5–8), values obtained from the experimental data are, at best, only estimates for those of any given patient. This problem, as well as the variations which exist among subjects, emphasizes the need to ob-

1

tain accurate plasma level measurements and to re-evaluate pharmacokinetic parameters for each patient. Review articles which list pharmacokinetic parameters for a number of drugs may be useful (6–9), but the reader is encouraged to seek out the original literature to determine the degree of intersubject variability and to evaluate the methodology and data from which such review material was obtained.

Plasma Concentration (Cp)

The plasma concentration (Cp) which is reported by the laboratory or calculated from a formula represents drug that is bound to plasma protein plus drug that is unbound or free. However, it is the free or unbound form of the drug that is in equilibrium with the receptor site and is the pharmacologically active moiety. Decreased plasma protein binding can present a problem in the interpretation of Cp for drugs which are highly protein bound because the usual ratio of free (active) drug to total drug concentration will be increased. In such cases, a greater pharmacologic effect can be expected for any given Cp.

In most cases the fraction of drug which is unbound is independent of the total drug concentration as long as saturation of the binding sites is not approached. Valproic acid (10) and salicylates (11) are important exceptions since concentrations in excess of protein binding capacity are commonly achieved with these drugs.

Two factors determine the degree of plasma protein binding. One is the binding affinity of the drug for the plasma proteins and the second is the number of binding sites available or the concentration of plasma protein. Acidic drugs such as salicyclate or phenytoin are usually bound to albumin (12,13). Basic drugs such as lidocaine or quinidine are usually bound to serum globulins, primarily alpha-1-acid glycoprotein (12,14,15). If the plasma protein concentration is decreased, the drug molecules which are released will not remain in the plasma exclusively, but will equilibrate with the tissue compartment, resulting in a minor increase in the free Cp as long as the drug's volume of distribution is relatively large (see Fig. 1).

The fraction of drug that is free is usually expressed as alpha (α):

$$\alpha = \frac{\text{free drug concentration}}{\text{total drug concentration}} \qquad \text{(Eq. 1)}$$

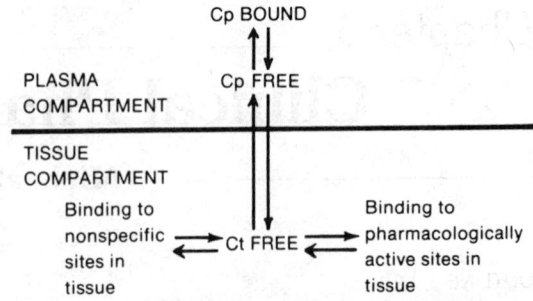

Figure 1. Equilibrium between free and bound drug concentrations. It is assumed that only Cp FREE can cross into the tissue compartment or site of pharmacologic activity.

The smaller alpha is, the greater will be the significance of altered plasma protein binding. In general, if alpha is normally less than or equal to 0.1 (ie, 10% or less free), there is a good possibility that protein binding changes will be significant. In such cases, the plasma concentration which will achieve a given therapeutic effect should be reassessed. If alpha is 0.5 or more, it is unlikely that protein binding changes will be important in the clinical setting.

Bioavailability (F)

Bioavailability (F) is the fraction of the parent compound which reaches the systemic circulation. Several factors influence the bioavailability of a drug.

Solubility. A drug must be both lipid and water soluble to be absorbed from the gastrointestinal tract. If a drug is too water soluble (eg, aminoglycosides) it cannot pass through the lipid membrane of the gastrointestinal (GI) tract and will not be orally available. Other drugs that are more lipid than water soluble (eg, griseofulvin and phenytoin) may have diminished or delayed absorption because they must first dissolve in the aqueous fluids of the GI tract before they can be absorbed (16,17). Drugs which have intermediate lipid-water solubilities are more likely to be completely bioavailable by the oral route if properly formulated (eg, theophylline).

Dosage Form and Route of Administration. The dosage form and route of administration may be important factors in determining the bioavailability of a drug. For example, the fraction of orally administered digoxin that is absorbed can vary not only with the manufacturer, but also with the dosage form. The average F for tablets is 0.7, while the F for digoxin elixir is 0.8 (18,19). Intravenous digoxin has an F of 1.0 because all of the drug reaches the systemic circulation.

First-Pass Effect. If a drug which is absorbed from the gastrointestinal tract is metabolized by the liver to a great extent before it reaches the systemic circulation (first-pass effect), oral bioavailability will be decreased. Lidocaine and propranolol are examples of drugs which undergo a large first-pass effect (20,21).

Salt Form. The salt form of a drug is another factor which determines how much drug will reach the systemic circulation. For example, theophylline has an F of 1.0. However, it is often administered as aminophylline which is 80 to 85% theophylline. The portion of the salt or ester of a drug which is the parent compound is represented by the letter S. The S for aminophylline is therefore 0.8 to 0.85. S can be determined by dividing the molecular weight of the parent drug by the molecular weight of the salt or ester form of the drug.

Rate of Administration (R_A)

The rate of drug administration is expressed by the following equation:

$$\text{Rate of Administration } (R_A) = \frac{(S)(F)(\text{Dose})}{\tau} \quad \text{(Eq. 2)}$$

where S and F are defined as above and τ (tau) is the dosing interval.

Volume of Distribution (Vd)

At steady state, drugs are distributed unequally between plasma and the various other fluids and tissues that make up the body, and the actual nature of this distribution is dependent upon the physicochemical properties of each drug. However, for practical purposes it is often assumed that the body is a single compartment in which drugs are uniformly distributed, and it is therefore assumed that the concentration of drug throughout the body is the same as in the plasma sample which is measured. The physicochemical properties of drugs are such that their volumes of distribution vary considerably. In fact, a drug may have such extensive tissue distribution that

its "apparent volume of distribution" greatly exceeds any conceivable volume in the body. The practical value of this fictitious "apparent volume of distribution" is that it allows the clinician to estimate the *loading dose* of a drug that would be required to rapidly achieve a desired plasma concentration.

The relationship between plasma concentration and volume of distribution is as follows:

$$Cp = \frac{Ab}{Vd} \quad \text{(Eq. 3)}$$

where Cp is the plasma concentration of the drug, Ab is the amount of drug in the body, and Vd is the apparent volume of distribution of the drug. Since Vd accounts for all of the drug in the body, it can be used to calculate the loading dose which would rapidly result in a desired plasma concentration:

$$\text{Loading Dose} = \frac{(Vd)(Cp)}{(S)(F)} \quad \text{(Eq. 4)}$$

where (S)(F) represent the fraction of the administered dose that will reach the systemic circulation.

For example, if one wished to calculate the loading dose of digoxin required to obtain a plasma concentration of 1.5 mcg/L for a 70 kg patient, the above formula would be used as follows. The apparent volume of digoxin is approximately 7.3 L/kg (22), or 511 L for this 70 kg individual (7.3 L/kg × 70 kg = 511 L). Assuming that digoxin tablets are to be used (F = 0.7, S = 1.0), the calculated loading dose would be:

$$\text{Loading Dose} = \frac{(Vd)(Cp)}{(S)(F)} \quad \text{(Eq. 4)}$$
$$= \frac{(511 \text{ L})(1.5 \text{ mcg/L})}{(1.0)(0.7)}$$
$$= 1095 \text{ mcg} = 1.095 \text{ mg}$$

The usual clinical approach would be to give the loading dose in divided doses (0.25 to 0.5 mg per dose) every six hours and observe the patient before each successive dose is administered. In addition, some clinicians frequently use a bioavailability factor greater than 0.7 for digoxin tablets to guard against overshooting the desired level.

If the patient already has some initial plasma

concentration (Cp observed), the above equation can be modified to calculate a loading dose which will produce a higher desired concentration (Cp desired):

$$\frac{\text{Loading}}{\text{Dose}} = \frac{(Vd)(Cp\ desired\ -\ Cp\ observed)}{(S)(F)} \quad (Eq.\ 5)$$

For example, if the above patient already had a measured steady state digoxin level of 1.0 mcg/L and 1.5 mcg/L were desired, the additional loading dose would be:

$$\frac{\text{Loading}}{\text{Dose}} = \frac{(511\ L)(1.5\ mcg/L\ -\ 1.0\ mcg/L)}{(1.0)(0.7)}$$

$$= 365\ mcg\ =\ 0.365\ mg$$

Two Compartment Model

Many pharmacokinetic calculations are based upon the premise that drugs are distributed into and eliminated from the body as though it were a single compartment. However, the pharmacokinetic behavior of many drugs does not lend itself to this model, and for them, it is more accurate to divide the body into two or more compartments.

The first compartment has a volume referred to as V_i or $V_{initial}$. This compartment equilibrates rapidly with administered drug and is usually made up of blood volume and those organs or tissues which have a high blood flow. The second compartment has a volume referred to as V_t or V_{tissue}. Administered drug distributes into V_t from V_i and eventually equilibrates with the second compartment. The half-time for the distribution phase (that is, the time for one-half of the drug to distribute from V_i into V_t) is referred to as the alpha (α) half-life, and the half-time for drug elimination from the body is referred to as the beta (β) half-life. The sum of V_i and V_t is the apparent volume of distribution (Vd). See Fig. 2.

If a drug does behave as though it distributes into two compartments, one could err in the calculation of a rapidly administered loading dose if the one-compartment model volume of distribution, Vd, were used. A loading dose calculated on the basis of Vd would result in an initial plasma concentration much higher than predicted because of the small initial volume of distribution.

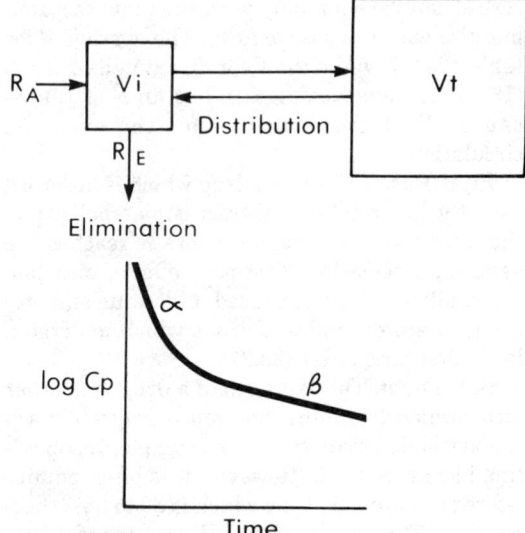

Figure 2. **Two Compartment Model.** Volumes of distribution for a two-compartment model. V_i is the initial volume of distribution. Note that drug administration and elimination (R_E) are assumed to occur in V_i. The lower graph shows how a drug administered into V_i follows a biphasic decay pattern. The initial decay half-life ($\alpha t\frac{1}{2}$) is usually due to drug being distributed into V_t. The second decay half-life ($\beta t\frac{1}{2}$) is usually due to drug being eliminated from the body.

If a drug's target organ behaves as though it were located in the first compartment, then toxicity may occur. This can be circumvented by first calculating a loading dose based on Vd. This dose can then be administered slowly to allow the drug to distribute from V_i into V_t, or the loading dose can be given in sufficiently small increments to prevent the Cp in V_i from exceeding some critical concentration. Examples of drugs which behave in this fashion are lidocaine and procainamide (23,24).

When a drug's target organ behaves as though it were located in the second compartment, toxicity is not a consequence of the initially high Cp. However, if plasma samples for these drugs are obtained before distribution into V_t is complete, the reported level will not reflect the drug concentration in the target organ and cannot be used to predict therapeutic or toxic effects of the drug. An example of a drug which behaves in this fashion is digoxin (25).

Clearance

Drugs are usually removed from the body at a rate which is proportional to their plasma concentration. Clearance may be thought of as the proportionality constant which makes the rate of drug elimination equal to the rate of drug administration at steady state. Clearance is the volume of blood which is completely cleared of a drug per unit of time. When the clearance of a drug is known, the *maintenance dose* required to sustain an average steady state plasma concentration can be calculated:

$$\text{Maintenance Dose} = \frac{(Cl)(Cpss\ ave)(\tau)}{(S)(F)} \quad \text{(Eq. 6)}$$

where Cl is clearance, Cpss ave is the average plasma concentration at steady state, and τ (tau) is the dosing interval. S and F represent the fraction of the dose which reaches the systemic circulation.

For example, if one wished to calculate the maintenance dose of phenobarbital required to produce a plasma concentration of 20 mg/L in a 65 kg individual, the above formula would be used as follows. First, one would need to know that the usual clearance of phenobarbital is 0.096 L/day/kg, or 6.24 L/day for this 65 kg individual (0.096 L/day/kg × 65 kg = 6.24 L/day). S and F can both be considered equal to 1.0 since the sodium in sodium phenobarbital is negligible and the drug is 100% absorbed. Therefore,

$$\text{Maintenance Dose} = \frac{(Cl)(Cpss\ ave)(\tau)}{(S)(F)} \quad \text{(Eq. 6)}$$

$$= \frac{(6.24\ \text{L/day})(20\ \text{mg/L})(1\ \text{day})}{(1.0)(1.0)}$$

$$= 124.8\ \text{mg (daily dose)}$$

This concept of clearance is applicable to most drugs. The rate of drug removal is proportional to the plasma concentration, and the concentration of drug diminishes logarithmically with time. Drugs which behave in this way are described as following first-order kinetics. However, a few drugs, phenytoin and salicylate being important examples, do not behave in this way. For these drugs clearance and volume of distribution are not fixed parameters. Therefore, equations which utilize clearance or volume of distribution as con-

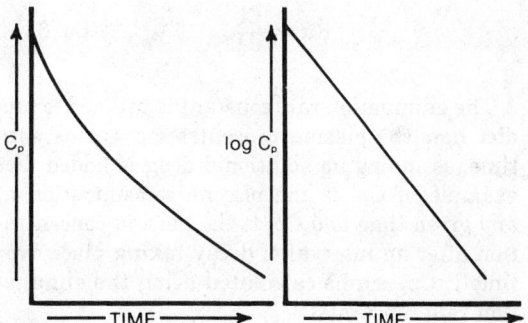

Figure 3. First order elimination when Cp or log Cp is plotted vs. time.

stant parameters are not applicable to these few drugs.

Half-life (t½)

For drugs which follow a first-order elimination process, the half-life is the time required for the plasma concentration of a drug or the total amount of drug in the body to decline by one-half. The half-life of a drug is important when one is considering questions involving time, such as "How long will it take a patient to reach steady state on a constant dosage regimen?" or "How long will it take for all of the drug to be eliminated from the body?" It may also be used to estimate the appropriate dosing interval or tau (τ) to be used during maintenance dose therapy.

It takes one half-life to reach 50% of steady state, two half-lives to reach 75%, three half-lives to reach 87.5%, and four half-lives to reach 93.75% of steady state. In most clinical situations, it is sufficient to wait three or four half-lives before steady state can be effectively assumed.

The half-life of a drug is dependent upon its volume of distribution and its clearance. This relationship is expressed by the following formula:

$$t\tfrac{1}{2} = \frac{0.693 Vd}{Cl} \quad \text{(Eq. 7)}$$

Elimination Rate Constant (Kd)

The elimination rate constant is the fraction of the volume of distribution which is cleared per unit of time. Like half-life, it is a function of the drug's volume of distribution and its clearance:

$$Kd = \frac{Cl}{Vd} \qquad \text{(Eq. 8)}$$

The elimination rate constant is utilized to predict how the plasma concentration varies with time, assuming no additional drug is added. For example, if Cp_1 is the plasma concentration at any given time and Cp_2 is the plasma concentration after an interval of decay taking place over time t, Cp_2 can be calculated using the elimination rate constant:

$$Cp_2 = (Cp_1)(e^{-Kdt}) \qquad \text{(Eq. 9)}$$

In this equation (e^{-Kdt}) is the fraction of the initial plasma concentration which is remaining at the end of the time interval t.

Evaluation of Renal Function

The daily production of creatinine, creatinine clearance, and serum creatinine is analogous to the relationship between maintenance dose, drug clearance and drug plasma concentration as expressed in Eq. 6:

$$\text{Maintenance Dose} = \frac{(Cl)(Cpss \ ave)(\tau)}{(S)(F)} \qquad \text{(Eq. 6)}$$

In the above equation, maintenance dose would be equivalent to the daily production of creatinine, Cl would correspond to the creatinine clearance (Cl_{Cr}) and Cpss ave would correspond to the steady state serum creatinine concentration (SrCr).

The usual creatinine clearance for a 70 kg adult is about 100–120 ml/min and the average production rate is 20 mg/kg/day. This clearance and production rate result in an average serum creatinine concentration of 1 mg/dl. As patients age, both the production and clearance of creatinine decrease. Therefore, elderly patients who have a normal serum creatinine concentration of 1 mg/dl may have a creatinine clearance which is much less than 100 ml/min.

There are a number of methods used to calculate creatinine clearance. Many of these use factors such as age, weight and sex to determine the expected production rate of creatinine. This value is then divided by the measured serum creatinine concentration to estimate the patient's creatinine clearance. One such method was developed by Cockcroft and Gault (26):

$$\frac{Cl_{Cr} \text{ for males}}{\text{(ml/min)}} = \frac{(140 - age)(weight)}{(72)(SrCr)} \qquad \text{(Eq. 10)}$$

$$\frac{Cl_{Cr} \text{ for females}}{\text{(ml/min)}} = \frac{(0.85)(140 - age)(weight)}{(72)(SrCr)}$$

The units for the above equation are as follows: weight in kg, age in years, SrCr in mg/dl and Cl_{Cr} in ml/min. Eq. 10 is reasonably accurate in predicting the creatinine clearance if the patient under consideration has a normal ratio of muscle mass to total body weight. The predicted creatinine clearance for obese or emaciated patients tends to be greater than the true value since these individuals tend to have a lower than average production of creatinine per kg of body weight. Also, when renal function is unstable and the serum creatinine is changing (ie, nonsteady-state), the predicted creatinine clearance may be under- or overestimated depending on whether the serum creatinine is rising or falling.

CLINICAL APPLICATIONS

1. T.M. is a 50-year-old 60 kg woman who was admitted to the coronary care unit with multiple premature ventricular contractions which occurred as the result of an acute myocardial infarction. She has a history of congestive heart failure and asthma.

Using the following pharmacokinetic parameters for lidocaine (27), calculate an appropriate loading and maintenance dose for T.M.

	$\alpha t\frac{1}{2}$ (min)	$\beta t\frac{1}{2}$ (hr)	Vi (L/kg)	Vd (L/kg)	Cl (ml/min/kg)
Normal	8.3	1.8	0.53	1.32	10
Heart failure	7.3	2.0	0.30	0.88	6.3
Liver disease	8.8	5.0	0.61	2.31	6.0

The distribution of lidocaine follows a two compartment model. Since the myocardium responds as though it is in the first compartment (Vi), the loading dose of lidocaine should be administered in a way which avoids toxic plasma levels in the first compartment before distribution is complete. This goal can be achieved by using the initial volume of distribution (Vi) in calculating the bolus dose. However, more than one loading bolus may be required, because plasma concentrations achieved by each loading bolus will decline rapidly to subtherapeutic concentrations as the drug is distributed into the larger final volume of distribution (Vd).

Using the value of 0.30 L/kg for T.M.'s initial volume of distribution, Vi would be 18.0 L in this 60 kg individual. The usual therapeutic range for lidocaine is 1 to 5 mg/L (mcg/ml); for the purpose of calculating the initial bolus dose a plasma concentration of 3 mg/L will be used. S and F can be assumed to be 1.0. Therefore, substituting Vi for Vd in Eq. 4, the loading dose would be calculated to be 54 mg:

$$\text{Loading Dose} = \frac{(Vi)(Cp)}{(S)(F)} \qquad \text{(Eq. 4)}$$

$$= \frac{(18.0 \text{ L})(3 \text{ mg/L})}{(1.0)(1.0)}$$

$$= 54 \text{ mg}$$

This bolus dose is compatible with the usual recommended dose of 1 to 2 mg/kg (28).

Eq. 6 can be used to calculate the maintenance dose. Since T.M. has congestive heart failure, her lidocaine clearance will be assumed to be 6.3 ml/min/kg or, expressed as L/min for her 60 kg of body weight, 0.378 L/min. Therefore, her maintenance infusion would be calculated as follows:

$$\text{Maintenance Dose} = \frac{(Cl)(Cpss \text{ ave})(\tau)}{(S)(F)} \qquad \text{(Eq. 6)}$$

$$= \frac{(0.378 \text{ L/min})(3 \text{ mg/L})(1 \text{ min})}{(1.0)(1.0)}$$

$$= 1.134 \text{ mg/min}$$

This maintenance infusion rate is compatible with the usual recommended rate of 1 to 4 mg/min (22,28). If more information about the severity of T.M.'s heart failure had been provided, the maintenance infusion could have been adjusted to the degree to which her cardiac output was compromised (29).

2. T.M.'s PVC's were abolished immediately after the loading dose was given. The maintenance infusion was then started, but 15 minutes later the PVC's recurred. What is an appropriate course of action?

The expected distribution or alpha half-life of lidocaine in this patient is 7.3 minutes, and the elimination or beta half-life is 2 hours. This early recurrence of the PVC's suggests that distribution of the initial bolus dose into the second compartment is the reason for loss of therapeutic effect. Therefore, an additional bolus dose should be given and the maintenance infusion should be left unchanged. If the PVC's had returned after several hours, it would be appropriate to administer a bolus dose and to increase the maintenance infusion as well.

3. On the following day, T.M. developed wheezing which required aminophylline therapy. She was given a 350 mg loading dose and started on a maintenance infusion of 40 mg/hr. Two hours after the loading dose, a theophylline level of 12 mg/L (mcg/ml) was obtained. Therapeutic concentrations of theophylline fall between 10–20 mg/L. Does this suggest that the maintenance infusion of 40 mg/hr is appropriate?

The half-life of theophylline in healthy nonsmokers is approximately 8 hours. In T.M., who has congestive heart failure, the half-life is likely to be doubled to approximately 16 hours. The plasma theophylline concentration of 12 mg/L was obtained two hours after the dose had been given, well within her approximate theophylline half-life. Drug levels which are drawn within one half-life of the time the dose is administered are primarily determined by the volume of distribution. Since only a small fraction of the drug has been eliminated at this point in time, plasma samples taken within one half-life are influenced very little by clearance. Therefore, no conclusion can be drawn from this reported plasma level with regard to the ultimate steady state plasma concentration of theophylline which will be achieved by her maintenance dose of 40 mg/hr.

The plasma concentration which would be expected after a loading dose and initiation of an infusion which has not yet reached steady state can be calculated with the following equation:

$$Cp = \left[\frac{(S)(F)(Dose)}{Vd} \times e^{-Kdt} \right] \qquad \text{(Eq. 11)}$$

$$+ \left[\frac{(S)(F)(Dose/\tau)}{Cl} \times 1 - e^{-Kdt} \right]$$

The first of the two principal terms in this equation accounts for the decaying loading dose and the second term accounts for drug which is accumulating from the infusion. Assuming the Vd to be 0.48 L/kg or 28.8 L for this 60 kg patient, and assuming that Cl is 0.02 L/hr/kg (half of the usual clearance because of her CHF) or 1.2 L/hr for her 60 kg of body weight (30), Kd can be calculated by use of Eq. 8:

$$Kd = \frac{Cl}{Vd} \qquad \text{(Eq. 8)}$$

$$= \frac{1.2 \text{ L/hr}}{28.8 \text{ L}}$$

$$= 0.042 \text{ hr}^{-1}$$

Substituting these pharmacokinetic parameters into the above equation, the plasma concentration that would be expected after two hours can be calculated:

$$Cp = \left[\frac{(0.85)(1.0)(350 \text{ mg})}{28.8 \text{ L}} \times e^{-(0.042)(2)} \right]$$

$$+ \left[\frac{(0.85)(1.0)(40 \text{ mg/hr})}{1.2 \text{ L/hr}} \times 1 - e^{-(0.042)(2)} \right]$$

$$= (10.3 \text{ mg/L})(0.92) + (28.3 \text{ mg/L})(1 - 0.92)$$

$$= 9.5 \text{ mg/L} + 2.3 \text{ mg/L}$$

$$= 11.8 \text{ mg/L}$$

This is very close to the observed concentration of 12 mg/L. Most of this calculated concentration of 11.8 mg/L is due to the loading dose which in turn is dependent upon the volume of distribution. When the above calculations are inspected, it can be seen that 9.5 mg/L of the total reported plasma concentration is due to the loading dose and 2.3 mg/L is due to the infusion. This indicates the volume of distribution was approximately correct, but it is still too early to determine whether or not the maintenance infusion, which is dependent upon clearance, is appropriate.

4. Fifteen hours after the initiation of aminophylline therapy, T.M. was doing well, and a second theophylline concentration was obtained. The reported concentration was 19 mg/L. Does this reported concentration indicate that the infusion rate of 40 mg/hr is appropriate?

Even though this plasma sample is taken prior to steady state (4 × 16 hr in this patient), it is useful in the clinical situation to obtain a plasma sample after approximately two times the *usual* half-life to determine if the drug concentration is higher or lower than would be expected. T.M. illustrates this principle in that her plasma concentration is already approaching the upper limits of normal, long before steady state has been achieved.

As in the previous question, the reported concentration can be compared with the concentration that would be expected. The calculation is the same as that used after two hours, except that t is increased to 15:

$$Cp = \left[\frac{(S)(F)(\text{Dose})}{Vd} \times e^{-Kdt} \right] \qquad \text{(Eq. 11)}$$

$$+ \left[\frac{(S)(F)(\text{Dose}/\tau)}{Cl} \times 1 - e^{-Kdt} \right]$$

$$= \left[\frac{(0.85)(1.0)(350 \text{ mg})}{28.8 \text{ L}} \times e^{-(0.042)(15)} \right]$$

$$+ \left[\frac{(0.85)(1.0)(40 \text{ mg/hr})}{1.2 \text{ L/hr}} \times 1 - e^{-(0.042)(15)} \right]$$

$$= (10.3 \text{ mg/L})(0.53) + (28.3 \text{ mg/L})(1 - 0.53)$$

$$= 5.5 \text{ mg/L} + 13.3 \text{ mg/L}$$

$$= 18.8 \text{ mg/L}$$

Inspecting the above calculations, it can be seen that 5.5 mg/L of the reported plasma concentration is due to the loading dose and 13.3 mg/L is due to the infusion. We now have a much better indication of the patient's clearance, and the similarity between the observed and predicted concentrations suggests that the clearance value used in the calculations is *approximately* correct. It is important to recognize that because the sample was obtained at about one actual half-life, the exact value of clearance is uncertain.

Using this clearance value, it is possible to predict a final steady state concentration of about 28 mg/L:

$$\text{Maintenance Dose} = \frac{(Cl)(\text{Cpss ave})(\tau)}{(S)(F)} \qquad \text{(Eq. 6)}$$

$$\text{Cpss ave} = \frac{(S)(F)(\text{Maintenance Dose}/\tau)}{Cl}$$

$$= \frac{(0.85)(1.0)(40 \text{ mg/hr})}{1.2 \text{ L/hr}}$$

$$= 28.3 \text{ mg/L}$$

Since the usually accepted therapeutic range for theophylline is 10 to 20 mg/L (mcg/ml), the current infusion rate of 40 mg/hr appears to be excessive. A new infusion rate that would maintain T.M.'s plasma concentration at 15 mg/L can be calculated using Eq. 6:

$$\text{Maintenance Dose} = \frac{(Cl)(Cpss\ ave)(\tau)}{(S)(F)} \quad \text{(Eq. 6)}$$

$$= \frac{(1.2\ L/hr)(15\ mg/L)(1\ hr)}{(0.85)(1.0)}$$

$$= 21\ mg/hr$$

This illustrates the usefulness of obtaining a drug concentration after approximately two of the usual half-lives of a drug to assess a maintenance regimen. (The usual half-life of theophylline is about 8 hours.) Plasma concentrations obtained at this time can be used to evaluate clearance. If the clearance is unusually low, a dosage adjustment at this time will prevent excessive accumulation, and future plasma level monitoring will aid in an accurate evaluation of the patient's theophylline pharmacokinetics.

5. Calculate a maintenance dose of aminophylline that will be appropriate for T.M. when she is able to take oral medications.

To minimize fluctuations in plasma levels between doses, the dosing interval should be shorter than the drug half-life. The half-life of theophylline in T.M. can be calculated as follows:

$$t_{1/2} = \frac{0.693 Vd}{Cl} \quad \text{(Eq. 7)}$$

$$= \frac{(0.693)(28.8\ L)}{1.2\ L/hr}$$

$$= 16.6\ hours$$

This half-life suggests that a dosing interval of 12 hours could be used even though it is somewhat longer than the usual dosing interval of six hours for aminophylline.

The dose which would be given every 12 hours can be calculated using Eq. 6:

$$\text{Maintenance Dose} = \frac{(Cl)(Cpss\ ave)(\tau)}{(S)(F)} \quad \text{(Eq. 6)}$$

$$= \frac{(1.2\ L/hr)(15\ mg/L)(12\ hr)}{(0.85)(1.0)}$$

$$= 254\ mg$$

$$= \text{approximately 250 mg}$$

The peak and trough concentrations that would be expected on this regimen can be estimated as follows:

$$Cpss\ max = \frac{\dfrac{(S)(F)(Dose)}{Vd}}{1 - e^{-Kd\tau}} \quad \text{(Eq. 12)}$$

$$= \frac{\dfrac{(0.85)(1.0)(250\ mg)}{28.8\ L}}{1 - e^{-(0.042)(12)}}$$

$$= 18.6\ mg/L$$

$$Cpss\ min = (Cpss\ max)(e^{-Kd\tau}) \quad \text{(Eq. 13)}$$

$$= (18.6\ mg/L)(e^{-(0.042)(12)})$$

$$= 11.23\ mg/L$$

These maximum and minimum plasma concentrations are within the therapeutic range, but other regimens could have been used, depending on the desired concentrations and the dosing interval selected.

6. When should a plasma sample for theophylline be obtained to evaluate T.M.'s oral aminophylline regimen?

Since the oral maintenance dose calculated for this patient was based upon the parenteral maintenance dose, the patient is theoretically at steady state and a level can be drawn after approximately one half-life or more on the oral regimen. If the oral maintenance dose had been substantially different from that used parenterally, a level would best be drawn after four or more half-lives.

In general, peak plasma levels are difficult to interpret, as they are subject to error if the actual peak occurs later than anticipated. Trough levels, on the other hand, will also be affected by absorption rate, but to a much lesser degree (see Fig. 4). Trough levels obtained just before the next dose are, therefore, more useful as a routine monitoring parameter in plasma level evaluation. Levels drawn at other times should be avoided unless there is a specific reason to do so (eg, in the case of an acute toxicity).

7. T.M. did well for the next three days, but then developed a fever. She had blood

cultures taken and was started on 100 mg of tobramycin infused over 30 minutes every 8 hours. T.M. still weighs 60 kg and has a serum creatinine of 2.1 mg/dl. Calculate the expected steady state "peak" concentration one hour after the initiation of a half-hour infusion and the steady state trough concentration.

In patients with normal renal function, the half-life for the aminoglycosides is usually about two hours; therefore, a significant amount of the drug may be eliminated from the body over the 30 minute infusion period of a dose. To predict a Cpss max for the aminoglycosides it is more appropriate to use Eq. 14 which is based upon an intermittent infusion model rather than Eq. 12 for Cpss max which is based upon a bolus model of administration.

$$Cpss = \frac{\dfrac{(S)(F)(Dose/t_{in})(1 - e^{-kdtin})}{Cl}}{1 - e^{-kd\tau}} \times (e^{-kdt2}) \qquad (Eq.\ 14)$$

Where τ is the time interval between each infusion, t_{in} is the actual duration of the intermittent infusion, t_2 is the number of hours since the end of the infusion and Cpss is the drug concentration t_2 hours following the completion of the infusion.

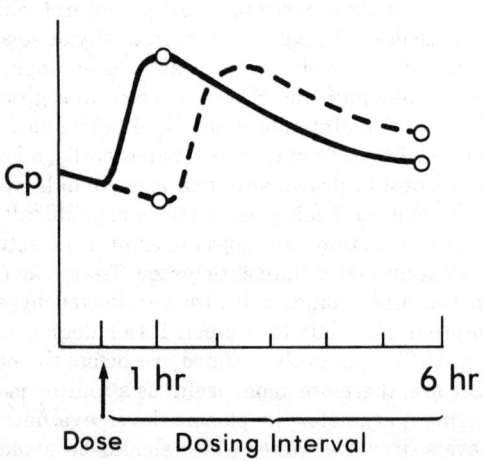

Figure 4. Schematic Representation of the Effect of Delayed Absorption (-----) on Plasma Level Measurements. Note the magnitude of error at one hour (theoretical time to reach Cpss max) as compared to six hours (Cpss min).

Eq. 14 is most appropriately used when the duration of the intermittent infusions approaches the half-life of the drug. If the half-life is much longer than the infusion time, the bolus model (Eq. 12) can be used. In this case Eq. 14 will be used for the purpose of illustration.

Conceptually, Eq. 14 can be broken down into several different components. $(S)(F)(Dose/t_{in})(1 - e^{-kdtin})/Cl$ represents the plasma concentration of a single infusion at the conclusion of the infusion (ie, 30 min after the initiation of the infusion). Dividing this value by $(1 - e^{-kd\tau})$ provides a steady state peak concentration produced by several intermittent infusion doses. Finally, multiplying this concentration by e^{-kdt2} provides the steady state concentration any time after the infusion has been discontinued (in this case 0.5 hrs following completion of the infusion).

Before Eq. 14 can be used, a variety of pharmacokinetic parameters for the aminoglycoside, tobramycin, must be calculated. The expected volume of distribution for the aminoglycosides is 0.25 L/kg (31,32) or 15 L for T.M. (0.25 L/kg × 60 kg). The clearance of aminoglycosides is approximately equal to the creatinine clearance (32,33). It can therefore be estimated for T.M. using Eq. 10 for women:

Cl_{Cr} for females (ml/min)

$$= \frac{(0.85)(140 - age)(weight)}{(72)(SrCr)}$$

$$= \frac{(0.85)(140 - 50)(60)}{(72)(2.1)}$$

$$= 30\ ml/min\ or\ 1.8\ L/hr$$

The half-life of tobramycin in T.M. can be estimated using Eq. 7:

$$t^{1/2} = \frac{(0.693)(Vd)}{Cl}$$

$$= \frac{(0.693)(15\ L)}{1.8\ L/hr}$$

$$= 5.8\ hr$$

The elimination rate constant can be estimated using Eq. 8:

$$Kd = \frac{Cl}{Vd}$$

$$= \frac{1.8 \text{ L/hr}}{15 \text{ L}}$$

$$= 0.12 \text{ hr}^{-1}$$

Using these calculated pharmacokinetic parameters and Eq. 14, the "peak" concentration of tobramycin one hour after the initiation of the infusion can be calculated:

$$Cpss = \frac{\dfrac{(1)(1)(100 \text{ mg/0.5 hr})(1 - e^{-(0.12)(0.5 \text{ hr})})}{1.8 \text{ L/hr}}}{1 - e^{-(0.12)(8 \text{ hr})}}$$

$$\times (e^{-(0.12)(0.5 \text{ hr})})$$

$$= \frac{(111.1 \text{ mg/L})(0.058)}{(1 - 0.38)} \times 0.94$$

$$= \frac{6.5 \text{ mg/L}}{0.62} \times 0.94$$

$$= (10.5 \text{ mg/L})(0.94)$$

$$= 9.9 \text{ mg/L}$$

Note that the true peak concentration would be at the end of the half-hour infusion, where t_2 would be 0 hrs. Most clinical studies refer to the "peak" as the concentration which occurs one hour after the dose or in this case one half-hour after the end of a half-hour infusion. If the plasma sample were obtained at the end of the half-hour infusion, the measured concentration could be much higher than the predicted concentration of 10.5 mg/L because of the two compartment volume of distribution and the fact that not all of the drug would have been fully distributed.

The trough concentration would be the peak concentration decayed to the time of the trough. In this case, with a dosing interval of 8 hours, the theoretical concentration of 10.5 mg/L could be decayed by the use of Eq. 9 for 7.5 hours:

$$Cp_2 = (Cp_1)(e^{-Kdt}) \qquad \text{(Eq. 9)}$$

$$= (10.5 \text{ mg/L})(e^{-(0.12)(7.5)})$$

$$= (10.5 \text{ mg/L})(0.41)$$

$$= 4.3 \text{ mg/L}$$

The trough concentration could also have been calculated by using Eq. 14 where t_2 would have been 7.5 hours.

If it is felt that the peak levels are too high or the trough levels are too low, the dose and/or the dosing interval could be adjusted in Eq. 14 until satisfactory peak and trough concentrations are achieved.

References

1. Winter ME: *Basic Clinical Pharmacokinetics,* Applied Therapeutics, Inc., San Francisco, 1980.
2. Evans WE et al: *Applied Pharmacokinetics: Principles of Therapeutic Drug Monitoring,* Applied Therapeutics, Inc., San Francisco, 1980.
3. Gibaldi M et al: *Pharmacokinetics,* Marcel Dekker, Inc., New York, 1980.
4. Roland M et al: *Clinical Pharmacokinetics: Concepts and Applications,* Lea and Febiger, Philadelphia, 1980.
5. Mitenko PA et al: Rational intravenous doses of theophylline, N Engl J Med. 1973; 289:600.
6. Pagliaro LA et al: Critical compilation of terminal half-lives, percent excreted unchanged, and changes of half-life in renal and hepatic dysfunction from studies in humans, with references. J Pharmacokinetics Biopharm. 1975; 3:333.
7. Welling PG et al: Predictions of drug dosage in patients with renal failure using data derived from normal subjects. Clin Pharmacol Ther. 1975; 18:45.
8. Benet LA et al: Design and optimization of dosage regimens; Pharmacokinetic data. In *The Pharmacologic Basis of Therapeutics,* Ed. by AG Gilman, LS Goodman, and A Gilman, McMillan Publishing Company, New York, 1980.
9. Chow MS et al: Pharmacokinetic data and drug monitoring: Antibiotics and antiarrhythmics. J Clin Pharmacol. 1975; 15:405.
10. Bowdle TA et al: Valproic acid dosage and plasma protein binding and clearance. Clin Pharmacol Ther. 1980; 28:486.
11. Furst DE et al: Salicylate clearance, the result of protein binding and metabolism. Clin Pharmacol Ther. 1979; 26:380.
12. Koch-Weser J et al: Binding of drugs to serum albumin. N Engl J Med. 1974; 290:706.
13. Odar-Cedarlof I et al: Kinetics of diphenylhydantoin in uremic patients: consequence of decreased protein binding. Eur J Clin Pharmacol. 1974; 7:31.
14. Piafsky KM: Disease-induced changes in the plasma binding of basic drugs. Clin Pharmacokinetics. 1980; 5:246.
15. Rutledge PA et al: Increased alpha-l-acid glycoprotein and lidocaine disposition in myocardial infarction. Ann Intern Med. 1980; 93:701.

16. Lin C et al: Absorption, metabolism and excretion of ^{14}C-griseofulvin in man. J Pharmacol Exper Ther. 1973; 187:415.

17. Jung O et al: Effect of dose on phenytoin absorption. Clin Pharmacol Ther. 1980; 28:479.

18. Huffman DH et al: Absorption of digoxin from different oral preparations in normal subjects during steady-state. Clin Pharmacol Ther. 1974; 16:310.

19. Johnson BE et al: A completely absorbed oral preparation of digoxin. Clin Pharmacol Ther. 1976; 19:746.

20. Reuning RH et al: Role of pharmacokinetics in drug dosage adjustment: Pharmacologic effect kinetics and apparent volume of distribution of digoxin. J Clin Pharmacol. 1973; 13:127.

21. Roland M: Drug administration and regimens. Ibid p 21.

22. Benowitz N: Clinical application of the pharmacokinetics of lidocaine. In *Cardiovascular Drug Therapy,* Edited by K Melmon, FM Davis, 1974 p 77.

23. Koch-Weser J: Pharmacokinetics of procainamide in man. Ann NY Acad Sci. 1971; 169:370.

24. Mitenko PA et al: Rapidly achieved plasma concentration plateaus with observations on theophylline. Clin Pharmacol Ther. 1972; 13:329.

25. Walsh FM et al: Significance of non-steady-state serum digoxin concentrations. Am J Clin Pathol. 1975; 63:446.

26. Cockcroft DW et al: Prediction of creatinine clearance from serum creatinine. Nephron. 1976; 16:31.

27. Thompson PD et al: Lidocaine pharmacokinetics in advanced heart failure, liver disease, and renal failure in humans. Ann Intern Med. 1973; 78:499.

28. Anderson JL et al: Anti-arrhythmic drugs: Clinical pharmacology and therapeutic uses. Drugs. 1978; 15:271.

29. Zito RA et al: Lidocaine kinetics predicted by indocyanine green clearance. N Engl J Med. 1978; 298:1160.

30. Powell JR et al: Theophylline disposition in acutely ill hospitalized patients. Am Rev Resp Dis. 1978; 118:229.

31. Sawchuk RJ et al: Pharmacokinetics of dosing regimens which utilize multiple intravenous infusions: Gentamicin in burn patients. J Pharmacokinetics Biopharm. 1976; 4:183.

32. Regamey C et al: Comparative pharmacokinetics of tobramycin and Gentamicin. Clin Pharmacol Ther. 1973; 14:396.

33. Gyselynek AM et al: Pharmacokinetics of gentamicin: distribution and plasma and renal clearance. J Infect Dis. 1971; 124 (suppl):70.

Chapter 2

Interpretation of Clinical Laboratory Tests

Gary H. Smith and Lloyd Y. Young

Several hundred laboratory tests are available to clinicians, and a comprehensive presentation of all these tests will not be attempted by this chapter. This chapter merely serves to introduce some of the basics of frequently ordered laboratory tests. Tests that are used to monitor specific diseases are presented in subsequent chapters. Likewise, many basic laboratory tests will be illustrated by case histories, questions, and answers in subsequent chapters rather than in this introductory chapter.

GENERAL PRINCIPLES

The serum, urine, and other fluids of patients are routinely analyzed; however, the cost of obtaining these data has significantly increased the overall cost of health care. Therefore, only those tests which will substantially benefit the patient should be ordered. There is little justification for frequent multi-organ baseline studies in the absence of any suspected problem.

Normal values. The results of clinical laboratory tests falling within a predetermined range of values are termed "normal" and those outside this range are called "abnormal." However, other factors must be taken into consideration. Sometimes age, sex, weight, height, time since last meal, drugs, or other factors may affect the range of normal values for a given test. It is important to note that normal limits are somewhat arbitrary, and abnormal laboratory values are not necessarily of diagnostic significance (see Question 5). Similarly, a normal value can actually be "abnormal" depending upon the disease state and conditions in the body (see Question 3).

Another important consideration with respect to normal values is that different clinical laboratories may use different methods for performing various tests which may produce differing ranges for normal values. Also, when a laboratory changes its methods or equipment, its normal values may change accordingly. Therefore, one should use the current normal value tables published by the laboratory when interpreting these tests and not those published in reference texts.

Laboratory Error. The possibility of laboratory error must always be considered when laboratory results do not correlate with clinical expectations. Common sources of laboratory error are as follows:

Spoiled Specimen. Improper handling, improper preservation, or undue delay in performing the test may invalidate test results. For example, if a blood sample is allowed to hemolyze, a spurious hyperkalemia may result because erythrocytes are rich in potassium as compared to plasma.

Specimen Taken at Wrong Time. The concentrations of substances in biological fluids can fluctuate depending upon the time of day, relationship to meals, and other factors. Thus, specimens obtained at improper times can yield misleading test results.

Incomplete Specimen. This is most likely to occur in studies requiring 24-hour urine collections because of the difficulty patients have in remembering to save the urine each time they void.

Faulty Reagents. Reagents which are improperly prepared or those which have deteriorated (more likely with infrequently ordered tests) may produce erroneous results.

Technical Errors. Laboratory personnel may make an error in reading an instrument or making a calculation. Patient names and samples may get interchanged, or results may be transcribed incorrectly.

Diagnostic and Therapeutic Procedures. Some diagnostic and therapeutic procedures can alter laboratory test results. For example, digital examination of the prostate can elevate serum acid phosphatase, and electrocardio-conversion can cause elevations in the serum creatine phosphokinase (CPK).

Diet. Certain foods contain substances which can appear in biological fluids and interfere with various laboratory tests.

Medication. Drugs can alter laboratory results by the following mechanisms (1):

a. Drugs can interfere with the testing procedure. For example, ascorbic acid can cause false negative results for urine glucose tested by the glucose-oxidase method.

b. Drugs can alter laboratory values by virtue of their pharmacological or toxicological properties. For example, thiazide diuretics can increase the serum uric acid concentration.

BLOOD CHEMISTRY

Sodium (135–145 mEq/Liter)

Sodium is the predominant cation of the extracellular fluid. Along with chloride, potassium, and water, it is important in establishing osmotic pressure relationships between intracellular and extracellular fluids. An increase in the serum sodium concentration may signify impaired sodium excretion or dehydration. Conversely, a decrease in the serum sodium concentration to less than normal values may reflect overhydration, abnormal sodium losses, or sodium starvation. Healthy individuals can maintain sodium balance easily; however, patients with kidney failure, heart failure, or pulmonary disease often have difficulty with sodium and water balance.

Hyponatremia may be related to dilution of serum sodium or to total body depletion of sodium. Dilutional hyponatremia occurs whenever the extracellular fluid compartment expands without an equivalent increase in sodium. This type is associated with cirrhosis, congestive heart failure, nephrosis, or the administration of osmotically active solutes such as albumin or mannitol. Hyponatremia which occurs as a result of sodium depletion presents as a low serum sodium in the absence of edema. Causes include mineralocorticoid deficiencies, sodium-wasting renal disease, and replacement of sodium-containing fluid losses with non-saline solutions. Since water moves freely across cell membranes in response to oncotic pressures, hyponatremia simply means that sodium is diluted throughout all body fluids.

Hypernatremia represents a state of relative water deficit and hence excessive concentrations of sodium in all body fluids (hypertonicity). Therefore, hypernatremia can be caused by the loss of pure water, the loss of hypotonic fluid, or by excessive sodium intake. Pure water loss is fairly uncommon except in the presence of diabetes insipidus. Fluid loss that occurs with gastroenteritis is the most common cause of hypotonic fluid loss in infants and in the very old (the "nursing home prune syndrome"). Excessive salt intoxication is usually accidental, or iatrogenic resulting from intravenous administration of hypertonic salt solutions.

The primary defense against hypertonicity is thirst and subsequent fluid intake. Therefore, hypernatremic syndromes usually occur in patients who are unable to drink sufficient fluids. Infants who cannot demand fluid or patients who are vomiting, comatose, or not allowed oral fluids are at greatest risk for the development of hypernatremia (2).

1. A 75-year-old woman was admitted to the hospital with a chief complaint of increasing shortness of breath and orthopnea over the past week. The patient has been previously treated for congestive heart failure but has not taken any medication over the past two weeks. The patient was noted to have severe (4+) pedal edema and to be in severe respiratory distress. A *stat* SMA-6 was ordered and revealed the following blood chemistries: Sodium 123 mEq/L (Normal: 135–145 mEq/L); Potassium 4.1 mEq/L (Normal: 3.5–5.0 mEq/L); Chloride 90 mEq/L (Normal: 100–106 mEq/L); Carbon Dioxide 28 mEq/L (Normal: 23–28 mEq/L); Blood Urea Nitrogen (BUN) 30 mg/dl (Normal: 7–20 mg/dl); Glucose 100 mg/dl (Normal: 70–110 mg/dl). Why shouldn't this patient with a serum concentration of 123 mEq/Liter be given sodium chloride to return her serum sodium value to normal?

Since mammalian cell membranes are freely permeable to water, all body fluids are in osmotic equilibrium, and changes in serum sodium concentration may be associated with major shifts of water into and out of cells. Therefore, the serum sodium concentration should not be used as an index of sodium need. Instead, it should only be used to detect disturbances of water balance, because the serum sodium concentration is a measure of body osmolality. The serum sodium concentration tells nothing directly about body sodium content.

In this particular patient with 4+ pedal edema and congestive heart failure, the concentration of sodium per liter of serum is probably low because the serum volume is increased relative to sodium. The usual treatment of this type of hyponatremia is salt and water restriction plus diuretics. See the chapters on Congestive Heart Failure and Fluid and Electrolyte Disorders for further discussion.

2. What are the advantages and relative costs of the SMA-12 and the SMA-6 which was ordered for this patient?

The SMA-6 and the SMA-12 are automated continuous flow analytic methods for blood chemistry analysis. Such tests have become increasingly "routine" procedures because they quickly provide basic information concerning vital organ function at relatively low cost. If abnormal values are noted, additional tests can be ordered to further investigate specific organ function.

The SMA-6 blood chemistry panel typically analyzes the sodium, potassium, chloride, CO_2, blood urea nitrogen (BUN), and glucose concentrations. Thus, this blood chemistry panel rapidly provides insights into the nature of this patient's serum electrolytes, acid-base status, renal function, and metabolic state. If an SMA-12 is ordered instead of the SMA-6 panel, six additional blood chemistry tests are performed. These six additional tests usually include a determination of the serum concentrations of albumin, total protein, bilirubin, alkaline phosphatase, calcium, and creatinine. The creatinine provides a more specific evaluation of renal function than the BUN, and some of the other added tests provide an evaluation of liver function. The SMA-12 blood chemistry panel has the advantage of providing these six additional tests for a minimal increase in cost ($19.25 compared with $17.50 for the SMA-6 at University Hospital, Seattle, Washington). Costs and the particular grouping of tests into an SMA-6 or SMA-12 panel vary with different clinical laboratories.

Although additional automated blood chemistry tests are relatively inexpensive, the probability of obtaining a false "abnormal" test result increases with the number of tests. For example, it has been calculated that about 65% of patients would have at least one abnormal test result if 20 tests were performed. Therefore, clinicians must interpret laboratory abnormalies with appropriate caution.

Potassium (3.5–5.0 mEq/Liter)

The potassium ion is the major intracellular cation present in the body. The body of a 70 kg man contains approximately 3500 milliequivalents of potassium. Only about 10% of this total body potassium is extracellular, and only about 50 milliequivalents are in the extracellular fluid. The serum potassium concentration, therefore, is not a good measure of total body potassium primarily because the bulk of potassium is sequestered within cells. On the other hand, intracellular potassium cannot be easily measured. Fortunately, the clinical manifestations of potassium deficiency (fatigue, drowsiness, dizziness, confusion, EKG changes, muscle weakness, and pain) correlate well with serum concentrations. Further, total body losses of potassium that are not reflected in decreases of the serum potassium are generally not of clinical significance.

Ordinarily, most potassium (about 40 to 90 mEq/day) is excreted from body via the urine. The potassium ion is freely filtered at the glomerulus of the kidney, and reabsorbed and tubularly secreted in the proximal and distal segments of the nephron, respectively. Thus, large osmotic diureses caused by mannitol or by the glucose load of an uncontrolled diabetic can cause *hypokalemia*. Vigorous diuresis induced by thiazide or loop diuretics commonly causes hypokalemia, as do diseases characterized by excessive mineralocorticoid activity.

The kidney has a limited ability to conserve potassium. Even when the potassium intake is reduced to zero, the urine will contain at least 5 to 20 mEq of potassium per 24 hours. Therefore, prolonged intravenous nutrition with potassium-free solutions in a patient who is unable to eat can also result in hypokalemia.

Protracted vomiting is another common cause of potassium depletion. Although the fluid secreted along most of the upper gastrointestinal tract contains only 5 to 20 mEq/L of potassium, this loss of potassium in conjunction with de-

creased food intake, loss of acid, loss of sodium, and the development of alkalosis all combine to produce hypokalemia. Severe diarrhea especially leads to potassium depletion because of the loss of large volumes of colonic fluid which contain up to 30 to 40 mEq/L of potassium.

Hyperkalemia most often occurs as the result of decreased renal excretion of potassium caused by acute renal failure, exogenous potassium ingestion, or excessive cellular breakdown (including hemolysis, burns, crush injuries, surgery, and infections).

Excesses or deficits of potassium primarily affect the excitability of nerve and muscle tissue. As a result, cardiac function can be severely affected. Potassium also affects certain enzyme systems, acid-base balance, as well as carbohydrate and protein metabolism.

3. A 27-year-old juvenile-onset diabetic was admitted to the hospital in diabetic coma with a blood sugar of 380 mg/dl (Normal: 70–110 mg/dl). Urine output was 135 ml/hr (Normal: 50 ml/hr) and the urine was 4+ positive for sugar and acetone. The chemistry results showed a blood pH of 7.21 and a serum potassium level of 4.1 mEq/L. Why should the clinician monitoring this patient be concerned about the "normal" potassium level?

Treatment of the patient's diabetic coma without supplemental potassium could result in a life-threatening hypokalemia with resulting cardiac arrest. When the pH of the blood is acidic, potassium shifts out of the cell due to increased intracellular hydrogen ion. Because this patient is acidotic, a higher than normal serum potassium level would be expected. However, because there has been a significant loss of total body potassium, the serum level appears normal. If the patient's acidosis and hyperglycemia are corrected without replacing potassium (both effects cause a shift of potassium into cells), severe hypokalemia may occur. See the chapter on Fluid and Electrolyte Disorders.

Chloride (100–106 mEq/Liter)

Chloride is the principal inorganic anion of the extracellular fluid and is important in the maintenance of acid-base balance. A decreased serum chloride concentration often accompanies metabolic alkalosis; whereas, an increased serum chloride concentration may be indicative of a hyperchloremic metabolic acidosis. The serum chloride, however, may also be slightly decreased in acidosis if organic acids or other acids are the primary cause of the acidosis. Clinically, *hyperchloremia* in the absence of metabolic acidosis is seldom encountered because chloride retention is usually accompanied by sodium and water retention. *Hypochloremia* may result from excessive gastrointestinal loss of chloride-rich fluid from vomiting, diarrhea, gastric suctioning, or intestinal fistulas. Since chloride ions are excreted renally with cations, hypochloremia may also develop during massive diuresis from any cause.

Generally, alteration in the serum concentration of chloride is seldom the primary indicator of a major medical problem. The serum chloride level per se has no real diagnostic significance. In fact, the only real reason for measuring the serum chloride is to validate the serum sodium concentration. The relationship between milliequivalents/liter of sodium, bicarbonate and chloride is as follows:

$$Cl^- + HCO_3^- + R = Na^+ \qquad (Eq.\ 1)$$

The R factor represents the contribution of unmeasured acids and normally has a numerical value of 10, although it may vary widely with different disease states. If the R fraction is established for a given patient by measuring the chloride, bicarbonate, and sodium concentration at the same time, then subsequent electrolyte measurements can be checked against each other because the R factor should remain fairly constant or at least change in a predictable manner (13).

4. The electrolyte values for the patient in Question 3 were as follows: Na 130 mEq/L, Cl 100 mEq/L, and HCO_3^- 20 mEq/L. The following evening's emergency laboratory results showed: Na 140 mEq/L, Cl 100 mEq/L, and HCO_3^- 20 mEq/L. Why is this second set of laboratory results suspicious?

The R fraction of this patient has suddenly increased from 10 to 20 and the R fraction should be fairly constant. Either there is a laboratory error in reporting these electrolyte values or else organic acids or other acids may be accumulating in this patient. In this particular case, the possibility of ketoacidosis should be considered because this patient is a brittle diabetic. Otherwise, one would have to question the validity of these electrolyte values.

Bicarbonate (23–28 mEq/Liter)

Bicarbonate in plasma is a component of the major buffer system by which the body regulates pH within physiological limits. Although there are several buffer systems in the body (including hemoglobin, phosphate, and protein), the most important in the extracellular fluid is the carbonic acid—sodium bicarbonate system. From a clinical standpoint, disturbances of acid-base balance can be considered in terms of imbalances in this system.

Combinations of weak acids and strong bases are called buffer systems because they resist changes in hydrogen ion concentration by binding and releasing H^+. For example, the base bicarbonate binds hydrogen ions and is converted to carbonic acid as follows:

$$HCO_3^- + H^+ \rightleftarrows H_2CO_3 \rightleftarrows H_2O + CO_2 \quad (Eq.\ 2)$$

Normally a ratio of one part of carbonic acid to twenty parts of bicarbonate is present in the extracellular fluid. This ratio is uniquely important and can best be appreciated when viewed in the context of the Henderson-Hasselbach equation, which is as follows:

$$pH = pka + \log \frac{[salt]}{[acid]} \qquad (Eq.\ 3)$$

$$= pKa + \log \frac{HCO_3^-}{H_2CO_3}$$

$$= 6.1 + \log \frac{20}{1} = 7.4$$

This equation unequivocally states that it is the *ratio* of HCO_3^- to H_2CO_3 (or pCO_2) and *not* the absolute value of either one which defines the pH or acid-base status of the patient. To accurately assess the acid-base status of the patient, two of the three variables (pH, pCO_2, bicarbonate) must be known. The bicarbonate concentration, by itself, does not determine a patient's acid-base balance.

Decreases in blood pH (acidosis) may be compensated for by either "blowing off" CO_2 from the lungs or by excreting H^+ in the urine. Increases in pH (alkalosis) result in compensatory retention of CO_2 by the lungs.

In clinical practice, the serum bicarbonate concentration is measured because the acid-base balance can be inferred if a patient has normal pulmonary function based upon past medical history and present bedside evaluation. For example, if a clinician can reasonably conclude that a patient's pCO_2 would not be greatly altered because of normal pulmonary function, an increase in measured serum bicarbonate concentration would most likely indicate alkalosis based upon the Henderson-Hasselbach equation. (The reader is referred to the chapter on Acid-Base Disorders for additional clinical examples.)

Calcium (9–11 mg/dl or 4.5–5.5 mEq/Liter)

The total calcium content of normal adult humans is 20 to 25 grams per kilogram of fat-free tissue, and about 44% of this calcium is in the body skeleton. About 1% of the skeletal calcium is freely exchangeable with that in the extracellular fluid. This reservoir serves to maintain a constant concentration of calcium in the plasma despite pronounced changes in the external balance of calcium. If the homeostatic factors (eg, parathyroid hormone, vitamin D, calcitonin) which regulate the calcium content of body fluid are intact, a patient may lose 25 to 30% of the total body calcium without a change in the concentration of calcium ion in the plasma.

About 40% of the calcium in the extracellular fluid is bound to plasma proteins (especially with albumin), 5 to 15% is complexed with phosphate and citrate, and about 45 to 55% is in the nonbound, ionized form. Most laboratories measure the total calcium concentration, although it is the free, ionized calcium level that is physiologically important and the form that is closely regulated.

A reduced calcium concentration, or *hypocalcemia*, usually implies a problem in either the production or response to parathyroid hormone or vitamin D. The abnormality in the parathyroid hormone system may be due to hypoparathyroidism, pseudohypoparathyroidism, or hypomagnesemia. The abnormality in the vitamin D system may be caused by decreased nutritional intake; decreased absorption of vitamin D because of gastrectomy, chronic pancreatitis, or small bowel disease; decreased production of 25-hydroxycholecalciferol because of liver disease; increased metabolism of 25-hydroxycholecalciferol because of enzyme stimulating drugs such as phenobarbital, phenytoin, and rifampin; or decreased production of 1,25-dihydroxycholecalciferol because of chronic renal disease.

Hypercalcemia may be due to malignancy, hyperparathyroidism, Paget's disease, milk-alkali syndrome, granulomatous disorders, thiazide diuretics, or vitamin D intoxication.

5. A 38-year-old male patient was admitted to General Hospital because of obtundation, somnolence, and severe alcoholic intoxication. Laboratory tests revealed the following abnormal results: albumin 1.1 gm/dl (Normal: 3.5–4.5 gm/dl) calcium 6.9 mg/dl (Normal: 9–11 mg/dl), total bilirubin 10.8 mg/dl (Normal: < 1.2 mg/dl), serum glutamic oxaloacetic transaminase 280 units/ml (Normal: 5–40 units/ml), and alkaline phosphatase 240 IU/L (Normal 13–39 IU/L). Why shouldn't this patient be treated with calcium gluconate?

This case presentation provides insufficient patient data to make a conclusion concerning treatment. Clinicians should not become so engrossed in the patient's "numbers" that the patient himself is overlooked. Always remember to *treat* the patient and *observe* laboratory tests; do not treat laboratory values. Furthermore, it should be recalled that serum calcium is partially bound to plasma proteins and that the serum concentration is dependent upon the concentration of these plasma proteins, particularly albumin. If the concentration of plasma proteins is low, the reported serum calcium will generally be less than the lower limit of normal. Although it would be best to measure ionized calcium, available instrumentation and methodology make it difficult to perform this measurement on a routine basis. In the absence of a direct measurement of ionized calcium, a useful way to estimate a corrected value for serum calcium in the presence of a low serum albumin is to use the rule that the total serum calcium will fall by 0.8 mg/dl for each decrement in serum albumin of 1.0 gm/dl. In this patient, the amount of available ionized calcium would be comparable to that available if his serum calcium were 9.2 mg/dl: (2.9 × 0.8 + 6.9). His serum albumin concentration is about 2.9 gm/dl less than "normal" (4.0 mg/dl − 1.1 mg/dl = 2.9 mg/dl). Because the corrected serum calcium is within the normal range, this patient should not receive calcium gluconate.

Phosphate (3.2–4.3 mg/dl)

Extracellular inorganic phosphate is the prime determinant of intracellular inorganic phosphate, which in turn is the cellular source of phosphate for ATP and phospholipid synthesis and an important factor in the regulation of nucleotide degradation. The extracellular fluid concentration of phosphate is in turn influenced by parathyroid hormone function, intestinal absorption, renal function, bone metabolism, and nutrition. *Hyperphosphatemia* is most commonly caused by renal insufficiency, although hypervitaminosis D and hypoparathyroidism are also significant causes. *Hypophosphatemia* can occur in various states of malabsorption but usually is due to renal phosphate losses caused by secondary hyperparathyroidism accompanying hypocalcemia and vitamin D malabsorption. Overuse of aluminum-containing antacid preparations is occasionally an iatrogenic cause of decreased serum phosphate concentrations. The common clinical syndromes associated with acute hypophosphatemia usually involve disorders of neuro-muscular function. The chapter entitled Kidney Diseases provides examples of disorders of phosphate metabolism.

Glucose (70–110 mg/dl)

The glucose concentration in extracellular fluid normally is closely regulated by homeostatic mechanisms to provide body tissues with a ready source of energy. The plasma glucose concentration is usually measured in either the fasting or postprandial state depending upon the type of information desired. Generally, normal glucose values refer to the plasma glucose concentration for the fasting state. The laboratory technique of blood sugar determinations must also be considered, because different methodologies vary in specificity and sensitivity to glucose. Hyperglycemia and hypoglycemia are nonspecific signs of abnormal glucose metabolism. Diabetes mellitus is the most common cause of hyperglycemia, and insufficient carbohydrate intake because of a missed meal in a patient receiving insulin or another hypoglycemic medication is the most common cause of hypoglycemia. The reader is referred to the chapter entitled Diabetes Mellitus for an indepth presentation of laboratory tests associated with abnormal glucose metabolism.

Uric Acid (3.0–7.0 mg/dl)

Uric acid is an end-product of nucleoprotein metabolism. It serves no biological function, is not metabolized, and must be excreted renally.

The rheumatological disorder, gout, is usually associated with increased serum concentrations of uric acid and deposits of monosodium urates. Elevated serum uric acid concentrations can result either from a decrease in renal excretion or from the excessive nucleoprotein turnover which accompanies neoplastic or myeloproliferative disorders. Low serum uric acid concentrations are inconsequential and usually are reflective of drugs which have hypouricemic activity. The determinants of the serum concentration of uric acid, the clinical implications of hyperuricemia, and the therapeutic management of uric acid metabolism disorders are presented in the chapter entitled Gout and Hyperuricemia.

Blood Urea Nitrogen, BUN (7–20 mg/dl)

Urea is an end-product of protein metabolism. It is produced solely by the liver, travels through the blood, and is excreted by the kidneys. Because the blood urea nitrogen is completely filtered at the glomerulus of the kidney, then reabsorbed and tubularly secreted within nephrons, the concentration of blood urea nitrogen (BUN) reflects renal function. Acute or chronic renal failure is the most common cause of an elevated BUN. Although the BUN is an excellent "screening" test for renal dysfunction, it is not sufficiently selective for quantifying the extent of renal disease. A number of factors other than renal function may influence the level of BUN. For example, unusually high protein intake or conditions which increase protein catabolism will tend to increase the BUN. Gastrointestinal bleeding or esophageal varices can elevate the BUN because the blood is converted by bacteria in the bowel to ammonia and urea nitrogen. The hydrational status of a patient may either increase or decrease the BUN because a water deficit would tend to concentrate the urea nitrogen and a water excess would dilute the urea nitrogen. Furthermore, the BUN may be decreased in the terminal stages of liver disease because of the inability of the liver to form urea.

6. Why is the BUN abnormal for the patient in Question 1?

The BUN in this patient is mildly elevated probably because she is unable to adequately perfuse her kidneys due to her heart failure. Furthermore, her renal function may be more severely compromised than one would anticipate from the slightly elevated BUN. The BUN probably has been diluted by her increased extracellular fluid volume. Therefore, further evaluation of this patient's renal status will be required.

Creatinine (0.5–1.3 mg/dl)

Creatinine is derived from creatine and phosphocreatine, a major constituent of muscle. Its rate of formation for a given individual is remarkably constant and is primarily determined by the individual's muscle mass or lean body weight. The serum creatinine level is therefore slightly higher in muscular subjects, but unlike the BUN level, it is less affected by exogenous factors. Once creatinine is released from muscle into plasma, it is excreted almost exclusively by the kidney by glomerular filtration. A decrease in the glomerular filtration rate would therefore result in an increase in the serum creatinine concentration. Thus, determination of the serum creatinine concentration is widely used in the clinical evaluation of patients with suspected renal disease.

A doubling of the serum creatinine roughly corresponds to a 50% reduction in the glomerular filtration rate. This general rule of thumb only holds for steady state creatinine levels (3,4).

7. The patient in Question 1 was given digoxin 0.25 mg/day, and a serum creatinine was ordered to further assess her renal function. The clinical laboratory determined that this patient's serum creatinine was 1.2 mg/dl. Since this laboratory test result is within normal limits, does it indicate normal renal function for this patient?

A serum creatinine of 1.2 mg/dl in this patient does not necessarily mean that she has normal renal function. As patients become older, their muscle mass represents a smaller proportion of their total weight, and creatinine production is decreased. Furthermore, the serum creatinine level in female patients is 0.2 to 0.4 mg/dl lower than in males. Because this patient is a 75-year-old female, a creatinine clearance determination would more accurately reflect her renal function status.

Creatinine Clearance (125 ml/min for men; 110 ml/min for women)

The clearance of any substance that is freely filtered at the glomerulus and is neither reabsorbed, secreted, synthesized, nor metabolized by the kidney is equal to the glomerular filtration

rate. Because creatinine meets these criteria, the clearance of creatinine should accurately reflect the glomerular filtration rate.

An accurate estimation of creatinine clearance is crucial to rational drug therapy because many drugs are partially or totally eliminated by the kidney. The creatinine clearance is the most accurate test of renal function. However, an accurate creatinine clearance is difficult to obtain clinically because it is based upon a 24-hour urine collection. Frequently, the urine collection is inaccurate because a portion is accidentally discarded, or the time of collection is shorter or longer than requested. An incomplete collection could result in a substantial underestimation of renal function. Furthermore, the method is time-consuming and expensive. As a result, several nomograms and formulas have been developed to provide estimates of creatinine clearances by utilizing measured serum creatinine values. The following formula is commonly used:

$$\text{Creatinine Clearance for males (ml/min/70 kg)} = \frac{98 - 0.8(\text{age} - 20)}{\text{serum creatinine}} \quad \text{(Eq. 4)}$$

This same formula must be adjusted by 90% to calculate creatinine clearances for females:

$$\text{Creatinine Clearance for females (ml/min/70 kg)} = 0.9 \left[\frac{98 - 0.8(\text{age} - 20)}{\text{serum creatinine}} \right] \quad \text{(Eq. 5)}$$

A comparative evaluation of various formulas which estimate creatinine clearance noted that all methods of calculation appeared to be equally reliable for patients with a serum creatinine in the 1.5 to 5.0 mg/dl range (17). However, the above formula substantially underestimated the creatinine clearance in patients with a serum creatinine of less than 1.5 mg/dl. The following method provided the best estimate of creatinine clearance over all ranges of renal function (17):

$$\text{Creatinine Clearance for males (ml/min/70 kg)} = \left[\frac{145 - \text{age}}{\text{serum creatinine}} \right] - 3 \quad \text{(Eq. 6)}$$

This particular formula must be adjusted by 85% to calculate creatinine clearance for females:

$$\text{Creatinine Clearance for females (ml/min/70 kg)} = 0.85\left[\left(\frac{145 - age}{serum\ creatinine}\right) - 3\right] \quad (Eq.\ 7)$$

For patients with liver dysfunction, all methods of calculating creatinine clearance from a serum creatinine value were associated with significant overprediction of creatinine clearance (17). Thus, methods for predicting creatinine clearance should not be used in patients with liver disease as a basis for the adjustment of drug dosages.

8. A 24-hour creatinine clearance determination was ordered for a 44-year-old, 50 kg male patient. The following data were returned from the clinical laboratory:

Total collection time: 24 hours
Urine volume: 1200 ml
Urine creatinine concentration: 42mg/dl
Serum creatinine: 1.5 mg/dl
Creatinine clearance:
   (Uncorrected)   23 ml/min
   (Corrected)   30 ml/min

Why should this patient's reported creatinine clearance be viewed with considerable suspicion?

Whenever creatinine clearance determinations are reported, clinicians should always verify the reliability of the test result before altering drug dosing schedules. The total amount of creatinine actually collected in the 24-hour period should be compared to the calculated amount of creatinine which is expected to be produced to determine whether the urine collection was complete.

$$(Eq.\ 8)$$

Amount of = (Urine Vol./24 hrs)(Urine Creatinine Conc.)
Creatinine = (1200 ml/24 hrs)(42 mg/100 ml)
Excreted   = 504 mg creatinine/24 hrs

The apparent creatinine production per day can be calculated by dividing the total amount of creatinine excreted by the patient's weight.

$$\text{Apparent Rate of Creatinine Production per Day} = \frac{\text{Amount of Creatinine Excreted}}{\text{Patient's Weight}} \quad (Eq.\ 9)$$

$$= \frac{504\ mg\ creatinine/24\ hrs}{50\ kg}$$

$$= 10.08\ mg/kg/day$$

Table 1.
EXPECTED DAILY CREATININE PRODUCTION FOR MALES

Age (Years)	Daily Creatinine Production (mg/kg/day)
20–29	24
30–39	22
40–49	20
50–59	19
60–69	17
70–79	14
80–89	12
90–99	9

Reproduced from Winter ME et al: *Basic Clinical Pharmacokinetics,* Applied Therapeutics, Inc., 1980, p 60.

This apparent rate of creatinine production of approximately 10 mg/kg/day is considerably less than the expected 20 mg/kg/day creatinine production for a 44-year-old male. See Table 1. Therefore, the collection of urine probably was incomplete, and the reported creatinine clearance is probably much less than the patient's actual creatinine clearance. However, if this patient has a very small muscle mass because of atrophy, cachexia, or age, the urine collection could be adequate and the reported creatinine clearance accurate.

As shown in this patient's laboratory test results, both uncorrected and corrected creatinine clearance values are reported by clinical laboratories. The "uncorrected" value usually represents the patient's actual creatinine clearance and the "corrected" value predicts what the patient's creatinine clearance would be if he or she were 1.73 m² or 70 kg (14).

Lactic Dehydrogenase, LDH
(70–210 IU/Liter)

The glycolytic enzyme, lactic dehydrogenase (LDH) catalyzes the interconversion of lactate and pyruvate and is present in nearly all metabolizing cells. It is present in especially high concentrations in heart, kidney, liver, and skeletal muscle, although it is also abundantly present in red cells and lung tissue. Thus, elevations of serum LDH levels can occur following diseases in many different organs and tissues. The diagnostic usefulness of serum LDH determinations, therefore, is somewhat compromised. However, there are five isoenzymes of LDH, and tissues contain varying proportions of these isoenzymes.

Studies of LDH isoenzyme levels in various diseases have revealed abnormal patterns reflecting the tissues involved. Therefore, chemical or electrophoretic separation of these isoenzymes can increase the diagnostic usefulness of serum LDH determinations. For example, the elevated serum LDH associated with myocardial infarction consists mostly of LDH_1 and LDH_2; whereas, with acute viral hepatitis, there is a greater proportion of LDH_4 and LDH_5. Unfortunately, these isoenzyme patterns are not necessarily typical of all myocardial or liver diseases; therefore, LDH isoenzyme patterns can only be used as an aid to the diagnosis, prognosis, and therapeutics of certain diseases.

Creatine Phosphokinase, CPK
(50–170 units/Liter)

Creatine phosphokinase is an enzyme which is found primarily in muscle tissue. It is the first enzyme to rise following an acute myocardial infarction and is also elevated following strenuous exercise or muscle injury. Intramuscular injections of irritating drugs such as digoxin, diazepam, chlorpromazine, phenytoin, and several antibiotics can elevate this enzyme and confuse diagnoses. Other drugs, such as amphotericin B and clofibrate can cause direct muscle damage and elevate CPK levels. However, the CK_2 or MB fraction of CPK is specific for cardiac muscle and when substantially elevated indicates myocardial damage.

Albumin (3.5–4.5 gm/dl)

Albumin is produced by the liver and, along with globulin (below), is a major determinant of colloidal osmotic pressure. Since albumin contributes approximately 80% of serum colloid osmotic pressure, edema and transudation of extracellular fluid commonly accompany hypoalbuminemic states. Decreased albumin concentrations may occur as the result of malnutrition or malabsorption, hepatic insufficiency, or kidney disease. The serum albumin concentration may be increased in dehydration, shock, and after the administration of large amounts of intravenous albumin. In addition to its diagnostic value, the serum albumin concentration is an important consideration in the dosing and evaluation of drugs which are highly bound to albumin (eg, phenytoin, diazepam, or salicylate).

Globulin (3.0–4.0 gm/dl)

Because globulin is not manufactured solely by the liver, the ratio of albumin to globulin (the A/G ratio) is changed in patients with liver disease. Changes in this ratio are due to decreased albumin concentration and a compensatory increase in globulin concentraton. In addition to maintaining osmotic pressure, globulins also function in a number of host defense capacities. Fractionated globulins such as IgG, IgM, or IgE are useful in the evaluation of immune disorders.

Serum Glutamic Oxaloacetic Transaminase, SGOT (5–40 units/ml)

The enzyme known as serum glutamic oxaloacetic acid (SGOT) is found in very large concentrations in heart and liver tissue, but only in moderate amounts in skeletal muscle, kidney, and pancreas. In cases of acute cellular injury to the heart or liver, the enzyme is released into the blood stream from the damaged cells and is presumably metabolized within the body. In clinical practice, SGOT determinations are used to evaluate myocardial injury and to diagnose and assess the prognosis of liver disease resulting from hepatocellular injury.

Serum SGOT values are markedly elevated in patients with acute hepatic necrosis caused by viral hepatitis or carbon tetrachloride poisoning. Patients with intrahepatic cholestasis, post-hepatic jaundice, or cirrhosis usually experience more moderate elevations of SGOT depending on the degree of cell necrosis taking place. Since SGOT determinations are especially useful in the early detection of viral or toxic hepatitis, they are commonly utilized in monitoring the hepatic status of patients exposed to hepatotoxic drugs.

Numerous studies indicate that 96–98% of patients with acute myocardial infarction have elevated SGOT levels. The typical enzyme pattern following an acute myocardial infarction is described in the Acute Myocardial Infarction chapter.

Serum Glutamic Pyruvic Transaminase, SGPT (5–40 units/ml)

The enzyme, serum glutamic pyruvic transaminase (SGPT) is found in essentially the same tissues which have high concentrations of SGOT. In liver diseases, serum SGPT elevations parallel those of SGOT, although slightly more acute hepatocellular parenchymal damage must occur to produce abnormal values. The SGPT is relatively more abundant in hepatic tissue versus cardiac tissue than SGOT; nevertheless, it is not as popular as the SGOT in monitoring liver deterioration because the liver still contains 3.5 times more SGOT than SGPT.

Alkaline Phosphatase
(2.0–4.5 Bodansky units/ml)

The alkaline phosphatases constitute a large group of isoenzymes which play important roles in the transport of sugar and phosphate. These isoenzymes of alkaline phosphatase have different physicochemical properties and originate from different tissues (eg, liver, bone, placenta, and intestine).

In normal adults, the circulating alkaline phosphatase is derived primarily from liver and bone. Although only small amounts of alkaline phosphatase are found in the normal liver, this enzyme is secreted into the bile, and its serum concentration increases substantially with mild intrahepatic or extrahepatic biliary obstruction. Thus, the presence of early bile duct abnormalities can result in alkaline phosphatase elevations before increases in the serum bilirubin are observed. The cholestatic jaundice produced by certain drugs such as chlorpromazine or sulfonamides can also cause elevation of this enzyme. Alkaline phosphatase determinations generally are not particularly useful in assessing the degree of hepatic impairment. In mild cases of acute liver cell damage, the alkaline phosphatase is seldom elevated, and even in cirrhosis the alkaline phosphatase serum concentration is variable and depends on the degree of hepatic decompensation and obstruction. However, the alkaline phosphatase is an excellent indicator of space-occupying lesions in the liver (5).

The osteoblasts in bone produce large amounts of alkaline phosphatase. Thus, alkaline phosphatase concentrations in serum are markedly increased in Paget's disease, hyperparathyroidism, osteogenic sarcoma, osteoblastic cancer metastatic to bone, and other conditions of pronounced osteoblastic activity. The alkaline phosphatase is physiologically elevated during periods of rapid bone growth in infancy, early childhood, or in healing bone fractures; it may also be elevated during pregnancy because of the contributions of the placenta and fetal bones.

Bilirubin (1.0 mg/dl for total bilirubin; 0.4 mg/dl for direct bilirubin)

Bilirubin is primarily a breakdown product of hemoglobin and is formed in the reticuloendothelial system (see Step 1 of Figure 1). It is then transferred into the blood (Step 2) where it is almost completely bound to serum albumin (Step 3). When the bilirubin arrives at the sinusoidal surface of the liver cells, the free fraction is rapidly taken up into the cell (Step 4) and converted primarily to bilirubin diglucuronide (Step 5). This conjugated form is then excreted in the bile (Step 6) and appears in the intestine where bacteria convert the majority of it to urobilinogen (Step 7). Most of the urobilinogen is destroyed or excreted in the feces (Step 13), but some is reabsorbed into the blood (Step 8). A portion of this small amount of urobilinogen in the blood is then reabsorbed into the liver (Step 9) and subsequently excreted into the bile (Step 12); the other portion is excreted into the urine (Step 10). The mechanism by which conjugated bilirubin in the liver cell is transferred to the blood (Step 14) is not well understood. However, in many types of liver disease the conjugated form of bilirubin (direct acting) is present in increased concentrations in the blood. When this concentration exceeds 0.2 to 0.4 mg/dl, bilirubin will begin to appear in the urine (Step 11). Unconjugated bilirubin (indirect acting) is water insoluble and is highly bound to serum albumin; both of these factors account for its lack of excretion in the urine (6).

9. A 42-year-old male with a two-year history of hypertension controlled with methyldopa was admitted to the hospital following an episode of orthostatic hypotension. Admitting laboratory results showed a hematocrit of 27%. Liver function tests were obtained because the patient had a long history of alcoholism and because of concern for methyldopa hepatotoxicity: Bilirubin (total) 3.5 mg/dl, Bilirubin (direct) 0.5 mg/dl, Alkaline phosphatase 3.0 Bodansky units, SGOT 42 units/ml, and SGPT 27 units/ml. Based upon the above information and Figure 1, what are three major causes of increased bilirubin in

adults, and what might be the most logical cause of increased bilirubin in this patient?

Hepatocellular damage. In conditions where the liver is unable to conjugate bilirubin, the total bilirubin will again rise out of proportion to the direct bilirubin. However, this patient's normal SGOT and SGPT values indicate that hepatocellular damage is not likely. Therefore, in the case

presented, a diagnosis of hepatocellular damage cannot be confirmed by the bilirubin levels alone.

Cholestasis. When an obstruction to bile flow occurs in the absence of severe liver impairment, the increase in total bilirubin will primarily be the result of an increase in direct or conjugated bilirubin. The alkaline phosphatase is useful in differentiating cholestasis from other forms of

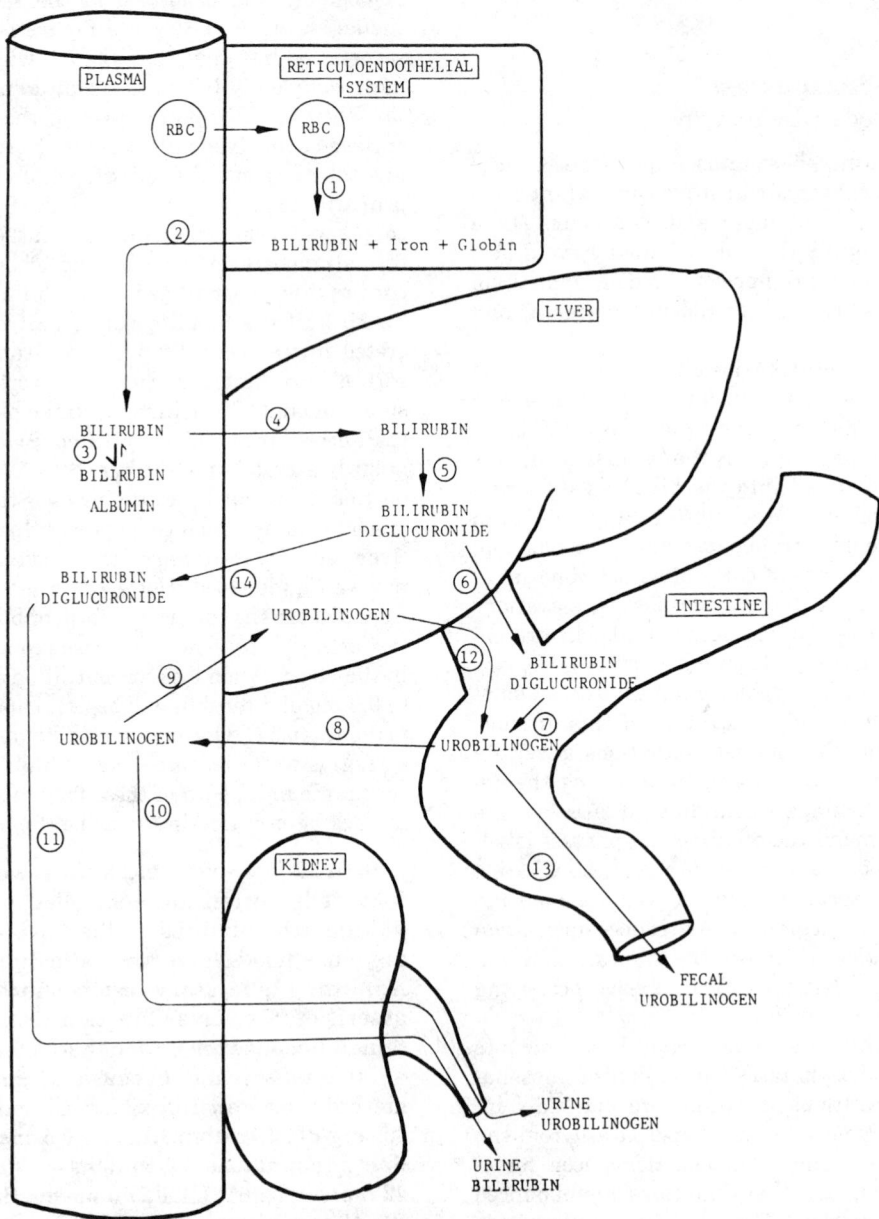

Figure 1. Bilirubin Metabolism.

jaundice. In this case, the normal values for alkaline phosphatase and direct bilirubin indicate that there is not a cholestatic component to this patient's problem.

Hemolysis. When erythrocytes are destroyed at a faster than normal rate, there is an increased formation of indirect bilirubin. If the liver is conjugating and eliminating bilirubin normally, the total bilirubin will increase out of proportion to the direct bilirubin. This was evident in the above case. Thus, the increased indirect bilirubin in this case is probably caused by hemolysis. Other tests can be ordered to confirm the diagnosis suggested by these routine liver function tests.

Acid Phosphatase (0.1–1.1 Bodansky units/ml)

The function of acid phosphatase is not well understood. This enzyme is present in high concentration in prostatic tissue, although a different acid phosphatase can also be found in erythrocytes and platelets. Significantly elevated serum levels of acid phosphatase occur in patients with metastatic carcinoma of the prostate. Patients with benign prostatic hypertrophy or prostatitis do not have increased serum concentrations of acid phosphatase, although slight elevations sometimes may be noticed after vigorous prostatic massage (7).

HEMATOLOGY

Red Blood Cells, RBC's (4.5–6.0 million/mm^3 for males; 4.0–5.5 million/mm^3 for females)

Red blood cells (RBC's) are produced in the bone marrow and released into the peripheral blood where they circulate for approximately 120 days before they are destroyed by the reticuloendothelial system. The function of RBC's is to transport oxygen to tissues.

Determination of the concentration of RBC's in the blood is required to detect anemia, to calculate red cell indices, or to calculate the hematocrit. For the purpose of monitoring quantitative changes in RBC's, the hematocrit and hemoglobin concentration generally are utilized.

Hematocrit; Packed Cell Volume (40–54% for males; 38–47% for females)

The hematocrit is determined by centrifuging a capillary tube of whole blood and comparing the height of the settled red cells to the height of the column of whole blood. The percentage of red cells to the blood volume is the hematocrit.

A decrease in hematocrit may result from bleeding, bone marrow suppressant effects of drugs, chronic diseases, genetic alterations in red cell morphology (sickle cell anemia), or from hemolysis. An increase in hematocrit may result from hemoconcentration, polycythemia vera, or polycythemia secondary to chronic hypoxia.

Hemoglobin (12.0–17.0 gm/dl for males; 11.0–15.0 gm/dl for females)

Hemoglobin is the oxygen-carrying compound contained in red blood cells. Therefore, the total hemoglobin concentration depends primarily upon the number of red cells in the blood sample, although it is also slightly influenced by the amount of hemoglobin in each red cell. The same medical conditions that increase or decrease the hematocrit or the number of RBC's affect the hemoglobin concentration in a similar fashion.

A hemoglobin determination is preferable to an RBC determination because it most directly reflects the oxygen transport capability of blood; however, the hematocrit is most commonly utilized clinically because it is technically simpler to perform (8).

Red Cell Indices (Wintrobe Indices)

Red cell indices are useful in the classification of anemias. These indices include the mean cell volume (MCV), the mean cell hemoglobin (MCH), and the mean cell hemoglobin concentration (MCHC). These indices are calculated as follows:

$$MCV = \frac{\text{hematocrit} \times 10}{\text{RBC count}_{actual} \times 10^{-6}} \qquad \text{(Eq. 10)}$$

$$= 90 \pm 8 \text{ cu microns}$$

$$MCH = \frac{\text{hemoglobin} \times 10}{\text{RBC} \times 10^{-6}} \qquad \text{(Eq. 11)}$$

$$= 30 \pm 3 \text{ picograms}$$

$$MCHC = \frac{\text{hemoglobin} \times 100}{\text{hematocrit}} \qquad \text{(Eq. 12)}$$

$$= \frac{MCH}{MCV} = 33 \pm 2 \text{ gm/dl}$$

The MCV detects changes in cell size. Therefore, descriptive terms such as *macrocytosis* or *microcytosis* can be used for abnormal MCV values. For example, a decreased MCV value would suggest a microcytic cell which may occur in iron deficiency anemia. A large MCV value would suggest a macrocytic cell which is commonly caused by a vitamin B-12 or folic acid deficiency anemia. Since the MCV may be normal in a patient with a "mixed" (microcytic and macrocytic) anemia, red cell indices cannot take the place of direct observation of a blood smear.

The MCHC is a more reliable index of red cell hemoglobin than the MCH. The former measures the concentration of hemoglobin in the average red blood cell; whereas, the latter measures the weight of hemoglobin in the average red cell. In normochromic anemias, changes in the size of red blood cells (MCV) are associated with corresponding changes in the weight of hemoglobin (MCH), but the concentration of hemoglobin (MCHC) remains normal (9).

Changes in the hemoglobin content of red cells alter the color of these cells. Thus, the terms hypochromic and normochromic are sometimes used to indicate, respectively, decreased or normal amounts of hemoglobin in cells. Hypochromic red cells are characteristic of an iron deficiency anemia, but hyperchromic cells are very rare (8).

10. A 58-year-old chronic alcoholic was admitted to the medical ward for observation following a barroom brawl. As part of the standard work-up, red blood cell indices were reported from the clinical laboratory as follows: MCV 108 cubic microns, MCH 38 picograms, MCHC 34 gm/dl. How should these indices be interpreted in this patient?

The MCH and MCV are both increased and the MCHC is usually normal in macrocytic anemias associated with vitamin B-12 or folic acid deficiency. The MCH is increased because the red blood cells have increased in size; however, the concentration of hemoglobin (MCHC) has not been changed. This characteristic picture is illustrated in the alcoholic patient described who most likely has a dietary folic acid deficiency. If this patient's indices were normal (normocytic, normochromic) and if anemia was present (decreased hemoglobin or hematocrit) then acute blood loss from his barroom brawl should be considered. If the anemia seems to be more chronic in nature, then alcohol bone marrow suppression should be considered. Refer to the chapter entitled Anemias for a thorough presentation on the topic of anemias and to the chapter entitled Alcohol Abuse for descriptions of the effects of alcohol on the red blood cell.

Reticulocytes (0.2–2.0% of red cells)

Reticulocytes are young blood cells which are not yet completely mature. The reticulocyte count, therefore, measures the rate of appearance of these new corpuscles into the circulating blood. Increased reticulocyte counts mean that an increased number of these red blood cells are being pushed into the blood stream in response to some stimulus. After hemorrhage or hemolysis, rapid red cell regeneration ensues and the reticulocyte count may be as high as 40%. Appropriate treatment of anemias caused by iron, vitamin B-12, or folic acid deficiencies should result in an increased reticulocyte count as well. If the reticulocyte count does not increase in response to replacement therapy, then the diagnosis or the treatment should be re-evaluated if the bone marrow is deemed competent. Furthermore, caution must be exercised in the interpretation of reticulocyte counts. Changes in the number of red blood cells will result in proportional changes in the reticulocyte count because the reticulocyte count is reported as a percentage of the number of red blood cells.

Erythrocyte Sedimentation Rate, ESR (0–20 mm/hour)

The sedimentation rate is the rate at which red blood cells settle to the bottom of a test tube through the forces of gravity. This test is nonspecific; the sedimentation rate is abnormally increased in acute and chronic inflammatory processes, acute and chronic infections, neoplasms, infarction, tissue necrosis, rheumatoid-collagen disease, dysproteinemias, nephritis, and even pregnancy. On the other hand, it is sometimes normal in diseases where it usually is abnormal, and even laboratory technique can substantially affect the sedimentation rate (7). Since many factors can enhance the settling rate of red blood cells, moderate to marked elevation of the sedimentation rate merely indicates a disease state. Nevertheless, the sedimentation rate is extremely useful in monitoring the activity or clinical course of certain diseases and to differentiate organic diseases from those of psychosomatic origin. This test is particularly valuable in following the course of rheumatoid arthritis, nephritis, tuberculosis, and rheumatic carditis.

White Blood Cells, WBC's
(4,000–11,000/mm^3)

White blood cells, unlike red blood cells and platelets, perform no physiological function within the vascular system. The blood merely serves as a transportation network which allows white cells to move into various body tissues and cavities. Nevertheless, in man, there are approximately 4,000–11,000 white blood cells per cubic millimeter of blood. Of these, neutrophils are the most common, followed in order of frequency by lymphocytes, monocytes, eosinophils, and basophils. The neutrophils, eosinophils, basophils, and monocytes are formed from stem cells in the bone marrow. Some lymphocytes are formed in the bone marrow, but most are formed in lymph nodes, thymus, and spleen. Also in the bone marrow, another type of leukocyte, the plasma cell, is observed. This entire system of white blood cells focuses on host defense; however, each of these types of cells has unique functions. Therefore, it is best to think of these cell types as individual types of cells rather than collectively as "leukocytes" (10).

Neutrophils. Neutrophils are important in defense against bacterial invasion and are usually the first white cells to gather in response to acute inflammation. The terms "polys," "segs," "PMN's," and sometimes "granulocytes" are synonymous with the term "neutrophil" in clinical practice. Additional neutrophil terminology is based upon the normal maturation sequence of this leukocyte in the bone marrow. The stem cell gives rise to the myeloblast, which then matures respectively into a promyelocyte, neutrophil myelocyte, neutrophil metamyelocyte, band neutrophil, and finally into a polymorphonuclear segmented neutrophil. Segmented neutrophils constitute 50–70% of circulating leukocytes, and band neutrophils usually represent about 3–5% of the total circulating white cells. Normally about 35% of the segmented neutrophils have two lobes, 41% have three lobes, and 20% have four or more lobes. This maturation process of neutrophils used to be diagrammed with the more immature neutrophils on the left progressing to the more mature forms on the right. Therefore, a "shift to the left" occurred when there were increased numbers of band neutrophils, other less mature neutrophils, and a lower average number of lobes of segmented cells in the blood (9).

Increased neutrophils or neutrophilia (> 8000 cells/mm^3) is most frequently caused by systemic or severe local bacterial infections. Viral infections are usually characterized by normal neutrophil counts or sometimes neutropenia. Tissue destruction (eg, burns, infarction, hemorrhage); inflammatory diseases (eg, acute gout, rheumatoid arthritis, hypersensitivity drug reactions); metabolic toxic states (eg, diabetic ketoacidosis, uremia, eclampsia); physiological response to stress (eg, physical exercise, childbirth); and drugs (eg, epinephrine, corticosteroids) can all cause significant neutrophilia.

Decreased neutrophils or neutropenia is defined as a neutrophil count of less than 2000 cells/mm^3. The term *agranulocytosis* has been used for severe neutropenia, and the risk of infection is substantial when the neutrophil count is less than 500 cells/mm^3. The most common causes of diminished neutrophil production are metastatic carcinoma, lymphoma, and drugs.

Lymphocytes. Lymphocytes constitute the second most common white cell in circulating blood. These white cells are essential to the immune defense system, as their primary function is to respond to antigens by initiating the immune response. The lymphocytes circulating in blood represent less than 5% of the total body pool. The vast majority of the lymphocytes are located in the spleen, lymph nodes, and other organized lymphatic tissue. There are two major types of lymphocytes. T-lymphocytes (thymic dependent) participate in cell mediated immune responses, and B-lymphocytes (bone-marrow derived) are responsible for humoral antibody responses. Therefore, diseases affecting lymphocytes primarily manifest themselves as immune deficiency disorders which render the patient unable to defend himself against normal pathogens or as autoimmune diseases in which immune responses are directed against the body's own cells (10).

Increased numbers of lymphocytes on a white count differential sometimes accompany viral infections such as infectious mononucleosis, mumps, and German measles. Occasionally, a relative lymphocytosis arises in various conditions in which there is neutropenia because the total lymphocytes have remained the same while the total neutrophils are declining (11).

Monocytes. Monocytes are formed in the bone marrow and transported by the blood to tissues where they mature into macrophages (12). Monocytosis may be observed in subacute bacterial endocarditis, malaria, tuberculosis, and during the recovery phase of some infections.

Eosinophils. Eosinophils seem to have the ability to inactivate mediators which are released from mast cells, thereby modifying reactions associated with IgE-mediated degranulation of mast cells. Eosinophils are also capable of damaging larval-tissue stages of some helminth parasites, especially *Schistosoma mansoni* (13). Therefore, it is not surprising that increased numbers of eosinophils are associated with allergic disorders such as bronchial asthma, urticaria, and drug hypersensitivity reactions as well as with parasitic infections. Eosinophilia also occurs with malignant disease, Hodgkin's disease, pernicious anemia, and some skin disorders.

Basophils. Basophils are poorly understood but an increase in basophils in blood is a useful diagnostic sign for certain diseases. In chronic myeloid leukemia, in myelofibrosis, and in polycythemia vera, an increase in basophils is common; however, it is not common in diseases which merely mimic these three diseases. A decrease in the number of basophils is generally not readily apparent because of the paucity of these cells in the blood (10).

11. A 45-year-old patient was admitted to General Hospital with a sustained high fever of 39.4° centigrade, shortness of breath, and pleurisy. He is coughing up rusty sputum and appears to be in acute distress. According to the patient, these symptoms appeared abruptly. The results of the WBC count and differential were reported from the laboratory as follows: Total white blood count 30,000, Neutrophils ("polys") 76%, Bands (stabs) 13%, Lymphocytes 10%, Monocytes 0, Eosinophils 1%, and Basophils 0. On the basis of this laboratory report and other findings, a diagnosis of pneumococcal pneumonia was made.

Why is this laboratory report consistent with bacterial infection?

White blood cells are the host's chief defense system, and the neutrophil is the main component of that system. Typically, in bacterial infections there is an increased WBC count, an increase in the proportion of neutrophils, and a "shift to the left." The percentage of other types of white cells is proportionately decreased because the number of neutrophils is increased.

As the infection progresses, the percentage of band cells may decrease, due to an increase in the number of neutrophils, which have a longer half-life. This decrease in bands does not necessarily indicate improvement. A decrease in the percentage of neutrophils with a drop in the total WBC count is characteristic of effective antibiotic therapy. Significant drops in the WBC count may be observed within the first 24 hours of antibiotic therapy.

12. H.A. is a 35-year-old patient who has been treated with dicloxacillin for seven days for a cellulitis of the left leg. On the eighth day the patient developed an urticarial rash consistent with an allergic reaction. An eosinophil count was obtained revealing 400 eosinophils/mm^3 (4%) in the peripheral blood. What does the eosinophil count contribute to this case?

Eosinophils are usually increased in allergic reactions to drugs and when coupled with a urticarial rash make the diagnosis of a drug-induced hypersensitivity fairly conclusive. Clinicians should become suspicious of an allergic drug reaction whenever the absolute eosinophil count exceeds 300 cells (3% of 10,000 WBC's). Eosinophils may increase before, after, or concurrent with other evidence of allergy such as a rash. An elevated count without evidence of allergy is not generally considered sufficient cause to discontinue a suspected medication. See Table 2 for other drugs implicated in eosinophilia.

URINALYSIS

A standard urinalysis begins with simple observation of the color and the gross general appearance of the urine specimen. The urine pH and specific gravity are then recorded. Formed elements in the urine are microscopically examined, and the urine is searched routinely for path-

Table 2.
DRUGS REPORTED TO HAVE CAUSED
EOSINOPHILIA [14-16]

Allopurinol	Erythromycin
Amoxicillin	Flucytosine
Amphotericin	Gold Salts
Ampicillin	Imipramine
Aspirin	Isoniazid
Carbamazepine	Meglumine Diatrizoate
Carbenicillin	Meglumine Iothalamate
Cephalosporins	Nitrofurantoin
Chloroquine	Pentazocine
Chlorpromazine	Phenacetin
Chlorpropamide	Phenylbutazone
Cloxacillin	Phenytoin
Desipramine	Quinidine
Dicloxacillin	Sodium Aminosalicylate
Doxycycline	Sulfonamide

ologically significant elements which are not normally present such as glucose, blood, ketones, and bile pigments.

Gross appearance of specimen. Urinalysis usually is performed on the concentrated, first-morning specimen to rule out effects of undue dilution due to water intake. The color of the urine may reveal clouds of crystals, bilirubin, blood, porphyrins, food or drug colorings, or melanin. The color should be slightly yellow depending upon the degree of dilution. The urine should not be red, brown, or dark orange in color. A red coloration may be imparted by blood, porphyria, or phenolphthalein from laxative use. A brown urine color may be caused by the acid hematin of blood or from melanin pigments. A dark orange color may be caused by the excessive excretion of urobilinogen or the effects of drugs such as rifampin or phenazopyridine.

Specimen pH. Urine is normally acidic when freshly produced. Alkaline urine may indicate an aged specimen, systemic alkalosis, failure of renal acidifying mechanisms, or infection in the urinary tract.

Specific gravity. A normal morning urine specimen should have a specific gravity between 1.020 and 1.025. The latter value reflects close to maximal concentrating ability by the kidney. Glomerular filtrate has a specific gravity of 1.010, and production of urine with such a low value, under conditions of restricted water intake, would indicate failure of renal concentrating mechanisms. Obviously, under situations of unre-

stricted water intake, specific gravity readings are difficult to interpret.

Protein. The healthy individual should excrete less than 0.1 gm protein per 24 hours. Protein in urine can result from a variety of renal and extra-renal causes but its presence always indicates the need for a careful evaluation of the patient. Protein in the urine is reported on a scale of 0 (30 mg/100 ml), 1+ (30–100 mg/100 ml), 2+ (100–300 mg/100 ml); 3+ (300–1000 mg/100 ml), and 4+ >(1000 mg/100 ml).

Microscopic examination. The urine sediment is examined for red cells, white cells, casts, yeast, crystals, and epithelial cells. *Red blood cells* should be absent in normal urine, although one RBC per high powered field (hpf) would still be considered in the normal range of acceptability. Bleeding or clotting disorders, some collagen diseases, and various bladder, urethral, and prostatic conditions may cause microscopic hematuria. In females, vaginal blood occasionally contaminates the urine specimen, but the presence of numerous squamous epithelial cells should be sufficient to alert clinicians to this artifact. *White blood cells* should be virtually absent in normal urine, although up to 5 WBC/hpf would still be in the normal range. The presence of white cells in the urine usually suggests an acute infection in the urinary tract. Some noninfectious inflammatory diseases of the kidney, ureter, or bladder may also contribute white cells to the urine sediment. *Casts* may be of various types but are basically composed of proteinaceous or fatty material which outline the shape of the renal tubules where they were deposited. Their significance varies and their presence must be interpreted in light of other factors related to the kidney and its function. Nevertheless, fatty casts, RBC casts, and WBC casts are always significant. Red cell casts usually suggest glomerular injury, and white cell casts suggest tubular injury. Hyaline or granular casts, however, only suggest some defect in factors which affect cast formation, and are therefore difficult to interpret. *Crystals* may originally appear as a cloud in the urine. Their formation is pH-dependent and they frequently appear only as the urine cools to room temperature. They also appear more commonly in concentrated urine. In acid urine, crystals may be uric acid or calcium oxalate; in alkaline urine they may be phosphates. Crystals per se are not highly significant, although they may reflect a tendency toward the formation of renal calculi.

ACKNOWLEDGMENT: The authors are grateful for the contributions of Drs. John T. Frank, Philip D. Hansten, and Mary Anne Koda-Kimble. Some of their material which appeared in earlier editions of this textbook has been included in this present chapter.

References

1. Hansten PD: *Drug Interactions,* 4th ed., Lea & Febiger, Philadelphia, 1980.
2. Scribner BH: Teaching syllabus for the course on Fluid and Electrolyte Balance, University of Washington, Seattle, 1969.
3. Kassirer J: Clinical evaluation of kidney function-glomerular function. N Engl J Med. 1971; 285:385.
4. Winter ME et al: *Basic Clinical Pharmacokinetics,* Applied Therapeutics, Inc., San Francisco, 1980, p 58.
5. Widmann FK: Goodale's *Clinical Interpretations of Laboratory Tests,* 8th Ed., F.A. Davis Company, Philadelphia, 1979.
6. Schmid R: Bilirubin metabolism in man. N Engl J Med. 1972; 285:703.
7. Ravel R: *Clinical Laboratory Medicine,* 2nd Ed., Yearbook Medical Publishers, Inc., Chicago, 1978.
8. Hillman RS and Finch CA: *Red Cell Manual,* 4th Ed., F.A. Davis Company, Philadelphia, 1974.
9. Henry JB (ed): Todd-Sanford-Davidsohn *Clinical Diagnosis and Management by Laboratory Methods,* 16th Ed., W.B. Saunders, Philadelphia, 1979.
10. Boggs DR and Winkelstein A: *White Cell Manual,* 3rd Ed., F.A. Davis Company, Philadelphia, 1974.
11. Bennington JL et al: *Laboratory Diagnosis,* MacMillan and Company, Toronto, 1970.
12. Cline MJ et al: Monocytes and macrophages: functions and diseases. Ann Intern Med. 1978; 88:78.
13. Butterworth AE and David JR: Eosinophil function. N Engl J Med. 1981; 304:154.
14. Swanson M and Cook R: *Drugs, Chemicals and Blood Dyscrasias.* Drug Intelligence Publications, Inc., Hamilton, IL, 1977.
15. Dukes MNG: Meyler's *Side Effects of Drugs,* volume 8, Excerpta Medica, Amsterdam, 1975.
16. Meyler L and Herxheimer A: *Side Effects of Drugs,* volume 7, Excerpta Medica, Amsterdam, 1972.
17. Hull JH et al: Influence of range of renal function and liver disease on predictability of creatinine clearance. Clin Pharmacol Ther. 1981; 29:516.

Chapter 3

Anxiety and Insomnia

Brian S. Katcher

Anxiety and its nocturnal manifestation, insomnia, are among the most prevalent symptoms seen in medical practice. Therefore, it is not surprising that the benzodiazepines, which are the safest and most effective drugs available for these conditions, are among the most commonly prescribed drugs. About 500 million people in the world have taken benzodiazepines since their introduction twenty years ago (1), and approximately 90% of the prescriptions for these drugs are written by non-psychiatrists (2).

Anxiety

A precise definition of anxiety is impossible, but the experience of anxiety is familiar to everyone and in most circumstances it cannot be considered pathological. Its manifestations include a diverse range of unpleasant mental and physical states including apprehension, irritability, nervousness, feelings of inadequacy, indecision, worry, tremor, insomnia, restlessness, headache, constipation, diarrhea, nausea, muscle tension, and palpitations.

A great variety of drugs have been used to treat anxiety, but the benzodiazepines are clearly the

31

drugs of choice. Specific benzodiazepine receptors in the brain have recently been described (3), suggesting the presence of endogenous benzodiazepine-like neurotransmitters analogous to the brain's morphine-like neurotransmitters. The benzodiazepines are more consistently effective, less likely to interact with other drugs, less likely to cause adverse effects, safer in overdose, and have less abuse potential than barbiturates and most other sedatives.

The number of prescriptions for benzodiazepine antianxiety drugs increased dramatically after their introduction in the early 1960's, and by 1975 it was predicted that if usage were to continue increasing at the then constant rate, everyone would be taking minor tranquilizers by the year 2000 (4). However, this trend has reversed and prescriptions for these drugs have declined (5). When the use of benzodiazepine antianxiety drugs was at its peak during 1973–1975, approximately 15% of the adults in the U.S. had taken these drugs during the previous year and about 6% of adults had taken them for as long as one month (6). The use of these drugs in Western Europe at that time was similarly high (7). Was this overuse and is the current trend toward lesser use an improvement? According to a nationwide household survey, approximately 30% of adults considered themselves as having high levels of psychic distress, yet only half of them took a single dose of medication for their problem and only 6% did so on a continuing basis (8). A related nationwide survey determined that patients have extremely conservative attitudes toward the use of these drugs (9). Several of the leading researchers in this field (1,5,10) interpret these and other recent data as indication that the benzodiazepines are not currently overused and may in fact be underused. Nevertheless, any CNS depressant possesses a potential for dependence, and the long term effectiveness of these drugs is unknown. Therefore, FDA labeling requirements advise against their use for the stress of everyday life and limit their indications to short term relief.

For those who respond to life's daily aggravations with unbearable anxiety or troublesome somatic complaints, psychoactive drug treatment is an option. Benzodiazepines are clearly effective in this regard but do not constitute a cure.

Insomnia

Individuals vary widely in their requirements for sleep. Although most adults average about seven and a half hours sleep per night, some healthy subjects require less than three hours; others require more than nine. Sleep tends to become shorter and more fragmented with age.

Insomnia is subjective. It is the individual's experience of difficulty in falling asleep and/or difficulty in staying asleep. Many health care professionals assume that patients who complain of insomnia can accurately describe their sleep. However, when this assumption was examined in sleep laboratory studies, surprising findings emerged. In many cases the actual sleep of patients complaining of insomnia is hardly disturbed, and there is an enormous overlap in the objective measures of sleep between insomniac patients and age-matched, normal controls (11). The beneficial effect, if any, of a hypnotic is typically a 10 to 20 minute reduction in the time needed to fall asleep and a 20 to 40 minute lengthening of the night's total sleep time. The importance of these effects is unclear at present (12).

The treatment of insomnia with hypnotics should be limited to specific short term situations such as transient emotional distress. Medical causes of insomnia, such as pain, nocturia, hypoxia, or pulmonary congestion, should receive more specific treatment. Severe psychiatric illnesses, such as schizophrenia or primary depression, often manifest with symptoms of insomnia. In these cases specific treatment with phenothiazines or tricyclic antidepressants is more rational than hypnotics which may cause further deterioration. Drug-induced causes of insomnia, such as caffeine, the early morning effects of a previous evening's excess with alcoholic beverages, or an evening dose of diuretic, are easily remedied without hypnotics.

Benzodiazepines

1. *Dosing.* **A.M. is a 28-year-old, 60 kg woman who complains of nervousness, insomnia, and general feelings of a lack of well being. A thorough physical examination revealed no objective signs of disease, and routine laboratory evaluations were within normal limits. She has taken no prescription medications within the past few years. She has smoked about one-half pack of cigarettes per day for the past eight years but recently she began smoking more than a pack a day, particularly during coffee breaks and at lunch. She drinks socially about once a week.**

Upon further questioning it became apparent that her symptoms began after her recent change in employment. After some discussion about the nature of her work and her feelings toward it she was given a prescription for diazepam (Valium) 5 mg, 20 tablets, "Take as directed. Not to be refilled." What information should A.M. receive as to when she should take her first dose of diazepam, the onset of effects, dosing intervals, and regularity of use?

She should take the first dose during the evening, at home. This will allow her to become acquainted with the effects of the drug and will help her sleep. The onset will occur quite rapidly, especially if she takes it on an empty stomach (13,14). This may cause a brief floating feeling or "buzz" which will dissipate in a few hours after redistribution of the drug occurs. After a few doses she will become accustomed to the acute effects and they will have only a minor effect on her performance.

The half-lives of diazepam and its principal metabolite, desmethyldiazepam, are both quite long, so if she were to take the same amount every day, it would require about one week before steady state would be reached. However, excess sedation from steadily rising blood levels probably will not occur. In fact, patients experiencing sedation early in the course of continuous therapy sometimes find that the sedative effects wane despite continually rising levels (15). Therefore, she should begin by taking one tablet each night for about a week, with full or half-tablet doses during the day as needed. Thereafter, she should take the drug only as needed. If she were to discontinue therapy after only one week, blood levels would slowly decline during the following week, thus providing a tapering effect.

An irregular dosing pattern is appropriate, since symptomatic effect is being titrated against clinical need. If she has any remaining tablets, she should not use them if she becomes pregnant, since diazepam may be teratogenic if taken early in pregnancy.

2. *Drug Interactions.* Is A.M. taking any drugs which might interact with diazepam?

She should be warned that alcohol will enhance the effects of diazepam. This combination results in higher diazepam levels (16) and greater psychomotor impairment than from alcohol alone (17). Occasional small amounts of alcohol will probably not cause problems unless she needs to drive or be alert for other reasons. Subjects who have taken diazepam for two weeks are less sensitive to the addition of alcohol than novice diazepam users, but when the doses of these two agents are high enough, substantial impairment occurs (17).

Cigarette smoking and coffee consumption will both decrease her response to diazepam, and either of these social drugs could be contributing to her problem. Smoking has been shown to impair sleep (18). Furthermore, sedation from benzodiazepines, a desired effect from her nighttime dose, is less likely to occur in smokers than in nonsmokers (19). Although not clearly established, smokers may have higher diazepam clearance rates than nonsmokers (20). Excessive coffee consumption has been suggested as a frequent cause of anxiety (21), and the stimulant effects of caffeine may offset the effects of her diazepam. Therefore, she should be informed of the effects of these drugs and encouraged to decrease their use. Other benzodiazepine drug interactions are presented in Table 1.

3. *Comparison of Benzodiazepines.* Why was diazepam prescribed for A.M.? What clinical advantages or disadvantages would the various other benzodiazepines offer in this situation? (Also see Table 2)

The various benzodiazepines are all quite similar from a pharmacological standpoint. They all have antianxiety, sedative-hypnotic, muscle relaxant, and anticonvulsant effects when given in appropriate dosage. The differences among these drugs lie in the way they are absorbed, distributed, and eliminated.

Diazepam (Valium) provides a rapid, intense effect which makes it an excellent choice both as a hypnotic and for "as needed" use. Furthermore, multiple dosing results in increasing blood levels of diazepam and desmethyldiazepam which provide long lasting antianxiety effect. These properties are ideal for this situation. *Chlordiazepoxide* (Librium) has long acting metabolites, but its onset effects are much less dramatic (22,23) which is a relative disadvantage for inducing sleep and for situational anxiety. On the other hand, chlordiazepoxide is available in generic form and is therefore less expensive. Its slower absorption and slower passage into the central nervous system (CNS) could be an advantage if abuse is considered a risk. Heroin addicts express a marked preference for diazepam over equipotent doses of chlordiazepoxide (24).

Table 1.
FACTORS WHICH MAY INFLUENCE BENZODIAZEPINE RESPONSE

Factor	Effect	Significance
age	The rate of absorption of chlordiazepoxide and both the rate and extent of absorption of clorazepate decrease with age (100,101). The half-lives of diazepam and chlordiazepoxide increase with age (20,34,36,100). The clearance of diazepam (20), desmethyldiazepam (25,37), and chlordiazepoxide (100) decrease with age in males. However, aging has little or no effect on the clearance of diazepam or desmethyldiazepam in females (20,25). The unbound or free fraction of diazepam increases with age in both males and females (20,34). These changes in pharmacokinetic parameters are not significant with oxazepam or lorazepam.	The elderly should receive lower doses of these drugs because they are more sensitive to their effects. Older subjects, especially males, are at risk for intoxication from repeated doses of long-acting benzodiazepines. For repeated dosing, oxazepam or lorazepam are preferable. (Also see Questions 8–10)
gender	The volumes of distribution of diazepam, desmethyldiazepam, and chlordiazepoxide are larger in young females than in young males (20,25,102). Males experience a much greater decrease in diazepam clearance with aging than females (20). The intrinsic clearance of desmethyldiazepam is higher in females of all ages than in males of all ages, and clearance declines with age in males but not in females (25). The intrinsic clearance of chlordiazepoxide is significantly less in young females than in young males, but this effect is offset by a much higher free fraction in females (102). Chlordiazepoxide requires further study in older females.	Older males are at greater risk for intoxication from repeated dosing with long-acting benzodiazepines than are older females. Older subjects of either gender should be dosed conservatively.
liver disease	The metabolism of diazepam, desmethyldiazepam, and chlordiazepoxide are impaired in liver disease (36,43,45). The metabolism of oxazepam and lorazepam is unaffected by liver disease (40,41,43). However, the half-life of lorazepam may be doubled in patients with cirrhosis because of a corresponding doubling in the volume of distribution (40).	For repeated dosing, oxazepam is safer than other benzodiazepines in patients with liver disease. (Also see Questions 11–12)
tobacco	see Question 2	
coffee	see Question 2	
alcohol	Ethanol decreases the clearance of diazepam and chlordiazepoxide, but not oxazepam or lorazepam (16,104,105). In addition, psychomotor impairment from benzodiazepines and alcohol is additive.	Alcohol and benzodiazepines cause additive psychomotor impairment. (Also see Question 2)

Table 1. (continued)
FACTORS WHICH MAY INFLUENCE BENZODIAZEPINE RESPONSE

Factor	Effect	Significance
disulfiram	Disulfiram decreases the clearance of diazepam and chlordiazepoxide by 40–50%; oxazepam clearance is not affected (105,106).	For repeated dosing, oxazepam or lorazepam may be the benzodiazepines of choice for patients who are taking disulfiram.
pregnancy	Serum albumin declines progressively during pregnancy and the free fraction of diazepam correspondingly increases, reaching a maximum just prior to delivery (103). In addition, benzodiazepines may be teratogenic early in pregnancy.	Increased maternal sensitivity to diazepam occurs during the last stages of pregnancy. Benzodiazepines may be teratogenic if given early in pregnancy.
cimetidine	Cimetidine decreases the clearance of diazepam, desmethyldiazepam, and chlordiazepoxide by 25 to 50%, but does not affect the clearance of oxazepam or lorazepam (107–110).	For repeated dosing, oxazepam or lorazepam are the benzodiazepines of choice for patients who are taking cimetidine.
anti-tuberculosis drugs	Isoniazid impairs the metabolism of diazepam, whereas rifampin induces the metabolism of diazepam. The clearance of diazepam is increased in patients receiving triple therapy with isoniazid, ethambutol, and rifampin (111).	Patients who are receiving antituberculosis therapy may respond to diazepam with lesser or more sedation than they did prior to therapy.
heparin	Heparin increases the circulating levels of free fatty acids which in turn displace benzodiazepines from their binding sites. The result is a 150–250% rise in the free fraction of diazepam, desmethyldiazepam, chlordiazepoxide, and oxazepam. The increases in free fraction were slightly smaller but still significant when subjects were fasting (112,113).	Benzodiazepine effects may be enhanced, but this has not been established. Some pharmacokinetic disposition determinants derived in studies which utilized heparin may be in error.
antacids	Antacids reduce the rate but not the extent of diazepam and chlordiazepoxide absorption (14,114). However, both the rate and extent of clorazepate absorption are decreased by antacids (115).	Decreased benzodiazepine effect.
birth control pills	Oral contraceptives increase the free concentration of chlordiazepoxide and cause a slight decrease in clearance of free chlordiazepoxide (102). Low-dose estrogen-containing oral contraceptives impair the clearance of diazepam and greatly increase its half-life (118).	Women receiving oral contraceptives may be more sensitive to the effects of some benzodiazepines; lower doses may be required.

Table 2.
COMPARISON OF BENZODIAZEPINES

Generic Name	Trade Name	Usual Dosage	Elimination Half-life	Active Metabolites	Speed of Onset After Single Dose
diazepam	Valium	5 mg tid	20–80 hr	desmethyldiazepam	very fast
chlordiazepoxide	Librium and various generics	10 mg tid	10–30 hr	several long acting metabolites, including desmethyldiazepam	intermediate
clorazepate	Tranxene	7.5 mg tid	50–200 hr	desmethyldiazepam (clorazepate is prodrug)	fast
	Tranxene SD	11.25 mg daily	50–200 hr	desmethyldiazepam (clorazepate is prodrug)	slow
prazepam	Centrax Verstran	10 mg bid	50–200 hr	desmethyldiazepam (prazepam is prodrug)	very slow
flurazepam	Dalmane	15 or 30 mg hs	more than 100 hr	desalkylflurazepam	intermediate
lorazepam	Ativan	1 mg bid	10–20 hr	none	intermediate
oxazepam	Serax	10 mg tid	5–10 hr	none	slow
temazepam	Restoril	15–30 mg hs	10–15 hr	insignificant	fast
triazolam	to be released	~0.6 mg hs	2–3 hr	insignificant	fast
alprazolam	Xanax	0.5 mg tid	12–15 hr	α-hydroxyalprazolam	_____
halazepam	Paxipam	40 mg tid	14 hr	desmethyldiazepam	_____

Also see Fig. 1 for metabolic relationships.

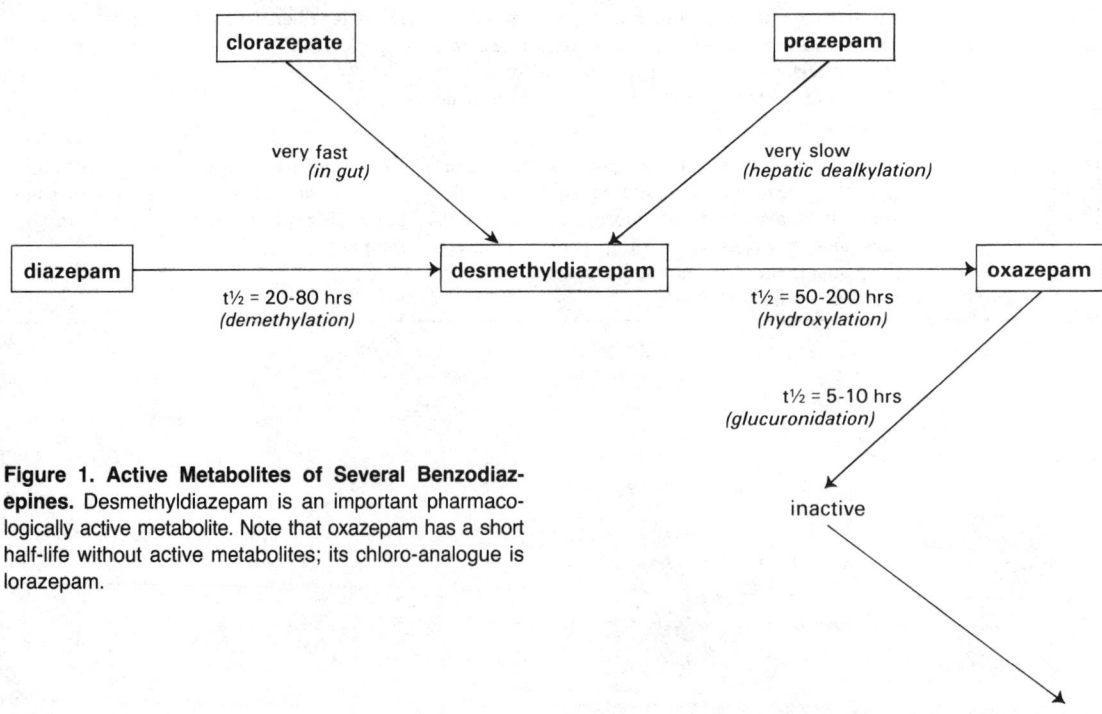

Figure 1. Active Metabolites of Several Benzodiazepines. Desmethyldiazepam is an important pharmacologically active metabolite. Note that oxazepam has a short half-life without active metabolites; its chloro-analogue is lorazepam.

Clorazepate (Tranzene) and *prazepam* (Centrax) are prodrugs or precursors for desmethyldiazepam (Fig. 1). Clorazepate is rapidly converted to desmethyldiazepam in the stomach and, like diazepam, has rapid onset effects that are terminated by redistribution. The single and multiple dose effects of clorazepate are similar to those of diazepam, making it an appropriate alternative for this patient. Prazepam is very slowly absorbed and requires hepatic dealkylation for activity. Because peak levels occur 11 to 20 hours after a dose (25), it is unsuitable for use as a hypnotic or for "as needed" use.

Flurazepam (Dalmane) could have been used to help A.M. sleep and its long acting metabolite would have provided antianxiety effects. Although this makes theoretical sense, some patients experience acute exacerbations of their anxiety during the day and this treatment would preclude daytime dosing.

Oxazepam (Serax) and *lorazepam* (Ativan) have shorter half-lives and inactive metabolites. While these properties are advantageous in older and debilitated patients, this woman is young and healthy. The lack of accumulation of active drug and metabolites on multiple dosing is a potential disadvantage here, since reappearance of symptoms soon after cessation of drug intake might foster dependence. Because of its poor absorption and slow passage into the CNS, oxazepam is often too slow in its effect to be useful for situational anxiety or for inducing sleep. (23,81,86,87). Peak levels generally occur at 2½–3 hours, but in some subjects this may be delayed by 8 hours (85). Despite its relatively short half-life (5 to 10 hours), oxazepam's sedative effects are fairly long lasting since it does not undergo extensive redistribution. Likewise, the duration of lorazepam's effects are dependent on its elimination half-life of 10 to 20 hours. Its rate of absorption falls between oxazepam and diazepam or clorazepate.

4. Benzodiazepines vs Other Sedative-Hypnotics. Dr. M. prefers to use meprobamate or phenobarbital when he prescribes antianxiety drugs. In his opinion the benzodiazepines are too expensive and not particularly effective. What information could be offered in response to these views?

When *phenobarbital* (134 mg daily mean), diazepam (20 mg daily mean), and placebo were compared in a double-blind multicenter comparison in 241 anxious, ambulatory patients, diazepam was superior to phenobarbital, and phenobarbital was only slightly more effective than placebo (26). An analysis of 26 controlled double-blind trials comparing *meprobamate* with placebo raised significant doubts as to its efficacy (27).

The explanation for this physician's clinical experience can be found in his attitudes toward these drugs. Placebo psychoactive agents produce about 50% successful response, compared to a 70% response for an effective drug when both are given with a neutral attitude. Since the placebo works as often as it fails, a prescriber's positive or negative attitude toward ineffective or slightly effective drugs can influence a patient's response to these agents.

Meprobamate can cause serious physiological dependence after doses of 3.2 to 6.4 gm per day for 40 or more days (29,30). Both phenobarbital and meprobamate are more hazardous in suicide attempts than the benzodiazepines. Finally, cost is not a significant issue since therapy should always be short term.

5. Parenteral Administration. A patient recovering from abdominal surgery had an acute anxiety reaction while his incision was being examined. Diazepam 10 mg intramuscularly (IM) has been ordered for this patient. Why is the IM route of administration inappropriate for diazepam?

The onset of effects will be too slow. Precipitation of diazepam at the injection site causes slow and incomplete absorption (46). Oral administration of diazepam results in faster and higher blood levels than the same dose given IM (47–49).

6. The intravenous route is deemed more appropriate for this situation. What precautions should be observed with intravenous (IV) diazepam administration?

Because of its poor solubility in water, diazepam for injection is formulated with 40% propylene glycol and 10% ethyl alcohol. Visible precipitation is noted when this formulation is injected at a rate of 5 mg/min into an IV line of 5% dextrose in water running at 20 ml/min or normal saline running at 15 ml/min (50). Diazepam should not be mixed with IV fluids but should be injected directly into the vein. The rate of administration should not exceed 5 mg/min to avoid the risk of propylene glycol induced hypotension and arrhythmias. Small veins, such as the dorsum of the hand or wrist, should be avoided because of the greater risk of thrombophlebitis (51).

7. Is slow absorption after IM administration a problem which is common to all injectable benzodiazepines?

Lorazepam is the only benzodiazepine which is rapidly absorbed after IM administration (52). Parenteral chlordiazepoxide is packaged as a powder which must be dissolved and reconstituted immediately prior to administration. When dissolved in the diluent packaged with the ampule, IM absorption of chlordiazepoxide is slower and less complete than the same dose given orally (53). IM absorption of chlordiazepoxide can be hastened and made more complete by dissolving the drug in normal saline (116). However, regardless of the diluent used, IM injection of chlordiazepoxide is painful, and onset of effect is slower than that obtained by oral or intravenous administration.

Elderly Patients

8. Mr. L. is a 72-year-old, 60 kg man who was admitted to the emergency room with superficial lacerations and bruises which occurred as the result of an automobile accident. The accident was apparently caused by Mr. L. A complete neurological exam revealed no abnormalities except for drowsiness and mild confusion. He had been taking no medication or other drugs except for diazepam 20 mg which he had taken nightly for the preceding two weeks. During this time he had increased muscle weakness, fatigue, and memory loss which he did not attribute to the drug. After a complete medical workup and 48 hours of observation he was discharged with instructions to discontinue his diazepam and not to drive for two weeks. His symptoms slowly improved while he was in the hospital, and within several days after discharge he felt fully recovered. What signs and symptoms in this case are consistent with diazepam intoxicaton?

Cardiovascular and other medical causes were apparently ruled out during his brief hospital stay, and the slow reversal of his symptoms upon discontinuation of the drug seem to confirm a diagnosis of diazepam intoxication. Decreased memory and motor function and increased fatigue were consistent effects among 20 elderly men who were given diazepam 12 mg daily for two weeks in a double-blind, placebo-controlled study

(31). Muscle weakness and excess sedation occur more frequently in the elderly than in young patients taking benzodiazepines (19,32).

9. Why did Mr. L. have such a profound response to moderate doses of diazepam?

First, older subjects are inherently more sensitive to the effects of sedatives and require lower doses and lower plasma levels than younger patients (33). At least part of this greater sensitivity can be explained on the basis of protein binding. The unbound fraction of diazepam is significantly higher in older subjects (20,34), and it is the unbound fraction which enters the CNS. Since diazepam is 98% protein bound, increases in the unbound fraction can be expected to be clinically significant (35).

Second, the half-life of diazepam is longer in older subjects (20,34,36). While there is considerable variation among individuals, it might, for example, be assumed that the half-life of diazepam in Mr. L. is 100 hours, a value which is two to three times longer than the half-life of diazepam in young adults. Assuming it requires four half-lives to achieve steady state concentrations, it would be 400 hours (16–17 days) before Mr. L. experiences the maximum cumulative effect of his nightly diazepam doses. Therefore, diazepam levels were still increasing when he had his automobile accident. Furthermore, the half-life of desmethyldiazepam is also prolonged in elderly men (25,37), and the cumulative effects of this active metabolite would also be delayed.

Thirdly, the clearance of diazepam is decreased by approximately one-half in elderly males (20). Since average steady state plasma concentrations are inversely related to clearance (35), this decrease in clearance will result in plasma concentrations which are twice that which would normally be achieved for any given dose. Furthermore, the clearance of desmethyldiazepam is also decreased in older men (25,37). These age-related decreases in diazepam and desmethyldiazepam clearance are significant in men but not in women (see Table 1).

10. If Mr. L. should require sedation in the future, what other benzodiazepines could be prescribed?

Diazepam could be used in smaller doses. However, the maximum cumulative effects of repeated doses would not be observed for two or more weeks. If these effects were excessive, reversal on discontinuation of diazepam would be slow. Similar precautions should be observed with other benzodiazepines which have long-acting, active metabolites (38).

The metabolism, distribution, and protein binding of *oxazepam* and *lorazepam* do not change significantly with age (39–42). Therefore, one of these drugs would be a good choice for Mr. L. Furthermore, since their half-lives are shorter, adverse effects from too high a dose with a multiple dosing schedule would appear sooner and reverse more quickly upon discontinuation of the drug. Both of these drugs are slowly absorbed with peak effects appearing after several hours. Although the half-life of oxazepam is somewhat shorter than that of lorazepam, it is the more slowly absorbed of the two. *Temazepam* might also be considered because of its short half-life and inactive metabolites. However, preliminary data suggest that its half-life is prolonged in the elderly and cumulative effects have been reported in such patients after repeated doses (117). Temazepam requires further study in older patients.

Liver Disease

11. G.N. is a 54-year-old, 70 kg, well-compensated cirrhotic male who complains of nervousness and restlessness. After ruling out impending hepatic coma and alcohol withdrawal as possible causes, an order for chlordiazepoxide 10 mg qid is written in his chart. His laboratory data include: total bilirubin 28 mg/dl (0.2 to 1.0), alkaline phosphatase 1200 IU/dl (30 to 85), SGOT 640 KU/dl (7 to 40), and albumin 4.2 gm/dl (3.6 to 5.0). Why might this dosage of chlordiazepoxide be excessive for G.N.?

The clearance of chlordiazepoxide is substantially decreased in patients with cirrhosis (mean 0.185 ml/min/kg in cirrhotics versus 0.54 ml/min/kg in normals), and the half-life is increased more than three-fold (43). Although tolerance develops to the sedative effects of benzodiazepines, there is a risk of intoxication from repeated dosing. Since chlordiazepoxide has been identified as a frequent precipitating cause of hepatic coma (44), it should be avoided.

12. Which benzodiazepines are preferred when needed for cirrhotic patients such as G.N. and why?

Quantitative recommendations for reduction

in the dosage of chlordiazepoxide cannot be made since the degree of impaired clearance cannot be correlated to any of the standard liver function tests (43). Similar impairment of metabolism in liver disease has been observed with diazepam and desmethyldiazepam (36,45).

The metabolism of *lorazepam* and *oxazepam* are not significantly impaired in liver disease (40,41,43). Diazepam, desmethyldiazepam, and chlordiazepoxide are all metabolized by oxidation. However, oxazepam and lorazepam are metabolized by glucuronidation, a process which is less impaired by hepatocellular disease than are metabolic processes catalyzed by other enzymes. Furthermore, the metabolites of oxazepam and lorazepam are inactive. Although either of these two drugs might seem appropriate for this patient, there is some basis for the use of oxazepam in this situation. One study demonstrated a doubling of lorazepam's half-life due to an increase in the volume of distribution in patients with cirrhosis (40). The mean half-life in these cirrhotics was 41 hours. Assuming this lorazepam half-life in G.N., maximal effects from repeated doses would be expected after 160 hours or nearly seven days (four half-lives). In contrast, the half-life of oxazepam is only slightly increased in cirrhotics (mean 5.6 hours in normals versus 7.1 hours in cirrhotics) (43). Consequently, the maximum cumulative effects from oxazepam could be observed after one day.

Respiratory Disease

13. A 65-year-old, 70 kg male with chronic obstructive pulmonary disease (COPD) is recovering from a severe upper respiratory infection. On the day before his planned discharge from the hospital he observes the first parts of a traumatic but successful treatment of a cardiac arrest in his roommate. He is now very anxious. His arterial blood gases are PO_2 65 mm Hg (normal 95–100) and PCO_2 50 mm Hg (normal 40). How hazardous are sedatives in this situation?

Although benzodiazepines cause less respiratory depression than other sedatives, their use in patients with respiratory disease must be approached with caution, since respiratory failure can be precipitated.

In a study of six patients with chronic obstructive pulmonary disease (COPD) whose mean PO_2

was 60 mm Hg and PCO_2 was 49 mm Hg, there was no change in pulmonary function or in arterial blood gases after five days of oral diazepam 10 mg qid (54). In ten patients with COPD who were given diazepam in doses of 0.11 mg/kg IV, respiratory depression was slight: the mean PO_2 fell from 67 to 65.6 mm Hg and the PCO_2 rose from 38 to 41.4 mm Hg (55). Large doses of diazepam, 0.5 mg/kg, in eighteen patients with COPD also produced slight respiratory depression: the mean PO_2 fell from 70 to 65 mm Hg and the PCO_2 rose from 43 to 49 mm Hg; these changes are comparable to those seen during sleep in this population (56). Although there was considerable variation in response among patients, these data suggest that a few oral doses of a benzodiazepine will be safe in this patient if he is carefully observed. Diazepam should be used for the initial dose because of its rapid onset. Oxazepam would be a good choice for subsequent doses, because its short half-life will allow effects to dissipate rapidly when it is stopped.

The hazard of respiratory depression from sedatives, including benzodiazepines, should not be dismissed. Benzodiazepines can cause significant deterioration in patients already in respiratory failure (57). Since hypoxia is a frequent cause of anxiety in obstructive pulmonary disease, these drugs should be administered only after pulmonary function has been evaluated.

Adverse Effects

14. *Adverse Behavioral Effects.* **M.L. has been taking chlordiazepoxide 10 mg three times a day for the past two weeks. During this time he has become increasingly argumentative with his wife, and at work he insulted his employer of ten years with unprecedented hostility. Could this be a drug effect?**

Yes. The drug should be discontinued. Isolated cases of hostility induced by chlordiazepoxide, clorazepate, and diazepam have been reported (58,59). Oxazepam appears to be free of this side effect (60–62). This hostility reaction is different from the behavioral disinhibition that may be caused by any sedating drug.

In animals this effect occurs with chlordiazepoxide and diazepam but not with pentobarbital (63). Chlordiazepoxide, but not oxazepam, increases hostility as an inner affective state (61,62,64,65). These increases in hostility require

sensitive psychological tests to be detected, but they are real and reproducible. Overt hostility is noted only in response to a frustrating stimulus.

However, reactions such as this are infrequent. For example, when chlordiazepoxide was compared with placebo in 225 anxious neurotic outpatients, chlordiazepoxide was significantly more effective in reducing hostile, irritable, and anxious symptomatology. None of the drug treated patients experienced hostility (66).

This behavioral side effect is rare, although subclinical tendencies may exist. The precise incidence is unknown.

15. *Benzodiazepine Withdrawal.* **T.M. has been taking diazepam 15 to 20 mg daily for the past three years. Will he experience withdrawal problems if he discontinues the drug? What precautions are necessary?**

Although it is unlikely that he will experience any withdrawal symptoms, he should taper his dose at a rate of 5 mg every other day to be safe. Like all sedative hypnotic drugs, the benzodiazepines can produce withdrawal symptoms after prolonged ingestion of unusually large doses (see chapter on Drug Abuse). However, there have been recent case reports of patients experiencing withdrawal symptoms after several years of treatment with usual therapeutic doses of diazepam and other benzodiazepines. These symptoms typically consist of dysphoria, sensory changes, hyperreflexia, diaphoresis, tremor, and agitation (67,68). In addition, seizures have occurred after abrupt discontinuation of the short acting benzodiazepines, lorazepam and oxazepam (69,70).

When they occur, withdrawal reactions after prolonged diazepam administration appear on the second or third day after discontinuation and are apparently related to the rate of decline of desmethyldiazepam levels (67,71). Propranolol may be useful in treating those symptoms associated with increased sympathetic outflow (68,71), but tapering T.M.'s diazepam dosage will prevent the appearance of symptoms. Preliminary data from a large scale study now in progress indicate that the risk of withdrawal symptoms in a patient such as T.M. is about 5% (10). As a precaution, continuous treatment with benzodiazepines should be limited to 20 weeks (1,10).

16. *Sleeping Pill Withdrawal Insomnia.* **E.W. is a 44-year-old woman who has a prescription for Nembutal 100 mg, #30, Sig: i hs**

for sleep. Her medication profile shows that she has been taking pentobarbital (Nembutal) or secobarbital (Seconal) at an average rate of two doses per night for the past two months. She explains that she is unable to sleep without medications, and that her sleeping problem began two months ago when she was hospitalized for a cholecystectomy. She continued the sleeping pills that were given to her on discharge from the hospital because they had helped her, and she felt they would insure the rest needed for a good recovery. She has stopped taking them on several occasions, but each time she has been plagued by difficulty in falling asleep and frequent wakenings. She has maintained a supply from several physicians at her insistence that normal sleep is impossible without them. What is a likely cause of this woman's sleep problem? How do hypnotics affect sleep?

The fact that E.W.'s sleeping difficulty began after she started using hypnotics is suggestive of sleeping pill withdrawal insomnia. This syndrome is well documented (72,73), but the incidence is unknown. Symptoms similar to those experienced by this patient have been produced in test subjects (72). The induction of this dependence can be understood by reviewing the way in which hypnotics affect sleep.

When normal sleep is studied in the laboratory with an electroencephalogram (EEG), the following patterns are noted. When the subject falls asleep, the EEG tracings are of low amplitude and high frequency (stage 1). As sleep progresses through stages 2, 3, and 4, the amplitude increases and the frequency decreases. Once stage 4 is reached, the pattern reverses through stages 3, 2, and 1. Return to stage 1 is usually followed by a period of rapid eye movements (REM). REM sleep is associated with dreaming and is sometimes referred to as D sleep. This entire cycle occurs over an interval of about 90 minutes and is repeated four or five times during a single night's sleep. Stage 4 is often absent in subsequent cycles; it also decreases with age. About 25% of normal sleep is spent in REM sleep (74).

Most hypnotics decrease REM sleep. Following repeated administration, this suppression is attenuated but remains below the baseline level. When the hypnotic is stopped, there is a marked increase in REM sleep well above the normal baseline levels. This REM rebound has been associated with increased dreaming, nightmares, and

frequent wakening (72–74). Patients experiencing these symptoms may continue to take hypnotics in an attempt to prevent insomnia and disturbed sleep caused by hypnotic withdrawal; thus, a sleeping pill habit is created.

REM rebound has been demonstrated after treatment with pentobarbital, glutethimide, methyprylon, and methaqualone 300 mg but not 150 mg (75,76). Flurazepam, diazepam, and chloral hydrate do not cause REM rebound (72,76–78).

17. How should E.W. be treated?

Once patients begin using hypnotics to suppress the insomnia caused by withdrawal, they are no longer effective. In fact, chronic users of hypnotics actually sleep worse than matched controls (11,73). Sleep laboratory studies have demonstrated that pentobarbital, secobarbital, glutethimide, and chloral hydrate begin to lose their effectiveness within a few nights and are ineffective after two weeks of continued use (11,79,80). Only flurazepam has been shown to affect sleep for as long as 28 nights of continuous use, and this demonstration of efficacy was limited to 10 insomniac subjects (11).

E.W.'s pentobarbital and secobarbital should be discontinued. However, since unpleasant effects will occur with abrupt withdrawal, flurazepam 30 mg should be substituted for about ten nights. Because of the long half-life of its active metabolites (50–100 hours), flurazepam will continue to be effective in promoting sleep for one or two nights after it is stopped. Thereafter the levels will slowly taper. Rebound insomnia does not occur after discontinuation of flurazepam (78). (Also see the chapter on Drug Abuse for a discussion of withdrawal of larger doses of barbiturates.)

18. Could any benzodiazepine have been used in this situation?

No. When five benzodiazepines were investigated in 15 sleep laboratory studies, it was found that the short- and intermediate-acting drugs produced withdrawal insomnia (78). Diazepam and flurazepam, which are long-acting, did not produce rebound insomnia. Although this study has been criticized on the basis that the patients may not have constituted a normal population (81), diazepam and flurazepam appear to be the benzodiazepines of choice for sedative/hypnotic withdrawal.

19. How might E.W.'s problem have been prevented?

This case illustrates the importance of monitoring and limiting the duration of hypnotic use. Patients who are encouraged to limit their hypnotic use are significantly more likely to do so than those who are given no instructions (11,82). Hypnotics which cause significant REM suppression and rebound should be avoided in outpatients.

20. *Sleeping Pill Hangover.* H.H. is a 40-year-old, 70 kg woman who has been having difficulty in falling asleep since last week when her husband was diagnosed with leukemia. A friend gave her a secobarbital 100 mg capsule, and although she slept well, she felt dizzy the next day. She reported this to her husband's physician who gave her a prescription for oxazepam 30 mg. The first night she took one capsule without apparent effect. The second night she took two. After much tossing and turning she finally fell asleep and slept late the following morning. That morning she was "spaced out" from the previous night's drug administration. She was subsequently given a prescription for diazepam 10 mg which was effective in inducing sleep without hangover on the following morning. Was her response to secobarbital unusual? Comment on the appropriateness of this drug in this situation.

Although secobarbital is traditionally categorized as a short- to intermediate-acting barbiturate, its half-life is 29 hours (83). Redistribution into body fat accounts for termination of its effect. Although 100 mg is a usual hypnotic dose, this dose was evidently too large for H.H. Substantial central nervous system levels apparently persisted during the following morning while redistribution was still occurring. Furthermore, the residual effects of barbiturates are more unpleasant than those of the benzodiazepines (84).

Rapid loss of effectiveness, risk of withdrawal insomnia, and severe toxicity in overdose make barbiturates and related drugs poor choices for outpatients.

21. Why was diazepam, but not oxazepam, effective in inducing sleep in this patient?

As discussed earlier, oxazepam is one of the most poorly absorbed benzodiazepines (23), and its absorption in H.H. was apparently too slow to induce sleep. Diazepam, on the other hand, is one of the most rapidly absorbed benzodiazepines (23). When various doses of oxazepam and diazepam were compared as hypnotics, it was found that oxazepam did not induce sleep while diazepam 5–10 mg was effective (81,86,87).

22. Why did H.H. experience a hangover from oxazepam but not from diazepam?

Delayed absorption of oxazepam is part of the answer to this question, but the difference in the way the two drugs are distributed is also important. Although the half-life of oxazepam is 5 to 10 hours, as compared to an expected diazepam half-life of approximately 45 hours in this woman, oxazepam does not undergo extensive redistribution. Therefore, termination of its effect is dependent on its half-life. Diazepam, on the other hand, undergoes rapid and extensive redistribution. For example, clinical effects generally begin about 15 minutes after oral administration of diazepam in fasting individuals; these effects reach maximal intensity after about 30 minutes, persist for another 30 minutes, and then decline over the next few hours (13). When oxazepam and diazepam were compared as hypnotics, it was found that 45 mg of oxazepam produced a morning hangover whereas 10 mg of diazepam did not (87); however, one cannot be certain that this was not simply a result of the large dose of oxazepam prescribed in the study.

23. Would chloral hydrate have been a reasonable alternative for this patient?

Chloral hydrate's reputation as a short-acting hypnotic is based on the relatively low potency of the 0.5 to 1.0 gm doses that are generally used. Chloral hydrate 1.0 gm is less effective than secobarbital 100 mg (88). Considering H.H.'s response to secobarbital, chloral hydrate probably would have produced the desired effects. However, because it rapidly loses its effect after a few nights (89) and is more toxic than benzodiazepines in overdose, it is not a good choice for outpatients.

24. What other drugs would have been appropriate for H.H?

Desmethyldiazepam administered as *clorazepate* is rapidly absorbed and undergoes redistribution such that residual sedation after six hours is minimal (90). *Triazolam* is a rapid-acting benzodiazepine with an extremely short half-life and inactive metabolites (91); it is available in Canada and will probably be released in the U.S. *Temazepam* has a relatively short half-life and inactive metabolites; 15 to 30 mg doses seldom produce residual effects (117). Any of these drugs would have been a good choice.

Although *flurazepam* 30 mg could have been used, it is less effective than diazepam for single night administration. It requires several nights of use to become maximally effective. Furthermore, morning-after effects are frequent with 30 mg doses, and 15 mg is only moderately effective (81,92).

25. *Oral Anticoagulant Interactions.* A 50 kg, 66-year-old woman is being stabilized on warfarin (Coumadin). It is noted that last night she inadvertently received a 100 mg dose of secobarbital. Will her prothrombin time be affected?

It is unlikely that this single dose will affect her prothrombin time. One or two doses of a barbiturate did not alter the prothrombin times of 27 patients taking oral anticoagulants (93). Secobarbital and pentobarbital are less potent stimulators of microsomal enzymes than phenobarbital (94); however, repeated doses of secobarbital significantly increase the rate of warfarin metabolism (95). Therefore, she should not receive further doses. Benzodiazepines and antihistamines do not interact with oral anticoagulants and can be used instead.

26. Would an antihistamine sedative be effective in helping the above patient sleep?

Diphenhydramine (Benadryl) 50 mg or hydroxyzine (Vistaril, Atarax) 50 mg are about as effective as 60 mg of pentobarbital (96,97), an appropriate dose for this woman. Thus, either of these drugs represent an appropriate choice for this situation, but should they fail to be effective, a benzodiazepine would be indicated.

Nonprescription Sedatives

27. A middle-aged man requests a nonprescription sedative to help him sleep. He has had difficulty in falling asleep ever since he was laid off his job two weeks ago. What non-prescription sedatives can be recommended?

Most nonprescription sleeping preparations contain pyrilamine maleate 25 mg (Nytol, Sleep-Eze, Sominex, Compoz), an antihistamine which has not been evaluated as a hypnotic. Most of these preparations formerly contained methapyrilene, an antihistamine which could not be distinguished from placebo in the induction of sleep (97,98) and which was removed from the market in 1979 because of possible carcinogenic properties. One can only guess as to the hypnotic potential of these pyrilamine-containing products. Dimenhydrinate (Dramamine), a salt of diphenhydramine, could be considered although it is not approved for this use. Products which contain small amounts of salicylate in addition to an antihistamine have no rational basis.

He could attempt a trial of a pyrilamine preparation, but nondrug approaches might be more beneficial. He should be encouraged to engage in a relaxing activity before bedtime and avoid the use of stimulants in the evening. He should not attempt to use alcohol as a hypnotic because it is not predictably effective and causes REM suppression and rebound. Adequate physical exercise during the day is also effective. He may be taking naps during the day and this could be contributing to his sleep difficulty at night. A warm bath or beverage in the evening may be beneficial. A hot milk beverage was more effective than a lactose placebo identified as a folk remedy in a sleep laboratory study; the beverage was effective in middle-aged subjects but not in younger subjects (99).

References

1. Ayd FJ: Social issues: misuse and abuse. Psychosomatics. 1980; 21(suppl):21.
2. Anon: Prescribing of minor tranquilizers. FDA Drug Bull. Feb 1980; 10:2.
3. Braestrup C et al: Benzodiazepine receptors. Arzneim-Forsch/Drug Res. 1980; 30:852.
4. Blackwell B: Minor tranquilizers: use, misuse or overuse? Psychosomatics. 1975; 16:28.
5. Hollister LE: A look at the issues. Psychosomatics. 1980; 21(suppl):4.
6. Parry HJ et al: National patterns of psychotherapeutic drug use. Arch Gen Psychiatry. 1973; 28:769.
7. Balter MB et al: Cross-national study of the extent of anti-anxiety/sedative drug use. N Engl J Med. 1974; 290:769.
8. Mellinger GD et al: Psychic distress, life crisis, and use

of psychotherapeutic medications. Arch Gen Psychiatry. 1978; 35:1045.

9. Manheimer DI et al: Popular attitudes and beliefs about tranquilizers. Am J Psychiatry. 1973; 130:1246.

10. Rickels K: Are benzodiazepines overused and abused? Br J Clin Pharmacol. 1981; 11(suppl):71S.

11. Institute of Medicine: *Sleeping Pills, Insomnia, and Medical Practice,* National Academy of Sciences, Washington, D.C., 1979.

12. Solomon F et al: Sleeping pills, insomnia, and medical practice. N Engl J Med. 1979; 300:803.

13. Hillestad L et al: Diazepam metabolism in normal man. I. Serum concentrations and clinical effects after intravenous, intramuscular, and oral administration. Clin Pharmacol Ther. 1974; 16:479.

14. Greenblatt DJ et al: Diazepam absorption: effect of antacids and food. Clin Pharmacol Ther. 1978; 24:600.

15. Hillestad L et al: Diazepam metabolism in normal man. II. Serum concentration and clinical effect after oral administration and cumulation. Clin Pharmacol Ther. 1974; 16:485.

16. Sellers EM et al: Intravenous diazepam and oral ethanol interaction. Clin Pharmacol Ther. 1980; 28:638.

17. Palva ES et al: Acute and subacute effects of diazepam on psychomotor skills: interaction with alcohol. Acta Pharmacol et Toxicol. 1979; 45:257.

18. Soldatos CR et al: Cigarette smoking associated with sleep difficulty. Science. 1980; 207:551.

19. Boston Collaborative Drug Surveillance Program: Clinical depression of the central nervous system due to chlordiazepoxide in relation to smoking and age. N Engl J Med. 1973; 288:277.

20. Greenblatt DJ et al: Diazepam disposition determinants. Clin Pharmacol Ther. 1980; 27:301.

21. Greden JF: Anxiety or caffeinism: a diagnostic dilemma. Am J Psychiatry. 1974; 131:1089.

22. Stanski DR et al: Plasma and cerebrospinal fluid concentrations of chlordiazepoxide and its metabolites in surgical patients. Clin Pharmacol Ther. 1976; 20:571.

23. Greenblatt DJ et al: Benzodiazepines: a summary of pharmacokinetic properties. Br J Clin Pharmacol. 1981; 11:11S.

24. Inaba DS: Personal communication. Haight Ashbury Free Medical Clinic, San Francisco.

25. Allen AD et al: Desmethyldiazepam kinetics in the elderly after oral prazepam. Clin Pharmacol Ther. 1980; 28:197.

26. Cohen J et al: Diazepam and phenobarbital in the treatment of anxiety: a controlled multicenter study using physician and patient rating scales. Curr Ther Res. 1976; 20:184.

27. Greenblatt DJ et al: Meprobamate: a study of irrational drug use. Am J Psychiatry. 1974; 131:1089.

28. Stone WN et al: Impact of psychosocial factors on the conduct of combined drug and psychotherapy research. Br J Psychiatry. 1975; 127:432.

29. Braun J et al: Anxiety, neurosis, depressive disorder and meprobamate addiction. West J Med. 1975; 123:115.

30. Haizlip TM et al: Meprobamate habituation. N Engl J Med. 1958; 258:1181.

31. Salzman C et al: Psychopharmacologic investigations in elderly volunteers: effect of diazepam in males. J Am Geriatrics Soc. 1975; 23:451.

32. Shader RI et al: *Psychotropic Drug Side Effects,* Williams & Wilkins, Baltimore, 1970.

33. Reidenberg MM et al: Relationship between diazepam dose, plasma level, age, and central nervous system depression. Clin Pharmacol Ther. 1978; 23:371.

34. Macklon AF et al: The effect of age on the pharmacokinetics of diazepam. Clin Sci. 1980; 59:479.

35. Winter ME: *Basic Clinical Pharmacokinetics,* Applied Therapeutics, Inc., San Francisco, 1980.

36. Klotz U et al: The effects of age and liver disease on the disposition and elimination of diazepam in adult man. J Clin Invest. 1975; 55:347.

37. Klotz U et al: Altered elimination of desmethyldiazepam in the elderly. Br J Clin Pharmacol. 1979; 7:119.

38. Greenblatt DJ et al: Effects of age and other drugs on benzodiazepine kinetics. Arzneim-Forsch/Drug Res. 1980; 30:886.

39. Greenblatt DJ et al: Lorazepam kinetics in the elderly. Clin Pharmacol Ther. 1979; 26:103.

40. Kraus JW et al: Effects of aging and liver disease on disposition of lorazepam. Clin Pharmacol Ther. 1978; 24:411.

41. Shull HJ et al: Normal disposition of oxazepam in acute viral hepatitis and cirrhosis. Ann Intern Med. 1976; 84:420.

42. Merlis S et al: The use of oxazepam in elderly patients. Dis Nerv Syst. 1975; 36:27.

43. Sellers EM: Chlordiazepoxide and oxazepam disposition in cirrhosis. Clin Pharmacol Ther. 1979; 26:240.

44. Fessel JM: An analysis of the causes and prevention of hepatic coma. Gastroenterology. 1972; 61:191.

45. Klotz U et al: Disposition of diazepam and its major metabolite desmethyldiazepam in patients with liver disease. Clin Pharmacol Ther. 1977; 21:430.

46. Greenblatt DJ et al: Intramuscular injection of drugs. N Engl J Med. 1976; 295:542.

47. Gamble JAS et al: Plasma diazepam levels after single dose oral and intramuscular administration. Anaesthesia. 1975; 30:164.

48. Kanto J: Plasma concentrations of diazepam and its metabolites after peroral, intramuscular, and rectal administration. Int J Clin Pharmacol. 1975; 12:427.

49. McCaughey W et al: Comparison of the sedative effects of diazepam given by the oral and intramuscular routes. Br J Anaesth. 1972; 44:901.

50. Kortila K et al: Polyethylene glycol as a solvent for diazepam: bioavailability and clinical effects after intramuscular administration, comparison of oral, intramuscular and rectal administration, and precipitation from intravenous solutions. Acta Pharmacol Toxicol. 1976; 39:104.

51. Landon DE et al: Thrombophlebitis with diazepam used intravenously. JAMA 1973; 223:184.

52. Greenblatt DJ et al: Pharmacokinetics and bioavailability of intravenous, intramuscular and oral lorazepam in humans. J Pharm Sci. 1979; 68:57.

53. Greenblatt DJ et al: Slow absorption of intramuscular chlordiazepoxide. N Engl J Med. 1974; 291:1116.

54. Kronenberg RS et al: The use of oral diazepam in patients with obstructive lung disease and hypercapnia. Ann Intern Med. 1975; 83:83.

55. Catchlove RFH et al: The effects of diazepam on respiration in patients with obstructive pulmonary disease. Anesthesiology. 1971; 34:14.

56. Rao S et al: Cardiopulmonary effects of diazepam. Clin Pharmacol Ther. 1973; 14:182.

57. Model DG: Effects of chlordiazepoxide in respiratory failure due to chronic bronchitis. Lancet. 1974; 2:869.

58. Hall RCW et al: Paradoxical reactions to benzodiazepines. Br J Clin Pharmacol. 1981; 11:99S.

59. Karch FE: Rage reaction associated with clorazepate dipotassium. Ann Intern Med. 1979; 91:61.

60. Salzman C et al: Is oxazepam associated with hostility? Dis Nerv Syst. 1975; 36:30.

61. Gardos G et al: Differential actions of chlordiazepoxide and oxazepam on hostility. Arch Gen Psychiatry. 1968; 18:757.

62. Kochanski GE et al: The differential effects of chlordiazepoxide and oxazepam on hostility in a small group setting. Am J Psychiatry. 1975; 132:861.

63. Leaf RC et al: Chlordiazepoxide- and diazepam-induced mouse killing in rats. Psychopharmacology. 1975; 44:23.

64. Salzman C et al: Chlordiazepoxide, expectation and hostility. Psychopharmacology. 1969; 14:38.

65. Salzman C et al: Chlordiazepoxide-induced hostility in a small group setting. Arch Gen Psychiatry. 1974; 31:401.

66. Rickels K et al: Chlordiazepoxide and hostility in anxious outpatients. Am J Psychiatry. 1974; 131:442.

67. Winokur A et al: Withdrawal reaction from long-term, low-dosage administration of diazepam. Arch Gen Psychiatry. 1980; 37:101.

68. Tyrer P et al: Benzodiazepine withdrawal symptoms and propranolol. Lancet. 1981; 1:520.

69. Howe JG: Lorazepam withdrawal seizures. Br J Med. 1980; 280:1163.

70. Mendelson G: Withdrawal symptoms after oxazepam. Lancet. 1978; 1:565.

71. Abernethy DR et al: Treatment of diazepam withdrawal syndrome with propranolol. Ann Intern Med. 1981; 94:354.

72. Kagan F et al: *Brook Lodge Conference on Hypnotics*, Spectrum Publications, New York, 1975.

73. Kales A et al: Chronic hypnotic drug use; ineffectiveness, drug-withdrawal insomnia, and dependence. JAMA. 1974; 227:513.

74. Kales A: Sleep disorders. N Engl J Med. 1974; 290:487.

75. Kales A et al: Hypnotics and altered sleep-dream patterns; all night EEG studies of glutethimide, methyprylon, and pentobarbital. Arch Gen Psychiatry. 1970; 23:211.

76. Kales A et al: All night EEG studies of chloral hydrate, flurazepam, and methaqualone. Arch Gen Psychiatry. 1970; 23:219.

77. Hartmann E et al: The effects of long-term administration of psychotropic drugs on human sleep: the effects of chloral hydrate. Psychopharmacology. 1973; 33:219.

78. Kales A et al: Rebound insomnia: a potential hazard following withdrawal of certain benzodiazepines. JAMA. 1979; 241:1692.

79. Kales A et al: Effectiveness of drugs with prolonged use: flurazepam and pentobarbital. Clin Pharmacol Ther. 1975; 18:356.

80. Kales A et al: Effectiveness of intermediate-term use of secobarbital. Clin Pharmacol Ther. 1976; 20:541.

81. Nicholson AN: The use of short- and long-acting hypnotics in clinical medicine. Br J Clin Pharmacol. 1981; 11:61S.

82. Clift AD: Factors leading to dependence on hypnotic drugs. Br J Med. 1972; 3:614.

83. Clifford JM et al: Absorption and clearance of secobarbital, heptabarbital, methaqualone, and ethinamate. Clin Pharmacol Ther. 1974; 16:376.

84. Bond JA et al: The residual effects of flurazepam. Psychopharmacology. 1973; 32:223.

85. Shader RI et al: The use of benzodiazepines in clinical practice. Br J Clin Pharmacol. 1981; 11:5S.

86. Stone BM: Diazepam and its hydroxylated metabolites: studies on sleep in healthy man. Br J Clin Pharmacol. 1979; 8:57S.

87. Clarke CH et al: Immediate and residual effects in man of the metabolites of diazepam. Br J Clin Pharmacol. 1978; 6:325.

88. Rickels K et al: A comparative controlled trial of seven hypnotic agents in medical and psychiatric inpatients. Am J Med Sci. 1963; 245:142.

89. Kales A et al: Hypnotic drugs and their effectiveness; all night EEG studies of insomniac subjects. Arch Gen Psychiatry. 1970; 23:226.

90. Greenblatt DJ: Pharmacokinetic comparisons. Psychosomatics. 1980; 21(suppl):9.

91. Eberts FS et al: Triazolam disposition. Clin Pharmacol Ther. 1981; 29:81.

92. Roth T et al: The differential effects of short- and long-acting benzodiazepines upon nocturnal sleep and daytime performance. Arzneim-Forsch/Drug Res. 1980; 30:891.

93. Samuelsson SM et al: Do barbiturates influence the prothrombin-proconvertin level during anticoagulant therapy? Scand J Clin Lab Invest. 1965; 17:73.

94. Valerino DM et al: Effects of various barbiturates on hepatic microsomal enzymes. Drug Metab Dispos. 1974; 2:448.

95. Robinson DS et al: Interaction of commonly prescribed drugs and warfarin. Ann Intern Med. 1970; 72:853.

96. Brown CR et al: The oral hypnotic bioassay of hydroxyzine and pentobarbital for nighttime sedation. J Clin Pharmacol. 1974; 14:210.

97. Teutsch G et al: Hypnotic efficacy of diphenhydramine, methapyrilene, and pentobarbital. Clin Pharmacol Ther. 1975; 17:195.

98. Calandre EP et al: Methapyrilene kinetics and dynamics. Clin Pharmacol Ther. 1981; 29:527.

99. Brezinova V et al: Sleep after a bedtime beverage. Br Med J. 1972; 2:431.

100. Shader RI et al: Absorption and disposition of chlordiazepoxide in young and elderly male volunteers. J Clin Pharmacol. 1977; 17:709.

101. Ochs HR et al: Effect of age and bilroth gastrectomy on absorption of desmethyldiazepam from clorazepate. Clin Pharmacol Ther. 1979; 26:449.

102. Roberts RK et al: Disposition of chlordiazepoxide: sex differences and effects of oral contraceptives. Clin Pharmacol Ther. 1979; 25:826.

103. Dean M et al: Serum protein binding of drugs during and after pregnancy in humans. Clin Pharmacol Ther. 1980; 28:253.

104. Desmond PV et al: Short-term ethanol administration impairs the elimination of chlordiazepoxide (Librium) in man. Eur J Clin Pharmacol. 1980; 18:275.

105. Sellers EM et al: Differential effects on benzodiazepine disposition by disulfiram and ethanol. Arzneim-Forsch/Drug Res. 1980; 30:882.

106. MacLeod SM et al: Interaction of disulfiram with benzodiazepines. Clin Pharmacol Ther. 1978; 24:583.

107. Klotz U et al: Delayed clearance of diazepam due to cimetidine. N Engl J Med. 1980; 302:1012.

108. Desmond PV et al: Cimetidine impairs the elimination of chlordiazepoxide (Librium) in humans. Ann Intern Med. 1980; 93:266.

109. Patwardhan RV et al: Cimetidine spares the glucuronidation of lorazepam and oxazepam. Gastroenterology. 1980; 79:912.

110. Klotz U et al: Influence of cimetidine on the pharmacokinetics of desmethyldiazepam and oxazepam. Eur J Clin Pharmacol. 1980; 18:517.

111. Ochs HR et al: Diazepam interaction with antituberculosis drugs. Clin Pharmacol Ther. 1981; 29:671.

112. Desmond PV et al: Effect of heparin administration on plasma binding of benzodiazepines. Br J Clin Pharmacol. 1980; 9:171.

113. Routledge PA et al: Diazepam and N-desmethyldiazepam redistribution after heparin. Clin Pharmacol Ther. 1980; 27:528.

114. Greenblatt DJ et al: Influence of magnesium and aluminum hydroxide mixture on chlordiazepoxide absorption. Clin Pharmacol Ther. 1976; 19:234.

115. Shader RI et al: Impaired absorption of desmethyldiazepam from clorazepate by magnesium aluminum hydroxide. Clin Pharmacol Ther. 1978; 24:308.

116. Morgan DD et al: Clinical pharmacokinetics of chlordiazepoxide in patients with alcoholic hepatitis. Eur J Clin Pharmacol. 1981; 19:279.

117. Heel RC et al: Temazepam: A review of pharmacological properties and therapeutic efficacy as a hypnotic. Drugs. 1981; 21:321.

118. Abernethy DR et al: Impairment of diazepam metabolism by low-dose estrogen-containing oral-contraceptive steroids. N Engl J Med. 1982; 306:791.

119. Fann WE et al: Pharmacology, efficacy, and adverse effects of halazepam, a new benzodiazepine. Pharmacotherapy. 1982; 2:72.

Chapter 4

Pain

Ronald P. Evens and James DuBe

Perception of Pain

Pain is an unpleasant sensation disturbing a patient's comfort, thought, sleep, or normal daily activity and is only symptomatic of an underlying disease process. It is influenced by attention, anxiety, fatigue, suggestion, prior conditioning, and a host of other psychological variables as well as the extent of tissue damage. Pain is the net effect of complex interactions of ascending and descending neurosystems with biochemical, physiological, psychological, and neocortical processes. By the time pain is perceived, it already has been submitted to the actions of many of these neurosystems (1–3).

Pain is a subjective experience. Therefore, it is the patient, not the clinician, who is the only one who can describe the intensity of pain. It has been said, "Pain is whatever the experiencing person says it is, existing wherever he/she says it does" (4). Thus, a patient's description of pain must be believed if clinicians wish to alleviate their patient's discomfort.

When obtaining a patient's subjective description of pain, clinicians may wish to organize their questions by use of a PQRST mnemonic (5). The letter P represents *palliative* or *precipitating* factors (eg, exertion, diet, emotion, stress, infections, antacids, and posture). The letter Q represents the *quality* of pain (eg, sharpness, dullness, knifelike, crushing, waxing, waning, or pulsating). The letter R represents *region* or *radiation* of pain (eg, substernal region radiating to the left arm). Many conditions may produce pain in the same regional area; eg, substernal pain may be secondary to angina pectoris, myocardial infarction, pleuritis, esophagitis, cholecystitis, bone fracture, or muscle strain. The letter S deals with the patient's *subjective* descriptions of the *severity* of the pain (eg, awakened at night by the pain, or takes the patient's breath away). The letter T concerns the *temporal* nature of the pain (eg, day or night, relationship to meals or activities, acute or chronic).

Pain Transmission

In the central nervous system (CNS) opiate receptors (OR) mediate analgesic activity (6–8). At least five characteristics can be attributed to these receptors. These opiate receptors are stereospecific for the levorotatory isomers of active compounds; dependent upon the strength of receptor binding for potency; blocked by opiate antagonists like naloxone; located in the areas of the brain which transmit and integrate pain sensory information; and capable of altering membrane ionic permeability and neuronal activity in the presence of agonist binding. Opiates like morphine bind to such receptors, eg, in the brainstem periaqueductal gray area (PAG), to stimulate and initiate the primary mechanism of CNS pain modulation (the descending pain suppression system).

Endorphins and enkephalins are normally occurring endogenous peptides which mimic morphine's pharmacologic actions (7,9–14). These endogenous opioids evoke the full spectrum of morphine-like properties in animals: analgesia, tolerance, dependence, withdrawal following chronic use, emotional changes, catatonia, temperature aberrations, and the salivation-shaking reaction.

Endorphins originate from the pituitary gland, especially the pars intermedius. Intrathecal endorphin administration produces analgesia in patients with intractable pain; its effects persist for over 24 hours and are accompanied by drowsiness.

Two pentapeptide *enkephalins* have been isolated from brain tissue. These enkephalins are considered to be inhibitory neurotransmitters which influence cationic membrane permeability and cyclic nucleotide activity. Their loci and actions are independent from endorphins. The anatomic sites for enkephalins usually are nerve terminals and axons in the CNS which deal with pain and related behavior.

The ascending spinal pain transmission system and the descending pain suppression system are depicted in Fig. 1 (7,15) which illustrates the following: PAG (brainstem site for stimulation of analgesia), substantia gelatinosa (Sg—spinal cord locus for initial integration of sensory information), trigeminal nucleus caudalis (Tnc—spinal cord area involved with pain stimuli), reticularis gigantocellularis nucleus (Rgc—medullary area for receipt of ascending pain transmission), amygdala (site for influencing emotional behavior), locus ceruleus (Lc), and others. A noxious event like pain first stimulates a peripheral receptor until a threshold level of activity is exceeded, at which time transmission of pain impulses is initiated (Position #1 in diagram). The impulses are dispatched along peripheral nerves to the spinal cord, and summation and facilitation, related to the extent of receptor stimulation, occur during the transmission process. The Sg in the dorsal horn of the spinal cord serves a preliminary integration function for sensory stimuli at Position #2. Then pain sensations are transmitted along ascending spinothalamic tracts in the spinal cord, including a medial spinal tract (Position #3), eventually culminating at the brain to result in pain perception (Position #5).

Inhibition of pain transmission is produced by three mechanisms (7,15). First, large fiber peripheral afferent (LFPA) neurons exert a segmental inhibitory action during ascending pain transmission at the spinal cord level (Position #2). Second, the lateral ascending spinothalamic tract modulates parallel medial tract pain transmission by inhibition at a thalamic level while pain impulses are ascending to the brain; the ventral-postero-lateral and -medial nuclei (VPL-VPM) of the thalamus suppress pain transmission (Position #4). The third and primary mechanism for pain modulation is a descending system which functions as a negative feedback loop from the medial tracts of the spinal cord (Position #3), through several brain centers in the midbrain and medulla (Positions #6 and #7), and back to the spinal cord at the Sg (Position #2). Mediators in this system include enkephalins, serotonin, and possibly catecholamines. Pain impulses travel to the brain through the ascending medial spinothalamic tract (Position #3) and activate the descending pain suppression neurons that extend to the Rgc nucleus in the medulla. From the Rgc nucleus, the PAG in the midbrain is then stimulated; this involves opiate receptors and enkephalins. The PAG is naloxone sensitive and opiate drugs activate the PAG midbrain center and enhance the negative feedback loop to reduce pain. The PAG, in turn, activates the nucleus raphe magnus (NRM) in the medulla, a serotonergic area, and also the reticularis magnocellularis nuclei (Rmc, a reticular formation area); the latter is non-serotonergic, non-enkephalergic, and naloxone insensitive. The locus ceruleus (Lc) is hypothesized to be an opiate withdrawal center with catecholamines (C) and opiate receptors involved in its activity. Other brain centers are involved in pain suppression (eg, the hypothalamus), but their roles have not been fully identified. The axonic projections of the medullary brain centers (NRM, Rmc) inhibit spinal pain transmissions at the Sg in the dorsal horn of the spinal cord (Location #2). Therefore, pain transmission is a dynamic system involving a major descending negative feedback loop which reduces ascending pain transmission.

Evaluation of Analgesic Efficacy

The measurement of pain is necessarily subjective because the sensation, transmission, perception, and reaction to pain are highly variable. Therefore, evaluation of analgesic efficacy is difficult. In a review of 15 double-blind clinical trials, placebos produced satisfactory pain relief in 35% ± 2% of 1082 patients. Furthermore, in one study, 52% of 199 patients with headaches were effectively treated with a placebo. Therefore, the following are major points to consider in evaluating analgesic studies (17–21):

a. A new analgesic should be tested against a placebo and a drug standard (eg, morphine sulfate 10 mg/70 kg or aspirin 600 mg).

b. Once analgesic efficacy has been established, equianalgesic doses must be employed when comparing side effects of any two agents.

c. The designs of clinical trials should be based upon double blinding and randomization to minimize bias.

d. The degree of pain relief should be determined by patients utilizing a standardized evaluative instrument such as a pain questionnaire which assesses the character and intensity of pain (22). Another evaluation instrument utilizes a 10 point line with descriptive terms such as "no pain" and "worst pain possible" at opposite ends of the continuum. With this latter instrument, the patient marks a point on the line before and after therapy; thereby quantifying the degree of pain relief. Supplemental analgesic intake and global assessments by clinicians are helpful as adjunctive evaluation tools.

e. The patient population should be large, homogeneous, and suffering from a similar type and degree of pain such as post-operative, post-partum, episiotomy, cancer, or headache pain.

f. Factors which alter pain perception and its relief should be minimized (eg, co-administration of central nervous system depressants, prior administration of other analgesics, sociological population differences).

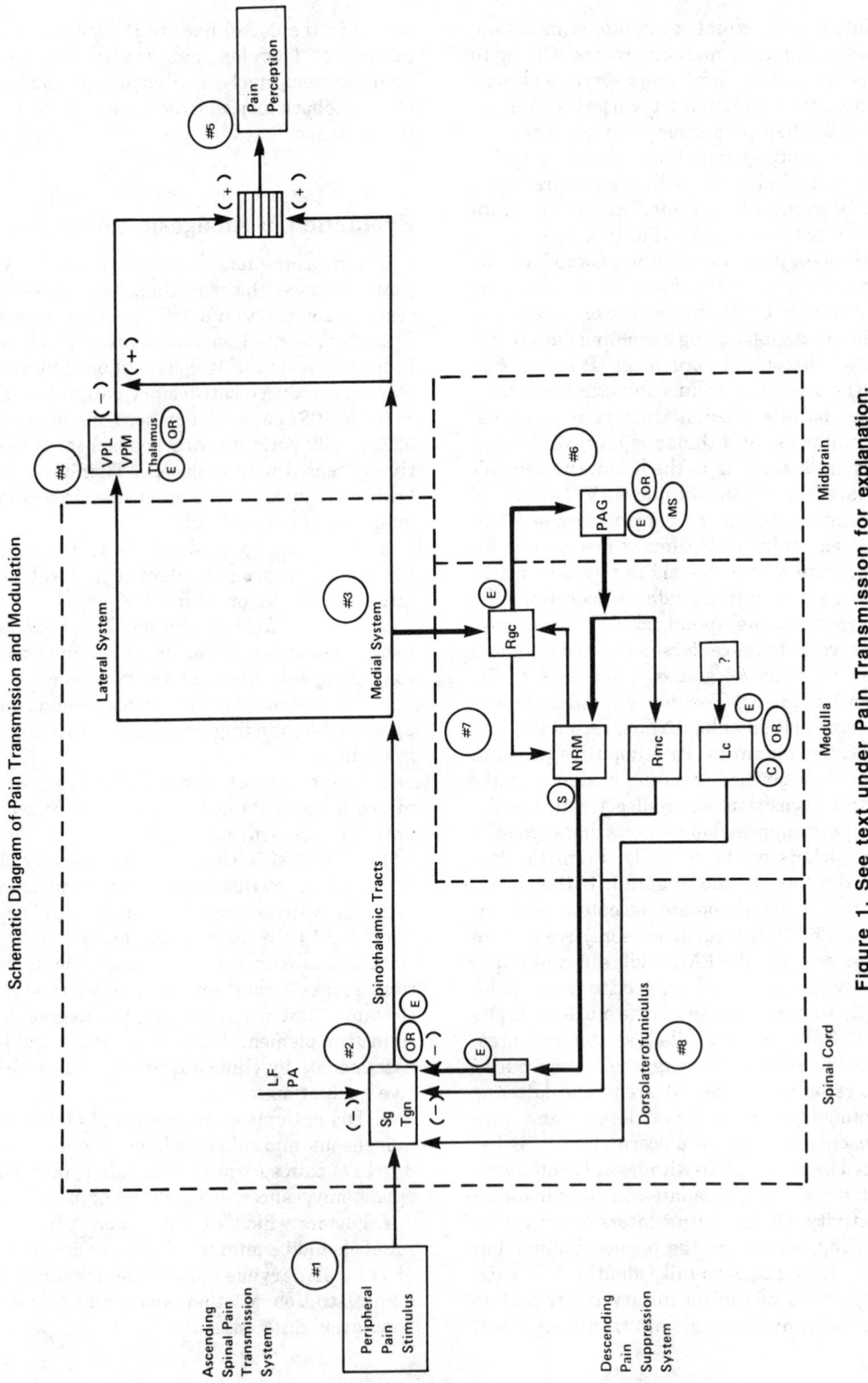

Figure 1. See text under Pain Transmission for explanation.

POTENT ANALGESICS

An intramuscular dose of 10 mg/70 kg of morphine sulfate can provide significant analgesia in two-thirds of patients with severe acute pain. A larger dose, 15 mg/70 kg, will provide pain relief for 75% of patients but will be accompanied by an increased incidence of side effects (17,23–25). Dosage requirements may vary with the severity of pain, response to pain, age, weight, and the presence of concomitant disease states. Thus, analgesic doses of morphine may range from less than 8 mg to 15 mg or more in acute pain, and doses as high as 800 mg per day have been required in treating cancer pain (17,23–25).

A 10 mg dose of morphine is the reference standard for evaluating the efficacy of other potent analgesics. Therefore, comparisons must be based upon equianalgesic doses.

1. Cancer Pain. B.B. is a 57-year-old woman with a diagnosis of ovarian carcinoma. Since the diagnosis several months ago, she had a total radical abdominal hysterectomy with bilateral salpingo-oophorectomy and resection of the small bowel and bladder. She received multiple courses of radiation therapy and chemotherapy. Her pain was reasonably well controlled until three weeks ago with Percodan (oxycodone 4.88 mg and aspirin 325 mg), two tablets every four hours. She consulted a neurosurgeon after the exacerbation of pain but declined to undergo a high thoracic cordotomy and increased her Percodan intake to three tablets every three hours. The pain in her left leg is severe, and she can walk with the aid of a cane only with great difficulty. She is now hospitalized for support and pain management. Why is cancer painful in such a patient?

A precise etiology for cancer pain has frustrated clinicians for some time. Nevertheless, the etiology of pain in patients with cancer has been categorized into three major syndromes, all of which may have occurred in this patient:

a. Pain caused by direct tumor infiltration of either bone, nerve, or hollow viscus;
b. Pain following surgery, chemotherapy or radiation; and
c. Pain that develops coincidentally with, but is unrelated to, cancer or cancer therapy.

2. What are the important differences between acute pain and chronic pain such as that experienced by this patient?

Acute pain is linear with a beginning and an end, even if poorly treated. Acute pain also has a purpose; it warns of a problem which requires attention. Chronic pain, however, is not linear. The patient often cannot remember an existence free of pain and is convinced that the pain will be present until he or she dies. Like a circle, it has no apparent beginning and no end. The suffering which accompanies chronic pain induces a sense of helplessness and hopelessness. Anticipation that the pain will be continuous leads to anxiety, depression and insomnia. These, in turn, accentuate the physical component of the pain. Such pain can become progressively more severe and cause relentless suffering. This suffering can accelerate the deterioration in the patient's physical and psychological condition that the disease itself causes. The pain is, however, not merely physical pain. The patient's pain has psychological, financial, interpersonal, and spiritual components, in addition to the physical component.

Some cancer patients, confronted with a dreaded disease and the possibility of impending death, respond with fear, resentment, anger, and frustration (36). Their anxiety is heightened by the fear of loss of social position, possible surgical mutilation, loss of dignity (self-control), and fear of uncontrollable pain. A full discussion of the psychologic and emotional aspects of cancer pain is beyond the scope of this chapter, but the successful treatment of a large percentage of these patients requires a multidisciplinary approach (37–39) not unlike that offered by hospices.

3. What general therapeutic guidelines should be followed for this cancer patient's pain?

Identify the cause. Effective treatment of cancer pain requires that pain be eliminated and prevented from recurring rather than treated when it becomes unbearable. Therefore, knowing the cause of the pain is helpful. For example, it would be irrational to treat the severe abdominal cramping pain of constipation with morphine.

Prevent pain. The elimination and prevention of recurring cancer pain is best accomplished by using analgesics at fixed time intervals rather than on an "as needed" basis. The data in Table 1 are helpful in accomplishing this goal.

Erase pain memory. When pain is prevented from recurring by the continual administration of analgesics, the fear of pain and the memory of pain diminish in the patient's mind, and he or she becomes more comfortable. The amount of analgesic needed should then gradually be decreased if possible (40).

Normal affect and unclouded sensorium. If the maintenance dose of narcotic analgesic is too high, the patient will be continually sedated and chemically bedridden. Patients, when given the choice of extinguishing the last trace of discomfort at the cost of some clouding of the sensorium, will almost invariably select full alertness and some pain (41).

Ease of administration. Orally administered analgesics allow a patient a greater degree of independence and control than parenteral administration. Regular parenteral administration can be difficult and painful in cachectic patients.

4. Why is Brompton's mixture not superior to other modes of treatment for this woman's cancer pain?

A narcotic mixture for oral administration in severe pain was formulated at the Brompton Chest Hospital in London in 1926 and was included in the *British Pharmaceutical Codex* by 1973. The mixture contained diamorphine (heroin) in a variable amount, cocaine 10 mg per dose, alcohol, chloroform water, and syrup (42). Because clinicians in the United States were precluded from using heroin, they formulated their own versions of *Brompton's mixture* by adding morphine or methadone instead of heroin, cocaine, and often a phenothiazine mixed in a variety of flavoring agents (43,44). Cancer pain was successfully treated in approximately 90% of patients using these Brompton's mixtures, and very little toler-

Table 1.

EQUIANALGESIC DOSES OF NARCOTIC ANALGESICS

Drug	Route	Average Dose (mg)	Average Duration (hr)
Alphaprodine (Nisentil)	SC	50	1
Butorphanol (Stadol)	IM, SC	2	3
Fentanyl (Sublimaze)	IV, IM, SC	0.2	1
Hydromorphone (Dilaudid)	PO	4	4
	IM, SC	2	4
	Rectal	6	4
Levorphanol (Levo-Dromoran)	PO	4	6
	SC	2	6
Meperidine (Demerol)	PO	300	3
	IM, SC	100	3
Methadone (Dolophine)	PO	20	6
	IM, SC	10	6
Morphine	PO	30	4
	IM, SC	10	4
Nalbuphine (Nubain)	IM, SC	10	4
Oxymorphone (Numorphan)	IM	1.5	4
	Rectal	4.5	4
Oxycodone (Percodan) (Tylox, Percocet)	PO	3 tablets	4
Pentazocine (Talwin)	IM	60	3
	PO	200	3

ance to the analgesic effect developed (40,46–48).

Although oral morphine is poorly absorbed, the analgesic effectiveness of heroin and morphine are comparable if the morphine dose is 1.5 times larger than the heroin dose (24). A double-blind crossover trial compared a standard Brompton's mixture containing morphine, cocaine, ethanol, syrup, and chloroform water to a flavored aqueous solution of morphine alone (49). Pain was measured by the pain intensity index of the McGill Pain Questionnaire, and an assessment of confusion, drowsiness and nausea was obtained from the patients, their relatives, and the nurses. No differences between the two products in pain relief, drowsiness, or other side effects were observed in the 44 patients with painful and advanced malignant diseases. Morphine oral solution is therefore an effective analgesic that avoids the expense or potential side effects of mixtures containing cocaine (50). Apparently, the "routinely scheduled" rather than the "as needed" use of narcotic analgesics probably accounts for much of the purported efficacy.

Oral morphine solution should be prescribed for this patient because Brompton's mixture is not superior.

5. What oral dose of morphine should be selected for this patient?

It is important to break the cycle of pain and have the patient pain-free as rapidly as possible. For this woman, an initial morphine dose of 40 mg every 3 hours should provide sufficient analgesia without unacceptable drowsiness or respiratory depression (24,25,49,51) (See Table 1). Her response to this medication should be carefully monitored one to two hours after her dose by utilizing a pain measurement instrument (see Evaluation of Analgesic Efficacy). If she is still uncomfortable after two hours, the dose should be increased by 50% (to 80 mg) and given at once. It must be emphasized that the response of the patient should be the primary criterion for determining the dose, and the kinetics of the agent should determine the dosing interval. Frequent reassessment of the patient's pain status and level of consciousness is essential.

When the pain has been relieved, the dose of morphine can often be decreased. Someone must assume responsibility for frequently monitoring the patient's level of awareness and presence or absence of pain. Dosage adjustment, once the pain has been controlled, should usually be made no more frequently than once a day.

6. Is tolerance or dependence to this large dose of morphine likely to occur?

Twycross (52) in reporting his experiences with heroin stated: a) There is no single optimal or maximum effective dose; b) The use of diamorphine does not, by itself, impair mental faculties; c) Tolerance is not a problem; d) Psychological dependence does not occur; and e) Physical dependence may occur, but does not prevent the downward adjustment of the dose when considered clinically feasible.

Although these statements pertain to heroin, there is little clinical difference between oral heroin (diacetylmorphine) and morphine provided allowance is made for the difference in potency. Of 115 patients who died of cancer and who received heroin for 12 weeks or longer, dose reductions were common and the median final dose was less than the median maximum dose (24,51–53).

7. The patient was discharged from the hospital with a prescription for oral morphine solution 20 mg every four hours. She has been relatively pain-free for about a month, but now returns to the clinic complaining of excessive morning sedation. She cannot reduce her morphine dose because the pain makes her too uncomfortable. What therapeutic intervention can be utilized to alleviate this patient's problem of excessive morning sedation?

Limited clinical data suggest that a morning dose of methylphenidate (Ritalin) or dextroamphetamine (Dexedrine) could relieve not only narcotic-induced drowsiness, but also potentiate analgesia (54). Less sleepiness has been associated with these combinations than with narcotic analgesics alone, and 10 mg doses of amphetamine combined with narcotic increased pain tolerance more than the narcotic alone in an artificial pain study (55). Although these studies involved only single doses, these agents should cause enough central nervous system stimulation to obviate morning drowsiness. The patient should try a morning dextroamphetamine dose of 5 mg to 20 mg. A somewhat smaller dose may be added around noon if the patient desires increased alertness in late afternoon and evening.

8. Three months later, B.B. is admitted to the hospital again. She now has a complete and inoperable bowel obstruction and has been placed on continual nasogastric suction. Her weight is now only 67 pounds. She

has been receiving 20 mg of morphine IM every three hours since her admission. Her pain is bothersome and her cachectic condition is not conducive to intramuscular injections. What would be a reasonable intravenous analgesic program for this patient?

A continuous intravenous infusion of morphine or meperidine is superior to intramuscular injections in maintaining a pain-free condition in cancer and surgical patients (56–58). In one study, six of eight children with cancer experienced complete pain control with 0.025–2.6 mg/kg/hr of morphine for 1–16 days (56).

This patient has been receiving 160 mg of morphine daily, which is about 7 mg per hour. A reasonable initial intravenous infusion dose of morphine would be 8 mg per hour since she is not now comfortable. A 200 mg dose of morphine can be added to 500 ml of 5% dextrose in water, and the solution should be infused intravenously at 20 ml per hour. In addition, an order should be written for a 4 mg intravenous bolus of morphine every hour as needed for signs of pain or discomfort.

The supplemental bolus doses of intravenous morphine will facilitate subsequent adjustments of the continuous infusion rate. At the end of a nursing work shift or at the end of a day, the number of milligrams of drug which were administered by constant infusion are added to 1.5 times the number of milligrams of drug used in supplemental bolus doses. This amount of drug is then divided by the elapsed interval of time. A new infusion rate can then be calculated. For example, if at the end of 6 hours the patient has received 5 supplemental doses of 4 mg each, then 6 hours × 8 mg per hour plus (1.5 × 5 doses of 4 mg) = 78 mg per 6 hours. The new infusion rate should then be 13 mg per hour, and the new as needed supplemental doses should be 6.5 mg (the amount of drug normally infused in 30 minutes) every hour.

Continual assessment of the patient and hourly dosage adjustments are probably superior to the method outlined above, but the above method may be more practical for the busy clinician.

9. S.C. is a 67-year-old man with advanced and now inoperable throat cancer. The patient is to receive orally 15 mg of morphine solution every four hours for pain, but he has been vomiting each dose despite seemingly adequate doses of phenothiazine. The patient is at home and does not wish to be institutionalized in order to receive parenteral analgesics. What can be done to relieve pain in this patient who vomits after oral morphine?

Morphine and its derivatives induce nausea and vomiting by stimulating the chemoreceptor trigger zone (CTZ). Although the CTZ is stimulated initially, subsequent doses of morphine generally suppress the vomiting center. Because the incidence of nausea (40%) and vomiting (15%) increases in ambulatory patients, it is generally agreed that a vestibular component is also involved (59,60). If the vomiting is vestibular in origin, instructing the patient to lie quietly, with as little head motion as possible for an hour or two, will often help. The nausea usually only persists for 48–72 hours.

Levorphanol (Levo-Dromoran) may case less nausea and vomiting with equianalgesic doses than other potent narcotic analgesics (26) and might be an alternative to morphine if the above recommendations are ineffective in modifying this patient's nausea and vomiting. An equipotent dose of levorphanol for this patient according to Table 1 would be 2 mg. The reported duration of action of levorphanol is longer than for most of the other potent narcotic analgesics, and it can be given every six hours instead of every 4 hours. These doses are for pain prevention and are not to be confused with doses which are ordered on an "as needed" basis for pain.

10. R.C. is a 67-year-old man with advanced lung cancer. He has received multiple courses of chemotherapy and radiation therapy with little success. The decision has been made to use methadone to treat this patient's pain. What are guidelines for the safe use of methadone in treating cancer pain?

Clinical experience with the use of methadone for the treatment of cancer pain has been favorable. In a recent trial, 11 of 14 patients experienced complete or almost complete pain relief with self-controlled dosing of 30–80 mg/day of methadone which was decreased to 10–40 mg/day one week later (64). The patient's physical and mental condition should be monitored closely, and clinicians should be aware of the prolonged drug half-life of methadone.

Methadone is 85% bound to serum proteins, and its average plasma half-life is about 23 hours with a range of 13 to 47 hours. Therefore, the drug probably is tightly bound and only slowly released from its binding sites (65,66). Plasma levels of methadone will continue to rise for 5 to 10 days after any increase in dose.

Unfortunately, analgesia is not related to the serum half-life, and multiple doses must be given each day. The absolute amount of methadone in plasma, although it undoubtedly affects sedation and respiratory depression, is not a factor in the magnitude of analgesic response. Rather, analgesic effects are observed only while plasma levels are elevated above a certain individualized pre-dose plasma level of methadone (65).

Most patients can be maintained on doses of methadone every 6 or 8 hours after pain control is achieved, but the drug often must be given every four hours or administered with another narcotic analgesic in the first day or two of therapy to control pain.

The necessity for frequent initial use of this agent can cause clinicians unfamiliar with the long half-life of methadone to adjust doses too frequently or to then maintain a patient at an inappropriately high dose after initial pain control is achieved. This can threaten the patient with dangerous drug accumulation (67). A scenario which is often repeated is one in which analgesia is obtained after two or three days of gradually increasing doses, and the patient is quite comfortable. On days four and five, the patient is increasingly more sedated and on day six alarmingly so. The drug is then discontinued or the narcotic antagonist, naloxone is administered. Suddenly, the patient is no longer sedated, but the pain has reappeared.

Elderly patients probably will require lower total daily doses of methadone. Twycross (25) recommends caution if using this drug in the elderly or extremely debilitated.

11. Three days later, the patient begins to complain of pain in his hip, an area where metastasis has been demonstrated by bone scan. Should the dose of methadone (10 mg every six hours) be increased?

The dose could be increased because pain from metastasis to bone is particularly distressing and difficult to treat. However, the most effective therapy for the relief of bone pain is radiation to the site of the pain. If additional radiation is unacceptable, prostaglandin inhibitors may be another reasonable alternative to increased doses of narcotics.

Osseous metastasis induces the production of prostaglandins which may cause osteolysis, sensitize free nerve endings, and augment pain perception. The non-steroidal anti-inflammatory drugs effectively decrease prostaglandin and endoperoxide production and may be useful in treating metastatic bone pain if administered on a scheduled, as opposed to an "as needed", basis. Usual analgesic doses are often effective but maximum therapeutic doses may be necessary. Some specialists in treating cancer pain advocate doses considerably larger than the manufacturers' recommendations (61–63).

12. Why should pentazocine (Talwin) not be used in treating cancer pain?

Mild oral analgesics should always be employed first in the treatment of cancer pain, but pentazocine is inferior to aspirin (68). The use of agonist-antagonists also should be avoided because of poor oral efficacy and because of the particularly disturbing nature of the psychotomimetic side effects in patients who are already fearful and anxious (see Question 17). Furthermore, pentazocine is a "ceiling" drug; doses cannot be greatly increased to treat increasing pain without greatly increasing the incidence and severity of side effects (27).

13. Why is meperidine so seldom prescribed for cancer pain management?

Meperidine has only a three hour half-life and perhaps an even shorter duration of action as an analgesic (26,69,70). Therefore, it is unsuitable for treatment of chronic pain. Furthermore, the demethylated metabolite of meperidine, normeperidine, accumulates in patients with cancer (71) and is known to cause apprehension, tremors, and seizures in these patients (72). This metabolite has only half the analgesic properties of meperidine and is twice as potent as a convulsant.

14. A 30-year-old male was admitted to the surgery ward with a chief complaint of severe peri-umbilical pain which was followed by nausea and vomiting. A diagnosis of acute appendicitis was made and the patient was scheduled for an emergency appendectomy.

The patient's past medical history was significant in that five years prior to admission (PTA) he had a goiter removed; he is currently treated with 0.2 mg thyroxine daily. He also had an acute psychotic episode eight

years PTA following the ingestion of LSD. He currently takes no drugs of abuse.

Following surgery, he was given 2 mg of morphine sulfate intravenously. Since he complained of itching along the arm, codeine 60 mg IM every four hours was ordered once he returned to the ward. This produced an itchy wheal at the site of injection and a generalized pruritus, and he was switched to meperidine 50 mg plus promethazine 50 mg every four to six hours prn pain. The next morning the meperidine and promethazine were discontinued because of this patient's history of drug abuse and substituted with pentazocine 60 mg IM every six hours prn pain. That evening the patient had to be restrained because he was found choking the patient who shared his room because he thought the man had turned into a gorilla.

If this patient is allergic to morphine and codeine, what alternative analgesics can be administered?

Narcotic agents can cause allergic-type reactions, although such occurrences are infrequent (26). Narcotics can also stimulate histamine release from mast cells (73) and cause a local wheal at the site of injection with burning and erythema (74). Itching can occur locally and, possibly, as a generalized effect as well. Systemic allergic symptoms are also possible.

If morphine allergy does exist, codeine should be avoided because both codeine and morphine are structurally similar phenanthrene derivatives. Codeine is methylmorphine, and about 10% of each codeine dose is demethylated to morphine. Meperidine (Demerol) and pentazocine (Talwin) are potent analgesics with substantially different chemical structures from morphine, and would most likely be safe in this patient.

15. Was the meperidine dose sufficient for this patient? Would narcotic addiction become a likely problem under these circumstances?

The addition of promethazine to an analgesic regimen is sometimes thought to potentiate or prolong the analgesia of meperidine, despite contradictory studies (see Question 16). The dose of meperidine itself, however, probably was inadequate for this patient, because a dose of 75–100 mg of meperidine is needed to provide the same degree of analgesia as 10 mg of morphine. Furthermore, the prescribed dosing interval was more consistent with the duration of action of morphine than meperidine (see Table 1).

In a survey by Marks and associates (76), a majority of physicians underestimated the effective dosage range, overestimated the duration of action, and exaggerated the dangers of addiction for medical inpatients receiving meperidine. Another study noted that nurses administered less than the prescribed amounts of narcotics to their patients and that 75% of these patients suffered moderate to marked distress (77). Patients should not suffer pain needlessly, as hospital-induced narcotic addiction is a rare problem. The Illinois State Drug Abuse Center showed that only three of 1900 cases of addiction were possible complications of previous medical treatment (76); and a Boston Collaborative Drug Study noted only 4 patients out of almost 12,000 who received narcotics had developed probable addiction (78). Furthermore, Saunders (79) and Twycross (53) have noted that the purported craving for narcotics, which occasionally is observed in cancer patients, is most likely due to inadequate analgesic doses of narcotics. Therefore, clinicians should not exercise undue caution in prescribing narcotic analgesics for fear of "addicting" patients in a hospital setting.

This paucity of cases does not mean to imply, however, that physical dependence does not occur in hospitalized patients. Approximately 50% of patients who receive therapeutic doses of narcotic analgesics several times daily for two to three weeks in a hospital setting will experience some mild degree of sleep disturbance and rhinorrhea after abrupt withdrawal of narcotic analgesics. However, these symptoms usually peak within 8–12 hours and usually are not recognized as being a consequence of narcotic administration. Therefore, physical dependence to narcotics frequently develops in hospital patients. However, physical dependence is not the same as addiction. In the hospital, narcotics are administered in a defined context and the patient does not have the same stimuli for addiction as in the nonmedical social setting where contact with friends, sights, and sounds associated with drug taking powerfully reinforce the rituals leading to abuse. The reader is referred to the chapter entitled Drug Abuse for additional discussions of addiction and physical dependence.

This patient's thyroid function should also be considered because hypothyroid individuals are said to be more sensitive, and hyperthyroid individuals less sensitive, to the analgesic and toxic effects of narcotics (26,86). This patient probably is clinically euthyroid, and the dose will not need adjustment if this is the case.

16. What might have been the rationale for the co-administration of promethazine with meperidine in this patient?

Promethazine (Phenergan) has a two-carbon side chain attached to its basic phenothiazine nucleus. As a result, it behaves pharmacologically more like an antihistamine than a neuroleptic. The promethazine, therefore, may have been prescribed for this patient's generalized pruritus. On the other hand, the promethazine probably was prescribed to enhance the action of meperidine. Phenothiazines are often administered concomitantly with narcotics to "enhance" analgesia. However, most claims of enhanced analgesia (53,87) are not supported by well designed studies (89) which meet the criteria described earlier in this chapter (see section entitled Evaluation of Analgesic Efficacy). Many of these studies lack double-blinding, a cross-over of patients, placebo control, or appropriate instruments capable of evaluating pain. Another problem in the design of studies evaluating the combination of a phenothiazine and a narcotic analgesic is the failure to differentiate between analgesia and sedation. Sedation is not necessarily indicative of analgesia.

All phenothiazines, with the exception of methotrimeprazine, initially have an anti-analgesic effect which may be followed by varying degrees of anti-analgesia or analgesia depending upon the phenothiazine. Promethazine, in particular, seems to have a significant anti-analgesic effect after one hour, and studies (135,136) suggest that it may not potentiate the analgesia produced by meperidine.

Dundee (88) divided the phenothiazines into three groups. Those with slight analgesic activity after one hour were, in general, those with a di-methylaminopropyl side chain. These include promazine (Sparine), triflupromazine (Vesprin), propiomazine (Largon), trimeprazine (Temaril), and methotrimeprazine (Levoprome). Promethazine (Phenergan) is an important exception. Those with a slight anti-analgesic effect after one hour were those with a piperazine side chain. These include perphenazine (Trilafon), prochlorperazine (Compazine), trifluperazine (Stelazine), thiethylperazine (Torecan). Those with significant anti-analgesia after one hour included thioridazine (Mellaril) and promethazine (Phenergan).

Therefore, the addition of promethazine to meperidine to enhance analgesia is not to be encouraged, especially because phenothiazines are known to enhance the hypotensive, sedative, and respiratory depressant effects of narcotic analgesics.

17. Could pentazocine have caused this patient's unusual behavior? What is the relative incidence of dysphoria secondary to pentazocine compared to alternative analgesics such as morphine, butorphanol and nalbuphine?

Numerous case reports describe visual and auditory hallucinations and other psychic reactions attributable to pentazocine following both oral and parenteral doses (96–101). Dysphoric hallucinations of multicolored flashing patterns or animals, with or without auditory changes, have been reported (98). Dysphoric side effects may be precipitated by only one or two doses. A survey of general medical and surgical patients receiving pentazocine showed 10/105 (9.5%) cases of hallucinations versus 0/71 matched control subjects. Vivid dreams also occurred in 10 of 105 patients (9.5%) taking pentazocine in comparison to 4 of 190 (2.1%) control subjects (101).

Pentazocine is associated with a higher incidence of psychotomimetic reactions than other potent analgesics. For example, hallucinations occurred in 7 of 49 patients (14%) who received 10 mg of intramuscular morphine as compared to 24 of 65 patients (37%) who received 40–50 mg of intramuscular pentazocine (96). In another trial, psychic changes occurred in 1.7% of patients receiving morphine versus 11.4% of pentazocine-treated patients (97). Butorphanol perhaps shares with pentazocine an equal propensity for inducing significant dysphoric responses. A two mg dose of butorphanol was associated with an 18% incidence of psychic disturbances and a 4 mg dose with a 33% incidence (27). In comparison, nalbuphine and other analgesics induce far less psychotomimetic effects than butorphanol or pentazocine (27).

18. *Obstetrical Pain.* A 28-year-old woman has been in labor for 10 hours and is experiencing hard, erratic contractions at 5–15 minute intervals. Her cervix is minimally dilated, suggesting that delivery is still several hours away. Her pain is severe and if continued may compromise her ability to assist in the labor and delivery process. Which potent

analgesics could be administered for the patient in this situation?

Central nervous system depressants should be avoided during labor, if possible, because they can compromise fetal vital functions. However, if an analgesic is deemed necessary, then an agent should be chosen which meets the following criteria: (a) provide adequate pain relief; (b) have little effect on the course or duration of labor; and (c) affect fetal vital signs minimally during labor and at birth (103–105). Meperidine more closely meets these criteria and as a result is frequently preferred over either morphine or methadone in obstetrics (108–110). Although meperidine seems to have only minimal residual effects on the neonate, adverse effects may still occur. For example, 4 of 35 neonates manifested some degree of respiratory depression following maternal analgesia with meperidine (113). Furthermore, according to an early neonatal neuro-behavior scale, meperidine broadly depressed most measured neonatal activities on the first and second days of life (115).

Nevertheless, if the contractions are very hard, erratic and prolonged early in the course of labor as in this patient, a short-acting analgesic like meperidine would be useful to blunt the labor pain and sedate the mother, so that she may regain control over her contractions and conserve her energy for the actual delivery. Butorphanol (114) and pentazocine (111–113) also have minimal effects on fetal and neonatal function and are reasonable alternatives to meperidine in this situation. These potent analgesics should be administered intramuscularly or subcutaneously because intravenous administration is associated with more neonatal and fetal depression (107). Should neonatal respiratory difficulties be manifested as a result of narcotic analgesics which were administered during labor, they can be reversed with the narcotic antagonist, naloxone (113,116).

19. *Myocardial Pain.* **A 65-year-old man with a history of angina pectoris has an acute myocardial infarction. Pentazocine 45 mg IV is prescribed. Why would another analgesic be preferred over pentazocine in this situation?**

This dose of pentazocine would be effective for analgesia in this situation (117); however, pentazocine has several hemodynamic effects which increase myocardial workload and oxygen con-

sumption. Parenteral doses of 30–60 mg increase the mean arterial pressure, left ventricular end diastolic pressure and, especially, pulmonary vascular pressures (118–123). In one study, the pulmonary artery pressure rose from 17.5 to 23.1 mm Hg in 10 acute myocardial infarction patients who received pentazocine (122). Furthermore, pentazocine can produce idiosyncratic hypotensive episodes, which could be disastrous in these patients (117). Preliminary data suggest that butorphanol similarly increases pulmonary vascular resistance and pulmonary artery pressure (124).

Morphine does not increase myocardial wall tension or oxygen consumption (117,123,125–128); decreases heart rate (126–127); does not affect cardiac dimensions (127); and only induces orthostatic changes in blood pressures minimally (118–129). Sedative and emetic effects of morphine and pentazocine are comparable (117, 123,125). Methadone and meperidine affect the cardiovascular system in a manner similar to morphine (122,125).

In summary, although all the above agents are effective analgesics, pentazocine causes greater cardiovascular toxicity and can exacerbate an acute myocardial infarction. Therefore, morphine remains the preferred agent (130,131). (Also see the chapter entitled Acute Myocardial Infarction.)

20. *Acute Trauma.* **A 24-year-old hemophiliac male is admitted to the emergency room with several minor lacerations, a possible concussion, shock secondary to internal bleeding, and painful hemarthrosis secondary to a motorcycle accident. Morphine sulfate 10 mg subcutaneously was ordered and he was transferred to the medical ward for further evaluation. There, the patient was given several units of blood and anti-hemophilic factor. He was also given 100 mg of meperidine intramuscularly every four hours as needed for pain. On the 25th hospital day, it was noted that the patient continued to use four to six doses of meperidine per day and it was decided to substitute pentazocine 80 mg every six hours as needed for pain. A review of his past drug history reveals chronic narcotic use for about 18 months for persistent pain in his joints. His recent past medical history also indicates continual mental depression related to his recurrent, long-term**

problems with his hemophilia. What was the danger in administering morphine to this patient shortly after he was admitted?

Narcotic analgesics are generally avoided in patients with head injury for the following reasons: (a) narcotic-induced pupillary changes, nausea, and general central nervous system clouding may mask or confuse the diagnosis; (b) head injury potentiates the respiratory depressant effects of narcotics; (c) narcotics induce carbon dioxide retention which in turn causes vasodilation of cerebral arteries and an increase in the intracranial pressure. This may be disastrous in a situation where cerebral spinal fluid pressure is already elevated (26,28,132).

21. What are dangers of administering pentazocine to this patient on day 25?

Although pentazocine is a mild narcotic antagonist (1/50 nalorphine), 80 mg has been known to precipitate abstinence in patients who have been given narcotics for chronic pain. If pentazocine is instituted, the dose should be increased gradually and the patient should be observed closely for symptoms of abstinence (27,133,134). If possible, the meperidine should be withdrawn gradually; a drug-free period of two days prior to the institution of pentazocine has also been suggested (26).

22. Are tricyclic antidepressants (TCA) useful as analgesic agents for chronic pain as in this patient?

Tricyclic antidepressants have been used experimentally at low to moderate doses as an adjunct to analgesics for pain control (141,142). These agents may alter psychological responses to pain, may have intrinsic analgesic activity, or may potentiate narcotic analgesics (143,144). European investigations note an 82% overall response rate to these agents (141). Imipramine relieved cancer and surgical pain in about 75–80% of patients, and doxepin relieved pain completely in about half of 16 depressed chronic pain patients (145). Tension headaches were also improved with 25–100 mg of doxepin (146). Adler (142) recommends imipramine 50–200 mg/day or amitriptyline 10–40 mg/day alone or in combination with fluphenazine. Other clinicians recommend amitriptyline, doxepin, or demethylated TCA for analgesic use (143). Although the present status of TCA in the treatment of pain is investigational, preliminary evidence is promising.

A TCA would be worthwhile to try in this patient with chronic pain and depression. Doxepin or imipramine can be initiated at low doses, eg, 25–50 mg/day, and gradually increased until a response is achieved.

23. *Biliary Colic.* A patient is admitted for severe, intermittent right upper quadrant pain accompanied by nausea, vomiting, and clay colored stools. The differential diagnosis is biliary colic versus acute pancreatitis. Two doses of morphine sulfate 10 mg IM four hours apart fail to ease the pain. What other potent analgesics are preferred in this situation?

Morphine and other narcotic analgesics produce spasm of smooth muscle, including the sphincter of Oddi, and increase intrabiliary pressures sufficiently to precipitate clinical problems. Furthermore, the resulting intraductal back pressure can increase the serum amylase by 5–10 times the control value and thereby complicate the diagnosis (151). A single 5 to 10 mg dose of morphine has induced biliary colic in several instances (147,148). Fentanyl also can increase biliary pressure (153); and intraoperative fentanyl during cholecystic surgery has caused abnormal cholangiography, non-passage of contrast medium from the bile duct to the duodenum, and unnecessary explorative surgeries (149,150).

Biliary pressures increase and spasms begin within five minutes of parenteral narcotics, peak within 20 to 60 minutes, and return to normal gradually over one to two hours (147,152,153,155). This timed sequence of events varies considerably (152,156), as do the severity, intensity, and duration of the biliary hypertension produced by different narcotic analgesics. Parenteral morphine can increase biliary pressure by 41–273% with doses of 10–15 mg (148,152,153); meperidine by 25–189% (148,152,153,155) with doses of 50–100 mg; and pentazocine by 10–114% (152,153,155) with 30–45 mg doses. Because the reported range of increased biliary pressures is so wide, it is unlikely that one narcotic has clear advantages over another in this regard. Also see chapter entitled Acute Cholecystitis.

24. *Liver Disease.* B.A. is a 54-year-old white male with alcoholic cirrhosis of the liver, severe ascites, and mild jaundice. His stools are generally benzidine positive and he occasionally has bright red blood per rectum

secondary to hemorrhoids. He was placed on oral lactulose for a flapping tremor and a decreased sensorium which developed when the protein content of his diet was increased. He is currently alert and receiving only a stool softener, spironolactone 200 mg/day, and lactulose. He develops severe right upper quadrant pain for which morphine sulfate is ordered. What must be considered when administering narcotics to this type of patient?

Morphine is metabolized in the liver and could accumulate in patients with decreased liver function. In patients with a history of hepatic encephalopathy, jaundice and ascites, or gastrointestinal bleeding complicating their liver disease, 8 mg of morphine sulfate can induce EEG changes similar to those which occur with impending hepatic encephalopathy. These changes cannot be correlated with alkalosis, hypokalemia or increased blood ammonia levels. The mechanism by which morphine induces these changes is unknown. Because morphine and other narcotic analgesics can induce hepatic coma, they are contraindicated in patients with signs of impending coma (26,157).

Meperidine is 95% metabolized, primarily through demethylation and deesterification in the liver at the rate of 10–22% per hour (158). In subjects without hepatic disease, the half-life is biphasic with a rapid alpha phase of 3.3–7.1 minutes and a slow beta phase of 3.1–3.7 hours following an IV dose (159).

In hepatic insufficiency, meperidine elimination is slowed considerably. Single IV doses of meperidine, usually 0.8 mg/kg, were given to normal subjects and patients with alcoholic cirrhosis or acute viral hepatitis in four separate studies (160–163). In each trial, the plasma clearance was reduced by 36% to 58%, and the elimination half-life was approximately doubled. Liver function tests did not correlate with plasma clearance. As hepatitis resolved, drug elimination returned to normal.

Pentazocine's clearance also is significantly influenced by hepatic disease. Plasma clearance was decreased 46% and half-life increased 72% (3.8 to 6.6 hours) in eight cirrhotic patients (162).

The bioavailability of oral narcotic analgesics also increases during active liver disease (162,163), because the metabolic first pass effect through the liver is reduced. Oral meperidine bioavailability increased 81% (162) and 40.4% (163) in two

studies of alcoholic cirrhotic patients. Pentazocine's bioavailability increased by 278% (162).

Therefore, prolonged and enhanced drug activity would be expected in patients with active liver disease. Doses should be lowered and the dosing interval expanded especially because these patients also are highly sensitive to central nervous system depressants.

25. *Respiratory Disease.* A 65-year-old man is admitted to the hospital with a broken hip. He has a history of chronic obstructive pulmonary disease and asthma. His respiratory signs include tachypnea, chronic cough, wheezing, shortness of breath, and dyspnea on exertion. His medical history includes several episodes of pneumonia. Morphine 10 mg IM is ordered to alleviate his severe hip pain. Why should morphine be used with caution in this patient? What are other alternative potent analgesics for this patient?

Morphine and all narcotic analgesics depress respiration in therapeutic doses and should be used cautiously in patients with compromised respiratory function (25,28,164). Narcotics decrease the rate of respiration, the tidal volume, and minute volume (26,59). Also, they suppress the respiratory response to increased carbon dioxide and hypoxia, which are both primary drives for ventilation in severely decompensated patients (165). Additionally, irregular and periodic breathing patterns are complications with narcotic analgesics (59). Furthermore, the involuntary cough reflex is depressed. Cough is a key factor in the expulsion of bronchial plugs which predispose patients to infections. Lastly, narcotics could precipitate bronchial constriction, theoretically, through the release of histamine.

The respiratory depression induced by other narcotic agents is comparable to that seen with equipotent doses of morphine (17,26,28,30). Preliminary anecdotal data, however, suggest that this respiratory depressive effect may plateau with the new analgesic, butorphanol (170–175). When the dose of butorphanol was increased from 2.0 mg to 4.0 mg in six normal subjects, a plateau effect was noted in the end tidal volume carbon dioxide versus minute volume curve. Butorphanol, nevertheless, has been associated with shortness of breath, dyspnea, and shallow respiration (174,175). Other preliminary data suggest that tolerance to respiratory depression may develop in patients using another new analgesic, nalbuphine (176–177). After four days of treatment with either nalbuphine or morphine, a carbon dioxide challenge equally suppressed the minute volume in both groups of patients; however, after seven days of treatment, the minute volume improved seven-fold in nalbuphine-treated patients while no improvement was noted in the morphine-treated group. This phenomenon of supposed tolerance to nalbuphine-induced respiratory depression needs considerable confirmation. Controversy concerning the respiratory depressive effects of pentazocine also arose during the early years of pentazocine use. However, now it is known that pentazocine also suppresses respirations to the same or greater extent than morphine (27,134,166,167).

Whether the respiratory depression is caused by morphine, pentazocine, butorphanol, or nalbuphine, the narcotic antagonist, naloxone, can reverse the respiratory difficulties caused by these agents. Unlike nalline or other narcotic antagonists, naloxone also will effectively antagonize pentazocine-induced respiratory depression (168,169). Mechanical ventilators usually are necessary until the narcotic's effects have waned.

Since this patient's pain is extremely severe, a low dose of any narcotic could be employed to make the pain more tolerable while closely monitoring respiratory function. If narcotic doses have to be increased to control pain, butorphanol (4 mg) and nalbuphine (15 mg) are reasonable alternatives because they may cause less respiratory depression. Another choice is methotrimeprazine, a phenothiazine with analgesic activity and less respiratory depression effects than morphine.

26. *Old Age.* J.S. is a 75-year-old man with extreme pain due to severe disabling osteoarthritis and vertebral disc degeneration. During an episode of acute back pain, an 8 mg dose of morphine produced complete relief to the surprise of the clinician. Characterize the response of older subjects to pain and to analgesics.

Aged patients experience greater relief of pain with analgesics. In a study of 712 patients receiving 10 mg of morphine or 20 mg of pentazocine, analgesia in patients over 50 years of age was superior to that experienced by younger subjects (178). In a comparative evaluation of 200 young subjects (20–30 years old) and aged patients (54–97 years old), artificial pain from a light dolorimeter resulted in significantly lower pain perception and higher reaction thresholds in the older patient sample (179). Total pain relief and duration of pain relief in 947 postoperative cancer patients was superior for older patients treated with morphine (180). Total pain relief was 37% greater for the oldest versus the youngest group. Furthermore, it has been demonstrated that older subjects achieve about two-fold higher plasma levels of meperidine after an IM or IV injection than do younger subjects (181,182). Physiological changes in the elderly, such as decreased lean body mass, lower plasma albumin, diminished renal clearance, reduced liver blood flow, and impaired metabolism (183), may account for this enhanced response to analgesics.

MILD ANALGESICS

It is commonly assumed that a 650 mg dose of *aspirin* produces maximum analgesia (68,184–186). However, there are studies which show an extension of the dose-response curve. In one study, increments of dose from 25 mg to 1800 mg increased the pain relief provided by aspirin for postpartum pain. Whether or not a significant increase in the incidence of side effects accompanied these high doses was not reported (187). Claims of superiority of one product over another on the basis of blood salicylate levels should be interpreted cautiously, because analgesic activity correlates better with blood acetylsalicylic acid levels than with blood salicylate concentrations (185,188).

In comparisons of aspirin 650 mg with other oral mild analgesics (68,184–186,189–195), codeine 60 mg, acetaminophen 650 mg, and aspirin or acetaminophen combined with propoxyphene provided comparable analgesia. Aspirin 650 mg in conjunction with 32 mg of codeine was superior to either of the components used alone.

The relative efficacy of *propoxyphene* is controversial and has been the subject of many studies. Two literature reviews of 25 double-blind propoxyphene studies concluded that 65 mg of propoxyphene was equivalent or inferior to acetaminophen 650 mg, aspirin 650 mg, or codeine 65 mg in the relief of cancer, postpartum, postoperative, or mixed painful situations (196,197).

Moertel and associates treated 57 ambulatory patients with mild to moderate cancer pain in a crossover comparison and determined that pain relief was achieved in 62% of patients receiving ASA 650 mg, 50% of patients receiving acetaminophen 650 mg, 60% of patients receiving codeine 60 mg, 43% of patients receiving propoxyphene 65 mg, and 32% of patients receiving a placebo; propoxyphene and placebo were statistically inferior to ASA (186). Acetaminophen 650 mg was superior to propoxyphene with regard to pain intensity score, relief from pain score, and global evaluation when used in the treatment of 100 women with episiotomy pain; acetaminophen was effective in 62% of the patients, whereas propoxyphene was effective in 34% (189).

The *non-steroidal anti-inflammatory drugs* provide analgesia equal to that of aspirin or acetaminophen. Pain is relieved in about 65–85% of treated patients. Post-partum episiotomy pain is controlled in about 75–85% of those treated with ibuprofen (198,199), naproxen (207), or fenoprofen (212,213). Dysmenorrheic pain is also relieved by ibuprofen (203,204) and naproxen (211). Dental pain is equally suppressed by ibuprofen (200,201), aspirin, or acetaminophen, and all of these agents are superior to propoxyphene.

Zomepirac 25–100 mg has been compared against a wide variety of analgesics (216–225). In general, successful analgesia can be achieved in about 50–80% of the patients. In situations associated with acute pain such as oral surgery (216,217), post-partum episiotomy (218), postoperative (219–222), and orthopedic pain (223), zomepirac is equal to or is superior to standard analgesics such as aspirin with codeine. In cancer pain (224) and orthopedic pain (225), zomepirac showed analgesic efficacy which was equal to or less than Percodan (aspirin plus oxycodone). Its side effects are less than those associated with aspirin, phenacetin, caffeine (APC) combinations with codeine (223).

In summary, the non-steroidal anti-inflammatory drugs are at least as effective as analgesics as acetaminophen or aspirin. Since their cost is far greater, however, their prime target population is patients intolerant to aspirin's gastric effects. Although zomepirac equals the aspirin plus codeine combination in analgesic efficacy, it has not been compared with other non-steroidal anti-inflammatory drugs.

27. *Gastrointestinal Side Effects from Aspirin.* A 43-year-old man with a history of peptic ulcer disease enters the emergency room with a chief complaint of severe upper abdominal distress and black stools. He describes a recent increase in aspirin intake of 16 tablets daily to control his severe headaches. Would buffered or enteric coated aspirin reduce the gastrointestinal adverse effects for this patient?

Aspirin has three major gastrointestinal effects which may or may not be related to one another: dyspepsia, occult blood loss, and acute gastrointestinal hemorrhage. This patient manifests the first two reactions.

Dyspepsia does not necessarily correlate with blood loss and occurs in one out of 15 patients taking aspirin, but only one out of 20 experiences this effect consistently (184). Ten to twenty percent of patients taking anti-inflammatory doses of aspirin experience dyspepsia (185). Since this effect is very likely due to local irritation from particulate ASA, ingestion of large quantities of warm water or antacids may alleviate this symptom in some patients. Both maneuvers increase the dissolution rate of the aspirin tablets.

Aspirin ingestion is associated with a 6- to 11-fold increase in daily gastrointestinal blood loss in normal subjects (226–230). When a 600 mg dose of ASA was given to normal subjects four times daily, 73% lost 5 cc of blood from the gastrointestinal tract each day, in comparison to 0.5 cc for a control group. Although there was little variation in the intraindividual daily blood loss caused by a given dose of aspirin, the variation between individuals was great; some individuals lost as much as 115 cc of blood after ingesting a similar dose of aspirin (231).

The amount of blood which is lost may be dose related. In one study, 300 mg four times daily produced an average daily blood loss of 4.6 cc, 600 mg four times daily produced an 8 cc loss, and 900 mg four times daily produced an 11.2 cc loss (231). Also, the same dose administered twice as frequently can increase the blood loss: ASA 600 mg qid produced a 4.3 cc blood loss; whereas, ASA 300 mg 8 times daily produced a 10.3 cc blood loss. The concomitant ingestion of alcohol also increases blood loss due to aspirin (232).

The amount of blood loss is apparently unrelated to the presence or absence of dyspepsia (233), a previous history of peptic ulcer disease, GI hemorrhage (234), or salicylate levels (231,235). However, in patients who are already bleeding, both aspirin and sodium salicylate can increase the amount of blood loss by 4- to 10-fold (234). Interestingly, the ingestion of aspirin with food or milk or the co-administration of corticosteroids does not alter the incidence or degree of occult blood loss (233).

The bleeding is primarily due to a local erosive effect of aspirin. Gastroscopic studies show local changes ranging from slight hyperemia to intense congestion with local hemorrhage and ulceration in as many as 100% of patients ingesting aspirin (235–238). Apparently, saturated solutions form around particles of ASA entrapped in the mucosal folds and promote cellular damage, mucosal erosion, and hemorrhage. Disruption of mucosal permeability has also been demonstrated following the gastric instillation of aspirin solution (239).

Occult blood loss can be almost eliminated by administering enteric-coated (E.C.) aspirin, but not by buffered aspirin (237,238). Submucosal hemorrhage in the stomach and duodenum was almost completely absent when E.C. aspirin 3.9 gm/day was given for 7 days, while buffered aspirin and plain aspirin caused equally large areas of abnormality (237). Chronic ingestion of E.C. aspirin over three months at anti-inflammatory doses also resulted in fewer mucosal erosions and ulcers than similar ingestion of buffered or plain aspirin (238). However, absorption of E.C. aspirin can be erratic or delayed, which is undesirable in patients seeking relief from acute pain (184,240).

Finally, acute gastrointestinal hemorrhage precipitated by aspirin is probably a phenomenon which is unrelated to its ability to cause dyspepsia or occult blood loss. Even though patients with a history of peptic ulcer disease do not necessarily exhibit more occult blood losses than the normal population, their susceptibility to massive hemorrhage precipitated by aspirin must always be considered (241,242).

28. *Platelet Effects from Aspirin.* A 35-year-old woman with hemophilia (factor VIII level of <1%) developed severe headaches and treated herself with three Anacin tablets as needed. Soon thereafter she noticed an increased frequency and severity of bruising following minor trauma. Why did this medi-cation cause bruising in this patient? What could be recommended for her headache?

The aspirin in this product inhibits platelet aggregation, depresses platelet adhesiveness, prolongs the bleeding time, and probably contributed to the easy bruisability observed by this patient.

Aspirin alters platelet function through irreversible acetylation of platelet membranes (243). This abolishes or severely delays the second wave of platelet aggregation stimulated by epinephrine, collagen or ADP; the first wave is unaltered (244–246). As little as 150 mg effectively acetylates all circulating platelets (247). The effect of a single dose is detectable for 7 days, which is the time required to turnover the platelet population.

Aspirin's effect on platelet function is reflected in a prolonged bleeding time. A two- to ten-fold increase has been observed following daily doses of 300–2925 mg of aspirin. Bleeding times remain prolonged for 4–10 days after cessation of therapy (249–251). Recent data suggest a plateau effect is seen in bleeding time with aspirin and there may even be a paradoxical reduction at high doses (251–254). For example, 1 gm and 3.9 gm doses produced increases in bleeding times of 194% vs 115%, respectively (255). However, this effect remains controversial and conflicting evidence exists (256). (The reader is referred to the chapter entitled Thrombosis for additional information on platelet function alterations.)

Individuals with bleeding disorders, such as this patient with a factor VIII deficiency, usually experience a two- to four-fold elevation in the bleeding time approximately two hours after aspirin administration (250,257). Severely hemophilic patients may exhibit an eight-fold prolongation in bleeding time following a single dose of 1000 mg of aspirin (250,258,259). Acetaminophen, propoxyphene, pentazocine, and codeine do not alter platelet function or bleeding times in hemophiliacs and can be considered for use in this patient (260–262).

29. *Hepatitis Due to Aspirin.* An 18-year-old woman with a diagnosis of rheumatoid arthritis was treated with 975 mg of aspirin four times a day with meals. Over the ensuing month, she complained of increasing nausea and abdominal tenderness. Antacids did not relieve the pain. A salicylate blood level was 33 mg/dl; a serum glutamic oxaloacetic transaminase level was 380 IU/ml; a serum pyruvic glutamic transaminase was 275 IU/ml; alkaline phosphatase was 190 IU/ml; and her bilirubin was normal. A liver biopsy showed hepatocellular swelling and necrosis. How compatible are the clinical data in this patient with aspirin-induced hepatotoxicity?

Toxic hepatitis due to aspirin primarily occurs in patients with juvenile rheumatoid arthritis (JRA) or systemic lupus erythematosus (SLE). These patients usually are receiving large anti-inflammatory doses of aspirin or have salicylate serum levels greater than 30 mg/dl. Since aspirin-induced hepatotoxicity is uncommon in patients who receive large anti-inflammatory doses of aspirin for the treatment of other connective tissue disorders, some believe that this hepatotoxicity simply may reflect a systemic manifestation of JRA or SLE. Nevertheless, eight clinical trials noted hepatic abnormalities in 25–66% of about 400 such children (254–272). Most of these children presented with only asymptomatic elevations in liver function tests, which by themselves may only implicate aspirin in the induction of transaminitis. However, six cases of severe hepatotoxicity were noted, and several cases of aspirin-induced hepatic encephalopathy have been reported in other pediatric patients (273). The seriously ill patients presented with nausea, vomiting, anorexia, and abdominal pain. Acute hepatocellular damage and necrosis were noted on liver biopsies. Discontinuation of the aspirin resulted in reversal of the hepatic abnormalities within one to two weeks, and rechallenge with aspirin resulted in a quicker and more severe reappearance of the hepatotoxicity.

This patient's symptomatology and clinical laboratory tests are compatible with aspirin-induced hepatitis. Although a definitive diagnosis cannot be made with the presented data, discontinuation of the aspirin for a few weeks is reasonable.

30. *Analgesic Nephritis.* A 68-year-old woman with a more than thirty-year history of chronic daily frontal headaches and backaches was recently admitted to the hospital for evaluation. Episodes of urinary tract infections have occurred almost twice yearly for five years. For the last six to twelve months, she suffered from malaise, weakness, and weight loss. Urinary frequency and nocturia are increasing problems. Urinalysis revealed a specific gravity of 1.010, 10–12 white blood cells and 3–5 red blood cells per high power field, and one plus albumin. Laboratory data showed a hemoglobin of 12 gm/dl, a white blood count of 9500/mm^3, SGOT of 85 IU/100 ml, a BUN of 32 mg/dl, a serum creatinine of 2.1 mg/dl, and normal electrolytes. An intravenous pyelogram indicated bilateral abnormal concentrating ability and obstruction. A drug history revealed chronic analgesic intake of about 10 tablets of aspirin, phenacetin, and caffeine per day for 20–30 years. A renal biopsy was performed, and a histologic examination showed extensive interstitial nephritis. Medullary tissue was congested with numerous inflammatory cells. Tubules were degenerating, atrophic, and scarring. How has this woman's analgesic use contributed to her kidney problem?

Analgesic abuse is a common cause of chronic interstitial nephritis (CIN) and accounts for over 100 new cases of CIN each year. Although most of these cases of CIN are caused by preparations containing aspirin and phenacetin in combination, case reports also have implicated aspirin, acetaminophen, and other oral analgesics individually (274–278). Investigators hypothesize that phenacetin and its metabolite, acetaminophen, accumulate in the renal medulla and cause oxidative breakdown of lipid cell membranes at this site. NADPH prevents this oxidative reaction and thereby protects the renal medulla. The salicylates, however, inhibit NADPH production by the hexose monophosphate shunt and, as a result, potentiate the nephritis induced by phenacetin. This hypothesis is compatible with analgesic nephropathy induced by both combination products as well as individual oral analgesics.

Analgesic-induced interstitial nephritis seems to be total-dose related, requiring a minimum cumulative dose of two to three kilograms of analgesics over a five year span. In this particular case, the patient consumed about 24.6 kg of aspirin in addition to about 17.0 kg of phenacetin over 30 years.

The prominent renal findings compatible with analgesic nephropathy include a history of urinary tract infections, abnormal urograms, papillary necrosis, pyuria, proteinuria, hematuria, azotemia, and an inability to concentrate urine. The pathology reports usually describe diffuse, particularly medullary, interstitial nephritis with lymphocytic and plasma cell infiltration; tubular basement membrane thickening; and degeneration of the collecting tubules and loops of Henle. Medullary papillae necrose, fibrose, calcify, and, eventually, slough off. The renal function generally improves when the analgesics are withdrawn; the presence of residual functional abnormalities depends on the extent of the tubular necrosis and fibrosis.

31. *Propoxyphene Overdose.* A 28-year-old woman with symptoms of lethargy following a suicide attempt with propoxyphene is brought into the emergency room by her husband. On physical examination, she presents with miosis, tachycardia (105 beats/minute), and a respiratory rate of 11/minute. What are the symptoms of propoxyphene intoxication? What is the treatment of choice?

The incidence of propoxyphene poisoning and death has increased from 2.7 deaths/million in 1969–72 to 7.7 deaths/million in 1973–1978 (284,285). This popular analgesic is a structural analog of methadone, and central nervous system depression is the predominant effect following the acute ingestion of large doses. The major manifestations of propoxyphene intoxication are lethargy, respiratory depression, miosis, tachycardia, coma, hypotension, and convulsions (279–283). A potentially lethal blood level is 0.2 mg/dl, which is about ten-fold higher than therapeutic levels (284,285).

Naloxone, a narcotic antagonist, reverses the symptoms of propoxyphene intoxication and does not produce adverse effects (280–283). The recommended dose of naloxone for this patient, as well as all narcotic overdose situations, is 0.005 mg/kg IV (165). A dose of 0.8 mg IV has induced pupillary dilatation, an increase in the respiratory rate from 2 to 20/minute, and consciousness within one minute (283). Single doses of 0.2 to 0.8 mg have similarly reversed the depression, but multiple doses are usually required to maintain the response (280–282). If a single 0.4 mg dose does not produce a rapid response, it should be repeated within minutes until reversal occurs (280,283). Up to 2.4 mg IV has been required to achieve a respiratory response; even then, subsequent doses were required within three hours to maintain consciousness (283).

32. Can an IV infusion of naloxone be utilized to treat the prolonged respiratory depression which accompanies overdoses of narcotic analgesics such as propoxyphene and methadone?

A 3.66 mcg/kg IV loading dose of naloxone followed by a constant IV infusion of 3.66 mcg/kg/hour for six hours effectively reversed the respiratory depression in seven healthy morphine treated adults (286). Likewise, naloxone infusion effectively treated a methadone overdose which occurred in a 17-year-old patient (287). In this patient, many intermittent doses of naloxone were needed over a 13-hour time period to reverse respiratory depression. Because of the recurrent relapses, naloxone (2 mg/500 ml 0.45% sodium chloride) was infused at a rate of 0.4 mg/30 minutes. A total dose of 12.4 mg was administered by infusion over a 12-hour period.

References

1. Melzack R: *The Puzzle of Pain,* New York Basic Books, Inc., New York 1, p 48.
2. Wall PD: The relation of injury to pain. Pain. 1979; 6:253.
3. Bonica JJ: The relation of injury to pain. Pain. 1979; 7:203.
4. McCaffery M: Current misconceptions about the relief of acute pain. In *Chronic Pain,* edited by B Crue, Spectrum Publications, New York, 1979, p 275.
5. Twycross RG: Pain and analgesics. Curr Med Res Opin. 1978; 5:497.
6. Snyder SH: Opiate receptors in the brain. N Engl J Med. 1977; 296:266.
7. Basbaum AI et al: Endogenous pain control mechanisms: review and hypothesis. Ann Neurol. 1978; 4:451.
8. Spector S: Opiate receptors and their clinical implications. Circ Res. 1980; 46 (Suppl. 1): I 138.
9. Verebey K et al: Endorphins in psychiatry. An overview and a hypothesis. Arch Gen Psych. 1978; 35:877.
10. Tregear GW et al: Enkephalin, endorphin, and the opiate receptor. Circ Res. 1980; 46 (Suppl. 1): I 142.
11. Duggan AW: Enkephalins as transmitters in the central nervous system. Circ Res. 1980; 46 (Suppl. 1): I 149.
12. Frohman LA: Endorphins and enkephalins: Neuroendocrine considerations. Hosp Form. 1980; 15:465.
13. Oyama T et al: Profound analgesic effects of beta-endorphin in man. Lancet. 1980; 1:122.
14. Gold MS et al: Clonidine in opiate withdrawal. Lancet. 1978; 1:929.

15. Iggo A: Peripheral and spinal "pain" mechanisms and their modulation. Adv Pain Res Ther. 1976; 1:381.

16. Beecher HK: The powerful placebo. JAMA. 1955; 159:1602.

17. Lasagna L: The clinical evaluation of morphine and its substitutes as analgesics. Pharmacol Rev. 1964; 16:47.

18. Loan WB et al: Strong analgesics: Pharmacological and therapeutic aspects. Drugs. 1973; 5:108.

19. Lutterbeck PM et al: Measurement of analgesic activity in man. Int J Clin Pharmacol. 1972; 6:315.

20. Sechzer PH: Demand method evaluation of analgesics. Curr Ther Res. 1976; 19:343.

21. Chapman CR: Measurement of pain: Problems and Issues. Adv Pain Res Ther. 1976; 1:345.

22. Melzack R: The McGill Pain Questionnaire: Major properties and scoring methods. Pain. 1975; 1:277.

23. Shimm DS et al: Medical management of chronic cancer pain. JAMA. 1979; 241:2409.

24. Twycross RG: Choice of a strong analgesic in terminal cancer: diamorphine or morphine? Pain. 1977; 3:93.

25. Twycross RG: Overview of analgesia. Adv Pain Res Ther. 1979; 2:617.

26. Jaffe HF et al: Narcotic analgesics and antagonists. In The Pharmacological Basis of Therapeutics, 6th Ed, edited by A Gilman et al, MacMillan Co., 1980; p 535, 569.

27. Houde RW: Analgesic effectiveness of the narcotic agonist-antagonists. Br J Clin Pharmacol. 1979; 7:297S.

28. Beaver WT: The pharmacologic basis for the choice of an analgesic. 1. Potent analgesics. Pharmacol Phys. 1970; 4:1.

29. Catalano RB: The medical approach to management of pain caused by cancer. Sem Oncol. 1975; 2:379.

30. Halpern LM et al: "Analgesics." In Drugs of Choice 1980–1981, edited by W Modell, CV Mosby Co, St. Louis, 1980, p 199.

31. Lewis JR: Evaluation of new analgesics butorphanol and nalbuphine. JAMA. 1980; 243:1465.

32. Vandam LD: Butorphanol. N Engl J Med. 1980; 302:381.

33. Foley KM: Pain. Syndromes in patients with cancer. Adv Pain Res Ther. 1979; 2:591.

34. Melzack R: The Puzzle of Pain, New York Basic Books, Inc, New York, 1973, p 142.

35. Lipman AG: Drug therapy in terminally ill patients. Am J Hosp Pharm. 1975; 32:270.

36. Chapman CR: Psychologic and behavioral aspects of cancer pain. Adv Pain Res Ther. 1979; 2:45.

37. Bonica JJ: Introduction to management of pain of advanced cancer. Adv Pain Res Ther. 1979; 2:115.

38. Saunder C: The nature and management of terminal pain and the hospice concept. Adv Pain Res Ther. 1979; 2:635.

39. Ford G: Terminal care from the viewpoint of the national health service. Adv Pain Res Ther. 1979; 2:653.

40. Mount BM et al: Use of the Brompton mixture in treating the chronic pain of malignant disease. Can Med Assoc J. 1976; 115:122.

41. Keeri-Szanto M: Drugs or Drums. What relieves postoperative pain? Pain. 1979; 6:217.

42. Wade A: Martindale: The Extra Pharmacopoeia, The Pharmaceutical Press, London, 1977, p 973.

43. Weintraub M: Potentiation of narcotic analgesics with central stimulant; The use of modified Brompton's mix-

ture. Clinical Pharmacology Reports, 1976; 5:9. A publication of the Univ. of Rochester, Dept. of Pharmacology and Toxicology.

44. Davis AJ: Brompton's cocktail: Making goodbyes possible. Am J Nurs. 1978; 78:611.

45. Way EL et al: The biological disposition of morphine and its surrogates—1. Bull WHO. 1961; 25:227.

46. Melzack R et al: The Brompton mixture: Effects on pain in cancer patients. Can Med Assoc J. 1976; 155:125.

47. Twycross RG: Clinical experience with diamorphine in advanced malignant disease. Int J Clin Pharmacol. 1974; 9:184.

48. Twycross RG et al: Euphoriant mixtures. Br Med J. 1973; 4:552.

49. Melzack R et al: The Brompton solution versus morphine solution given orally: effects on pain. Can Med Assoc J. 1979; 120:435.

50. Twycross RG: The Brompton Cocktail. Adv Pain Res Ther. 1979; 2:291.

51. Twycross RG et al: Long-term use of morphine in advanced cancer. Adv Pain Res Ther. 1976; 1:653.

52. Twycross RG: Clinical experience with diamorphine in advanced malignant disease. Int J Clin Pharmacol. 1974; 9:184.

53. Twycross RG et al: Relief of pain. In The Management of Terminal Disease, edited by CM Saunder et al, Year Book Med., London, 1978, p 65.

54. Forrest Jr WH et al: Dextroamphetamine with morphine for the treatment of postoperative pain. N Engl J Med. 1977; 296:712.

55. Webb SS et al: Toward the development of a potent, nonsedating, oral analgesic. Psychopharmacol. 1978; 60:25.

56. Miser AW et al: Continuous intravenous infusion of morphine sulfate for control of severe pain in children with terminal malignancy. J Pediatr. 1980; 96:930.

57. Bryan-Brown CW et al: Decremental morphine infusion for postoperative pain. Crit Care Med. 1980; 8:233.

58. Church JJ: Continuous narcotic infusions for relief of postoperative pain. Br Med J. 1979; 1:977.

59. Anonymous: Narcotic analgesics—II. Adverse effects. Br Med J. 1970; 2:587.

60. Gutner LB et al: The effects of potent analgesics upon vestibular function. J Clin Invest. 1952; 31:259.

61. Twycross RG: Bone pain in advanced cancer. In Topics in Therapeutics, Vol 4, edited by DW Vere et al, Turnbridge Wells, 1978, p 94.

62. Gerbershagen HV: Non-narcotic analgesics. Adv Pain Res Ther. 1979; 2:255.

63. Moncada S et al: Interaction between anti-inflammatory drugs and inflammatory mediators: a reference to products of arachidonic acid metabolism. Agents Actions. 1977; (Suppl. 3): 141.

64. Säwe J: Patient-controlled dose regimen of methadone for chronic cancer pain. Br Med J. 1981; 1:771.

65. Verbely K et al: Methadone in man: Pharmacokinetic and excretion studies in acute 2nd chronic treatments. Clin Pharmacol Ther. 1975; 18:180.

66. Olsen GD: Methadone binding to human plasma proteins. Clin Pharmacol Ther. 1973; 14:338.

67. Ettinger DS et al: Important clinical pharmacologic considerations in the use of methadone in cancer patients. Can Treat Rep. 1979; 63:457.

68. Moertel CG et al: Relief of pain by oral medications. JAMA. 1974; 229:55.

69. Mather LE et al: Meperidine kinetics in man. Intravenous injection in surgical patients and volunteers. Clin Pharmacol Ther. 1975; 17:21.

70. Stambaugh JE et al: The clinical pharmacology of meperidine—comparison of routes of administration. J Clin Pharmacol. 1976; 16:245.

71. Szeto HH et al: Accumulation of nonmeperidine, an active metabolite of meperidine, in patients with renal failure or cancer. Ann Intern Med. 1977; 86:738.

72. Reidenberg MM: A metabolite of meperidine that accumulates and causes central nervous system irritability. Hosp Pharm. 1978; 13:339.

73. Doenicke A et al: Histamine liberation and anaphylactic reactions after I.V. narcotics. Anaesthesist. 1970; 19:413.

74. Cromwell TA et al: Hypersensitivity to intravenous morphine sulfate. Plast Recon Surg. 1974; 54:224.

75. Voorhorst R et al: Four cases of recurrent pseudo-scarlet fever caused by phenanthrene alkaloids with a 6-hydroxy group (codeine and morphine). Ann Allergy. 1980; 44:116.

76. Marks RM et al: Undertreatment of medical inpatients with narcotic analgesics. Ann Intern Med. 1973; 78:173.

77. Cohen FL: Postsurgical pain relief: patients' status and nurses' medication choices. Pain. 1980; 9:265.

78. Porter J et al: Addiction rate in patients treated with narcotics. N Engl J Med. 1980; 302:123.

79. Saunders C: Control of pain in terminal cancer. Nursing Times. 1976; 72:1134.

80. Himmelsbach CK: Studies of the addiction liability of Demerol. J Pharmacol Exper Ther. 1942; 75:64.

81. Himmelsbach DK: Further studies of the addiction liability of Demerol. J Pharmacol Exper Ther. 1943; 79:5.

82. Wiedner H: Addiction to meperidine hydrochloride. JAMA. 1946; 132:1066.

83. Noth PH et al: Demerol: A new synthetic analgetic spasmolytic and sedative agent 1. Clinical observations. Ann Intern Med. 1944; 21:17.

84. Parkhouse J et al: *Analgesic Drugs,* Blackwell Scientific Publications, London, 1979, p 24.

85. Becker CE et al: Alcohol and Drug Abuse. In *Clinical Pharmacology: Basic Principles in Therapeutics,* edited by KK Melmon et al, MacMillan Publ Co., N.Y., 1978, p 1015.

86. Benedict EB: Morphine in myxedema. JAMA. 1930; 94:1916.

87. Mount BM: Narcotic analgesics in the treatment of pain of advanced malignant disease. In *The RVH Manual on Palliative/Hospice Care,* edited by I Ajemian et al, Arno Press, New York, 1980, p 148.

88. Dundee JW et al: Alterations in response to somatic pain associated with anaesthesia. XV. Further studies with phenothiazine derivatives and similar drugs. Br J Anaesth. 1963; 35:597.

89. McGee JL et al: Phenothiazine analgesia—fact or fantasy? Am J Hosp Pharm. 1979; 36:633.

90. Beaver WT et al: A comparison of the analgesic effects of methotrimeprazine and morphine in patients with cancer. Clin Pharmacol Ther. 1966; 7:436.

91. Helrich M et al: Circulatory response to tilting following methotrimeprazine and morphine in man. Anesthesiology. 1964; 25:662.

92. Pearson JW et al: Effect of methotrimeprazine in respiration. Anesthesiology. 1963; 24:38.

93. Ayd FJ: A survey of drug-induced extrapyramidal reactions. JAMA. 1961; 175:1054.

94. Lambersten CJ et al: The separate and combined respiratory effects of chlorpromazine and meperidine in normal men controlled at 46 mm Hg alveolar pCO_2. J Pharm Exper Ther. 1961; 131:381.

95. Houde RW et al: Analgetic power of chlorpromazine alone and in combination with morphine. Fed Proc. 1955; 14:353.

96. Alexander JI et al: Central nervous system effects of pentazocine. Br Med J. 1974; 2:224.

97. Bellville JW et al: Evaluating side effects of analgesics in a cooperative clinical study. Clin Pharmacol Ther. 1968; 9:303.

98. Hansbrough ET: Hallucinations following pentazocine. Missouri Med. 1970; 67:602.

99. Hemphill RE: Hallucinations from pentazocine. S Afr Med J. 1973; 47:1984.

100. Kane FR et al: Mental and emotional disturbance with pentazocine use. Southern Med J. 1975; 68:808.

101. Taylor M et al: Psychotomimetic effects of pentazocine and dihydrocodeine tartrate. Br Med J. 1978; 2:1198.

102. Elliott JP et al: Butorphanol and meperidine compared with acute ureteral colic. J Urol. 1979; 122:455.

103. Pearson JW: Analgesia for obstetric and gynecologic patients. Mod Treat. 1968; 5:1164.

104. Ricciarelli EAM et al: Opioids and obstetrics. Clin Obstet Gynecol. 1974; 17:259.

105. Steel GC: Obstetric analgesia. Int Anesth Clin. 1973; 11:75.

106. Morrison JC et al: Metabolites of meperidine in the fetal and maternal serum. Am J Obstet Gynecol. 1976; 126:997.

107. Nation RL: Drug kinetics in childbirth. Clin Pharmacokinetics. 1980; 5:340.

108. DeVoe SJ et al: Effects of meperidine on uterine contractility. Am J Obstet Gynecol. 1969; 105:1004.

109. Riffel HD et al: Effects of meperidine and promethazine during labor. Obstet Gynecol. 1973; 42:738.

110. Sliom CM: Analgesia during labor: A comparison between dihydrocodeine and pethidine. S Afr Med J. 1970; 44:317.

111. Levy DL: Obstetric analgesia. Pentazocine and meperidine in normal primiparous labor. Obstet Gynecol. 1971; 38:907.

112. Mowat J et al: Comparison of pentazocine and pethidine in labour. Br Med J. 1970; 2:757.

113. Refstad SO et al: Ventilatory depressions of the newborn of women receiving pethidine or pentazocine. Br J Anaesth. 1980; 52:265.

114. Maduska AL et al: A double-blind comparison of butorphanol and meperidine in labour: Maternal pain relief and effect on the newborn. Can Anaesth Soc J. 1978; 25:398.

115. Hodgkinson R et al: Double-blind comparison of the neurobehavior of neonates following the administration of different doses of meperidine to the mother. Can Anaesth Soc J. 1978; 25:405.

116. Weiner PC: Effects of naloxone on pethidine-induced neonatal depression. Part II—Intramuscular naloxone. Br Med J. 1977; 2:229.

117. Grossman JA et al: A clinical trial of pentazocine an-
     algesia in acute myocardial infarction and acute coro-
     nary insufficiency. Curr Ther Res. 1971; 13:505.
118. Jewitt DE et al: Increased pulmonary arterial pres-
     sures after pentazocine in myocardial infarction. Br Med
     J. 1970; 1:795.
119. Jewitt DE et al: Cardiovascular effects of pentazocine
     in patients with acute myocardial infarction. Br Heart
     J. 1971; 33:145.
120. Miller HC et al: Effect of pentazocine on pulmonary
     circulation. Lancet. 1972; 2:1167.
121. Scott ME et al: Circulatory effects of IV pentazocine in
     patients with acute myocardial infarction. Curr Ther
     Res. 1971; 13:81.
122. Lee G et al: Comparative effects of morphine, meperi-
     dine and pentazocine on circulatory dynamics in pa-
     tients with acute myocardial infarction. Am J Med. 1976;
     60:949.
123. Alderman EL et al: Hemodynamic effects of morphine
     and pentazocine differ in cardiac patients. N Engl J
     Med. 1972; 287:623.
124. Popio KA et al: Hemodynamic and respiratory effects
     of morphine and butorphanol. Clin Pharmacol Ther.
     1973; 23:281.
125. Scott ME et al: Effects of diamorphine, methadone,
     morphine and pentazocine in patients with suspected
     acute myocardial infarction. Lancet. 1969; 1:1065.
126. Timmis AD et al: Haemodynamic effects of intravenous
     morphine in patients with acute myocardial infarction
     complicated by severe left ventricular failure. Br Med
     J. 1980; 1:980.
127. Ryan WF et al: Effects of morphine on left ventricular
     dimensions and function in patients with previous my-
     ocardial infarction. Clin Cardiol. 1979; 2:417.
128. Gould L et al: Hemodynamic effects of morphine in car-
     diac disease. J Clin Pharmacol. 1978; 18:448.
129. Grendahl H et al: The effect of morphine on blood pres-
     sure and cardiac output in patients with acute myocar-
     dial infarction. Acta Med Scand. 1969; 186:515.
130. Alderman EL: Analgesics in the acute phase of my-
     ocardial infarction. JAMA. 1974; 229:1646.
131. Kerr F et al: Analgesic in myocardial infarction. Br
     Heart J. 1974; 36:117.
132. Keats AS: Effect of nalorphine and morphine on the
     cerebral spinal fluid pressure in man (Abstract 1228).
     Fed Proc. 1954; 13:374.
133. Beaver WT et al: A comparison of the analgesic effects
     of pentazocine and morphine in patients with cancer.
     Clin Pharmacol Ther. 1966; 7:740.
134. Martin WR: Opioid antagonists. Pharmacol Rev. 1967;
     19:463.
135. Keats AS et al: "Potentiation" of meperidine by pro-
     methazine. Anesthesiology. 1961; 22:34.
136. McQuitty FM: Relief of pain in labour. J Obstet Gy-
     naecol Br Commonw. 1967; 74:925.
137. Washton AM et al: Clonidine for outpatient opiate de-
     toxification. Lancet. 1980; 17:1078.
138. Gold MS et al: Effect of methadone dosage on clonidine
     detoxification efficacy. Am J Psychiatry. 1980; 137:375.
139. Gold MS et al: Opiate withdrawal using clonidine. JAMA.
     1980; 243:343.
140. Gold MS et al: Noradrenergic hyperactivity in opiate
     withdrawal supported by clonidine reversal of opiate
     withdrawal. Am J Psychiatry 1979; 136:100.

141. Kocher R: The use of psychotropic drugs in the treat-
     ment of chronic, severe pains. Eur Neurol. 1976; 14:458.
142. Adler RH: Psychotropic agents in the management of
     chronic pain. J Human Stress. 1978; 4:13.
143. Budd K: Psychotropic drugs in the treatment of chronic
     pain. Anaesthesia. 1978; 33:531.
144. Merskey H et al: The treatment of chronic pain with
     psychoactive drugs. Postgrad Med J. 1972; 58:594.
145. Ward NG et al: The effectiveness of tricyclic antide-
     pressants in the treatment of coexisting pain and
     depression. Pain. 1979; 7:331.
146. Morland TJ et al: Doxepin in the prophylactic treat-
     ment of mixed 'vascular' and tension headache. Head-
     ache. 1979; 19:382.
147. Lang DW et al: Naloxone reversal of morphine-induced
     biliary colic. Anesth Analg. 1980; 59:617.
148. Gaensler EA et al: A comparative study of the action
     of demerol and opium alkaloids in relation to biliary
     spasm. Surgery. 1948; 23:211.
149. McCammon RL et al: Naloxone reversal of choledo-
     choduodenal sphincter spasm associated with narcotic
     administration. Anesthesiology. 1978; 48:437.
150. Chessick KC et al: Spasm and operative cholangiog-
     raphy. Arch Surg. 1975; 110:53.
151. Nossell HL: The effect of morphine on the serum and
     urine amylase and the sphincter of Oddi. Gastroenter-
     ology. 1955; 29:409.
152. Economou G et al: A cross-over comparison of the effect
     of morphine, pethidine, pentazocine, and phenazocine
     on biliary pressure. Gut. 1971; 12:218.
153. Radnay PA et al: The effect of equi-analgesic doses of
     fentanyl, morphine, meperidine and pentazocine on
     common bile duct pressure. Anaesthesist. 1980; 29:26.
154. Hopton DS et al: Action of various new analgesic drugs
     on the human common bile duct. Gut. 1967; 8:296.
155. Greenstein AJ et al: A comparative study of pentazo-
     cine and meperidine on the biliary passage pressure.
     Am J Gastroenterol. 1972; 58:417.
156. Danhof IE: Pentazocine effect on gastrointestinal motor
     function in man. Am J Gastroenterol. 1967; 48:295.
157. Jackson GL et al: Analgesic properties of mixtures of
     chlorpromazine with morphine and meperidine. Ann
     Intern Med. 1956; 45:640.
158. Burns JJ et al: The physiological disposition and fate
     of meperidine in man and a method for its estimation
     in plasma. J Pharmacol Exper Ther. 1955; 114:289.
159. Mather LE et al: Meperidine kinetics in man. Intra-
     venous injection in surgical patients and volunteers.
     Clin Pharmacol Ther. 1975; 17:21.
160. Klotz U et al: The effect of cirrhosis on the disposition
     and elimination of meperidine in man. Clin Pharmacol
     Ther. 1974; 16:667.
161. McHorse TS et al: Effect of acute viral hepatitis in man
     on the disposition and elimination of meperidine. Gas-
     troenterology. 1975; 68:775.
162. Neal EA et al: Enhanced bioavailability and decreased
     clearance of analgesics in patients with cirrhosis. Gas-
     troenterology. 1979; 77:96.
163. Pond SM et al: Bioavailability and clearance of meper-
     idine in patients with chronic liver disease. Clin Phar-
     macol Ther. 1979; 25:242.
164. Weil JV et al: Diminished ventilatory response to hy-
     poxia and hypercapnia after morphine in normal man.
     N Engl J Med. 1975; 292:1103.

165. Driesbach RH: *Handbook of Poisoning,* 10th Ed, Lange Medical Publications, Los Altos, Ca. 1980, p 320.

166. Keats AS et al: Studies of analgesic drugs. VIII. A narcotic antagonist analgesic without psychotomimetic effects. J Pharmacol Exper Ther. 1964; 143:157.

167. Keats AS et al: Respiratory effects of narcotic antagonists. J Pharmacol Exper Ther. 1966; 151:126.

168. Kallos T et al: Naloxone reversal of pentazocine-induced respiratory depression (letter). JAMA. 1968; 204:932.

169. Telford J et al: Narcotic and narcotic antagonist mixtures (review). Anesthesiology. 1961; 22:465.

170. Nagashima H et al: Respiratory and circulatory effects of intravenous butorphanol and morphine. Clin Pharmacol Ther. 1976; 19:738.

171. Popio KA et al: Hemodynamic and respiratory effects of morphine and butorphanol. Clin Pharmacol Ther. 1978; 23:281.

172. Kalman T et al: Respiratory effects of butorphanol. Clin Pharmacol Ther. 1977; 21:107.

173. Kallos T et al: Respiratory effects of butorphanol and pethidine. Anaesthesia. 1979; 34:633.

174. Lippmann M et al: Analgesic onset time of intravenous butorphanol in postsurgical patients: a placebo-controlled study. Curr Ther Res. 1977; 22:276.

175. Kliman A et al: Clinical experience with intramuscular butorphanol for the treatment of chronic pain syndromes. Curr Ther Res. 1977; 22:105.

176. Elliott HW et al: A double-blind controlled study of the pharmacological effects of nalbuphine (EN-2234A). J Med. 1970; 1:74.

177. Fragen RJ et al: Acute intravenous premedication with nalbuphine. Anesth Analg. 1977; 56:808.

178. Belleville JW et al: Influence of age on pain relief from analgesics. JAMA. 1971; 217:1835.

179. Sherman ED et al: Sensitivity to pain in the aged. Can Med Assoc J. 1960; 83:944.

180. Kaiko RF: Age and morphine analgesia in cancer patients with postoperative pain. Clin Pharmacol Ther. 1980; 23:823.

181. Chan K et al: The effect of ageing on plasma pethidine concentration. Br J Clin Pharmacol. 1975; 2:297.

182. Berkowitz BA et al: The disposition of morphine in surgical patients. Clin Pharmacol Ther. 1975; 17:629.

183. Vestal RE: Drug use in the elderly: A review of problems and special considerations. Drugs. 1978; 16:358.

184. Beaver WT: Mild analgesics: A review of their clinical pharmacology, part I. Am J Med Sci. 1965; 250:577.

185. Beaver WT: Mild analgesics: A review of their clinical pharmacology, part II. Am J Med Sci. 1966; 251:576.

186. Moertel CG et al: A comparative evaluation of marketed analgesic drugs. N Engl J Med. 1972; 286:813.

187. Parkhouse J et al: The clinical dose response to aspirin. Br J Anaesthesiol. 1968; 40:433.

188. Hicklin JA: Relationship of plasma salicylate levels to pain relief with two different salicylates. Curr Med Res Opin. 1978; 5:572.

189. Hopkinson III JA et al: Acetaminophen versus propoxyphene hydrochloride for relief of pain in episiotomy patients. J Clin Pharmacol. 1973; 13:251.

190. Koch-Weser J: Acetaminophen. N Engl J Med. 1976; 295:1297.

191. Miller RR: Propoxyphene: A review. Am J Hosp Pharm. 1977; 34:413.

192. Hollister LE: Effective use of analgesic drugs. Ann Rev Med. 1977; 27:431.

193. Messick RT: Evaluation of acetaminophen, propoxyphene, and their combination in office practice. J Clin Pharmacol. 1979; 19:227.

194. Cooper SA: Comparative analgesic efficacies of aspirin and acetaminophen. Arch Intern Med. 1981; 141:282.

195. Beaver WT: Aspirin and acetaminophen as constituents of analgesic combinations. Arch Intern Med. 1981; 141:293.

196. Miller RR et al: Propoxyphene hydrochloride: A critical review. JAMA. 1970; 213:996.

197. O'Brien JR: Effects of salicylates on human platelets. Lancet. 1968; 1:779.

198. Hopkinson JH III: Ibuprofen versus propoxyphene hydrochloride and placebo in the relief of postepisiotomy pain. Curr Ther Res. 1980; 27:55.

199. Bloomfield SS et al: Comparative efficacy of ibuprofen and aspirin in episiotomy pain. Clin Pharmacol Ther. 1974; 15:565.

200. Iles JD: Relief of postoperative pain by ibuprofen: A report of two studies. Can J Surg. 1980; 23:288.

201. Dionne RA et al: Evaluation of preoperative ibuprofen for postoperative pain after removal of third molars. Oral Surg. 1978; 45:851.

202. Rondeau PL et al: Dental surgery pain analgesic. Can Dent Assoc J. 1980; 46:433.

203. Morrison JC et al: Analgesic efficacy of ibuprofen for treatment of primary dysmenorrhea. Southern Med J. 1980; 73:999.

204. Larkin RM et al: Dysmenorrhea: treatment with an antiprostaglandin. Obstet Gynecol. 1979; 54:456.

205. Stetson JB et al: Analgesic activity of oral naproxen in patients with postoperative pain. Scand J Rheum. 1973; 2 (Suppl 2):50.

206. Mahler DL et al: Assay of aspirin and naproxen analgesia. Clin Pharmacol Ther. 1976; 19:18.

207. Bloomfield SS et al: Naproxen, aspirin, and codeine in postpartum uterine pain. Clin Pharmacol Ther. 1977; 21:414.

208. Filtzer HS: A double-blind randomized comparison of naproxen sodium, acetaminophen and pentazocine in postoperative pain. Curr Ther Res. 1980; 27:293.

209. Ruedy J et al: A comparison of the analgesic efficacy of naproxen and propoxyphene in patients with pain after orthopedic surgery. Scand J Rheum. 1973; 2 (Suppl 2):56.

210. Ruedy J: A comparison of the analgesic efficacy of naproxen and acetylsalicylic acid-codeine in patients with pain after dental surgery. Scand J Rheum. 1973; 2 (Suppl 2):60.

211. Hamann GO: Severe, primary dysmenorrhea treated with naproxen. A prospective, double-blind, crossover investigation. Prostaglandins. 1980; 19:651.

212. Gruber CM: Evaluating interactions between fenoprofen and propoxyphene: analgesia and adverse reports by postepisiotomy patients. J Clin Pharmacol. 1976; 16:407.

213. Sechzer PH: Evaluation of fenoprofen as a postoperative analgesic. Curr Ther Res. 1977; 21:137.

214. Davie IT et al: Comparative assessment of fenoprofen and paracetamol given in combination for pain after surgery. Br J Anaesth. 1978; 50:931.

215. Sunshine A et al: A comparative analgesic study of propoxyphene, fenoprofen, the combination of propoxy-

phene and fenoprofen, aspirin, and placebo. J Clin Pharmacol. 1978; 18:556.

216. Cooper SA: Efficacy of zomepirac in oral surgical pain. J Clin Pharmacol. 1980; 20:230.

217. Mehlisch DR et al: Clinical comparison of zomepirac with APC/codeine combination in the treatment of pain following oral surgery. J Clin Pharmacol. 1980; 20:271.

218. Messer RH et al: Clinical evaluation of zomepirac and APC with codeine in the treatment of postpartum episiotomy pain. J Clin Pharmacol. 1980; 20:279.

219. Baird WM et al: Comparison of zomepirac, APC with codeine, codeine and placebo in the treatment of moderate and severe postoperative pain. J Clin Pharmacol. 1980; 20:243.

220. DeAndrade JR et al: Clinical comparison of zomepirac with pentazocine in the treatment of postoperative pain. J Clin Pharmacol. 1980; 20:293.

221. Wallenstein SL et al: Relative analgesic potency of oral zomepirac and intramuscular morphine in cancer patients with postoperative pain. J Clin Pharmacol. 1980; 20:250.

222. Forrest WH: Oral zomepirac and intramuscular morphine in postoperative pain. J Clin Pharmacol. 1980; 20:259.

223. Mayer TG et al: Clinical evaluation of zomepirac in the treatment of acute orthopedic pain. J Clin Pharmacol. 1980; 20:285.

224. Stambaugh JE et al: Double-blind comparisons of zomepirac and oxycodone with APC in cancer pain. J Clin Pharmacol. 1980; 20:261.

225. McMillen JI et al: Treatment of chronic orthopedic pain with zomepirac. J Clin Pharmacol. 1980; 20:385.

226. Beirne JA et al: Gastrointestinal blood loss caused by tolmetin, aspirin, and indomethacin. Clin Pharmacol Ther. 1974; 16:821.

227. Leonards JR et al: Effect of pharmaceutical formulation on gastrointestinal bleeding from aspirin tablets. Arch Intern Med. 1972; 129:457.

228. Leonards JR et al: Gastrointestinal blood loss from aspirin and sodium salicylate tablets in man. Clin Pharmacol Ther. 1973; 14:62.

229. Leonards JR et al: Gastrointestinal blood loss during prolonged aspirin administration. N Engl J Med. 1973; 289:1020.

230. Silverstein FE et al: Upper gastrointestinal tract bleeding. Arch Intern Med. 1981; 141:322.

231. Pierson RN et al: Aspirin and GI bleeding, chromate blood loss studies. Am J Med. 1961; 31:259.

232. Goulston K et al: Alcohol, aspirin and GI bleeding. Br Med J. 1968; 4:664.

233. Scott JT et al: Studies of GI bleeding caused by corticosteroids, salicylates, and other analgesics. Quart J Med. 1961; 30:167.

234. Grossman MI et al: Fecal blood loss produced by oral and IV administration of various salicylates. Gastroenterology. 1961; 40:383.

235. Holt PR: Measurement of GI blood loss in subjects taking aspirin. J Lab Clin Med. 1960; 56:717.

236. Hahn KJ et al: Morphology of gastrointestinal effects of aspirin. Clin Pharmacol Ther. 1975; 17:330.

237. Lanza FL et al: Endoscopic evaluation of the effects of aspirin, buffered aspirin, and enteric coated aspirin on gastric and duodenal mucosa. N Engl J Med. 1980; 303:136.

238. Silvoso GR et al: Incidence of gastric lesions in patients with rheumatic disease on chronic aspirin therapy. Ann Intern Med. 1979; 91:517.

239. Smith BM et al: Permeability of the human gastric mucosa. Alteration by acetylsalicylic acid and ethanol. N Engl J Med. 1971; 285:716.

240. Canada AT et al: The bioavailability of enteric-coated acetylsalicylic acid: a comparative study in rheumatoid arthritis, part I. Curr Ther Res. 1975; 18:727.

241. Shambaugh Jr GE: Gastric bleeding and aspirin. JAMA. 1971; 218:1573.

242. Jick H: Effects of aspirin and acetaminophen in gastrointestinal hemorrhage. Arch Intern Med. 1981; 141:316.

243. Mielke Jr CH: Comparative effects of aspirin on hemostasis. Arch Intern Med. 1981; 141:305.

244. Sutor AH et al: Effect of aspirin, sodium salicylate and acetaminophen on bleeding. Mayo Clin Proc. 1971; 46:178.

245. Mielke Jr CH et al: Aspirin as an antiplatelet agent: Template bleeding time as a monitor of therapy. Am J Clin Path. 1973; 59:236.

246. Piccioretti MJ et al: Effects of aspirin on platelet aggregation as a function of dosage and time. Clin Pharmacol Ther. 1980; 27:803.

247. Masotti G et al: Differential inhibition of prostacyclin production and platelet aggregation by aspirin. Lancet. 1979; 2:1213.

248. Stuart RK: Platelet function studies in human being receiving 300 mg of aspirin per day. J Lab Clin Med. 1970; 75:463.

249. Hirsh J et al: Relation between bleeding time and platelet connective tissue reaction after aspirin. Blood. 1973; 41:369.

250. Kaneshiro MM et al: Bleeding time after aspirin in disorders of intrinsic clotting. N Engl J Med. 1969; 281:1039.

251. Treacher D et al: Aspirin and bleeding-time. Lancet. 1978; 2:1378.

252. O'Grady J et al: Aspirin: a paradoxical effect on bleeding-time. Lancet. 1978; 1:780.

253. Rajah SM et al: Aspirin and bleeding-time. Lancet. 1978; 2:1104.

254. Jorgensen KA et al: Aspirin and bleeding-time: dependency of age. Lancet. 1979; 2:302.

255. Godal HC et al: Aspirin and bleeding-time. Lancet. 1979; 1:1236.

256. Praga C et al: Effect of aspirin on platelet aggregation and bleeding-time in haemophilia and Von Willibrand's disease. Acta Med Scand. (Suppl) 1971; 525:219.

257. Quick AJ: Salicylates and bleeding: The aspirin tolerance test. Am J Med Sci. 1966; 252:265.

258. Quick AJ: Acetylsalicylic acid as a diagnostic aid in hemostasis. Am J Med Sci. 1967; 254:392.

259. Binder RA et al: Treatment of pain in hemophilia. Am J Dis Child. 1974; 127:371.

260. Kasper CK et al: Bleeding times and platelet aggregation after analgesics in hemophilia. Ann Intern Med. 1972; 77:189.

261. Mielke Jr CH et al: Use of aspirin or acetaminophen in haemophilia. N Engl J Med. 1970; 282:1270.

262. Kanada SA et al: Aspirin hepatotoxicity. Am J Hosp Pharm. 1978; 35:330.

263. Schaller JG: Chronic salicylate administration in juvenile rheumatoid arthritis: aspirin "hepatitis" and its clinical significance. Pediatrics. 1978; 62 (Suppl):916.

264. Zimmerman HJ: Effects of aspirin and acetaminophen on the liver. Arch Intern Med. 1981; 141:333.

265. Manso C et al: Effect of aspirin administration on serum glutamic oxaloacetic and glutamic pyruvic transaminases in children. Proc Soc Exp Biol Med. 1956; 93:84.

266. Russell AS et al: Serum transaminases during salicylate therapy. Br Med J. 1971; 2:428.

267. Iancu T: Serum transaminases and salicylate therapy. Br Med J. 1972; 2:167.

268. Rich RR et al: Salicylate hepatotoxicity in patients with juvenile rheumatoid arthritis. Arthritis Rheum. 1973; 16:1.

269. Athreya BH et al: Aspirin-induced hepatotoxicity in juvenile rheumatoid arthritis. Arthritis Rheum. 1975; 18:347.

270. Miller JJ et al: Correlations between transaminase concentrations and serum salicylate concentrations in juvenile rheumatoid arthritis. Arthritis Rheum. 1976; 19:115.

271. Rachelefsky GS et al: Serum enzyme abnormalities in juvenile rheumatoid arthritis. Pediatrics. 1976; 58:730.

272. Bernstein BH et al: Aspirin-induced hepatotoxicity and its effect on juvenile rheumatoid arthritis. Am J Dis Child. 1977; 131:659.

273. Ulshen MH et al: Hepatotoxicity with encephalopathy associated with aspirin therapy in rheumatoid arthritis. J Pediatr. 1978; 93:1034.

274. Murray T et al: Analgesic abuse and renal disease. Ann Rev Med. 1975; 26:537.

275. Dubach UC: Nephropathies due to analgesics. Contrib Nephrol. 1978; 10:30.

276. Shelley JH: Pharmacological mechanisms of analgesic nephropathy. Kidney Int. 1978; 13:15.

277. Murray TG et al: Analgesic-associated nephropathy in the USA: epidemiologic, clinical and pathogenetic features. Kidney Int. 1978; 13:64.

278. Schreiner GE et al: Clinical analgesic nephropathy. Arch Intern Med. 1981; 141:349.

279. Young DJ: Propoxyphene suicides. Report of nine cases. Arch Intern Med. 1972; 129:62.

280. Kersh ES: Treatment of propoxyphene overdosage with naloxone. Chest. 1973; 63:112.

281. Lovejoy FH et al: The management of propoxyphene poisoning. J Pediatr. 1974; 85:98.

282. Tarala R et al: Treatment of dextropropoxyphene poisoning. Br Med J. 1973; 2:550.

283. Vlasses PH et al: Naloxone for propoxyphene overdosage. JAMA. 1974; 229:1167.

Chapter 5

Fever

— Louis C. Littlefield —

NORMAL THERMOREGULATORY MECHANISMS

Under normal conditions body temperature is controlled about a specific "set-point" temperature by neuronal regulatory mechanisms within the hypothalamus and is the summation of heat production and heat dissipation. The preoptic area and adjacent regions of the anterior hypothalamus contain heat sensitive receptors and neurons which are capable of altering physiologic processes to increase heat loss and decrease heat production in response to hyperthermia. In contrast, when cold receptors in the posterior hypothalamus are stimulated, signals are transmitted to the hypothalamic temperature control center to increase heat production and decrease heat dissipation (1).

Although the terms fever and hyperthermia have been used interchangeably in the past, recently they have been differentiated into distinct pathophysiologic entities (2). *Fever* is defined as an elevated thermoregulatory set-point to which physiologic processes are altered to increase body temperature. *Hyperthermia* describes a condition whereby the patient's thermoregulatory set-point may be normal but abnormal physiologic processes exist to produce an elevated body temperature.

Pathophysiology

Fever. Fever is believed to result from a pyrogen-mediated elevation in the set-point temperature. While exogenous pyrogens, such as live viruses, bacterial endotoxins and antigen-antibody complexes may act directly to increase body temperature, most experimental evidence suggests that these substances produce fever through the action of intermediary biochemical entities. These intermediary substances are endogenous pyrogens that are synthesized and released from bone marrow-derived phagocytic cells which have been activated by exogenous pyrogens. Endogenous pyrogens are produced by neutrophils, monocytes, eosinophils, alveolar macrophages, Kupffer cells and other fixed macrophages (3). Once released, endogenous pyrogens act upon the hypothalamic thermoregulatory center to increase the set-point temperature possibly through induction of prostaglandin synthesis and activation of cyclic-AMP (4). The body responds by increasing heat production and decreasing heat dissipation. A primary motor center in the posterior hypothalamus produces shivering which increases skeletal muscle tone throughout the body. This results in increased thermal energy. Heat conservation occurs primarily through decreased cutaneous blood flow which prevents the conduction of body heat from central compartments to the surrounding environment. Cutaneous vasoconstriction also reduces sweating thereby decreasing evaporative water loss and heat dissipation.

Hyperthermia. Hyperthermia results from increased heat production and/or decreased heat dissipation similar to fever; however, it differs in that there is no alteration in the set-point temperature. Heat stroke is an example of hyperthermia in which overexertion in an excessively hot and humid environment results in increased heat production under conditions where heat dissipation cannot occur (5). The risk of life-threatening hyperthermia is even greater if large amounts of fluid loss through sweating occur. Hyperthermia attributable to increased metabolic rate may accompany endocrinological disorders such as thyrotoxicosis and pheochromocytoma (6). Hypothalamic lesions secondary to stroke, neurosurgical procedures or tumors may impair thermoregulatory mechanisms such that patients cannot adapt to environmental temperature fluctuations. When ingested in toxic doses, a number of drugs have been associated with hyperthermia. Examples include LSD, cocaine, amphetamines, salicylates, anticholinergics and tricyclic antidepressants (7). Even in usual pharmacological doses, anticholinergic drugs may increase the risk of exercise-induced hyperthermia by blocking sweat gland secretions (8). Another drug-induced alteration of thermoregulatory function has been reported in a few patients receiving inhalation anesthetics and muscle relaxants commonly employed in surgery. The term malignant hyperthermia has been used to describe this pharmacogenetic myopathy which can produce tremendous heat production in anesthetized patients (9).

Clinical Assessment

From the previous definitions and examples of altered thermoregulatory mechanisms, it is apparent that an elevation of body temperature requires a careful history, physical examination and diagnostic evaluation to determine the underlying cause.

Diurnal Temperature Variations. In all normal persons there exists a diurnal temperature variation: the peak occurs in the late afternoon or early evening and the nadir occurs in the early morning between three and five o'clock (10). This variation in body temperature appears to be independent of sleep habits and eating or working patterns, although exercise and emotional stress have been shown to produce significant temperature elevations.

Clinical Definition of Fever. The average oral temperature recording is 37°C although the normal range may vary between 36.5 to 37.5°C in older children and adults, and may be even higher in infants (11). Therefore, the clinical definition of fever is generally accepted to be an oral temperature above 37°C. If rectal temperatures are properly recorded, the readings are generally 0.5°C higher than oral temperatures, whereas axillary temperatures are generally 0.5°C lower than oral readings (12).

Methods of Measurement. The most accurate body temperature is measured rectally. Axillary temperatures may be less accurate than rectal temperatures although safer and easier to measure. For the patient who is fully cooperative and does not have an acute respiratory illness, oral temperature recordings may be the most convenient. Accurate and consistent body temperature measurements can be obtained by following simple guidelines. First, due to the variability in accuracy between thermometers of different manufacturers, it is suggested that, whenever feasible, the same thermometer be used throughout a patient's illness. Rectal temperatures should be obtained by inserting a security bulb thermometer 5 cm (2 inches) into the patient's rectum for a period of three minutes. Accurate oral temperature recordings generally require five to ten minutes. During this time the patient should not breathe through the mouth to avoid spuriously low values. Also, it is important to remind patients not to take an oral temperature just after the mouth has been artificially heated or cooled. Axillary temperatures should be recorded after the thermometer has been in place for three to five minutes.

Efficacy of Skin Thermometers. A recently marketed skin thermometer (Clinitemp®), consisting of thermophototropic esters of cholesterol that change color over a specific temperature range, has been evaluated in one study and found to be inaccurate (13). Of thirty patients found to be febrile by an electronic thermometer, the skin thermometer detected fever in only thirteen (43%). Although the skin thermometer performed better in patients with high fevers, the authors stated that there may be an appreciable risk of undetected serious illness if this temperature measuring device is the only method used.

Factors Affecting Treatment Decisions. Although the role of fever during infectious processes has been studied extensively, it is not well established whether fever is an essential host defense mechanism or a normal biological response to infection (14). *In vitro,* elevated temperatures have been shown to produce unfavorable growth conditions for certain bacteria and viruses (15,16); however, there is no solid evidence, *in vivo,* that fever enhances host defense against infection (17). Therefore, the decision to treat fever is often based upon factors, such as the attitudes of the patient and prescriber, the patient's age, past medical history and concurrent symptoms, and the diagnostic plan. The importance of these factors will be illustrated in the ensuing cases.

1. The mother of an 18-month-old, 26 lb child calls for advice regarding the treatment of her child's high fever. She states that the child was well until mid-afternoon at which time she noticed that he felt warm. A rectal temperature taken ten minutes ago was 40.9°C. The mother called the child's pediatrician who was not immediately available. The mother states that she is worried that the child's temperature may continue to rise and result in permanent damage. Is this mother's concern valid? How should this child's febrile illness be treated?

Harmful Effects of Fever. This mother's concern regarding the harmful effects of fever is one shared by many parents. A recent study revealed that 46% of parents believed that brain damage could result from high fever which the large majority defined as a temperature greater than 40°C (18). Forty-eight percent of parents believed that, if untreated, a child's temperature may continue to rise to 41.7°C and above. From these results, it is apparent that many parents are poorly informed and overly concerned about febrile illnesses in their children.

Several studies involving both ambulatory and hospitalized pediatric patients have shown that fevers accompanying common pediatric infections in otherwise normal patients seldom exceed 41.1°C (19–22). Patients with central nervous system infections, underlying chronic brain damage, brain tumors or an impaired capacity to dissipate heat are at greater risk for developing extreme hyperpyrexia (20,21). Other than personal discomfort and increased insensible water loss, fever rarely produces any permanent harm to the patient except in patients suffering from heat stroke (23). Even in this condition, the body temperature must generally exceed 41.1°C before neurological damage occurs. Fever-triggered seizures remain a concern of the pediatrician since about 4% of children will experience at least one febrile seizure during early childhood (24). In this instance, both the absolute temperature recording and the rate of temperature rise appear to be critical factors in producing the seizure. Whether or not simple febrile seizures lead to permanent neurological sequelae remains controversial.

General Management Principles. The initial step in handling this situation is to assure the mother that her child's high fever is not likely to produce serious consequences. The next step would be to recommend methods by which the child's temperature can be reduced. Since the child's temperature is above 40°C, it is reasonable to recommend both general and specific measures by which heat production can be decreased and heat dissipation can be increased. General measures include providing an adequate amount of fluid intake to replace increased insensible water losses and removing excessive clothes and blankets. The environment should be kept at room temperature (26°C) to facilitate heat dissipation.

Specific Antipyretic Measures. Specific measures include administration of an oral antipyretic and topical sponging. When these two modalities are used in combination, it is important that the oral antipyretic be given prior to topical sponging to lower the hypothalamic set-point temperature (17). If sponging is employed before the set-point temperature is reduced, its effect is generally of short duration and accompanied by shivering. The choice between aspirin and acetaminophen is generally based upon concurrent diseases, side effects, product formulations and cost since several well-controlled studies have shown that these two agents are comparable with respect to onset, peak, duration and intensity of action when administered in equal doses.

Topical sponging with tepid water has been shown to be a safe and effective means of lowering body temperature (25). Although ice water and hydroalcoholic solutions have been used alone and in combination with oral antipyretics, these modalities have been associated with a greater amount of personal discomfort than tepid water. In addition, the toxic potential of topically applied alcohol solutions is sufficient to avoid their use in febrile patients (26–28).

Antipyretic dosage. A variety of pediatric dosage schedules for orally administered aspirin and acetaminophen based upon age, body surface area and body weight appear in the literature. Although the pharmacokinetic characteristics of these two drugs differ significantly, clinical studies have shown that the effective antipyretic doses are quite similar (29–33). A recent review of aspirin dosage recommendations suggests that body weight provides an effective and uniformly consistent criterion for calculating pediatric antipyretic doses (34). Although age provides a more convenient means of estimating aspirin dosage, the nonlinear relationship between age and body weight results in non-uniform dosage recommendations when this criterion is used. In contrast, body surface area provides a reliable dosage estimate through ten years of age; however, it is often impractical to determine accurately.

Therefore, oral administration of aspirin or acetaminophen at a dose of 10–15 mg/kg body weight every four hours as needed up to a maximum daily dose of 65 mg/kg should be recommended for this patient. If aspirin is used, the mother should be instructed to avoid exceeding the maximum dosage recommendations since the early signs and symptoms of therapeutic salicylate intoxication (nausea, vomiting, irritability, hyperpnea and hyperthermia) (37) may closely resemble the clinical manifestations of the disease for which the drug is being used.

Rectal administration of antipyretics is commonly employed despite the paucity of information regarding bioavailability and clinical response. A study by Nowak and associates reported that both the rate and total amount of aspirin absorbed from a suppository dosage form was less than that reported for oral dosage forms (35). A general trend which was noted in the study was that a rectal retention time of five hours or less resulted in a total urinary salicylate recovery of 54–64%, while a retention time greater than ten hours resulted in a total urinary salicylate recovery of 82–98%. Variations in the amount of acetaminophen absorbed from commercially available suppository vehicles have also been reported (36). At equivalent mg/kg doses, the oral dosage formulations produce higher serum levels and result in a greater total amount absorbed than is reported for rectal suppositories. Although some effect may be derived from rectal antipyretic administration, the decreased rate and amount absorbed may result in an unpredictable therapeutic response.

2. *Combined Aspirin and Acetaminophen.* While making rounds on the pediatric floor you notice that one pediatrician has begun

writing antipyretic orders as follows: aspirin every four hours alternating with acetaminophen every four hours prn T > 39°C. Is there any advantage to the use of these two agents in this manner?

A study reported by Steele and associates demonstrated that the simultaneous administration of acetaminophen and aspirin produced a more sustained antipyretic effect than either agent alone (31). In this single dose study of 120 pediatric patients, there were no apparent differences between the three treatment groups (A—aspirin alone, B—acetaminophen alone, C—combined therapy) in the first two hours of observation. However, four to six hours after antipyretic administration, group C's temperatures were still suppressed whereas groups A and B were noted to have gradual increases in body temperature. The authors suggest that since aspirin and acetaminophen are eliminated, in part, by similar metabolic pathways, the additive antipyretic effect may reflect accumulation of one of the drugs. Although Levy and Yamada demonstrated a competitive inhibition between acetaminophen and salicylamide biotransformation (38), orally administered salicylic acid and acetaminophen did not produce the same effect (39). Therefore, other explanations must be sought to explain the sustained effect reported following the simultaneous administration of these two drugs.

While it has been suggested that the simultaneous administration of aspirin and acetaminophen may reduce the toxic potential of aspirin since doses could be given less frequently, a more simplistic approach would be to eliminate aspirin altogether. The sustained effect from simultaneous administration of these agents has not been demonstrated in a controlled study where the drugs are administered on an alternating schedule. Therefore, this alternating antipyretic schedule cannot be advocated until cost and risk versus benefit can be determined.

3. *Treatment of Newborn.* A 10-day-old child has been admitted to the hospital with the diagnoses of dehydration and possible sepsis. The child became lethargic, increasingly irritable and anorectic over the last twelve hours. At the time of physical examination the child was fully clothed and wrapped in two heavy blankets. His vital signs included a temperature of 39.3°C, pulse of 140/min, and a respiratory rate of 40/min. The mucous membranes were dry and the child's skin was described as mottled with decreased turgor. How should this patient's febrile illness be managed?

This patient's clinical presentation illustrates several commonly encountered problems in newborn infants. Since the clinical manifestations of overwhelming infection may be subtle during the newborn period (40), the child's history of lethargy, irritability and decreased appetite indicates the need for a complete septic workup, including blood, urine and cerebrospinal fluid cultures. Heavy clothing and blankets may elevate body temperature by interfering with heat dissipation. Simple measures such as removal of the child's blankets and clothes in an environment which is at normal room temperature may be sufficient to produce a reduction in body temperature. The patient's vital signs and physical findings are compatible with dehydration; therefore, rehydration at approximately twice the normal maintenance fluid intake is important to restore intravascular volume and increase cutaneous blood flow. This will also facilitate this patient's capacity to dissipate heat. Additionally, appropriate antibiotic coverage pending receipt of the culture results is indicated.

If the child's body temperature remains elevated subsequent to these measures, then more specific antipyretic therapy should be considered. In this case, a cooling blanket is preferred over an oral antipyretic due to the decreased ability of the newborn to eliminate aspirin or acetaminophen. Studies of newborn infants whose mothers had received aspirin just prior to delivery indicate that the neonate's salicylate clearance is decreased due to immature liver and renal function (41).

Similarly, a study of twelve healthy full-term infants two to three days of age demonstrates that the elimination rate constant for acetaminophen (mean = 0.208 hr^{-1}) (42) is decreased as compared to that reported for adults (mean = 0.315 to 0.368 hr^{-1}) (43–45). In a second study of three full-term infants one to two days of age, the biological half-life of acetaminophen was not increased significantly, although decreased acetaminophen glucuronide formation and increased acetaminophen sulfate formation as reported by Levy and associates was confirmed (46).

From the above data, it may be concluded that a single dose of acetaminophen or aspirin may be given to neonates; however, repeated doses would be difficult to schedule without knowledge of the precise elimination rate characteristics. Therefore, a safer reduction and control of body temperature may be obtained through the use of a cooling blanket.

4. *Allergic Rhinitis and Asthma.* A 23-year-old male with allergic rhinitis and bronchial asthma asks whether he should take aspirin or acetaminophen for a fever secondary to cellulitis. The patient has no history of acute allergic symptoms following previous aspirin administration.

A number of factors have been implicated in precipitating acute airway obstruction in asthmatic patients; among these are aspirin and other nonsteroidal anti-inflammatory agents (47). Other manifestations of aspirin sensitivity may include urticaria, angioedema, vasomotor rhinitis, purpura and abdominal cramps (48–51). Asthmatic episodes may occur within minutes after ingestion of aspirin-containing products and may range in severity from mild, brief exacerbations to severe protracted attacks accompanied by cyanosis, coma and rarely, death (52–54). Recent literature evaluating the incidence of aspirin sensitivity indicates that as many as 28% of children and 16% of adults with asthma may show a significant deterioration of pulmonary function testing following aspirin ingestion (55,56).

Several studies have examined the effects of acetaminophen ingestion upon asthma symptoms. The majority of patients given acetaminophen have not developed increased respiratory symptoms or airway obstruction (57–59). However, acetaminophen-induced bronchospasm was reported in twelve of forty-two patients with an unequivocal history of aspirin sensitivity (60).

Since this patient has taken aspirin without experiencing detectable symptoms it is possible that its use during the current illness would not produce any acute symptoms. On the other hand, this patient's history suggests that acetaminophen may be the safer agent to use since there is a decreased likelihood that it would produce a decrease in pulmonary function.

5. *Salicylate Overdosage.* A 43-year-old female with a "flu syndrome" calls complaining of stomach upset, myalgia and fever which have persisted over the last three days. During this time the patient has been taking aspirin, 650 mg every three to four hours and Pepto-Bismol, two ounces every four hours. Over the last twenty-four hours the patient has developed ringing in her ears and an increased severity of symptoms. What would you recommend for this patient?

The immediate consideration from this patient's history is the possibility of a therapeutic salicylate intoxication. Pepto-Bismol contains 1.75% bismuth subsalicylate which is a readily absorbable form of salicylate (61). The daily ingestion of twelve ounces provides a salicylate content equivalent to 3.9 gms of aspirin. This amount, in combination with the 3.9 to 5.2 gms of aspirin taken for fever and myalgia, may constitute an excessive dose. Discontinuation of these products may help relieve some of the persistent symptoms which this patient is experiencing. If the symptoms persist or intensify during the next twenty-four hours, the patient should be seen for further evaluation. Additionally, the patient should be instructed to avoid any other OTC cold or fever products which may contain salicylates.

6. *Malignant Hyperthermia.* A 68-year-old male was admitted to the hospital for surgical decompressive laminectomy. The previous medical history revealed the patient to be in good general health, without illness other than chronic intractable lumbar pain. There was no previous history of major surgery. Preoperative medications included diazepam (Valium) 10 mg, meperidine (Demerol) 75 mg and atropine 0.6 mg, administered one hour before surgery. The patient arrived in the operating room with normal vital signs: blood pressure 120/80, pulse 84/min, respiratory rate 16/min, temperature 37.3°C. He was given 2 mg of d-tubocurarine followed by 300 mg of thiopental (Pentothal) and 80 mg of succinylcholine (Anectine) intravenously. No trismus was noted on intubation, but immediately thereafter the patient became increasingly difficult to ventilate and the extremities became rigid. The blood pressure rose to 220/100, the pulse increased to 140/min and the temperature increased to 39.4°C over the next five minutes. An arterial blood gas on 50% oxygen demonstrated a pO_2 of 156, a pCO_2 of 58 and a pH of 7.16. Although anesthesia was discontinued, the patient's temperature continued to rise over the next five minutes to 41.1°C. What is the most likely cause of this patient's acute problems and how should he be treated?

This patient's response to anesthesia induction is consistent with the syndrome of malignant hyperthermia (MH). MH has an estimated incidence ranging from one in 14,000 to one in 40,000 operations with general anesthesia (62,63). MH, a life-threatening complication, occurs in susceptible patients upon exposure to potent anesthetics and muscle relaxants. The susceptibility to MH is inherited, apparently as an autosomal dominant trait which produces a generalized skeletal muscle membrane abnormality. When the abnormal membrane is exposed to a triggering agent, there is a rapid, excessive release of calcium into the myoplasm which produces the primary clinical features of the syndrome (64).

The presenting signs of MH vary depending upon whether or not succinylcholine has been administered during anesthesia induction (65). If succinylcholine is given to a susceptible individual, profound muscle rigidity ensues. If MH is recognized after the first dose, recovery within twenty-four hours is usually uneventful except for a mild fever and muscle enzyme elevation. On the other hand, if MH is undetected and additional doses of succinylcholine are administered, intensification of muscle rigidity may occur.

When succinylcholine is not given during induction, the earliest presenting sign of MH is usually a tachyarrhythmia although other dysrhythmias have also been reported. Additional early signs may include a generalized erythematous flush followed by cyanotic mottling, hypertension or an unstable blood pressure and tachypnea.

Late manifestations of MH may include sustained muscle rigidity progressing to rigor mortis, severe and rapidly progressing hyperthermia, bleeding, and left ventricular failure. Biochemical changes which occur include respiratory and metabolic acidosis secondary to hypercapnia and lactic acid accumulation, hyperkalemia, hypercalcemia, hyperphosphatemia, thrombocytopenia, decreased serum fibrinogen and Factor VIII levels and elevated CPK, LDH and SGOT.

The successful management of MH is, in the main, dependent upon early recognition of the condition and prompt intervention. The initial treatment should include discontinuation of anesthesia, administration of 100% oxygen, hyperventilation, institution of cooling measures and correction of acid-base and electrolyte disturbances (63). Vigorous cooling measures may be required and have included surface cooling with ice, gastric and rectal lavage with iced saline solutions and intravenous administration of iced saline solutions.

Concurrently, consideration should be given to controlling dysrhythmias and skeletal muscle rigidity. Intravenous procainamide (Pronestyl) in a dose of 15 mg/kg body weight infused over ten minutes has been recommended for control of tachyarrhythmias. Intravenous dantrolene sodium (Dantrium) has been employed (66,67) and recently marketed for controlling the muscle rigidity. Dantrolene appears to act directly on the contractile mechanism of skeletal muscle to interfere with the release of calcium from the sarcoplasmic reticulum (68). The drug is administered by rapid IV push in an initial dose of 1 mg/kg body weight followed by repetitive doses until symptoms subside or a maximum of 10 mg/kg has been administered. Oral doses of 1–2 mg/kg four times a day for one to three days may be necessary to control recurrences. To date, no significant adverse effects have been reported with short-term use.

7. *Reye's Syndrome.* A 4½-year-old female is admitted to the hospital with the tentative diagnosis of Reye's Syndrome. The child had an upper respiratory tract infection one week prior to admission during which time the mother administered several doses of aspirin for fever. The child began vomiting about twenty-four hours prior to admission and subsequently became increasingly lethargic. Approximately three hours prior to admission the patient had a generalized tonic-clonic seizure which lasted about twenty minutes at which time the child was brought to the emergency room by ambulance. Initial diagnostic evaluation revealed an increased serum ammonia, increased liver function tests and a decreased serum glucose. On admission the child was febrile (T–39.4°C). There is some concern regarding the use of aspirin and acetaminophen in this patient. Can naproxen (Naprosyn) be used as an antipyretic instead?

Reye's Syndrome. The concern regarding the use of aspirin and acetaminophen is valid because of the possible relationship between oral antipyretics and the pathogenesis of Reye's Syndrome and because the clearance of these drugs is, in part, influenced by hepatic function.

Despite the numerous reports describing the clinical manifestations of Reye's Syndrome which culminates in encephalopathy and fatty degeneration of the liver, the pathogenesis of this disease remains an enigma (69). Since the prodrome is characterized by a viral-like illness, antipyretics are often administered. Recent epidemiological studies have attempted to examine whether aspirin consumption during antecedent illness may play a role in the development of Reye's Syndrome (70). In seven children with Reye's Syndrome reported by Starko, an association between the amount of aspirin ingested and the severity of the clinical manifestations was noted although the amount of salicylates taken by the children was not excessive. Based upon this and earlier reports, the Centers for Disease Control and the Food and Drug Administration have advised caution regarding the use of oral antipyretics in viral illnesses associated with vomiting because of the suspicion that these drugs may contribute to the pathogenesis of Reye's Syndrome (71,72).

Naproxen. The use of naproxen as an alternative to aspirin and acetaminophen is reasonable based upon its reported antipyretic effectiveness. In a double blind study of 109 children, naproxen 7.5 mg/kg was comparable to aspirin 15 mg/kg with respect to temperature reduction over the first four hours of observation (73). A major difference between the two drugs was noted after four hours in that body temperature began to rise in the aspirin treated patients whereas it remained suppressed for up to twelve hours in the naproxen treated patients. A dose-response relationship for naproxen was evident in that a dosage of 2.5 mg/kg was only slightly better than placebo during the first seven hours and considerably less effective than aspirin or high dose naproxen during the first four hours.

Regardless of its efficacy, before recommending naproxen for this patient one should consider its elimination pathways and the overall management of Reye's Syndrome in terms of temperature regulation. Only about 10% of naproxen is excreted unchanged in the urine; the remainder is excreted as either conjugated or desmethyl metabolites (74). Therefore, hepatic dysfunction accompanying Reye's Syndrome may also significantly reduce the clearance of naproxen. Since patients with Reye's Syndrome frequently have increased intracranial pressure, hypothermia is generally employed to reduce the metabolic needs of the brain and to reduce cerebral edema through reduction of systemic blood pressure (75). Because a body temperature between 32°C to 37°C is required to achieve these goals, the use of mechanical cooling devices is preferred over oral antipyretics which are effective in reducing body temperature only to within the near normal range.

8. *Pregnancy.* A 26-year-old pregnant female who is within a few days of delivery calls to determine whether or not it is acceptable for her to take aspirin for fever and a "head cold."

The answer to this question requires examination of the effects of aspirin upon the mother and fetus. The effects of aspirin upon the duration of human gestation and labor have been reported in a retrospective study of 103 patients who took daily salicylate doses in excess of 3,250 mg for the last six months of gestation (76). This study revealed that those women who took aspirin had gestational periods which were seven to ten days longer than the control group's, labor times which were approximately five hours longer than the control group's, and increased estimated blood loss at the time of delivery. Similar findings were also reported by Collins and Turner (77).

Two separate studies have reported suppression of collagen-induced platelet aggregation in 80% to 100% of newborn infants whose mothers ingested aspirin within seven days of delivery (78,79). This platelet effect coupled with aspirin's ability to interfere with prothrombin synthesis adds a risk factor to both the mother and fetus. Another factor to consider is the ability of the salicylates to displace bilirubin from albumin binding sites, resulting in increased concentrations of free bilirubin in the neonate's serum (80). Maternal ingestion of aspirin and other prostaglandin synthetase inhibitors has been also implicated as a causative factor in the development of persistent pulmonary hypertension (PPHN) in neonates (81). The patency of the ductus arteriosus in utero is, in part, dependent upon the availability of vasoactive prostaglandins. Inhibition of prostaglandin synthesis results in constriction of the ductus arteriosus and an increase in pulmonary arterial pressure. Since PPHN may be associated with increased fetal mortality and increased neonatal morbidity and mortality, the avoidance of agents which decrease prostaglandin synthesis seems justified.

Since acetaminophen has not been associated with any of the previously described unwanted effects on the mother or fetus, it would serve as an acceptable alternative for the symptomatic treatment of this patient.

9. *G6PD Deficiency.* A 19-year-old black male is seeking advice regarding an antipyretic/analgesic agent for the treatment of a febrile illness. Further questioning of the patient reveals that he has a glucose-6-phosphate dehydrogenase (G6PD) deficiency.

Hemolytic disease involving a deficiency of G6PD occurs in about 13% of black males and about 2% of black females (82). In general, these patients are susceptible to the development of a hemolytic anemia following the ingestion of drugs with oxidant properties. Until recently, aspirin has been reported to be a hemolytic agent in patients with erythrocyte G6PD deficiency (83–85). Criticism of previously reported cases of aspirin-induced RBC hemolysis has been raised by Glader who commented that infections and other clinical conditions known to produce RBC hemolysis are often present in those patients receiving salicylates (86).

In vitro and *in vivo* studies with aspirin and its oxidant metabolite, gentisic acid, confirmed that gentisic acid possesses oxidant activity but only at concentrations which would be produced with blood salicylate levels of 500–3500 mg/dl. Similarly, salicylate concentrations of up to 350 mg/dl have no apparent effect on G6PD deficient cells. To support the *in vitro* data, Glader challenged twenty-two patients with G6PD deficiency with a four-day course of aspirin in doses of 50 mg/kg/day and found no evidence of increased hemolysis.

Acetaminophen's effects on G6PD deficient RBC's have also been studied and the results indicate that it does not increase the rate of RBC hemolysis (87). Therefore, this patient could take either aspirin or acetaminophen for symptomatic relief.

References

1. Benzinger TH: Clinical temperature: New physiological basis. JAMA. 1969; 209:1200.
2. Kluger MJ: Fever. Pediatrics. 1980; 66:720.
3. Atkins E: Pathogenesis of fever. Physiol Rev. 1960; 40:580.
4. Willies GH et al: The effect of sodium salicylate on dibutyryl cyclic AMP fever in the conscious rabbit. Neuropharmacology. 1976; 15:9.
5. Musacchia XJ: Fever and hyperthermia. Federation Proceedings. 1979; 38:27.
6. Sitt JT: Fever versus hyperthermia. Federation Proceedings. 1979; 38:39.
7. Holdcroft A: Body Temperature Control. In *Anaesthesia, Surgery and Intensive Care,* Bailliere Tindall, London, 1980, p 79.
8. Weiner N: Atropine, scopolamine and related antimuscarinic drugs. In *The Pharmacological Basis of Therapeutics,* 6th ed, edited by AG Gilman, LS Goodman and A Gilman, MacMillian, New York, 1980, p 126.
9. Britt BA et al: Hereditary aspects of malignant hyperthermia. Can Anaesth Soc J. 1969; 16:89.
10. Dinarello CA et al: Pathogenesis of fever in man. N Engl J Med. 1978; 298:607.
11. Iliff A et al: Pulse rate, respiratory rate and body temperature of children between two months and 18 years of age. Child Develop. 1952; 23:238.
12. Steele RW: Fever. In *Pediatric Therapy,* 5th ed, edited by HC Shirkey, CV Mosby, St. Louis, 1975, p 331.
13. Reisinger KS et al: Inaccuracy of the Clinitemp® skin thermometer. Pediatrics. 1979; 64:4.
14. Klastersky J et al: Is suppression of fever or hypothermia useful in experimental and clinical infectious disease? J Infec Dis. 1970; 128:81.
15. Enders JF et al: Studies on the natural immunity to pneumococcus type III. I: The capacity of pneumococcus type III to grow at 41°C and their virulence for rabbits. J Exp Med. 1936; 64:7.
16. Walter DL et al: Factors influencing host-virus interaction. III: Further studies on the alteration of Coxsackie virus infection in adult mice by environmental temperature. J Immunol. 1958; 80:39.
17. Stern RC: Pathophysiologic basis for symptomatic treatment of fever. Pediatrics. 1977; 59:92.
18. Schmitt BD: Fever phobia: Misconceptions of parents about fevers. Am J Dis Child. 1980; 134:176.
19. Tomlinson WA: High fever: Experience in private practice. Am J Dis Child. 1975; 129:693.
20. McCarthy PL et al: Hyperpyrexia in children. Am J Child. 1976; 130:849.
21. Akerren Y: On hyperpyretic conditions during infancy and childhood. Acta Pediatr. 1943; 31:1.
22. DuBois EF: Why are fever temperatures over 106°F rare? Am J Med Sci. 1948; 217:361.
23. Knochel JP: Environmental heat illness. Arch Intern Med. 1974; 133:841.
24. Millichap JG: A critical evaluation of febrile seizures. J Pediatr. 1960; 56:364.
25. Steele RW et al: Evaluation of sponging and of oral antipyretic therapy to reduce fever. J Pediatr. 1970; 77:824.
26. McFadden SW et al: Coma produced by topical application of isopropranol. Pediatrics. 1969; 43:622.
27. Senz EH et al: Coma in a child following use of isopropyl alcohol in sponging. J Pediatr. 1958; 53:323.
28. Garrison RF: Acute poisoning from use of isopropyl alcohol in tepid sponging. JAMA. 1958; 152:317.

29. Hunter J: Study of antipyretic therapy in current use. Arch Dis Child. 1973; 48:313.

30. Eden AN et al: Clinical comparison of three antipyretic agents. Am J Dis Child. 1967; 114:284.

31. Steele RW et al: Oral antipyretic therapy: Evaluation of aspirin-acetaminophen combination. Am J Dis Child. 1972; 123:204.

32. Tarlin L et al: A comparison of the antipyretic effectiveness of acetaminophen and aspirin. Am J Dis Child. 1972; 124:880.

33. Colgan MT et al: The comparative antipyretic effect of N-acetyl-P-aminophenol and acetylsalicylic acid. J Pediatr. 1957; 50:552.

34. Done AK et al: Aspirin dosage for infants and children. J Pediatr. 1979; 95:617.

35. Nowak MM et al: Rectal absorption from aspirin suppositories in children and adults. Pediatrics. 1974; 54:23.

36. Pagay SN et al: Effect of vehicle dielectric properties on rectal absorption of acetaminophen. J Pharm Sci. 1971; 60:600.

37. Temple AR: Pathophysiology of aspirin overdosage toxicity, with implications for management. Pediatrics. 1978; 62 (suppl):873.

38. Levy G et al: Drug biotransformation interactions in man. III: Acetaminophen and salicylamide. J Pharm Sci. 1971; 60:215.

39. Levy G et al: Drug biotransformation interactions in man. V: Acetaminophen and salicylic acid. J Pharm Sci. 1971; 60:608.

40. Klein JO et al: An introduction to infections of the fetus and newborn infant. In *Infectious Diseases of the Fetus and Newborn Infant,* edited by JS Remington and JO Klein, WB Saunders Co, Philadelphia, 1976, p 22.

41. Levy G et al: Kinetics of salicylate elimination by newborn infants of mothers who ingested aspirin before delivery. Pediatrics. 1974; 53:201.

42. Levy G et al: Pharmacokinetics of acetaminophen in the human neonate: Formation of acetaminophen glucuronide and sulfate in relation to plasma bilirubin concentration and d-glucaric acid excretion. Pediatrics. 1975; 55:818.

43. Nelson E et al: Kinetics of the metabolism of acetaminophen by humans. J Pharm Sci. 1963; 52:864.

44. Cummings AJ et al: A kinetic study of drug elimination: The excretion of paracetamol and its metabolites in man. Br J Pharm. 1976; 29:150.

45. Prescott LF et al: The comparative metabolism of phenacetin and N-acetyl-P-aminophenol in man, with particular reference to effects on the kidney. Clin Pharmacol Ther. 1968; 9:605.

46. Miller RP et al: Acetaminophen elimination kinetics in neonates, children, and adults. Clin Pharmacol Ther. 1976; 19:284.

47. Weinberger M: Analgesic sensitivity in children with asthma. Pediatrics. 1978; 62(suppl):910.

48. Prickman LE et al: Hypersensitivity to acetylsalicylic acid (aspirin). JAMA. 1937; 108:445.

49. Friedlaender S et al: Aspirin allergy: Its relationship to chronic intractable asthma. Ann Intern Med. 1947; 26:734.

50. Walton CHA et al: Aspirin allergy. Can Med Asso J. 1957; 76:1016.

51. Moore-Robinson M et al: Effect of salicylates in urticaria. Br Med J. 1967; 4:262.

52. Lamson RW et al: Some untoward effects of acetylsalicylic acid. JAMA. 1932; 99:107.

53. Dysart BR: Death following ingestion of five grains of acetylsalicylic acid. JAMA. 1933; 101:446.

54. Francis N et al: Death from ten grains of aspirin. J Allergy. 1935; 6:504.

55. McDonald JR et al: Aspirin intolerance in asthma. J Allergy Clin Immunol. 1972; 50:198.

56. Rachelefsky GS et al: Aspirin intolerance in chronic childhood asthma: Detected by oral challenge. Pediatrics. 1975; 56:443.

57. Samter M et al: Intolerance to aspirin: Clinical studies and consideration of its pathogenesis. Ann Intern Med. 1968; 68:975.

58. Szczeklik A et al: Aspirin-induced asthma. J Allergy Clin Immunol. 1976; 58:10.

59. Szczeklik A et al: Relationship of inhibition of prostaglandin biosynthesis by analgesics to asthma attacks in aspirin-sensitive patients. Br Med J. 1975; 1:67.

60. Delaney JC: The diagnosis of aspirin idiosyncrasy by analgesic challenge. Clin Allergy. 1976; 6:177.

61. Anonymous: Salicylate in Pepto-Bismol. Med Let Drugs Ther. 1980; 22:63.

62. Anonymous: Dantroline for malignant hyperthermia during anesthesia. Med Let Drugs Ther. 1980; 22:61.

63. Ryan JF: Treatment of acute hyperthermia crisis. International Anesthesiology Clinics. 1979; 17:153.

64. Britt BA: Etiology and pathophysiology of malignant hyperthermia. Federation Proceedings. 1979; 38:44.

65. Steward DJ: Malignant hyperthermia—The acute crisis. International Anesthesiology Clinics. 1979; 17:1.

66. Friesen CM et al: Successful use of dantrolene sodium in human malignant hyperthermia syndrome: A case report. Can Anaesth Soc J. 1979; 26:319.

67. Liebenschutz F et al: Increased carbon dioxide production in two patients with malignant hyperpyrexia and its control by dantrolene. Br J Anaesth. 1979; 51:899.

68. Putney JW et al: Site of action of dantrolene in frog sartorius muscle. J Pharmacol Exper Ther. 1974; 189:202.

69. Shaywitz BA et al: Monitoring and management of increased intracranial pressure in Reye's Syndrome: Results in 29 children. Pediatrics. 1980; 66:198.

70. Starko KM et al: Reye's Syndrome and salicylate use. Pediatrics. 1980; 66:859.

71. Anonymous: Followup on Reye's Syndrome—United States. Morbidity and Mortality Weekly Reports. 1980; 29:321.

72. Anonymous: Reye's Syndrome—Ohio, Michigan. Morbidity and Mortality Weekly Reports. 1980; 29:532.

73. Cashman TM et al: Comparative effects of naproxen and aspirin on fever in children. J Pediatr. 1979; 95:626.

74. Segre EJ: Naproxen metabolism in man. J Clin Pharmacol. 1975; 15:316.

75. Batzdorf U: The management of cerebral edema in pediatrics practice. Pediatrics. 1976; 58:78.

76. Levis RB et al: Influence of acetylsalicylic acid, an inhibitor of prostaglandin synthesis, on the duration of human gestation and labor. Lancet. 1973; 2:1149.

77. Collins E et al: Salicylates and pregnancy. Lancet. 1973; 2:1494.

78. Corby DG: The effects of antenatal drug administration on aggregation of platelets of newborn infants. J Pediatr. 1971; 79:307.

79. Bleyer WA et al: Studies on the detection of adverse drug reactions in the newborn. II: The effects of prenatal aspirin on newborn hemostasis. JAMA. 1970; 213:2049.

80. Maisels MJ: Bilirubin: On understanding and influencing its metabolism in the newborn infant. Pediatr Clin North Am. 1972; 19:447.

81. Perkin RM et al: Serum salicylate levels and right-to-left ductus shunts in newborn infants with persistent pulmonary hypertension. J Pediatr. 1980; 96:72.

82. Pearson HA: Enzymatic defects of the red cells. In *Nelson Textbook of Pediatrics* 11th ed, edited by VC Vaughn, RJ McKay and RE Behrman, WB Saunders Co, Philadelphia, 1979, p 1384.

83. Hochstein P: Glucose-6-phosphate dehydrogenase deficiency: Mechanisms of drug-induced hemolysis. Exp Eye Res. 1971; 11:389.

84. Kellermeyer RW et al: Hemolytic effect of therapeutic drugs: Clinical considerations of the Primaquine-type hemolysis. JAMA. 1962; 180:128.

85. Swanson M: Drugs, chemicals and hemolysis. Drug Intell Clin Pharm. 1973; 7:6.

86. Glader BE: Evaluation of the hemolytic role of aspirin in glucose-6-phosphate dehydrogenase deficiency. J Pediatr. 1976; 89:1027.

87. Fraser IM et al: Effects of drugs and drug metabolites on erythrocytes from normal and glucose-6-phosphate dehydrogenase-deficient individuals. Ann N Y Acad Sci. 1968; 151:777.

Chapter 6

Nausea and Vomiting

Philip E. Johnston

Nausea is a subjective feeling of discomfort of the stomach accompanied with a propensity to vomit, tightness of the epigastric area, noticeable widening of the throat, and various parasympathetically mediated events. Pupil dilation, tachycardia or bradycardia, skin pallor, tachypnea, increased perspiration, salivation, anorexia, hypotension, headache, drowsiness, and lassitude may all be present. Duodenal tone initially decreases, stomach motility decreases, then duodenal tone gradually increases and causes reflux of duodenal contents into the stomach (2–4). Vomiting may or may not proceed from this point.

Vomiting is a more dramatic event than nausea, is more likely to have an underlying cause, and is a more significant symptom of underlying disease. Vomiting is defined as a forceful expulsion of gastric contents. The gastric fundus and gastroesophageal sphincter relax, intra-abdominal pressure increases due to contraction of the abdominal wall and diaphragm, and the pylorus contracts. These events cause the gastric and duodenal contents to project with accelerating speed through the dilated esophagus and through the oral cavity. Reflex closure of the epiglottis and the soft palate prevent aspiration of the vomitus and entry into the nasopharynx (2,4,5).

Vomiting can be due to various causes including infection, neoplasm, radiation, uremia, pregnancy, anesthesia, severe pain, and adverse reaction to drug therapy. Various clinical characteristics are useful in differentiating among possible causes of vomiting. For example, vomiting in the morning is often associated with the morning sickness of pregnancy, alcoholic gastritis, or uremia; while vomiting experienced shortly after eating is commonly associated with pylorospasm or gastritis. Vomiting of large amounts of undigested food 4–6 hours after eating suggests gastric retention which is common in patients with gastric atony or pyloric obstruction and which is often associated with visible peristaltic movement from left to right across the epigastric area. A putrid or fecal odor of vomitus may signify bacterial influence on food material and might reflect lower bowel fistula or obstruction (2). Bile, while commonly seen in prolonged vomiting, is not significant unless it appears in large quantities over a long period of time. When this occurs, there may be an obstruction of the bowel below the ampulla of vater (2). Blood in the vomitus signifies esophageal, gastric, or duodenal bleeding. Rupture of the cardio-esophageal junction (Mallory-Weiss syndrome) occurs most often in a setting of alcohol abuse, and life-threatening

Table 1.

CAUSES OF NAUSEA AND VOMITING

I. Abdominal Emergencies
   acute appendicitis
   acute cholecystitis
   acute peritonitis
   intestinal obstruction

II. Chronic Indigestion

III. Acute Systemic Infections
   viral, bacterial, or parasitic
   intestinal disease
   viral hepatitis

IV. Central Nervous System Disorders
   increased intracranial pressure
   otitis interna (labyrinthitis)
   nonsuppurative disease of the labyrinth
      (Meniere's syndrome)
   migraine headache
   generalized body wasting (tabetic crisis)
   hypotension and syncope

V. Drugs
   levodopa
   aspirin
   antibiotics
   digitalis glycosides
   quinidine
   theophylline
   opiates
   nitrogen mustards and other cancer
      chemotherapeutic agents
   oral contraceptives
   many drug metabolites

VI. Cardiovascular Disorders
   myocardial infarction
   congestive heart failure

VII. Endocrine Disorders
   diabetes
   adrenal insufficiency
   pregnancy

VIII. Psychogenic Stimuli
   anorexia nervosa
   mental association

IX. Uremia

blood loss can result (2,3). Vomited blood may be red or coffee ground in appearance. Bright red blood is most likely fresh and can be from tears or ulcerations of the mouth, esophagus, stomach, or duodenum. Blood exposed for any reasonable time to gastric acid will be coffee ground in appearance, having been changed to acid hematin.

Pathophysiology

The physiological aspects of nausea and vomiting are not fully understood and present knowledge is based primarily upon animal experiments. It is known that specific centers in the medulla transmit stimuli and initiate nausea or vomiting, and that the stomach, duodenum, and other tissue respond to these stimuli (1).

Initiation of vomiting ultimately involves the vomiting center (VC) which consists of a nucleus of cells located in the reticular formation of the medulla. In close proximity to this VC is another nucleus of cells called the chemoreceptor trigger zone (CTZ). The CTZ receives input from the cerebral cortex, hypothalamus, vestibular apparatus, and is also capable of reacting to non-neural, blood-borne stimuli such as bacterial toxins and drugs. The VC receives input from the CTZ and from the afferent fibers of the gastrointestinal tract via the vagus. Thus, the act of vomiting can be initiated in either of two ways. First, the CTZ, receiving cortical, vestibular, hypothalamic, or chemical stimuli, activates the vomiting center which, in turn, sends impulses down the vagal efferents to the gastrointestinal (GI) tract. Secondly, the vomiting center can be activated without CTZ mediation, by vagal stimulation through irritation of mucosal receptors in the GI tract.

Propagation of emesis involves an enormously complex coordination of skeletal and smooth muscle. Not by coincidence then, the vomiting center is surrounded by the centers for inspiratory and spastic respiration, the vasomotor center, the vestibular, and the salivary centers. Apparently, this intimate association allows perfect coordination to occur. It may also explain why vomiting is an all or none response which cannot be aborted by most physiologic or pharmacologic manipulations. Consequently, termination of vomiting depends solely on the removal or interruption of stimuli reaching the CTZ or vomiting center.

Although this model (101) is over thirty years old, surprisingly little new information has been

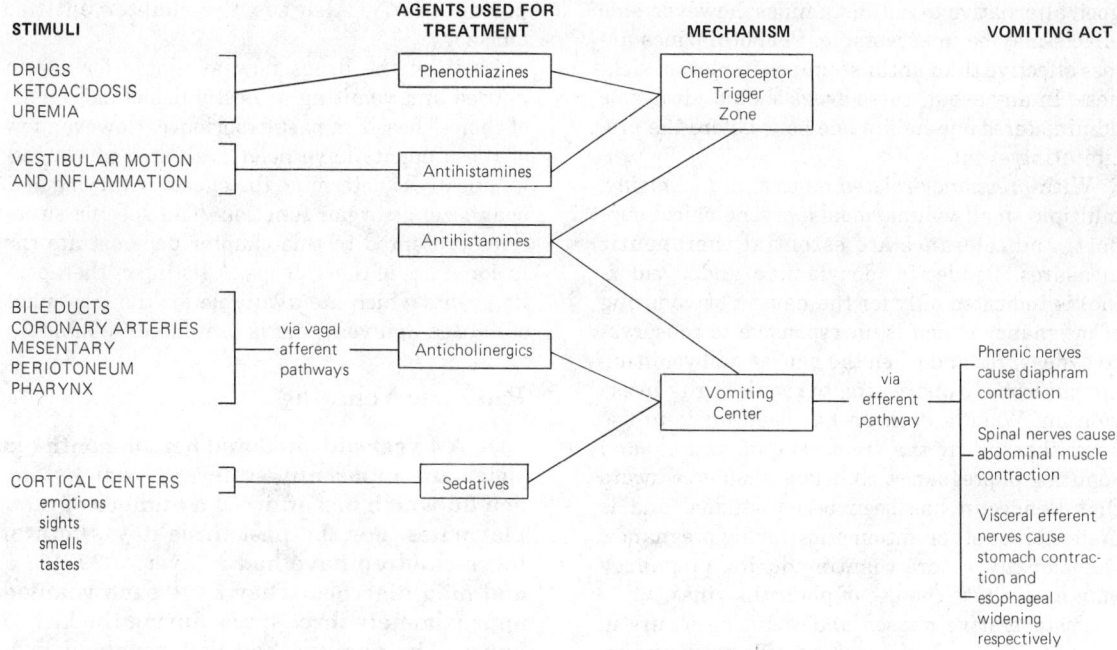

Figure 1. Causes, Treatments and Mechanisms of Vomiting.

uncovered since. If these mechanisms are accepted, then pharmacologic agents capable of depressing sensitivity of the CTZ and/or vomiting center to chemical or neural stimuli or blocking afferent impulses through selective anticholinergic action, will in theory be therapeutically effective antiemetics.

Treatment

Treatment should be directed toward correction of the underlying cause of vomiting; however, since this is not always possible, palliative treatment with antiemetic drugs is often indicated.

The benefits gained from preventing emesis are a reduction in the risks of aspiration and electrolyte abnormalities, as well as alleviation of the obvious distress that accompanies vomiting. Unfortunately, the antiemetic agents available today are less than ideal for the control of vomiting, both in effectiveness and in absence of toxicity. As a result, the risks versus benefits of antiemetic therapy must be weighed carefully.

Nausea and vomiting associated with *gastritis* and *gastroenteritis* can many times be treated effectively and safely by dietary manipulations.

Phosphorated carbohydrate solutions (Emetrol, Especol), which supposedly relieve nausea and vomiting by a direct local action on the wall of the gastrointestinal tract, or antihistamines such as dimenhydrinate (Dramamine), meclizine (Bonine), or cyclizine (Marezine) may be required. For severe vomiting, benzquinamide (Emete-Con) or phenothiazines such as thiethylperazine (Torecan) or prochlorperazine (Compazine) may be necessary.

In *children,* nausea and vomiting is more common and usually less indicative of severe disease than in adults. However, with prolonged, profuse, or projectile vomiting, medical attention should be sought to discover the underlying cause before instituting symptomatic treatment, especially in the infant. Fluid and electrolyte replacement can be critical in the vomiting infant.

Motion sickness is most appropriately treated with an antihistamine. While none of the antihistamines have significant advantages over the others, it could be beneficial to switch to another antihistamine should one agent be found ineffective because patients vary in their response to individual antihistamines. Scopolamine alone or in combination with sympathomimetics can be a good alternative to antihistamines; however, side effects may be unacceptable. Phenothiazines are less effective than antihistamines in motion sickness. In any event, these drugs should always be administered one-half to one hour before the precipitating event.

With *pregnancy-related nausea and vomiting,* multiple small volume meals, psychological support, and tolerance are essential therapeutic measures. Bendectin (doxylamine and pyridoxine) is indicated only for the nausea or vomiting of pregnancy which is unresponsive to conservative measures and when the nausea and vomiting are sufficiently distressing to require drug intervention. When a decision has been made to use drug therapy in the treatment of nausea and vomiting of pregnancy, clinicians should be aware that Bendectin has been better studied and is preferable to other antiemetics during pregnancy. Occasionally, severe vomiting during pregnancy may necessitate the use of phenothiazines.

Postoperative nausea and vomiting occurs in one of five patients. Benzquinamide, various phenothiazines, haloperidol (Haldol), and metoclopramide (Reglan) are effective for this condition. Benzquinamide has few side effects and perhaps beneficial hemodynamic and respiratory effects. Phenothiazines, on the other hand, may cause central nervous system depression and respiratory depression, either alone or in conjunction with narcotic or parasympatholytic use. Metoclopramide has not been approved for this use.

Narcotic-induced nausea and vomiting results from direct CTZ stimulation and increased sensitization of the vestibular area. This generally occurs with low or initial doses of the narcotic and does not generally require treatment. If treatment becomes necessary, benzquinamide may be most useful because it does not potentiate narcotic-induced hypotension or respiratory depression. Phenothiazines may be particularly effective when combined with antihistamines because this combination would tend to block both the CTZ and vestibular components.

Cancer chemotherapeutic agents, especially cisplatin, can cause nausea and vomiting. Prophylactic treatment with phenothiazines, haloperidol, metoclopramide and delta-9-tetrahydrocannabinol (THC) have all been shown to be somewhat beneficial. However, THC is not readily available. *Radiation*-induced nausea and vomiting is responsive to phenothiazines and halo-

peridol (5–7). Also see the chapter entitled Oncology.

Many of the drugs now available for use in nausea and vomiting are established as "agents of choice" based on past experience. However, few of these agents have been evaluated pharmacokinetically to determine the effects of varying age, body size, or organ function. The specific situations presented in this chapter demonstrate the rational use of these drugs. A listing of therapeutic agents which are available for the treatment of nausea and vomiting is presented in Table 2.

Pediatric Vomiting

1. A 4-year-old child and her 10-month-old sister are apparently suffering from a stomach flu which has afflicted a number of their playmates. For the past three days, both of these children have had a fever of 99–100°F and mild diarrhea. They have each vomited approximately three times during the last 36 hours. The vomitus has had no blood in it and the children appear to be otherwise free of discomfort. Except for dry mouth, pallor, dry lips, and sluggishness, the 10-month-old seems to be in the same clinical condition as her older sister. What therapeutic interventions should be initiated for the nausea and vomiting of these two children?

Assuming these children have been essentially healthy and have not recently made abrupt dietary changes prior to this episode, they are most likely suffering from a self-limited gastroenteritis. The older child is not in any apparent danger of excessive fluid loss or electrolyte problems if her condition continues to gradually improve over the next 12–24 hours. However, small servings of carbonated beverages along with a liquid diet of gelatin, warm weak tea, Pedialyte, or Gatorade in frequent, small amounts (1–2 oz per hour) as tolerated may help to alleviate some of the discomfort of vomiting. This hypoosmolar diet will replenish some of the fluid loss and prevent unwanted stimulation of the gastric or bowel mucosa. Electrolyte mixtures have no unique value and may be dangerous if overused (11,12).

The younger child presents with a more urgent problem. This child should be referred immediately to a physician for evaluation, because fluids represent a greater percentage of body weight in infants than in older children. This infant exhib-

Table 2.

AVAILABLE ANTIEMETIC AGENTS (8,9)

Drug Name	Commercial Name(s)	Adult Dosage Regimen*	Pediatric Dosage Regimen*	Dosage Form(s)	Drug Status
Concentrated Syrups					
Invert Sugar	Emetrol			OL	OTC
Levulose/Dextrose	Especol			OL	OTC
Antihistamines					
Buclizine	Bucladin-S softabs	N & V: 50 mg by mouth three times daily Motion Sickness: 50 mg ½ hr before travel then every 4 to 6 hours		**	
Cyclizine	Marezine	50 mg by mouth or intramuscularly every 4 to 6 hours	*Less than 6 yrs*: one-fourth of adult dose; *6 to 10 yrs*: one-half of adult dose	T,S,I	T = OTC S,I = L
Dimehydrinate	Dramamine	50 mg every 4 to 6 hours	*Less than 8 yrs*: Individualized; *8 to 12 yrs*: 25–50 mg three times daily	OL,T,S,I	OL, T = OTC S, I = L
	Eldodram	same	same	T	OTC
	Trav-Arex	same	same	T	OTC
	Ram	same	same	T	OTC
Diphenhydramine	Benadryl	50 mg orally or intramuscularly 3 to 4 times daily	*Under 20 pounds*: 6.25 to 12.5 mg orally or intramuscularly 3 or 4 times daily; *20 pounds or more*: 12.5 to 25 mg orally or intramuscularly 3 or 4 times daily	OL,C,I	OL, C = OTC, I = L
	BAX	same	same	OL,C	OTC
Doxylamine with Pyridoxine	Bendectin	10 mg orally at onset and 10 to 20 mg orally at bedtime		T	L
Hydroxyzine	Vistaril	25 to 100 mg orally or intramuscularly 3 to 4 times daily	*Under 6 yrs*: 50 mg per day orally or intramuscularly in divided doses; *6 yrs and over*: 50 to 100 mg per day orally or intramuscularly in divided doses	OL,C,I	L
	Atarax	same	same	OL,T	L
Meclizine	Antivert	25–50 mg orally or intramuscularly every 4 to 6 hours		T**	L
	Bonine	same		T**	OTC
	Vertrol	same		T	OTC

Table 2. (continued)

AVAILABLE ANTIEMETIC AGENTS (8,9)

Drug Name	Commercial Name(s)	Adult Dosage Regimen*	Pediatric Dosage Regimen*	Dosage Form(s)	Drug Status
Phenothiazines					
Chlorpromazine	Thorazine	10–25 mg orally every 4 to 6 hours or 25 mg intramuscularly every 4 to 6 hours or 100 mg rectally every 6 to 8 hours	0.25 mg per pound body weight orally or intramuscularly every 4 to 6 hours	OL,T, S,I***	L
	Prormapar	same	same	T	L
	Chlor-PZ	same	same	T	L
Perphenazine	Trilafon	8 to 16 mg daily orally in divided doses or 5 mg intramuscularly		T,I****	L
Prochlorperazine	Compazine	5 to 10 mg orally or intramuscularly 3 to 4 times daily (limit 40 mg/day)	Not recommended for those under 20 pounds; *20–29 pounds*: 2.5 mg 1 or 2 times daily (limit 7.5 mg/day); *30–39 pounds*: 2.5 mg 2 to 3 times daily (limit 10 mg/day); *40–85 pounds*: 2.5 mg 3 times daily (limit 15 mg/day)	OL,T, S,I***	L
Promethazine	Phenergan	25 mg every 4 to 6 hours	12.5–25 mg every 4 to 6 hours	OL,T, S,I**	L
	Remsed	same	same	T	L
Thiethylperazine	Torecan	10 to 30 mg orally three times daily or intramuscularly 2 ml up to three times a day		T,S,I	L
Triflupromazine	Vesprin			OL,T,I	L
Other					
Benzquinamide	Emete-Con	50 mg intramuscularly (repeat in 1 hour if needed) then 50 mg every 3 to 4 hours; or 25 mg intravenously (1 ml/min), then 25 mg intramuscularly thereafter		I	L
Dipenidol	Vontrol	25–50 mg orally every 4 hours as needed or 20–40 mg intramuscularly	*Children less than 6 months or 25 pounds*: none; 0.4 mg/pound orally or 0.2 mg/pound intramuscularly every four hours	T,I	L
Haloperidol	Haldol	1 to 2 mg orally or intramuscularly			LX

Table 2. (continued)

AVAILABLE ANTIEMETIC AGENTS (8,9)

Drug Name	Commercial Name(s)	Adult Dosage Regimen*	Pediatric Dosage Regimen*	Dosage Form(s)	Drug Status
Metoclopramide	Reglan	10 mg 3–4 times daily 15–30 minutes before meals not to exceed 60 mg per day	*Children less than six years*: 0.1 mg/kg three times per day; *children 6 to 14 years*: 2.5–5 mg three times daily	T,I	LX
Scopolamine	Transderm-V	1 pad postauricularly every 3 days		Transdermal pad	L
Trimethobenzamide	Tigan	250 mg orally 3–4 times daily or 200 mg rectally 3–4 times daily	*30–90 pounds*: 100 to 200 mg orally 3–4 times daily or 100–200 mg rectally 3–4 times daily	C,S,I	L

*Dose for treatment of nausea and vomiting (check drug insert for more information)
**Chewable tablet also
***Timed release capsule and oral concentrate also available
****Timed release tablet and oral concentrate also available

OL	Oral liquid	OTC	Over-the-counter
T	Tablet	L	Legend (on Prescription)
S	Suppository	LX	Legend; not approved for nausea and vomiting
I	Injection		

ited several signs of dehydration including lethargy and dry mucous membranes. Her dry skin and membranes may also be due to her fever and breathing through her mouth. For a more detailed presentation of dehydration in children, see the chapters entitled Fluids and Electrolyte Disorders and Pediatric Therapy.

Motion Sickness

2. Mrs. Roberts has refilled her son's prescription for dimenhydrinate 25 mg every six hours as needed for motion sickness while boating. His prescription was written six years ago when he was twelve years of age. Although the drug has been effective over this period of time, its effectiveness has been waning. What factors might account for his decreasing success with this drug and how should he prevent future motion sickness while boating?

If the medication does not work as well, it may be due to several factors. The boy has become an adult and probably needs to increase the dose of dimenhydrinate up to 50 mg every four to six hours. Furthermore, he may not be taking this medication appropriately. In order to be the most effective, the medication should be ingested 30 to 60 minutes prior to the activity which is likely to produce motion sickness. Antiemetics which are given after nausea and vomiting have begun will not abort the attack or alleviate further episodes. Also, another antihistamine such as cyclizine (Marezine) or meclizine (Bonine, Antivert) could be tried because individuals may vary in their response to various antihistamines. Dimenhydrinate and these other antihistamines may be purchased without a prescription. The patient should be advised that a change to a larger dose of dimenhydrinate or switching to another agent may cause drowsiness, dizziness, tinnitus, inability to concentrate, cycloplegia, dry mouth, or blurred vision. Finally, he should be advised to avoid taking these drugs with alcohol and other central nervous system depressants to avoid potential boating or driving accidents (9,14,15).

3. What therapeutic alternatives are available for this patient should his motion sickness fail to respond to antihistamines?

Scopolamine, in doses of 0.6 mg po initially, followed by 0.3 mg every six hours would be more effective and would also be more likely to produce undesirable anticholinergic effects (14). A transdermal product has been developed which delivers scopolamine at a continuous rate through intact skin (17,20,21). Transdermal Therapeutic System-scopolamine (TTS-scopolamine, Transderm-V) is applied postauricularly and delivers scopolamine at a rate of 3 to 10 mcg/hr for three days. It appears to be effective and side effects are generally minimal or well-tolerated. This preparation is available only on prescription.

Sympathomimetics such as ephedrine or amphetamine are effective in motion sickness but are most effective when combined with anticholinergics or antihistamines. Since motion sickness most likely is regulated by both acetylcholine- and norepinephrine-mediated centers, such combination therapy is rational (1).

Patients vary markedly in their response to stimuli which may produce motion sickness and in their response to treatment. Therefore, changing from one agent to another is appropriate when therapeutic failure occurs (18,21).

4. Why are antihistamines and sympathomimetics preferred over phenothiazines such as Compazine for the treatment of the nausea and vomiting of motion sickness?

Motion sickness appears to be a result of stimulation of the labyrinth system and subsequent transmission of this stimulus through a balanced network of cholinergic and adrenergic fibers to the vestibular network located near the vomiting center (19). When there is strong stimulation, the vestibular nucleus is bombarded with an abnormal number of impulses which could radiate through the adjacent cholinergic-mediated reticular system to the vomiting center. Thus, drugs which inhibit the cholinergic-mediated spread of impulses from the vestibular nucleus to the vomiting center should be effective in the treatment of motion sickness (113). Indeed, all of the drugs effective in the treatment of motion sickness possess significant anticholinergic properties as evidenced by their common side effects of dry mouth, cycloplegia, tachycardia, constipation, and sedation. The effectiveness of antihistamines in motion sickness is, therefore, probably due to their anticholinergic properties because drugs with greater ability to block histamine than diphenhydramine afford no protection against motion sickness (114). Although some phenothiazines have minor anticholinergic effects and can block apomorphine-induced emesis, they generally are ineffective in the treatment of motion sickness.

The efficacy of the amphetamines can be explained by the theoretical balance between sympathetic and parasympathetic fibers terminating on the vestibular nucleus. Presumably, motion sickness can be prevented if the norepinephrine-mediated system is favored because it appears to shunt vestibular impulses away from the vomiting center. This phenomenon may be due to the fact that anatomical sympathetic fibers from the vestibular nucleus pass by the vomiting center at a greater distance than do the cholinergic fibers. In any case, a supra-additive effect is achieved when an anticholinergic is given together with an amphetamine (1).

5. Do patients on lengthy ocean cruises develop tolerance to antihistamines when taken for prolonged periods of time for motion sickness?

Patients usually develop tolerance to the motion rather than to the drug (1,18,19). Military personnel exposed to slow rotation rooms developed motion sickness more frequently and sooner in the early stages of training as compared to later stages of training. Furthermore, smaller doses of medication were needed to prevent episodes of motion sickness in the later stages of training (18). Therefore, only short-term treatment is usually needed to prevent motion sickness even when patients are exposed to prolonged motion. If a patient continues to suffer from motion sickness, further evaluation would be prudent.

Morning Sickness

6. A 21-year-old female who is six weeks pregnant reported daily episodes of vomiting. Her obstetrician ordered a standard urinalysis, SMA-12, and a complete blood count with differential. The patient then was counseled to eat smaller, more frequent meals rich in carbohydrates, and was given a prescription for Bendectin to be taken every six hours for nausea and vomiting. What is the most likely cause of this patient's nausea and vomiting?

This patient appears to be suffering from nausea and vomiting of early pregnancy, or morning sickness. Nausea with or without vomiting occurs in 50–80% of pregnancies during the sixth to fourteenth weeks of gestation (21–25). By the twentieth week of gestation, morning sickness will afflict only about 10% of patients and it generally subsides by the end of gestation (16,26). Although nausea usually occurs in the morning and subsides by mid-day, it may appear at other times or be persistent. The vomiting associated with morning sickness is not usually significant in volume or complicated by dehydration.

7. What is the physiological basis for the morning sickness of pregnancy?

An increased gastric emptying time due to a generalized decrease in smooth muscle tone of the gastric mucosa, displacement of the entire gastrointestinal tract, decreased hydrochloric acid release, and increased estrogen levels may all contribute to the nausea and vomiting of early pregnancy (23,26). Increased estrogen serum concentrations may initiate vomiting via the CTZ. Estrogen serum levels tend to be high during the third and fourth weeks of the menstrual cycle in some women who experience nausea and vomiting at this time. Furthermore, oral contraceptives with high estrogen content, estrogen replacement therapy, and estrogen chemotherapy of some carcinomas also are associated with nausea and vomiting. Nevertheless, the precise cause of morning sickness remains unknown. Neurological, endocrine, metabolic, and psychological factors have all been proposed (102).

8. Nausea and vomiting are symptoms which may be associated with illnesses. What are some possible causes of nausea and vomiting which are not associated with this patient's pregnancy?

Gastroenteritis, gastritis, ulcerative colitis, urinary tract infection, and bowel obstruction are a few possible causes of nausea and vomiting. Severe vomiting also may be associated with cerebral tumor, appendicitis, or hepatitis. This patient is only in her sixth week of pregnancy, but vomiting late in pregnancy can be associated with the onset of labor, eclampsia, or intrahepatic cholestasis (23,25).

9. How should this patient's morning sickness be treated?

Drugs were commonly used to treat morning sickness until 1961 when thalidomide was found to be teratogenic. Understandably, the use of drugs in pregnancy, especially for mild nausea and vomiting, has fallen sharply in recent years. Reassurance, sympathy, and understanding are now the mainstays in the therapy of mild morning sickness (23,26). When nausea becomes frequent, many women empirically treat themselves with weak tea, cola, ice chips, or crackers, and occasionally with phosphorated syrups such as Emetrol or Especol (27). These syrups may affect gastric emptying and further complicate nausea and vomiting (28–30). Nevertheless, such simple therapeutic measures are not apt to affect the fetus, and the physician's suggestion regarding small, frequent, high carbohydrate meals is a good one (23).

When conservative management of nausea and vomiting in pregnancy has failed and when symptoms are sufficiently distressing to require drug intervention, most physicians prescribe doxylamine/pyridoxine (Bendectin). Although hydroxyzine (Vistaril) (32), promethazine (Phenergan) (31), trimethobenzamide (Tigan) (21), dimenhydrinate (28), meclizine (31), cyclizine (31), and chlorpromazine (Thorazine) have been used for morning sickness, Bendectin has been better studied and is preferable to other antiemetics for use in pregnancy (27). If Bendectin is unsuccessful, another antihistamine such as meclizine should be prescribed. If necessary, phenothiazines can be prescribed subsequently; however, potential benefits must be weighed against the risk of side effects to both mother and fetus.

10. If the early morning nausea and vomiting which afflicts the above pregnant patient is not controlled by conservative management, then Bendectin is to be used. What is the teratogenic potential of antihistaminic drugs such as Bendectin?

An estimated 10 to 25% of pregnant women in the United States receive prescriptions for Bendectin, usually in the first trimester (27). Because of a highly publicized legal case involving a child with birth defects whose mother took Bendectin during gestation, there has been considerable public interest surrounding this drug.

Doxylamine/pyridoxine has been associated with more than 80 cases of teratogenicity in the United States and another 50 cases worldwide (33). These single and multiple case reports include cleft lip (33), cleft palate (33), long bone deformities of the leg (34–36), missing leg (36), abdominal contents born externally (omphalocele) (36), absent fingers (34), heart defects (37), Poland's anomaly (38), and other intestinal defects (39). However, birth defects also occur without drugs, and whether or not doxylamine/pyridoxine was the cause of these reported defects is unknown.

More recent and more convincing studies suggest that doxylamine/pyridoxine is not teratogenic (41–43,45). However, the nature of epidemiologic studies for the evaluation of birth defects is such that small increases in the overall malformation rate may remain undetected, and epidemiologic study of doxylamine/pyridoxine is continuing (27).

Other antihistamines are not approved for use in pregnancy (14). Meclizine and cyclizine were thought to be teratogenic in humans (28,31) but subsequent study refuted this conclusion (26). Indeed, in 1966 the FDA required that meclizine and cyclizine carry labels warning against their use in pregnant women based on teratogenicity studies in animals. However, subsequent epidemiologic studies have shown no increase in embryo deaths or malformed children born to women using these drugs during pregnancy and consequently the FDA warning has since been removed (103). Promethazine (40) and trimethobenzamide (21) have been associated with an increased rate of fetal malformation, but these associations were not of statistical significance.

In summary, no antinauseant drug can be conclusively proclaimed free of teratogenic effect, but the use of doxylamine/pyridoxine in more than twenty million pregnancies without fetal abnormality (33) suggests that it is the safest drug choice in this situation.

Post-Surgery

11. A 38-year-old female is to undergo surgery for a hysterectomy tomorrow morning and is to receive a pre-operative injection of meperidine 50 mg, atropine 0.4 mg, and hydroxyzine 50 mg. The patient is concerned about nausea post-operatively because of similar problems with past surgeries. Would prophylaxis with an antiemetic be appropriate for this patient?

Vomiting occurs in 20–25% of surgical patients who do not receive antiemetics (46). The nature of the surgery, duration of surgery, choice of anesthetic, and the use of pre-operative medications all influence post-surgical nausea and vomiting. If vomiting does occur and if antiemetics are not contraindicated, antihistamines such as cyclizine (Marezine), piperazine phenothiazines such as thiethylperazine (Torecan) or prochlorperazine (Compazine), or benzquinamide (Emete-Con) can be utilized. However, these antiemetics should not be routinely used prophylactically because of potential adverse effects. Some antiemetics, when used alone or in combination with anesthetics, narcotics, or pre-operative medications, may depress respiration or blood pressure, cause extrapyramidal side effects, or increase post-surgical recovery time. Underlying patient disease states such as chronic obstructive pulmonary disease, asthma, or congestive heart failure may increase the risks of morbidity when antiemetics are used. Therefore, this patient should not receive prophylactic antiemetics. Furthermore, this patient will be receiving hydroxyzine (Vistaril) as part of her pre-operative medications. Hydroxyzine does have antihistaminic and anticholinergic properties and may be somewhat useful in preventing post-surgical nausea and vomiting.

12. If this patient were to develop post-surgical nausea and vomiting, which phenothiazine would be the most appropriate for empirical antiemetic therapy?

Clinically, the antiemetic activity of all the phenothiazines is equal in the treatment of nausea and vomiting due to infection, uremia, cancer, radiation, anesthesia, or drug toxicity (104–110). Therefore, the choice of phenothiazine for initial antiemetic therapy must be determined on the basis of relative potentials for side effects at equipotent doses.

Although the list of phenothiazine adverse effects is long, examination of the clinical studies using these drugs as antiemetics reveals that only sedation, hypotension, and extrapyramidal effects are of significant consequence. Sedation is reported in 50–80% of the patients receiving aliphatic phenothiazines as antiemetics, with chlorpromazine causing the highest incidence (106,111,112). Hypotension occurs with the next greatest frequency, again with chlorpromazine being the greatest offender (111,112). Although this side effect is rare with the piperazine analogs (prochlorperazine and thiethylperazine), the concomitant use of a narcotic increases the incidence to that of chlorpromazine alone. Although relatively rare at antiemetic doses, extrapyramidal effects occur more frequently with the more potent piperazine phenothiazines, perphenazine and fluphenazine (105,110), and the risk of this effect eliminates the use of agents as first-line, empirical antiemetic therapy.

On the basis of these observations, the recommended phenothiazines for initial antiemetic therapy in situations where the duration of therapy is expected to be short are prochlorperazine and thiethylperazine. If chronic therapy is planned, chlorpromazine may be considered as well because tolerance appears to develop to the sedative and hypotensive effects of this agent (111).

13. What type of post-surgical patients with nausea and vomiting would benefit more from benzquinamide (Emete-Con) than prochlorperazine (Compazine)?

Benzquinamide (Emete-Con) is a non-phenothiazine antiemetic which challenges the role of the phenothiazines in the control of post-surgical vomiting. When comparing such a drug with phenothiazines, both its efficacy and its safety must be considered. It should be equally capable of preventing or controlling emesis and, more importantly, should not lower the blood pressure, prolong sleeping time, or depress respirations to the same extent as the phenothiazines.

When clinical trials compared 100 mg doses of benzquinamide to 10 mg doses of prochlorperazine, benzquinamide was significantly more effective in preventing apomorphine-induced vomiting and in blocking the CTZ. It also had a more rapid onset of action and caused virtually no adverse effects (50). In comparisons of benzquinamide to perphenazine in the treatment of post-surgical vomiting, benzquinamide was slightly more effective and caused fewer episodes of somnolence (51). In two other comparative studies, benzquinamide was more effective than prochlorperazine (48) and thiethylperazine (Torecan) (52). In all of these studies (48–52), benzquinamide did not cause hypotension or extrapyramidal adverse effects. Therefore, benzquinamide might be preferred over phenothiazines when treating post-surgical vomiting in patients who have a history of cardiovascular disease.

Two studies compared the respiratory depressant effects of benzquinamide and prochlorperazine, with and without meperidine, by examining their effect on the CO_2 stimulation test (72,74). The well known respiratory depressant action of meperidine was demonstrated, as was the supra-additive effect of prochlorperazine combined with meperidine. No respiratory depression was caused by benzquinamide, and that observed following the administration of benzquinamide and meperidine was less than that seen with meperidine alone. Therefore, benzquinamide also would seem to be the antiemetic of choice in post-surgical patients with nausea and vomiting induced by narcotic analgesics, because unlike phenothiazines, it does not potentiate narcotic-induced hypotension or respiratory depression (71–74). Likewise, it would seem that benzquinamide would be preferred over phenothiazines in vomiting post-surgical patients with a history of pulmonary disease. However, benzquinamide is more costly than prochlorperazine and is only available parenterally. Furthermore, enthusiastic early studies need the tincture of time and extended clinical use to validate apparent advantages.

Narcotic-Induced

14. A patient who had three wisdom teeth extracted 24 hours ago has been experiencing severe nausea since this morning when she began taking acetaminophen with codeine tablets. She vomited two hours after the first dose and is still nauseated, although the nausea and vomiting seem to come and go. What is the most likely cause of this patient's nausea and vomiting?

Although there are many possible causes of nausea and vomiting in this patient, she most likely is experiencing narcotic-induced vomiting because of the temporal association between these events. Nausea and vomiting associated with the anesthetic or with the swallowing of blood from the dental procedure would have occurred soon after oral surgery, and other causes such as uremia, pregnancy, or gastroenteritis are unrealistic with this patient history. Medications other than narcotic analgesics also are associated with nausea and vomiting (see Table 1) and need to be considered in this patient's differential diagnosis. Nevertheless, this patient's vomiting is consistent with reports that narcotic analgesics induce vomiting shortly after initiation of therapy and that the vomiting diminishes when the narcotic achieves therapeutic concentrations (66).

Codeine and other morphine analogs have profound and complicated effects on the CTZ and on the vomiting center. These drugs can induce nausea and vomiting by stimulating the CTZ when therapy is initiated. However, once therapeutic drug levels are achieved, these drugs also can inhibit nausea and vomiting by suppressing the vomiting center. Thus, patients using these drugs on an "as needed" basis may experience nausea after each dose, but patients who use these narcotics for pain relief at regular time intervals may not experience nausea or vomiting. These opposing effects might account for the waxing and waning pattern of this patient's episodes of nausea and vomiting.

In addition to stimulatory effects on the CTZ and inhibitory effects on the vomiting center, narcotics also can increase the sensitivity of the vomiting center to vestibular stimulation (66,67). Indeed, nausea and vomiting from narcotic analgesics are relatively uncommon in recumbent patients as opposed to those who are ambulatory such as this patient. Clinically, most hospitalized patients seem to be affected by narcotic-induced nausea and vomiting most commonly at a time when they first begin to walk again and at a time when the dosing interval of their narcotic analgesic is lengthened. This clinical observation perhaps could be explained by the stimulatory effects of these analgesics on the CTZ and the vestibular nucleus.

Cancer Patients

15. A 63-year-old male with prostatic carcinoma is undergoing chemotherapy with cisplatin. Previous radiation treatments did not cause this patient much difficulty with nausea and vomiting; however, cisplatin treatments cause considerable vomiting which usually begins within three hours of his treatment and continues for 10 to 12 hours. Intramuscular prochlorperazine (Compazine) 10 mg every four hours lessens the vomiting but does not totally relieve it as it did when he was undergoing radiation therapy. Why is this patient having less relief with prochlorperazine than in the past?

Radiation therapy and cancer chemotherapy are simply different therapeutic modalities and affect patients differently. Radiation therapy is associated with about a 10% incidence of nausea or vomiting, while drugs such as cisplatin or doxorubicin are associated with a considerably higher incidence of nausea and vomiting. Therefore, this patient should be expected to respond less well to prochlorperazine during chemotherapy as compared to radiation therapy. Phenothiazines like prochlorperazine selectively inhibit the CTZ and possibly the VC as well (75) and only are effective for the treatment of mild to moderate nausea and vomiting. (The reader should refer to the chapter entitled Oncology for a more detailed discourse on the management of nausea or vomiting which is associated with cancer chemotherapy.)

16. Would haloperidol or tetrahydrocannabinol (THC) be effective alternatives for this patient's cisplatin-induced vomiting?

Haloperidol has been recommended as an alternative to prochlorperazine for the treatment of drug-induced nausea and vomiting (75,82). A 1–2 mg intramuscular dose of haloperidol can decrease nausea and vomiting by 60% and a trial would be worthwhile in this patient. However, this drug is not currently approved for this use and additional clinical trials are needed to clarify its role in the therapeutic armamentarium for nausea and vomiting.

Tetrahydrocannabinol (THC) has been studied extensively and clearly is effective in treating refractory vomiting induced by cancer chemotherapy (79–81, 84–87). Doses of 10–15 mg/m^2 before, during, and after chemotherapy significantly decreased nausea and vomiting in large percentages of patients during clinical trials. This investigational drug is available upon special request in a cigarette or capsule dosage in selected medical institutions in various areas of the country. Doses up to 15 mg/m^2 occasionally caused euphoria (79,84,85), drowsiness (84), fear (80,86,87), anxiety (80), panic (86), visual hallucinations (80,86), severe distortion of time (80), or paranoid ideation (86,87). In most cases these side effects resolved within three hours. (For additional information on THC, see the chapter entitled Oncology as well as the chapter entitled Drug Abuse.)

ACKNOWLEDGMENT: The contributions of Dr. Scott Matthiesen are sincerely appreciated. Portions of his work which appeared in an earlier edition of this textbook have been included into this present chapter.

References

1. Wood CD: A theory of motion sickness based on pharmacological reactions. Clin Pharmacol Ther. 1970; 11:621.
2. Isselbacher KJ: Anorexia, nausea, and vomiting. In *Harrison's Principles of Internal Medicine*, 9th ed, edited by KJ Isselbacher, RD Adams, EB Braunwald, RG Petersdorf and JD Wilson, McGraw-Hill, Inc, New York, 1980, p 198.
3. Brooks FP: Nausea and vomiting. In *Gastrointestinal Pathophysiology*, 2nd ed, edited by FP Brooks, Oxford University Press, New York, 1978, p 22.
4. Lumsden K et al: The act of vomiting in man. Gut. 1969; 10:173.
5. Feldman M et al: Vomiting. In *Gastrointestinal Disease: Pathophysiology, Diagnosis, Management,* 2nd ed, edited by MH Sleisenger and JS Fordtran, WB Saunders, Philadelphia, 1978, p 200.
6. Sallan SE et al: Antiemetics. In *Handbook of Drug Therapy,* edited by RR Miller and DJ Greenblatt, Elsevier, New York, 1979, p 1060.
7. Schwinghammer T: Antiemetics: choosing from the alternatives. Hosp Form. 1980; 15:38.
8. *American Drug Index*, 25th ed, edited by NF Billups, JB Lippincott Co, Philadelphia, 1981.
9. Wyman JB et al: The vomiting patient. Am Fam Physician. 1980; 21:139.
10. *Physicians' Desk Reference,* 35th ed., Medical Economics Co, Oradell, NJ, 1981.
11. Silverberg M et al: Vomiting. In *Pediatric Therapy,* 5th ed, edited by HC Shirkey, CV Mosby, St. Louis, 1975, p 347.
12. Davidson M et al: Acute and chronic diarrhea. In *Pediatric Therapy,* 5th ed, edited by HC Shirkey, CV Mosby, St. Louis, 1975, p 631.
13. Ginsburg CM et al: Evaluation of Trimethobenzamide (Tigan) suppositories for treatment of nausea and vomiting in children. J Pediatr. 1980; 96:767.
14. Oderda GM et al: Emetic and antiemetic products. In *Handbook of Nonprescription Drugs,* 6th ed, edited by LL Corrigan and J Welsh, American Pharmaceutical Association, Washington, 1979, p 55.
15. Cirillo VJ et al: Pharmacology and therapeutic use of antihistamines. AJHP. 1976; 33:1200.
16. Gibbs D: Diseases of the alimentary system nausea and vomiting. Br Med J. 1976; 2:1489.
17. Shaw JE et al: Clinical pharmacology of scopolamine. Clin Pharmacol Ther. 1976; 19:115.
18. Graybiel A et al: Human assay of antimotion sickness drugs. Aviat Space Environ Med. 1975; 46:1107.
19. Wood CD: Antimotion sickness and antiemetic drugs. Drugs. 1979; 17:471.
20. Shaw JE et al: Transdermally administered scopolamine for prevention of motion sickness in a vertical oscillator. Clin Pharmacol Ther. 1977; 21:117.
21. Graybiel A et al: Prevention of experimental motion sickness by scopolamine absorbed through the skin. Aviat Space Environ Med. 1976; 47:1096.
22. Wheatley D: Treatment of pregnancy sickness. Br J Obstet Gynacol. 1977; 84:444.
23. Biggs JSG: Treatment of gastrointestinal disorders of pregnancy. Drugs. 1980; 19:70.
24. Huff PS: Safety of drug therapy for nausea and vomiting of pregnancy. J Fam Prac. 1980; 11:969.
25. Biggs JSG: Vomiting in pregnancy: causes and management. Drugs. 1975; 9:299.
26. Yerushalmy J et al: Evaluation of the teratogenic effect of meclizine in man. Am J Obstet Gyn. 1965; 93:553.
27. Anon. Indications for Bendectin narrowed. FDA Drug Bulletin. March 1981.
28. Mellin GW et al: Meclozine and foetal abnormalities. Lancet. 1963; 1:233.
29. Elias E et al: The slowing of gastric emptying by monosaccharides and disaccharides in test meals. J Physiol. 1968; 194:317.
30. Hunt JN et al: The slowing of gastric emptying by nine acids. J Physiol. 1969; 201:161.
31. Nelson MM et al: Association between drugs administered during pregnancy and congenital abnormalities of the fetus. Br Med J. 1971; 1:523.
32. Selcuk E et al: Double-blind evaluation of hydroxyzine as an antiemetic in pregnancy. J Reprod Med. 1971; 7:35.
33. Dickson JH: Congenital deformities associated with Bendectin. Can Med Assoc J. 1977; 117:721.
34. Patterson DC: Congenital deformities. Can Med Assoc J. 1969; 101:175.
35. Patterson DC: Congenital deformities associated with Bendectin. Can Med Assoc J. 1977; 116:1348.
36. Donnor D et al: Unusual fetal malformations after antiemetics in early pregnancy. Br Med J. 1978; 1:690.
37. Rothman KJ et al: Exogenous hormones and other drug exposures of children with congenital heart disease. Am J Epidem. 1979; 109:433.
38. Menzies CJG: Fetal malformation after Debendox treatment in early pregnancy. Br Med J. 1978; 1:925.
39. Mellor S: Fetal malformation after Debendox treatment in early pregnancy. Br Med J. 1978; 1:1055.
40. Kullander S: A prospective study of drugs and pregnancy: antiemetic drugs. Acta Obstet Gynecol Scand. 1976; 55:105.
41. Mitchell AA et al: Birth defects related to Bendectin use in pregnancy I. oral clefts and cardiac defects. JAMA. 1981; 245:2311.
42. Cordero JF et al: Is Bendectin a teratogen? JAMA. 1981; 245:2307.
43. Shapiro S et al: Antenatal exposure to doxylamine succinate and dicyclomine hydrochloride (Bendectin) in relation to congenital malformations, perinatal mortality rate, birth weight and intelligence quotient score. Am J Obstet Gynecol. 1977; 128:480.
44. Slone D et al: Antenatal exposure to the phenothiazines in relation to congenital malformation, perinatal mortality rate, birth weight, and intelligence quotient score. Am J Obstet Gynecol. 1977; 128:486.
45. Jick H et al: First-trimester drug use and congenital disorders. JAMA. 1981; 246:343.
46. Braly BE et al: The use of intramuscular perphenazine to control postoperative vomiting. Am J Surg. 1961; 102:120.

47. Scurr CF et al: Trials of perphenazine in the prevention of post-operative vomiting. Br Med J. 1958; 1:922.

48. Finn H et al: Antiemetic efficacy of benzquinamide. NY State J Med 1971; 71:651.

49. Medoff J: A double-blind evaluation of the anti-emetic efficacy of benzquinamide, prochlorperazine and trimethobenzamide in office practice. Curr Ther Res. 1970; 12:706.

50. Klein RL et al: Inhibition of apomorphine-induced vomiting by benzquinamide. Clin Pharmacol Ther. 1970; 11:530.

51. Larrauri RM: Benzquinamide parenteral for the treatment of post-operative nausea and vomiting. Curr Ther Res. 1969; 11:118.

52. Lutz H et al: Antiemetic effect of benzquinamide in post-operative vomiting. Curr Ther Res. 1972; 14:178.

53. Korttila K et al: Comparison of domperidone, droperidol, and metoclopramide in the prevention and treatment of nausea and vomiting after balanced anesthesia. Anesth Analg. 1979; 58:396.

54. Zegveld C et al: Domperidone in the treatment of post-operative vomiting: a double-blind multicenter study. Anesth Analg. 1978; 57:700.

55. Handley AJ: Metoclopramide in the prevention of post-operative nausea and vomiting. Br J Clin Prac. 1967; 21:460.

56. Clarke RSJ et al: Side effects of anti-emetics: results of a class experiment. Eur J Pharmacol. 1971; 14:291.

57. Dundee JW et al: Studies of drugs given before anesthesia XXIII: metoclopramide. Br J Anaesth. 1974; 46:509.

58. Tornetta FJ: Clinical studies with the new antiemetic, metoclopramide. Anesth Analg. 1969; 48:198.

59. Schulze-Delrieu K: Metoclopramide. Gastroenterology. 1979; 77:768.

60. Shields KG et al: Antiemetic effectiveness of haloperidol in human volunteers challenged with apomorphine. Anesth Analg. 1971; 50:1017.

61. Tornetta FJ: Double-blind evaluation of haloperidol for antiemetic activity. Anesth Analg. 1972; 51:964.

62. Barton MD et al: The use of haloperidol for treatment of postoperative nausea and vomiting—a double-blind placebo controlled trial. Anesthesiology 1975; 42:508.

63. Christman RS et al: Low-dose haloperidol as antiemetic treatment in gastrointestinal disorders: a double-blind study. Curr Ther Res. 1974; 16:1171.

64. Wolfson B et al: Investigation of the usefulness of trimethobenzamide (Tigan) for the prevention of postoperative nausea and vomiting. Anesth Analg. 1962; 41:172.

65. Moertel CG et al: Controlled clinical studies of orally administered antiemetic drugs. Gastroenterology. 1967; 57:262.

66. Ancillary therapy. In Manual of Oncology Therapeutics, edited by K See-Lasley and RJ Ignoffo, CV Mosby, St Louis, 1981, p 310.

67. Gutner LB et al: The effects of potent analgesics upon vestibular function. J Clin Invest. 1952; 31:259.

68. Lasagna L: The clinical evaluation of morphine and its substitutes as analgesics. Pharmacol Rev. 1964; 16:47.

69. Pinder RM: Metoclopramide: a review of its pharmacological properties and clinical use. Drugs. 1976; 12:81.

70. Burstein CL: Benzquinamide: cardiovascular stimulant useful during general anesthesia. Anesth Analg. 1963; 42:429.

71. Burstein CL: Respiratory effects of benzquinamide during anesthesia. Anesth Analg. 1963; 42:435.

72. Mull TD et al: Comparison of the ventilatory effects of two antiemetics, benzquinamide and prochlorperazine. Anesthesiology. 1974; 40:581.

73. Sciabine A et al: Some cardiovascular actions of benzquinamide. J Pharmacol Exp Ther. 1964; 144:131.

74. Steen SN et al: The effects of benzquinamide and prochlorperazine, separately and combined, on the human respiratory center. Anesthesiol 1972; 36:519.

75. Frytak S et al: Management of nausea and vomiting in the cancer patient. JAMA. 1981; 245:393.

76. Movan C et al: Incidence of nausea and vomiting with cytotoxic chemotherapy: a prospective randomized trial of antiemetics. Br Med J. 1979; 1:1323.

77. Hurley JD et al: Trimethobenzamide HCI in the treatment of nausea and vomiting associated with antineoplastic chemotherapy. J Clin Pharmacol. 1980; 20:352.

78. Moertel CG et al: A controlled clinical evaluation of antiemetic drugs. JAMA 1963; 186:116.

79. Sallen SE et al: Antiemetics in patients receiving chemotherapy for cancer: a randomized comparison of delta-9-tetrahydrocannabinol and prochlorperazine. N Engl J Med. 1980; 302:135.

80. Lucas VS et al: Delta-9-tetrahydrocannabinol for refractory vomiting induced by cancer chemotherapy. JAMA. 1980; 243:1241.

81. Chang AE et al: Delta-9-tetrahydrocannabinol as an antiemetic in cancer patients receiving high-dose methotrexate. Ann Intern Med. 1979; 91:819.

82. Neidhart JA et al: Specific antiemetics for specific cancer chemotherapeutic agents: haloperidol versus benzquinamide. Cancer. 1981; 47:1439.

83. Plotkin DA et al: Haloperidol in the treatment of nausea and vomiting due to cytotoxic drug administration. Cur Ther Res. 1973; 15:599.

84. Ekert H et al: Amelioration of cancer chemotherapy-induced nausea and vomiting by delta-9-tetrahydrocannabinol. Med J Aust. 1979; 2:657.

85. Frytak S et al: Delta-9-tetrahydrocannabinol as an antiemetic for patients receiving cancer chemotherapy. Ann Intern Med. 1979; 91:825.

86. Sallen SE et al: Antiemetic effect of delta-9-tetrahydrocannabinol in patients receiving cancer chemotherapy. N Engl J Med. 1975; 293:795.

87. Orr LE et al: Antiemetic effect of tetrahydrocannabinol compared nausea and emesis. Arch Intern Med. 1980; 140:1431.

88. Nahas GG: Marihuana-Deceptive Weed, Raven Press, New York, 1975, p 176.

89. Baker JJ et al: Nabilone as an antiemetic. N Engl J Med. 1979; 301:728.

90. Grossman B et al: Droperidol prevents nausea and vomiting from cis-platinum. N Engl J Med. 1979; 301:47.

91. Lee BJ: Methylprednisolone as an antiemetic. N Engl J Med. 1981; 304:486.

92. Rich MW et al: Methylprednisolone as an antiemetic drug during cancer chemotherapy—a pilot study. Gynecol Oncol. 1980; 9:193.

93. Kahn T et al: A single dose of metoclopramide in the control of vomiting from cis-dichlorodiammine-platinum (II) in man. Cancer Treat Rep. 1978; 62:1106.

94. Herman TS et al: Superiority of nabilone over prochlorperazine as an antiemetic in patients receiving cancer chemotherapy. N Engl J Med. 1979; 300:1295.

95. Steel N et al: Double-blind comparison of the antie-metic effects of nabilone and prochlorperazine on chemotherapy-induced emesis. Proc Am Soc Clin Oncol. 1979; 20:337.

96. Sawicka J et al: Transdermal therapeutic system sco-polamine: prevention of vomiting associated with can-cer chemotherapy. Proc Am Soc Clin Oncol. 1977; 18:302.

97. Reyntieus A: Domeperidone as an antiemetic; sum-mary of research reports. Postgrad Med J. 1979; 55:50.

98. Stoll BA et al: Radiation sickness an analysis of over 1000 controlled drug trials. Br Med J. 1962; 2:507.

99. Stryker JA et al: Ibuprofen (Motrin) prophylaxis during pelvic irradiation. Proc Am Soc Clin Oncol. 1979; 20:294.

100. Cooper JR et al: Control of radiation-induced emesis with promethazine, cimetidine, thiethylperazine, or na-loxone. Am J Vet Res. 1979; 40:1057.

101. Borrison HL et al: Physiology and pharmacology of vomiting. Pharmacol Rev. 1953; 5:193.

102. Fairwheather DVI: Nausea and vomiting in pregnancy. Am J Obstet Gyn. 1968; 102:135.

103. The Federal Register: 1975; 40:12935 (March 21).

104. Browne E et al: Vomiting mechanisms: trial of a new antiemetic—thiethylperazine. South Med J. 1961; 54:593.

105. Homburger F: Perphenazine as an antiemetic in cancer and other diseases. JAMA. 1958; 167:1240.

106. Homburger F et al: Chlorpromazine in nausea and vomiting due to cancer. N Engl J Med. 1954; 251:820.

107. Laffen RJ: Comparison of fluphenazine with other phe-nothiazines in inhibiting apomorphine induced vomit-ing. J Pharmacol Exp Ther. 1961; 131:130.

108. Smithy G et al: Prochlorperazine for the treatment of nausea and vomiting in patients with cancer and other diseases. N Engl J Med. 1957; 256:27.

109. Taylor C et al: Thiethylperazine: a clinical investiga-tion of a new antiemetic drug. Can Anesth Soc J. 1963; 10:51.

110. Weiss S et al: Symptomatic relief of nausea and vom-iting with perphenazine; a preliminary report. Am J Gastroent. 1958; 29:173.

111. Mayer JH: Chlorpromazine as a therapeutic agent. Arch Intern Med. 1955; 95:202.

112. Stephens CR et al: Control of nausea and vomiting with chlorpromazine: incidence of side effects. Arch Intern Med. 1955; 96:794.

113. Jaju BP et al: Effects of belladonna alkaloids on the vestibular system. Am J Physiol. 1970; 21:1248.

114. Chin HI et al: Motion sickness. Pharmacol Rev. 1955; 7:33.

Chapter 7

Constipation and Diarrhea

Linda L. Hart

All people complain of abnormalities in bowel function at one time or another. In addition, some individuals are preoccupied with the size, frequency, and consistency of their stools. As a result, many Americans utilize medications to regulate bowel function on a regular although irrational basis.

One individual's diarrhea can be another's constipation. Normal defecatory patterns vary from three stools per day to three stools per week (1). The average time between stools in healthy males is usually about 27 hours (2).

Constipation is defined as infrequent, incomplete, or painful evacuation of feces (4). *Diarrhea* is defined as increased frequency and/or fluid content of bowel movements (5). Since normal patterns of defecation and people's perception of bowel function vary, a careful and detailed history must be obtained to define any alteration in bowel hab-

its. The present complaint should be differentiated from the normal pattern of bowel movements for that individual.

Normal Colonic Physiology

About 2 liters per day of digestive residue and fluid pass from the small intestine to the colon. Approximately 90% of the fluid is reabsorbed along with certain components of the residue, leaving only about 200 grams, including 150 ml of water, to be eliminated as stool (5).

The colon is innervated by both parasympathetic and noradrenergic fibers, but it is the parasympathetic system which controls colonic motility. Basal colonic activity is nonpropulsive. Contractions of circular muscles move the contents back and forth over short distances. Propulsive movements result from parasympathetic stimulation and move contents at a forward movement rate of 5 cm/hr. Massive peristalsis begins in the right or transverse colon and rapidly moves the contents to the sigmoid and rectum. These massive contractions occur several times per day, are associated with eating or gastric emptying, and are usually strongest after breakfast. This may explain why many people move their bowels following breakfast (5,6).

Defecation is normally triggered by distention of the rectum. Nerve impulses from spinal reflexes and the brain stimulate contraction of the rectum which increases the pressure within the rectum. The simultaneous contraction of the internal and relaxation of the external anal sphincters, combined with increased intraabdominal pressure, result in evacuation. Defecation is a voluntary act and may be inhibited by voluntary contraction of the pelvic diaphragm and external anal sphincter. Resisting defecation on a routine basis can lead to chronic rectal distention, decreased afferent impulses from the rectum, lax motor tone, and chronic constipation (5).

Diagnosis

Constipation. A history is necessary to establish the extent, onset, and duration of the constipation and characteristics of the stool. Drugs should be excluded as contributing factors. Digi-

tal examination of the rectum or proctoscopy may be required. A barium enema may be indicated (4,5,9).

Diarrhea. In all cases of diarrhea, a detailed history of the illness including onset and duration of the diarrhea, characteristics of the stool, and associated symptoms is required. The recent administration of drugs, particularly antibiotics, or changes in diet should be considered as potential causes. Blood or pus in the stool indicate inflammation or infection. Stool culture may be diagnostic. Parasites or their eggs may be seen in an appropriately prepared stool specimen. Barium enema and sigmoidoscopy are sometimes necessary to determine the cause of diarrhea (5,7).

Laxatives

In the past, laxatives have been classified as stool softeners (or emollients), bulk-forming, saline, and stimulant (or irritant). More recently, stimulant laxatives have been classified as contact laxatives, because their action is on the intestinal wall. Table 1 lists safe and effective laxatives (9). Lactulose is an alternative laxative which is effective but expensive (10). Lactulose should be administered with caution since it can cause serious fluid loss, dehydration, and hypernatremia (11). Sorbitol is less effective than lactulose (8).

Table 1.

SAFE AND EFFECTIVE LAXATIVES

Stool Softeners	Bulk-Forming	Saline	Contact
glycerin 3 gm	psyllium 10–30 gm	magnesium citrate 11–18 gm	castor oil 15–60 ml
sorbitol 120 ml 30%	cellulose 4–6 gm	magnesium hydroxide 2.4–4.8 gm	bisacodyl 10–15 mg
docusate 100–300 mg	dietary bran	magnesium sulfate 10–50 gm	aloe 120–150 mg
	karaya gum 5–10 gm	disodium phosphate 1.9–3.8*gm	cascara
	polycarbophil	monosodium phosphate 8.3–16.6*gm	aromatic fluid extract 15–60 ml
	malt soup extract 4–12 gm	sodium biphosphate 9.6–19.2*gm	cascara sagrada fluid extract 1 ml
		sodium phosphate 3.6–7.2*gm	cascara sagrada extract 300 mg
			casantranol 30–90 mg
			danthron 15–150 mg
			senna
			senna leaf powder 2 gm
			senna fluid extract 2 ml
		*higher oral dose is also the rectal dose	senna syrup 8 ml
			sennosides A & B 12–36 mg
			senna pod concentrate 1–4 ml
			phenolphthalein 30–100 mg
			dehydrocholic acid 750–1500 mg

Onset of Effect. The stool softeners or bulk-forming laxatives, if taken regularly, will result in elimination of a soft, formed stool in one to three days. Contact laxatives usually result in a soft or semifluid bowel movement in 6 to 8 hours. Saline laxatives in full doses cause a watery evacuation in 1 to 3 hours (8).

Antidiarrheals

Opiates (narcotics) are safe and effective as antidiarrheal agents in acute self-limiting diarrhea (9). Various preparations of opium are available; camphorated tincture of opium (paregoric) is most commonly utilized. The recommended adult dose of paregoric is 5–10 ml qid (12). Paregoric is available in some states without a prescription. Other narcotics such as codeine 15 to 30 mg po q6h or diphenoxylate 2.5 to 5 mg qid can also be used to treat diarrhea in an adult; these require a prescription in all states. Since diarrhea may be a defense mechanism to rid the body of infecting organisms, the use of antimotility agents in the treatment of acute diarrhea has been questioned (13,14).

In 1975, the FDA panel on OTC antidiarrheal agents (10) was unable to classify other agents as safe and effective because of the lack of relevant scientific evidence. These include:

Absorbents: activated attapulgite, activated charcoal, kaolin, and pectin.

Anticholinergics: atropine, homatropine, and hyoscyamine.

Astringents: hydrated alumina powder, bismuth salts, calcium hydroxide, phenylsalicylate, and zinc phenosulfonate.

Other ingredients: calcium carbonate, Lactobacilli acidophilus and bulgaricus, sodium carboxymethylcellulose, and bismuth subsalicylate.

Kaopectate, which contains 25% kaolin and 1% pectin, causes stools to be more formed but has no effect on stool frequency, weight, or water content in children with diarrhea (15). The results of several other studies (15–18) suggest that neither kaolin, pectin, charcoal, nor lactobacillus can be recommended as being efficacious.

CONSTIPATION

1. *Simple or Drug-Induced Constipation.* H.C. is an obese 58-year-old male who complains of constipation. He has had only one bowel movement in seven days which contrasts with his usual one bowel movement every third day. He does not complain of nausea, vomiting, or abdominal or rectal pain. There is no blood or pus in the stools. He recently changed jobs and began making long business trips. He eats most of his meals at fast food restaurants or bars. He takes a number of medications: chlorpheniramine maleate 12 mg bid for allergic rhinitis, hydrochlorothiazide 50 mg bid and clonidine 0.3 mg bid for hypertension, imipramine 300 mg hs which he began taking two weeks ago for depression, and aluminum hydroxide gel or calcium carbonate tablets for indigestion.

What predisposing factors for constipation are present in H.C.'s history?

Constipation is frequently caused by psychological stress or alterations in daily routine such as that which can occur during travel. H.C. recently changed jobs and began making business trips. A diet low in fiber, lack of exercise, and decreased water intake also commonly contribute to constipation. H.C.'s dietary history suggests that some counseling may be appropriate.

Constipation can also be drug-induced. Drugs to consider include narcotic analgesics, anticholinergics, diuretics, and various inorganic ions such as iron, aluminium, and calcium. H.C. is taking an antihistamine and a tricyclic antidepressant which are constipating because of their anticholinergic properties. Anticholinergics retard the massive propulsive contractions which move feces over long distances or move large volumes of material. Constipation is a frequent side effect among patients treated with tricyclic antidepressants. H.C. is being treated with several inorganic ions which can cause constipation. These include aluminum and calcium which have astringent properties. A number of cases of intestinal obstruction caused by antacid tablets and gels have been reported (21–23). A magnesium-containing antacid could be substituted. Clonidine also causes constipation, and one case of ileus has been attributed to this agent (24).

2. What are general contraindications for laxative use and is a laxative contraindicated for this patient?

All laxatives are contraindicated in patients with cramps, colic, nausea, vomiting, or other symptoms of appendicitis or in any case of undiagnosed abdominal pain (9). Pain may be caused by inflammation of the colon wall or peritoneum. With peritoneal inflammation, there is sharp localized pain, abdominal guarding, and rebound tenderness. Fever and leukocytosis may or may not be present (25).

This patient does not appear to have any of the contraindications for laxative use, and the use of a laxative appears to be appropriate for this patient.

3. What laxative should be recommended for H.C.?

A contact laxative or a small dose of a saline laxative could be recommended. See Table 1. However, certain products should not be recommended because of his history of hypertension. The sodium content of some laxatives may be important in this patient; oral phosphate solutions, for example, contain 4.83 mEq of sodium per ml. Stool softeners or bulk-forming laxatives would not be satisfactory because of their slow onset of action.

4. What instructions should H.C. receive about his laxative treatment? What subsequent treatment should be recommended?

All contact laxatives may cause gripping, intestinal cramps, increased mucus secretion, and excess fluid and electrolyte loss. Saline laxatives are systemically absorbed and may cause serious electrolyte disturbances and water loss if used frequently (9). For specific adverse reactions, see Question 7.

The patient should be warned about the dangers of laxative habituation and educated concerning proper bowel habits. A high fiber diet, increased fluid intake, and increased exercise should be recommended. If simple measures do not alleviate the problem, the patient should be evaluated for more complicated causes of constipation.

5. High Fiber Diet. How should he increase the fiber in his diet? He has heard that high fiber diet cures a number of diseases; what are the legitimate claims for a high fiber diet in this patient?

An increase in dietary fiber is a natural and inexpensive way to treat and prevent constipation, and H.C. would probably benefit from increasing the amount of fiber in his diet. A diet which contains 50 grams (range: 30 to 60 gm) of dietary fiber should be prescribed. Unrefined car-

bohydrates such as whole grains should replace refined carbohydrates. Plenty of fruits and vegetables, preferably uncooked, should be eaten. Coarsely ground bran could be used as a food supplement. One tablespoonful mixed with food three times a week should be begun and increased as tolerated. The rapid introduction of bran into the diet may cause flatulence (26). Wheat bran is contraindicated in celiac disease (28). A high fiber diet is lower in calories per volume than traditional diets. Therefore, a high fiber diet may prevent future constipation and help him loose weight.

Dietary fiber has been proposed as a cure for constipation and irritable bowel syndrome and for prevention of hemorrhoids, appendicitis (29), colon cancer (30,31), hiatal hernia, diverticulosis (32,33), gallstones, and as an adjuvant for treatment of diabetes, hypercholesterolemia (34) and obesity (35). There is no clear evidence that dietary fiber prevents any chronic disease including colonic cancer (26,35,36). The low fiber diet of western civilization is also a diet high in animal fats, proteins, and concentrated carbohydrates. The cause and effect relationship is more complex than lack of fiber alone (26).

6. Laxative Abuse. P.H. is a 63-year-old woman who complains of diarrhea, dry skin with severe pruritus and rash, cough, skeletal pain in her hips, and tremor. She admits to extensive laxative use. She has taken 10 Correctol (docusate and phenolphthalein) and 5 Senokot (senna) tablets daily for the past 15 years. She also takes mineral oil 30 ml at bedtime, one bottle of magnesium citrate per week, and various other laxatives. Occasionally she uses Fleet (phosphate) enemas and Ducolax (bisacodyl) suppositories. She takes no other medication.

On physical examination, she was observed to be thin and in mild distress. Severe generalized eczematous dermatitis and hyperpigmentation were present on her forearms. Numerous ecchymoses and decreased skin tugor were also noted.

Abnormal laboratory findings were as follows: Sodium 145 mEq/L (nl 135–145 mEq/L), Potassium 2.9 mEq/L (nl 3.5–5.0 mEq/L), Calcium 7.9 mg/dl (nl 8.5–10 mg/dl), Magnesium 2.8 mEq/L (nl 1.5–2.0 mEq/L), Phosphate 4.7 mg/dl (nl 3.0–4.5 mg/dl), Albumin 3.0 mg/dl (nl 3.6–5.0 mg/dl), Creatinine 2.9 mg/dl (nl 0.6–1.5 mg/dl), BUN 48 mg/dl (nl 8–25 mg/dl), Hematocrit 33% (nl 37–48%), and Hemoglobin 10 gm/dl (nl 12–16 gm/dl).

Urinalysis showed a two plus proteinuria. Neither glucose nor ketones were present in the urine.

A stool examination was positive for phenolphthalein and negative for ova or parasites. Stool culture was negative. There were few white blood cells but many red blood cells in the stool sample.

Sigmoidoscopy demonstrated a grossly inflamed rectum with diffuse dark pigmentation of the colon wall.

After barium enema, a dilated terminal ileum, contracted cecum, loss of haustral markings, and areas of strictures were noted.

Colon biopsy demonstrated atrophy of smooth muscle and excess submucosal adipose tissue.

What is the subjective and objective evidence that P.H. has "cathartic colon?"

The abnormal barium enema findings associated with cathartic colon are predominantly right-sided as noted above; severe ulceration is usually not seen. Pathologically, there is loss of innervation and thickening of the muscularis mucosae in addition to the findings that were seen on biopsy. The anthraquinone laxatives such as senna and cascara cause a pigmentation of the bowel wall (melanosis coli) which is associated with degeneration of the myenteric plexus (37,38,39).

"Cathartic colon" has been described in patients who have chronically ingested contact laxatives in very large doses for 15 to 40 years; other types of laxatives have not been implicated. The doses that P.H. claims to have ingested are consistent with cathartic colon. The history is frequently underestimated in these patients.

7. What other adverse effects of chronic laxative abuse may be manifested in P.H.?

Specific adverse effects of laxatives depend upon the ingredients ingested (40). P.H. has severe dermatitis and pruritus. Fixed drug eruptions, erythema multiforme, Steven Johnson's syndrome, and lupus erythematosus have been attributed to phenolphthalein (41,42). This agent can also cause albuminuria and a red color in alkaline urine; P.H. has proteinuria. Mineral oil is sometimes aspirated by those with swallowing abnormalities and/or abnormalities of consciousness. Such aspiration can cause lipoid pneumonia which is frequently an asymptomatic condition that is found by routine chest radiography and at autopsy (43,44). P.H. complains of a cough and needs a chest x-ray to rule out this problem. Phenolphthalein and mineral oil have been reported to cause osteomalacia (44,45). This is consistent with P.H.'s complaints of skeletal pain in her hips and low serum calcium. Although P.H. does not claim to have ingested calomel, she has renal impairment, dermatitis, colitis and tremor which, along with dementia, is consistent with mercury intoxication (46,47).

Chronic laxative ingestion may cause dehydration and electrolyte disturbances. Hypernatremia (11,48), hypokalemia (49–52), hypocalcemia (51,53–56), and hyperphosphatemia (57–59) have resulted from laxative use and abuse and all are present in P.H. Usually infants and young children (53,54,57,58), patients with renal disease (54), and those with gastrointestinal disorders such as Hirschsprung's disease and imperforate anus (48,59) appear to be predisposed to these adverse effects. P.H. appears to have renal disease.

The use of laxatives can lead to malabsorption and steatorrhea (60). P.H. has a low serum albumin and evidence of fat soluble vitamin deficiencies including dry skin, ecchymoses, low serum calcium, and skeletal pain.

Factitious diarrhea may be due to laxative ingestion (61–64). P.H. presents with diarrhea and a stool that is positive for phenolphthalein.

8. How should P.H. be treated for her laxative abuse?

The patient who has been chronically ingesting laxatives must be educated concerning proper bowel function, the lack of harmful effects of infrequent bowel movements, and the adverse effects of laxative ingestion. The patient should develop a morning routine that allows her to sit on the toilet for 10 to 15 minutes after breakfast without interruption. A high fiber diet should be prescribed along with exercise and increased fluid intake. The doses of laxatives should gradually be reduced. If needed, tap water enemas can be used intermittently until normal bowel function returns. Success of the bowel retraining program is often poor, because it depends upon the willingness of the patient to discontinue laxative ingestion (65).

9. Irritable Bowel Syndrome (IBS). T.L. is a 34-year-old female advertising executive

who complains of chronic constipation which has troubled her for the past seven years. She has severe lower abdominal cramping which is relieved by defecation. Her stools are hard, fragmented (pellet-like), and usually coated with mucus. Sometimes, if her schedule is very busy, she has watery diarrhea that interrupts her morning appointments. At other times she has no gastrointestinal complaints at all. Her appetite is normal and she has not lost any weight. She is frequently nervous or depressed.

Physical examination and laboratory reports were unremarkable. Sigmoidoscopy, barium enema, and stool examination revealed no pathology.

What is the subjective and objective evidence for irritable bowel syndrome in this patient?

The pain in irritable bowel syndrome is usually intermittent and crampy and is located in the lower abdomen. Passage of flatus or stool will relieve the pain. The spastic constipation may alternate with diarrhea. The diarrhea is usually not associated with any pain, and the stools may be watery or pasty. The diarrhea usually consists of three to four bowel movements in the morning with no complaints for the rest of the day; nocturnal diarrhea is rare. Exacerbations and remissions are common in the long history of IBS. The physical examination is within normal limits and there is no evidence of physical deterioration. T.L. has these typical findings of IBS. There are no clear, reproducible criteria for the diagnosis of IBS. The diagnosis is made from the history and the absence of other findings on examination (66,67). The abnormality in IBS is disordered colon motility which may be demonstrated by manometery, although this is rarely necessary (67–69). These patients may have significant psychological disturbances with depressive, hysteric, or obsessive-compulsive traits.

IBS, which is a very common gastrointestinal disorder, may represent a population of patients who are overly concerned with bowel symptoms and who are very bowel conscious. They may abuse laxatives, thereby distorting the history and aggravating the condition (25,65,67).

10. How should this patient's IBS be treated?

Initial treatment involves reassuring the patient that she does not have a life-threatening disorder. Information about IBS should be given to the patient with particular emphasis on the relationship of the symptoms to stress. The patient should not be told that the disorder is psychological or that "her problem is all in her head." If the patient were well adjusted prior to the onset of symptoms, information and education may be all that is required for treatment. There is no diet or drug that will be effective in all patients with IBS. Therefore, after patient education is completed, various treatments may be tried. Since the disease is relatively benign and is chronic, the treatment should be free of serious side effects (66,67).

Some patients with IBS respond favorably to a high fiber diet. Harvey et al reported a decrease in symptoms in patients who were treated with a high fiber diet (70). However, Søltoft et al found bran to be without benefit in IBS (71). A high fiber diet should be prescribed for T.L. and a bulk-forming laxative (see Table 1) may be tried if the high fiber diet is not effective.

Anticholinergics, usually in combination with a tranquilizer, are frequently prescribed for the symptoms of IBS, although evidence of efficacy is lacking. A 1975 review of 400 papers on eighteen of the most commonly prescribed oral anticholinergic agents failed to reveal any well-controlled trials showing that these drugs are effective for IBS (73). Since that time Sullivan et al conducted a double blind trial in 10 patients with IBS and found that colonic motility was somewhat normalized after a single dose of propantheline (68). Rhodes et al also reported 10 of 15 IBS patients were subjectively helped "some" or "a lot" with the combination of 30 mg phenobarbital and 8 mg belladonna (74). An anticholinergic such as propantheline 15 mg tid could be recommended for T.L. if all other maneuvers are ineffective. The therapeutic endpoint should be defined before initiating therapy and the patient monitored for adverse effects.

Neuroleptics and tranquilizers cannot be recommended because of the potential for serious side effects. However, treatment of any existing emotional problems may improve IBS. Relaxation, hypnosis, and biofeedback may benefit patients with IBS (76) and could be recommended as alternative therapy.

11. Colon Examination. D.G. is a 55-year-old male with diverticulosis who is scheduled for a sigmoidoscopy and barium enema

for evaluation of his continued constipation. **What is the best laxative regimen to prepare this patient for these studies?**

The colon must be cleaned before examination by sigmoidoscopy or barium enema. The regimen should be efficacious and cause the patient the least discomfort possible. Various regimens have been advocated.

Meisel et al compared the effects of oral mannitol, saline enemas, phosphate enemas, and rectal bisacodyl on the rectal mucosa. In this double blind study, the rectal mucosa of volunteers treated with either saline enemas or oral mannitol could not be distinguished from normal mucosa. Both phosphate enemas and bisacodyl in either suppository or rectal solution caused mucosal hyperemia and obliteration of vasculature in all subjects. Increased mucosal friability was seen in four patients treated with bisacodyl and in one patient who was given phosphate enemas. The epithelial surface, as seen on rectal biopsy, was disrupted in those treated with bisacodyl (80). Therefore, it should be kept in mind that bowel preparation may result in abnormalities on examination, although these would be more important in a patient with inflammatory bowel disease than in this patient.

Castor oil has been traditionally used to prepare patients for barium enema. Castor oil, through its action on the small intestine, results in complete evacuation of the bowel in 2 hours (9). This rapid onset of action precludes bedtime use. The emulsified form of castor oil is a more palatable alternative, but in one study 120 ml of castor oil emulsion (Neoloid) was not as effective as 60 ml of plain castor oil (81). Patients who take castor oil are also given "enemas until clear" just prior to the examination. In a study of 102 patients, 40% were unable to retain any enema solution, 60% required three or more enemas, and only 25% of the study films were considered excellent (82). The enema itself may cause hyperemic changes in the mucosa and increase mucus secretion. Therefore it is recommended that the examination not be performed until at least 30 minutes after the last enema (83). Rectal irritation lasting as long as three weeks after soap enemas has been reported, as has anaphylaxis, rectal gangrene, and serious fluid loss secondary to acute colitis (84). It is recommended that soap enemas not be used. Profuse bleeding, laceration of internal hemorrhoids, and suppuration has been attributed to self-administration of concentrated enemas (85). This regimen of castor oil and enemas should not be recommended.

Another regimen that is used to prepare patients for barium enema examination is known as the hydration technique (86,87) and is recommended for D.G. The patient is placed on a clear liquid diet 24 to 48 hours prior to the examination. With lunch or dinner on the day prior to the study, the patient is given 11 to 14 oz of magnesium citrate. At bedtime the patient is given bisacodyl 10 to 20 mg orally. The enteric coated tablets should not be chewed and should not be taken within one hour of antacids or milk. The effect of oral bisacodyl occurs in 6 to 12 hours. A bisacodyl suppository is inserted on the morning of the study one hour prior to the examination. The effect of rectal bisacodyl is seen in 15 to 60 minutes. The patient drinks a glassful of liquid every hour during the preparation. This regimen has been found superior to castor oil and enemas; 85% of radiologic examinations were rated as good (86) and 55% of films were rated as excellent (87). All patients complained of cramps with castor oil and expressed a dislike of the enemas (86).

A patient who has had a barium enema should be given a contact or saline laxative after the procedure to prevent impaction of the barium. Milk of magnesia 30 ml is effective. Fluid intake should also be increased if it is not contraindicated by other medical problems.

12. *Prophylaxis for Constipation.* J.F. is a 65-year-old man who suffered a myocardial infarction three days ago and is being routinely treated in the Coronary Care Unit. His other medical problems include diabetes mellitus, hypertension, congestive heart failure, and chronic renal failure.

Should J.F. be treated to prevent constipation? If so, what laxative would be appropriate?

Patients with a recent myocardial infarction (MI) may require a laxative to prevent constipation. Defecation alters hemodynamics, and straining at stool may be dangerous if a thrombus is present in the heart or the deep veins of the legs. Deaths from emboli, ventricular rupture, and cardiogenic shock have been attributed to straining in patients with a recent MI (88). Bowel movements usually do not occur and are not encouraged during the first three days after an MI. Although there are no controlled studies to support the practice, patients with a recent MI are routinely placed on laxatives.

No well controlled trials support the choice of one laxative over another in these patients, but only mild laxatives should be used. An uncontrolled trial indicates that docusate 240 mg daily provides excellent results in post-MI patients (88). A bulk forming laxative could be used instead, but the sodium and glucose content must be considered for this patient. For example, Metamucil Effervescent contains more than 250 mg of sodium per dose and can not be recommended. In contrast, the amount of sodium in docusate is insignificant. Metamucil and L.A. Formula contain 50% glucose and would not be a good choice in this patient with diabetes. Effersyllium and Konsyl are bulk forming laxatives which do not contain excessive amounts of sodium or glucose. Milk of magnesia is frequently prescribed, but approximately 15 to 30% of magnesium is absorbed and toxicity could occur in this patient with renal failure (9). Oral phosphate laxatives contain 12.45 mEq of phosphate per ml and the enemas contain 4.15 mEq/ml. Phosphate enemas and laxatives have been reported to cause hyperphosphatemia and hypocalcemia in patients with renal failure (54,56).

13. Docusate 100 mg bid was ordered for J.F. and two days later he complained of constipation. Is this an effective dosage?

Although docusate 200 mg daily is usually effective (90,91), poor response has been reported (89). The maximal effects of docusate are seen in three days (8). If necessary, the dosage can be increased to 400 mg daily and adjusted at three day intervals.

14. *Constipation in a Pregnant Patient with Hemorrhoids*. R.M. is in the eighth month of a healthy pregnancy. She now complains of constipation and painful external hemorrhoids. Her medications include prenatal vitamins and ferrous sulfate. Should her constipation be treated? If so, what laxative would be appropriate?

Constipation is a common complaint during pregnancy, and a laxative should be recommended for R.M. In pregnancy, hormones decrease smooth muscle tone in the large bowel and the pressure of the uterus may delay or inhibit emptying of the bowel or inhibit contraction of abdominal muscles and the diaphragm. Hemorrhoids, a common complication of pregnancy, and painful anal lesions associated with them may cause voluntary suppression of the defecatory urge

(102). Iron therapy may also be contributing to R.M.'s constipation.

Stool softeners or bulk laxatives can be used but contact or strong laxatives should be avoided (102). Podophyllin may be teratogenic (103,104). The recommended laxative should be continued into the postpartum period when constipation is caused by ileus secondary to bowel dilation in a decompressed abdomen, perineal pain, and laxness of the anal sphincter and abdominal muscles (102). Laxatives which are secreted into breast milk may result in diarrhea in the infant. Phenolphthalein and the anthraquinones have been reported to cause this unwanted effect (105–108).

Patients with anorectal disease (hemorrhoids, fissures, or fistulas) should take a stool softener or a bulk-forming agent when a laxative is indicated. A psyllium or cellulose product could be recommended. Patients with anal disease should avoid mineral oil, because the bacteria-laden oily film that coats the rectum has been implicated in causing infection and delaying healing in rectal lesions (44).

15. *Constipation in the Elderly*. M.N., a 73-year-old woman, is a debilitated nursing home resident who complains of chronic constipation. Her stools are small, hard, and difficult to pass. She is not receiving any medication which might contribute to her constipation. What factors predispose the elderly to constipation? How should her constipation be treated?

Individuals do not necessarily become constipated with age (113,114), but patients who are immobile may not have the same increase in propulsive colon activity after meals that occurs in physically active individuals (6). Muscle tone decreases with aging, and in some debilitated patients muscle atrophy prevents evacuation of feces (117). The amount of rectal distention required to produce rectal discomfort increases with age (118).

In this patient with small, hard stools which are difficult to pass, a high fiber diet is indicated. A bulk-forming laxative may be used temporarily or chronically if her diet cannot be changed. The clinician could recommend Effersyllium or Metamucil one tablespoonful in water or fruit juice twice daily with instructions to drink additional liquids. The laxative effect of the bulk-forming agents begins in 12 to 24 hours, but a full effect may not be seen for three days. The stool that is produced is soft and formed, unlike the watery stool some patients expect with laxative use. The patient should also be warned that flatulence is likely to occur at the beginning of therapy, and increased fluid intake may relieve this side effect (8).

There is no scientific evidence to justify the choice of one bulk-forming agent over any other product in this class. Important factors to consider include taste, palatability, cost, convenience, and ingredient restrictions such as sodium or glucose (see Question 12).

Stool softeners are not of much value in elderly patients with hypotonic constipation. The colon in these patients is full of putty-like stool which cannot be evacuated. Those who do not respond adequately to high fiber diet and/or bulk laxatives may require a contact laxative in addition (111,112). Cascara sagrada fluid extract 5 ml, bisacodyl 5–10 mg, danthron 75 mg, or senna 12 mg may be given, but all will cause cramping (8).

16. *Laxative Drug Interactions.* **Laxatives are used by many of the residents of the nursing home where the above patient resides. What laxative drug interactions have been reported?**

Cellulose derivatives are reported to bind digitalis, nitrofurantoin, and salicylates, but the clinical significance of this interaction is unknown (9).

Mineral oil may decrease the absorption of fat soluble vitamins. A dose of mineral oil greater than 2.5 ml given with meals significantly decreases the plasma level of vitamin A (97). Daily ingestion of 15 to 30 ml of mineral for one to two weeks resulted in decreased prothrombin levels in a third of the patients studied in one trial (98). The timing of the dose in relation to meals was not stated.

Docusate enhances the absorption of mineral oil which has been associated with granuloma formation in lymph nodes, the liver, and intestinal mucosa (44). The concomitant ingestion of these two agents is not recommended.

Laxative ingestion that produces diarrhea may interfere with absorption of isoniazid, oral anticoagulants, and sulfonamides (101).

DIARRHEA

17. *Diarrhea in Infants.* **A 15-month-old infant with severe diarrhea caused by viral gastroenteritis was treated with fluid and electrolyte replacement. The parent asks if Lomotil (diphenoxylate with atropine) can be prescribed for the child.**

The administration of Lomotil to infants and young children is dangerous. The drug may decrease the frequency of bowel movements without decreasing the fluid and electrolyte loss into the bowel. This may decrease the awareness of the need to compensate for these losses (122). The anticholinergic effects of urinary retention, dry mucous membranes, thirst, and flushing can occur in children even with the small doses of atropine contained in Lomotil (122). Serious poisonings have occurred with ingestions of less than ten tablets of Lomotil (123).

Specific recommendations for fluid and electrolyte replacement in infants with diarrhea are presented in the chapter on Pediatric Therapy.

18. *Traveler's Diarrhea.* **R.K. and his family are planning a trip to Mexico. They have heard of a variety of recommendations for traveler's diarrhea. What advice should be given and what drugs have been used?**

They should be advised to avoid tap water, iced beverages, and uncooked foods. Bottled carbonated beverages, beer, and boiled water are safe.

Fluid and Electrolyte Replacement. Should traveler's diarrhea occur, fluid and electrolyte replacement is the most important treatment. A solution which contains 3.5 gm NaCl, 2.5 gm $NaHCO_3$, 1.5 gm KCl, and 20 gm glucose per liter is available in some countries and is useful for oral rehydration (121). Canned fruit juices or carbonated beverages with added salt and bicarbonate can be used if electrolyte solution is unavailable. A two glass method for rehydration is as follows (132):

Glass I

orange or apple juice	8 oz
honey or corn syrup	1/2 tsp
salt	1 pinch

Glass II

boiled or carbonated water	8 oz
$NaHCO_3$	1/4 tsp

Glasses I and II are alternated. Additional water (carbonated or boiled) is taken as desired.

Bismuth Subsalicylate. Bismuth Subsalicylate (Pepto-Bismol) has been found to decrease the number of stools and provide relief of nausea and abdominal pain in traveler's diarrhea, but water content and weight of the stools and vomiting are not affected (135). The active moiety in this preparation has not been identified. Bismuth inhibits the action of castor oil in mice (136), and acetylsalicylate has been claimed effective in radiation-induced diarrhea (137) and infantile diarrhea (138). The doses required, 30–60 ml every 30 minutes for eight doses result in therapeutic concentrations of salicylate. Therefore, patients who are already taking large doses of salicylate or drugs that may be affected by salicylate (eg, uricosurics, oral anticoagulants) should not take bismuth subsalicylate (139). Large doses of bismuth subsalicylate suspension (60 ml qid) also have been shown effective in decreasing the incidence of traveler's diarrhea (149), but most individuals will find this prophylactic treatment inconvenient.

Antimotility Agents. Antimotility agents such as Lomotil, Imodium, and paregoric should be avoided. These agents may delay the clearance of infecting organisms and should never be used for more than three days or by persons with a fever or with blood or pus in the stools. Nevertheless, these agents may relieve abdominal cramps and decrease the inconvenience of frequent visits to the toilet (132).

Iodochlorhydroxyquin. Clioquinol or iodochlorhydroxyquin (Enterovioform) is one of the family of halogenated hydroxyquinolines. This drug is no longer available in the United States but is available in other countries, frequently without a prescription. Except for one poorly designed study, there is no evidence that this drug is of any therapeutic or prophylactic benefit in traveler's diarrhea (133). The use of halogenated hydroxyquinolines has been associated with the development of a dose-related peripheral neuropathy and/or myelopathy (140). The epidemiological data describing subacute myeloptic neuropathy and its occurrence outside of Japan had been debated (141,142), but this toxicity has been documented in other countries (142,143). Because of lack of evidence of efficacy in traveler's diarrhea and possible toxicity, it is recommended that this drug not be used.

Antibiotics. Enteropathogenic *Escherichia coli* (EPEC) is the pathogen isolated in 50 to 75% of cases of traveler's diarrhea. Other infectious agents such as *Salmonella, Shigella, giardia,* and enteroviruses may also be involved. Antibiotics are not indicated unless *Shigella* are isolated (133,134).

Although prophylactic doxycycline may be effective in preventing traveler's diarrhea, it should not be recommended for R.K. and his family. Prophylactic doxycycline has been found effective in double-blind, controlled trials in Kenya and Morocco (145). This treatment is less likely to be effective in countries where EPEC are less sensitive to tetracyclines. For example, 45% of EPEC are reported to be resistant to tetracyclines in the Philippines, Korea, and Indonesia (145). Prophylactic doxycycline therapy may predispose travelers to infections with *Shigella* and *Salmonella,* although there is no evidence in man for the latter (147,148). Furthermore, doxycycline may cause photosensitization, and most of the countries where prophylaxis might be considered are tropical. Finally, there is fear that widespread use of doxycycline prophylaxis in travelers will increase the number of organisms which are resistant to tetracyclines (145,146).

19. *Lactase Deficiency.* **F.P. is a 22-year-old Black male who developed bloating, crampy abdominal pain, flatulence, and diarrhea after meals. He related the onset of symptoms to the ingestion of milk, although he had drunk milk as a child without problems. He was diagnosed as having lactase deficiency and given appropriate dietary instructions. What predisposing factors for lactase deficiency does F.P. have and what mechanisms are involved?**

F.P. is Black and the deficiency, which is probably hereditary, occurs in 60 to 90% of Blacks and Asians. It also occurs in 60 to 70% of Jews, others of Mediterranean ancestry, and American Indians. The prevalence of lactase deficiency among Caucasians in the United States is between 10 to 20%. Adults with lactase deficiency are able to tolerate milk as infants, and the symptoms usually develop during adolescence or early adulthood as in this patient. Lactase deficiency is not an allergic or hypersensitivity reaction to milk proteins. Disaccharidases in the intestinal brush border split sugar molecules to moieties that can be absorbed. Fermentation of the lactose by colonic bacteria produces short chain fatty acids and lactic acid. The accumulation of nonabsorbable molecules in the lumen inhibits water and electrolyte absorption, thereby causing an osmotic diarrhea. The symptoms of lactase deficiency are those described by the patient. Lactase deficiency also occurs in inflammatory bowel disease and temporarily after viral gastroenteritis (150,151).

20. How should his lactase deficiency diarrhea be treated?

The treatment of diarrhea due to lactase deficiency is elimination of milk and certain milk products from the diet. The patient should avoid all milk products until his symptoms subside. He then may reintroduce small quantities of milk into his diet. The amount of milk necessary to produce symptoms may be from 1 to 4 glassfuls. Lact Aid is a yeast-derived beta-galactosidase in a glycerin vehicle which converts lactose to glucose and galactose. The product, which is added to milk prior to drinking, is available in pharmacies and specialty food stores or from Sugar Lo Company, P.O. Box 1100, Pleasantville, N.J., 08232.

21. *Viral Gastroenteritis.* J.S. is a 30-year-old woman with viral gastroenteritis. How should her diarrhea be treated?

Viral gastroenteritis produces acute self-limiting diarrhea. Treatment should consist only of rest and oral fluids in otherwise healthy individuals. Serious morbidity is seen only in infants or the elderly.

Bismuth subsalicylate suspension may be of limited benefit. In a clinical trial in volunteers inoculated with parovirus, 30 ml every thirty minutes for eight doses decreased the severity and duration of abdominal cramps and the duration of the GI symptoms, but the number, weight, and water content of the stools were not affected (169).

22. J.S. was given a prescription for loperamide (Imodium) to make her more comfortable. How does loperamide differ from diphenoxylate with atropine (Lomotil) or codeine? When should antimotility drugs such as these be avoided?

Like diphenoxylate, paregoric, or codeine, loperamide inhibits peristaltic activity by acting on the circular and longitudinal muscles of the intestinal wall. Its activity is similar to diphenoxylate with atropine (Lomotil) or codeine (171–175).

Antimotility agents are contraindicated in patients with infectious diarrhea caused by organisms that may invade the mucosa (13,14) and in patients with pseudomembranous colitis (176). Toxic megacolon can occur in patients with ulcerative colitis who are treated with antimotility drugs (177,178). These drugs should not be used in infants or children.

References

1. Connell AM et al: Variations in bowel habits in two population samples. Br Med J. 1965; 2:1095.
2. Rendtorff RC et al: Stool patterns of healthy adult males. Dis Colon Rectum. 1967; 10:222.
3. Pelot D et al: Constipation of prolonged duration. Am J Gastroenterology. 1975; 63:252.
4. Devroede G: Constipation: Mechanisms and management. In *Gastrointestinal Diseases,* 2nd ed, edited by MN Sleisenger and JS Fordtran, WB Saunders, Philadelphia, 1978, p 368.
5. Goldfinger SE: Constipation, diarrhea, and disturbances of anorectal function. In *Harrison's Principles of Internal Medicine,* 9th ed, edited by KJ Isselbacher, RD Adams, E Braunwald, RG Petersdorf and JD Wilson, McGraw Hill Book Company, New York, 1980, p 198.
6. Holdstock DJ: Propulsion (mass movements) in the human colon and its relationship to meals and somatic activity. Gut. 1970; 11:91.
7. Krejs GH et al: Physiology and pathophysiology of ion and water movements in the human intestine. In *Gastrointestinal Diseases,* 2nd ed, edited by MH Sleisenger and JS Fordtran, WB Saunders, Philadephia, 1978, p 213.
8. Fingl E: Laxatives and cathartics. In the *Pharmacologic Basis of Therapeutics,* 6th ed, edited by AG Gilman, LS Goodman and A Gilman, Macmillan, New York, 1980; p 1002.
9. Proposal to establish monographs for OTC laxative, antidiarrheal, emetic and antiemetic products. Federal Register. 1975; 40:12902.
10. Lactulose (Chronulac) for constipation. Med Lett Drugs Ther. 1980; 22:2.
11. Kaupe et al: Hypernatremia after administration of lactulose. Ann Intern Med. 1977; 86:745.
12. Jaffe JH et al: Opiod analgesics and antagonists. In *The Pharmacologic Basis of Therapeutics,* 6th ed, edited by AG Gilman, LS Goodman, and A Gilman, The MacMillan Co, New York, 1980, p 494.
13. Dupont HL et al: Adverse effect of Lomotil therapy in shigellosis. JAMA. 1973; 226:1525.

14. Dupont HL et al: Lomotil therapy of induced shigellosis. Clin Res. 1973; 21:598.

15. Portnoy BL et al: Antidiarrheal agents in the treatment of acute diarrhea in children. JAMA. 1976; 236:844.

16. Limaye AS: Comparison of Lomotil with Pectokab in furazolidone treated infective diarrhea. Curr Therap Res. 1980; 28:80.

17. Alestig K et al: Acute nonspecific diarrhea studies on the use of charcoal, kaolin-pectin, and diphenoxylate. Practitioner. 1979; 222:859.

18. Pearce JL et al: Controlled trial of orally administered lactobacilli in acute infantile diarrhea. J Pediatr. 1974; 84:261.

19. Diamond S: Amitriptyline in the treatment of gastrointestinal diseases. Psychosomat. 1964; 5:221.

20. Connell PH: Stimulant and antidepressant drugs in *Side Effects of Drugs*, Vol VI, edited by L Meyler and A Herxheimer, The Williams and Wilkins Co., Baltimore and Excerpta Medica Foundation, Amsterdam, 1968, p 10.

21. Ghose MK et al: Spontaneous colonic perforation; a complication in a hemodialysis patient. JAMA. 1970; 214; 145.

22. Brettschneider L et al: Intestinal obstruction due to antacid gels. Gastroenterology. 1965; 49:291.

23. Potyk D: Intestinal obstruction from impacted antacid tablets. N Engl J Med. 1970; 283:134.

24. Bauer GE et al: Pseudoobstruction due to clonidine. Br Med J. 1976; 1:169.

25. Lamont JT et al: Diseases of the colon and rectum. In *Harrison's Principles of Internal Medicine*, 9th ed, edited by KJ Isselbacher, RD Adams, E Braunwald, RG Petersdorf and JD Wilson, McGraw Hill Book Company, New York, 1980, p 1419.

26. Mendeloff AI: Dietary fiber and human health. N Engl J Med. 1977; 297:811.

27. Southgate DAT et al: A guide to calculating intakes of dietary fiber. J Hum Nutr. 1976; 30:303.

28. Thompson WG: Laxatives, clinical pharmacology and rational use. Drugs. 1980;19:49.

29. Burkitt DP: The aetiology of appendicitis. Br J Surg. 1971; 58:695.

30. Burkitt DP: Possible relationships between bowel cancer and dietary habits. Proc Roy Soc Med. 1971; 64:964.

31. Irving D et al: Fiber and cancer of the colon. Br J Cancer. 1973; 28:462.

32. Painter NS et al: Unprocessed bran in treatment of diverticular disease of the colon. Br Med J. 1972; 2:137.

33. Painter NS et al: Diverticular disease of the colon, a deficiency disease of western civilization. Br Med J. 1971; 2:450.

34. Jenkins DJA et al: Effect of pectin, guar gum and wheat fiber on serum cholesterol. Lancet. 1975; 1:116.

35. Pomare EW: Dietary fiber: When is it worth a trial? Drugs. 1977; 14:213.

36. Mendeloff AL: A critique of fiber deficiency. Am J Dig Dis. 1976; 21:109.

37. Plum GE et al: Prolonged cathartic abuse resulting in roentgen evidence suggestive of enterocolitis. Am J Roentgen. 1960; 83:919.

38. Urso FP et al: The cathartic colon. Radiology. 1975; 116:557.

39. Clain J et al: Cathartic colon with unusual histological features. S Afr Med J. 1974; 48:216.

40. Salden CE: Effects of purgative abuse. Roy Soc Med Pro. 1972; 65:288.

41. Lewin KJB: Phenolphthalein reactions simulating disseminated (systemic) lupus erythematosus. Lancet. 1962; 2:461.

42. Savin JA: Current causes of fixed drug eruptions. Br J Dermatol. 1970; 83:546.

43. Frieman DG: Oil aspiration (lipoid) pneumonia in adults, a study of 47 cases. Arch Intern Med. 1940; 66:11.

44. Becker GL: The case against mineral oil. Am J Dig Dis. 1952; 19:344.

45. Frame B et al: Osteomalacia induced by laxative (phenolphthalein) ingestion. Arch Intern Med. 1971; 128:794.

46. Davis LE et al: Central nervous system intoxication from mecurous chloride laxatives. Arch Neurol. 1974; 30:428.

47. Wands JR et al: Chronic inorganic mercury poisoning due to laxative abuse. Am J Med. 1974; 57:92.

48. Fonkalsrud E et al: Hypernatremic dehydration from hypertonic enemas in congenital megacolon. JAMA. 1969; 199:584.

49. Schwartz WB et al: Metabolic and renal studies in chronic potassium depletion resulting from overuse of laxatives. J Clin Invest. 1953; 32:258.

50. Gossian W et al: Surreptitious laxation and hypokalemia. Ann Intern Med. 1972; 76:671.

51. Goldfinger P: Hypokalemia metabolic acidosis and hypocalcemic tetany in a patient taking laxatives. J Mt Sinai Hosp. 1969; 36:113.

52. Fleischer N et al: Chronic laxative-induced hyperaldosteronism and hypokalemia simulating Bartter's syndrome. Ann Intern Med. 1969; 70:791.

53. Honig P et al: Hypocalcemic tetany following hypertonic phosphate enemas. Clin Pediatr (Phila). 1975; 14:7.

54. Chesney RW: Tetany following phosphate enemas in chronic renal disease. Am J Dis Chil. 1974; 127:584.

55. Sotos JD et al: Hypocalcemia coma following two pediatric phosphate enemas. Pediatrics. 1977; 60:305.

56. McConnell TN: Fatal hypocalcemia from phosphate absorption from laxative preparations. JAMA. 1971; 216:147.

57. Levitt M et al: Inorganic phosphate (laxative) poisoning resulting in tetany in an infant. J Pediatr. 1973; 82:481.

58. Smith M et al: Coma in infant due to hypertonic sodium phosphate medications. J Pediatr. 1973; 82:481.

59. Moseley PK et al: Fluid and serum electrolyte disturbances as a complication of enemas in Hirschsprung's disease. Am J Dis Chil. 1968; 115:714.

60. Heizer WD et al: Protein-losing gastroenteropathy and malabsorption associated with factitious diarrhea. Ann Intern Med. 1968; 68:839.

61. Kramer P et al: Factitious diarrhea induced by phenolphthalein. Arch Intern Med. 1964; 114:634.

62. Bumin JJ: Factitious diarrhea. Ann Intern Med. 1958; 48:1328.

63. Love DR et al: An unusual case of self-induced electrolyte depletion. Gut. 1971; 12:184.

64. Cummings JH et al: Laxative-induced diarrhea, a continuing clinical problem. Br Med J. 1974; 1:537.

65. Heffernon EW: Medical management of chronic constipation. Modern Treatment. 1971; 8:870.

66. Almy TP: Wrestling with the irritable colon. Med Clin North Am. 1978; 62:203.

67. Almy TP: Irritable bowel syndrome. In *Gastrointestinal Diseases*, 2nd ed, edited by MH Sleisenger and JS Fordtran, WB Saunders, Philadelphia, 1978, p 1585.

68. Sullivan MA et al: Colonic myoelectrical activity in irritable bowel syndrome. N Engl J Med. 1978; 298:878.

69. Harvey RF: Effect of cholecystokinin on colonic motility and symptoms in patients with irritable bowel syndrome. Lancet. 1973; 1:1.

70. Harvey RF et al: Effects of increased dietary fibre on intestinal transit. Lancet. 1973; 1:1278.

71. Søltoft S et al: A double-blind trial on the effect of wheat bran on symptoms of irritable bowel syndrome. Lancet. 1976; 1:270.

72. Katz LJ et al: A clinical evaluation of certain bulk and irritant laxatives. Gastroenterology. 1952; 20:149.

73. Ivey KJ: Are anticholinergics of use in irritable colon syndrome? Gastroenterology. 1975; 68:1300.

74. Rhodes JB et al: Controlled clinical trial of sedative-anticholinergic drugs in patients with irritable bowel syndrome. J Clin Pharmacol. 1978. 18:340.

75. Ritchie JA et al: Comparison of various treatments for irritable bowel syndrome. Br Med J. 1980; 281:1317.

76. Schuster MM: Operant conditioning in gastrointestinal dysfunction. Hosp Pract. 1974; 9:135.

77. Almy TP et al: Diverticular disease of the colon. N Engl J Med. 1980; 302:324.

78. Barbezat GO: Rational treatment of diverticular disease. Drugs. 1980; 19:63.

79. Brodribb AJM et al: Diverticular disease: three studies. II. Treatment with bran. Br Med J. 1976; 1:425.

80. Meisel JL et al: Human rectal mucosa, proctoscopic and morphologic changes caused by laxatives. Gastroenterology. 1977; 72:1274.

81. Thoeni RF et al: The state of radiographic technique in the examination of the colon in a survey. Radiology. 1978; 127:317.

82. Padilla G et al: Variables affecting the preparation of the bowel for radiologic examination. Nurs Rev. 1972; 21:305.

83. Devroede G et al: Effects of hypertonic enemas on rectal mucosa. Ann of Roy Coll Phys and Surgeons Canada. 1975; 8:27.

84. Pike BF et al: Soap colitis. N Engl J Med. 1971; 285; 271.

85. Turrell R: Lacerations to anorectum incident to enema. Archives of Surg. 1960; 81:953.

86. Barnes MR: How to get a clean colon with less effort. Radiology. 1968; 91:948.

87. Dodds WJ et al: Evaluations of colon cleansing regimens. Am J Roentgenol. 1977; 128:57.

88. Dennison AD: Use of dioctyl sodium sulfosuccinate in cardiovascular disease correction of bowel function. Am J Cardiol. 1958; 1:400.

89. Goodman J et al: Dioctyl sodium sulfosuccinate—an ineffective prophylactic laxative. J Chron Dis. 1976; 29:59.

90. Hyland CM et al: DSS as a laxative in the elderly. Practitioner. 1968; 200:698.

91. Phelps DK: Effect of DSS on bowel function in mental patients. J Indiana State Med Assoc. 1958; 51:646.

92. Dujoune CA et al: Toxicity of a hepatotoxic laxative preparation in tissue culture and excretion in bile in man. Clin Pharmacol Ther. 1972; 13:602.

93. Mallory A et al: Oxyphenisatin and chronic active hepatitis. N Engl J Med. 1971; 285:1266.

94. Reynolds TB et al: Chronic active and lupoid hepatitis caused by a laxative, oxyphenisatin. N Engl J Med. 1971; 285:813.

95. Tolman KG et al: Possible hepatotoxicity of Doxidan. Ann Intern Med. 1976; 84:290.

96. Cochran KM et al: Laxatives and gastric mucosal damage, the danger of DSS (abstract). Gut. 1977; 18:422.

97. Steigman FH et al: Critical levels of mineral oil affecting the absorption of vitamin A. Gastroenterology. 1952; 20:287.

98. Javert ET et al: Prothrombin concentration and mineral oil. Am J Obstet Gynecol. 1941; 42:409.

99. Sinclair, L: Rickets from liquid paraffin. Lancet. 1967; 1:792.

100. Prescott LF: Pharmacokinetic drug interaction. Lancet. 1969; 2:1239.

101. Hansten PD: Drug Interactions, 4th ed, Lea & Febiger, Philadelphia, 1979.

102. Biggs JSG et al: Treatment of gastrointestinal disorders of pregnancy. Drugs. 1980; 19:70.

103. Joneja MG et al: Effects of vinblastine and podophyllin on DBA mouse fetuses. Toxicol and Appl Pharmacol. 1974; 27:408.

104. Chamberland MJ et al: Toxic effect of podophyllin application in pregnancy. Br Med J. 1972; 3:391.

105. Anderson PO: Drugs and breast feeding. Seminars in Perinatology. 1979; 3:271.

106. Wilson JT et al: Drug excretion in human breast milk. Clin Pharmacokinetics. 1980; 5:1.

107. Greenhalf NJ et al: Laxatives in the treatment of constipation of pregnant and breast feeding mothers. Practitioner. 1973; 210:259.

108. Mundow L: Danthron/poloxalkol and placebo in puerpural constipation. Br J Clin Pract. 1975; 29:95.

109. Souter WA: Bolus obstruction of gut after use of hydrophilic colloid laxatives. Br Med J. 1965; 1:166.

110. Sandeman DR et al: Oesophageal obstruction due to hydroscopic gum laxative. Lancet. 1980; 1:364.

111. Palmer ED: Presbycolon problems in nursing homes. JAMA. 1976; 235:1150.

112. Brocklehurst JC: The large bowel. In Textbook of Geriatric Medicine and Gerontology, 2nd ed, edited by JC Brocklehurst, Churchill Livingstone, Edinburgh, London, NY. 1978. p 368.

113. Wesselius-De Caspris A: Treatment of chronic constipation with lactulose syrup. Gut. 1968; 9:84.

114. Milne JS et al: Bowel habits in older people. Gerontol Clin. 1972; 14:56.

115. Brocklehurst JC et al: A study of faecal stasis in old age and use of Dobanex in its prevention. Gerontol Clin. 1969; 11:293.

116. Hinton JM et al: A new method of studying gut transit times using radio-opaque markers. Gut 1969; 10:842.

117. Bank S: The aetiology, diagnosis and treatment of constipation and diarrhea in geriatric patients. S Afr Med J. 1977; 51:409.

118. Newman HF et al: Physiologic factors affecting defecatory sensation. J Am Geriat Soc. 1974; 22:553.

119. Blacklow NR et al: Viral gastroenteritis. N Engl J Med. 1981; 304:397.

120. Nalin DR et al: Comparison of sucrose with glucose in oral therapy of infant diarrhea. Lancet. 1978; 2:277.

121. Chaterjee A et al: Oral rehydration in infant diarrhea. Arch Dis Childhood. 1980; 55:376.

122. Lomotil for diarrhea in children. Med Let Drug Ther. 1975; 17:104.

123. Penfold D et al: Overdose from Lomotil. Br Med J. 1977; 2:1401.

124. Caplan LH et al: Antidiarrheal drug effect simulating intestinal obstruction. Am J Gastroent. 1964; 42:540.

125. Ryder RW et al: Infantile diarrhea produced by heat-stable enterogenic Escherichia coli. N Engl J Med. 1976; 295:849.

126. Ulsher MH et al: Pathogenesis of Escherichia coli gastroenteritis in man: another mechanism. N Engl J Med. 1980; 302:99.

127. McCracken GH et al: Antimicrobial therapy in infants and children. Part II. Therapy of infectious conditions. J Pediatr. 1978; 93:357.

128. Dupont HL: Enteropathogenic organisms. Med Clin North Am. 1978; 62:945.

129. Yoshikawa TT et al: Salmonellosis. West J Med. 1980; 133:408.

130. Beard CM et al: Lack of evidence of cancer due to use of metronidazole. N Engl J Med. 1979; 301:519.

131. Freedman GD: Cancer after metronidazole (letter). N Engl J Med. 1980; 302:519.

132. *Health information for international travel 1980* published as a supplement to the Morbidity and Mortality Weekly Report, US Department of Health and Human Services, Center for Disease Control, Atlanta, Georgia.

133. Merson MH et al: Traveler's diarrhea. JAMA. 1975; 234:201.

134. Traveler's diarrhea. Med Let Drug Ther. 1979; 21:41.

135. Dupont HL et al: Symptomatic treatment of diarrhea with bismuth subsalicylate among students attending a Mexican University. Gastroenterology. 1977; 73:715.

136. Goldenberg MM et al: The antidiarrheal effect of bismuth subsalicylate in the mouse and the rat. Am J Dig Dis. 1975; 20:955.

137. Mennie AJ et al: Treatment of radiation induced gastrointestinal distress with acetylsalicylate. Lancet. 1975; 2:942.

138. Burke V et al: Reduction by aspirin of intestinal fluid loss in acute childhood gastroenteritis. Lancet. 1980; 1329.

139. Salicylate in Pepto Bismol. Med Let Drug Ther. 1980; 22:63.

140. Oakley GP: The neurotoxicity of halogenated hydroxyquinolines. JAMA. 1973; 225:395.

141. Asao M: Clioquinol and S.M.O.N. Reanalysis of original data. Lancet. 1979; 1:446.

142. Baumagartner G et al: Neurotoxicity of halogenated hydroxyquinolines: Clinical analysis of cases reported outside of Japan. J Neurosurg Psychiat. 1979; 42:1073.

143. Hansson O et al: Neurotoxicity of oxyquinolines. Lancet. 1980; 1:1253.

144. Sack DA et al: Prophylactic doxycycline for traveler's diarrhea. N Engl J Med. 1978; 298:758.

145. Sack RB et al: Prophylactic doxycycline for traveler's diarrhea. Gastroenterology. 1979; 76:1368.

146. Guerrant RL et al: Doxycycline for traveler's diarrhea: risks and benefits. N Engl J Med. 1978; 299:1412.

147. Hentges DJ: Enteropathogen normal flora interactions. Am J Clin Nutr. 1970; 23:1451.

148. Bohnhoff M et al: Resistance of mouse intestinal tract to experimental salmonella infections. J Exp Med. 1964; 120:805.

149. Dupont HL et al: Prevention of traveler's diarrhea. JAMA. 1980; 243:237.

150. Bayless TM et al: Lactose intolerance and milk drinking habits. Gastroenterology. 1971; 60:605.

151. Greenberger NJ et al: Disorders of absorption. In *Harrison's Principles of Internal Medicine.* 9th ed, edited by KJ Isselbacher, RD Adams, E Braunwald, RG Petersdorf and JD Wilson, McGraw Hill Book Company, New York, 1980, p 1393.

152. Ruddell WJJ et al: Severe diarrhea due to small intestinal colonization during cimetidine treatment. Br Med J. 1980; 281:273.

153. Gifford LM et al: Cimetidine postmarketing outpatient surveillance program. JAMA. 1980; 243:1532.

154. Meyer JH: Chronic morbidity after ulcer surgery. In *Gastrointestinal Diseases,* 2nd ed, edited by MH Sleisenger and JS Fordtran, WB Saunders, Philadelphia, 1978, p 947.

155. Johnson LP et al: Treatment of dumping with serotonin antagonists. JAMA. 1962; 180:493.

156. Ayulo JA: Cholestyramine in post-vagotomy syndrome. Am J Gastroenterol. 1972; 57:207.

157. Stebbins GG et al: Clinical use of cholestyramine resin in diarrhea of various etiologies. Drug Intell Clin Pharm. 1978; 12:272.

158. Roseman DM et al: Systemic disease and the gut. In *Gastrointestinal Diseases,* 2nd ed, edited by MH Sleisenger and JS Fordtran, WB Saunders, Philadelphia, 1978, p 454.

159. Condon JR: Cholestyramine in diabetic and post-vagotomy diarrhea. Br Med J. 1973; 4:423.

160. Bass JW et al: Adverse effects of orally administered ampicillin. J Pediatr. 1973; 83:106.

161. Tedesco FJ: Ampicillin associated diarrhea, a prospective study. Am J Dig Dis. 1975; 20:295.

162. Klein K: Hypotensive drugs. In *Side Effects of Drugs,* Vol VI, edited by L Meyer and Hercheimer, The Williams and Wilkins Co. Baltimore and Excerpta Medica Foundation, Amsterdam; 1968, p 207.

163. Ferguson RK et al: Patient acceptance of guanethidine as therapy for mild to moderate hypertension. Circulation. 1976; 54:32.

164. Bell GD: Drugs used in the management of gall stones. In *Side Effects of Drugs,* Annual 2, edited by MNG Dukes, Excerpta Medica, Amsterdam. 1978, p 300.

165. Prescott LF: Antiinflammatory agents and drugs used in rheumatism and gout. In *Side Effects of Drugs,* Annual 1, edited by MNG Dukes, Excerpta Medica, Amsterdam. 1977; p 90.

166. Carpenter CCJ: Acute infectious diarrheal disease and bacterial food poisoning. In *Harrison's Principles of Internal Medicine,* 9th ed, KJ Isselbacher, RD Adams, E Braunwald, RG Petersdorf and JD Wilson. McGraw Hill Book Company, New York, 1980, p 586.

167. Blaser MJ: Campylobacter enteritis: Clinical and epidemiologic features. Ann Intern Med. 1979; 91:179.

168. Lambert JR et al: Campylobacter enteritis. Ann Intern Med. 1979; 91:929.

169. Steinhoff MC et al: Bismuth subsalicylate therapy of viral gastroenteritis. Gastroenterology. 1980; 78:1485.

170. Heel RC et al: Loperamide, new antidiarrheal. Drugs. 1978; 15:33.

171. Jaffe G: A comparison of Lomotil and Imodium in acute nonspecific diarrhea. J Internat Med Res. 1977; 5:9.

172. Cornett JD et al: A double-blind comparative evaluation of loperamide versus diphenoxylate with atropine in acute diarrhea. Curr Ther Res. 1977; 21:629.

173. Palmer KR et al: Double-blind cross-over study comparing loperamide, codeine and diphenoxylate in the treatment of chronic diarrhea. Gastroenterology. 1980; 79:1272.

174. Pelemans W et al: A double-blind crossover comparison of loperamide with diphenoxylate in symptomatic treatment of chronic diarrhea. Gastroenterology. 1976; 70:1030.

175. Shee CD et al: Loperamide, diphenoxylate and codeine phosphate in chronic diarrhea. Br Med J. 1980; 280:254.

176. Novak E et al: Unfavorable effect of atrophine-diphenoxylate therapy in lincomycin caused diarrhea. JAMA. 1976; 235:1451.

177. Brown JW: Toxic megacolon associated with loperamide therapy. JAMA. 1979; 24:501.

178. Norland CC et al: Toxic dilation of colon. Med. 1969; 48:229.

Chapter 8

Essential Hypertension

Thomas H. Wiser

Hypertension is the most common adult medical problem in the industrialized world. The World Health Organization estimates that 8 to 18% of adults have blood pressures greater than 95 mm Hg diastolic and/or 160 mm Hg systolic (7). Approximately 35 million Americans are hypertensive as defined by these criteria, and another 25 million have diastolic blood pressures between 90 and 95 mm Hg (8).

In general, it can be stated that the greater the elevation in systolic or diastolic blood pressure, the greater the risk of cardiovascular morbidity and mortality. The following arbitrary stratification of hypertension by diastolic blood pressure has become conventional: *Mild* - 90 to 104 mm Hg, *Moderate* - 105 to 114 mm Hg, and *Severe* - 115 mm Hg and greater (3). Hypertension can also be classified by extent of organ damage (Table 1).

Etiology. Known or secondary causes can be identified in about 6 to 10% of those with hypertension (10–13); the secondary causes of hypertension are listed in Table 2. The majority of individuals with hypertension present with essential or primary hypertension which has no established cause. Although, by definition, the cause

of essential hypertension is unknown, a variety of neural and humoral changes have been implicated (see Pathophysiology, below) (7,14–17). Because of its prevalence, essential hypertension will be the focus of this chapter.

Pathophysiology. Arterial blood pressure is a highly integrated and complex system regulated by a number of variables. Very simply stated using basic hydrodynamic laws, mean arterial pressure (MAP) equals cardiac output (CO) times total peripheral resistance (TPR):

$$MAP = CO \times TPR$$

Cardiac output is defined as the volume of blood in liters pumped by the heart per minute. Total peripheral resistance is defined as the resistance to the flow of blood exerted by the vascular bed. These two variables, CO and TPR, are in turn regulated by numerous hemodynamic, neural, and humoral factors that are thoroughly discussed elsewhere (14,15).

Early in the course of essential hypertension, patients have an increased heart rate, elevated cardiac output, and normal or subnormal total peripheral resistance. As the hypertension be-

Table 1.

CLASSIFICATION OF HYPERTENSION BY ORGAN DAMAGE*

Stage I
No objective signs of organic changes are evident.

Stage II
At least one of the following signs of organ involvement is present:
1. Left ventricular hypertrophy on physical examination, chest x-ray, electrocardiography, echocardiography.
2. Generalized and focal narrowing of the retinal arteries.
3. Proteinuria and/or slight elevation of plasma creatinine concentration.

Stage III
Both signs and symptoms have appeared as a result of damage to various organs from hypertensive disease. These include:
1. Heart: Left ventricular failure.
2. Brain: Cerebral, cerebellar, or brain stem hemorrhage; hypertensive encephalopathy.
3. Optic Fundi: Retinal hemorrhage and exudates with or without papilledema.
4. Other conditions frequently present in Stage III but less clearly a direct consequence of high blood pressure include:
   – Angina
   – Myocardial infarction
   – Intracranial arterial thrombosis
   – Dissecting aneurysm
   – Arterial occlusive disease
   – Renal failure

*Criteria used by the World Health Organization.

comes well-established, cardiac output returns to normal and peripheral resistance elevates. This resistance is particularly noticed in the kidneys as documented by the development of nephrosclerosis, a fall in glomerular filtration rate, and a deterioration in overall renal function. As total peripheral resistance progresses, the heart shows evidence of hyperfunction resulting in left ventricular hypertrophy. Eventually, cardiac output gradually falls, leading to cardiac decompensation (14,15). (Also see Question 3.)

It has been speculated that neural changes or neurogenic factors play a role in the development of hypertension. However, increased sympathetic outflow from vasomotor centers or increased catecholamine concentrations have not been documented in comparison with age-matched controls. Nevertheless, antihypertensive medicines that suppress adrenergic functions are effective in treating essential hypertension.

A variety of humoral changes have also been implicated in essential hypertension; among the most important of these are renin-angiotensin, antidiuretic hormone, prostaglandins, and the kallikrein/kinin system (7,14–17). The renin-angiotensin system has been the most extensively studied. Renin is an enzyme secreted from the juxtaglomerular apparatus in response to a drop in blood pressure, blood volume, or sodium concentration. Renin converts circulating renin substrate to the decapeptide, angiotensin I. During passage through the pulmonary circulation, a converting enzyme lyses angiotensin I into angiotensin II which causes vasoconstriction and aldosterone release; this, in turn, results in sodium retention, intravascular volume expansion, and

increased blood pressure (15,16). A variety of substances are known to affect renin release, including sodium, potassium, angiotensin II, catecholamines, estrogens, adrenal steroids and ADH (17). If renin activity is measured in patients with essential hypertension, approximately one-third will have lower than normal values and 10–15% will have higher than normal values. Laragh and co-workers classified hypertensive patients on the basis of high, normal, or low plasma renin activity (PRA). It is postulated that patients with essential hypertension may have a) normal to high PRA with contracted plasma volume and increased sympathetic drive or b) low PRA with expanded plasma volume and particular responsiveness to diuretic therapy. In addition, PRA and angiotensin II levels or secretion are inversely related to age in essential hypertension. Long-term studies are needed to substantiate PRA subgroup theories or to determine whether these differences are merely time-dependent.

In summary, research in the field of pathophysiology of hypertension indicates several multifactorial variables, none being more important than the others as a single cause. The eventual outcome of this research has vast implications, however, in determining appropriate antihypertensive agent selection and disease prevention.

Evaluation

1. G.P. is a 50-year-old black man who is referred to the Primary Care Clinic for evaluation of high blood pressure noted on routine screening. His only complaint is the presence of a pounding occipital morning headache. Hypertension was detected four years ago and treated with a weight reducing diet and sodium restriction. A gradual 15 pound weight gain was noted over the past 12–18 months. He also had peptic ulcer 10 years ago. His father had hypertension and died of a heart attack at age 59. His mother died of a stroke at age 62 and was an insulin dependent diabetic. He has a 20 pack per year history of cigarette smoking. He believes his elevated blood pressure has been caused by anxiety over his recent loss of employment.

Physical examination revealed a well developed, overweight black man who appeared his stated age and was in no acute distress. His height was 175 cm and his weight

Table 2.

CAUSES OF SECONDARY HYPERTENSION

I.	Renal Disease (such as):	
	A. Renoparenchymal disease.	
	B. Renovascular disease.	
II.	Coarctation of the Aorta	
III.	Primary Aldosteronism	
IV.	Cushing's Syndrome	
V.	Pheochromocytoma	
VI.	Iatrogenic (such as):	
	A. Oral contraceptives	
	B. Anorectics	
	C. Alcohol	
VII.	Pregnancy	

was 107 kg. Blood pressures were as follows: 170/120 mm Hg (right arm) and 176/122 mm Hg (left arm) while sitting; 168/120 mm Hg (right arm) and 172/118 mm Hg (left arm) while standing. His pulse was 75 beats per minute and regular. Funduscopic examination revealed mild arteriolar narrowing, sharp disks, and no exudates or hemorrhages. The remainder of the physical examination was within normal limits.

Laboratory examination revealed the following: serum electrolytes within normal limits, BUN 30 mg/dl (nl 8–25 mg/dl), serum creatinine 2.0 mg/dl (nl 0.6–1.5 mg/dl), serum uric acid 12 mg/dl (nl 3–7 mg/dl), serum glucose 90 mg/dl (nl 70–110 mg/dl), hematocrit 42% (nl 45–52%), and mildly elevated fasting cholesterol and triglycerides. Urinalysis revealed one-plus proteinuria.

Electrocardiogram revealed mild left ventricular hypertrophy by voltage criteria. Chest x-ray showed left ventricular hypertrophy with a 17/32 cm cardiac thoracic ratio.

What symptoms of essential hypertension are manifested in G.P.?

Hypertension is usually not associated with any symptoms, unless the blood pressure elevation is severe or target organs are affected. Although G.P.'s pounding, occipital headache, which is present in the morning and wears off as the day progresses, is considered a classic symptom (18), others have evaluated the occurrence of headache and other signs and symptoms in mild and moderately severe hypertension and demonstrated no correlation (19).

2. *Data Base*. What additional laboratory data or diagnostic evaluation for secondary hypertension should be obtained for G.P. at this time?

It is recommended by the Joint National Committee on Detection, Evaluation and Treatment of High Blood Pressure (3) and others (5,6,7,20) that most patients receive an evaluation as shown in Table 3. Since secondary hypertension is infrequent, special evaluation designed to identify causes of secondary hypertension (Table 2) should be limited to the following clinical circumstances: patients refractory to drug therapy, young patients (under 35 years of age) with moderate or severe hypertension, patients with a clinical clue suggesting a secondary form of hypertension, previously well-controlled hypertensive patients whose blood pressure rises and patients with accelerated or malignant hypertension. G.P. does not meet any of these criteria and does not require a further diagnostic evaluation for secondary hypertension.

Table 3.

HYPERTENSIVE DATA BASE

Routine hypertensive initial data base should minimally include (3,5,6,7,20):

I.   *History*
  A. Family history of hypertension and its complications
  B. History of cardiovascular or cerebrovascular, or renal disease, or diabetes mellitus
  C. Known duration and levels of elevated blood pressure
  D. Results and side effects from previous treatment
  E. Drugs or substances which may influence blood pressure, eg contraceptive pills, corticosteroids, licorice
  F. Smoking habits
  G. Sodium intake
  H. Alcohol intake

II. *Physical Examination*
  A. Two or more blood pressure measurements in both arms with the patient seated and standing.
  B. Height and weight
  C. Funduscopic examination for arteriolar narrowing, hemorrhages, exudates and papilledema
  D. Examination of the neck for carotid bruits and distended veins
  E. Examination of the heart for rate, size, precordial heave, murmurs, arrhythmias and gallops
  F. Examination of the abdomen for bruits, large kidneys or dilation of the aorta
  G. Examination of the extremities for diminished or absent peripheral pulses
  H. Neurologic examination

III. *Laboratory Tests*
  A. Urinalysis, including testing for protein, blood and glucose
  B. Serum potassium
  C. Serum creatinine
  D. Serum cholesterol
  E. Serum glucose
  F. Serum uric acid
  G. Electrocardiogram
  H. Hematocrit
  I. Chest roentgenogram (if warranted)

3. *End Organ Effects.* How are the major organs of the body adversely affected by hypertension, and how can these adverse effects be subjectively and objectively monitored in G.P.?

The morbid events associated with hypertension are increased risk of stroke, ischemic heart disease, renal failure, and congestive heart failure (25–27).

Effects on the Brain. Hypertension, unequivocally more than any other factor, predisposes individuals to the development of atherothrombotic brain infarcts which are the most common variety of stroke (29–32). With long-standing hypertension, multiple large infarcts or hemorrhages can cause brain tissue destruction. Fifty percent of all brain infarctions occur in 20% of the adult hypertensive population (33). With accelerated hypertension, encephalopathy, cerebral edema, infarcts, and hemorrhages appear rapidly. It is estimated that the risk of stroke is five times higher in hypertensives as compared to normotensives (29), and the mortality rate from stroke is four to five times higher in blacks than in whites (32). Cerebrovascular accidents are probably responsible for up to 10 to 15% of deaths attributed to hypertension. Hypertensives are also prone to cardiovascular complications (see below) which in turn are associated with increased risk of brain infarction (33). Because morbid central nervous system events are often all or none phenomena, it is difficult to evaluate progressive neurologic damage. Therefore, prevention of strokes becomes a goal for the treatment of hypertension.

Effects on the Heart. A number of long-term studies have confirmed the relationship of hypertension to accelerated atherosclerosis and coronary artery disease. Left ventricular hypertrophy occurs as a result of cardiac compensation for the excessive workload on the left ventricle which must pump the usual amount of blood against an increased peripheral resistance. This increased heart size and subsequent increased myocardial oxygen requirement may exceed the capacity of the coronary circulation and result in angina pectoris. Myocardial infarction and congestive heart failure account for the majority of deaths secondary to hypertension (34). Furthermore, the mortality rate from hypertensive heart disease is substantially higher in blacks than in whites.

Since cardiovascular complications from uncontrolled hypertension are usually slowly progressive events, G.P. should be monitored for subjective and objective evidence of ischemic heart disease and congestive heart failure. This includes chest pain or discomfort, shortness of breath, paroxysmal nocturnal dyspnea, pedal edema, nocturia, cardiomegaly, and increasing left ventricular hypertrophy.

Effects on the Kidney. Abnormalities in renal function usually do not occur until late in the course of mild to moderate essential hypertension. The degree of impairment varies and some reduction of glomerular filtration rate is present in patients with severe hypertension (14,34). Renal complications include a) accelerated atherosclerosis of the renal arteries, b) nephrosclerosis, and c) necrotizing arteriolar fibrinoid changes in malignant hypertension. The first occurs without high blood pressure but occurs prematurely in the presence of an elevated pressure. The second produces a slowly progressive renal impairment and renal failure in rare instances. The third is diagnostic of accelerated hypertension and occurs with retinal hemorrhages and exudates (with or without papilledema) and requires prompt treatment. Like the cardiovascular complications of uncontrolled hypertension, renal complications, eg, nephrosclerosis and chronic renal failure, are usually slowly progressive events. G.P. should be monitored for evidence of worsening renal function as demonstrated by nocturia, polyuria, rising blood urea nitrogen and creatinine, and the appearance or progression of proteinuria.

Effects on the Eye. Disturbances in vision can be due to cerebral lesions but are usually due to hemorrhage into the retina or vitreous humor. Retinal lesions can produce scotomata and blurred vision. Even blindness may occur in the presence of papilledema (34–36).

The *Keith-Wagener* (KW) classification of hypertensive retinopathy commonly is used to provide a simple method for serial evaluation of the hypertensive patient. Repeated eye examinations can be used to observe the progression of hypertensive vascular effects, because the retina is the only tissue in which the arterioles can be examined directly.

KW I—Minimal arteriolar narrowing.
KW II—AV nicking and above: Generally indicates chronic hypertension of 10 years duration or more.
KW III—Hemorrhages, exudates, and above: Generally indicates accelerated phase of hypertension.

KW IV—Papilledema and above: Generally indicates malignant hypertension. Therapy is urgent. The term "malignant" is used because mortality is 100% within two years if the patient is not treated (34).

G.P.'s current eye ground findings are compatible with long standing hypertension; therefore, G.P. should be monitored for visual complaints and periodic funduscopic examinations should be performed to evaluate progression or change in the disease process.

4. What evidence of end organ damage is manifested by G.P. and is this reversible with good anti-hypertensive treatment?

G.P. has the following evidence of hypertension end organ damage: Grade I KW changes, cardiomegaly, mildly elevated BUN and creatinine, proteinuria, and no evidence of a morbid event.

Severe retinopathy (Grade III or IV KW changes) will resolve with successful anti-hypertensive therapy. Grade I or II KW changes may be reversed in young hypertensives, while older patients demonstrate less reversal. Because of G.P.'s age and duration of hypertension, reversal of his retinopathy is unlikely to occur.

Successful control of G.P.'s blood pressure may result in objective evidence of a decrease in left ventricular hypertrophy both on electrocardiogram and chest x-ray examination.

Proteinuria noted in G.P.'s urinalysis is important for two reasons: a) The kidney is a main site of target organ damage in long standing or malignant hypertension, and b) Renovascular disease may be a cause of secondary hypertension. Regardless, the proteinuria requires an evaluation, ie, 24 hour quantitative urinary collection for protein and perhaps an intravenous pyelogram. The borderline renal dysfunction and elevated serum uric acid are also signs of mild target organ damage. These findings require periodic monitoring to evaluate the progression of the disease.

5. Risk Factors. Does G.P. have any of the major cardiovascular risk factors which predispose toward hypertension or enhance his risk of myocardial infarction?

Several of the most important risk factors for predicting coronary artery disease are positive family history, elevated blood pressure, smoking, elevated blood lipids, excess weight, and excess sodium chloride intake.

G.P.'s *family history* is highly suggestive of familial hypertension. The concept of genetic influences on blood pressure regulation is well established (37,38) and clinicians recognize that hypertension and its complications commonly occur in families. Although familial aggregation of blood pressure is well documented in children of natural families (39), such a correlation is not as strong in adopted children (40). It is estimated that a child with two hypertensive parents has a 60% chance of becoming hypertensive (41). Nevertheless, it should be noted that families share not only common genes but also a common environment. It is reasonable, therefore, to conclude that hypertension is determined by genetic factors which in turn are modified by various environmental factors such as weight, blood lipids, and high salt intake (42–44).

G.P.'s *history of uncontrolled hypertension* is a significant risk factor for ischemic heart disease. Numerous prospective studies have demonstrated a two-fold increase in coronary disease among hypertensives as compared with normotensive individuals.

Smoking is a cardiovascular risk factor whose severity is directly related to the daily number of cigarettes smoked. The mortality rates from coronary disease among men age 45–54 who smoke more than 20 cigarettes a day are three times higher than similar aged non-smokers (45). The Center for Disease Control estimates that 25% of approximately 649,540 heart disease deaths in the United States each year are the result of cigarette smoking (46). Cigarette smoking also increases epinephrine and norepinephrine release, as well as systolic and diastolic blood pressures. In one study, the mean systolic pressures increased from 108 mm Hg to a maximum of 120 mm Hg and the mean diastolic pressures increased from 67 mm Hg to a maximum of 70 mm Hg during smoking. Control groups were not similarly affected (47).

G.P. also has mildly *elevated cholesterol and triglyceride levels.* The role of cholesterol and other lipids as major cardiovascular risk factors is significant (49–53). See the chapter on Hyperlipidemias.

The risk of combinations of high blood pressure, smoking, and elevated serum lipids are additive. Men between the ages of 30 and 59 with hypertension as the only risk factor are twice as likely to die over the next 10 years as men with no risk factors. When either hypercholesterolemia or smoking are added, the risk of death is tripled over the next 10 years. When hypertension is combined with both smoking and elevated lipids, the risk of death over the next 10 years is five times higher (49).

In addition to its relationship to serum lipids, *excess weight* (obesity) demonstrates a very close correlation to high blood pressure. The prevalence and incidence of hypertension has been shown to increase with increased weight (40,43,54,55,56). There are few well-documented studies, however, that demonstrate significant lowering of blood pressure (BP) when weight reduction alone is utilized as treatment. A recent study (55) divided 107 patients into three groups: a) weight reduction diet (800–1200 calories), b) antihypertensive therapy or c) a combination of diet and medication. All patients were encouraged not to restrict their salt intake. The results of the study suggested that weight loss of approximately 20 pounds lowered blood pressure by a mean of 25/20 mm Hg, and normal BP was attained in 75% of patients. In combination with medications, weight loss produced even a greater decrease in blood pressure. However, numerous other studies have demonstrated that only a small percentage of patients can lose weight, maintain that loss, and reduce blood pressure more than 5% (40,43,54,56). Most clinicians confirm this finding. The pragmatic approach to weight reduction is to recommend a weight reduction program together with other therapy and, after weight reduction is achieved and maintained, reduce other therapy gradually to determine if weight reduction alone is sufficient to maintain normotensive levels.

The data base for G.P. is unclear on his current *salt intake.* The results of epidemiological studies suggest an association between dietary salt intake and blood pressure (43,57,58). Sodium content in arteriolar walls may be instrumental in the degree of vasoconstriction. Most clinicians recommend adding no salt to food and avoiding salty food, although the efficacy is unproven and compliance is low.

G.P. has a number of risk factors that would increase the likelihood of a morbid cardiovascular event. The family history of hypertension, diabetes, stroke and early death together with his obesity, dietary indiscretion, smoking, increased lipids, and hypertension are all significant findings. Not only does G.P. need treatment for his high blood pressure, but behavior modification regarding the other risk factors must be instituted.

6. *Patient Education.* What information about high blood pressure and its treatment should be given to this patient?

A plethora of studies and articles on hypertensive patient education are readily available in the literature (59–71). The Joint National Committee on Detection, Evaluation, and Treatment of Hypertension (3) recommends that patients a) know the benefits and possible adverse effects of therapy, and understand that b) their blood pressure exceeds normal limits; c) hypertension is often asymptomatic and perceived symptoms do not reliably indicate blood pressure levels; d) uncontrolled high blood pressure has serious consequences; e) prolonged follow-up and therapy are necessary; and f) therapy will not cure but should control high blood pressure.

The goal of patient education is to gain the patient's cooperation, motivate him/her to accept long-term therapy, and to ensure his/her understanding of the illness and its treatment. Factors highly associated with the patient's motivation and cooperation are a) patient-provider interactions, b) social support, c) simplified therapeutic regimens and d) identification and correction of erroneous health beliefs. Based upon the "health belief model" (59) it has been shown that a person is more likely to take action or change behavior in regards to a health problem if he/she believes that a) the illness or condition is serious, b) he/she is susceptible to the problem and its consequences, c) compliance with therapy is likely to be effective, d) he/she believes that he/she can be sick without symptoms, and e) he/she encounters a tolerable number of difficulties in compliance with the therapy.

G.P.'s association of hypertension and anxiety over his recent loss of employment is an example of an erroneous belief that hypertension is synonymous with nervous tension or is caused by nervous tension. G.P. needs to understand that hypertension is a chronic disease that may require lifelong treatment. Hypertension may be aggravated by anxiety or tension but is not necessarily caused by anxiety or tension. Some experts feel that hypertension is a misnomer because patients equate the word hypertension with tension. Therefore, the term high blood pressure should be used in emphasizing this point to G.P. during the patient education session. Patient education makes a significant contribution to therapeutic outcomes (62–67,69).

7. *Therapeutic Objectives.* What are the therapeutic objectives for G.P. and hypertensive patients in general?

Reduction of elevated blood pressure, whatever the cause, unequivocally lowers morbidity and mortality. The Veterans Administration's classic study of 143 men with initial diastolic pressures averaging 115 through 129 mm Hg had to be terminated because of the high incidence of morbidity in the untreated hypertensive group. Of the 70 untreated patients, 38% developed a complication in less than 16 months as compared to only 3% of the treated hypertensives (218). Four deaths out of 70 patients (5.7%) and severe complications such as myocardial infarction, cerebral thrombosis, congestive heart failure, transient ischemic attacks, cerebral hemorrhage, increasing azotemia, and grade IV retinopathy occurred in the placebo-treated group. Only two serious complications occurred in all of the 73 treated patients.

Phase II of the Veterans Administration Study Group followed 380 male hypertensives with diastolic blood pressures averaging 90–114 mm Hg. In this study, treatment decreased the risk of morbidity over a five year period from 55% to 18% (27). The majority of patients who benefited from treatment either had systolic pressures above 164 mm Hg or diastolic pressures above 104 mm Hg. Hypertensives with diastolic pressures ranging from 90 to 104 mm Hg did not benefit as dramatically perhaps because end-organ complications appear considerably more slowly, and longer term follow-up would be necessary to uncover such sequelae. In general, the higher the pre-treatment blood pressure, the greater the benefit of treatment. Therapy effectively allays the development of congestive heart failure, stroke, and other hypertensive complications, but is relatively ineffective in preventing the atherosclerotic complications of coronary heart disease (26,27).

Data from the Hypertension, Detection and Follow-up Program (HDFP) demonstrates that setting a specific therapeutic goal for each patient is important (28). The specific goal for all HDFP patients was lowering of blood pressure to at least 140/90 mm Hg. For those patients with initial diastolic pressures of 100 mm Hg or less, the goal was even more rigorous: 10 mm Hg below entry diastolic pressure. Even though the Veterans Administration Cooperation Study Group on Hypertensive Agents demonstrated in 1972 that drug therapy was effective in preventing stroke, renal failure, and heart failure in men with moderate to severe hypertension, it was not clear to what extent these findings could generally be applied to the population at large, or to women, minorities, the young or patients with "mild" hypertension, ie diastolic pressures between 90 and 105 mm Hg. The results of this study confirm without doubt that treatment of mild hypertension is beneficial in the general population with possible exceptions as discussed later.

The HDFP study was not designed as a placebo-controlled trial on ethical grounds, because the VA data previously demonstrated the significant benefits of treatment. HDFP compared systematic, optimum drug therapy offered in special clinics with routine care available in 14 community sites. The 10,500 hypertensive participants were randomly assigned to the special centers or referred to their usual sources of medical care.

Patients at the HDFP centers received a standardized stepped-care program of uninterrupted drug therapy. These patients received free care, drugs, and transportation to the health centers which facilitated treatment compliance. Nonphysician health professionals were utilized to minimize expense and waiting time. A variety of compliance-promotion techniques were also used. Counseling emphasized drug compliance, but also included attention to other risk factors such as smoking, excess sodium intake, and overweight.

The HDFP data show that systematic effective treatment may reduce premature deaths by 20% in patients with diastolic pressures between 90 and 104 mm Hg. Like the special care group, the referred group experienced a substantial overall decrease in mean blood pressure during the five-year treatment period, but not by as much as the special care group. This treatment (lowering blood pressure to the therapeutic objective) was effective in blacks, men, women, and for persons aged 30–49, 50–59, and 60–69 at entry.

A reduction in overall mortality was not demonstrated in patients below the age of 50 years with mild hypertension, most likely because of the short duration of the trial. Smith and co-workers, however, demonstrated that treatment of younger patients with mild hypertension reduced the incidence of complications such as stroke, congestive heart failure, left ventricular hypertrophy, and progressive rise of blood pressure (72).

The analysis of data from the HDFP trial will continue to be evaluated for several years. In addition, results from the European Working Party on High Blood Pressure in the Elderly; National Heart, Lung and Blood Institute Study Group Evaluating Treatment of Mild Hypertension; Medical Research Council Working Party on Mild to Moderate Hypertension, the Mayo Three Community Hypertension Control Program and others will provide the final results and conclusions. Until such time, the Joint National Committee recommends that the initial goal of antihypertensive therapy is to achieve and maintain diastolic pressures at less than 90 mm Hg or the lowest diastolic pressure consistent with safety and tolerance.

The goal of therapy for G.P. is ultimately to prevent premature death and hypertensive morbidity. This goal is achievable if elevated blood pressures are lowered and maintained at acceptable levels. However, the need to maintain normal blood pressure must be balanced against potential drug toxicities and unnecessary or intolerable adverse drug effects. It is counterproductive to expect G.P. to tolerate incapacitating or uncomfortable side effects simply to treat an essentially asymptomatic disease.

Treatment

8. What methods are available to treat G.P.'s high blood pressure?

Non-Drug Therapy. Several studies have documented blood pressure lowering with weight reduction or moderate control of sodium intake (40,43,44,54–58). Large clinical trials are needed to confirm the effectiveness and compliance to such interventions. In general, weight reduction and sodium control are considered adjunctive measures. After weight reduction and/or sodium control is achieved, pharmacotherapy may gradually be reduced or eliminated if normotensive levels are maintained.

Behavioral methods, ie, biofeedback, psychotherapy, meditation (or other relaxation techniques), and regular exercise are considered experimental and cannot be recommended for long-term control of hypertension (3,43). Several investigators have advocated regular practice of such interventions (44,73–78). Patient adherence to these life-style modifications is not certain and no data demonstrating reduction of cardiovascular mortality and morbidity are present. Because these interventions are inexpensive and probably safe, encouragement would be appropriate if such practices are embraced by the patient.

Drug Therapy. The Joint National Committee on Detection, Evaluation and Treatment of High Blood Pressure recommends a "stepped care" approach to the management of hypertension (3). The basic principle of stepped care is as follows: initiate therapy with a small dose of an antihypertensive drug, increase the dose of that drug, and then add, sequentially, one drug after another as needed. Each drug is administered in gradually increasing doses until the therapeutic objective of normal blood pressure is attained or intolerable adverse effects develop or the maximum dose is reached. (See Table 5)

Sedatives, tranquilizers, and anti-anxiety agents are not included, because they are not effective in lowering blood pressure (3). Phenobarbital demonstrates no greater blood pressure reduction than placebo (79). There are no data demonstrating consistent hypotensive effects from the benzodiazepines or other anti-anxiety agents.

The first step of treatment is the initiation of diuretics together with the previously discussed dietary instructions. Diuretics remain the cornerstone of hypertensive therapy because: a) They have a low incidence of adverse effects, b) 70% of the adult hypertensive population will respond to diuretics alone, c) diuretics potentiate the hypotensive activity of the nondiuretic antihypertensive agents, and d) diuretics are often the least expensive of antihypertensive agents (80). The recommended dosage ranges are shown in Table 4.

9. What drug therapy should be initiated to treat G.P.'s high blood pressure?

For the reasons outlined above, diuretics are most often used as step-1 agents for the treatment of hypertension. This is especially true in black hypertensives like G.P. who seem to have more of a volume dependent hypertension and therefore respond dramatically to diuretics. Beta blockers, on the other hand, have been used extensively in Europe as step-1 agents with good results. Beta blockers may be indicated as first line drugs in patients who have hyperkinetic hypertension, cardiac arrhythmias, or angina (see Question 15). Nevertheless, diuretic therapy seems most appropriate for G.P.'s hypertension.

10. *Diuretic Selection.* Which diuretic should be given to G.P. and how much of a reduction in blood pressure is expected?

Thiazide and thiazide-related agents are generally considered the most efficacious antihypertensive diuretic compounds (80–86). An overall average expected decrease in systolic and diastolic blood pressure is approximately 20/10 mm Hg (Range: 3/2–32/21 mm Hg) (86). When compared with furosemide, a loop diuretic, hydrochlorothiazide consistently lowers blood pressure more effectively (87–89). More frequent dosing and higher total doses of furosemide may be required to produce blood pressure reduction comparable to 50 mg of hydrochlorothiazide administered twice daily. These higher dosage

requirements not only increase cost but may adversely affect compliance. In general, furosemide is reserved for hypertensive patients with impaired renal function or those with resistant hypertension (3,80,81,84,85).

Potassium-sparing diuretics (triamterene and spironolactone) are most often reserved for patients with hypokalemia from diuretic-induced hyperaldosteronism (3,80). Triamterene alone is not recommended in the treatment of essential hypertension since it produces only a slight reduction in blood pressure (91,92). Spironolactone may be as efficacious as thiazides or loop diuretics in low-renin hypertension, but hydrochlorothiazide is as effective in these patients and produces fewer side effects (80,81).

G.P.'s renal function tests suggest a mild reduction in renal function. This does not preclude the use of thiazides. Hydrochlorothiazide 50 mg bid would be appropriate. Hydrochlorothiazide is

Table 4.

DIURETIC USE IN HYPERTENSION

		Dose Range (mg/Day)	Duration of Action (Hours)
I.	**Thiazides and Thiazide Derivatives**		
	Bendroflumethiazide	5–20	18–24
	Benzthiazide	50–200	12–18
	Chlorothiazide	500–1,000	6–12
	Chlorthalidone	25–50	48–72
	Cyclothiazide	1–2	18–24
	Flumethiazide	500–1,000	6–12
	Hydrochlorothiazide	50–100	12
	Hydroflumethiazide	50–100	12–24
	Methyclothiazide	2.5–5	24
	Metolazone	2.5–10	12–24
	Polythiazide	2–4	24–36
	Quinethazone	50–100	18–24
	Trichlormethiazide	2–4	24
II.	**Non-thiazide Diuretic Agent**		
	Furosemide*	80–320	4–6
III.	**Potassium-Sparing Diuretics****		
	Spironolactone	50–100	24 ***
	Triamterene	50–150	12–16 ***

*Not usually a step-1 drug; especially useful in renal insufficiency or resistant cases.
**Not usually a step-1 drug; usually used in combination with one of the thiazide diuretics.
***Diuresis begins at two hours; peaks at eight hours.

the least expensive antihypertensive agent (especially if prescribed generically), has been the most widely studied, and it is most often recommended. This twice daily regimen will accommodate the addition of most step-2 agents, if required. Individual response is variable; it may normalize G.P.'s blood pressure or have only a minimal effect which can only be determined after two weeks of therapy.

11. After two weeks of hydrochlorothiazide treatment, G.P. returned to clinic for evaluation of treatment. He had no complaints; in fact, his headache had resolved. His blood pressure was 150/100 mm Hg without orthostasis. His weight was 105.5 kg. Pertinent laboratory findings were: Serum potassium—normal (although a 0.5 mEq/L drop was noted), serum glucose—normal (unchanged) and serum uric acid—13 mg/dl.

Comment on the routine monitoring of diuretic therapy for high blood pressure.

The reduction in G.P.'s blood pressure is compatible with the expected pharmacologic response to hydrochlorothiazide. The weight loss is most likely related to the decreased extracellular fluid loss. The orthostatic blood pressure measurement is an important monitoring parameter to assure volume loss was not excessive. The alleviation of the patient's headache may be related to the reduction in blood pressure or simply resolution of a tension headache or other self-limiting phenomenon.

Potassium. Serum potassium reductions are not uncommon with thiazide or loop diuretics. The reported incidence of hypokalemia in ambulatory hypertensive patients is 0–60% for thiazide-type diuretics and 4–14% for furosemide (86). Thiazide-type and loop diuretics both have the potential for causing hypokalemic-induced cardiac ar-

Table 5.

STEPPED-CARE REGIMENS

Step 1:	Diuretic[1]	
	+	
Step 2:	Adrenergic Inhibiting Agents[2]	
Clonidine	Metoprolol	Propranolol
Methyldopa	Nadolol	Rauwolfia alkaloids
	Prazosin[3]	
	+	
Step 3:	Hydralazine Vasodilator[4]	
	+	
Step 4:	Additional Adrenergic Inhibiting Agent Guanethidine[5]	

[1]Thiazide-type diuretics are drugs of choice. Loop diuretics are reserved for selected patients. Potassium-sparing agents may be used in combination with thiazide diuretics. Some clinicians utilize B-adrenergic blocking agents as step-1 drug therapy with the addition of diuretics if control is not achieved.

[2]Adrenergic inhibiting agents are listed in *alphabetical* order. This does not indicate preferential order of usage. Clinical experience with Nadolol is limited.

[3]The post-synaptic alpha-receptor-blocking effects of prazosin appear to be more prominent than its vasodilator effects, thus encouraging its inclusion as a step-2 drug. Prazosin may be used in a step-3 drug if it has not been added in step-2.

[4]Minoxidil is reserved only for selected patients and should not be considered a step-3 drug.

[5]Guanethidine is a potent agent but may be used in small doses as a step-2 agent.

rhythmias. Most often the hypokalemia is mild, resulting in mean decrease in serum potassium of 0.1–0.6 mEq/L (88,93). The commonly debated question is whether or not this reduction is clinically significant. Some authors even argue the value of serum potassium levels since 98% of total body potassium is intracellular. Serum potassium is affected by numerous variables such as total body weight, state of hydration, and pH of the serum. On the other hand, the clinical manifestations of potassium deficiency (weakness and EKG changes) correlate better with serum concentrations than with the total amount in the body (94).

In general, healthy, ambulatory patients with mild hypokalemia require no treatment unless the serum potassium value falls below an acceptable lower limit, usually somewhere between 2.7–3.5 mEq/L or if symptoms occur. In addition, one should consider either adding a potassium sparing agent or a potassium salt (preferably potassium chloride) prophylactically in patients who might be particularly susceptible to potassium depletion (provided renal function is intact), eg a) concomitant digoxin or corticosteroid therapy, b) patients with poor dietary potassium intake and/or excessive sodium ingestion, c) previous episodes of documented hypokalemia, d) patients refractory to diuretic therapy secondary to hyperaldosteronism, e) cirrhotic patients, and f) diabetic patients (because hypokalemia may accelerate glucose intolerance).

Most of the diuretic-induced potassium losses occur within the first month or two of therapy (88,93,96). If diet and drug compliance remain constant, serum potassium levels usually remain stable thereafter. Every patient, however, must be evaluated on an individual basis, and periodic serum potassium levels should arbitrarily be obtained as determined by the primary provider after the initial two month monitoring period.

Diuretic-induced hypokalemia is a dose-related phenomenon (97,98,99). For example, Tweeddale and co-workers demonstrated that 25 mg of chlorthalidone lowered serum potassium levels approximately 0.4 mEq/L and 100 mg of chlorthalidone produced a 0.9 mEq/L reduction when measured after an eight week period of drug administration.

Hypokalemia, if it does occur, can be corrected with oral potassium chloride in liquid preparations or slow release potassium chloride tablets,

as well as with the potassium sparing diuretics, spironolactone or triamterene. If spironolactone is chosen, 50 to 100 mg daily is usually adequate for most mild cases of potassium insufficiency resulting from 100 mg/day doses of hydrochlorothiazide or its equivalent. Triamterene daily doses should be 100 to 200 mg. Although triamterene is usually less expensive than spironolactone, unlike spironolactone, it is without significant antihypertensive properties. Both spironolactone and triamterene should be used with extreme caution in patients receiving concomitant potassium supplements and in patients with renal dysfunction, because hyperkalemia can occur. Furthermore, individual patient responses to the potassium conserving actions of these two agents are not always predictable, and moderately severe hypokalemia would best be corrected with potassium chloride.

Potassium-rich foods such as dried fruits, fresh bananas, and orange juice are expensive, high in calories, high in sugar, and usually inadequate for all but the very mildest cases of hypokalemia. Diabetics, obese hypertensives, and other overweight patients should not be encouraged to utilize these foods as potassium supplements without due consideration for the above factors.

Reports of hyperkalemia resulting from abuse of salt substitutes (100) has led to speculation concerning the use of such substitutes as viable therapeutic agents. One teaspoonful of Morton's LITE-SALT contains about 37 mEq of potassium and 3.0 grams of sodium chloride (101). When used in conjunction with other true salt substitutes like Neocurtasal or Adolph's Salt Substitute, this form of potassium supplementation is not only palatable but inexpensive. The LITE-SALT can be used at the dining table, and the salt substitutes can be used in cooking and can be sprinkled over a dinner salad as well. Patients with renal impairment, cardiac failure, or patients receiving spironolactone and triamterene must be cautioned concerning the use of salt substitutes (102).

It is apparent that G.P. does not require potassium supplementation at this time. A repeat serum potassium value in one or two months would be appropriate. Alternatively, his serum potassium can be monitored in a problem-oriented manner, ie onset of generalized weakness or a concurrent potassium losing condition such as diarrhea.

Uric Acid. The second most commonly encountered adverse effect of thiazide-type and loop diuretics is hyperuricemia. Although the mechanism of hyperuricemia is not clear, it may involve an increased reabsorption of uric acid in the proximal convoluted tubule of the kidney. Some investigators propose that there is a decrease in tubular secretion or an increase in post-secretory reabsorption of uric acid (103). The resultant hyperuricemia, regardless of the mechanism, is usually persistent. The serum uric acid returns to pretreatment levels only when the diuretic is stopped. Actual gout occurs in patients with diuretic-induced hyperuricemia but is very unpredictable and is speculated to be significant only in patients with hereditary predisposition (85). In the absence of overt gout, diuretic-induced hyperuricemia is considered harmless and requires no treatment. A history of gout or the development of gout is not considered a contraindication since the hyperuricemia responds to treatment with probenecid or allopurinol. Routine prophylactic use of uric acid lowering agents is unwarranted and unnecessary. In general, 50–100 mg of hydrochlorothiazide, 80 mg of furosemide or 100 mg of chlorthalidone produce 1–2 mg/dl elevation in serum uric acid and these effects are dose-related (87,88,97,98). Spironolactone and triamterene do not cause hyperuricemia.

G.P. requires an evaluation of his elevated serum uric acid, ie a thorough review of his family history for gout and 24 hour urine collection for quantification of his uric acid. This is particularly important in view of G.P.'s mild renal impairment as the cause of the uric acid pathogenesis. Since hyperuricemia is a separate problem requiring evaluation and management and because of the importance of diuretic therapy in hypertension, the hydrochlorothiazide should be continued.

Glucose. The third most common adverse effect of thiazide-type and loop diuretics is hyperglycemia. Although abnormalities in carbohydrate metabolism associated with the use of thiazide and loop diuretics are widely reported in the literature, there have been conflicting reports concerning the relative degree of hyperglycemia caused by each of these drugs and the clinical significance of chemically-induced hyperglycemia both in normal and in diabetic patients. While no studies have definitely resolved this question, it is clear that thiazide and loop diuretics worsen glucose tolerance and precipitate

diabetes within usual therapeutic doses in patients with overt and subclinical disease (104–109). Some investigators have noted no glucose intolerance with furosemide or conclude that glucose intolerance occurs to a lesser extent with furosemide than with thiazides (80,106,107,109). Amery and co-workers conclude that the diabetogenic effect may be more pronounced in the elderly population (108).

Diabetes is not a contraindication to the use of these agents. Often there is no perceptible effect on the diabetes, and when effects do occur, they can usually be managed by altering the diet or by increasing the dose of insulin. Rarely, thiazide diuretics induce severe hyperglycemia, requiring large doses of insulin for control. When this occurs, it may be advisable to try another type of diuretic such as furosemide.

G.P. is at risk for diuretic-induced hyperglycemia because of his family history and genetic predisposition. Periodic fasting blood glucose levels, patient education regarding signs and symptoms of hyperglycemia, and dietary education to obtain weight reduction will obviate or minimize this problem.

Cholesterol and Triglycerides. The thiazide diuretics (110,112,113) chlorthalidone (111–113), and, theoretically, furosemide are associated with increases in serum cholesterol and triglycerides. In one study, a mean increase in serum cholesterol of 11 mg/dl occurred in 39 diuretic-treated patients on a special diet. Although this increase was not large, it appears more dramatic when compared to the 11 mg/dl mean *decrease* in serum cholesterol which occurred in the 35 patients in the control group. The diuretic-treated group also demonstrated a 34 mg/dl increase in serum triglyceride concentration. In general, total plasma cholesterol increases about 6 to 8% and triglycerides increase about 15 to 17% during treatment with thiazide-type diuretics. These changes cannot be explained by hemoconcentration, and the mechanism remains a mystery. Since elevated serum lipids are associated epidemiologically with coronary heart disease, these mean serum lipid increases could possibly offset the benefit gained from lowering blood pressure in an otherwise healthy young person. It recently has been found that a specific cholesterol-lowering diet largely prevents this increase in serum lipids (113). Until further evidence, it seems prudent to advise young persons in particular to reduce weight. The primary provider may prescribe a cholesterol-lowering diet and periodically monitor blood lipid levels in patients with a strong family history of lipid abnormalities or premature death, or in obese patients.

Since G.P. has a family history of hypertension (premature death of his father) and is overweight, a lipid evaluation would be appropriate, and dietary intervention should be provided if abnormalities are noted.

12. *Plasma Renin Activity.* In the referral process it was discovered that G.P. had a normal plasma renin level. Comment on the value of plasma renin activity in predicting severity of hypertensive disease or identifying appropriate therapeutic treatment.

In 1972, Laragh and co-workers (16,118) grouped essential hypertensive patients into different categories based upon renin and aldosterone determinations. Of 219 essential hypertensives, 27% had subnormal plasma renin activity, 57% had normal renin activity, and 16% had abnormally high renin activity. This discovery pointed out that essential hypertension is not a homogeneous disease. Even further, it was suggested that the high renin group exhibited a higher incidence of complications, eg strokes, myocardial infarctions, azotemia, proteinuria, hypokalemia, funduscopic abnormalities, and higher mean diastolic pressures.

Other investigators have also grouped essential hypertensives into similar categories consisting of low, normal, or high renin activity, approximating the percentages of Laragh's groupings. There is, however, a growing body of evidence to suggest a dissociation between reduction in plasma renin activity and the lowering of arterial pressure and, even more importantly, that low doses of propranolol are required to suppress renin activity and substantially larger doses are required to lower blood pressure (119–123). As a result, Laragh's multitude of publications have been carefully re-evaluated and constructively criticized (124). Despite much intensive research and debate, the precise relationship between plasma renin activity (PRA) and hypertension prognosis and/or treatment is unclear. Most evidence suggests no significant relationship.

13. *Step-2 Therapy Selection.* Since the therapeutic objective for G.P. has not been reached, reserpine 0.1 mg once a day was added to his regimen. How is a step-2 agent

chosen? Was the choice of reserpine appropriate for this patient?

Several second-step agents are currently available (see Table 5). Using the stepped-care approach, the primary provider selects a step-2 agent at the usual starting dose and increases gradually to a maximum dose or development of side effects. If blood pressure continues to remain elevated, a step-3 drug is added in a similar manner and so on.

Adequate doses of any of the step-2 agents have essentially similar blood pressure lowering effects when used with a step-1 diuretic in recommended doses. In selecting a step-2 drug, several guidelines should be considered. First, no specific antihypertensive drug is best for all patients, and there is no way to predict the antihypertensive response that a given agent will produce in an individual patient. Therefore, previous adverse reactions should be identified. The clinician should also seek out patient-related variables that might preclude the use of certain agents or require close monitoring for appearance of a particular side effect that would be likely to occur in the patient being treated (see Table 6). Also, regimens which require once a day or twice a day therapy are more likely to be complied with. Furthermore, the cost of therapies should be considered. The clinician should use antihypertensive agents that he/she is confident and competent in using. And finally, antihypertensive agents with multiple indications or benefits should be used when possible. For example, patients with congestive heart failure may receive additional benefits from thiazides. Similarly, those with angina will receive additional benefit from treatment with propranolol (80,81,83,114–117).

Reserpine is a reasonable choice for G.P. for a variety of reasons. The VA study (26,27) and the HDFP study (28) are two classic large clinical trials that substantiated the value of hypertension therapy, and both studies utilized reserpine in a large number of their patients. It is long acting, inexpensive, and can be given once a day. It is not effective in moderate or severe hypertension, but G.P. has only to lower his blood pressure by another 10 to 15 mm Hg in order to achieve control, and this is within the realm of reserpine's effectiveness. G.P. has no known allergies or previous reactions to antihypertensive medicines. In addition G.P. has no patient-related variables (see Table 6) which would preclude its use with the possible exception of a history of peptic ulcer 10 years ago.

Table 6.

CONTRAINDICATIONS AND SIDE-EFFECTS OF ANTIHYPERTENSIVE AGENTS
(Modified from Wollam et al, 83)

Drug	Side-effects		Contraindications[2]
	Innocuous, but sometimes annoying	Harmful or potentially harmful	
Oral diuretics			
a) Thiazide type	Increased urination (onset of therapy), Weakness, Muscle cramps, Hyperuricemia (sometimes with gout), Gastrointestinal disturbances.	Hypokalemia, Hyponatremia[1], Hyperglycemia, Hypercalcemia[1], Azotemia[1], Skin rash[1], Photosensitivity[1], Purpura[1], Marrow depression[1], Lithium toxicity[1] (patients on lithium therapy).	Persistent anuria/ oliguria, Advanced renal failure Hyponatremia.
b) Spironolactone	Hirsutism, Menstrual irregularities, Gynecomastia, Gastrointestinal disturbances.	Hyperkalemia[1], Hyponatremia[1].	Renal failure, Hyperkalemia, Hyponatremia.
Reserpine	Bradycardia, Lethargy, Lassitude, Sexual difficulty, Diarrhea, Nasal congestion.	Depression[1], Activation of peptic ulcer[1], Parkinsonian state[1].	Depression (past or present), Active peptic ulcer, Parkinsonism.
Methyldopa	Drowsiness, Lethargy, Dry mouth, Sexual difficulty, + Direct Coombs' test, Nasal congestion.	Abnormal liver function tests, Hepatitis[1], Drug fever[1], Hemolytic anemia[1], Retroperitoneal fibrosis[1], Skin rash[1], Orthostatic hypotension, Depression[1].	Coombs' positive, Hemolytic anemia, Hepatic disease.
Guanethidine	Bradycardia, Exercise hypotension, Diarrhea (especially following meals), Weakness, Retrograde ejaculation or impotence, Nasal congestion.	Orthostatic hypotension (potentially harmful in patients with cerebral or myocardial ischemia and advanced renal insufficiency), Drug sensitivity (rare)[1].	Interacts with tricyclic antidepressants and sympathomimetic amines.

1 Usually requires cessation of therapy, at least temporarily.
2 Hypersensitivity is obviously a contraindication to any drug and will not be repeated for each.
3 Some of these side-effects are modified or absent with other β-blocking agents due to differences in pharmacological properties (CNS effects and aggravation of arterial insufficiency are more common with propranolol than with other β-blockers).
4 These side-effects are often minimized or prevented by the co-administration of a β-blocker.

Table 6. (continued)

Drug	Side-effects		Contraindications[2]
	Innocuous, but sometimes annoying	Harmful or potentially harmful	
Propranolol[3]	Bradycardia, Weakness, Lethargy, Gastrointestinal disturbances.	Congestive heart failure (only in patients with diminished cardiac reserve), Bronchospasm[1] (in patients with asthmatic propensity), Hypoglycemia[1] (propranolol can mask the warning symptoms in insulin dependent diabetics), Aggravation of arterial insufficiency[1] (in patients with peripheral occlusive arterial disease), Nightmares[1], Insomnia[1], Hallucinations[1], Depression[1], Hyperglycemia, Hyperosmolar coma[1].	Bronchial asthma, Second or third degree heart block, Congestive heart failure (unless due to an arrhythmia amenable to therapy with propranolol or controlled hypertension), 'Brittle' diabetes mellitus.
Minoxidil	Tachycardia[4], Hypertrichosis, Initial rise in plasma renin activity.	Salt/water retention (can lead to congestive heart failure or pulmonary edema), Pericardial effusion, Profound orthostatic hypotension with guanethidine.	Advanced renal disease, Limited to patients unresponsive to usual therapy, Pheochromocytoma.
Clonidine	Dry mouth, Drowsiness, Lethargy, Sexual difficulty, Gastrointestinal disturbances, Constipation.	'Rebound hypertension', Parotid pain[1].	Hypotensive activity is reversed with tricyclic antidepressants.
Hydralazine	Tachycardia[4], Palpitation[4], Headache[4], Flushing[4], Nasal congestion, Gastrointestinal disturbances.	Aggravation of angina[1,4], Precipitation of congestive failure in patients with myocardial disease[1], Lupus-like syndrome[1], Drug fever[1], Skin rash[1].	Symptomatic arteriosclerotic heart disease (unless used with propranolol).
Prazosin	Headache, Palpitation, Drowsiness, Dizziness, Nausea.	Sudden collapse and loss of consciousness related to orthostatic hypotension (usually after initial dose; minimize by always using low first dose at bedtime).	None[2].

Reserpine can cause gastrointestinal ulcerations by stimulating excessive secretions of hydrochloric acid. This parasympathetic-mediated secretory response is dose-related and usually occurs when reserpine is given parenterally or in very large oral doses (128,129). In standard doses, oral reserpine does not stimulate gastric secretion significantly. Moser (130) claims that ulceration is almost non-existent with the small doses commonly used in the treatment of mild hypertension. Hollister (131) noted only three cases of ulcers among six hundred patients receiving large doses of rauwolfia preparations. Nevertheless, some patients may be unusually sensitive to rauwolfia compounds, because perforation and hemorrhage have occurred with reserpine doses of less than 1.0 mg per day (132). Thus, it is best to avoid reserpine in patients with active gastrointestinal problems.

14. *Reserpine Carcinogenicity.* In discussing the use of reserpine with G.P., he stated that he read a newspaper article linking reserpine to cancer. What assurances can be offered?

In 1974 reports from the Boston Collaborative Drug Surveillance Program (BCDSP), Oxford University, and the University of Helsinki suggested that the statistical risk of breast cancer was three times greater in reserpine-treated women over 50 years of age who received this drug for more than one year than in women not taking reserpine (133,134,135). Unfortunately, all three studies were performed by retrospective chart reviews, thereby minimizing the value of case controls. Also, these three studies can be criticized because of inborn patient selection biases. Patients with breast cancer may simply have had better accessibility to health care facilities, because patients in higher socio-economic classes are known to have a higher incidence of breast cancer. Other epidemiological risk factors were also not considered. Although three independent studies seem to represent confirmatory findings, closer consideration uncovers a strong possibility of investigator bias, because the BCDSP requested close colleagues from Oxford and Helsinki to confirm their findings. These studies have not been confirmed, and actually have been refuted (136). Approximately one year later an editorial written in the Lancet retracted the hard line suggestion that "use of these drugs (rauwolfia derivatives) should be restricted." The Lancet went on to say the "lack of consistent, specific association makes a causal relationship less likely . . . ." Their final statement was "when suspicion falls on a drug of proven value, caution is right, but rejection should await hard evidence."

A recent communication to participants in the National High Blood Pressure Education Program (137), made the following points: a) An FDA advisory committee (June, 1979) determined that the current evidence does not warrant labeling changes in the drug (reserpine), b) the risk to life from untreated hypertension far exceeds the potential risk of breast cancer, c) it is reasonable that those persons prescribing reserpine and using reserpine continue with usual practice until more definitive information becomes available, and d) no drug is without risk, especially when it is used on a chronic basis.

Popular lay magazines and newspapers have dramatized reserpine's association with cancer because of the popularity of the subject. Patients should be informed of the controversy to avoid provider-patient conflict, and a mutual decision regarding its use can be reached. Side effects which are commonly encountered during reserpine therapy are listed in Table 6.

G.P. elected not to take reserpine. Instead, he was given methyldopa in gradually increasing doses over the next two visits, and his blood pressure was subsequently controlled at 130/86 mm Hg without orthostasis by a dosage of 500 mg bid.

15. *Beta-Blocking Drugs.* A.K. is a 30-year-old white woman recently found to have elevated blood pressures during her routine gynecological exam. Her hypertension was confirmed by her internist who observed average blood pressure of 150/115 mm Hg and a concomitant resting pulse rate of 96 beats per minute with occasional palpitations. EKG documented a normal sinus rhythm. She was diagnosed as having hyperkinetic hypertension. Her other medical problems include stable diabetes mellitus controlled with 30 units of NPH U-100 insulin and a duodenal ulcer two months ago that responded to cimetidine treatment; she is currently receiving cimetidine 400 mg hs as prophylaxis. She was started on propranolol 20 mg bid for hypertension.

Is propranolol more efficacious than other beta-blocking agents? Why was propranolol prescribed without diuretic therapy?

Current evidence suggests that all beta-blockers have similar antihypertensive activity when administered in equipotent doses (83,115,117). It has also been demonstrated that patients not responding to one beta-blocker generally fail to respond to others (154). Other beta-blockers are currently available for use in hypertension in the U.S. (metoprolol, nadolol, and atenolol).

Propranolol was first noted to reduce the blood pressure of hypertensive patients in 1964 (152). Beta-blocking agents subsequently became widely used in Europe as antihypertensives; as many as 70–80% of European hypertensives receive these drugs (117,153). Propranolol use in the U.S. has also become significant since its approval as an antihypertensive in 1976. The clinical advantages of beta-blocking agents in the treatment of hypertension include low capacity for postural hypotension, prolonged effect (requiring only once or twice daily administration), blood pressure reduction in the supine position, minimal exercise hypotension, no effect on sexual function, and little or no central nervous system slowing (83,115,155,156).

Although beta-blockers are widely used as step-1 antihypertensives in Europe, they are generally considered step-2 agents in the U.S. Nevertheless, A.K.'s hyperkinetic hypertension (see below) makes propranolol appropriate for initial therapy. If the therapeutic objective is not met with propranolol alone, a diuretic may be given with additive results (169).

The following clinical circumstances warrant high consideration for beta-blockade therapy:

Patients with co-existing angina pectoris. This is the ideal clinical setting for the use of propranolol or nadolol (metoprolol is not approved for use in angina), because they improve overall myocardial oxygen balance in patients with ischemic heart disease by decreasing heart rate, contractility, and systemic blood pressure.

Patients with hyperkinetic essential hypertension. Infrequently in young patients with essential hypertension, the elevated blood pressure is due to increased cardiac output and presence of a hyperkinetic state. These patients may even complain of palpitations. Propranolol has been shown to reduce their pulse rate and lower their blood pressure (3,83,155,157). In addition, plasma renin activity is higher in young patients. This may suggest why blood pressure reduction is significantly greater in 25- to 35-year-olds than in patients above age 55 (153).

Patients with certain co-existing cardiac arrhythmias. Propranolol only (in U.S.) has been approved for a variety of supraventricular and ventricular arrhythmias. In addition, it is useful in patients with Barlow's syndrome or idiopathic hypertrophic subaortic stenosis (IHSS), also known as hypertrophic obstructive cardiomyopathy (83,155).

Patients receiving tricyclic antidepressants. Guanethidine, clonidine, reserpine, and methyldopa may have their hypotensive activity reduced or negated by tricyclic antidepressants (80,83,158). Propranolol is not blocked by these agents, but depression has been rarely associated with propranolol and caution must be exercised (83,159).

Patients with a variety of less common co-existing problems, ie migraine headaches, essential tremors, pheochromocytoma, or hyperthyroidism may receive symptomatic relief of cardiovascular symptoms with propranolol while surgical or appropriate medical treatment is initiated or begins to take effect (164,165).

16. *Dosing of Beta-Blockers.* **Is the dosing of propranolol in A.K. compatible with the pharmacokinetic characteristics of propranolol? Are these characteristics different from the other beta-blockers?**

The efficacy of beta-blocking agents and particularly propranolol is well established. Therapeutic responses, however, are observed at widely varying doses. Hypertensive control with propranolol can be achieved with doses varying from 40 mg to 2000 mg per day. Clinicians therefore must titrate the dose to each patient very carefully.

This wide variation in dose response is apparently due to inter-individual differences in propranolol kinetics. Identical doses of propranolol in different individuals have been reported to produce up to a 20-fold range in steady state plasma concentrations (170–173). This wide variation was recently disputed by Walle and co-workers who felt that previous studies demonstrating wide variability were inadequately controlled (ie, no evidence existed that plasma concentrations were actually drawn at steady-state, documentation of compliance was inadequate, or assay specificity was inadequate) (174). In order to obviate these variables they obtained peak (2 hr) and trough (6 hr) plasma concentrations at carefully established steady-state conditions in 46 heterogeneous patients with hypertensive or coronary disease, carefully documented compliance, and measured propranolol levels with a molecularly specific gas chromatography-mass spectrometry technique employing stable isotope-labeled propranolol as the internal standard. Their results demonstrated that plasma propranolol (ng/ml) was linearly related to dose over the range 160 to 960 mg. A maximum 3-fold variation was observed at the 40 mg dose level and decreased linearly with dose to a 1.3-fold variation at doses exceeding 600 mg per day.

Variables which explain the need for higher doses of propranolol compared to other beta-blocking agents include differences in bioavailability, protein binding, and receptor-site affinity. In general, beta-blocking agents are well absorbed from the gut. Significant differences, however, exist between these agents in the extent of their metabolism in the liver ("first-pass" phenomenon) as can be seen in Table 7. As much as 70% of propranolol is extracted by the liver making it 30% bioavailable (165,175,176). Secondly, propranolol is significantly bound to plasma protein, and this contributes further to inter-individual dosage variations and the need for higher doses than similar drugs with lower protein binding. Thirdly, the affinity of beta-blockers for the two types of beta-receptors is a relative and not absolute difference which partially explains the lower doses required with metoprolol compared to propranolol. Metoprolol is a relatively selective beta-1-adrenergic antagonist, while propranolol is equally beta-1 and beta-2 antagonistic (80). Nadolol, like propranolol, blocks both cardiac (beta-1) and bronchial (beta-2) adrenergic receptors equally. Unlike propranolol and metoprolol, which are metabolized by the liver, nadolol is excreted unchanged in the urine and accumulates as renal function becomes impaired (166). In conclusion, clinical potency is directly related to bioavailability and receptor-site affinity and inversely related to protein binding and metabolism and excretion. Nadolol has been promoted on the basis of its long half-life, 17–24 hours, requiring only once a day administration (166). Recently, however, Watson and co-workers demonstrated that metoprolol and propranolol produce sustained blood pressure reduction for 24 hours with chronic

Table 7.

COMPARISON OF COMMONLY USED BETA-BLOCKING AGENTS

	Metoprolol	Nadolol	Propranolol
Absorption (%)	>95	~30	>90
Bioavailability (%)	40 – 50	~30	~30
Protein Binding (%)	10 – 12	30	90 – 95
Elimination half-life (hours)	3 – 4	14 – 24	3.5 – 6
Predominate Route of elimination	Hepatic metabolism	Renal* excretion	Hepatic metabolism
% Dose Excreted unchanged	3	>90	<1
Active Metabolites	No	No	Yes
Approved indications	HBP	HBP Angina	HBP Angina Arrythmias Migraine**
Frequency of administration	Twice daily	Once daily	Two to four times daily

* – half-life prolonged in patients with renal dysfunction
** – prophylaxis only

once daily administrations (167). The starting propranolol dose and bid regimen is appropriate for A.K. Stepwise increments and careful clinical monitoring are needed.

17. What patient-related variables does A.K. exhibit which may predispose her to beta-blockade toxicity? What subjective and objective monitoring parameters and/or intervention procedures are appropriate?

Child-bearing Age. Assurance of appropriate birth control measures should be obtained from A.K. Several authors have reported growth retardation and poor fetal response to the stress of labor in propranolol-treated patients (159,168). The lack of evidence supporting the safe use of propranolol in pregnancy should be discussed, and future plans for pregnancy should take hypertensive therapy into account.

Diabetes. A.K.'s insulin-dependent diabetes mellitus represents a significant patient-related variable for a variety of reasons. Beta-blocking agents may mask some premonitory symptoms of impending hypoglycemia which are largely due to sympathetic discharge, eg palpitations (tachycardia) and tremor. Hypoglycemia-induced sweating is not inhibited by beta-blockade and may even be prolonged (180). In addition, several authors suggest that beta-blocking agents seem to adversely affect the glucose recovery from insulin-induced hypoglycemia, such that hypoglycemia seems to be enhanced (80,180). Of equal, if not greater significance, is the dramatic rise in blood pressure noted with propranolol and other nonselective beta-blockers during these hypoglycemic episodes. This occurs despite the presence of a bradycardia and may be explained by increased catecholamine output stimulating the vascular alpha receptors while the vasodilatory beta-2 receptors are blocked. The cardioselective beta-1 metoprolol does not cause bradycardia during hypoglycemia and produces minimal blood pressure elevation presumably because the alpha mediated effect of catecholamines is opposed by the vasodilatory beta-2 effect (250).

Therefore, A.K. requires increased diabetic education and monitoring. Investigation regarding previous hypoglycemic reactions is warranted (ie, how often do they occur, what signs or symptoms does she develop, and how does she treat them?). Patient education should emphasize increased caution for periods of potentially low glucose levels. She should also be aware of increased sweating as a key symptom of hypoglycemia. Metoprolol should be considered as an alternative.

Cimetidine Interaction. Cimetidine use by A.K. also represents a patient-related variable to be considered with propranolol use. Therapeutic doses of cimetidine (300 mg four times daily) reduce liver blood flow and inhibit metabolism, causing a significant reduction in the clearance of oral propranolol (251). Prophylactic dosing of cimetidine in A.K. does not contraindicate the administration of propranolol but does require increased monitoring of propranolol's pharmacologic effect. If cimetidine is discontinued, the opposite effect would be expected, and monitoring for decreased propranolol efficacy should be performed.

18. *Hydralazine with Propranolol.* A.L., a 54-year-old woman, was referred to Hypertension Clinic for evaluation and management. She has had hypertension for nine years and over the past three years has noted increasing exertional dyspnea and fatigue. Treatment with digoxin 0.25 mg daily, furosemide 80 mg daily, and propranolol 80 mg bid resulted in some improvement, but she still was unable to complete her housework or walk slowly for more than two or three blocks. She has remained clinically stable for the past several months. At the clinic visit her blood pressure was 160/110 mm Hg; pulse was 80 beats per minute and regular. Jugular venous pressure was normal, and the lung fields were clear. Cardiac examination showed a sustained apical pulse in the anterior axillary line in the sixth intercostal space. An S₃ gallop was noted. Chest roentgenogram showed cardiomegaly. Electrocardiogram showed left ventricular hypertrophy. Serum electrolytes, hemogram, and renal function data were within normal limits. The impression was mild to moderate decompensated congestive heart failure that would most likely improve with adequate blood pressure therapy. A trial of hydralazine was begun. The patient responded favorably over the next several months on an eventual dose of 200 mg bid. She was able to perform all her housework and able to walk two miles on level ground with only mild fatigue.

Why was the combination of propranolol and hydralazine used for treatment of A.L.'s hypertension?

How should therapy be monitored?

Since the vast majority of hypertensive patients manifest an abnormal elevation of systemic vascular resistance, a logical approach to antihypertensive therapy would be to use drugs which lower blood pressure by direct dilation of the arterial bed. Vasodilator drugs such as hydralazine and minoxidil directly relax arteriolar smooth muscle and have far greater effects on resistance than on capacitance vessels. These agents not only reduce the increased peripheral vascular resistance characteristics of hypertension, but do so without producing the significant postural hypotension, weakness, lethargy, and sexual dysfunction which are so commonly observed with sympatholytic agents. The antihypertensive effect achieved by these agents, however, is limited by reflex increases in sympathetic discharge that increase heart rate and cardiac output inappropriately. Thus, hydralazine is said to be contraindicated in patients with a myocardial infarction or angina pectoris. In order to offset the cardiac stimulating properties of hydralazine, reserpine or guanethidine are oftentimes administered concomitantly, because in high doses, these agents cause a bradycardia and a decrease in cardiac output. However, these sympatholytic agents cause generalized sympathoplegia that interferes with reflex mechanisms necessary to maintain blood pressure during postural changes and exercise (187).

Since propranolol inhibits cardiac adrenergic stimulation, decreases cardiac output, and is an effective antihypertensive agent, it is logical to combine beta-blockade with a vasodilating drug. The combination of propranolol and hydralazine was evaluated in 23 patients on a stabilized diuretic regimen with moderate to severe, difficult to control, essential hypertension. Propranolol was initiated first in doses of 20 mg every six hours and then increased to 40 mg every six hours after two days in most patients. Beta-blockade was confirmed by an isoproterenol infusion test, and then hydralazine was added to therapy in an initial dose of 25 mg every six hours which was increased to a maximum of 400 mg per day. Propranolol lowered the mean supine blood pressure from 188/118 to 162/102 mm Hg and lowered the heart rate from 94 to 72 beats per minute. Addition of hydralazine further reduced the mean supine blood pressure to 134/88 mm Hg. Only two patients failed to achieve diastolic pressures lower than 100 mm Hg on this combination therapy, yet their diastolic pressures were lowered by 31 and

41 mm Hg. The effective antihypertensive action was not associated with postural hypotension, tachycardia, other hemodynamic disturbances, impairment of renal function, or adverse symptoms in any patient (187).

Similar dramatic responses in blood pressures were obtained when propranolol was used in combination with the newer vasodilator, minoxidil (188). Moreover, a comparative study of minoxidil and hydralazine in combination with beta-blockers and diuretics demonstrated greater therapeutic efficacy with minoxidil (189). However, because minoxidil is more likely to produce side effects, the combination of hydralazine and propranolol is preferred.

In addition to being an effective combination drug to use with propranolol, hydralazine has the added benefit of arteriolar dilation (afterload reduction), blood pressure reduction, and improved cardiac performance which obviously improved A.L.'s decompensated congestive heart.

As a singular agent, hydralazine only modestly lowers blood pressure, approximately 10 to 15 mm Hg systolic and 8 to 10 mm Hg diastolic. However, when used in conjunction with diuretics and sympatholytic agents, these effects may be doubled (80,193). Therefore, the Joint National Committee recommends hydralazine as a step-3 agent. Hydralazine may be administered twice daily (194), using stepped-care principles up to a maximum dose of 200 mg per day. It was recently reported that administration of hydralazine with food may double or triple its bioavailability (195). Hydralazine may be particularly useful in maintaining renal function in hypertensive patients with renal insufficiency or in improving cardiac output in hypertensive patients with congestive heart failure (80,194). As with all vasodilator therapy, hydralazine may cause sodium and fluid retention, increased heart rate (which may aggravate ischemic heart disease), and headache (117).

A.L. should be informed about routine administration of hydralazine with food. She should take it in a similar manner each day (ie, always with food or always without food) and educated as to the reason. Her pulse rate and history of chest pain should be evaluated at each visit. A new complaint of headache, weight gain, or new onset of edema should evoke the consideration of hydralazine-induced sodium and fluid retention in addition to other causes. Hydralazine has been associated with systemic lupus erythematosus and requires appropriate monitoring in A.L. (see following question).

19. *Hydralazine-Induced Lupus.* Nine months after A.L. had been on hydralazine therapy she walked into clinic complaining of multiple joint aches and pains, generalized weakness, a gradual 5 pound weight loss, and a rash. Suspecting drug-induced lupus, the primary provider obtained a fluorescent antinuclear antibody and LE preparation which were both positive. What subjective and objective data does A.L. have which are compatible with drug-induced lupus syndrome? What will happen if the hydralazine is discontinued?

Hydralazine was first noted in 1953 to induce a syndrome clinically and serologically similar to systemic lupus erythematosus (SLE). Since then, more than 200 cases have been reported. Hydralazine-induced lupus develops in 8 to 13% of patients receiving relatively large doses. This observation led to the initial recommendation that hydralazine dosages be maintained below 400 mg/day to minimize this toxicity. However, Alarcon-Segovia and associates (190) reported nineteen patients who developed lupus even though their doses were less than 200 mg per day. SLE has occurred following dosages as small as 75 mg daily for less than one month. Nevertheless, the consensus remains that the likelihood of developing lupus as a result of hydralazine increases with large doses and with long duration of therapy. A possible contributing factor to hydralazine-induced lupus is the rate at which the drug is metabolized. Hahn and co-workers (191) report that the patients in their series who developed hydralazine lupus were slow acetylators of the drug.

The clinical manifestations of hydralazine-induced lupus resemble those of SLE and include polyarthritis, fever, dermatitis, lymphadenopathy, hepatosplenomegaly, serositis, antinuclear antibodies, leukopenia, and LE cells (191). However, unlike spontaneously occurring SLE, nephritis, central nervous system involvement, and cardiac manifestations are uncommon in hydralazine-induced SLE (192).

A.L. has many of the signs and symptoms of hydralazine-induced SLE. No comment was made regarding nodes, hepatosplenomegaly, or leukopenia. A complete blood count and thorough liver, spleen, and node exam should be performed and documented qualitatively and quantitatively (along with the other signs and symptoms) so that the course of the phenomenon can be appropriately followed to assure remission. Circulating antibodies to hydralazine have been reported, suggesting that hydralazine-induced lupus is, in part, a hypersensitivity response (191). As with all drug-induced cases of lupus, clinical manifestations are generally reversible upon cessation of hydralazine therapy. In most cases the symptoms subside rapidly and totally within 48 hours, never to recur. Rarely, clinical manifestations may continue seven to eight years after the drug is stopped. Occasionally, prolonged and complete remissions of hypertension follow toxicity, so A.L.'s blood pressure should be closely monitored (252). In addition A.L. should be informed of the remission process and reassured that the arthritis is not deforming.

The antinuclear antibody titer usually becomes positive after the second or third month and rises in subsequent months. The LE preparations begin to be positive at about the sixth month. These tests become abnormal before clinical symptoms occur which is opposite of the usual SLE disease process. Following drug discontinuation, the LE cell preparation becomes negative within a few months, but the fluorescent antinuclear antibody titer remains high for a period of months to several years (252).

Although absence of renal disease with drug-induced SLE is noted, isolated case reports of central nervous system or renal disease have appeared. Follow-up neurological and renal function tests should be performed to assure absence of these processes in A.L.

20. *Prazosin.* Three months later A.L. noted complete remission of the symptom complex induced by hydralazine. Gradual reappearance of her cardiac decompensation (as previously noted) and hypertension occurred. Would prazosin be a reasonable antihypertensive to add to her regimen?

A.L. has congestive heart failure (CHF) and reduction of blood pressure is paramount as shown by her previous response. Prazosin is an appropriate choice for this patient. Miller and co-workers (203,205) first studied the use of prazosin in patients with CHF. Prior to the introduction of prazosin, hydralazine was used in combination with long-acting nitrates for refractory or severe CHF. Hydralazine lowered systemic resistance and raised cardiac output but failed to lower left ventricular filling pressure. The long-acting nitrates reduced left ventricular preload but failed to enhance cardiac output. Miller and associates theorized that prazosin might serve both functions and documented benefits in 10 patients with severe CHF. Patients with CHF maintain a cardiac output that functions on a depressed Frank-Starling curve as a result of increased ventricular filling pressures (preload) and cardiac impedance (afterload). A reduction in preload and afterload decreases the workload of the heart and improves cardiac output; therefore, the Starling curve is shifted towards normal. However, the chronic effects of prazosin on CHF are less clear. Awan, Miller and associates (204) went on to document the long-term efficacy of prazosin by demonstrating improvement by echocardiography, exercise tolerance (treadmill), and ventricular function (cardiac catheterization) after two weeks of therapy and observed continued symptomatic improvement (New York Heart Association functional class) for two to four months. Subsequent studies by different cohorts demonstrate conflicting results. Some studies demonstrate continued objective CHF improvement after 6 to 12 weeks of therapy with prazosin that are usually less than initial results (206,207). Others demonstrate loss of CHF effect by the fifth dose despite adequate blood pressure control (208,209). Further studies are needed to resolve this issue. If prazosin therapy is instituted for hypertension in patients with borderline or fulminant CHF, careful CHF as well as blood pressure monitoring is required to assure response and maintenance of effect. Tolerance to the antihypertensive effects has not been reported in long-term studies (196,198). A.L. is currently taking furosemide and propranolol for hypertension; prazosin is a logical addition to this combination which has been suggested as an effective regimen in severe hypertension treatment (200). Prazosin will not affect ANA titers or produce drug-induced lupus syndrome in A.L. (210).

21. *Cessation of Antihypertensive Therapy.* B.W. is a 38-year-old school teacher who has been taking clonidine 0.2 mg twice daily for two weeks along with hydrochlorothiazide 100 mg daily. Her severely elevated blood pressure (180/120 mm Hg) has returned to normal (140/90 mm Hg); however, she has been somnolent at work and continually has a dry mouth with accompanying parotid gland pain. She related her discomfort to her medica-

tions and discontinued them. Twenty-four hours later, she become restless, agitated, developed headaches, insomnia, and began sweating. Upon visiting the local emergency room, she was again hypertensive (170/115 mm Hg).

What is the most likely cause of B.W.'s symptoms? How should her problems be treated in the emergency room?

The most troublesome side effects of clonidine are sedation and dry mouth which occur in as many as half the patients treated. These side effects may be profound and require discontinuation of clonidine.

The most significant adverse effect reported with clonidine is rebound hypertension. A great deal has been written about this potentially serious and frequently unrecognized syndrome (217–223). There seem to be three basic responses to the sudden cessation of any antihypertensive treatment: a) Normotension for several days, then a slow rise in blood pressure to pretreatment values, b) same as "a" but with significant development of signs and symptoms of sympathetic overactivity such as nervousness, agitation, sweating, headache, palpitation, insomnia, or nausea, and c) rapid rise in blood pressure, approaching pretreatment levels, within hours after discontinuation of treatment. This rapid increase is referred to as *rebound hypertension;* on occasion the blood pressure clearly exceeds the highest previously known blood pressure reading and is termed overshoot. The development of severe morbidity or mortality from rebound hypertension has caused much alarm and concern (218,219,224). The incidence of rebound hypertension is difficult to estimate since most studies are retrospective case reports. However, the incidence is considered by most to be small in view of the prevalence of hypertension and the infrequency of the reports. Prospective studies have been done on clonidine specifically (223), and out of a total of 97 patients, all failed to demonstrate an overshoot phenomenon. Many mechanisms have been suggested, such as increased levels of circulating norepinephrine, increased sensitivity to norepinephrine, decreased vagal function, increased oxygen demand, and increased renin-angiotensin activity, but no mechanism has been proven.

B.W. requires a thorough cardiovascular evaluation. Reinstitution of her previous medications is logical if no end-organ damage is present (ie, encephalopathy, congestive heart failure, arrhythmias, angina, or renal damage). Bedrest (and possibly mild sedation) is usually the only treatment necessary for patients with symptoms and no significant BP elevation. The presence of end-organ damage requires a problem-oriented therapeutic approach.

The essence of the issue of abrupt cessation of clonidine or any antihypertensive therapy is patient education emphasizing the following: a) the syndrome exists but is a rare phenomenon, b) it is preventable, so providers and patients should be aware of it (particularly patients with pre-existing angina, arrhythmias, severe hypertension, or a history of a myocardial infarction), c) reinstitution of the previously administered agent will remedy most episodes, and d) reduction of antihypertensives should be gradual (7–14 days) when needed.

22. Clonidine-Drug Combinations. Clonidine 0.2 mg bid and hydrochlorothiazide 50 mg bid were reinstituted in the emergency room. Is this a rational combination of drugs? What clonidine-drug combinations should be avoided?

The exact mechanism of clonidine's activity is complex. Clonidine can be considered a prototype of centrally acting antihypertensive agents. It is both a partial alpha-adrenergic agonist and a partial alpha-adrenergic antagonist depending on the region of the hypothalamus; both actions, however, inhibit sympathetic outflow from the vasomotor center.

Clonidine is most effective when combined with a diuretic, since it may cause some salt and water retention. The initial dosing should start at 0.1 mg bid and be increased at weekly or biweekly intervals by 0.1 to 0.2 mg daily. Although the manufacturer's recommended maximum dose is 2.4 mg, 0.4 to 0.8 mg per day usually suffice. It is an effective step-2 agent with a diuretic for mild or moderate hypertension. Clonidine can be added to beta-blocking agents or vasodilators with increased effects. Clonidine and methyldopa have similar central mechanisms of actions and this combination offers no advantage. In addition, concomitant use of reserpine or guanethidine seems illogical.

23. Should long-term clonidine treatment be continued in B.W.?

Because of her extreme discomfort during clonidine therapy and the impairment of mental alertness needed by her profession, clonidine should be gradually tapered with the addition of another antihypertensive from a different category. A beta-blocker with or without a vasodilator would be appropriate alternatives.

24. Guanethidine. W.S., a 60-year-old male, was found to have blood pressures in the range of 165/105 mm Hg. There was no evidence of secondary hypertension. Except for some AV nicking, there was no evidence of end organ damage. He was treated initially with hydrochlorothiazide 50 mg bid with minimal response. Guanethidine 10 mg daily was then added, and the dosage was slowly increased at monthly intervals until five months later when his blood pressure was controlled with guanethidine 50 mg daily in addition to hydrochlorothiazide 50 mg bid.

Was the dosing of guanethidine in W.S. compatible with its general pharmacologic and pharmacokinetic characteristics? How often can the dose of guanethidine be increased?

Guanethidine concentrates in the neurosecretory granules in post-ganglionic sympathetic nerve endings. At this site, it depletes norepinephrine from storage granules and blocks norepinephrine release upon physiologic nerve stimulation (225). The net result of these actions is inhibition of sympathetic reflexes, with a resultant decrease in blood pressure due primarily to venous pooling.

Oral absorption of guanethidine ranges from 3 to 60% (226,227). Approximately 30% of the absorbed drug is excreted unchanged renally, and 60% appears in the urine as inactive metabolites. While individual responses vary greatly, serum plasma levels of 8 ng/ml usually correlate well with effective antihypertensive responses. Individual differences in dosage requirements may be due to variations in absorption, metabolism, distribution, or excretion patterns (228). The estimated serum half-life is five days (83). Guanethidine has a long onset of action; minimal effects may be seen within three days while maximal effects may take three to six weeks.

Although methods for administering loading doses in hospitalized patients appear effective (229,230), such an approach is inappropriate for the treatment of ambulant patients. The more conservative use of 10 to 12.5 mg initial doses, adjusted to the patient's response in 10 to 12.5 mg increments every one to two weeks is more rational. When combined with effective diuretic therapy, 25 to 50 mg daily is the usual therapeutic dose, although up to 400 mg may be needed in patients with severe hypertension (117).

The time it took to reach the therapeutic objective for W.S. was nearly 6 months. In retrospect, control could probably have been obtained sooner with more frequent visits and dosage increments (every two weeks rather than every four weeks). However, several factors favor the way W.S. was treated: Hypertension is a chronic disease which requires chronic treatment, gradual dosage increments minimize adverse effects, and the risks of morbidity and mortality are reduced as blood pressure decreases. Six months for blood pressure control was a reasonable expectation for this patient who was not experiencing any end organ effects from his moderate essential hypertension.

25. W.S. returned to clinic three months later with his blood pressure out of control. It was discovered that he had been started on amitriptyline for a depression caused by an impending marriage dissolution. How should this current blood pressure problem be approached?

Guanethidine-Tricyclic Antidepressant Interaction. Norepinephrine is synthesized from tyrosine and is stored in intra-axonal granules which protect it from inactivation by monoamine oxidase (MAO). Following a stimulus, norepinephrine is released from nerve terminals into the synaptic cleft where it can then initiate a synaptic transmission. After release, norepinephrine is either inactivated by circulating catechol-o-methyl transferase (COMT), or is recaptured and transported back into the storage granules by an amine concentrating pump mechanism located in the neuronal membrane. This specialized re-uptake mechanism is not entirely specific, and the storage granules will accept other amines if they have a betahydroxyl or a dihydroxybenzene group (231). Thus, other amines such as tyramine, amphetamine, ephedrine, and guanethidine share this re-uptake pump.

Drugs like guanethidine block adrenergic neurons because they are concentrated within them by this membrane transport system. The necessity of this transport system for guanethidine's antihypertensive activity is demonstrated by the loss of guanethidine's effectiveness when its uptake is inhibited. This is the basis of the significant drug-drug interaction with amitriptyline, because tricyclic antidepressants block this amine uptake and thereby antagonize the antihypertensive effect of guanethidine (232). All tricyclic antidepressants can antagonize the antihypertensive effects of guanethidine within two days. This effect persists for four to five days after discontinuing antidepressants.

Sexual Dysfunction. Guanethidine is associated with significant sexual dysfunction and this should be investigated as a possible cause of his depression. Guanethidine can interfere with sexual performance in a large percentage of patients by causing impotence or failure of ejaculation. It has been claimed that 63% of men studied have this side effect (233). Vejlsgaard (234) reports this side effect in twelve out of forty patients (34%); Nies (117) states that the sexual impotence is less common than delayed or retrograde ejaculation, which may be intolerable.

During a thorough evaluation it was discovered that W.S. was not experiencing adverse effects and was compliant to the guanethidine. It was concluded that the amitriptyline-guanethidine interaction was clinically significant. The amitriptyline was discontinued because the depression was reactive in nature, and tricyclic antidepressant therapy was not needed. W.S.'s blood pressure control returned at the next visit.

26. *Guanethidine Side Effects.* Two years later W.S. returned to clinic with his blood pressure controlled on the same regimen. Because his blood glucose was 120 mg/dl (normal: 70–110 mg/dl), hydrochlorothiazide was discontinued. Two weeks later, his blood pressure rose to 160/100 mm Hg and a five pound weight gain was noted. Hydrochlorothiazide therapy was reinstituted and the guanethidine dose was increased to 75 mg/ daily. Within one week, his blood pressure dropped to 140/76 mm Hg. He experienced fainting spells upon arising too quickly and developed explosive diarrhea as well. How could these symptoms be alleviated?

Like all non-diuretic antihypertensive agents, guanethidine produces sodium and fluid retention which results in some loss of antihypertensive activity (235). Therefore, guanethidine should always be administered concurrently with a diuretic.

Due to its peripheral venous pooling action, guanethidine commonly produces orthostatic hypotension characterized by dizziness, light-headedness, weakness and, occasionally, fainting. In order to minimize this problem, doses should be slowly titrated to the patient's level of tolerance (see Question 24). Individuals who are physically active, the elderly, and patients who have autonomic insufficiency (eg, some diabetics) are particularly vulnerable. Techniques for minimizing this problem include arising slowly from sitting or prone positions and flexing one's arms and legs prior to standing. Potentiating factors include ingestion of vasodilating chemicals such as alcohol, entering a warm room, vigorous exercise, prolonged standing, hot showers, or acute exposure to heat. Patients should be cautioned about these factors when guanethidine therapy is initiated and when doses are increased.

The sympatholytic action of guanethidine often results in a relative excess of parasympathetic innervation of the gastrointestinal (GI) tract. As a result of this imbalance, GI motility is increased and loose stools or explosive diarrhea may occur. Possible methods of correction include dividing a single daily dose into two doses, or adding small doses of an anticholinergic agent.

In this case, the dose of guanethidine should not have been increased prior to assessing the effect of the reinstituted hydrochlorothiazide. The effects of thiazides on blood glucose are discussed in Question 11. Vigorous lowering of blood pressure, especially in the elderly, may precipitate strokes or myocardial infarctions.

27. Minoxidil. C.R. is a 57-year-old black man with a ten year history of essential hypertension. Despite therapy with hydrochlorothiazide 50 mg bid and propranolol 120 mg bid, his blood pressure is 160/110 mm Hg. Compliance was documented by history and consistent medication refills. Laboratory findings were unremarkable. His pulse was 60 beats per minute and regular. Funduscopic examination revealed grade-I KW changes. Chest x-ray demonstrated borderline cardiomegaly. IVP and renin studies were normal. Minoxidil 10 mg daily was added to his drug therapy and a clinic appointment was made for the following week. Why was minoxidil selected for this patient? How should therapy be monitored?

Since he is apparently not responding to the combination of a thiazide and a beta-blocker, the addition of another antihypertensive with a different mechanism of action is appropriate. The benefits of minoxidil in combination with propranolol were discussed in Question 18. The initial dose may be increased by 5–10 mg every three to seven days until the desired reduction in blood pressure is attained. Most patients respond to 40 mg per day or less; the maximum approved daily dose is 100 mg.

Vasodilation from minoxidil administration activates the peripheral sympathetic nervous system through stimulation of carotid and aortic baroreceptors. This action, in turn, causes renin release, tachycardia, and increased cardiac output. These effects remain as long as minoxidil therapy is continued and for the most part may be offset by concomitant administration of propranolol. Sodium and fluid retention with minoxidil is significant and is largely due to redistribution of renal blood flow, resulting in increased sodium reabsorption in the proximal convoluted tubule.

Perhaps the most common adverse effect is hypertrichosis, increased hair growth. Although this effect is also referred to as hirsutism, it is not associated with any endocrine abnormality. It commonly develops during the first several weeks of therapy in about 80% of the patients taking minoxidil. Fine and short hairs become darker and thicker on the pinna of the ear, above the eyebrows, over the temples, or in the sideburn areas. With continued administration, hair growth occurs on the arms, legs, chest, back and scalp. The hair growth may be controlled by shaving or use of dipilatories (238–240).

Because C.R. has borderline cardiomegaly, careful monitoring for development of congestive heart failure is mandatory. In addition, thorough monitoring for ischemic complications is warranted. Minoxidil has been associated with the development of angina, presumably due to increased heart rate and cardiac output, and the resultant increases in myocardial oxygen demand.

28. Fluid Retention and Cardiac Effects from Minoxidil. The dose of minoxidil was gradually increased to 40 mg daily and C.R.'s blood pressure was controlled to 145/85 mm Hg without orthostasis. However, three months later C.R. returned to the clinic complaining of shortness of breath. In addition, a 13 kg weight gain, S_3 gallop, bibasilar rales

3+ pedal edema, and EKG changes (non-specific ST-T wave changes and T wave inversion) were noted. He was admitted to the hospital, minoxidil was discontinued, and furosemide 80 mg was ordered. An echocardiogram was ordered. Comment on his current treatment.

Fluid retention, manifested by weight gain and edema, is a common adverse effect of minoxidil therapy. Although pre-existing congestive heart failure may improve when minoxidil therapy is administered, substantial fluid retention can precipitate or worsen congestive heart failure. Severe fluid retention secondary to minoxidil often responds to the addition of furosemide, particularly in high doses (244,245–247). If high dose furosemide fails to remove the fluid accumulation, minoxidil should be stopped. Treatment with digoxin is not effective unless decompensated heart failure is already present. Pericardial effusions have also occurred in patients on minoxidil therapy (245,247). The echocardiogram is being performed to assure that pericardial effusion has not occurred.

Reversible EKG abnormalities occur in a large proportion of patients (90%) shortly after starting minoxidil therapy (248,249). These EKG findings are often non-specific T-wave changes consisting of flattening or inversion and range from slight to marked (249). The EKG changes noted in this patient are of little diagnostic value.

29. *Captopril.* **C.R.'s fluid retention and congestive heart failure responded well to furosemide and discontinuation of minoxidil. His EKG changes returned to normal. It was decided not to resume therapy with minoxidil. Instead, captopril is being considered as an addition to C.R.'s therapy. How does captopril lower blood pressure? Would it be an appropriate choice for this patient?**

Captopril was approved for use as an antihypertensive in May 1981. It is indicated for the treatment of hypertensive patients who failed to respond satisfactorily or developed unacceptable side effects on multidrug regimens. It is believed that captopril produces its effect by inhibiting angiotensin converting enzyme (ACE) (253–257). ACE increases blood pressure by several mechanisms: a) ACE converts angiotensin I to angiotensin II, a potent vasoconstrictor, b) ACE indirectly produces more angiotensin II which is a stimulus of aldosterone release, increasing sodium retention and intravascular volume, and c) it inactivates bradykinin, a potent vasodilator. Therefore inhibition of ACE should produce a lowering of blood pressure. Other mechanisms involving kinins and prostaglandins have also been suggested (254,256,257).

Captopril appears appropriate for C.R. for several reasons. First, captopril has been shown to be effective in combination with propranolol and hydrochlorothiazide (253–255). This is logical since these drugs all lower blood pressure by different mechanisms. Also, diuretic agents generally stimulate the renin-angiotensin system, and this effect would be prevented by captopril use. Furthermore, chronic use of captopril increases stroke volume, cardiac output, and oxygen consumption and has been shown to be useful in congestive heart failure (258–260).

30. *Monitoring of Captopril Therapy.* **Captopril 25 mg bid was added to C.R.'s regimen. He is scheduled to return in two weeks for evaluation. What subjective and objective data should be obtained at this time?**

As with the initiation of any new antihypertensive medicine, compliance should be assessed. A maculopapular rash on the upper extremities and trunk occurs in about 10% of patients within the first 4 weeks of therapy, and C.R. should be questioned for this adverse effect. Taste impairment occurs in about 7% of patients and is manifested as an alteration or loss of taste perception. In some cases dysguesia (or aguesia) is severe and is accompanied with significant weight loss. This phenomenon usually occurs within the first three months and resolves in 4–12 weeks with continued therapy (253,254). Orthostatic blood pressure measurements should be obtained. Captopril usually reduces blood pressure to the same extent in both the supine and upright positions; orthostasis may occur in fluid or sodium depleted patients. Proteinuria associated with captopril has been shown to occur in about 1% of the patients and is rarely accompanied with elevated serum creatinine or BUN values. Proteinuria most often occurs within the first eight months and mostly in patients with pre-existing renal disease. C.R. should have urinary protein estimates using a dipstick prior to the initiation of captopril and monthly thereafter (254,261).

C.R.'s blood pressure after initiation of captopril 25 md tid was 145/100 mm Hg. The captopril was increased to 50 mg tid with subsequent normal blood pressures.

31. *Hypertension in the Elderly.* R.K., a 69-year-old man, was found to have a blood pressure of 184/96 mm Hg on routine physical examination and this elevated blood pressure was confirmed on two subsequent follow-up visits. The physical exam was unremarkable except for some early funduscopic changes. The EKG and routine blood and urine studies showed nothing unusual.

After four weeks of treatment with hydrochlorothiazide 50 mg daily, his blood pressure was 165/92 mm Hg and the dosage was increased to 50 mg bid. Two months later the patient was admitted to the hospital for extreme weakness. Hypokalemia and severe dehydration were observed, and appropriate treatment with fluid and electrolytes was instituted. In view of R.K.'s age, did his elevated blood pressure warrant treatment?

Many clinicians and investigators would advocate treatment (262–264,266). Either systolic or diastolic hypertension is a risk factor for cardiovascular morbidity and mortality in older persons. Furthermore, treatment reduces the morbidity and mortality in elderly patients. Twenty-two percent of those in the Hypertension Detection and Follow-up Program (28) were 60–69 years of age, and the benefit to these patients in terms of reduced morbidity and mortality was as positive as it was for younger patients. A specially designed trial entitled European Working Party on High Blood Pressure in the Elderly

(EWPHE) has already demonstrated that both systolic and diastolic blood pressure can safely be lowered with the empirical use of diuretics and methyldopa. The beneficial effects, if any, on morbidity and mortality have not yet been reported since the EWPHE trial is still in progress (268).

32. *Treatment of Essential Hypertension in the Elderly.* Comment on R.K.'s diuretic therapy.

The elderly are more sensitive to both the therapeutic and toxic effects of diuretics. Routine serum electrolytes should have been performed on R.K. Dosages above 25 mg bid of hydrochlorothiazide are probably not needed. If blood pressure is not adequately controlled with these doses, a step-2 agent can be added. It must be recognized that low blood volume, reduced baroreceptor reflex activity, decreased liver and renal function, decreased serum protein, altered distribution, and the presence of other drugs may serve to increase responsiveness to antihypertensive therapy. Therefore, therapy should begin with low dosages that should be increased gradually over weeks rather than days. It is established that diuretics are effective in these patients. Propranolol, however, may (262,263,266) or may not (263,269,270) be effective in the elderly. Methyldopa would be an appropriate choice for R.K. The starting dosage should be 125 mg bid to avoid drowsiness and orthostatic hypotension.

References

1. Kirkendall WM (Chairman) et al: American heart association recommendations for human blood pressure determination by sphygmomanometer. Circulation. 1980; 62:1146.
2. Rose GA et al: A sphygmomanometer for epidemiologists. Lancet. 1964; 1:296.
3. Krishan I (Chairman) et al: The 1980 report of the joint national committee on detection, evaluation, and treatment of high blood pressure. Arch Intern Med. 1980; 140:1280.
4. Perry HM (Chairman): Recommendations for a national high blood pressure program data base for effective antihypertensive therapy. Report of Task Force I, DHEW Publication No. (NIH) 75-593. Bethesda, Maryland. U.S. Department of Health, Education and Welfare, 1973.
5. Report of the Joint National Committee on Detection, Evaluation, and Treatment of High Blood Pressure: A Cooperative Study. JAMA. 1977; 237:255.
6. Hawthorne EW et al: Mild hypertension—appropriate diagnostic work-up. Ann NY Acad Sci. 1978; 304:363.
7. Gross F (Chairman) et al: Arterial hypertension. World Health Organization Technical Report Series (628), WHO, Geneva, 1978.
8. Stamler J et al: Hypertension screening of 1 million Americans. JAMA. 1976; 235(21):2299.
9. Levy RI: 5-year study shows systematic hypertension care saves lives. J Cardiovas Med. 1980; 5(3):209.
10. Gifford RW: Evaluation of the hypertensive patient with emphasis on detecting curable causes. Millbank Memorial Fund Quarterly. 1969; 47:170.
11. Laragh JH: Evaluation and care of the hypertensive patient. Am J Med. 1972; 52:565.
12. Ferguson RK: Cost and yield of the hypertensive evaluation. Ann Intern Med. 1975; 82:761.
13. Wilhelmsen L et al: Prevalence of primary and secondary hypertension. Am Heart J. 1977; 97(4):543.

14. Dollery CT: Arterial hypertension. In *Cecil, Textbook of Medicine,* 15th ed, edited by PB Beeson, W McDermott and JB Wyngaarden, WB Saunders, Philadelphia, 1979, p 1199.

15. Tarazi RC and Gifford RW: Systemic arterial pressure. In *Pathologic Physiology, Mechanisms of Disease,* 6th ed, edited by WA Sodeman and TM Sodeman, WB Saunders, Philadelphia, 1979, p 198.

16. Laragh JH et al: Renin, angiotensin and aldosterone systems in pathogenesis and management of hypertensive vascular disease. Am J Med. 1972; 52:633.

17. Sullivan JM: Physiologic and biochemical profile of hypertension for rational clinical management. Adv Int Med. 1978; 23:219

18. UCLA Conference: Hypertension, primary and secondary. Ann Intern Med. 1971; 75:761.

19. Weiss NS: Relation of high blood pressure to headache, epistaxis and selected other symptoms. N Engl J Med. 1972; 287:631.

20. Caris TN: Initial evaluation of patients with hypertension: an office procedure. So Med J. 1978; 71:403.

21. Ayers CR: Standards for quality care of hypertensive patients in offices and hospital practice. Am J Cardiol. 1973; 32:533.

22. Stamey TA: Unilateral renal disease causing hypertension. JAMA. 1976; 35:2340.

23. Hunt JC and Strong CG: Renovascular hypertension, mechanisms, natural history and treatment. Am J Cardiol. 1973; 32:562.

24. Kincaid-Smith P: Renal disease and hypertension. Med Clin North Am. 1977; 61:611.

25. Kannel WB et al: Blood pressure and risk of coronary heart disease: the Framingham study. Dis Chest. 1969; 56:43.

26. Veterans Administration Cooperative Study Group on Antihypertensive Agents: Effects of treatment on morbidity in hypertension II: results in patients with diastolic blood pressures averaging 90 through 114 mm Hg. JAMA. 1970; 213:1143.

27. Veterans Administration Cooperative Study Group on Antihypertensive Agents: Effects of treatment on morbidity in hypertension: results in patients with diastolic pressures averaging 115 through 129 mm Hg. 1967; 202:1028.

28. Five-year findings of the Hypertension Detection and Follow-up Program, Hypertension, Detection and Follow-up Program Cooperative. JAMA. 1979; 242:2562.

29. Kannel WB et al: Epidemiologic assessment of the role of blood pressure in stroke, the Framingham study. JAMA. 1970; 214:301.

30. Conomy JP: Impact of arterial hypertension on the brain. Postgrad Med. 1980; 68:86.

31. Rabkin SW et al: The relation of blood pressure to stroke prognosis. Ann Intern Med. 1978; 89:15.

32. Smith WM: Epidemiology of hypertension. Med Clin North Am. 1977; 61:467.

33. Kannel WB et al: Hypertension and cardiac impairments increase stroke risk. Geriatrics. 1978; 33:71.

34. Engelman K et al: Elevation of arterial pressure. In *Harrison's Principles of Internal Medicine,* Chapter 34, 8th ed, McGraw-Hill, New York, 1977, p 188.

35. Gilmore HR: The treatment of chronic hypertension. Med Clin North Am. 1971; 55:317.

36. Pickering G: Chapters 8,15,17,20. In *High Blood Pressure,* 2nd ed, J and A Churchill Ltd, 1968.

37. Platt R: Heredity in hypertension. Lancet. 1963; 1:889.

38. Schweitzer MD et al: Genetic factors in primary hypertension and coronary disease. J Chron Dis. 1962; 45:1093.

39. Zinner SH et al: Familial aggregation blood pressure in children. N Engl J Med. 1971; 284:401.

40. Smith WM: Epidemiology of hypertension. Med Clin North Am. 1977; 61:467.

41. Schoenberger JA: Management of essential hypertension. Med Clin North Am. 1971; 55:11.

42. Kawasaki T et al: The effect of high sodium and low sodium intake on blood pressure and other related variables in human subjects with idiopathic hypertension. Am J Med. 1978; 64:193.

43. Black HR: Non-pharmacologic therapy for hypertension. Am J Med. 1979; 66:837.

44. Shapiro AP et al: Non-pharmacologic treatment of hypertension. Ann NY Acad Sci. 1978; 304:222.

45. Lew EA: High blood pressure, other risk factors and longevity: the insurance point of view. Am J Med. 1973; 55:281.

46. Center for Disease Control: The effects of smoking on health. Morbid Mortal Weekly Report. 1977; 26:145.

47. Cryer PE et al: Norepinephrine and epinephrine release and adrenergic medication of smoking-associated hemodynamic and metabolic effects. N Engl J Med. 1976; 295:573.

48. Lefkowitz RJ: Smoking, catecholamines and the heart. N Engl J Med. 1976; 295:615.

49. Inter-Society Commission for Heart Disease Resources. Atherosclerosis Study Group and Epidemiology Study Group. Primary Prevention of the Atherosclerotic Diseases. In *Cardiovascular Diseases—Guidelines for Prevention and Care,* edited by Wright IS and Fredrickson DT, US Government Printing Office, Washington, DC, 1974, p 15.

50. Gordon T et al: High density lipoprotein as a protective factor against coronary artery disease. The Framingham Study. Am J Med. 1977; 62:707.

51. Wallace RB et al: Alterations of plasma high-density lipoprotein cholesterol levels associated with consumption of selected medications. Circulation. 1980; 62(Suppl IV):77.

52. Leven P et al: Effect of propranolol and prazosin on blood lipids. Lancet. 1980; 11:4.

53. Grimm RH et al: Effects of thiazide diuretics on plasma lipids and lipoproteins in mildy hypertensive patients. Ann Intern Med. 1981; 94:7.

54. Kannel WB et al: The relation of adiposity to blood pressure and development of hypertension: The Framingham Study. Ann Intern Med. 1967; 67:48.

55. Reisin E et al: Effect of weight loss without salt restriction on the reduction of blood pressure in overweight patients. N Engl J Med. 1978; 298:1.

56. Tyroler HA et al: Weight and hypertension: Evans County Studies of Blacks and Whites. In *Epidemiology and Control of Blood Pressure,* edited by O Paul, New York, 1975.

57. Freis ED: Salt, volume, and prevention of hypertension. Circulation. 1976; 53:589.

58. Dahl LK: Salt and hypertension. Am J Clin Nutr. 1972; 25:231.

59. Rosenstock IM: Why people use health services. Part II. Milbank and Memorial Fund Quarterly. 1966; 44:94.

60. Becker MH: Sociobehavioral determinants of compliance. In *Compliance with Therapeutic Regimens,* edited by DL Sackett and RB Haynes, The Johns Hopkins University Press, Baltimore, 1976, p 40.

61. Sackett DL: The magnitude of compliance and noncompliance. In *Compliance with Therapeutic Regimens,* edited by DL Sackett and RB Haynes, The Johns Hopkins University Press, Baltimore, 1976, p 9.

62. Schulman BA: Active patient orientation and outcomes in hypertensive treatment: application of a socio-organizational perspective. Med Care. 1979; 17:267.

63. Levine DM et al: Health education for hypertensive patients. JAMA. 1979; 241:1700.

64. Levy RI et al: What does the public know about high blood pressure? Am Pharm. 1979; 19:39.

65. Bloom JR et al: From screening to seeking care: removing obstacles in hypertension control. Prev Med. 1979; 8:500.

66. Deeds SG (Chairman) et al: Patient behavior for blood pressure control. Guidelines for professionals. JAMA 1979; 241(23):2534.

67. Rehder TL et al: Improving medication compliance by counseling and special prescription container. Am J Hosp Pharm. 1980; 37:379.

68. Schoof CS: Hypertension: common questions patients ask. Am J Nurs. 1980; 80:926.

69. Webb PA: Effectiveness of patient education and psychosocial counseling in promoting compliance and control among hypertensive patients. J Fam Pract. 1980; 10:1047.

70. McCombs J et al: Critical patient behaviors in high blood pressure control. Cardiovasc Nurs. 1980; 16:19.

71. Bullen MU: What patients with hypertension should know about their medication. Drugs. 1980; 19:373.

72. Smith WM: Treatment of mild hypertension: results of a ten year intervention trial. Circ Res. 1977; 40(Suppl 1):98.

73. Shapiro AP et al: Behavioral methods in the treatment of hypertension. Ann Intern Med. 1977; 86:626.

74. Hill O: The psychological management of psychosomatic diseases. Br J Psychiatry. 1977; 136:113.

75. Schwartz GE: Biofeedback and cardiovascular self-regulation: neurophysiological mechanisms. Prog Brain Res. 1977; 47:317.

76. Shapiro DH et al: Meditation and psychotherapeutic effects. Arch Gen Psych. 1978; 35:294.

77. Pollack AA et al: Limitations of transcendental meditation in the treatment of essential hypertension. Lancet. 1977; 1:71.

78. Stone RA et al: Psychotherapeutic control of hypertension. N Engl J Med. 1976; 294:80.

79. Chesrow E et al: Comparison of mebutamate, phenobarbital and placebo with essential hypertension. Am J Med Sci. 1966; 251:166.

80. Blaschke TF et al: Antihypertensive agents and the drug therapy of hypertension. In *The Pharmacological Basis of Therapeutics,* 6th ed, edited by AG Gilman, LS Goodman and A Gilman, Macmillan Publishing Co, New York, 1980, p 793.

81. Gerber JG et al: Antihypertensive pharmacology. West J Med. 1980; 132:430.

82. Tarazi RC et al: Long-term thiazide therapy in essential hypertension - evidence for persistent alteration in plasma volume and renin activity. Circulation. 1970; 41:709.

83. Wollam GL et al: Antihypertensive drugs: clinical pharmacology and therapeutic use. Drugs. 1977; 14:420.

84. Frazier HS and Yager H: The clinical use of diuretics. N Engl J Med. 1973; 288:455.

85. Gifford RW: A guide to the practical use of diuretics. JAMA. 1976; 235:1980.

86. McMahon FG: Thiazides, In *Management of Essential Hypertension,* Futura Publishing Co, New York, 1978; p 23.

87. Araoye MA et al: Furosemide compared with hydrochlorothiazide, long-term treatment of hypertension. JAMA. 1978; 240:1863.

88. Finnerty FA et al: Long-term effects of furosemide and hydrochlorothiazide in patients with essential hypertension. Angiology. 1977; 28(2):125.

89. Holland OB et al: Antihypertensive comparisons of furosemide with hydrochlorothiazide for black patients. Arch Intern Med. 1979; 139:1015.

90. Mroczek WJ et al: Large dose furosemide therapy for hypertension. Am J Cardiol. 1974; 33:546.

91. Cranston WI et al: Effect of triamterene on elevated arterial pressure. Am Heart J. 1965; 68:455.

92. Morin Y et al: Triamterene: clinical studies in arterial hypertension. Am Heart J. 1965; 69:195.

93. Schwartz AB and Swartz CD: Dosage of potassium chloride elixir to correct thiazide-induced hypokalemia. JAMA. 1974; 230(5):702.

94. Kosman ME: Management of potassium problems during long-term diuretic therapy. JAMA. 1974; 230:743.

95. Ramsay LE and Ramsay MH: Rational potassium prescribing. Practitioner. 1977; 219:529.

96. Kohvakka A et al: Maintenance of potassium balance during diuretic therapy. Acta Med Scand. 1979; 205:319.

97. Tweeddale MG et al: Antihypertensive and biochemical effects of chlorthalidone. Clin Pharmacol Ther. 1977; 22:519.

98. Finnerty FA: a double-blind study of chlorthalidone and hydrochlorothiazide in an outpatient population of moderate hypertensives. Angiology. 1976; 27:738.

99. Wilson TW et al: Effect of dosage regimen on natriuretic response to furosemide. Clin Pharmacol Ther. 1975; 18:165.

100. Haddad A et al: Potassium in salt substitutes. N Engl J Med. 1975; 292:1082.

101. Cummins RO et al: Potassium in salt substitutes. N Engl J Med. 1975; 292:1082.

102. Riddiough MA: Preventing, detecting and managing adverse reactions to antihypertensive agents in the ambulant patient with essential hypertension. Am J Hosp Pharm. 1977; 34:465.

103. Bennett WM et al: Efficacy and saftey of metolazone in renal failure and nephrotic syndrome. J Clin Pharm. 1973; 13:357.

104. Cowley AJ et al: Diabetes and therapy with potent diuretics. Lancet. 1978; 1:154.

105. Anderson BE et al: A comparison of the effects of hydrochlorothiazide and of furosemide in the treatment of hypertensive patients. Quart J Med. 1971; 160:541.

106. Kohner EM et al: The effects of oral diuretic therapy on glucose tolerance. Lancet. 1971; 1:986.

107. Kaldor A et al: Diabetogenic effect or oral diuretics in asymptomatic diabetics. Int J Clin Pharm Biopharm. 1975; 11:232.

108. Amery A et al: Glucose intolerance during diuretic therapy. Lancet. 1978; 1:681.

109. Lewis PJ et al: Deterioration of glucose tolerance in hypertensive patients on prolonged diuretic treatment. Lancet. 1976; 1:564.

110. Ames RP et al: Elevation of serum lipids during diuretic therapy of hypertension. Am J Med. 1976; 64:748.

111. Ames RP et al: Increase in serum lipids during treatment of hypertension with chlorthalidone. Lancet. 1976; 1:721.

112. Wallace RB et al: Alterations of plasma high-density lipoprotein cholesterol levels associated with consumption of selected medications. Circulation. 1980; 62(Suppl IV):77.

113. Grimm RH et al: Effects of thiazide diuretics on plasma lipids and lipoproteins in mildly hypertensive patients. Ann Intern Med. 1981; 94:7.

114. Dollery CT: Pharmacological basis for combination therapy of hypertension. Ann Rev Pharmacol Toxicol. 1977; 17:311.

115. Simpson FO: Principles of drug treatment for hypertension: indications for treatment and for selection of drug. Pharmcol Ther. 1979; 7:153.

116. Feigenbaum LZ: Drug choice for treatment of hypertension at 'Step 2'. West J Med. 1979; 130:391.

117. Nies AS: Clinical pharmacology of antihypertensive drugs. Med Clin North Am. 1977; 61:675.

118. Buhler FR et al: Propranolol inhibition of renin secretion: a specific approach to diagnosis and treatment of renin-dependent hypertensive diseases. N Engl J Med. 1972; 287:1209.

119. Bravo EL et al: On the mechanism of suppressed plasma renin activity during beta-adrenergic blockade with propranolol. J Lab Clin Med. 1974; 83:119.

120. Anavekar SN et al: The relationship of plasma levels of pindolol in hypertensive patients of effects on blood pressure, plasma renin, and plasma noradrenaline levels. Clin Exper Pharm Physiol. 1975; 2:203.

121. Woods JW et al: Renin profiling in hypertension and its use in treatment with propranolol and chlorthalidone. N Engl J Med. 1976; 294:1137.

122. Mookerjee S et al: Hemodynamic and plasma renin effects of propranolol in essential hypertension. Arch Intern Med. 1977; 137:290.

123. Bravo EL et al: Dissociation between renin and arterial pressure responses to beta-adrenergic blockade in human essential hypertension. Circ Res. 1975; 36(Suppl. 1):241.

124. Kaplan NM: The prognostic implications of plasma renin in essential hypertension. JAMA. 1975; 231:167.

125. Goodwin FK et al: Depressions following reserpine: a re-evaluation. Semin Psychiat. 1971; 3:435.

126. Simpson FO: Hypertension and depression and their treatment. Aust NZ J Psychiat. 1973; 7:133.

127. Pfeiffer HJ et al: Clinical toxicity of reserpine in hospitalized patients. Am J Med Sci. 1976; 271:269.

128. Kirsner JB et al: The effect of reserpine upon basal gastric secretion in man. Arch Intern Med. 1957; 99:390.

129. Roth JL: Role of drugs in the production of gastrointestinal ulcer. JAMA. 1964; 187:418.

130. Moser M: Use and abuse of antihypertensive drugs. Gen Pract. 1967; 35:87.

131. Hollister LE: Hematemesis and melena complicating treatment with rauwolfia alkaloids. Arch Intern Med. 1957; 99:218.

132. West WO: Perforation and hemorrhage from duodenal ulcer during the administration of rauwolfia serpentina: report of five cases. Ann Intern Med. 1958; 48:1033.

133. Armstrong B et al: Retrospective study of the association between use of rauwolfia derivatives and breast cancer in English women. Lancet. 1974; 2:672.

134. Boston Collaborative Drug Surveillance Program: Reserpine and breast cancer. Lancet. 1974; 2:669.

135. Heinonen OP et al: Reserpine use in relation to breast cancer. Lancet. 1974; 2:675.

136. Mack TM et al: Reserpine and breast cancer in a retirement community. N Engl J Med. 1975; 292:1366.

137. Ward GW (editorial): Reserpine—the facts as we know them. Info Memo. 1979; 17:1.

138. Oates JA: Antihypertensive drugs that impair adrenergic neuron function. Pharmacol for Physicians. 1967; 1:1.

139. Glontz GE et al: Methyldopa fever. Arch Intern Med. 1968; 122:445.

140. Cacace CG et al: Alpha-methyldopa hepatitis. Drug Intell Clin Pharm. 1976; 10:144.

141. Maddrey WC et al: Severe hepatitis from methyldopa. Gastroenterology. 1975; 68:351.

142. Thomas E et al: Spectrum of methyldopa liver injury. Am J Gastroent. 1977; 68:125.

143. Miller AC et al: Methyldopa-induced granulomatous hepatitis. JAMA. 1976; 234:2001.

144. Schweitzer IL et al: Acute submassive hepatic necrosis due to methyldopa. Gastroenterology. 1974; 66:1203.

145. Hoyumpa AM Jr et al: Methyldopa hepatitis. Am J Dig Dis. 1973; 18:213.

146. Klatskin G: Toxic and drug-induced hepatitis. In *Diseases of the Liver,* 4th ed, edited by L Schiff, JB Lippincott, Philadelphia, 1975; 604.

147. Wallerstein RO: Ch 9: Blood. In *Current Diagnosis and Treatment,* 12th ed, edited by MA Krupp and MJ Chafton, Lange Medical Publication, Los Altos, 1973, p 262.

148. Carstairs KC et al: Incidence of a positive direct Coomb's test in patients on alphamethyldopa. Lancet. 1966; 2:133.

149. Louis WJ: Methyldopa and hemolytic anemia. Med J Aust. 1967; 2:104.

150. deTorregrosa MV et al: Coombs' positive drug-induced hemolytic anemia. Am J Clin Path. 1970; 53:490.

151. Worlledge SM et al: Autoimmune hemolytic anemia associated with alphamethyldopa. Lancet. 1966; 2:135.

152. Prichard BNC et al: The use of propranolol in the treatment of hypertension. Br Med J. 1964; 2:725.

153. Stumpe KO et al: Clinical aspects of beta-blockers in hypertension. Cardiology. 1980; 66(Suppl. 1):36.

154. Morgan TO et al: A comparison of beta-adrenergic blocking drugs in the treatment of hypertension. Postgrad Med. 1974; 50:253.

155. Lubbe WF: Clinical usefulness of the beta-adrenergic antagonists. S Afr Med J. 1978; 54:139.

156. O'Brien ET: Advantages and disadvantages of beta-adrenergic blocking drugs in hypertension. Angiology. 1978; 29:332.

157. McMahon FG: Ch 11: Propranolol. In *Management of Essential Hypertension,* Futura Pub Co, New York, 1978, p 291.

158. Bayne L et al: Ch 21: Antihypertensive drugs. In *Meyler's Side Effects of Drugs,* 9th ed, edited by MNG Dukes, Excerpta Medica, Amsterdam, 1980, p 317.

159. Carruthers SG: Ch 19: Antianginal and beta-adrenoceptor blocking drugs. In *Meyler's Side Effects of Drugs,* 9th ed, edited by MNG Dukes, Excerpta Medica, Amsterdam, 1980, p 295.

160. The Medical Letter on Drugs and Therapeutics: Propranolol for the prevention of migraine headaches. Med Let Drugs Ther. 1979; 21:77.

161. Winkler GF et al: Efficacy of chronic propranolol in action tremors of the familial, senile or essential varieties. N Engl J Med. 1974; 290:984.

162. Ljung O: Treatment of essential tremor with metoprolol (Letter). N Engl J Med. 1979; 301:1005.

163. Riley T et al: Metoprolol for essential tremor (Letter). N Engl J Med. 1979; 301:663.

164. Frishman W et al: Clinical Pharmacology of the new beta-adrenergic blocking drugs. Part 3: Comparative clinical experience and new therapeutic applications. Am Heart J. 1979; 98:119.

165. Weiner N: Drugs that inhibit adrenergic nerves and block adrenergic receptors. In *The Pharmacological Basis of Therapeutics,* 6th ed, edited by AG Gilman et al, Macmillan Publishing Co, New York, 1980, p 176.

166. Heel RC et al: Nadolol: a review of its pharmacological properties and therapeutic efficacy in hypertension and angina pectoris. Drugs. 1980; 20:1.

167. Watson RDS et al: Influence of once daily administration of beta-adrenoceptor antagonists on arterial pressure and its variability. Lancet. 1979; 1:1210.

168. Reed RL et al: Propranolol therapy throughout pregnancy: a case report. Anesth Analg. 1977; 53:214.

169. Veterans Administration Cooperative Study Group on Antihypertensive Agents: Propranolol in the treatment of essential hypertension. JAMA. 1977; 237:2303.

170. Esler M et al: Pathophysiologic and pharmacokinetic determinants of the antihypertensive response to propranolol. Clin Pharmacol Ther. 1977; 22:299.

171. Pine M et al: Correlation of plasma propranolol concentration with therapeutic response in patients with angina pectoris. 1975; 52:886.

172. Lehtonen A et al: Plasma concentrations of propranolol in patients with essential hypertension. Eur J Clin Pharmacol. 1977; 11:155.

173. Chidsey CA et al: Studies of the absorption and removal of propranolol in hypertensive patients during therapy. Circulation. 1975; 52:313.

174. Walle T et al: The predictable relationship between plasma levels and dose during chronic propranolol therapy. Clin Pharmacol Ther. 1978; 24:668.

175. Louis WJ et al: Use of adrenoceptor-blocking agents in hypertension. Cardiology. 1980; 66(Suppl 1):28.

176. Evans GH et al: Disposition of propranolol: drug accumulation and steady state concentrations during chronic oral administration in man. Clin Pharmacol Ther. 1973; 14:487.

177. Myers MG et al: Sudden withdrawal of propranolol in patients with angina pectoris. Chest. 1977; 71:1.

178. Oka Y et al: Clinical Pharmacology of the new beta-adrenergic blocking drugs. Part 10. Beta-adrenoceptor blockade and coronary artery surgery. Am Heart J. 1980; 99:255.

179. Koch-Weser J: Metoprolol. N Engl J Med. 1979; 301:698.

180. Hansten PD: Beta-blocking agents and antidiabetic drugs. Drug Intell Clin Pharm. 1980; 14:46.

181. Brogden RN et al: Metoprolol: a review of its pharmacological properties and therapeutic efficacy in hypertension and angina. Drugs. 1977; 14:321.

182. The Medical Letter on Drugs and Therapeutics: Metoprolol (Lopressor). Med Let Drugs Ther. 1978; 20:97.

183. Sullivan JM et al: Beta-adrenergic blockade in essential hypertension. Reduced renin release despite renal vasoconstriction. Circ Res. 1976; 39:532.

184. Falch DK et al: Renal plasma flow and cardiac output during hydralazine and propranolol treatment in essential hypertension. Scan J Clin Lab Invest. 1978; 38:143.

185. O'Connor DT et al: Renal perfusion changes during treatment of essential hypertension: Prazosin versus propranolol. J Cardiovasc Pharm. 1979; 1:S38.

186. Bauer JH et al: The long term effect of propranolol therapy on renal function. Am J Med. 1979; 66:405.

187. Zacest R et al: Treatment of essential hypertension with combined vasodilation and beta-adrenergic blockade. N Engl J Med. 1972; 286:617.

188. Gilmore E et al: Treatment of essential hypertension with a new vasodilator in combination with beta-adrenergic blockade. N Engl J Med. 1970; 282:521.

189. Gottlieb TB et al: Combined therapy with vasodilator drugs and beta-adrenergic blockade. Circulation. 1972; 45:571.

190. Alarcon-Sergovia et al: Clinical and experimental studies on the hydralazine syndrome and its relationship to systemic lupus erythematosus. Medicine. 1967; 46:1.

191. Hahn BH et al: Immune responses to hydralazine and nuclear antigens in hydralazine-induced lupus erythematosus. Ann Intern Med. 1972; 76:365.

192. Carey RM et al: Pericardial tamponade: a major manifestation of hydralazine-induced lupus syndrome. Am J Med. 1973; 54:84.

193. McMahon FG: Chap 7: Hydralazine. In *Management of Essential Hypertension,* Futura, New York, 1978, p 209.

194. Cooper I: Maintenance treatment of moderate hypertension with b.i.d. hydralazine. Curr Ther Res. 1976; 20:579.

195. Melander A et al: Enhancement of hydralazine bioavailability by food. Clin Pharmacol Ther. 1977; 22:104.

196. Graham RM et al: Prazosin. N Engl J Med. 1979; 300:232.

197. Lowenstein J et al: Prazosin: mechanism of action and role in antihypertensive therapy. Cardiovasc Med. 1979; 4:885.

198. Brodgen RN et al: Prazosin: a review of its pharmacological properties and therapeutic efficacy in hypertension. Drugs. 1977; 14:163.

199. Stokes GS et al: Prazosin: new alpha-adrenergic blocking agent in treatment of hypertension. Cardiovasc Med. 1978; 3:41.

200. Schirger A et al: Prazosin—new hypertensive agent. JAMA. 1977; 237:989.

201. Hayes JM: Prazosin in severe hypertension. Med J Aust. 1977; (Suppl)2:30.

202. Curtis JA et al: Use of prazosin in management of hypertension in patients with chronic renal failure and in renal transplant recipients. Br Med J. 1975; 4:432.

203. Miller RR et al: Sustained reduction of cardiac impedance and preload in congestive heart failure with the antihypertensive vasodilator and prazosin. N Eng J Med. 1977; 297:303.

204. Awan NA et al: Comparison of effects of nitroprusside and prazosin on left ventricular function and the peripheral circulation in chronic refractory congestive heart failure. Circulation. 1978; 57:152.

205. Awan AA et al: Efficacy of ambulatory systemic vasodilator therapy with oral prazosin in chronic refractory heart failure. Circulation. 1977; 56:346.

206. Aronow WS et al: Effect of prazosin versus placebo on chronic left ventricular heart failure. Circulation. 1979; 59:344.

207. Goldman SA et al: Improved exercise ejection fraction with long-term prazosin therapy in patients with heart failure. Am J Med. 1980; 68:36.

208. Arnold SB et al: Attenuation of prazosin on cardiac output in chronic heart failure. Ann Intern Med. 1979; 91:345.

209. Elkayam V et al: Marked early attenuation of hemodynamic effects of oral prazosin therapy in chronic congestive heart failure. Am J Cardiol. 1979; 44:540.

210. Wilson JD et al: Influence of prazosin on the development of antinuclear antibodies in hypertensive patients. Clin Pharmacol Ther. 1979; 26:209.

211. Isaac L: Clonidine in the central nervous system: site and mechanism of hypotensive action. J Cardiovasc Pharmacol. 1980; 2(Suppl):S5.

212. Lowenstein J: Clonidine. Ann Intern Med. 1980; 92:74.

213. Fyhrquist F et al: Plasma renin activity, blood pressure and sodium excretion during treatment with clonidine. Acta Med Scand. 1975; 197:457.

214. Lowenthal DT: Pharmacokinetics of clonidine. J Cardiovasc Pharmacol. 1980; 2(Suppl 1):S29.

215. Pettinger W: Pharmacology of clonidine. J Cardiovasc Pharmacol. 1980; 2(Suppl 1):S21.

216. Wood RA: The therapeutic uses of clonidine. Scot Med J. 1979; 24:226.

217. Goldberg AD et al: Blood pressure and heart rate and withdrawal of antihypertensive drugs. Br Med J. 1977; 1:1243.

218. Horwitz D et al: Effects of methyldopa in fifty hypertensive patients. Clin Pharmacol. 1967; 8:224.

219. Hansson L et al: Blood pressure crisis following withdrawal of clonidine. Am Heart J. 1973; 85:605.

220. Whitsett TL et al: Abrupt cessation of clonidine administration: a prospective study. Am J Cardiol. 1978; 41:1285.

221. Hubbel FA et al: Adverse effects of sudden withdrawal of antihypertensive medication. Postgrad Med. 1980; 68:129.

222. Garbus SB et al: The abrupt discontinuation of antihypertensive treatment. J Clin Pharmacol. 1979; 19:476.

223. Weber MA: Discontinuation syndrome following cessation of treatment with clonidine and other antihypertensive agents. J Cardiovasc Pharmacol. 1980; 2(Suppl 1):S73.

224. Miller RR et al: Propranolol-withdrawal hypertension. N Engl J Med. 1975; 293:416.

225. Melmon KL: The clinical pharmacology of commonly used antihypertensive drugs In *Cardiovascular Drug Therapy,* edited by KL Melmon, F.A. Davis Co, Philadelphia, 1974, p 175.

226. McMartin C et al: The absorption and metabolism of guanethidine in hypertensive patients requiring different doses of the drug. Clin Pharmacol Ther. 1971; 12:73.

227. Rahn KH et al: Comparison of antihypertensive efficacy, intestinal absorption, and excretion of guanethidine in hypertensive patients. Clin Pharmacol Ther. 1969; 10:858.

228. Walter IE et al: The relationship of plasma guanethidine levels to adrenergic blockage. Clin Pharmacol Ther. 1975; 18:571.

229. Shand DG et al: A loading-maintenance regimen for more rapid initiation of the effect of guanethidine. Clin Pharmacol Ther 1975; 18:139.

230. McAllister RG: Guanethidine in antihypertensive therapy: experience with an oral loading regimen. J Clin Pharmacol. 1975; 15:771.

231. Nies AS et al: Recent concepts in the clinical pharmacology of antihypertensive agents. West J Med. 1967; 106:388.

232. Meyer JF et al: Insidious and prolonged antagonism of guanethidine by amitriptyline. JAMA. 1970; 213:1487.

233. Beckman H: *Dilemmas in Drug Therapy,* W.B. Saunders Co, Philadelphia, 1967, 176.

234. Vejlsgaard V et al: Double-blind trial of four antihypertensive drugs. Br Med J. 1967; 2:598.

235. Smith AJ: Clinical features of fluid retention complicating treatment with guanethidine. Circulation. 1965; 31:485.

236. Lowenthal DT et al: Pharmacology and pharmacokinetics of minoxidil. J Cardiovasc Pharmacol. 1980; 2(Suppl 2):S93.

237. The Medical Letter on Drugs and Therapeutics: Minoxidil (Loniten) Med Let Drugs Ther. 1980; 22:21.

238. Pettinger WA: Minoxidil and the treatment of severe hypertension. N Engl J Med. 1980; 303:922.

239. Miller DD et al: Evaluation of minoxidil. Am J Hosp Pharm. 1980; 37:808.

240. Canaday B: Minoxidil. South Med J. 1980; 73:59.

241. Gottlieb TB et al: Pharmacokinetic studies of minoxidil. Clin Pharmacol Ther. 1972; 13:436.

242. Bennett WM et al: Efficacy of minoxidil in the treatment of severe hypertension in systemic disorders. J Cardiovasc Pharmacol. 1980; 2(Suppl 2):S142.

243. Wells JO: Unusual cases of resistance to minoxidil therapy. J Cardiovasc Pharmacol. 1980; 2(Suppl 1):S228.

244. Dormois JC et al: Minoxidil in severe hypertension: value when conventional drugs have failed. Am Heart J. 1975; 90:360.

245. Campese VM et al: Treatment of severe hypertension with minoxidil: advantages and limitations. J Clin Pharmacol. 1979; 19:231.

246. Mitchell HC et al: Long-term treatment of refractory hypertensive patients with minoxidil. JAMA. 1978; 239:2131.

247. Wilburn RL et al: Long-term treatment of severe hypertension with minoxidil, propranolol and furosemide. Circulation. 1975; 52:706.

248. Kosman ME: Evaluation of a new antihypertensive agent: minoxidil. JAMA. 1980; 244:73.

249. Hall D et al: Serial electrocardiographic changes during long-term treatment of severe hypertension with minoxidil. J Cardiovasc Pharmacol. 1980; 2(Suppl 2):S200.

250. Lloyd-Mostyn RH et al; Modification by propranolol of cardiovascular effects of induced hypoglycemia. Lancet. 1975; 1:1213.

251. Feely J et al: Reduction of liver blood flow and propranolol metabolism by cimetidine. N Engl J Med. 1981; 304:692.

252. Perry HM: Late toxicity to hydralazine resembling systemic lupus erythematosus or rheumatoid arthritis. Am J Med. 1973; 54:58.

253. The Medical Letter on Drugs and Therapeutics: Drugs for hypertension. Med Let Drugs Ther. 1981; 23:45.

254. Heel RC et al: Captopril: a preliminary review of its pharmacological properties and therapeutic efficacy. Drugs. 1980; 20:409.

255. Ferguson RK et al: Captopril in severe treatment-resistant hypertension. Am Heart J. 1980; 99:579.

256. Gavras H et al: Antihypertensive effect of the oral angiotensin converting-enzyme inhibitor SQ 14225 in Man. N Engl J Med. 1978; 298:991.

257. Brunner HR et al: Oral angiotensin converting enzyme inhibitor in long-term treatment of hypertensive patients. Ann Intern Med. 1979; 90:19.

258. Tarazi RC et al: Renin, aldosterone and cardiac decompensation: studies with an oral converting enzyme inhibitor in heart failure. Am J Cardiol. 1979; 44:1013.

259. Levine TB et al: Acute and long-term response to an oral converting enzyme inhibitor, captopril, in congestive heart failure. Circulation. 1980; 62:35.

260. Faxon DP et al: Angiotensin inhibition in severe heart failure: acute central and limb hemodynamic effects of captopril with observations on sustained oral therapy. Am Heart J. 1981; 101:548.

261. Case DB et al: Proteinuria during long-term captopril therapy. JAMA. 1980; 244:346.

262. Kirkendall WM et al: Hypertension in the elderly. Arch Intern Med. 1980; 140:1155.

263. O'Malley K et al: Management of hypertension in the elderly. N Engl J Med. 1980; 302:1397.

264. Ostfeld AM: Elderly hypertensive patient, epidemiologic review. NY State J Med. 1978; 78:1125.

265. Chobanian AV: Therapeutic decision-making in systolic hypertension. Geriatrics. 1981; 36:36.

266. Niarchos AP et al: Hypertension in the elderly. Mod Concepts Cardiovas Dis. 1980; Part I, 49:43, Part II, 49:49.

267. The Medical Letter on Drugs and Therapeutics: Drugs in the elderly. Med Let Drug Ther. 1979; 21:43.

268. Amery A et al: Antihypertensive therapy in elderly patients: pilot trial of the European working party on high blood pressure in the elderly. Gerontology. 1977; 23:426.

269. Drayer JIM et al: Hypertension in the elderly: a new understanding. Drug Therapy. 1981; 11:91.

270. Drayer JIM et al: Unexpected pressor responses to propranolol in essential hypertension. Am J Med. 1976; 60:897.

Chapter 9

Hypertensive Emergencies

Robert Michocki

Signs and Symptoms. Symptoms associated with hypertensive crisis are highly variable and result from damage to specific organ systems. The primary sites of damage are the central nervous system, heart, kidneys, and eyes. Therefore, symptoms of hypertensive crisis merely reflect the degree of injury of these organ systems.

Central nervous system (CNS) damage may present solely as a severe headache or can be accompanied by dizziness, nausea, vomiting, and anorexia. Mental confusion with apprehension is indicative of more severe disease, as is nystagmus, localized weakness, or a positive Babinski sign. CNS damage may be rapidly progressive and result in coma or death. If a cerebrovascular accident has occurred, slurred speech or motor paralysis may be present.

Cardiac complications of hypertensive crisis may be manifested by congestive heart failure or angina pectoris. Myocardial infarction may also be precipitated.

Ocular symptomatology of hypertensive crisis is usually related to changes in visual acuity.

Complaints of blurring of vision or loss of eyesight are frequently associated with the funduscopic findings of hemorrhages, exudates, and sometimes papilledema.

Renal complications are generally noted by laboratory examination and may include hematuria, proteinuria, pyelonephritis, as well as an elevated serum BUN and creatinine (2,29).

The term hypertensive crisis (emergency) refers to a clinical situation in which a marked elevation of arterial pressure, if not treated promptly, carries a high rate of morbidity and mortality. These episodes are usually characterized by an acute and marked elevation of arterial pressure, arteriolar spasm, necrotizing arteriolitis, and secondary organ damage. Hypertensive emergencies generally occur in patients with pheochromocytoma, renal vascular disease, or accelerated essential hypertension. Acute life-threatening elevations of blood pressure can also occur in previously normotensive individuals during the course of acute glomerulonephritis, head injury, severe burns, eclampsia, or in patients receiving monoamine oxidase inhibitors who ingest foods rich in tyramine (1–9).

Rapid, severe blood pressure elevation is not always the hallmark of a hypertensive emergency. Indeed, even moderate elevations of arterial pressure in the context of a variety of disease states demand prompt treatment. Specific examples include acute left ventricular failure, intracranial hemorrhage, dissecting aortic aneurysm, and post-operative bleeding at suture sites.

Hypertensive emergencies rarely develop in previously normotensive patients. Most commonly, they complicate the accelerated phase of poorly controlled chronic hypertension (2,5,10). Before effective modes of treatment for hypertension were available, it was estimated that 1–7% of hypertensive patients progressed to an accelerated phase (11,12). Currently it is estimated that less than 1% of hypertensives now progress to this phase (13). Hypertensive emergencies occur more frequently in blacks than whites (14–16), and it has been suggested that this could be due to late presentation or inadequate therapy (17). A greater frequency in the 40- to 60-year age range and a slight predominance of males over females has also been observed (11,12,18,19).

Malignant hypertension is best described as a clinical syndrome characterized by necrotizing arteriolitis, markedly elevated blood pressure, severe retinopathy (ie, a Keith-Wagener Classification of III or IV), renal failure, and a rapidly deteriorating clinical course (20,26–28).

Accelerated hypertension is a term used to describe a clinical picture that is similar to malignant hypertension but which differs in that it has a less rapidly progressive course (3,26). It has also been considered a forerunner of malignant hypertension (20). Often, the terms malignant and accelerated hypertension are used synonymously (2,7,10,20,30).

Treatment. Hypertensive emergencies require immediate hospitalization and administration of medications to reduce arterial pressure. Effective therapy greatly improves the prognosis, reverses symptoms, and arrests the progression of end-organ damage. Treatment reverses the vascular changes in the eyes and slows or arrests the progressive deterioration in renal function. Treatment of malignant hypertension may transiently worsen renal function. However, after two to three months of adequate medical therapy, renal function may gradually improve to the usual pre-malignant level of renal insufficiency or to a new,

slightly deteriorated level (32,33). Whether treatment can completely reverse end-organ damage is related to two factors, how soon treatment is begun and the extent of damage at the initiation of therapy. Without treatment, the two-year mortality approaches 90% (12,19,33).

There are two fundamental concepts in the management of hypertensive emergencies (5). The first is that immediate and intensive therapy is required and takes precedence over time-consuming diagnostic procedures. Secondly, the choice of drugs will depend on how their time course of action, hemodynamic and metabolic effects meet the needs of a crisis situation. If encephalopathy, acute left ventricular failure, dissecting aortic aneurysm, or other serious conditions are present, the blood pressure should be promptly lowered with parenteral antihypertensive medications such as nitroprusside, trimethaphan, or diazoxide. If a slower blood pressure reduction over several hours or days is acceptable, parenteral hydralazine or methyldopa may be used.

Goals of Therapy. The rate of blood pressure lowering must be individualized. Too rapid a decrease can reduce blood flow to the brain and kidneys and could precipitate a stroke. This is especially true in the elderly and those suffering from cardiovascular disease. In addition, patients who have chronically elevated blood pressures are less likely to tolerate abrupt reductions in their blood pressures, and the amount of reduction appropriate for these patients is somewhat less. Although there are no absolute guidelines, a reduction of 5 to 10 mm Hg every 5 to 10 minutes to a diastolic pressure of 100 mm Hg is an appropriate therapeutic endpoint for most patients.

1. M.R. is a 55-year-old black male who presents to the emergency room with a three-day history of progressively increasing shortness of breath. Over the past two days he developed a severe headache unrelieved by aspirin, substernal chest pain, anorexia, and nausea.

His past medical history includes a five-year history of angina which two months prior to admission resulted in hospitalization for an acute inferior myocardial infarction. He is currently being followed in the renal clinic for chronic renal failure. He has been taking furosemide, hydralazine, propranolol, and methyldopa, but discontinued these medications on his own three weeks ago.

Physical examination reveals an anxious-appearing, elderly black male who is alert, oriented, and in moderate respiratory distress. His vital signs include a pulse rate of 125/min, a respiratory rate of 36/min, a blood pressure of 220/145 mm Hg without orthostasis, and a normal body temperature. Funduscopic examination shows arteriolar narrowing and A-V nicking without hemorrhages, exudates, or papilledema. There is no jugular venous distension. Bilateral carotid bruits are present. Chest examination reveals decreased breath sounds with bilateral rales extending to the tip of the scapula. The heart is displaced 2 cm left of the mid-clavicular line with no thrills or heaves. The rhythm is regular with an S_3 and an S_4 gallop; no murmurs are noted. The remainder of his examination is within normal limits.

Significant laboratory values include the following: Na 142 mEq/L; K 5.5 mEq/L; Cl 101 mEq/L; HCO_3 15 mEq/L; blood urea nitrogen (BUN) 95 mg/dl; creatinine 5.0 mg/dl; hematocrit 33%; hemoglobin 11.5 gm/dl; WBC and differential are within normal limits. A urinalysis shows 1+ hemoglobin and 1+ protein. Microscopic examination of the urine reveals 5–10 red blood cells per high powered field and no casts. Arterial blood gases on room air reveal a pO_2 of 55, pCO_2 of 32, and a pH of 7.28.

An electrocardiogram demonstrates a sinus tachycardia and left ventricular hypertrophy. The chest x-ray shows moderate cardiomegaly and bilateral fluffy infiltrates.

What aspects of this patient's history are consistent with the diagnosis of malignant hypertension?

As discussed earlier, malignant hypertension occurs most frequently in blacks, males and individuals between the ages of 40 and 60. This patient meets all of the characteristics of this population group. Furthermore, many individuals who present with malignant hypertension have a recent history of discontinuing the use of their antihypertensives as is the case with M.R.

The recent onset of a severe headache, nausea, and vomiting are consistent with central nervous system signs of severe hypertension, as are the acute onset of angina (substernal pain) and congestive heart failure (shortness of breath, increased pulse and respiratory rate, cardiomegaly, and chest x-ray findings of pulmonary edema).

The absence of signs of right heart failure such as jugular venous distension or hepatomegaly suggest an acute onset of congestive heart failure caused by hypertension as opposed to a gradual worsening of chronic heart failure.

The patient has a history of chronic renal failure, and his relatively high BUN to creatinine ratio suggests that there is also a pre-renal component to his renal dysfunction which may be due to the acute rise in blood pressure as well as the congestive heart failure. The urinary sediment is relatively unimpressive at this time, especially in light of his history.

Ocular complications are absent in this patient.

2. Which antihypertensive agent should be specifically avoided in M.R.? Why?

Antihypertensive medications which cause cardiostimulation should be avoided because this patient has severe coronary artery disease and has recently had an acute myocardial infarction.

Diazoxide is a potent, rapid-acting hypotensive agent that is closely related to the thiazide group of drugs. The hypotensive action is caused by a reduction in peripheral vascular resistance through direct relaxation of arterioles. As arterial pressure is lowered, baroreceptor reflexes are activated, leading to cardiac stimulation with increased heart rate, stroke volume, and cardiac output (94). Because of the *cardiostimulating effect,* the use of diazoxide could potentially be dangerous in patients such as M.R. with ischemic heart disease, and its use should be avoided. An early report indicated that 50% of the patients receiving diazoxide for hypertensive emergencies had significant ST and T wave changes after its use (95). Chest discomfort developed in several patients, suggesting myocardial ischemia, and other investigators have reported an association between myocardial infarction and the use of diazoxide (97).

There are other reasons why diazoxide should be avoided or used cautiously in M.R. Although diazoxide has a thiazide-like structure, it causes significant *sodium and water retention* which could be deleterious in a patient such as M.R. with severe congestive heart failure and pulmonary edema (94,126–129). The exact mechanism for this effect is not known, but it may be through an activation of the renin system or a direct antinatriuretic effect on the renal tubules (129). It is generally recommended that a potent diuretic such as furosemide be administered prior to the administration of diazoxide.

M.R. also has *renal failure* and there is some evidence that smaller doses of diazoxide must be used in this situation. This is most likely related to decreased protein binding which produces higher levels of free or active drug and a corresponding increase in hypotensive effect (107–108).

Even though there is no uric acid level reported, it is likely that M.R. has elevated levels associated with his chronic renal failure. Diazoxide decreases urate excretion and *increases uric acid levels* (109–111). In patients with normal renal function this effect can be reversed with the use of probenecid. In this patient, allopurinol or dialysis would have to be used to lower serum uric acid levels if they became extraordinarily high.

3. Considering M.R.'s medical history, which antihypertensive agent should be used?

M.R.'s arterial pressure should be lowered with parenteral medications which have a rapid onset of action. Nitroprusside (Nipride) and trimethaphan (Arfonad) both decrease total peripheral resistance rapidly with minimal effect on myocardial oxygen consumption and heart rate. Of these two agents, nitroprusside is usually preferred, because rapid tolerance develops to trimethaphan's hypotensive action and its use is associated with many side effects (see Question 11).

Nitroprusside has many pharmacologic effects which should favor M.R.'s condition. It dilates both venous and arterial vessels. Thus, it increases venous capacitance and decreases the venous return or preload on the heart. A decrease in the pulmonary capillary wedge pressure and ventricular filling pressure ultimately will improve M.R.'s pulmonary edema. Afterload is also decreased as a result of the arterial dilating effects. The net effect of this action is an increase in cardiac output, a reduction in arterial pressure, and an increase in tissue perfusion (34–38).

4. *Administration of Nitroprusside.* How should nitroprusside be prepared and administered? What dose should be used initially?

Because of its extreme potency, sodium nitroprusside must be prepared in exact concentrations and administered at precisely calculated rates. Sodium nitroprusside is supplied in units of 50 mg of lyophilized powder. The powder is reconstituted with two to three ml of 5% dextrose in water which produces a brownish solution. The

contents of the vial are then added to 500 ml of 5% dextrose in water (D5W) to produce a solution for intravenous administration with a drug concentration of 100 mcg per ml (36,39).

Because nitroprusside decomposes upon exposure to light, the solution should be shielded by wrapping the container with the metal foil provided in each package (40,41). It has been suggested that solutions of sodium nitroprusside be discarded four hours after reconstitution (40,42,43). However, others have reported the stability, protected from light, to be from 12–24 hours (44) or longer (45,46). Decomposition of the solution results in a highly colored solution of orange (4), dark brown (4), or blue (40,41,47). A blue color indicates almost complete degradation (47).

Effective infusion rates range from 0.5–8.0 mcg/kg/min (4,20). For this patient, an infusion of nitroprusside should be initiated at a rate of 0.5 mcg/kg/min, using a microdrip regulator or an infusion pump. The dose should be increased slowly by 0.5 mcg/kg/min every five minutes until the desired pressure is achieved (39,48). A maximum infusion rate of 10 mcg/kg/min has been recommended (49,50), but the dose must be individualized according to patient response and signs or symptoms of toxicity.

5. A nitroprusside infusion of 0.5 mcg/kg/min is started. What is the goal of therapy?

M.R.'s arterial pressure should be reduced to near normal levels; however, because M.R. has renal failure and cerebral occlusive disease (carotid bruits), excessive reduction of blood pressure should be avoided. This will also favor recovery of his renal function to pre-crisis status (9). As stated earlier, even though an increase in the BUN and creatinine may occur during antihypertensive therapy, these elevations are usually transitory and reflect hemodynamic alterations rather than progressive renal disease (51).

An excessive reduction of blood pressure in the presence of stenosis of major cerebral vessels may decrease cerebral blood flow and produce strokes (2) or other neurological complications (58–61). Normal cerebral blood flow remains relatively constant over a wide range of systemic blood pressures through autoregulatory mechanisms (52). However, there is evidence that the blood pressure required to maintain cerebral perfusion is higher in hypertensive patients than it is for normotensive individuals (55–57). If M.R.'s blood pressure is reduced excessively, cerebral blood flow may decrease sharply. Therefore, a diastolic blood pressure of 100–105 mm Hg would be a reasonable initial therapeutic goal for M.R. If hypotension does occur, nitroprusside should be discontinued and M.R.'s feet should be elevated.

6. *Nitroprusside Toxicity.* **The patient is treated with nitroprusside for 48 hours. Over the past 24 hours, the infusion has been tapered to 1 mcg/kg/min, and oral antihypertensive therapy has been initiated. What are the major side effects associated with nitroprusside and what indices of toxicity should be monitored? Should hydroxycobalamin be given to prevent nitroprusside toxicity?**

A major concern when using sodium nitroprusside is toxicity which may result from the accumulation of its metabolic by-products, cyanide and thiocyanate. Sodium nitroprusside reacts with free or intracellular hemoglobin by a nonenzymatic oxidation reaction. A ferrous ion from hemoglobin is transferred to nitroprusside, leading to the formation of methemoglobin and an unstable nitroprusside radical. Five cyanide ions are liberated from this unstable radical and one of these reacts with methemoglobin to form cyanmethemoglobin. The remaining cyanide ions are either converted to thiocyanate by the rhodanase enzyme system or bind to tissue cytochrome oxidase (62,63). Cyanide is liberated rapidly (64), and the amount released is directly related to the size of the dose (65). The majority of the total blood cyanide is contained within the erythrocytes, and since erythrocyte cyanide is firmly bound, the freely diffusable plasma cyanide is probably the main determinant of toxicity (66).

Although *cyanide toxicity* is relatively rare, several deaths have been reported following the use of sodium nitroprusside (67–73). Cyanide toxicity is more likely to occur in patients who receive high doses because of apparent resistance to the drug (38,68,72,74).

Two experimental approaches have been used to reduce cyanide toxicity during nitroprusside infusions. The concurrent administration of a continuous infusion of hydroxycobalamin (25 mg/hr) lowers red blood cell and plasma cyanide concentrations (75). The hydroxycobalamin combines with cyanide to form cyanocobalamin, which is nontoxic and excreted in the urine. Cyanide poisoning has also been prevented by the concurrent administration of sodium thiosulfate which is a sulfate donor for rhodanase; this reduces the level of circulating cyanide (76).

Since cyanide toxicity occurs rarely, the empiric use of hydroxycobalamin or thiosulfate is not necessary in M.R. The duration of nitroprusside therapy has been short, and he has been adequately maintained on relatively normal doses.

Cyanide toxicity can be detected early by monitoring M.R.'s metabolic status. The development of a metabolic acidosis is an early indicator of toxicity, because the progressive inactivation of cytochrome oxidase by cyanide results in an increase in anaerobic glycolysis. The development of a metabolic acidosis accompanied by an increase in the blood lactate or lactate-pyruvate ratio and an increase in the mixed venous blood oxygen tension would be early signs of cyanide toxicity (63,72,76–78). Serum thiocyanate levels are of no value in detecting the onset of cyanide toxicity. If toxicity develops, the infusion should be stopped, and appropriate therapy for cyanide intoxication should be instituted.

Sodium nitroprusside is more likely to produce *thiocyanate toxicity.* Although this is also rare, patients with renal failure (such as M.R.) who receive prolonged infusions are particularly susceptible (79–81). The conversion of cyanide to thiocyanate proceeds relatively slowly and thiocyanate levels rise gradually in proportion to the dose and duration of administration (65,82–85). On the basis of pharmacokinetic calculations, a total daily dose up to 125 mg is non-toxic in a patient with normal renal function. If the total daily dose is 250 mg, intoxication may be expected after approximately ten days; if it is 500 mg, a toxic level of thiocyanate can be reached within three to four days. A total daily dose of 1000 mg per day of nitroprusside may produce toxicity within 24–48 hours (85).

Thiocyanate causes a neurotoxic syndrome which is manifested by toxic psychosis, hyperreflexia, confusion, weakness, tinnitus, seizures, and coma (30,38,86). Prolonged exposure to thiocyanate can suppress thyroid function through inhibition of iodine uptake and binding by the thyroid (87). Thiocyanate toxicity is rare, but it is recommended that blood levels of thiocyanate be measured if the nitroprusside infusion exceeds three or four days (9). Nitroprusside should be discontinued if serum thiocyanate levels exceed 10–12 mg/dl (9,36,88,89), although some patients have tolerated levels of 20 mg/dl without adverse effects (90). Thiocyanate is readily removed by hemodialysis, and intermittent dialysis has been used to decrease thiocyanate levels during prolonged infusions (81).

For M.R., the potential for thiocyanate toxicity is greater than cyanide toxicity because of his underlying renal disease. If a prolonged course of therapy had been necessary, serum thiocyanate levels would have been monitored. However, since the infusion is being tapered and the expected duration of treatment is less than seventy-two hours, thiocyanate levels are not needed at this time.

Other side effects which have been associated with nitroprusside therapy include nausea, vomiting, diaphoresis, nasal stuffiness, muscular twitching, dizziness, and weakness. These effects are usually acute and occur when nitroprusside is administered too rapidly. They can be reversed by decreasing the rate of the infusion (42,91–93).

7. R.N., a 32-year-old black female, is admitted to the hospital with a two-day history of nausea, blurred vision, confusion, and an intractable generalized headache. The past medical history is remarkable for diabetes mellitus controlled by diet. Physical examination reveals an alert but disoriented black female with a blood pressure of 220/160 mm Hg without orthostasis and a pulse of 110/min. There is no evidence of heart failure, but the neurological examination reveals an altered mental status. Serum electrolytes, blood urea nitrogen, creatinine, a urinalysis, chest x-ray, and electrocardiogram are within normal limits. The plasma glucose is 275 mg/dl. The assessment at this time is hypertensive encephalopathy, and diazoxide is ordered. Are any special precautions required in the use of diazoxide in R.N.?

Diazoxide induces a significant rise in blood glucose. Several mechanisms have been postulated, including a direct increase in catecholamine levels, decreased peripheral glucose utilization, and direct inhibition of insulin release (98). However, the predominant and most important effect of diazoxide is its inhibition of insulin secretion from pancreatic beta cells (98–101). Although hyperglycemia occurs frequently, it is usually mild and does not preclude the use of the drug. In one study of 700 patients treated with diazoxide, a mild transitory elevation of serum glucose occurred in 40% of the non-diabetics, and

in 75% of diabetic subjects, one to four hours after treatment was initiated (102). In another study, of 41 patients who received diazoxide, the mean glucose values increased by only 6 mg/dl during the first 48 hours (96).

In this patient with a history of diabetes, blood glucose levels should be monitored. If necessary, treatment with insulin or oral hypoglycemics may be required. Failure to recognize and treat significant hyperglycemia may result in ketoacidosis or hyperglycemic hyperosmolar coma (103–106). This occurs most frequently in patients with renal failure, adult onset diabetes mellitus, liver disease, and patients recovering from general anesthesia.

8. *Diazoxide Administration.* How should diazoxide be administered to achieve an optimal hypotensive response?

Originally, it was thought necessary to administer diazoxide as an intravenous bolus (5 mg/kg or 300 mg in less than 30 seconds) to achieve an optimal hypotensive response (112-117). Theoretically, this method of administration produced a higher concentration of "unbound" or "free" diazoxide which activated the vasodilator receptors on the arterioles. However, some authors have challenged this conventional method of administration, and recent studies suggest that diazoxide can be administered effectively by intermittent injection (118-121), slow injection (122), or by intravenous infusion (123-125).

Earlier, it was thought that while the slow rate of administration was ineffective in patients with accelerated hypertension, patients with chronic hypertension responded equally well to rapid and slow administration (115). However, this has been disputed by others who have demonstrated that patients in hypertensive crisis respond equally well to diazoxide administered by slow infusion (15 mg/min) and rapid intravenous administration (less than 10 seconds) (125). Intermittent injections of smaller doses of diazoxide (150 mg every 5-20 minutes) have also been effective in patients with elevated diastolic pressures (119-121). All of these alternative methods should be used in an attempt to avoid the neurological or cardiovascular complications associated with a rapid and large decline in blood pressure. Even though it has not been proven that these methods will minimize such consequences, all measures which could potentially avoid these side effects should be used. In general, diazoxide should only be used in those instances where nitroprusside or a combination of nitroprusside and propranolol are contraindicated.

Diazoxide should always be given undiluted into a peripheral vein using caution to avoid extravasation. The high alkalinity of the solution (pH 11.6) can cause severe local pain and cellulitis. In the case of extravasation, conservative local therapy of the infiltrated area is adequate. Neither necrosis or sloughing has been reported.

9. The patient is given 300 mg of diazoxide by intravenous injection over 30 seconds. When will the maximum hypotensive effect occur and how long will this persist? What should be done if there is no substantial decrease in the blood pressure after 30 minutes?

The hypotensive effects of diazoxide begin within one minute and maximum effects occur within two to five minutes (113,117). Over the next 20 minutes, the blood pressure gradually increases because of a reflex increase in heart rate and cardiac output. The patient should remain recumbent for 15-30 minutes following the injection of each dose of diazoxide, and the blood pressure should be monitored every 5 minutes for the first 30 minutes. The duration of action is variable in that the blood pressure gradually increases to the pretreatment level in 3-15 hours (113,115,117). If the patient fails to respond to the first dose, a second dose should be given after 30 minutes. In one study (96), repeated injections of diazoxide were required 35% of the time. Ten percent of the doses administered were transiently effective and 55% were effective.

10. *Dissection of the Aorta.* A 68-year-old white male with a long history of hypertension, asthma, and noncompliance presents to the local emergency room complaining of the sudden onset of severe sharp diffuse chest pain which radiates to the back between the shoulder blades. Significant findings on physical examination include a pulse of 100 beats/minute, a blood pressure of 200/120 mm Hg, grade II K-W changes, clear lungs, and an S_4 without murmurs. The laboratory data were unremarkable. The electrocardiogram was interpreted as sinus tachycardia with left ventricular hypertrophy, but no acute changes were noted. Chest x-ray was significant for widening of the mediastinum. An emergency aortogram revealed a dissection at the arch of the aorta. What antihypertensive medication would be most appropriate for this patient and why?

The ultimate treatment for dissection of the aorta depends on its location and severity; however, the first principle of therapy is to control any existing hypertension with agents that do not increase the force of cardiac contraction (130). This lessens the force that the cardiac impulse transmits to the dissecting aneurysm.

Trimethaphan alone and sodium nitroprusside in combination with propranolol are the preferred drug regimens (2). Both decrease the blood pressure, venous return, and cardiac contractility. The concurrent administration of a beta blocking agent with nitroprusside is desirable since the latter may induce reflex tachycardia in response to the vasodilation (36). Palmer et al (48) have documented progression of aortic dissection under combined nitroprusside-propranolol therapy and advocate the return to trimethaphan as the agent of choice. Others also agree that trimethaphan is the drug of choice in the hypertensive patient with an aortic dissection (8,9,30,130). Diazoxide and hydralazine should be avoided because they increase stroke volume and left ventricular ejection rate. These effects augment the pulsatile flow and accentuate the sharpness of the pulse wave (131) which increases mechanical stress on the aortic wall and may lead to further dissection.

The drug of first choice in this patient is trimethaphan. Although a combination of nitroprusside and propranolol has been used successfully in the antihypertensive treatment of dissecting aortic aneurysms, this patient's past medical history of asthma would preclude the use of propranolol.

11. *Trimethaphan.* How should trimethaphan be administered, and what indices of toxicity should be monitored?

Trimethaphan is a ganglionic blocking drug that inhibits sympathetic nervous influences on the arterioles, veins, and the heart. The hypotensive effect is immediate, and because minor changes in the infusion rate can produce dramatic changes in blood pressure, the rate must be carefully regulated (preferably by a constant infusion pump), and the blood pressure must be monitored continuously.

The drug is usually prepared in a concentration of 500 mg per liter of 5% dextrose in water. The infusion rate is initiated at 0.5 to 1.0 mg/min and is increased incrementally at intervals of 3-5 minutes until the desired response is obtained. The hypotensive effect is most pronounced when the patient is upright, and it is often necessary to elevate the head of the bed to achieve an optimal effect. Therapy with oral antihypertensive agents should begin simultaneously, and an attempt should be made to discontinue the ganglionic blocker within 48 hours before significant tolerance renders the patient resistant to its action.

Toxicity is common and is related to trimethaphan's parasympathetic inhibition of the nervous system. Urinary retention often occurs with prolonged therapy, necessitating placement of an indwelling catheter. Constipation and paralytic ileus may occur as well as paralysis of visual accommodation. Severe hypotension following administration of trimethaphan may last for 10-15 minutes. To correct the hypotension, the infusion should be discontinued and the patient should be placed in a Trendelenburg position.

References

1. deCarvolho JG et al: Treatment of hypertensive emergencies. Drug Ther. 1979; 9:107.
2. Koch-Weser J: Hypertensive emergencies. N Engl J Med. 1974; 290:211.
3. Mailloux LU: Management of hypertensive emergencies. NY State J Med. 1977; 77:1290.
4. Keith TA: Hypertensive crisis: Recognition and management. JAMA. 1977; 237:1570.
5. Guazzi MD: Treatment of special forms of hypertension. In *The Treatment of Hypertension*, edited by E Freis, University Park Press, Baltimore, 1978, p 115.
6. Kincaid-Smith P: Malignant hypertension: Mechanisms and Management. Pharmac Ther. 1980; 9:245.
7. Rabin EZ: Malignant hypertension. Can Med Assoc J. 1978; 118:941.
8. Anon: Drugs for rapidly lowering blood pressure. Drug Therapy Bull. 1979; 17:61.
9. AMA Committee on Hypertension: Treatment of malignant hypertension and hypertensive emergencies. JAMA. 1974; 228:1673.
10. Segal JL: Hypertensive emergencies. Postgrad J Med. 1980; 68:107.
11. Perera GA: The accelerated form of hypertension: A unique entity? Trans Assoc Am Phy. 1958; 71:62.
12. Kincaid-Smith P et al: The clinical course and pathology of hypertension with papilloedema (malignant hypertension). Quart J Med. 1958; 27:117.
13. Dranov J et al: Malignant hypertension-current modes of therapy. Arch Intern Med. 1974; 133:791.
14. Sokolow M et al: Five year survival of consecutive patients with malignant hypertension treated with antihypertensive agents. Am J Cardiol. 1960; 6:858.
15. Freis ED: Age, race, sex, and other indices of risk in hypertension. Am J Med. 1973; 55:275.
16. Entwisle G: Target organ damage in black hypertensives. Circulation. 1977; 55:792.
17. Lee TH: Malignant hypertension. Declining mortality rate in New York City, 1958 to 1974. NY State J Med. 1978; 78:1389.
18. Heptinstall RH: Malignant hypertension: A study of 51 cases. J Pathol. 1953; 65:423.
19. Schottstaedt WF et al: The natural history and cause of malignant hypertension with papilledema. Am Heart J. 1953; 45:331.
20. Mroczek W: Malignant hypertension. Angiology. 1977; 28:444.
21. Volhard F et al: Die Brightsche Nierenkranheit. Springer-Verlag, Berlin 1914.
22. Keith NM et al: Some different types of essential hypertension: their course and prognosis. Am J Med Sci. 1939; 197:332.
23. McMichael J et al: Methonium treatment of severe and malignant hypertension. J Chron Dis. 1955; 1:527.
24. Perera GA: Hypertensive vascular disease: Description and natural history. J Chron Dis. 1955; 1:33.
25. Onesti G: The malignant phase of essential hypertension. In *Hypertension: Mechanisms and Management*, edited by G Onesti, K Kim, and J Moyer, Grune and Stratton, New York, 1973, p 207.
26. Susin M et al: Essential malignant hypertension. NY State J Med. 1978; 78:54.
27. Moore MA: Hypertensive emergencies. Am Fam Physician, 1980; 21:141.
28. Schoenberger A: Accelerated hypertension. J Tenn Med Assoc. 1977; 70:102.
29. Moser M: When hypertension is an emergency. Drug Ther. 1976; 6:6.
30. Becker CE et al: Hypertensive emergencies. Med Clin North Am. 1979; 63:127.
31. Curry CL et al: Current treatment of malignant hypertension. JAMA. 1975; 232:1367.
32. Woods JW et al: Management of malignant hypertension complicated by renal insufficiency. N Engl J Med. 1967; 277:57.
33. Mroczek WJ et al: The value of aggressive therapy in the hypertensive patient with azotemia. Circulation. 1969; 40:893.
34. Schlant RC et al: Studies on the acute cardiovascular effects of intravenous sodium nitroprusside. Am J Cardiol. 1962; 9:51.
35. Page IH et al: Cardiovascular actions of sodium nitroprusside in animals and hypertensive patients. Circulation. 1955; 11:188.
36. Palmer RF et al: Sodium nitroprusside. N Engl J Med. 1975; 292:294.
37. Tuzel IH: Sodium nitroprusside: A review of its clinical effectiveness as a hypotensive agent. J Clin Pharmacol. 1974; 14:494.

38. Cohn JN et al: Nitroprusside. Ann Intern Med. 1979; 91:752.

39. Kohli RK et al: Treating acute hypertensive crisis with sodium nitroprusside. Am Fam Physician. 1977; 15:141.

40. Tourville J: Sodium nitroprusside. Drug Intell Clin Pharm. 1975; 9:361.

41. Anon: Sodium nitroprusside in anesthesia. Br Med J. 1975; 2:524.

42. Romankiewicz JA: Pharmacology and clinical use of drugs used in hypertensive emergencies. Am J Hosp Pharm. 1977; 34:185.

43. Opie LH: Vasodilator drugs. Lancet. 1980; 1:966.

44. Anon: Sodium nitroprusside for hypertensive crisis. Med Let Drugs Ther. 1975; 17:82.

45. Anderson RA et al: Stability of sodium nitroprusside infusions. Aust J Pharm Sci. 1972; 1:45.

46. Schumacher GE: Sodium nitroprusside injection. Am J Hosp Pharm. 1966; 23:532.

47. Hargrave RE: Degradation of solutions of sodium nitroprusside. J Hosp Pharm. 1974; 32:188.

48. Palmer RF et al: Nitroprusside and aortic dissecting aneurysms. N Engl J Med. 1976; 294:1403.

49. Reves JG et al: Therapeutic use of sodium nitroprusside and an automated method of administration. Int Anesthesiol Clin. 1978; 16:51.

50. Katz RL: Dose limits to acute nitroprusside therapy challenged. Anesthesiology. 1977; 47:395.

51. Finnerty FA: Malignant hypertension. Am Heart J. 1974; 88:265.

52. Ram CV: Hypertensive encephalopathy: recognition and management. Arch Intern Med. 1978; 138:1851.

53. Johnson PC: Review of previous studies and current theories of autoregulation. Circ Res. 1964; 14-15 (suppl):1.

54. Cowley AW: The concept of autoregulation of total blood flow and its role in hypertension. Am J Med. 1980; 68:906.

55. Finnerty FA et al: Cerebral hemodynamics during cerebral ischemia induced by acute hypertension. J Clin Invest. 1954; 33:1227.

56. Strandgaard S: Autoregulation of cerebral blood flow in hypertensive patients: the modifying influence of prolonged antihypertensive treatment on the tolerance to acute, drug-induced hypotension. Circulation. 1976; 53:720.

57. Strandgaard S et al: Autoregulation of brain circulation in severe arterial hypertension. Br Med J. 1973; 1:507.

58. Hulse JA et al: Blindness and paraplegia in severe childhood hypertension. Lancet. 1979; 2:553.

59. Pryor JS et al: Blindness and malignant hypertension. Lancet. 1979; 2:803.

60. Graham DI: Ischaemic brain damage of cerebral perfusion failure type after treatment of severe hypertension. Br Med J. 1975; 4:739.

61. Ledingham JG et al: Cerebral complications in the treatment of accelerated hypertension. Quart J Med. 1979; 48:25.

62. Smith RP et al: Nitroprusside produces cyanide poisoning via a reaction with hemoglobin. J Pharmacol Exper Ther. 1974; 191:557.

63. Tinker JH et al: Sodium nitroprusside: pharmacology, toxicology, and therapeutics. Anesthesiology. 1976; 45:340.

64. Vesey CJ et al: Nitroprusside and cyanide. Br J Anaesth. 1975; 47:1115.

65. Vesey CJ et al: Cyanide and thiocyanate concentrations following nitroprusside infusion in man. Br J Anaesth. 1976; 48:651.

66. Vesey CJ et al: Red cell cyanide. J Pharm Pharmacol. 1978; 30:20.

67. Lazarus-Barlow P et al: Fatal cases of poisoning with sodium nitroprusside. Br Med J. 1941; 2:407.

68. Macrae WR et al: Severe metabolic acidosis following hypertension induced with sodium nitroprusside. Br J Anaesth. 1974; 46:795.

69. Jack RD: Toxicity of sodium nitroprusside. Br J Anaesth. 1974; 46:952.

70. Merrifield AJ et al: Toxicity of sodium nitroprusside. Br J Anaesth. 1974; 46:324.

71. Davies DW et al: A sudden death associated with the use of sodium nitroprusside for induction of hypotension during anaesthesia. Can Anaesth Soc J. 1975; 22:547.

72. Rauscher LA et al: Nitroprusside toxicity in a renal transplant patient. Anesthesiology. 1978; 49:428.

73. Montoliu J et al: Fatal hypotension in normal dose nitroprusside therapy. Am Heart J. 1979; 97:541.

74. McDowall DG et al: The toxicity of sodium nitroprusside. Br J Anaesth. 1974; 46:327.

75. Cottrell JE et al: Prevention of nitroprusside-induced cyanide toxicity with hydroxycobalamin. N Engl J Med. 1978; 298:809.

76. Michenfelder JD et al: Cyanide toxicity and thiosulfate protection during chronic administration of sodium nitroprusside in the dog: correlation with a human case. Anesthesiology. 1977; 47:441.

77. Fahmy NR: Consumption of vitamin B-12 during nitroprusside administration. Anesth Analg. 1980; 59:538.

78. Anon: Controlled intravascular sodium nitroprusside treatment. Br Med J. 1978; 2:784.

79. Page IH et al: Cardiovascular actions of sodium nitroprusside in animals and hypertensive patients. Circulation. 1955; 11:188.

80. Nickerson M et al: Renal excretion of thiocyanate. J Lab Clin Med. 1951; 38:194.

81. Danzig LE: Dynamics of thiocyanate dialysis. N Engl J Med. 1954; 252:49.

82. DuCailar J et al: Nitroprusside, its metabolites and red cell function. Can Anaesth Soc J. 1978; 25:92.

83. Japp H et al: Toxizitat und Konzentration von thiocyanat im serum bei der therapie mit natrium-nitroprussid. Schweiz Med WSCHR. 1978; 108:1987.

84. Bogusz M et al: Blood cyanide and thiocyanate concentrations after administration of sodium nitroprusside as hypotensive agent in neurosurgery. Clin Chem. 1979; 25:60.

85. Schulz V et al: Thiozyanat-vergiftung bei der antihypertensiven therapie mit natrium-nitroprussid. Klin WSCHR. 1978; 56:355.

86. Barnett HJ et al: Thiocyanate psychosis. JAMA. 1951; 147:1554.

87. Nourok DS et al: Hypothyroidism following prolonged nitroprusside therapy. Am J Med Sci. 1964; 248:129.

88. Cole P: The safe use of sodium nitroprusside. Anaesthesia. 1978; 33:473.

89. Ahearn DJ et al: Treatment of malignant hypertension with sodium nitroprusside. Arch Intern Med. 1974; 133:187.

90. Lupatkin WL et al: Prolonged use of sodium nitroprusside. J Pediatr. 1978; 92:1032.

91. Cacace L et al: Treatment of hypertensive emergencies with sodium nitroprusside. Drug Intell Clin Pharm. 1970; 4:187.

92. Gifford RW: Hypertensive emergencies and their treatment. Med Clin North Am. 1961; 45:441.

93. Tuzel I: Nitroprusside: A review of its clinical effectiveness as a hypotensive agent. J Clin Pharmacol. 1974; 14:494.

94. Koch-Weser J: Diazoxide. N Engl J Med. 1976; 294:1271.

95. Kanada S et al: Angina-like syndrome with diazoxide therapy for hypertensive crisis. Ann Intern Med. 1976; 84:696.

96. McDonald WJ et al: Intravenous diazoxide therapy in hypertensive crisis. Am J Cardiol. 1977; 40:409.

97. Kumar GK et al: Side effects of diazoxide. JAMA. 1976; 235:275.

98. Speight TM et al: Diazoxide: A review of its pharmacological properties and therapeutic use in hypertensive crisis. Drugs. 1971; 2:78.

99. Fajans SS et al: Further studies on diazoxide suppression of insulin release from abnormal and normal islet tissue in man. Ann NY Acad Sci. 1968; 150:261.

100. Porte D: Inhibition of insulin release by diazoxide and its relation to catecholamine effect in man. Ann NY Acad Sci. 1968; 150:281.

101. Tabachnick II et al: Mechanism of diazoxide hyperglycemia in animals. Ann NY Acad Sci. 1968; 150:204.

102. Finnerty F: Hyperglycemia after diazoxide administration. N Engl J Med. 1971; 285:1487.

103. Updike SJ et al: Acute diabetic ketoacidosis-a complication of intravenous diazoxide treatment for refractory hypertension. N Engl J Med. 1969; 280:768.

104. Charles MA et al: Nonketoacidic hyperglycemia and coma during intravenous diazoxide therapy in uremia. Diabetes. 1971; 20:501.

105. Shin B et al: Hyperglycemic hyperosmolar nonketotic coma following diazoxide anesthesia and operation. Anesth Analg. 1977; 56:506.

106. Harrison B et al: Severe nonketotic hyperglycemia precoma in a hypertensive patient receiving diazoxide. Lancet. 1972; 2:599.

107. O'Malley K et al: Decreased plasma protein binding of diazoxide in uremia. Clin Pharmacol Ther. 1975; 18:53.

108. Pearson RM et al: Renal function, protein binding and pharmacological response to diazoxide. Br J Clin Pharmacol. 1976; 3:169.

109. Lockwood CH et al: Diazoxide therapy in hypertension. Am J Med Sci. 1963; 246:312.

110. Thompson GR et al: The effects of intravenous diazoxide, non-diuretic thiazide, upon blood pressure, electrolyte and uric acid secretion. Michigan Med. 1966; 65:17.

111. Thompson GR: The effect of diazoxide, potassium chloride, and ammonium chloride on serum and urinary uric acid. Arthritis Rheum. 1965; 8:830.

112. Sellers EM et al: Influence of intravenous injection rate on protein binding and vascular activity of diazoxide. Ann NY Acad Sci. 1973; 226:319.

113. Finnerty FA et al: Clinical evaluation of diazoxide. A new treatment for hypertension. Circulation. 1963; 28:203.

114. Freis ED: Hypertensive crisis. JAMA. 1969; 208:338.

115. Mroczek WM et al: The importance of the rapid administration of diazoxide in accelerated hypertension. N Engl J Med. 1971; 285:603.

116. Kosman ME: Evaluation of diazoxide. JAMA. 1973; 224:1422.

117. Hamby WM et al: Intravenous use of diazoxide in the treatment of severe hypertension. Circulation. 1968; 37:169.

118. Velasco M et al: A new technique for safe and effective control of hypertension with intravenous diazoxide. Curr Ther Res. 1976; 19:185.

119. Boerth RC et al: Dose-response relation of diazoxide in children with hypertension. Circulation. 1977; 56:1062.

120. Wilson DJ et al: Control of severe hypertension with pulse doses of diazoxide. J Clin Pharmacol Ther. 1978; 23:135.

121. Ram CV et al: Individual titration of diazoxide dosage in the treatment of severe hypertension. Am J Cardiol. 1979; 43:627.

122. Waugh WH: Efficacy of slow injection of diazoxide in accelerated hypertension. NC Med J. 1977; 38:448.

123. Crout JR et al: Intravenous diazoxide in hypertension. Clin Res. 1970; 18:337.

124. Johnson BF et al: The influence of rate of injection upon the effects of diazoxide. Am J Med Sci. 1972; 273:481.

125. Thien TA et al: Diazoxide infusion in severe hypertension and hypertensive crisis. Clin Pharmacol Ther. 1979; 25:795.

126. Finnerty FA: Hypertensive encephalopathy. Am Heart J. 1968; 75:559.

127. Koch-Weser J: Vasodilator drugs in the treatment of hypertension. Arch Intern Med. 1974; 133:1017.

128. Moser M: Diazoxide: An effective vasodilator in accelerated hypertension. Am Heart J. 1974; 87:791.

129. Bartorelli C et al: Hypotensive and renal effects of diazoxide-a sodium-retaining benzothiadiazine compound. Circulation. 1963; 27:895.

130. Friedman S: The evaluation and treatment of patients with arterial aneurysms. Med Clin North Am. 1981; 65:83.

131. Paulissian R: Diazoxide. Int Anesthesiol Clin. 1978; 16:201.

Chapter 10

Congestive Heart Failure

Wayne A. Kradjan and Mary Anne Koda-Kimble

Congestive heart failure (CHF) results when the left, right, or both ventricles fail to pump sufficient blood to meet the body's needs. An estimated two million people in the United States currently have CHF and 2 to 5 cases per 1000 persons are diagnosed yearly. There is a clear correlation between the incidence of CHF and both sex and age. The Framingham Heart Disease Epidemiology Study (1) reported an annual rate of 2.3 and 1.4 cases per 1000 males and females, respectively. By the sixth decade, the incidence among men is five times that of the fourth decade. It is apparent that as the size of the geriatric population increases, CHF will become a more frequently encountered clinical entity. Despite early diagnosis and optimal medical management by today's standards, the prognosis of these patients is not much better than it is for those with cancer. In the Framingham study, 60% of men and 40% of women died within five years of the diagnosis of CHF.

ETIOLOGY

There are two major types of heart failure. *High output failure* occurs when the heart fails to pump enough blood to meet the metabolic demands of the tissues. This may occur in hyperthyroid patients whose metabolic demands are greater than normal or in severely anemic patients whose tissues require a greater volume of blood to supply normal metabolic needs. *Low output (congestive) failure* is the more common of the two and will be the major emphasis of this discussion. This form occurs when the heart is unable to pump all of the blood with which it is presented. Whereas a normal *ejection fraction* (EF, percent of ventricular volume expelled during systole) is greater than 60%, a person with serious CHF may have an EF as low as 20 to 30%. Increased cardiac workload and impaired myocardial contractility are important factors which contribute to the development of CHF.

Cardiac Workload. There are two components which contribute to the left ventricular workload: preload and afterload.

Preload (2–4) is a term used to describe forces acting on the *venous* side of the circulation to affect myocardial wall tension. The relationship is as follows: as venous return increases, the volume of blood in the left ventricle increases. This increased volume raises the pressure within the ventricle (left ventricular end diastolic pressure—LVEDP) which in turn increases the "stretch" or wall tension of the ventricle. The volume and pressure in the ventricle are greatest at the end of diastole when filling of the ventricle is complete and least at the end of systole when the ventricle has been maximally emptied. Venous dilation and decreased venous volume diminish preload, while venous constriction and increased venous volume increase preload.

An elevated preload will aggravate congestive heart failure. This can occur following the rapid administration of blood plasma expanders and osmotic diuretics or by the administration of large amounts of sodium or sodium-retaining agents. A malfunctioning aortic valve which results in regurgitation of blood into the left ventricle can also increase the volume of blood which must be pumped. A malfunctioning mitral valve may cause retrograde ejection of blood from the left ventricle into the left atrium with a resultant decrease in ejection fraction. By the same token, if the left heart fails and ventricular blood is ejected less effectively, the volume of blood retained in the ventricle is increased and preload is elevated.

Afterload (2–4) strictly defined is the tension developed in the ventricular wall as contraction (systole) occurs. The tension developed during contraction relates to intraventricular pressure, ventricular diameter, and wall thickness. More simply, afterload is regulated by the resistance or impedance against which the ventricle must pump during its ejection and is chiefly determined by arterial blood pressure. Hypertension, atherosclerotic disease, or a narrow aortic valve increase arterial impedence (afterload), thereby increasing the workload on the heart. Hypertension is a major etiologic factor in the development of CHF. The Framingham group (1) found that 75% of patients who developed congestive heart failure had prior histories of hypertension. In another study, the risk of developing CHF was six times greater for hypertensive than for normotensive patients (5).

Contractility. Contractility is the inherent strength and speed of contraction of the myocardium (cardiac muscle) and is independent of preload and afterload. Beta sympathetic tone is one determinant of contractility. Myocardial contractility is decreased when there are diminished or poorly functioning myocardial fibers. This usually results from primary cardiac disease of which rheumatic heart disease, coronary artery disease, myocardial infarction, and persistent arrhythmias are examples. *Cardiomyopathy,* a non-specific term referring to a generalized deterioration of myocardial muscle function, may also produce CHF. Occasionally, drugs such as propranolol or daunomycin induce CHF by decreasing myocardial contractility.

Drug-Induced CHF. Drugs which produce expansion of the intravascular volume or decrease cardiac contractility should be avoided or used with caution in patients with congestive heart failure. Drugs may produce volume expansion by increasing retention of sodium and water by the kidney, by increasing the intravascular osmotic pressure and thereby causing a redistribution of interstitial and intracellular water into intravascular space, or by increasing total body sodium and water from their high sodium content. Only rarely have such drug effects been quantitated. In many cases one can only rely on what is known about the pharmacology of the drug and on scattered case reports. Drugs which adversely affect cardiac contractility may do so either by directly affecting the cardiac muscle or by interfering with the sympathetic nervous system.

Amphetamines. Smith et al report a case of amphetamine-induced cardiomyopathy manifested as severe CHF in a 45-year-old female. The patient had a history of depression, narcolepsy, and cataplexy for which she was treated with high dose dextroamphetamine (100 mg/day; 2 mg/kg) intermittently for five years and continuously for seven years. An attempt to withdraw the amphetamine resulted in deterioration of her cardiac status. The authors point to the similarity between this case and the myocarditis associated with pheochromocytoma and refer to ischemia and myocardial hypertrophy induced by sympathomimetic amines in animals (12).

Androgens. Sodium retention and edema may result from the chronic administration of these substances.

Beta blocking agents. (Propranolol, timolol, metoprolol, atenolol, nadolol). All of these agents have negative inotropic and negative chronotropic effects on the heart. See the Angina chapter and Question 2.

Daunomycin. This cancer chemotherapeutic agent, used in the treatment of acute myelocytic leukemia, has a direct, dose-related cardiotoxic effect that may occur several months after therapy has been terminated (average 80 days) (13,14). Electrocardiographic changes may occur at the time of or soon after drug administration, but these are not predictive of the long-term, therapy-resistant congestive heart failure that may subsequently occur. Initially, when high doses were used (greater than 35 mg/kg or 950 mg/m^2), the incidence of cardiotoxicity was estimated to be 10%. When daunomycin doses were confined to less than 600 mg/m^2, the incidence dropped to less than 3% in a group of 2000 patients (15). An analysis of 5,613 patients receiving daunomycin revealed that the incidence of cardiomyopathy was 1.5% at a total dose of 600 mg/m^2 and 12% at a dose of 1000 mg/m^2. Children appear to be more susceptible to this effect; the overall incidence among children was 1.6%, and the incidence among adults was 0.6% (14). Fatality may be as high as 80%.

Diazoxide. The mechanism by which this drug induces sodium and water retention has not been clarified, but it may increase the proximal tubular reabsorption of sodium (16,17). Potent, loop diuretics are frequently used in conjunction with this agent to prevent volume expansion, edema, weight gain, CHF, and resistance to its hypotensive effects.

Disopyramide. Previously controlled CHF may be exacerbated by the negative inotropic effect of disopyramide. Although this is a relatively infrequent occurrence, its potential must be considered when treating a person with concurrent CHF and arrhythmias. In one series, 16% of patients developed acute CHF within 48 hours of beginning disopyramide therapy (18).

Estrogens. These agents frequently produce sodium retention, edema, and weight gain.

Table 1.

SODIUM CONTENT OF MEDICINALS—
SELECTED ADULT MEDICATIONS WITH AN
EXTRAORDINARILY HIGH SODIUM CONTENT (50 MG/DOSE)

Drug	Unit	mg Na$^+$/unit*
Parenteral products		
Amcillin S	1 gm injection	62
Dynapen	63 mg/ml	67
Geopen	5 gm	680
Keflin	1 gm vial	62
Methicillin	1 gm vial	55
Omnipen-N	2 gm vial	124
Penbritin-S	1 gm vial	66
Pen-G Sodium (Squibb)	5 million unit vial	233
Polycillin	1 gm vial	68
Principen N	1 gm injection	70
Prostaphlin	4 gm vial	144
Staphcillin	1 gm vial	61
Unipen Injection	1 gm vial	73
Oral liquids		
Dristan Cough Formula	5 ml	59
Phenergan Expectorant (Plain or VC)	5 ml	51
Phospho-Soda	5 ml	554
Vicks Cough Syrup	5 ml	54
Vicks Formula 44 Syrup	5 ml	68
Oral solid dosage forms		
Alka Seltzer	1 tab	521
Bisodol Powder	10 gm	1540
Bromo Seltzer	80 gm capful	717
Erythrocin Filmtab	250 mg	70
Fizrin	1 packet	673
Kayexelate Powder	15 gm	550
Nervine Effervescent	1 tab	544
Panteric Granules	1 teaspoonful	161
Pasna-pak Granules	6 gm packet	600
Pasna Tri-pak Granules	5.5 gm packet	490
Rolaids	1 tab	53
Sal Hepatica	1 rounded teaspoonful	1000
Sodium Salicylate	10 grain tab	97
Food supplements		
Carnation Slender	10 oz. can	440
Lytren	1 oz.	189
Meritene Powder	1 oz.	113
Vivonex 100	6 doses	2385
Miscellaneous		
Fleets Enema	4.5 oz.	5000**

*23 mg Na$^+$ = 1 mEq
**Average absorption = 275 − 400 mg/enema

Glucocorticoids. Those with significant mineralocorticoid effects cause sodium retention through stimulation of sodium reabsorption in exchange for potassium in the distal convoluted tubule of the kidney. Those with minimal mineralocorticoid effects (eg, prednisone in low to moderate doses or dexamethasone) should be used in preference to hydrocortisone in CHF patients.

Guanethidine. See Question 2.

Licorice. Glycerrhyzic acid and a related compound, carbenoxolone, closely resemble the mineralocorticoids in structure and have been used experimentally in the treatment of peptic ulcer disease. They induce cardiac asthma or edema in up to 20% of the patients in whom they are used (19,19a). Symptomatic CHF has been produced after the ingestion of 700 gm of licorice over a period of one week (19).

Lithium carbonate. Although the diuretic effect of this agent is well known, it is occasionally associated with sodium retention, edema, and, rarely, CHF (20,20a). It is important to note that a low sodium diet may result in retention of lithium (21).

Methyldopa. See Question 2.

Minoxidil. See Question 2.

Osmotic agents. The rapid intravenous administration of slowly diffusable substances capable of exerting osmotic activity may result in acute volume overload and the exacerbation of congestive heart disease. Such agents include mannitol, albumin, urea, hypertonic glucose, and/or saline.

Phenylbutazone. See Question 2.

Salicylates. Large, anti-inflammatory doses of aspirin can cause vasodilation and dilution of blood with tissue fluids resulting in a decreased hematocrit and increased blood volume. These doses also cause sodium retention by a mechanism yet to be elucidated. This may become clinically significant in arthritics taking large, chronic doses of aspirin who also have underlying carditis (22). In a series of 50 arthritic patients, 9 (18%) developed symptoms of congestive heart failure after 3–8 days of therapy. Six of these cases were mild and of short duration (23). Salicylates containing large amounts of sodium (eg, effervescent products) should also be avoided in CHF.

Sodium-Containing Drugs. See Table 1 (24).

PATHOGENESIS

When the heart begins to fail, the body activates several complex compensatory mechanisms in an attempt to maintain cardiac output and oxygenation of vital organs (25). These include cardiac (ventricular) dilation, cardiac hypertrophy, increased sympathetic tone, and sodium and water retention. An understanding of these compensatory mechanisms is essential to the understanding of the signs and symptoms of congestive heart failure.

Cardiac dilation results when the ventricles fail to pump the entire volume of blood with which they are presented. If the rate at which blood is delivered (preload) remains the same, but the rate at which it is pumped to other tissues diminishes, it is apparent that a residual amount of blood will begin to accumulate in the ventricles. Thus, end diastolic volume increases, myocardial fibers are stretched, and the ventricle(s) become dilated.

The Frank-Starling ventricular function curve (Fig. 1) implies a curvilinear relationship between left ventricular myocardial muscle fiber

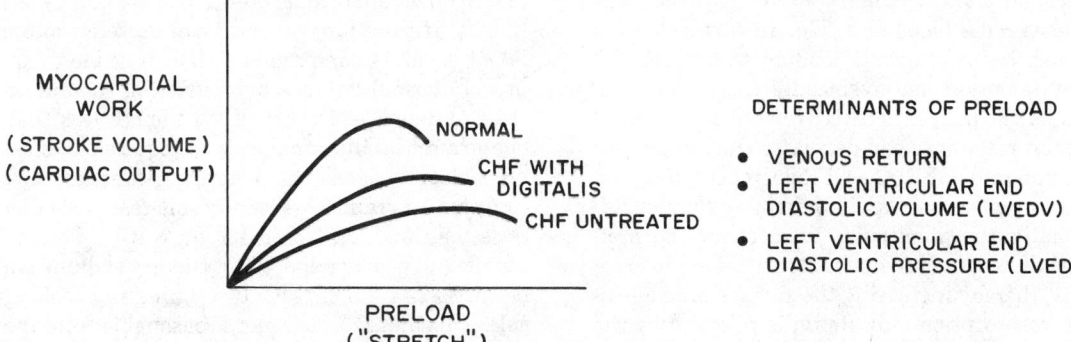

Figure 1. Representation of Frank-Starling ventricular function curve.

"stretch" (wall tension) and myocardial work. As stretch increases, the volume of blood ejected with each systolic contraction *(stroke volume)* increases. In congestive heart failure, the work capacity for any degree of stretch is diminished. A simple analogy may be drawn using a balloon. The more air you blow into a balloon, the more it stretches and, if released, the more it flies around a room. As the balloon gets old, it loses its elasticity and thus has less recoil when stretched. Similarly, dilation of the ventricles may initially serve as an effective compensating mechanism, but it becomes inadequate as the elastic limits of the myocardial muscle fibers are reached. Theoretically, as cardiac dilatation progresses beyond a certain point, cardiac output could decrease (descending limb of the Starling Curve), but this is rarely observed clinically.

Cardiac hypertrophy is a long-term adaptation to an increased diastolic volume and represents an absolute increase in myocardial muscle mass. Cardiac hypertrophy should not be confused with cardiac dilation.

An important relationship to remember is that cardiac output (CO) is the product of ventricular stroke volume (SV) and heart rate (HR). A diminished stroke volume or cardiac output results in decreased tissue perfusion which in turn causes a reflex *activation of the sympathetic autonomic nervous system (SANS)*. The inotropic (increased contractility) and chronotropic (increased heart rate) effects of the SANS may initially maintain near normal cardiac output, thus preserving perfusion of vital organs such as the CNS and myocardium. However, SANS-mediated vasoconstriction in the skin and the gastrointestinal and renal circulation decreases perfusion of these organs.

Both the decreased cardiac output of CHF and vasoconstriction secondary to sympathetic tone decrease renal blood flow. This in turn sets off a complex chain of events leading to sodium and water retention and eventually *increased blood volume.* The increased SANS tone increases renal vascular resistance and decreases the glomerular filtration rate (GFR). As GFR decreases, more sodium is reabsorbed in the proximal tubule. Additionally, the glomerular filtrate may be preferentially shunted to nephrons with long loops of Henle, thereby increasing the surface area for sodium reabsorption (25). Renin is released by the kidney in response to decreased renal perfusion, leading to a corresponding increase in angioten-

sin formation. Angiotensin has two effects favoring sodium and water retention: its vasoconstricting effects may further decrease GFR, and it stimulates the adrenals to secrete aldosterone, a hormone which increases sodium reabsorption in the distal tubule. A diminished effective circulating plasma volume also stimulates the release of antidiuretic hormone (ADH) from the pituitary, resulting in the subsequent retention of free water in the renal collecting ducts.

TREATMENT

The medical management of congestive heart failure includes correction of underlying disease states (eg, hypertension), bed rest, a sodium-restricted diet, diuretics, and digitalis glycosides. More recently, vasodilators and, in some instances, inotropic agents have been used to manage CHF unresponsive to traditional therapy. The ultimate goal of therapy is to abolish disabling symptoms and improve the quality of the patient's life. None of the aforementioned measures are curative, and it has been dishearteningly demonstrated that despite treatment, the five-year survival of CHF patients is not prolonged (5).

Bedrest. Bedrest and restricted physical activity decrease the metabolic demands of the failing heart and minimize gravitational forces contributing to the formation of edema. Renal perfusion is also increased in the prone position, resulting in diuresis and eventual mobilization of edema fluid. Edema can also be minimized by use of elastic hosiery that increase interstitial pressure and help mobilize fluid into vascular spaces.

Sodium-Restricted Diet. A sodium-restricted diet should be instituted to decrease blood volume and to offset abnormal retention of sodium by the kidney. If the kidney's ability to excrete sodium is not severely compromised, it is possible to approach normal balance by restricting sodium intake to match excretion. Even though less than one gram of sodium chloride is required to meet physiologic needs, the average American diet contains 10 grams. A severely salt-restricted diet (less than 500 mg Na or 1.3 gm NaCl) is unpalatable and poorly adhered to. Dietary sodium can be cut to 2–4 gm of NaCl by eliminating cooking salt. This diet is much more reasonable from the patient's point of view; it is more palatable and therefore more easily adhered to. It is convenient to remember that 1 gram of sodium is equivalent to 2.5 grams of salt (NaCl) and that one level teaspoonful of salt weighs approximately 6 grams. 1 mEq of Na = 23 mg. 1 gm Na = 43 mEq Na. 1 gm NaCl = 17 mEq Na.

Diuretics. Diuretic therapy is usually necessary in advanced CHF or when sodium restriction fails to control volume overload. By enhancing renal excretion of sodium and water, diuretics diminish vascular volume, thus relieving ventricular and pulmonary congestion and decreasing peripheral edema. Initially, the goal of diuretic therapy is symptomatic relief of CHF by removing volume without causing intravascular depletion. Once excess volume is removed, therapy is aimed at maintaining sodium balance and preventing reaccumulation of new fluid while at the same time avoiding dehydration. The rate at which edema fluid can be removed is limited by its rate of mobilization from the interstitial to the intravascular fluid compartment. If diuresis is too vigorous, intravascular volume depletion may result. A weight loss exceeding 1 kg per day is to be avoided except in extreme cases of acute pulmonary edema.

Digitalis. Digitalis has two major pharmacologic actions on the heart. The first, and most important to the treatment of CHF, is that of increasing the force of contraction of both the normal and abnormal heart (positive inotropic effect). The second is to decrease the conduction velocity and prolong the refractory period of the AV node. This AV node blocking effect prolongs the PR interval and is the basis for the use of digitalis in atrial arrhythmias. (See the chapter on Cardiac Arrhythmias.) Coupled with the inotropic effect of digitalis is a propensity to increase the automaticity and irritability and decrease the refractory period of the atrial and ventricular myocardium which predisposes the patient to a multitude of ectopic beats and arrhythmias (26–28).

Since digitalis increases the force of contraction of the failing heart, cardiac output is increased and the compensatory mechanisms are reversed. End diastolic volume is decreased, heart size is reduced, and elevated venous pressure and pulmonary congestion are relieved. As tissue perfusion improves, sympathetic tone is lowered toward normal levels resulting in a diuresis and a drop in heart rate. Because it improves the primary defect which leads to the development of the syndrome, digitalis represents a rational choice in the pharmacologic management of congestive heart failure (29,30). Nonetheless, the role of digitalis in CHF therapy has recently been challenged (see Question 3) (31,32).

Vasodilators. Drugs such as hydralazine, nitroprusside, and prazosin are potent arterial dilating agents that can provide symptomatic relief of CHF by decreasing arterial impedence (afterload) to left ventricular outflow. Nitroprusside, nitrates, and possibly prazosin also have venous dilating properties that decrease left ventricular congestion (preload). Their exact role in the management of CHF is yet to be defined. At this time they are primarily reserved for use in those persons with far-advanced CHF refractory to diuretic and digitalis therapy. However, they are also effective agents in mild to moderate CHF and may receive increased use by those clinicians wishing to avoid the risks of digitalis therapy. Nifedipine is a calcium antagonist with arterial vasodilating and antispasmodic properties. It too may be used as an afterload reducing agent in CHF, but its applicability may be diminished by its mild negative inotropic effect. (See Questions 26–28 for a more detailed discussion on the use of vasodilators).

Captopril is a unique agent that may have a future role in the therapy of CHF. By inhibiting the activation of angiotensin II, it has both afterload reducing properties (by blocking angiotensin-mediated vasoconstriction) and volume reducing potential (by inhibiting activation of aldosterone). It appears to be effective, but its use is limited by significant side effects (see Question 29).

Other Inotropic Agents. Digitalis derivatives are the only orally available inotropic agents in common use. Recent doubt about their clinical effectiveness and concern over their potential for toxicity point to the need for identification of useful alternatives. Intravenously-administered sympathomimetic derivatives such as dopamine and dobutamine are frequently used in acute cardiac emergencies such as after myocardial infarction or cardiac arrest. Intravenous amrinone is a non-sympathomimetic inotropic agent undergoing clinical trials.

Diuretic Therapy (38–41)

The kidney serves to provide the only realistic route of sodium elimination. Glomerular filtration and tubular reabsorption are the major determinants of sodium content in the urine. All of the sodium present in the blood is filtered at the glomerulus (25,000 mEq/24 hr). Under most circumstances, all but a very small fraction (ie, approximately 1%) of the filtered sodium and water is reabsorbed. See Fig. 2.

Under normal conditions, the proximal tubule reabsorbs 60 to 70% of the filtered sodium load. At this site, water is passively and isotonically reabsorbed along an osmotic gradient created by active sodium reabsorption. Chloride is also passively reabsorbed down a negative electrochemical gradient formed secondary to sodium reabsorption. Therefore, no dilutional or concentrational changes occur in the proximal tubule; the filtrate remains isotonic and isosmotic. However, a compositional change does occur here. As a result of the carbonic anhydrase-mediated secretion of hydrogen ion in exchange for sodium ions, approximately 90% of filtered bicarbonate will be reabsorbed as carbon dioxide along with sodium in this segment of the nephron.

Because of the large reabsorptive capacity of the proximal tubule, this site has a major role in regulating extracellular fluid volume. Proximal tubule reabsorption remains nearly constant despite moderate changes in glomerular filtration rate (GFR). However, if marked reductions in GFR occur, fractional sodium and water reabsorption by the proximal tubule increases. Thus, poor renal perfusion, which is often noted in cardiac failure, can lead to sodium retention.

In the ascending limb of the loop of Henle, another 20 to 25% of the filtered sodium load is reabsorbed. Sodium and chloride are passively reabsorbed in the thin segment of the ascending loop. In the thick portion of this segment (also called the "cortical or diluting segment" or "distal portion of the ascending loop"), chloride is actively reabsorbed, and sodium passively follows the electrochemical gradient that is created. Because this portion of the tubule is relatively impermeable to water, the medullary interstitium becomes hypertonic and the filtrate becomes increasingly hypotonic as it approaches the distal

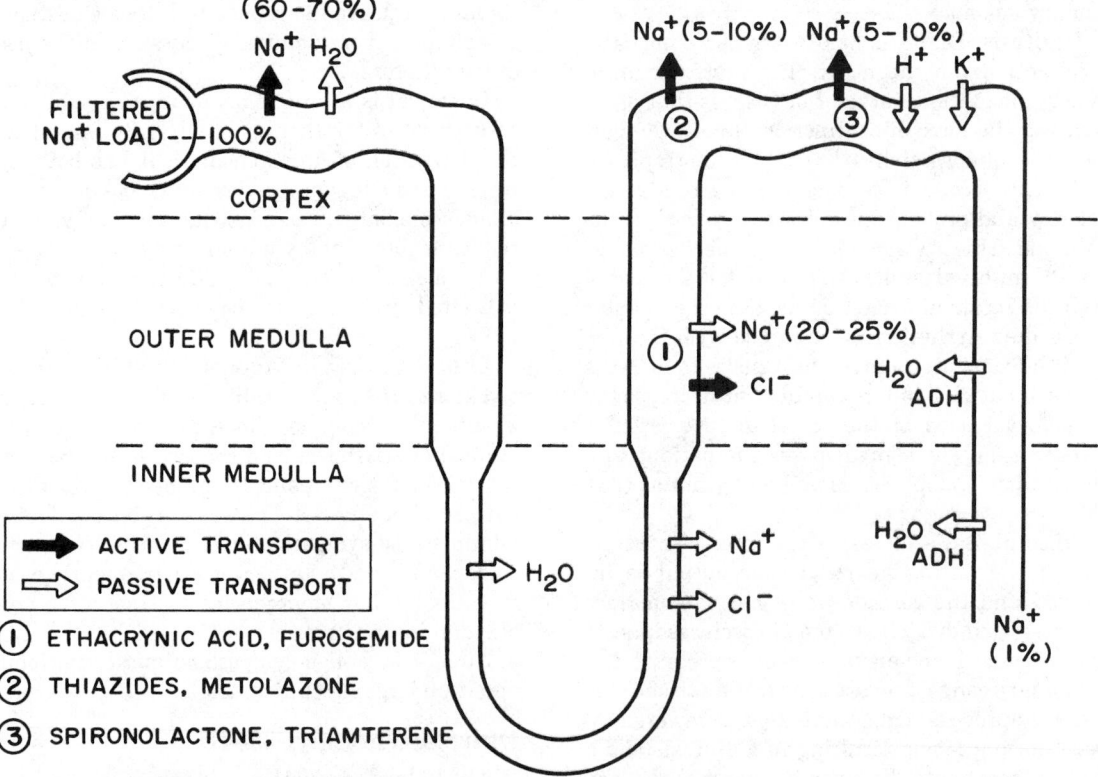

Figure 2. Probable sites of sodium reabsorption and diuretic action in the nephron.

tubule. The production of hypotonic filtrate in this portion of the segment is also referred to as the production of "free water."

In contrast, the descending limb of the loop of Henle is permeable to water. Therefore, in this portion of the nephron, equilibration with the hypertonic medullary interstitium reduces the filtrate volume and results in the production of an increasingly hypertonic filtrate toward the tip of the loop. This gradient of increasing medullary osmolality created by the counter-current mechanism of the loop of Henle ultimately provides the driving force for the formation of concentrated urine in the presence of antidiuretic hormone (ADH). In the absence of ADH, the hypotonic filtrate generated by the ascending loop of Henle is passed through the collecting ducts and excreted as dilute urine. To summarize, this segment of the nephron contributes significantly to sodium homeostasis and provides a mechanism for urinary dilution or concentration.

At the distal tubule, the remaining 5 to 10% of the filtered sodium load is actively filtered in exchange for potassium and hydrogen ion. The efficiency of sodium reabsorption in the distal tubule is governed to a large extent by the mineralocorticoid aldosterone.

The final reabsorptive site through which the filtrate must pass is the collecting duct where antidiuretic hormone (ADH) acts to increase water absorption without sodium. The susceptibility of this portion of the tubule to ADH is important to the maintenance of serum osmolality. Water reabsorption is enhanced via ADH stimulation in hypertonic states and excess water is eliminated in hypotonic states. The former situation produces a hypertonic urine, and the latter a hypotonic urine.

Sites of Diuretic Action. Based on the knowledge of where a diuretic exerts its major effect along the kidney tubule, it is possible to predict its relative potency and electrolyte imbalances which are likely to result from its use.

The more proximal the site of action, the more potent will be the diuretic effect. None of the diuretics exerts its major effect at the proximal tubule where a majority of the filtered sodium is reabsorbed. Therefore, furosemide and ethacrynic acid, which inhibit sodium reabsorption in the proximal portion of the ascending loop of Henle, are the most potent diuretics. The thiazide diuretics inhibit sodium reabsorption at the distal

portion of the ascending loop and are 1/6 to 1/8 as potent as the "loop" diuretics. Finally, spironolactone and triamterene, which exert their effects at the distal tubule, are the least potent diuretics. See Table 2.

Another generalization which can be made is that any diuretic which acts proximally to the distal tubule may potentially produce hypokalemia and alkalosis. This occurs because more sodium is presented to the distal tubule where sodium is exchanged for potassium and hydrogen ion. In contrast, spironolactone and triamterene, which inhibit sodium at the distal tubule, will produce potassium retention.

Spironolactone and Triamterene. Used alone, the potassium sparing diuretics, spironolactone, triamterene, and amiloride are minimally effective in the treatment of symptomatic edema (42). However, their effects are additive with other diuretics, and they are often used as adjunctive therapy to counterbalance potassium loss from thiazide or loop diuretics (38,43). Spironolactone is a competitive receptor site antagonist of aldosterone in the distal tubule and may be specifically indicated for those patients with hyperaldosteronism secondary to decreased renal perfusion. These patients are identified by urinary electrolyte screening as evidenced by high urine potassium excretion and diminished or absent urine sodium excretion. Doses as high as 200 to 400 mg per day may be required to induce natriuresis. In contrast to spironolactone, triamterene and amiloride conserve potassium by a direct action on sodium and potassium transport processes in the distal renal tubular cells. Despite its lack of specificity for aldosterone inhibition, triamterene is effective clinically and frequently prescribed be-

Table 2.

RELATIVE POTENCY OF DIURETICS

Drug	Percent of Filtered Sodium Load Excreted
Furosemide and ethacrynic acid	15–25%
Metolazone	10–15%
Thiazides and chlorthalidone	5–10%
Spironolactone and triamterene	2–3%
No drug (normal)	1%

cause of its lower cost and more rapid onset of action than spironolactone.

It may take two or three days for the initial effects of spironolactone to be observed and several more days for maximal response. Part of the delay in action with spironolactone may be due to its conversion to an active metabolite, canrenone, which accounts for approximately 72% of the drug's anti-mineralocorticoid activity. The liver is the major site of transformation of both triamterene and spironolactone as well as canrenone. Five-day urinary excretion data account for only 14 to 31% of an administered dose of spironolactone (44,45). The elimination half-life of canrenone ranges from 13.5 to 24 hours in normal subjects (44–49) and is dose-related; it was 19.2 hours following a single daily spironolactone dose of 200 mg and 12.5 hours when the same amount was divided into four daily doses (49). Canrenone's half-life is prolonged in patients with chronic liver disease (59 hours, range 32 to 105 hours) or congestive heart failure (37 hours, range 19 to 48 hours) (46). However, the total daily dose requires no adjustment in these patients since plasma canrenone levels do not differ significantly from those in normal subjects, despite changes in the elimination half-life (46). No correlation has been made between plasma canrenone levels and liver function tests (47).

Triamterene is incompletely absorbed from the gastrointestinal tract. The drug has a short half-life of 1.5 to 2.5 hours. Total body clearance is high because of rapid and extensive metabolism by the liver. Both the parent compound and the metabolite undergo biliary and renal excretion. As with spironolactone, the hepatic metabolism of triamterene may be altered in patients with cirrhosis (50,51). The diuretic effect of triamterene begins within two to three hours of its administration, and its maximum duration is 12 to 16 hours.

As with clinical effectiveness, little difference exists between triamterene and spironolactone with regard to side effects. The major adverse reactions to both agents are gastrointestinal distress and hyperkalemia (52). The latter may be aggravated by concurrent potassium supplementation or use of potassium-containing salt substitutes. Long-term (several weeks to years) use of spironolactone is associated with a relatively high incidence of breast swelling (gynecomastia) (53–56). This condition is related to the estrogenic structure of spironolactone, and the effect may be more pronounced with concurrent digitalis therapy or cirrhosis (55,56). Other hormonal side effects seen with spironolactone include decreased libido, impotence, and semen abnormalities (57–59). In females, breast soreness and enlargement, chloasma and menstrual irregularities have been reported (60). An initial association of spironolactone with breast cancer in women (61) has not been confirmed by subsequent follow-up studies (62). By inhibiting dihydrofolate reductase, triamterene may occasionally induce a megaloblastic (folate deficiency) anemia. This has usually been reported in patients with alcoholic liver disease (63–65). In summary, spironolactone and triamterene are essentially interchangeable. Both play only a minor role in the overall therapy of CHF. They are useful only in those who cannot tolerate potassium supplementation and remain hypokalemic with other diuretic therapy.

Thiazides. Thiazide diuretics, especially hydrochlorothiazide, are commonly prescribed because of proven clinical effectiveness in mild to moderate CHF and low cost. They are frequently associated with bothersome side effects, but they pose less potential for overdiuresis than do the loop diuretics. Despite claims of superiority of different products by pharmaceutical companies, the only difference between the various thiazide diuretics is in the recommended dosage and duration of action (38,40) (Table 3). Hydrochlorothiazide is the least expensive of all the agents and has rapid absorption and good bioavailability, even among generic preparations (48,66). Chlorothiazide was recently shown to have limited bioavailability; a 500 mg dose given as a single tablet, a 500 mg dose given as two 250 mg tablets, and a 250 mg dose given as a single tablet all deliver a similar amount of drug (about 50 mg) to the systemic circulation (66a). Chlorthalidone (actually a quinazoline derivative) is the longest-acting agent. It is advocated by some that the long-acting compounds be given on an intermittent schedule, for example every other day or every third day, to minimize side effects. On the other hand, this may create compliance problems if the patient forgets when the last dose was taken. Once-daily therapy is probably the ideal way to dose these agents. Nighttime dosing should be avoided to prevent nocturia. Whatever regimen is chosen, it must be individualized to the patient's response. All of the thiazides are excreted unchanged in the urine by both glomerular filtration and active proximal tubular secretion (48). Their effects are markedly diminished in states of compromised renal function.

Predictable side effects of all of the diuretics are volume depletion, hypotension, dizziness, hypokalemia, hyperuricemia, and hyperglycemia (38,40,67). These effects are discussed more fully in Question 4. Other less common side effects include gastrointestinal disturbances, skin rashes (note: these drugs may cross-react with other sulfonamide derivatives), photosensitivity, immune thrombocytopenia, pancreatitis, and cholecystitis. In contrast to loop diuretics, thiazides may cause hypercalcemia through a parathyroid hormone-like effect.

Metolazone. Metolazone is a long-acting quinazoline sulfonamide diuretic. Like the thiazides, it is thought to inhibit sodium reabsorption in the cortical diluting segment of the ascending loop of Henle or in the early distal tubule. It may also block proximal tubular sodium reabsorption, even though it has little, if any, inhibitory effect on carbonic anhydrase (68–71). Metolazone in large doses (up to 150 mg/day) can induce diuresis in patients with markedly reduced glomerular filtration rates (72–75). In normal volunteers, the natriuretic response to metolazone is associated with less kaliuresis than an equivalent natriuretic response to thiazides (68–70). Nevertheless, hypokalemia frequently occurs during metolazone therapy, and the overall incidence does not appear to differ significantly from that associated with the thiazide diuretics (69,71,76,77).

Furosemide and Ethacrynic Acid. The effectiveness of diuretics is dependent upon the amount of sodium delivered to their site of action in the kidney and the patient's renal function. Proximal tubular reabsorption of sodium is increased in patients with severe CHF when renal blood flow is compromised, rendering thiazide diuretics, which act primarily at the distal tubule, minimally effective. In these cases, the use of furosemide or ethacrynic acid, which work more proximally than the thiazides, should be considered. In addition, loop diuretics and metolazone are the only agents which may be effective in the presence of any significant degree of renal failure (serum creatinine 3–8 mg/dl). Besides its activity in the ascending limb of the loop of Henle, furosemide may have vasodilating properties that decrease renal vascular resistance and may enhance sodium excretion by shifting renal blood flow from the long juxtamedullary nephrons to shorter superficial nephrons. In pulmonary edema, the initial beneficial effects of furosemide may be due more to dilation of venous capacitance ves-

Table 3.

THIAZIDE AND THIAZIDE TYPE DIURETICS

Generic Name	Trade Name	Equivalent Dose	Duration of Action	Daily Dose	Doses Per Day
Benzthiazide	Exna	50 mg	6–12 hr	50–200 mg	1–2
Bendroflumethiazide	Naturetin	5 mg	18–24 hr	2.5–20 mg	1–2
Chlorothiazide	Diuril	500 mg	6–12 hr	250–1000 mg	1–2
Chlorthalidone	Hygroton	50 mg	48–72 hr	50–100 mg	1**
Cyclothiazide	Anhydron	2 mg	12 hr	2–6 mg	1–2
Hydrochlorothiazide	Esidrex, Oretic Hydrodiuril	50 mg	12 hr	25–100 mg	1–2
Hydroflumethiazide	Saluron	50 mg	12 hr	50–100 mg	1–2
Methychlorthiazide	Enduron	5 mg	18–24 hr	2.5–20 mg	1
Metolazone	Diulo, Zaroxyln	5 mg	18–24 hr	2.5–20 mg	1
Polythiazide	Renese	2 mg	36 hr	1–4 mg	1
Quinethazone	Hydromox	50 mg	18–24 hr	50–100 mg	1–2
Trichloromethiazide	Metahydrin, Naqua	2 mg	24 hr	1–4 mg	1–2

**Chlorthalidone may be given every other day.

sels (decreasing preload) than to its diuretic properties (78).

The diuresis which follows an intravenous injection of furosemide or ethacrynic acid begins within 5 minutes, peaks within the first 30 minutes, and is usually complete within two hours. Intramuscular administration results in a somewhat slower onset of action. Natriuresis usually begins 30 to 60 minutes after oral administration of furosemide; diuresis peaks within the first or second hour and lasts for six to eight hours (38,40,50). A 40 mg dose of furosemide is essentially equal to 50 mg of ethacrynic acid.

Major side effects of furosemide and ethacrynic acid are similar to those of the thiazides, including electrolyte disturbances, hyperuricemia, and glucose intolerance. Volume depletion, hypotension and secondary azotemia can result with vigorous diuresis. Both may cause a calcium diuresis, an opposite effect to that seen with thiazides. Both ethacrynic acid and furosemide may cause ototoxicity, especially with large intravenous doses. The incidence appears to be less with furosemide, and several persons have experienced irreversible and complete hearing loss after ethacrynic acid. Gastrointestinal irritation and bleeding are significantly higher with ethacrynic acid than with furosemide (86). From a practical standpoint, ethacrynic acid is harder to administer parenterally since it requires reconstitution by the pharmacy.

Refractoriness to Furosemide. Occasionally patients with severe CHF and/or renal impairment develop a refractoriness to the effects of furosemide, requiring up to a gram or more per day. Switching from furosemide to ethacrynic acid may overcome the problem, or a combination of diuretics may be tried. The most effective combinations are those which combine diuretics that work on two different parts of the tubule. For example, a loop diuretic that works on the ascending limb of the loop of Henle is added to a thiazide that further blocks sodium reabsorption in the distal tubule. Metolazone has been documented to have a synergistic effect with furosemide in several poorly-controlled studies (87–90). While literature for thiazide diuretics is not available, clinical experience has shown that hydrochlorothiazide plus furosemide is frequently effective at much less cost than metolazone. Because of the long action of metolazone, its combination with furosemide may result in a greater than predicted

diuresis and electrolyte loss. Hydrochlorothiazide with its shorter action may be a safer drug. A small dose of hydrochlorothiazide (50 mg) or metolazone (5 mg) is first added to the furosemide therapy, doubling the dose of the non-loop diuretic every 24 hours until the desired diuretic response is achieved. If the synergism desired is seen with the first dose, the dose of the loop diuretic should be decreased. Careful monitoring of weight, urine output, blood pressure, and BUN is required.

Digitalis Therapy

All of the digitalis glycosides increase cardiac output and reverse the compensatory mechanisms in CHF as described above. However, major pharmacokinetic differences exist among the various digitalis preparations.

Digoxin. Digoxin is a polar glycoside which is adequately but incompletely absorbed. Variability in the bioavailability of digoxin preparations has been the subject of several reports (234–241). Differences in methodology, sampling time and standards used for comparison make the studies difficult to compare directly and lead to conflicting conclusions. Nevertheless, it is possible to make some generalizations. The intramuscular route has equal or slightly less bioavailability than the intravenous route, with a relative fraction of drug available (F) varying from 0.7 to 1.0 (235,242,243). The F of the solution varies from 0.65 to 0.9 (236,239,240,243–245); that of the elixir is 0.65 to 0.77 (235); and that of the tablets varies from 0.5 to 0.9 (235,239,240) with an average F of 0.65 for the tablets. It has also been demonstrated that the bioavailability of oral tablets may vary from manufacturer to manufacturer (237,239), and even from lot to lot (237). In some instances there may only be a difference in the *rate* of absorption and not necessarily the *extent* of absorption. It appears that there is a correlation between dissolution rate and bioavailability of some products (239,241), while other products lack content uniformity. Current FDA batch certification considers drug dissolution only. Until better criteria can be defined, it is suggested that the clinician use the Lanoxin brand of digoxin.

The rapid onset of action (30–60 minutes) of digoxin corresponds with peak plasma levels. Maximum effects from a single dose are observed 5–6 hours after drug administration, a time at which drug distribution in the body is complete.

Digoxin has a volume of distribution of 290 L/m^2 or approximately 7.3 to 10 L/kg of lean body weight (246,247). Only 23% is protein bound (28,29,246), but the volume of distribution may be significantly decreased in renal failure (see Question 21) (246). A serum level of 1.0 to 2.0 ng/ml (mcg/L) is generally considered to be therapeutic (see Question 13).

Digoxin's half-life of 1.6 to 2.0 days (36–40 hours) is intermediate between that of ouabain and digitoxin and reflects elimination primarily by first order kinetics (28,246,248). In the presence of renal impairment, the half-life of digoxin is prolonged, reaching 4.4 days or more in total anuria (235). The renal clearance of digoxin in ml/min is about equal to or a little less than creatinine clearance. Many have the erroneous impression that non-renal excretion of digoxin is unimportant. In fact, anywhere from 20–40% of a given digoxin dose is excreted non-renally, either as metabolites or in the feces (29,246,249), corresponding to a non-renal clearance of 40–60 ml/min. In a few individuals, up to 55% of a dose is eliminated as metabolite, primarily as inactive dihydrodigoxin. Very little digoxin (6.8%) enters the enterohepatic circulation, and its metabolism has been found to be unaltered in patients with cirrhosis (250).

Jelliffe presents digoxin elimination in a slightly different context by describing the *percent elimination in 24 hours* (245). By plotting creatinine clearance versus percent of drug eliminated per day (Fig. 3), he found a linear relationship between 24 hour drug excretion and renal function. As can be seen from the figure, the best fit equation of the line (y = b + mx) is:

$$\text{\% eliminated per day} = 14 + \frac{Cl_{Cr}}{5} \quad \text{(Eq. 1)}$$

where the *y intercept* (b), representing non-renal elimination, is 14% and the *slope of the line* (m), representing that portion of daily elimination dependent upon renal elimination, is 1/5. At a creatinine clearance of 100 ml/min, the percent eliminated per day is 35%, whereas at a creatinine clearance of 0 (ie, anuria), the percent eliminated per day is 14%, all via non-renal clearance mechanisms.

Digoxin has become the most widely used digitalis glycoside. This is because of its relatively short action compared to other digitalis products,

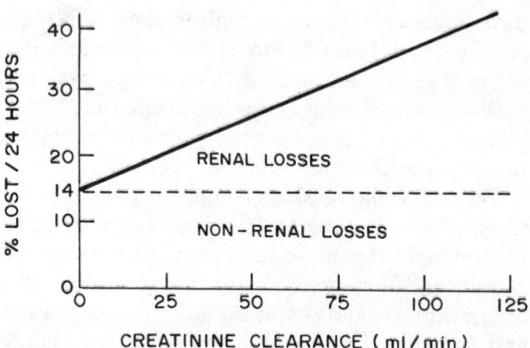

Figure 3. Relationship of digoxin elimination to renal function.

its convenient once-daily dosage regimen, and because its pharmacologic and pharmacokinetic properties are so well described. Although it is dependent in part upon the kidney for elimination and thus requires dosage manipulation with declining renal function, many practitioners still consider it the drug of choice in uremia because a sound scientific knowledge base exists for appropriate dosage alteration.

Digitoxin. Digitoxin is the least polar and most lipid soluble of the glycosides. It has the slowest onset of action (1–2 hours) and peak effect (4–12 hours) and the longest half-life (5–7 days) of all the digitalis glycosides (28,244,251). Only 11.4% of the total body stores are eliminated daily (252). It is more completely absorbed (100%) than is digoxin and undergoes enterohepatic circulation to a greater degree (26%). Digitoxin is 90–95% protein bound (28,244,251). Its elimination occurs primarily via hepatic metabolism and renal excretion of metabolic by-products, 92% of which are inactive and 8% of which are active. Digoxin is the major active metabolite, but because the conversion half-life of digitoxin to digoxin is short in relationship to the elimination half-life of digoxin, little digoxin accumulation occurs. Although never specifically reported, diminished liver function (eg, chronic active hepatitis) may predispose to digitoxin toxicity.

Use of digitoxin compared to digoxin has diminished. This is primarily due to its long half-life which means that several weeks may be required before the full effects are seen if no loading dose is given. There may also be a long delay before toxicity appears, and once toxicity appears it may take a week or longer to dissipate. Some have advocated the use of digitoxin, especially in patients with renal failure, since renal excretion of the drug is minimal (253). Conversely, patients with hepatic disease or taking drugs that affect biliary recirculation may be prone to digitoxin toxicity (see Question 18).

Digitalis leaf USP is composed primarily of three glycosides: digitoxin, gitoxin, and gitalin. Digitoxin is the most important of these compounds and is responsible for the majority of the pharmacologic activity of the mixture. The onset and duration of action of digitalis leaf are therefore identical to that of digitoxin. The use of powdered digitalis leaf has been largely replaced by the purified crystalline preparations (digoxin, digitoxin). More accurate standardization of active drug content and an insignificant difference in cost have made these latter preparations the agents of choice.

Ouabain has the most rapid onset (5–10 minutes) and shortest half-life (21 hours) of the digitalis glycosides. Its peak effects occur in 30–120 minutes. Ouabain is absorbed very poorly from the gastrointestinal tract and is therefore only available for intravenous use. Like all the digitalis glycosides, its elimination from the body follows first-order kinetics. Because the kidneys comprise the primary route of excretion for ouabain, a decrease in renal function will result in a decrease in its rate of elimination and a prolonged half-life (28). The kinetics of ouabain in patients with varying degrees of renal dysfunction have not been extensively studied, and definitive data are not available. It might be best, therefore, to avoid its use in such patients.

The clinical situations in which ouabain would be the glycoside of choice are rather limited. The time to onset of action and peak effect following an intravenous dose of ouabain are not a great deal shorter than is that for digoxin. In most circumstances where prompt action is required, digoxin will suffice. Ouabain is the agent of choice in the relatively rare case where a few minute's delay in increasing cardiac output would be life-threatening.

1. A.J. is a 58-year-old male who was admitted with a chief complaint of increasing shortness of breath (SOB) and an 8 kg weight gain. Approximately two years prior to admission, he noted the onset of dyspnea on exertion (DOE) after one flight of stairs, orthopnea, and ankle edema. Since that time, the patient's symptoms progressed in spite of intermittent hydrochlorothiazide therapy. Approximately three weeks prior to admission, he noted the onset of episodic bouts of paroxysmal nocturnal dyspnea (PND). Since then he has only been able to sleep in a sitting position. In the past three weeks, the patient has noted a productive cough, nocturia (2–3 times/night), and a mild, dependent edema.

A.J.'s other medical problems include a four-year history of peptic ulcer disease, a two-year history of rheumatoid arthritis which has been managed with phenylbutazone, chronic headaches, and hypertension which has been poorly controlled with guanethidine and propranolol. There is also a strong family history for diabetes melitus.

Physical examination revealed a dyspneic, cyanotic, tachycardic male with a blood pressure of 160/100 mm Hg, a pulse of 100/min, and a respiratory rate of 28/min. He was 5'11" and 78 kg. His neck veins were distended. On cardiac examination an S_3 gallop was heard; point of maximal impulse (PMI) was at the sixth intercostal space (ICS) 12 cm from the midsternal line (MSL). His liver was enlarged and tender to palpation, and a positive hepatojugular reflex (HJR) was observed. He was noted to have 3+ pitting edema of the extremities and sacral edema. Chest examination revealed inspiratory rales and rhonchi bilaterally.

The medication history revealed the following: *Present medications:* Hydrochlorothiazide 50 mg bid; propranolol 80 mg tid; guanethidine 50 mg daily; phenylbutazone 100 mg qid; Maalox 30cc alternating with Amphogel, 30 cc q 2 hr while awake. *Allergies:* None. He claims no dietary restrictions.

Admitting laboratory values included the following (normal values are in parentheses): Hematocrit 41.4% (40–45); White Blood Cell Count 5300/mm³ (5–10,000); Sodium 132 mEq/L (136–144); Potassium 3.2 mEq/L (3.5–5.3); Chloride 90 mEq/L (96–106); Bicarbonate 30 mEq/L (23–28); Magnesium 1.2 mEq/L (1.7–2.7); Fasting Blood Sugar 120 mg/dl (65–110); Uric Acid 8.0 mg/dl (3.5–7.0); Blood Urea Nitrogen 40 mg/dl (10–20); Creatinine 0.8 mg/dl (0.5–1.2); Alk Phos 120 U (40–80); SGOT 100 U (40). The chest x-ray showed bilateral pleural effusions and cardiomegaly.

What signs, symptoms, and laboratory abnormalities of CHF are exhibited by A.J.? Relate them to the pathogenesis of the disease and to left or right heart failure.

The signs and symptoms of congestive heart failure (CHF) observed in A.J. are easily visualized if one recalls that the work of the left ventricle is the major determinant of cardiac output and that blood flows from the left ventricle into the arterial system, through capillaries, into the venous system and back into the right heart. From the right heart the blood circulates through the pulmonary tree and back into the left ventricle. Thus, left heart failure causes primarily pulmonary symptoms due to back up of blood into the lungs, while right sided failure causes mostly signs of systemic venous congestion. Although left ventricular failure usually develops first, most patients, including A.J., present with signs of combined left and right-sided failure.

Signs and Symptoms of Left Heart Failure. *Weakness, fatigue,* and *cyanosis* result from a decreased cardiac output and compromised tissue perfusion.

If the left heart is not completely emptied, blood backs up into the pulmonary circulation. *Shortness of breath (SOB), dyspnea on exertion (DOE),* a productive cough, rales, pleural effusions on chest x-ray, and cyanosis all result from pulmonary congestion. Pulmonary symptoms are aggravated in the reclining position which minimizes the gravitational effects on excess fluids in the extremities and improves venous return to the heart and lungs. Shortness of breath in the prone position *(orthopnea)* is often quantified by the number of pillows the patient must lay upon to sleep comfortably. In the case of A.J., he eventually could only sleep sitting upright. *Paroxysmal nocturnal dyspnea (PND)* or cardiac asthma is characterized by severe shortness of breath which awakens the patient from sleep and is alleviated by an upright position. It results from pulmonary vascular congestion which has advanced to pulmonary edema and bronchospasm while the patient sleeps.

Left ventricular hypertrophy (LVH) and *cardiac dilation* are caused by an increased end diastolic volume. These effects are observed on the chest x-ray as an enlarged heart silhouette. The point of maximal impulse (PMI) corresponds to the apex of the left ventricle and is visualized as an external pulsation on the left chest. It is displaced laterally or downward from its normal location at the 5th intercostal space (ICS), less than 10 cm from the midsternal line (MSL). An S_3 gallop rhythm denotes a third heart sound often heard in close time proximity to the second heart sound (closing of the aortic and pulmonary valves) in CHF. The cause of this extra heart sound is not clearly understood but is thought to be an extra ventricular "kick" to increase cardiac output. *Tachycardia* is due to compensatory increases in sympathetic tone.

Weight gain and *edema* reflect sodium and water retention resulting from decreased renal perfusion (see Pathogenesis). As renal blood flow and GFR decrease, a disproportionate amount of blood urea nitrogen (BUN) may be retained. This phenomenon is termed *pre-renal azotemia* and may be detected by an elevated BUN to serum creatinine ratio of greater than 20:1. Pre-renal azotemia may also be caused by dehydration and overuse of diuretics. Frequency of urination at night *(nocturia)* is due to enhanced perfusion of the kidney when the patient is lying down.

Signs and Symptoms of Right Heart Failure. The signs and symptoms of right-sided heart failure can be related to either hypervolemia or the back-up of blood from the right ventricle into the peripheral venous circulation. The overall effect is the development of systemic *venous hypertension.*

Dependent pitting edema results from increased venous and capillary hydrostatic pressure, causing a redistribution of fluid from the intravascular to interstitial spaces. Ankle and pretibial edema are common findings in ambulatory patients (ie, with prolonged standing or sitting), because fluid tends to localize in the dependent portions of the body secondary to gravitational forces. *Sacral edema* may be present in patients at bed rest. Edema is grossly quantified on a 1+ (minimal) to 4+ (severe) scale. A.J. has 3+ pitting edema.

Hepatomegaly, hepatic tenderness, and ascites (fluid in the abdomen) arise from hepatic venous congestion and increased portal vein pressure. Metabolism of drugs highly dependent upon the liver for body elimination may be notably impaired by both the backward venous congestion of the liver from right-sided failure and by the decreased arterial perfusion of the liver from left-sided failure.

Congestion of the gastrointestinal tract makes the patient *anorexic.*

Neck vein distention, primarily seen as jugular venous distention (JVD), denotes the presence of an elevated jugular venous pressure (JVP). How high the neck veins are distended while the patient is lying down and how much his head has to be raised before the JVD disappears give the physician a rough estimate of the patient's central venous pressure (CVP). Applying pressure to the liver may cause further distention of the neck veins if hepatic venous congestion is present. This phenomenon is termed the *hepatojugular reflex* (HJR).

2. What factors contributed to the etiology of A.J.'s heart failure?

A.J.'s age of 58 puts him in a high-risk category for development of cardiovascular disease (see introduction). He is especially vulnerable to heart failure because of his poorly-controlled *hypertension* which places an increased afterload on his left ventricle.

As pointed out above (see Etiology), there are many drugs that may potentially precipitate or aggravate congestive heart failure. A.J. was receiving several agents that may have contributed to his CHF, the most significant of which was *propranolol*. All beta adrenergic blocking drugs decrease myocardial contractility and slow the heart rate. Both of these factors compromise the ability of the heart to empty effectively. Since propranolol-induced CHF is a frequently encountered clinical problem, the clinician must always weigh the risks versus benefits in prescribing beta blockers for hypertension or angina in a patient with CHF. If the CHF is well compensated by other therapy, a beta blocker may be tried as long as the patient is closely monitored for signs of worsening failure (eg, shortness of breath, ankle edema, weight gain). Even topically applied beta blocking drugs (eg, timolol eye drops for glaucoma) may cause systemic toxicity in sensitive patients (6).

Another of A.J.'s drugs, *guanethidine,* is a sympatholytic agent that theoretically may deprive the failing heart of the sympathetic drive required to maintain cardiac output. This in turn could diminish glomerular filtration rate and increase sodium retention (7,8). However, exacerbation of CHF does not appear to be a clinically significant problem with this agent. Methyldopa is also a mild sympatholytic agent, but it should pose even less of a hazard than guanethidine.

Both the *phenylbutazone* used for A.J.'s ar-

thritis and *antacids* may contribute to sodium overload. Phenylbutazone has well-documented renally-mediated sodium-retaining properties, increasing the blood volume by up to 50% in some individuals. Several cases of CHF which have been exacerbated by this drug are reported in the literature (9). Other non-steroidal anti-inflammatory agents such as ibuprofen and naproxen also have sodium-retaining properties (10); see the Rheumatic Diseases chapter. Antacids do not cause sodium retention, but may contribute to volume overload by the physical presence of large quantities of sodium in the manufactured product. Clinicians should be aware that many pharmaceutical manufacturers (including the manufacturers of Maalox, Mylanta, and Riopan) have changed their antacid formulations to minimize the sodium content. Unless large daily quantities of antacids are consumed, they are probably of little concern to the CHF patient.

On admission to the hospital, both A.J.'s hypertension and CHF were poorly controlled and he had gained 8 kg in weight. He needs increased diuresis, probably with a loop diuretic, although careful attention must be paid to his low serum potassium. Propranolol must be discontinued. Guanethidine should probably be discontinued as well, although blood pressure is high in face of fairly large doses (assuming good compliance). The phenylbutazone dose is also high. This drug should be withheld and replaced with another anti-inflammatory agent with less sodium-retaining properties such as naproxen. If hypertension is not controlled with a loop diuretic alone, a drug which has only mild sodium-retaining properties, such as hydralazine, prazosin, clonidine, or methyldopa, may be tried. Minoxidil would be useful only if the hypertension is refractory to other agents. It is a potent inducer of sodium retention and edema and must be used concurrently with a loop diuretic (11).

Finally, it is possible that A.J.'s *diet* contains a considerable excess of sodium from foods such as canned soups and vegetables, potato chips, or overzealous use of the salt shaker at meal time. He should be instructed on a low sodium (eg, 2 grams per day) diet. If salt substitutes are used he should be warned that they are high in potassium and may cause hyperkalema if used concurrently with potassium supplements or potassium sparing diuretics.

3. Bedrest and a 1 gm sodium diet were ordered. Which is the drug of first choice for A.J., digitalis or diuretics?

Correction of the underlying defect is the most rational approach to the treatment of any disease. Therefore, digitalis, which traditionally has been claimed to improve cardiac contractility, cardiac output, and renal perfusion should represent the rational drug of first choice in the pharmacologic management of congestive heart failure. However, the primary role of digitalis in the management of CHF in patients with normal sinus rhythm has recently been questioned. Cohn et al (31) studied eight patients (four with cardiomyopathy, four with ischemic heart disease) after administration of two 0.5 mg intravenous doses of digoxin given 2 hours apart. There was no consistent increase in cardiac output or decrease in pulmonary arterial pressure during a 4-hour observation period, suggesting minimal beneficial effect of the drug. This study is limited by a small sample size and use of short-term therapy. The findings cannot be extrapolated to chronic drug use or to other causes of CHF such as aortic and mitral valve defects, volume overload, or atrial arrhythmias. The authors conclude that while many previous studies have consistently demonstrated enhancement of myocardial contractility in pharmacologic tissue studies, an improvement in cardiac function in an intact heart may be less predictable. Similarly, Hutcheon et al (32), in studying 15 patients, found that treatment with vigorous diuresis was as effective as diuresis plus digitalis in controlling the symptoms of CHF.

Conversely, Arnold and associates (33) claim that oral digoxin has value in the long-term therapy of CHF. They studied nine patients with chronic congestive heart failure (due to idiopathic cardiomyopathy or ischemic heart disease) who were in normal sinus rhythm and had been receiving continuous oral digoxin therapy for at least two months prior to the study. Baseline cardiac function tests were performed while the patients were taking digoxin. Therapy was then discontinued and the patients were monitored weekly for six to seven weeks. At the end of the observation period, 1 mg of digoxin was infused and hemodynamic testing was repeated. Upon withdrawal of digoxin, pulmonary capillary wedge pressure increased significantly and the cardiac index decreased, suggesting a deterioration in left ventricular function. Four patients had to be hospitalized after drug withdrawal. Acute infusion of 1 mg of digoxin at the end of the study restored the hemodynamic values to those observed during long-term digoxin therapy. Follow-up studies to determine if improvement was maintained with continued oral dosing were not performed.

It should be emphasized that the studies discussed above were all performed in patients with normal sinus rhythmn. Atrial arrhythmias, especially atrial fibrillation or flutter, frequently herald congestive heart failure or may precipitate cardiac congestion. Digitalis is the drug of choice under these circumstances because its AV blocking effect controls the ventricular response and its inotropic effect reverses the underlying cause of the atrial arrhythmia (34).

The evidence regarding digitalis effectiveness is controversial and has divided clinicians' opinions (35–37). One group claims that digitalis is the logical first drug of choice for CHF of any cause, while others claim its usefulness is limited by an unacceptably high rate of side effects with minimal effectiveness and should be reserved only for those patients with coexisting atrial arrhythmias. Whichever approach to therapy one wishes to accept, all clinicians agree that excessive volume increases the workload of a compromised heart and that diuretics are an integral part of therapy. This is especially true if volume overload is symptomatic (eg, pulmonary congestion, venous stasis and thrombosis of the extremities) as it is in A.J. However, it is important to emphasize that vigorous diuretic therapy carries the risk of volume depletion and diminished cardiac output.

The final decision as to whether diuretics or digitalis should be the first drug of choice is highly individualized based upon many patient factors and clinicians' opinions. In the case of A.J., who is in biventricular failure, a reasonable approach to management is to initiate both increased diuresis, probably with a loop diuretic, and cautious digitalization (using digoxin) since he has not responded well to diuretics in the past. He will also require a potassium supplement, because he is already hypokalemic and therefore predisposed to possible digitalis toxicity. Since he is in normal sinus rhythm, he will not require large doses of digitalis.

4. Adverse Diuretic Effects. Examine A.J.'s laboratory values (Question 1). Can any of the abnormal values be attributed to the hy-

drochlorothiazide A.J. has been taking? What is the significance of these abnormalities?

Hyponatremia. The first abnormality noted is a marginally low serum sodium of 132 mEq/L. It must be clearly understood that a low serum sodium is not necessarily a sign of overdiuresis. The serum sodium reported by the laboratory is the *concentration* of sodium in the serum. A person may be markedly overdiuresed (dehydrated) with a large body deficit of sodium, but if that sodium were lost isotonically, the serum sodium concentration will be normal. Conversely, a person such as A.J. may be volume overloaded (edema and hypertension) indicating excessive body sodium, but the serum sodium concentration may be normal or even low. Hyponatremia (low serum sodium concentration) is a reflection of a dilutional effect of sodium by extra free water in the plasma. The most frequent cause of dilutional hyponatremia is excess antidiuretic hormone (ADH) production or excessive water drinking (ie, non-electrolyte containing fluids). Persons on severely sodium-restricted diets or who are markedly overdiuresed and who are then given salt-free fluids or who have compensatory ADH release by the body may become hyponatremic. The exact cause of hyponatremia in A.J. is unknown.

Dilutional hyponatremia, resembling the syndrome of inappropriate antidiuretic hormone (SIADH) secretion, has been described following treatment with thiazide and loop diuretics (91–100). Patients with congestive heart failure or hepatic cirrhosis are more likely to develop this diuretic-induced dilutional hyponatremia because of pre-existing defects in free water clearance. Strict low sodium diets and excessive fluid intake further enhance the risk. Additionally, impaired free water clearance can result in acute symptomatic hyponatremia in psychogenic water drinkers receiving thiazide diuretics (91,92,97,99).

Severe hyponatremia with serum sodiums ranging from 91 to 120 mEq/L was attributed to diuretics by Fichman (95). Twenty-five patients with diuretic-induced hyponatremia had a syndrome which was indistinguishable from SIADH except that alkalosis and hypokalemia were also present (as seen in this patient). The diuretics implicated in this study included a variety of thiazide derivatives, furosemide (Lasix), and chlorthalidone (Hygroton) in conventional doses. Within 3 to 10 days after discontinuation of therapy, the hyponatremia disappeared and the ability to excrete a water load returned to normal.

Repetitive episodes of hyponatremia occurred within 2 to 12 days after the reinstitution of these diuretics. An elevated ADH activity was noted in all 10 patients with diuretic-related hyponatremia in whom ADH activity was measured. Treatment of dilutional hyponatremia includes fluid restriction and discontinuation of the offending diuretic agent (38). A.J.'s marginally low serum sodium does not contraindicate continued diuretic therapy.

Hypokalemia. A.J. has a serum potassium of 3.2 mEq/L. Hypokalemia reflecting total body potassium depletion is a side effect of the thiazides and loop diuretics. It is primarily caused by an exchange of sodium for potassium in the distal tubule. The urinary excretion of potassium is enhanced by: (a) an increased rate of delivery of sodium to the distal tubule; (b) diuretic-related chloride loss and alkalosis; and (c) increased aldosterone secretion secondary to either the disease state or diuretic-induced volume depletion (101–109). Also see the chapters on Fluid and Electrolyte Disorders and Acid-Base Disorders.

The actual incidence and significance of diuretic-induced hypokalemia is a clouded issue. Using a definition of hypokalemia as a serum potassium less than 3.5 mEq/L, the incidence is small, being observed in 15–40% of patients receiving 50–100 mg hydrochlorothiazide (105,109). If one accepts serum levels above 3.0 mEq/L as normal, the incidence is even lower. Unfortunately, experts cannot agree on the definition of hypokalemia. In a large clinical study Davidson and Surawicz (110) found little evidence, clinical or ECG, to suggest that a serum potassium level between 3.0 and 3.5 mEq/L was harmful. Similar findings have been presented by other investigators (111,112). On the other hand, Steiness et al showed increased ectopic activity in those persons with serum levels between 3.0 and 3.5 mEq/L (113). Perhaps more important than serum levels is the measurement of actual tissue and body stores of potassium. Davidson et al found only a 3–5% deficit of total body potassium in a group of diuretic-treated patients (109). This deficit did not differ significantly from that found in a control group of subjects not taking diuretics.

One must also take into account the serum potassium concentration in patients before therapy as well as the actual degree of fall in serum potassium. The incidence of hypokalemia is usually less in patients with heart failure than in patients with hypertension, because the patients with heart failure have a higher serum potassium concentration before treatment (108). A subgroup of CHF patients with poor renal blood flow and secondary hyperaldosteronism may have more hypokalemia. In cirrhosis, the serum potassium values tend to be even lower before treatment, and these individuals are more susceptible to diuretic-induced hypokalemia. The opposite is true in renal failure where there is a tendency toward hyperkalemia in the absence of diuretic therapy.

It is interesting to note that the degree of hypokalemia produced by furosemide may be less than that produced by thiazides (103,108,114). This seems paradoxical when one considers that furosemide blocks tubular reabsorption of sodium to a greater degree than thiazides, allowing more sodium to be presented to the distal tubule for exchange with potassium and hydrogen ions. The reason for this anomaly is not well explained. It may be due to the fact that furosemide's activity is of shorter duration than the thiazides, allowing for more recovery of potassium between doses.

A.J.'s serum potassium of 3.2 mEq/L falls in that grey area between 3.0 and 3.5 mEq/L. While the risk may be low, he will be receiving increased doses of diuretics over the next several days and started on digoxin. Since low serum potassium levels predispose to digitalis toxicity (see Question 19), potassium replacement is warranted for A.J. Choice of agent and proper doses are discussed in Question 5.

Hypochloremic alkalosis. A.J.'s low serum chloride of 90 mEq/L concurrent with an elevated serum bicarbonate (total CO_2) of 30 mEq/L signify hypochloremia with a metabolic alkalosis. When sodium is reabsorbed, electroneutrality must be maintained by the concomitant reabsorption of an anion or the tubular secretion of a cation. Since chloride is readily reabsorbable and is abundant, considerable sodium reabsorption is accompanied by the concomitant reabsorption of chloride. Likewise, a sodium diuresis results in a chloride diuresis.

Under normal conditions urinary excretion of chloride is consistently greater than that of sodium, because the distal nephron allows for the reabsorption of sodium in "exchange" for the tubular secretion of potassium and hydrogen ions. Since there is no net change in electroneutrality, chloride does not accompany the reabsorbed sodium and is therefore excreted (115,116).

Diuretic-induced alkalosis is generally associated with hypochloremia, although it need not be.

Alkalosis can occur as the result of a shrinking extracellular fluid compartment along with normal renal bicarbonate reabsorption.

Since diuretic therapy is aimed at an increased sodium excretion, concomitant chloruresis is unavoidable. Morever, diuretic programs often include salt restriction which further decrease chloride intake. Also see the chapter on Acid-Base Disorders.

The therapy of both hypochloremia and metabolic alkalosis is potassium chloride replacement. Under unusual circumstances either ammonium chloride or a dilute hydrochloric acid infusion may be required.

Hypomagnesemia. A serum magnesium level of 1.2 mEq/L is observed in A.J. This could either be a result of magnesium diuresis induced by his diuretic therapy or binding of magnesium ions in the intestines by his antacids, causing malabsorption of magnesium. The problem of antacid binding is more important with aluminum hydroxide than with a mixed aluminum-magnesium hydroxide preparation. Severe hypomagnesemia can lead to somnolence, muscle spasms, a decreased seizure threshold, and cardiac arrhythmias (117–118). These effects are similar to those seen with hypocalcemia and hyperkalemia. Some investigators have claimed that many of the arrhythmias previously ascribed to diuretic-induced hypokalemia were actually due to diuretic-induced hypomagnesemia (119–120). Concurrent hypokalemia and hypomagnesemia can be especially dangerous. A.J. should be given 1 gm of $MgSO_4$ intravenously and observed for changes in his magnesium level. If needed, he could be given oral supplements of magnesium such as milk of magnesia. One ampule of hydrated magnesium sulfate provides 79 mg or 8.12 mEq of Mg^{++}. One teaspoonful (5 cc) of milk of magnesia provides 165 mg (13.8 mEq Mg^{++}). This small of a dose should not cause diarrhea, but because of varied oral absorption, it may not provide adequate replacement.

Hyperglycemia. It can be seen that A.J. has a fasting blood sugar of 120 mg/dl. This is only a small elevation in blood sugar over normal and in fact may be normal if the sample was not taken in the fasting state. It also may represent a stress-related diabetic reaction.

Hyperglycemia and glucose intolerance have been reported to occur during treatment with thiazide diuretics (121–126). Mild to moderate rises in fasting blood sugar (FBS) commonly occur within the first several weeks of thiazide administration in diabetic, as well as prediabetic patients. Since A.J. has a family history of diabetes, he is especially at risk. Occasionally, elevations in FBS may be more pronounced with increases as great as 350 mg%. In some patients, discontinuation of thiazides may be necessary, or alternatively, the addition of hypoglycemic agents may be required to control blood glucose levels. Although diabetic and prediabetic patients are more prone to the diabetogenic effects of thiazides, significant carbohydrate disturbances may also become evident in nondiabetic patients after several years of chronic thiazide treatment (121,122,124,125).

Hyperosmolar nonketotic coma associated with marked hyperglycemia has also been reported as a serious sequela of thiazide's diabetogenic effects. Elderly, late onset diabetics appear to be at greatest risk. The incidence of hyperosmolar nonketotic coma is very low, but the mortality rate ranges between 20 to 40% (125,127,128).

The exact mechanism of diuretic-induced carbohydrate intolerance is unknown, but a number of possibilities exist. These include impaired pancreatic insulin release, extrapancreatic effects on glucose utilization, and thiazide-related changes in catecholamine release affecting carbohydrate metabolism. Impaired insulin release caused by thiazide-induced hypokalemia and decreased peripheral glucose utilization have also been suggested as mechanisms. Potassium replacement has reportedly reversed the hyperglycemic effect of thiazides; however, the association of hypokalemia and thiazide hyperglycemia has not been consistently demonstrated (121,123).

Furosemide (122,125,129–133), ethacrynic acid, and triamterene (134–135) have also been reported to affect carbohydrate metabolism. However, the effects of these drugs on blood sugar and glucose tolerance appear to be weaker and less consistent than those seen with thiazides. Nonetheless, in certain patients, the diabetogenic effect of these diuretic agents can be significant as evidenced by the fact that hyperosmolar nonketotic coma has been reported in patients treated with furosemide (130,132).

At this time A.J.'s blood sugar needs further monitoring, but no specific therapy is required.

Hyperuricemia. Diuretics have been implicated as a cause of hyperuricemia in over 20% of patients with this condition (67). In addition, more than 50% of diuretic-treated patients with essen-

tial hypertension are hyperuricemic. Increases of 1 to 2 mg/dl in uric acid levels are common during thiazide administration, although 4 to 5 mg/dl elevations have been reported. A.J. shows an increase of 1 mg/dl.

Diuretic-induced hyperuricemia is due to decreased excretion of urates as well as extracellular fluid volume contraction. Replacement of urinary sodium and fluid losses abolishes the hyperuricemia caused by the diuretics. Although moderate elevations in plasma uric acid are common during chronic diuretic treatment, the development of acute gouty arthritis is relatively rare; however, it is not known whether these patients are at risk of developing gouty nephropathy.

The majority of patients who develop elevated uric acid levels during treatment with diuretic agents will remain asymptomatic and need not be treated. Only those with uric acid levels persistently greater than 10.0 mg/dl (SMA 12/60 autoanalyzer), as well as those with a history of gout or a familial predisposition should be considered for treatment with urate lowering agents. Although treatment of asymptomatic hyperuricemia may be initiated to prevent the complications of elevated uric acid, there is no clearcut evidence that asymptomatic hyperuricemia alone is harmful (136,137). Also see the chapter on Gout and Hyperuricemia.

Azotemia. Our patient has an elevated BUN (40 mg/dl), but a normal serum creatinine (0.8 mg/dl). Normally, a BUN to creatinine ratio of 10–20:1 is seen. Progressive renal failure is characterized by an elevation of both BUN and creatinine. A disproportionately elevated BUN to creatinine is indicative of *pre-renal azotemia*. The major causes of pre-renal azotemia are dehydration or poor renal perfusion. Dehydration with subsequent pre-renal azotemia is not an uncommon consequence of excessive diuretic therapy. In the case of A.J., his laboratory values reflect pre-renal azotemia, but his edematous state and elevated blood pressure rule against dehydration. The most probable cause of his azotemia is decreased renal blood flow from uncompensated CHF. Diuretics should not be withheld and, in fact, judicious diuresis and improvement of his CHF may help to lower his BUN. Prolonged overdiuresis and dehydration may cause renal ischemia leading to true renal damage. In this case the serum creatinine will also begin to rise.

Liver Function. The elevated alkaline phosphatase and SGOT seen in A.J.'s laboratory values are probably not indicative of any drug-related toxicity. Although cholestatic jaundice has been reported with thiazide diuretics, the elevated liver function tests are most likely due to hepatic congestion from right-sided heart failure.

5. Potassium Supplementation. The physician gave A.J. three 20 mEq doses of potassium chloride intravenously. This raised his serum potassium to 3.9 mEq/L. Should he receive prophylactic potassium supplementation? What is the best drug and appropriate dose?

As discussed in the previous question, potassium supplementation is not required in all patients receiving diuretics. Patients should be monitored frequently in the first few months of diuretic therapy to determine their potassium requirements. Prophylactic or therapeutic potassium replacement should be given only when the therapeutic gains of treatment are balanced against its risks (223). A fall in serum potassium concentration may be seen within hours of the first dose of a diuretic, and the maximum fall is usually reached by the end of the first week of treatment. When diuretics are stopped it may take several weeks for the serum potassium to return to normal (101,102,104–108). Therefore, we can be fairly certain that A.J.'s admitting potassium level of 3.2 mEq/L reflects the nadir of his response to hydrochlorothiazide. His response to potassium supplementation shows that his hypokalemia will be easy to control. It might be argued that he should be observed for a few days and not given supplements, but because his diuresis is to be increased and digitalis therapy begun, potassium supplementation is warranted.

Potassium replacement may consist of dietary supplementation with potassium-containing foods, pharmacologic replacement with various oral potassium salts, or use of potassium-sparing diuretics. Table 4 lists the potassium content of selected foods (224). Inclusion of these foods in the patient's diet may be all that is required to maintain potassium balance, especially in the 60–90% of people who are not prone to hypokalemia in the first place. Unfortunately, the food products listed are expensive and many are high in sodium which makes them hard to use in people with low salt diets. The potassium content of salt substitutes is also included in Table 4. Patients using these products liberally may get adequate potassium replacement and, in fact, they can contrib-

Table 4.

POTASSIUM CONTENT OF SELECTED FOODS AND SALT SUBSTITUTES

Food	Quantity	Potassium content (mg, approx.)*
Meats		
Hamburger	3 oz.	290
Beef chuck	3 oz.	310
Beef round	3 oz.	340
Rib roast	3 oz.	290
Chicken fryer	4 oz.	710
Turkey	4 oz.	350
Vegetables		
Sweet corn	1 cup	230
Lima beans	1 cup	520
Tomato	1 medium	340
Brussels sprouts	1 cup	300
Spinach	1 cup	600
Artichoke	1 medium	210
Fruits		
Banana	1 medium	630
Orange	1 medium	360
Apricot	3 medium	500
Dates	1 cup	1390
Cantaloupe	½ melon	820
Raisins	1 cup	1150
Grapefruit	1 cup	380
Watermelon	½ slice	380
Peach	1 medium	180
Juices		
Orange	8 oz.	440
Grapefruit	8 oz.	370
Prune	8 oz.	620
Pineapple	8 oz.	340

Salt substitutes (one teaspoonful is approximately 5 gm of salt substitute)

Adolph's salt substitute	1 gm	333
Neocurtasal	1 gm	487
Cosalt	1 gm	476
Diasal	1 gm	442
Nusalt	1 gm	405
Morton Salt substitute	1 gm	493
Morton light salt	1 gm	233**

*39 mg K⁺ = 1 mEq
**Morton light salt also contains 550 mg of sodium per gram of product.

ute to hyperkalemia. Some patients object to the taste of salt substitutes. It should be noted that Morton Light Salt is not sodium free, a fact that is overlooked by many patients.

If potassium replacements are used, no other product than *potassium chloride* should be used. All potassium-wasting diuretics may cause hypochloremic alkalosis (see Question 4) and if the chloride ion is not replaced, alkalosis and hypokalemia will not be reversed, even if large quantities of potassium are given (116). Therefore, the use of potassium agents which are converted to bicarbonate *in vivo* [potassium gluconate (Kaon), potassium citrate (K-Lyte), or the combination of potassium acetate, potassium bicarbonate, and potassium citrate (Potassium Triplex)] will have very little effect on diuretic-induced hypokalemia if hypochloremic alkalosis is present. These more palatable preparations may be effectively used to replace potassium deficits only if hypochloremic alkalosis is not present (104,105,115).

One of the major problems of potassium chloride supplementation is patient non-compliance due to the unpalatable taste of most liquid preparations. Sometimes the problem can be alleviated by mixing solutions of potassium chloride in fruit juices (eg, orange, grapefruit, or grape) or by trying somewhat more expensive potassium chloride effervescent tablets or powders which partially alter the taste. Use of low sodium tomato juice or a tomato juice-flavored product (KATO) has high patient acceptance despite its high cost. Diluting potassium chloride solutions reduces gastrointestinal upset which is a common complaint.

Slow K and Kaon-Cl are slow release solid dosage forms of potassium chloride crystals imbedded in a wax matrix. They are equal to potassium chloride solutions in bioavailability and are associated with less gastrointestinal bleeding and ulceration than enteric-coated potassium tablets (231). Although esophageal ulceration and stricture, as well as gastric and small bowel ulceration have been reported with the wax-matrix slow release potassium preparations (225–230), the incidence is less than that associated with enteric coated tablets (151). The major drawback to the use of the wax matrix products is high cost and the large number of tablets needed per day. Kaon-Cl only contains 500 mg (6.7 mEq) KCl per tablet and Slow K has 600 mg (8 mEq) per tablet. Newer products contain 10 mEq per tablet (eg, K-tabs)

and 12.5 mEq (Klotrix). Slow release potassium tablets should be avoided in patients with impaired gastrointestinal mobility (101), and enteric-coated potassium tablets should be avoided at all times.

It is difficult to predict the dose of potassium chloride that will be required to maintain proper potassium balance. Many patients do well with 20 mEq per day, but it is questionable how many of these need any supplements at all. People with well-documented hypokalemia may require anywhere from 20–120 mEq of KCl per day (105,109,232). Those patients with disease states associated with high circulating aldosterone levels require doses of potassium in excess of 60 mEq/day (101,104,105,233).

Because of palatability and cost problems with KCl, the potassium sparing diuretics, spironolactone, triamterene, and amiloride have received increased use. They are clearly effective and one recent review concludes that they are more effective in preventing or correcting the fall in serum potassium than potassium supplements. However, this was a retrospective review and one cannot assess comparability of doses or compliance. Nonetheless, these agents reduce urinary potassium losses and minimize alkalosis as well as providing edema-mobilizing properties. A very popular combination is Dyazide which contains triamterene plus hydrochlorothiazide. While this is effective in the majority of cases, its cost is only warranted if a thiazide alone caused unwanted hypokalemia. One should also be aware that the dose of hydrochlorothiazide in Dyazide is small (25 mg) and therefore large doses are required for maximal diuresis. Hyperkalemia is the major toxicity from both triamterene and spironolactone and may occur even when they are used in combination with potassium-wasting diuretics. As a general rule, potassium-sparing diuretics and KCl should not be used together. However, their combined use may be warranted in those patients requiring over 60 mEq per day of KCl. Judicious monitoring is necessary, bearing in mind the slow onset of spironolactone's effects.

6. *Furosemide.* It is decided to begin furosemide therapy for A.J. What route, dose, and dosing schedule should be used?

Clinicians commonly experience erratic responses to furosemide, especially in persons with severe CHF or diminished renal function. Some patients respond promptly and vigorously to small oral doses, while others require massive intravenous doses to achieve only a minimal diuresis. Part of these differences can be explained by the pharmacokinetics of the drug as summarized by Cutler and Blair (79). Compared to intravenous dosing, oral absorption is erratic and incomplete, averaging 50–60% in healthy subjects and 43–46% in those with renal failure. When taken with a meal, absorption is delayed because of slowed gastric emptying, but the total amount absorbed does not differ significantly from that in fasting states. It has been claimed that absorption, and therefore effectiveness, of furosemide will be further diminished in CHF due to edema of the bowel and decreased splanchnic blood flow. This has been partially refuted by Greither et al who showed an average bioavailability of 61% in CHF patients, the same as in normals. However, there was a wide variability in absorption (34–80%) and a delay of up to 30 minutes before drug appeared in the plasma (80).

One might therefore imply that intravenous therapy would be the preferred route, giving a better response for any given dose. Surprisingly, this is not the case. It has been shown in both normal volunteers and in patients with CHF that total daily fluid and electrolyte loss after oral therapy and parenteral therapy are comparable. The major difference is in the time course of response. During the first two hours, diuresis from the intravenous dose far exceeds that from the oral therapy, but by 4–6 hours the total urinary output is equivalent (80–82). Therefore, considering the marked cost differential between oral and parenteral furosemide, there seems to be little clinical advantage in using intravenous therapy. Exceptions to the rule are those patients with severe pulmonary edema who need acute symptomatic relief and those patients who have failed adequate oral challenge.

Another controversy exists as to whether furosemide should be given as a once-daily dose or in multiple doses. The drug's short half-life of 4–6 hours would imply the need for multiple dosing. Two authors observed equivalent daily diuresis from the same dose given as either single or divided doses (83,84), while another investigator found better effects from divided doses (85). Since evening and nighttime doses of diuretics frequently disturb patients' sleep patterns because of nocturnal diuresis, the total daily dose should usually be given as a single morning dose. For those patients with symptomatic nocturnal edema, 2/3 of the dose can be given in the morning and 1/3 in the late afternoon or, if necessary, at night.

Since A.J. is not in acute distress, oral therapy is warranted. A typical regimen is to begin with 20–80 mg of furosemide as a single dose and monitor for responsiveness. If the desired diuresis is not obtained, the dosage can be increased in 40–80 mg increments over the next several days to a total daily dose of 320–600 mg per day.

7. A.J. is begun on 80 mg of furosemide each morning and KCl elixir 20 mEq twice daily. How should his therapy be monitored?

He needs to be monitored for both an improvement in his CHF and for the presence of side effects. Subjectively, one should monitor for a decrease in pulmonary distress and an increase in exercise tolerance, demonstrating control of CHF. Objective monitoring parameters for disease control include weight loss (ideal is 0.5–1 kg/day), a decrease in edema, flattening of neck veins, and disappearance of the S_3 gallop and rales. Since A.J. has hypertension, his blood pressure also requires monitoring. Dizziness and weakness are subjective indices of volume depletion, hypotension, or potassium loss. Muscle cramps and abdominal pain may indicate rapid changes in electrolyte balance. Objectively, a lowering of the blood pressure, especially upon standing, and a rising BUN (pre-renal azotemia) signify overdiuresis. As discussed in Question 4, serum sodium, potassium, chloride, bicarbonate, glucose, and uric acid should be routinely monitored. Quizzing the patient as to the time of onset of diuresis and the duration of the diuretic effect help to develop the most convenient schedule for the patient. If a poor diuretic response is noted, urinary sodium and potassium measurements should be done to detect possible hyperaldosteronism. If the potassium excretion exceeds sodium excretion, spironolactone should be begun and the potassium supplement discontinued after several days.

8. *Digitalis Therapy.* A.J. is to receive digitalis. What baseline information is important to obtain prior to its administration? How should this patient be managed prior to the administration of digitalis?

Before a patient is given digitalis, it is essential to ascertain whether or not he has taken any form of the drug within the past two to three weeks. Dissipation of digitalis activity may require days to weeks depending upon the half-life of the particular preparation ingested. It is apparent that if a loading dose is required it will have to be decreased if the patient already has some digitalis remaining in his body (see Question 24 for sample calculations). According to A.J.'s history, he has never taken any digitalis preparations.

Cardiac arrhythmias may be the only sign of digitalis toxicity. Therefore, a baseline electrocardiogram is essential if the clinician is to distinguish between digitalis toxicity and a cardiac arrhythmia from underlying heart disease should an arrhythmia occur. Our patient has no EKG abnormalities.

Finally, the clinician should be cognizant of the presence of any disease states, drugs, or physiologic disturbances which could increase the patient's susceptibility to digitalis intoxication (see Question 19). A.J.'s low serum potassium has already been corrected by IV potassium supplementation. Renal function (BUN and serum creatinine) should also be evaluated since many digitalis preparations are dependent upon the kidney for their elimination. A.J. has an elevated BUN from poor renal perfusion, but his serum creatinine is normal, signifying good underlying renal function. He should be at little risk for excessive digitalis accumulation, and his BUN may correct itself as the CHF is controlled.

9. Which digitalis glycoside should A.J. receive? Can he be started with a properly chosen maintenance dose, or is a loading (digitalizing) dose necessary?

Considering the factors discussed in the introduction, digoxin is the drug of choice for A.J. He is relatively young and has no renal dysfunction to impair elimination of digoxin. Compared to digitoxin, digoxin is relatively rapid in onset, reaching a therapeutic plateau sooner whether or not a loading dose is used.

Slow initiation of therapy with maintenance doses of digoxin in lieu of a loading dose is considered the method of choice for ambulatory or non-acutely ill patients with normal renal function (254). Slow digitalization with maintenance doses does not require continuous monitoring of the patient and is thus suitable to the outpatient setting.

The main disadvantage to foregoing a loading dose is that a considerable length of time is required to accumulate maximum body glycoside stores and to achieve therapeutic effects. The length of time required to achieve 92% of plateau concentrations of a drug administered on a routine basis at maintenance doses is four half-lives. Thus, a patient with normal renal function placed on a daily dose of 0.25 mg of digoxin will require about seven days to reach maximum glycoside concentrations (4×1.8 days = 7.2 days). If the same patient were anephric ($t\frac{1}{2}$ = 4.4 days) it would take 17 days to reach plateau, and the maximum concentration would be approximately $2\frac{1}{2}$ times that of a normal patient receiving the same dose. If digitoxin were administered in such a manner it would require approximately 25 days to reach steady-state in patients with normal kidney function and up to 45 days for patients with renal insufficiency.

When using the slow method of digitalization, the clinician should avoid increasing doses before maximum effects are observed. For example, it would be fallacious to increase a patient's maintenance dose after three days if no clinical improvement were observed. Slow digitalization also means that the time to onset of toxic signs may be delayed and go unrecognized if the patient is at home.

Our patient (A.J.) is in moderate to severe CHF. It would be possible to treat him without a loading dose, but since he is hospitalized he can be safely given a more rapid digitalizing course. This will give him more rapid relief of symptoms and allow his doctor to better assess the value of digitalis.

10. *Calculation of the Loading Dose.* What would be an appropriate loading dose of digoxin for A.J.?

Not infrequently, the clinician will arbitrarily choose a digoxin loading dose based upon his or her clinical experience. The usual range of empirical loading doses is 0.5–1.5 mg. A more appropriate method of determining a loading dose is based on the patient's *lean* body weight. Jelliffe (255) notes that *oral* digitalizing doses ranging from 0.01–0.02 mg/kg produce therapeutic levels and carry a minimal risk for toxicity. The lower range (0.01 mg/kg) may be used for mild CHF, while the upper range (0.02 mg/kg) may be required for control of ventricular rate in atrial fibrillation (247). Intravenous loading doses should be lower than oral doses, taking into account the poor absorption (65%) of oral digoxin.

Since our patient has moderate to severe CHF, an intermediate loading dose of 0.015 mg/kg may be used. His admitting weight is 78 kg, but we know that he has gained 8 kg since the onset of his CHF. This represents fluid weight and not lean body mass. Therefore, a more appropriate estimate of his weight is 70 kg. For obese patients, lean body mass may be estimated from tables based upon the patient's age, height and frame size.

A.J.'s oral digitalizing dose = 0.015 mg/kg × 70 kg = 1.05 mg. For convenience, an oral dose of 1.0 mg could be given. The equivalent parenteral dose is 0.7 mg.

Alternatively, the loading dose can be calculated based upon pharmacokinetic principles (256). It will be recalled that immediately after a rapidly-administered intravenous loading dose (ie, before any drug elimination has occurred), the total amount of drug in the body (Ab) is equal to the loading dose (LD). The amount of drug in the body is related to the volume of distribution (Vd) and plasma level (Cp) of the drug by the following relationship:

$$Ab = (Vd)(Cp) \qquad \text{(Eq. 2)}$$

Substituting the loading dose for Ab and taking into account the fraction of drug absorbed (F), the equation may be rewritten as:

$$\text{Oral LD} = \frac{(Vd)(Cp)}{(F)} \qquad \text{(Eq. 3)}$$

By arbitrarily choosing a plasma (serum) level one wishes to achieve (eg, 1.5 mcg/L) and using data from Table 5 for Vd, a loading dose can be calculated for the sample patient:

$$
\begin{aligned}
\text{Oral LD} &= \frac{(Vd)(Cp)}{F} \\
&= \frac{(7.3 \text{ L/kg} \times 70 \text{ kg})(1.5 \text{ mcg/L})}{0.65} \\
&= 1179 \text{ mcg} \\
&= \text{approximately } 1.25 \text{ mg}
\end{aligned}
$$

The equivalent parenteral dose is:

$$
\begin{aligned}
\text{IV LD} &= (\text{Oral LD})(0.65) \\
&= (1179 \text{ mcg})(0.65) \\
&= 0.77 \text{ mg}
\end{aligned}
$$

Table 5.

PHARMACOKINETIC SUMMARY—DIGOXIN

Half-life (t½)	
Normal	1.6–2 days
Renal failure	4.4 days or more
Bioavailability (F)	
Tablets	0.65 (0.5–0.9)
Elixir	0.77
Volume of distribution (Vd)	
Normal	7.3 L/kg or 290 L/m^2
Renal failure	4.7 L/kg
Clearance (Cl)	
Normal	1.02 Cl$_{Cr}$ + 57 ml/min
Renal failure	0.88 Cl$_{Cr}$ + 23 ml/min
Usual safe digitalizing dose	0.015 mg/kg (0.01–0.020 mg/kg)
Therapeutic serum concentration	1.0–2.0 ng/ml (mcg/L)

11. *Administration of the Loading Dose.* It is decided to give the patient a 1.0 mg oral loading dose. How rapidly should he be digitalized?

Administration of the total loading dose of digoxin in divided doses over a 12–24 hour period is the method of choice for hospitalized patients. This method minimizes toxicity but allows for rapid achievement of the maximum therapeutic effect. The patient can be evaluated for toxicity and efficacy prior to receiving each portion of the total loading dose. If toxicity develops or the therapeutic goal is achieved before all of the loading dose is given, the remainder of the doses are withheld.

The usual procedure is to give 50% of the loading dose to start (eg, 0.50 mg for our patient), with the remaining 50% of the loading dose split into two equal doses (eg, 0.25 mg each for our patient) at 6–8 hour intervals. Separating each fraction of the digitalizing dose by 6–8 hours allows for complete tissue distribution and observation of the full clinical effects of the preceding dose (256). Since digitalization is given over a 12-hour period, some drug elimination occurs between doses. Therefore, the actual amount of drug in the body is somewhat less than the desired 1.0 mg.

12. *Selection of a Maintenance Dose.* Determine the appropriate maintenance dose of digoxin for this patient.

The usual maintenance doses for digoxin range from 0.125 mg to 0.5 mg per day, with the most common dose being 0.25 mg per day. Equivalent doses of digitoxin are 0.005–0.2 mg per day (usually 0.1 mg/day). Smaller doses of digoxin (but not digitoxin) are given to patients with impaired excretion rates (eg, renal failure, older patients, or small body size). At one extreme, a totally anuric patient may receive only 0.125 mg every other day, while at the other extreme, patients with atrial fibrillation may need up to 0.75 mg per day (247). Because of the long half-life of both digoxin and digitoxin, most patients are given a single daily dose. Twice-daily dosing is occasionally used with larger doses.

Since A.J. is of average body size and has normal kidney function, an empirical approach would be to maintain him on 0.25 mg of digoxin per day. Pharmacokinetic principles can be applied to obtain more rational dosing. The principle that must be remembered is that for any drug the maintenance dose (MD) is simply that dose which replaces the amount of drug eliminated (lost) from the body during one dosing interval, tau (τ). For digoxin the dosing interval is usually 24 hours and, as presented in the introduction, it is possible to estimate the percent of total body stores (drug in the body; Ab) which are lost per day by the equation:

$$\text{\% eliminated daily} = 14 + \frac{\text{Cl}_{\text{Cr}}}{5} \qquad \text{(Eq. 1)}$$

Since A.J.'s renal function is normal, we can assume his Cl_{Cr} is 100 ml/min, giving him a percent of drug eliminated per day of 34%.

The *amount* of drug lost per day (ie, the desired dose) is then calculated by multiplying the maximum amount of drug you wish to achieve in the body after each dose (ie, Ab) by the *percent* lost per day. As in calculating the loading dose (Question 10), the desired Ab can be estimated by multiplying the desired plasma (serum) level (eg, 1.5 mcg/L) by the volume of distribution. Therefore, the equation defining an oral maintenance dose is:

$$\text{Oral MD} = \frac{(\text{Ab})(\text{\% eliminated daily})}{F} \qquad \text{(Eq. 4)}$$

$$= \frac{(\text{Vd})(\text{Cp})(\text{\% eliminated daily})}{F} \qquad \text{(Eq. 5)}$$

If a loading dose has already been calculated, Equation 5 can be simplified to:

$$\text{Oral MD} = (\text{Oral LD})(\text{\% eliminated daily}) \qquad \text{(Eq. 6)}$$

Note that the fraction absorbed term is not included in Equation 6 since it was already used to calculate the oral loading dose. If an IV loading dose is used to calculate the oral maintenance dose, then F needs to be included in Equation 6:

$$\text{Oral MD} = \frac{(\text{IV LD})(\text{\% eliminated daily})}{F} \qquad \text{(Eq. 7)}$$

For A.J., we calculated an oral loading dose of 1.18 mg (based on a desired serum level of 1.5 mcg/L). Using Equation 6, his maintenance dose would be:

$$\text{Oral MD} = (\text{Oral Ld})(\text{\% eliminated daily})$$
$$= (1.18 \text{ mg})(34\%)$$
$$= 0.40 \text{ mg}$$

Since one is limited by the tablet sizes of digoxin that are available (0.125, 0.25 and 0.5 mg), the maintenance dose for A.J. would be 0.375 mg per day.

The daily dose of digoxin may also be calculated by estimating its clearance rate from the body. Clearance (Cl) is equal to the product of the elimination rate constant (Kd) and the volume of distribution (Vd):

$$\text{Cl} = (\text{Kd})(\text{Vd}) \qquad \text{(Eq. 8)}$$

From basic pharmacokinetic principles it is known that Kd is equal to $0.693/t\frac{1}{2}$. If it is assumed that A.J. has a normal digoxin $t\frac{1}{2}$ of 1.8 days and an average Vd of 7.3 L/kg, his clearance would be:

$$\text{Cl} = \frac{0.693(\text{Vd})}{t\frac{1}{2}}$$
$$= \frac{0.693(7.3 \text{ L/kg} \times 70 \text{ kg})}{1.8 \text{ days}} \qquad \text{(Eq. 9)}$$
$$= 196.7 \text{ L/day}$$

Another method of estimating digoxin clearance is to use equations derived by Sheiner et al (257) from pooled data from several hundred patients:

$$Cl_{digoxin} = 1.02 \, (Cl_{Cr}) + 57 \text{ ml/min} \quad \text{(Eq. 10)}$$

where $1.02 \, (Cl_{Cr})$ represents the renal clearance of digoxin and 57 ml/min represents the metabolic clearance of digoxin for a 70 kg man. The equation must be adjusted in patients with severe CHF to account for decreased renal and hepatic perfusion. The adjusted equation is:

$$Cl_{digoxin} = 0.88 \, (Cl_{Cr}) + 23 \text{ ml/min} \quad \text{(Eq. 11)}$$

For A.J., who is not in severe CHF, we can use Equation 10:

$$
\begin{aligned}
Cl_{digoxin} &= 1.02 \, (Cl_{Cr}) + 57 \text{ ml/min} \\
&= 1.02 \, (100 \text{ ml/min}) + 57 \text{ ml/min} \\
&= 159 \text{ ml/min} \\
&= 230 \text{ L/day}
\end{aligned}
$$

Once clearance is determined, the maintenance dose is calculated using the general pharmacokinetic equation:

$$MD = \frac{(Cl)(Cpss \ ave)(\tau)}{F} \quad \text{(Eq. 12)}$$

where Cpss ave is the average desired plasma level at steady state. Using the clearance value obtained from Equation 9:

$$
\begin{aligned}
MD &= \frac{(Cl)(Cpss \ ave)(\tau)}{F} \\
&= \frac{(197 \text{ L/day})(1.5 \text{ mcg/L})(1 \text{ day})}{0.65} \\
&= 0.45 \text{ mg/day}
\end{aligned}
$$

Using the clearance value obtained from Sheiner et al's method (Equation 10):

$$
\begin{aligned}
MD &= \frac{(Cl)(Cpss \ ave)(\tau)}{F} \\
&= \frac{(230 \text{ L/day})(1.5 \text{ mcg/L})(1 \text{ day})}{0.65} \\
&= 0.53 \text{ mg/day}
\end{aligned}
$$

It is apparent that there is some discrepancy in the various methods used to calculate the maintenance dose (0.40 vs 0.45 vs 0.53 mg).

The principle used by Sheiner et al to calculate clearance appears to be the most valid since it eliminates the need to estimate the volume of distribution which can vary widely among patients (258–260). Jelliffe's approach is fallacious in that it inherently assumes that the Vd for all subjects is constant, and it is now recognized that Vd's vary, especially in patients with renal failure. However, in general, his formula gives a reasonable first estimate in the clinical setting because his methods are derived from data garnered from congestive heart failure patients with and without renal failure rather than from healthy subjects. Based on these pharmacokinetic methods, A.J. could be given either a 0.375 or 0.5 mg dose daily. It is probably best to start at the lower dose and assess his needs after 1–2 weeks of therapy.

13. *Monitoring Therapy.* A.J. is begun on 0.375 mg per day of digoxin. How should his digitalis therapy be monitored? How useful are digoxin serum levels in monitoring therapy?

There is no clear therapeutic endpoint for digitalis therapy. Non-specific ECG changes (ST depression, T wave abnormalities, and shortening of the QT interval) correlate poorly with both toxic and therapeutic effects of the drug (26,28,29). Although digoxin and digitoxin serum levels are readily available from most clinical laboratories, a "therapeutic level" has *not* been clearly defined. A common goal of clinicians is to maintain a digoxin level of 1–2 mcg/L (ng/ml) (234,236,237, 261,262). Corresponding levels for digitoxin are 15–25 mcg/L (251). Unfortunately, a small number of patients will develop signs of toxicity with concentrations of digoxin below 1 mcg/L, especially if hypokalemia is also present (247). On the other hand, if supraventricular arrhythmias are being treated, a level of 2–4 mcg/L may be required to control the ventricular rate. Ingelfinger and Goldman (263) concluded that digoxin levels are frequently over-used and cannot be relied upon to clearly separate toxic from non-toxic patients. Serum levels may be used as a *guide* in confirming suspected toxicity or in explaining a poor therapeutic response, but *clinical evaluation* ultimately remains the best therapeutic guide. Another frequent error which is made when evaluating digoxin serum levels is to obtain a level prior to complete tissue distribution. A level drawn less than 6–8 hours after the last dose may be falsely elevated. Serum levels which are obtained just before a dose are considered most reliable (256).

Clinical monitoring is the key to evaluating adequacy of digitalis therapy. As A.J. begins to improve, he will become less dyspneic and will complain less of orthopnea; venous distension and signs of pulmonary congestion will diminish or disappear; diuresis (monitored through urinary output and weight loss) may increase; and a diminished heart rate may be observed. The response of heart rate to digitalis may be variable depending upon the patient's underlying disease. Since bradycardia and other rhythm disturbances may herald digitalis toxicity, daily monitoring of A.J.'s pulse will be needed until his condition and serum levels have reached a steady-state. Ankle edema does not mobilize immediately and is a poor therapeutic endpoint (26,28).

14. After 10 days on a maintenance dose of 0.375 mg, a serum digoxin level was drawn just prior to that day's administration. The serum level was reported as 0.7 mcg/L, and A.J. was discharged on the same dose with instructions to return to the clinic in two weeks. Examination in the outpatient clinic revealed that he had become progressively dyspneic and edematous since his hospital discharge. A "stat" serum digoxin level drawn at this time was 0.3 mcg/L. The serum level was drawn at 3 p.m. and the patient had taken his dose of digoxin at 8 a.m. What are some possible explanations for these events?

As stated in Question 13, serum levels are not an absolute guide to monitoring digitalis therapy. However, in this case, the decrease in serum levels are accompanied by a corresponding increase in symptoms of CHF. We can be reasonably sure of the accuracy of the serum concentration measured because it was drawn at the appropriate time (ie, at steady-state and at least 6–8 hours after the last dose) and the patient's responses are compatible with the level reported. However, wherever doubt exists as to the reliability of a reported serum level, the lab should be asked to repeat the measurement.

Patient compliance must definitely be taken into consideration. Weintraub et al (264) determined that the mean serum digoxin concentration for non-compliant patients was 0.7 ng/ml while that for compliant patients was 1.2 ng/ml. Scheiner et al (265) found that serum digoxin levels were lower in out-patients than in in-patients. They postulate that this difference may be attributable to poor compliance. Thirty-four percent of the patients in Weintraub's study were non-compliant, but this was felt to be a conservative figure since the patient's word was taken as fact. Those patients taking two or more drugs were less likely to comply. It is possible that A.J. is a poor complier since his blood pressure was out of control on his first admission, although this could also have been related to his new onset of CHF. He should be carefully counseled on proper use of his medications.

Digoxin bioavailability should also be considered. Since the prescription was written generically, it is possible that the patient received a less bioavailable brand than Lanoxin the last time he filled his prescription. His dispensing records should be checked to see if he received Lanoxin brand of digoxin (see introduction). Administration of digoxin with *meals* affects the rate, but not the extent of absorption (266,267). That is, the peak concentrations are lower and delayed, but the steady-state serum concentrations are equivalent.

Alteration of the absorption of digoxin following oral administration in patients with *malabsorption syndromes* has been studied (268). It was found that poor and erratic absorption occurred in patients with malabsorption states such as sprue, short-bowel syndrome, and rapid intestinal transit. Mean steady-state serum levels for 0.25 mg digoxin daily were significantly less than those of controls (0.4 vs 1.2 ng/ml). This difference was even more significant in view of the fact that the malabsorbers had a much lower mean body weight (268). Hall et al (269) also studied digoxin bioavailability in malabsorptive states but were unable to demonstrate large differences in serum digoxin concentrations. Their patients were administered a more soluble form of digoxin, and their malabsorbers had poorer renal function than did the controls.

Altered digoxin metabolism is rare but should be considered. Luchi et al (270) report a patient who required 1.0–2.0 mg digoxin daily to control atrial fibrillation. Although her half-life for digoxin was the same as the controls, she metabolized a greater percent of digoxin to cardio-inactive products.

Concurrent metabolic abnormalities may decrease the responsiveness to digoxin. *Hypocalcemia* has been reported as a cause of digitalis resistance (271) as has *hyperthyroidism* (256,272) (see chapter on Diseases of the Thyroid).

15. *Digoxin-Quinidine Interaction.* It was found that A.J. had been taking his digoxin only sporadically. After being counseled on the importance of good compliance, he was restarted on 0.375 mg per day. He did well for the next six months until he noted the onset of palpitations in his chest which were diagnosed by electrocardiogram as atrial fibrillation. A digoxin level drawn at that time was 1.6 mcg/L, but all other laboratory tests were normal. He was begun on quinidine sulfate at a dose of 200 mg qid with rapid resolution of the atrial fibrillation. Four days later, during a follow-up clinic visit, he was noted to have a bradycardia with a pulse rate of 50. He also complained of nausea, dizziness, and weakness. His digoxin level was 2.9 ng/ml. Could the quinidine be contributing to the apparent digitalis toxicity in A.J.?

Quinidine and digoxin are frequently used adjunctively in the treatment of atrial fibrillation: digoxin to control ventricular response by decreasing AV node conduction and quinidine to decrease atrial irritability. Recent reports show that over 90% of patients previously stabilized on digoxin and who are subsequently begun on quinidine experience an average 2–2.5-fold increase in serum digoxin levels (273–277). The actual magnitude of effect is highly variable, but may be dependent on the dose of quinidine administered. Very little change is seen with quinidine doses of less than 500 mg per day. Serum digoxin concentrations usually begin to rise within 24 hours of starting quinidine and reach a new steady-state in about five days. Conversely, upon discontinuing quinidine, digoxin concentration returns to pre-quinidine levels in about five days.

The mechanism of the interaction is still in part speculative. The original reports hypothesized a displacement of digoxin from tissue binding sites (274,275), but this was not verified by Doering (278). A more consistent observation has been a decrease in renal clearance of digoxin, but without a concurrent decrease in creatinine clearance, leading to a possible explanation of impaired tubular secretion of digoxin (277–279). However, since very little digoxin is normally cleared by tubular secretion, Holford speculates that quinidine may decrease the non-renal clearance of digoxin as well (280). Hager et al (279) showed no appreciable change in digoxin half-life in six patients, but they did observe a 35% decrease in total body digoxin clearance, a 30% decrease in renal digoxin clearance, and a 30% decrease in apparent volume of distribution. It may be that the initial effect is a displacement from the tissue binding sites followed by a more sustained impairment of renal clearance. The half-life does not change, since the changes in distribution and clearance tend to counter-balance each other.

While there is little doubt that quinidine will increase digoxin levels, there is not a consensus as to the clinical implications of the interaction. Leahey (275) described GI toxicity in 89% of his patients and cardiac irritability in 29%, while others (274,278,279) describe a very small percentage of subjects with side effects. It is possible that some of the GI toxicities are related to the quinidine rather than digoxin, but 10 of Leahey's patients had decreased side effects when digoxin was stopped or the dose reduced.

It has been suggested that the dose of digoxin be reduced by 50% when adding quinidine (278,281). Unfortunately, this does not take into account the variability in the magnitude of the interaction (282). One patient may have no increase in serum digoxin concentration while another may have a 3–5-fold increase. Others have suggested no dosage modification, but instead close digoxin monitoring and measurement of digoxin levels.

Since neither procainamide nor disopyramide have the interaction potential seen with quinidine (278,283), they may be better alternative drugs. The effect of quinidine on digitoxin is not clear. Fenster et al showed a prolonged half-life and decreased clearance of digitoxin (284), while others have found no appreciable interaction (285). A.J.'s physician decided to place him on disopyramide and discontinue quinidine. This led to good control of the atrial fibrillation and a reversal of the digitalis toxicity.

16. *Digitalis-Drug Interactions.* Are there any other potential drug interactions with digoxin present in A.J.'s therapy? Name other

drug interactions that have been reported to occur with either digoxin or digitoxin.

Antacids and *kaolin-pectin* decreased the bioavailability of a single dose of digoxin (0.75 mg) in normal subjects (286). Sixty ml doses of aluminum hydroxide, magnesium hydroxide, magnesium trisilicate, and kaolin-pectin taken concurrently with tablets of digoxin (Lanoxin) decreased the six-day total urinary excretion. The percentages of total dose recovered were as follows: control—40%; aluminum hydroxide—30.7%; magnesium hydroxide—27%; magnesium trisilicate—29%; and kaolin-pectin—23%. Since A.J. has a history of taking Maalox for his ulcer symptoms, he should be counseled to avoid antacids within one or two hours before a dose of digoxin or within one hour afterward.

Bowel hypermotility secondary to *laxatives* may result in low steady-state digoxin levels. A single case is reported in the studies of Heizer et al (268).

The effect of *neomycin* on digoxin absorption was studied by Lindenbaum et al (287). They found that single doses of neomycin (0.1–3 gm) administered in conjunction with digoxin delayed and depressed peak serum concentrations. Steady-state serum concentrations of digoxin when administered daily with 2 gm neomycin for eight days were significantly lower than those achieved when digoxin was given alone (eg, 0.82 ng/ml vs 0.58 ng/ml).

Non-absorbable *bile acid binding resins* (cholestyramine, colestipol) bind both digoxin and digitoxin. Digoxin does not bind as extensively as does digitoxin, probably because digitoxin undergoes greater enterohepatic recycling than digoxin (288,289). Administration of both digoxin and digitoxin should precede that of the resin by 1½ hours.

Metoclopramide may decrease digoxin bioavailability by increasing gastrointestinal transit time, but this is only significant for slowly absorbed products (290). Lanoxin is not affected. Conversely, *propantheline* may slightly increase digoxin bioavailability by slowing gastrointestinal transit (290).

Digitoxin Interactions. Digitoxin differs from digoxin in several respects (see introduction). These differences become important when considering drug interactions with digitalis preparations. Unlike digoxin, a significant fraction of digitoxin is metabolized to more polar compounds which are readily excreted into urine and bile. Thus, drugs which induce hepatic enzymes (eg, phen-

ylbutazone, phenytoin, phenobarbital, and rifampin) can theoretically increase the metabolic degradation rate of digitoxin. Solomon et al (291) noted that steady-state serum levels of digitoxin were lower in two patients. One was ingesting phenylbutazone, the other phenytoin along with digitoxin. The ingestion of phenobarbital (60 mg tid × 12 weeks) lowered serum digitoxin levels by 50%. Doses of 60 mg qid for eight weeks decreased the plasma half-life by 24%. Patients taking any of these drugs in combination with digitoxin may require higher doses of the latter. Conversely, if these drugs are discontinued, the patient should be monitored for emerging digitalis toxicity.

Digitoxin is protein bound to a greater degree than digoxin (79% vs 23%) (28). *In vitro* experiments have demonstrated that high concentrations of drugs which also have a high affinity for albumin (phenylbutazone, clofibrate, warfarin, tolbutamide, sulfadimethoxine) are capable of displacing digitoxin from plasma proteins. However, therapeutic doses of these drugs do not produce levels which displace digitoxin to a significant extent (242).

Twenty-five percent of a given dose of digitoxin enters the enterohepatic circulation (244). Thus drugs which interrupt enterohepatic recycling by binding digitoxin in the GI tract and preventing its reabsorption may shorten its half-life and lower steady-state serum concentrations of the drug. On this basis, anion exchange resins (colestipol and cholestyramine) have been administered to patients who have taken overdoses of digitoxin (288). These investigators found that the administration of colestipol (10 gm initially followed by 5 gm every 6 hours) shortened the plasma half-life of digitoxin from 9.3 days to an average of 2.75 days. Additionally, clinical signs of toxicity disappeared in 24–30 hours in treated patients, whereas symptoms of toxicity persisted for three days in the untreated controls. Cholestyramine would be expected to have effects similar to those of colestipol but to a lesser degree. *In vitro* studies indicate that duodenal juice decreases the binding capacity of cholestyramine for digitoxin. Sulfasalazine (293) and phenytoin (294) have also been reported to decrease the bioavailability of digoxin.

17. *Intramuscular Digoxin.* One year later A.J. was admitted for elective cholecystectomy. His CHF was still well controlled on

digoxin 0.375 mg daily. After surgery, he was placed on an NPO regimen and given digoxin by the intramuscular (IM) route. On hospital day three he experienced severe pressing chest pain which radiated to his left arm. An ECG was performed and serial serum enzymes were ordered to rule out MI. An elevated CPK was noted, but all other enzymes and the ECG were normal. Comment on the postoperative use of IM digoxin in this patient. What would you recommend?

Patients who are hospitalized and placed on a nothing by mouth (NPO) regimen are frequently given medications by the parenteral route. While many drugs are well absorbed after IM injections, there is evidence for delayed or incomplete absorption of intramuscular digoxin; its availability appears intermediate between that of IV and PO digoxin (235,242). Peak serum levels following IM injections are lower and occur later than comparable oral doses (243); serum-tissue equilibration requires 10–12 hours as opposed to the 6 hours required for the oral route.

Greenblatt (295) noted that IM injection of undiluted digoxin was consistently followed by intense muscular pain and fasciculations. Pain was disabling for two hours and subsided over the next several hours; however, local tenderness and pain on motion persisted for two days.

Digoxin-induced creatine phosphokinase (CPK) elevations are of great importance in this patient. Although any IM injection can cause mild elevations of serum CPK, digoxin can increase control levels by 15–17 times 8 hours after its injection (295). A.J. has probably not had an MI, but patients have been falsely diagnosed as having an MI from CPK elevations due to IM injections.

Based on the above considerations it can be concluded that there are few indications for the use of IM digoxin. If IM injections must be given (for example patients on prolonged NPO regimens in whom no IV lines are established) the dose should be reduced to 80% of the previous oral dose.

The intravenous route is the preferred parenteral method of administration for A.J. The urinary recovery of digoxin is 17% higher from IV injection when compared to an IM injection of an equivalent dose. However, caution is warranted when digoxin is given intravenously. His maintenance dose will have to be reduced by 30% to approximately 0.25 mg per day. Too rapid administration may result in acute myocardial toxicity

caused by a direct effect of the drug. Additionally, the commercially available preparation contains 40% propylene glycol which may also result in acute myocardial depression with rapid administration. It is therefore recommended that the commercial preparation be given at a maximum rate of 1 cc per minute, or preferably that it be diluted with 10 cc of normal saline for injection and then administered as a slow infusion (295). A.J. should be switched back to his usual oral regimen as soon as possible.

18. *Digitalis Toxicity.* **Digoxin was prescribed for a 70-year-old male with mild congestive heart failure. The label on his prescription bottle instructed him to take one tablet (0.25 mg) twice daily for three days and one tablet daily thereafter. Ten days later the patient returned to clinic complaining of extreme fatigue, anorexia, nausea, and a "funny" heart beat. Close questioning and a "tablet count" disclosed that the patient failed to decrease his digoxin to 0.25 mg daily. An ECG revealed multiple PVCs and second degree AV block. A "stat" digoxin serum level was 2.8 ng/ml. Are the patient's signs and symptoms consistent with digitalis toxicity? What are some other adverse effects of digitalis?**

The clinical presentation of digitalis toxicity is highly unpredictable. In some cases, only a high serum digoxin level without any appreciable adverse effects is the only clue to possible digitalis toxicity. In other patients, such as the one described above, a multitude of symptoms may be present including both noncardiac signs (eg, gastrointestinal complaints) and rhythm disturbances (eg, palpitation, heart block, arrhythmias).

The most important adverse effects are those relating to the heart. One must avoid the false impression that gastrointestinal or other noncardiac signs will precede cardiac toxicity. In fact, cardiac symptoms may precede noncardiac symptoms of digitalis toxicity in up to 47% of cases. Frequently (26–66%), nonspecific arrhythmias may be the only manifestation of toxicity (296,297) with estimates that rhythm disturbances occur in 80–90% of all digitalis toxic patients (298).

Almost all known *arrhythmias* can occur as a result of digoxin toxicity. Decreased conduction velocity through the atrioventricular node is manifested as a prolonged PR interval (1st degree AV block) and is seen in many patients with therapeutic levels of digitalis. However, as exemplified in Question 15, higher concentrations of digitalis can impair conduction and result in bradycardia or a variable block (2nd degree AV block). A complete AV block (3rd degree AV block) results in dissociation of the atrial and ventricular rates with a very slow idioventricular rate predominating. Increased automaticity of the atria can cause multifocal atrial tachycardia (MAT) with block, paroxysmal atrial tachycardia (PAT) with block, or atrial fibrillation. Ventricular arrhythmias (as seen in this patient) are among the most common rhythm disturbances caused by digitalis toxicity and include premature ventricular contractions (PVCs), bigeminy (every other beat is a PVC), multifocal PVCs, and tachycardia. Comprehensive reviews are available on the topic of digitalis-induced arrhythmias (26,298,299).

Vague *gastrointestinal symptoms* characteristic of digitalis toxicity may be difficult to evaluate since anorexia and nausea are also part of the clinical picture of congestive heart failure. Beller et al (300) observed an equal frequency of anorexia and nausea in both toxic and nontoxic patients. Even more frustrating is the fact that digitalis toxicity may occasionally present as progressive congestive heart failure.

Recent studies indicate that *CNS symptoms* of digitalis toxicity may be common. Chronic digitalis intoxication resulting from misformulation was observed in 179 patients (296). Acute extreme fatigue was a complaint in 95% of these patients. Approximately 80% experienced weakness of the arms and legs and 65% suffered from psychic disturbances occurring in the form of nightmares, agitation, listlessness, and hallucinations. Visual disturbances were observed in 95% of these patients. Hazy vision, difficulty in reading and difficulty in red-green color perception were frequently present. Other complaints included glitterings, dark or moving spots, photophobia, and yellow-green vision. Disturbances in color vision returned to normal two or three weeks following discontinuation of digitalis.

Prospective studies show a good correlation between *serum digoxin levels* and toxicity. Eighty-seven percent of digitalis-toxic patients had levels greater than 2 mcg/L and 90% of the nontoxic patients had levels of less than 2 mcg/L. However, because a significant overlap between toxic and therapeutic levels exists, serum level determinations are currently most useful as an aid in confirming suspected digitalis toxicity and in in-

dividualizing dosing regimens so that toxicity is avoided (262,300).

Allergic reactions to digitalis are rare as is thrombocytopenia secondary to digitoxin. Unilateral or bilateral *gynecomastia* is often observed during chronic digoxin administration and is reversible upon withdrawal of the drug. This latter effect may occur in addition to the gynecomastia seen with spironolactone.

19. *Factors Predisposing to Digitalis Toxicity.* **A 64-year-old alcoholic male is admitted to the hospital with a three-day history of epigastric pain radiating to the back and associated with nausea and vomiting. The patient also has cirrhosis of the liver and mild CHF well controlled with hydrochlorothiazide 50 mg bid and digoxin 0.25 mg daily. He has a three-year history of severe rheumatoid arthritis which is moderately relieved with hydrocortisone 50 mg tid. Since the initial impression was acute pancreatitis, the patient was placed on nasogastric suction and 3 liters of D5¼NS daily. The following evening the laboratory report disclosed the following: Sodium 136 mEq/L (136–144); Potassium 2.3 mEq/L (3.5–5.3); Chloride 90 mEq/L (96–106); Bicarbonate 32 mEq/L (23–28); Magnesium 1.3 mEq/L (1.7–2.7); Creatinine 0.8 mg/dl (0.5–1.2); SGOT 80 U (40); Alkaline Phosphatase 130 U (80); Amylase 1200 U (4–25); Digoxin 1.8 mcg/L; Creatinine Clearance 100 ml/min (104–125). An electrocardiogram showed occasional PVCs and runs of bigeminy.**

What factors predispose this patient to digitalis toxicity?

This is an example of a subtle presentation of digitalis toxicity. The serum level is in the high end of the therapeutic range. Nevertheless he shows clinical signs of digitalis toxicity (eg, PVCs and bigeminy). His renal function is normal, so digoxin excretion should not be markedly altered. The major contribution to toxicity in this patient is *hypokalemia*. The association between digitalis toxicity and hypokalemia is well recognized. Jelliffe (301) has observed that twice as much digitalis is required to produce toxicity in patients with a serum potassium of 5 mEq/L than in those with a serum potassium of 3 mEq/L. Therefore, drugs, diseases, and medical maneuvers which induce hypokalemia or drop a serum potassium from elevated to normal levels may unmask existing digitalis toxicity or allow toxicity to occur at lower doses. The mechanism of this potentiation is unclear; however, a low serum potassium has been observed to increase the uptake of digitalis by the myocardial tissue (302).

The patient is taking hydrochlorothiazide. All diuretics, with the exception of triamterene and spironolactone, may cause hypokalemia through kaliuresis. (See the introduction and Question 4) In addition, hydrocortisone will promote potassium excretion at the distal portion of the renal tubule. He should be switched to an equivalent dose of prednisone or another glucocorticoid with less mineralocorticoid effect. Similarly, diseases in which mineralocorticoid activity is high (eg, Cushing's disease, hyperaldosteronism) also are associated with low serum potassium levels.

Other causes of hypokalemia in this patient include vomiting and nasogastric suction. Gastrointestinal secretions contain potassium in concentrations as high as 8–10 mEq/L. Similarly, hypokalemia can result from diarrheal losses including drug-induced diarrhea (eg, ampicillin, quinidine).

The patient is in *metabolic alkalosis* (HCO_3 = 32) as a result of the diuretic therapy, vomiting, and nasogastric suctioning of hydrogen ion. Alkalosis results in the redistribution of potassium intracellularly and an increased renal excretion of potassium, thus potentiating effects of hypokalemia (see the chapter on Acid-Base Disorders). In addition, alkalosis in and of itself has been associated with an increased incidence of digitalis toxicity. Brater et al (303) attribute this to an intracellular depletion of potassium due to increased urinary excretion and a relative increase in the ratio of extracellular to intracellular potassium. This has the same effect on the membrane potential as digoxin.

Another metabolic problem arising in this patient that may contribute to digitalis toxicity is *hypomagnesemia*. The causes are the same as for hypokalemia including diuretic therapy, nasogastric suction losses, and, in addition, there is a high incidence of hypomagnesemia among chronic alcoholics. The observation of hypomagnesemia in the absence of hypokalemia in four digitalis-toxic patients prompted an animal study to test the effect of this electrolyte imbalance on digitalis toxicity. The toxic dose of acetylstrophanthidin in dogs was decreased when the serum

magnesium was reduced by hemodialysis (304). The prevalence of hypomagnesemia is higher in digitalis-toxic patients (305), and magnesium sulfate has been used successfully in the treatment of digitalis toxicity (306). The long-term administration of magnesium-free fluids (eg, hyperalimentation), diuretics, amphotericin B, and hemodialysis have also been associated with hypomagnesemia (307).

Although not illustrated by this patient, it should be noted that *hypercalcemia* may theoretically predispose patients to digitalis toxicity. The electrical and contractile effects of calcium on the myocardium are similar to those of digitalis. For this reason, rapid intravenous infusions of calcium may facilitate the development of digitalis toxicity, and normal or low doses of digitalis may induce toxicity in patients with hypercalcemia (eg, hyperparathyroidism or metastatic cancer). The clinical significance of calcium-induced digitalis toxicity has been questioned by Lown et al (308). There have been no reports of digitalis toxicity secondary to the oral administration of calcium-containing products. Nonetheless, if a patient in whom digitalis toxicity is suspected should have a cardiac arrest, administration of calcium is probably contraindicated.

Age may be an important predisposing factor in the production of digitalis toxicity in this patient. The same intravenous dose of digoxin administered to elderly and young patients produced higher serum concentrations of digoxin in the elderly. Ewy et al (309) propose that the higher levels and prolonged half-life observed in these patients are due to diminished renal clearance of the drug and the smaller body size of this population. It is important to emphasize that although the serum creatinine of the elderly patients (average age 77 years) was within normal limits, the mean creatinine clearance (56 ml/min) was approximately half that observed in the younger patients.

The response to digitalis may also be altered in the very young. Levine et al (310) have recommended the use of lower doses in premature infants and neonates (less than one month of age). Toxic arrhythmias were observed when infants tested during the first 72 hours of life were given doses of digoxin comparable to those recommended for children and older infants. This may be due to the decreased renal function normally observed in newborns. Their studies demonstrate that the absorption, tissue fixation and/or excretion of digoxin in infants are similar to that of adults. They point out, however, that infants excrete a smaller percentage of digoxin metabolites than do adults.

20. Treatment of Digitalis Toxicity. How should the above patient's digitalis toxicity (see Question 19) be treated?

Withhold Digitalis. For many patients without life-threatening arrhythmias or major electrolyte imbalances, simple withdrawal of digitalis may be the only treatment required. Although it may take five half-lives for the drug to be totally eliminated from the body, by one to two half-lives the serum level will have dropped to a safe level in most individuals. This would be 2–3 days for digoxin and up to a week for digitoxin.

Potassium. Our subject does not have markedly elevated digoxin levels so his ectopy should disappear rapidly with drug withdrawal. His major problem is related to his hypokalemia which must be corrected. As a general rule, potassium administration should be considered in any patient with digitalis-induced ectopic beats who has low or normal serum potassium levels. The oral route of administration is usually adequate and should be used unless the patient cannot take medications by mouth. The following precautions should be considered when potassium is used to treat digitalis toxicity: (a) Potassium should be administered with caution in patients who have conduction disturbances characterized by second degree or complete atrioventricular (AV) block. Potassium also depresses conduction velocity in the AV node, and its use may result in an augmentation of this cardiac arrhythmia. (b) Toxic doses of digitalis inhibit the uptake of potassium by myocardial, skeletal muscle, and liver cells. For this reason, these patients may occasionally develop refractory hyperkalemia; large doses of potassium should be administered cautiously. (c) Because potassium is eliminated by the kidneys, excessive potassium loads should be avoided in patients with compromised renal function. (d) Cardiac arrhythmias have been observed following the rapid intravenous administration of concentrated potassium solutions.

If digitalis-induced arrhythmias are severe enough to warrant intravenously administered potassium, the maximum recommended rate of administration is 40 mEq/hr (preferably 10 mEq/hr) at a concentration which does not exceed 80–100 mEq/L. A total of several hundred mEq of potassium may be required to replete body stores. Our patient has a fairly significant potassium deficit, with potentially dangerous arrhythmias, but no contraindications to potassium therapy. He should receive 80–120 mEq of intravenous potassium over the next 24 hours and then be switched to an appropriate oral dose. He should be monitored for signs and symptoms of potassium toxicity with frequent ECG tracings (tall, peaked T waves; prolonged PR interval) and serum potassium determinations.

Antiarrhythmics. Virtually all of the antiarrhythmic agents have been used to treat digitalis-induced arrhythmias. Intravenous lidocaine, phenytoin, and propranolol have been used with the greatest success (26). Lidocaine and phenytoin have a theoretical advantage over propranolol and quinidine-like agents in that they do not further depress AV conduction. For our patient, potassium replacement will probably be all that is required. However because of his bigeminy, lidocaine could be given for a few hours until he has been given sufficient potassium supplementation.

Although lidocaine has an elimination half-life of approximately two hours, an initial IV bolus may last only 10–20 minutes because of rapid tissue distribution. Generally, the drug is administered as a constant infusion (1–4 mg/min) following an initial bolus dose of 50–100 mg (1 mg/kg). Caution should be exercised in patients with congestive heart failure since it has been demonstrated that the volume of distribution and plasma clearance of lidocaine may be decreased in these patients (311). Elimination half-life and time to reach plateau are therefore prolonged and symptoms of lidocaine toxicity may not be evident for several hours (two to three half-lives). See the chapters on Cardiac Arrhythmias and Clinical Pharmacokinetics.

Reports regarding the efficacy of phenytoin as an antiarrhythmic agent have been variable; however, the drug appears to be particularly efficacious in the suppression of digitalis-induced tachyarrhythmias with or without first or second degree AV block. A loading dose of one gram or more (in divided doses) may be required during the first 12 to 24 hours. Thereafter, the patient may be maintained at doses of 300–600 mg daily. The diluent for parenteral phenytoin contains 40% propylene glycol which is cardiotoxic (312); for this reason phenytoin should not be administered at a rate which exceeds 50 mg/min. Phenytoin is soluble in saline but not in D_5W and can be administered by intravenous infusion only if the concentration does not exceed 1 mg/ml and the pH is greater than 10.0 (313).

Intravenous propranolol has been useful in abolishing digitalis-induced atrial tachycardia with AV block and ventricular premature contractions. One to three mg should be given at a rate of 1 mg/min with careful ECG monitoring. A similar dose may be repeated after two minutes, but further doses should be withheld for four hours. Unlike phenytoin and lidocaine, propranolol depresses conduction velocity and may therefore augment AV and intraventricular block. It should not be used in asthmatic patients since it may induce bronchoconstriction and it may exacerbate the underlying CHF. Should profound bradycardia occur, atropine may be used to counter this effect.

Procainamide and quinidine have been used less frequently because their intravenous administration is associated with hypotension and cardiotoxicity. Since conduction velocity is diminished by both of these drugs, their use should be avoided when AV or intraventricular block is present. See the chapter on Cardiac Arrhythmias.

Other agents which are used less frequently because of unpredictable or toxic effects or limited availability include EDTA (a calcium chelating agent), magnesium (306), cholestyramine (288), and specific digoxin antibodies (314). Peritoneal and hemodialysis are ineffective in removing digoxin from the body, but charcoal hemoperfusion may be used for life-threatening overdoses in patients with renal failure (315).

21. Dosing of Digoxin in Renal Failure. An 84-year-old female is admitted to the hospital in acute distress with breathlessness, markedly distended neck veins and in atrial fibrillation. She has been an insulin-dependent diabetic for 35 years, and she has had progressively deteriorating renal function but has never required hemodialysis. She has no previous cardiac history. Her only home medication is 30 units NPH insulin per day. Pertinent admitting laboratory values and physical examination reveal: Sodium 140 mEq/L; Potassium 5.1 mEq/L; Chloride 101 mEq/L; Bicarbonate 24 mEq/L; Glucose (fasting) 180 mg/dl; BUN 48 mg/dl; Creatinine 3.8 mg/

dl; Weight 82 kg; Height 5'6"; Pulse 118 beats/min and irregular.

She is given furosemide 80 mg IV and 20 mEq of potassium with each dose of furosemide. Because of her distress, it is decided to give her an intravenous loading dose of digoxin. Calculate the loading dose for this patient. Do any alterations have to be made in the loading dose because of her decreased renal function?

From a theoretical basis, loading doses for renally excreted drugs do not have to be altered in renal failure because a loading dose only fills up the body tissue stores and is independent of elimination (245,256). However, the volume of distribution (Vd) for digoxin may vary tremendously in patients with renal failure (Cl_{cr} less than 25 ml/min). Koup et al (258) observed volumes of distribution ranging from 195–489 L/1.73 m^2 in seven renal failure patients. Reunig et al (259) calculated volumes of distribution for renal failure patients reported in the literature and found a range of 230 to 380 L/1.78 m^2, 30–50% less than that observed in subjects with normal renal function. An average value for Vd of 330 L/70 kg or 4.7 L/kg in renal failure patients may be used.

As the volume of distribution decreases, the theoretical loading dose also decreases. Unfortunately, it is usually not possible to know what a given patient's volume of distribution really is until the drug has already been given and serum levels are measured. A recent report of 22 renal failure patients showed no toxicity using an intravenous loading dose of digoxin of 0.01 mg/kg (316).

Using the adjusted value for Vd, we can use a modification of Equation 3 (Question 10) for calculating a loading dose for this patient:

$$\text{Intravenous Loading Dose} = (Vd)(Cp) \quad \text{(Eq. 13)}$$

We will again assume a desired Cp of 1.5 mcg/L. In calculating Vd, we must correct the patient's weight to ideal body weight (IBW) since she is obese (82 kg) (317).

IBW (males)
$$= 50 \text{ kg} + 2.3 \text{ kg/inch over 5 feet} \quad \text{(Eq. 14)}$$

IBW (females)
$$= 45.5 \text{ kg} + 2.3 \text{ kg/inch over 5 feet} \quad \text{(Eq. 15)}$$

For this patient:

$$IBW = 45.5 \text{ kg} + 2.3 \text{ kg (6'')} = 59.3 \text{ kg}$$

Therefore, her loading dose will be:

$$
\begin{aligned}
\text{Intravenous LD} &= (Vd)(Cp) \\
&= (4.7 \text{ L/kg})(59.3 \text{ kg})(1.5 \text{ mcg/L}) \\
&= 417 \text{ mcg}
\end{aligned}
$$

This loading dose is considerably smaller than that calculated in Question 10. This is because we assumed a smaller volume of distribution and because the dose is given intravenously, not orally. She should be given either 0.4 or 0.5 mg intravenously to start and then reassessed at 6–8 hours. If at this time she is still in atrial fibrillation, an extra 0.125 mg could be safely given.

22. Calculate a maintenance dose for this patient.

The principles for calculating a maintenance dose are the same as those used in Question 12. The major difference is that the effect of her age and renal function on digoxin clearance must be taken into account. Both of these factors will slow drug elimination necessitating a reduced maintenance dose. Rather than repeating all of the methods described in Question 12, only the method of Jelliffe (Eq. 1, 5, and 6) will be used. The reader is encouraged to apply the patient data to the method of Scheiner (Eq. 10–12) as well.

The first step is to make an estimate of the patient's creatinine clearance. While several methods are available, we will use the method of Cockcroft and Gault (318):

$$Cl_{Cr} \text{ (males)} = \frac{IBW (140 - \text{age})}{72 \, S_{Cr}} \qquad \text{(Eq. 16)}$$

$$Cl_{Cr} \text{ (females)} = 0.85 \, Cl_{Cr} \text{ (males)} \qquad \text{(Eq. 17)}$$

For our patient:

$$Cl_{Cr} = 0.85 \, \frac{59.3 \text{ kg} (140 - 84 \text{ years})}{72 (3.8 \text{ mg/dl})}$$
$$= 10.31 \text{ ml/min}$$

As can be seen, the creatinine clearance is markedly depressed. Likewise, the percent of digoxin eliminated per day is substantially reduced:

$$\% \text{ eliminated daily} = 14\% + \frac{Cl_{Cr}}{5} \qquad \text{(Eq. 1)}$$
$$= 14\% + \frac{10.3 \text{ ml/min}}{5}$$
$$= 16\%$$

Instead of the normal 34–36% of drug being eliminated per day, only 16% is eliminated. The required oral maintenance dose is:

$$
\begin{aligned}
\text{Oral MD} &= \frac{(Vd)(Cp)(\% \text{ eliminated daily})}{F} \qquad \text{(Eq. 5)} \\
&= \frac{(4.7 \text{ L/kg})(59.3 \text{ kg})(1.50 \text{ mcg/L})(.16)}{0.65} \\
&= 102.9 \text{ mcg} \\
&= 0.10 \text{ mg}
\end{aligned}
$$

This dose can be given in one of two ways: 0.125 mg every day using tablets or 0.1 mg per day using a pediatric elixir. The last method is more exact but is inconvenient. The elixir may also be absorbed better than the tablets.

23. Digoxin Dosage Adjustment. A 50-year-old, 55 kg female with normal renal function has been given digoxin 0.125 mg daily for ten days. She continues to have debilitating symptoms of CHF. Estimate her serum digoxin concentration. If we wish to increase her serum concentration to 1.2 ng/ml, what will her new maintenance dose be?

Since this patient has been taking the same dose of digoxin for ten days and since her renal function is normal, her digoxin level should be at steady state. A simple way to estimate her plasma level is to first estimate her total body stores (Ab) of digoxin by rearranging Equation 4 from Question 12:

$$
\begin{aligned}
Ab &= \frac{(F)(\text{Oral MD})}{\% \text{ eliminated daily}} \qquad \text{(Eq. 18)} \\
&= \frac{0.65 (0.125 \text{ mg})}{35\%} \\
&= 0.232 \text{ mg}
\end{aligned}
$$

Then, using Equation 2 from Question 10 and assuming an average value of 7.3 L/kg for Vd, the plasma level is calculated:

$$Cp = \frac{Ab}{Vd}$$

$$= \frac{0.232 \text{ mg}}{(7.3 \text{ L/kg})(55 \text{ kg})}$$

$$= 0.58 \text{ mcg/L (ng/ml)}$$

An alternative way of estimating the serum digoxin level is by using clearance data, thus eliminating the need to estimate Vd. Since this patient is in decompensated CHF, the method of choice for calculating digoxin clearance is to use Scheiner's equation (see Question 12) that accounts for decreased clearance in CHF:

$$Cl_{digoxin} = 0.88 \, (Cl_{Cr}) + 23 \text{ ml/min} \qquad \text{(Eq. 11)}$$

$$= [0.88(100 \text{ ml/min}) + 23 \text{ ml/min}]\frac{(55 \text{ kg})}{(70 \text{ kg})}$$

$$= 87.2 \text{ ml/min}$$

$$= 125.6 \text{ L/day}$$

Note that since Scheiner's equations are based on 70 kg body weight, the clearance value was adjusted for the patient's weight of 55 kg. Once the clearance is known we can calculate the average steady state serum level by rearranging Equation 12 (Question 12):

$$Cpss \text{ ave} = \frac{(F)(MD)}{(\tau)(Cl)} \qquad \text{(Eq. 19)}$$

$$= \frac{(0.65)(125 \text{ mcg})}{(1 \text{ day})(125.6 \text{ L/d})}$$

$$= 0.65 \text{ mcg/L (ng/ml)}$$

Both methods are in agreement in estimating a plasma level of approximately 0.6 mcg/L. According to Equation 19, a plasma level is proportional to the dose and the fraction of the drug absorbed and inversely proportional to drug clearance and dosing interval. If we assume no immediate change in the patient's clinical status, three of the variables (F, τ, and Cl) remain constant. Therefore, to increase her serum concentration to 1.2 ng/ml, one would simply double her maintenance dose. This is determined by setting up a proportionality equation:

$$\frac{\text{Current MD}}{\text{Current Cpss ave}} = \frac{\text{New MD}}{\text{Desired Cpss ave}} \qquad \text{(Eq. 20)}$$

If a more rapid response is desired, the patient could be given a loading dose to attain the higher serum concentration. Assuming the patient's current digoxin level is 0.6 mcg/L and the desired level is 1.2 mcg/L, a net increase of 0.6 mcg/L must be achieved. Using Equation 3 from Question 10, the new oral loading dose can be estimated:

$$Oral \text{ LD} = \frac{(Vd)(Cp)}{F}$$

$$= \frac{(7.3 \text{ L/kg})(55 \text{ kg})(.6 \text{ mcg/ml})}{0.65}$$

$$= 370 \text{ mcg}$$

$$= 0.370 \text{ mg}$$

24. Partial Loading Dose. A 70-kg male whose CHF has been well controlled with digoxin 0.5 mg daily for two years is admitted with a three-day history of intestinal flu. The patient is treated with fluid and electrolyte replacement. The patient has not taken digoxin for four days. On the morning of hospital day two, it is decided to digitalize the patient to his former level. Calculate his current body stores of digoxin (Ab). What would the loading dose for this patient be? His creatinine clearance is 100 ml/min.

Using Equation 18 from Question 23, it is possible to calculate the maximum body stores of digoxin in the body at steady state before the patient discontinued his therapy. This patient has normal renal function, so the percent eliminated per day is 35%.

$$Ab \text{ max} = \frac{(F)(MD)}{\% \text{ eliminated daily}}$$

$$= \frac{(0.65)(0.5 \text{ mg})}{(0.35)}$$

$$= 0.96 \text{ mg}$$

To calculate the amount of drug remaining in his body four days after discontinuing therapy, we could use the formula that describes the exponential elimination of a drug excreted by first order kinetics:

$$Ab = (Ab_{max})(e^{-kdt}) \qquad \text{(Eq. 21)}$$

where (e^{-kdt}) represents the fraction of drug remaining after time (t). Assuming a normal digoxin t½ of 1.6 days, kd can be calculated from the relationship:

$$kd = \frac{0.693}{t½} \qquad \text{(Eq. 23)}$$

$$= \frac{.693}{1.6 \text{ days}}$$

$$= 0.43 \text{ days}$$

Substituting:

$$Ab = (Ab_{max})(e^{-kdt})$$

$$= (0.96 \text{ mg})e^{(-0.43 \text{ days}-1 \times 4 \text{ days})}$$

$$= 0.17 \text{ mg}$$

More simply, we could draw a line on semilog paper which represents the elimination of digoxin in this patient (see Fig. 4). After 1 day, 65% remains; after 4 days, only 18% remains. Therefore:

$$Ab = (Ab \text{ max})(\text{Fraction of drug remaining})$$

$$= (0.96 \text{ mg})(18\%)$$

$$= 0.17 \text{ mg} \qquad \text{(Eq. 23)}$$

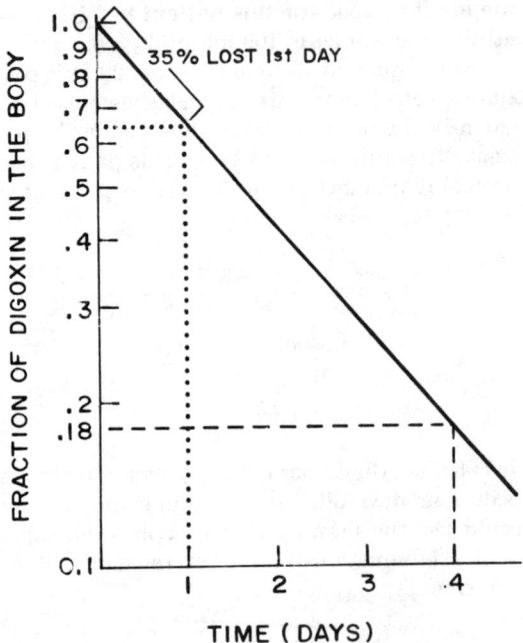

Figure 4. Graph representing the elimination of digoxin for a patient with normal renal function.

The loading dose for this patient would then be the difference between Ab max and the amount in the body at 4 days:

$$0.96 \text{ mg} - 0.17 \text{ mg} = 0.79 \text{ mg}$$

Two oral doses of 0.5 mg administered 6 hours apart will approximate the calculated loading dose considering the fact that oral digoxin is not completely available. At the end of each 6 hour period, the patient should be evaluated for symptoms of digitalis toxicity. In 6 hours absorption and tissue distribution should be virtually complete so that one should be able to observe the full effects of the dose. Thereafter, his previous maintenance dose of 0.5 mg per day can be continued.

25. *Severe CHF.* L.M. a 50-year-old man, was admitted with severe, progressive and debilitating symptoms of congestive heart failure. The patient's history was significant in that his father and two brothers succumbed to heart attacks shortly after the age of forty. The patient had a 12-year history of CHF which was symptomatic despite treatment with full therapeutic doses of digoxin and furosemide. He had no history of hypertension, but previous studies suggested a diagnosis of cardiomyopathy. Over the previous eight months L.M.'s DOE became progressively worse, and for the month prior to admission he was confined to bed because of extreme fatigue. He awoke once or twice nightly with PND.

Physical examination revealed a dyspneic, cyanotic male in apparent distress, but with no complaints of chest pain. The blood pressure was 100/66 mm Hg and his pulse was 105/min. Marked jugular venous distension, bilateral rales, hepatomegaly, and 3+ peripheral edema were also observed. Chest x-ray revealed marked cardiomegaly and pulmonary congestion. The patient was admitted to the coronary care unit where a Swan-Ganz catheter was passed from an antecubital vein to the pulmonary artery. Prior to therapy, the patient's pulmonary-capillary pressure was 27 mm Hg and his cardiac index was 1.9 L/min–m². Intravenous nitroprusside was initiated at a dose of 16 mcg/min and eventually increased to 200 mcg/

min. At this dose, the patient's pulmonary-capillary pressure decreased to 15 mm Hg and his cardiac index increased to 2.5 L/min–m². He was eventually discharged on digoxin 0.375 mg daily, furosemide 80 mg bid, spironolactone 50 mg bid, nitroglycerin ointment 2 inches q 4 h, and hydralazine 75 mg qid. What was the importance of obtaining a pulmonary-capillary pressure and cardiac index in this patient? To what other hemodynamic measurements do these correspond?

Severe congestive heart failure which is resistant to conventional therapy occurs in association with intrinsic myocardial failure (eg, myocardial infarction and cardiomyopathy). In its most severe form, this failure is characterized by an increased pulmonary-capillary pressure (PCP) and a decreased cardiac output as illustrated by this patient. The *pulmonary-capillary pressure* (or pulmonary wedge pressure—PWP) is the hydrostatic pressure which forces fluids from the pulmonary vascular space into the interstitial or intra-alveolar spaces (319). It is measured by inflating a balloon at the tip of a Swan-Ganz catheter wedged into a pulmonary capillary and is a good index of left ventricular pressure in the absence of mitral valvular disease. Other terms or measurements which generally correspond to the PWP are left ventricular filling pressure (LFP or LVFP), left ventricular end diastolic pressure (LVEDP), left atrial pressure, and pulmonary vein pressure. These values reflect the preload on the heart and are primarily influenced by venous return, cardiac output, and less frequently mitral or aortic valve insufficiency. The normal PCP is 5 to 12 mm Hg. Clinically, the onset of pulmonary congestion occurs at 18 to 20 mm Hg; moderate pulmonary congestion is present at a level of 25 or 30 mm Hg, and the onset of pulmonary edema occurs at values greater than 30 mm Hg (319,320). L.M. had a PCP of 27 mm of Hg and had marked symptoms of CHF, but without frank pulmonary edema.

The *cardiac index* is cardiac output (stroke volume × heart rate) which has been corrected for body surface area and is measured by a thermodilution technique described elsewhere (319). Symptoms of decreased perfusion to the kidneys, brain, and skin are consequences of a diminished cardiac output. A normal value is 2.7 to 4.3 L/min/m²; subclinical hypoperfusion occurs at 2.2

to 2.7 L/min/m²; and cardiogenic shock is associated with a cardiac index of less than 1.8 L/min/m². The cardiac index in L.M. was 1.9 L/min/m² which puts him in an emergency status category.

The objective of therapy is to decrease the PCP and increase the stroke volume or cardiac output in patients such as L.M.

26. What was the rationale for nitroprusside therapy in L.M.? What doses are used? What are the hazards of this type of therapy?

Vasodilating drugs that decrease afterload and/or preload are becoming increasingly more important in the therapy of severe congestive heart failure (2–4, 321). They are generally used in patients who continue to be symptomatic after maximal doses of diuretics and digitalis. Some cardiologists will initiate vasodilator therapy in place of digitalis, believing that digitalis has greater toxic potential than therapeutic benefit (see Question 3).

Three general categories of vasodilators have been used: Those drugs that primarily dilate arterial vessels and in so doing decrease the afterload or impedance to left ventricular afterflow (eg, hydralazine); those that dilate venous vessels, thereby increasing venous capacity and decreasing venous return (preload) to the heart (eg, nitrates); and those with mixed arterial and venous effects (eg, nitroprusside and possibly prazosin). The benefits gained from afterload reduction generally outweigh those from preload reduction, but combined afterload and preload reduction is often beneficial. Decreased peripheral vascular resistance from arterial vasodilation may potentially cause hypotension and a reflex increase in heart rate. However, this is infrequently seen in patients with congestive heart failure since any decrease in blood pressure is counterbalanced by a comparable increase in cardiac output (321). Similarly, excessive preload reduction can cause postural hypotension from peripheral pooling of blood in the lower extremities and deficient ventricular filling, causing less blood to be available for ventricular ejection. The overall response in any given patient is determined by his baseline arterial and venous pressure, volume status, and renal function. Also see the chapter on Intensive Care Therapeutics.

Nitroprusside dilates both arterial and venous vessels; thus, it has the theoretical advantage of decreasing both afterload and preload (2–4,

320–322). Its major disadvantage is that it must be given by continuous intravenous infusion, and it is unstable in the presence of heat and light after reconstitution.

The major hazard associated with nitroprusside use is a sudden, profound hypotension which will decrease cardiac output. This occurred in three out of 43 patients in one study and was reversed in five to ten minutes by discontinuing the nitroprusside and elevating the patient's feet (321). Nitroprusside may also decrease cardiac output and increase heart rate in patients with cardiac failure associated with a normal or low pulmonary-capillary pressure. Another concern with regard to all vasodilator therapy is that when decreasing the arterial pressure, coronary perfusion may also be decreased and the area of ischemia increased in patients with recent myocardial infarction. Chatterjee and Parmley (321) have reviewed this extensively and present evidence which argues to the contrary. However, since the effects of vasodilators on myocardial ischemia are not actually known, they suggest that the use of nitroprusside therapy be reserved for congestive heart failure patients with a pulmonary-capillary pressure greater than 18 mm Hg and with a mean arterial pressure (diastolic + 1/3 the pulse pressure) of greater than 60 mm Hg. Other toxic effects of nitroprusside relating to cyanide and thiocyanate toxicity are discussed in the chapters on Hypertensive Emergencies and Intensive Care Therapeutics.

Since severe hypotension is of major concern, patients should be initiated on small doses of nitroprusside (6–20 mcg/min) which are increased slowly (3–6 mcg/min to a maximum of 800 mcg/min) until a decrease in the PCP or arterial pressure is observed (321,322). When stopping nitroprusside therapy, a slow taper is recommended since a rebound increase in CHF has been observed 10 to 30 minutes after drug withdrawal (323).

27. Compare and contrast other vasodilators which are used parenterally to treat refractory congestive heart failure.

L.M. only received nitroprusside parenterally. He responded well and needed no other therapy. However, other parenteral products can be tried if nitroprusside fails.

Nitroglycerin (NTG) is given intravenously for severe chest pain or CHF following a myocardial infarction (324–327). Until recently, all nitroglycerin solutions had to be prepared extemporaneously. Now three manufacturers make available concentrated solutions of NTG for reconstitution. Tridil (American Critical Care) and Nitrobid (Marion Labs) come in 10 ml ampules containing 5 mg/ml, while Nitrostat (Parke-Davis) is available in a 10 ml ampule containing 0.8 mg/ml. One to two ampules of the concentrated drug are diluted in 250–500 ml of 5% dextrose or saline. Caution must be exercised in noting which manufacturer's product was used since the Parke Davis product will give a smaller drug concentration than the other two preparations. Glass bottles must be used since plastic bags may absorb large quantities of the nitroglycerin (326). It has also been recognized that from 40–80% of the drug may bind to standard intravenous administration sets (327a). All of the manufacturers provide special administration sets that will not bind the drug and one must be careful not to interchange administration sets when changing IV bottles to prevent erratic patient responses to the drug.

The dose of nitroglycerin to administer is confused by the fact that dosing recommendations made in the literature (324–327) are from studies where standard administration sets were used, while the manufacturer's labeling is based upon use of administration sets that do not bind the drug. With the commercially available products, the recommended starting dose is 5 mcg/min. This corresponds to approximately 20–25 mcg/min in the literature. Incremental increases of the infusion rate of 5–10 mcg/min may be made every 3–5 minutes until the desired response (a 25% decrease in PCP) or a maximum of 200 mcg/minute is achieved (324,325). Over half of the patients treated will achieve clinical benefit at infusion rates of 15–94 mcg/min with corresponding nitrate plasma levels of 1.2–11.1 mcg/L. The remaining patients either require very high infusion rates or appear to be resistant to NTG. It is unknown if this resistance is due to vascular insensitivity or an underlying near-maximal peripheral venous distension in these patients (325). Nitroglycerin primarily affects the venous capacitance vessels with a slight effect on the arterial bed. The pulmonary-capillary pressure or left ventricular filling pressure (preload) is reduced in patients with a PCP greater than 18 mm Hg. However, because it may only slightly decrease or have no effect on afterload, cardiac output may remain unchanged or increase only slightly. Nitroglycerin may actually decrease cardiac output in some patients by reducing the left ventricular filling pressure to less than 15 mm Hg (152). Overall, nitroglycerin is most useful in those patients whose primary problem is one of pulmonary congestion with a high preload.

Phentolamine is a short-acting, alpha-adrenergic blocking agent which predominantly affects the arterial vessels, but also increases venous capacitance. Like nitroprusside, it is most likely to increase the cardiac output in patients with elevated left ventricular filling pressures. The usual dose is an intravenous infusion of 0.2–2.0 mg/min. Unlike nitroprusside, 80% of patients with CHF treated with phentolamine develop an increased heart rate and increased myocardial oxygen consumption, which is of major concern in patients with ischemic heart disease (319). For this reason, nitroprusside is generally favored over phentolamine.

Trimethaphan, a ganglionic blocker, has been used infrequently because it can produce profound postural hypotension. It apparently decreases pulmonary wedge pressure without increasing the heart rate, but produces no increase in cardiac output (321).

28. Once L.M. was controlled with nitroprusside therapy, he was placed on nitroglycerin ointment and hydralazine. Why were both hydralazine and nitroglycerin used? What other vasodilating agents are available for ambulatory congestive heart failure patients unresponsive to conventional therapy?

Various forms of nitrates have been used (328,329). Sublingual administration of *nitroglycerin* is limited by its brief hemodynamic effects which only last from 20–60 minutes. Timed release capsular forms of nitroglycerin have been shown to produce a prolonged (4–8 hr) response in angina if the dose exceeds 6.5 mg, but little information is available on their use in congestive heart failure. More attention has been given to *nitroglycerin ointment* which also has prolonged hemodynamic effects (3–5 hr). Like the other nitrates, it decreases pulmonary and systemic venous pressures and LVFP, but has a variable effect on cardiac output. An apparent lack of response in some patients may be related to poor peripheral circulation and poor absorption of NTG from the ointment (319,330,331). The dose may be titrated using 1–4 inches of 2% NTG applied to the skin of the chest, back, or thigh. Effects should be observed within 15–30 minutes.

If a response is not observed after 30 minutes, another application can be made. The site of application should be rotated to decrease inflammatory reactions. One advantage of NTG ointment over oral forms of nitrates is that if the patient becomes hypotensive (systolic BP less than 100 mg Hg) or develops a tachycardia (heart rate greater than 100) or severe headaches, it can be wiped off with rapid resolution of effect. This makes the ointment an ideal agent for use in the hospital. At the time of the writing of this chapter, three manufacturers (Ciba, Key, Searle) released various forms of impregnated disks designed to slowly release a fixed amount of NTG via dermal absorption. Literature is not available to allow comparison of these products to the ointment form of nitroglycerin. See the chapter on Angina for a more detailed discussion on the application of NTG ointment.

Because of the short duration of response with sublingual nitroglycerin, increasing attention has been focused on sublingual and oral *isosorbide dinitrate* (328,329). Sublingual isosorbide is well absorbed and bypasses first-pass metabolism. Its onset is rapid (about five minutes), but its effects are relatively short (1–3 hours) (321,332,333). The usual starting dose is 5 mg every 4–6 hours, but doses may be titrated up to 20 mg. These larger doses are associated with longer beneficial effects (eg, 3 hours), but are also accompanied by a high frequency of intolerable headaches and hypotension. Previous claims of a poor response to orally administered isosorbide because of a large first-pass metabolic effect have been refuted with a better understanding of drug kinetics (326, 328,334,335). If a large enough oral dose is given, the metabolic capacity of the liver is overwhelmed and beneficial effects are seen. The onset is slow after oral doses (15–30 minutes), but the length of activity may be slightly longer than after sublingual therapy (4–6 hours). It must be fully appreciated that oral doses of 5 mg are probably ineffective, with at least 10 mg being the smallest starting dose, then titrating to as high as 20–80 mg every 4–6 hours. With both sublingual and oral nitrates, the best dose is that which provides the desired beneficial effect with the least side effects. The major effect of oral nitrates is to decrease left ventricular filling pressure, but the effect on cardiac output is variable. The oral compound reverses cardiac output in patients with control LVFPs of greater than 20 mm Hg. The effects on cardiac output are more short-lived (3 hours) than those on LVFP which indicates that a small arterial (afterload) effect may also be occurring (334).

Non-nitrate vasodilators include *hydralazine, minoxidil, prazosin,* and *nifedipine.* Hydralazine and minoxidil primarily affect the arterial bed and thus only reduce afterload. Hydralazine (50–100 mg every six hours) is the most frequently used agent. These doses exceed those used in hypertension; afterload reduction is usually not apparent with smaller doses (336–338). For example, our patient, L.M., required 75 mg qid. The tachycardia and hypotension that are frequently observed in hypertensive patients are minor or absent when treating CHF since the increased cardiac output overrides the vasodilatory effect (336). Prazosin has been claimed to be the ideal agent in that it affects both the venous and arterial beds and thus decreases the LVFP (preload) as well as arterial impedance (afterload) (4,339–341). It is less likely to cause tachycardia than hydralazine. Single oral doses of 1 to 10 mg of prazosin have an onset of action of one hour, and the effects persist up to 6 hours (339,340). The first dose of prazosin should always be given under direct medical supervision since syncope following the initial dose has been reported. The initial enthusiasm for prazosin has been tempered by the observation of decreased response (tachyphylaxis) with chronic dosing (342,343), although other clinicians have shown the benefits to continue for two weeks (340,344) or more. The beneficial effects of hydralazine appear to be sustained with chronic therapy (344a). Long term side effects of hydralazine include a lupus-like syndrome and peripheral neuropathies.

Nifedipine is a potent vasodilator that acts as a calcium flux antagonist. It is primarily indicated as an anti-anginal agent, especially in variant angina caused by coronary artery vasospasm. Because of its vasodilator properties, it has been studied in primary pulmonary hypertension and in CHF (345–347). Limited data show nifedipine to be effective in increasing the cardiac index and decreasing total systemic vascular resistance. However, its use may be limited by a negative inotropic effect which is the result of inhibition of calcium influx into heart muscle cells. In this case a paradoxical worsening of CHF will be seen. When given in a dose of 20 mg three times daily, the major limiting side effects are nausea, hypotension, and dizziness. Capsules of

nifedipine may either be swallowed or chewed for a more rapid sublingual effect.

L.M. was discharged with both hydralazine and nitroglycerin ointment. It has been observed that by combining a primary preload reducing agent (eg, nitrates) with a primary afterload reducing agent (hydralazine), complementary effects can be obtained. This combination has been used successfully when one or both of the other agents has failed by itself (348–352).

29. A 62-year-old male was admitted to the coronary care unit with a two-day history of breathlessness which necessitated sleeping upright in a chair and prevented him from walking to the bathroom. Physical examination showed 4+ pitting edema of the legs, scrotal and sacral edema, and markedly distended neck veins with a CVP of 26 mm Hg. Urine output was less than 20 ml per hour, blood urea nitrogen was 48 mg/dl, serum creatinine was 2.0 mg/dl, and serum potassium was 3.2 mEq/L. Home medications which had been faithfully administered by the patient's wife included digoxin 0.25 mg/day, furosemide 240 mg/day, KCl 40 mEq/day, hydralazine 100 mg every six hours, and isosorbide dinitrate 20 mg every four hours. A 100 mg IV bolus of furosemide in the emergency room resulted in a urine output of 600 ml over two hours, but with a subsequent rise of the BUN to 65 mg/dl. Finally, the patient was begun on captopril 25 mg three times daily. Within two hours the patient was breathing easier, his CVP was down to 16 mm Hg, and he was diuresing briskly. He was discharged to home one week later with mild SOB on exertion, 2+ ankle edema, and improved renal function. Discharge medications included furosemide 120 mg/day, captopril 50 mg tid, and isosorbide dinitrate 20 mg q 6 h.

What is the role of captopril in the treatment of congestive heart failure?

The enzyme *renin* is released by the kidney when renal perfusion pressure is decreased. Renin acts to convert a substrate present in the blood called *angiotensinogen* into the inactive decapeptide, *angiotensin I.* Angiotensin I is further metabolized to the active decapeptide, *angiotensin II,* under the influence of circulating *angiotensin-converting-enzyme.* Angiotensin II is a potent vasoconstrictor and also stimulates aldosterone release by the adrenals. Activation of the renin-angiotensin-aldosterone system may be responsible for the increase in systemic vascular resistance often seen in severe cardiac failure.

Several drugs that interfere with the renin-angiotensin system are effective antihypertensive agents (353–355) and may reduce vascular resistance in congestive heart failure (353, 355–362). The first drug, saralasin, is a competitive antagonist of angiotensin II, but its use is limited by the need for parenteral administration (355). Teprotide (SQ 20881) (359,360) and captopril (353–355,358,361,362) both act by antagonizing angiotensin-converting-enzyme, causing a build-up of inactive angiotensin I and a marked reduction in the production of angiotension II and aldosterone. Although the major effect of teprotide and captopril seems to be mediated via angiotensin II inhibition, evidence is conflicting as to whether measurement of renin or angiotensin II levels before therapy have any predictive value (354). Angiotensin-converting-enzyme (also called kinase II) is also responsible for degradation of bradykinin and other vasodilatory substances. Thus the beneficial effects of teprotide and captopril may be partially due to the accumulation of kinins, but this effect is poorly documented.

Captopril is the only orally active agent in this class of drugs and has recently been released with a primary indication as an antihypertensive. However, it holds promise in the treatment of CHF, producing beneficial effects in patients similar to this case who have failed traditional therapy including other vasodilators. Davis et al (361) studied the effects of single doses of captopril ranging from 25 to 150 mg in 10 subjects with severe CHF. In all subjects the drug increased cardiac index, decreased pulmonary capillary wedge pressure, and decreased systemic vascular resistance. The results suggest that captopril reduces both preload and afterload. The optimal single dose was 25 mg in six patients, 50 mg in one, 100 mg in two, and 150 mg in one. Three subjects did not receive the 150 mg dose because of hypotension from smaller doses. Hemodynamic changes usually began within 30 minutes of oral captopril, peaked at 90 minutes and returned to baseline by 3–4 hours. Dzau and his colleagues (358) studied eight patients with severe (functional class IV) congestive heart failure that persisted despite treatment with digoxin, maximum doses of diuretics (often limited by azotemia), and large doses

of vasodilators. Within two hours of administering a loading dose of 5–25 mg of oral captopril (titrated to a fall in diastolic pressure of 10 mm Hg), the cardiac index increased from a baseline of 1.6 L/min to 2.2 L/min, pulmonary-capillary wedge pressure fell from a mean of 28 mm Hg to 18 mm Hg. All patients were symptomatically improved. After a stabilization period of 10–20 days, seven of the patients were discharged home for continuous therapy at doses of 25–150 mg three times daily. In all cases diuretic therapy was reduced and it was possible to discontinue other vasodilators. In most subjects, beneficial effects were maintained over a six month follow-up period with improved exercise capacity, decreased hospitalizations, and improved renal function. However, radiologic signs of improvement in pulmonary congestion were minor, and there was no decrease in heart size.

Unfortunately, captopril is not without significant side effects (353,358,363–365). Up to 15% of subjects develop skin eruptions or fever (363). These effects occur mainly at higher dose (average 683 mg per day) and resolve with discontinuation of the drug or by using lower doses (below 225 mg per day). Skin reactions may be edematous, urticarial, erythematous, maculopapular, or morbilliform. The fact that the rashes disappear with continued therapy in some patients suggests that they may be due to potentiation of kinin-mediated skin reactions. Transient loss of taste, tachycardia, and hypotension are also common. Because of antagonism of aldosterone by these drugs, hyperkalemia may be observed, especially if existing potassium therapy is not altered (364). For example, in the case history cited, the patient was taking 40 mEq of potassium per day before hospitalization and had a low serum potassium. He was discharged home with no potassium supplement and a normal serum potassium despite an increased diuretic response. Proteinuria, a transient rise in serum creatinine, agranulocytosis, and one case of fatal pancytopenia (365) have also been attributed to captopril therapy.

30. B.J. is a 60-year-old male admitted to the hospital with severe, crushing substernal chest pain after a domestic quarrel at home. He has a history of occasional chest pain for the last three years treated with prn sublingual nitroglycerin. The admitting impression is an acute myocardial infarction. Over the

next three hours he becomes less alert, hypotensive, diaphoretic, and has a thready pulse. Wedge pressure is elevated to 27 mm Hg, and a chest x-ray shows pulmonary edema. He is diagnosed as having cardiogenic shock. He does not have atrial fibrillation.

Should he be given digitalis? Are there other positive inotropic agents that can be used in place of digitalis? (Also see the chapter on Intensive Care Therapeutics.)

Digitalis has been documented to have an inotropic effect after myocardial infarction, but its use in the immediate peri-infarction period may be deleterious. This issue is best summarized in an editorial review by Marcus (34). A digitalis-induced increase in contractility may be prevented from causing an increase in stroke volume and a decrease in left ventricular filling pressure by several mechanisms. First, enhanced contractility may increase bulging of ischemic or infarcted segments, thereby dissipating the inotropic effect that it exerts on the undamaged myocardium. Secondly, digitalis exerts a direct arteriolar vasoconstrictive effect after a rapid (less than 10 minutes) IV injection. This may cause an increase in afterload and thus aggravate left ventricular failure and increase myocardial oxygen consumption.

Digitalis should not be given to patients with myocardial infarction who are not in cardiac failure because it may increase infarct size. In patients with mild to moderate CHF persisting for several days after an MI, digitalis may exert a minimal but significant increase in ejection fraction without an increase in infarct size (366). In severe heart failure or cardiogenic shock, digitalis is not the initial drug of choice due to the delay in its time to peak action and its possible deleterious effect on the peri-infarction area. Nevertheless, it may have a role in the subsequent chronic treatment of CHF.

The patient in the case presented fits into the latter category of cardiogenic shock. At this stage of his treatment, digitalis is to be avoided. Other agents are more effective with less chance of extending the infarct. Beta adrenergic agonists such as *isoproterenol* have been used in cardiogenic shock, but are of limited value due to a high incidence of arrhythmias (367). Another sympathomimetic agent, *dopamine* (368) is a precursor in the endogenous synthesis of norepinephrine,

stimulating the myocardium both directly and indirectly by enhancing the release of norepinephrine stores. In low doses (eg, continuous IV infusion of less than 10 mcg/kg/min), dopamine has the unique property of stimulating vasodilatory dopamine receptors in the kidney resulting in a decreased afterload. Larger doses act more like norepinephrine with a predominant vasoconstrictive effect. Unfortunately, the effect of dopamine on cardiac output is variable. By itself, dopamine has little direct cardiotonic effect.

Further modification of the chemical structure of isoproterenol resulted in the synthesis of *dobutamine* (369,370). This agent acts directly on beta adrenergic receptors of the heart and has a predominant inotropic effect and a relatively small chronotropic effect. Therefore, its use is associated with fewer arrhythmias than isoproterenol as long as the dose is less than 20 mcg/kg/min. Cardiac output rises, and ventricular diastolic pressure tends to fall. Total peripheral arterial resistance is slightly reduced, and arterial pressure is not greatly changed. Dobutamine is less potent than norepinephrine as a peripheral vasoconstrictor and does not act on dopamine receptors in the kidney to produce renal vasodilation. In one study comparing dobutamine to IV digoxin in cardiogenic shock, dobutamine was consistently more effective than digoxin in increasing cardiac output (371). The main drawback to dobutamine is that because of its short half-life (372), it must be given by continous IV infusion. The usual dose is 2.5–15 mcg/kg/min. Approximately 10% of patients receiving dobutamine in clinical studies have had heart rate increases of 30 beats per minute or more, and about 7.5% have had an increase in systolic blood pressure of 50 mm Hg or higher (369). These effects can be managed by decreasing the infusion rate. Other side effects in 1–3% of patients include nausea, headache, anginal pain, palpation, and shortness of breath.

Amrinone (373–376) is a nonsympathomimetic agent with a direct cardiac stimulatory effect that has shown promise in severe CHF refractory to traditional therapy. Chemically, amrinone is a biperiden derivative. Its mechanism of positive inotropic activity is unknown, but it is not blocked by propranolol, nor does it affect cyclic AMP, phosphodiesterase, or Na^+-K^+-dependent ATP. Initial studies in humans (373–374), have used intravenous pushes or infusions at doses of 1.8 – 3.5 mg/kg leading to an onset of action in 3–5 minutes with a substantial reduction in LVEDP and an increase in cardiac index. Little effect was noted on heart rate or blood pressure, and the only side effects reported were minor irritations at the IV injection site. Continuous infusions of amrinone at 40 mcg/kg/min for one hour and then 10 mcg/kg/min for 24 hours showed continuous benefit without tachyphylaxis (375). A preliminary trial (376) using single doses of oral amrinone in nine patients resistant to digitalis, diuretics, and vasodilating agents showed a 50% improvement in left ventricular ejection fraction that peaked at 1–3 hours and lasted for 4–6 hours. Doses varied from 1.6 to 4.0 mg/kg. With continued therapy (2–9 weeks), six of nine subjects experienced subjective improvement in CHF symptoms. However, side effects were frequent. Two subjects developed thrombocytopenia, one accompanied by fever and the other by nephrogenic diabetes insipidus. Long-term effects and the development of tachyphylaxis have not been studied.

APPENDIX: INFREQUENT REACTIONS TO THIAZIDE AND LOOP DIURETICS

Dermatologic Reactions. Thiazide-induced skin eruptions are rarely reported. They include non-specific rashes, photosensitivity, and necrotizing vasculitis. All appear to be allergic in nature and not dose-dependent.

Due to the sulfonamide component of the thiazide chemical structure, there is a possibility of cross reactivity with sulfonamide antibiotics. Some investigators believe that the metabolites of the antibacterial sulfonamides, rather than the parent compound, are responsible for skin lesions and hypersensitivity reactions. Since sulfonamides are acetylated and oxidized to varying extents, it is possible for a patient to become allergic to one antibacterial sulfonamide and not another. One study showed that the cross-sensitivity between different antibacterial sulfonamides was approximately 17% (138). Therefore, the cross-sensitivity between chemically different sulfonamides such as the thiazide diuretics and sulfisoxazole should be practically nil. It would probably be safe to administer furosemide or a thiazide to a patient who had previously experienced a mild rash from an antibacterial sulfonamide, provided that the patient is closely monitored. Ethacrynic acid does not contain a sulfa radical and may be used in a patient who proves to be cross-sensitive.

High-dose furosemide treatment regimens have been implicated as a cause of epidermolysis bullosa (139–141). In one study, twelve of 56 patients with chronic renal failure who were treated with 0.5 to 2.0 grams/day of furosemide developed bullous dermatoses (140). Bullous pemphigoid lesions and erythema multiforme have also been reported after standard doses of furosemide (142–44). The interval between the onset of furosemide treatment and the appearance of bullae is variable. Bullae may not become evident for as long as three years after the initiation of furosemide therapy. Clinically, the bullae vary in size and are easily ruptured; the intravesicular fluid is clear and the surrounding tissue is not involved. Bullous eruptions primarily occur in areas exposed to light, such as the dorsal aspect of the hands and feet, which may indicate that furosemide acts as a photosensitizing agent. This theory is also supported by the fact that a higher incidence of furosemide-induced bullae has been reported in the summer months (140). At present it is not clear whether a toxic or allergic mechanism is responsible for furosemide photosensitization. The bullae can persist for a few weeks to several months. They ultimately heal without scarring, and, in many cases, even with continued furosemide use (139–141).

Although the clinical presentation of the skin lesions described in these patients is similar to that of porphyria cutanea tarda, blood and urine screens for porphyria have been uniformly negative (139–141). Finally, bullous dermatosis resembling porphyria cutanea tarda has also occurred in patients undergoing hemodialysis who were not receiving furosemide (145,146). Therefore, the exact role of furosemide in the production of a porphyria cutanea tarda-like syndrome in hemodialysis patients remains to be determined.

Calcium. Thiazide diuretics have two major effects on calcium homeostasis: hypercalcemia and hypocalciuria. They increase both total and ionized serum calcium in normal subjects and in patients with various diseases (147–156). Perhaps because of feedback inhibition on parathyroid hormone (PTH) secretion, these elevations of serum calcium are usually transient even with continued treatment, and they rarely reach levels of clinical significance. However, symptomatic hypercalcemia secondary to thiazides can occur, especially in patients with metabolic bone diseases.

In contrast to the transient effects seen in most patients, thiazide administration commonly causes a sustained hypercalcemia in patients with primary hyperparathyroidism, probably because PTH secretion is not suppressed in response to increases in serum calcium (147,148,156).

Thiazide-induced hypercalcemia may be related to hemoconcentration and reduced calcium excretion (147,150). However, these mechanisms are not solely responsible. The increase in total and ionized plasma calcium may also be due to thiazide-induced release of calcium from bone into the extracellular fluid and may be caused by enhancement of the action of PTH or vitamin D (150,153–155). Hyperparathyroidism has been observed in six hypertensive patients undergoing chronic thiazide treatment (157). In addition, a high prevalence of hypercalcemia and primary hyperparathyroidism was found on routine medical health screening in patients receiving thiazide (148). Although these studies, as well as experimental investigations in animals, raise the possibility that thiazides may stimulate parathyroid gland hyperplasia (156), studies on PTH levels in thiazide-treated patients have shown either no change (155) or a decrease in PTH levels (158). Therefore, it is not clear whether thiazides may in fact induce hyperparathyroidism or only unmask underlying aberrations in parathyroid function.

The chronic administration of thiazides and thiazide-type diuretics can reduce urinary calcium excretion. The hypocalciuric effect of thiazides usually begins within two to three days following initiation of drug treatment and may occur in normal patients, patients with hypercalciuria, and in patients with hyperparathyroidism (147,149,152–154,156,159,160). This action of thiazides has been used successfully to prevent calcium nephrolithiasis and renal calculi formation (156,159–161).

There are other factors which contribute to this hypocalciuric effect. For example, the vast majority of hypoparathyroid patients have a blunted or absent hypocalciuric response to thiazide diuretics. This occurs despite extracellular fluid volume depletion and suggests that the presence of parathyroid hormone is essential for the hypocalciuric action of thiazides. Although thiazides enhance the hypocalciuric effect of circulating parathyroid hormone (PTH) on the renal tubules (147,149,152–154,156), a direct effect of thiazides on the renal tubule cannot be ruled out (156,162).

Conversely, furosemide increases renal calcium excretion (163–165). The calciuric effect of furosemide can best be explained by the fact that a large percentage of the filtered sodium and calcium load is reabsorbed in the loop of Henle. By inhibiting active chloride transport in the loop of Henle, furosemide causes an increase in the excretion of both sodium and calcium. This calciuric action is usually transient, because shrinkage of the extracellular fluid volume following furosemide diuresis leads to enhanced proximal tubular reabsorption of sodium and water, as well as calcium.

Acute hypocalcemia does not occur in most patients receiving furosemide, probably because increased parathyroid hormone secretion secondary to furosemide-induced calciuria maintains serum calcium levels within normal limits (158,166). However, tetany has been reported following furosemide administration in patients with impaired parathyroid hormone function (163). Furosemide-induced hypercalcemia has also been reported (167). The clinical significance of this latter finding remains to be determined.

Ototoxicity. Ototoxicity, primarily affecting the auditory component, is a serious complication of ethacrynic acid (168–175) and furosemide (168,174,176–181) therapy. These sensorineuronal hearing losses may be transient (170,172–173,175,179–181), or permanent (171,173,176–178). With rare exception, diuretic-induced ototoxicity is limited to patients with renal insufficiency receiving rapid intravenous injections of moderate to large doses of either drug. Wigund et al (181) observed mild to severe transient hearing losses in 8 to 16 uremic patients receiving a furosemide infusion of 25 mg/min for 40 minutes and recommended slower infusions. Other ototoxic drugs, especially the aminoglycoside antibiotics, can potentiate the ototoxic effects of the loop duretics (171,172,174,182,183).

Bilateral hearing loss usually occurs within 5 to 30 minutes following intravenous administration of either loop diuretic (169–172,179,180). Concurrent complaints include vertigo, tinnitus, or a fullness in the ears (173,177,178). In some cases, hearing impairment may not occur immediately (173,177,178). Insidious hearing losses that have gradually progressed for up to 6 months have been reported in six transplant patients (five children) following varying doses of oral and parenteral furosemide (177).

The etiology of this drug-induced ototoxicity is still debatable. Reproducible morphologic and functional changes in the stria vascularis which is responsible for the ionic concentrations of the endolymph can be produced by administering ethnacrynic acid to animals (184–187). Cochlear damage in both laboratory animals and in humans has also been demonstrated (171, 183,185,188).

Fortunately, the auditory complications of ethacrynic acid and furosemide are relatively rare. The Boston Collaborative Drug Surveillance Program noted that only 2 out of 165 patients (12 per 1,000) who received intravenous ethacrynic acid developed transient deafness (168), and no cases of ototoxicity occurred in over 2,300 hospitalized patients who received either oral or parenteral furosemide (189). However, a higher incidence of ototoxicity has been reported in patients with renal impairment. In a seven year prospective study of 602 hemodialysis and renal transplant patients, 107 (17.6%) demonstrated appreciable hearing losses during the observation period (174). In 71 patients the event which precipitated the hearing loss was identified. Furosemide and ethacrynic acid, alone (14 patients) or in combination with aminoglycoside antibiotics (8 patients) were the most frequent cause of hearing loss in these patients. Ototoxicity almost always occurred following rapid and repeated administration of these drugs. It was also evident from this and other studies (190) that in any given patient with renal disease, multiple factors may combine to produce a hearing deficit.

Pancreatitis and Cholecystitis. Acute hemorrhagic necrotizing pancreatitis is a rare complication of thiazide diuretics (191–195) and chlorthalidone (196). A number of fatalities have been reported (192–195). The overall incidence of thiazide-induced pancreatitis appears to be low. However, 1.0 to 2.0 gm/day of chlorothiazide can cause a 1½-to-2-fold increase in serum amylase levels in 50% of patients (98).

Several case reports also implicate furosemide as a cause of acute pancreatitis (191,199–202). In two separate cases, drug rechallenge clearly identified furosemide as the causative agent (200,201).

In one study, diuretic intake was substantially more frequent among patients with acute pancreatitis than among other patients of the same age and sex (26 versus 11%) (191). Although the results of this study indicate that diuretics may induce acute pancreatitis, the clinical conditions in which diuretics were used could not be ruled out as possible etiologic factors. Rosenberg et al (203) noted an association between thiazide use and an increased incidence of cholecystitis during routine screening of data from a case control drug surveillance program. However, a follow-up study found no association between thiazides and cholecystitis (204).

Hyperlipidemia. An increase in serum lipids has been described in hypertensive patients undergoing treatment with thiazide and thiazide-type diuretics (205–209). The reported rise in lipid levels may become evident as soon as the first week of diuretic treatment and apparently persists (207). The mechanisms by which thiazides affect lipid metabolism are not known.

Hematologic. The thiazide and thiazide-type diuretics can cause thrombocytopenia (210–214). A low platelet count is usually the sole hematologic abnormality, but on occasion neutropenia or agranulocytosis may also be present (213,214). In most cases, thrombocytopenia is associated with purpura, although purpura in the absence of thrombocytopenia has been reported as well (215,216).

The time course from the initiation of thiazide treatment to the development of thrombocytopenia varies. Thrombocytopenia usually becomes clinically evident one week to several months after initiation of diuretic treatment, although as many as nine months may pass before thrombocytopenia is discovered. Platelet counts return to normal following withdrawal of thiazide diuretics.

In a retrospective study (212), 19 of 71 patients (26%) receiving diuretics (5 thiazides, 14 chlorthalidone) developed asymptomatic thrombocytopenia with platelet counts of less than $100,000/mm^3$ as compared to only 4 of 93 (4%) cardiac patients not receiving diuretics. The thrombocytopenia may be related to dosage and duration of diuretic therapy. Further evidence for toxic myelosuppression is the finding of a hypoplastic marrow with decreased megakaryocytes in several cases in which thrombocytopenia was associated with other blood dyscrasias (213). However, several other reports implicate an immunologic mechanism as the cause of thiazide-induced thrombocytopenia (210,211,217). Circulating IgM globulin was identified in one case (211). The possibility that there are two mechanisms by which thiazides cause thrombocytopenia cannot be ruled out.

Neutropenia (213,218–220), agranulocytosis (214, 221),and immune hemolytic anemia (222) are other blood dyscrasias which have been associated with thiazide and thiazide-type diuretic treatment.

References

1. McKee PA et al: The natural history of congestive heart failure; The Framingham Study. N Engl J Med. 1971; 285:1441.

2. Cohn J et al: Vasodilator therapy of cardiac failure (2 parts). N Engl J Med. 1977; 269:917.

3. Shah PK: Ventricular unloading in the management of heart disease: role of vasodilators (2 parts). Am Heart J. 1977; 93:256 and 403.

4. Lakier J et al: Rationale and use of vasodilators in the management of congestive heart failure. Am Heart J. 1977; 97:519.

5. Kannel WB et al: Role of blood pressure in the development of congestive heart failure. The Framingham Study. N Engl J Med. 1972; 287:781.

6. Linkewich J et al: Bradycardia and congestive heart failure associated with ocular timolol maleate. Am J Hosp Pharm. 1981; 38:699.

7. Well JV et al: Plasma volume expansion resulting from interference with adrenergic function in normal man. Circulation. 1978; 37:54.

8. Smith AJ: Clinical features of fluid retention complicating treatment with guanethidine. Circulation. 1965; 31:485.

9. Sperling I: Adverse reactions with long term use of phenylbutazone and oxyphenbutazone. Lancet. 1969; 2:535.

10. Schooley R et al: Edema associated with ibuprofen therapy. JAMA. 1977; 237:1716.

11. Miller D et al: Evaluation of minoxodil. Am J Hosp Pharm. 1980; 37:808.

12. Smith HJ et al: Cardiomyopathy associated with amphetamine administration. Am Heart J. 1976; 91:792.

13. Halazan JF et al: Daunorubicin cardiac toxicity in children with ALL. Cancer. 1974; 33:545.

14. VonHoff DD et al: Daunomycin-induced cardiotoxicity in children and adults. A review of 110 cases. Am J Med. 1977; 62:200.

15. Bernard J et al: Treatment of acute leukemias. Semin Hematol. 1972; 9:181.

16. Bartorelli C et al: Hypertensive and renal effects of diazoxide, a sodium retaining benzothiadiazine compound. Circ. 1963; 27:895.

17. Thomsom AE et al: Clinical observations on an antihypertensive chlorothiazide analogue devoid of diuretic activity. Can Med Assoc J. 1962; 78:306.

18. Podrid P et al: Congestive heart failure caused by oral disopyramide. N Engl J Med. 1980; 300:614.

19. Chamerlain TJ: Licorice poisoning, pseudoaldosteronism and heart failure. JAMA. 1970; 283:1150.

19a. Piper DW et al: Medical management of peptic ulcer. Drugs. 1972; 3:834.

20. Bigger JT et al: Digitalis toxicity: drug interactions promoting toxicity and the management of toxicity. Semin in Drug Treat. 1972; 2:147.

20a. Stancer HC et al: Lithium carbonate and oedema (Letter). 1971; 2:985.

21. Platman ST et al: Lithium retention and excretion. The effect of sodium and fluid intake. Arch Gen Psychiatry. 1969; 20:285.

22. Tainter MI and Ferris AJ: Aspirin in modern therapy. Bayer Co., N.Y., 1969.

23. Beaver WT: Mild analgesics, a review of their clinical pharmacology, Part I. Am J Cardiol. 1974; 33:225.

24. Diet Committee of the San Francisco Heart Association in cooperation with the U.C. Hospital Pharmacy: Sodium in medicinals. San Francisco Heart Association, San Francisco, 1973.

25. Brod J: Pathogenesis of cardiac edema. Br Med J. 1972; 1:222.

26. Chung EK: The current status of digitalis therapy. Mod Treat. 1971; 8:643.

27. Hoffman BF et al: Effects of digitalis on electrical activity of cardiac fibers. Progr Cardiovasc Dis. 1964; 7:226.

28. Smith TW et al: Medical progress; digitalis (four part series). N Engl J Med. 1973; 288:719,942;289:945,1063.

29. Bresnahan J et al: Digitalis glycosides. Mayo Clin Proc. 1979; 54:675.

30. Smith TW: Digitalis glycosides (second of two parts). N Engl J Med. 1973; 288:942.

31. Cohn K et al: Variability of hemodynamic responses to acute digitalization in chronic cardiac failure due to cardiomyopathy and coronary artery disease. Am J Cardiol. 1975; 35:461.

32. Hutcheon D et al: The role of furosemide alone and in combination with digoxin in the relief of symptoms of congestive heart failure. J Clin Pharmacol. 1980; 20:59.

33. Arnold S et al: Long-term digitalis therapy improves left ventricular function in heart failure. N Engl J Med. 1980; 303:1443.

34. Marcus F: Editorial. Use of digitalis in acute myocardial infarction. Circulation. 1980; 62:17.

35. Spector R: Digitalis therapy in heart failure: a rational approach. J Clin Pharmacol. 1979; 19:692.

36. Shapiro W: Digitalis update. Arch Intern Med. 1981; 141:17.

37. Selzer A: Digitalis in cardiac failure. Do benefits justify risk? Arch Intern Med. 1981; 141:18.

38. Davis L and Wilson G: Diuretics, mechanism of action and clinical application. Drugs. 1975; 9:178.

39. Burg MB: Tubular chloride transport and the mode of action of some diuretics. Kidney Internat. 1976; 9:189.

40. Frazier HD et al: The clinical use of diuretics – parts 1 and 2. N Engl J Med. 1973; 228:246 and 455.

41. Earley LE et al: Edema formation and the use of diuretics. Calif Med. 1971; 114:56.

42. Brest AN et al: Clinical selection of diuretic drugs in the management of congestive heart failure. Am J Cardiol. 1968; 22:168.

43. Gussin RF: Potassium sparing diuretics. J Clin Pharmacol. 1977; 17:651.

44. Karim A et al: Spironolactone, I: Disposition and metabolism. Clin Pharmacol Ther. 1976; 19:158.

45. Sadee W et al: Pharmacokinetics of spironolactone, canrenone and canrenoate-K in humans. J Pharmacol Exper Ther. 1973; 185:686.

46. Jackson J et al: Elimination of canrenone in congestive heart failure and chronic liver disease. Eur J Clin Pharmacol. 1977; 11:177.

47. Sadee W et al: Multiple dose kinetics of spironolactone and canrenoate potassium in cardiac and hepatic failure. Eur J Clin Pharmacol. 1974; 7:195.

48. Beermann B et al: Clinical pharmacokinetics of diuretics. Clin Pharmacokinetics 1980; 5:221.

49. Karim A et al: Spironolactone III: canrenone maximum and minimum steady state plasma levels. Clin Pharmacol Ther. 1976; 19:177.

50. Beyer KH: The pharmacologic basis for modern diuretic therapy. Ration Drug Ther. 1978; 12:1.

51. Pruitt AW et al: Variations in the fate of triamterene. Clin Pharmacol Ther. 1977; 21:610.

52. Greenblatt D et al: Adverse reactions to spironolactone. JAMA. 1973; 225:40.

53. Loriaux DL et al: Spironolactone and endocrine dysfunction. Ann Intern Med. 1976; 85:630.

54. Huffman D et al: Gynecomastia induced in normal male by spironolactone. Clin Pharmacol Ther. 1978; 24:465.

55. Rose L et al: Pathophysiology of spironolactone-induced gynecomastia. Ann Intern Med. 1977; 87:398.

56. Carlson H: Gynecomastia. N Engl J Med. 1980; 303:795.

57. Caminos-Torres R et al: Gynecomastia and semen abnormalities induced by spironolactone in normal men. J Clin Endocrinol Metab. 1977; 45:255.

58. Greenblatt DJ et al: Gynecomastia and impotence complication of spironolactone therapy. JAMA. 1973; 223:82.

59. Zarren HS et al: Unilateral gynecomastia and impotence during low dose spironolactone administration in men. Milit Med. 1975; 140:417.

60. Levitt JL: Spironolactone therapy and amenorrhea. JAMA. 1970; 211:2014.

61. Loube SD et al: Breast cancer associated with administration of spironolactone. Lancet. 1975; 1:1428.

62. Jick H et al: Breast cancer and spironolactone. Lancet. 1975; 2:368.

63. Chang JC et al: Effect of triamterene on nucleic acid synthesis. Clin Pharmacol Ther. 1972; 13:372.

64. Corcino J et al: Mechanism of triamterene-induced megaloblastosis. Ann Intern Med. 1970; 73:419.

65. Lieherman FL et al: Megaloblastic anemia possibly induced by triamterene in patients with alcoholic cirrhosis. Ann Intern Med. 1968; 68:168.

66. Meyer M et al: Bioavailability monograph-hydrochlorothiazide. J Am Phrm Assn. 1976; 16:47.

66a. Anon.: Bioavailability problem with chlorothiazide. FDA Bulletin. 1981; 11:44.

67. Riddiough M: Preventing, detecting and managing adverse reactions of antihypertensive agents. Am J Hosp Pharm. 1977; 34:465.

68. Bennett WB et al: Comparison of intravenous chlorothiazide and metolazone in normal man. Curr Ther Res. 1977; 22:326.

69. Puschett JB et al: Comparative study of the effects of metolazone and other diuretics on potassium excretion. Clin Pharmacol Ther. 1974; 15:397.

70. Steinmuller SR et al: Effects of metolazone in man: Comparison with chlorothiazide. Kidney Internat. 1972; 1:169.

71. Stern A: Metolazone, a diuretic agent. Am Heart J. 1976; 91:262.

72. Bennett WM et al: Efficacy and safety of metolazone in renal failure and the nephrotic syndrome. J Clin Pharmacol. 1973; 13:357.

73. Craswell PW et al: Use of metolazone, a new diuretic in patients with renal disease. Nephron. 1973; 12:63.

74. Dargie HJ et al: High dosage metolazone in chronic renal failure. Br Med J. 1972; 4:196.

75. Schoones R et al: Evaluation of metolazone: new diuretic in chronic renal disease. NY State Med J. 1971; 71:566.

76. Fotiu S et al: Antihypertensive efficacy of metolazone. Clin Pharmacol Ther. 1974; 16:318.

77. Levey BA et al: Biochemical and clinical effects of metolazone in congestive heart failure. Curr Ther Res. 1975; 18:641.

78. Dikshit K et al: Renal and extra renal hemodynamic effects of furosemide in congestive heart failure after acute myocardial infarction. N Engl J Med. 1973; 288:1087.

79. Cutler R and Blair A: Clinical pharmacokinetics of furosemide. Clin Pharmacokinetics. 1979; 4:279.

80. Greither A et al: Pharmacokinetics of furosemide in patients with congestive heart failure. Pharmacology. 1979; 19:121.

81. Kelly M et al: Pharmacokinetics of orally administered furosemide. Clin Pharmacol Ther. 1979; 15:178.

82. Kelly M et al: A comparison of the diuretic response to oral and intravenous furosemide in diuretic resistant patients. Curr Ther Res. 1977; 21:1.

83. McKenzie I: A clinical trial of furosemide (Lasix). Med J. Aust. 1960; 879.

84. Stallings S et al: Comparison of natriuretic and diuretic effects of single and divided doses of furosemide. Am J Hosp Pharm. 1979; 36:68.

85. Wilson T et al: Effect of dosage regimen and natriuretic response to furosemide. Clin Pharmacol Ther. 1976; 18:165.

86. Stone D et al: Intravenously given ethacrynic acid and gastrointestinal bleeding. JAMA. 1969; 209:1668.

87. Asscher A: Treatment of furosemide resistant edema by the addition of metolazone. Clinical Trials J. 1974; 11:134.

88. Venkata C: Treatment of loop diuretic resistant edema by the addition of metolazone. Curr Ther Res. 1977; 22:686.

89. Epstein M et al: Potentiation of furosemide by metolazone in refractory edema. Curr Ther Res. 1977; 21:656.

90. Gunstone RF et al: Clinical experience with metolazone in 52 African patients: synergy with furosemide. Postgrad Med J. 1971; 47:789.

91. Beresford HR: Polydipsia, hydrochlorothiazide, and water intoxication. JAMA. 1970; 214:879.

92. Day JO: Water intoxication in psychogenic water drinkers taking thiazide diuretics. South Med J. 1977; 70:572.

93. DeRubertis FR et al: Complications of diuretic therapy: severe alkalosis and syndrome resembling inappropriate secretion of antidiuretic hormone. Metabolism. 1970; 19:709.

94. Earley LE et al: The mechanism of antidiuresis associated with the administration of hydrochlorothiazide in patients with vasopressin resistant diabetes insipidus. J Clin Invest. 1962; 41:1988.

95. Fichman MP et al: Diuretic-induced hyponatremia. Ann Intern Med. 1971; 75:853.

96. Fuisz RE et al: Diuretic-induced hyponatremia and sustained antidiuresis. Am J Med. 1962; 33:783.

97. Gossain VV et al: Drug-induced hyponatremia in psychogenic polydipsia. Postgrad Med J. 1976; 52:720.

98. Grantham JJ et al: Asymptomatic hyponatremia and bronchogenic carcinoma: the deleterious effects of diuretics. Am J Med Sci. 1965; 249:273.

99. Kennedy RM et al: Profound hyponatremia resulting from a thiazide-induced decrease in urinary diluting capacity in a patient with primary polydipsia. N Engl J Med. 1970; 282:1185.

100. Mataverde AQ et al: Hydrochlorothiazide-induced water intoxication in myxedema. JAMA. 1974; 230:1014.

101. Kassier JP et al: Diuretics and potassium metabolism: a reassessment of the need, effectiveness and safety of potassium therapy. Kidney Internat. 1977; 11:505.

102. Lawson OH et al: Potassium supplements in patients receiving long-term diuretics for oedema. Quart J Med. 1976; 45:469.

103. Manner RJ et al: Prevalence of hypokalemia in diuretic therapy. Clin Med. 1972 (Nov); 15.

104. Morgan TO: Clinical use of potassium supplements and potassium sparing diuretics. Drug. 1973; 6:222.

105. Kosman ME: Management of potassium problems during long-term diuretic therapy. JAMA. 1974; 230:743.

106. Kunau RT et al: Disorders of hypo- and hyperkalemia. Clin Nephrol. 1977; 7:173.

107. Morgan DB et al: Potassium depletion in heart failure and its relation to long-term treatment with diuretics. Postgrad Med J. 1978; 54:72.

108. Morgan DB and Davidson: Hypokalemia and diuretics: analysis of publications. Br Med J. 1980; 1:905.

109. Davidson C et al: Effect of long-term diuretic treatment on body potassium in heart disease. Lancet. 1976; 2:1044.

110. Davidson S and Surawicz B: Ectopic beats and atrioventricular conduction disturbances. Arch Intern Med. 1967; 120:280.

111. Healey JJ et al: A comparison of diuretic induced potassium losses in normal and abnormal subjects. Irish J Med Sci. 1968; 1:115.

112. Leemhuis MP et al: Effects of chlorthalidone on serum and total body potassium in hypertensive patients. Acta Med Scand. 1976; 200:37.

113. Steiness E et al: Cardiac arrhythmias induced by hypokalemia and potassium loss during maintenance digoxin therapy. Br Heart J. 1976; 38:167.

114. Finnerty FA et al: Long-term effects of furosemide and hydrochlorothiazide in patients with essential hypertension. Angiology. 1977; 28:125.

115. Kassier JP et al: The critical role of chloride in the correction of hypokalemic alkalosis in men. Am J Med. 1965; 38:172.

116. Schwartz WB: Pathogenesis and replacement of diuretic-induced potassium and chloride loss. Ann NY Acad Sci. 1965; 139:506.

117. Dyckner T: Serum magnesium in acute myocardial infarction. Acta Med Scand. 1979; 206:137.

118. Loeb HS et al: Paroxysmal ventricular fibrillation in two patients with hypomagnesemia. Circulation. 1968; 37:210.

119. Chadda KD et al: Hypomagnesemia and refractory cardiac arrhythmia in a non-digitalized patient. Am J Cardiol. 1973; 31:98.

120. Seller RH: The role of magnesium in digitalis toxicity. Am Heart J. 1971; 82:551.

121. Amery A et al: Glucose intolerance during diuretic therapy. Lancet. 1978; 1:681.

122. Breckenridge A et al: Glucose tolerance in hypertensive patients on long-term diuretic therapy. Lancet. 1967; 1:61.

123. Chazan IA et al: Etiological factors in thiazide-induced or aggravated diabetes mellitus. Diabetes. 1965; 14:132.

124. Kohner EM et al: Effect of diuretic therapy on glucose tolerance in hypertensive patients. Lancet. 1971; 1:986.

125. Lewis PJ et al: Deterioration of glucose tolerance in hypertensive patients on prolonged diuretic treatment. Lancet. 1976; 1:564.

126. McFarland KF et al: Changes in the fasting blood sugar after hydrochlorothiazide and potassium supplementation. J Clin Pharmacol. 1977; 17:13.

127. Curtis J et al: Chlorthalidone-induced hyperosmolar hyperglycemic nonketotic coma. JAMA. 1972; 220:1592.

128. Gerich JE et al: Clinical and metabolic characteristics of hyperosmolar nonketotic coma. Diabetes. 1971; 20:228.

129. Jackson WP et al: Effect of furosemide on carbohydrate metabolism, blood pressure, and other modalities: a comparison with chlorothiazide. Br Med J. 1966; 2:333.

130. Lavender S et al: Nonketotic hyperosmolar coma and furosemide therapy. Diabetes. 1974; 23:247.

131. Mustala O et al: Comparison of the diabetogenic effects of chlorothiazide and furosemide. Ann Med Fenn. 1965; 54:75.

132. Tasker PRW et al: Nonketotic diabetic precoma associated with high-dose furosemide therapy. Br Med J. 1976; 1:626.

133. Walsh CH et al: A study of the effect of furosemide on carbohydrate metabolism in diabetic subjects. J Irish Med Assn. 1974; 67:18.

134. Anderson QO et al: Carbohydrate metabolism during treatment with chlorthalidone and ethacrynic acid. Br Med J. 1968; 2:798.

135. Feldman E et al: Ethacrynic acid: a non-diabetogenic diuretic. Dis Chest. 1967; 51:282.

136. Steele TH: Diuretic-induced hyperuricemia. Clinics Rheumat Dis. 1977; 3:37.

137. Liang MH et al: Asymptomatic hyperuricemia, the case for conservative management. Ann Intern Med. 1978; 88:166.

138. Dowling HF et al: Toxic reactions accompanying second courses of sulfonamides in patients developing toxic reactions during a previous course. Ann Intern Med. 1946; 24:629.

139. Burry JN et al: Phototoxic blisters from high furosemide dosage. Br J Dermatol. 1976; 94:495.

140. Heydenreich G et al: Bullous dermatosis among patients with chronic renal failure on high dose furosemide. Acta Med Scand. 1974; 202:61.

141. Kennedy AC et al: Acquired epidermolysis bullosa due to high dose furosemide. Br Med J. 1976; 1:1509.

142. Ebringer A et al: Bullous haemorrhagic eruption associated with furosemide. Med J Aust. 1969; 1:768.

143. Fellner MJ et al: Occurrence of bullous pemphigoid after furosemide therapy. Arch Dermatol. 1976; 112:75.

144. Gibson TP et al: Erythema multiforme and furosemide therapy. JAMA. 1970; 212:1709.

145. Brivet F et al: Porphyria cutanea tarda-like syndrome in hemodialyzed patients. Nephron. 1978; 20:258.

146. Gilchrest B et al: Bullous dermatosis of hemodialysis. Ann Intern Med. 1975; 83:480.

147. Brickman AS et al: Changes in serum and urinary calcium during treatment with hydrochlorothiazide: Studies on mechanisms. J Clin Invest. 1972; 51:945.

148. Christensson T et al: Hypercalcemia and primary hyperparathyroidism. Arch Intern Med. 1977; 137:1138.

149. Duarte CG et al: Thiazide-induced hypercalcemia. N Engl J Med. 1971; 284:828.

150. Koppel MH et al: Thiazide-induced rise in serum calcium and magnesium in patients on maintenance hemodialysis. Ann Intern Med. 1970; 72:895.

151. Lindy S et al: Serum calcium and phosphorous in patients treated with thiazides and furosemide. Acta Med Scand. 1973; 194:319.

152. Middler S et al: Thiazide diuretics and calcium metabolism. Metabolism. 1973; 22:139.

153. Parfitt AM: The interactions of thiazide diuretics with parathyroid hormone and vitamin D. J Clin Invest. 1972; 51:1879.

154. Parfill AM: Thiazide-induced hypercalcemia vitamin D-treated hypoparathyroidism. Ann Intern Med. 1972; 77:557.

155. Stote RM et al: Hydrochlorothiazide effects on serum calcium and immunoreactive parathyroid hormone concentrations. Ann Intern Med. 1972; 77:587.

156. Yendt ER et al: Prevention of calcium stones with thiazides. Kidney Internat. 1978; 13:397.

157. Paloyan E et al: Hyperparathyroidism coexisting with hypertension and prolonged thiazide administration. JAMA. 1969; 210:1243.

158. Coe FL et al: Evidence for secondary hyperparathyroidism in idiopathic hypercalciuria. J Clin Invest. 1973; 52:134.

159. Ehrig U et al: Effect of long-term thiazide therapy on intestinal calcium absorption in patients with recurrent renal calculi. Metabolism. 1974; 23:139.

160. Yendt ER et al: The use of thiazides in the prevention of renal calculi. Can Med Assoc J. 1970; 102:614.

161. Coe FL: Treated and untreated recurrent calcium nephrolithiasis in patients with idiopathic hypercalciuria, hyperuricosuria, or no metabolic disorder. Ann Intern Med. 1977; 87:404.

162. Costanzo LS et al: On the hypocalciuric action of chlorothiazide. J Clin Invest. 1974; 54:628.

163. Gabow PA et al: Furosemide-induced reduction in ionized calcium in hypoparathyroid patients. Ann Intern Med. 1977; 86:579.

164. Suki WN et al: Acute treatment of hypercalcemia with furosemide. N Engl J Med. 1970; 283:836.

165. Toft H et al: Effect of furosemide administration on calcium excretion. Br Med J. 1971; 1:437.

166. McElligott M: Effect of furosemide on serum calcium. Irish J Med Sci. 1971; 140:410.

167. Chandler PT et al: Increased serum calcium levels induced by furosemide. South Med J. 1977; 70:571.

168. Boston Collaborative Drug Surveillance Program: Drug-induced deafness. JAMA. 1973; 224:515.

169. Cooperman LB et al: Toxicity of ethacrynic acid and furosemide. Am Heart J. 1973; 85:831.

170. Hanzelik E et al: Deafness after ethacrynic acid. Lancet. 1969; 1:416.

171. Matz GJ et al: Ototoxicity of ethacrynic acid. Arch Otolaryngol. 1969; 90:60.

172. Meriwether WD et al: Deafness following standard intravenous dose of ethacrynic acid. JAMA. 1971; 216:795.

173. Pillay VKG et al: Transient and permanent deafness following treatment with ethacrynic acid in renal failure. Lancet. 1969; 1:77.

174. Quick CA: Hearing loss in patients with dialysis and renal transplants. Ann Otol. 1976; 85:776.

175. Schneider WJ et al: Acute transient hearing loss after ethacrynic acid therapy. Arch Intern Med. 1966; 117:715.

176. Lloyd-Mostyn RH et al: Ototoxicity of intravenous furosemide. Lancet. 1971; 2:1156.

177. Quick CA et al: Permanent deafness associated with furosemide administration. Ann Otol. 1975; 84:94.

178. Rifkin SI et al: Deafness associated with oral furosemide. South Med J. 1978; 71:86.

179. Schwartz GH et al: Ototoxicity induced by furosemide. N Engl J Med. 1970; 282:1413.

180. Venkateswaran PS: Transient deafness from high doses of furosemide. Br Med J. 1971; 4:113.

181. Wigand ME et al: Ototoxic side-effects of high doses of furosemide in patients with uremia. Postgrad Med J. 1971; 47 (Apr Suppl):54.

182. Johnson AH et al: Kanamycin ototoxicity—possible potentiation by other drugs. South Med J. 1970; 63:511.

183. Mathog RH et al: Ototoxicity of ethacrynic acid and aminoglycoside antibiotics in uremia. N Engl J Med. 1969; 280:1223.

184. Bosher SK et al: The effects of ethacrynic acid upon the cochlear endolymph and the stria vascularis. Acta Otolaryngol. 1973; 75:184.

185. Brummett RE et al: The delayed effects of ethacrynic acid on the stria vascularis of the guinea pig. Acta Otolaryngol. 1977; 83:98.

186. Prazma J et al: Ototoxicity of ethacrynic acid. Arch Otolaryngol. 1972; 95:448.

187. Quick CA et al: Early changes in the cochlear duct from ethacrynic acid: An electron microscopic evaluation. Laryngoscope. 1970; 80:854.

188. Brummett RE et al: Cochlear damage resulting from kanamycin and furosemide. Acta Otolaryngol. 1975; 80:86.

189. Greenblatt DJ et al: Clinical toxicity of furosemide in hospitalized patients. Am Heart J. 1977; 94:6.

190. Johnson DW et al: Hearing function and chronic renal failure. Ann Otol. 1976; 85:43.

191. Bourke JB et al: Drug-associated primary acute pancreatitis. Lancet. 1978; 1:706.

192. Johnston DH et al: Acute pancreatitis. JAMA. 1959; 170:2054.

193. Minkowitz S et al: Fatal hemorrhagic pancreatitis following chlorothiazide administration in pregnancy. Obstet Gynecol. 1964; 24:332.

194. Shanklin DR: Pancreatic atrophy apparently secondary to hydrochlorothiazide. N Engl J Med. 1966; 266:1097.

195. Wenger J et al: Acute pancreatitis related to hydrochlorothiazide therapy. Gastroenterology. 1964; 46:768.

196. Jones MF et al: Acute hemorrhagic pancreatitis associated with administration of chlorthalidone. N Engl J Med. 1962; 267:1029.

197. Diamond MT: Hyperglycemic hyperosmolar coma associated with hydrochlorothiazide and pancreatitis. NY State J Med. 1972; 72:1741.

198. Cornish AL et al: Effects of chlorothiazide on the pancreas. N Engl J Med. 1961; 265:673.

199. Buchanan N et al: Furosemide-induced pancreatitis. Br Med J. 1977; 2:1417.

200. Call T et al: Acute pancreatitis secondary to furosemide with associated hyperlipidemia. Am J Dig Dis. 1977; 22:835.

201. Jones PE et al: Furosemide-induced pancreatitis. Br Med J. 1975; 1:133.

202. Wilson AE et al: Acute pancreatitis associated with furosemide therapy. Lancet. 1967; 1:105.

203. Rosenberg L et al: Thiazide and acute cholecystitis. N Engl J Med. 1980; 303:546.

204. Porter J et al: Acute cholecystitis and thiazides. N Engl J Med. 1981; 304:954.

205. Grimm R et al: Effects of thiazide diuretics on plasma lipids and lipoproteins in mildly hypertensive patients. Ann Intern Med. 1981; 94:7.

206. Ames RP et al: Increase in serum-lipids during treatment of hypertension with chlorthalidone. Lancet. 1976; 1:721.

207. Ames RP et al: Elevation of serum lipid levels during diuretic therapy of hypertension. Am J Med. 1976; 61:748.

208. Helgeland A et al: Serum triglycerides and serum uric acid in untreated and thiazide-treated patients with mild hypertension. Am J Med. 1978; 64:34.

209. Schnaper H et al: Chlorthalidone and serum cholesterol. Lancet. 1977; 2:295.

210. Bettman JW: Drug hypersensitivity purpuras. Arch Intern Med. 1963; 112:840.

211. Eisner EV et al: Hydrochlorothiazide dependent thrombocytopenia due to IgM antibody. JAMA. 1971; 215:480.

212. Kutti J et al: The frequency of thrombocytopenia in patients with heart disease treated with oral diuretics. Acta Med Scand. 1968; 183:245.

213. Sprivastava G et al: Thiazide-induced bone-marrow aplasia. Indian J Pediatr. 1967; 34:407.

214. Zuckerman AM et al: Agranulocytosis with thrombocytopenia following chlorothiazide therapy. Br Med J. 1958; 2:1338.

215. Fitzgerald EW: Fatal glomerulonephritis complicating allergic purpura due to chlorothiazide. Arch Intern Med. 1960; 105:305.

216. Horowitz HI et al: A thrombocytopenia purpura caused by chlorthiazide. NY State J Med. 1959; 59:1117.

217. Gesink MH et al: Thrombocytopenia purpura associated with hydrochlorothiazide therapy. JAMA. 1960; 172:556.

218. Neaverson MA: Neutropenia due to chlorthalidone. Lancet. 1964; 2:208.

219. Schotland MG et al: Neutropenia in an infant secondary to hydrochlorothiazide therapy. Pediatrics. 1963; 31:754.

220. Turner NA et al: Neutropenia associated with chlorthalidone therapy. Med J Aust. 1964; 1:361.

221. Klein M: Agranulocytosis secondary to chlorthalidone therapy. JAMA. 1963; 184:310.

222. Vila JM et al: Thiazide-induced immune hemolytic anemia. JAMA. 1976; 236:1723.

223. Hutcheon D: Benefit risk factors associated with supplemental potassium therapy. J Clin Phrmacol. 1976; 16:85.

224. McRae MP: Foods high in potassium. Hosp Pharm. 1979; 14:730.

225. Farquaharson-Roberts MA et al: Perforation of small bowel due to slow release potassium chloride (slow-K). Br Med J. 1975; 3:206.

226. Howie AD et al: Slow release potassium chloride treatment. Br Med J. 1975; 2:176.

227. Learmonth I et al: Potassium stricture of the upper alimentary tract. Lancet. 1976; 1:251.

228. McCall AJ: Slow-K ulceration of oesophagus with aneurysmal left atrium. Br Med J. 1975; 3:238.

229. McMahon FG et al: Gastric ulceration after "Slow-K". N Engl Med. 1976; 295:733.

230. Rider JA et al: Potassium chloride preparations and fecal blood loss. JAMA. 1975; 231:836.

231. Ben-ishay D et al: Bioavailability of potassium from a slow release tablet. Clin Pharmacol Ther. 1973; 14:250.

232. Schwartz A et al: Dosage of potassium chloride elixir to correct thiazide-induced hypokalemia. JAMA. 1974; 230:702.

233. Ramsay LE et al: Factors influencing serum potassium in treated hypertension. Quart J Med. 1977; 46:401.

234. Wagner JG: Appraisal of digoxin bioavailability and pharmacokinetics in relation to cardiac therapy. Am Heart J. 1974; 88:133.

235. Greenblatt DJ et al: Evaluation of digoxin bioavailability in single-dose studies. N Engl J Med. 1973; 289:651.

236. Huffman DH et al: Absorption of digoxin from different oral preparations in normal subjects during steady state. Clin Pharmacol Ther. 1974; 16:310.

237. Lindenbaum J et al: Variation in biologic availability of digoxin from four preparations. N Engl J Med. 1971; 285:1344.

238. Sorby DL et al: On the evaluation of biologic availability of digoxin from tablets. Drug Intell Clin Pharm. 1973; 7:79.

239. Wagner JG et al: Equivalence lack in digoxin plasma levels. JAMA. 1973; 224:199.

240. Huffman DH: Absorption of digoxin from different oral preparations. JAMA. 1972; 22:957.

241. Steiness E et al: Bioavailability of digoxin tablets. Clin Pharmacol Ther. 1973; 14:949.

242. Brown DD et al: Plasma digoxin levels in normal human volunteers following chronic oral and intramuscular digoxin. J Lab Clin Med. 1973; 82:201.

243. Doherty JE et al: Studies following intramuscular tritiated digoxin in human subjects. Am J Cardiol. 1965; 15:170.

244. Doherty JE: Digitalis glycosides: Pharmacokinetics and their clinical implications. Ann Intern Med. 1973; 79:229.

245. Jelliffe RW et al: A nomogram for digoxin therapy. Am J Med. 1974; 57:63.

246. Aronson Clinical Pharmacokinetics of Digoxin 1980. Clin Pharmacokinetics. 1980; 5:137.

247. Clayton B: Reduction of digitalis glycoside intoxication by rational dosing procedure. Am J Hosp Pharm. 1974; 31:855.

248. Koup JR et al: Pharmacokinetics of digoxin in normal subjects after intravenous bolus and infusion doses. J Pharmacokinetics Biopharm. 1975; 3:181.

249. Peters U et al: Digoxin metabolism in patients. Arch Intern Med. 1978; 138:1074.

250. Marcus RI et al: The metabolism of digoxin in cirrhotic patients. Gastroenterology. 1964; 47:517.

251. Perrier D et al: Clinical pharmacokinetics of digitoxin. Clin Pharmacokinetics. 1977; 2:292.

252. Jelliffe RW et al: An improved method of digitoxin therapy. Ann Intern Med. 1970; 72:453.

253. Rasmussen K et al: Digitoxin kinetics in patients with impaired renal function. Clin Pharmacol Ther. 1972; 13:6.

254. Marcus FI et al: Administration of tritiated digoxin with and without a loading dose. A metabolic study. Circulation. 1966; 34:865.

255. Jelliffe RW et al: Reduction of digitalis toxicity by computer assisted glycosides dosage regimens. Ann Intern Med. 1972; 77:891.

256. Winter M et al: *Basic Clinical Pharmacokinetics*, 1st edition, edited by Winter M, with Katcher B, Koda-Kimble M. Applied Therapeutics Inc, San Francisco. 1980; p 5,71.

257. Sheiner LB et al: Estimation of population characteristics of pharmacokinetic parameters from routine clinical data. J Pharmacokinetics Biopharm. 1977; 5:445.

258. Koup JR et al: Digoxin pharmacokinetics: role of renal failure in dosage regimen design. Clin Pharmacol Ther. 1975; 18:9.

259. Reunig RH et al: Role of pharmacokinetics in drug dosage adjustment 1. Pharmacologic effect kinetics and apparent volume of distribution of digoxin. J Clin Pharmacol. 1973; 13:4.

260. Jusko W et al: Pharmacokinetic design of digoxin dosage regimen in relation to renal function. J Clin Pharmacol. 1974; 14:525.

261. Butler VP: Digoxin: immunologic approaches to measurement and reversal of toxicity. N Engl J Med. 1970; 283:1150.

262. Smith TW et al: Determination of therapeutic and toxic serum digoxin concentrations by radioimmunoassay. N Engl J Med. 1973; 288:942.

263. Inglefinger J et al: The serum digitalis concentration does it diagnosis digitalis toxicity? N Engl J Med. 1976; 294:897.

264. Weintraub M et al: Compliance as a determinant of serum digoxin concentration. JAMA. 1973; 224:481.

265. Sheiner LB et al: Differences in serum digoxin concentrations between outpatients and inpatients; an effect of compliance? Clin Pharmacol Ther. 1974; 15:239.

266. Sanchez N et al: Pharmacokinetics of digoxin: interpreting bioavailability. Br Med J. 1973; 4:132.

267. White RJ et al: Plasma concentrations of digoxin after oral administration in the fasting and postprandial state. Br Med J. 1971; 1:380.

268. Heizer WD et al: Absorption of digoxin in patients with malabsorption syndromes. N Engl J Med. 1971; 285:257.

269. Hall WH et al: Tritiated digoxin XXII. Absorption and excretion in malabsorption syndromes. Am J Med. 1974; 56:437.

270. Luchi RJ et al: Unusually large digitalis requirements; a study of altered digoxin metabolism. Am J Med. 1968; 37:263.

271. Chopra D et al: Insensitivity to digoxin associated with hypocalcemia. N Engl J Med. 1977; 297:917.

272. Shenfield G: Influence of thyroid dysfunction on drug pharmacokinetics. Clin Pharmacokinetics. 1981; 6:275.

273. Dahlquist R et al: Effect of quinidine on plasma concentration and real clearance of digoxin. Br J Clin Pharmacol. 1980; 9:413.

274. Ejivson G et al: Effect of quinidine on plasma concentration of digoxin. Br Med J. 1978; 1:279.

275. Leahey E et al: Interaction between quinidine and digoxin. JAMA. 1980; 240:533.

276. Leahey F et al: Enhanced cardiac effect of digoxin during quinidine treatment. Arch Intern Med. 1979; 139:519.

277. Mungall D et al: Effects of quinidine on serum digoxin concentration. Ann Intern Med. 1980; 93:689.

278. Doering W et al: Quinidine-digoxin interaction: pharmacokinetics, underlying mechanism and clinical implications. N Engl J Med. 1979; 301:400.

279. Hager W et al: Digoxin-quinidine interaction, pharmacokinetic evaluation. N Engl J Med. 1979; 300:1238.

280. Holford N et al: The quinidine digoxin interaction. N Engl J Med. 1980; 302:864.

281. Burkle W et al: Effect of quinidine on serum digoxin concentrations. Am J Hosp Pharm. 1979; 36:968.

282. Bigger J et al: The quinidine-digoxin interaction: what do we know about it? N Engl J Med. 1979; 301:779.

283. Leahey E et al: The effect of quinidine and other oral antiarrhythmic drugs on serum digoxin: a prospective study. Ann Intern Med. 1980; 92:605.

284. Fenster P et al: Digitoxin-quinidine interaction: pharmacokinetic evaluation. Ann Intern Med. 1980; 93:698.

285. Ochs H et al: Noninteraction of digitoxin and quinidine. N Engl J Med. 1980; 303:672.

286. Brown DD et al: Decreased bioavailability of digoxin due to antacids and kaolin-pectin. N Engl J Med. 1976; 295:1035.

287. Lindenbaum J et al: Impairment of digoxin absorption by neomycin. Clin Res. 1970; 20:410.

288. Banzano G et al: Digitalis intoxication. Treatment with a new steroid binding resin. JAMA. 1972; 220:828.

289. Hall WH et al: Effect of cholestyramine on digoxin absorption and excretion in man. Am J Cardiol. 1977; 39:213.

290. Manninen V et al: Altered absorption of digoxin in patients given propantheline and metoclopramide. Lancet. 1973; 1:398.

291. Solomon HM et al: Interactions between digitoxin and other drugs in man. Am Heart J. 1972; 83:277.

292. Bigger J et al: Digitalis toxicity–drug interactions promoting toxicity and the management of toxicity. Semin In Drug Treat. 1972; 2:147.

293. Juhl RP et al: Effects of sulfasalazine on digoxin bioavailability. Clin Pharmacol Ther. 1976; 20:387.

294. Sahiri K et al: Mechanism of diphenylhydantoin (DPH) induced decrease of serum digoxin levels. Clin Res. 1974; 22:321A.

295. Greenblatt DJ et al: Pain and CPK elevation after intramuscular digoxin. N Engl J Med. 1973; 288:689.

296. Lely AH et al: Non cardiac symptoms of digitalis intoxication. Am Heart J. 1972; 83:149.

297. Rodensky PL et al: Observations on digitalis intoxication. Arch Intern Med. 1961; 108:61.

298. Chung EK: Digitalis-induced cardiac arrhythmias. Am Heart J. 1970; 8:643.

299. Seltzer A et al: Production, recognition and treatment of digitalis toxicity. Calif Med. 1970; 79:57.

300. Beller GA et al: Digitalis intoxication. A prospective clinical study with serum level correlations. N Engl J Med. 1971; 284:989.

301. Jelliffe RW: Factors to consider in planning digoxin therapy. J Chron Dis. 1971; 24:407.

302. Prindle KH Jr et al: Influence of extracellular potassium concentration on myocardial uptake and inotropic effect of tritiated digoxin. Circ Res. 1971; 28:337.

303. Brater C et al: Digoxin toxicity in patients with normokalemic potassium depletion. Clin Pharmacol Ther. 1977; 22:21.

304. Seller RH et al: Digitalis toxicity and hypomagnesemia. Am Heart J. 1970; 79:57.

305. Beller Ga et al: Correlation of serum magnesium levels and cardiac digitalis intoxication. Am J Cardiol. 1974; 33:225.

306. Singh RB et al: Hypomagnesemia in relation to digoxin intoxication in children. Am Heart J. 1976; 92:144.

307. Wacker WE et al: Magnesium metabolism (3 parts). N Engl J Med. 1968; 278:658,712,722.

308. Lown B et al: Digitalis, electrolytes and the surgical patient. Am J Cardiol. 1960; 6:309.

309. Ewy GA et al: Digoxin metabolism in the elderly. Circulation. 1969; 39:449.

310. Levine OR et al: Digitalis dosage in premature infants. Pediatrics. 1972; 29:18.

311. Thomson PD et al: Lidocaine pharmacokinetics in advanced heart failure, liver disease and renal failure. Ann Intern Med. 1973; 78:499.

312. Louis S et al: The cardiocirculatory changes caused by intravenous dilantin and its solvent. Am Heart J. 1967; 74:523.

313. Bauman J et al: Phenytoin crystallization in intravenous fluids. Drug Intell Clin Pharm. 1977; 11:646.

314. Smith TW et al: Reversal of advanced digoxin intoxication with Fab fragments of digoxin-specific antibodies. N Engl J Med. 1976; 294:797.

315. Marbury T et al: Advanced digoxin toxicity in renal failure; treatment with charcoal hemoperfusion. South Med J. 1979; 72:279.

316. Gault M et al: Loading doses of digoxin in renal failure. Br J Clin Pharmacol. 1980; 9:593.

317. Devine BJ: Gentamicin therapy. Drug Intell Clin Pharm. 1974; 8:650.

318. Cockcroft DW and Gault MH: Prediction of creatinine clearance from serum creatinine. Nephron. 1976; 16:31.

319. Forrester JS et al: Medical therapy of acute myocardial infarction by application of hemodynamic subsets (2 parts). N Engl J Med. 1976; 295:1356.

320. Gorlin R: Practical cardiac hemodynamics. N Engl J Med. 1977; 269:203.

321. Chatterjee K et al: Combination vasodilator therapy for severe chronic congestive heart failure. Progr Cardiovasc Dis. 1977; 19:301.

322. Guiha N et al: Treatment of refractory heart failure with infusion of nitroprusside. N Engl J Med. 1974; 291:587.

323. Packer M et al: Rebound hemodynamic events after the abrupt withdrawal of nitroprusside in patients with severe congestive heart failure. N Engl J Med. 1979; 301:1193.

324. Hill N et al: Intravenous nitroglycerin–a review of pharmacology, indications, therapeutic effects and complications. Chest. 1981; 79:1.

325. Armstrong P et al: Pharmacokinetic–hemodynamic studies of intravenous nitroglycerin. Circulation. 1980; 62:160.

326. McNiff B et al: Potency and stability of extemporaneous nitroglycerin infusions. Am J Hosp Pharm. 1979; 36:173.

327. Fung H: Potency and stability of extemporaneously prepared nitroglycerin intravenous solutions. Am J Hosp Pharm. 1978; 35:528.

327a. Baaske D: Administration set suitable for use with intravenous nitroglycerin. Am J Hosp Pharm. 1982; 39:121.

328. Abrams J et al: Usefulness of long acting nitrates in cardiovascular disease. Am J Med. 1978; 64:183.

329. Warren S et al: Nitroglycerin and nitrate ester. Am J Med. 1978; 65:53.

330. Armstrong PW et al: Nitroglycerin ointment in acute myocardial infarction. Am J Cardiol. 1976; 38:474.

331. Taylor W et al: Hemodynamic effects of nitroglycerin ointment in congestive heart failure. Am J Cardiol. 1976; 38:469.

332. Mantle JA et al: Isosorbide dinitrate for the relief of severe heart failure after myocardial infarction. Am J Cardiol. 1976; 37:263.

333. Gray R et al: Hemodynamic and metabolic effects of isosorbide dinitrate in chronic congestive heart failure. Am Heart J. 1975; 90:346.

334. Vyssnabb W et al: Orally administered isosorbide dinitrate in patients with and without left ventricular failure due to acute myocardial infarction. Am J Cardiol. 1977; 39:91.

335. Franciosa JA et al: Hemodynamic effects of orally administered isosorbide dinitrate in patients with congestive heart failure. Circulation. 1974; 50:1020.

336. Chatterjee K et al: Oral hydralazine therapy for chronic refractory heart failure. Circulation. 1976; 54:879.

337. Packer M et al: Hemodynamic evaluation of hydralazine dosage in refractory heart failure. Clin Pharmacol Ther. 1980; 27:337.

338. Greenberg B et al: Beneficial effects of hydralazine on severe mitral regurgitation. Circulation. 1978; 58:273.

339. Miller RR et al: Sustained reduction of cardiac impedence and preload in congestive heart failure with the antihypertensive vasodilator prazosin. N Engl J Med. 1977; 297:303.

340. Awan N et al: Clinical pharmacology and therapeutic application of prazosin in acute and chronic refractory congestive heart failure. Am J Med. 1978; 65:146.

341. Mehta J et al: Comparative hemodynamic effects of intravenous nitroprusside and oral prazosin in refractory heart failure. Am J Cardiol. 1978; 41:925.

342. Packer M et al: Hemodynamic and clinical tachyphylaxis to prazosin mediated afterload reduction in severe congestive heart failure. Circulation. 1979; 59:531.

343. Desch C et al: Development of pharmacologic tolerance to prazosin in congestive heart failure. Am J Cardiol. 1979; 44:1178.

344. Colucci W et al: Long term therapy of heart failure with prazosin. Am J Cardiol. 1980; 45:337.

344a. Massie B et al: Long term vasodilator therapy for heart failure. Circulation. 1981; 63:269.

345. Matsumoto S et al: Hemodynamic effects of nifedipine in congestive heart failure. Am J Cardiol. 1980; 46:476.

346. Brooks N et al: Unpredictable response to nifedipine in severe cardiac failure. Br Med J. 1980; 281:324.

347. Lorell B et al: Improved diastolic function and systolic performance in hypertrophic cardiomyopathy after nifedipine. N Engl J Med. 1980; 303:801.

348. Chatterjee K et al: Combination vasodilator therapy for severe chronic congestive heart failure. Ann Intern Med. 1976; 85:467.

349. Pierpont G et al: Combined oral hydralazine-nitrate therapy in left ventricular failure. Chest. 1978; 73:8.

350. Chatterjee K et al: Long term outpatient vasodilator therapy of congestive heart failure. Am J Med. 1978; 65:134.

351. Massie B et al: Hemodynamic advantage of combined administration of hydralazine orally and nitrates nonparenterally in the vasodilator therapy of chronic heart failure. Am J Cardiol. 1977; 40:794.

352. Franciosa J et al: Immediate effects of hydralazine-isosorbide dinitrate combination on exercise capacity and exercise hemodynamics in patients with left ventricular failure. Circulation. 1979; 59:1085.

353. Heel RC et al: Captopril–a preliminary review of its pharmacologic properties and therapeutic efficacy. Drugs. 1980; 20:409.

354. Ferguson R et al: Captopril in severe treatment-resistant hypertension. Am Heart J. 1980; 99:579.

355. Atkinson A and Robertson J: Captopril in the treatment of clinical hypertension and cardiac failure. Lancet. 1979; 11:836.

356. Faxon DP et al: Angiotensin inhibition in severe heart failure. Am Heart J. 1981; 101:548.

357. Awan NA et al: Efficacy of oral angiotensin-converting enzyme inhibition with captopril therapy in severe chronic normotensive congestive heart failure. Am Heart J. 1981; 101:22.

358. Dzau V et al: Sustained effectiveness of converting-enzyme inhibition in patients with severe congestive heart failure. N Engl J Med. 1980; 302:1373.

359. Curtiss C et al: Role of the renin-angiotensin system in the systemic vasoconstriction of chronic congestive heart failure. Circulation. 1978; 58:763.

360. Gavras H et al: Angiotensin converting enzyme inhibition in patients with chronic congestive heart failure. Circulation. 1978; 58:770.

361. Davis R et al: Treatment of chronic congestive heart failure with captopril, an oral inhibitor of angiotensin-converting enzyme. N Engl J Med. 1979; 301:117.

362. Turin G et al: Improvement of chronic congestive heart failure by oral captopril. Lancet. 1979; 1:1213.

363. Wilkin J et al: The captopril induced eruption. Arch Dermatol. 1980; 116:902.

364. Warren S et al: Hyperkalemia resulting from captopril administration. JAMA. 1980; 244:2551.

365. Gavras I et al: Fatal pancytopenia associated with the use of captopril. Ann Intern Med. 1981; 94:58.

366. Morrison J et al: Digitalis and myocardial infarction in men. Circulation. 1980; 62:8.

367. Gunnar R et al: Ineffectiveness of isoproterenol in shock due to acute myocardial infarction. JAMA. 1967; 202:1124.

368. Goldberg L: Dopamine–clinical uses of an endogenous catecholamine. N Engl J Med. 1974; 291:707.

369. Sonnenblick E et al: Dobutamine–a new synthetic cardioactive sympathetic amine. N Engl J Med. 1979; 300:17.

370. Park C et al: Dobutamine–a new agent for the management of cardiac decompensation. Drug Intell Clin Pharm. 1979; 13:728.

371. Goldstein R et al: A comparison of digoxin and dobutamine in patients with acute infarction and cardiac failure. N Engl J Med. 1980; 303:846.

372. Kates R et al: Dobutamine pharmacokinetics in severe heart failure. Clin Pharmacol Ther. 1978; 24:537.

373. LeJemtel T et al: Amrinone; a non glycosidic, non adrenergic cardiotonic agent effective in the treatment of intractable myocardial failure. Circulation. 1979; 59:1098.

374. Benotti J et al: Hemodynamic assessment of amrinone. N Engl J Med. 1978; 299:1373.

375. Klein NA et al: Amrinone for congestive heart failure. Am J Cardiol. 1981; 48:170.

376. Wynne J et al: Oral amrinone in refractory congestive heart failure. Am J Cardiol. 1980; 45:1245.

Chapter 11

Cardiac Arrhythmias

Mark A. Gill

Conduction Pathway. The treatment of cardiac arrhythmias requires a synthesis of drug knowledge with electrophysiology and anatomy. The electrical system of the heart consists of intrinsic pacemakers and conduction tissues. A diagram of the heart which depicts the pathways for conduction is provided in Fig. 1.

The rate of electrical firing of the heart is determined by the most rapid pacemaker. Spontaneous electrical firing or automaticity can occur anywhere in the heart under certain conditions; however, the sino-atrial node (S-A node) which has the most rapid intrinsic rate (60–100 per minute) normally serves as the major pacemaker.

Firing of the S-A node initiates atrial contraction. The electrical impulse is conducted through the atria via internodal tracts to the atrio-ventricular node (A-V node) located near the coronary sinus between the left and right atria. The A-V node has pacemaker properties but normally coordinates atrial and ventricular contraction.

The conduction system in the ventricles is more elaborate than that in the atria since the muscle mass is larger. Rapid and effective excitation is critical since ventricular contraction is the major determinant of cardiac output. Fibers leaving the A-V node are called the Bundle of His and separate into the bundle branches which traverse the septum between the ventricles. The final conducting components of the ventricles are the Purkinje fibers which emanate from the bundle branches to stimulate ventricular contraction.

Pathophysiology of Arrhythmias. Arrhythmias are the result of abnormalities in electri-

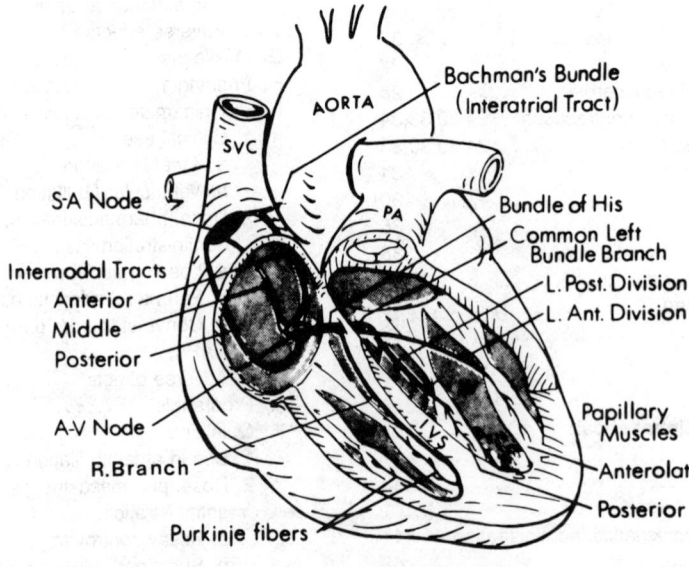

Figure 1. Electrical System of the Heart.

cal generation (eg, ectopic tachyarrhythmias) or in electrical conduction (eg, re-entrant arrhythmias) (1). There may also be situations where ectopic and re-entrant rhythms occur simultaneously.

Ectopic arrhythmias often develop in latent pacemaker tissues that have developed an accelerated rate of electrical firing. In addition, other tissues which normally have no pacemaker activity may be stimulated to develop automaticity. Stimuli for these processes include local hypoxia, stretch, edema, and catecholamines. On the other hand, *re-entrant rhythms* involve dissociation in the progression of electrical current through adjacent fibers. The dissociation can be visualized in Fig. 2, where damage to one of two bifurcating fibers causes a unidirectional block of impulse conduction. The original impulse then continues through one fiber and completes the circuit through the second fiber which is now no longer refractory. This reciprocating current may perpetuate an arrhythmia.

Normal Electrophysiology. The mechanisms of action for antiarrhythmic agents are based upon alterations in the action potential. The normal action potential is separated into five phases. (See Fig. 3.) The initial phase is Phase 0, which is the sudden depolarization after a threshold has been reached. *Phase 0* is dependent upon ionic fluxes of sodium and calcium. Sodium transfer is rapid and produces a fast response. Calcium exchange occurs more slowly and its transfer is referred to

as the slow response. *Phase 1* is a period of rapid repolarization and may be produced by the cessation of sodium transfer. The plateau of the action potential is *Phase 2,* with the current maintained mostly by calcium flow. The repolarization of the cell in *Phase 3* is produced by potassium moving out of the cell. *Phase 4* is a spontaneous depolarization produced by a sodium leak. Automaticity occurs when the slope of the depolarization phase is increased such that the threshold (X) is reached independently of other tissues. Non-pacemaker tissue has a slower rise of Phase 4 and cannot reach threshold without stimulation from pacemaker tissue.

Antiarrhythmic Drugs. The antiarrhythmic drugs may be classified according to their effects on the action potential. The several schemes for categorizing these drugs seem to change as new drugs with different mechanisms are introduced. One scheme separates drugs into four classes. See Table 1 (1).

Group I drugs are local anesthetics whose dominant electrophysiological effect is depression of Phase 0 of the action potential. This depression is mediated through blockade of the fast sodium influx. This group of drugs reduce automaticity and prolong the effective refractory period; however, they do not significantly alter the resting membrane potential or the action potential duration. This group includes drugs like quinidine, procainamide, N-acetyl-procainamide (NAPA),

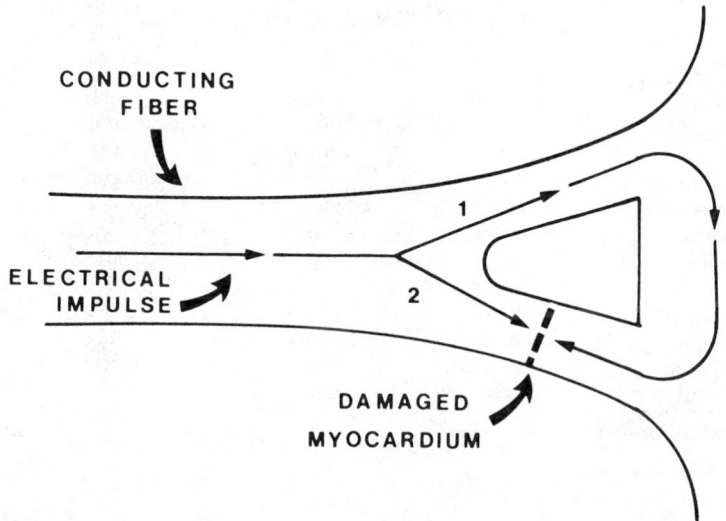

Figure 2. Electrical Conduction Through Myocardial Fibers Exhibiting Re-entry.

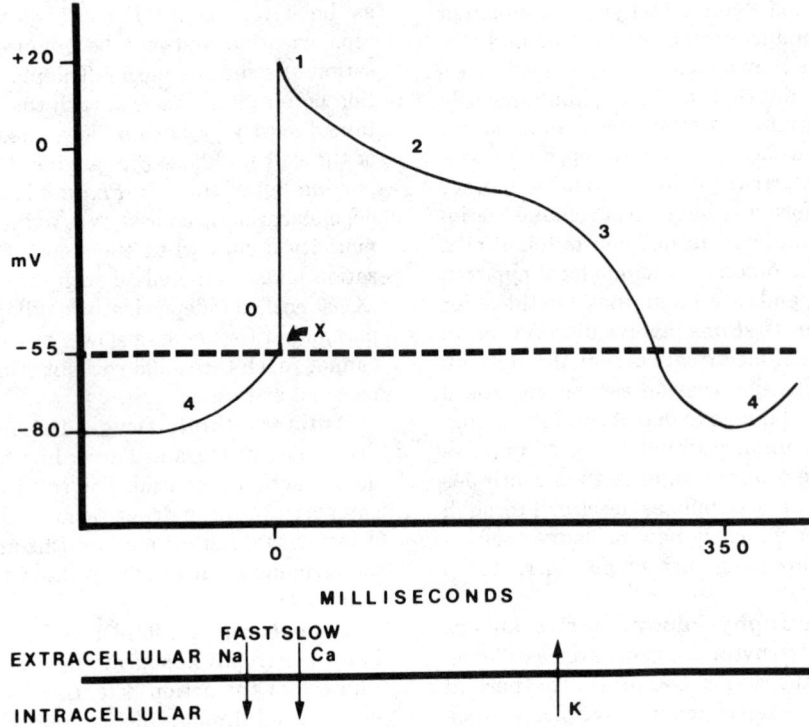

Figure 3. Normal Action Potential. X = Electrical Threshold. Below the action potential are the corresponding electrolyte shifts that produce the electrical current.

Table 1.

CLASSIFICATION OF ANTIARRHYTHMIC DRUGS[1]

Group	Drug	Fast Response	APD*	Beta Block	Slow Response
I	Quinidine	major	minor	minor	0
	Procainamide	major	minor	0	0
	NAPA	major	minor	0	0
	Phenytoin	major	minor	0	0
	Disopyramide	major	minor	0	0
	Mexiletine	major	0	0	0
	Tocainide	major	0	0	0
	Lidocaine	major	0	0	0
II	Propranolol	minor	minor	major	0
III	Bretylium	minor	major	minor	0
	Amiodarone	minor	major	minor	0
IV	Verapamil	minor	minor	0	major

*APD = Action Potential Duration

lidocaine, phenytoin, disopyramide, mexiletine, and tocainide. These drugs have varying but minor effects on the duration of the action potential; their primary effect is depression of membrane responsiveness.

Inhibitors of the sympathetic nervous system comprise *Group II.* Beta blockade reduces the slope of Phase 4 of the action potential. In higher concentrations these drugs are membrane depressants, but this effect is felt to be minor.

Group III drugs produce a prolongation of repolarization (Phase 3). Bretylium and the investigational coronary vasodilator amiodarone have their major activity in lengthening the duration of the action potential. Since the repolarization phase is lengthened, the effective refractory period is consequently prolonged.

Calcium antagonists are in *Group IV.* Stretch and hypoxia in cardiac tissues may inactivate the sodium mediated fast response and allow the slow response, through calcium, to emerge. Slow response activity may produce re-entry and automaticity. These abnormalities are effectively abolished by calcium antagonists.

Verapamil. Verapamil may be used as a Group IV antiarrhythmic. The primary electrophysiologic effects of verapamil include a delay in atrioventricular conduction and depression of sinus node frequency. As such, the P-R interval is prolonged. The QRS and Q-T intervals are unchanged, suggesting that verapamil does not impede intraventricular conduction (21).

In general, the clinical utility of verapamil is limited to atrial tachyarrhythmias; its effects on ventricular arrhythmias are negligible. Verapamil exerts a dramatic effect in supraventricular tachycardia, with rapid and predictable reversion in 80–100% of cases. Normal sinus rhythm (NSR) is achieved within 2–5 minutes after an injection of 3–10 mg. This response contrasts with a 56% success rate using intravenous beta blockers (23). Most of the clinical experience using verapamil is based on atrial fibrillation. (See Questions 6 and 7). Oral verapamil has also been shown to be effective in controlling the ventricular rate during exercise in patients treated with digitalis (26). However, verapamil may increase serum digoxin concentrations, and the combination has produced asystole (27).

The electrocardiogram (ECG) provides the basis for diagnosing an arrhythmia. As seen in Fig. 4, the ECG is commonly separated into various wave components that reflect conduction through specific tisues.

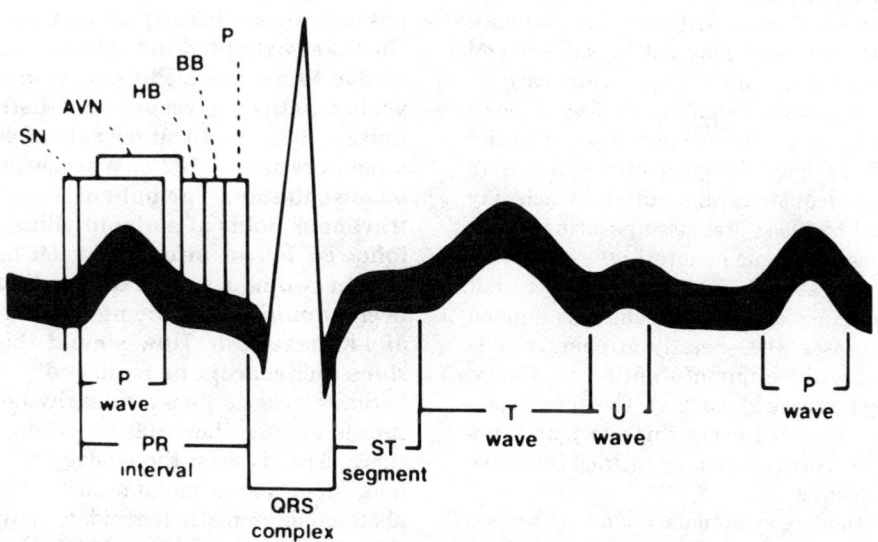

Figure 4. Electrocardiogram. The P wave is atrial depolarization. The PR interval is formed from the firing of the S-A node (SN) and conduction through the A-V node (AVN), Bundle of His (HB), the Bundle branches (BB), and Purkinje fibers (P). The QRS complex is ventricular depolarization. The S-T segment is the refractory period. The T wave is ventricular repolarization.

Sinus Bradycardia

1. **59-year-old male was admitted to the coronary care unit with a chief complaint of severe chest pain which was relieved by three nitroglycerin tablets. The pain radiated from the sternum up the neck and down his left arm and was associated with nausea, diaphoresis and shortness of breath. On admission the patient was in acute distress, obtunded, and cyanotic. His blood pressure was 90/10 mm Hg. The ECG showed sinus bradycardia (30 beats/min) with ST segment depression. Does this patient require anti-arrhythmic treatment? What would you recommend?**

A logical first step in determining the need for, and type of anti-arrhythmic therapy depends on the expected morbidity and mortality associated with the arrhythmia. Clearly the patient, not the electrocardiogram, should be treated. Sinus bradycardia is a rhythm emanating from the S-A node with a rate of less than 60 beats/min which is caused by a decrease in S-A node automaticity and a defect in impulse formation. This arrhythmia is seen in approximately 40% of patients with infarction of the right coronary artery (the artery that perfuses the S-A node) (2).

This patient deserves treatment since his cardiac output is not sufficient to maintain a normal blood pressure and tissue perfusion. Maintenance of a normal rate alone may not be sufficient to improve cardiac output if significant cardiac damage has occurred. *Atropine* is the drug of choice and should be given intravenously in an initial dose of 0.6–1.0 mg. The goal of therapy is to maintain an adequate cardiac output (which may be evaluated by blood pressure and urinary output or by hemodynamic monitoring) as well as a normal heart rate. Animal data indicate that atropine may increase ischemic changes if given in excessive doses (3). Generally, atropine may be repeated every three minutes until a maximum dose of 2 mg has been given (2,4). The appropriate dose may be repeated every three to four hours as needed (5). (Also see chapter entitled Intensive Care Therapeutics.)

If the patient is symptomatic and still has a rate of less than 45 beats/min after adequate doses of atropine, a temporary transvenous artificial cardiac pacemaker should be inserted. In addition to maintaining a normal rate, artificial pacing suppresses ventricular ectopic beats that fre-

quently appear when the automaticity of the S-A node falls below the intrinsic automaticity of the ventricles (4).

Isoproterenol may be used to treat bradycardia only if other measures have failed or are not available. It has several drawbacks in that excessive doses may increase ventricular irritability and induce ventricular tachyarrhythmias. In addition, isoproterenol increases myocardial oxygen consumption which may increase the infarct size (6). Isoproterenol should be administered as a constant infusion at a rate of 1–4 mcg/min.

The infarct is the most likely cause for this patient's bradycardia; however, digitalis intoxication should be considered in all cases of bradycardia. Sinus bradycardia is seen in approximately 4% of patients with digitalis-induced arrhythmias (7). A comprehensive drug history should be taken and a serum concentration of the drug obtained. The management of digitalis-induced bradycardia is similar to that outlined above. Additionally, digitalis should be discontinued and potassium given if the patient is hypokalemic.

Sinus Tachycardia

2. **A 24-year-old female is admitted with a chief complaint of shortness of breath. She has a ten-year history of asthma for which she takes oxtriphylline 400 mg qid and prednisone 10 mg daily. Physical examination reveals a patient in respiratory distress with a pulse of 90, a respiratory rate of 40/min, and a temperature of 102°F. Wheezes were heard on auscultation. The patient was given an intravenous bolus of aminophylline, 5.6 mg/kg, followed by an infusion of 0.9 mg/kg/hour. Within two hours after the loading dose had been administered, the nurses noted a pulse of 140 beats/min. How should this patient's sinus tachycardia be managed?**

Sinus tachycardia is a sinus rhythm except the rate is greater than 100 beats/min. Its significance depends upon the etiology of the arrhythmia. Anxiety or stimulants such as caffeine, amphetamine, or methylphenidate may produce a sinus tachycardia. This is generally benign and requires no treatment other than removal of the offending agent(s).

This patient could be exhibiting aminophylline toxicity. Most young, otherwise healthy asthmatics can tolerate this arrhythmia with careful observation. The aminophylline does not necessarily need to be stopped or decreased unless there is a potential for more dangerous complications. In addition, the fever may indicate an infection which may also contribute to the tachycardia.

Some patients may not tolerate an increase in heart rate such as this. For example, the tachycardia could increase myocardial oxygen consumption and exacerbate angina pectoris. Also, a rapid heart rate limits ventricular filling and thus reduces cardiac output. Therefore, in some patients the risk of the arrhythmia may outweigh the benefits of aminophylline for bronchodilation. Propranolol is generally used to treat sinus tachycardia but it should be avoided in this patient since it may exacerbate the bronchospasm.

Atrial Fibrillation

3. A 45-year-old 60 kg female is admitted to the hospital with palpitations as the chief complaint. The prior medical history revealed that the patient had rheumatic fever at age 9. On physical examination the patient was noted to have an irregular pulse of about 130 beats/min. The point of maximum impulse (PMI) was displaced to the mid-axillary line at the sixth intercostal space, and the apical rate was 170 beats/min. The lungs were clear, but a murmur was noted. The ECG was read as atrial fibrillation. What is atrial fibrillation? Why is digitalis considered the drug of choice?

Atrial fibrillation is an irregularly, irregular rhythm originating from ectopic atrial foci at a rate of 400–650 beats/min. However, since the A-V node prevents the majority of these impulses from stimulating the ventricles, the ventricular rate is significantly less. Atrial fibrillation is the second most common arrhythmia after premature ventricular contractions and is frequently associated with rheumatic heart disease.

Digitalis is considered the drug of choice for atrial fibrillation because it is the only drug that can reduce the ventricular rate and simultaneously reduce the major consequence of the arrhythmia, congestive heart failure (8).

Digitalis increases the force of myocardial contraction and decreases A-V conduction as reflected by a prolonged P-R interval. Intraventricular conduction is not affected (ie, the QRS complex

is not altered). Digitalis also prolongs the refractory period (repolarization) of the A-V node; this effect is most apparent when digitalis is used in the treatment of rapid atrial rates. There is an increase in ectopic impulse formation which occurs in all areas of the heart except the S-A node; this effect is usually seen in the Purkinje fibers. Finally, digitalis decreases the rate of S-A node impulse formation. There are two mechanisms for this phenomenon: Vagal stimulation which can be reversed by atropine occurs with lower doses, and there is also a direct effect that is not blocked by atropine.

Reflex vagal stimulation, depression of the S-A node, prolongation of the A-V nodal refractory period, and slowing of A-V conduction brought about by digitalis form the basis for the use of this drug in the treatment of supraventricular tachyarrhythmias—that is, arrhythmias originating in the S-A node or atria. Digitalis may hyperpolarize cells in the atrium and decrease the slope of phase 4 which would suppress atrial ectopic beats (9). However, conversion to normal sinus rhythm (NSR) with digitalis occurs infrequently.

4. What are the goals of therapy in the treatment of atrial fibrillation? How is therapy monitored?

The primary goal of therapy is to slow the rate of ventricular contraction so that diastolic filling is increased and cardiac output is improved. Generally a ventricular rate of 100 beats/min is arbitrarily set as a therapeutic goal. This rate should be based upon a pulse obtained at the apex of the heart or by electrocardiogram rather than at the radial artery since all of the ventricular beats may not be transmitted to the periphery. This pulse deficit (ie, ventricular rate minus radial artery pulse) is often used as a guide in therapy. As the ventricular rate falls and effective contractions develop this deficit should fall towards zero. Note that the pulse deficit on admission is 40 beats/min (170 – 130). Since the heart consumes oxygen for these ineffectual beats, susceptible patients may experience myocardial ischemia or congestive heart failure. Objective and symptomatic relief is the ultimate goal; drug intoxication can result from overzealous treatment of the rate alone. Improved pulmonary, renal and cerebral function will also give clues to increased cardiac output.

The second goal in the treatment of atrial fibrillation is to convert the arrhythmia to NSR with electrocardioversion, quinidine, or procainamide. It is important that patients who are to receive quinidine for atrial fibrillation be digitalized first to produce some degree of A-V block. This is necessary because the vagolytic effects of quinidine may actually enhance A-V conduction in these patients and increase the ventricular rate. The recent onset of the arrhythmia and the apparent absence of congestive heart failure would suggest that this patient has a good chance of converting; however, the displaced PMI may indicate left ventricular hypertrophy which makes conversion less likely (10,11).

5. A 50-year-old male is admitted for fever and mental confusion. Vital signs include a pulse of 140 beats/min, a temperature of 102°F, a respiratory rate of 35/min, and a blood pressure of 160/90 mm Hg. A chest x-ray (CXR) revealed an infiltrate in the right lower lobe and a normal sized heart. The ECG was read as atrial fibrillation. Two hours after digoxin 0.5 mg was given by intravenous push, the rate remained at 130–140 beats/min, and an additional 0.5 mg was given intravenously. One hour later, another 0.25 mg digoxin was given, since the rate was 130 beats/min. Two hours later, the rate is still rapid at 125 beats/min. Should additional doses of digoxin be given?

Clinically, it appears that higher doses of digoxin are required for atrial fibrillation than for congestive heart failure (12). Several studies reveal that neither the total dose nor serum digoxin level are useful indicators of response in the treatment of atrial fibrillation (13,14,15). A modest, mean digoxin level of 1.4 ng/ml has been observed in patients with controlled atrial fibrillation (13). (See Table 2 for generally accepted

therapeutic drug levels). Goldman et al (14) noted that in patients with acute illnesses (such as this patient's infection), doses of digoxin which produced toxicity did not control the ventricular response. An arterial blood gas would be helpful in this patient, since hypoxia (secondary to the pulmonary infection) may predispose him to digitalis toxicity (16).

It is still too early to conclude that digoxin is ineffective in this patient, since at least four hours are required before digoxin is distributed into cardiac tissue (17). In fact, distribution may be delayed in some subjects for 12 hours (18).

Control of the infection and correction of any acid-base or electrolyte abnormality may allow digoxin to control the ventricular response without the risk of digoxin toxicity. See the chapter on Congestive Heart Failure for discussion of digoxin dosing.

6. Digoxin is ineffective in the patient described above. What additional maneuvers are possible?

Beta blockers such as propranolol have been used either alone or in combination with digoxin after digoxin alone has failed (19). Generally, this use has been in patients without congestive heart failure. However, since many patients with atrial fibrillation also are in failure, propranolol has limited usefulness.

The combination of *propranolol and quinidine* has been studied in chronic atrial fibrillation (20). Using low doses of each drug, conversion to normal sinus rhythm was achieved more readily with the combination than with an individual agent. Fewer side effects were encountered with the combination than with quinidine alone.

Patients unresponsive to conventional therapy might benefit from *verapamil,* a synthetic papav-

Table 2.

COMMONLY ACCEPTED THERAPEUTIC PLASMA CONCENTRATIONS

Drug	Therapeutic Range	Reference
Digoxin	0.9–2.0 ng/ml	13
Quinidine	2–5 mcg/ml	70
Procainamide	4–8 mcg/ml	80
NAPA	9.4–19.5 mcg/ml	89
Phenytoin	10–20 mcg/ml	140
Disopyramide	2–5 mcg/ml	47
Lidocaine	1–6 mcg/ml	102

erine derivative. Sinus rhythm is restored in only 15% of cases (24). However, verapamil will effectively increase A-V block and slow the ventricular rate even in patients unresponsive to digitalis. Patients with congestive heart failure are more resistant and may require higher doses (25).

7. It is decided to start the patient on verapamil. By what route should it be administered? What dose should be used? Summarize the adverse effects which may be associated with its use.

Verapamil is well absorbed orally but undergoes first-pass liver metabolism. As a result, oral doses must be 8–10 times the intravenous dose. The drug is 90% protein bound and has a bi-exponential disposition with an alpha phase lasting 18–35 minutes followed by a beta elimination half-life of 3–7 hours. Intravenous doses of verapamil produce electrocardiographic changes in 1–2 minutes. Its effect peaks in 10–15 minutes and lasts six hours. The response to an oral dose may occur in 30 minutes (22).

Verapamil should be administered intravenously to this patient to achieve a rapid onset of action. The intravenous dose of verapamil in the treatment of atrial arrhythmias is 0.075 mg/kg or 4.5 mg for this 60 kg patient. This dose should be infused over 60 seconds, although it may be given over 10–15 seconds in an emergency. If the response is poor after 30 minutes, the dose may be repeated to a maximum dose of 10 mg. The loading dose may be followed by a constant infusion of 0.005 mg/kg/min or 0.3 mg/min in this patient (21).

The overall incidence of adverse reactions to verapamil is 9% with severe toxicity seen in 1% (21). The most common effect after a parenteral dose is a transient and mild fall in blood pressure; more severe hypotension, bradycardia, AV block, ventricular fibrillation and asystole are reported with the combination of beta blockers and verapamil. Verapamil may have variable effects in patients with heart failure with or without infarction. Even though afterload reduction may improve left ventricular performance (28), and reversal of the arrhythmia may improve the cardiac index, heart failure is considered a contraindication to the use of verapamil (21).

8. A 30-year-old male patient with a long history of hyperthyroidism controlled with methimazole failed to refill his medications. **He came to the emergency room complaining of nervousness, insomnia, and a throbbing sensation in his chest. The ECG indicated atrial fibrillation and he was treated with digoxin without success. Explain. Propranolol is to be used. Is it likely to be effective in this patient? What route and dose are appropriate, and what side effects should be anticipated?**

Atrial fibrillation associated with hyperthyroidism has been reported to be refractory to digoxin (13). This observed resistance may be due to the fact that when equivalent doses of digoxin are administered to hyperthyroid and euthyroid individuals, lower plasma levels occur in the hyperthyroid subjects. Doherty et al (29) suggested that a larger volume of distribution could account for the lower digoxin concentration since they did not observe any alteration in the elimination half-life in the hyperthyroid individuals. Croxson et al (30) discounted this theory since they observed a shorter digoxin half-life in hyperthyroid patients and associated this with an increased glomerular filtration rate. In any case, these patients are unlikely to respond to normal doses of digoxin until their hyperthyroid state is corrected.

Propranolol may be the drug of choice to treat atrial fibrillation induced by hyperthyroidism if there is no evidence of congestive heart failure. Propranolol slows A-V conduction but has little direct effect on atrial tissue (31). Although propranolol has antiarrhythmic properties, it rarely converts atrial fibrillation to normal sinus rhythm when used alone. When used in conjunction with quinidine, 64.8% of patients will convert (8).

This patient may be treated with intravenous propranolol to rapidly reduce the ventricular rate and associated symptoms of hyperthyroidism. An intravenous dose of 0.5–0.75 mg propranolol may be repeated every two minutes up to a maximum of 0.1 mg/kg. Alternatively a total dose of 0.1 mg/kg may be diluted in 50–100 ml D5W and infused over ten minutes (31). The patient should be monitored closely as these doses are given, since decreased cardiac output is more likely to occur early in therapy (32). Propranolol given to patients with arrhythmias and severe congestive heart failure has been associated with improvement in the cardiac index. Apparently in these situations the antiarrhythmic properties predominated while the negative inotropic effects were minimal (33).

Once the ventricular rate is controlled with intravenous therapy, the drug may be given orally. Oral doses are larger than IV doses because of first-pass metabolism after oral administration (34). This extraction process varies significantly among patients as evidenced by a twenty-fold difference in peak serum levels observed after the administration of equivalent oral doses to several subjects (35). This patient may be switched to an oral dose of 10 mg every four to six hours. This may be increased each day by 10 mg per dose until the ventricular rate is maintained at 100 beats/min or the patient develops other evidence of propranolol toxicity. Of course, treatment of the underlying cause of the arrhythmia, the patient's thyroid disease, should be resumed.

The Boston Collaborative Drug Surveillance Program reported a 9.4% incidence of side effects associated with the use of propranolol (36). Reactions are most commonly related to the central nervous system and include fatigue, hallucinations, weakness, insomnia, and nightmares. Yet, when avoided in patients with obvious contraindications, propranolol is considered to be the antiarrhythmic agent with the fewest side effects (1).

9. R.R., a 68-year-old, 50 kg female, was admitted with a chief complaint of shortness of breath. She was diagnosed as having atrial fibrillation and was digitalized. Although the apical rate is 80 beats/min, she is still in atrial fibrillation. What are the possibilities of converting the atrial fibrillation to normal sinus rhythm (NSR)? Describe the various approaches which may be used to make this conversion.

Digitalis alone very rarely converts atrial fibrillation to NSR. The methods for conversion are neither completely effective nor without risk. The mortality rate for electrical conversion is reported to be two percent (20), and in a patient without underlying cardiovascular disease this risk may not be justifiable. This patient does, however, present with complaints that require hospitalization and the potential for conversion is greater now than it will be at a later date (20).

Electrical stimulation is a more rapid and effective method of conversion than is the use of drugs (11). Yet electric shock may abruptly release catecholamines and induce arrhythmias, especially in the presence of digitalis (37). The rhythm is converted 80–90% of the time (38); however, atrial fibrillation will recur in 72% of patients within one year (39). Quinidine is an alternative to electric shock for cardioversion and has a variable response rate of 59–82% (40,41).

Quinidine

10. The patient described above responded to electrocardioversion without complications. Should she be placed on antiarrhythmic drugs chronically? Which drugs are used?

Chronic administration of quinidine prevents the recurrence of atrial fibrillation in only 10–20% of patients (42) and there are some studies which indicate that quinidine may have no effect at all on the recurrence of atrial fibrillation (43). However, it is worthwhile to try to prevent recurrence since effective atrial contraction may improve cardiac output by 30% (44). There is some morbidity associated with the chronic use of quinidine since 30% of patients may develop side effects severe enough to require discontinuation of the drug (45).

Because this arrhythmia compromises the patient's limited cardiac reserve, arrhythmia suppression is probably indicated, but patients must be monitored carefully for adverse drug reactions.

11. The patient is placed on a maintenance dose of quinidine sulfate, 200 mg every 6 hours. Would this dose maintain a therapeutic level in this patient?

To determine if this dosage will maintain a therapeutic concentration, one can estimate the steady-state trough concentration (Cpss min) which will be produced:

$$\text{Cpss min} = \frac{(S)(F)(\text{Dose})/Vd}{1 - e^{-Kd\tau}} \times e^{-Kd\tau} \qquad (\text{Eq. 1})$$

where τ is the dosing interval and Kd is the elimination rate constant. The elimination rate constant can be estimated from the clearance of quinidine which in healthy subjects is 2–5 ml/min/kg. It is reduced in the elderly and in patients with cirrhosis and congestive heart failure (65). Assuming the clearance in this elderly patient is 3 ml/min/kg or 9 L/hr, the Kd can be estimated to be 0.06 hr^{-1}:

$$Kd = \frac{Cl}{Vd} \qquad \text{(Eq. 2)}$$

$$= \frac{9 \text{ L/hr}}{(3 \text{ L/kg})(50 \text{ kg})}$$

$$= 0.06 \text{ hr}^{-1}$$

Using Eq. 1, it can be estimated that the trough concentration will be within the therapeutic range for the specific assay: 1.76 mcg/ml. Therefore, the maintenance dose of 200 mg every 6 hours should adequately maintain the patient:

$$Cpss \text{ min} =$$

$$\frac{(0.82)(0.7)(200 \text{ mg})/(3 \text{ L/kg})(50 \text{ kg})}{1 - e^{-(0.06/hr)(6 \text{ hr})}} \times e^{-(0.06/hr)(6 \text{ hr})}$$

$$= 1.76 \text{ mcg/ml}$$

12. How can ECG changes be used to monitor the toxic effects of quinidine? Do they correlate with serum levels?

Changes in the QRS complex (ie, conduction velocity through the ventricles) correlate most closely with quinidine levels (60). Heissenbuttel et al (61) reported that widening of the QRS complex begins when serum levels reach 2 mcg/ml using a non-specific assay. In addition, there was progressive widening as the quinidine levels rose. The Q-T interval or refractory period also increased but did not correlate as well with the serum level as did changes in the QRS. Other investigators have noted a more pronounced effect of quinidine on the Q-T interval than the QRS (62).

A widening of the QRS of more than 25% (ie, greater than 0.14 sec) should be taken as a warning that toxic levels are being approached. Increases in the QRS complex of 50% or more are often followed by ventricular fibrillation. Most clinicians avoid QRS widening of more than 25%, and few, if any, are willing to continue treatment if there is more than a 50% change in the QRS (61).

13. A 50-year-old male with rheumatic heart disease has been treated with quinidine sulfate 400 mg qid for six months for chronic atrial fibrillation. On repeated visits to the clinic his quinidine plasma levels have been 1 mcg/ml (normal: 2–5 mcg/ml). The patient complains that he cannot find the time at work to take his midday doses. How can the regimen be manipulated to fit into the patient's lifestyle? What is the appropriate dosing interval for quinidine sulfate?

This patient's compliance may be improved through the use of a sustained release (SR) form of quinidine. Single dose studies have shown that the peak serum concentration produced by equivalent doses of the sustained release form of quinidine gluconate is lower and delayed in comparison to that produced by quinidine sulfate. This is caused by the slower absorption rate and lower bioavailability (60% vs 70%) (51). However, multiple dose trials comparing the SR gluconate given every 12 hours with the sulfate salt given every 6 hours have shown the interdose fluctuation of steady-state peaks and troughs to be nearly identical. One and one-half tablets (486 mg) of the quinidine gluconate taken every 12 hours would provide approximately the same amount of quinidine as quinidine sulfate 400 mg qid (52).

Another possible option in this patient is to increase the dose and dosing interval of quinidine sulfate (same total daily dose). Although quinidine sulfate is routinely given every six hours, recent studies employing the high pressure liquid chromatography (HPLC) assay show wide individual variation in quinidine elimination half-life. It may be as short as 2.2 hours in some individuals or as long as 49.5 hours in patients with congestive heart failure or severe liver impairment (53). The six-hour dosing interval is based upon the mean half-life which varies from 4.5 hours (53) to 7.3 hours (54). This wide variation in half-life points to the importance of tailoring the quinidine dose to each individual by monitoring the heart rate, ECG, and plasma concentrations.

14. K.C. is a 65-year-old, 50 kg female who is admitted to the hospital for assessment and treatment of ileus. On physical examination her pulse is noted to be 130/min and irregular. She has had a history of atrial fibrillation which was previously controlled with digoxin 0.25 mg daily and quinidine sulfate 200 mg qid. She has not taken either of these agents for the past 3 months. She also has deteriorating renal function and the last reported creatinine clearance was 25 ml/min. It is planned to reinstitute digoxin and quinidine parenterally. The effect of renal func-

tion and quinidine on digoxin kinetics are known and that drug will be dosed accordingly. (See chapter on Congestive Heart Failure.) How should the quinidine be given? Will her renal function affect the dose of quinidine?

The bioavailability of quinidine sulfate is approximately 70% after undergoing some first-pass hepatic extraction (65). Thus, any parenteral dose should be reduced in relation to an oral dose. Since different salt forms of the drug are used in the parenteral preparations, some additional adjustment is necessary. Quinidine sulfate is generally given orally (83% quinidine) and quinidine gluconate is generally given parenterally (62% quinidine). The following equation may be used to calculate the equivalent parenteral dose of quinidine for this patient (155):

$$\text{Dose of New Salt Form} = \frac{(S)(F)(\text{Dose of Current Dose Form})}{(S)(F \text{ of New Dose Form})}$$

$$= \frac{(0.83)(0.70)(200 \text{ mg})}{(0.62)(1)} \quad \text{(Eq. 3)}$$

$$= 187 \text{ quinidine gluconate q 6 h}$$

The intramuscular injection of quinidine is painful and produces local muscle damage. Also, absorption is erratic and only 85–90% complete (66). Intravenous administration is more reliable but has not been used routinely because of the cardiovascular toxicity associated with this route. However, recent studies indicate that adverse effects are minimal when the gluconate salt is administered slowly at a rate of 0.3–0.4 mg/kg/min IV (67,68). Since intravenous quinidine may produce severe hypotension, this patient should be placed in a coronary care unit where her electrocardiogram, heart rate, and blood pressure can be monitored constantly.

Although an early study indicated that the half-life of quinidine was prolonged in patients with renal failure (69), a more recent study shows no influence of renal failure on the half-life of quinidine (70). The conflicting findings of these two studies can be explained by the assay methodology used by each group. Early quinidine studies used a fluorometric assay which measures metabolites and quinidine contaminants (71). More recent studies use high pressure liquid chromatography (HPLC) which is a more specific assay (72,73). Studies using the fluorometric technique measure a prolonged quinidine elimination in pa-

tients with renal failure since the elimination of renally excreted quinidine metabolites is retarded. Therefore, no dosage adjustment appears to be necessary when quinidine is given to patients in renal failure. However, since some of the quinidine metabolites may contribute to the toxic and therapeutic effects of quinidine, the ECG and blood pressure should be monitored closely in these patients.

15. An 80-year-old female patient with moderately severe congestive heart failure (CHF) uncontrolled by diuretics is placed on quinidine for prophylaxis of atrial fibrillation (400 mg qid). What factors present in this patient might alter the clearance and therefore the dose of quinidine?

Both congestive heart failure and the patient's age may alter quinidine clearance. Only two studies address the impact of heart failure on the pharmacokinetics of quinidine. Kesseler et al (70) reported no change in the elimination half-life in patients with heart failure. Ueda et al (74) confirmed this but found that the volume of distribution and clearance of quinidine were reduced by heart failure.

There are no guidelines for the adjustment of quinidine dose in patients with CHF because the number of patients studied is too small to correlate cardiac output or severity of heart failure with the clearance of quinidine. In addition, there is such wide inter-patient variability in quinidine clearance that normals overlap with heart failure patients. The mean quinidine clearance observed by Ueda et al (54,73,74) suggests that the maintenance dose should be reduced by about 32% in patients with congestive heart failure.

This patient's age may also affect the dose of quinidine. Elderly subjects have significantly prolonged elimination half-lives and a reduced total clearance of quinidine as compared to young controls (75). Since age and heart failure may have additive effects on quinidine clearance, this patient should be started on a relatively low dose of quinidine sulfate (eg, 200 mg qid) and closely evaluated for quinidine efficacy and toxicity.

16. A patient with alcoholic liver disease who has been taking quinidine sulfate 300 mg qid for one month complains of diarrhea at a clinic visit. A trough quinidine level is drawn and is reported to be 8 mcg/ml (normal: 2–5 mcg/ml) by fluorometric assay with

double extraction. How should this patient be managed? What is the meaning of the high quinidine level?

Quinidine is extensively metabolized by the liver, and cirrhotics are known to have prolonged elimination half-lives. Cirrhotics also have an increased volume of distribution of quinidine because of decreased protein binding (76). This decreased protein binding allows more quinidine to exist in the free (active) state which results in a greater pharmacologic effect and higher assay levels. For both of these reasons, it is recommended that low doses of quinidine (eg, 200 mg qid) be used in patients with liver disease (65).

The diarrhea may reflect local irritation secondary to the quinidine and not necessarily the high serum level. Aluminum hydroxide gel has been used to manage the gastrointestinal side effects of quinidine without affecting the drug's absorption or elimination (79). Alternatively, the patient can be switched to a sustained release product which has a lower incidence of gastrointestinal problems (see Question 17). There is also the possibility that reduction of the dose to 200 mg qid will be associated with a resolution of the diarrhea.

The quinidine level reported for this patient is high. In spite of the fact that the fluorometric assay measures both unchanged quinidine and its metabolites, this level probably reflects an excess level of parent compound because the patient's metabolism is impaired. Several assay methods are used by laboratories reporting quinidine levels. The protein precipitation method is the simplest, least reliable fluorometric assay in that it measures considerable amounts of quinidine metabolites and contaminants. The fluorometric assay with double extraction used by the patient's laboratory is more specific than the protein precipitation method. Originally, the therapeutic range for quinidine using this method was 2–8 mcg/ml (77). However, over the years the upper limit of the therapeutic range has decreased to 5 mcg/ml (70). The therapeutic range for the specific HPLC assay has not been established, but a range of 2–3 mcg/ml has been suggested by Drayer et al (78).

17. A patient who was successfully cardioverted was placed on quinidine sulfate 400 mg qid. Two weeks later he returned to clinic complaining of diarrhea. The quinidine sulfate was discontinued and quinidine polygalacturonate (Cardioquin) was ordered to decrease the gastrointestinal (GI) side effects. Comment.

Nausea, vomiting, diarrhea, and anorexia are the most common side effects of quinidine and it is not clear whether they are caused by a central effect of quinidine or by local irritation. Even though many patients complain of diarrhea early in quinidine therapy, most become tolerant to this side effect. Should the symptoms become severe, the patient should be evaluated and treated for electrolyte and acid-base imbalances. If necessary, bothersome diarrhea may be controlled on a short term basis with small doses of opiates or diphenoxylate.

Gerstenbleth (49) found that the polygalacturonate (PG) salt did produce fewer GI side effects. The incidence of side effects was reduced from 56% to 13% when 270 mg of the PG salt was given in place of 200 mg of the sulfate. Both drugs were similarly successful in converting arrhythmias back to normal sinus rhythm. The amount of quinidine in the two dosage forms is approximately the same, but the PG salt is less soluble and releases free quinidine more slowly, producing fewer side effects. Evidence that all of the quinidine from the PG salt is completely absorbed from the GI tract is lacking since blood levels were not measured in this particular study and it was not shown that comparable quinidine levels were achieved by both salt forms.

Others (50) have shown that equivalent doses of the PG salt produce much lower blood levels than the sulfate after seven days of a multiple dosing schedule. The substantial cost difference between the two drugs is also an important consideration, since patients can remain on quinidine for a long period of time.

18. A bruise is noted on the forehead of a patient who has been taking quinidine for the past three months. When questioned about this bruise the patient says that he "passed out" and hit his head as he fell. He has fainted on several occasions since he started taking quinidine, but he was told not to worry because the drug causes the "veins to dilate" and makes the blood pressure go down. He was told that if he felt faint, he should just lie down. Is this "quinidine syncope?" What is the mechanism by which syncope occurs?

How is it treated? What are some other cardiovascular side effects of quinidine?

The patient's problem could be "quinidine syncope," but there is no way to ascertain this unless evidence of ventricular arrhythmias can be documented at the time of his syncopal episodes. Quinidine syncope is caused by drug-induced changes in ventricular rhythm (tachycardias and fibrillation) which decrease cardiac output and cause a loss of consciousness or "syncope." Pallor, muscular twitching, seizures and apnea may also occur.

The drugs of choice to treat quinidine-induced arrhythmias include lidocaine or phenytoin; however, these are often not as effective as external cardiac massage, DC shock, or pacemakers. For those ventricular arrhythmias secondary to quinidine syncope that are refractory to lidocaine and defibrillation, bretylium may be used successfully (59); this may be related to the electrophysiologic antagonism of quinidine by bretylium (58). Needless to say, quinidine must be discontinued in these cases. This is the most serious side effect of quinidine and can result in sudden death if left unrecognized (55,56).

Quinidine may also be hazardous in patients with compromised cardiac output since it also produces a dose-related hypotension by alpha adrenergic blockade and has a direct negative inotropic effect (57).

19. A patient was hospitalized for atrial fibrillation, cardioverted, and placed on quinidine. Four days following his discharge from the hospital he developed a fever with no signs or symptoms of infection. Quinidine is the only medication he is taking. Could the fever be drug-related?

This is a typical reaction to quinidine. Fever most commonly occurs 3–20 days after the drug is initiated and is usually accompanied by other signs of an allergic reaction such as a maculopapular or urticarial rash or thrombocytopenia. There are no apparent signs of allergy in this patient but this is not inconsistent with quinidine fever. Symptoms generally resolve spontaneously once the quinidine is discontinued and no further intervention is required. The patient may be treated with another antiarrhythmic agent such as procainamide.

20. A 65-year-old male with a history of deep vein thrombophlebitis has been taking warfarin for the past two months. He is now experiencing a few PVC's. The plan is to treat these with quinidine 200 mg qid. Comment.

The anticoagulant effect or depression of the prothrombin complex by quinidine or quinine is well known. Koch-Weser (63) reports that patients developed hematuria, conjunctival hemorrhages, guaiac positive stools, hematomas, and epistaxis 6–10 days after the initiation of quinidine in doses of 200 mg qid when begun in combination with warfarin. Changes in the prothrombin time have been noted by the second or third day. This patient is obviously a candidate for such a reaction. An appropriate solution would be to check the prothrombin time in two or three days, caution the patient about symptoms of excessive anticoagulation, and reduce the dose of warfarin if necessary. Another option is to use an alternate antiarrhythmic agent such as procainamide.

There are two proposed mechanisms for this interaction. Since quinidine is highly protein bound, drug-displacement or competition for binding sites is a postulated mechanism. However, quinidine is an organic base and warfarin is an organic acid, and they are most likely bound to different sites on the protein molecule; this would tend to negate the displacement theory. The second postulated mechanism is that quinidine may be a direct antagonist of vitamin K (64).

Procainamide

21. A 64-year-old 60 kg male with a history of chronic glomerulonephritis is admitted to the hospital for work-up and evaluation of a gall bladder problem. On physical examination his pulse is noted to be 135 beats/min and irregular. He has had a history of atrial fibrillation which was successfully cardioverted and maintained on procainamide 250 mg qid; however, the procainamide was discontinued three months ago when he ran out of his medication. Because the patient can take nothing by mouth, the plan is to initiate parenteral procainamide and convert him to oral procainamide when all of the necessary tests are completed. The patient's creatinine clearance is 15 ml/min. Calculate an intravenous loading dose and maintenance dose for this patient.

The *loading dose* for procainamide is determined by the volume of distribution (2 L/kg) and the desired therapeutic plasma concentration (4–8 mg/L) (80,81,155). The volume of distribution is decreased by 25% in patients with congestive heart failure (80), but this patient has no signs or symptoms consistent with heart failure at this time. Using a desired procainamide concentration of 6 mg/L, the loading dose may be calculated as follows:

$$\text{Loading Dose} = \frac{(Vd)(Cp)}{(S)(F)} \qquad \text{(Eq. 4)}$$

where Vd is the volume of distribution, Cp is the desired plasma level, S is the fraction of the administered salt which is the active moiety (0.82 for the HCl salt), and F is the bioavailability.

$$\text{Loading Dose} = \frac{(2 \text{ L/kg})(60 \text{ kg})(6 \text{ mg/L})}{(0.82)(1)}$$

$$= 878 \text{ mg or approximately 800 mg}$$

This loading dose may be administered by small repeated boluses or by infusion. The rate of administration is critical in both cases to avoid acute toxicities. Small boluses of 100 mg may be given over two minutes and repeated every 5 minutes. The rate of administration should never exceed 25–50 mg/min. The boluses are repeated until sustained therapeutic control is achieved, the total loading dose of 800 mg has been administered, or toxicity is encountered. Alternatively, the total dose of 800 mg can by given in a "piggyback" IV bottle over one hour (83).

To maintain the procainamide level at 6 mg/L once the loading dose has been administered, a maintenance infusion must be given. The usual maintenance infusion for procainamide is between 1.48 and 2.96 mg/kg/hr (84). A more specific maintenance dose may be calculated for this patient by adjusting the procainamide clearance to the patient's renal function. The normal procainamide clearance is about 540 ml/min (80); 50% (270 ml/min) is cleared metabolically and 50% (270 ml/min) is cleared renally. If one assumes that a normal creatinine clearance is 100 ml/min, this patient has only 15% of his renal function remaining. His total clearance could then be estimated to be 310 ml/min or 18.6 L/hr if his metabolic clearance is unchanged. The maintenance dose would then be about 136 mg/hr or 2.26 mg/kg/hr (155).

$$\frac{\text{Maintenance Dose}}{\text{(mg/hr)}} = \frac{(Cl)(Cpss \text{ ave})(\tau)}{(S)(F)} \qquad \text{(Eq. 5)}$$

where Cl is clearance, Cpss ave is the average steady state plasma concentration, τ is the dosing interval, S is the fraction of the administered salt which is the active moiety, and F is the bioavailability.

$$\frac{\text{Maintenance Dose}}{\text{(mg/hr)}} = \frac{(18.6 \text{ L/hr})(6 \text{ mg/L})(1 \text{ hr})}{(0.82)(1)}$$

$$= 136 \text{ mg/hr or 2.26 mg/kg/hr}$$

22. All of the necessary tests are completed and the patient is taken off oral restriction. The plan is to discontinue his IV's and place him on oral procainamide. Calculate an oral dose of procainamide which will maintain an average steady state plasma concentration of 6 mg/L and which will not exceed a level of 8 mg/L.

Conversion of the parenteral dose of procainamide to the oral dose is based upon the bioavailability which is reported to be between 75% and 95%; ten percent of patients may absorb less than one-half of the oral dose (81). If bioavailability of 85% is assumed, the hourly oral dose will be 153 mg/hr (130 mg/hr ÷ 0.85). If no more than a 50% change in the plasma level is desired within the dosing interval (ie, 4–8 mg/L), the drug should be administered every half-life. For this patient, the procainamide half-life would be about 5 hours.

$$t\frac{1}{2} = \frac{(0.693)(Vd)}{Cl} \qquad \text{(Eq. 6)}$$

$$= \frac{(0.693)(120 \text{ L})}{18.6 \text{ L/hr}}$$

$$= 4.47 \text{ or approximately 5 hours}$$

If a dosing interval of 4 hours is selected, a dose of 600 mg (4 hr × 150 mg/hr) should maintain procainamide levels in the therapeutic range of 4–8 mg/L. This dose is higher than those traditionally administered (250–500 mg q 3–4 hours) and seems especially high in a patient with renal failure. This may be based upon the fact that the active metabolite, NAPA, accounts for some of the pharmacologic effect and is not considered in the calculation. Alternatively, the empiric doses used may actually produce therapeutic levels in patients who also have some heart failure, since the clearance of procainamide appears to be reduced in these patients (84). In view of all of these considerations, it is reasonable to initiate this patient on a slightly lower than calculated dose (eg 500 mg every 4 hours) and to closely monitor his ECG, plasma levels, and therapeutic response.

23. How should the toxic effects of procainamide be monitored in this patient? Do serum levels correlate with the toxic effects of procainamide?

Procainamide toxicities include gastrointestinal distress, weakness, mild to serious hypotension, a wide QRS interval, ventricular conduction disturbances, and arrhythmias. The ECG changes are similar to those produced by quinidine. Below levels of 12 mg/L cardiovascular toxicities are rare; however, these are quite common at levels above 16 mg/L using the fluorometric assay (80). Signs and symptoms of procainamide-induced systemic lupus erythematosus must also be considered with chronic therapy. See Question 26.

24. A patient with chronic PVC's has been placed on procainamide 500 mg every six hours. On a clinic visit one month later his procainamide level is reported to be 3 mcg/ml and his NAPA level is 16 mcg/ml. The patient is normotensive and without complaints with the exception of increased nervousness and nausea. He continues to have occasional runs of 3–4 PVC's per minute. Comment on the patient's drug levels. Compare NAPA with procainamide with regard to its pharmacokinetics, antiarrhythmic activity, and toxicity. What are the signs and symptoms of NAPA toxicity? How should this patient be managed?

The amount of procainamide which is converted to NAPA varies between 12–25% and is determined by the patient's acetylation phenotype (129,130). Patients who are fast acetylators convert the largest percent of procainamide to NAPA. The steady-state distribution volumes are similar for both compounds (130). Whereas varying renal function produces only small changes in procainamide's half-life, NAPA's half-life increases tremendously from a normal value of approximately 6 hours (130) to 42 hours in anephric patients (131).

This patient's procainamide level is below the therapeutic range of 4–8 mcg/ml (80) which might explain the persistence of the PVC's. In any given patient the pharmacologic effect of NAPA may be additive or antagonistic (89), because the electrophysiologic effects of NAPA are different from those of procainamide (132,133). It is consistent that a beneficial response to procainamide is not predictive of a response to NAPA (89).

The therapeutic range for NAPA is still under investigation. In the treatment of PVC's, NAPA has been used alone with a 70% or greater reduction in arrhythmia frequency; efficacy was associated with levels of 9.4–19.5 mcg/ml in one study (89) and 10–24 mcg/ml in another (134). Therefore, this patient has a NAPA level that is within the therapeutic range, but this has apparently not compensated for the subtherapeutic procainamide concentration. In contrast to this patient, steady-state NAPA levels during chronic procainamide therapy are frequently below the therapeutic range (78,89). However, azotemic patients may have NAPA levels within or beyond the therapeutic range (78).

As illustrated by this patient, one-half of those with therapeutic plasma concentrations of NAPA develop adverse reactions (89). Gastrointestinal symptoms such as nausea and abdominal pain are common as are dizziness, nervousness, and blurred vision. These uniformly disappear if the dose is decreased or the drug discontinued, although the symptoms will often resolve even if the dose is maintained (134). Hemodynamic changes induced by NAPA differ from those caused by procainamide. Mild increases in blood pressure and decreases in heart rate are seen. NAPA produces prolongation in the Q-Tc duration without changing the PR and QRS intervals. The lack of cardiovascular toxicity even with high NAPA serum levels contrasts with the hypotension induced by procainamide.

The PVC's in this patient may not require treatment. They apparently are not compromising the patient's cardiovascular status or predisposing him to more serious arrhythmias. The procainamide should be discontinued and the patient observed for increased arrhythmia frequency and cardiovascular stability.

25. A patient who was hospitalized for a myocardial infarction developed several episodes of ventricular fibrillation that responded to electric shock. Procainamide was given in 100 mg bolus doses to prevent re-

currence; the total dose required was 1250 mg. Plasma levels of procainamide and NAPA obtained two hours later were 12.5 mcg/ml and 1.0 mcg/ml respectively. Are high doses of procainamide usually required for the prophylactic therapy of ventricular fibrillation? Do NAPA levels contribute to the pharmacologic effect? What side effects might be anticipated in this patient if he continued to take procainamide?

The use of conventional doses of procainamide has not been particularly effective in the prevention of electrically-induced ventricular tachyarrhythmias (149). However, larger doses of procainamide (500–1200 mg every 4 hours) were effective in preventing such arrhythmias in 14/16 patients. This ability to inhibit recurrence was dose-dependent, and the efficacy correlated with plasma levels beyond the usual therapeutic range (mean plasma level of 13.6 mcg/ml). However, these investigators were unable to show that successful prophylactic therapy was dependent on the maintenance of these high levels.

Acutely, NAPA probably contributes little to suppression of the arrhythmia since levels are low during the loading dose phase. This is illustrated by this patient. Chronically, high doses of procainamide result in high NAPA levels which may contribute to the antiarrhythmic activity. However, ventricular tachycardia recurred in one patient who had a plasma procainamide level of 5 mcg/ml and a NAPA level of 51.4 mcg/ml. Therefore, therapeutic NAPA levels cannot be relied upon in patients with low procainamide levels.

Toxicity such as hypotension or Q-Tc prolongation were not observed acutely in patients receiving high doses of procainamide in this situation. However, chronic high dose therapy produced gastrointestinal effects in 12.5% of the patients and drug-induced lupus in 25%. (150)

26. A.X. is a 54-year-old female with a long history of systemic lupus erythematosus (SLE) and recurrent, debilitating paroxysmal atrial tachycardia. What is the risk of administering procainamide to this patient? Characterize procainamide-induced lupus. What role could NAPA play (if available) in such a patient?

Twenty-nine percent of patients who take therapeutic doses of procainamide on a chronic basis will develop a reversible lupus-like syndrome characterized by arthralgias, myalgias, fevers, pleuritis, and pericarditis (85). Although the risk of developing this syndrome is minimal if procainamide is taken on a short term basis (86), symptoms may occur as early as two weeks and as late as two years after therapy is initiated (87). The syndrome is believed to be caused by the parent compound since slow acetylators have a higher risk of developing the syndrome. The incidence of positive laboratory tests (eg antinuclear antibody, ANA and LE cells) without other symptoms is substantially higher (86,88). It has been estimated that 83% of patients will develop positive serologic tests. Since many of these patients may never become symptomatic, these findings are not particularly useful monitoring parameters and should not be used as the sole criterion to determine whether procainamide should be discontinued. These tests revert to normal when the drug is discontinued. The drug-induced syndrome also differs significantly from the idiopathic form of SLE in that there is not a higher incidence in females and it is rarely complicated by leukopenia, anemia, thrombocytopenia, hypergammaglobulinemia, or renal failure (87).

It could be argued that since the syndromes differ substantially in their presentations, procainamide is not likely to exacerbate the pre-existing, idiopathic form. However, there are two main reasons to avoid the use of procainamide in this patient. First, her arrhythmia is recurrent, and it is likely that she will need to take procainamide chronically; this will increase the risk of developing the syndrome. Secondly, the drug-induced complication is monitored on the basis of symptoms and since arthralgias, myalgias, fever, and pleuritis are all common symptoms of the idiopathic form, it would be virtually impossible to differentiate between the two forms without serologic testing. Since quinidine has the same basic effects on the myocardium, it is a reasonable alternative to procainamide for this patient.

NAPA when used alone has a lower incidence of elevated ANA titers than procainamide (89). In fact, NAPA has been used in patients who have developed procainamide-induced lupus without exacerbating either the titers or symptoms. There is the risk of exposing NAPA-treated patients to small amounts of procainamide since 2.8% of NAPA is deacetylated (90). Theoretically, patients with renal failure would be exposed to the greatest amount of procainamide while receiving

NAPA. Until there is further study, NAPA should be avoided in patients with procainamide-induced lupus who also have impaired renal function.

AV Block

27. Quinidine was to be administered to a patient with atrial fibrillation by slow intravenous infusion; however, the infusion device malfunctioned and delivered the entire dose over two minutes. The patient is no longer in atrial fibrillation but has a sinus rhythm with a rate of 80 and first degree atrioventricular (AV) block. What is AV block? How should this patient be treated?

There are three types of AV block. First degree AV block is a delay in impulse conduction through the AV node and is characterized by a P-R interval greater than 0.21 seconds. All atrial impulses will be conducted as long as the AV node has completed the repolarization process from the previous impulse. Second degree AV block is characterized by a block of some of the atrial impulses so that a ventricular response is not elicited following every atrial beat. In this case some of the P waves produced by atrial depolarization would not be followed by a QRS complex on the ECG. Second degree AV block is characterized as being either Mobitz Type I or Mobitz Type II. Mobitz Type I AV block is usually due to increased vagal tone or drug therapy such as digitalis and usually requires no treatment other than elimination of the precipitating factor. Mobitz Type II may at times be difficult to distinguish from Type I; yet, it is a more serious condition in that syncopal attacks associated with ventricular fibrillation occur commonly in these patients. Most patients with Type II will eventually develop complete or third degree block if they survive previous episodes of syncopy and ventricular fibrillation. In third degree block none of the atrial depolarizations are transmitted to the ventricles; consequently the ventricles are paced by ectopic foci or ventricular pacemakers. Although patients with third degree heart block can sustain an adequate cardiac output, they are subject to the risk of ventricular arrhythmias and cardiovascular collapse.

The drugs most commonly used for AV block are catecholamines, such as isoproterenol or possibly epinephrine (92,93). An artificial electrical pacemaker may also be appropriate. It should be noted that the administration of drugs such as

quinidine, procainamide, disopyramide, or potassium to patients with a high degree of AV block may increase the block and suppress the ventricular pacemakers, resulting in cardiac standstill (92). If the patient is being paced electrically, the above mentioned agents may be used.

This patient has only first degree AV block (a direct effect of quinidine) and has sufficient cardiac output. In this situation quinidine should be discontinued until the AV block resolves. Once this occurs and the quinidine plasma levels have declined, the drug may be reinstituted.

PAT with Block

28. A 65-year-old female admitted in congestive heart failure was initially treated with furosemide 80 mg IV and digoxin 1.0 mg. Approximately four hours later after she had diuresed 2.5 liters she developed a rapid pulse. An ECG showed an irregular rhythm with a rate from 120–200 which was interpreted as paroxysmal atrial tachycardia (PAT) with block. The laboratory reported a serum potassium of 2.9 mEq/L and a plasma digoxin level of 2.8 ng/ml. What is the etiology of the arrhythmia and the treatment?

PAT with block induced by digitalis is a dangerous arrhythmia that has a mortality rate of 28–58% (94,95). Until proven otherwise, this arrhythmia should be considered to be a symptom of digitalis toxicity in a patient taking digitalis. The presence of a high digoxin level and hypokalemia in this patient both make digitalis toxicity highly likely. The digoxin and furosemide should be discontinued immediately. Potassium, the drug of choice for PAT due to digoxin, typically slows the atrial rate, improves AV conduction and converts the arrhythmia to NSR (96). However, it must be administered carefully since high levels of potassium may actually enhance AV block.

PVC's

29. A patient with a well documented myocardial infarction (MI) develops unifocal premature ventricular contractions (PVC's) at a rate of 25 per minute. Should this arrhythmia be treated? How?

PVC's are ectopic beats originating in the ventricles. PVC's are the most common arrhythmia and comprise 40–80% of all arrhythmias which occur following an MI (97). Isolated PVC's are probably benign but may be predecessors of the frequently fatal ventricular tachycardia, flutter or fibrillation. Studies evaluating the prophylactic effects of procainamide, quinidine and lidocaine in the treatment of PVC's do not demonstrate a significant lowering of the mortality rates of the treated group (98,99). Lidocaine and procainamide have comparable antiarrhythmic efficacy for PVC's (100,101). However, lidocaine is the drug of choice for PVC's following an MI (8) because procainamide produces more depression of myocardial contractility, AV conduction and peripheral resistance (100).

Lidocaine

30. A 30-year-old 70 kg man admitted for an abdominal stab wound has become hypotensive from excessive blood loss. His ECG shows multifocal PVC's. Should this arrhythmia be treated? How?

The increased work load on the heart to maintain tissue perfusion coupled with myocardial hypoxia probably contribute to ventricular irritability in this patient. Nasal oxygen and blood transfusions will benefit this patient more than an antiarrhythmic; however, the presence of multifocal PVC's indicates that there are several ectopic foci. Multifocal PVC's are ectopic beats of differing morphology. PVC's that interrupt the T wave, are multifocal in origin, which occur in a series of two or more, or exceed a frequency of five per minute should be treated with lidocaine.

Lidocaine should be administered to produce levels of 1–6 mcg/ml (102). This is usually accomplished by the administration of one or more bolus injections followed by an infusion. Although an infusion can be initiated without loading doses, steady-state therapeutic levels may not be reached for approximately six hours since the elimination half-life for lidocaine in normal subjects is 100 minutes (103). The size of each bolus is governed by the relatively small volume of the central compartment, since the myocardium behaves as though it were located in this compartment (see chapter on Clinical Pharmacokinetics for an explanation of two-compartment models) (155). The average central compartment volume is 0.5 L/kg (104). This volume may be reduced to 0.3 L/kg in patients with congestive heart failure and in-

creased to 0.6 L/kg in patients with chronic liver disease (103). The volume of the central compartment can be used in the Eq. 4 to determine the size of each bolus:

$$\frac{\text{Loading}}{\text{Dose}} = \frac{(Vd)(Cp)}{(S)(F)} \qquad \text{(Eq. 4)}$$

$$= \frac{(0.5 \text{ L/kg})(70 \text{ kg})(3 \text{ mg/L})}{(1)(1)}$$

$$= 105 \text{ mg or approximately } 100 \text{ mg}$$

A 100 mg bolus given over 1–2 minutes should produce a level of 3 mg/L in the central compartment. If an alpha or distribution half-life of 8 minutes is assumed, a second bolus of 50 mg may be given in 10 minutes if there is a recurrence of the PVC's. Another 50 mg bolus may be given 10 minutes thereafter if necessary (105).

If the patient has normal cardiac output, it may be assumed that each 10 mcg/kg/min of a lidocaine maintenance infusion will produce a level of 1 mcg/ml. If it is desired to maintain a level of 3 mcg/ml, the patient should be placed on a maintenance infusion of 30 mcg/kg/min or 2 mg/min.

31. A patient is admitted to the CCU with a chief complaint of chest pain. The ECG is consistent with an MI but otherwise indicates a normal sinus rhythm. The patient was started on prophylactic lidocaine. Discuss the dosing of lidocaine in an MI.

In 40% of MI patients there is inadequate warning of dangerous ventricular tachyarrhythmias (119). Thus lidocaine has been recommended as prophylaxis after an MI. Cardiac output is frequently decreased after an MI and this may require the use of lower than usual doses of lidocaine (103). It appears that both the clearance and volume of distribution are decreased to about 60% of their usual values, indicating that both the loading and maintenance doses should be reduced (120). It is interesting to note that because both the volume of distribution and clearance are reduced by the same magnitude, the elimination half-time will remain unchanged. Many intensive care units are capable of measuring cardiac output which may be applied to published nomograms for estimating dosing requirements of lidocaine (105). In the absence of these sophisticated techniques, modest doses of lidocaine should be used with careful monitoring of side effects. It should be remembered that side effects which occur during the maintenance infusion may take several hours to dissipate, as the elimination half-life (100 minutes) rather than the distribution half-life (10 minutes) will be the primary factor in determining the rate with which the plasma level will be decreasing (121).

32. A 50-year-old, 70 kg male is admitted to the hospital from a nursing home because of mental confusion. He has a long history of alcoholism and is diagnosed as having developed the hepato-renal syndrome. On the tenth hospital day he developed multifocal PVC's associated with an acute upper gastrointestinal bleeding episode. A lidocaine infusion of 4 mg/min is planned. Comment on the dose of lidocaine in this patient.

The volume of distribution for lidocaine is increased and the hepatic clearance is decreased in patients with hepatic disease. This results in a prolonged elimination half-life of approximately 300 minutes (120). Therefore, therapeutic concentrations may not be achieved for several hours unless a loading or bolus dose is administered. Since the volume of distribution is probably increased in this patient, a larger total loading dose may be required. However, in most cases, the usual bolus dose of 50–100 mg is given and additional injections of one-half the usual amount are administered if the arrhythmia reappears within 10–30 minutes.

The maintenance infusion of 4 mg/min or 57 mcg/kg/min may be too high for this patient in view of the fact that his hepatic clearance of lidocaine may be decreased. This dose would be expected to produce a steady state plasma concentration of 5.7 mcg/ml in a patient with normal cardiac function (see Question 30). Since there is no reliable way to quantify the degree of liver dysfunction, this patient should be started on a low dose infusion of 30 mcg/kg/min or less and carefully monitored over the next 20–24 hours (ie 3–5 half-lives of 300 minutes).

Signs of central nervous system lidocaine-related toxicities should be monitored. Dizziness, drowsiness, paresthesias, visual disturbances, and euphoria may be seen at the higher end of the therapeutic range, while confusion, dysarthria, psychoses, coma, respiratory failure and seizures may occur at levels above 6 mcg/ml (122).

In this patient lidocaine plasma levels should also be monitored since many of the symptoms of lidocaine toxicity will be difficult to identify in a patient such as this with pre-existing confusion.

No additional dose adjustments will have to be made for the patient's renal dysfunction, since less than 10% of lidocaine is excreted unchanged in the urine and there appear to be no alterations in the volume of distribution or clearance of this drug in the presence of renal failure.

33. An 83-year-old woman with frequent coupled PVC's has been receiving lidocaine by constant infusion at a rate of 3 mg/min for 30 hours. Approximately 12 hours after therapy was initiated, the lidocaine level was 5 mcg/ml. The patient is asymptomatic and has no history of coronary artery disease. Should her PVC's be treated?

The decision to treat this patient's PVC's is a difficult one. Even though coupled PVC's may precipitate ventricular fibrillation, the incidence of ventricular fibrillation decreases with advancing age. For example ventricular fibrillation following a myocardial infarction (MI) is one-half as common in patients over 50 years of age (123). Another consideration in this decision is the fact that lidocaine toxicity is more likely to occur in elderly patients. In one study, lidocaine toxicity was three times more frequent in those over 60 years of age (126). This patient is asymptomatic, has no heart disease and probably requires no suppression. Alternatively, her PVC's could be moderately suppressed (see Question 34). If she were asymptomatic but had a history of heart disease and she had more than 30 PVC's per hour, she would definitely require suppressive therapy.

34. A decision is made to maintain lidocaine therapy. What are the endpoints of therapy?

The endpoint used for the treatment of PVC's is controversial and varies from study to study. A reduction in the frequency of PVC's by 75% or more from the baseline or placebo period is used as an endpoint in many studies. However, this method is limited by the fluctuating nature of PVC frequency and has not been correlated with a decrease in patient morbidity or mortality. Assessment of the mortality rate from sudden death is difficult in that the mortality rate of MI patients following discharge is low (10–20%) and long follow-up periods are required. A more attractive method of monitoring suppressive antiarrhythmic therapy has been proposed by Lown et al (124). They use an arbitrary rating scale to evaluate PVC's and attempt to use drugs to achieve a low rating by converting the patient from ectopic beats that may precipitate fatal ventricular tachyarrhythmias to less malignant PVC's or none at all. In this 83-year-old patient, a reasonable goal would be to achieve a rating of 1 or 2:

    0 = no PVC's
    1 = occasional, isolated (30/hour)
    2 = frequent (greater than 30/hour)
    3 = multiform
    4 = repetitive (couplets or salvos)
    5 = early (interrupting the T wave)

It should be emphasized that a change in rating may not necessarily decrease the mortality rate.

35. Does the lidocaine level drawn at 12 hours represent a steady-state level? What precautions must be taken in patients receiving prolonged infusions of lidocaine?

Even patients with heart failure or liver disease should achieve steady-state after 12 hours of uninterrupted lidocaine infusion (105). At least, this is what the pharmacokinetic data obtained using lidocaine infusions of 12 hours or less would suggest. Nevertheless, after 30 hours, levels which are considerably higher than those measured at a theoretical "steady-state" have been observed by investigators studying uncomplicated myocardial infarction patients receiving lidocaine infusions for 30 or more hours. The prolonged half-life in these patients (3.2–4.3 hours) and progressive accumulation after 6–12 hours suggest that prolonged infusions are associated with impaired elimination. It has therefore been recommended that the rate of infusion of lidocaine be reduced by one-half after the first 24 hours (127,128).

36. Discuss the pharmacokinetics and activity of tocainide and mexiletine, investigational drugs which show promise in the treatment of PVC's and other ventricular arrhythmias.

Tocainide. Research into lidocaine congeners has produced an oral agent with good bioavailability and efficacy: tocainide. Lidocaine has a high hepatic extraction ratio after it is administered orally and is therefore poorly available by that route. Tocainide is a primary amine which does not undergo initial N-de-ethylation, as does lidocaine, and the oral bioavailability approaches 100% (106). Oral absorption is rapid with peak plasma levels occurring at about one hour. Approximately 40% of tocainide is eliminated unchanged by the kidneys (107); the remainder is metabolized to glucuronide conjugate (108). The long elimination half-life of 10–17.5 hours (109) may mean that the drug can be administered less frequently than currently available oral agents.

Tocainide has been used primarily in the treatment of ventricular arrhythmias. It appears to be more effective than quinidine in the management of PVC's. One study demonstrated an efficacy rate of 75% for tocainide as compared with a rate of 46% for quinidine and 11% for placebo (110). An even higher success rate has been reported in uncontrolled studies (111).

The effective plasma concentration for tocainide remains to be determined. Some patients respond to levels as low as 3.5 mcg/ml, while others require levels of 14.6 mcg/ml. Greater than 70% reduction of PVC's may require levels above 6 mcg/ml (109), but toxicity usually limits increasing the drug level beyond 10 mcg/ml (111). Although its half-life suggests the possibility of a 12-hour dosing interval, an increase in ectopic beats at the end of the dosing interval and toxicity produced by peak levels following a 12-hourly dose must be considered (112). Doses range from 400–600 mg every 8–12 hours.

Toxicity may limit the value of tocainide for chronic use in that adverse effects occur in 64–70% of patients receiving the drug (110,113). The most common minor symptoms include anorexia, nausea, and vomiting that may be transient. Persistent adverse symptoms include lightheadedness, incoordination, tremor, confusion, and paresthesias. There have been no consistent changes in blood pressure, heart rate, or ECG interval changes. One patient on tocainide had a relapse of procainamide-induced lupus (111).

Mexiletine, another lidocaine congener, has an oral bioavailability of 88%, and peak levels appear in 2–4 hours; however, absorption may be delayed and incomplete in patients who have suffered a myocardial infarction. Intravenous injection of the drug results in extensive tissue distribution involving three compartments and a large volume of distribution of 600 L or more. Mexiletine is extensively metabolized; only 8% is excreted unchanged in the urine. The elimination half-life is 10.4 hours in healthy subjects and 16.7 hours in cardiac patients. (116)

Mexiletine has little effect on the normal sinus node, although patients with the sick sinus syndrome have developed severe bradycardia. Since this drug does not alter atrial refractoriness, it has not been effective in the treatment of atrial flutter or fibrillation. The primary utility of mexiletine has been in the prophylaxis of ventricular arrhythmias and in the treatment of arrhythmias unresponsive to lidocaine. Arrhythmias may recur in as many as 72% of patients who have suffered an MI after lidocaine is discontinued; mexiletine and procainamide appear to be equally effective in the management of these late ventricular arrhythmias. Oral mexiletine has been found to be as effective as procainamide in the reduction of PVC's but with fewer side effects. (114,115)

An intravenous loading dose regimen of 150–250 mg over 2–5 minutes followed by an infusion of 250 mg over thirty minutes, and another dose of 250 mg over 2.5 hours has been used. This can be followed by a maintenance infusion of 1 mg/min (116). Oral doses of 200–300 mg every eight hours will produce therapeutic blood levels of 0.75–2.0 mcg/ml in 67% of patients (117).

An early sign of mexiletine toxicity is a fine tremor of the hands; this progresses to dizziness, blurred vision, dysarthrias, diplopia, ataxia, nystagmus, and confusion as the levels increase. Although mexiletine generally produces only slight changes in blood pressure and cardiac function, hypotension, sinus bradycardia, atrial fibrillation, and widened QRS complexes may occur (118).

Disopyramide

37. A patient with chronic atrial fibrillation has been electrically converted. The patient has been treated in the past with quinidine and procainamide with poor results due to toxicity and noncompliance. Disopyramide is being considered. Is disopyramide likely to be effective in this patient? What toxicities can be expected if the drug is used?

Disopyramide 100–200 mg qid can be used as an alternative oral antiarrhythmic agent for patients who fail to respond to quinidine and procainamide or who cannot take these agents for other reasons. Disopyramide was originally approved for use for the treatment of ventricular

arrhythmias, but it appears to be as effective as quinidine in the treatment of atrial fibrillation (48).

Disopyramide may have a lower incidence of side effects than quinidine. In one double blind study comparing these two drugs, the incidence of side effects associated with quinidine was 36%, versus 10% for patients taking disopyramide. Nevertheless, other studies report a substantial incidence of side effects related to disopyramide, many of which are related to the dose-dependent anticholinergic properties of this drug. Urinary retention occurs in 10–20% of patients, while dry mouth is reported in up to 40% of patients (46). Gastrointestinal disturbances including diarrhea, nausea, and vomiting which may limit the acceptance of the other antiarrhythmics occur in 8% of disopyramide-treated patients. Disopyramide produces little prolongation of the P-R, Q-T or QRS intervals (47). In most patients receiving usual doses, disopyramide does not alter the heart rate, cardiac output or arterial pressure; however, the drug does have important negative inotropic effects, and acute heart failure has been precipitated in some patients (See Questions 38 and 39).

38. A patient with chronic renal failure (creatinine clearance 25 ml/min) who is to be admitted for an elective cholecystectomy next week is noted to have 4–5 PVC's/min at an office visit. The patient says she is "allergic" to quinidine and has a history of procainamide-induced lupus erythematosus. Is disopyramide likely to be effective in suppressing the PVC's? Describe its pharmacokinetic characteristics and suggest a dose for this patient.

Disopyramide is approved for use for ventricular arrhythmias and has been effective in reducing ventricular tachycardia, ventricular fibrillation, infarct extension, and mortality in patients with myocardial infarction (135). It appears to be effective in patients unresponsive to lidocaine (136). In this patient, the PVC's should be controlled prior to surgery to prevent intraoperative arrhythmias. If the PVC's had been noted on admission, the treatment of choice would have been lidocaine; however, since the patient will not be undergoing surgery for one week, it is appropriate to initiate an oral antiarrhythmic agent such as disopyramide.

Disopyramide is 78% bioavailable, and a single dose produces peak levels in 3.8 hours. The volume of distribution varies from 20–89 liters. Metabolism occurs to some extent, but 71% of unchanged drug is eliminated renally. The elimination half-life in normal subjects is 4.4–8.2 hours; this increases to 8.3–43 hours (46) in patients with renal dysfunction. The suggested therapeutic range is 2–5 mcg/ml (47).

The standard loading dose is 300 mg. This is reduced to 200 mg in patients with heart failure, hepatic disease, or patients such as this with renal failure. The usual maintenance is 150 mg every 6 hours. This may be increased to 200 mg every 6 hours (maximum) if there is no response to the lower dose. A maintenance dose of 100 mg every 6 hours is recommended for patients with cardiac decompensation, liver disease, or moderate renal failure.

Severe renal failure requires a change in the dosing interval from 6 hours to 10, 20, or 30 hours in patients with creatinine clearances of 15–40, 5–15, or 1–5 ml/min respectively (46). For this patient, 150 mg every 10 hours is a reasonable maintenance dose. A loading dose of 200 mg can be given initially.

39. A 50-year-old patient with long-standing coronary artery disease was placed on disopyramide for occasional PVC's. He was subsequently brought into the emergency room where he was found to be unresponsive and cyanotic. His blood pressure was unobtainable and the electrocardiogram showed intermittent runs of ventricular fibrillation with a sinus rhythm. Physical examination revealed anasarca. Could this patient's condition have been induced by disopyramide? How should the patient be managed?

Cases of disopyramide-induced ventricular arrhythmias have been reported (151). Typically there is prolongation of the QT interval without change in the QRS complex, but syncope is not always present. Ventricular fibrillation may occur after only a few doses or after several months of therapy. The arrhythmias usually resolve after discontinuation of the disopyramide; however, there may be considerable delay. In these instances lidocaine, propranolol, phenytoin, and procainamide have been used, but the drug of choice has not been determined.

Disopyramide has also produced cardiogenic shock without concomitant ventricular arrhythmias (152). Dopamine and nitroprusside were used successfully to reverse the shock. See the chapter entitled Intensive Care Therapeutics for a detailed discussion of the use of these drugs in the therapy of cardiogenic shock.

The edema observed in this patient may also be induced by disopyramide. In a prospective analysis of 100 patients receiving disopyramide, Podrid et al (153) reported that the overall risk of developing congestive heart failure while taking this agent was 16%. A prior history of CHF definitely predisposed patients to this effect in that 55% of patients with controlled CHF developed heart failure while taking this drug. Still, some patients developed heart failure without any prior evidence of CHF. Disopyramide-induced heart failure does not appear to be dose-related and may develop acutely after taking disopyramide; however, it is more commonly associated with chronic administration. Symptoms resolve one to four days after the drug is discontinued, but digitalis and diuretics may be used for symptomatic patients. For more severe cases (illustrated by this patient), inotropic agents and vasodilators are indicated (see the chapter entitled Intensive Care Therapeutics). The frequency and severity of the negative inotropic effect associated with disopyramide appear greater than that associated with other antiarrhythmics, even propranolol (154), prompting some clinicians to favor other drugs.

Ventricular Tachycardia

40. A 56-year-old, 70 kg male is admitted to the emergency room with a history of having ingested ten 0.25 mg digoxin tablets five hours prior to admission. An ECG shows ventricular tachycardia, and it is decided to institute phenytoin. Is this an appropriate drug to use in the treatment of this arrhythmia? What dose and route of administration should be used? How should the patient be monitored?

Digitalis-induced ventricular tachycardia occurs in 10% of patients with digitalis-induced arrhythmias and is associated with a 60–100% mortality rate. Generally, electric shock is the treatment of choice for ventricular tachycardia; however, it should be avoided in patients who have high levels of digitalis because it may precipitate ventricular flutter or fibrillation in these individuals (137). Both lidocaine and phenytoin have been used to treat digitalis-induced arrhythmias, but phenytoin is considered by some to be the drug of choice (137). Although phenytoin is generally most effective in the treatment of ventricular arrhythmias, it appears to be effective in the treatment of both ventricular and atrial arrhythmias induced by high doses of digitalis (137–139).

The intravenous (IV) route of administration for phenytoin is recommended because results are much more predictable. The intramuscular route is not advised because the absorption, although complete, may be slow and erratic. When phenytoin is given by the IV route it should be infused at a maximum rate of 50 mg/min to avoid cardiotoxicity associated with the diluent, propylene glycol (139a). Intravenous administration also poses some compatibility problems which are discussed in the chapter on Epilepsy.

The total loading dose of phenytoin is approximately 1 gram. Usually this is administered as four 250 mg boluses at a rate of 50 mg/min every hour. As an alternative, Bigger (140) recommends a dose of 100 mg IV every 5 minutes until an effect is seen. It should be noted that the arrhythmia may recur 20–30 minutes after the initial administration of phenytoin boluses. This is related to the distribution of phenytoin from plasma into the tissues. Subsequent maintenance doses of 300 to 400 mg of phenytoin daily administered orally or parenterally usually maintain therapeutic concentrations.

As the bolus doses are administered, careful attention should be paid to the appearance of toxicities and serum phenytoin levels which correlate with both the toxic and therapeutic effects of the drug. Seventy percent of arrhythmias respond to levels of 10–18 mcg/ml while 20% respond to levels of 2–10 mcg/ml. Side effects almost always occur at levels above 20 mcg/ml. Levels of 20, 30, 40 mcg/ml classically correspond with nystagmus, ataxia and dysarthria, and mental confusion, respectively (141).

41. A 70 kg patient who was admitted to the coronary care unit is currently hypotensive secondary to an episode of ventricular tachycardia which is unresponsive to electrical cardioversion and lidocaine. Bretylium is currently being considered. Is bretylium likely to be effective in the treatment of this arrhythmia? What is its mechanism of action, and what are its pharmacokinetic character-

istics? What dose should be administered and by what route?

Bretylium is currently approved for use in the treatment of life-threatening ventricular arrhythmias that have failed to respond to lidocaine and procainamide. Several studies indicate the bretylium is approximately 70% effective in the treatment of such arrhythmias (142), and it is therefore reasonable to use in this patient.

Bretylium is taken up by the adrenergic nerve terminal where it initially releases then inhibits the release and re-uptake of norepinephrine. The sympathomimetic action lasts 20–30 minutes after administration and may produce hypertension and dysrhythmia. This initial adrenergic stimulating activity may also precipitate more serious arrhythmias in patients with digitalis toxicity. The sympathetic blockade ultimately increases receptor sensitivity to catecholamines. Bretylium inhibits re-entry rhythms by prolonging the action potential duration of normal tissues to that of surrounding infarcted tissue. In contrast to other agents used to treat ventricular arrhythmias, it does not depress automaticity or slow conduction. (144)

Bretylium is eliminated unchanged by the kidneys, and its half-life varies widely between 4.2–16.9 hours. The elimination is multiphasic and does not follow first-order kinetics (146).

Bretylium is available for parenteral use only and may be given intramuscularly (IM) or intravenously (IV). The usual dose of 5–10 mg/kg may be administered undiluted by rapid IV injection. The usual response occurs within minutes, and if there is no effect after 15–30 minutes, the dose may be repeated to a total of 30 mg/kg. To maintain arrhythmia suppression, bretylium may be infused at a rate of 1–2 mg/min or injected over 8–10 minutes in a dose of 5–10 mg/kg every 6–8 hours. A maximum daily dose of 30 mg/kg/day is suggested (144). The intramuscular administration has an onset of action of 15 minutes, a maximum activity of 2–3 hours, and a duration of action of 10–20 hours (145).

42. The patient described above was given 500 mg of bretylium by IV push over 10 seconds. The ventricular tachycardia resolved in 30 minutes; however, the patient complained of nausea shortly after the injection. After sinus rhythm was restored the patient's blood pressure dropped from 110/70 to 90/65 mm Hg. What side effects must be an-

ticipated when bretylium is administered? How can they be avoided and treated if they occur? Is this patient exhibiting signs and symptoms of bretylium toxicity?

Bretylium is generally well tolerated. In clinical trials the drug was discontinued because of toxicity in 6–8% of patients (142). Nausea and vomiting are unusual except when the drug is given by rapid injection as in this patient. This suggests that this side effect could be minimized by infusing bolus doses of the drug over several minutes.

Initially hypertension and tachyarrhythmias secondary to the release of norepinephrine may be observed; however, hypotension is more common. A fall in arterial blood pressure which is usually less than 20 mm Hg (as in this patient) is observed in two-thirds of the individuals receiving this agent one hour after injection (147).

The hypotension is primarily orthostatic and can usually be reversed or minimized by placing the patient in a recumbent position. Excessive hypotension can be treated with intravenous fluids; vasopressors may also be used, but because adrenergic terminals may be supersensitive to the catecholamines, low doses should be administered. Dopamine, for example, has been used successfully in a dose of 0.7 mcg/kg/min (148). This patient should be placed in a recumbent or reverse Trendelenberg position if he is symptomatic from the hypotension. His mentation and peripheral perfusion should be assessed to determine if pressor agents are indicated.

It is of interest that unlike other antiarrhythmics, bretylium has no negative inotropic effects on the heart, and the afterload reduction produced by the hypotension may actually benefit patients with left ventricular failure.

References

1. Singh BN: Rational basis of antiarrhythmic therapy: Clinical pharmacology of commonly used antiarrhythmic drugs. Angiol. 1978; 29:206.
2. Nevins MA et al: The treatment of acute myocardial infarction. Med Clin North Am. 1974; 38:435.
3. Epstein S et al: The early phase of myocardial infarction: Pharmacologic aspects of therapy. Ann Intern Med. 1973; 78:818.
4. Cooper JA et al: Atropine in the treatment of cardiac disease. Am Heart J. 1969; 78:124.
5. Thomas M et al: Effect of atropine on bradycardia and hypotension in acute myocardial infarction. Br Heart J. 1966; 28:409.
6. Marako PR et al: Factors influencing infarct size in experimental coronary artery occlusions. Circulation. 1971; 43:67.
7. Fisch C: Digitalis intoxication. JAMA. 1971; 216:1770.
8. Warner H: Therapy of common arrhythmias. Med Clin North Am. 1974; 58:995.
9. Rosen MR et al: Electrophysiology and pharmacology of cardiac arrhythmias and toxic effect of digitalis. Am Heart J. 1975; 89:391.
10. Hillestad L et al: Quinidine in maintenance of sinus rhythm after electro-conversion of chronic atrial fibrillation, a controlled clinical study. Br Heart J. 1971; 33:518.
11. Hall JI et al: Factors affecting cardioversion of atrial arrhythmias with special reference to quinidine. Br Heart J. 1968; 30:84.
12. Jelliffe RW: A mathematical analysis of digitalis kinetics in patients with normal and reduced renal function. Math Bio. 1967; 1:305.
13. Chamberlain DA et al: Plasma digoxin concentrations in patients with atrial fibrillation. Br Med J. 1970; 3:429.
14. Goldman S et al: Inefficacy of "therapeutic" serum levels of digoxin controlling the ventricular rate in atrial fibrillation. Am J Cardiol. 1975; 35:651.
15. Redfors A: Plasma digoxin concentration—its relation to digoxin dosage and clinical effects in patients with atrial fibrillation. Br Heart J. 1972; 34:383.
16. Smith TW: Digitalis toxicity: Epidemiology and clinical use of serum concentration measurements. Am J Med. 1975; 58:470.
17. Shapiro W et al: Relationship of plasma digitoxin and digoxin to cardiac response following intravenous digitalization in man. Circulation. 1970; 42:1065.
18. Reuning RH et al: Role of pharmacokinetics in drug dosage adjustment. J Clin Pharmacol. 1973; 13:127.
19. David D et al: Inefficacy of digitalis in the control of heart rate in patients with chronic atrial fibrillation: Beneficial effect of an added beta adrenergic blocking agent. Am J Cardiol. 1979; 44:1378.
20. Levi GF et al: Combined treatment of atrial fibrillation with quinidine and beta blockers. Am Heart J. 1972; 34:911.
21. Singh BN et al: Verapamil: A review of its pharmacological properties and therapeutic use. Drugs. 1978; 15:169.
22. Schomerus M et al: Physiologic disposition of verapamil in man. Cardiovasc Res. 1976; 10:605.
23. Gibson D et al: The use of beta adrenergic receptor blocking drugs in dysarrhythmias. Progr Cardiovasc Dis. 1969; 12:16.
24. Aronow WS et al: Verapamil in atrial fibrillation and atrial flutter. Clin Pharmacol Ther. 1979; 26:578.
25. Dominic J et al: Verapamil plasma levels and ventricular rate response in patients with atrial fibrillation and flutter. Clin Pharmacol Ther. 1979; 26:710.

26. Klein HO et al: Effects of oral verapamil in treatment of chronic atrial fibrillation. Arch Intern Med. 1979; 139:747.

27. Klein HO et al: Verapamil-digoxin interaction. N Engl J Med. 1980; 303:160.

28. Ferlinz J et al: Effects of verapamil on myocardial performance in coronary disease. Circulation. 1979; 59:313.

29. Doherty JE et al: Digoxin metabolism in hypo and hyper thyroidism, studies with tritiated digoxin. Ann Intern Med. 1966; 64:489.

30. Croxson MS et al: Serum digoxin in patients with thyroid disease. Br Med J. 1975; 236:566.

31. Singh BN et al: Beta adrenergic receptor blocking drugs in cardiac arrhythmias. Drugs. 1974; 7:426.

32. Prichard BN et al: Treatment of hypertension with propranolol. Br Med J. 1969; 1:7.

33. Lemberg L et al: The use of propranolol in arrhythmias complicating acute myocardial infarction. Am Heart J. 1970; 80:479.

34. Evans GH et al: Disposition of propranolol. Clin Pharmacol Ther. 1973; 14:487.

35. Shand DG: Pharmacokinetic properties of beta adrenergic blocking drugs. Drugs. 1974; 7:39.

36. Greenblatt DJ et al: Adverse reactions to beta adrenergic receptor blocking drugs. Drugs. 1974; 7:118.

37. Lown B: Electrical reversion of cardiac arrhythmias. Br Heart J. 1967; 29:469.

38. Radford MD et al: Long-term results of D.C. reversion of atrial fibrillation. Br Heart J. 1968; 30:91.

39. Sjelky PS et al: Maintenance of sinus rhythm after atrial defibrillation. Br Heart J. 1970; 32:741.

40. Cramer G: Early and late results of conversion of atrial fibrillation with quinidine. Acta Med Scand. 1968; S490:5.

41. Goldman MJ: The management of chronic atrial fibrillation: Indications for and methods of conversion to sinus rhythm. Progr Cardiovasc Dis. 1960; 2:465.

42. Sokolow M et al: The clinical pharmacology and use of quinidine in heart disease. Progr Cardiovasc Dis. 1961; 33:316.

43. Oram S et al: Further experience of electrical conversion of atrial fibrillation to sinus rhythm; analysis of one hundred patients. Lancet. 1964; 1:1294.

44. McIntosh HD et al: The hemodynamic consequences of arrhythmias. Progr Cardiovasc Dis. 1966; 8:330.

45. Lown B et al: Approaches to sudden death from coronary heart disease. Circulation. 1971; 44:130.

46. Heel RC et al: Disopyramide: A review of its pharmacological properties and therapeutic use in treating cardiac arrhythmias. Drugs. 1978; 15:331.

47. Koch-Weser J: Disopyramide. N Engl J Med. 1979; 300:957.

48. Hartel G et al: Disopyramide in the prevention of recurrence of atrial fibrillation after electroconversion. Clin Pharmacol Ther. 1974; 15:551.

49. Gerstenbleth T et al: Quinidine utilization in cardiac arrhythmias. N Y State J Med. 1966; 66:701.

50. Goldberg WM: The relationship of dosage schedules to blood level of quinidine using all available quinidine preparations. Can Med Assoc J. 1964; 91:991.

51. Woo E et al: Short and long acting oral quinidine preparations. Angiol. 1978; 29:243.

52. Collste P et al: Quinidine dosage, with special reference to oral loading dose schedule. Br J Clin Pharmacol. 1979; 7:293.

53. Carliner NH et al: Quinidine therapy in hospitalized patients with ventricular arrhythmias. Am Heart J. 1979; 98:708.

54. Ueda CT et al: Disposition kinetics of quinidine. Clin Pharmacol Ther. 1976; 19:30.

55. Miller DS et al: Quinidine-induced recurrent ventricular fibrillation (quinidine syncope). South Med J. 1971; 64:597.

56. Selzer A et al: Quinidine syncope: Paroxysmal ventricular fibrillation occurring during treatment of chronic atrial arrhythmias. Circulation. 1964; 30:617.

57. Mason DT et al: The clinical pharmacology and therapeutic applications of the antiarrhythmic drugs. Clin Pharmacol Ther. 1970; 11:460.

58. de Acevedo IM et al: Electrophysiologic antagonism of quinidine and bretylium tosylate. Am J Cardiol. 1974; 33:633.

59. Van Der Ark CR et al: Quinidine syncope: A report of successful treatment with bretylium tosylate. J Thorac Cardiovasc Surg. 1976; 72:464.

60. Cho YW: Quantitative correlation of plasma and myocardial quinidine concentrations with biochemical and electrocardiographic changes. Am Heart J. 1973; 85:648.

61. Heissenbuttel RH et al: The effect of oral quinidine on intraventricular conduction in man: Correlation of plasma quinidine with changes in QRS duration. Am Heart J. 1970; 80:453.

62. Feldman A et al: The effect of quinidine sulfate on QRS duration and QT and systolic time intervals in man. J Clin Pharmacol. 1977; 17:134.

63. Koch-Weser J: Quinidine-induced hypoprothrombinemic hemorrhage in patients on chronic warfarin therapy. Ann Intern Med. 1968; 68:511.

64. Koch-Weser J: Drug interactions with coumarin anticoagulants. N Engl J Med. 1971; 285:487.

65. Ochs HR et al: Clinical pharmacokinetics of quinidine. Clin Pharmacokinetics. 1980; 5:150.

66. Greenblatt DJ et al: Pharmacokinetics of quinidine in humans after intravenous, intramuscular and oral administration. J Pharmacol Exper Ther. 1977; 202:365.

67. Hirschfeld DS et al: Clinical and electrophysiologic effects of intravenous quinidine in man. Circulation. 1974; 50:S230.

68. Ochs HR et al: Intravenous quinidine: Pharmacokinetic properties and effects on left ventricular performance in humans. Am Heart J. 1980; 99:468.

69. Bellet S et al: Relation between serum quinidine levels and renal function. Am J Cardiol. 1971; 27:368.

70. Kessler KM et al: Quinidine elimination in patients with congestive heart failure or poor renal function. N Engl J Med. 1974; 290:706.

71. Cramer G et al: Quantitative determination of quinidine in plasma. Scand J Clin Lab Invest. 1963; 15:553.

72. Guentert TW et al: Divergence in pharmacokinetic parameters of quinidine obtained by specific and nonspecific assay methods. J Pharmacokinetics Biopharm. 1979; 7:303.

73. Ueda CT et al: Absolute quinidine bioavailability. Clin Pharmacol Ther. 1976; 20:260.

74. Ueda CT et al: Quinidine kinetics in congestive heart failure. Clin Pharmacol Ther. 1978; 23:158.

75. Ochs HR et al: Reduced quinidine clearance in elderly persons. Am J Cardiol. 1978; 42:481.

76. Kessler KM et al: Quinidine pharmacokinetics in patients with cirrhosis or receiving propranolol. Am Heart J. 1978; 96:627.

77. Edgar AL et al: Experiences with the photofluorometric determination of quinidine in blood. J Lab Clin Med. 1950; 36:478.

78. Drayer DE et al: Steady state serum levels of quinidine and active metabolites in cardiac patients with varying degrees of renal function. Clin Pharmacol Ther. 1978; 24:32.

79. Romankiewicz JA et al: The noninterference of aluminum hydroxide gel with quinidine sulfate absorption: An approach to control quinidine-induced diarrhea. Am Heart J. 1978; 96:518.

80. Koch-Weser J et al: Procainamide dosage schedules, plasma concentrations and clinical effects. JAMA. 1971; 215:1454.

81. Koch-Weser J: Pharmacokinetics of procainamide in man. Ann NY Acad Sc. 1971; 179:370.

82. Giardiona E et al: Intermittent intravenous procainamide to treat ventricular arrhythmias. Ann Intern Med. 1973; 78:183.

83. Lima JJ et al: Pharmacokinetic approach to intravenous procainamide therapy. Eur J Clin Pharmacol. 1978; 13:303.

84. Lima JJ et al: Safety and efficacy of procainamide infusions. Am J Cardiol. 1979; 43:98.

85. Henningsen NC et al: Effects of long term treatment with procainamide, a prospective study with special regard to ANF and SLE in fast and slow acetylators. Acta Med Scand. 1975; 198:475.

86. Kosowsky BD et al: Long term use of procainamide following acute myocardial infarction. Circulation. 1973; 47:1204.

87. Sheldon JHS et al: Procainamide induced systemic lupus erythematosus. Ann Rheum Dis. 1970; 29:236.

88. Klajman A et al: Occurrence, immunoglobulin pattern and specificity of antinuclear bodies in sera of procainamide treated patients. Clin Exp Immunol. 1970; 7:641.

89. Roden DM et al: Antiarrhythmic efficacy, pharmacokinetics and safety of N-acetylprocainamide in human subjects: Comparison with procainamide. Am J Cardiol. 1980; 46:463.

90. Stec GP et al: Kinetics of N-acetylprocainamide deacetylation. Clin Pharmacol Ther. 1980; 28:659.

91. Moss AJ: Use of edrophonium in evaluation of supraventricular tachycardias. Am J Cardiol. 1966; 17:58.

92. Sobel B et al: Cardiac dysrrhythmias. In *Harrison's Principles of Internal Medicine,* 8th ed., edited by G Thorn et al, McGraw-Hill Co., New York, 1977, p 1187.

93. Sokolow M et al: Conduction defects. In *Clinical Cardiology,* Larne Medical, Los Altos, 1977, p 421.

94. Bigger JT et al: Digitalis toxicity: Drug interactions promoting toxicity and the management of toxicity. Semin Drug Treatment. 1972; 2:147.

95. Chung EK: Digitalis induced cardiac arrhythmias. Am Heart J. 1970; 79:845.

96. Lown B et al: Paroxysmal atrial tachycardias with block. Circulation. 1960; 21:129.

97. Metzler LE et al: The incidence of arrhythmias associated with acute myocardial infarction. Progr Cardiovasc Dis. 1966; 9:50.

98. Koch-Weser et al: Antiarrhythmic prophylaxis with procainamide in acute myocardial infarction. N Engl J Med. 1969; 281:1253.

99. Pitt A et al: Lidocaine prophylaxis to patients with acute myocardial infarction. Lancet. 1971; 1:612.

100. Bigger JT et al: The use of procainamide and lidocaine in the treatment of cardiac arrhythmias. Progr Cardiovasc Dis. 1969; 1:515.

101. Schwartz MI et al: Comparative antiarrhythmic effects of intravenously administered lidocaine and procainamide and orally administered quinidine. Am J Cardiol. 1970; 26:520.

102. Gianelli R et al: Effect of lidocaine on ventricular arrhythmias in patients with coronary heart disease. N Engl J Med. 1967; 277:1215.

103. Thomson PD et al: The influence of heart failure, liver disease and renal failure on the disposition of lidocaine in man. Am Heart J. 1971; 82:417.

104. Rowland M et al: Disposition kinetics of lidocaine in normal subjects. Ann NY Acad Sci. 1977; 179:383.

105. Benowitz N: Clinical applications of the pharmacokinetics of lidocaine. Cardiovasc Drug Ther. 1969; 1:515.

106. Lalka D et al: Kinetics of the oral antiarrhythmic lidocaine congener, tocainide. Clin Pharmacol Ther. 1976; 19:757.

107. McDevitt DG et al: Antiarrhythmic effects of a lidocaine congener, tocainide, 2-amino-2', 6'-propionoxylidide, in man. Clin Pharmacol Ther. 1976; 19:396.

108. Elvin AT et al: Tocainide kinetics and metabolism: Effects of phenobarbital and substrates for glucuronyl transferase. Clin Pharmacol Ther. 1980; 28:652.

109. Winkle RA et al: Clinical efficacy and pharmacokinetics of a new orally effective antiarrhythmic, tocainide. Circulation. 1976; 54:884.

110. Wasenmiller JE et al: Effect of tocainide and quinidine on premature ventricular contractions. Clin Pharmacol Ther. 1980; 28:431.

111. Winkle RA et al: Long-term tocainide therapy for ventricular arrhythmias. Circulation. 1978; 57:1008.

112. Woolsley RL et al: Suppression of ventricular ectopic depolarizations by tocainide. Circulation. 1977; 56:980.

113. Ryan W et al: Efficacy of a new oral agent (tocainide) in the acute treatment of refractory ventricular arrhythmias. Am J Cardiol. 1979; 43:285.

114. Jewitt DE et al: Comparative antiarrhythmic efficacy of mexiletine, procainamide and tolamolol in patients with symptomatic ventricular arrhythmias. Postgrad Med J. 1977; S53:158.

115. Campbel RWF et al: Comparison of procainamide and mexiletine in prevention of ventricular arrhythmias after acute myocardial infarction. Lancet. 1975; 1:1257.

116. Prescott LF et al: Absorption, distribution and elimination of mexiletine. Postgrad Med J. 1977; S53:50.

117. Pottage A: Oral dosage schedules for mexiletine. Postgrad Med J. 1977; S53:155.

118. Chew CYC et al: Mexiletine: A review of its pharmacological properties and therapeutic efficacy in arrhythmias. Drugs. 1979; 17:161.

119. Dhurhandhar RJ et al: Primary ventricular fibrillation complicating acute myocardial infarction. Am J Cardiol. 1971; 27:347.

120. Thomson PD et al: Lidocaine pharmacokinetics in advanced heart failure, liver disease, and renal failure in humans. Ann Intern Med. 1973; 78:499.

121. Collinsworth KA et al: The clinical pharmacology of lidocaine as an antiarrhythmic drug. Circulation. 1974; 50:1217.

122. Selden R et al: Central nervous system toxicity induced by lidocaine. JAMA. 1967; 201:908.

123. Lie KI et al: Characteristics and predictability of primary ventricular fibrillation. Eur J Cardiol. 1974; 1:379.

124. Lown B et al: Management of patients with malignant ventricular arrhythmias. Am J Cardiol. 1977; 39:910.

125. Wilhesmsson C et al: Reduction of sudden death after acute myocardial infarction by treatment with alprenolol. Lancet. 1974; 2:1157.

126. Lie KI et al: Lidocaine in the prevention of primary ventricular fibrillation. N Engl J Med. 1974; 291:1324.

127. Prescott LF et al: Impaired lidocaine metabolism in patients with myocardial infarction and cardiac failure. Br Med J. 1976; 1:939.

128. Lelorier J et al: Pharmacokinetics of lidocaine after prolonged intravenous infusions in uncomplicated myocardial infarctions. Ann Intern Med. 1977; 87:800.

129. Gibson TP et al: Acetylation of procainamide in man and its relationship to isonicotinic acid hydrazide acetylation phenotype. Clin Pharmacol Ther. 1975; 17:395.

130. Dutcher JS et al: Procainamide and N-acetylprocainamide kinetics investigated simultaneously with stable isotope methodology. Clin Pharmacol Ther. 1977; 22:447.

131. Stec GP et al: N-acetylprocainamide pharmacokinetics in functionally anephric patients before and after perturbation by hemodialysis. Clin Pharmacol Ther. 1979; 26:618.

132. Dangman KH et al: Effects of N-acetylprocainamide on cardiac purkinje fibers. Pharmacol. 1978; 20:150.

133. Jaillon P et al: Electrophysiologic comparative study of procainamide and N-acetylprocainamide in anesthetized dogs: Concentration-response relationships. Circulation. 1979; 60:1385.

134. Kluger J et al: The clinical pharmacology and antiarrhythmic efficacy of acetylprocainamide in patients with arrhythmias. Am J Cardiol. 1980; 45:1250.

135. Kidner PH et al: The effects of disopyramide in the prevention of ventricular irritability following acute myocardial infarction. J Irish Med Assoc. 1977; 70S14:22.

136. Sbarbaro J et al: Suppression of ventricular arrhythmias with intravenous disopyramide and lidocaine: Efficacy comparison in a randomized trial. Am J Cardiol. 1979; 44:513.

137. Chung EK: Digitalis induced cardiac arrhythmias. Am Heart J. 1970; 79:845.

138. Dreifus LS et al: Current status of diphenylhydantoin. Am Heart J. 1970; 30:709.

138a. Mercer EN et al: The current status of diphenylhydantoin in heart disease. Ann Intern Med. 1967; 60:1084.

139. Eddy JD et al: Treatment of cardiac arrhythmias with phenytoin. Br Med J. 1969; 270:273.

139a. Louis S et al: The cardiocirculatory changes caused by intravenous Dilantin and its solvent. Am Heart J. 1967; 74:523.

140. Bigger JT et al: Relationship between the plasma level of diphenylhydantoin and its cardiac antiarrhythmic effects. Circulation. 1968; 38:363.

141. Kutt H et al: Diphenylhydantoin metabolism, blood levels and toxicity. Arch Neurol. 1964; 11:642.

142. Koch-Weser J: Drug Therapy: Bretylium. N Engl J Med. 1979; 300:473.

143. Gillis RA et al: Deleterious effects of bretylium in cats with digitalis induced ventricular tachycardia. Circulation. 1973; 47:974.

144. Heissen-Buttel et al: Bretylium tosylate: A newly available antiarrhythmic drug for ventricular arrhythmias. Ann Intern Med. 1979; 91:229.

145. Bryan CK et al: Bretylium tosylate: A review. Am J Hosp Pharm. 1979; 36:1189.

146. Romhilt DW et al: Evaluation of bretylium for the treatment of premature ventricular contractions. Circulation. 1972; 45:800.

147. Bernstein JG et al: Effectiveness of bretylium tosylate against refractory ventricular arrhythmias. Circulation. 1972; 45:1024.

148. Luomanmaki K et al: Bretylium tosylate. Arch Intern Med. 1975; 135:515.

149. Wellens HJJ et al: Effect of procainamide, propranolol, and verapamil on mechanism of tachycardia in patients with chronic recurrent tachycardia. Am J Cardiol. 1977; 40:579.

150. Greenspan AM et al: Large dose procainamide therapy for ventricular tachyarrhythmia. Am J Cardiol. 1980; 46:453.

151. Nicholson WJ et al: Disopyramide-induced ventricular fibrillation. Am J Cardiol. 1979; 43:1053.

152. Stony JR et al: Cardiogenic shock and disopyramide phosphate. JAMA. 1979; 242:654.

153. Podrid PJ et al: Congestive heart failure caused by oral disopyramide. N Engl J Med. 1980; 302:614.

154. Stephen SA: Unwanted effects of propranolol. Am J Cardiol. 1966; 18:463.

155. Winter ME: *Basic Clinical Pharmacokinetics,* Applied Therapeutics, Inc., San Francisco, 1980.

Chapter 12

Angina Pectoris

Barbara L. Greenberg and Moses S. Chow

Angina pectoris, a clinical syndrome characterized by chest pain due to transient myocardial ischemia, results when the metabolic demands of the heart for oxygen exceed the ability of diseased coronary arteries to supply adequate blood flow to the myocardium.

Pathogenesis

The most common cause of angina pectoris is coronary atherosclerotic heart disease, a pathological condition of the coronary arteries characterized by atheromatous lesions which thicken and harden vessel walls (1). These lesions narrow

245

the coronary vessel wall lumen and reduce blood flow to the myocardium. Although atherosclerotic coronary arteries usually provide adequate blood flow during rest or moderate activity, stenotic arteries cannot supply the extra oxygenated blood required by the heart during exercise or other stress. This imbalance of supply and demand results in myocardial ischemia and chest pain. Further complications can occur if the atherosclerotic lesions progress, causing complete occlusion of blood flow. Coronary artery vasospasm (transient narrowing of the coronary) may cause some types of angina and myocardial infarction (2). Ross (3) provides a more comprehensive review of the various theories related to the pathogenesis of atherosclerosis.

Myocardial oxygen demand, referred to as myocardial oxygen consumption or MVO_2, is determined by several physiologic factors (4,5). Many of the drugs used to treat angina are designed to alter these physiologic determinants. The most important determinant of myocardial oxygen consumption is the tension created in the myocardial muscle wall. Because both the volume of blood inside the ventricle and the systolic pressure created in the ventricle influence the intramyocardial tension, a drug that elevates systolic pressure augments intramyocardial wall tension and raises oxygen demand. Heart rate also affects oxygen demand. Any drug or physiologic stimulus that increases heart rate, without influencing the other factors, elevates oxygen consumption. The third major determinant of oxygen demand is contractility. An increase in the inotropic state of the heart usually elevates oxygen consumption.

Goals of Therapy

The goals in treatment of angina pectoris are: to relieve symptoms, to improve the quality of life, to prevent complications such as sudden death, myocardial infarction and arrhythmias, and to increase life expectancy. Risk factors for atherosclerotic cardiovascular disease have been identified, and modifying these risks may enhance life expectancy. Drug therapy centers around alleviating symptoms to allow a more normal lifestyle.

Stable Angina

1. T.P., a 57-year-old, hard-driving, male bank executive, was hospitalized to evaluate his chest pain. He visited his private physi-cian regularly for three months prior to admission complaining of a dull, heavy, squeezing substernal chest pain that occasionally radiated to the left shoulder and arm and lasted only a few minutes. The chest pain usually occurred during exertion and subsided when he rested. T.P. was 6 feet tall, weighed 250 pounds, had hypertension for seven years, and smoked one pack of cigarettes a day for 20 years. His father died of a heart attack at the age of 49, and his brother had hypertension for ten years.

T.P.'s admission electrocardiogram showed no abnormalities. His serum cholesterol and triglycerides were elevated. Other clinical laboratory tests were normal. During his graded treadmill exercise test, ST segment depression appeared after 4 minutes. The chest pain that occurred during the test responded well to nitroglycerin. The physicians diagnosed stable angina pectoris, most likely secondary to coronary artery disease.

What signs and symptoms of angina pectoris did this patient manifest?

T.P.'s dull, heavy, squeezing substernal chest pain that radiated to his left sholder and arm is typical of angina. The pain may radiate also to the back, neck, or lower jaw. A patient with angina often describes this discomfort as gripping, pressing, boring, choking, or squeezing rather than calling this sensation pain. T.P. had a classic pattern of pain; it occurred with exertion and subsided with rest or when the precipitating cause was discontinued. Although his electrocardiogram was normal when he was resting, the chest pain and ST segment depression induced by his graded exercise test indicated myocardial ischemia.

2. What are the risk factors associated with coronary atherosclerotic heart disease, and which of these did T.P. have?

Studies of the natural history of coronary atherosclerosis indicate a relationship between the development of the disease and certain characteristics of lifestyle and medical history. These characteristics are termed risk factors. The risk factors associated with atherosclerotic heart disease are cigarette smoking, elevated serum lipids, family history of premature atherosclerosis, hypertension, obesity, a hard-driving (Type A) personality, male gender, advanced age, diabetes mellitus, and a sedentary lifestyle (6–8). Because patient T.P. had the first seven of these risk factors, he was at greater risk than the general population for developing atherosclerotic heart disease.

3. What changes in daily activities would decrease the number of angina episodes this patient experiences or would help prevent the progression of coronary atherosclerosis?

Although some risk factors are unalterable (ie, age, sex, and family history), modifying those risk factors that can be changed may slow the progression of atherosclerotic heart disease, and possibly extend life expectancy (6,8,9). T.P. should stop smoking cigarettes and begin a diet that will achieve ideal body weight and lower blood lipid concentrations. If possible, his daily activities should be structured to avoid emotional stress, and he should take regular vacations from work. His hypertension should be treated to maintain normal blood pressures (10). A graduated exercise program would increase his exercise tolerance and decrease the incidence of chest pain (11).

Certain daily activities enhance the likelihood of chest pain because they increase myocardial oxygen demand and reduce exercise capacity (12). These activities include intense exertion (shoveling snow, running), exposure to very cold weather or hot humid weather, eating large meals, and emotional stress. T.P. should avoid these activities.

Some beverages and over-the-counter medications may aggravate angina. The clinician should take a careful drug history and encourage T.P. to refrain from taking common cold medications that contain sympathomimetics, diet medications with stimulants or thyroid derivatives, and caffeinated beverages such as coffee, tea, and colas (13).

4. T.P. has stable angina. Compare this type of angina with the other presentations of angina.

Stable angina is the classical angina; it is precipitated by physical activity and relieved by rest or nitroglycerin. *Unstable angina* comprises a group of syndromes ranging from stable angina to myocardial infarction. Subgroups of unstable angina include: angina of recent onset (less than 4 weeks), angina at rest, and stable angina with a changing pattern (14,15). Unstable angina was once termed "crescendo angina" and "impending myocardial infarction" because any increase in frequency or severity of angina may indicate a worsening of the disease or a myocardial infarction. *Nocturnal angina* or angina decubitus may

occur during recumbency when congestive heart failure complicates coronary artery disease. *Prinzmetal's variant angina* refers to angina at rest associated with ST segment elevation. Prinzmetal's angina is discussed in more detail in Questions 35 to 41.

Nitroglycerin

5. T.P.'s physician prescribed sublingual nitroglycerin 0.6 mg prn chest pain. What are the mechanisms of action of nitroglycerin in the treatment of angina?

Although the mechanism of action of nitroglycerin is not understood completely, its therapeutic benefit is probably due to actions on both the peripheral circulation and the coronary blood flow. The primary effect of nitroglycerin is relaxation of vascular smooth muscle, especially of the peripheral veins (16). Dilation of the venous system increases venous capacitance resulting in pooling of blood in the peripheral veins which decreases venous return to the heart and diminishes myocardial preload. Arteriolar relaxation causes a mild decrease in systemic arterial and mean blood pressures by lowering peripheral resistance which reduces ventricular afterload. These effects on the capacitance and resistance vessels result in a decrease in myocardial wall tension (a major determinant of myocardial oxygen consumption) thereby decreasing the oxygen demands of the heart muscle (12,17,18). Although a reflex rise in heart rate and contractility tend to increase myocardial oxygen consumption, the hemodynamic changes caused by nitroglycerin have a net beneficial effect on the myocardium (19,20,21,22).

Although nitroglycerin causes generalized dilation of coronary arteries in normal subjects who do not have coronary artery disease, the effects of nitroglycerin in patients with atherosclerotic coronary arteries are less clear. Nitroglycerin injected directly into coronary arteries did not relieve pacing-induced angina in patients with coronary artery disease (23). This finding is consistent with the theory that coronary arteries which are narrowed and stiffened by atherosclerotic plaques cannot dilate in response to nitroglycerin (18).

Other recent evidence suggests that nitroglycerin can affect coronary artery circulation. In animals, nitroglycerin induces a redistribution of coronary blood flow to ischemic subendocardium (24). Studies in patients with coronary atherosclerosis suggest that nitroglycerin can both dilate coronary arteries and improve collateral circulation, even in the presence of severe major coronary artery stenosis (25–28). Nitroglycerin also dramatically reverses angina caused by coronary artery vasospasm (29,30).

It has not been established whether the antianginal efficacy of nitroglycerin is due primarily to its action on the peripheral vasculature or to its effect on coronary artery blood flow. The relative contribution of each of these actions probably depends upon the degree of coronary stenosis, the presence of collateral blood vessels, and the ability of the coronary vessels to dilate in each individual patient.

6. When should T.P. use sublingual nitroglycerin?

Immediately upon experiencing chest pain T.P. should sit down and dissolve one tablet under his tongue (not swallow it). Nitroglycerin is well established as an effective treatment of angina pectoris. Sublingual nitroglycerin rapidly relieves chest pain, usually within 3 to 5 minutes, making it ideally suited for treatment of acute angina (31). No more than three tablets should be taken over a 15-minute period. Continued chest pain may indicate a myocardial infarction (32,33).

T.P. can take nitroglycerin prophylactically 5 to 10 minutes before activities that he knows trigger his angina attacks (eg, sexual intercourse). In addition to relieving chest pain, nitroglycerin may help prevent an angina attack. When tested using standardized exercise protocols, sublingual nitroglycerin improved exercise tolerance at 45 and 60 minutes (34–36).

7. Nitroglycerin relieved T.P.'s chest pain after the exercise test. What clinical data, in addition to a favorable response to nitroglycerin, are needed to diagnose angina pectoris?

Nitroglycerin aids in the diagnosis of angina (31,37), because nitroglycerin rapidly relieves the chest pain associated with most forms of angina. However, to confirm the diagnosis other findings must be present, such as a history of pain on exertion, lessening of pain with rest, and electrocardiographic changes. Diffuse esophageal spasm may cause acute chest pain similar to angina (38,39). Because nitroglycerin also relieves the pain associated with diffuse esophageal spasm, a response to nitroglycerin alone may indicate either condition. Accordingly, a response to nitroglycerin should be considered along with other clinical findings to confirm the diagnosis of angina.

8. *Side Effects.* After T.P. took one sublingual nitroglycerin 0.6 mg, he experienced a severe pounding and fullness in his head. He refused to use nitroglycerin again because the headache was worse than his chest pain. What would reduce the likelihood of nitroglycerin-induced headaches in T.P.?

T.P.'s first dose of 0.6 mg was too large and probably caused his headache. The ideal dose for nitroglycerin is one that relieves angina pain in 3 to 5 minutes but does not produce headache or hypotension. In individuals first starting nitroglycerin treatment, a lower strength tablet, preferably 0.3 mg, often is sufficient and less likely to cause unpleasant side effects. If this dose still produces a headache, a trial dose of 0.15 mg may be worthwhile.

Headaches, the most common side effect of nitroglycerin, are usually of short duration (5 minutes) and seldom last more than 20 minutes in patients with coronary artery disease (31,40). Often described as a pounding fullness, these headaches create a problem clinically when patients are hesitant to take their nitroglycerin prophylactically or even during episodes of chest pain. Because tolerance to headaches often develops with subsequent therapy, the use of mild oral analgesics such as aspirin or acetaminophen during the first few weeks of therapy is helpful.

9. What instructions about the other common side effects of nitroglycerin should be given to this patient?

Dizziness and syncope are other undesirable effects of nitroglycerin (31). These side effects, which result from a rapid lowering of blood pressure, occur more frequently in elderly patients and in patients taking other vasodilators or antihypertensive drugs. To avoid the symptoms of postural hypotension and its attendant reflex tachycardia, the patient should sit down when taking sublingual nitroglycerin. If the dizziness is excessive, the patient should elevate his or her feet 12 inches (32,33). If systemic hypotension is severe enough to compromise coronary or cerebral circulation, the dose of nitroglycerin must be reduced; if this approach is not possible, other antianginal agents should be used.

Minor gastrointestinal symptoms are reported (40,41). These do not require any special treatment.

10. *Plasma Monitoring.* What is the value of plasma concentrations of nitroglycerin in dosing nitroglycerin in this patient?

Due to the lack of studies that correlate plasma concentrations of nitroglycerin with its ability to prevent angina attacks, the clinical response of each individual patient is more reliable than plasma concentrations for determining the optimal dose of nitroglycerin. Nitroglycerin is difficult to assay because it is volatile and small therapeutic blood concentrations persist in the serum for only a short time. Recently, analytical methods sufficiently sensitive to detect nitroglycerin in blood have been developed (42–44).

The results of a pharmacokinetic analysis (42) of nitroglycerin 0.6 mg given sublingually to 10 normal subjects indicated that nitroglycerin appeared in the plasma at 0.5 minutes, reached a peak of 2.3 ng/ml at 2 minutes, and was barely detectable at 20 minutes. In these normal subjects, changes in heart rate and systolic blood pressure paralleled the plasma concentrations. Another study (43) involving normal subjects and patients with unstable angina or acute myocardial infarction found that blood pressure responses did not correlate with nitroglycerin plasma concentrations. Because circulatory changes do not necessarily correlate with antianginal effects, these hemodynamic changes do not directly apply to dosing of angina patients.

11. *Storage and Handling.* What instructions should T.P. receive regarding proper storage and handling of nitroglycerin?

T.P. should be warned to keep his sublingual nitroglycerin tablets in the original container to prevent loss of potency. The cotton filler should be discarded after initial opening of the bottle. Immediately after each use, the cap should be closed tightly. The drug should not be stored in the inside pocket of clothes, in an automobile glove compartment, near a fireplace, or in other hot humid locations. Patients should not put bottles containing nitroglycerin in the refrigerator (45). A fresh, potent nitroglycerin tablet will produce a burning sensation under the tongue when administered sublingually (46). Headache, if it occurs, is another indication of potency.

Time, light, heat, air, and moisture inactivate nitroglycerin. The drug should be stored in an amber glass container with a tight fitting screw cap. Nitroglycerin stored for 201 days in amber or clear glass vials lost 5% of its potency; in polystyrene vials, 14 to 29% was lost; and in pill boxes, 72% was lost. Storage in strip-packaging resulted in a 47 to 90% loss of potency after 52 days (47). Storing nitroglycerin with large amounts of cotton filler, or with other tablets or capsules is undesirable. When nitroglycerin was stored in a glass vial with a large amount of cotton filler, only 33% of its activity remained after one week (48). Two aspirin tablets absorbed 400 mcg of nitroglycerin when the drugs were stored together for a month (49).

Nitroglycerin is a volatile liquid prepared in a tablet form. At 70°F, 400 mcg nitroglycerin supplies enough vapor to fill a 3 dram prescription vial over 10,000 times (49). Even if all the vapor escapes each time the bottle is opened, the loss is not significant. If the bottle is not closed tightly, however, the vapor can escape continuously, resulting in a constant loss of the drug. Dispensing nitroglycerin in bottles containing 25 tablets, rather than 100 tablets, decreases the probability of using tablets that have lost their potency.

Long-Acting Nitrates

12. H.S., a 64-year-old woman with stable angina pectoris, takes sublingual nitroglycerin prn for her chest pain. Because she must use over eight tablets a day to control her angina, her physician would like to prescribe a longer acting nitrate.

How can the efficacy and duration of action of "long-acting" nitrates be evaluated?

Although longer acting preparations of nitroglycerin and other nitrates enjoy wide use, the value of these preparations remains controversial. Reports concerning the efficacy of long-acting nitrates contain conflicting results. Some reports evaluating nitrates use questionable study methods to determine antianginal efficacy and duration of action (50–52). When evaluating the information about these drugs clinicians should understand the relative merits of the various study methods.

Reports concerning the antianginal efficacy and duration of action of nitrates evaluate various aspects of their therapeutic effects, including: a) lowering angina attack rate, b) hemodynamic response, and c) enhancing exercise tolerance. Many studies lack a placebo trial, or are not blinded. Because there is a significant placebo effect in the treatment of angina, a double-blind placebo trial is a necessary part of a well designed study (53).

Studies in which patients evaluate the frequency, duration, and intensity of their angina attacks while taking long-acting preparations provide information pertinent to the clinical setting. Because the daily activities and pain perception of patients can vary, studies that evaluate angina attack rate may contain bias. These clinical studies provide "soft data," but lack objective evidence of antianginal activity (51).

Some studies describe the extent and duration of circulatory changes produced by various nitrates. Although these contain objective measures of the intensity and duration of hemodynamic effects, the results of these studies do not evaluate antianginal efficacy directly. The hemodynamic effects of nitrates do not necessarily correlate with their antianginal activity (50). Some hemodynamic changes improve angina (eg, decreased systolic blood pressure) while other changes may aggravate it (eg, increased heart rate). Thus, duration of a hemodynamic response may suggest, but does not directly measure, the duration of antianginal effect.

Protocols using standardized exercise tests that reproducibly induce chest pain in patients with stable angina at the same workload provide reliable objective evidence concerning the efficacy and duration of antianginal activity (54). If an agent improves exercise performance compared to placebo, the agent is effective in the treatment of angina. Serial exercise tests can be performed after a dose is given to determine the duration of action of an agent. Further, because blood pressure and heart rate can be measured when chest pain occurs, estimates of oxygen consumption based upon the pressure-rate product can be made during an exercise test.

13. Which long-acting preparation of nitroglycerin could be used to treat patient H.S.? How should it be used?

Nitroglycerin ointment has sustained antianginal efficacy and would provide H.S. with long-acting prophylaxis. Reichek et al (55), in a carefully designed study, showed that nitroglycerin ointment improved exercise capacity in patients with stable angina for at least 3 hours. They also observed a concurrent reduction of electrocardiographic evidence of ischemia, decrease in systolic blood pressure, and increase in heart rate.

Several subsequent studies have demonstrated similar prolonged antianginal activity from topical nitroglycerin (56–59). The onset of action of the two percent nitroglycerin ointment in lanolin base is about 30 minutes.

In patients with congestive heart failure, nitroglycerin ointment achieved plasma concentrations of 3.1 ng/ml and 8.9 ng/ml at doses of 1 to 2 inches, and 4 inches, respectively. These concentrations were maintained for at least 4 hours (60).

The initial dose of nitroglycerin ointment is 0.5 inch squeezed from the tube onto a dose measuring applicator and spread onto the skin without massaging or rubbing. Every four hours the amount of ointment should be increased by 0.5 inch, and this process repeated until the optimal dose is reached, ie, the largest amount of ointment that does not produce a headache. If headache or severe hypotension occurs at a given dose, the amount of ointment should be decreased by 0.5 inch. Residual ointment left on the skin from a previous dose should be removed before a subsequent dose is applied. Nurses who apply the ointment should avoid contact with their own skin by using gloves or by using the applicator.

There is little information concerning the best method to apply the ointment (61). The number of square inches to which the ointment is applied (62), the site of application (63), and the type of covering all influence the rate and extent of nitroglycerin absorption. Several different methods have been recommended; they range from use of a 6 by 6 inch area covered with plastic wrap (55) to placing the measured dose directly on the skin and covering with the applicator. The patient should decide the site, the amount of skin on which the ointment is applied, and the type of covering that is most comfortable and convenient. Many patients prefer the chest site covered with plastic to avoid staining clothes. If any of these factors are changed drastically in the same patient (eg, a patient stabilized on a 2.5 inch dose using applicator paper suddenly spreads the same amount of ointment over a 36 square inch area), severe hypotension could result. Accordingly, the patient should alter the method of application only under medical supervision.

Sustained release nitroglycerin tablets (64) *and capsules* (65) are effective in decreasing the number of angina episodes and increasing exercise tolerance. However, these oral preparations do not enjoy wide use in the United States.

14. H.S. developed headaches after using 0.5 inch of nitroglycerin ointment. She would not use the ointment because she found it messy to apply. What other nitroglycerin preparation could she use?

Transdermal nitroglycerin patches could also be used to treat H.S. (179). The patches, which are applied to the skin like a bandage, release nitroglycerin from a drug reservoir.

Most of the information about these new transdermal delivery systems comes from the manufacturers of these products (see Table 1). The manufacturers claim that the patches protect patients from angina for at least 24 hours, allowing once daily dosing. Compared to the ointment, the patches are easier to apply and allow more consistent dosage application. However, more trials testing the efficacy of the patches must be completed before these products can be recommended as the universal solution to the problem of long-acting antianginal therapy.

The cost of the transdermal patches may deter their popularity. One 60-gram tube of nitroglycerin, which lasts about 14 to 19 days when applied 1 inch four times a day (180), costs considerably less than a two-week supply of transdermal patches.

The labeling of the transdermal patches causes confusion among patients and health care profes-sionals. Ciba labels the dosage size of the patch in terms of the amount of nitroglycerin delivered over 24 hours (181). Key Pharmaceuticals designates the dosage size by the surface area of the patches (182). And Searle Laboratories labels their patches with the amount of nitroglycerin contained within the patch (183). The amount of nitroglycerin delivered in 24 hours appears to be the most important consideration when selecting these transdermal patches, but further data are needed before any other comparisons can be made.

Even though the three transdermal patches appear similar, they should not be used interchangeably (184). The physical and chemical properties of the delivery systems differ among the products. The amount of nitroglycerin and the release pattern of the drug into the circulation may differ from patch to patch and from patient to patient. At present, no data are available comparing the three manufacturers' patches with respect to time of onset and duration of action, therapeutic efficacy, drug release patterns, adhesion, skin irritation, and side effects.

The dosing of the nitroglycerin patches remains empiric. When H.S. begins using transdermal nitroglycerin patches, she should use the smallest dose size, expressed as mg of drug released over 24 hours. She should be monitored for relief of symptoms, as well as for headache and

Table 1.

TRANSDERMAL NITROGLYCERIN PATCHES*

Product Name	Manufacturer	Surface Area (cm²)	Nitroglycerin Content (mg)	Nitroglycerin Delivered Over 24 Hours (mg)
Transderm-Nitro 5	Ciba	10	25	5.0
Transderm-Nitro 10	Ciba	20	50	10.0
Nitro-Dur 5	Key	5	26	2.5
Nitro-Dur 10	Key	10	51	5.0
Nitro-Dur 15	Key	15	77	7.5
Nitro-Dur 20	Key	20	104	10.0
Nitro-Dur 30	Key	30	154	15.0
Nitrodisc 16	Searle	8	16	—**
Nitrodisc 32	Searle	16	32	—**

*Adapted from Dasta et al (179)

**The actual amount of nitroglycerin released from the Searle patches is not published. A representative of the company said verbally that about 5 mg/24 hours was released from Nitrodisc 16, and 10 mg/24 hours from Nitrodisc 32.

hypotension. The dose can be increased by adding more patches or by using a larger size patch. The largest patch size that relieves angina without causing headaches or hypotension should be used. If H.S. cannot tolerate the smallest size patch by one manufacturer, a patch by another manufacturer can be tried.

Even in patients previously stabilized on nitroglycerin ointment, clinical response must be used as a guide when they are changed to the transdermal patches. Although preliminary data in normal subjects suggest that two patches that deliver 5 mg per 24 hours are equivalent to one half inch of nitroglycerin applied every 8 hours (181), these results cannot be extrapolated to the patient with angina. Generally, patients who have used nitroglycerin ointment or other long-acting nitrates, may start with a larger size patch, e.g. 10 mg per 24 hours. Patient H.S. appears to be very sensitive to nitroglycerin ointment, and therapy should be initiated with a smaller patch size, for example 2.5 or 5.0 mg per 24 hours.

Patients may apply the transdermal nitroglycerin patch to any hairfree skin area except to the distal parts of the extremities. Many patients find the upper arm or chest convenient. Skin areas with scars, calluses, skin folds, irritation, or skin damage should be avoided because variable absorption may occur in such areas. The patches should be applied once daily at the same time each day, preferably at bedtime. The site of application should be changed each day. Patients should wash their hands after applying the transdermal patch, to remove any nitroglycerin they may have contacted on their hands. Health care professionals should remind patients to remove the protective peel strip that covers the nitroglycerin patch before adhering the patch to the skin. Because the adhesive properties differ among the products, patients must consult the patient product insert to determine whether the patch will remain on the skin during bathing or swimming.

15. H.S. complained of dizziness and orthostatic hypotension after applying the smallest nitroglycerin transdermal patch available. How effective would sublingual isosorbide dinitrate 5 mg every six hours be for patient H.S.?

Sublingual isosorbide dinitrate probably is no more effective than the sublingual nitroglycerin H.S. is already taking. Despite claims that sublingual isosorbide dinitrate is a long-acting ni-

trate preparation, little evidence in the literature supports claims of prolonged action.

Goldstein et al (34), using standard exercise testing, determined that sublingual isosorbide dinitrate increased exercise capacity and had a duration of action similar to sublingual nitroglycerin. Based on a double-blind crossover study, Aronow et al (66) concluded that sublingual isosorbide dinitrate was no more effective than placebo in treating angina pectoris. Steele et al (67) demonstrated that this preparation provided protection against pacing-induced angina for up to 65 minutes. Klaus et al (68) found that sublingual isosorbide dinitrate enhanced exercise performance at 45 minutes, but not at 100 minutes. Thus, sublingual isosorbide dinitrate has a relatively short duration of action.

16. Would chewable isosorbide dinitrate be a better choice?

Chewable isosorbide dinitrate is similar to the sublingual preparation because the patient chews the tablet and retains the particles in his or her mouth. Hurwitz et al (69) found that chewable isosorbide dinitrate was no better than placebo in improving performance during standardized exercise tests. Kattus et al (70) developed a unique exercise protocol in which the patients did not stop exercising when they experienced angina, but took the medication and continued walking on the exercise treadmill. Kattus found that the onset of action and peak effects of chewable isosorbide dinitrate occurred at 108 seconds and 315 seconds, respectively; nitroglycerin's onset and peak effect occurred at 75 seconds and 190 seconds, respectively. The results of a subsequent study by Kattus et al (36), using a similar protocol, demonstrated that 5 mg chewable isosorbide dinitrate protected patients from exercise-induced angina for 2.5 to 3.0 hours after the drug was administered. The differences between the results of the work by Hurwitz and Kattus may be due to the different exercise testing protocols. However, even if the work by Kattus is more indicative of the effectiveness of isosorbide dinitrate in the clinical setting, the three-hour protection demonstrated does not justify dosing chewable isosorbide dinitrate every 6 to 8 hours.

17. How effective would oral isosorbide dinitrate be for the treatment of patient H.S.'s angina?

The results of studies evaluating the antianginal efficacy of *oral isosorbide dinitrate* are more encouraging than the results of studies using the sublingual or chewable forms. Danahy et al demonstrated that oral isosorbide dinitrate in doses of 20 to 50 mg (mean 29 mg) increased exercise performance 3 hours after administration, but not at 5 hours, when given as a single dose (71) and after chronic use (35). Other studies of oral doses ranging from 7.5 mg to 50 mg confirmed that the antianginal efficacy of isosorbide dinitrate lasted for at least 3 hours (72–74). The 40 mg capsule of isosorbide dinitrate increased exercise tolerance for up to 6 hours after administration (75).

Thadani et al (76) evaluated the duration of action and peak plasma concentrations obtained from several doses of oral isosorbide dinitrate. They found that the oral dosage form had long-acting antianginal effects, and that plasma concentrations did not correlate with these effects. Each single dose of 15, 30, 60, and 120 mg produced an increase in exercise tolerance that began within 1 hour and lasted for 8 hours. The effects on exercise performance were not dose dependent; the 15 mg dose produced improvement similar to the 30, 60, and 120 mg doses. The time course and peak concentrations of the drug varied widely among the patients. The average peak plasma concentrations were 6.8, 14.3, 17.5, and 26.0 ng/ml after 15, 30, 60, and 120 mg, respectively.

Thadani (76) also found that the reduction in systolic blood pressure was dose-dependent. Because the hypotensive side effects became more pronounced with increasing dosage, but the antianginal effects did not increase with dose, the lowest effective dose of oral isosorbide dinitrate should be used. Severe orthostatic hypotension can occur even at low doses (76); therefore, the initial dose should be 10 mg every 6 to 8 hours. If the 10 mg dose does not provide protection, it may be increased gradually up to 60 mg. The side effects of isosorbide dinitrate are similar to those of nitroglycerin: headache, lightheadedness, and hypotension (35,40,74,76).

18. What other nitrate preparations provide long-acting antianginal protection?

The antianginal effects of other "long-acting" nitrates, such as *pentaerythritol tetranitrate* and *erythrityl tetranitrate*, are not as well documented as the effects of isosorbide dinitrate. The limited objective data available indicate that when these nitrates are given sublingually, they do im-

prove exercise performance, but the duration of this action is similar to the duration of effect of sublingual nitroglycerin (68). Little objective data document the effectiveness of oral pentaerythritol tetranitrate and oral erythrityl tetranitrate. However, the wide use of these agents suggests they may be effective when given orally.

The dose needed to control a patient's symptoms may be larger than the dose recommended by the manufacturer; in addition, the dosages required by different patients vary considerably (32,77). Thus, the dose must be titrated individually for each patient to provide a maximum therapeutic effect while avoiding excessive hypotension.

19. *Tolerance.* H.S. was stabilized on 40 mg oral isosorbide dinitrate every six hours. Will she develop tolerance to the effects of isosorbide dinitrate or other nitrates?

Although the question of developing tolerance to nitrates is not completely answered, evidence in the literature indicates that patient H.S. should expect to receive continued therapeutic benefit from her isosorbide dinitrate without increasing the dose with time. If she suffers an acute angina attack, sublingual nitroglycerin should relieve her chest pain.

Several studies using high-dose chronic nitrate therapy showed that nitrates did not lose their effectiveness in treatment of angina with time (34,35,55,64,65,75). Further, chronic treatment with nitrates did not decrease the ability of nitroglycerin to improve exercise performance (35,55,72,78).

Tolerance commonly develops to some actions of a drug, but not to others. While the studies cited above reported that tolerance does not develop to the antianginal effects of nitrates, tolerance and cross-tolerance develop to the effects on blood pressure and heart rate. Chronic use of long-acting nitrates caused an attenuation of the hypotensive and tachycardic responses to the drugs (35,79). Thadani et al (80) found that the changes in the blood pressure and heart rate induced by large doses of oral isosorbide dinitrate were significantly higher after the first dose than those induced after chronic therapy. Because plasma concentrations of isosorbide dinitrate are higher after sustained therapy than during the acute dosing, tolerance is due to decreased responsiveness of the end organ site, rather than to increased metabolism of the drug. Thadani et al

(80) also reported that cross-tolerance to the blood pressure and heart rate effects of nitroglycerin developed in less than one week with isosorbide dinitrate 15 mg every six hours. Headaches, which commonly occur early in nitrate treatment, subside with continued therapy (81), indicating that tolerance also develops to the effects on the cerebral vasculature.

20. What instructions should patient H.S. receive about nitrate dependence and stopping her medication suddenly?

It is not yet established whether patients on high-dose, long-term nitrate therapy develop dependence to nitrates. Most information concerning dependence relates to chronic exposure of industrial workers to nitrates while manufacturing explosives (81). Workers exposed to very high concentrations of nitrates during the work week developed symptoms of ischemic heart disease on weekends. There are reports of myocardial infarctions and sudden deaths in munitions workers who were withdrawn from industrial exposure. Lange et al (82) hypothesized that chronic nitrate-induced vasodilation evokes homeostatic vasoconstriction, and the constriction persists during the withdrawal from nitrates, resulting in myocardial ischemia. It is not clear whether the development of dependence in industrial workers is relevant to the clinical setting in which patients with angina receive much lower doses of nitrates. Because the consequences of a possible withdrawal syndrome (accelerated angina, myocardial infarction, or sudden death) are very serious, H.S. should be told not to stop her long-acting nitrate suddenly (81).

Beta-Adrenergic Blocking Agents

21. M.T., a 65-year-old man with angina, was treated with nitroglycerin 0.4 mg prn for 1 year. One month ago he experienced increasing frequency of chest pain. His cardiologist prescribed propranolol 10 mg every six hours in addition to his nitroglycerin. Why was propranolol used to treat M.T.?

Because M.T.'s angina became more severe, and he required more than nitroglycerin to control his chest pain, propranolol was an appropriate choice. Subjective and objective evidence demonstrate the beneficial effects of this drug. In adequate doses propranolol reduced the number of anginal episodes, shortened the duration of pain, lowered nitroglycerin consumption, decreased heart rate, improved ST segment changes, and enhanced exercise performance (83–85). The benefit of long-term (5-8 years) use of propranolol is also documented (86).

22. How does propranolol affect myocardial oxygen consumption?

Propranolol reduces myocardial oxygen consumption by decreasing heart rate, contractility, and the development of left ventricular tension (83,87,88). On the other hand, propranolol increases myocardial oxygen consumption by increasing the ventricular ejection period and end-diastolic pressure (87,88). However, the net effect of propranolol is to reduce myocardial oxygen consumption (88).

23. *Dosing.* What is the optimum dose of propranolol for patient M.T.?

The initial dose of propranolol is 10 mg tid or qid. This dose should be increased gradually in increments of 40 mg per day every 3 to 7 days until (a) the desired clinical response is obtained, (b) the pulse rate falls to 55-60 beats per minute, or (c) undesirable effects occur (89–91). The effective dose varies with individual patients. For mild angina, a small dose, eg, 10 mg tid, may be adequate. Although doses as high as 2000 mg have been used, the average dose is around 160 mg per day (91).

24. B.L. was maintained on propranolol 40 mg four times a day. A week ago his physician changed the dosage to 80 mg two times a day. What is the duration of action of propranolol?

Thadani et al (92) studied the duration of action of propranolol following both acute and sustained therapy. Using exercise-induced angina as the end point, the onset of action occurred within one hour, and the effect persisted for 12 hours, with either 80 or 160 mg doses. A similar time course of action was observed for heart rate, systolic blood pressure, and rate-pressure product.

25. How effective is propranolol twice a day compared to four times a day?

A well designed comparative study assessing subjective and objective parameters determined that propranolol given twice daily was as effective in the treatment of angina as propranolol given four times a day (93).

26. *Plasma Monitoring.* What is the role of plasma propranolol concentrations in monitoring patient B.L.'s angina therapy?

Plasma propranolol concentrations are not useful for monitoring the therapeutic efficacy of its antianginal effect (94). Patients receiving either 80 or 160 mg propranolol exhibited wide variations in plasma propranolol concentrations. In addition, the time course and intensity of action did not correlate with dose and/or plasma concentration (92). The chapter entitled *Essential Hypertension* contains additional information about plasma propranolol concentrations and propranolol's adverse effects.

27. *Prior to Surgery.* A.C. has been taking propranolol 80 mg qid, nitroglycerin ointment 3 inches qid, and more than 10 tablets of sublingual nitroglycerin a day. Despite good compliance and appropriate use of these drugs, he still experiences chest pains. Cardiac catheterization and a coronary angiogram revealed an adequately functioning ventricle with 90% occlusion of the right coronary artery and 75% occlusion of his left circumflex artery. He is scheduled for aortocoronary saphenous vein bypass surgery. What changes, if any, are needed in A.C.'s propranolol therapy before surgery?

In the past 10 years, recommendations regarding the treatment of patients on chronic propranolol therapy have varied a great deal. Initially, Viljoen et al (95) recommended complete withdrawal of propranolol two weeks prior to coronary artery bypass surgery due to myocardial depression attributed to beta-adrenergic blockade and interaction with general anesthesia. Faulkner et al (96) studied propranolol concentrations after chronic therapy and found that the drug could not be detected in plasma or left atrium 36 to 48 hours after discontinuation of propranolol. Therefore, they recommended withdrawal of propranolol 48 hours prior to surgery.

Recently, Oka et al (97) showed clearly that continuing propranolol up to the time of surgery resulted in a lower incidence of postoperative supraventricular arrhythmias and a smaller increase in heart rate-blood pressure product during intubation than occurred after abrupt withdrawal of the drug either 48 hours or 10 hours prior to surgery. Other researchers observed fewer arrhythmias and less intraoperative ischemia in patients continued on propranolol than in patients who had propranolol abruptly discontinued 24 hours prior to surgery (98,99). Further, sudden propranolol withdrawal can cause rebound ischemic events in patients with coronary artery disease (100,101). Therefore, propranolol therapy should be maintained up to the time of surgery.

28. *Comparison of Beta-Blockers.* Z.M.T., a 69-year-old man, experienced more frequent attacks of angina despite therapy consisting of nitroglycerin 0.4 mg sublingual prn, isosorbide dinitrate 40 mg po qid, and theophylline slow-release tablets (Theo-dur) 300 mg q 12 h for asthma. To better control his angina medically, a beta-adrenergic blocking agent is being considered. How can one best select an appropriate beta-adrenergic blocking agent for Z.M.T.?

Other than propranolol, the only beta-blocker presently approved for the treatment of angina pectoris in the United States is nadolol. However, oxprenolol, alprenolol, pindolol, sotalol, timolol, acebutolol, practolol, atenolol, and metoprolol are effective for angina.

The beta-adrenergic blocking drugs differ in pharmacologic action, side effects, and pharmacokinetics. Table 2 summarizes the cardioselectivity, major route of elimination, half-life ($t\frac{1}{2}$), and intrinsic sympathomimetic activity (ISA), (indicator of adrenergic agonist activity) of these agents.

Aside from consideration of availability and pharmacokinetics, the choice of a particular beta-blocker depends on the patient's other medical problems. For example, in patients with concurrent heart failure, drugs with partial ISA might have an advantage; on the other hand, in patients such as Z.M.T. with concurrent asthma, a cardioselective beta-blocker is preferred. Cardioselectivity, however, is not absolute, and all beta-adrenergic blocking agents must be used with extreme caution in asthmatics.

29. What are the advantages for patient Z.M.T. of using the combination of a nitrate and a beta-adrenergic blocking agent?

When a nitrate and a beta-adrenergic blocker are used together, certain cardiac effects are complementary. The increase in heart rate induced by the nitrate is offset by the bradycardic effect of the beta-blocker. The increase in ejection time and the increase in ventricular volume produced by beta-blockers are opposed by nitrates (83,12).

In general, the combination provides a beneficial hemodynamic action (104).

Although the combination of nitroglycerin and propranolol provides a beneficial effect in most patients with angina pectoris, some patients may receive no benefit. Russek et al (105) observed that the combination improved pain, ST depression, and exercise capacity. Battock et al (106) found that the combination resulted in a greater overall clinical improvement, although the combination did not improve exercise performance more than either drug used alone. However, Aronow et al (107) observed no advantage with combination therapy.

Calcium Channel Blocking Agents

30. Patient Z.M.T. was not able to tolerate the beta-adrenergic blocker after an initial trial. How useful are calcium channel blocking agents in the treatment of angina?

Calcium channel blocking agents, a new category of drugs sometimes called calcium antagonists, include nifedipine, verapamil, perhexiline, diltiazem, prenylamine, fendiline, and methoxyverapamil (108,109). These agents are most useful for the treatment of variant angina (109). Nifedipine has been studied most extensively. Hugenboltz et al showed that intracoronary injection of nifedipine reversed coronary spasm in patients (110). Nifedipine also decreased the frequency of angina attacks and prevented malignant ventricular arrhythmias and conduction

disturbances associated with episodes of variant angina (109,111,112). In addition, the drug neither decreased exercise performance nor adversely affected left ventricular function in patients with Prinzmetal's angina (113).

Calcium channel blockers are also effective in the treatment of classical angina and unstable angina when used alone or in combination with nitrates or beta-adrenergic blocking agents (109,114,115).

31. What are the proposed mechanisms of action of calcium channel blocking agents?

The calcium channel blocking agents cause coronary arterial dilation, peripheral arterial dilation, and a negative inotropic effect. These hemodynamic effects may decrease myocardial oxygen consumption and abolish inappropriate coronary vasoconstriction in classical angina (109). The calcium channel blocking agents also reverse coronary artery spasm in patients with variant angina. Such an effect may be related to an inhibitory action on calcium ions involved in cardiac and smooth muscle contraction. The precise biochemical mechanism, however, has not been determined (116).

32. What are the doses, pharmacokinetics, and major side effects of the calcium channel blocking agents?

Table 3 shows the usual effective doses for angina, routes of elimination, t½, protein binding, and major side effects of four calcium channel blocking agents.

Table 2.

PROPERTIES OF BETA-ADRENERGIC AGENTS*

Drug	ISA**	Cardioselectivity	Elimination	Half-life (hr)
Acebutolol	+	+	non-renal	2.9
Alprenolol	+	−	non-renal	2.7
Atenolol	−	+	40% renal	6.1
Metoprolol	−	+	non-renal	3.2
Nadolol	−	−	41-71% renal	14.1
Oxprenolol	+	−	non-renal	1.6
Pindolol	+	−	50% renal	2.2
Practolol	+	+	mostly renal	11.0
Propranolol	−	−	non-renal	2–6
Sotalol	−	−	75% renal	14.0
Timolol	−	−	non-renal	4.9

*Adapted from Frishman (102) and Ritschel (103)

**ISA = Intrinsic Sympathomimetic Activity

Table 3.

CALCIUM CHANNEL BLOCKING AGENTS*

	Usual Dosage	Route of Elimination	Half-life (hr)	Plasma Protein Binding	Side Effects
Nifedipine	Initially 10 mg tid Maximum 120 mg daily	liver metabolism	4–5	90%	Headache, hypotension, flushing, digital dysesthesia, leg edema
Verapamil	80–120 mg tid to qid	liver metabolism	3–7	90%	Constipation, headache, vertigo, hypotension, AV conduction disturbances
Diltiazem	30–60 mg q 8 h	liver metabolism	4	80%	Headache, dizziness, flushing, AV conduction disturbances
Perhexiline	Initially 100 mg bid Maintenance: 150– 200 mg bid	liver metabolism	2–6 days	90%	Elevation of liver enzymes, abnormal glucose metabolism

*Adapted from Stone et al (109)

Other Drugs

33. What other drugs are used for the treatment of angina pectoris?

Digitalis and diuretics are useful in the treatment of nocturnal angina. Nocturnal angina, which may occur when patients with congestive heart failure assume the recumbent position, may be due to the shift of peripheral fluid and elevation of left ventricular end diastolic volume (117). Diuretics and digitalis decrease left ventricular volume and thus may be helpful in nocturnal angina associated with recumbency (12,117).

A new long-acting vasodilator, molsidomine, prolongs exercise duration in patients with angina (118,119). More studies are needed to establish the effectiveness of this drug.

Coronary vasodilators such as dipyridamole, papaverine, and ethaverine are advocated for the treatment of angina pectoris. At present, the efficacy of these agents has not been adequately demonstrated (117). Whether the long-term use of these drugs has any beneficial effect on the development of coronary collateral vessels in humans has not been determined.

Sedatives are important adjuncts in the management of certain patients with angina. Benzodiazepines are helpful in those individuals whose emotional responses must be curbed to control their angina (90).

Drug-Induced Angina

34. A 60-year-old man with vascular headaches experienced an episode of chest pain shortly after taking 1 mg of ergotamine tartrate. What is the reason for his chest pain? What other drugs can induce angina?

Ergotamine and other ergot alkaloids produce vasoconstriction and coronary artery vasospasm which can induce angina (120).

Methysergide, a serotonin antagonist and an ergot derivative, can induce or exacerbate angina-like symptoms at normal doses (4–6 mg per day). The chest pain is usually reversible when the drug is discontinued. The incidence of methysergide-induced angina is probably less than 1% (121,122).

Hydralazine-induced angina pectoris is well documented (123–125). This drug increases cardiac output and heart rate, thereby increasing oxygen demand, and may precipitate or exacerbate angina pectoris. Hydralazine can produce myocardial ischemia independent of changes in heart rate by decreasing the coronary perfusion pressure gradient (125). The angina symptoms from hydralazine may be accompanied by electrocardiographic changes manifested by ST segment depression and QRS and T wave alterations (123). These changes are more common in patients with coronary artery disease. The incidence of hydralazine-induced angina in the hypertensive patients is about 7%; it is much less if a cardiodepressive agent is also used with hydralazine (123).

Digitalis-induced angina occurred in 15 out of 179 patients suffering from digitoxin intoxication (126). However, in normal doses, digitalis therapy for congestive heart failure usually does not induce angina. The overall hemodynamic effects of the drug may result in a decrease in myocardial oxygen consumption in angina patients (127).

Diazoxide, an antihypertensive drug, can cause an angina-like syndrome. Patients receiving diazoxide developed ST-T changes and substernal discomfort probably related to the sudden drop of blood pressure (128–130). Thus, hypertensive crisis in patients with coronary artery disease preferably should be treated with nitroprusside.

Large doses of *sympathomimetic agents* and *thyroid* preparations may precipitate angina pectoris. Less frequently, insulin, fat emulsions for parenteral nutrition, and prazosin may induce angina (131,132).

Prinzmetal's Variant Angina

Prinzmetal's angina, originally described in 1959 (133), is a variant form of angina that occurs at rest; it is unlike stable angina which is precipitated by exercise or stress. The attacks are often cyclic and recur at the same time of day, commonly in the early morning. Electrocardiograms taken during attacks usually show ST segment elevation, indicating more severe transmural myocardial ischemia than occurs in stable angina which is associated with ST depression (134). Serious arrhythmias, including ventricular tachycardia and AV block, may accompany Prinzmetal's angina (134–136).

The cause of Prinzmetal's angina is coronary artery spasm (30,136–138) which is a transient, reversible, subtotal or total narrowing of a major coronary artery. Before an attack there is no increase in myocardial oxygen demand; the myocardial ischemia leading to chest pain is secondary to a decreased supply of oxygen through the constricted vessel. This differs from stable angina which is caused by an increase in oxygen demand during exertion in the face of a stable, though inadequate, oxygen supply from a coronary artery narrowed by atherosclerosis.

The pathogenesis of coronary vasospasm leading to Prinzmetal's angina is not clear. Altered alpha-adrenergic activity is implicated because

spasm occurs when epinephrine and propranolol are given together, and spasm can be reversed by phenoxybenzamine (139–141). When atherosclerotic coronary heart disease accompanies Prinzmetal's angina, the spasm often occurs at the site of an atheromatous lesion; thus, atherosclerosis and spasm may be related (142–145). Vasoactive substances released from platelets have also been implicated in the production of vasospasm (143).

35. C.V., a 38-year-old male construction worker, was hospitalized for evaluation of chest pain that had been waking him about 3 AM in the morning several times a week for the past month. The pain was severe, substernal, and not relieved by change of position. It did not recur during his daily activities at heavy construction. He had no risk factors for atherosclerotic heart disease. The admission electrocardiogram was normal, as were serum electrolyte and cardiac enzyme concentrations. Sublingual nitroglycerin relieved the chest pain he experienced at 4 AM on the first two mornings in the hospital. On the second hospital day his graded exercise test was negative. On the third hospital day coronary angiography revealed no significant stenosis of his coronary arteries. An ergonovine provocative test was performed while he remained in the cardiac catheterization laboratory. A 0.05 mg dose of intravenous ergonovine produced no response. After ergonovine 0.1 mg was injected, C.V. experienced the same quality chest pain he usually had in the early morning, his electrocardiogram showed ST segment elevation in leads II, III, and aVF, and an angiogram showed intense focal narrowing of the right coronary artery. Sublingual nitroglycerin 0.4 mg was given every 3 minutes. The pain subsided and the electrocardiogram returned to normal after the third dose. The physicians diagnosed Prinzmetal's angina.

Why was a provocative test indicated for C.V.?

The cause of chest pain in C.V. was in doubt before the provocative test. His pain occurred spontaneously, and the electrocardiogram did not document ST segment changes. He also had no evidence of atherosclerotic disease. It was important to establish if his pain was related to unstable angina, coronary artery spasm or noncardiac causes because each of these disorders requires different treatment. A provocative test uses a stimulus, usually a drug, that is known to induce coronary artery vasospasm in patients with Prinzmetal's variant angina. Provocative testing is used to diagnose coronary artery spasm in patients who have normal coronary arteries and a negative exercise test, and in whom the cause of chest pain at rest cannot be determined because there is no electrocardiogram acquired during chest pain (146–149).

36. What is the usual procedure involved in an ergonovine provocative test?

The agent most commonly used in a provocative test is ergonovine maleate. When given intravenously, it induces a spasm of the affected coronary artery in patients with Prinzmetal's (146,147,150–154). During the test, the patient is monitored for symptoms of chest pain, and an electrocardiogram is taken to record ST segment changes and to detect any arrhythmias that might occur. If the test is performed in the cardiac catheterization laboratory, the spasm is visualized using coronary angiography. After the spasm is documented, it is reversed with a vasodilator, usually nitroglycerin. Because the ergonovine provocative test is relatively new, there is no standardization of the test. For more details concerning the different provocative testing procedures the reader is directed to references 146 to 157.

37. Which drugs reverse the coronary artery spasm induced by ergonovine in this patient?

Ergonovine provokes a coronary artery spasm similar to the vasospasm that occurs spontaneously in Prinzmetal's angina (155), and similar arrhythmias occur in both situations (146–149,157). To reverse the vasospasm, sublingual nitroglycerin 0.4 mg repeated every 3 to 5 minutes is administered as soon as the spasm is detected. If this does not reverse the spasm, nitroglycerin is given intravenously (147,151,157) or directly into the coronary artery (148,156). Unremitting spasm can cause transmural myocardial ischemia and malignant arrhythmias (156). Cardiac resuscitation drugs and equipment should be available in the case of life threatening arrhythmias or cardiac arrest.

38. What drug treatment should patient C.V. receive when he has an acute attack of Prinzmetal's angina?

C.V. should use sublingual nitroglycerin immediately whenever he experiences chest pain. Sublingual nitroglycerin in doses of 0.3 to 0.6 mg promptly reverses the chest pain and electrocardiographic changes associated with coronary artery spasm. Because nitroglycerin reversed the spasm during his provocative test, nitroglycerin probably will be effective for C.V.

39. Which long-acting nitrates should patient C.V. use to prevent his chest pain?

Because C.V.'s Prinzmetal's angina frequently occurs in the early morning, he will need a long-acting prophylactic agent. This is a difficult therapeutic problem. There are very few well designed trials evaluating the efficacy of agents in Prinzmetal's variant angina. Coronary artery vasospasm occurs spontaneously, and Prinzmetal's angina may remit with time, making it difficult to design a study using patients with a stable condition. Therefore, many of the therapeutic recommendations concerning nitrates are based upon the studies of efficacy and duration of action in patients with stable angina.

Although long-acting nitrates, such as isosorbide dinitrate, are often used in the treatment of Prinzmetal's angina, the results of nitrate therapy can be disappointing (158–160). However, isosorbide dinitrate given by continuous intravenous infusion, to assure adequate plasma concentrations, decreased the number of vasospastic episodes in coronary care unit patients (161). The relatively poor performance of non-parenteral isosorbide dinitrate preparations is probably due to their inability to maintain adequate plasma concentrations for sustained periods.

Nitroglycerin ointment applied at bedtime should be more effective (162). C.V. should use nitroglycerin ointment, starting with 0.5 inch, at bedtime for prophylaxis of his attacks. Nitroglycerin transdermal patches (see Question 14) may also provide C.V. with relief overnight and through the next day. If C.V. prefers not to use a topical nitroglycerin preparation, an alternative would be isosorbide dinitrate given in doses large enough and frequent enough to provide protection. Very large doses or sustained release capsules may be necessary to prevent attacks at night.

40. How effective is propranolol as a long-acting medication for Prinzmetal's variant angina?

Present medical treatment of Prinzmetal's angina avoids propranolol (162–164). Theoretically, propranolol blocks the beta-adrenergic receptors that mediate vasodilation, potentiating the effects of vasoconstricting stimuli. Although propranolol may benefit some patients (165,166), many investigators describe an increase in severity and frequency of coronary artery vasospasm with propranolol administration (135,141).

41. Which calcium channel blocking agents are useful in the treatment of coronary artery spasm?

The action of calcium channel blocking agents on coronary artery smooth muscle makes them ideally suited for treatment of Prinzmetal's angina. Successful treatment of coronary artery vasospasm is reported with nifedipine (159,160,167–172), diltiazem (162,168,173,174), and verapamil (143,175–177). The reports of perhexilene use (171,178) in Prinzmetal's angina indicate variable success. For more information concerning calcium channel blocking agents see Questions 30 to 32.

References

1. Hurst JW et al: Definitions and classification of coronary atherosclerotic heart disease. In *The Heart,* 4th ed, edited by JW Hurst, McGraw-Hill Book Co, New York, 1978, p 1094.

2. Maseri A et al: Significance of spasm in the pathogenesis of ischemic heart disease. Am J Cardiol. 1979; 44:788.

3. Ross R et al: The pathogenesis of atherosclerosis. N Engl J Med. 1976; 295:369 & 420.

4. Sonnenblick EH et al: Oxygen consumption of the heart: Physiological principles and clinical implications. Mod Concepts Cardiovasc Dis. 1971; 40:9.

5. Braunwald E: Control of myocardial oxygen consumption. Physiologic and clinical considerations. Am J Cardiol. 1971; 27:416.

6. DiGirolamo M et al: Etiology of coronary atherosclerosis. In *The Heart,* 4th ed, edited by JW Hurst, McGraw-Hill Book Co, New York, 1978, p 1103.

7. Brand RJ et al: Multivariate prediction of coronary heart disease in the Western Collaborative Group Study compared to the findings of the Framingham Study. Circulation. 1976; 53:348.

8. American Heart Association: Risk factors and coronary disease. Circulation. 1980; 62:449A.

9. Ross RS: Ischemic heart disease: An overview. Am J Cardiol. 1975; 36:496.

10. Sostman HD et al: Contemporary medical management of stable angina pectoris. Am Heart J. 1978; 95:775.

11. Esptein SE et al: Angina pectoris: Pathophysiology, evaluation, and treatment. Ann Intern Med. 1971; 75:263.

12. Goldstein RE et al: Medical management of patients with angina pectoris. Progr Cardiovasc Dis. 1972; 14:360.

13. Aronow WS et al: The medical treatment of angina pectoris IX. The medical management of angina pectoris. Am Heart J. 1973; 85:275.

14. Conti CR et al: Unstable angina pectoris: Morbidity and mortality in 57 consecutive patients evaluated angiographically. Am J Cardiol. 1973; 32:745.

15. Plotnick GD: Approach to the management of unstable angina. Am Heart J. 1979; 98:243.

16. Mason DT et al: The effects of nitroglycerin and amyl nitrite on arteriolar and venous tone in the human forearm. Circulation. 1965; 32:755.

17. DeMaria AN et al: Effects of nitroglycerin on left ventricular cavitary size and cardiac performance determined by ultrasound in man. Am J Med. 1974; 57:754.

18. Mason DT et al: Actions of the nitrites on the peripheral circulation and myocardial oxygen consumption: Significance in the relief of angina pectoris. Chest. 1971; 59:296.

19. Sharma B et al: Left ventricular function during spontaneous angina pectoris: Effect of sublingual nitroglycerin. Am J Cardiol. 1980; 46:34.

20. Slutsky R et al: Effect of sublingual nitroglycerin on left ventricular function at rest and during spontaneous angina pectoris: Assessment with a radionuclide approach. Am J Cardiol. 1979; 44:1365.

21. Greenberg H et al: Effects of nitroglycerin on the major determinants of myocardial oxygen consumption: An angiographic and hemodynamic assessment. Am J Cardiol. 1975; 36:426.

22. Parker JO et al: The effect of nitroglycerin on coronary blood flow and the hemodynamic response to exercise in coronary artery disease. Am J Cardiol. 1971; 27:59.

23. Ganz W et al: Failure of intracoronary nitroglycerin to alleviate pacing-induced angina. Circulation. 1972; 46:880.

24. Winbury MM: Redistribution of left ventricular blood flow produced by nitroglycerin: An example of integration of the macro- and microcirculation. Circ Res. 1971; 28/29 (suppl 1):I-140.

25. Klein RC et al: Evaluation of the effects of systemic nitroglycerin on perfusion of ischemic myocardium in coronary heart disease assessed intraoperatively by antegrade blood flow through intact saphenous vein bypass grafts. Am Heart J. 1981; 101:292.

26. Cohn PF et al: Effect of sublingually administered nitroglycerin on regional myocardial blood flow in patients with coronary artery disease. Am J Cardiol. 1977; 39:672.

27. Goldstein RE et al: Intraoperative coronary collateral function in patients with coronary occlusive disease: Nitroglycerin responsiveness and angiographic correlations. Circulation. 1974; 49:298.

28. Feldman RL et al: Coronary arterial responses to graded doses of nitroglycerin. Am J Cardiol. 1979; 43:91.

29. Hillis LD et al: Coronary-artery spasm. N Engl J Med. 1978; 299:695.

30. Oliva PB et al: Coronary arterial spasm in Prinzmetal angina: Documentation by coronary arteriography. N Engl J Med. 1973; 288:745.

31. Horwitz LD et al: Clinical response to nitroglycerin as a diagnostic test for coronary artery disease. Am J Cardiol. 1972; 29:149.

32. Warren SE et al: Nitroglycerin and nitrate esters. Am J Med. 1978; 65:53.

33. Aronow WS: Clinical use of nitrates: I. Nitrates as antianginal drugs. Mod Concepts Cardiovasc Dis. 1979; 48:31.

34. Goldstein RE et al: Clinical and circulatory effects of isosorbide dinitrate: Comparison with nitroglycerin. Circulation. 1971; 43:629.

35. Danahy DT et al: Hemodynamics and antianginal effects of high dose oral isosorbide dinitrate after chronic use. Circulation. 1977; 56:205.

36. Kattus AA et al: Comparison of placebo, nitroglycerin, and isosorbide dinitrate for effectiveness of relief of angina and duration of action. Chest. 1979; 75:17.

37. Levine HJ: Difficult problems in the diagnosis of chest pain. Am Heart J. 1980; 100:108.

38. Orlando RC et al: Clinical and manometric effects of nitroglycerin in diffuse esophageal spasm. N Engl J Med. 1973; 289:23.

39. Swamy N: Esophageal spasm: Clinical and manometric response to nitroglycerine and long acting nitrates. Gastroenterology. 1977; 72:23.

40. Miller RR: Antianginal agents. In *Drug Effects in Hospitalized Patients,* edited by RR Miller and DJ Greenblatt, Wiley Biomedical Publc, New York, 1976, p 55.

41. Carruthers SG: Antianginal and beta-adrenoceptor blocking drugs. In *Meyler's Side Effects of Drugs,* Vol 9, edited by MNG Dukes, Exerpta Medica, Princeton, 1980, p 301.

42. Armstrong PW et al: Blood levels after sublingual nitroglycerin. Circulation. 1979; 59:585.

43. Wei JY et al: Quantitative determination of trinitroglycerin in human plasma. Circulation. 1979; 59:588.

44. Yap PSK et al: Improved GLC determination of plasma nitroglycerin concentrations. J Pharm Sci. 1978; 67:582.

45. Stephenson RE: Nitroglycerin tablets not to be refrigerated (letter). Am J Hosp Pharm. 1980; 37:794.

46. Copelan HW: Burning sensation and potency of nitroglycerin sublingually. JAMA. 1972; 219:176.

47. Edelman BA et al: The stability of hypodermic tablets of nitroglycerin packaged in dispensing containers. J Am Pharm Assoc. 1971; NS11:30.

48. Shangraw RF: Unstable nitroglycerin tablets (letter). N Engl J Med. 1972; 286:950.

49. Shangraw RF et al: New developments in the manufacture and packaging of nitroglycerin tablets. J Am Pharm Assoc. 1972; NS12:633.

50. Goldstein RE et al: Nitrates in the prophylactic treatment of angina pectoris. Circulation. 1973; 48:917.

51. Tremblay G et al: Quantification pitfalls in comparative studies of antianginal therapies. Am Heart J. 1975; 89:521.

52. Aronow WS: The medical treatment of angina pectoris: II. Design of an antianginal drug study. Am Heart J. 1972; 84:132.

53. Benson H et al: Angina pectoris and the placebo effect. N Engl J Med. 1979; 300:1424.

54. Redwood DR et al: Importance of the design of an exercise protocol in the evaluation of patients with angina pectoris. Circulation. 1971; 43:618.

55. Reichek N et al: Sustained effects of nitroglycerin ointment in patients with angina pectoris. Circulation. 1974; 50:348.

56. Davidov ME et al: The effect of nitroglycerin ointment on the exercise capacity in patients with angina pectoris. Angiology. 1976; 27:205.

57. Parker JO et al: Effect of nitroglycerin ointment on the clinical and hemodynamic response to exercise. Am J Cardiol. 1976; 38:162.

58. Karsh DL et al: Prolonged benefit of nitroglycerin ointment on exercise tolerance in patients with angina pectoris. Am Heart J. 1978; 96:587.

59. Salem HH et al: Glycerly trinitrate ointment in angina pectoris. Postgrad Med J. 1979; 55:874.

60. Armstrong PW et al: Pharmacokinetic-hemodynamic studies of nitroglycerin ointment in congestive heart failure. Am J Cardiol. 1980; 48:670.

61. Adkison HW: Standardized regimen for applying nitroglycerin ointment. Am J Cardiol. 1977; 40:143.

62. Meister SG et al: Sustained hemodynamic action of nitroglycerin ointment. Br Heart J. 1976; 38:1031.

63. Hansen MS et al: Relative effectiveness of nitroglycerin ointment according to site of application. Heart & Lung. 1979; 8:716.

64. Winsor T et al: Oral nitroglycerin as a prophylactic antianginal drug: Clinical, physiologic, and statistical evidence of efficacy based on a three-phase experimental design. Am Heart J. 1975; 90:611.

65. Davidov ME et al: Effect of sustained release nitroglycerin capsules on anginal frequency and exercise capacity: A double-blind evaluation. Angiology. 1977; 28:181.

66. Aronow WS et al: Sublingual isosorbide dinitrate therapy versus sublingual placebo in angina pectoris. Circulation. 1970; 41:869.

67. Steele RJ et al: Effects of isosorbide dinitrate on the response to atrial pacing in coronary heart disease. Am J Cardiol. 1975; 36:206.

68. Klaus AP et al: Comparative evaluation of sublingual long-acting nitrates. Circulation. 1973; 48:519.

69. Hurwitz L et al: Isosorbide dinitrate and cardiovascular adaptation to exercise. Chest. 1976; 69:10.

70. Kattus AA et al: Effectiveness of isosorbide dinitrate and nitroglycerin in relieving angina pectoris during uninterrupted exercise. Chest. 1975; 67:640.

71. Danahy DT et al: Sustained hemodynamic and antianginal effect of high dose oral isosorbide dinitrate. Circulation. 1977; 55:381.

72. Lee G et al: Effects of long-term oral administration of isosorbide dinitrate on the antianginal response to nitroglycerin. Absence of nitrate cross-tolerance and self-tolerance shown by exercise testing. Am J Cardiol. 1978; 41:82.

73. Markis JE et al: Sustained effect of orally administered isosorbide dinitrate on exercise performance of patients with angina pectoris. Am J Cardiol. 1979; 43:265.

74. Glancy DL et al: Effect of swallowed isosorbide dinitrate on blood pressure, heart rate and exercise capacity in patients with coronary artery disease. Am J Med. 1977; 62:39.

75. Lee G et al: Antianginal efficacy of oral therapy with isosorbide dinitrate capsules: Prolonged benefit shown by exercise testing in patients with ischemic heart disease. Chest. 1978; 73:327.

76. Thadani U et al: Oral isosorbide dinitrate in the treatment of angina pectoris: Dose-response relationship and duration of action during acute therapy. Circulation. 1980; 62:491.

77. Abrams J: Nitroglycerin and long-acting nitrates. N Engl J Med. 1980; 302:1234.

78. Aronow WS et al: Evaluation of nitroglycerin in angina in patients on isosorbide dinitrate. Circulation. 1970; 42:61.

79. Schelling JL et al: A study of cross-tolerance to circulatory effects of organic nitrates. Clin Pharmacol Ther. 1966; 8:256.

80. Thadani U et al: Tolerance to the circulatory effects of oral isosorbide dinitrate: Rate of development and cross-tolerance to glyceryl trinitrate. Circulation. 1980; 61:526.

81. Abrams J: Nitrate tolerance and dependence. Am Heart J. 1980; 99:113.

82. Lange RL et al: Nonatheromatous ischemic heart disease following withdrawal from chronic industrial nitroglycerin exposure. Circulation. 1972; 46:666.

83. Elliot WC et al: Beta-adrenergic blocking agents for the treatment of angina pectoris. Progr Cardiovasc Dis. 1969; 12:83.

84. Prichard BNC: Propranolol in the treatment of angina: a review. Postgrad Med J. 1976; 52(suppl 4):35.

85. Miller RR et al: Efficacy of beta adrenergic blockade in coronary heart disease: Propranolol in angina pectoris. Clin Pharmacol Ther. 1975; 18:598.

86. Warren SG et al: Long-term propranolol therapy for angina pectoris. Am J Cardiol. 1976; 37:420.

87. Robinson BF: Mechanism of action of beta-blocking drugs in angina pectoris: A review. Postgrad Med J. 1976; 52(suppl 4):43.

88. Wolfson S et al: Cardiovascular pharmacology of propranolol in man. Circulation. 1969; 40:501.

89. Lesch M et al: Pharmacological therapy of angina pectoris. Mod Concepts Cardiovasc Dis. 1973; 42:5.

90. Logue RB et al: Medical management of angina pectoris. Circulation. 1972; 46:1132.

91. Inderal prescribing information. *Physicians' Desk Reference* 1981; 613.

92. Thadani U et al: Propranolol in the treatment of angina pectoris. Comparison of duration of action in acute and sustained oral therapy. Circulation. 1979; 59:571.

93. Thadani U et al: Propranolol in angina pectoris: Comparison of therapy given two and four times daily. Am J Cardiol. 1980; 46:117.

94. Chidsey C et al: The use of drug concentration measurements in studies of the therapeutic response to propranolol. Postgrad Med J. 1976; 52(suppl 4):26.

95. Viljoen JF et al: Propranolol and cardiac surgery. J Thorac Cardiovasc Surg. 1972; 64:826.

96. Faulkner SL et al: Time required for complete recovery from chronic propranolol therapy. N Engl J Med. 1973; 289:607.

97. Oka Y et al: Clinical pharmacology of the new beta-adrenergic blocking drugs. Part 10. Beta-adrenergic blockade and coronary artery surgery. Am Heart J. 1980; 99:255.

98. Boudoulas H et al: Beneficial effect of continuation of propranolol through coronary bypass surgery. Clin Cardiol. 1979; 2:87.

99. Slogoff S et al: Preoperative propranolol therapy and aortocoronary bypass operation. JAMA. 1978; 240:1487.

100. Alderman EL et al: Coronary artery syndromes after sudden propranolol withdrawal. Ann Intern Med. 1974; 81:625.

101. Miller RR et al: Propranolol-withdrawal rebound phenomenon: Exacerbation of coronary events after abrupt cessation of antianginal therapy. N Engl J Med. 1975; 293:416.

102. Frishman W et al: Clinical pharmacology of the new beta-adrenergic blocking drugs. Part 3. Comparative clinical experience and new therapeutic applications. Am Heart J. 1979; 98:119.

103. Ritschel WA: Compilation of pharmacokinetic parameters of beta-adrenergic blocking agents. Drug Intell Clin Pharm. 1980; 14:746.

104. Wiener L et al: Hemodynamic effects of nitroglycerin, propranolol, and their combination in coronary heart disease. Circulation. 1969; 39:623.

105. Russek HI: Propranolol and isosorbide dinitrate synergism in angina pectoris. Am J Cardiol. 1968; 21:44.

106. Battock DJ et al: Effects of propranolol and isosorbide dinitrate on exercise performance and adrenergic activity in patients with angina pectoris. Circulation. 1969; 39:157.

107. Aronow WS et al: Propranolol combined with isosorbide dinitrate versus placebo in angina pectoris. N Engl J Med. 1969; 280:847.

108. Zsoter TT: Calcium antagonists. Am Heart J. 1980; 99:805.

109. Stone PH et al: Calcium channel blocking agents in the treatment of cardiovascular disorders. Part II: Hemodynamic effects and clinical applications. Ann Intern Med. 1980; 93:886.

110. Hugenholtz PG et al: Nifedipine in the treatment of unstable angina, coronary spasm and myocardial ischemia. Am J Cardiol. 1981; 47:163.

111. Johnson SM et al: A comparison of verapamil and nifedipine in patients with Prinzmetal's variant angina pectoris (abstract). Am J Cardiol. 1981; 47:398.

112. Bertrand ME et al: Treatment of Prinzmetal's variant angina. Role of medical treatment with nifedipine and surgical coronary revascularization combined with plexectomy. Am J Cardiol. 1981; 47:174.

113. Johnson SM et al: Effects of verapamil and nifedipine on left ventricular function in patients with Prinzmetal's variant angina (abstract). Am J Cardiol. 1981; 47:394.

114. Johnson SM et al: Double-blind, randomized, placebo-controlled comparison of propranolol and verapamil in patients with stable, exertional angina pectoris (abstract). Am J Cardiol. 1981; 47:463.

115. Hagemeijer F: Benefits of added nifedipine in unstable angina persisting despite beta blockade and isosorbide dinitrate (abstract). Am J Cardiol. 1981; 47:399.

116. Zelis R et al: "Calcium influx blockers" and vascular smooth muscle: Do we really understand the mechanism? Ann Intern Med. 1981; 94:124.

117. Aronow WS: The medical treatment of angina pectoris. VIII. Miscellaneous antianginal drugs. Am Heart J. 1973; 85:132.

118. Takeshita A et al: Long-lasting effect of oral molsyn-domine on exercise performance. A new antianginal agent. Circulation. 1977; 55:401.

119. Majid PA et al: Molsidomine in the treatment of patients with angina pectoris: Acute hemodynamic effects and clinical efficacy. N Engl J Med. 1980; 302:1.

120. Wendkos MH: The antianginal effect of rapidly acting nitrates in subjects with ergot-induced angina. Am J Med Sci. 1967; 253:39.

121. Graham JR: Methysergide for prevention of headache. N Engl J Med. 1964; 270:67.

122. Hudgson P et al: Methysergide and coronary-artery disease. Lancet. 1967; 1:444.

123. Moyer JH et al: Hydralazine in the treatment of hypertension. Med Clin N Am. 1961; 45:375.

124. Schirger A et al: Pharmacology and clinical use of hydralazine in the treatment of diastolic hypertension. Am J Cardiol. 1962; 9:854.

125. Packer M et al: Hydralazine-induced ischemia without tachycardia: The importance of coronary perfusion pressure gradients. Am J Cardiol. 1978; 41:398.

126. Lely AH et al: Large-scale digitoxin intoxication. Br Med J. 1970; 3:737.

127. Sharma B et al: Clinical electrocardiographic and haemodynamic effects of digitalis (ouabain) in angina pectoris. Br Heart J. 1972; 34:631.

128. Kanada SA et al: Angina-like syndrome with diazoxide therapy for hypertensive crisis. Ann Intern Med. 1976; 84:696.

129. Kumar GK et al: Side effects of diazoxide. JAMA. 1976; 235:275.

130. O'Brien KP et al: Intravenous diazoxide in treatment of hypertension associated with recent myocardial infarction. Br Med J. 1975; 4:74.

131. Meyler L (Eds.) et al: Side effects of drugs, Vol. VII. A survey of unwanted effects of drugs reported in 1968-71. Exerpta Medica, Amsterdam. 1972; p 579.

132. Charness ME et al: Exacerbation of angina pectoris by prazosin. Southern Med J. 1979; 72:1213.

133. Prinzmetal M et al: Angina pectoris. I. A variant form of angina pectoris. Am J Med. 1959; 27:375.

134. Selzer A et al: Clinical syndrome of variant angina with normal coronary arteriogram. N Engl J Med. 1976; 295:1343.

135. Robertson D et al: Variant angina pectoris: Investigation of indexes of sympathetic nervous system function. Am J Cardiol. 1979; 43:1080.

136. Wiener L et al: Spectrum of coronary arterial spasm. Clinical angiographic and myocardial metabolic experience in 29 cases. Am J Cardiol. 1976; 38:945.

137. Maseri A et al: Coronary artery spasm as a cause of acute myocardial ischemia in man. Chest. 1975; 68:625.

138. Meller J et al: Coronary arterial spasm in Prinzmetal's angina: A proved hypothesis. Am J Cardiol. 1976; 37:938.

139. Ricci DR et al: Altered adrenergic activity in coronary arterial spasm. Insight into mechanism based on study of coronary hemodynamics and the electrocardiogram. Am J Cardiol. 1979; 43:1073.

140. Yasue H et al: Prinzmetal's variant form of angina as a manifestation of alpha-adrenergic receptor-mediated coronary artery spasm: Documentation by coronary arteriography. Am Heart J. 1976; 91:148.

141. Yasue H et al: Role of autonomic nervous system in the pathogenesis of Prinzmetal's variant form of angina. Circulation. 1974; 50:534.

142. Maseri A et al: Variant angina: One aspect of a continuous spectrum of vasospastic myocardial ischemia. Pathogenetic mechanisms, estimated incidence and clinical and coronary arteriographic findings in 138 patients. Am J Cardiol. 1978; 42:1019.

143. Yasue H: Pathophysiology and treatment of coronary arterial spasm. Chest. 1980; 78:216.

144. Marzilli M et al: Some clinical considerations regarding the relation of coronary vasospasm to coronary atherosclerosis: A hypothetical pathogenesis. Am J Cardiol. 1980; 45:882.

145. MacAlpin RN: Relation of coronary arterial spasm to sites of organic stenosis. Am J Cardiol. 1980; 46:143.

146. Heupler FA et al: Ergonovine maleate provocative test for coronary arterial spasm. Am J Cardiol. 1978; 41:631.

147. Waters DD et al: Ergonovine testing in a coronary care unit. Am J Cardiol. 1980; 46:922.

148. Heupler FA: Provocative testing for coronary arterial spasm: Risk, method and rationale. Am J Cardiol. 1980; 46:335.

149. Nelson C et al: Provocative testing for coronary arterial spasm: Rationale, risk and clinical illustrations. Am J Cardiol. 1977; 40:624.

150. Feldman RL et al: Regional coronary hemodynamic effects of ergonovine in patients with and without variant angina. Circulation. 1980; 62:149.

151. Cipriano PR et al: The effects of ergonovine maleate on coronary arterial size. Circulation. 1979; 59:82.

152. Curry RC et al: Hemodynamic and myocardial metabolic effects of ergonovine in patients with chest pain. Circulation. 1978; 58:648.

153. Curry RC et al: Effects of ergonovine in patients with and without coronary artery disease. Circulation. 1977; 56:803.

154. Schroeder JS et al: Provocation of coronary spasm with ergonovine maleate. New test with results in 57 patients undergoing coronary arteriography. Am J Cardiol. 1977; 40:487.

155. Curry RC et al: Similarities of ergonovine-induced and spontaneous attacks of variant angina. Circulation. 1979; 59:307.

156. Buxton A et al: Refractory ergonovine-induced coronary vasospasm: Importance of intracoronary nitroglycerin. Am J Cardiol. 1980; 46:329.

157. Sobol SM et al: Ventricular fibrillation during ergonovine maleate provocation of coronary arterial spasm. Am J Cardiol. 1980; 45:718.

158. Maseri A et al: Coronary vasospasm as a possible cause of myocardial infarction. A conclusion derived from the study of 'preinfarction' angina. N Engl J Med. 1978; 299:1271.

159. Heupler FA et al: Nifedipine therapy for refractory coronary arterial spasm. Am J Cardiol. 1979; 44:798.

160. Antman E et al: Nifedipine therapy for coronary-artery spasm: Experience in 127 patients. N Engl J Med. 1980; 302:1269.

161. Distante A et al: Management of vasospastic angina at rest with continuous infusion of isosorbide dinitrate. A double crossover study in a coronary care unit. Am J Cardiol. 1979; 44:533.

162. Schroeder JS et al: Medical therapy of Prinzmetal's variant angina. Chest. 1980; 78(suppl):231.

163. Luchi RJ et al: Coronary artery spasm. Ann Intern Med. 1979; 91:441.

164. Conti CR et al: Coronary artery spasm and myocardial ischemia. Mod Concepts Cardiovasc Dis. 1980; 49:1.

165. Guazzi M et al: Clinical, electrocardiographic, and haemodynamic effects of long-term use of propranolol in Prinzmetal's variant angina pectoris. Br Heart J. 1971; 33:889.

166. Guazzi M et al: Treatment of spontaneous angina pectoris with beta blocking agents. A clinical, electrocardiographic, and haemodynamic appraisal. Br Heart J. 1975; 37:1235.

167. Bertrand ME et al: Treatment of Prinzmetal's variant angina. Role of medical treatment with nifedipine and surgical coronary revascularization combined with plexectomy. Am J Cardiol. 1981; 47:174.

168. Yasue H et al: Exertional angina pectoris caused by coronary arterial spasm: Effects of various drugs. Am J Cardiol. 1979; 43:647.

169. Gunther S et al: Therapy of coronary vasoconstriction in patients with coronary artery disease. Am J Cardiol. 1981; 47:157.

170. Goldberg S et al: Nifedipine in the treatment of Prinzmetal's (variant) angina. Am J Cardiol. 1979; 44:804.

171. Theroux P et al: Provocative testing with ergonovine to evaluate the efficacy of treatment with calcium antagonists in variant angina. Circulation. 1979; 60:504.

172. Previtali M et al: Treatment of angina at rest with nifedipine: A short-term controlled study. Am J Cardiol. 1980; 45:825.

173. Yasue H et al: Circadian variation of exercise capacity in patients with Prinzmetal's variant angina: Role of exercise-induced coronary arterial spasm. Circulation. 1979; 59:938.

174. Rosenthal SJ et al: Efficacy of diltiazem for control of symptoms of coronary arterial spasm. Am J Cardiol. 1980; 46:1027.

175. Solberg LE et al: Prinzmetal's variant angina—response to verapamil. Mayo Clin Proc. 1978; 53:256.

176. Parodi O et al: Management of unstable angina at rest by verapamil. A double-blind cross-over study in coronary care unit. Br Heart J. 1979; 41:167.

177. Henry PD: Comparative pharmacology of calcium antagonist: nifedipine, verapamil and diltiazem. Am J Cardiol. 1980; 46:1047.

178. Raabe DS: Treatment of variant angina pectoris with perhexilene maleate. Chest. 1979; 75:152.

179. Dasta JF et al: Topical nitroglycerin: A new twist to an old standby. Am Pharm. 1982; NS22:85.

180. Hodge RH et al: How long does a tube of nitroglycerin ointment last? Ann Intern Med. 1980; 93:373.

181. Transderm-Nitro product information, Ciba Pharmaceutical Company, Summit, New Jersey, 1981.

182. Nitrodisc product information, Searle Pharmaceuticals, Chicago, Illinois, 1982.

183. Nitro-Dur product information, Key Pharmaceuticals, Miami, Florida, 1981.

184. Shaw JE: Transdermal NTG: Raising some issues. Am Pharm. 1982; NS22:227.

Chapter 13

Acute Myocardial Infarction

Barbara L. Greenberg

Pathophysiology. Acute myocardial infarctions occur primarily in patients with significant coronary artery stenosis secondary to atherosclerosis. Acute obstruction of a coronary artery occludes blood flow to the dependent myocardial tissue. The exact pathogenesis of coronary artery occlusion is not completely understood. Proposed causes of obstruction include: coronary artery thrombosis, rupture of an atherosclerotic plaque resulting in hemorrhage into the coronary artery, platelet aggregates adhering to the endothelium of atherosclerotic arteries, and coronary artery spasm (1,2).

Regardless of the etiology of the occlusion, lack of blood supply results in ischemic changes in the myocardial tissue. These ischemic changes are reversible if blood supply returns to the tissue. However, if hypoxia persists, irreversible cell necrosis occurs, resulting in myocardial infarction. Irreversible damage probably starts about 2 hours after the onset of symptoms of myocardial infarction (3). Cell necrosis may continue for 6 to 24 hours.

Surrounding the core zone of infarcted tissue, there is an ischemic "twilight" zone, or border zone, in which the blood supply is compromised but not occluded. This area is in jeopardy of infarcting if the balance of oxygen supply and de-

mand is not maintained. The size of infarction may be increased by factors that decrease oxygen supply (eg, hypotension, thrombus formation, spasm) or increase oxygen demand (eg, tachycardia, hypertension). Metabolic factors that inhibit cell respiration and cause membrane damage, such as increased circulating free fatty acids, may also increase infarct size (3).

During the infarction process, the heart is susceptible to electrical and mechanical instability. Arrhythmias are frequent, and pump failure may occur if damage to the ventricular wall is extensive.

The following case illustrates the treatment of an uncomplicated acute myocardial infarction. The complications that may accompany myocardial infarction are discussed elsewhere in this textbook. For more information concerning the sequelae of myocardial infarction the reader is directed to the chapters on Congestive Heart Failure, Cardiac Arrhythmias, and Intensive Care Therapeutics.

1. B.F., a 54-year-old, 130 lb female accountant arrived at the hospital via life squad. Her chief complaint was severe chest pain that felt like a heavy weight on her chest. About six months prior to admission B.F. developed angina pectoris that was treated with

sublingual nitroglycerin and oral isosorbide dinitrate. On the day of admission she experienced severe "crushing," substernal chest pain that radiated to her left elbow, accompanied by diaphoresis and nausea. When her chest pain persisted for over one hour despite taking 5 nitroglycerin tablets, she called the life squad. In the ambulance her blood pressure was 115/85 mm Hg and her heart rate was 75/min. She arrived at the hospital about three hours after her chest pain began.

B.F. has no past medical history of diabetes or hypertension. She began menopause at age 52, has a 20-pack-year smoking history, and drinks alcohol occasionally. Her mother died at age 68 of a cerebrovascular accident; her 78-year-old father has a history of two myocardial infarctions. Her sister, age 52, is in good health.

In the emergency room B.F.'s blood pressure was 110/80 mm Hg and her heart rate was 80/min. An ECG revealed ST segment elevations in leads II, III and aVF. Because she was very anxious about her chest pain, she was given diazepam 10 mg intramuscularly and transferred to the coronary care unit with a diagnosis of suspected acute myocardial infarction.

In the coronary care unit her physical examination was unremarkable, revealing no signs of heart failure. After an intravenous line was established, she was given morphine sulfate 4 mg IV to control her chest pain. The chest pain continued and she was given morphine 8 mg IV 15 minutes later. Twenty minutes after the second morphine injection her heart rate was 65/min, her blood pressure was 90/75 mm Hg, and her pain was gone. Other medications included lidocaine 100 mg IV push followed by 2 mg/min infusion, diazepam 5 mg po q6h, and docusate calcium 240 mg qd.

An ECG taken during the second day of her hospital stay demonstrated Q waves in leads II, III, and aVF and deepening T waves in these same leads. The patterns of ECG changes confirmed the diagnosis of acute myocardial infarction. The lidocaine infusion was discontinued after 48 hours, and no arrhythmias occurred during the four days she was in the coronary care unit.

Her cardiac enzyme concentrations dur-

ing the first three days of her admission were as follows:

	Admission	12 hr	24 hr	36 hr	48 hr	72 hr
CPK	38	432	640	580	529	456
SGOT	42	58	136	124	98	96
LDH	95	103	122	156	183	204

What subjective and objective evidence is compatible with the diagnosis of myocardial infarction in this patient?

The diagnosis of myocardial infarction requires at least two of the following: history of characteristic chest pain; ECG changes consistent with myocardial damage; and an elevation in the concentrations of cardiac enzymes (4).

Chest Pain. B.F.'s chest pain was typical of a patient with acute myocardial infarction. The pain is commonly described by patients as "deep," "crushing," "squeezing," or "heavy." Although usually located in the center of the chest, the pain can radiate to the jaw or arms. Unlike the pain of angina pectoris, the chest discomfort is not relieved by rest or nitroglycerin. Patients describe the pain of infarction as more severe than angina, often accompanied by feeling of impending doom. Other symptoms that can occur with acute myocardial infarction are weakness, diaphoresis, nausea, vomiting, and extreme anxiety (5).

Electrocardiogram (ECG). B.F.'s ECG demonstrates the pattern associated with acute myocardial infarction: Q waves; ST segment elevation; and T wave inversion (6,7). The pattern of these changes reflects the stages of myocardial damage occurring after occlusion of a coronary artery. The diagnosis includes assessment of the progressive, day to day ECG changes. ST segment elevation, which represents myocardial injury, appears early. T wave inversion, caused by myocardial ischemia, becomes evident as the ST segment elevation returns to baseline. The Q wave, which represents irreversible damage and necrosis of the myocardium, may occur early or progress over several days.

Enzymes. The three enzymes measured to confirm a diagnosis of acute myocardial infarction are creatine phosphokinase (CPK), serum glutamic oxaloacetic transaminase (SGOT) and lactic dehydrogenase (LDH). Ischemic destruction of the myocardial cells releases large quantities of these intracellular enzymes into the systemic circulation. Because these enzymes are released at different rates following infarction, the time course of the enzyme concentrations is of diagnostic importance (5). Typically, the CPK peaks at one day and returns to normal levels after two days. B.F.'s CPK concentrations are not reliable because she received an IM injection that released CPK from her muscle tissue. The CPK could have been fractionated to isolate levels of the CPK-MB isoenzyme which is specific for myocardial tissue. The SGOT concentrations usually peak at 24–48 hours and return to normal in 4 to 5 days. The concentration of LDH peaks at 48–72 hours and may persist for up to 14 days. The LDH can be fractionated; the LDH_1 isoenzyme, which is specific for cardiac tissue, increases before the total LDH in patients with myocardial infarction and is a more sensitive indicator than total LDH.

2. Why was B.F. given morphine sulfate? Were the route and dose appropriate?

Morphine is the drug of choice for relief of the pain associated with acute myocardial infarction (5,7–9). In addition to its potent analgesic action, morphine induces a euphoria that helps diminish the anxiety often associated with infarction. Morphine also dilates peripheral vessels, causing a decrease in both peripheral resistance and venous tone. These cardiovascular effects decrease cardiac work load and tend to lower myocardial oxygen consumption (9–14).

In patients with a myocardial infarction, the intravenous route is preferred because of its rapid onset of action and assured absorption. To minimize the orthostatic hypotension and bradycardia that can complicate morphine therapy after an acute myocardial infarction, small doses of 1 to 4 mg should be used. Therefore, B.F., who was initially given 4 mg of morphine sulfate intravenously, was dosed appropriately.

3. What is the goal of morphine therapy in B.F? How should she be managed if the pain is not relieved?

The goal of morphine therapy in the treatment of acute myocardial infarction is to relieve pain without inducing hypotension, bradycardia, or respiratory depression. Because the pain can be severe, more than one dose of morphine may be needed to relieve the pain. Morphine doses should be repeated until the pain subsides, but the patient must be monitored after each dose for signs of respiratory difficulty and hypotension. Because hypotension occurs more commonly in the sitting or standing positions, B.F. should remain in the recumbent position after she receives morphine.

Repeated doses of morphine should remain small (1 to 4 mg) to minimize risks of hypotension. Further, because the peak respiratory depressant effects occur within 10 minutes after intravenous administration, doses should be separated by at least 10 to 15 minutes.

B.F. was given a second dose of morphine sulfate 20 minutes after her initial dose. Although the time interval between doses was appropriate, the dose of 8 mg was large, resulting in a lowered heart rate and blood pressure. This could have been prevented had a smaller dose been given.

4. If B.F. had been unable to tolerate morphine, what alternative analgesic could have been used? Are there any analgesics which are contraindicated in the setting of acute myocardial infarction?

Meperidine is effective in relieving the pain associated with myocardial infarction and is the preferred alternative to morphine (5,7,15). Although *pentazocine* also reduces the pain associated with an acute myocardial infarction (16–18), it increases blood pressure through vasoconstriction and thereby increases cardiac work and myocardial oxygen consumption (10,13,19,20). Both of these effects may exacerbate myocardial ischemia; it also has a negative intropic effect. For all of these reasons, pentazocine is contraindicated in patients with acute myocardial infarction.

5. Patient B.F. received diazepam 10 mg IM in the emergency room. What evidence supports the use of anxiolytic agents like diazepam in the routine management of acute myocardial infarctions?

Diazepam and other benzodiazepines mildly sedate patients and decrease the anxiety associated with chest pain (7,15,21). Anxiety can augment catecholamine release, which increases cardiac work and thereby extends the size of the infarction; anxiety may also increase the likelihood of malignant tachyarrhythmias. Melsom et al (22) reported that diazepam 10 mg IV followed by 15 mg po tid for 3 days had beneficial effects in patients with myocardial infarction. There was a decrease in the signs and symptoms of anxiety, a reduced frequency and severity of arrhythmias, and a smaller amount of analgesic usage in acute myocardial infarction patients treated with diazepam compared to a control group that received no anxiolytic medication.

These results were not confirmed in a placebo-controlled, double-blind study by Dixon et al (23) who used diazepam 10 mg po q 6 h for 3 days after acute myocardial infarction. Dixon found no significant difference between treatment and control groups in the degree of anxiety experienced by the patients, although the drug-treated patients had more severe drowsiness. The same number of patients in each group experienced arrhythmias.

Differences in study design may account for the conflicting results of these two studies. Dixon randomly assigned 172 acute myocardial infarction patients to drug or placebo treated groups. Melsom had a control group, but did not mention a placebo or a blinding procedure. Also, Melsom administered an initial dose of 10 mg IV; thus, the concentrations of diazepam in his patients on the first day were higher than the concentrations reported in Dixon's study.

A long history of clinical success attests to the benefit of mild sedation after acute myocardial infarction. Accordingly, anxiolytics, such as diazepam, are routinely prescribed for the management of myocardial infarction.

6. B.F. received 10 mg of diazepam IM in the emergency room. Was this an appropriate route of administration?

Oral diazepam results in faster and more complete absorption than does intramuscular administration (24). Intramuscular injections are painful. Furthermore, they destroy muscle tissue resulting in a release of CPK enzyme into the circulation (25,26) which may ultimately cause difficulty in diagnosing myocardial infarction. For these reasons, oral diazepam would have been the preferred route of administration of diazepam.

7. Patient B.F. received intravenous lidocaine in the hospital even though she had no arrhythmias. Why?

Ventricular fibrillation causes a significant number of deaths after acute myocardial infarction, especially in patients like B.F. who are less than 70 years of age (27–30). Fibrillation is most common in the first 6 to 12 hours after the infarction, but seldom occurs beyond 48 hours. Although "warning arrhythmias" (frequent premature ventricular contractions, R-on-T contractions, or multifocal beats, etc.) may pre-cede some episodes of ventricular fibrillation, about 25–50% of the patients experiencing ventricular fibrillation have no prodromal arrhythmias (27–29). Further, even if these warning arrhythmias do occur, they may precede fibrillation by only a matter of minutes, making it difficult to institute antiarrhythmic therapy before the more serious arrhythmia occurs. Therefore, routine prophylactic antiarrhythmic therapy is indicated in all myocardial infarction patients to prevent these lethal arrhythmias.

Lidocaine is the agent used most extensively to prevent ventricular fibrillation after an acute myocardial infarction. Lie et al (31) in a placebo-controlled, double-blind study demonstrated that lidocaine 100 mg IV followed by an infusion of 3 mg/min for 48 hours prevented primary ventricular fibrillation when it was given to patients within 6 hours of the onset of symptoms of acute myocardial infarction. Nine of the 105 patients receiving placebo experienced primary ventricular fibrillation, one of whom died. None of the patients receiving lidocaine experienced fibrillation.

The doses of lidocaine used for prophylaxis are the same as those used to treat arrhythmias therapeutically. See chapter on Cardiac Arrhythmias for more details concerning the proper dosing of lidocaine.

8. Patient B.F. did not receive prophylactic lidocaine in the ambulance on her way to the hospital. Why isn't prophylactic intramuscular lidocaine routinely given to acute myocardial infarction patients?

Over one-half of the deaths associated with acute myocardial infarction occur before arrival at the hospital. The primary cause of these deaths is ventricular fibrillation (29). Several investigators have suggested that the administration of intramuscular antiarrhythmic therapy to all patients suspected of having acute myocardial infarction before they arrive at the hospital would decrease the "prehospital" phase mortality. It has not been established, however, that this maneuver is clearly beneficial.

Valentine et al (32) studied the effect of lidocaine 300 mg IM given before hospitalization on the mortality associated with acute myocardial infarction. When compared to placebo, IM lidocaine did decrease the number of deaths that occurred 2 hours after injection. Unfortunately, their study suffered from design defects; in particular, neither myocardial infarction nor ventricular arrhythmias were adequately documented in the study population. Lie et al (33) found that lidocaine 300 mg was not effective in preventing primary ventricular fibrillation one hour after intramuscular injection. They suggest that 300 mg did not provide concentrations high enough to prevent ventricular fibrillation. Zener et al (34) reported that a dose of 6 mg/kg injected into the intradeltoid muscle provided therapeutic blood concentrations within 30 minutes. These concentrations remained over 1.5 mcg/ml for more than 2 hours. The results of the studies by Lie and Zener (33,34) indicate that larger intramuscular doses of lidocaine may be effective in preventing ventricular fibrillation. Further testing of intramuscular lidocaine is needed before specific recommendations can be made.

9. B.F. was not given any anticoagulants during her hospitalization. What are the indications for anticoagulation after an acute myocardial infarction?

The routine care of uncomplicated acute myocardial infarction does not include anticoagulation. Such therapy is reserved for patients who have a high risk of developing venous or arterial thrombi. Risk factors for thrombosis following an acute myocardial infarction include heart failure, shock, prolonged bedrest, and a history of thromboembolic disease. B.F. did not experience complications after her myocardial infarction, and prolonged bedrest was not necessary. Because she was not in a high risk group for the development of either arterial or venous thrombi, anticoagulation was not indicated.

Advocates of anticoagulation for all patients with acute myocardial infarction claim this therapy will decrease mortality associated with myocardial infarction by: preventing pulmonary embolism and deep vein thrombosis of the leg; reducing arterial embolization of cardiac mural thrombi; decreasing the extent of myocardial necrosis; and lowering the recurrence rate of infarction (35). Unfortunately, evidence supporting these claims is lacking. The incidence of thromboembolic complications after an acute myocardial infarction currently is lower than it was in the 1940's and 1950's. The present aggressive approach to post-infarction therapy includes early ambulation which decreases the risks of embolization. Contemporary reports (36,37) suggesting benefits from anticoagulation are fraught with

problems in methodology and statistical analysis (38,39).

10. How could drugs reduce the size of the myocardial infarction in this patient?

Myocardial damage after an infarction begins with reversible ischemic changes that evolve to irreversible myocardial cell necrosis. Drugs that interrupt the infarction process during the reversible ischemic phase can reduce the size of myocardial infarction. These drugs are most effective in salvaging the myocardial tissue in the ischemic border zone surrounding the core area of infarction (40). This zone is in jeopardy of infarction because of poor perfusion after coronary occlusion, increased oxygen demands resulting from myocardial infarction (eg, tachycardia, hypertension), and metabolic changes that enhance myocardial cell damage (eg, elevated free fatty acid concentrations) (3). Table 1 lists some of the agents that reduce myocardial infarction size and their proposed mechanisms of action.

Much of the information concerning these agents is based upon animal studies. Therapeutic intervention to reduce myocardial infarction size is presently investigational in humans and cannot be recommended for routine use in uncomplicated acute mycoardial infarction. This therapy holds great promise as a method of limiting myocardial damage and heart failure after coronary occlusion. Opie (3,41) and Maroko et al (42,43) provide more detailed reviews of this topic.

Table 1.

AGENTS THAT REDUCE MYOCARDIAL INFARCT SIZE*

Drug	Proposed Mechanism
Propranolol	Decreases heart rate, blood pressure, contractility, and afterload
	Improves tissue metabolism
	Decreases microvascular damage
Nitrates	Decreases blood pressure, preload, and afterload
	Improves coronary blood flow
Hyaluronidase	Improves coronary blood flow
Glucose-Insulin-Potassium	Improves tissue metabolism
	Improves contractility without extending infarct size

*Adapted from Opie (41)

11. What role do thrombolytic agents play in the treatment of this patient?

The use of thrombolytic agents, such as streptokinase and urokinase, in the treatment of acute myocardial infarction is presently investigational. Thrombolytics activate plasminogen and initiate clot lysis. They can decrease the extent of necrosis by preventing the formation of primary or secondary thrombi in the microcirculation near the occluded coronary vessel (44,45). Although some studies suggested that intravenous thrombolytic agents reduced mortality after an acute myocardial infarction, other reports indicated no benefit (44,46). There is not enough information available at present to recommend the routine use of intravenous thrombolysis (45).

Selective intracoronary thrombolysis, a recently developed procedure, recannulates an occluded vessel by injecting thrombolytics directly into the occluded coronary artery. Selective intracoronary thrombolysis with streptokinase reopened coronary vessels when it was administered within a few hours of myocardial infarction (47–51). Although further study is needed, available data indicate that this procedure may decrease infarct size or even prevent myocardial necrosis.

12. B.F. did not take an antiplatelet agent after she was discharged from the hospital. What evidence supports the use of antiplatelet agents in the prevention of reinfarction?

Interest in antiplatelet therapy in patients with atherosclerotic coronary heart disease began when the Boston Collaborative Drug Surveillance Program noted that patients taking aspirin regularly were less likely to have fatal myocardial infarctions (52,53). This finding stimulated research concerning the protective effect of antiplatelet therapy on myocardial infarction mortality. Several large, randomized, placebo-controlled, double-blind trials evaluated the effects of aspirin in patients with atherosclerosis. Although aspirin tended to reduce mortality, the differences between the aspirin treated and placebo groups were not statistically significant (54–58). The Aspirin Myocardial Infarction Study (AMIS) found no difference in the mortality rate in patients receiving aspirin 1 gm/day compared to patients receiving placebo (59). However, the patients taking aspirin had a greater incidence of gastrointestinal complaints. Because definitive proof of the benefit of aspirin is lacking, aspirin is not used routinely after acute myocardial infarction.

The Persantine-Aspirin Reinfarction Study (PARIS) randomized myocardial infarction patients into three treatment groups: aspirin 324 mg tid plus dipyridamole 75 mg tid, aspirin 324 mg tid alone, and placebo tablet tid (60). Again, the results suggested a lower mortality rate in both drug treated groups, but the differences did not reach statistical significance.

A major investigation concerning the ability of sulfinpyrazone to prevent reinfarction, Anturane Reinfarction Trial (ART), reported that sulfinpyrazone prevented sudden cardiac death when given to patients one to six months after acute myocardial infarction (61). Although the design of the ART was elaborate (62,63), the Food and Drug Administration did not approve the use of sulfinpyrazone to prevent myocardial infarction. Reviewers of the study (64) noted significant problems with the trial, especially regarding the classification of the causes of death and the exclusion of some patients from the trial after they had entered the study. Further analysis of the results of the ART (65) and additional trials are needed before sulfinpyrazone can be recommended routinely to prevent reinfarction. (Also see the chapter entitled Thrombosis.)

References

1. Willerson JT et al: Cause and course of acute myocardial infarction. Am J Med. 1980; 69:903.
2. Oliva PB: Pathophysiology of acute myocardial infarction. Ann Intern Med. 1981; 94:236.
3. Opie LH: Myocardial infarct size. Part 1. Basic considerations. Am Heart J. 1980; 100:355.
4. Hurst JW et al: The clinical recognition and management of coronary atherosclerotic heart disease. In *The Heart,* 4th ed, edited by JW Hurst, McGraw-Hill Book Co, New York, 1978, p 1156.
5. Braunwald E et al: Acute myocardial infarction. In *Harrison's Principles of Internal Medicine,* 9th ed, edited by KJ Isselbacher, McGraw-Hill Book Co, San Francisco, 1980, p 1125.
6. Marriott HJL: Myocardial infarction. In *Practical Electrocardiography,* 6th ed, Williams & Wilkins Co, Baltimore, 1977, p 232.
7. Wenger NK et al: Management of the patient with myocardial infarction. DM. 1979; 25:1.
8. Kerr F et al: Analgesia in myocardial infarction. Br Heart J. 1974; 36:117.
9. Alderman EL: Analgesics in the acute phase of myocardial infarction. JAMA. 1974; 229:1646.
10. Alderman EL et al: Hemodynamic effects of morphine and pentazocine differ in cardiac patients. N Engl J Med. 1972; 287:623.
11. Eckerhoff JE et al: The effects of narcotics and antagonists upon respiration and circulation in man. A review. Clin Pharmacol Ther. 1960; 1:483.
12. Lowenstein E et al: Cardiovascular response to large doses of intravenous morphine in man. N Engl J Med. 1969; 281:1389.
13. Lee G et al: Comparative effects of morphine, meperidine and pentazocine on cardiocirculatory dynamics in patients with acute myocardial infarction. Am J Med. 1976; 60:949.
14. Timmis AD et al: Haemodynamic effects of intravenous morphine in patients with acute myocardial infarction complicated by severe left ventricular failure. Br Med J. 1980; 1:980.
15. Gazes PC et al: Bedside management of acute myocardial infarction. Am Heart J. 1979; 97:782.
16. Miller HC et al: Effect of pentazocine on pulmonary circulation. Lancet. 1972; 2:1167.
17. Rettig G et al: Hemodynamic effects of pentazocine in acute myocardial infarction. Jpn Heart J. 1979; 20:253.
18. Scott ME et al: Circulatory effects of intravenous pentazocine in patients with acute myocardial infarction. Curr Ther Res. 1971; 13:81.
19. Jewitt DE et al: Cardiovascular effects of pentazocine in patients with acute myocardial infarction. Br Heart J. 1971; 33:145.
20. Jewitt DE et al: Increased pulmonary arterial pressures after pentazocine in myocardial infarction. Br Med J. 1970; 1:795.
21. Côté P et al: Therapeutic implications of diazepam in patients with elevated left ventricular filling pressure. Am Heart J. 1976; 91:747.
22. Melsom M et al: Diazepam in acute myocardial infarction. Clinical effects and effects on catecholamines, free fatty acids, and cortisol. Br Heart J. 1976; 38:804.
23. Dixon RA et al: Diazepam in immediate post-myocardial infarct period. A double-blind trial. Br Heart J. 1980; 43:535.
24. Hillestad L et al: Diazepam metabolism in normal man 1. Serum concentrations and clinical effects after intravenous, intramuscular, and oral administration. Clin Pharmacol Ther. 1974; 16:479.
25. Greenblatt DJ et al: Serum creatine phosphokinase concentrations after intramuscular chlordiazepoxide and its solvent. J Clin Pharmacol. 1976; 16:118.
26. Hansten PD: Drugs which may elevate serum creatine phosphokinase. In *Drug Interactions,* 4th ed, Lea & Febiger, Philadelphia, 1979, p 340.
27. Ribner HS et al: Lidocaine prophylaxis against ventricular fibrillation in acute myocardial infarction. Progr Cardiovasc Dis. 1979; 21:287.
28. Harrison DC: Should lidocaine be administered routinely to all patients after acute myocardial infarction? Circulation. 1978; 58:581.
29. Noneman JW et al: Lidocaine prophylaxis in acute myocardial infarction. Medicine (Baltimore). 1978; 57:501.
30. Resnekov L et al: Prevention of ventricular rhythm disturbances in patients with acute myocardial infarction. Am Heart J. 1979; 98:653.
31. Lie KI et al: Lidocaine in the prevention of primary ventricular fibrillation. A double-blind, randomized study of 212 consecutive patients. N Engl J Med. 1974; 291:1324.
32. Valentine PA et al: Lidocaine in the prevention of sudden death in the pre-hospital phase of acute infarction. N Engl J Med. 1974; 291:1327.
33. Lie KI et al: Efficacy of lidocaine in preventing primary ventricular fibrillation within 1 hour after 300 mg intramuscular injection. A double-blind, randomized study of 300 hospitalized patients with acute myocardial infarction. Am J Cardiol. 1978; 42:486.
34. Zener J et al: Blood lidocaine levels and kinetics following high-dose intramuscular administration. Circulation. 1973; 47:984.
35. Frishman WH et al: Anticoagulation in myocardial infarction: Modern approach to an old problem. Am J Cardiol. 1979; 43:1207.
36. Chalmers TC et al: Evidence favoring the use of anticoagulants in the hospital phase of acute myocardial infarction. N Engl J Med. 1977; 297:1091.
37. Szklo M et al: Additional data favoring use of anticoagulant therapy in myocardial infarction. A population-based study. JAMA. 1979; 242:1261.
38. Selzer A: Use of anticoagulant agents in acute myocardial infarction: Statistics or clinical judgement? Am J Cardiol. 1978; 41:1315.
39. Goldman L et al: Anticoagulants and myocardial infarction. The problems of pooling, drowning, and floating. Ann Intern Med. 1979; 90:92.
40. Karlsberg RP et al: Reduction of myocardial infarct size. Approach for the 1980s. Arch Intern Med. 1980; 140:616.
41. Opie LH: Myocardial infarct size. Part 2. Comparison of anti-infarct effects of beta-blockade, glucose-insulin-potassium, nitrates, and hyaluronidase. Am Heart J. 1980; 100:531.
42. Maroko PR et al: Modification of myocardial infarction size after coronary occlusion. Ann Intern Med. 1973; 79:720.

43. Maroko PR et al: Infarct size reduction: A critical review. Adv Cardiol. 1980; 27:127.

44. Duckert F: Thrombolytic therapy in myocardial infarction. Progr Cardiovasc Dis. 1979; 21:342.

45. Sullivan JM: Streptokinase and myocardial infarction. N Engl J Med. 1979; 301:836.

46. European Cooperative Study Group: Streptokinase in acute myocardial infarction. N Engl Med J. 1979; 301:797.

47. Mathey DG et al: Nonsurgical coronary artery recanalization in acute transmural myocardial infarction. Circulation. 1981; 63:489.

48. Rentrop P et al: Selective intracoronary thrombolysis in acute myocardial infarction and unstable angina pectoris. Circulation. 1981; 63:307.

49. Ganz W et al: Intracoronary thrombolysis in evolving myocardial infarction. Am Heart J. 1981; 101:4.

50. Reduto LA et al: Lysis of coronary artery thrombosis with intracoronary streptokinase in acute myocardial infarction. (Abstract). Am J Cardiol. 1981; 47:493.

51. Schuler G et al: Intracoronary streptokinase in acute myocardial infarction: Assessment by T1-201 scintigraphy. (Abstract). Am J Cardiol. 1981; 47:493.

52. Boston Collaborative Drug Surveillance Group: Regular aspirin intake and acute myocardial infarction. Br Med J. 1974; 1:440.

53. Jick H et al: Regular aspirin use and myocardial infarction. Br Med J. 1976; 1:1057.

54. Elwood PC et al: A randomized controlled trial of acetyl salicylic acid in the secondary preventio of mortality from myocardial infarction. Br Med J. 1974; 1:436.

55. Coronary Drug Project Research Group: Aspirin in coronary heart disease. J Chron Dis. 1976; 29:625.

56. Elwood PC et al: Aspirin and secondary mortality after myocardial infarction. Lancet. 1979; 2:1313.

57. McNicol GP: Antiplatelet drugs in the secondary prevention of myocardial infarction. Lancet. 1980; 2:736.

58. Fuster V et al: Antithrombotic therapy: Role of platelet-inhibitor drugs. III. Management of arterial thromboembolic and atherosclerotic disease (third of three parts). Mayo Clin Proc. 1981; 56:265.

59. Aspirin Myocardial Infarction Study Research Group: A randomized, controlled trial of aspirin in persons recovered from myocardial infarction. JAMA. 1980; 243:661.

60. Persantine-Aspirin Reinfarction Study Research Group: Persantine and aspirin in coronary heart disease. Circulation. 1980; 62:449.

61. Anturane Reinfarction Trial Research Group: Sulfinpyrazone in the prevention of sudden death after myocardial infarction. N Engl J Med. 1980; 302:250.

62. Anturane Reinfarction Trial Research Group: Sulfinpyrazone in the prevention of cardiac death after myocardial infarction: The Anturane Reinfarction Trial. N Engl J Med. 1978; 298:289.

63. Sherry S: Drug trials in myocardial infarction. Lessons to be learned from the Anturane Reinfarction Trial. Eur J Clin Pharmacol. 1980; 17:401.

64. Temple R et al: The FDA's critique of the Anturane Reinfarction Trial. N Engl J Med. 1980; 303:1488.

65. Relman AS: Sulfinpyrazone after myocardial infarction: No decision yet. N Engl J Med. 1980; 303:1476.

Chapter 14

Intensive Care Therapeutics

Charles C. Depew and R. Jon Auricchio

ABBREVIATIONS

ABG	=	arterial blood gases
BP	=	blood pressure
BSA	=	body surface area
CI	=	cardiac index
CNS	=	central nervous system
CO	=	cardiac output
COP	=	colloid osmotic pressure
CVP	=	central venous pressure
CXR	=	chest x-ray
EKG	=	electrocardiogram
FFP	=	fresh frozen plasma
HCT	=	hematocrit
HES	=	hydroxyethyl starch
HR	=	heart rate
ICU	=	intensive care unit
LVEDP	=	left ventricular end diastolic pressure
LVSWI	=	left ventricular stroke work index
MAP	=	mean arterial pressure
MI	=	myocardial infarction
MVO_2	=	myocardial oxygen demand
NE	=	norepinephrine
P	=	pulse
PAD	=	pulmonary artery diastolic
PAP	=	pulmonary artery pressure
PCWP	=	pulmonary capillary wedge pressure
PMH	=	past medical history
PPF	=	plasma protein fraction
PRBC	=	packed red blood cells
PTA	=	prior to admission
RAP	=	right atrial pressure
RR	=	respiratory rate
SV	=	stroke volume
SVI	=	stroke volume index
TPVR	=	total peripheral vascular resistance
U/O	=	urine output
UTI	=	urinary tract infection

SHOCK

Shock is defined as an acute pathophysiologic syndrome in which vital organs are inadequately perfused. If the shock state is prolonged, transcapillary exchange of essential substrates and oxygen is hindered, resulting in cellular impairment. Cellular injury results from the disruption of intracellular mitochondria and lysosomes, and from disablement of enzymatic processes. As a compensatory response, the cells shift into anerobic glycolysis in order to generate a high energy phosphate supply for vital organs. Tissue hypoxia ensues and lactic acid accumulates (1). This lack of adequate tissue perfusion for maintenance of aerobic metabolism is crucial to the development of the shock syndrome.

It should be emphasized that inadequate delivery of oxygen and nutrients to tissues is not necessarily associated with hypotension and, conversely, hypotension does not necessarily indicate inadequate tissue perfusion. Shock may occur with a normal blood pressure, and hypotension may occur without shock.

The physiological defect which underlies the shock state is acute circulatory failure with reduction of effective blood flow to the skin, muscle, brain, kidneys, heart, and other vital organs (2). The concept of effective blood flow is important because cardiac output is normal or increased in hyperdynamic septic shock, but due to anatomic and physiologic shunting, oxygen is unavailable to the nutrient capillary beds.

Initial hemodynamic states vary according to the etiology of the shock. In fact, seven different hemodynamic defects of the circulatory system may account for the acute perfusion failure and the clinical signs of shock: (a) excessive resistance in the arterial circuit; (b) shunting of blood through arteriovenous communications; (c) excessive resistance in the post capillary venous bed;

(d) pooling of blood in a dilated venous capacitance bed; (e) reduction in blood volume; (f) failure of the heart to serve as an effective pump or (g) obstruction to the mainstream of flow through the circulatory system (3). Once shock is diagnosed and the primary hemodynamic defect assessed, therapy is then directed at correcting the underlying hemodynamic abnormality. Regardless of the etiology, therapy of shock must include early correction of any cardiac dysfunction because the shock state can be perpetuated by a developing cardiac lesion even if the initiating event (eg, hemorrhage) has been corrected.

The classic shock syndrome is characterized by a coldness and moistness of the skin, hyperventilation, tachycardia, collapse of superficial veins, thready pulse, oliguria, anxiety, confusion, and restlessness. These signs and symptoms may not be present concurrently and usually occur late in the course of shock relative to biochemical changes. Thus, it is important to monitor vital signs, intracardiac pressures, urinary output, cardiac output, ventilatory status, metabolic derangements, sensorium, and derived hemodynamic indices of patients in shock.

Shock can be divided into six main categories (see Table 1). At any given time, one form of shock may take on the characteristics and sequelae of another.

Hypovolemic shock is caused by a decrease in intravascular volume and is associated with a blood volume deficit of 15% to 25%. The blood volume deficit may be a result of hemorrhage, blood and plasma sequestration in body cavities, or excessive vomiting, diarrhea, or diuresis. This loss of intravascular volume results in a low cardiac output and reflexly increases sympathetic nervous system outflow in an attempt to maintain intravascular perfusion pressure. The heightened sympathetic response increases peripheral vascular resistance and redistributes vascular volume from the peripheral to the central circulation. Thus, the tachycardia, cold clammy skin, and oliguria can be attributed to the sympathetic excess. The confusion, anxiety, and restlessness often exhibited by patients in moderate to severe hypovolemic shock are attributable to poor central nervous system perfusion.

Hypovolemic shock can be divided into three stages. *Stage I* of hypovolemic shock results from a blood volume deficit of up to 10% (500 ml). At this stage, cardiac output and arterial pressure are maintained and the patient is usually asymptomatic. *Stage II* occurs when blood loss is 15–25%. In stage II, cardiac output and blood pressure are markedly reduced, and typical symptoms include tachycardia, tachypnea, pallor, diaphoresis, oliguria, apprehension, and restlessness. *Stage III* occurs when the blood volume deficit is greater than 25%. In this stage, the circulatory system deteriorates rapidly as the cardiac output, blood pressure, and tissue perfusion become markedly reduced. If circulatory blood volume is not restored promptly, myocardial depression, anoxia, hypercapnia, lactic acidosis, increased capillary permeability, and disseminated intravascular coagulation develop. Prolonged hypotension may cause such severe organ damage that shock may continue despite replacement of the lost in-

Table 1.

CLASSIFICATION OF SHOCK STATE AND COMMON ETIOLOGIC FACTORS

1. Hypovolemic Shock
   A. Blood loss due to hemorrhage, intrathoracic or intraabdominal sequestration.
   B. Plasma loss due to burns and third space accumulation.
   C. Fluid loss due to diarrhea, vomiting, diabetes mellitus, diabetes inspidus, diabetic keto acidosis, overuse of diuretics.

2. Cardiogenic Shock
   A. Arrhythmias
   B. Myocardial infarction
   C. Heart failure with low cardiac output
   D. Post cardiopulmonary bypass surgery

3. Septic Shock
   A. Gram negative septicemia
   B. Gram positive septicemia

4. Obstruction to Blood Flow
   A. Pericardial tamponade
   B. Pulmonary embolus
   C. Dissecting aortic aneurysm
   D. Intracardiac ball valve thrombus

5. Neurogenic Shock
   A. Drug induced: ganglionic blockade, spinal anesthesia, drug overdose
   B. Spinal cord injury

6. Other
   A. Anaphylaxis
   B. Endocrine: Addison's disease, myxedema, hypoglycemia

travascular volume (21). The shock state may proceed through all three stages gradually or develop abruptly.

Treatment of patients with hypovolemic shock requires replacement of intravascular volume with fluids or blood products. If the cardiac output remains low despite adequate fluid replacement, and if the elevated central venous pressure and pulmonary artery pressures are indicative of myocardial depression, inotropic agents may be helpful in supporting cardiac function.

Cardiogenic shock results when the heart fails to serve as an effective pump to maintain tissue perfusion. Acute myocardial infarction is the most common cause of cardiogenic shock. About 15% of hospitalized patients with acute myocardial infarction develop shock and about 75 to 80% of these cases are fatal (4). Cardiogenic shock may also result from arrhythmias such as ventricular tachycardia or fibrillation, which impair cardiac output, or from depressed cardiac function following cardiopulmonary artery bypass surgery.

Most patients in cardiogenic shock have low cardiac output, hypotension, tachycardia, and the typical signs of inadequate tissue perfusion such as cool clammy skin, decreased urine output, and central nervous system changes. Hypoxemia occurs because of pulmonary arteriovenous shunting through inadequately ventilated areas of the lung.

Unlike hypovolemic shock, the reflex activation of the sympathetic nervous system in patients experiencing shock from acute myocardial infarction may not result in increased peripheral vascular resistance. Approximately half of the patients with acute myocardial infarction and shock have a normal or low peripheral vascular resistance (5,6). These patients are less likely to have cool clammy skin and their prognosis is better than patients having a high peripheral vascular resistance. It is important that hemodynamic monitoring be provided to distinguish between various clinical presentations of acute myocardial infarction with shock because different treatment approaches will be required. Cardiogenic shock following acute myocardial infarction must also be differentiated from that of a depressed cardiac output following coronary artery bypass surgery. Therapeutic interventions which decrease coronary perfusion pressure or increase myocardial oxygen demand could extend the area of myocardial necrosis and must be approached with extreme caution.

In "shocky" patients with depressed cardiac output following coronary artery bypass surgery, the problem is not usually due to a specific myocardial lesion and interventions which may increase myocardial oxygen demand are not as hazardous. In this situation, maintaining peripheral perfusion is as important as maintaining coronary perfusion in shock following acute myocardial infarction.

Septic shock occurs when invasion by microorganisms causes circulatory insufficiency and inadequate tissue perfusion. Although gram-negative organisms account for the majority of the cases of septic shock, gram-positive cocci, clostridia, viruses, rickettsia, and fungi account for some cases (7).

Gram-positive shock is not well described in the literature, although septic shock associated with gram-positive organisms has been reported (136,137). Gram-negative bacteremic shock usually arises as a secondary disease or as a complication during hospitalization for another illness. In the majority of patients, gram-negative shock is precipitated by manipulative procedures such as bladder catheterization or genitourinary tract surgery. Other usual sites of access into the bloodstream include the gastrointestinal and pulmonary systems, the skin, and uterus. Predisposition to gram-negative sepsis includes serious underlying diseases, instrumentation, immunosuppressive agents, surgery, abdominal abcesses, trauma, burns, manipulation of infected wounds, and intravascular lines (7–9).

Most patients experiencing gram-negative shock experience chills followed by a spiking fever, tachycardia, tachypnea, hypotension, and signs of central nervous system hypoperfusion within 2–24 hours after the occurrence of gram-negative bacteremia. Hemodynamic changes in septic shock can be divided into two stages. The early stage is referred to as a hyperdynamic phase or "warm shock" and is characterized by a marked decrease in total peripheral vascular resistance, high or normal cardiac output, low blood pressure, wide pulse pressure, and warm dry skin. In some circumstances the cardiac output may decrease because of large amounts of blood which pool in the splanchnic circulation or because of fluid which leaves the vascular space as a result of capillary leak. The hemodynamic changes and alterations in vascular permeability in this first stage of shock are thought by some investigators to result from the effect of bacterial endotoxin (8,9,10).

Gram-negative endotoxin is a macromolecule composed of a polysaccharide outer layer and a phospholipid inner layer (138). The endotoxin is liberated from the cell wall of gram-negative bacteria at the time of bacterial death and enters the circulation. Hess and associates (8) suggest that the endotoxin initially induces release of histamines, bradykinins, prostaglandins, and endorphins into the circulation. These mediators decrease peripheral vascular resistance and reflexly increase cardiac output. If the cardiac output or tissue perfusion cannot be maintained at this early stage of septic shock, a later, more lethal stage, referred to as the hypodynamic phase or "cold state," may develop. This second stage of septic shock is characterized by the classical signs of cold extremities, elevated peripheral vascular resistance, low cardiac output, hypotension, oliguria, respiratory difficulties, signs of central nervous system hypoperfusion, anaerobic metabolism, and lactic acidosis (7,11).

The progression to the later stage of septic shock is both complex and controversial. It appears that venous capacitance is increased with pooling of blood in the hepato-splanchnic vasculature. This relative hypovolemia, in addition to the loss of plasma volume to the interstitial tissue because of marked capillary permeability, leads to a decrease in venous return and reduction in cardiac output. The decreased cardiac output stimulates the sympathoadrenal system and increases the level of circulating catecholamines. As a consequence, total peripheral and pulmonary vascular resistance increase, resulting in ventilation/perfusion defects and subsequent hypoxia.

The increase in peripheral vascular resistance is more pronounced on the venous side of the circulation than on the arterial side. This favors an increase in the capillary hydrostatic pressure, vascular fluid movement into the interstitial space, and a further reduction in cardiac output. These events, along with activation of the renin-angiotensin-aldosterone system because of impaired renal blood flow, lead to tissue hypoperfusion, which results in systemic acidosis. The combination of acidosis and myocardial depressant-like factors further depresses the myocardium and cardiac output. As this cycle of events accelerates, a high resistance-low output situation, which can lead to death, becomes established.

The lower the cardiac output, the more likely progressive lactic acidemia will develop and result in a fatal outcome (139–141). Cardiac index and survival are closely correlated (141). Failure to maintain cardiac output in the early stages of shock has been associated with a mortality rate of 80%.

Maintaining adequate vascular volume with fluids to prevent the "cold state" of septic shock is of primary importance until the underlying cause of bacterial invasion can be removed and/or treated with appropriate antibiotics. Although sympathomimetic agents are often needed for additional cardiovascular support, their effect on outcome is not known.

Obstruction to blood flow (eg, pericardial tamponade, pulmonary embolus, dissecting aortic aneurysm, or malfunctioning cardiac valves) also may induce a shock state. Pericardial tamponade, from severe constrictive pericarditis or failure of clot removal following heart surgery, often requires surgical intervention to relieve the ventricular compression that is compromising cardiac output. Adrenergic agents and maintenance of vascular volume may be necessary until the primary defect can be corrected surgically. Pulmonary embolism requires anticoagulant therapy to prevent further embolization and subsequent respiratory compromise or heart failure. A rapidly dissecting aortic aneurysm requires surgical intervention to prevent cardiovascular collapse. In this situation, induced hypotension with trimethophan (Arfonad) is often needed prior to surgery to prevent generation of high aortic systolic pressure which may potentiate aortic dissection. When the mainstream of blood flow is severely impeded by malfunctioning heart valves, open heart surgery for artificial valve replacement is necessary.

Neurogenic shock is uncommon and is usually precipitated by pharmacologic blockade or injury to the sympathetic nervous system. Neurogenic shock is most often caused by spinal anesthesia which induces a relative hypovolemia due to arterial and venous vasodilation. The relative hypovolemia decreases the blood pressure; the cardiac output may remain normal or increase. Elevation of the patient's lower extremities and administration of fluids to fill the expanded vascular space may reverse the perfusion failure. If these measures do not reverse the hypotension, an adrenergic agonist such as phenylephrine, metaraminol, or ephedrine sulfate can increase arterial resistance and elevate arterial perfusion pressure.

There are many etiologies of shock, although hypovolemic and cardiogenic shock are the most common. Hemodynamic changes which accompany shock result from a combination of an inciting event and sympathetic reflex responses. Changes in plasma levels of angiotensin, vasopressin, insulin, glucagon, histamine, endorphins, and prostaglandins also might be involved in the shock syndrome. Early recognition and early treatment of shock will affect the survival of patients. Hemodynamic monitoring with a pulmonary artery catheter helps to differentiate the various types of shock states and guide therapeutic interventions. Until the primary cause of shock can be resolved, maintenance of coronary and tissue perfusion with fluids, appropriate vasoactive drugs, and other supportive measures are the mainstays in the therapy of shock.

HEMODYNAMIC MONITORING

Monitoring the hemodynamic parameters of critically ill patients has become extremely important in the assessment of certain cardiovascular conditions and in the evaluation of therapeutic interventions which affect blood volume, blood pressure, or blood flow. Hemodynamic monitoring has been made easier with the development of the Swan-Ganz catheter, which can measure central venous and pulmonary artery pressures. However, it is important to stress that in any individual patient, prediction of hemodynamic responses to pharmacologic agents is not always absolute.

There are several versions of the Swan-Ganz catheter, but the one most commonly used is a quadruple-lumen thermodilution catheter (12). The catheter is inserted into a peripheral vein— usually the internal jugular or subclavian—and is advanced into the superior vena cava. Once in the superior vena cava, a 1.5 ml balloon, located 1 cm from the tip of the catheter, is inflated with air and the catheter advanced into the right atrium, through the tricuspid valve, into the right ventricle and then into the pulmonary artery, where the balloon lodges in a branch of the pulmonary artery of equal diameter. The catheter in

this position with the balloon inflated is in the "wedge" position. Figure 1 shows the anatomical position of the catheter and the different pressure tracings as it is advanced through the right side of the heart into a branch of the pulmonary artery and wedged. The pattern of the pressure tracing indicates the location of the catheter. After insertion of the catheter, the balloon is only intermittently inflated to obtain the pulmonary capillary wedge position. If inflated for prolonged periods, pulmonary infarction can occur due to obstruction of blood flow. The catheter is attached to transducers which provide for continuous monitoring of intracardiac and pulmonary pressures via an oscilloscope or digital display.

One lumen terminates at the distal tip of the catheter within a branch of the pulmonary artery; when the balloon is inflated, the pulmonary capillary wedge pressure (PCWP) is measured. A second lumen terminates in the right atrium and measures atrial pressures. This second lumen also serves as a portal of entry for both the administration of drugs and for the administration of iced solutions which are used to compute cardiac output. The third lumen contains the electrical leads for the thermistor which is positioned at the catheter surface 4 cm proximal to its tip. This allows determination of cardiac output by the thermodilution technique (13). A known quantity and temperature of solution is injected into the second lumen and the resultant change in pulmonary artery blood temperature is measured by the thermistor in the third lumen. Cardiac output is determined electronically by a bedside analog computer using the change in pulmonary artery blood temperature and a thermistor calibration

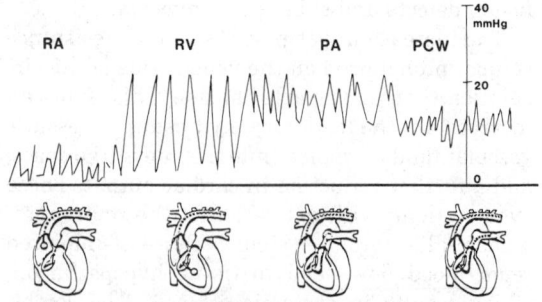

Figure 1. Placement of Swan-Ganz Catheter with Corresponding Pulmonary Artery Tracing. RA = right atrium; RV = right ventricle; PA = pulmonary artery; PCW = pulmonary capillary wedge pressure.

factor. This method measures output of the right side of the heart, which is normally equal to the left side in absence of intracardiac shunts. The fourth lumen serves to inflate and deflate the 1.5 ml capacity balloon.

Right Atrial Pressure (RAP). The RAP as measured by the Swan-Ganz catheter is 2–6 mm Hg in the normal heart. Central Venous Pressure (CVP) is measured by inserting a long polyethylene catheter into the superior vena cava or right atrium, and is normally about 4–8 cm H_2O. RAP varies with respiration and should be measured at the level of the right atrium. For all practical purposes, the CVP and RAP can be used interchangeably.

RAP reflects the filling pressure of the right heart. Vascular capacitance, circulating blood volume, and cardiac pump action maintain RAP. A low RAP is usually secondary to hypovolemia. An elevated RAP signifies increased intravascular volume, right ventricular failure, tricuspid regurgitation, pulmonary embolus, pulmonary hypertension, obstructive airway disease with cor pulmonale, or pericardial tamponade. In tamponade the left ventricular filling pressure is also elevated to the same degree as the right atrial pressure. In diastole when the tricuspid valve is open, the superior vena cava, right atrium, and right ventricle become a common chamber. An increase in right ventricular volume for whatever reason is reflected by a rise in RAP. Alterations in cardiovascular performance of the right and left side of the heart can produce significantly different right and left ventricular function curves resulting from unequal action and efficiency (14,15). An increase in RAP may not reflect left heart failure until the failure is severe enough to generate a systolic pulmonary artery pressure greater than 40 mm Hg.

Pulmonary Artery Pressure (PAP). Normal PAP ranges from 15 to 30 mm Hg systolic and 5 to 12 mm Hg diastolic. The PAP is elevated when pulmonary vascular resistance is increased, such as in pulmonary embolus, pulmonary hypertension, or obstructive lung disease. A low circulating blood volume results in a low PAP. In Figure 1, the pulmonary artery diastolic (PAD) pressure is approximately equal to the PCWP in the absence of any increase in pulmonary vascular resistance. The PAD can be used in place of the PCWP as an indication of left side heart function when the pulmonary vascular resistance is nor-

mal. However, with elevated pulmonary vascular resistance, the PAD pressure is substantially elevated over the PCWP and may not be a useful indication of left sided status.

Pulmonary Capillary Wedge Pressure (PCWP). PCWP provides an indication of the filling pressure in the left side of the heart. It approximates the left ventricular end diastolic pressure (LVEDP) and normally is about 5–12 mm Hg. When a branch of the pulmonary artery is occluded with the inflated balloon, the pressure distal to the balloon is measured and is equivalent to a phase-delayed, amplitude-damped left atrial pressure. When the balloon is deflated, the measured pressure represents flow from the right ventricle as noted above. The PCWP reflects pulmonary capillary hydrostatic pressure. Elevations in the PCWP generally indicate pulmonary congestion, because the hydrostatic pressure in the pulmonary venous vasculature is the major factor which forces fluid out of the pulmonary venous bed into the intra-alveolar and interstitial spaces.

With a normal functioning mitral valve, the pulmonary venous bed, left atrium, and left ventricle become a common chamber during diastole. Therefore, an increase in left ventricular volume is reflected by an increase in PCWP. This information can be used to evaluate left heart status according to the Starling ventricular function curve (16). Starling's "Law of the Heart" states that the strength of cardiac contraction, hence cardiac output, is proportional to myocardial fiber length (or ventricular volume) at the onset of contraction. This proportionality is maintained as long as physiologic limits of myocardial fiber contraction are not exceeded. Viewed in another manner, cardiac output is proportional to myocardial fiber length as long as the ventricular filling pressure does not exceed 20 mm Hg (Figure 2). PCWP is elevated in left ventricular failure, mitral insufficiency, pericardial tamponade, increased intravascular volume (preload), and increased total peripheral vascular resistance (afterload) (17).

Parameters which reflect cardiovascular function can be derived from the hemodynamic measurements from the Swan-Ganz catheter as listed in Table 2. *Cardiac index* (CI) is the cardiac output per square meter of body surface area. This measurement allows for comparing cardiac outputs of different sized persons. The same is true for *stroke volume index* (SVI).

Table 2.

NORMAL HEMODYNAMIC VALUES AND DERIVED INDICES

		Normal Value	Units
BP S/D/M	Blood Pressure Systolic/Diastolic/Mean	120/80/93	mm Hg
CO	Cardiac Output	4–6	Liters/min.
RAP	Right Atrial Pressure (mean)	2–6	mm Hg
PAP S/D/M	Pulmonary Artery Pressure Systolic/Diastolic/Mean	25/12/16	mm Hg
PCWP	Pulmonary Capillary Wedge Pressure (mean)	5–12	mm Hg
CI	Cardiac Index $CI = \dfrac{CO}{Body\ Surface\ Area}$	2.5–3.5	Liters/min/m^2
SV	Stroke Volume $SV = \dfrac{CO}{Heart\ Rate}$	60–80	ml/beat
SVI	Stroke Volume Index $SVI = \dfrac{SV}{Body\ Surface\ Area}$	30–50	ml/beat/m^2
PVR	Pulmonary Vascular Resistance $PVR = \dfrac{MPAP - PCWP}{CO} \times 80$	<200	dynes·sec·cm^{-5}
TPVR	Total Peripheral Vascular Resistance $TPVR = \dfrac{MBP - RAP}{CO} \times 80$	900–1400	dynes·sec·cm^{-5}
LVSWI	Left Ventricular Stroke Work Index $LVSWI = (MBP - PCWP)\ (SVI)\ (.0136)$	35–80	gm-m/m^2/beat

The *stroke volume* (SV) is the amount of blood ejected from the ventricle with each myocardial contraction. When cardiac output is increased by therapeutic maneuvers, it is important to know if the increase was due to an inotropic (stroke volume) or chronotropic response (heart rate). Cardiac output is equal to the stroke volume multiplied by the heart rate.

The *pulmonary vascular resistance* (PVR) and *total peripheral vascular resistance* (TPVR) are determined by the change in pressure divided by the flow (Δ pressure/cardiac output = resistance). It is important to realize that therapeutic maneuvers which alter total peripheral vascular resistance do not indicate a resistance change in any specific vascular bed, such as the renal or splanchnic vascular beds; changes in TPVR reflect the overall change.

The *left ventricular stroke work index* (LVSWI) provides an indication of left ventricular contractility which takes into account preload, afterload, and cardiac output. The constant 0.0136 is the specific weight of mercury conversion factor which changes mm Hg·ml into gram·meters. Elevation in left ventricular stroke work index can be achieved by changes in preload, afterload, and contractility.

In summary, a single catheter in the right side of the heart provides considerable data for continuous diagnostic and therapeutic assessment.

Changes in intracardiac pressures, pulmonary pressures, and cardiac output can be monitored continuously. These hemodynamic measurements can be used to calculate cardiovascular performance indices (Table 2) which can guide specific therapeutic interventions with inotropic, vasopressor, and vasodilator agents, as well as with diuretics and fluids.

HYPOVOLEMIC SHOCK

Hemorrhage

1. J.B., a 32-year-old male, is brought to the emergency room with a gunshot wound to the abdomen. External blood loss and internal hemorrhage are significant. His systolic blood pressure (by cuff) is 60 mm Hg; his pulse is thready and greater than 140 beats/minute; respirations are shallow and at a rate of 40/minute. His skin is cool and clammy to touch, and he is combative and disoriented to time and place. What is this patient's physiological response to the hypovolemic shock?

J.B. has lost significant amounts of intravascular fluid from both the gunshot wound and from the sequestration of large amounts of fluid in and around the injured cells. He is presently in hypovolemic shock, and cardiac dysfunction will become an additional complication if his shock state is prolonged.

The major hemodynamic abnormality in hypovolemic shock is decreased venous return to the heart and a low cardiac output. When the PCWP (representing venous return) is low, cardiac output is also low (Fig. 2). In view of this patient's low cardiac output, his low systolic blood pressure of 60 mm Hg is not unexpected. Arterial blood pressure is directly proportional to cardiac output and is inversely proportional to total peripheral vascular resistance (TPVR). Therefore, in order to maintain an adequate arterial pressure when the cardiac output is decreased, TPVR generally will increase because of a baroreceptor reflex response. This reflex activation of the sympathetic nervous system constricts the arteriolar bed, increases myocardial contractility, and increases the heart rate (18,19). Thus, this patient's increased heart rate of 140 beats/minute and his cool clammy skin suggest sympathetic nervous system reflex activation.

This patient's blood loss also tends to cause fluid to move from the interstitial space into the vascular space in order to preserve circulating volume (20). Additionally, increased amounts of antidiuretic hormone, renin, and aldosterone are secreted. Furthermore, blood flow is directed away from nutrient capillary beds and kidneys in order to maintain perfusion of the heart and brain. During prolonged intense vasoconstriction, this redistribution in blood flow results in inadequate tissue oxygenation. Anerobic metabolism ensues and metabolic acidosis with a compensatory respiratory alkalosis develops. Systemic hypotension has developed in this patient because the increase in TPVR is insufficient to compensate for the marked reduction in cardiac output. Patients in shock who fail to develop an appropriate tachycardia have a poorer prognosis.

2. What is the most important therapeutic intervention in the initial treatment of this patient?

In addition to maintaining the patency of airways, the primary therapeutic consideration in this patient is fluid replacement with blood products, crystalloid solutions, or colloid solutions. Early complete correction of hypovolemia prevents the later complications of shock such as "shock lung," myocardial depression, or acute renal failure.

Initially, crystalloids or colloids are usually used to reestablish intravascular volume, because blood products are often not immediately available. In this patient, fluid replacement with crystalloids or colloids should be administered at a wide-open infusion rate until blood pressure is restored. Whole blood or packed red blood cells should be given to restore the hematocrit to at least 30%. Maintenance of a hematocrit in the range of 30 to 35% is adequate to support oxygen transport to the tissues and at the same time optimize blood flow by limiting viscosity and hemagglutination (22). If the hematocrit is less than 25%, cardiac output must increase to deliver the same amount of oxygen to the tissues. When cardiac output is limited because of severe volume loss or pump failure in conjunction with a less than optimal hematocrit, tissue oxygenation is compromised.

3. Several minutes after his arrival in the emergency room, this patient became comatose. He was intubated to improve oxygen delivery and to prevent aspiration. Over the next

20 minutes, 1.5 L of Ringer's Lactate and 1 unit of whole blood were administered in an attempt to stabilize him for surgery. Would a nonlactated solution have been a better choice?

Ringer's Lactate (RL) is designed to simulate intravascular plasma electrolyte concentration. It contains 27 mEq/L of lactate which is metabolized to bicarbonate in patients with a normal circulation and normal liver function. Infusion of lactate might compound preexisting metabolic acidosis in patients with compromised hepatic blood flow if unmetabolized lactate could be converted to lactic acid. In actuality, no differences in serum pH, electrolytes, lactate, or clinical course were noted in surgical patients who received either Ringer's Lactate or normal saline (25). Acidosis was decreased and survival rates were improved in patients who received either Ringer's Lactate or normal saline in addition to blood as compared to patients who received blood alone (23,24).

Most emergency room clinicians use normal saline (NS) and Ringer's Lactate interchangeably, as neither solution appears to be superior to the other. A buffered solution without lactate can easily be made by adding two 50 ml ampules of 8.4 percent sodium bicarbonate to one liter of D5/0.2 NS or 0.2 NS. Overcorrecting acute acidosis with systemic alkalinization may increase oxyhemoglobin affinity and lead to severe metabolic alkalosis.

4. A "stat" blood chemistry drawn prior to the infusion of the Ringer's Lactate revealed a hematocrit of 21%. Patient J.B. will require large amounts of blood replacement prior to and during surgery. What potential hematologic problems should the clinician anticipate?

Banked *blood* which is stored for more than 24 hours is deficient in platelets and clotting factors V and VIII. Furthermore, the patient's own clotting factors are also decreased by a dilutional effect and by consumption. The patient is therefore at risk for coagulation disorders if he receives large amounts of stored blood (26,27). *Fresh frozen plasma* (FFP) contains clotting factors V and VIII and should be administered to patients receiving large amounts of whole blood or packed red blood cells. Platelet transfusions may also be necessary to control bleeding when the platelet count is severely low.

Stored whole blood is also acidic and may contain large amounts of potassium which potentiates myocardial depression. Levels of 2,3-DPG (diphosphoglycerate) in stored blood can also be depressed, impairing tissue oxygenation (28,29). *Packed red blood cells* (PRBC) are safer than whole blood because they contain less sodium and potassium, are less antigenic, and are less likely to cause hepatitis (30).

PRBC and FFP would be appropriate blood replacement products for J.B. This patient's prothrombin time and activated partial thromboplastin time should be monitored to assess clotting factor status.

Postoperative Hypovolemia

5. R.M. is a 75-year-old male who has undergone triple vessel coronary artery bypass grafting. He weighs 80 kg, his body surface area (BSA) is 2 m², and he has a history of mild hypertension (BP 160/100 mm Hg) which is controlled with diuretic therapy. One hour postoperatively he is seen in the surgical intensive care unit with the following hemodynamic profile: BP (S/D/M) 80/40/53 mm Hg; P 130 beats/minute; CO 3 L/min; RAP 2 mm Hg; PAD 8 mm Hg; PCWP 4 mm Hg; Urine output 10 ml/hr; HCT 30%; Chest tube drainage 150 ml/hr; ABG's: (intubated: FiO₂ 0.5) pO₂ 150, pCO₂ 24, pH 7.43.

From the hemodynamic profile, is R.M. hypovolemic or experiencing pump failure?

This patient's decreased blood pressure, PCWP, CO, and urine output along with his increased pulse rate suggest hypovolemia. The increased pulse rate is a sympathetic compensatory response. The decreased CO and PCWP indicate decreased venous return (preload) to the heart. Urine output has declined and probably reflects a compensatory drop in renal perfusion to preserve intravascular volume. The foley catheter should be checked for proper functioning before the low urine output is credited to decreased renal perfusion. The most likely explanation for the hypovolemia is inadequate fluid administration intraoperatively and postoperatively. This patient needs intravascular volume replacement.

6. How will replacement of the intravascular volume improve cardiac output?

Starling's "Law of the Heart" implies that the volume of blood returned to the heart (preload) is the main determinant of volume pumped by the heart. Therefore, as venous return is increased, the cardiac output also will increase, albeit within physiological limitations (Fig. 2). The PCWP, which is an approximation of left ventricular end diastolic pressure (LVEDP), can be used as a guide for assessing venous return or preload to the left ventricle. The PCWP, however, does not correlate well with LVEDP in the presence of mitral stenosis or patients with severe pulmonary hypertension.

A ventricular function curve can be constructed by plotting a measure of cardiac pumping action (cardiac output, stroke volume, or stroke work index) against a measure of volume returning to the left heart (PCWP). A change in preload will move the ventricular output upward or downward along a given curve (Fig. 2). Thus, volume replacement is the first choice of therapy in either relative or absolute hypovolemic situations.

7. R.M. is given a 200 ml bolus of normal saline over five minutes, resulting in the following hemodynamic profile: BP 95/60/75 mm Hg, P 115 beats/minute, CO 3.3 L/min, RAP 4 mm Hg, PAD 10 mm Hg, PCWP 6 mm Hg.

In view of this patient's increased cardiac output and improved hemodynamic profile, has his volume deficit been adequately corrected?

Although a cardiac output of 3.3 L/min may seem adequate, R.M. weighs 80 kg and has a body

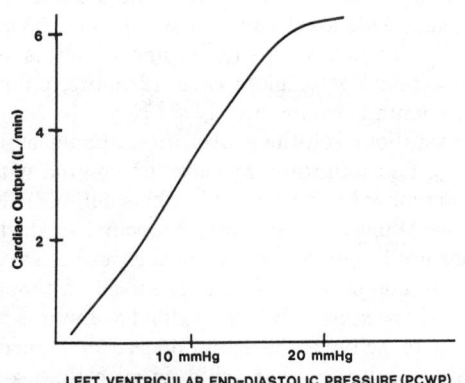

Figure 2. Ventricular Function Curve in A Normal Heart Demonstrating Starling's Law of The Heart. As LVEDP is increased (volume return to the heart) myocardial fiber shortening enhances contraction and therefore cardiac output. Beyond a filling pressure of 15–20 mm Hg, cardiac output does not improve significantly because the volume has exceeded the physiologic limit of which myocardial fibers can handle.

surface area of 2 m². Therefore, the cardiac index is only 1.65 L/min/m², which is less than the 2.5 L/min/m² needed for adequate tissue perfusion (32). This patient is still on the lower end of the ventricular function curve and still needs additional fluid. The optimal preload (PCWP) to achieve a maximal stroke volume in most patients is 12–18 mm Hg (32), although in an occasional patient the preload can be pushed higher to maximize the cardiac output when evidence of pulmonary congestion is absent.

The best guidelines for administering a fluid challenge to suspected hypovolemic patients are based upon changes in RAP and PCWP values rather than upon the absolute values themselves. According to the "7-3 Rule" for PCWP, an increase in the PCWP or PAD of more than 7 mm Hg following infusion of 200 ml of normal saline over ten minutes reflects left ventricular distress. If the baseline pressure is not increased by more than 3 mm Hg after ten minutes of fluid infusion or if it decreases to less than this value over a subsequent ten minute rest period, a second aliquot of fluid is given and the "7-3 Rule" is applied again. The "5-2" rule for RAP or CVP uses the CVP values of 5 and 2 cm H₂O or an absolute RAP value not exceeding 15 mm Hg in the same manner as the "7-3" rule. If the CVP or PCWP rise abruptly as the fluid is given, the intravenous infusion rate should be slowed (7). This patient's PCWP increased from 4 mm Hg to 6 mm Hg. Because his baseline PCWP has not increased by more than 3 mm Hg, a second fluid challenge would be appropriate.

Generally, a PCWP of less than 10 mm Hg suggests hypovolemia and a PCWP of 20 mm Hg or higher suggests left ventricular overload or left ventricular failure. Therefore, patient R.M. should continue to receive fluid until a PCWP of 15–18 mm Hg or a cardiac index greater than 2.5 L/min/m² is achieved. PRBC's and FFP should be given as necessary to replace red cells and clotting factors.

8. R.M. has required 600 ml normal saline and 1 unit PRBC's over 1½ hours to maintain the following hemodynamic profile: BP 115/60/90 mm Hg, P 100 beats/minute, CO 4.5 L/min, RAP 10 mm Hg, PAD 21 mm Hg, PCWP 15 mm Hg, Urine output 50 ml/hr, Hct 33%, Na 130 mEq/L, Cl 90 mEq/L, K 4.2 mEq/L, HCO₃ 22 mEq/L.

The following IV fluids are ordered: "D5½NS at 50 ml/hr or intake = urine output. If the blood pressure decreases to less than 100 mm Hg systolic, or if the cardiac output decreases to less than 4 L/min, or if the PCWP decreases to less than 15 mm Hg, 5% albumin (250 ml) is to be administered over 30 minutes times 2." Why is the 5% albumin colloid solution for this patient more, or less, appropriate than an order for a crystalloid solution?

Colloid solutions contain molecules such as albumin which are relatively impermeable to the vascular membrane. In plasma, albumin is the natural colloid which maintains fluid in the vascular space and which is responsible for approximately two-thirds of the colloid oncotic pressure. Intravenous serum albumin solutions are available in a 5% or 25% concentration and are prepared from human blood or plasma. The 5% solution (250 ml) is iso-oncotic with human plasma. The 25% solution osmotically draws about 3.5 times the volume infused into the vascular space from a well-hydrated extravascular space. Both the 5% and 25% solutions contain 130–160 mEq/L of sodium and are no longer referred to as "salt poor" (30,34). Administration of the 25% solution delivers a large amount of protein in a small volume of fluid. Therefore, it is most useful in correcting hypoproteinemia or intravascular hypovolemia in patients with excess interstitial water. Either the 5% or the 25% solution can be used in postoperative hypotension, acute traumatic shock, severe thermal injuries, or as a pump prime for cardiopulmonary bypass (35). For volume replacement, albumin solutions are given in amounts necessary to keep arterial pressure, CVP, and PCWP at reasonable levels.

Human plasma protein fraction (PPF) is a 5% solution containing 85% albumin. PPF is reported to contain vasoactive kinins which can cause hypotensive reactions when administered at rates greater than 10–15 ml/min (36–38). PPF offers no advantage over 5% albumin. Synthetic colloid solutions include the dextrans and hydroxyethyl starch.

Crystalloids are electrolyte containing solutions of water and/or dextrose. Saline or Ringer's Lactate are most commonly used to increase intravascular volume and replace interstitial water. The distribution of saline between the intravascular and extravascular compartment is determined by the net forces of colloid oncotic pressures and hydrostatic pressures both inside and outside the capillary vascular space. In normal patients, approximately one-fourth of the infused volume remains in the intravascular space; whereas, in critically ill patients as little as 9% is retained in the intravascular space (39). The major advantage of crystalloids over colloids is a substantial savings in cost.

Two views have emerged as to the correct type of fluid for volume replacement or expansion. Proponents of colloid or albumin administration contend that increasing intravascular oncotic pressure (colloid osmotic pressure) will keep a greater proportion of the fluid in the intravascular compartment. This will reduce fluid requirements by about 50%, prevent overexpansion of interstital water content, and decrease the risk of pulmonary edema (24,40–45).

According to proponents of the colloid regimen, maintenance of colloid osmotic pressure (COP) is necessary to prevent fluid extravasation into the pulmonary interstitium (45,53,54). This concept is based on Starling's law which states that the force responsible for movement of fluid across the pulmonary vessel wall is the net force of colloid oncotic pressure minus the hydrostatic pressure or its equivalent PCWP. The normal COP is 25 mm Hg and the normal PCWP is 12 mm Hg; thus, a net of 13 mm Hg intravascular force favors fluid retention in the vascular space. A COP - PCWP gradient of less than 6 mm Hg is associated with a higher incidence of pulmonary edema (45,53,54). If the difference between COP and PCWP is less than 3 mm Hg for more than 12 hours, pulmonary edema is common.

Crystalloid solutions also are capable of restoring and maintaining vascular volume without detrimental pulmonary effects (46–48). Effective volume expansion can be accomplished with either fluid regimen, and in most cases both crystalloid and colloid solutions are used. Although at least twice as much crystalloid volume is required to achieve the same degree of hemodynamic stability as that achieved with the use of colloids, the major concern focuses on which fluid regimen will minimally damage the lung through pulmonary edema.

In a baboon shock model, intravascular lung water was substantially increased following resuscitation with colloid but was not changed after resuscitation with Ringer's Lactate (49). Supposedly, albumin extravasation increased tissue on-cotic pressure, resulting in pulmonary edema. Several investigators (43,46,48) suggest that in clinical situations where an "albumin leak" may be present (eg, acute respiratory distress syn-drome or severe sepsis), pulmonary edema can result from fluid being drawn into the interstitial spaces where the leaked albumin has accumu-lated. As a result, the lymphatic system, which is a major pathway for water and albumin clear-ance from the pulmonary interstitium, is over-whelmed (50–52).

In summary, clinical studies have not clearly substantiated which fluid regimen presents the least risk for development of pulmonary edema. Studies differ with respect to population size, cri-teria for assessing pulmonary edema, shock ver-sus non-shock patients, amount and type of in-travenous fluids administered. Many patients also received both colloid and crystalloid solutions to replenish intravascular volume.

The question of whether the 5% albumin so-lution is better for R.M. than a simple crystalloid solution is difficult to answer. Certainly if R.M. is hypoalbuminemic and the COP - PCWP gra-dient is less than 6 mm Hg, albumin 5% may be indicated for further fluid resuscitive measures. As long as R.M. does not show signs of adult res-piratory distress syndrome (ARDS) or sepsis, al-bumin could be given safely for its oncotic effect.

9. What advantages do the synthetic col-loid volume expanders such as the dextrans and hydroxyethyl starch (HES) offer over the more traditional colloidal solution of albumin?

The *dextrans* are glucose polymers with aver-age molecular weights of 40,000 (range 10,000–90,000) and 70,000 (range 20,000–200,000). Dex-tran 40 is available as a 10% solution in D5W or normal saline. Dextran 70 is available as a 6% solution in D5W or normal saline. Molecules less than 55,000 molecular weight are excreted by the kidneys; whereas, larger molecules are elimi-nated by the reticuloendothelial system (50). Plasma volume expansion with dextran 40 lasts 3–4 hours; whereas, volume expansion with dex-tran 70 lasts longer due to the slower excretion rate (58,60,61). Dextrans are limited by the amount that can be administered. The first day's total dose should not exceed 20 ml/kg and 10 ml/kg every day thereafter. Duration of therapy is limited to a maximum of five days (58).

Cross matching of blood should be done prior to the administration of dextrans, because dex-tran interferes with the laboratory process. Al-teration of coagulation status by interference with platelet adhesiveness is a problem in postopera-tive and hemorrhagic shock patients. Dextran is also reported to decrease fibrinogen levels, thus increasing the potential for hemorrhage (58,62,63).

Renal failure has been reported both clinically and experimentally with dextran use (58,61). When large doses of dextran are infused before adequate renal perfusion has been established, changes in renal tubules resembling osmotic ne-phrosis can occur. Dextran 40 should not be used (64) if the urine output is less than 25 ml/hr and the urine specific gravity is more than 1.030. Al-lergic reactions including anaphylaxis have also been reported (58,61).

Hydroxyethyl starch (HES) is a highly graded glucose polymer made from amylopectin. The av-erage molecular weight is 450,000 (10,000–1,000,000). HES is available as a 6% solution in normal saline. Molecules less than 70,000 molec-ular weight are eliminated via the reticuloendo-thelial system (65,66). HES expands plasma vol-ume to the same degree as dextran 70, but the duration of action is about twice as long (59).

Problems associated with HES include ele-vated erythrocyte sedimentation rate (67), ele-vated serum amylase level (68), and allergic re-actions (69), although these are not as frequent as those associated with the dextrans.

The synthetic colloids offer no advantage over albumin solutions with the exception of cost. The greater frequency and number of adverse effects associated with their use may not be acceptable in terms of cost savings. HES is still relatively new in the United States; thus, the lack of fa-miliarity with this product limits its use.

CARDIOGENIC SHOCK

Postoperative Cardiac Failure

10. J.J., a 50-year-old female, has just undergone coronary artery bypass graft sur-gery (3 vessels) and is now in the intensive care unit. Her body weight is 60 kg, and her body surface area is 1.5 m². Past medical his-tory includes one anterior wall myocardial infarction 6 months PTA; unstable angina treated with nitrates and propranolol 80 mg

qid; and hypertension poorly controlled with diuretics. Her hemodynamic profile 30 minutes postoperatively is as follows: BP 100/60/72 mm Hg; P 115 beats/minute (sinus rhythm); CO 3.0 L/minute; CI 2.0 L/min/m²; RAP 14 mm Hg; PAD 25 mm Hg; PCWP 22 mm Hg; ABG's (FiO₂ .80): pO₂ 110, pCO₂ 34, pH 7.38; RR 12 breaths/minute; Urine Output (U/O) 20 ml/hr; Chest tube drainage 120 ml/hr. What assessment of fluid balance can be made from the above profile?

The rapid pulse, low urine output, and low mean arterial pressure (MAP) suggest volume depletion; however, the elevated PCWP and decreased CO also suggest pump failure. The chest x-ray and sputum from endotracheal suctioning should be examined for signs of pulmonary edema. The cardiac index (CI) is 2.0 L/min/m² which, in the presence of a PCWP greater than 18 mm Hg, can be a poor prognostic sign (31,32). An elevated PCWP of greater than 18 mm Hg is associated with pulmonary edema and a CI of less than 2.2 L/min/m² is indicative of hypoperfusion.

The hemodynamic profile of this patient in conjunction with her recent acute myocardial infarction is associated with a mortality rate up to 51% (31,32). A blood sample should be sent to the laboratory for cardiac enzyme analysis and an EKG should be obtained to rule out a myocardial infarction.

Further analysis reveals the following derived hemodynamic parameters (see Table 2): SV 26 ml/beat, SVI 17 ml/beat/m², TPVR 1546 dynes·sec·cm⁻⁵, LVSWI 12 gm-m/m²/beat.

The left ventricular stroke work index (LVSWI) reflects cardiac performance and tissue perfusion. Total peripheral vascular resistance (TPVR) is elevated in response to a depressed cardiac output in order to maintain arterial pressure (MAP = CO × TPVR). A mean arterial pressure (MAP) of at least 65 mm Hg is desired to maintain coronary blood flow to prevent development of ischemic areas in the myocardium.

Construction of a ventricular function curve with LVSWI indicating cardiac performance and PCWP, a measure of preload, shows J.J.'s hemodynamic status is on the flat portion of a depressed curve (Fig. 3).

In summary, it appears that J.J. is not volume depleted, although the patient's fluid intake and output (I's and O's) should be monitored to confirm the values.

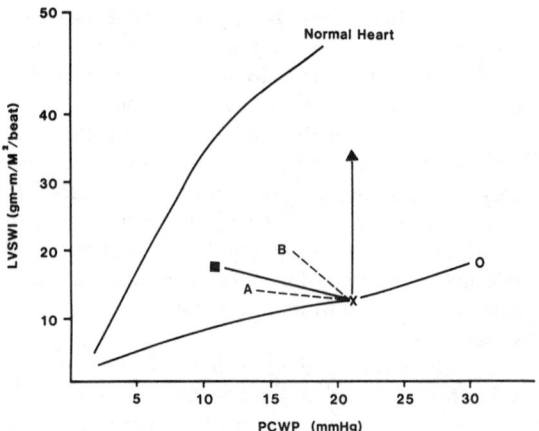

Figure 3. Ventricular Function Curve for J.J. O = Fluid challenge; ■ = Vasodilator; ▲ = Inotropic agent; A = Isoproterenol at .02 mcg/kg/min; B = Dobutamine at 5 mcg/kg/min; X = Pre-treatment.

11. The chest x-ray does not show signs of pulmonary edema, although atelectasis is present in the right lower lobe. The EKG shows ST-T wave changes but no indication of acute myocardial infarction when compared with the preoperative EKG. Cardiac enzymes are pending. Recalibration of the monitors confirms the elevated PCWP and RAP. Improvement of cardiac output is desired to increase perfusion to the kidneys. Using the above hemodynamic parameters, what therapeutic interventions are available to achieve this goal, and how would these affect this patient's ventricular function curve?

Three therapeutic interventions are available.

Fluid Challenge. First, preload can be further increased in hopes of increasing cardiac output. However, the PCWP is already 22 mm Hg, and increases above 18–20 mm Hg usually do not result in further benefit (31,32,70,71). If a fluid challenge is attempted, no more than 50 ml of normal saline or 5% albumin should be given without careful evaluation. If the PCWP rises, but the cardiac output does not improve, the infusion should be discontinued. The major risk associated with this maneuver is the potential exacerbation of myocardial ischemia. If the PCWP (preload) is raised without appreciably improving cardiac output, left ventricular wall tension, a major determinant of myocardial oxygen requirements, will be increased (72). There is also the risk of precipitating pulmonary edema.

Vasodilator. The second consideration would be the administration of a peripheral vasodilator to reduce afterload, thus improving forward output from the left ventricle. The purpose of vasodilator therapy is to decrease pulmonary venous congestion by lowering the PCWP and to improve cardiac output by decreasing the resistance to left ventricular ejection (32,72–74). In patients without cardiac failure, blood pressure is primarily maintained by systemic vascular tone, and the left ventricle operates on the steep ascending limb of the Starling curve. In this situation, any reduction of aortic impedance is of little importance (75). However, with left ventricular failure, arterial resistance is elevated and cardiac output becomes increasingly dependent on resistance to outflow from the left ventricle (76). By shifting the ventricular function curve up and to the left, cardiac performance can be improved at a lower filling pressure (Fig. 3). Lowering the filling pressure decreases myocardial oxygen consumption. This patient has left ventricular failure and an elevated PCWP and TPVR, and these are the hemodynamic variables which usually are predictive of a beneficial response to vasodilator therapy (70,72,77,78). The major risk of vasodilator therapy in this patient is a further reduction of an already low mean arterial pressure. This could reduce coronary perfusion pressure, thereby exacerbating or producing myocardial ischemia.

Inotropic Agent. The third consideration is the use of a rapidly acting inotropic agent to increase contractility. This intervention shifts the ventricular function curve upward and slightly to the left. The disadvantage of this intervention is that improved cardiac output is not accomplished without increasing myocardial oxygen demand (increased MVO_2). Depending on the agent selected, three of the determinants of MVO_2 could be elevated: heart rate, contractility, and systolic wall tension (32). Therefore, inotropic support is directed at establishing or maintaining a reasonable arterial pressure, insuring adequate tissue perfusion, and improving cardiac output.

In summary, the most appropriate therapeutic intervention in J.J. at this time would be inotropic support. Her pulmonary capillary wedge pressure (preload) is maximized; thus, a fluid bolus would increase the potential for pulmonary edema.

Although this patient's TPVR is slightly elevated, her blood pressure is low and a peripheral vasodilator would be risky at this point. Thus, inotropic support aimed at improving cardiac output, and hence tissue perfusion, is the therapeutic intervention which is least likely to cause problems.

12. Isoproterenol was chosen for this patient because of its potent inotropic properties. How would the pharmacologic properties of isoproterenol affect this patient's hemodynamics?

Isoproterenol (Isuprel) stimulates both B_1 (heart) and B_2 (peripheral) adrenergic receptors. It is the most potent inotropic agent available. It increases the rate and strength of myocardial contraction and relaxes smooth muscles in arterioles, bronchioles, the uterus, stomach, intestine, and bladder (79). Isoproterenol also improves cardiac output through an increase in both heart rate and stroke volume ($CO = HR \times SV$). Its stimulation of $beta_2$-adrenergic receptors decreases TPVR, especially in the skeletal muscle and mesenteric vascular beds. The net effect of inotropic stimulation and decreased TPVR is that systolic pressure often increases but diastolic pressure decreases, resulting in no change or a decrease in the mean arterial pressure. The lowered TPVR could contribute to improvement of the cardiac output, but the increased flow in skeletal muscle may shunt blood flow away from the kidney (79). The decrease in diastolic pressure could also be detrimental to coronary blood flow. Isoproterenol also generates ectopic beats and shortens the atrioventricular conduction time (3,79).

In summary, isoproterenol should be used cautiously in patient J.J. because it may cause arrhythmias, accelerate heart rate, redistribute blood flow, and increase myocardial oxygen demand. The acceleration in heart rate along with a drop in diastolic pressure will lower coronary perfusion pressure and, in time, possibly accentuate myocardial ischemia. Although isoproterenol is a potent inotropic agent, its major use is limited to severe bradyarrhythmias unresponsive to atropine, reversal of beta blockade, or cautious use in heart failure with valvular insufficiency (80).

13. Isoproterenol (2 mg/500 ml D5W) was administered at a rate of 10 drops/minute and

later increased to 20 drops/minute. The following hemodynamic profile was produced.

10 drops/min (0.01 mcg/kg/min)	20 drops/min (0.02 mcg/kg/min)
BP 110/55/73 mm Hg	120/50/73 mm Hg
P 123 beats/min	137 beats/min
RAP 12 mm Hg	10 mm Hg
PCWP 18 mm Hg	16 mm Hg
CO 3.4 L/min	3.8 L/min
CI 2.2 L/min/m²	2.5 L/min/m²
SV 28 ml/beat	28 ml/beat
TPVR 1435 dynes·sec·cm⁻⁵	1326 dynes·sec·cm⁻⁵
LVSWI 13.5 gm-m/m²/beat	14 gm-m/m²/beat

Has myocardial performance been improved in this patient?

As can be seen, the improved CO is due to the increased heart rate because SV has not increased significantly from base line (26 ml/beat) prior to the isoproterenol. Myocardial oxygen demand has increased due to the elevated heart rate and no benefit has been gained since myocardial performance (LVSWI) was not significantly improved (12 to 14 gm-m/m²/beat).

14. What other intravenous inotropic agents are available and what are their pharmacologic differences?

Dopamine (Intropin), dobutamine (Dobutrex), and epinephrine are the other commonly employed inotropic agents for cardiac failure associated with hypotension. Each has unique pharmacologic effects on vascular beds and cardiac stimulation (Table 3).

Dopamine, a precursor of norepinephrine, has inotropic, chronotropic, and vasoactive properties, all of which are dose dependent (81). At 1–3 mcg/kg/min, dopamine stimulates dopaminergic receptors in the splanchnic and renal vascular beds, producing vasodilation and improved blood flow (81,82). The vasodilation is not blocked by propranolol, but is antagonized by dopaminergic blocking agents such as the butyrophenones and phenothiazines (81,83,84). Depending on the laboratory preparation, animal model, or clinical state of the patient, dopamine in low doses will slightly increase contractility but usually not alter heart rate or TPVR significantly. The improved cardiac performance is by direct stimulation of beta₁-adrenergic receptors and indirectly

through release of norepinephrine (81,82). This effect can be blocked by propranolol (79).

At 5–20 mcg/kg/min, more beta₁-adrenergic receptors are stimulated, increasing stroke volume and heart rate. At this dosage, the vasodilation of peripheral blood vessels is unpredictable and dependent upon the net interactions of beta₁-adrenergic stimulation, alpha-adrenergic stimulation, and reflex mechanisms (81,83,85,86). Mean arterial pressure and pulmonary capillary wedge pressure will usually rise (86,87). At doses greater than 15–20 mcg/kg/min, dopamine primarily stimulates peripheral alpha-adrenergic receptors. TPVR often increases and renal blood flow may be decreased. Cardiac irritability is not unusual and the overall myocardial oxygen demand is increased (83,84,88–90). The increase in TPVR limits cardiac output; thus, infusion rates should be limited to 10–15 mcg/kg/min if possible.

Dobutamine, a derivative of isoproterenol, directly stimulates beta₁-adrenergic receptors. It also stimulates beta₂-adrenergic and alpha-adrenergic receptors, albeit to a lesser degree (see Table 3) (91). Slight vasoconstriction occurs with low doses because of the alpha stimulation, and vasodilation is apparent with larger doses because of the beta₂-adrenergic stimulation. Phenoxybenzamine blocks the alpha adrenergic response, and propranolol blocks the beta₂ response (91,92).

In patients with heart failure, 2.5–15.0 mcg/kg/min of dobutamine increases cardiac output and decreases the PCWP and TPVR. There is no direct effect on renal blood flow (93–97). In Class IV (NYHA) cardiac failure patients, cardiac output and stroke volume increase linearly, and PCWP and TPVR decrease linearly with increasing dobutamine concentrations.

The inotropic effect of dobutamine will significantly improve cardiac output, but the relative advantage of dobutamine over other inotropic agents is controversial. Three studies compared dobutamine with isoproterenol in postoperative open heart surgery patients in various degrees of cardiac failure (93,95,98). The results of these studies indicate that dobutamine has a slight advantage over isoproterenol because of less chronotropic effects. TPVR which decreased with dobutamine in these studies may be due to direct beta₂-adrenergic stimulation or to a reflex response to the increased cardiac output (99).

In a cross-over study of dopamine and dobutamine in 13 patients with congestive heart fail-

Table 3.
INOTROPIC AGENTS AND VASOPRESSORS

Drug	Usual Dose (IV Infusion)	Receptor Specificity			Pharmacological Effect				Hemodynamic Effect*				Usual Concentration of Infusion	Central Vs Peripheral Administration
		Alpha	Beta₁	Beta₂	VD	VC	INT	CHT	MAP	CO	PCWP	TPVR		
Dobutamine	2.5–15.0 mcg/kg/min	+	+++	+	++		+++	+	↔	↑	↓	↓	1–2 mg/ml	C,P
Dopamine**	1–3 mcg/kg/min (renal) 5–15 mcg/kg/min (heart) 15–20 mcg/kg/min (heart) (PV)	(low dose) (high dose) + +++	++ ++	+	+	+++	++	++	↑	↑	↑	↑	800–1600 mcg/ml	C
Epinephrine	.01–1 mcg/kg/min Highly variable—titrate to effect.	(low dose) + (high dose) +++	+++ ++	++	++	++++	+++	++	↑	↑	↓	↓	4–8 mcg/ml	C
Isoproterenol	.02–1 mcg/kg/min		++++	+++	+++		+++	+++	↓	↑	↓	↓	4–8 mcg/ml	P
Metaraminol	1.5–10 mcg/kg/min Highly variable—titrate to effect.	++	+			++	+	+	↑	↔	↑	↑	.2–.4 mg/ml	C
Norepinephrine	2–10 mcg/min Highly variable—titrate to effect.	++++	+			+++	+++	+	↑	↔	↑	↑	16–32 mcg/ml	C
Phenylephrine	Highly variable—titrate to effect.	+++				+++			↑	↔	↑	↑	40–80 mcg/ml	C

*As infusion rate increased hemodynamic direction changes.
**Dopamine at 1–3 mcg/kg/ml stimulates dopaminergic receptors in the renal vasculature.

Key:
PV = peripheral vasculature, VD = vasodilatation,
VC = vasoconstriction, INT = inotropic,
CHT = chronotropic, MAP = mean arterial pressure,
CO = cardiac output, C = central, P = peripheral.

ure, dobutamine at 2.5–10.0 mcg/kg/min increased cardiac index and stroke volume (94). PCWP and TPVR decreased, and there was no change in heart rate. Dopamine increased the cardiac index at doses of 4 mcg/kg/min, but did not increase the cardiac index at doses of 6–8 mcg/kg/min without also significantly increasing heart rate. Dopamine also increased the PCWP at doses greater than 4 mcg/kg/min and lowered TPVR only with infusions of less than 6 mcg/kg/min. During a 24-hour maintenance infusion of each drug (dopamine at 3.7–4.0 mcg/kg/min and dobutamine at 7.3–7.7 mcg/kg/min), only dobutamine maintained a significant increase in stroke volume, cardiac output, urine flow, and creatinine clearance.

The dose response curves of inotropic support were evaluated in postoperative open heart surgery patients (87). Dobutamine was compared to isoproterenol in one group of patients, and dobutamine was compared to dopamine in another group of patients. All three drugs elevated cardiac index substantially, and the improvement was primarily a function of an increased heart rate. Dobutamine increased heart rate significantly more than dopamine at an infusion rate of 10 mcg/kg/min for both drugs. Unlike the study by Leier et al (94), dopamine did not raise the TPVR at doses greater than 6 mcg/kg/min.

Epinephrine is a well-known inotropic and vasopressor agent, although clinical studies comparing the drug with other inotropic agents are scarce. Epinephrine stimulates alpha, beta$_1$-adrenergic, and beta$_2$-adrenergic receptors and enhances cardiac output by increasing both heart rate and contractility. Various vascular beds respond differently to epinephrine because of differences in receptor abundance. The blood vessels to the skin, mucosa, and kidney constrict in response to alpha-adrenergic receptor stimulation, while vessels in skeletal muscle vasodilate in response to beta$_2$-adrenergic receptor stimulation. The beta$_2$-adrenergic receptors are activated by smaller doses of epinephrine than are the alpha receptors. Thus, a biphasic response in systemic vascular resistance is observed with increasing doses. Vasodilation occurs with small doses; vasoconstriction occurs with larger doses (79,100). The receptor specificities of various inotropic and vasopressor agents are noted in Table 3.

In 34 patients with low cardiac output syndrome following cardiopulmonary bypass, dopa-

mine and dobutamine were administered in doses of 5, 10, and 15 mcg/kg/min and compared to epinephrine at 0.04 mcg/kg/min (101). Although all three drugs significantly improved the cardiac index, dopamine had the greatest effect. The mean arterial pressure was increased to the same degree by all three of these medications, and the heart rate was increased 7–13% by all three agents. Epinephrine did not alter the TPVR significantly from baseline, indicating that alpha and beta effects balanced each other at an infusion rate of 0.04 mcg/kg/min; however, the pulse pressure was increased by 75%. Although all three of these drugs are suitable for inotropic support, this inordinately high systolic pressure could be detrimental to aortic valve replacement due to stress on the sutures (101).

In summary, the pure beta$_1$-adrenergic and beta$_2$-adrenergic agonist, isoproterenol, is used mainly for reversal of bradyarrhythmias. Potential hazards associated with its use include lowering of peripheral vascular resistance and tachyarrythmias. The effects of dopamine are dose dependent. Improved renal blood flow is achieved with dopamine doses of 1–3 mcg/kg/min, and improved cardiac performance is achieved at doses of 3–15 mcg/kg/min. At doses greater than 15–20 mcg/kg/min, alpha effects predominate and may potentially decrease renal blood and adversely affect cardiac output. Dopamine doses of this magnitude have variable effects on PCWP, TPVR, and heart rate.

Dobutamine's major action is on beta$_1$-adrenergic receptors, although it also minimally affects beta$_2$- and alpha-adrenergic receptors. Cardiac output increases linearly with dobutamine doses; whereas, TPVR and PCWP decrease linearly with the dose. Dobutamine may not increase heart rate, although tachycardia appears to be more of a problem than originally described. A significant decrease in TPVR is also observed in a number of patients especially at doses of dobutamine which are greater than 10 mcg/kg/min. Epinephrine infusion has been studied the least in a clinical setting. Vasodilation predominates with small doses of epinephrine, and vasoconstriction predominates with large doses. Cardiac output is improved because of epinephrine's chronotropic and inotropic effect. The effect of epinephrine on TPVR, PCWP, and mean arterial pressure depends upon the infusion rate.

Investigations of these vasopressor and inotropic agents often involve non-shock or stable patients with moderate to severe cardiac failure. Therefore, comparisons of these agents are difficult. Although the pharmacology of these drugs is well-known, patient response is sometimes unpredictable. Careful hemodynamic monitoring is needed to guide the selection and dose of the drug to be given.

15. Isoproterenol has not been of benefit to this patient and is to be discontinued. Would dopamine or dobutamine be most appropriate for patient J.J.?

J.J.'s baseline hemodynamic parameters included a PCWP of 22 mm Hg, a TPVR of 1546, and a CI of 2.0. Dopamine can elevate PCWP, and its ability to increase the TPVR is dependent upon the dose. Dobutamine lowers the PCWP and TPVR in most patients. Since it is desirable in this patient to decrease TPVR and exert inotropic support, dobutamine would be the most appropriate agent.

16. Dobutamine is started at 5 mcg/kg/min resulting in the following hemodynamic profile.

	Baseline	Dobutamine (5 mcg/kg/min)
BP	100/60/72 mm Hg	100/55/73 mm Hg
P	115 beats/min	112 beats/min
PCWP	22 mm Hg	17 mm Hg
RAP	14 mm Hg	12 mm Hg
CO	3.0 L/min	3.8 L/min
TPVR	1546 dynes·sec·cm^{-5}	1284 dynes·sec·cm^{-5}
SV	26 ml/beat	34 ml/beat
LVSWI	12 gm-m/m^2/beat	17 gm-m/m^2/beat

Has dobutamine improved cardiac performance in this patient without detrimental effects to the myocardium? (See Fig. 3.)

Dobutamine has improved cardiac output without altering heart rate. Both the TPVR and PCWP have been reduced. Therefore, three of four major determinants of myocardial oxygen consumption have been favorably changed, enhancing myocardial performance. Because the heart rate has not increased, a trial of dobutamine at 7.5 mcg/kg/min is warranted to determine whether or not further benefits can be obtained (eg, a further decrease in TPVR and an improved CO).

Myocardial Infarction

17. D.T., a 42-year-old male weighing 72 kg and having a body surface area of 1.8 m^2, is brought to the emergency room complaining of severe chest pain unrelieved by sublingual nitroglycerin. He is disoriented, showing signs of labored breathing, and his skin is cold and clammy. The EKG is consistent with an acute myocardial infarction; there are 10–15 PVC's/minute with occasional coupling. BP by cuff is 90/40 mm Hg; P 90 beats/min; RR 30 respirations/min; ABG's: pO$_2$ 60, pCO$_2$ 30, pH 7.32; Stat electrolytes: Na 142 mEq/L, K 4.2 mEq/L, Cl 98 mEq/L, HCO$_3$ 24 mEq/L; Cardiac enzymes are sent for analysis.

D.T. is given 10 mg IV morphine and 60 mg IV furosemide. He is given a 150 mg bolus of lidocaine followed by a 3 mg/min infusion resulting in suppression of the PVC's to less than 3/minute. What other immediate steps must be taken to stabilize the patient and what are the therapeutic goals?

The arterial pressure must be maintained to provide adequate coronary perfusion. Coronary blood flow is dependent upon coronary perfusion pressure and the diastolic time interval. Shortening the diastolic time interval (eg, tachycardia) or lowering coronary perfusion pressure by decreasing the mean aortic pressure can adversely influence the course of an acute MI. Tissue necrosis will expand around the ischemic zone of infarction if myocardial tissue oxygen demands are not met (102). If the mean aortic pressure is less than 65 mm Hg, the perfusion pressure gradient (aortic diastolic pressure—left ventricular end diastolic pressure) is insufficient for optimal coronary blood flow. Blood flow is redistributed away from the subendocardial layer to the epicardial layers resulting in a further decrease in contractile force (70). However, elevation of the mean aortic pressure above 80 mm Hg is unnecessary because coronary blood flow is not significantly changed, but energy expenditure is.

Other immediate steps that need be taken in patient D.T. include oxygen and ventilatory support if needed. Other goals of therapy include relief of pulmonary congestion and improvement of hypoperfusion.

18. Insertion of an arterial line and a pulmonary artery catheter reveal the following:

BP 95/40/58 mm Hg, P 90 beats/min, CO 3.6 L/min, CI 2.0 L/min/m^2, SV 40 ml/beat, RAP 4 mm Hg, PAD 20 mm Hg, PCWP 14 mm Hg, and LVSWI 17.5.

Based on the above parameters, how should D.T. be further evaluated and treated? Would a vasopressor, inotropic agent, or fluid challenge be indicated at this time?

Treatment of acute myocardial infarction with pump failure can be based on hemodynamic subsets as indicated in Table 4 (31,32). Patients in subset I (SI) require little intervention except for oxygen, bedrest, sedation, morphine for chest pain, and appropriate drugs for tachycardia, bradycardia, and hypertension. Patients in subset II (SII) have an adequate cardiac index (CI) but also have evidence of pulmonary congestion (elevated PCWP) and are best treated with furosemide or ethacrynic acid. When blood pressure is also elevated, a vasodilator can be used. Patients in subset III (SIII) are hypoperfused (CI < 2.2) without pulmonary congestion and require volume expansion to a PCWP of 18 mm Hg. If a depressed CI persists after volume expansion, an inotropic agent may be necessary to enhance contractility or heart rate if the resting heart rate is below 50–70 beats per minute. Patients in subset IV (SIV) are the most difficult to treat and have the highest mortality. With both pulmonary congestion and hypoperfusion, therapy often includes a combination of diuretics, inotropic agents, and vasodilators.

The subset classifications must be used only as guidelines because not all patients with a CI < 2.2 or PCWP > 18 will present clinically with hypoperfusion and pulmonary congestion.

From the clinical presentation of disorientation, and cold clammy skin in the presence of a CI < 2.2, patient D.T. appears to be in cardiogenic shock. True cardiogenic shock is defined as 40 to 50% destruction of the left ventricular myocardium (103). The CI is usually < 2.2 and the PCWP is usually > 18. Fifty percent of AMI patients with shock have a low or normal TPVR. Patients in whom the TPVR is elevated have a poorer prognosis (104). D.T. has a CI < 2.2, but the PCWP is 14 mm Hg. This might be explained by the administration of furosemide and morphine prior to insertion of the pulmonary artery catheter. Both furosemide and morphine produce venous pooling through dilation, thereby lowering the PCWP.

Having assessed the hemodynamic parameters, a fluid challenge is a reasonable therapeutic intervention with which to begin. Although hypovolemia is uncommon in the setting of an acute

Table 4.

HEMODYNAMIC SUBSETS IN ACUTE MYOCARDIAL INFARCTION

	Subset I (SI)	Subset (SII)	Subset (III)	Subset (IV)
Pulmonary congestion (PCWP > 18mm Hg)	No	Yes	No	Yes
Peripheral hypoperfusion (CI < 2.3 L/min/m^2)	No	No	Yes	Yes
Percent mortality based on clinical signs	1	11	18	60
Percent mortality based on hemodynamic signs	3	9	23	51
Therapy	Usually no specific therapy required.	Diuretics. Digitalis when diuretics ineffective.	Volume expansion. Pacing when slow heart rate present.	Vasodilators, vasopressors, inotropic agents depending on hemodynamic measurements.

Adapted From: Forrester et al., Am J Med 1978; 65:173.

MI, the overzealous use of diuretics can be hazardous.

19. After two fluid challenges of 250 ml of normal saline, D.T. has the following hemodynamic profile: BP 100/60/73 mm Hg; P 83 beats/min; CO 4.2 L/min; CI 2.3 L/min/m²; SV 50 ml/beat; SVI 28 ml/beat/m²; RAP 10 mm Hg; PCWP 18 mm Hg; TPVR 1200 dynes·sec·cm⁻⁵; LVSWI 21 gm-m/m²/beat; Urine output 60 ml/hr; ABG's (O₂ by face mask): pO₂ 90, pCO₂ 34, pH 7.38; RR 18.

D.T. no longer complains of chest pain and is more alert and oriented. Are further drug interventions necessary at this time?

D.T. appears to have stabilized. All hemodynamic parameters and ABG's are reasonable. His fluid balance should be maintained, but no other drug interventions are necessary at this time. The lidocaine infusion should also be reassessed for benefit and risk.

20. No other therapy was initiated and fluid intake was equal to urine output in this patient. Two hours later D.T. has the following hemodynamic profile: BP 85/45/58 mm Hg; H 90 beats/min; CO 3.4 L/min; CI 1.8 L/min/m²; SV 38 ml/beat; SVI 21 ml/beat/m²; RAP 14 mm Hg; PAD 30 mm Hg; PCWP 24 mm Hg; TPVR 1035 dynes·sec·cm⁻⁵; LVSWI 10 gm-m/m²/beat; ABG's (O₂ by mask): pO₂ 50, pCO₂ 50, pH 7.28, HCO₃ 16; RR 28 breaths/min (shallow); Urine output 10 ml over past 30 minutes; Chest x-ray suggests pulmonary edema; EKG 2–5 PVC's/min; CNS status—confused, anxious, combative.

D.T. is intubated and given ventilatory support. Furosemide 40 mg every 6 hours is begun to improve urine output and decrease preload (PCWP). Dopamine is ordered to improve contractility, increase renal perfusion, and lower PCWP. Is this therapeutic maneuver appropriate at this time? How would the dopamine infusion be initiated?

D.T. has deteriorated and is now in SIV with cardiogenic shock probably as a result of an extension of the infarcted ventricle. Recalibration of the bedside monitor is advisable to confirm the readings. Initiating administration of an inotropic agent with vasopressor properties is appropriate to improve cardiac output and tissue perfusion. It will also elevate mean aortic pressure which will improve coronary blood flow. Hopefully, by increasing cardiac contractility, renal perfusion will improve and the PCWP will be lowered, thereby alleviating pulmonary edema. The direct vasodilating effect of dopamine on the renal vasculature would be an additional benefit.

Dopamine 200 mg is diluted in 250 ml D5W to provide a concentration of 800 mcg/ml. The usual dopamine infusion rate is started at 1–5 mcg/kg/min depending on the clinical status of the patient; however, for this patient with a CI of 1.8 and a MAP of 58, a starting dose of 3–4 mcg/kg/min is reasonable. Doses can be adjusted every 10–15 minutes until the desired effect is achieved; however, alpha effects may begin to predominate at doses greater than 15–20 mcg/kg/min.

The infusion is administered through a central venous line to avoid the consequences of peripheral intravenous extravasation. Use of an infusion pump device is preferable to a continuous intravenous infusion by gravity drip because the latter is subject to alteration in the delivery rate with changes in the patient's position or the height at which the IV bag or bottle is hung.

Most intravenous tubing sets deliver 60 drops/min or 60 ml/hr. The number of drops/min which will deliver 3 mcg/kg/min of dopamine can be calculated as follows:

$$\text{Drops/min} = 3 \text{ mcg/kg/min} \times 72 \text{ kg BW}$$
$$\times \frac{1 \text{ ml}}{800 \text{ mcg}} \times \frac{60 \text{ drops}}{\text{ml}}$$

$$= 16 \text{ drops/min}$$

21. D.T. requires 6.0 mcg/kg/min of dopamine to maintain a BP of 115/50/71 mm Hg 30 minutes after beginning the infusion. Other hemodynamic parameters include: P 105 beats/min; CO 5.0 L/min; CI 2.8 L/min/m²; SV 48 ml/beat; SVI 27 ml/beat/m²; RAP 12 mm Hg; PAD 30 mm Hg; PCWP 24 mm Hg; TPVR 944 dynes·sec·cm⁻⁵; LVSWI 17.25 gm-m/m²/beat; Urine output 30 ml over 30 minutes. This patient's blood pressure and cardiac output have been improved considerably. How has this affected myocardial oxygen requirements (MVO₂)?

Heart rate, contractility, preload, and afterload are the major determinants of MVO₂ (31,72). Stroke volume or stroke index is an indirect measurement of contractility. Preload (venous return) is governed by change in intravascular volume and myocardial contractility. Afterload (myocardial wall tension) is determined by systolic pressure and the radius of the ventricle. In turn, the systolic pressure is governed by impedance to outflow from the left ventricle. Peripheral vascular resistance in the arterial bed and compliance in the larger arteries determine impedance. The left ventricular radius is determined by left ventricular volume or venous return. Therefore, in the clinical setting, MVO_2 can be influenced by changes in heart rate, PCWP which approximates left ventricular end diastolic pressure, contractility, and peripheral vascular resistance.

In this case, dopamine has increased heart rate and contractility. PCWP has not been changed and TPVR has declined by only 13%. The net effect on MVO_2 cannot be determined unless myocardial lactate production and oxygen extraction are measured, and these are rarely measured in the clinical setting (105).

Dopamine administered at an average infusion rate of 17 mcg/kg/min to eight patients with cardiogenic shock secondary to myocardial infarction improved CI, raised MAP and heart rate, and lowered TPVR and PCWP (89). However, myocardial metabolism deteriorated in five patients as indicated by an elevated myocardial lactate production and oxygen extraction.

The net effect of dopamine on MVO_2 in D.T. is unknown, but most likely MVO_2 has increased. Certainly the cautious use of inotropic agents is warranted in patients with acute myocardial infarction since ischemia can be expanded. In emergency situations complicated by cardiogenic shock, the acute use of inotropic agents is definitely warranted to preserve coronary artery and tissue perfusion.

22. Would dobutamine offer any advantage over dopamine in augmenting the cardiac output without increasing the MVO_2?

It is generally assumed that all inotropic agents increase MVO_2. Animal studies have produced conflicting results, and human studies are insufficient to determine the effect of dobutamine on MVO_2.

Tuttle (106) suggests that dobutamine will not increase the infarct size in dog experiments. Others (107) have shown that after experimental coronary artery embolization in dogs, dobutamine increased left ventricular function at the expense of a 23% increase in MVO_2.

Gillespie et al (108) administered dobutamine to patients with acute myocardial infarction and found no increase in myocardial injury compared with a control group as determined by cardiac enzyme studies. However, Myer et al (109) advise clinicians to use dobutamine cautiously in patients with severe coronary artery disease because it may provoke uneven myocardial perfusion.

In the case of D.T., dobutamine would be a reasonable alternative. Dobutamine improves cardiac output and lowers the PCWP and TPVR in most patients; a change in the heart rate is unpredictable. D.T.'s PCWP (24 mm Hg) has not been affected by dopamine and furosemide; therefore, dobutamine may be useful. The TPVR is somewhat low; thus, cautious use is advised. Mean arterial pressure must also be followed closely in order to preserve coronary perfusion pressure. It has been the authors' experience that dobutamine reduces mean arterial pressure more than studies indicate. (Whether MVO_2 will be improved by dobutamine is unpredictable.)

Another alternative would be to leave the dopamine at 6 mcg/kg/min and increase the dose of furosemide in an attempt to improve urine output and lower the PCWP.

23. How would dobutamine infusion be initiated in D.T., who is already receiving dopamine at 6 mcg/kg/min?

After preparation of a 1000 mcg/ml solution, the dobutamine can be administered at an infusion rate of 2–3 mcg/kg/min. As the dobutamine infusion rate is increased every 15–20 minutes by 2 mcg/kg/min, the dopamine infusion could be decreased by a similar rate depending on heart rate and blood pressure. If the urine output is less than 0.5 ml/kg/hour, the dopamine infusion could be reduced to 1–2 mcg/kg/min to improve renal blood flow, and dobutamine could be adjusted to maintain a sufficient cardiac output and blood pressure. Dopamine should be administered through a central venous line, whereas dobutamine can be given in a peripheral vein. If peripheral lines are unavailable, both agents can be infused into the same central line via a "Y" connector site. The dobutamine solution will turn a light pink color several hours after mixing, but this will not alter potency or stability according to the manufacturer.

24. D.D., a 70-year-old female weighing 80 kg and having a body surface area of 2.0 m², is admitted to the ICU via the emergency room with the diagnosis of acute anterior wall MI.

Her PMH is significant for coronary artery disease, chronic atrial fibrillation, and one anterior wall MI six months PTA. Medications include digoxin 0.125 mg qd, quinidine 200 mg q 6 h, furosemide 40 mg bid, KCl 20 mEq qd, Isordil 10 mg PO q 6 h, and sublingual nitroglycerin as needed.

ABG's in the ER: (O_2 by mask), pO_2 50, pCO_2 70, pH 7.18; Temp: 38.1°C; Na 140 mEq/L; K 5.0 mEq/L; Cl 100 mEq/L; HCO_3 15 mEq/L.

One ampule of sodium bicarbonate was given in the emergency room and a dopamine drip was started.

D.D. was intubated and given ventilatory support. Upon admission to the ICU, D.D. has the following vital signs on a dopamine infusion of 30 mcg/kg/min: BP 80/30/45 mm Hg; P 110 beats/min; RR 30 breaths/min; U/O at the time of catheterization: 100 ml; ABG's (FiO_2 .80): pO_2 110, pCO_2 42, pH 7.30.

A Swan-Ganz catheter is inserted and the following hemodynamic parameters are obtained: CO 4.0 L/min; CI 2.0 L/min/m^2; SV 36 ml/beat; SVI 18 ml/beat/m^2; RAP 10 mm Hg; PCWP 16 mm Hg; TPVR 700; LVSWI 7.1 gm-m/m^2/beat.

Why is patient D.D. unresponsive to the peripheral vascular effects of dopamine?

Although dopamine at 30 mcg/kg/min has sustained a reasonable cardiac output, the MAP is not elevated and the TPVR is slightly low for what would be expected at this high infusion rate. It is extremely important to increase the MAP to 60–65 mm Hg to ensure coronary perfusion. Acid-base imbalances are a major cause of unresponsiveness to the pressor effects of sympathomimetics (109–111). Reversal of acidosis and hypoxia are necessary to achieve a greater therapeutic response. Other factors associated with a blunted response to catecholamines are sepsis, intravascular volume depletion, and the prior use of catecholamine blocking or depleting drugs. D.D.'s acid-base imbalance should be corrected and her blood, urine, and sputum should be sent for cultures.

Some patients do not respond to sympathomimetics with enhanced cardiac output. As infarct size increases, there may not be enough functional myocardium to respond to the inotropic agent and the remaining viable myocardium is already functioning at near maximal potential (31). The prognosis is poor for these patients.

25. D.D. is continued on dopamine at 30 mcg/kg/min and is given 200 ml of 5% albumin over 10 minutes as well as 50 mEq of sodium bicarbonate. The following hemodynamic profile results: BP 80/40/53 mm Hg; P 115 beats/min; CO 4.5 L/min; CI 2.25 L/min/m^2; SV 39 ml/beat; RAP 14 mm Hg; PCWP 24 mm Hg; TPVR 690 dynes·sec·cm^{-5}; LVSWI 7.8 gm-m/m^2/beat; Urine output 0; ABG's (FiO_2 .80): pO_2 100, pCO_2 40, pH 7.38; RR 24.

The volume load has increased PCWP without significantly affecting the patient's blood pressure or the cardiac output. The TPVR is low, and the LVSWI indicates a very poorly functioning myocardium. Arterial blood pressure should be stabilized to at least 90–100 mm Hg systolic. What therapeutic agents in Table 3 can be used in this situation?

Norepinephrine (Levophed) can elevate the blood pressure when severe hypotension exists in conjunction with a low TPVR (30,80,112,113). Norepinephrine (NE) is identical to the neurotransmitter released from sympathetic nerve endings. Small norepinephrine doses stimulate beta$_1$-adrenergic receptors in the heart, but less than epinephrine. Large norepinephrine doses stimulate alpha-adrenergic receptors resulting in arterial and venous vascoconstriction. An infusion rate of 10 mcg/min of norepinephrine in man results in the following: both systolic and diastolic pressures increase with a slightly widened pulse pressure; cardiac output is unchanged or may decline due to a reflex vagal response that tends to slow the heart rate; stroke volume is slightly increased; peripheral vascular resistance is increased due to vasoconstriction; venous tone is increased and renal glomerular filtration is unchanged, unless arterial vasoconstriction is severe enough to reduce renal blood flow; and myocardial blood flow is enhanced by an elevated coronary perfusion pressure (3,114). Tachyphylaxis has occurred (79).

Any deficit in plasma volume should be corrected before or as NE is administered. The initial dose of NE can be administered as a 1–2 mcg/min infusion by diluting 4–8 mg into 500 ml of D5W. The infusion must be through a central line because local tissue necrosis will result if extravasation occurs in a peripheral line.

The infusion should be titrated upward until a systolic pressure of 90–100 mm Hg is established. The lowest infusion rate which will attain an adequate blood pressure should be employed because large doses may lead to ventricular irritability, cardiac depression (increased afterload), impaired renal blood flow, intravascular volume depletion, and reflex vagal slowing of the heart (3,102).

Metaraminol (Aramine) is similar to NE with regard to selectivity of alpha and beta receptors, although it acts both directly and indirectly by releasing NE from adrenergic nerve endings. Metaraminol is a weaker vasoconstrictor than NE on both resistance and capacitance vessels. Prolonged infusions can deplete NE stores in adrenergic nerve endings, although responsiveness can be restored by discontinuing metaraminol and infusing NE (3,79,110,114).

In hypotensive patients with clinical features of shock, metaraminol can increase cardiac output and TPVR simultaneously. Increases in dose can increase the TPVR without affecting the cardiac output (79,114).

A continuous infusion can be administered by diluting 50–100 mg of metaraminol in 500 ml D5W. The infusion can be initiated at 10 drops/minute and is titrated upward to the desired response. Metaraminol can also be given intramuscularly or subcutaneously, although these routes are very rarely utilized.

Phenylephrine (Neo-Synephrine) is a pure alpha agonist without beta-adrenergic properties. Based upon our personal experience, phenylephrine is much less likely to decrease renal blood flow and urine output than norepinephrine. Its vasoconstricting action is also milder than NE's and is limited to the peripheral vascular system, although there is some evidence that stimulation of alpha-adrenergic receptors in the heart will increase the myocardial contractile force (83). The alpha-adrenergic effects will increase peripheral vascular resistance and may also increase workload on the heart (increased afterload). Furthermore, it increases capillary hydrostatic pressure, leading to a net loss of fluid into the interstitial space, and as a consequence venous return is decreased. These actions potentiate a decline in cardiac output, and the reflex bradycardia further reduces cardiac output (3). An infusion rate of 10–15 drops/minute can be initiated following the dilution of 10–20 mg in 500 ml D5W. The infusion rate is titrated upward to achieve the desired response.

26. D.D.'s blood pressure is now 80/40 mm Hg and is unresponsive to both dopamine 30 mcg/kg/min and a volume load. Which of the above therapeutic agents would be the most appropriate in this situation?

The first consideration would be to decide if the dopamine dose could be increased to achieve more vasoconstriction. The heart rate is already 115/beats/min, and further increases would put the patient at risk for dangerous arrhythmias, especially in a patient prone to metabolic acidosis.

Since D.D. has no evidence of pulmonary edema, her preload could be further augmented with another fluid challenge. The risks are increased workload on the heart, development of pulmonary congestion, and increased myocardial oxygen requirements.

Metaraminol, with its alpha-adrenergic properties, could be initiated, but responsiveness may be blunted because dopamine may have already depleted NE from the adrenergic nerve endings.

Phenylephrine would raise the blood pressure, but it could also cause a reflex slowing of the heart rate. If the cardiac output is reduced as a result of supraventricular tachycardia (HR > 150), phenylephrine could be used to slow the rate, improve ventricular filling, and thereby elevate cardiac output and blood pressure.

Norepinephrine, with its vasoconstrictive properties plus some beta$_1$ inotropic effects, or phenylephrine would be the drugs of choice for this patient in this situation. The norepinephrine infusion could be initiated at 2–3 mcg/min and titrated upward by 1–2 mcg/min every 3–5 minutes until a systolic blood pressure of 90–100 mm Hg or a mean arterial pressure of 60 mm Hg is achieved. The major drawback is that renal blood flow may decrease. In D.D., with essentially no urine output, any further insult to the kidney could be detrimental.

27. How will norepinephrine affect coronary blood flow in D.D.?

Theoretically, the rise in diastolic pressure will improve coronary perfusion and myocardial oxygen supply and compensate for the increased oxygen demand caused by the increased afterload, contractility, and heart rate. In patients with coronary artery disease, such as D.D., the level of diastolic pressure needed to achieve adequate coronary perfusion cannot be determined. At each stenosis within the coronary artery, the pressure gradient falls so that the perfusion pressure needed to supply ischemic myocardium is unknown (31).

28. Norepinephrine is titrated to 15 mcg/min over 10 minutes and dopamine is continued at 30 mcg/kg/min. The following hemodynamic profile is obtained two hours later: BP 90/60/70 mm Hg; P 110 beats/min; CO 5.2 L/min; CI 2.6 L/min/m^2; SV 47 ml/beat; SVI 23.5 ml/beat/m^2; RAP 18 mm Hg; PCWP 28 mm Hg; TPVR 800 dynes·sec·cm^{-5}; LVSWI 13.4 gm-m/m^2/beat; Urine output 15 ml/hr, unresponsive to furosemide 200 mg IV.

The dopamine and norepinephrine are being administered through the same central intravenous line. Is there a problem in administering the drugs in this fashion?

Compatibility data of intravenous admixtures are derived from studies in which different agents are mixed in the same containers of D5W or other intravenous solutions. Studies of two or more agents infused into a common section of intravenous tubing and assayed for potency or structural changes are not available. It has been the authors' experience that the following drugs can be administered into a common intravenous line in any combination without visual changes (color or precipitate) and without sudden changes in the pharmacologic action of the drug: lidocaine, procainamide, bretyllium, epinephrine, norepinephrine, dopamine, and dobutamine. This should not be followed as a standard of practice. However, when multiple intravenous sites of administration are unavailable, these drugs can be given together within a short length of IV tubing to support the patient. None of these agents should be mixed in the same containers because they will all be administered at different rates. Dopamine loses stability in alkaline solutions and should probably not be exposed to alkaline drugs in "Y" connector sites of intravenous tubing.

29. D.D. has required dopamine and norepinephrine for six hours. Two attempts to wean the dopamine have been unsuccessful. Urine output is 15 ml/hr and is unresponsive to additional doses (240 mg and 400 mg) of IV furosemide. There are no neurological deficits in D.D., and she remains on ventilatory support. An intraaortic balloon pump (IABP) is being considered in an attempt to wean D.D. from vasopressors so that she can proceed to coronary artery arteriography. How can the IABP improve pump function and lessen inotropic and vasopressor support?

The intraaortic balloon pump is designed to improve coronary perfusion and reduce afterload, thus relieving myocardial ischemia. A 30 or 40 ml balloon catheter is inserted into the femoral artery and advanced to just below the arch of the aorta. Balloon inflation and deflation are synchronized with the EKG to inflate during diastole (after the aortic valve closes) and deflate at the onset of systole. The inflated balloon in diastole will increase coronary perfusion by elevating the mean aortic pressure. The rapid deflation of the balloon at the onset of systole will decrease systolic blood pressure, thus reducing afterload and improving cardiac ejection.

Cardiovascular function can be temporarily stabilized, although recovery from shock has not been promising (115,116). In a small randomized study (117), IABP insertion 4.8 to 13.7 hours following a transmural myocardial infarction did not limit infarction size and did not improve survival in comparison to therapy with diuretics and vasoactive agents. Recovery with IABP assistance most often occurs in conjunction with surgical intervention for repair of aneurysms, mechanical defects, or coronary artery bypass grafting (80,118). There are no studies which indicate the extent to which the dose of vasoactive agents can be reduced prior to surgery while simultaneously maintaining IABP assistance.

If D.D. decides to undergo surgery, an IABP should be inserted and coronary arteriographic studies should be performed.

30. M.L., a 68-year-old male weighing 55 kg, is scheduled for an elective cholecystectomy. His body surface area is 1.6 m^2, and his medical history includes adult onset diabetes mellitus (AODM) treated with 20 units NPH insulin each morning and hypertension treated with methyldopa 250 mg qid and furosemide 20 mg tid. Past medical history includes an anterior wall myocardial infarction ten years ago.

On the morning of surgery, M.L. is observed to be severely short of breath and is experiencing dull chest pain. He is oriented to name but not date or place. Vital signs are as follows: BP 140/76 mm Hg; P 84 (weak) beats/min; RR 22 (shallow) breaths/min; EKG

shows changes consistent with acute myocardial infarction. M.L. is admitted to the CCU to rule out myocardial infarction. An arterial line and Swan-Ganz catheter are inserted, revealing the following: BP 130/70/90 mm Hg; P 90 beats/min; CO 3 L/min; CI 1.8 L/min/m^2; SV 33 ml/beat; SVI 21 ml/beat/m^2; RAP 24 mm Hg; PAPD 36 mm Hg; PCWP 33 mm Hg; TPVR 1760 dynes·sec·cm^{-5}; LVSWI 16 gm-m/m^2/beat; ABG's: pO$_2$ 50, pCO$_2$ 50, pH 7.34; Stat electrolytes WNL; CXR: suggestive of pulmonary edema; Cardiac enzymes are sent for analysis.

M.L. appears to have suffered an acute MI and is in pulmonary edema. Morphine sulfate (MS) 5 mg IV and furosemide 40 mg IV are administered to M.L. His trachea is intubated and he is administered 100% oxygen.

Fifteen minutes after administration of the MS and furosemide, the following parameters are obtained: BP 115/65/80 mm Hg; P 94 beats/min; CO 3.2 L/min; CI 2.0 L/min/m^2; SVI 21 ml/beat/m^2; RAP 16 mm Hg; PCWP 26 mm Hg; TPVR 1600 dynes·sec·cm^{-5}; LVSWI 15.5 gm-m/m^2/beat.

Why has the PCWP declined and cardiac output remained essentially unchanged? (See Fig. 4.)

Furosemide and possibly morphine sulfate (MS) are venous vasodilators. Venous capacitance is increased, thus decreasing venous return (preload). Fluid is redistributed away from the lungs, thus lowering the PCWP (119,120). The diuretic effect from furosemide will also lower preload, but the vasodilating action often precedes the diuresis. Left ventricular filling pressure is reduced within five minutes and this effect peaks at 15 minutes after furosemide administration (120).

Morphine sulfate is also an arterial vasodilator; furosemide is not (32). In patients with a severely depressed cardiac output in conjunction with elevated TPVR, morphine could potentially improve cardiac output by lowering the TPVR. Furosemide does not affect cardiac output or stroke volume and may actually decrease it if left ventricular end diastolic volume is excessively reduced (Fig. 4). Both agents contributed to the reduced PCWP in this patient.

31. M.L.'s cardiac function is still severely depressed. Based on the above parameters, should an inotropic agent or a peripheral vasodilator be used at this point?

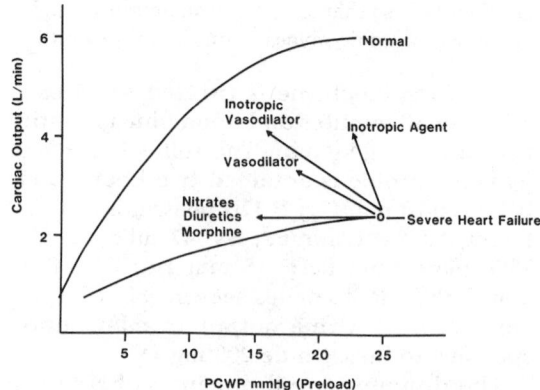

Figure 4. Ventricular Function Curve. Effects of various agents on cardiac output and PCWP.

The inotropic agent would improve cardiac output at the expense of increased heart rate and contractility, and the PCWP and TPVR may or may not improve. The TPVR is currently 1600 and any further increase would add to the workload on the heart.

A peripheral vasodilator such as nitroprusside, which has both arterial and venous vasodilatory properties, would decrease pulmonary venous congestion by lowering preload, and would increase cardiac output by decreasing the resistance to left ventricular ejection. Therefore, two of the major determinants of myocardial oxygen demand can be lowered. Meanwhile, the contractility will be unaltered and the heart rate may increase slightly (32,121–123). The objective of vasodilator therapy in acute heart failure is to improve cardiac output by lowering peripheral vascular resistance while maintaining a reasonable blood pressure (BP = CO × TPVR). Whether nitroprusside will decrease myocardial ischemia is controversial and unclear (124).

M.L. has a PCWP which is greater than 15 mm Hg and an elevated TPVR. He is not hypotensive but he is in left ventricular failure; therefore, he meets the criteria necessary for implementation of nitroprusside therapy in acute heart failure (32,72,125).

32. Would a nitroglycerin infusion offer any advantage over nitroprusside in M.L. who has an elevated PCWP of 26 mm Hg and a depressed cardiac output of 3.2 L/min?

Nitroglycerin (NTG) directly relaxes the systemic venous vascular system. As a result, venous capacitance increases, with a marked reduction of left ventricular filling pressure, left ventricular volume, and cardiac work (126,127). In contrast to nitroprusside, which has a relatively balanced effect on both preload and afterload, sustained NTG administration lowers preload to a much greater extent than afterload. Cardiac output is usually unaffected or may even be reduced (Fig. 4) (124,128).

Since M.L. could benefit from both afterload and preload reduction, nitroprusside is the agent of choice. The only advantage NTG might offer is the possible reduction of infarct size, although experimentally this is unproven. NTG infusion significantly reduces ST segment elevations in patients with left ventricular impairment (129–131). Moreover, nitroprusside could worsen ischemia by dilating vessels to nonischemic myocardium at the same time that aortic pressure is lowered (30). Thus, blood flow may be directed away from the ischemic area. Further studies are needed to clarify the effects of both nitroprusside and NTG on infarct size in patients with severe left ventricular failure following an acute MI.

33. What would be an appropriate nitroprusside infusion rate for patient M.L.?

Most patients require between 0.5–3.0 mcg/kg/min of nitroprusside to achieve therapeutic benefit; however, the initial infusion rate should be no more than 0.5 mcg/kg/min. Mason (72) recommends that the systolic blood pressure be maintained above 90 mm Hg at all times and that the PCWP be maintained between 15–18 mm Hg. If M.L.'s heart rate increases beyond 105–110/min, the infusion rate should be lowered. The TPVR and CO must also be monitored throughout to evaluate change in cardiac function.

34. Fifteen minutes after beginning M.L. on nitroprusside at 0.5 mcg/kg/min, the following hemodynamic profile is obtained: BP 120/60/80 mm Hg; P 96 beats/min; CO 3.7 L/min; CI 2.3 L/min/m²; SV 38.5 ml/beat; SVI 24 ml/beat/m²; RAP 14 mm Hg; PCWP 21 mm Hg; TPVR 1427 dynes·sec·cm⁻⁵; LVSWI 19 gm-m/m²/beat. Has nitroprusside exerted a therapeutic effect in M.L.?

M.L.'s cardiac output has increased by 14%, his PCWP has been lowered by 19%, and his heart rate and mean arterial pressure have remained unchanged. The TPVR has dropped 11% and LVSWI has increased by 19%. Thus, nitroprus-

side has improved perfusion by lowering afterload and has further lessened workload on the heart by lowering preload. The overall net benefit at this point appears to be improved cardiac status without an increase in myocardial oxygen demand. The patient's arterial blood gases, urine output, and clinical status must also be evaluated.

35. Should the nitroprusside infusion be gradually increased to achieve greater systemic perfusion?

The hemodynamic parameters in this patient have improved; however, the TPVR and PCWP are still elevated and it would be desirable to further reduce afterload and preload. The duration of action of nitroprusside is 2–3 minutes; thus, any adverse effect which may occur can be rapidly corrected by decreasing the infusion rate. Therefore, further improvement in cardiac performance can be attempted without great risk.

The answer to this question must be based on the clinical status of the patient as well as the hemodynamic measurements. If M.L. does not have clinical signs of hypoperfusion, his ABG's are good, and if his urine output is greater than 0.5 ml/kg/hr, then maintenance of nitroprusside at 0.5 mcg/kg/min is reasonable while attempting to further lower the PCWP with the careful use of diuretics. If M.L. still has clinical signs of hypoperfusion and if his urine output is inadequate, then the nitroprusside infusion could be cautiously increased to further reduce afterload and preload.

36. Over the next four hours M.L.'s urine output declined to less than 20 ml/hr despite the administration of 200 mg and 400 mg IV furosemide. Nitroprusside was maintained at 0.5 mcg/kg/min. The following observations were made: BP 105/50/68 mm Hg; P 90 beats/min; CO 3.0 L/min; CI 1.9 L/min/m²; SV 33 ml/beat; RAP 12 mm Hg; PADP 29 mm Hg; PCWP 24 mm Hg; TPVR 1490 dynes·sec·cm⁻⁵; LVSWI 12.5 gm-m/m²/beat; ABG's (FiO₂ .60): pO₂ 90, pCO₂ 40, pH 7.36; EKG 6–12 PVC's/minute with occasional bigeminy and trigeminy.

Lidocaine 100 mg bolus plus a 2 mg/min infusion were started to suppress the PVC's. Would an increase in the nitroprusside infusion be reasonable at this point?

Before the nitroprusside dose is adjusted, sufficient time (5–10 minutes) should be allowed to determine if lidocaine will suppress the PVC's. If the PVC's are responsible for the drop in blood pressure and cardiac output, then lidocaine might reverse this trend. A serum potassium level should also be checked immediately.

37. Lidocaine suppressed the PVC's to less than 2/minute. Thereafter, the following were noted: BP 110/60/76 mm Hg; P 95 beats/min; CO 3.2 L/min; CI 2.0 L/min/m^2; SV 34 ml/beat; RAP 14 mm Hg; PAD 31 mm Hg; PCWP 24 mm Hg; TPVR 1550 dynes·sec·cm^{-5}; LVSWI 15 gm-m/m^2/beat; Urine output less than 20 ml/hr; ABG's (FiO$_2$ .6): pO$_2$ 90, pCO$_2$ 42, pH 7.34; CXR — increased signs of pulmonary congestion and edema; CNS — lethargic, responds to loud verbal commands.

M.L.'s cardiac state is still depressed and his urine output is inadequate. What therapeutic maneuvers could be initiated at this time and what would be the expected result?

M.L. has been unresponsive to 200 mg and 400 mg IV furosemide. The dose of furosemide could be increased to 800 mg to improve urine output and to lower the PCWP, but this would take considerable time before beneficial results would be noted.

The nitroprusside infusion rate could be gradually increased if the increments are no more than 0.25 mcg/kg/min, although the heart rate and blood pressure may or may not change. M.L.'s blood pressure is somewhat low; his TPVR is elevated. A reduction in TPVR (afterload) by nitroprusside would improve cardiac output and improve renal perfusion. Not only does the increase in cardiac output improve renal perfusion, but nitroprusside may also directly vasodilate the renal vasculature and improve renal perfusion if intravascular volume is well maintained (133). Adequate coronary perfusion also must be maintained in a patient with suspected acute myocardial infarction that is several hours old.

A third alternative would be to supplement the nitroprusside infusion with dopamine or epinephrine. Inotropic support would enhance contractility and maintain arterial pressure with the nitroprusside on board. Changes in heart rate, TPVR, and PCWP would depend on the agent selected and the dose. Since M.L. has declining renal function in addition to poor cardiac status and does not show signs of hypovolemia, dopamine at 2–5 mcg/kg/min would be the best agent with which to begin therapy. The dopamine would enhance cardiac support and would produce the beneficial dopaminergic effects on the renal vasculature. The

risk associated with this maneuver is an increased myocardial oxygen demand. After the dopamine is started at 2 mcg/kg/min, both agents should be titrated to achieve the optimal cardiac output with the least adverse effect on arterial pressure and heart rate. Dosages only should be adjusted one agent at a time.

A fourth alternative would be to add dobutamines to nitroprusside or to use dobutamine alone. Dobutamine would give inotropic support and increase afterload reduction beyond that produced by the nitroprusside. This would require careful titration because the maintenance of coronary perfusion is of utmost importance. Preload would also be reduced to a greater extent than that produced by either agent alone. The disadvantage of this combination is that dobutamine does not directly vasodilate the renal vasculature as does dopamine. Dobutamine could be initiated at 2–3 mcg/kg/min and the dosage titrated upward if necessary. The heart rate should not be allowed to increase above 115 beats/min, and PCWP should not drop below 12–15 mm Hg.

Dobutamine alone and nitroprusside plus dopamine in eight acute myocardial infarction patients (134) improved the cardiac index and lowered the left ventricular filling pressure and TPVR to similar degrees. The mean arterial pressure was slightly higher in patients on dobutamine alone. Apparently, the only advantage of dobutamine over the combined use of dopamine and nitroprusside was the administration of a single agent.

In the case of M.L. the nitroprusside/dopamine combination would be acceptable because his urine output is markedly reduced.

38. Over the next two hours dopamine and nitroprusside are titrated to 3.2 mcg/kg/min and 1.2 mcg/kg/min respectively. The following profile is obtained: BP 115/50/71 mm Hg; P 100 beats/min; CO 4.7 L/min; CI 2.9 L/min/m^2; SV 47 ml/beat; SVI 29 ml/beat/m^2; RAP 10 mm Hg; PCWP 20 mm Hg; TPVR 1038 dynes·sec·cm^{-5}; LVSWI 20 gm-m/m^2/beat; ABG's (FiO$_2$ .50): pO$_2$ 85, pCO$_2$ 35, pH 7.42; Urine output 60 ml/hr.

The dopamine and nitroprusside were continued at the same infusion rates, and furosemide 40 mg IV every six hours was added for the pulmonary edema. If the hemodynamic parameters are maintained for the next

12 hours, how should these infusions be discontinued in this patient?

There are no established guidelines for weaning intravenous vasodilators or inotropic agents. The rapidity at which these solutions can be discontinued often depends on the experience of the nurse, familiarity with the drugs, and knowledge of the drugs' effects on the cardiovascular system. Unstable patients in severe cardiogenic or septic shock who require high infusion rates often need hours to days to be weaned from these drugs.

Nitroprusside for afterload therapy should be weaned slowly over several hours, because the mean arterial pressure, PCWP, heart rate, and TPVR can rebound dramatically 10–30 minutes after abrupt withdrawal of the infusion (135). If the TPVR increases during the weaning process, oral afterload reducing agents may be initiated before the nitroprusside is completely withdrawn. In patient M.L., the nitroprusside infusion can be decreased 0.25 mcg/kg/min each hour.

Specific guidelines for weaning infusions of pressors and inotropic agents must be written for the nursing staff. Guidelines appropriate for M.L. would be: wean dopamine by 0.5 mcg/kg/min each hour; check all hemodynamic parameters fifteen minutes after each reduction of the infusion rate, and notify the physician if the MAP < 65 or > 80 mm Hg; PCWP < 12 or > 22 mm Hg; TPVR < 900 or > 1200 dynes·sec·cm^{-5}; CO < 4.0 L/min. If the patient's hemodynamic status deteriorates during the weaning process, the infusion rates will require readjustment.

SEPTIC SHOCK

39. S.B. is a 58-year-old female who weighs 65 kg and has a body surface area of 1.6 m^2. She underwent aortic valve replacement 13 days ago for treatment of severe aortic stenosis. Postoperative recovery has been complicated by the following sequence of events. Four hours after the initial surgical procedure, correction of surgically induced bleeding was needed. Respiratory support with a ventilator was required for the next three days, as was cardiovascular support with dopamine 2–10 mcg/kg/min. Four days postoperatively, S.B. developed a *Escherichia coli* urinary tract infection which was successfully treated with ampicillin 1 gm every 6 hours for 5 days. S.B. also received a five-day

course of cefamandole at this time for valve replacement prophylaxis. S.B.'s major problem has been failure of the sternal wound to heal properly. On postoperative day 12, the sternal wound was noticed to be severely inflamed and the granulation process impaired. Pus was extruded from the wound upon compression. A Gram's stain from the wound showed gram-positive cocci as well as gram-negative rods, and wound specimens were sent for cultures. S.B. had a fever of 38.2°C and a total white blood cell count of 17,000 with 60% neutrophils and 25% bands. She again was started on cefamandole 1 gm every 4 hours.

On the morning of postoperative day 13, the patient began to complain of chills, and a spiking fever to 39.2°C was noted. Pertinent physical findings included a blood pressure of 130/70 mm Hg, heart rate of 110 beats/min, and a respiratory rate of 28 breaths/min. S.B. complained of right upper quadrant pain. Bowel sounds were absent. The cardiac examination was normal. Chest x-ray showed atelectasis on the right lower base. Laboratory analysis revealed the following: Na 134 mEq/L; Cl 95 mEq/L; K 4.2 mEq/L; HCO$_3$ 22 mEq/L; BUN 22 mg/dl; Creatinine 1.0 mg/dl; T. Bilirubin 2.0 mg/dl; alkaline phosphatase 13.5 Bodansky units/ml; SGOT 30 units/ml; LDH 200 IU/L; WBC 12,000 with 55% neutrophils and 30% bands; Urine output was 400 ml/8 hours. Gentamicin 80 mg every 8 hours was begun after sputum, blood, wound, and urine cultures were obtained. Acetaminophen suppositories were ordered for temperature greater than 39°C.

Six hours later, S.B. was noted to be anxious, restless, and confused with a respiratory rate of 30 breaths/min. Blood pressure by cuff was 100/40 mm Hg with a heart rate of 140 beats/min. Temperature was 39.2°C. Stat blood chemistries showed: Na 138 mEq/L; Cl 97 mEq/L; K 4.0 mEq/L; HCO$_3$ 18 mEq/L; Glucose 210 mg/dl; BUN 24 mg/dl; Creatinine 0.8 mg/dl; WBC 16,000; ABG's (room air): pO$_2$ 65, pCO$_2$ 24, pH 7.30.

One ampule of sodium bicarbonate (50 mEq) was given and normal saline was started at 200 ml/hr. One-hundred percent O$_2$ by mask was begun at 8 L/minute. A pulmonary artery catheter and arterial line were inserted and the following hemodynamic parameters obtained: BP 90/40/56 mm Hg; HR 142 beats/min (sinus tachycardia with occasional PAC's); CO 8.2 L/min; CI 5.1 L/min/m^2; SV 58 ml/beat; SVI 36 ml/beat/m^2; PAP 24/10/15 mm Hg; RAP 8 mm Hg; PCWP 4 mm Hg; TPVR 468 dynes·sec·cm^{-5}; PVR 107 dynes·sec·cm^{-5}; Urine output by foley 40 ml/hr.

What is the most likely etiology and stage of sepsis in this patient?

According to S.B.'s hemodynamic profile and clinical presentation of confusion, anxiety, chills, spiking fever, and hypotension, early septic shock is present. Her elevated cardiac index and low TPVR indicate that she is in the hyperdynamic phase of septic shock. Maintenance of a high cardiac output with volume replacement is essential to prevent progression to a low output—high resistant state and myocardial depression. Although volume infusion could substantially increase venous return as measured by LVEDP, cardiac output and stroke work may not increase once the low output—high resistant state is established (142).

Pseudomonas and *Staphylococci* would be the most likely pathogens because the most obvious source of sepsis in S.B. is the sternal wound infection. Pathogenic organisms from this patient's gastrointestinal tract (eg, *Escherichia coli, Klebsiella,* and anaerobes) also must be considered because the increased total bilirubin to 2.0 mg/dl in conjunction with the increased alkaline phosphatase, right upper quadrant pain, and absent bowel sounds suggest possible biliary obstruction or stasis. Development of cholestasis after a major procedure is not uncommon (143). Other possibile foci of infection include the urinary tract (recent history of *E.coli* urinary tract infection), intravascular lines, and the pulmonary system. Table 5 lists the most likely pathogens which are usually associated with specific sites of infection.

40. What are the immediate goals of therapy in S.B. and how can achievement of those goals be assessed?

Hemodynamic Status. Immediate attention must be given to this patient's hemodynamic status. S.B.'s elevated cardiac output must be main-

Table 5.
USUAL SITE OF INFECTION*

Organism	Site
Escherichia coli	Urinary tract, abdominal abscess, peritonitis
Klebsiella species	Lung, abdominal wound, intravenous line, urinary tract
Enterobacter species	Contaminated blood products or intravenous fluids, intravenous lines, urinary tract, intravascular pressure monitoring equipment
Serratia species	Peritoneal catheter, intravenous line, urinary tract, lung, intravascular pressure monitoring equipment.
Pseudomonas aeruginosa	Lung, urinary tract, cutaneous wound, intravenous line
Bacteroides species	Subphrenic abscess, abdominal wound, decubiti
Erwinia species	Intravenous infusion set
Acinetobacter species	Intravenous line
Citrobacter species	Urinary tract

*Gleckman: S Med J 1981; 74:335.

tained with volume expansion in an attempt to halt the development of progression of poor tissue perfusion, because a decreased cardiac index decreases the chances of survival. Specifically, survival improves when the cardiac index is maintained above 3.1 L/min/m² (11). The mean arterial pressure also should be maintained at greater than 65 mm Hg, because a decrease in coronary flow is a major contributing factor to the development of myocardial failure in endotoxin shock (144–146).

S.B. has a cardiac output of 8.2 L/min, a PCWP of 4 mm Hg, a TPVR of 468 dynes·sec·cm^{-5}, and a MAP of 56 mm Hg. These hemodynamic parameters should be monitored during volume expansion. Urine output is not a reliable indicator of hemodynamic status in early septic shock because some patients will be oliguric and others will put out large volumes of urine (147). S.B. should be administered fluid challenges with normal saline to increase the PCWP to 8–12 mm Hg. Hopefully this will maintain the CO through the Starling mechanism and thus increase the MAP (BP = CO x TPVR). Also, pulmonary function must be examined closely because non-cardiogenic pulmonary edema commonly develops in septic shock. Finally, assessments of the patient's sensorium and urine output also provide insights into the adequacy of volume expansion. A favorable response to fluid therapy should improve the sensorium, and the urine output should be more than 0.5 ml/kg/hour.

Ventilation. In addition to volume expansion, a second and equally important treatment goal is the provision of adequate ventilation. In the later phase of septic shock, an increase in pulmonary vascular resistance results in ventilation/perfusion defects and a high incidence of respiratory failure and mortality (8,148). S.B. has a respiratory rate of 30 breaths/min, a pO₂ of 65 mm Hg, pCO₂ of 24 mm Hg, and pH of 7.3 on room air. S.B. appears to have a mixed metabolic acidosis and respiratory alkalosis acid-base disorder (149). If the arterial pO₂ decreases to less than 60 mm Hg in conjunction with an elevated respiratory rate (> 30 breaths per minute), intubation and mechanical ventilation with the use of positive end expiratory pressure (PEEP) is usually indicated.

Antibiotics. The third immediate treatment goal is initiation of antibiotics after blood, urine, sputum, and wound cultures have been taken. S.B. has a prosthetic aortic valve and is highly sus-

ceptible for development of acute bacterial endocarditis in the setting of a nonhealing sternal wound and recent urinary tract infection. Until cultures and sensitivities are available to guide antibiotic therapy, empiric broad spectrum bactericidal parenteral antibiotics should be administered. The choice of antibiotics depends on the clinical setting and most likely source of sepsis. The three potential primary foci of infection in this patient are the urinary tract, the sternal wound, and the biliary tract. The most likely pathogens include: *E. coli* from the urinary tract; *Staphylococcus aureus, enterococcus,* and *Pseudomonas aeruginosa* from the sternal wound; and *E. coli, Klebsiella pneumoniae,* and *Bacteroides fragilis* from the biliary tract. An aminoglycoside in combination with ampicillin, clindamycin, and penicillinase-resistant penicillin such as nafcillin would cover these suspected organisms. Once the pathogen is identified, unnecessary antibiotics can be discontinued. (See the Endocarditis chapter for antibiotic dosing and sensitivities.) A decrease in the white blood cell count without a left shift, defervescence, and stabilization of hemodynamic parameters would indicate the pathogens are initially sensitive to the antibiotics chosen.

Surgical Evaluation. The fourth immediate treatment goal is surgical evaluation for drainage of S.B.'s sternal wound and debridement of necrotic tissue. Gall bladder studies might be considered when S.B. is stabilized to rule out biliary obstruction. Surgical intervention is often necessary to eliminate persistent foci of bacteremia.

41. Gentamicin 80 mg every 8 hours is to be continued, and nafcillin 2 gm every 4 hours, clindamycin 600 mg every 6 hours, and ampicillin 1 gm every 4 hours are to be added pending culture and sensitivity results. In addition to continuing intravenous normal saline at 200 ml/hr, S.B. is given a 500 ml bolus of normal saline over the next 15 minutes along with 2 gm of methylprednisolone sodium succinate (Solu-Medrol). What is the evidence that high dose corticosteroids decrease mortality in septic shock?

The therapeutic efficacy of corticosteroids in the management septic shock has not been established because of poorly designed studies in human subjects (150). However, in animal studies, protection from the full development of the shock and improvement in survival are provided when steroids are administered early in the course of shock (158,159). Perhaps this discrepancy between increased survival in animals and lack of therapeutic benefit in humans is because corticosteroids are administered in human subjects only after the septic shock syndrome is fully developed.

The strongest argument for high dose corticosteroid therapy in septic shock is provided by a two-part prospective and retrospective 8-year study which evaluated the effects of dexamethasone, methylprednisolone, or saline on mortality rate (153). In the prospective portion, 172 patients with blood culture positive septic shock were treated with antibiotics and either an intravenous bolus of saline, 3 mg/kg of intravenous dexamethasone, or 30 mg/kg of intravenous methylprednisolone. This bolus dose could be repeated once after 4 hours if needed. Mortality was 38.4% in the saline-treated group, 11.6% in the methylprednisolone group, and 9.3% in the dexamethasone group. The retrospective portion of this study, involving 378 patients, noted that 14% of the patients receiving corticosteroids died, as contrasted with 47.5% of patients not receiving steroids. In both parts of the study, treatment groups were comparable in age, severity of shock, and underlying disease. There was no significant difference in complications (gastrointestinal bleeding, non-ketotic hyperosmolar diabetes, and acute psychosis) between the steroid and non-steroid treated groups. Although the mortality differences are impressive between the steroid treated and non-steroid treated groups, several questions and criticisms remain unanswered. At what stage of treatment were the corticosteroids started? How frequently was a second dose given? What criteria were used to determine if a second dose was needed? What circulatory support (volume replacement and/or vasoactive amines) was given to each group and how frequently? Which group of patients required more or less surgical intervention to drain or eradicate a septic focus? Chloramphenicol was given during the first three years of the study; the combination of gentamicin and clindamycin was administered in last five years of the study. Patients in the latter half of the study probably received more generalized care. It is unknown whether the answers to these criticisms and questions would have affected the outcome of this study.

In a more recent retrospective study, 4.0 gm/day of hydrocortisone (or its equivalent) did not increase survival and, in fact, was associated with a significant increase in fatality rates (162).

Proposed corticosteroid actions in septic shock include: increased cardiac output with improved tissue perfusion, decreased peripheral vascular resistance, decreased coagulopathies, anticomplement activity, and stabilization of lysosomal and capillary membranes. The evidence may favor corticosteroid stabilization of capillary membranes (10). It appears that endotoxin activates the production of complement products C3, C5, and C5a within the intravascular compartment. These complement products are vasodilators themselves and also activate polymorphonuclear leukocytes (PMN's). The activated PMN's adhere to other PMN's and to vascular endothelium, subsequently releasing arachidonic acid derivatives, cytotoxic products of molecular oxygen, and lysosomal enzymes. These produce additional local vasoactive effects on the microvasculature as well as substantial endothelial cytotoxicity, resulting in capillary leaks. In vitro, high concentrations of glucocorticoids inhibit complement-induced PMN aggregation and the cytotoxic effects on endothelial cells (154–156). Furthermore, some patients with sepsis have a remarkable decrease in pulmonary-capillary leakage after a large dose of a corticosteroid.

In summary, the use of high dose corticosteroids in septic shock is still considered controversial. Animal studies suggest that early use may be beneficial in reducing mortality. One large clinical study provides strong evidence that corticosteroids reduce mortality, but important questions have not been answered regarding other treatment the study population may have received (153). Most clinicians choose methylprednisolone over dexamethasone when giving steroids for septic shock, although no significant differences in survival have been shown in clinical trials. It is apparent that a prospective, randomized study is still needed to clarify whether high-dose corticosteroids are useful in patients with early septic shock.

42. S.B. has received 800 ml of normal saline as fluid challenges over the past 45 minutes. The following hemodynamic parameters are obtained: BP 80/38/52 mm Hg; HR 125 beats/min; CO 8.0 L/min; CI 5.0 L/min/m^2; SV 64 ml/beat; SVI 40 ml/beat/m^2; RAP 15 mm Hg; PCWP 10 mm Hg; PAP 32/18/23 mm Hg;

TPVR 370 dynes·sec·cm^{-5}; PVR 130 dynes· sec·cm^{-5}; Urine output 80 ml/hr; ABG's (100 percent O_2 by mask): pO_2 60, pCO_2 30, pH 7.31; Respiratory rate 36 breaths/min; Mental status: confused and anxious; Pulmonary exam— No rales or ronchi; Chest x-ray shows atelectasis on the right lower base; Cardiac examination—within normal limits. Why is an inotropic agent indicated for this patient at this time?

S.B. is still in the hyperdynamic phase of septic shock, as would be expected. Despite maintenance of the cardiac output and urine output via fluid resuscitation, S.B.'s blood pressure and peripheral vascular resistance has fallen. The pulmonary examination and chest x-ray are not suggestive of pulmonary congestion or edema. The pulmonary capillary wedge pressure has been increased from 4 mm Hg to 10 mm Hg with a net fluid intake of 720 ml normal saline. Therefore, S.B. could receive further fluid to maintain intravascular volume. But until enough fluid can be administered, it is important to preserve cerebral and coronary artery perfusion pressure. The coronary artery perfusion gradient (aortic diastolic pressure—pulmonary capillary wedge pressure) has declined from 36 mm Hg to 28 mm Hg in the past 45 minutes and, as a result, has severely limited oxygen supply to the myocardium despite a pO_2 of 60 mm Hg. Inotropic support would be indicated at this time along with intubation, artificial ventilation, and continued fluid administration.

43. What inotropic agent would be appropriate in S.B. at this time?

Controlled comparative studies have not established clearly which inotropic agent or vasopressor is the best for treatment of septic shock. Indeed, it is unknown whether these agents improve over-all survival (11,158). Vasopressors, or inotropic agents with vasopressor properties, are to be avoided if possible in the cold stage of septic shock because they theoretically could intensify the already elevated sympathetic tone and limit tissue perfusion even further.

In one comparison of norepinephrine, dopamine, or isoproterenol in 50 patients with bacteremic shock, dopamine produced the most favorable response (142). Dopamine elevated the cardiac output and maintained the mean arterial pressure, although neither dopamine or norepinephrine improved the survival rate of patients in septic shock (8). Dopamine may be the better drug due to its ability to increase renal and mesenteric vascular blood flow (7,159,160).

In the case of S.B., dopamine would be an appropriate inotropic agent. Blood pressure would be increased by elevation of both the cardiac output and peripheral vascular resistance. Dopamine could have variable effects on PCWP, depending on the infusion rate.

44. What would be a reasonable therapeutic end-point of inotropic therapy for this patient at this time?

The goal of dopamine therapy would be to increase the MAP to 60–65 mm Hg or until vascular volume could be adequately maintained with fluids alone. A 3–5 mcg/kg/min initial infusion rate which is increased upward every 5–10 minutes as needed would be reasonable for this patient. Once the blood pressure is stabilized with additional fluids, the dopamine infusion rate could be discontinued or slowed to 2–3 mcg/kg/min, which is a rate still compatible with enhanced renal vascular blood flow. The wedge pressure should not be increased beyond 15–18 mm Hg because patients in septic shock are very vulnerable to pulmonary edema from adult respiratory distress syndrome.

45. When would vasopressors be indicated for this patient?

If inotropic agents such as dopamine or epinephrine cannot maintain a satisfactory mean arterial pressure with a cardiac output greater than 10 L/min, then vasopressors may be useful. If the cardiac output is less than 10 L/min, further inotropic support is reasonable.

Studies which compare vasopressor agents in the treatment of septic shock are not available, but norepinephrine and phenylephrine are the most commonly used. Our personal clinical experience suggests that norepinephrine is a much more potent vasoconstrictor than phenylephrine, but it also has a much greater potential for decreasing renal blood flow and lowering urine output. The dosages of these agents are titrated upwards to maintain a mean arterial pressure of 60–65 mm Hg. It would also be reasonable to maintain the dopamine infusion rate at 2–3 mcg/kg/min for this patient when vasopressor support is needed in order to facilitate renal blood flow.

46. S.B. is given 250 ml of normal saline over the next ten minutes. Dopamine is begun and the dosage is gradually increased to 12 mcg/kg/min in order to stabilize her blood pressure. S.B. is intubated and ventilatory support initiated at an F_iO_2 of 100% at a rate of 12 breaths/minute. The maintenance IV rate is adjusted to 125 ml/hr of D5/¼NS.

Thirty minutes later the following hemodynamic parameters are obtained: BP 110/62/78 mm Hg; HR 110 beats/min; CO 8.8 L/min; CI 5.5 L/min/m²; SV 80 ml/beat; SVI 50 ml/beat/m²; RAP 20 mm Hg; PCWP 16 mm Hg; PAP 42/26/31 mm Hg; TPVR 527 dynes·sec·cm⁻⁵; PVR 136 dynes·sec·cm⁻⁵; Urine output: 20 ml over last 30 minutes; ABG's (F_iO_2 100%): pO_2 220, pCO_2 38, pH 7.38; Mental status: oriented to name and place; Pulmonary examination: rales in both lower lobes. What are the therapeutic goals over the next 24 hours?

The hemodynamic goal over the next 24 hours is to maintain perfusion pressure to vital organs by adjusting fluid intake and inotropic support and to balance cardiac output, peripheral resistance, and intravascular volume. S.B. is currently requiring dopamine at 12 mcg/kg/min and fluid at 125 ml/hr to maintain a MAP greater than 70 mm Hg, a CI of 5.5 L/min/M², and a TPVR of 527 dynes·sec·cm⁻⁵. The PCWP has been increased from 4 to 16 mm Hg over the past two hours because of fluid challenges and dopamine. Early signs of pulmonary congestion have appeared as noted by rales heard over both lower lung fields. Therefore, the PCWP probably has been increased as high as S.B. can tolerate at this point. Further fluid challenges might aggravate the pulmonary congestion, especially because an increase in pulmonary capillary leakage is possible in sepsis.

It is also important to note that the dopamine infusion rate is sufficient to induce alpha-adrenergic vasoconstriction, thus mimicking the later phase of septic shock. Although the peripheral vascular resistance is not very high (527 dynes·sec·cm⁻⁵), TPVR does not represent the vascular resistance of a specific vascular bed. Therefore, renal function must be evaluated closely.

In this patient, the fluid infusion rate should try to maintain the PCWP between 12–16 mm Hg, the RAP less than 20 mm Hg, and the urine output greater than 0.5 ml/kg/hr. If the PCWP is in the suggested range and the urine output drops below 0.5 ml/kg/hr for more than 1½-2 hours, then a loop-diuretic would be appropriate.

While the IV fluid infusion rate is being established, the dopamine infusion rate should be decreased to less than 10 mcg/kg/min to avoid its alpha-adrenergic effects. Some patients can be weaned off dopamine in a few hours; others require days or even weeks before they cease to be dopamine dependent. The MAP should be maintained between 60–65 mm Hg while the dopamine is being tapered. A reasonable approach would be to decrease the dopamine infusion rate by 2–3 mcg/kg/min every 1–2 hours if tolerated. The dopamine infusion can be maintained at 2–3 mcg/kg/min because of the beneficial effects on renal perfusion at this dosage.

Adjustment of ventilatory support is also important in S.B. She has a pO_2 of 220 on 100% F_iO_2; thus a decrease in the F_iO_2 is indicated in order to prevent oxygen toxicity. Weaning down the F_iO_2 to less than 50% if tolerated with the use of positive end expiratory pressure over the next several hours would be appropriate.

Surgical evaluation of the sternal wound for drainage and debridement and a surgical evaluation of the abdomen also should be obtained because both the total bilirubin and alkaline phosphatase are elevated in addition to absent bowel sounds. Elimination of possible septic foci is extremely important.

47. What other potential problems should be anticipated in septic shock?

There are several potential problems that must be anticipated in sepsis. "Shock lung" is common in bacteremic shock. The pulmonary insufficiency is associated with pulmonary congestion, atelectasis, and edema with ventilation-perfusion abnormalities (161). In some patients it is very difficult not to amplify this condition when a large amount of fluid is needed for stabilizing hemodynamic abnormalities.

Coagulation abnormalities and thrombocytopenia are commonly observed in septic patients. In a recent retrospective study of 612 patients with gram-negative bacteremia, 10% had evidence of disseminated intravascular coagulation (DIC) (162). Use of fresh frozen plasma, whole blood, platelets, or cryoprecipitate is often necessary to restore clotting function until the underlying infection can be eliminated.

Other problems that require attention include fever control, acid-base disturbances, declining renal function, and nutritional support.

PULMONARY EDEMA

Pathophysiology

The basic problem in pulmonary edema, regardless of etiology, is an increase in extravascular fluid in the interstitium or alveoli of the lung. Normally, the small amount of fluid which moves from the pulmonary capillaries into the interstitial space is drained via the lymphatic system (163). If filtration of fluid into the interstitium exceeds the capability of the lymphatics to remove it, excess fluid accumulates first in the interstitium and eventually in the alveoli and alveolar ducts. Ultimately, pulmonary surfactant is inactivated, alveoli collapse (congestive atelectasis), and perfusion of these alveoli which are unable to participate in gas exchange results in hypoxemia.

Fluid movement across capillary membranes is regulated by opposing hydrostatic and oncotic pressures in the pulmonary capillaries and interstitium.

There are essentially two kinds of edema: Edema due to increased filtration pressure (P) resulting from either elevated capillary hydrostatic pressure (cardiogenic) or decreased protein oncotic pressure and edema due to increased capillary permeability (non-cardiogenic). Depending on the state of the pulmonary vascular bed and integrity of the capillary endothelium, interstitial fluid begins to accumulate when the pulmonary venous pressure exceeds 25 mm Hg, such as in the variety of clinical conditions listed in Table 6. The higher the pressure, the more rapid the accumulation of fluid. Pulmonary capillary pressure may be estimated by the pulmonary venous or wedge pressure (31).

Adult respiratory distress syndrome (ARDS) is one of several synonyms used to describe a clinical syndrome characterized by severe respiratory distress, tachypnea, refractory hypoxemia, diffuse alveolar and interstitial infiltrates on radiography, and decreased lung compliance. Other terms used to describe this condition include shock lung, primary pulmonary edema, non-cardiogenic pulmonary edema, adult hyaline membrane disease, and wet lung.

Although a variety of clinical conditions have been associated with the development of ARDS (Table 6), the primary physiologic and morphologic defect appears to be a diffuse metabolic malfunction of the alveolar capillary membrane. This most commonly involves the endothelial-interstitial complex, resulting in increased capillary permeability (capillary leak) to water and protein. Fluid moves into the interstitial space, causing swelling of the interstitia. This reduces the lung volume at which alveolar distensibility becomes limited, resulting in an acute restrictive process and decreased pulmonary compliance. Regional lung units are underventilated (ventilation-perfusion mismatch) and arterial hypoxemia develops. Eventually there is destruction of the alveolar epithelium with leakage of fluid into the alveolar space. Damaged alveolar epithelial cells result in a malfunctioning surfactant system with alveolar collapse, loss of residual volume, and increasing intrapulmonary shunting leading to further lowering of the arterial oxygen tension (refractory hypoxemia). In contrast to cardiogenic pulmonary edema, pulmonary capillary hydrostatic pressure is usually normal. The capillary-interstitial oncotic gradient is lost as protein moves from the intravascular to the interstitial space. As protein osmotic pressure decreases, the force opposing capillary hydrostatic pressure also declines and fluid moves across the capillary membrane. One of the hallmarks of ARDS is pulmonary edema with a normal PCWP. In both cardiogenic and noncardiogenic pulmonary edema, the hydrostatic pressure forces fluid from the pulmonary capillaries into the interstitial and intra-alveolar spaces.

Treatment

All drugs used in the treatment of pulmonary edema decrease left ventricular diastolic pressure by affecting one of three variables: 1) *increasing myocardial contractility,* thereby shifting to a new ventricular function curve that allows an increased stroke volume at lower filling pressures; 2) *afterload reduction,* allowing more effective ventricular ejection; and 3) *preload reduction,* allowing decreased venous return.

Ventilatory Support. Placing the patient in an upright sitting position will decrease the work of breathing and increase vital capacity (164). In

Table 6.

CAUSES OF PULMONARY EDEMA

Increased Filtration Pressure	Increased Permeability
Hypoproteinemia	Infection
Nephrosis	Gram-negative sepsis
Hepatic disease	Viral pneumonia
	Cytomegalovirus
Left ventricular failure	
Mitral stenosis	Trauma
Myocardial infarction	Fat emboli
Arrhythmias	Lung contusion
Volume overload	Nonthoracic trauma
Hypertension	Head injury
	Aspiration
	Gastric
	Fresh and salt water
	Hydrocarbons
	Drug Overdose
	Narcotics
	Barbiturates
	Inhaled Toxins
	Oxygen
	Smoke
	Phosgene

addition, the upright position will help reduce pulmonary congestion by decreasing venous return, which in turn lowers pulmonary blood volume. Oxygen therapy will raise hemoglobin saturation and help prevent tissue hypoxia. Delivery by mask or nasal cannula usually provides adequate amounts of oxygen, and flow is increased until the patient's pO_2 is maintained above 60 mm Hg. In severe respiratory depression, intubation with mechanical ventilation may be necessary.

Narcotics. *Morphine* has been used to treat cardiogenic pulmonary edema for many years and is especially useful in patients with concomitant pain due to MI or who are severely agitated. Traditionally, the beneficial effects of morphine have been attributed to systemic venodilation with pooling of blood in the peripheral capacitance bed (165,166). Recent studies have failed to show changes in PCWP or peripheral venous pooling of a magnitude which would relieve pulmonary edema (167,168), suggesting that other mechanisms may account for the observed beneficial effects. Through its narcotic action, morphine calms patients in distress, reduces the work of breath-

ing and perhaps, through a central mechanism of action, decreases sympathetic outflow affecting vascular tone. Generally, opioids cause a decrease in arterial pressure when given intravenously. This hypotensive action results from a peripheral vasodilation in part due to histamine release (169) and a reduction in sympathetic nervous system activity.

Recent studies evaluating narcotic-induced hemodynamics in patients with acute pulmonary edema (168), acute myocardial infarction (167), and coronary artery disease (170) have failed to show significant changes in heart rate, O_2 consumption, cardiac index, or stroke volume, although morphine decreases these parameters slightly. Pulmonary capillary wedge pressure remains unchanged with morphine and meperidine.

Meperidine is structurally dissimilar to morphine and is not cross allergenic. It also possesses the same favorable hemodynamic profile. For these reasons, meperidine would be the drug of choice in morphine-allergic cardiac patients.

Diuretics. *Furosemide* is frequently used in acute pulmonary edema to reduce pulmonary capillary pressure. This reduction in PCWP is usually accompanied by little if any change in cardiac output or heart rate (119,171), a desirable feature in patients with compromised coronary circulation. Patients usually respond within minutes of an intravenous injection, before any significant diuresis occurs. The initial reduction in the PCWP is due to an increase in venous capacitance rather than diuresis which accounts for the later (after about one hour) secondary fall in capillary pressure (120).

The dose used to treat pulmonary edema varies and in part depends on the degree of renal blood flow. If renal blood flow is decreased, a larger dose will be needed to achieve a diuretic response. Some authors recommend an initial dose of 40 mg IV in patients with good renal function who have not received previous diuretic therapy (172). Larger doses (60–80 mg) are used in patients currently receiving diuretics. Other authors have used starting doses of 0.5 to 1 mg/kg (120,173). A decrease in PCWP is usually observed within 5–15 minutes, and diuresis occurs 2–30 minutes after IV injection.

Vasodilators. Vasodilators rapidly improve pulmonary edema by decreasing preload, afterload, or both.

Nitroprusside lowers systemic vascular resistance (afterload) and increases venous capacitance (preload) (174). The combined effects reduce pulmonary capillary pressure and usually elevate cardiac output. Nitroprusside also reduces myocardial oxygen demand in ischemic heart disease (125). However, some authors have suggested that it may shift perfusion from ischemic to normal myocardium and is potentially harmful (132). Still other studies indicate a beneficial effect on ischemic myocardium (175,176). Nevertheless, nitroprusside is remarkably effective in reducing pulmonary edema, especially in patients with coexistent systemic hypertension. The disadvantages of this agent are that it must be given as an intravenous infusion, thus requiring infusion pumps and, preferably, hemodynamic monitoring.

The dose varies depending on the clinical circumstances and is adjusted to achieve an optimal reduction in PCWP (15–18 mm Hg) while elevating the CO and maintaining arterial pressures between 90–100 mm Hg. Patients with arterial hypotension may also benefit from nitroprusside. Chatterjee et al (125) have shown that the response to vasodilators is determined by the infusion rate and follows a three step progression. Low doses increase CO, decrease the PCWP, and have little effect on the arterial pressure. With increasing doses, there is a further increase in the CO and a reduction of the PCWP, but with a concomitant fall in arterial pressure. Higher infusion rates eventually result in profound vasodilation leading to reduction in CO, PCWP, and arterial pressure. A reasonable approach is to start with a low dose of 10–20 mcg/min and increase it by increments of 5 mcg/min every 5 minutes until optimal hemodynamics are achieved or the systemic arterial pressure falls below 90 mm Hg.

Nitroglycerin rapidly reduces the PCWP, predominantly by its effect on preload. Reduction in preload is a result of increased venous capacitance (174), leading to marked diminution of left-ventricular filling pressures and a reduction in ventricular volume and work. Nitroglycerin also reduces afterload by dilating arterioles (177), but this effect is less prominent than the venodilation and is accompanied by minimal augmentation of CO, especially in comparison to nitroprusside. Improvement in perfusion of ischemic myocardium (178) and increases in coronary collateral flow (179) also are associated with nitroglycerin therapy. In hypotensive patients, administration of nitroglycerin may be detrimental because further reduction in coronary perfusion pressure can enhance myocardial ischemia.

Both intravenous and sublingual routes of nitroglycerin administration can be used to treat acute pulmonary edema (127,180). Disadvantages of the oral route include erratic buccal absorption, which in some cases can lead to a marked reduction in arterial pressure. In addition, excessive reductions in preload may reduce cardiac output (128). A commercially available intravenous preparation (Tridil) has recently been marketed in the concentration of 5 mg/ml. The drug must be diluted in either 5% dextrose in water or 0.9% sodium chloride for injection prior to administration. An infusion containing 200 mcg/ml may be prepared by adding 1 ampule (50 mg) to 250 ml or 2 ampules to 500 ml of diluent. Polyvinylchloride containers and infusion sets should be avoided because of the problem of absorption of nitroglycerin into the plastic. Dosages used to treat pulmonary edema have ranged from 0.8 mg to 2.4 mg sublingually, and 10 to 200 mcg/min intravenously. The onset of action begins within minutes after sublingual or intravenous administration. The duration of action is approximately one hour after sublingual administration and about forty minutes after intravenous administration. As with most drugs, a reasonable approach to therapy is to start with low doses and to increase the dose slowly to achieve optimal hemodynamic effects.

Phentolamine, a pure alpha-adrenergic blocking agent, has also been used to decrease left ventricular filling pressure. Beneficial effects result from direct vascular smooth muscle relaxation, resulting in decreases in preload and afterload. However, phentolamine reduces afterload more than preload because it predominantly affects resistance vessels. In patients with left ventricular dysfunction, phentolamine increases the ejection fraction and cardiac output and decreases left ventricular filling pressure (181). Tachycardia and hypotension may complicate therapy, especially when larger doses are employed. The average dose used in cardiac failure is 0.75 mg/min (range 0.1 to 3 mg/min).

Inotropic Agents. Inotropic agents are useful in managing pulmonary edema especially when cardiac output is too low to maintain peripheral perfusion.

Digitalis gylcosides are helpful in the management of mild congestive heart failure. They are particularly useful in patients whose pulmonary edema is secondary to mitral stenosis accompanied by atrial fibrillation or other supraventricular tachycardias with fast ventricular rates in which shortened diastolic filling times have caused increased left atrial pressure (182). The use of digitalis glycosides in acute cardiogenic pulmonary edema is limited by: a) relative lack of efficiency in this situation (72,183); b) potentiation of their toxicity by hypoxemia (184); c) their potential for increasing myocardial ischemia (185).

Dopamine and *dobutamine* are the drugs of choice when an inotropic agent is indicated. Although equally effective in increasing cardiac output, dobutamine produces a greater reduction of pulmonary capillary pressure compared to dopamine for a similar improvement in cardiac output (186). Cardiac irritability and the propensity for arrhythmia production may be less with dobutamine. Dobutamine is less chronotropic than dopamine, making it particularly useful in the setting of acute myocardial infarction.

Theophylline compounds have been advocated

for use in pulmonary edema primarily when there is a significant bronchospastic component. Beneficial effects have been attributed to the drug's mild inotropic, diuretic, and venodilation properties. However, use of the drug is limited by its propensity for inducing supraventricular tachyarrhythmias and its chronotropic action, which increase myocardial oxygen demand.

Cardiogenic Pulmonary Edema

48. M.B. is a 65-year-old male who comes to the emergency room with severe shortness of breath and a productive cough. Earlier in the evening he had severe substernal chest pain lasting two hours which was not relieved by nitroglycerin.

His past history is significant for an acute inferior myocardial infarction two years prior to admission, a coronary artery bypass graft two years prior to admission, and a history of hypertension for the past ten years treated with Lasix 40 mg bid. He is allergic to morphine.

Physical examination reveals a well-nourished white male looking older than his stated age in severe respiratory distress with a cough productive of pink frothy sputum. On cardiac examination there were no murmurs, but a S_3 gallop was present. The pulse was 110 beats/minute, rapid, and thready. Neck veins were distended, but there was no organomegaly or peripheral edema. On chest examination there were bilateral wet rales extending one-third of the way up the chest. The skin was cool and moist, and the lower extremities were cyanotic. Vital signs were as follows: temperature 100.1°F; respiratory rate 30/minute; pulse 110 beats/minute; blood pressure (supine) 100/60 mm Hg. Laboratory results on admission disclosed the following: arterial blood gases pO_2 55, pCO_2 48, pH 7.30. Chest x-ray showed prominent vascular markings especially in the upper lobes, Kerley B lines (engorged interlobular septae), and diffuse alveolar infiltrates. The heart was markedly enlarged.

What kind of pulmonary edema does this patient most likely have and what subjective and objective data support it?

This patient has pulmonary edema which is cardiac in origin. Subjectively, the patient presents complaining of SOB which results from inadequate gas exchange due to fluid filling the alveoli. In addition, the presence of severe substernal chest pain and the patient's past medical history of having had an MI with subsequent bypass surgery suggest an already compromised left ventricle further compromised by an evolving acute MI. The 10-year history of hypertension puts the patient at risk of developing CHF and adds additional support for the diagnosis of a cardiogenic origin.

Objectively, the data also support cardiogenic pulmonary edema. The chest x-ray shows an enlarged heart characteristic of CHF. As the left ventricle fails and becomes dilated, the pulmonary capillary pressure rises, dilating the blood vessels and favoring fluid movement into the interstitium and alveoli (vascular markings, Kerley B lines, alveolar infiltrates, bilateral wet rales). The inability of the fluid filled alveoli to exchange gas efficiently results in hypoxemia ($pO_2 = 55$) and hypercapnia ($pCO_2 = 48$) with the resulting respiratory acidosis ($pH = 7.3$). In contrast to the previously held notion that patients with acute pulmonary edema secondary to left ventricular failure have respiratory alkalosis and no metabolic abnormality, new data suggest that a large percentage of patients have a combined respiratory and metabolic acidosis (187,188). Physiologically, the body tries to maintain homeostasis by: a) increasing respirations ($R = 30$) in an attempt to improve oxygenation and remove CO_2 and b) improve tissue perfusion by increasing CO through elevation of heart rate (pulse = 110, rapid and thready) and contractility.

49. Since this patient was allergic to morphine, pentazocine (Talwin) was ordered. Was this a reasonable alternative?

Unlike morphine and meperidine, pentazocine significantly increases the pulmonary capillary wedge, systolic, and diastolic pressures. Aortic pressures (systolic and diastolic) increase significantly when pentazocine is infused and remain unchanged or slightly decreased when morphine or meperidine are infused. In addition, echocardiographic analysis of left ventricular function in patients receiving pentazocine (167), as well as animal data (189), suggest the drug has marked negative inotropic properties. This is not found with morphine or meperidine.

The use of pentazocine as an alternative drug

in this patient is inappropriate for several reasons. First, by increasing systemic blood pressure, pulmonary artery pressure, and left ventricular filling pressure, both preload and afterload are increased, enhancing myocardial oxygen demand. This patient has an acute MI and compromised coronary circulation, indicating imbalance between myocardial oxygen requirements and delivery. Augmentation of O_2 demand will exacerbate myocardial ischemia and extend necrosis. Second, this patient's left ventricle is already compromised from his heart disease. Further depression of an already failing ventricle will make his CHF worse and increase pulmonary edema. Third, increasing the left ventricular and capillary wedge pressures increases capillary hydrostatic pressure, forcing more fluid out of the vascular compartment into the lung interstitium.

50. Should narcotics be administered to treat this patient's pulmonary edema?

Narcotic administration can be detrimental under some clinical circumstances. All narcotics possess respiratory depressant effects and when given in normal clinical doses decrease both tidal volume and respiratory rate (190). This may be particularly detrimental in patients with decreased respiratory reserve or who are hypoxic and hypercapnic (especially COPD). Although respiratory depression may be reversed with naloxone (Narcan), ventricular tachyarrhythmias (190) and arterial hypertension (191) have been reported after its use. Both situations are potentially harmful, especially in patients with myocardial infarction where the balance between myocardial oxygen demand and supply is already inadequate (see the chapter on Acute Myocardial Infarction).

Administration of narcotics to patients with myocardial infarction has been associated with unpredictable effects on heart rate and blood pressure (193). Similarly, patients who are hypovolemic or hypoxemic may have a profound hypotensive response when given opioids (194,195). Although patients with pulmonary edema are generally not fluid depleted, patients whose pulmonary edema was complicated by hypovolemia have been reported (196).

This patient presents in acute pulmonary edema secondary to a myocardial infarction. Blood gas analysis shows the patient to be hypoxic and hypercapnic. Although respiratory depression is a concern, judicious use of morphine in combination with oxygen in patients with pulmonary edema and elevated pCO_2 usually does not lead to impaired oxygenation (187). Therefore, hypercapnia per se is not an absolute contraindication to opiate use. More significantly, this patient is hypotensive (BP = 100/60 mm Hg) and hypoxic, both of which weigh in favor of avoiding narcotics. In addition, our patient is not severely agitated or having chest pain. Thus, the need for narcotics can be questioned. In view of the above considerations and the availability of other potentially less dangerous drugs known to be effective in the treatment of pulmonary edema, it would be appropriate not to administer narcotics to this patient.

51. M.B. was immediately transferred to the intensive care unit where a Swan-Ganz catheter was inserted for hemodynamic monitoring. Physical examination at this time showed the patient to be in respiratory distress. Lung examination again revealed bilateral wet rales with diffuse scattered wheezes bilaterally. Extremities are now warm with no evidence of cyanosis. The patient is receiving oxygen 6 L/min by nasal cannula. Urine output is 5 ml/hr. PCWP 35 mm Hg, CI 2.7 L/min, Na 141 mEq/L, K 4.2 mEq/L, Cl 98 mEq/L, pH 7.3, PO_2 55, PCO_2 48 on room air. What are the goals of therapy for this patient?

This man is in severe respiratory distress, has a markedly elevated pulmonary capillary pressure and is hypotensive. Goals of treatment are to a) acutely improve ventilation and correct the altered arterial blood gases, reduce the elevated capillary wedge pressure, and improve tissue perfusion by enhancing cardiac output and contractility; b) second, attention should be directed towards identifying any precipitating factors (for example, acute MI, tachyarrhythmias, fluid overloading, infection, pulmonary embolism, thyrotoxicosis, severe anemia and instituting treatment if possible; c) third, direct attention to any underlying conditions not already clear and correct them if possible (eg, valvular insufficiency).

52. Which drug(s) should be used to treat this patient's pulmonary edema?

The choice of therapy must be tailored to the individual clinical situation and should be made after considering the severity of the pulmonary edema, nature of the underlying disease, and presence or absence of tissue hypoperfusion. Hemodynamic monitoring is useful in assessment of patients and monitoring drug therapy.

Generally, patients may be placed into one of two general categories: those with peripheral hypoperfusion and those without. In cases without hypoperfusion (low cardiac index), rapid reduction of pulmonary capillary pressure can be achieved with a wide margin of safety by employing diuretic agents such as furosemide. Vasodilator drugs such as nitrates or nitroprusside are also useful, especially in patients with elevated arterial pressure. In patients with hypoperfusion, the goal is not only to reduce pulmonary capillary pressure but also to increase cardiac output. In this circumstance, drugs which reduce afterload, such as nitroprusside or phentolamine, may be useful providing that arterial pressure can be maintained at a level of 90 mm Hg or greater. In the situation where arterial pressure drops below this value, inotropic agents are used either alone or in combination with a vasodilator.

Upon admission to the intensive care unit M.B. had an elevated pulmonary capillary wedge pressure (35 mm Hg) and a marginally depressed cardiac index (2.7 L/min). His blood pressure was low but stable. Diuretics would be expected to rapidly relieve pulmonary congestion by lowering the capillary pressure and would produce little if any change in cardiac output. Furosemide is readily available in the ICU, requires no preparation, and is easily administered intravenously. This patient's cardiac index is depressed, but not to the point of severely compromising peripheral perfusion which would favor the use of an inotropic agent such as dobutamine or dopamine. Nitroprusside will lower the PCWP, rapidly relieving pulmonary congestion and perhaps enhance cardiac output. However, in view of the fact that this patient's blood pressure is already low, cardiac output is not severely depressed and is stable, and peripheral perfusion is adequate, the administration of a drug requiring special preparation, infusion pumps, and close monitoring to titrate the dose may be withheld in favor of other agents which are effective and easy to administer. Phentolamine would be potentially harmful because of the existing hypotension and compromised coronary blood flow. Similarly, aminophylline, with its positive chronotropic effects, may have deleterious effects in this patient with coronary artery insufficiency. Nitrates are potentially useful.

Again, the patient has existing hypotension which could be exacerbated. Oral nitrates are easily administered, but erratic absorption and unpredictable effects make them somewhat of a problem to use. Furosemide is a reasonable choice for initial therapy of this patient because of the expected favorable response and the ease with which the drug may be administered. Furosemide 40 mg IV should be given; if there is no response, the dose should be increased or the use of other agents should be entertained.

53. Thirty minutes after the administration of furosemide, no response was observed. What other therapeutic interventions may be appropriate?

Failure to respond to furosemide is not uncommon with the first dose, especially if the patient has previously been receiving the drug. Clinically, one tends to use larger initial doses in patients who have been on chronic diuretic therapy or who appear to be in severe respiratory distress. If a response (eg, as manifested by clinical improvement in shortness of breath or urine output) is not observed, it is common practice to double the dose. If a response is still not observed, one can administer additional furosemide, add an additional diuretic such as metolazone or mannitol to potentiate the action of furosemide, or administer vasodilators. In our experience, the addition of metolazone in a dose of 5 to 10 mg produces a diuretic response within thirty minutes in patients previously unresponsive to furosemide alone. This synergistic effect has been suggested by several authors (197) and may in part be related to matolazone's ability to block proximal tubular sodium reabsorption (198).

DIABETIC KETOACIDOSIS

54. J.L. is a 25-year-old, 60 kg, female, insulin-dependent diabetic on 24 units NPH plus 10 units of regular insulin every morning, who presents to the Emergency Room (E.R.) complaining of abdominal tenderness, nausea, and vomiting. According to her family, J.L. was feeling well until last evening when she awoke with nausea, vomiting, diarrhea, and chills. She continued to have nausea and did not eat breakfast. Since she had not eaten, she omitted her usual morning insulin dose.

There was no improvement, and the nausea, diarrhea, and vomiting continued. The patient became lethargic and was brought to the E.R.

Past medical history includes an eight-year history of insulin-dependent diabetes which was first diagnosed at age 17.

Physical examination reveals an ill-appearing female who is lethargic but responsive. Examination of the head, eyes, ears, nose, and throat (HEENT) is within normal limits, although the mucous membranes are dry. The lungs are clear; respirations are deep; inspirations are labored; and a fruity odor is noticeable on her breath. Cardiac examination reveals a regular rhythm with no gallops and a grade 2/6 mid-systolic murmur at the left lateral sternal border. In the supine position, the pulse rate is 115 beats/minute and the blood pressure is 105/60 mm Hg. In the upright position, the pulse increased to 140 beats/minute and the blood pressure dropped to 85/40 mm Hg. The respiratory rate is 20/minute. On abdominal examination there are some increased bowel sounds and some mild diffuse tenderness. Examination of her extremities reveals no clubbing, cyanosis, or edema.

Laboratory results on admission at approximately 4 A.M. disclosed the following: blood glucose 750 mg/dl; Na 148 mEq/L; K 5.4 mEq/L; Cl 106 mEq/L; HCO_3 3 mEq/L; creatinine 2.0 mg/dl; hemoglobin 14.7 gm/dl; hematocrit 49%; WBC 7.9 x 10^3 with 3% bands, 70% polys, and 27% lymphs; serum ketones were moderate at 1:10 dilution. The urinalysis showed 2% glucose, moderate ketones, pH 5.5, specific gravity 1.029, WBC 0–3/hpf, RBC 0–3, no bacteria, and no casts. The arterial blood gas results were as follows: pH 7.05, pCO_2 20, pO_2 120.

This patient was diagnosed as having acute diabetic ketoacidosis (DKA) and transferred to the ICU for treatment. What supports the diagnosis of DKA in this patient?

The fact that J.L. is an insulin-dependent diabetic puts her at risk for developing ketoacidosis. Absolute or relative insulin deficiency promotes lipolysis in peripheral tissues, elevating free fatty acids which are converted to β-hydroxybutyrate, acetoacetic acid, and acetone in the liver. Primary factors responsible for the acidosis are a lack of insulin and an excess of glucagon which

enhances liver ketogenesis and impairs peripheral ketone utilization (199,200). Although this
process is prevented by insulin administration,
this patient falsely assumed that her morning dose
should be omitted, thereby favoring the development of ketoacidosis.

Stress of any nature may contribute to the development of DKA by stimulating release of insulin counter-regulatory hormones such as glucagon, catecholamines, glucocorticoids, and growth
hormone. Exactly how these agents favor a ke-
toacidotic state is controversial but has been extensively reviewed by Schade and co-workers (201).
Common stress factors include infection, pregnancy, pancreatitis, trauma, hyperthyroidism, and
acute M.I. This patient presented with symptoms
of nausea, vomiting, diarrhea, and chills suggestive of an acute viral gastroenteritis.

Patients with DKA generally have moderate
to high serum glucose levels (BG 750 mg/dl) caused
by decreased peripheral utilization and increased
production (gluconeogenesis). Consequently, serum
osmolality increases, shifting fluid from the intracellular to the intravascular compartment.
Glomerular filtration of glucose is increased, exceeding its tubular rate of reabsorption and resulting in excessive urinary losses of glucose,
water, sodium, and potassium (urine 2% glucose).
In addition, fluid and electrolyte losses are also
enhanced in this patient because of vomiting and
diarrhea. Eventually, as losses exceed input, the
patient becomes dehydrated (dry mucous membranes) and intravascular volume decreases (increased hematocrit secondary to hemoconcentration). Confirmatory evidence of this is suggested
by the presence of orthostatic changes in blood
pressure (105/60 mm Hg supine changes to 85/45
mm Hg upright) and heart rate (115 beats/min
supine changes to 140 beats/min upright). In an
effort to maintain declining arterial pressure,
cardiac output is increased by elevation of heart
rate (pulse 115 beats/min).

Objective evidence of excessive ketone production includes moderate amounts of urine ketones,
positive plasma ketones at 1:10 dilution, and the
characteristic fruity odor of acetone on the breath.
As plasma levels of these organic acids rise, normal body buffers and compensatory respiratory
mechanisms are overwhelmed. Serum pH (7.05)
and bicarbonate levels (HCO_3 3 mEq/L) drop and
the respiratory rate is increased, leading to hypocapnia (pCO_2 20) in an effort to compensate for
the metabolic acidosis.

**55. Treatment of DKA is aimed at revers-
ing altered tissue metabolism, replacement of
fluid and electrolyte losses, and removal of
any concurrent aggravating conditions. How
should fluid and electrolyte replacement be
managed in this patient?**

Patients presenting with DKA have significant fluid losses. Depending on the relative water
to solute loss, volume contraction can be isotonic,
hypotonic, or hypertonic, with serum sodium values being normal, low, or elevated. The usual fluid
deficit approximates 6 to 10 L, or 10% of body
weight (202). The loss of total body sodium (not
represented by serum sodium) can be extensive
due to glucose-induced osmotic diuresis and insulin deficiency (203). Human studies examining
insulin's role in renal excretion of electrolytes
suggest it increases sodium reabsorption at the
level of the diluting segment in the ascending
loop of Henle (206). Therefore, lack of insulin would
favor enhanced sodium excretion. Total body sodium is usually depleted by 7 to 10 mEq/kg of
body weight (204,205). A point to remember when
assessing serum sodium is that false low values
may be reported as a result of hyperglycemia and
hypertriglyceridemia. A corrected value may be
obtained by adding 1.6–2 mEq/L to the observed
value for every 100 mg/dl above 200 mg/dl serum
glucose (206,207) (see Fluid and Electrolyte Disorders chapter).

The choice of fluid for initial treatment has
been controversial. Some authors recommend hypotonic saline on the basis that water loss is relatively greater than that of salt as a consequence
of osmotic diuresis (202). Other clinicians favor
isotonic saline for several reasons. First, since patients generally have a pronounced fluid deficit,
protecting intravascular volume and preventing
shock is a consideration. Fluid movement out of
the intravascular space may accompany the use
of hypotonic fluids, and the treatment of hyperglycemia decreases osmolality and further compromises circulating blood volume. Isotonic saline, by remaining intravascularly, would be
expected to maintain blood volume. Second, development of cerebral edema during treatment,
albeit rare, is a severe and often fatal consequence (208). In the face of sustained hyperglycemia, the brain is able to produce intracellular
osmotically active substances to restore cellular
hydration to normal. Although originally thought
to be sorbitol, the identity of these substances
remains obscure (209,210), and their role in the

development of cerebral edema is also unclear. One possibility is that rapid reduction in serum glucose widens the CSF/plasma osmotic gradient, causing fluid to move intracellularly and resulting in edema. Patients with significant hyponatremia may be at particular risk. Rapid lowering of glucose in these patients, coupled with inadequate restoration of serum sodium, may actually produce hypo-osmolar serum and hence intracellular fluid movement (211). At present, most clinicians agree that normal saline is the initial fluid of choice (204,205,208).

This patient has evidence of significant fluid loss (dry mucous membranes, orthostatic drop in blood pressure, elevated heart rate). A rough calculation (10% times 70 kg = 7 L) indicates that approximately seven liters of fluid will be needed. Rapid infusion of one liter of normal saline over 30 to 60 minutes is appropriate. If blood pressure normalizes, a second liter of saline should be infused over the next 2 hours. When blood pressure and serum sodium are normal, fluids can be switched to hypotonic half-normal saline at a rate of 300–350 ml/hr. When the serum glucose approaches 300 mg/dl, solutions should be changed to D5½NS to prevent a too rapid reduction in plasma osmolality and hypoglycemia. The use of a D5½NS solution also allows for continued insulin administration which is required for reduction of ketoacids and resolution of the acidosis. These fluid recommendations apply to adolescents and adults with previously normal renal and myocardial function. In the elderly or those with compromised renal or myocardial function, fluid administration should be titrated against central venous pressure.

56. What role do potassium and phosphate have in treatment of DKA and how should they be administered to this patient?

Potassium. Potassium balance is markedly altered in DKA because of combined urinary and gastrointestinal losses. Invariably, total body potassium is depleted; however, the serum potassium concentration may be high, normal, or low depending on the degree of acidosis and volume contraction (212). Usual potassium deficits in this situation average 3–5 mEq/kg of body weight (204,211). Thus, this patient will need approximately 200–350 mEq of potassium to replenish stores. In patients whose initial serum potassium concentrations are elevated, supplementation is withheld for the first hour or until serum levels

begin to drop to avoid hyperkalemia. However, low serum potassium in the face of pronounced acidosis suggests severe potassium depletion requiring early aggressive therapy to prevent life-threatening hypokalemia during treatment (from dilution, urinary losses, correction of acidosis, and insulin-mediated cellular uptake). In those cases, initial intravenous solutions should contain from 20–60 mEq of supplemental potassium.

Admission laboratory data reveal a slightly elevated serum creatinine, suggesting compromised renal function (most likely pre-renal azotemia). This in conjunction with a high normal serum potassium concentration weighs in favor of withholding supplementation until serum levels begin to decline and urine output increases. Potassium levels generally begin to decrease in 1–2 hours, but bicarbonate therapy may facilitate a more rapid decline. If repeat determinations indicate that the serum potassium concentration is decreasing, 20–40 mEq may be added to the intravenous infusion.

Phosphorus. The use of phosphorus in treating DKA has received much attention in the past few years. Phosphate is lost during the development of hyperglycemia and ketoacidosis as a result of increased tissue catabolism, impaired cellular uptake, and enhanced renal excretion (211). Although body stores may be depleted, serum levels may initially appear normal (204). As treatment continues, phosphate serum concentrations may drop rapidly to concentrations of 1 mg/100 ml or less (213,214). The consequences of profound hypophosphatemia include decreased cardiac output, hemolysis, altered mental status, and tissue hypoxia (215,216). Most attention has focused on phosphorus deficiency leading to decreased erythrocyte 2,3-DPG concentrations and the consequences of altered hemoglobin affinity for oxygen. Lowered erythrocyte 2,3-DPG levels shift the oxygen-hemoglobin dissociation curve to the left, thereby increasing the affinity of hemoglobin for oxygen and decreasing oxygen delivery to tissues. Although definitive data on the role of phosphorus therapy in DKA are lacking, animal data suggest that its deficiency produces a state of insulin deficiency (185). It is reasonable, in view of the theoretical benefits, to provide part of the potassium replacement as the phosphate salt. For this patient, administration of 20 mEq K_2HPO_4 for three doses is appropriate.

Overzealous phosphate replacement has resulted in several reports of hypomagnesemia and hypocalcemia (218,219). In all of these cases, potassium was replenished entirely as the phosphate salt. The available preparation of potassium phosphate contains 66 mEq of potassium and phosphorus per vial (15 cc). Using this preparation for replacing the potassium deficit (200–350 mEq for our patient) would result in administration of large amounts of PO_4. The amount of phosphate which should be administered has not been clearly established. Some authors recommend about 65–130 mEq of phosphorous for patients with severe DKA (220,221). Our approach is to add one half the potassium replacement as the phosphate salt for a total dose of 60 mEq PO_4. Subsequent phosphate in our experience is rarely required but may be administered based upon serum phosphate determinations.

57. In view of this patient's acidosis (pH = 7.05, HCO_3^- = 3) should bicarbonate be administered, and if so, how much?

Sodium Bicarbonate. The use of sodium bicarbonate in diabetic ketoacidosis has been controversial. Most investigators discourage its routine use (204,205), reserving it for patients with severe acidemia or those in clinical shock. Severe acidosis per se can be life-threatening through its deleterious effects on vascular tone (vascular collapse and shock). Additionally, acidemia may contribute to insulin resistance. On the other hand, overly aggressive use of alkali is to be discouraged because the majority of patients recover without it, and because there are several undesirable features of sodium bicarbonate. Some real and some theoretical disadvantages of sodium bicarbonate are listed in Table 7. Furthermore, bicarbonate administration can mask continuing acidosis and remove the serum bicarbonate as an index of recovery.

Most clinicians agree that bicarbonate administration is probably justified if the serum pH is 7.1 or below. A general guideline is to administer 1 ampule (45.5 mEq) of bicarbonate if the pH is between 7.0 and 7.1. If the pH is below 7.0, two to three ampules may be administered.

This patient's acidosis is fairly severe, judging by the serum pH of 7.05, bicarbonate of 3 (normal 26), and the presence of Kussmaul respirations (rapid deep breathing). Therefore, administration of 1 ampule sodium bicarbonate either by infusion or by IV push is appropriate. If bicarbonate is to be added to the IV fluids, ½NS should be used to prevent administration of hyperosmolar

fluids. Additional bicarbonate is administered only if a repeat pH remains below 7.1.

58. The major treatment modality for diabetic ketoacidosis is insulin administration. What would be an appropriate insulin dosage and route of administration for this patient?

The appropriate dose of insulin in the management of DKA has been the topic of considerable debate in the past decade. Treatment of this disorder has traditionally been with relatively large insulin doses of 50–200 U every 2–4 hours. These doses were presumably required because of the phenomenon of "insulin resistance." Only in the past ten years have data been gathered suggesting that lower doses can be used with equal efficacy and possibly less morbidity. In the early 1970's, small doses of insulin were administered either by continuous intravenous infusion or intramuscularly to treat diabetic ketoacidosis (222–225). Alberti et al (222) showed good results using initial intramuscular injections of 10–20 U/hour of regular insulin followed by additional injections of 10 U/hour. Similar results were reported in subsequent studies (225–228). Low dose intravenous insulin also was successful in the treatment of diabetic ketoacidosis and even lower loading doses (2–12 U) were used (223–22).

Table 7.

HAZARDS ASSOCIATED WITH EXCESS BICARBONATE ADMINISTRATION

1. Alkalosis with increasing insulin resistence

2. Cardiac arrhythmias associated with hypokalemia

3. Paradoxical CNS acidosis; diffusion of bicarbonate across blood-brain-barrier is slow; rapid increase in serum pH depresses respiratory center resulting in hypoventilation and increases CO_2 which diffuses rapidly into the CSF causing CNS acidosis.

4. Tetany: increased binding of free Ca^{++} to albumin resulting in low free serum Ca^{++}

5. Shift of the oxygen-hemoglobin dissociation curve to the left reducing oxygen availability to tissues.

6. Severe hypokalemia resulting from increased renal loss because of enhanced potassium/hydrogen exchange in the renal tubule and movement of potassium into cells previously blocked by the acidosis.

Despite differences in study design, similar observations were noted by all investigators studying the low dose insulin regimen. Serum glucose declines at a fairly constant rate of approximately 75 to 100 mg/dl/hr, and large insulin doses do not cause a more rapid decline. Correction of the acidosis lags behind that of serum glucose, usually by several hours. Low dose intravenous and intramuscular regimens appear to be equally effective in resolution of hyperglycemia and acidosis. Low dose regimens are associated with considerably less hypoglycemia and hypokalemia than regimens which use large doses of insulin.

Although some clinicians opposed low dose insulin therapy on the grounds that few randomized, prospective trials comparing high and low dose regimens had been conducted (229), several comparative trials have shown low dose therapy to be equally as effective as large doses of insulin.

Ideally, the goal of insulin therapy is to provide peripheral target tissues with sufficient insulin to reverse the metabolic alterations which lead to hyperglycemia and ketosis. It is now fairly well established that insulin concentrations in the range of 20–200 mu/ml produce a maximal biological effect (234,235). Doses of 5–10 U/hr regular insulin intramuscularly are associated with levels ranging from 64 to 92 mu/ml (222,226). Other studies using average intravenous insulin doses of 2–7 mu/hr also produced plasma insulin concentrations comparable to the above (223, 225,234).

Continuous insulin infusion is usually preferred because intravenous delivery rapidly establishes effective blood insulin levels which can be maintained or altered almost instantaneously. It also avoids potential erratic absorption due to tissue deposits which might occur with subcutaneous or intramuscular injections, especially in patients who are severely volume depleted. An IV bolus of 0.1 U/kg can be given and is followed by an infusion of 0.1 U/kg/hr. Thus, for this patient a bolus of 6 U followed by infusion of 6 U/hr would be appropriate. The insulin infusion should be kept separate from the fluids being used to replace volume. An insulin concentration of 1 U/10 ml can be obtained by adding 50 U of regular insulin to 500 ml of normal saline. The administration rate can be adjusted to deliver the desired amount of insulin which may be piggybacked into the replacement fluid tubing. If the plasma glucose remains unchanged after two

hours, the infusion rate is doubled. The use of standard regimens simplifies management but should not lead to a false sense of security. Individualization of therapy and close monitoring of the patient are essential components of treatment.

59. Is the absorption of insulin onto intravenous bottles and infusion sets of clinical significance?

The magnitude of insulin adsorption to glassware and plastic tubing appears to vary with the concentration of insulin and the duration of the infusion and ranges from 20 to 70% (235–238). Although the addition of human serum albumin in a concentration of 1.25–3.5 mg/ml to the insulin mixtures decreases insulin adsorption to 5% or less (235,237), the high price of human serum albumin makes this approach unrealistic. Furthermore, insulin infusions without the addition of protein have resulted in significant insulin serum concentrations (223–225,234). Thus, the clinical significance of insulin adsorption is questionable. This problem can be minimized without the addition of protein by running 50 to 100 ml of a solution containing 5 U/100 ml or greater of insulin through the tubing before connecting it to the patient (237). Clinicians should be aware of the potential decrease in bioavailability and monitor the patient for the appropriate response.

60. This patient was treated with fluids, electrolytes, bicarbonate and insulin as discussed in previous questions. Laboratory and clinical data three hours after therapy were as follows: pH 7.17, blood glucose 505 mg/dl, K 3.8 mEq/L, HCO₃ 11 mEq/L, creatinine 3.1 mg/dl, and serum ketones strongly positive at 1:40. The BP was 120/70 mm Hg with no orthostatic changes. Urine output over the past three hours has been 500 ml. Comparing the above data to those obtained on admission, serum ketones have increased from moderate at 1:10 to strongly positive at 1:40. Should this patient receive more insulin in view of this increasing ketosis?

The assumption that ketosis is worse because of increased serum ketones is incorrect. In DKA, lack of insulin causes accelerated oxidation of fatty acids (generated from lipolysis), resulting in the formation of excess acetyl CoA and NADH. Acetyl CoA can be decarboxylated to acetone or undergo a reduction reaction with NADH, producing beta-hydroxybutyrate. Since the latter participates in an equilibrium reaction [Aceto-acetate + NADH + H $\rightleftharpoons$ betahydroxybutyrate + NAD], the excess NADH drives the reaction to the right, increasing the betahydroxybutyrate concentration. Therefore, betahydroxybutyrate may become the most abundant acid present in serum.

Quantitative tests for serum ketones are not routinely available in most hospitals. Therefore, qualitative tests using the nitroprusside reaction (Acetest tablet, Ketostix strip) are routinely used to measure ketones. Nitroprusside reacts with acetoacetate and acetone. (Acetone is only 1/20 as reactive as acetoacetate on a molar basis). It does not react with betahydroxybutyrate, the primary ketone; hence, serum ketones may be low when ketosis is most predominant. However, during treatment with insulin, lipolysis and fatty acid oxidation decrease, regenerating NAD and shifting the reaction back in favor of acetoacetate. The nitroprusside reaction may then show a stronger ketone reaction than recorded before treatment, as illustrated by this patient whose ketone test changed from 1:10 to 1:40. In view of the above data, increasing pH, declining blood sugar, and increasing HCO_3, this patient is responding appropriately and no change in insulin dosage is indicated.

61. Examination of the laboratory data on admission and in the previous question shows the serum creatinine rising from 2.0 mg/dl to 3.1 mg/dl. How do you interpret this change?

Creatinine elevation in patients with DKA is not uncommon and usually results from volume depletion-induced prerenal azotemia. As volume is replaced and urine output increases, the serum creatinine returns to normal. In this patient, however, the serum creatinine rose by 2 mg/dl despite the fact that volume replacement was adequate enough to restore urine output. This finding suggests that something other than volume is responsible for the elevated creatinine. Molitch et al (239) recently reported a false elevation of serum creatinine in DKA. Their patient displayed a serum creatinine of 3.2 mg/dl as measured by the automated Technicon method. When remeasured by a more specific manual method, the level was 1 mg/dl, suggesting the presence of a substance which interferes with the automated assay. Subsequent analysis of samples to which acetoacetate, betahydroxybutyrate, or both were added confirmed that acetoacetate was the inter-fering chromogen. The magnitude of rise of the serum creatinine concentration varied depending on the automated assay which was used (Technicon or Beckman) and the concentration of the acetoacetate. Generally, serum creatinine concentration is increased by 1 to 2 mg/dl which is in agreement with other data in the literature (240,241).

This patient's serum creatinine of 3.1 mg/dl was measured at a time when the serum acetoacetate concentration may have been increasing due to insulin therapy (see Question 60). Subsequent creatinine assays in this patient were normal, as were urinary sediment and electrolytes. Because no evidence of renal disease was noted on repeat testing and in view of the fact that the serum creatinine returned to normal, the creatinine of 3.1 mg/dl probably was indeed a result of laboratory interference.

Treatment Summary

Upon admission at 1600 hours, fluids and insulin were administered. One liter (L) of normal saline (NS) was administered over one hour and was followed by a second liter of NS over the next two hours. One ampule (50 mEq) of sodium bicarbonate was also administered initially. An 8 unit intravenous (IV) bolus of regular insulin was given and followed with a constant IV infusion at 8 units/hour (100 units of regular insulin in 1 L NS to run at 80 cc/hour in a separate line).

1900 Hours. Laboratory results were as follows: blood glucose 505 mg/dl, K 3.8 mEq/L, creatinine 3.1 mg/dl, serum ketones strongly positive in a 1:40 dilution, pH 7.17, and HCO_3 11 mEq/L. The urine output over the past three hours was 500 cc. The blood pressure was 120/70 mm Hg with no orthostatic changes.

A continuous IV infusion of NS with 20 mEq/L of K-Phos and 20 mEq/L of KCl was administered at a rate of 333 ml/hr. Regular insulin was continued at a constant IV infusion of 8 units/hr.

2200 Hours. Laboratory results included: pH 7.21, blood glucose 385 mg/dl, K 3.4 mEq/L, and Na 151 mEq/L. The continuous IV infusion of ½ NS with 20 mEq/L of K-Phos and 20 mEq/L of KCl was slowed to a rate of 250 cc/hr, and the insulin infusion was slowed to 6 units/hr.

0200 Hours of Second Hospital Day. The blood glucose was 235 mg/dl and the potassium was 3.5 mEq/L. The IV infusion was changed to 5% Dextrose in water (D5W) with 20 mEq/L of K-Phos and 20 mEq/L of KCL and was administered at a rate of 250 cc/hr. The IV infusion of regular insulin was decreased to 4 units/hr.

0600 Hours of Second Hospital Day. The patient began to feel better and started taking full oral liquids. The laboratory reported: blood glucose 237 mg/dl, K 4.3 mEq/L, Na 147 mEq/L, HCO₃ 16 mEq/L, pH 7.32, creatinine 1.3 mg/dl, serum ketones were moderate, and the urine was 2 + for glucose. The K-Phos was deleted and the constant IV infusion of D5W with 20 mEq/L of KCl was decreased to 200 cc/hr. The regular insulin was continued at 4 units/hr.

1800 Hours of Second Hospital Day. The laboratory results were: blood glucose 175 mg/dl, K 4.6 mEq/L, Na 144 mEq/L, and the urine was 1 + for glucose and contained moderate amounts of ketones. The IV fluids and insulin were discontinued and a regular insulin rainbow coverage was given throughout the night.

0600 Hours of Third Hospital Day. The laboratory results were: blood glucose 207 mg/dl, K 3.9 mEq/L, Na 141 mEq/L, HCO₃ 21 mEq/L, creatinine 0.6 mg/dl, and the urine was positive for trace amounts of ketones and 2 + for glucose. The patient was given her usual dose of NPH insulin and regular insulin subcutaneously and was sent home.

CARDIOPULMONARY ARREST

62. A.A. is a 63-year-old male who was admitted to the coronary care unit twelve hours ago with an acute inferior myocardial infarction. The nurse taking care of him observes the following rhythm:

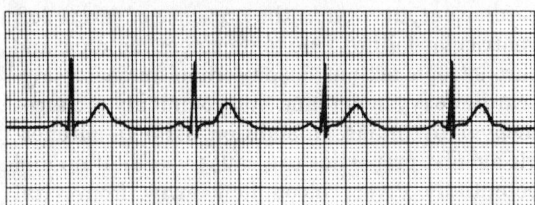

Is drug therapy indicated for this arrhythmia?

The above rhythm is regular with P waves preceding each QRS complex, and the PR interval is normal and constant with a rate of 50 beats/minute. The dysrhythmia is sinus bradycardia. It occurs commonly in the early course of inferior myocardial infarctions. The goal of treatment is to increase heart rate to a level which maintains an adequate cardiac output in order to perfuse vital organs. The concern in treating sinus bradycardia stems from the potential of drugs to cause marked acceleration of heart rate. Since heart rate is a major determinant of myocardial oxygen demand, a marked increase in heart rate carries the risk of worsening ischemia or extending infarct size.

In the setting of acute myocardial infarction, bradydysrhythmias (ventricular rate less than 60 beats/minute) should be treated only when accompanied by hypotension or premature ventricular contractions, or when the rate falls to less than 50 beats/minute in the absence of hypotension or ectopy (242). Thus, before a decision can be made regarding treatment for this patient, one must recognize the rhythm disturbance and acquire additional clinical information.

Assuming treatment is indicated, atropine would be the drug of choice. Its anticholinergic action blocks the vagal effect on the SA and AV nodes, resulting in enhanced SA nodal discharge and increased conduction through AV nodal tissue. A minimum dose of 0.5 mg of atropine should be administered undiluted intravenously over 20–30 seconds. Smaller doses administered slowly should be avoided because they have been associated with paradoxical bradycardia (243). The initial dose may be repeated every five minutes until the heart rate is between 60–100 beats/minute or until a total dose of 2 mg is reached. It is important to remember that atropine can cause the pupils to become fixed and dilated, a finding which may be misleading on neurological examination.

63. Evaluation of A.A. revealed a blood pressure of 70/40 mm Hg accompanied by obtundation. Atropine 0.5 mg was administered. Heart rate increased to 75 beats/minute, blood pressure increased to 110/70 mm Hg, and his mental status improved. The patient's rhythm remained stable for 30 minutes when the following rhythm was recorded. A.A. was symptom free at this time.

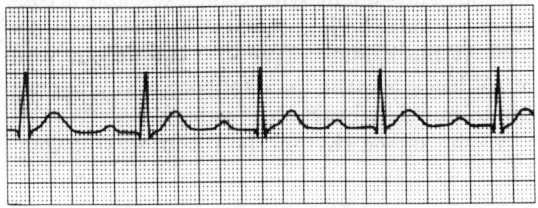

Should additional atropine be administered?

Examination of this rhythm shows it to be regular, with a normal rate (60–100 beats/minute), and P waves precede each normal QRS complex. However, the PR interval is prolonged to greater than 0.21 seconds and is unchanged. This is first degree AV block and represents a slowing of conduction from the atria to the ventricle. First degree AV block is significant in that it may indicate the presence of underlying cardiac disease or toxicity from digitalis, quinidine or procainamide. It may warn of the development of more advanced forms of AV block (Mobitz I and II). No treatment is indicated for first degree heart block, but close monitoring for rhythm disturbances is appropriate.

64. No additional atropine was administered to A.A. and his rhythm remained stable, converting back to normal sinus rhythm. Twenty minutes later the following rhythm strip was observed.

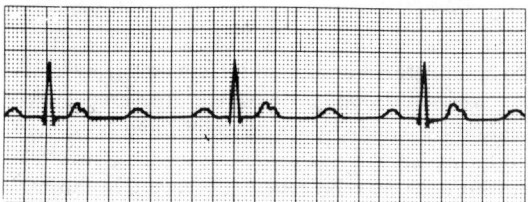

A bolus of atropine 0.5 mg was administered without result. The dose was repeated and the following rhythm developed.

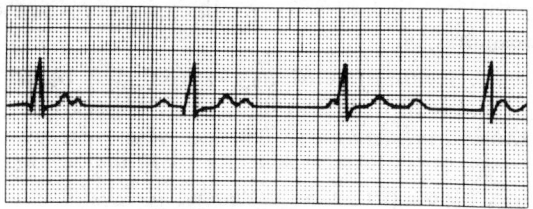

Was atropine the appropriate therapy for this patient?

The first rhythm showed P waves occurring without subsequent QRS complexes and a constant prolonged PR interval. This is second degree AV block, Mobitz type II. It is a serious form of AV block because the likelihood of it progressing to complete heart block is high.

In the second rhythm the PR interval is completely variable and nonrelated to the QRS complex. Atria and ventricles are beating independently of one another, indicating third degree or complete heart block.

Treatment of the above arrhythmias requires insertion of a pacemaker. The mortality rate from complete heart block without pacemaker therapy ranges from 40 to 100% (244,245). However, drug therapy is indicated as a temporary measure to maintain a ventricular rate of 60 beats/minute or greater, especially if there is accompanying hypotension or signs of inadequate cerebral blood flow. Atropine is an appropriate choice to decrease the degree of AV block and increase the ventricular rate.

65. A.A.'s ventricular rate remained at 40 beats/minute despite two boluses of atropine 0.5 mg. Blood pressure had now dropped to 70/30 mm Hg, and the patient was confused and becoming less responsive. What drug should be administered at this point while waiting for pacemaker placement?

Although additional atropine may be administered up to a total dose of 2 mg, the deterioration of the patient and the lack of response to atropine support the decision to begin a more potent drug. Isoproterenol is indicated for immediate control of hemodynamically significant bradycardia due to heart block resistant to atropine. Structurally, it is related to epinephrine and is the most potent cardiac stimulant available. However, unlike epinephrine it is a pure beta-adrenergic receptor agonist. It stimulates firing of the SA node and increases conduction through the AV node. Generally, there is an increase in cardiac output even in the presence of severe left ventricular failure. Due to its potent inotropic and chronotropic actions, isoproterenol increases myocardial oxygen demand and commonly produces tachyarrhythmias. In addition, its beta-adrenergic agonist properties can cause vasodilation and potentially divert blood flow away from vital organs.

Isoproterenol is administered as a continuous infusion at rates of 2–20 mcg/minute, titrated according to heart rate and rhythm response. A high infusion rate may be needed at the beginning of therapy. The infusion is prepared by mixing one ampule (1 mg) in 500 ml or 250 ml of 5% dextrose in water to achieve concentrations of 2 mcg/ml and 4 mcg/ml respectively.

66. An isoproterenol infusion was begun, resulting in an increased ventricular rate to 85 beats/minute. A.A.'s mental status had improved and the BP was 100/50 mm Hg. Suddenly A.A. became unresponsive with no audible or palpable blood pressure. A code "5" was called. What steps need to be performed initially in a cardiopulmonary arrest?

When a cardiopulmonary arrest occurs, it is imperative that basic life support be instituted as rapidly as possible to prevent development of severe acidosis and hypoxemia. Untreated cardiac arrest usually results in irreversible central nervous system damage within four minutes. After establishing unresponsiveness and calling for help, the patient must be placed in the horizontal position on a hard surface so that external chest compression will be maximally effective. If the patient is in bed, a board should be placed under the back. The airway should be opened by gently tilting the head backward. If the patient is not breathing, one should administer four quick full breaths by blowing into the patient's mouth. In the absence of a pulse, chest compression to provide artificial circulation alternating with artificial breathing in the ratio of 15 compressions to two breaths if one person is present or 5 compressions to one breath if two rescuers are available. This procedure is continued until equipment and personnel able to deliver advanced life support arrive. At this point, a cuffed endotracheal tube may be inserted and oxygen-enriched artificial ventilation by mask begun. An intravenous line should be established for administration of drugs and fluids to aid in maintaining an effective cardiac rhythm. Electrodes should be placed for rhythm recognition.

In the hospital setting, such as the coronary care unit where patients are monitored and defibrillation equipment and personnel capable of delivering advanced life support are immediately available, the sequence of events may be slightly different. If cardiopulmonary resuscitation is instituted rapidly following cardiac arrest and/or a defibrillator is readily available, immediate countershock is the therapy of choice because the rhythm most often responsible for cardiac arrest is ventricular fibrillation or ventricular tachy-

cardia. Under these circumstances, the need to start an infusion first and administer drugs is not indicated since countershock can be rapidly delivered before excessive hypoxemia or acidosis develop.

67. A.A. displayed the following rhythm:

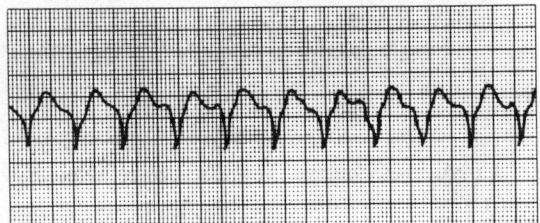

How should he be treated?

The rhythm is regular at a rate of approximately 150 beats/minute. There are no discernible P waves, which are probably lost in the QRS complex. The QRS interval is widened. This dysrhythmia is ventricular tachycardia and is a serious development because it may degenerate to ventricular fibrillation. Treatment involves the use of antiarrhythmic drugs, such as lidocaine, procainamide and bretyllium, and/or cardioversion. The exact approach depends upon the clinical circumstance. If the patient is hemodynamically stable, lidocaine should be administered. When the patient is hypotensive or unresponsive, immediate cardioversion may be employed.

Treatment of this patient would include discontinuation of the isoproterenol infusion and immediate countershock. If a supraventricular rhythm is restored or ventricular tachycardia persists, a lidocaine bolus of 1 mg/kg should be administered, followed by an infusion of 1–4 mg/minute to establish a steady suppressive concentration in the blood. The infusion is prepared by adding 1 gm of lidocaine to 500 ml or 250 ml of 5% dextrose in water, providing a concentration of 2 mg/ml or 4 mg/ml. It may be necessary to readminister subsequent loading doses to the patient within 3–5 minute intervals; however, lidocaine's biphasic half-life must be considered. (For details of electrophysiologic effects and pharmacokinetics of lidocaine, see the chapter on Cardiac Arrhythmias.) Cumulative loading doses in excess of 300 mg should be used with caution because of the danger of drug toxicity.

68. A.A. was immediately cardioverted and went into a supraventricular tachycardia. A bolus of lidocaine 100 mg was administered and an infusion of 2 mg/minute was started. The supraventricular tachycardia suddenly changed to the following:

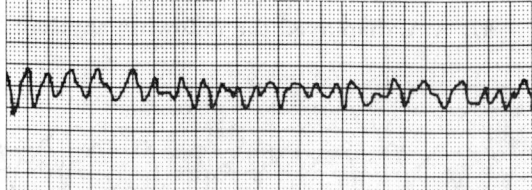

Cardiopulmonary resuscitation was begun and blood gases were ordered. A second cardioversion was attempted but was not successful in changing the rhythm. What drugs may be used to help convert this rhythm?

This rhythm is completely and totally irregular. There are no identifiable P waves or QRS complexes. The rhythm is ventricular fibrillation and is the most disorganized of all the arrhythmias. There is no effective cardiac output in patients with ventricular fibrillation. Prompt treatment is essential because it is universally fatal if allowed to persist.

Treatment of ventricular fibrillation includes DC countershock, antiarrhythmic drugs, epinephrine, and sodium bicarbonate. Initially, countershock is the treatment of choice. If this fails, administration of an antiarrhythmic drug followed by cardioversion is appropriate. Although lidocaine is often the antiarrhythmic selected because of proven efficacy and because of familiarity of dose, bretylium may be just as effective (246).

Recommendations for bretylium dosage vary, but 5–10 mg/kg is an appropriate first dose. Administration is by rapid undiluted intravenous injection over 5–10 seconds during a cardiopulmonary arrest. Boluses of 10 mg/kg repeated at 15–30 minute intervals to a total dose of 30 mg/kg may be given in refractory cases.

When an antiarrhythmic medication and cardioversion fail to convert ventricular fibrillation, epinephrine alone or in combination with bicarbonate (if the serum pH is low) may be tried. Exactly how epinephrine works in this disorder is unknown. Pharmacologically, it stimulates both alpha- and beta-adrenergic receptors which probably mediate its beneficial effects (247).

Administration of epinephrine enhances automaticity and conduction, increases the force of ventricular contraction, and increases systemic vascular resistance. The latter action elevates perfusion pressure during chest compression, which may augment coronary artery blood flow (248). It often is administered to convert fine ventricular fibrillation to coarse ventricular fibrillation, which is more amenable to DC cardioversion. The dosage given is 0.5–1 mg of the 1:10,000 dilution by intravenous push. The dosage can be repeated at five minute intervals if needed. When no response is seen and/or the function of the intravenous line is questionable or not yet established, epinephrine may be given by direct instillation into the tracheobronchial tree via the endotracheal tube (249,250). Direct intracardiac injection may also be used but is less desirable because of the hazards of coronary artery laceration, tamponade, and pneumothorax.

69. A.A. was given a second lidocaine bolus of 100 mg and then cardioverted with no result. Epinephrine, 5 ml of a 1:10000 solution (0.5 mg), was then administered and cardioversion repeated. Normal sinus rhythm was briefly restored and immediately degenerated back to ventricular fibrillation. Blood gas analysis was now available and showed: pH 7.20, pO$_2$ 65, pCO$_2$ 38, and HCO$_3$ 14.5.

How should these blood gases be interpreted? What treatment is indicated?

The blood gases show A.A. to have a significant metabolic acidosis. Acidosis develops rapidly during cardiopulmonary arrest from hypoventilation and the accumulation of fixed acids, especially lactic acid which is a product of anaerobic metabolism (251,252). Assisted ventilation and effective cardiac compression to maintain cardiac output are the major treatments in preventing the development of severe refractory acidemia during a cardiopulmonary arrest. A.A.'s blood gases indicate that ventilation is adequate (normal pCO$_2$) but that cardiac output is inadequate to perfuse peripheral tissues (low pH, low HCO$_3$). One should consider poor performance of chest compression as a cause of acidosis and check for the presence of a pulse when CPR is being performed.

In addition to CPR, the metabolic component of the acidosis should be treated with sodium bicarbonate to keep the arterial pH near normal.

Alkali therapy is important because reversal of acidosis may: a) increase the electrical threshold required to produce ventricular fibrillation (253), b) increase ventricular contractile force and thus, cardiac output (254), c) restore cardiovascular responsiveness to catecholamines (255), and d) improve the success rate of electrical countershock in terminating ventricular fibrillation (251).

Current standards recommend that bicarbonate therapy be administered in accordance to the results of arterial blood pH and pCO_2 measurements (242). However, blood gas measurements are not always available, and administration of bicarbonate must often be empirical. In such situations, 1 mEq/kg can be administered initially followed by 0.5 mEq/kg every ten minutes of continued arrest (242). In general, no more than two ampules should be given initially without knowledge of the serum pH.

Overzealous use of alkali runs the risk of changing metabolic acidosis to metabolic alkalosis, as well as producing a hyperosmolar state. Both have been associated with high mortality (256). Other consequences of excess bicarbonate include hypokalemia, tissue hypoxia from increased oxygen-hemoglobin affinity, and the potentiation of cerebral acidosis.

70. A.A. was given one 50 ml ampule of sodium bicarbonate and another 0.5 mg of epinephrine. The pulse was checked to assess the adequacy of chest compression. CPR was continued for two minutes to circulate the drugs and another cardioversion was attempted. The ventricular fibrillation was converted to a supraventricular tachycardia which quickly changed back to ventricular fibrillation, then coverted to asystole. Blood gases were repeated. Is this rhythm treatable?

The development of asystole carries a poor prognosis for resuscitation. Severe metabolic imbalances should be ruled out as a contributory factor and CPR continued. Ventricular asystole has traditionally been treated with epinephrine 0.5 mg intravenously along with bicarbonate, if needed. The goal of epinephrine administration is to stimulate normal and ectopic foci in an attempt to restore normal sinus rhythm or to convert asystole to ventricular fibrillation, which may be electrically defibrillated. Electric cardioversion of asystole is of no benefit.

Asystole unresponsive to bicarbonate and ep-inephrine may be responsive to calcium chloride. Calcium increases ventricular contraction and enhances automaticity, thereby making it potentially useful in restoring an electrical rhythm. Calcium should be avoided if digitalis toxicity is suspected and used cautiously if a patient has been receiving digitalis because of the risk of potentiating digitalis toxic rhythms. If hyperkalemia is present or suspected, calcium often reverses the abnormal rhythm while measures are undertaken to lower the serum potassium level. Although there are three different salt forms of calcium available, the chloride salt is preferred in adults. It should be administered by intravenous injection over 30 seconds when used in asystole. The dosage is 500 mg–1 gm (5–10 cc of 10% solution) and may be repeated at 3–5 minute intervals.

New data suggest that atropine may be useful in treating asystole (257). Its use is based on the premise that high levels of parasympathetic tone inhibit supraventricular and ventricular pacemaker activity. Therefore, anticholinergic or parasympatholytic drugs, by blocking vagal activity, may be of benefit. The dosage is 1 mg intravenously repeated in 30 to 60 seconds to a total dose of 2–4 mg. When all else fails, ventricular pacing using a transvenous or transthoracic pacemaker may be tried.

71. Blood gas data showed the pH to be 7.32. One ampule of calcium chloride (1 gm) was administered with no effect. Atropine was then administered and after a total dose 2 mg had been given, a supraventricular rhythm was restored but without the presence of a pulse. The patient was in electromechanical dissociation. How might this patient be treated?

Electromechanical dissociation, like asystole, carries a grave prognosis for recovery. Treatment of this disorder is similar to that outlined for asystole with the exception of atropine and pacemaker insertion (see Fig. 5).

In those instances where ventricular fibrillation and asystole are successfully terminated, it is not uncommon for the patient to become hypotensive. Fluids and inotropic and vasopressor support are often necessary. Guidelines for choice of agent and administration are the same as those discussed in previous cases, with the occasional exception that larger doses or infusion rates are

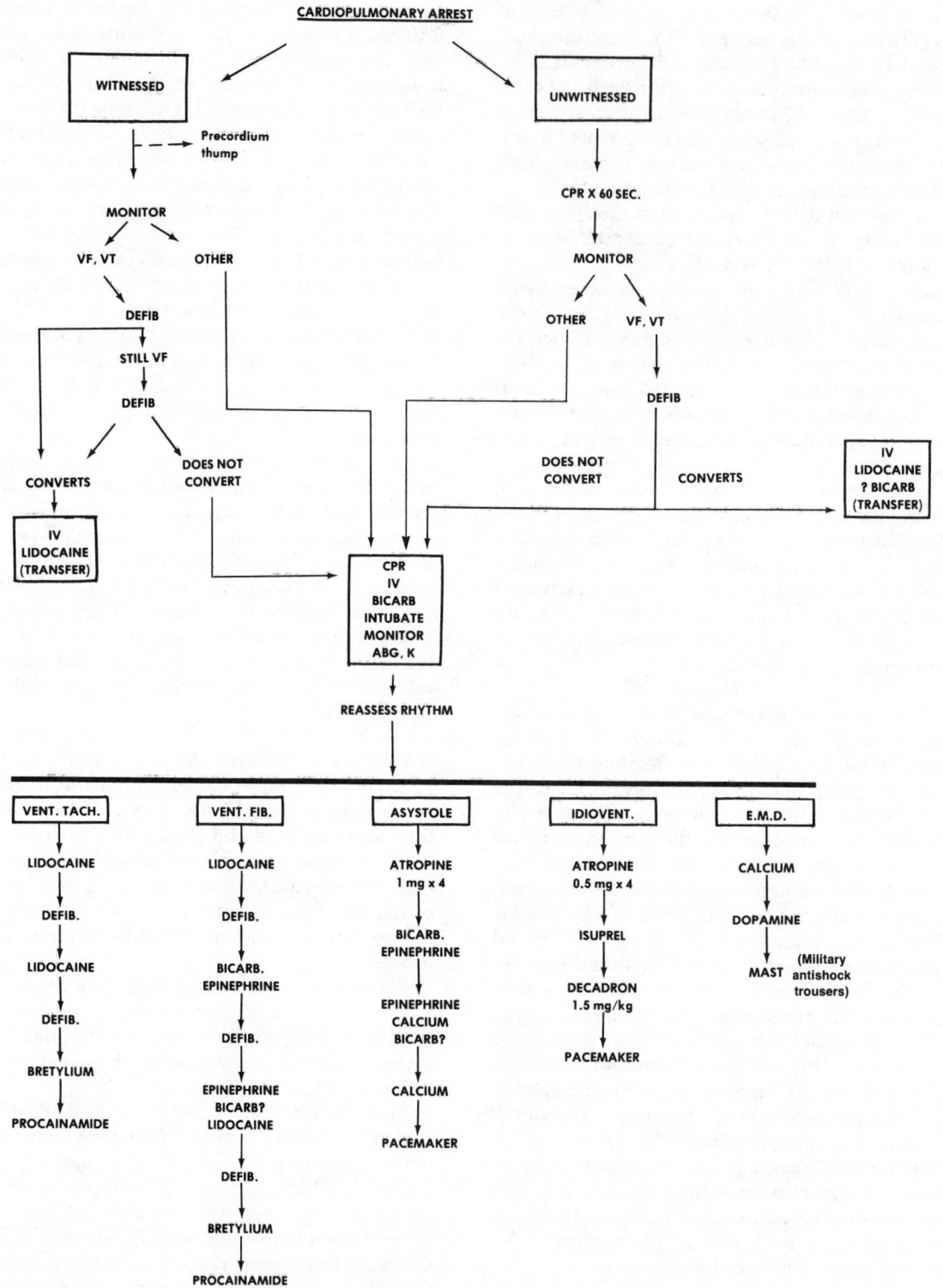

Figure 5. Algorithm for Drug Use During Cardiopulmonary Arrest.

Table 8.

COMMONLY USED CARDIOPULMONARY RESUSCITATION DRUGS

Drug	Dose	Rationale/Indications	Comments
Atropine	0.5–1 mg IV push over 20–30 seconds. Repeated at 3–5 minute intervals up to total of 2 mg. **Pediatric:** 0.02 mg/kg.	Blocks parasympathetic activity due to excessive vagal activity. Useful in: sinus bradycardia, heart block, asystole.	Must be given rapidly to avoid paradoxical vagal activity. Do not give when heart rate ⁓ 60 beats/minute.
Bretyllium	Initial dose 5–10 mg/kg IV push for ventricular fibrillation. Dilute in 50 ml D5W and infuse over ten minutes for ventricular tachycardia. May repeat in ten minutes up to total of 30 mg/kg. Continuous infusion 1–2 mg/min. Intermittent infusion 5–10 mg/kg every 6–8 hours.	Ventricular tachycardia and fibrillation unresponsive to lidocaine. Works best just prior to defibrillation.	Questionable use in digitalis toxicity. Catecholamine release initially followed by hypotension.
Calcium Chloride	**Cardiac arrest:** 1 gm IV over 30 seconds. May repeat in 3–5 minutes 2–3 times. **Hyperkalemic-induced arrhythmias:** 500 mg IV over 2–4 minutes repeat PRN. **Pediatric:** 15 mg/kg	Cardiac stimulant. Improves force of ventricular contraction. Useful in asystole, electrical mechanical dissociation, hyperkalemia.	Avoid in digitalis toxicity. Flush lines before and after administration. Do not mix with bicarbonate.
Epinephrine	0.5–1 mg IV push (1:10,000 dilution). May be repeated in 3–5 minutes. **Infusion:** 1–5 mcg/minute or titrate to desired effect.	Cardiac stimulant. Inotropic and chronotropic response. Increases peripheral vascular resistance. Useful in: Asystole, electromechanical dissociation, ventricular fibrillation.	Infusion: give in central line if possible.
Isoproterenol	0.5–5 mcg/minute by IV infusion only.	Inotropic and chronotropic support. Useful in bradydysrhythmias.	Caution: hypotension, tachyarrhythmias.
Lidocaine	I mg/kg IV bolus over 30–60 seconds. Repeat 0.5 mg/kg if needed. **Infusion:** 1–4 mg/minute.	Suppression of ventricular arrhythmias: Ventricular fibrillation, ventricular tachycardia. Ventricular arrhythmias associated with digitalis toxicity.	Decrease loading dose by one-half in heart failure and/or liver failure.
Procainamide	100 mg IV push over 2–5 minutes every five minutes up to 1 gm. **Infusion:** 1–6 mg/min.	Ventricular arrhythmias unresponsive to lidocaine.	Limit loading dose to 0.5 gm in heart failure. Decrease infusion by one-half in renal failure. Caution: hypotension; avoid in tricyclic antidepressant or phenothiazine overdose.
Sodium Bicarbonate	1 mEq/kg IV push over 30–60 seconds. 0.5 mEq/kg every 10 minutes of continued arrest depending on arterial blood gases. **Pediatric:** 1–2 mEq/kg initially followed by 1 mEq/kg every ten minutes.	Reverses metabolic acidosis in shock. DKA, severe hypotension, and cardiac arrest. Restores responsiveness to catecholamines and improves response to defibrillation.	Use cautiously in the presence of hypokalemia. Flush lines before and after use.

used initially, then titrated downward as the patient continues to improve. In addition, Figure 5 provides a general guideline for drug usage during a cardiac arrest situation and is presented in algorithmic form. Additional references on cardiopulmonary resuscitation are provided at the end of the chapter (258–268).

References

1. Weil MH et al: Experimental and clinical studies on lactate and pyruvate as indicators of the severity of acute circulatory failure (shock). Circulation. 1970; 41:989.
2. Weil M: Current understanding of mechanisms and treatment of circulatory shock caused by bacterial infections. Ann of Clin Reser. 1977; 9:181.
3. Weil MH et al: Treatment of circulatory shock: use of sympathomimetic and related vasoactive agents. JAMA. 1975; 321:1280.
4. Houston M: Diagnosis and treatment of shock. S Med J. 1980; 73:477.
5. Shillingford JP et al: Cardiovascular and pulmonary changes in patients with acute myocardial infarction treated in an intensive care unit. Am J Cardiol. 1967; 20:484.
6. Gunnar RM et al: Hemodynamic studies in shock with myocardial infarction. In *Shock In Myocardial Infarction,* Gunnar RM, Loeb HS, Rahimtoula (eds), New York, Grune and Stratton, 1974; pp 113–130.
7. Shubin H et al: Bacterial Shock. JAMA. 1976; 235:421.
8. Hess ML et al: Spectrum of cardiovascular function during gram-negative sepsis. Progr Cardiovasc Dis. 1981; 23:279.
9. Gleckman R et al: Gram-negative bacteremic shock: pathophysiology, clinical features, and treatment. S Med J. 1981; 74:335.
10. Sheagren J: Septic shock and corticosteroids, editorial. N Engl J Med. 1981; 305:456.
11. Weil MH et al: Cardiac output in bacterial shock. Am J Med. 1978; 64:920.
12. Swan HJC et al: Catheterization of the heart in man with use of a flow-directed balloon-tipped catheter. N Engl J Med. 1970; 283:447.
13. Ganz W et al: A new technique for measurement of cardiac output by thermodilution in man. Am J Cardiol. 1971; 27:392.
14. James PM et al: Central venous pressure monitoring: misinterpretations, abuses, indications and a new technic. Ann Surg. 1972; 175:693.
15. Archer G et al: Long-term pulmonary artery pressure monitoring in the management of the critically ill. Ann Surg. 1974; 180:747.
16. Braunwald E et al: Studies on Starling's law of the heart. IV. Observations on the hemodynamic functions of the left atrium in man. Circulation. 1961; 24:633.
17. Gorlin R: Current concepts in cardiology: practical cardiac hemodynamics. N Engl J Med. 1977; 296:203.
18. Forsyth RP et al: Redistribution of cardiac output during hemorrhage in the unanesthetized monkey. Circ Res. 1970; 27:311.
19. Slater G et al: Sequential changes in the distribution of cardiac output in various stages of experimental hemorrhagic shock. Surgery. 1973; 73:714.
20. Moss GS et al: Traumatic shock in man. N Engl J Med. 1974; 290:724.
21. Zweifach BW et al: The interplay of central and peripheral factors in irreversible hemorrhagic shock. Progr Cardiovasc Dis. 1975; 18:147.
22. Grindon AJ: The use of packed red blood cells. JAMA. 1976; 235:389.
23. Baue AE et al: Hemodynamic and metabolic effects of Ringer's lactate solution in hemorrhagic shock. Ann Surg. 1967; 166:29.
24. Shoemaker WC: Comparison of the relative effectiveness of whole blood transfusions and various types of fluid therapy in resuscitation. Crit Care Med. 1976; 4:71.
25. Lowery BD et al: Electrolyte solutions in resuscitation in human hemorrhagic shock. Surg Gynecol Obstet. 1971; 133:273.
26. Westphal RG: Rational alternatives to the use of whole blood. Ann Intern Med. 1972; 20:987.
27. Lim R et al. Platelet response and coagulation changes following massive blood replacement. J Trauma. 1973; 13:577.
28. Shires GT et al: Fluid resuscitation in the severely injured. Surg Clin North Am. 1973; 53:1341.
29. Sugerman et al: The basis of defective oxygen delivery from stored blood. Surg Gynecol Obstet. 1970; 13:733.
30. Buchanan EC: Blood and blood substitutes for treating hemorrhagic shock. Am J Hosp Pharm. 1977; 34:631.
31. Forrester JS et al: Medical therapy of acute myocardial infarction by application of hemodynamic subsets, part I and II: N Engl J Med. 1976; 295:1356 and 1404.
32. Forrester JS et al: Hospital treatment of congestive heart failure, management according to hemodynamic profiles. Am J Med. 1978; 65:173.
33. Shubin H et al: Bacterial shock. JAMA. 1976; 235:421.
34. Rothschild M et al: Albumin synthesis. N Engl J Med. 1972; 286:14.
35. Tullis JL: Albumin, background and use. JAMA. 1977; 237:355 and 460.
36. Bland JHL et al: Vasodilator effects of commercial 5% plasma protein fraction solutions. JAMA. 1973; 224:1721.
37. Alving B et al: Hypotension associated with pre-kallikren activator in PPF. N Engl J Med. 1978; 299:66.
38. FDA Drug Bulletin: Adverse reactions to PPF. 1977; 7(4):20.
39. Shoemaker WC: Effects of transfusion on surviving and non-surviving post-operative patients. Surg Gynecol Obstet. 1976; 142:33.
40. Skillman JJ et al: Pulmonary arteriovenous admixture improvement with albumin and diuresis. Am J Surg. 1970; 119:440.
41. da Luz PL et al: Pulmonary edema related to changes in colloid osmotic and pulmonary wedge pressure in patients with acute myocardial infarction. Circulation. 1975; 51:350.

42. Skillman JJ: The role of albumin and oncotically active fluids in shock. Crit Care Med. 1976; 4:55.

43. Shoemaker WC et al: Critique of crystalloid versus colloid therapy in shock lung. Crit Care Med. 1979; 7:117.

44. Virgilio RW et al: Balanced electrolyte solutions: experimental and clinical studies. Crit Care Med. 1979; 7:98.

45. Weil MH et al: Colloid oncotic pressure: clinical significance. Crit Care Med. 1979; 7:113.

46. Weaver DW et al: Pulmonary effects of albumin resuscitation for severe hypovolemic shock. Arch Surg. 1978; 113:387.

47. Moss GS: An argument in favor of electrolyte solution for early resuscitation. Surg Clin North Am. 1972; 52:3.

48. Lowe RJ et al: Crystalloid vs colloid in the etiology of pulmonary failure after trauma; a randomized trial in man. Surgery. 1977; 81:676.

49. Holcroft JW et al: Extravascular lung water following hemorrhagic shock in the baboon: comparison between resuscitation with ringers lactate and plasmanate. Ann Surg. 1974; 180:408.

50. Holcroft et al: Pulmonary extravasation of albumin during and after hemorrhagic shock in baboons. J Surg Res. 1975; 18:91.

51. Staub N et al: "State of the Art" Review: Pathogenesis of pulmonary edema. Am Rev Resp Dis. 1974; 109:358.

52. Stein L et al: Pulmonary edema during volume infusion. Circulation. 1975; 52:483.

53. Weil et al: Relationship between colloid osmotic pressure and pulmonary artery wedge pressure in patients with acute cardio-respiratory failure. Am J Med. 1978; 64:643.

54. Weil MH et al: New concepts in the diagnosis and fluid treatment of circulatory shock. Anesth Analgesia. 1979; 58:124.

55. Virgilio RW et al: Crystalloid vs colloid resuscitation: is one better than the other? Surgery. 1979; 85:129.

56. Jelenko C et al: Studies in shock and resuscitation, I: Use of a hypertonic, albumin containing fluid demand regimen (HALFD) in resuscitation. Crit Care Med. 1979; 7:157.

57. Jelenko C et al: Shock and resuscitation III, accurate refractometric COP determinations in hypovolemia treated with HALFD. J Am Coll Emergency Physicians. 1979; 8:253.

58. Data JL et al: Dextran 40. Ann Intern Med. 1974; 81:500.

59. Thompson WL et al: Intravascular persistence, tissue storage, and excretion of hydroxyethyl starch. Surg Gynecol Obstet. 1970; 131:965.

60. Moffitt EA: Blood substitutes. Can Anaes Soc J. 1975; 22:12.

61. Buchanan EC: Blood and blood substitutes for treating hemorrhagic shock. Am J Hosp Pharm. 1977; 34:631.

62. Murray S et al. Low molecular weight dextran and matching by enzyme technics. Transfusion. 1971; 11:378.

63. Atik M: Dextran 40 and dextran 70: A review. Arch Surg. 1967; 94:664.

64. Thomas JM et al: Dextran 40 in the treatment of peripheral vascular disease. Arch Surg. 1973; 106:138.

65. Mishler J et al: HES, an agent for hypovolemic shock treatment. J Surg Res. 1977; 23:239.

66. Boon J et al: Intravascular persistence of HES in man. Br J Surg Res. 1976; 8:497.

67. Metcalf W et al: A clinical physiologic study of hydroxyethyl starch. Surg Gynecol Obstet. 1970.

68. Kohler H et al: HES induced macroamylassemia. Int J Clin Pharmacol. 1977; 15:428.

69. Ring J et al: Incidence and severity of anaphylactoid reactions to colloid volume substitutes. Lancet. 1977; 1:466.

70. Shine KI et al: Aspects of the management of shock. Ann Intern Med. 1980; 93:723.

71. Johnson SA et al: Treatment of shock in myocardial infarction. JAMA. 1977; 237:2106.

72. Mason DT: Afterload reduction and cardiac performance, physiologic basis of systemic vasodilators as a new approach to treatment of CHF. Am J Med. 1978; 65:106.

73. Chatterjee K: Vasodilator therapy for heart failure. Ann Intern Med. 1975; 83:421.

74. Chatterjee K et al: Vasodilator therapy in heart failure. Progr Cardiovasc Dis. 1977; 19:131.

75. Mason DT: Alterations of hemodynamics and myocardial mechanics in patients with congestive heart failure. Progr Cardiovasc Dis. 1970; 12:507.

76. Mason DT: Ventricular afterload reduction therapy in management of congestive heart failure. Clin Cardiol. 1978; 2:55.

77. Cohn JN et al: Vasodilator therapy of cardiac failure. N Engl J Med. 1977; 297:254.

78. Miller RR et al. Clinical use of sodium nitroprusside in chronic ischemic heart disease. Circulation. 1975; 51:328.

79. Smith NT et al: The use and misuse of pressor agents. Anesthesiology. 1970; 33:58.

80. Gunnar RM et al: Management of acute myocardial infarction and accelerating angina. Progr Cardiovasc Dis. 1979; 22:1.

81. Goldberg L et al: Newer catecholamines for treatment of heart failure and shock: an update on dopamine and a first look at dobutamine. Progr Cardiovasc Dis. 1977; 19:327.

82. Goldberg LI: Cardiovascular and renal actions of dopamine: potential clinical applications. Pharmacological Reviews. 1972; 24:1.

83. Goldberg LI: Dopamine—clinical use of an endogenous catecholamine. N Engl J Med. 1974; 291:707.

84. Goldberg LI: The dopamine vascular receptor. Biochemical Pharmacology. 1975; 24:651.

85. Winslow EJ et al: Hemodynamic studies and results of therapy in 50 patients with bacteremic shock. Am J Med. 1973; 54:421.

86. Leier CV: Comparative systemic and regional hemodynamic effects of dopamine and dobutamine in patients with cardiomyopathic heart failure. Circulation. 1978; 58:466.

87. Chamberlain JA et al: Dobutamine, isoprenaline, and dopamine in patients after open heart surgery. Intern Care Med. 1980; 7:5.

88. Loeb HS et al: Acute hemodynamic effects of dopamine in patients with shock. Circulation. 1971; 44:163.

89. Mueller HS et al: Effect of dopamine on hemodynamic and myocardial metabolism in shock following acute myocardial infarction in man. Circulation. 1978; 57:361.

90. Robie NW et al: Comparative systemic and regional hemodynamic effects of dopamine and dobutamine. Am Heart J. 1975; 90:340.

91. Tuttle RR et al: Dobutamine, development of a new catecholamine to selectively increase cardiac contractility. Circulation Research. 1975; 36:185.

92. Robie NW et al: In vivo analysis of adrenergic receptor activity of dobutamine. Circulation Research. 1974; 34:663.

93. Tinker JH et al: Dobutamine for inotropic support during emergence from cardiopulmonary bypass. Anesthesiology. 1976; 44:281.

94. Leier CV et al: The relationship between plasma dobutamine concentrations and cardiovascular responses in cardiac failure. Am J Med. 1979; 66:238.

95. Sakamoto T et al: Hemodynamic effects of dobutamine in patients following open heart surgery. Circulation. 1977; 55:525.

96. Akhtar N et al: Hemodynamic effect of dobutamine in patients with severe heart failure. Am J Cardiol. 1975; 36:202.

97. Bergegovich J. Hemodynamic effects of a new inotropic agent (dobutamine) in chronic cardiac failure. Br Heart J. 1975; 37:629.

98. Kersting F et al: A comparison of cardiovascular effects of dobutamine and isoprenaline after open heart surgery. Br Heart J. 1976; 38:622.

99. Mikulic E et al: Comparative hemodynamic effects of inotropic and vasodilator drugs in severe heart failure. Circulation. 1977; 56:528.

100. Weiner N: Norepinephrine, epinephrine, and the sympathomimetic amines. In *The Pharmacologic Basis of Therapeutics*, 6th ed, edited by A Goodman, LS Goodman, and A Gilman, Macmillian, New York, 1980, p 138.

101. Steen PA et al: Efficacy of dopamine, dobutamine, and epinephrine during emergence from cardiopulmonary bypass in man. Circulation. 1978; 57:378.

102. Braunwald E: Limitations of infarct size. Current Problems in Cardiology. 1978; 3:10.

103. Krone RJ et al: Surgical correction of cardiogenic shock. Arch Intern Med. 1976; 136:1186.

104. Gunnar RM et al: Hemodynamic studies in shock with myocardial infarction. In *Shock in Myocardial Infarction*, edited by RM Gunnar, HS Loeb, and SH Rahimtoula, Grune and Straton, New York, 1974, p 113.

105. Mueller HS et al: Hemodynamics, coronary blood flow and myocardial metabolism in coronary shock: Response to 1-Norepinephrine and isoproterenol. J Clin Invest. 1970; 49:1885.

106. Tuttle RR et al: The effect of dobutamine on cardiac oxygen balance, regional blood flow, and infarction severity after coronary artery narrowing in dogs. Circulation Research. 1977; 4:357.

107. Cohn J et al: Selection of a vasodilator, inotropic or combined therapy for management of heart failure. Am J Med, 1978; 65:181.

108. Gillespie TA et al: Effects of dobutamine in patients with acute myocardial infarction. Am J Cardiol. 1977; 39:588.

109. Meyer SL et al: Influence of dobutamine on hemodynamics and coronary blood flow in patients with and without coronary artery disease. Am J Cardiol. 1976; 38:103.

110. Tarazi RC: Sympathomimetic agents in the treatment of shock. Ann Intern Med. 1974; 81:364.

111. Safar P: Cardiopulmonary and cerebral resuscitation including emergency airway control. In *Principles and Practice of Emergency Medicine*, edited by GR Schwartz, P Safar, JH Stone, PB Storey, and DK Wagner, Saunders, Philadelphia, 1978, p 177.

112. Mueller HS: Shock following acute myocardial infarction: assessment, pathophysiology, and therapy. CVP. 1980; June/July:19.

113. Kuhn LA: Management of shock following acute myocardial infarction. I. Drug Therapy. Am Heart J. 1978; 95:529.

114. Dymond DS: Inotropic agents. In *Drugs for Heart Disease,* edited by J Hamer, Yearbook Medical, Chicago, 1979, p 318.

115. Schedt S et al: Intra-aortic balloon. Counterpulsation in cardiogenic shock. Report of a co-operative clinical trial. N Engl J Med. 1973; 288:979.

116. Mueller HS et al: Intra-aortic counterpulsation in treatment of myocardial infarction shock. Experience in 51 patients. Circ Shock. 1978; 5:210.

117. O'Rourke MF et al: Randomized controlled trial of intra-aortic balloon counterpulsation in early myocardial infarction with acute heart failure. Am J Cardiol. 1981; 47:815.

118. Johnson SA et al: Treatment of cardiogenic shock in myocardial infarction by intra-aortic balloon counterpulsation and surgery. Am J Med. 1977; 62:687.

119. Kiely J et al: The role of furosemide in the treatment of left ventricular dysfunction associated with acute myocardial infarction. Circulation. 1973; 48:581.

120. Dikshit K et al: Renal and extrarenal hemodynamic effects of furosemide in congestive heart failure after myocardial infarction. N Engl J Med. 1973; 288:1087.

121. Mason DT et al: Treatment of acute and chronic congestive heart failure by vasodilator-afterload reduction. Arch Intern Med. 1980; 140:1577.

122. Raabe DS: Combined therapy with digoxin and nitroprusside in heart failure complicating acute myocardial infarction. Am J Cardiol. 1979; 43:990.

123. Cohn JN et al: Selection of vasodilator, inotropic or combined therapy for the management of heart failure. Am J Med. 1978; 65:181.

124. Cohn JN et al: Nitroprusside. Ann Intern Med. 1979; 91:752.

125. Chattergee K et al: Hemodynamic and metabolic response to vasodilator therapy in acute myocardial infarction. Circulation. 1973; 48:1183.

126. Hempelmann G et al: Changes in hemodynamic parameters, inotropic state, and myocardial oxygen consumption owing to intravenous application of nitroglycerin. J Thorac Cardiovasc Surg. 1977; 73:836.

127. Hill NS et al: Intravenous nitroglycerin. Chest. 1981; 79:69.

128. Williams DO et al: Hemodynamic effects of nitroglycerin in acute myocardial infarction. Decrease in ventricular preload at the expense of cardiac output. Circulation. 1975; 51:421.

129. Flaherty JT et al: Intravenous nitroglycerin in acute myocardial infarction. Circulation. 1975; 51:132.

130. Flaherty JT et al: Effect of intravenous nitroglycerin on left ventricular function and ST segment changes in acute myocardial infarction. Br Heart J. 1976; 38:612.

131. Come PC et al: Reversal by phenylephrine of the beneficial effects of intravenous nitroglycerin in patients with acute myocardial infarction. N Engl J Med. 1975; 293:1003.

132. Mann T et al: Effect of nitroprusside on regional myocardial blood flow in coronary artery disease. Circulation. 1978; 57:732.

133. Maseda J et al: The renal effects of sodium nitroprusside in post-operative cardiac surgical patients. Anesthesiology. 1981; 54:284.

134. Keung ECH et al: Dobutamine therapy in acute myocardial infarction. JAMA. 1981; 245:144.

135. Packer M et al: Rebound hemodynamic events after the abrupt withdrawal of nitroprusside in patients with severe chronic heart failure. N Engl J Med. 1979; 301:1193.

136. Kwaan HM et al: Differences in the mechanism of shock caused by bacterial infections. Surg Gynecol Obstet. 1969; 128:37.

137. Guenter CA et al: Comparison of septic shock due to gram-negative and gram-positive organisms. Proc Soc Exp Biol Med. 1970; 134:780.

138. Shands SJ: Evidence for a bilayer structure in gram-negative lipopolysaccharide: Relationship to toxicity. Infect Immun. 1971; 4:167.

139. Clowes GH et al: Circulating factors in the etiology of pulmonary insufficiency and right heart failure accompanying severe sepsis. Ann Surg. 1970; 171:663.

140. Shoemaker WC: Cardiorespiratory patterns in complicated and uncomplicated septic shock. Ann Surg. 1971; 174:119.

141. Nishijima H et al: Hemodynamic and metabolic studies on shock associated with gram-negative bacteremia. Medicine. 1973; 52:287.

142. Winslow EJ et al: Hemodynamic studies and results of therapy in 50 patients with bacteremic shock. Am J Med. 1973; 54:421.

143. Keighley MRB: Septicaemia and biliary tract obstruction. Scott Med J. 1978; 23:253.

144. Bruni FD et al: Endotoxin and myocardial failure: Role of the myofibril and venous return. Am J Physiol. 1978; 235:H150.

145. Bohrs CT et al: Coronary blood flow alterations in endotoxin shock and the response to dipyridamole. Circ Shock. 1976; 3:281.

146. Dunn MJ et al: The role of assisted circulation in the management of endotoxin shock. Ann Thorac Surg. 1974; 17:574.

147. Rosenberg IK et al: Renal insufficiency after trauma and sepsis. Arch Surg. 103:175.

148. Siegel JH et al: Ventilation: perfusion maldistribution secondary to the hyperdynamic cardiovascular state as the major cause of increased pulmonary shunting in human sepsis. J Trauma. 1979; 19:432.

149. Blair E: Acid-base balance in bacteremic shock. Arch Intern Med. 1971; 127:731.

150. Weitzman S et al: Clinical trials design in studies of corticosteroids for bacterial infections. Ann Intern Med. 1976; 81:36.

151. Hinshaw LB et al: Survival of primates in LD_{100} septic shock following steroid/antibiotic therapy. J Surg Res. 1980; 28:151.

152. Hinshaw LB et al: Recovery from lethal Escherichia coli shock in dogs. Surg Gynecol Obstet. 1979; 149:545.

153. Schumer W: Steroids in the treatment of clinical septic shock. Ann Surg. 1976; 184:333.

154. Hammerschmidt DE et al: Corticosteroids inhibit complement-induced granulocyte aggregation: a possible mechanism for their efficacy in shock states. J Clin Invest. 1979; 63:798.

155. Skubitz KM et al: Corticosteroids block binding of chemotactic peptide to its receptor on granulocytes and cause disaggregation of granulocyte aggregates in vitro. J Clin Invest. 1981; 68:13.

156. Sacks T et al: Oxygen radicals mediate endothelial cell damage by complement-stimulated granulocytes: an in vitro model of immune vascular damage. J Clin Invest. 1978; 61:1161.

157. Sibbald WJ et al: Alveo-capillary permeability in human septic ARDS: effect of high-dose corticosteroid therapy. Chest. 1981; 79:133.

158. Ledingham IM et al: Propsective study of the treatment of septic shock. Lancet. 1978; 2:1194.

159. Samii K et al: Hemodynamic effects of dopamine in septic shock with and without acute renal failure. Arch Surg. 1978; 113:1414.

160. Regnier B et al: Comparative haemodynamic effects of dopamine and dobutamine in septic shock. Intern Care Med. 1979; 5:115.

161. Clowes GHA et al: Septic lung and shock lung in man. Ann Surg. 1975; 181:681.

162. Kreger BE et al: Gram-negative bacteremia IV. Re-evaluation of clinical features and treatment in 612 patients. Am J Med. 1980; 68:344.

163. Staub NC: The pathogenesis of pulmonary edema. Progr Cardiovasc Dis. 1980; 23:53.

164. Ramirez A et al: Cardiac decompensation. N Engl J Med. 1974; 290:499.

165. Vasko JS et al: Mechanisms of action of morphine in the treatment of experimental pulmonary edema. Am J Cardiol. 1966; 18:876.

166. Felis R et al: The cardiovascular effects of morphine: the peripheral capacitance and resistance vessels in human subjects. J Clin Invest. 1974; 54:1247.

167. Lee G et al: Comparative effects of morphine, meperidine and pentazocine on cardiocirculatory dynamics in patients with acute myocardial infarction. Am J Med. 1976; 60:949.

168. Vismara LA et al: The effects of morphine on venous tone in patients with acute pulmonary edema. Circulation. 1976; 54:335.

169. Eckenhoff JE et al: The effects of narcotics and antagonists upon respiration and circulation in man. A review. Clin Pharmacol Ther. 1960; 1:483.

170. Alderman EL et al: Hemodynamic effects of morphine and pentazocine differ in cardiac patients. N Engl J Med. 1972; 287:623.

171. Mond H et al: Hemodynamic effects of furosemide in patients suspected of having acute myocardial infarction. Br Heart J. 1974; 36:44.

172. Davidov M et al: Intravenous administration of furosemide in heart failure. JAMA. 1967; 200:120.

173. Biddle T et al: Effect of furosemide on hemodynamics and lung water in acute pulmonary edema secondary to myocardial infarction. Am J Cardiol. 1979; 43:86.

174. Miller R et al: Pharmacological mechanisms for left ventricular unloading in clinical congestive heart failure: differential effects of nitroprusside, phentolamine and nitroglycerine on cardiac function and peripheral circulation. Cir Res. 1976; 39:127.

175. Awan N et al: Reduction of ST segment elevation in patients with acute myocardial infarction. Am J Cardiol. 1976; 38:435.

176. Da Luz et al: Hemodynamic and metabolic effects of sodium nitroprusside on the performance and metabolism of regional ischemic myocardium. Circulation. 1975; 52:400.

177. Strauer BE et al: Ventricular function and coronary hemodynamics after intravenous nitroglycerine in coronary artery disease.

178. Horowitz LD et al: Effects of nitroglycerine on regional myocardial blood flow in coronary artery disease. J Clin Invest. 1977; 50:1578.

179. Cohen MV et al: The effects of nitroglycerin on coronary collaterals and myocardial contractility. J Clin Invest. 1973; 52;2836.

180. Bussman WD et al: Effect of sublingual nitroglycerine in emergency treatment of severe pulmonary edema. Am J Cardiol. 1978; 41:931.

181. Perret C et al: Phentolamine for vasodilator therapy in left ventricular failure complicating acute myocardial infarction. Br Heart J. 1975; 37:640.

182. Ingram RH et al: Pulmonary edema: cardiogenic and noncardiogenic forms. In *Heart Disease: A Textbook of Cardiovascular Medicine,* Braunwald E, Philadelphia, W.B. Saunders Co, 1980.

183. Bleifield W et al: New and traditional therapy of congestive heart failure. Am J Med. 1978; 65:203.

184. Green LH et al: The use of digitalis in patients with pulmonary disease. Ann Intern Med. 1977; 87:459.

185. Marcus FI. Use of digitalis in acute myocardial infarction. Circulation. 1980; 62:17.

186. Stoner JD et al: Comparison of dobutamine and dopamine in treatment of severe heart failure. Br Heart J. 1977; 39:536.

187. Aberman A et al: The metabolic and respiratory acidosis of acute pulmonary edema. Ann Intern Med. 1972; 76:173.

188. Fulop M et al: Lactic acidosis in pulmonary edema due to left ventricular failure. Ann Intern Med. 1973; 79:180.

189. Amsterdam EA et al: Effects of narcotic analgesics on myocardial contractile function: greater depressant action of pentazocine than morphine or meperidine. Clin Res. 1976; 24:251.

190. Nunn JF: *Applied Respiratory Physiology,* 2nd ed, London, Butterworths, 1977.

191. Michaelis LL et al: Ventricular irritability associated with the use of naloxone hydrochloride: two case reports and laboratory assessment of the effect of the drug on cardiac excitability. Ann Thorac Surg. 1974; 18:608.

192. Tanaka GY: Hypertensive reaction to naloxone. JAMA. 1974; 228:25.

193. Thomas M et al: Hemodynamic effects of morphine in patients with acute myocardial infarction. Br Heart J. 1965; 27:863.

194. Wood-Smith FG et al: *Drugs in Anesthetic Practice,* 4th ed, London, Butterworth, 1973.

195. Malcom AD et al: Cardiocirculatory effects of strong analgesic agents. In *Pain: New Perspectives in Measurement and Management,* Harcus AW, Smith R, Whittle B, eds, Edinburgh, Churchill Livingstone, 1977.

196. Figueras J et al: Hypovolemia and hypotension complicating management of acute pulmonary edema. Am J Cardiol. 1979; 44:1349.

197. Epstein M et al: Potentiation of furosemide by metolazone in refractory edema. Curr Ther Res. 1977; 21:656.

198. Gunstone RF et al: Clinical experience with metolazone in 52 African patients: Synergy with furosemide. Postgrad Med J. 1971; 47:789.

199. McGarry JD et al: Ketogenesis and its regulation. Am J Med. 1976; 61:9.

200. Sherwin RS et al: Effect of diabetes mellitus and insulin on the turnover and metabolic responses to ketones in man. Diabetes. 1976; 25:776.

201. Schade DS et al: The controversy concerning counterregulatory hormone secretion. A hypothesis for the prevention of diabetic ketoacidosis? Diabetes. 1977; 26:596.

202. Felig P: Diabetic Ketoacidosis. N Engl J Med. 1974; 290:1360.

203. DeFronzo RA et al: The effect of insulin on renal handling of sodium, potassium, calcium and phosphate in man. J Clin Invest. 1975; 55:845.

204. Banik SB et al: Diabetic ketoacidosis and coma. Med Clin North Am. 1981; 65:117.

205. Taylor AL: Diabetic ketoacidosis: reassessment of therapeutic truths. Postgrad Med. 1980; 68:161.

206. Katz MA: Hyperglycemia-induced hyponatremia—calculation of expected serum sodium depression. N Engl J Med. 1973; 289:843.

207. Fuise RE: Hyponatremia. Medicine. 1963; 42:149.

208. Duck SC: Cerebral edema complicating therapy for diabetic ketoacidosis. Diabetes. 1976; 25:111.

209. Prockop LD: Hyperglycemia, polyol accumulation, and increased intracranial pressure. Arch Neurol. 1971; 25:126.

210. Arieff AI: Studies on the mechanisms of cerebral edema in diabetic comas. J Clin Invest. 1973; 52:571.

211. Kriisberg RA: Diabetic ketoacidosis: new concepts and trends in pathogenesis and treatment. Ann Intern Med. 1978; 88:681.

212. Martin HE et al: The fluid and electrolyte therapy of severe diabetic acidosis and ketosis. Am J Med. 1956; 20:376.

213. Franks M et al: Metabolic studies in diabetic acidosis. II the effect of the administration of sodium phosphate. Arch Intern Med. 1948; 81:42.

214. Kanter Y et al: 2, 3-Diphosphoglycerate, nucleotide phosphate and organic and inorganic phosphate levels during the early phases of diabetic ketoacidosis. Diabetes. 1977; 26:429.

215. Martin DW et al: Hypophosphatemia. West J Med. 1975; 122:482.

216. Knochel VP: Hypophosphatemia. West J Med. 1981; 134:15.

217. Harter HR et al: The relative role of calcium, phosphorus and parathyroid hormone in glucose and tolbutamide-mediated insulin release. J Clin Invest. 1976; 58:359.

218. Winter RJ et al: Induction of hypocalcemia and hypomagnesemia by phosphate therapy. Am J Med. 1979; 67:897.

219. Zipf WB et al: Hypocalcemia, hypomagnesemia and transient hypoparathyroidism during therapy with potassium phosphate in diabetic ketoacidosis. Diabetes Care. 1979; 2:265.

220. Keller U et al: Prevention of hypophosphatemia by phosphate infusion during treatment of diabetic ketoacidosis and hyperosmolar coma. Diabetes. 1980; 29:87.

221. Barsotti MM. Potassium phosphate and potassium chloride in the treatment of DKA. Diabetes Care. 1980; 3:569.

222. Alberti KGMM et al: Small doses of intramuscular insulin in the treatment of diabetic "coma." Lancet. 1973; 2:515.

223. Kidson W et al: Treatment of severe diabetes mellitus by insulin infusion. Br Med J. 1974; 2:691.

224. Sample PF et al: Continuous intravenous infusions of small doses of insulin in treatment of diabetic ketoacidosis. Br Med J. 1974; 2:694.

225. Page MM et al: Treatment of diabetic coma with continuous low-dose infusion of insulin. Br Med J. 1974; 2:687.

226. Kitabchi AE et al: The efficacy of low-dose versus conventional therapy of insulin for treatment of diabetic ketoacidosis. Ann Intern Med. 1976; 84:633.

227. Soler NG et al: Comparative study of different insulin regimens in management of diabetic ketoacidosis. Lancet. 1975; 2:1221.

228. Fisher JN et al: Diabetic ketoacidosis: low-dose therapy by various routes. N Engl J Med. 1977; 297:238.

229. Madison LL: Low-dose insulin: a plea for caution. N Engl J Med. 1976; 294:393.

230. Edwards GA et al: Effectiveness of low-dose continuous insulin infusion in diabetic ketoacidosis. J Pediatr. 1977; 91:701.

231. Heber D et al: Low-dose continuous insulin therapy for diabetic ketoacidosis. Prospective comparison with conventional insulin therapy. Arch Intern Med. 1977; 137:377.

232. Morris LR et al: Efficacy of low-dose insulin therapy for severely obtunded patients in diabetic ketoacidosis. Diabetes Care. 1980; 3:53.

233. Burghen GA et al: Comparison of high-dose and low-dose insulin by continuous intravenous infusion in the treatment of diabetic ketoacidosis in children. Diabetes Care. 1980; 3:15.

234. Shade DS et al: Dose response to insulin in man. Differential effects on glucose and ketone body regulation. J Clin Endocrinol Metab. 1977; 44:1038.

235. Guerra SMO et al: Comparison of the effectiveness of various routes of insulin injection: insulin levels and glucose response in normal subjects. J Clin Endocrinol Metab. 1976; 42:869.

236. Hirsch JL et al: Clinical significance of insulin absorption by polyvinylchloride infusions systems. Am J Hosp Pharm. 1977; 34:583.

237. Peterson L et al: Insulin absorbence to polyvinylchloride surfaces with implications for constant infusion therapy. Diabetes. 1976; 25:72.

238. Petty G et al: Insulin absorption by glass infusion bottles, polyvinylchloride infusion containers and intravenous tubing. Anesth. 1974; 40:400.

239. Molitch ME et al: Spurious serum creatinine elevations in ketoacidosis. Ann Intern Med. 1980; 93:280.

240. Watkins IJ: The effect of ketone bodies on the determination of creatinine. Clin Chem Octa. 1967; 18:191.

241. Soldin SJ et al: The effect of bilirubin and ketones on reaction rate methods for the measurement of creatinine. Clin Biochem. 1978; 11:82.

242. Anon: Standards and guidelines for cardiopulmonary resuscitation and emergency cardiac care. JAMA. 1980; 244:453.

243. Das G et al: New observations on the effects of atropine on the sinoatrial and atrioventricular nodes in man. Am J Cardiol. 1975; 36:281.

244. Courter SR et al. Advanced atrioventricular block in acute myocardial infarction. Circulation. 1963; 27:1034.

245. Bruce RA et al. Treatment of asystole or heart block during acute myocardial infarction with electrode catheter pacing. Am Heart J. 1965; 69:460.

246. Haynes RE et al. Comparison of Bretylium Tosylate and Lidocaine in Management of Out of Hospital Ventricular Fibrillation: A Randomized Clinical Trial. Am J Cardiol. 1981; 48:353.

247. Redding JS et al. Resuscitation from ventricular fibrillation. JAMA. 1968; 203:255.

248. Livesay JJ et al. Optimizing myocardial supply/demand balance with alpha-adrenergic drugs during cardiopulmonary resuscitation. J Thorac Cardiovasc Surg. 1978; 76:244.

249. Roberts JR et al: Endotracheal epinephrine in cardiorespiratory collapse. J Am Col Emergency Phys. 1979; 8:515.

250. Roberts JR et al: Blood levels following intravenous and endotracheal epinephrine administration. J Am Col Emergency Phys. 1979; 8:53.

251. Fillmore SJ et al: Serial blood gas studies during cardiopulmonary resuscitation. Ann Intern Med. 1970; 72:465.

252. Stewart JSS et al: Cardiac arrest and acidosis. Lancet. 1962; 2:964.

253. Gerst PH et al: A quantitative evaluation of the effects of acidosis and alkalosis upon the ventricular fibrillation threshold. Surgery. 1966; 59:1050.

254. Marsigliz JC et al: Relevance of beta receptor blockade to negative inotropic effect induced by metabolic acidosis. Cardiovasc Res. 1973; 7:336.

255. Thrower WB et al: Acid-base derangements and myocardial contractibility. Effects as a complication of shock. Am Med Assoc Arch Surg. 1961; 82:56.

256. Mattor JA et al: Cardiac arrest in the critically ill. II. Hyperosmolal states following cardiac arrest. Am J Med. 1974; 56:162.

257. Brown DC et al: Asystole and its treatment: the possible role of the parasympathetic nervous system in cardiac arrest. J Am Col Emergency Phys. 1979; 8:448.

258. Bigger JT et al: Management of cardiac problems in the intensive care unit. Med Clin North Am. 1971; 55:1183.

259. Bishop RL et al: Sodium bicarbonate administration during cardiac arrest; effect on arterial pH, pCO_2, and osmolality. JAMA. 1976; 235:506.

260. Cohen MR et al: Definitive therapy in cardiopulmonary resuscitation; part 2. Hosp Pharm. 1974; 9:208.

261. Escher DJW et al: Emergency treatment of cardiac arrhythmias. JAMA. 1970; 214:2028.

262. Goldberg AH: Cardiopulmonary arrest. Med Intelligence. 1974; 290:381.

263. Greenblatt DJ et al: Pharmacotherapy of cardiopulmonary arrest. Am J Hosp Pharm. 1976; 33:579.

264. Harner RH et al: Resistant ventricular tachycardias and recurrent cardiac arrest. Chest. 1977; 24:426.

265. Heissenbutter RH: Bretylium tosylate: A newly available antiarrhythmic drug for ventricular arrhythmias. Ann Intern Med. 1979; 91:229.

266. McIntyre KM et al: Pathophysiologic syndromes of cardiopulmonary resuscitation. Arch Intern Med. 1978; 138:1130.

267. Rotman M et al: Bradyarrhythmias in acute myocardial infarction. Circulation. 1972; 45:703.

268. Zoll PM: Rational use of the drugs for cardiac arrest and after cardiac resuscitation. Am J Cardiol. 1971; 27:645.

Chapter 15

Thrombosis

Steven R. Kayser

Arterial and venous thromboembolism contribute to many of the leading causes of death in the United States. In addition, adverse reactions to oral anticoagulants are frequent causes of hospital admissions. It is important to consider the risks of adverse reaction whenever anticoagulants are utilized. In order to minimize this risk, a working understanding of the pharmacology of anticoagulants, the physiologic and pathologic processes of blood coagulation, and their laboratory evaluation is essential.

In recent years there have been several significant therapeutic additions to the treatment of thromboembolic events. Fibrinolytic agents such as urokinase and streptokinase facilitate the dissolution of emboli. Drugs which inhibit platelet activity have been found useful for selected indications. And finally, a better understanding of heparin and the oral anticoagulants now allows more effective treatment of thromboembolic disease.

When selecting and evaluating a course of antithrombotic therapy, there are several general principles to consider. Among these, one should: (a) Consider the indication for therapy. When did the event occur? Is it likely to respond to the proposed course of therapy? (b) Consider the anticipated duration of therapy. Is it likely that the course of therapy will be appropriate for a particular patient's condition? (c) Clearly define the expected therapeutic objectives and endpoints and consider the risks of the proposed therapy and the risks of failing to treat. (d) Consider other conditions present in the patient which might deter his response to therapy. (e) Consider the presence of other drugs and whether they present a risk to therapy. If so, what alternatives are there? (f) Consider any changes which may occur in any of the above factors over time. Consider not only those factors which might affect a course of therapy, but which might affect subsequent recurrence of disease following a course of therapy.

Clot Formation

The formation of a firm fibrin clot is the result of a complex series of events. Tissue injury, with release of adenosine diphosphate (ADP), thrombin, or epinephrine, or exposure of collagen and other subendothelial surfaces, may stimulate the initial adhesion of platelets. Subsequent granular release of additional ADP causes circulating platelets to adhere to those already adherent, producing platelet aggregates (1) (see Fig. 1).

Activation of phospholipase in the platelet membrane leads to splitting of arachidonic acid from platelet membrane phospholipid. Arachidonic acid is the precursor of several prostaglandins which may affect platelet function. Thromboxane A_2 (TXA_2), the most potent inducer of platelet release and aggregation known, is synthesized in the presence of an enzyme found in platelet microsomes. Prostacyclin A_2 (pGI_2), an inhibitor of platelet aggregation, is synthesized by an enzyme found in arteries and veins.

The initial control of thrombogenesis is thus a result of a balance between stimulation of aggregation by several different mechanisms and inhibition by prostacyclin.

Transformation of the platelet plug to a permanent fibrin clot is achieved through activation of the extrinsic or intrinsic blood clotting system (see Fig. 2).

Each of the clotting factors exists in the blood in the inactive form and must be converted to an active (a) or enzymatic form before further clotting is stimulated. Injury to blood vessels or surface contact of collagen initiates the intrinsic pathway by stimulating the activation of factor XII. Activated factor XII then stimulates the conversion of factor XI to its active form, which then stimulates the activation of factor IX. Activated factor IX, in the presence of calcium, phospholipids (platelet factor III), and factor VIII, stimulates the conversion of factor X to its active form. Activated factor X, in the presence of Ca^{++}, phospholipid (platelet factor III), and factor V, stimulates the conversion of prothrombin (factor II) to thrombin (factor IIa) (2).

The conversion of prothrombin to thrombin may also be achieved through the extrinsic clotting pathway. The release of material extrinsic to the blood, such as tissue extract or tissue thromboplastin, activates factor VII, which stimulates the activation of factor X. Factor X thus occupies a central position at the junction of the extrinsic and intrinsic systems.

Thrombin, which is generated by either pathway, stimulates the conversion of fibrinogen to fibrin in the presence of ionized calcium. The initial soluble fibrin clot is further converted to an insoluble fibrin polymer when factor XIII is activated by thrombin (3). In addition to stimulating the conversion of fibrinogen to fibrin, thrombin stimulates further platelet aggregation and potentiates the activity of factors V, VIIa, VIII, and Xa.

Once thrombin is formed, it is partly removed by absorption into fibrin. This, plus other naturally occurring inhibitors of clotting factors, plays a role in localizing fibrin formation to the sites of injury and in maintaining the fluidity of circulating blood. Agents have been identified in normal blood which inhibit the activated forms of factors II, X, XI, and XII (4). The deposition of fibrin is also associated with activation of plasmin or fibrinolysin, a fibrinolytic enzyme which also prevents excessive coagulation (see Fig. 3).

Pathologic thrombi are often referred to as white thrombi or red thrombi. *White thrombi,* or arterial thrombi, are composed primarily of platelets, although they also contain fibrin and occasional leukocytes (5). They generally occur in areas of rapid blood flow and are formed in response to an injured or abnormal vessel wall.

Red thrombi, or stasis thrombi, are primarily found in the venous circulation and are almost entirely composed of fibrin and erythrocytes. They have a small platelet head, and they form in areas of stasis when dilution of activated blood coagulation factors by blood flow is prevented.

The selection of an antithrombotic agent may thus be influenced by the type of thrombus which is to be treated. Streptokinase, urokinase, heparin, and the coumarins are presently used to treat both white and red thrombi. Drugs altering platelet function have been investigated for their role in the prevention of thromboembolic disease associated with white emboli.

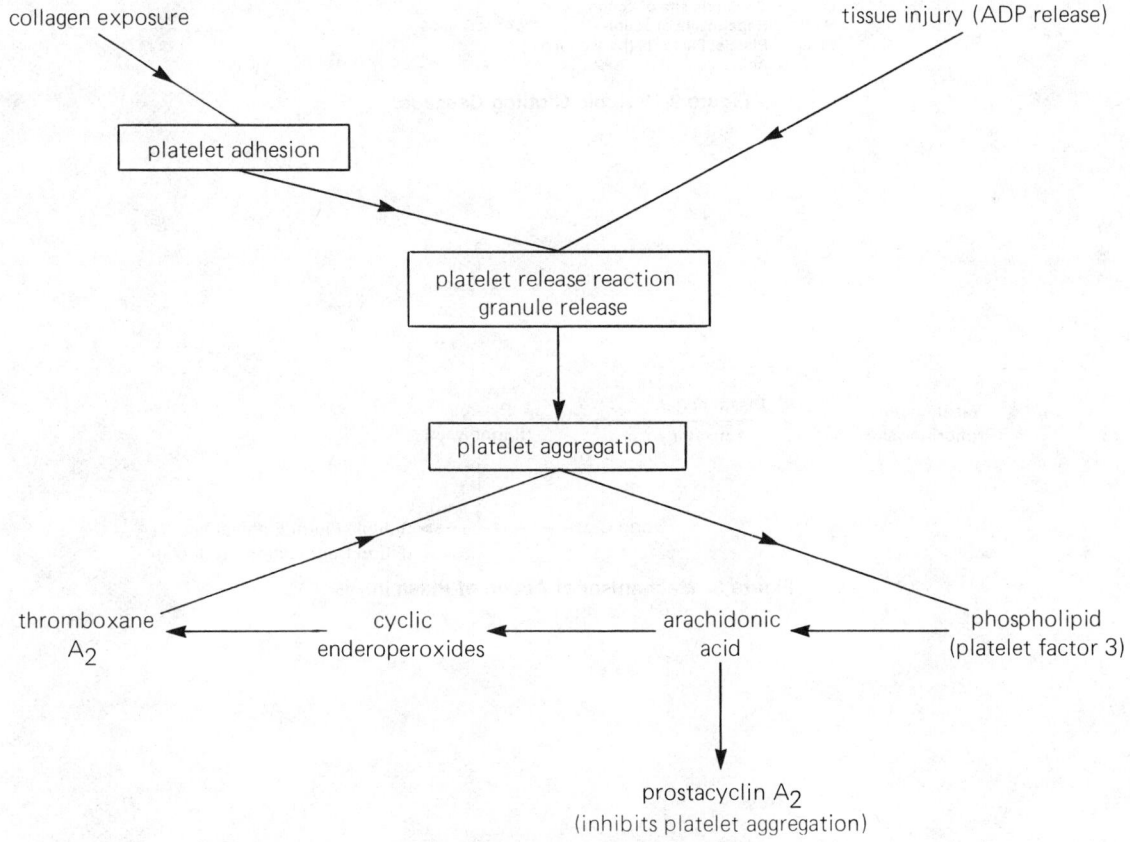

Figure 1. Formation of Platelet Plug.

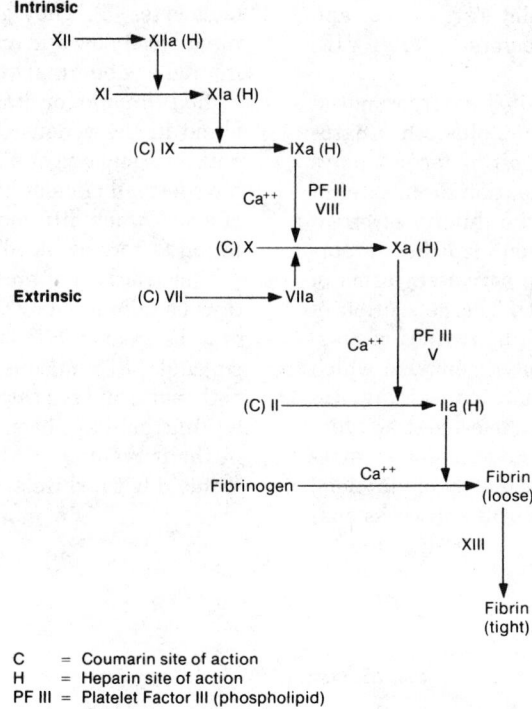

C = Coumarin site of action
H = Heparin site of action
PF III = Platelet Factor III (phospholipid)
a = Activated

Figure 2. Soluble Clotting Cascade.

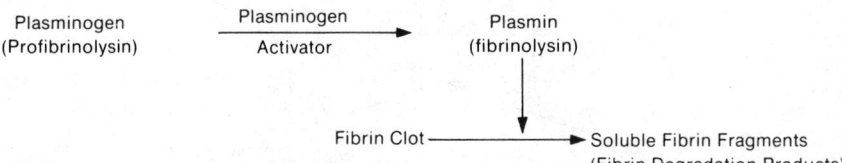

Figure 3. Mechanism of Action of Plasmin.

Anticoagulant Pharmacology

Heparin. Heparin is a rapid-acting anticoagulant that is effective only when administered parenterally (18). It prevents clot formation by accelerating the action of a naturally occurring inhibitor of thrombin, antithrombin III. The resulting conformational change in antithrombin III leads to rapid inhibition of thrombin (19,20). Antithrombin also neutralizes the activated forms of factors XII, XI, IX, X, and probably VII, and this effect is also accelerated by heparin. The effect that heparin has on platelets may vary. Heparin has been reported to increase, decrease, or have no effect on platelet activity. It has been claimed that platelets in normal subjects given heparin obtained from beef lung showed slower aggregation than those from subjects who had been given heparin obtained from hog mucosa (21). However, this has been disputed (22). While the effect of heparin *in vivo* on platelets is debatable (19,23), there does not appear to be conclusive evidence indicating a therapeutic advantage for one source over another.

The anticoagulant half-life of heparin is 1½ hours (24,25). Following intravenous administration of heparin, an anticoagulant effect is noted immediately. Heparin is primarily metabolized in the liver, and only a small fraction is eliminated unchanged in the urine (26). Heparin may be administered intravenously or subcutaneously. Intramuscular administration should be avoided because of the potential for hematoma formation (27).

Heparin therapy is aimed at achieving a clotting time which is 1½ to 2½ the control value. Several tests may be used, but the APTT or ACT tests offer the best correlation for control of heparin therapy (15,16) (Table 1).

Oral Anticoagulants. Vitamin K is essential for the hepatic synthesis of four circulating proteins required for the formation of a clot (28). These factors are II, VII, IX, and X.

It was originally proposed that vitamin K and the coumarins act as simple competitive antagonists (29,30). The interaction is more complex than this, despite the fact that within a limited dosage range, the effect of either substance can overcome the effect of the other. The vitamin K-dependent clotting factors synthesized in the presence of oral anticoagulants are antigenically similar to those synthesized in the absence of anticoagulants; however, they lack biologic activity because of their inability to bind calcium ions (31–33).

During the process of activation, vitamin K is oxidized to vitamin K oxide (epoxide). In the normal non-anticoagulated individual, vitamin K oxide is in reversible equilibrium with vitamin K. Oral anticoagulants act by interfering with the cyclic interconversion of vitamin K and vitamin K oxide (epoxide) (28). The accumulation of vitamin K oxide reduces the effective concentration of vitamin K and prevents the synthesis of normal prothrombin (factor II). Abnormal coumarin-induced forms of factors IX and X have also been identified.

Warfarin is completely absorbed in the upper gastrointestinal tract by passive diffusion. However, bishydroxycoumarin is poorly and variably absorbed; 15 to 30% is recovered in the stool as unchanged drug (34,35). Peak absorption of both warfarin and bishydroxycoumarin occurs in 60 to 120 minutes (36). The volume of distribution (Vd) for warfarin and high doses of bishydroxycoumarin is about the same: 12.5% of body weight. This small volume of distribution is consistent with the extensive binding of warfarin to albumin, since it is equivalent to the Vd for albumin, or 2.6 times the plasma volume.

The mean half-life of warfarin is 42 hours and is independent of dose. In contrast, the half-life of bishydroxycoumarin is 24 hours and is dependent upon the plasma concentration (35). Both warfarin and bishydroxycoumarin are highly protein bound; warfarin is approximately 99% bound to serum albumin (262). Nevertheless, no apparent relationship exists between the extent of protein binding of warfarin and the concentration of albumin or total protein in the serum (37). Furthermore, among individuals there appears to be no correlation between the prothrombin time and the dose of warfarin, total warfarin concentration, or free warfarin concentration.

The coumarins are metabolized in the hepatic microsomes by mixed function oxidase enzymes. Warfarin is administered as a racemate containing equal parts of the enantiomers R(+)-warfarin and S(−)-warfarin. The S-isomer is approximately five times more potent as an anticoagulant than is the R-isomer (38). S-warfarin is oxidized to 7-hydroxywarfarin and reduced to an alcohol 2 (RS alcohol), whereas R-warfarin is metabolized primarily by reduction to alcohol 1 (RS alcohol). Both racemates are metabolized to 6-hydroxywarfarin in small amounts. The warfarin alcohols have minimal anticoagulant activity and are excreted renally (39–42). The hydroxylated products are inactive and are eliminated only by metabolism.

The reason why the R and S isomers differ in potency is unclear. Differences in permeability or affinity to the receptor site may account for the differing potencies. The half-life of the R-isomer is 45 hours, and the half-life of the S-isomer is 33 hours. They both have the same volumes of distribution (40).

Drugs, such as phenylbutazone (38), metronidazole, and trimethoprim-sulfamethoxazole (209), interact with warfarin stereoselectively. They inhibit the S-isomer but have no effect on the R-isomer. Long-term warfarin therapy in thrombotic disease may be made safer in the future by the administration of the R-isomer alone since it does not appear to interact with other drugs to the same extent as the racemic mixture.

Tests Used to Monitor Antithrombotic Therapy

The **bleeding time** is a measure of platelet aggregation and capillary contraction; it is of little value in monitoring anticoagulant therapy (6) or antiplatelet drug therapy. Simple clotting factor deficiencies result in a normal bleeding time. The normal bleeding time is 2½–7 minutes.

The **whole blood clotting time (WBCT)**, or **Lee-White clotting time**, is now used infrequently because it lacks sensitivity. It is usually normal in the presence of factor VII deficiency. It is an insensitive measure of prothrombin deficiency and is only moderately sensitive in measuring thromboplastin generation or fibrin formation (7). The clotting time by this method depends greatly on the size and types of tubes used, the temperature, degree of agitation, type of blood used (i.e., venous or capillary), and the skill of the laboratory technician. The normal clotting time is less than 15 minutes (18). (See Table 1.)

The **prothrombin time (PT)** of Quick (8) is prolonged by deficiencies of factors V, VII, X, and II; by low levels of fibrinogen; and by high levels of heparin (9). It reflects alterations in the extrinsic system and the common clotting pathway, but not the intrinsic system. The normal prothrombin time is 12 ± 0.5 seconds. An individual patient's prothrombin time is compared to a control or standard curve determined by various dilutions of commercially available thromboplastin. Therapeutic prothrombin times are in the range of 1½ to 2½ times the control value. Prothrombin times have also been reported as percent activity (10). This should be avoided because of the risk of confusing a percentage activity with prothrombin time in seconds. The prothrombin time is very sensitive to changes in factor VII, and because factor VII has the shortest half-life

Table 1.

TESTS USED TO MONITOR ANTICOAGULANT THERAPY

Test	Factors Measured	Normal Value*	Drug Monitored
WBCT (Lee-White)	All except VII	9–14 min	Heparin
Prothrombin Time (PT)	II, V, VII, X	12 ± 0.5 sec	Warfarin
Partial Thromboplastin Time (PTT)	All except VII	60–85 sec	Warfarin, Heparin[+]
Activated Partial Thromboplastin Time (APTT)	All except VII	24–36 sec	Warfarin, Heparin[+]
Activated Coagulation Time (ACT)	All except VII	80–130 sec	Heparin

*University of California, San Francisco

[+]Primary drug monitored

of the clotting factors affected by warfarin, the prothrombin time serves as an effective means for monitoring the response to warfarin.

The **partial thromboplastin time (PTT)** reflects deficiencies of all the plasma coagulation factors except factors VII and XIII (11) and thus measures deficiencies in the intrinsic pathway. Since the test is performed with platelet-poor plasma, it does not reflect the role of platelets in clotting. It has been used to measure the response to oral anticoagulants (12), but it is not very sensitive to heparin (13). It is primarily used to screen for deficiencies in clotting factors of the intrinsic system in patients being considered for oral anticoagulant therapy. The normal PTT is 60 to 85 seconds. If platelets are present, or if the test is performed more than one hour after collection, values that are unexpectedly low may be observed (14).

The **activated partial thromboplastin time (APTT)** is sensitive to deficiencies of all the plasma coagulation factors except factors VII and XIII. It is generally a more sensitive test than the PTT, and it is widely used to monitor heparin therapy (15). The APTT correlates well with the Lee-White clotting test but is more sensitive. Its advantage over the Lee-White method is that it can be performed within a few minutes. This test, like the PTT, is performed with platelet-poor plasma; thus it does not reflect the activity of platelets. Normal values for the APTT may vary but are usually between 24 and 36 seconds. Therapeutic values are 1½ to 2½ times the control APTT.

The **activated coagulation time (ACT)** of whole blood measures all of the factors except factor VII; its sensitivity to factors V and II has not been established. Since it is a whole blood test, it reflects the role of platelets in coagulation. The test is used to monitor heparin therapy and can be performed at the bedside (16,17). Normal values are 80 to 130 seconds (see Table 1).

The **thrombin time** is a test used to determine fibrinogen concentration and is useful in detecting the presence of fibrin and fibrinogen degradation products. The time required for a patient's plasma to clot after the addition of thrombin is compared to that of a normal plasma control. A value of 3 seconds or more longer than the control is considered abnormal. Since deficiencies of thrombin or the presence of fibrin or fibrinogen degradation products may prolong it, it is useful in assessing fibrinolytic status (14).

HEPARIN AND WARFARIN

1. *Pulmonary Embolus.* M.S. is a 38-year-old, 70 kg male with a 5-year history of ulcerative colitis. During his present hospitalization for treatment of bowel disease, he developed a swollen left calf which was painful and warm. This swelling gradually increased, affecting the entire left leg to the groin. Several days later he noted the onset of right-sided pleuritic chest pain without shortness of breath or hemoptysis.

Past medical history included a gastric ulcer in 1966 treated medically without recurrence. Physical examination revealed a pleasant, obese male with an enlarged left leg and mild to moderate tenderness in the entire leg. Chest examination revealed a loud P_2. Vital signs showed a blood pressure of 150/85 mmHg, a pulse of 100 beats/min, and a respiratory rate which was 22/min and regular.

Laboratory data revealed a hematocrit of 26.7% (normal 42–52%), erythrocyte sedimentation rate of 91 mm/hr (normal 1–13 mm/hr), arterial blood gases (on room air) as follows: pO_2 72 mmHg (75–100), pCO_2 35 mmHg (35–45), pH 7.48 (7.35–7.45). Chest X-ray and lung scan were highly suggestive of pulmonary embolism. An angiogram was not performed. ECG showed sinus tachycardia. Venogram was positive for the presence of defects in the ileofemoral artery.

Coagulation tests included a prothrombin time of 11.2 seconds (11.5–12.5), activated partial thromboplastin time of 28 seconds (24–36), activated clotting time of 90 seconds (80–130), and a platelet count of 248,000/mm³ (150,000–350,000).

What subjective and objective evidence in this patient are compatible with a pulmonary embolus?

The clinical diagnosis of pulmonary embolism is often difficult to make because of the nonspecificity of symptoms. Experience from the Urokinase Pulmonary Embolism Trial and the Urokinase-Streptokinase Embolism Trial has provided some helpful guidelines in utilizing the history and physical examination in establishing the presence of acute pulmonary embolism in patients without preexisting cardiac or pulmonary disease. The most frequently observed symptoms were dyspnea (84%), pleuritic pain (74%), apprehension (63%), and cough (50%). Hemoptysis occurred in only 28%. The signs most frequently observed were tachypnea at a rate of 20/min or more (85%), tachycardia of 100 beats/min or more (58%), accentuated pulmonary component of the second heart sound (57%), and rales (56%). Deep venous thrombosis was present in 41% of patients (44). A combination of these signs and symptoms provides further evidence for acute pulmonary embolism. Based on these criteria, documentation exists for the presence of pulmonary embolism in M.S.

Lung scans and pulmonary angiograms are useful laboratory procedures in documenting the presence of pulmonary embolism. A positive lung scan (M.S. had one highly suggestive of pulmonary embolism) and a positive pulmonary angiogram would confirm the presence of a pulmonary embolism. In any case, when a diagnosis of pulmonary embolism or deep venous thrombosis of the thigh or ileo-femoral region is suspected, heparin should be initiated since it does not interfere with the measures used in diagnosis and it helps to ensure more rapid anticoagulation if the diagnosis is confirmed.

2. What measures might have prevented the development of pulmonary embolus in this patient?

There are many risk factors for the development of deep venous thrombosis and pulmonary embolism. Most of them are the result of trauma to the vessel wall, abnormalities of circulating blood, or stasis. Injury is of course best prevented by proper attention to avoiding trauma in susceptible patients. Stasis may occur secondary to prolonged bedrest, obesity, recent surgery, or sitting in one position, such as in a car, for a prolonged time. Wearing of supportive stockings or occasional moving about of the limbs as well as early ambulation of post-surgical patients are useful in preventing stasis. Hypercoagulability may occur as a result of certain medical problems. Prevention with low-dose heparin is discussed in Question 10.

In the case of M.S., elevation of his legs, the wearing of support stockings, and ambulation all may have been helpful in preventing the subsequent pulmonary embolism.

3. What additional baseline laboratory data should be obtained, and what precautions should be undertaken prior to administration of anticoagulants to this patient?

In addition to those parameters already obtained, one should obtain a complete blood count, urinalysis, stool sample for occult blood, liver function panel, and type and crossmatch of blood. It is extremely important, not only in the acute management, but in the long-term management to have baselines upon which to compare parameters likely to be used in monitoring therapy.

4. *Initiation of Heparin Therapy.* How should heparin therapy be initiated in M.S.?

Heparin should be administered immediately when there is a high suspicion that a pulmonary embolism has occurred (45). Intravenous doses of 5,000 to 15,000 units of heparin are administered after baseline clotting tests are obtained (46). Initial heparin resistance may exist that is partially due to the release of platelet factor 4, a protein within platelets that neutralizes heparin and is released during a thrombotic event (47). Larger doses of the drug may be necessary to overcome the enhanced platelet-thrombin interaction (48).

Once the initial drug is administered, continuous infusions of heparin may be started. A minimum heparin dose of 35–50 units/kg is required to anticoagulate blood to a clinically desirable level (24). Since the patient weighs 70 kg, it will be necessary to maintain a level of 2,450 to 3,500 units in the body at all times. Because the half-life of heparin is 1½ hours, the infusion can be started at the rate of 1,225 to 1,750 units every 1½ hours, or 900–1,200 units every hour, after an initial loading dose. Therapy should be monitored closely; any deviation in laboratory control can be adjusted by altering the rate of infusion. The heparin solution should be administered through a constant infusion pump or controller, not by gravity flow, in order to avoid changes in the flow rate due to altered patient position and to minimize the chance of nursing error.

Because there is an initial insensitivity to heparin treatment of pulmonary embolism (49), a return to normal sensitivity and a decrease in dose requirement should be anticipated over time. Frequent (at least daily) laboratory assessment of clotting tests will enable detection of these changes.

In addition to assessment of clotting tests, resolution of symptoms (both from history and physical examination), blood gases, and other laboratory tests (lung scan, stool guaiac, urinalysis, CBC) should be monitored. Observation of infusion sites and venipunctures for oozing of blood is also important.

Heparin therapy in this patient must be approached with extreme care because of his ulcerative colitis. Fibrinolytic agents, contraindicated in him, would be a good choice in another patient with his symptoms.

5. How effective are the use of coagulation tests in monitoring the therapeutic and toxic effects of anticoagulation? What degree of prolongation is desireable?

Most clinicians feel that it is necessary to monitor coagulation tests so that embolism and hemorrhage can be prevented (51–54). However, some clinicians do not agree and consider testing to be superfluous. Early studies indicated that maintenance of clotting times in excess of twice control provided optimal protection against experimentally-induced thrombi in dogs (55,62).

Several investigations have shown that a continuous infusion of heparin (in doses which maintain the APTT between 1½ and 2½ times the control level) safely and effectively prevents venous thromboembolism (15,56). This method of administration also decreases the incidence of hemorrhage (57–59), although agreement is not universal.

Sevitt and Innes (60) studied patients who were being treated with oral anticoagulants to prevent thromboembolism. When they compared the prothrombin times of those patients who were treated successfully to those patients who were not, they found that prothrombin values which were less than two times the control correlated with treatment failure. Successful therapy correlated with prothrombin values greater than two times the control; however, no therapeutic advantage was observed when prothrombin times were greater than three times the control value.

Hemorrhage from anticoagulation is frequently, but not always, associated with excessive hypoprothrombinemia. A review of hemorrhagic complications secondary to anticoagulant therapy by Coon and Willis (61) revealed that more than two thirds of all hemorrhagic complications occurred when the PT was more than two times baseline activity. They concluded that while fewer thromboembolic complications occur when prothrombin times are maintained at twice normal or more, this is also the range associated with a greater incidence of hemorrhage. However, the

morbidity and mortality associated with hemorrhage are far less than that associated with inadequately treated thromboembolic disease.

In conclusion, it is reasonable to control anticoagulant therapy with an appropriate laboratory test, because the response to a given dose of heparin or warfarin can generally be correlated with a specific value. Maintenance of the selected clotting parameter between 1½ and 2½ times the control value appears to provide the greatest protection against embolization with minimal risk of hemorrhage. However, even in this range, bleeding complications cannot always be avoided, especially in postoperative patients.

6. Besides observing for signs and symptoms of bleeding, what subjective and objective parameters should be monitored for adverse heparin side effects?

The development of osteoporosis has been associated with the administration of more than 10,000 units of heparin for six months or longer (80,81). The size of the dose appears to be more important than the duration of therapy. The incidence of osteoporosis as a result of anticoagulant therapy is low, and this condition may reflect the more common use of oral coumarin anticoagulants (rather than heparin) in the long-term treatment of thromboembolic disease.

Other problems of heparin therapy include generalized hypersensitivity reactions such as rhinitis, urticaria, conjunctivitis, and a reversible temporal alopecia (82).

Heparin may interfere with aldosterone secretion and cause hypoaldosteronism (83). This can occur in healthy and edematous salt-restricted patients who receive 30,000–40,000 units of heparin per day. It usually takes four to five days for this rare side effect to become apparent and a corresponding time for aldosterone levels to return to normal. These patients should be monitored for elevated serum potassium levels.

Thrombocytopenia secondary to heparin administration was first recognized in the early 1960's. Recently it has been reported with increased frequency in patients receiving heparin of bovine lung source (84–90). It characteristically occurs after 3 to 12 days of therapy, is unrelated to dose, may be related to complement-mediated platelet injury, and resolves 3 to 5 days after heparin is discontinued. Since thrombocytopenia increases the risk for bleeding in patients already receiving an anticoagulant, it is important to carefully look for its occurrence with frequent platelet counts and blood smears.

7. *Duration of Therapy.* How long should anticoagulant therapy be continued in this patient?

Little agreement exists regarding the duration of anticoagulant therapy in the treatment of pulmonary embolism. Most studies which have looked at this problem have been uncontrolled or have looked retrospectively at patients over a time when diagnostic criteria and techniques were changing. Available evidence indicates that therapy should continue six weeks to six months after the embolic event (50,63,64). If there is no past history of venous thromboembolism, no recurrent thrombotic tendency, and no continuing predisposing cause, it is unnecessary to continue treatment beyond six weeks. If any of these, or any other risk factors exist, treatment may then be indicated for longer.

Anticoagulants should be continued in M.S. until he has become fully ambulatory and there is evidence of resolution (eg, return of blood gases to normal and normalization of chest X-ray and lung scan). If leg swelling should continue, he may be at risk for further stasis-induced clotting, and therapy may need to be continued for a longer period; lifetime therapy may even be required.

8. *Switching to Warfarin Therapy.* In order to provide adequate treatment for M.S.'s pulmonary embolus, oral anticoagulant therapy is planned. What is the best method for switching this patient from heparin to warfarin?

Heparin therapy should be continued for 7 to 10 days following a pulmonary embolus. Since the onset of warfarin's anticoagulant effect is delayed, both heparin and warfarin may be given simultaneously from the first day, or alternatively warfarin may be started on the third to the fifth day of heparin therapy (91).

Heparin and maintenance doses of warfarin are administered concurrently until a therapeutic prothrombin time is reached. However, care must be taken to measure the prothrombin time when heparin's effect is at a minimum, since heparin may interfere with determination of the one-stage prothrombin time (91). When heparin is administered on an intermittent basis, the prothrombin time should be measured just before the next dose of heparin. With continuous-infusion heparin, the

prothrombin time may be monitored at any time during the infusion. There may be a prolongation of one or two seconds in the prothrombin time during continuous infusion (57). Low-dose subcutaneous heparin may cause transient prolongation in the PT, but only immediately after administration.

Administration of warfarin from the first day of heparinization, or as soon as the patient is stable, would be the preferred method for M.S. This would shorten the overall time required to achieve a therapeutic prothrombin time.

9. Should M.S. receive an initial loading dose of warfarin?

As previously described, warfarin interferes with the synthesis of clotting factors. Its onset of activity is dependent upon its own pharmacokinetics and upon the rate of elimination of already circulating clotting factors since warfarin has no effect on these. The half-lives of the four vitamin K-dependent clotting factors are 5 hours for factor VII, 60 hours for factor II, and 20–40 hours for factors IX and X (93).

Studies using a traditional loading dose (1.5 mg/kg) versus a maintenance dose (10 or 15 mg daily) have shown that in the first 48 hours there is less factor VII activity with a loading dose and also a greater prolongation of the prothrombin time (94). Factor VII is not only the vitamin K-dependent clotting factor with the shortest half-life but is also the factor to which the prothrombin time is most sensitive. Rapid prolongation of the prothrombin time really only reflects rapid depletion of this factor and does not reflect adequate protection from thromboembolism, since it has been shown that factors IX and X are more important in the pathogenesis of thromboembolic disease (95,96). Additionally, the study comparing dosage regimens shows that there are no significant differences between the methods with respect to maximum suppression of any of the four factors.

Administration of 10 mg warfarin per day would be the regimen of choice for M.S. He should be followed closely with daily prothrombin times in order to recognize any unusual sensitivity to warfarin. If there is a rapid prolongation of the prothrombin time (greater than 2–3 seconds per day) the dosage must be decreased or withheld.

10. *Low-Dose Heparin.* Because M.S.'s ulcerative colitis presents an increased risk for

bleeding, the question of low-dose subcutaneous heparin is raised. What is the basis for this regimen, and would it be appropriate for this patient?

The majority of low-dose heparin studies have focused on surgical procedures. Patients are at a higher risk for deep venous thrombosis during the postoperative period and continue to be at risk until at least the seventh postoperative day (65). Studies using ^{125}I fibrinogen have shown that approximately 20–30% of all surgical patients, 40–50% of elderly surgical patients, and more than 50% of patients who undergo hip-nailing procedures or prostatectomies develop postoperative venous thrombosis (66).

Some have postulated that if the hypercoagulable state that occurs in the postoperative period can be prevented, embolism can be prevented (65,66,68). This theory serves as the basis for the administration of low-dose subcutaneous heparin to prevent venous thrombosis. The International Multicenter Trial, published in 1975, provides strong evidence for the efficacy of this procedure (68). While the design of the trial may be criticized, the results do show clinically significant benefits in reduction of venous thrombosis and pulmonary embolism with low doses of subcutaneous heparin. Furthermore, this form of heparin therapy is associated with a small, generally insignificant risk of bleeding (66,69).

Low-dose heparin is most effective for elective gynecological or abdomino-thoracic surgery (66,75). Prevention of venous thromboembolism with low-dose heparin is less effective after hip fracture (66), elective hip surgery (74), or prostatic surgery. Low-dose heparin may also be useful in prophylaxis of venous thromboembolism in certain high-risk medical patients (67,71,72).

The use of heparin in low subcutaneous doses augments the activity of an inhibitor of activated factor X (69). This inhibitor of factor Xa, or anti-Xa, is probably the same as antithrombin III (73).

The protocols for low-dose heparin generally recommend that 5000 units of heparin be administered subcutaneously from 2 to 12 hours preoperatively and that this dose be continued every 8 to 12 hours for five to seven days post-operatively, or until the patient is fully mobile. APTT values indicate that the clotting time is moderately elevated for approximately five hours after 5,000 units of heparin has been administered subcutaneously (66).

When heparin is administered subcutaneously (usually in the fat of the abdomen), it is important that the area of injection not be traumatized because of the risk for bleeding. Heparin should not be administered intramuscularly because of the risk of hematoma formation.

Low-dose heparin therapy has been compared with adjusted dose warfarin therapy in the treatment of deep-vein thrombosis (DVT) and pulmonary embolism (PE), but conflicting results have been obtained (74,77). In a trial which included both non-surgical and surgical patients (74), none of the warfarin- or heparin-treated patients with calf-vein thrombosis developed recurrence. Forty-seven percent of the group with proximal-vein thrombosis receiving heparin developed recurrence versus no recurrences in the patients treated with warfarin. A study in medical patients (77) showed no difference in recurrence rate (undefined location of clot) between the heparin- and warfarin-treated groups. A recent study of 106 patients with venographically diagnosed proximal deep-vein thrombosis evaluated the role of adjusted-dose subcutaneous heparin therapy for three months versus warfarin therapy for three months. Patients were randomly assigned to treatment groups after 14 days of conventional high-dose intravenous heparin therapy. Subcutaneous heparin doses (every 12 hours) were established in the hospital. The dose shown to maintain the mid-interval APTT at 1½ times the control value was subsequently administered without further laboratory control. Neither group had a thromboembolic event during therapy. Bleeding occurred nine times more often in patients who received warfarin (3 major, 6 minor events) (264).

The freedom from bleeding in patients given low-dose heparin is advantageous. However, the risk of thrombocytopenia, the need for frequent injection, and the cost are disadvantages. More careful control of warfarin may help reduce the incidence of bleeding.

The results of these studies are encouraging, but several questions remain unanswered, particularly the efficacy of subcutaneous heparin in the treatment of pulmonary embolism.

The use of low-dose heparin would be a desirable regimen in M.S. because of his risk for hemorrhage. However, this therapy should not be used until its efficacy is proven in the treatment of pulmonary embolism.

11. Change in Prothrombin Time. Institution of warfarin therapy during M.S.'s hospital stay resulted in the following response:

Day	1	2	3	4	5	
PT(sec)	10.8	11.2	14.8	15.9	18.2	
Dose (mg)	10	10	10	7.5	7.5	

Day	6	7	8	9	10	11
PT(sec)	18.8	19.6	22.3	23.4	23.2	22.6
Dose (mg)	7.5	7.5	7.5	7.5	7.5	7.5

On day 11 he was discharged with the following medications: warfarin 7.5 mg every evening, ampicillin 500 mg every six hours, prednisone 5 mg every morning, ferrous sulfate 325 mg three times daily, and furosemide 40 mg every morning. On his first clinic appointment ten days after his hospital discharge, his prothrombin time is 17.1 seconds. Why has his prothrombin time decreased when it appeared to be stable prior to discharge? How should his therapy be altered?

Many variables can alter the response to warfarin. *Diets* rich in vitamin K may antagonize the effects of warfarin. Acquired warfarin resistance has been described in a patient on a weight reducing, high vegetable content diet. Daily ingestion of 1,277 mcg of vitamin K resulted in warfarin requirements of 30–35 mg to achieve prothrombin times in the 16 second range. Foods high in vitamin K include cauliflower, beans, spinach, rice, pork, fish and some cheeses (97,98). Nutritional supplements such as En-Sure and Osmolite also contain vitamin K, but the quantities have been decreased so that antagonism is less likely to occur (99,100). Questioning M.S. should help to identify whether this is a concern in his altered response. Unless there has been a sudden change in his diet, this is unlikely to account for the decreased prothrombin time.

Poor absorption can contribute to resistance. However, the fact that M.S. responded initially rules this out as a likely factor. When it is considered as a possibility, intravenous administration of warfarin can be utilized to document poor oral absorption (97).

Alterations in metabolism, either intrinsic or extrinsic may account for altered response. Patients have been described who exhibit increased clearance of both warfarin and phenindione (101).

This is usually more important with initiation of therapy than in a patient known to be stable previously. Drugs may extrinsically interact with warfarin and decrease the warfarin effect. These are discussed in the section of this chapter dealing with drug interactions. Neither of these factors is apparent in M.S. Hereditary resistance has also been identified in several families but is not relevant in the case of M.S. (102,103).

An *increased rate of clearance* of warfarin was observed in alcoholics who had a prothrombin content of 100% before warfarin was given. Since single doses were given, the significance of this effect must be substantiated with chronic dosing (104). Ingestion of 300 ml of fortified wine by normal volunteers anticoagulated with warfarin had no effect on the anticoagulant response (105).

Numerous *other factors,* such as myxedema (106), hyperthyroidism (107), and hypercholesterolemia (108) have been observed to alter response in some patients but not all.

Probably the single most likely reason for changes in response is *inadequate or inappropriate compliance,* and this is the most likely cause of the observed change in M.S.'s prothrombin time. Certainly one should eliminate drug interactions, including nonprescription drugs, as a possible cause.

When a patient appears to be unresponsive to warfarin, the dose should not be altered every day. Since the drug has a half-life of 42 hours, it takes a while before a new steady state is reached. When changing a maintenance dose, it takes six days to achieve 90% and 12 days to achieve 99% of the new steady state. In addition, changes in clotting factors occur slowly (see Introduction). Frequent dosing changes make evaluation of response difficult. M.S.'s warfarin dosage could be increased to 7.5 mg every other day alternating with 10 mg every other day; the prothrombin time should be checked in one week and the dosage adjusted accordingly. Increments greater than 25% of the weekly requirement should generally be avoided.

12. Hemorrhage Risk During Heparin Therapy. V.R. is a 65-year-old woman who developed acute onset of right leg pain and swelling after a long automobile journey. Deep-venous thrombosis was diagnosed, and full-dose heparin therapy was initiated. Her only other medical problem was bursitis of the left shoulder for which she had been taking ibuprofen (Motrin) 400 mg four times daily for the past year. What factors present in this patient increase her risk of bleeding during heparin therapy?

A number of risk factors for bleeding due to heparin have been identified (109). Age greater than 60, particularly in females, has been observed to be accompanied by more bleeding (59). Although not applicable to V.R., severely ill patients, patients with a history of alcohol intake, and patients who receive aspirin are also at a greater risk for bleeding.

Because of its effects on platelets and the gastrointestinal mucosa, ibuprofen may increase her risk of bleeding, and its necessity during this period should be re-evaluated. Her heparin therapy should be monitored carefully.

13. Heparin Overdose. On the sixth day of heparin therapy, V.R. inadvertently received 25,000 units of heparin over one hour. The infusion was stopped. Within one-half hour she became diaphoretic and hypotensive. Bright red blood was noted upon rectal examination, and a large retroperitoneal mass was noted. How should she be managed?

V.R. has definite signs of hemorrhage from the gastrointestinal tract, a site associated with considerable mortality. The heparin should be discontinued immediately, and treatment should include maintenance of fluid volume and replacement of clotting factors. Unlike albumin, *fresh whole blood* or *fresh frozen plasma* provide clotting factors and are preferred in this situation (78). If hemorrhage had not been present and the only manifestation of the overdose had been a prolonged clotting time, administration of the heparin could have been simply discontinued and the effects would clear in a few hours.

Protamine sulfate has been utilized to inactivate heparin by forming an inactive protamine-heparin complex. Protamine has a rapid onset of action and its effect lasts for about two hours. It is most useful immediately after heparin administration and is infused as a 1% solution in a dosage of 1 mg per 100 units of heparin. Response to therapy can be followed by a return of the clotting tests to baseline. There appears to be little risk of excessive protamine inducing an anticoagulant effect itself (79).

The appropriate management of this patient would include immediate discontinuation of hep-

arin, followed by fresh frozen plasma or whole blood. Additionally, protamine sulfate might be a useful adjunct in this patient. Since it has been one-half hour since heparin was administered and the effect of heparin has already started to decline, the dosage of protamine should be decreased (46).

14. Warfarin Overdose. A patient who had been taking warfarin for six months with good laboratory control noted a slight pink color in his urine. In the emergency room, a prothrombin time of 36 seconds was reported. Upon careful questioning, he admitted taking an extra dose two days previously. His hematocrit and hemoglobin were both within normal limits, as were his vital signs. A stool guaiac was negative. However, urinalysis revealed more than 50 red blood cells per high powered field. How can the effect of warfarin be reversed? How should this patient be managed?

Hematuria may be an early sign of more serious bleeding, but in most cases this condition is associated with minor bleeding episodes. In a reliable patient, discontinuing the warfarin until the prothrombin time returns to a therapeutic level usually suffices, although a more rapid return to normal can be accomplished if vitamin K and/or fresh frozen plasma are administered.

Vitamin K. Phytonadione is the only vitamin K that should be used (124). Its effects are more specific and more rapid because of the presence of a phytol side chain which is lacking in the menadione derivatives. Administration of 10 mg phytonadione (vitamin K) orally, subcutaneously, or intravenously will return the prothrombin time to normal within 4 to 24 hours in a case of minor hemorrhage (124–127). Intramuscular administration provides a site for bleeding and should be avoided. Intravenous administration should be slow, at a rate not exceeding 1 mg per minute to avoid flushing of the face, constriction of the chest, and vascular collapse. If this should occur, administration of epinephrine may be indicated as well as other standard measures to support blood pressure and maintenance of an airway.

Fresh Frozen Plasma. If vitamin K is administered, warfarin therapy may be ineffective for 7–14 days because of the development of relative resistance (128). If transient reversal is desired and indicated, fresh frozen plasma 200–400 ml is the treatment of choice. This will decrease the prothrombin time for 4–6 hours (128–130). This is particularly useful in patients requiring short-term discontinuation of therapy in order to undergo minor surgical procedures.

Since this patient appears only to be bleeding into the urine and he is hemodynamically stable, withholding his warfarin until the prothrombin time returns to the therapeutic range would be the proper treatment. He should be counseled regarding the importance of accurate compliance.

15. How great is the risk of hemorrhage during anticoagulant therapy, and what are the most common sites of bleeding?

In a survey of more than 2400 courses of anticoagulant therapy (61), hemorrhage occurred in 8% of the patients. In 2.5% of the patients studied, hemorrhage was of sufficient magnitude to require termination of therapy. The remaining episodes of bleeding (5.5%) were considered minor and required alteration of dose, but not discontinuation of therapy. The most common site of major hemorrhage in this series was the gastrointestinal tract. This was followed by vaginal bleeding, wound bleeding, and severe epistaxis. The most common site of minor bleeding was the genitourinary tract. This was followed by epistaxis, then gastrointestinal bleeding.

During long-term anticoagulant therapy, serious hemorrhagic complications most commonly occur intracranially and in the gastrointestinal tract (114,115). In fact, 90% of the serious hemorrhage episodes that are crippling or fatal are caused by bleeding at these sites. Although hypertension does not appear to increase the risk of hemorrhage in a patient on anticoagulants, its presence does make hemorrhage worse if it occurs. Gastrointestinal hemorrhage occurs more frequently and is more severe in patients receiving anticoagulants; it is frequently associated with underlying lesions (eg, ulcers) and can occur within the therapeutic range of laboratory control (114).

Minor hemorrhage is usually due to capillary breaks and includes purpura, hematomas, episcleral hemorrhage, epistaxis, and hematuria (116–118). There seems to be no correlation between minor bleeding and serious bleeding.

Unusual sites of bleeding have included intrapulmonary hemorrhage (119), hemorrhage into the pericardial space (119), intestinal hemorrhage resulting in obstruction (120), adrenal hemorrhage, hemarthroses, and retroperitoneal hemorrhage (121).

Although this list is by no means complete, and there are other reports and figures for incidence of hemorrhage (122,123), generalizations can be made. Major hemorrhage appears to occur in 2.3% of all courses of anticoagulant therapy, while minor hemorrhage occurs in approximately 4.5%. Bleeding can occur even when laboratory parameters are within the therapeutically accepted range.

16. A 26-year-old woman is taking warfarin for a thromboembolic episode which was attributed to oral contraceptives. How would warfarin affect her menstrual flow?

Menstrual flow may be increased and prolonged in patients on anticoagulants. However, unless there is some underlying pathology of the reproductive tract which would make this condition a great risk, it is of little significance (110). The patient should be advised to have her prothrombin times checked monthly and she should watch for an unusual increase in blood loss. Should there be unusually heavy or excessively prolonged bleeding, or breakthrough bleeding, gynecologic evaluation should be obtained because of the risk of a latent organic lesion (111).

17. *Pregnancy.* A 30-year-old woman has been taking warfarin for continuing therapy of a resolved pulmonary embolus. She has just learned she is pregnant. What effects might warfarin have on the fetus? Is heparin a safer alternative drug in this situation?

Coumarin anticoagulants cross the placental barrier and may place the fetus at risk for hemorrhage and teratogenic effects (112,113). Approximately one-sixth of pregnancies which included exposure to coumarins resulted in abnormal liveborn infants, one-sixth in abortion or stillbirth, and two-thirds in apparently normal infants. Abnormalities include stippled calcifications and nasal cartilage hypoplasia and occurred in infants born to mothers receiving warfarin during the sixth to ninth weeks of gestation. Other abnormalities, such as central nervous system and eye abnormalities, are more likely to occur following later exposure to warfarin.

Because heparin does not cross the placental barrier, it was once considered a good alternative to coumarins. Heparin has not been shown, however, to be associated with a significantly better outcome of pregnancy. Of 135 published cases reviewed, one-eighth of infants were stillborn, one-fifth were premature (one-third of whom died), and two-thirds were normal (113).

Patients who become pregnant while receiving warfarin should be informed of the risks of continued anticoagulation to the fetus, as well as the risk to themselves of discontinuing anticoagulation. Women of child-bearing age who require anticoagulation should be counseled in some form of contraception to prevent the need for considering termination of pregnancy. Heparin no longer seems to be the safe alternative it was once thought to be.

This patient obviously requires counseling regarding continuation of her therapy.

18. *Anticoagulant Prophylaxis prior to Cardioversion.* **M.K. is a 45-year-old woman with a history of rheumatic heart disease who was seen in cardiac clinic because of a rapid heart beat and general lack of energy. She was diagnosed as being in atrial fibrillation with a rapid ventricular response. Elective cardioversion was planned. Should she be anticoagulated prior to this procedure?**

Atrial fibrillation has been shown by autopsy studies to increase significantly the risk of systemic arterial embolism in patients with mitral valve disease (132). This indirect evidence has not been confirmed by recent observations, although early reports of a 30% incidence of systemic embolism have been quoted.

Despite the controversy regarding the actual overall incidence of emboli, several groups of patients are at greater risk for developing systemic emboli. These include patients with rheumatic valvular disease, idiopathic hypertrophic subaortic stenosis, cardiomyopathy, or a history of previous emboli (133,134).

The risk of embolism following cardioversion without anticoagulation is usually reported to be 1.5–3.0% (135). In some series the risk of embolism has been reduced to zero with anticoagulation.

This patient would appear to fall into a category of patients at greater risk of embolism because of her history of rheumatic heart disease. Anticoagulation should be initiated prior to cardioversion, with heparin if immediate cardioversion is required, or with warfarin if a suitable time period exists in order for it to become effective. Because the risk of embolism is still high for three to four weeks after cardioversion, anticoagulation should be continued for this time period.

Another question which arises is the prophylaxis of patients who have atrial fibrillation but do not require defibrillation or have been unsuccessfully cardioverted. The answer is less clear. If there is a previous history of emboli, most clinicians would anticoagulate. In the absence of a history of emboli, many clinicians would consider the risk of bleeding to be greater than the risk of embolization (136). This decision can be influenced by many different variables; for example, close anticoagulant supervision should decrease the risk of bleeding.

19. *Anticoagulant Prophylaxis after Myocardial Infarction.* **A patient has just suffered his first acute myocardial infarction. In addition to the usual protocol, it is decided that he will be treated with heparin and then warfarin. What evidence supports the use of anticoagulants after myocardial infarction?**

General disagreement still exists regarding the value of long-term anticoagulation in the treatment of myocardial infarction (137,138). Many early studies failed to meet the criteria for adequate trial design (139–141). Some studies which have met the criteria for a good trial (142,143), including a recent study from the Netherlands (144), do report a decreased mortality in anticoagulant-treated patients. The incidence of strokes and non-fatal systemic emboli may also be decreased with anticoagulants (144–147), although the risk of hemorrhage is higher. Several questions regarding the introduction of bias into the Netherlands study have been raised, and while its results are encouraging, further evidence must be presented before long-term anticoagulation can be recommended.

A method which may be preferred, although it likewise has not been unequivocally shown to be useful, is low-dose heparin prophylaxis during hospitalization (148). Because of the risk of embolization with bed-rest along with the potential development of ventricular wall mural thrombi, this method, which is associated with a very low risk of bleeding, may be the method of choice and would be a good recommendation in this patient. (Also see Question 10.)

ANTIPLATELET DRUGS

Arachidonic acid is a precursor of the prostaglandins which are involved in blood coagulation (149). It is released from membrane phospholipids following an appropriate stimulus and is metabolized by several enzyme systems. It is metabolized by cyclo-oxygenase to the unstable endoperoxides pGH_2 and PGG_2, which in turn are metabolized to pGI_2 (prostacyclin) and TXA_2 (thromboxane A_2). Prostacyclin is a potent inhibitor of platelet aggregation and a vasodilator. Thromboxane A_2 is a potent stimulator of platelet aggregation and a vasoconstrictor. Prostacyclin is found predominantly in the walls of arteries and veins, and thromboxane A_2 is found in platelets.

Drugs may inhibit platelet function by a number of different mechanisms (150). Aspirin, indomethacin, and sulfinpyrazone inhibit the arachidonate pathway. *Aspirin* irreversibly inhibits the ability of platelets to form thromboxane A_2 by acetylating platelet cyclo-oxygenase. This effect persists for the life of the platelets. The action of aspirin on vessel wall prostacyclin is temporary, presumably because vessel walls can synthesize cyclo-oxygenase while platelets cannot. The effect of aspirin is also dose-dependent. Low doses of aspirin (80–150 mg) inhibit thromboxane A_2 as well as prostacyclin, but the effect on thromboxane A_2 persists much longer (151,152). Larger doses of aspirin (300 mg or greater) may inhibit platelet wall and vessel wall cyclo-oxygenase activity. The ability of other salicylates to inhibit platelet function by inhibition of the arachidonate pathway has not been adequately studied, although animal studies indicate that salicylic acid has little effect on cyclo-oxygenase (153).

Sulfinpyrazone and *indomethacin* produce an effect on platelets that is reversible and only persists as long as the drug is present in the serum. Sulfinpyrazone also prolongs platelet survival, an effect not shared by aspirin.

Dipyridamole inhibits platelet function by inhibiting phosphodiesterase with a resultant increase in platelet cyclic AMP levels. Dipyridamole has other effects on platelet function; its beneficial effect in patients with prosthetic heart valves is related to its ability to restore normal platelet survival (162), and it is a vasodilator.

Intravenous dextran is also a promising drug in prevention of venous thromboembolism. It affects not only platelet function but also decreases blood viscosity and affects the susceptibility of fibrin clots to lysis.

Therapeutic Applications

The therapeutic role of drugs which affect platelet function has been investigated by several groups over the last few years. Part of the stimulus for these studies has been the recognition that patients with some diseases, such as coronary artery disease, diabetes, and hyperlipidemia, have increased platelet activation and secretion (154,155). The major conditions which have been studied are: coronary heart disease, cerebrovascular disease, venous thromboembolic disease, and patients with prosthetic heart valves.

Myocardial Infarction. The results of trials investigating the role of antiplatelet drugs in secondary prevention of myocardial infarction are reminiscent of the trials of anticoagulants in the prevention of recurrent myocardial infarction. Despite the completion of the Aspirin Myocardial Infarction Study (AMIS), the Anturane Reinfarction Study (ART), the Persantin-Aspirin Reinfarction Study (PARIS), and several European studies, no antiplatelet drug has been demonstrated to reduce mortality, recurrent infarction, or cardiac mortality in patients who have had an MI. Sulfinpyrazone may decrease the incidence of sudden death, but this is still unresolved because of questions of the final analysis (156).

Transient Ischemic Attacks. Aspirin in doses of 325 mg qid, has been shown to reduce the incidence of stroke and death (157). However, this protection was afforded only to men with a previous history of transient cerebral ischemia. It is not clear why there is a predilection for males. Other antiplatelet agents have not been effective in this context.

Venous Thrombosis. Evidence is promising, but inconclusive, for the usefulness of aspirin in reducing the incidence of venous thrombosis in some groups of surgical patients. The evidence is best for patients undergoing hip surgery, although results are mixed (158,159).

Prosthetic Heart Valves. Patients with prosthetic heart valves (particularly ball valves) have a considerable risk of developing arterial emboli despite adequate anticoagulation (160). A combination of oral anticoagulants and aspirin (161) or dipyridamole (162) has been shown to offer better protection against arterial thromboembolism, but the risk of gastrointestinal bleeding is greater, particularly with the combination of aspirin and oral anticoagulants. Therefore, patients who receive this combination should be monitored closely, and their stools should be checked for the presence of blood.

FIBRINOLYTIC AGENTS

Streptokinase (SK) and urokinase (UK) are capable of inducing thrombolytic activity. They have the advantage over heparin and warfarin of directly dissolving emboli rather than merely preventing their extension. The development of streptokinase and urokinase was hoped to decrease mortality from pulmonary emboli and deep venous thrombosis as well as decrease the morbidity from pulmonary hypertension and the postphlebitic syndrome.

Results of national cooperative trials have documented the efficacy of these agents in bringing about clot dissolution in both arterial and venous thromboembolic disease (164–167). Despite this documentation, the use of these agents has been slowly accepted, for several reasons. Therapy with streptokinase and urokinase has been shown to help resolve the physiologic abnormalities caused by pulmonary emboli, but this therapy has not been shown to reduce mortality. Furthermore, reports of significant hemorrhage have also diminished the enthusiasm of clinicians.

Both streptokinase and urokinase activate the nonspecific proteolytic enzyme, plasmin, through conversion of its inactive precursor, plasminogen. (See Fig. 3.) Streptokinase activates plasmin by first combining with plasminogen in an equimolar concentration. This activator complex is then capable of converting plasminogen to plasmin. Urokinase stimulates plasmin production directly by cleavage of plasminogen.

Streptokinase and urokinase share equal efficacy in fibrinolytic therapy but have numerous differences as outlined in Table 2. Urokinase is the preferred fibrinolytic agent in patients who have a high anti-streptococcal antibody titer. Frequent adverse reactions to streptokinase include allergic reactions (15%) and mild fever (33%); these reactions are much less frequent with urokinase (166,167).

20. C.C. is a 51-year-old male who was admitted to the hospital after two hours of severe pleuritic chest pain. Blood gases obtained in the emergency room revealed severe respiratory distress. He was intubated and started on heparin. An emergency lung scan and a pulmonary angiogram were both positive for massive pulmonary embolism.

Laboratory values obtained prior to the administration of heparin included: Platelets

Table 2.

DIFFERENCES BETWEEN UROKINASE AND STREPTOKINASE

	Urokinase	Streptokinase
Source	human fetal culture or human urine	streptococci (group c)
Antigenic	no	yes
Pyrogenic	+	+ +
T½	11–16 min	10–12 min
Loading Dose	4400 CTA units/kg or 2000 CTA units/lb over 10 min	250,000 units over 20–30 min (standard dose)
Maintenance Dose	4400 μ/kg/hr or 2000 μ/lb/hr × 12–24 hr	100,000 μ/hr + 24–72 hr
Cost	expensive	tolerable
Stability	refrigerate	room temp
Retreatment	as needed	usually 2–6 months

272,000/mm^3 (nl 150,000–350,000/mm^3), Activated Partial Thromboplastin Time (APTT) 27.1 sec (nl 24–36 sec), Prothrombin Time (PT) 11.6 sec (nl 11.5–12.5 sec), Thrombin Time 15.6 sec (nl 16–20 sec), Fibrinogen 283 mg/dl (nl 200–450 mg/dl), Hematocrit 45.5% (nl 45–52%), Hemoglobin 14.7 gm/dl (nl 13–18 gm/dl).

Are fibrinolytic agents indicated in the treatment of C.C.'s pulmonary embolus?

Acute treatment with urokinase or streptokinase, followed by traditional anticoagulant therapy, has been compared with conventional treatment with heparin and warfarin in patients with pulmonary emboli (164,165,168,169). In the patients who were treated initially with urokinase and streptokinase, there was accelerated resolution of pulmonary emboli. This was documented by greater acute improvement of angiographic abnormalities and perfusion defects and restoration towards normal cardiopulmonary hemodynamics. The differences between urokinase, streptokinase, and heparin were not statistically significant as the patients' courses progressed, and there was no difference in mortality. Fibrinolytic therapy should therefore be reserved for patients with emboli unresponsive to traditional therapy or those with marked impairment of cardiorespiratory function. It would be appropriate therapy for C.C. because of his severe respiratory compromise and decompensation.

21. In what other clinical circumstances is the use of fibrinolytic agents warranted?

The approved indications for fibrinolytic therapy are massive pulmonary embolism, deep venous thrombosis, and the clearing of vascular access devices and shunts.

Treatment of proximal deep vein thrombosis with fibrinolytic agents has been documented to more rapidly lyse the clot and prevent venous valvular damage and subsequent venous hypertension in the lower extremities (168).

Intracoronary infusion of streptokinase has been reported to restore coronary circulation following acute occlusion. Its overall role in preservation of the ischemic myocardium or prevention of infarction has not yet been established (170–172). Similarly, the role of systemic fibrinolysis following acute infarction has been studied; preliminary results are inconclusive and conflicting (173,174).

22. How should fibrinolytic therapy be initiated in C.C., and how should it be monitored?

Before beginning infusions of streptokinase or urokinase, the thrombin time, prothrombin time, activated partial thromboplastin time, hematocrit, and platelet count should be obtained, as was done in C.C.

Heparin therapy should be discontinued immediately. It was reasonable to start the patient on heparin initially since it does not interfere with the diagnosis of pulmonary embolism and does provide a headstart in therapy if the diagnosis is confirmed. However, since fibrinolysis is indicated, heparin should be stopped. Ideally, fibrinolytic therapy should not be started until the APTT returns to twice control or less.

Administration of standard doses of fibrinolytic agents achieves a "lytic" state in 95% of cases. Standard dosing of urokinase involves a loading dose of 2000 units/lb over 10 minutes followed by continuous infusion of 2000 units/lb/hour for 12 hours (175,176,178). Streptokinase is started with a loading dose of 250,000 units over 30 minutes followed by 100,000 units/hr for 24–72 hours. Occasionally when SK is begun, a "lytic" state may not be accomplished with standard doses because of the presence of a high titer of anti-streptococcal antibody. In this case urokinase should be instituted. Following fibrinolytic therapy, and when the APTT has returned to twice baseline, heparin therapy is instituted and followed by warfarin.

During fibrinolytic therapy, the thrombin time or a PTT should be obtained four to six hours after initiation in order to confirm that a "lytic" state has been obtained; there is no correlation between the degree of prolongation of the clotting test and clot lysis or bleeding. Subsequent tests should only be obtained to document the presence of a "lytic" state.

23. How great is C.C.'s risk of bleeding during fibrinolytic therapy? How can this risk be minimized?

The incidence of major bleeding (hematocrit drop of 5–9%) during treatment with urokinase or streptokinase appears to be about 8–9% (177,179). Patient selection is extremely important. Not only should the indication for treatment be appropriate, but the presence of unacceptable risk factors must be considered. Patients with a history within the previous 10 days of major surgery, external cardiac massage, biopsies in inaccessible locations, intracranial disorders, active major bleeding sites, or postpartum state should not be treated with these agents. Relative minor contraindications include bacterial endocarditis, recent minor trauma, high likelihood of left heart thrombus, pregnancy, age over 75 years, and diabetic hemorrhagic retinopathy (176,177). In order to minimize bleeding, invasive procedures should be avoided unless absolutely essential, and other trauma should be avoided. Antiplatelet agents should not be administered.

If uncontrollable bleeding should occur during thrombolytic therapy, the infusion should be terminated. Transfusion with packed cells or whole blood may also be used.

DISSEMINATED INTRAVASCULAR COAGULATION

24. A.K. is a 70-year-old white female who was admitted to the coronary care unit after a suicide attempt with amitriptyline. She required intubation and ventilator support upon admission. Attempts at extubation resulted in aspiration with subsequent sepsis. In addition, she developed adult respiratory distress syndrome (ARDS). Because of the sudden onset of bright red blood per rectum and bright red blood through her naso-gastric tube, a coagulation screen was ordered. All coagulation studies had been normal on admission. Now the results showed: Platelets 43,000/mm³ (nl 150,000–350,000), Prothrombin Time 21.6 sec (nl 11.5–2.5), Activated Partial Thromboplastin Time 69 sec (nl 24–36), Fibrin Degradation Products 80 mcg/ml (nl 0–10), Fibrinogen 206 mg/dl (nl 200–400), and Protamine Sulfate strongly positive (nl negative). Her WBC was 23,000/mm³ with 98% polys. Therapy was instituted with triple antibiotics while awaiting culture reports.

What subjective and objective evidence in this patient are compatible with the assessment of disseminated intravascular coagulation?

Laboratory evidence of disseminated intravascular coagulation (DIC) is manifested by an increase in the prothrombin time, partial thromboplastin time, and thrombin time. The platelet count and fibrinogen level are low, and the protamine sulfate test is positive due to the presence of a circulating fibrin isomer and fibrin degradation products. A peripheral smear, although not performed, may show red blood cells which are fragmented because of circulation across fibrin strands which bridge the lumen of the blood vessel.

The presence of bright red blood per rectum and through her naso-gastric tube is secondary to the coagulation abnormalities and is also consistent with DIC.

25. How can the abnormal hematological picture be explained by the pathophysiology of DIC?

Activation of the coagulation and fibrinolytic system results in microvascular coagulation and deposition of fibrin in the microcirculation. Subsequent hemorrhage occurs secondary to consumption of platelets and clotting factors. Stimulation of the fibrinolytic system in response to fibrin generation results in the formation of fibrin and fibrinogen degradation products. These breakdown products inhibit the further polymerization of fibrin and inhibit normal platelet function (180,181) (Fig. 4).

Microvascular congestion may result in ischemic tissue damage, particularly to the kidneys, adrenal glands, and skin. Shock is another manifestation of acute DIC, and thus this syndrome represents a true clinical emergency (181,182).

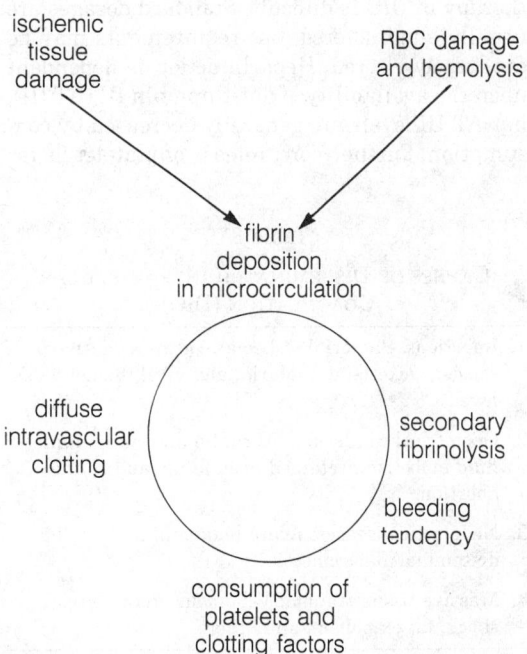

Figure 4. Disseminated Intravascular Coagulation.

26. What event(s) may have precipitated the development of DIC in this patient?

Pathologic activation of the coagulation and fibrinolytic system may occur in response to many different stimuli (Table 3). The resulting syndrome, disseminated intravascular coagulation (DIC), also known as consumption coagulopathy or the defibrination syndrome, is an important intermediary of disease (184,185). The most likely stimulus for DIC in this patient is a combination of sepsis and perhaps tissue trauma induced by hypoxemia and acidosis following her respiratory compromise.

27. What would be a reasonable treatment plan for this patient's DIC?

Treatment of DIC should be directed toward alleviation of the underlying cause; without this, the stimulus for continued clotting and bleeding exists. Restitution of normal or adequate hemostatic function generally occurs with appropriate treatment; however, administration of fresh frozen plasma, vitamin K, or platelets may be useful when the DIC is improving.

Heparin therapy has been advocated by some clinicians, but remains controversial. Heparin treatment is advocated on the premise that prevention of further intravascular generation of thrombin will result in decreased deposition of fibrin in the microvasculature. Control of heparin therapy in DIC is difficult. Standard dosages are usually administered, but requirements may be drastically altered. Heparin action is dependent upon the availability of antithrombin III (AT III), but AT III levels are generally decreased by consumption. Furthermore, release of platelet factor

4 by disintegrating platelets may also alter heparin response by antagonism of its effect. Other anticoagulant drugs such as the coumarins are not indicated because of their slow onset of action. A decrease in fibrin degradation products is perhaps the most useful tool in assessing response to heparin therapy since traditional tests are already prolonged.

Treatment with heparin was considered but not used in A.K. because of the conflicting evidence for its role in the treatment of DIC. It was concluded that antibiotic therapy directed towards sepsis and continued respiratory support were more specifically indicated. She did respond to these measures with resolution of her DIC. She unfortunately died following continued respiratory deterioration.

APPENDIX: DRUG INTERACTIONS WITH ORAL ANTICOAGULANTS

Alcohol, Ethyl (104,105,251)

Mechanism. Not clear (see characteristics).

Characteristics. Unclear. Increased clearance of warfarin from the serum of chronic alcoholic patients has been reported. However, both acute enhancement of anticoagulant response (in non-alcoholic patients) and no effect (in normal subjects) have also been reported.

Recommendation. Avoid alcohol because of unpredictable effect, gastric irritant potential, antiplatelet effect, and risk of injury if intoxicated.

Allopurinol (197,220,221)

Mechanism. Decreased elimination of bishydroxycoumarin and warfarin by an undocumented mechanism.

Characteristics. Questionably significant increase in anticoagulant effect. Described in patients and normal volunteers. Does not occur in all subjects, therefore of unpredictable significance. Generally occurs after several days of therapy.

Recommendation. May be used with coumarins, but requires close monitoring of PT.

Anabolic Steroids (222,223)

Mechanism. Affinity at receptor site may be increased. Not firmly established.

Characteristics. Questionably significant increase in anticoagulant effect. Reported with oxymetholone, norethandrolone and methyltestosterone. Occurs with warfarin and bishydroxycoumarins.

Recommendation. Avoid.

Table 3.

CAUSES OF DISSEMINATED INTRAVASCULAR COAGULATION (DIC)

1. Infections: Bacterial (especially gram-negative sepsis), rickettsial, malaria, and viral; hemorrhage; fever.

2. Obstetrical conditions: Abruptio placenta, amniotic fluid embolism, retained dead fetus, and saline abortion.

3. Neoplastic diseases: Acute leukemia and disseminated carcinoma.

4. Massive tissue trauma: Venomous snake bites, shock, fat embolism, and others.

Table 4.

MECHANISMS OF DRUG INTERACTIONS WITH COUMARIN ANTICOAGULANTS (185–190)

Pharmacodynamic Interactions

Interaction Site	Example
1. Site of action of coumarins	Vitamin K
2. Synthesis of clotting factors	Contraceptive steroids
3. Clotting factor catabolism	Thyroxine
4. Hemostatic process	Antiplatelet drugs

Pharmacokinetic Interactions

Interaction Site	Example
1. Bioavailability	Cholestyramine
2. Protein binding	Phenylbutazone
3. Increased metabolism	Phenobarbital
4. Decreased metabolism	Metronidazole
5. Altered excretion	

Barbiturates (235–242)

Mechanism. Increased metabolism of warfarin secondary to enzyme induction. The onset and duration are dependent upon the specific barbiturate.

Characteristics. Clinically significant decrease in anticoagulant effect. Reported with secobarbital, pentobarbital, amobarbital, butabarbital, aprobarbital, heptabarbital, and phenobarbital. The interaction is predictable and has been observed in normal subjects and in patients.

Recommendation. Benzodiazepines are the best alternatives.

Carbamazepine (243,244)

Mechanism. Unclear; may be hepatic microsomal enzyme induction.

Characteristics. Clinically significant decrease in anticoagulant effect. Reported with warfarin in patients. Onset is not clearly described, but appears to require several days.

Recommendation. Other appropriate anticonvulsant medications may also interact with warfarin. Monitor concomitant use carefully.

Chloral Hydrate (224–230)

Mechanism. Plasma protein binding displacement of warfarin from binding sites by trichloroacetic acid, a metabolite of chloral hydrate and also triclofos. Reported with bishydroxycoumarin as well.

Characteristics. Questionably significant increase in anticoagulant effect. Interaction occurs during first 4–7 days and disappears with continued exposure. There

may be mild prolongation of the PT which is of little clinical significance. Studied in patients.

Recommendation. Use a benzodiazepine.

Cholestyramine (248–250)

Mechanism. Many mechanisms have been described including decreased absorption of anticoagulants from the GI tract and decreased enterohepatic circulation.

Characteristics. Clinically significant decrease in anticoagulant effect. Studied in normal healthy subjects; it occurs with simultaneous administration as well as with dosing separated by several hours. Occurs with warfarin and phenprocoumon.

Recommendations. If both drugs must be administered, they should be separated by the longest dosing interval possible.

Cimetidine (192–195)

Mechanism. Probably inhibits warfarin metabolism. Occurs with other oral anticoagulants as well.

Characteristics. Clinically significant increase in anticoagulant effect. Described in normal volunteers and patients. Occurs within the first few days of concomitant therapy and may increase PT by 20% or more.

Recommendation. Avoid cimetidine; use antacids. Use anticoagulants cautiously in patients with a history of GI bleeding.

Clofibrate (196–198)

Mechanism. Pharmacodynamically-mediated enhancement of warfarin anticoagulant response which appears to involve the S-isomer.

Characteristics. Clinically significant increase in anticoagulant effect. Interaction occurs within first few days of combined therapy in normal volunteers.

Recommendation. Avoid.

Disulfiram (199–201)

Mechanism. Stereoselective interaction with warfarin S-isomer; probably a dynamic interaction in which there is an effect on the hypoprothrombinemic mechanism of the liver.

Characteristics. Clinically significant increase in anticoagulant effect. Studied in normal subjects after single and multiple doses. Reported in two patients.

Recommendation. Avoid.

Glucagon (202)

Mechanism. Not clearly established. May be direct depression of vitamin K-dependent clotting factors, or altered affinity of receptors resulting in increased response.

Characteristics. Clinically significant increase in anticoagulant effect. May occur after several days of therapy. Although observations have been limited, it is more predictable with doses greater than 25 mg. Described in patients.

Recommendation. Avoid.

Indomethacin (233,234)

Mechanism. No direct effect on warfarin pharmacodynamics, but potent inhibitor of platelet function and strongly ulcerogenic.

Characteristics. Questionably significant increase in anticoagulant effect. Studies in normal volunteers reveal no interaction. Case observation showed prolonged PT, but more likely due to loading dose of warfarin.

Recommendation. Avoid because of ulcerogenic agents. Ibuprofen is the most reasonable alternative.

Metronidazole (43,203)

Mechanism. Stereoselective inhibition of S-isomer metabolism.

Characteristics. Clinically significant increase in anticoagulant effect. Studied in normal volunteers after single and multiple doses of warfarin. Interaction occurs within 48 hours. Reported in a patient receiving 750 mg per day of metronidazole.

Recommendation. Use other appropriate anti-infective agents.

Non-Steroidal Anti-Inflammatory Agents (252–261)

1. All non-steroidal anti-inflammatory agents may affect normal platelet function. Comparing the concentration at which there is 50% inhibition of collagen-induced platelet aggregation, the most potent inhibitor is zomepirac, followed by indomethacin, tolmetin, aspirin, naproxen, flufenamic acid, ibuprofen, and phenylbutazone.

2. All non-steroidal anti-inflammatory agents may cause gastic irritation and should be used with caution in anticoagulated patients.

3. Some non-steroidal anti-inflammatory agents have been studied for their ability to interact directly with oral anticoagulants: (Also see Indomethacin, Phenylbutazone, and Salicylates.)

Diclofenac—No clinically significant interaction with warfarin.

Diflunisal—Loss of anticoagulant effect when diflunisal discontinued in normal subjects. Unknown mechanism and unknown effect when diflunisal added to anticoagulant regimen.

Fenbufen—Minor, non-significant (1.9 sec) potentiation of warfarin.

Ibuprofen—No interaction.

Naproxen—No effect on anticoagulant activity of warfarin in healthy volunteers.

Sulindac—Conflicting reports. No interaction ob-

served in healthy volunteers but two isolated case reports in patients.

Tolmetin—No interaction.

Phenylbutazone and Oxyphenbutazone (38,204,205)

Mechanism. Stereoselective inhibition of warfarin S-isomer metabolism. There also is protein binding displacement.

Characteristics. Clinically significant increase in anticoagulant effect. Has been described in patients and normal volunteers. The potentiation occurs within several days and may persist for up to 4–10 days after discontinuation of phenylbutazone or oxyphenbutazone.

Recommendation. There is no ideal non-steroidal anti-inflammatory agent. The most reasonable alternative is ibuprofen.

Phenytoin (231,232)

Mechanism. May be stereoselective inhibition of warfarin metabolism, but exact mechanism has not been documented.

Characteristics. Questionably significant increase in anticoagulant effect. Described in two patients stabilized on warfarin who demonstrated a 30% increase in PT.

Recommendation. Follow concomitant therapy with frequent PT's, especially in patients receiving phenytoin loading doses.

Rifampin (245–247)

Mechanism. Enhancement of warfarin metabolism and elimination. Also reported with phenprocoumon and acenocoumarol. Exact mechanism not clearly established.

Characteristics. Clinically significant decrease in anticoagulant effect. Effect appears within 5–7 days of initiation of rifampin and persists for a similar length of time following withdrawal.

Recommendation. Monitor concomitant use carefully.

Salicylates (213–218)

Mechanism. Multiple risks of concomitant administration: (a) Direct hypoprothrombinemic effect with large doses (greater than 3 gm per day). (b) Antiplatelet effect of acetylsalicylic acid (ASA). (c) Ulcerogenic potential.

Characteristics. Clinically significant increase in anticoagulant effect. Antiplatelet activity of ASA may occur with very low doses. Severity of ulcerogenic effect varies among individuals, but all show some blood loss.

Recommendation. All but the anti-inflammatory effects of ASA may be substituted for with acetaminophen. For anti-inflammatory action substitute with ibuprofen. When ASA is used as an antiplatelet drug in combination with warfarin, careful monitoring must be employed.

Sulfinpyrazone (206–208,263)

Mechanism. Sulfinpyrazone stereoselectively augments the effect of racemic warfarin by reducing the metabolic clearance of S-warfarin. Protein binding displacement may occur as well.

Characteristics. Clinically significant increase in anticoagulant effect. Generally appears within first week of therapy. May be observed sooner with daily monitoring. Observations have been made in patients.

Recommendation. Use alternative antiplatelet agents if continued antiplatelet therapy is indicated. Avoid the combination of SPZ/warfarin.

Sulfonamides (209–212)

Mechanism. Reported with TMP/SMX, sulfisoxazole, and sulfamethizole. Stereoselective inhibition of warfarin S-isomer metabolism by TMP-SMX. Protein binding displacement may also occur initially.

Characteristics. Clinically significant increase in anticoagulant effect. Studied in both patients and normal subjects. Potentiation may occur within 48 hours.

Recommendation. Avoid sulfonamide or sulfonamide-containing products; use appropriate alternative anti-infectives (eg, ampicillin).

Thyroid (198,219)

Mechanism. Catabolism of vitamin K-dependent clotting factors appears to be accelerated.

Characteristics. Clinically significant increase in anticoagulant effect. Described in hyperthyroid patients. Described with both D-thyroxine and L-thyroxine in normal volunteers and some patients.

Recommendation. Carefully monitor anticoagulated patients in whom thyroid preparations are added or withdrawn.

References

1. Didisheim P et al: Actions and clinical status of platelet-suppressive agents. Semin Hematol. 1978; 15:55.
2. Bennett B et al: The normal coagulation mechanism. Med Clin North Am. 1972; 56:96.
3. Finlayson JS: Crosslinking of fibrin. Sem Thromb Hemostasis. 1974; 1:33.
4. Bennett B et al: Blood coagulation mechanism. Clin Hematol. 1973; 2:3.
5. Salzman EW et al: Reduction in venous thromboembolism by agents affecting platelet function. N Engl J Med. 1971; 284:1287.
6. Bowie EJW et al: Evaluation of the hemostatic mechanism. Med Clin North Am. 1970; 54:889.
7. Ravel R: *Blood Coagulation in Clinical Laboratory Medicine, Application of Laboratory Data,* 2nd ed., Year Book Medical Publishers, Inc., 1973, p 80.
8. Quick AJ: Clinical interpretation of the one-stage prothrombin time. Circulation. 1961; 24:1422.
9. Quick AJ: Detection and diagnosis of hemorrhagic states. JAMA. 1966; 197:418.
10. Didisheim R: Tests of blood coagulation and hemostasis I. The prothrombin time. JAMA. 1966; 196:33.
11. MacAuley MA et al: Relationship of the partial thromboplastin time to the Lee-White coagulation time. Am J Clin Path. 1968; 50:403.
12. Struver GD et al: The partial thromboplastin time (cephalin time) in anticoagulant therapy. Am J Clin Path. 1962; 38:473.
13. Rapaport SL et al: Clotting factor assays on plasma from patients receiving intramuscular or subcutaneous heparin. Am J Med Sci. 1957; 234:678.
14. Hougie C: Recalcification time test and its modifications (PTT, APTT and expanded PTT). In *Hematology,* Williams WJ et al (Ed), McGraw Hill, New York, 1972, p 1400–1407.
15. Basu D et al: A prospective study of the value of monitoring heparin treatment with the activated partial thromboplastin time. N Engl J Med. 1972; 287:324.
16. Hattersly PG: Activated coagulation time of whole blood. JAMA. 1966; 196:436.
17. Hattersly PG: The activated coagulation time of whole blood as a routine pre-operative screening test. Calif Med. 1971; 114:15.
18. Douglas AS et al: Anticoagulant and thrombolytic therapy. Clin Hematol. 1973; 2:175.
19. Rosenberg RD: Heparin action. Circulation. 1974; 49:603.
20. Rosenberg RD: Actions and interactions of antithrombin and heparin. N Engl J Med. 1975; 292:146.
21. Novak E et al: A comparative study of the effect of lung and gut heparins on platelet aggregation and protamine neutralization in man. Clin Med. 1972; 79:22.
22. Silverglade A: Biological equivalence of beef lung and hog mucosal heparins. Curr Ther Res. 1975; 18:91.
23. O'Brien JR: Heparin and platelets. Curr Ther Res. 1975; 18:79.
24. Estes JW: The fate of heparin in the body. Curr Ther Res. 1975; 18:45.
25. Estes JW et al: A retrospective study of the pharmacokinetics of heparin. Clin Pharmacol Ther. 1969; 10:329.
26. Coon WW: Some recent developments in the pharmacology of heparin. J Clin Pharmacol. 1979; 19:337.
27. Griffith GC et al: The clinical usage of heparin. Am J Cardiol. 1964; 14:39.
28. Woolf IL et al: Vitamin K and warfarin metabolism, function, and interaction. Am J Med. 1972; 53:261.
29. Coon WW et al: Some aspects of the pharmacology of oral anticoagulants. Clin Pharmacol Ther. 1970; 11:312.
30. O'Reilly RA: Vitamin K and oral anticoagulant drugs as competitive antagonists in man. Pharmacol. 1972; 7:149.

31. Suttie JW: Oral anticoagulant therapy: The biosynthetic basis. Semin Hematol. 1977; 14:365.

32. Jackson CM et al: Recent developments in understanding the mechanism of vitamin K and vitamin K-antagonist drug action and the consequences of vitamin K action in blood coagulation. Prog Hematol. 1977; 10:333.

33. Stenflo J: Vitamin K, prothrombin and gamma-carboxyglutamic acid. N Engl J Med. 1977; 296:624.

34. O'Reilly RA et al: Studies on the coumarin anticoagulant drugs: the pharmacodynamics of warfarin in man. J Clin Invest. 1963; 42:1543.

35. O'Reilly RA et al: Studies on the coumarin anticoagulant drugs: a comparison of the pharmacodynamics of dicoumarol and warfarin in man. Thromb Diath Hemorrh. 1964; 11:1.

36. Breckenridge A et al: Kinetics of warfarin absorption in man. Clin Pharmacol Ther. 1973; 14:955.

37. Yacobi A et al: Serum protein binding as a determinant of warfarin body clearance and anticoagulant effect. Clin Pharmacol Ther. 1976; 19:552.

38. Lewis RJ et al: Warfarin. Stereochemical aspects of its metabolism and the interaction with phenylbutazone. J Clin Invest. 1974; 53:1607.

39. Chan KK et al: Absolute configuration of the four warfarin alcohols. J Med Chem. 1972; 15:1265.

40. Hewick DS et al: Plasma half-lives, plasma metabolites and anticoagulant efficacies of the enantiomers of warfarin in man. J Pharm Pharmacol. 1973; 25:458.

41. Lewis RJ et al: The metabolic fate of warfarin studies on the metabolites in plasma. Ann NY Acad Sci. 1971; 179:205.

42. Lewis RJ et al: Warfarin metabolites: the anticoagulant activity and pharmacology of warfarin alcohols. J Lab Clin Med. 1973; 81:915.

43. O'Reilly RA: The stereoselective interaction of warfarin and metronidazole in man. N Engl J Med. 1976; 295:354.

44. Stein PD et al: History and physical examination in acute pulmonary embolism in patients without preexisting cardiac or pulmonary disease. Am J Cardiol. 1981; 47:223.

45. Tibutt DA et al: Pulmonary embolism: Current therapeutic concepts. Drugs. 1976; 11:161.

46. Gallus AS et al: Antithrombotic drugs. Part II. Drugs. 1976; 12:132.

47. Nath H et al: Platelet factor 4-antiheparin protein releasable from platelets. Purification and properties. J Lab Clin Med. 1973; 82:754.

48. Thomas DP: Therapeutic role of heparin in acute pulmonary embolism. Curr Ther Res. 1975; 18:21.

49. Hirsh J et al: Heparin kinetics in venous thrombosis and pulmonary embolism. Circulation. 1976; 53:691.

50. O'Sullivan EF et al: Heparin in the treatment of venous thromboembolic disease: administration, control, and results. Med J Aust. 1968; 2:153.

51. Engelberg J: The clinical use of heparin. Curr Ther Res. 1975; 18:34.

52. Genton E et al: Observations in anticoagulant and thrombolytic therapy in pulmonary embolism. Progr Cardiavasc Dis. 1975; 17:335.

53. Sassahara AA: Therapy for pulmonary embolism. JAMA. 1974; 229:1795.

54. Wessler S et al: Anticoagulant therapy—1974. JAMA. 1974; 8:757.

55. Wessler S et al: Studies in intravascular coagulation IV. The effect of heparin and dicumarol on serum-induced venous thrombus. Circulation. 1955; 12:553.

56. Hirsh J: The value of monitoring heparin therapy in the prevention of occurrence in patients with venous thromboembolic disease. Thromb Diath Haemorrh. 1973; 56:181 (suppl).

57. Salzman EW et al: Management of heparin therapy. Controlled prospective trial. N Engl J Med. 1975; 292:1046.

58. Glazier RL et al: Randomized prospective trial of continuous vs intermittent heparin therapy. JAMA. 1976; 236:1365.

59. Mant MJ: Hemorrhagic complications of heparin therapy. Lancet. 1977; 1:1133.

60. Sevitt S et al: Prothrombin time and thrombotest in injured patients on prophylactic anticoagulant therapy. Lancet. 1964; 1:124.

61. Coon WW et al: Hemorrhagic complications of anticoagulant therapy. Arch Intern Med. 1976; 133:386.

62. Carey LC et al: Comparative effects of dicumarol, tranexan, and heparin on thrombus propagation. Ann Surg. 1960; 152:919.

63. Coon WW et al: Recurrence of venous thromboembolism. Surgery. 1973; 73:823.

64. Acheson L et al: Venous thromboses, duration of anticoagulant therapy (letter). N Engl J Med. 1975; 293:879.

65. Sharnoff JG: Results in the prophylaxis of postoperative thromboembolism. Surg Gynecol Obstet. 1966; 123:303.

66. Hume M et al: 1125 fibrinogen and the prevention of venous thrombosis. Arch Surg. 1973; 107:803.

67. Gallus AS et al: Prevention of venous thrombosis with small, subcutaneous doses of heparin. JAMA. 1976; 235:1980.

68. Kakkar VV et al: Prevention of fatal postoperative pulmonary embolism by low doses of heparin. An international multicentre trial. Lancet. 1975; 3:45.

69. Wessler S et al: Theory and practice of minidose heparin in surgical patients. A status report. Circulation. 1973; 47:4.

70. Gurewich V et al: Hemostatic effects of uniform, low-dose subcutaneous heparin in surgical patients. Arch Intern Med. 1978; 138:41.

71. McCarthy ST et al: Low-dose heparin as a prophylaxis against deep-venous thrombosis after acute stroke. Lancet. 1977; 2:800.

72. Wray T et al: Prophylactic anticoagulant therapy in the prevention of calf-vein thrombosis after myocardial infarction. N Engl J Med. 1973; 288:815.

73. Yin ET et al: Identity of plasma-activated factor X inhibitor with antithrombin III and heparin co-factor. J Biol Chem. 1971; 216:3712.

74. Bynum LJ et al: Low-dose heparin therapy in the long-term management of venous thromboembolism. Am J Med. 1979; 47:553.

75. Hampson WGJ: Failure of low-dose heparin to prevent deep-vein thrombosis after hip replacement arthroplasty. Lancet. 1974; 4:1.

76. Clagett GP et al: Prevention of venous thromboembolism in surgical patients. N Engl J Med. 1974; 290:93.

77. Hull R et al: Warfarin sodium versus low dose heparin in the long-term treatment of venous thrombosis. N Engl J Med. 1979; 301:855.

78. Westphal RG: Rational alternatives to the use of whole blood. Ann Intern Med. 1972; 76:987.

79. Ellison N et al: Is protamine a clinically important anticoagulant? Anesthesiology. 1971; 35:621.

80. Griffith GC et al: Heparin osteoporosis. JAMA. 1965; 193:85.

81. Jaffe MD et al: Multiple fractures associated with long-term sodium heparin therapy. JAMA. 1965; 193:158.

82. Zinn WJ: Side reactions of heparin in clinical practice. Am J Cardiol. 1964; 14:36.

83. Wilson ID et al: Selective hypoaldosteronism after prolonged heparin administration. Am J Med. 1964; 36:635.

84. Babcok RB et al: Heparin-induced immune thrombocytopenia. N Engl J Med. 1976; 295:237.

85. Bell WR et al: Thrombocytopenia occurring during the administration of heparin. A prospective study in 52 patients. Ann Intern Med. 1976; 85:155.

86. Fratantoni JC et al: Heparin-induced thrombocytopenia: confirmation of diagnosis with in vitro methods. Blood. 1975; 45:395.

87. Rhodes GR et al: Heparin-induced thrombocytopenia with thrombotic and hemorrhagic manifestations. Surg Gynecol Obstet. 1973; 136:409.

88. Powers PJ et al: Thrombocytopenia found uncommonly during heparin therapy. JAMA. 1979; 241:2396.

89. Cines DB et al: Heparin-associated thrombocytopenia. N Engl J Med. 1980; 303:788.

90. Bell WR et al: Heparin-associated thrombocytopenia: A comparison of three heparin preparations. N Engl J Med. 1980; 303:902.

91. Genton E: Guidelines for heparin therapy. Ann Intern Med. 1974; 80:77.

92. Moser KM et al: Effect of heparin on the one-stage prothrombin time. Ann Intern Med. 1967; 66:1207.

93. Kazmier FJ et al: Effect of oral anticoagulants on factors VII, IX, X, and II. Arch Intern Med. 1965; 115:667.

94. O'Reilly RA et al: Studies on coumarin anticoagulant drugs. Initiation of warfarin therapy without a loading dose. Circulation. 1968; 38:169.

95. Hoak JC et al: The antithrombotic properties of coumarin drugs. Ann Intern Med. 1961; 54:73.

96. Wessler S: Thrombosis in the presence of vascular stasis. Am J Med. 1962; 33:648.

97. O'Reilly RA et al: Determinants of the response to oral anticoagulant drugs in man. Pharmacol Rev. 1970; 22:35.

98. Qureshi GD et al: Acquired warfarin resistance and weight-reducing diet. Arch Intern Med. 1981; 141:507.

99. Lee M et al: Warfarin resistance and vitamin K. Ann Intern Med. 1981; 94:140.

100. O'Reilly RA et al: "Resistance" to warfarin due to unrecognized vitamin K supplementation. N Engl J Med. 1980; 303:160.

101. Lewis RJ et al: Warfarin resistance. Am J Med. 1967; 42:620.

102. O'Reilly RA et al: Hereditary transmission of exceptional resistance to coumarin anticoagulant drugs. First reported kindred. N Engl J Med. 1964; 271:809.

103. O'Reilly RA: Hereditary resistance to oral anticoagulant drugs: a second reported kindred. Clin Res. 1969; 17:317.

104. Kater RMH et al: Increased rate of clearance of drugs from the circulation of alcoholics. Am J Med Sci. 1969; 258:35.

105. O'Reilly RA: Lack of effect of fortified wine ingested during fasting and anticoagulant therapy. Arch Intern Med. 1981; 141:458.

106. Rice AJ et al: Decreased sensitivity to warfarin in patients with myxedema. Am J Med Sci. 1971; 262:211.

107. Loelinger EA et al: The biological disappearance rate of prothrombin factors VII, IX, and X from plasma in hypothyroidism, hyperthyroidism, and during fever. Thromb Diath Haemorrh. 1964: 10:267.

108. Pyorala K: Coumarin anticoagulant requirement in relation to serum cholesterol and triglyceride level. Acta Med Scand. 1968; 183:437.

109. Walker AM: Predictors of bleeding during heparin therapy. JAMA. 1980; 244:1209.

110. Alexander B et al: A guide to anticoagulant therapy. Circulation. 1961; 34:123.

111. Zweifer AJ: Relation of prothrombin concentration to bleeding during oral anticoagulant therapy. Its importance in detection of latent organic lesions. N Engl J Med. 1962; 267:283.

112. Stevenson RE et al: Hazards of oral anticoagulation during pregnancy. JAMA. 1980; 243:1549.

113. Hall J et al: Maternal and fetal sequelae of anticoagulation during pregnancy. Am J Med. 1980; 68:122.

114. Askey JM: Hemorrhage during long-term anticoagulant drug therapy, Part II: gastrointestinal hemorrhage. Calif Med. 1966; 104:88.

115. Askey JM: Hemorrhage during long-term anticoagulant drug therapy, Part I: Intracranial hemorrhage. Calif Med. 1966; 104:6.

116. Askey JM: Hemorrhage during long-term anticoagulant drug therapy, Part III: The relationship of minor to serious bleeding. Calif Med. 1966; 104:175.

117. Askey JM: Hemorrhage during long-term anticoagulant drug therapy, Part IV: Selection and management of patients. Calif Med. 1966; 104:284.

118. Askey JM: Hemorrhage during long-term anticoagulant drug therapy, Part V: Unusual bleeding episodes. Calif Med. 1966; 104:377.

119. Reussi C et al: Unusual complications in the course of anticoagulant therapy. Am J Med. 1969; 46:460.

120. Miller RL: Hemopericardium with use of oral anticoagulant therapy. JAMA. 1969; 209:1362.

121. Crisler C et al: Intestinal obstruction in patients receiving anticoagulants. Med Clin North Am. 1970; 50:1009.

122. Macon WL et al: Significant complications of anticoagulant therapy. Surg. 1970; 68:571.

123. Kelton JG: Bleeding associated with antithrombotic therapy. Semin Hematol. 1980; 17:259.

124. Udall JA: Don't use the wrong vitamin K. Calif Med. 1966; 112:65.

125. Gamble JR et al: Clinical comparison of vitamin K_1 and water soluble vitamin K. Arch Intern Med. 1955; 95:52.

126. Shoshkes M et al: Vitamin K_1 in treatment of bishydroxycoumarin-induced hypoprothrombinemia, comparison of intravenous and intramuscular administration. JAMA. 1956; 161:1145.

127. Taberner DA et al: Comparison of prothrombin complex concentrate and vitamin K_1 in oral anticoagulant reversal. Br Med J. 1976; 1:83.

128. Wright IS: Anticoagulant therapy—practical management. Am Heart J. 1969; 77:280.

129. Gazzard BG et al: The use of fresh frozen plasma or a concentrate of factor IX as replacement therapy before liver biopsy. Gut. 1975; 6:621.

130. Manucci PM et al: Correction of abnormal coagulation in chronic liver disease by combined use of fresh frozen plasma and prothrombin complex concentrates. Lancet. 1976; 2:542.

131. Spector I et al: Effect of plasma transfusions on the prothrombin time and clotting factors in liver disease. N Engl J Med. 1966; 275:1052.

132. Hinton RC et al: Influence of etiology of atrial fibrillation in incidence of systemic embolism. Am J Cardiol. 1977; 40:509.

133. Morris DC et al: Atrial fibrillation. Curr Prob Cardiol. 1980; 5:1.

134. Resnekov L: Present status of electroversion in the management of cardiac dysrhythmias. Circulation. 1973: 47:1356.

135. DeSilva RA et al: Cardioversion and defibrillation. Am Heart J. 1980; 100:881.

136. Easton JD et al: Management of cerebral embolism of cardiac origin. Stroke. 1980; 11:433.

137. Modan B et al: The case for anticoagulants in acute myocardial infarction. Arch Intern Med. 1976; 136:1230.

138. Rogel S et al: Anticoagulants in ischemic heart disease. Arch Intern Med. 1976; 136:1229.

139. Feinstein AR: More blood for the anticoagulant battle. N Engl J Med. 1975; 292:1400.

140. Gifford RH et al: A critique of methodology in studies of anticoagulant therapy for acute myocardial infarction. N Engl J Med. 1969; 280:351.

141. Gross H et al: Anticoagulant therapy in myocardial infarction, an overview of methodology. Am J Med. 1972; 52:421.

142. Modan B et al: Reduction of hospital mortality from acute myocardial infarction by anticoagulant therapy. N Engl J Med. 1975; 292:1359.

143. Tonascia J: Retrospective evidence favoring use of anticoagulants for myocardial infarction. N Engl J Med. 1975; 292:1362.

144. Tijssen JG et al: A double-blind trial to assess long-term oral anticoagulant therapy in elderly patients after myocardial infarction. Report of the sixty plus reinfarction study research group. Lancet. 1980; 2:989.

145. Cooperative Clinical Trial: Anticoagulants in acute myocardial infarction. JAMA. 1973; 225:724.

146. Drapkin A et al: Anticoagulant therapy after acute myocardial infarction. Relation of therapeutic benefit to patient's age, sex, and severity of infarction. JAMA. 1972; 222:541.

147. Working Party Report: Assessment of short-term anticoagulant administration after cardiac infarction. Br Med J. 1969; 1:335.

148. Gallus AS et al: Small subcutaneous doses of heparin in prevention of venous thrombosis. N Engl J Med. 1973; 288:11.

149. Moncada S et al: Arachidonic acid metabolites and the interactions between platelets and blood-vessel walls. N Engl J Med. 1979; 300:1142.

150. Packham MA et al: Pharmacology of platelet-affecting drugs. Circulation. 1980; 62:26 (suppl V).

151. Preston FE et al: Inhibition of prostacyclin and platelet thromboxane A_2 after low-dose aspirin. N Engl J Med. 1981; 304:76.

152. Paccioretti MJ et al: Effects of aspirin on platelet aggregation as a function of dosage and time. Clin Pharmacol Ther. 1980; 27:803.

153. Vargaftig BB: Salicylic acid fails to inhibit generation of thromboxane A_2 activity in platelets after in vivo administration to the rat. J Pharm Pharmacol. 1978; 30:101.

154. Sobel M et al: Circulating platelet products in unstable angina pectoris. Circulation. 1981; 63:300.

155. Fuster V et al: Current concepts of thrombogenesis. Role of platelets. Mayo Clin Proc. 1981; 56:102.

156. Fuster V et al: Management of arterial thromboembolic and atherosclerotic disease. Mayo Clin Proc. 1981; 56:265.

157. Canadian Cooperative Study Group: A randomized trial of aspirin and sulfinpyrazone in threatened stroke. N Engl J Med. 1978; 299:53.

158. Harris WH et al: Aspirin prophylaxis of venous thromboembolism after total hip replacement. N Engl J Med. 1977; 297:1246.

159. McKenna R et al: Prevention of venous thromboembolism after total knee replacement by high-dose aspirin or intermittent calf and thigh compression. Br Med J. 1980; 1:514.

160. Dale J et al: Prevention of arterial thromboembolism with acetylsalicylic acid. A controlled clinical study in patients with aortic ball valves. Am Heart J. 1977; 94:101.

161. Altman R et al: Aspirin and prophylaxis of thromboembolic complications in patients with substitute heart valves. J Thorac Cardiovasc Surg. 1976; 72:127.

162. Sullivan JM et al: Pharmacologic control of thromboembolic complications of cardiac valve replacement. N Engl J Med. 1971; 284:1391.

163. Harker LA et al: Studies of platelet and fibrinogen kinetics in patients with prosthetic heart valves. N Engl J Med. 1970; 283:1302.

164. Urokinase-streptokinase embolism trial: phase 1 results: a cooperative study. JAMA. 1970; 214:2163.

165. Urokinase-streptokinase embolism trial: phase 2 results: a cooperative study. JAMA. 1974; 229:1606.

166. Bell WR: Thrombolytic therapy: A comparison between urokinase and streptokinase. From a national cooperative study. Semin Thromb Hemostas. 1975; 2:1.

167. Bell WR et al: Guidelines for the use of thrombolytic agents. N Engl J Med. 1979; 301:1266.

168. Marder VJ: Guidelines for thrombolytic therapy of deep-vein thrombosis. Progr Cardiavasc Dis. 1979; 21:327.

169. Genton E: Thrombolytic therapy of pulmonary thromboembolism. Progr Cardiovasc Dis. 1979; 21:333.

170. Mathey DG et al: Nonsurgical coronary artery recanalization in acute transmural myocardial infarction. Circulation. 1981; 63:489.

171. Ganz W et al: Intracoronary thrombolysis in evolving myocardial infarction. Am Heart J. 1981; 101:4.

172. Rentrop R et al: Selective intracoronary thrombolysis in acute myocardial infarction and unstable angina pectoris. Circulation. 1981; 63:307.

173. Duckert F: Thrombolytic therapy in myocardial infarction. Progr Cardiovasc Dis. 1979; 21:342.

174. Verstrate M: Streptokinase in acute myocardial infarction. European Cooperative Study Group for Streptokinase Treatment in acute myocardial infarction. N Engl J Med. 1979; 301:797.

175. Anon: Streptokinase and Urokinase. Med Let Drugs Ther. 1978; 20:37.

176. Marder VJ: The use of thrombolytic agents: Choice of patient, drug administration, laboratory monitoring. Ann Intern Med. 1979; 90:802.

177. National Institutes of Health Consensus Development Conference: Thrombolytic therapy in thrombosis. Ann Intern Med. 1980; 93:141.

178. Stambaugh RL et al: Therapeutic use of thrombolytic agents. Am J Hosp Pharm. 1981; 38:817.

179. Marder VJ: Are we using fibrinolytic agents often enough? Ann Intern Med. 1980; 93:136.

180. Heene DL: Disseminated intravascular coagulation: Evaluation of therapeutic approaches. Semin Throm Hemostas. 1977; 3:268.

181. Sharp AA: Diagnosis and management of disseminated intravascular coagulation. Br Med Bull. 1977; 33:265.

182. Yoshikawa T et al: Infection and disseminated intravascular coagulation. Medicine. 1971; 50:237.

183. Mant MJ et al: Disseminated intravascular coagulation. A reappraisal of its pathophysiology, clinical significance, and therapy based on 47 patients. Am J Med. 1979; 67:557.

184. Deykin D: The clinical challenge of disseminated intravascular coagulation. N Engl J Med. 1970; 283:636.

185. Owen CA et al: Chronic intravascular coagulation and fibrinolysis (ICF) syndromes (DIC). Semin Thromb Hemostas. 1977; 3:268.

186. Hansten PD: *Drug Interactions,* 2nd ed. Lea & Febiger, Phila., 1973.

187. MacLeaod SM et al: Pharmacodynamic and pharmacokinetic drug interactions with coumarin anticoagulants. Drugs. 1976; 11:461.

188. Sigell LT et al: Drug interactions with anticoagulants. JAMA. 1970; 214:2035.

189. Koch-Weser J et al: Drug interactions in cardiovascular therapy. Am Heart J. 1975; 90:93.

190. Williams JRB et al: Effect of concomitantly administered drugs on the control of long term anticoagulant therapy. Quart J Med. 1976; 45:63.

191. Koch-Weser J et al: Drug interactions with coumarin anticoagulants. N Engl J Med. 1971; 285:487, 547.

192. Hind AC: Cimetidine and oral anticoagulants. Br Med J. 1978; 2:1367.

193. Serling MJ et al: Cimetidine: Interactions with oral anticoagulants in man. Lancet. 1979; 2:327.

194. Wallin BA et al: Cimetidine and effect of warfarin. Ann Intern Med. 1979; 90:993.

195. Silver BA et al: Potentiation of the hypoprothrombinemic effect of warfarin. Ann Intern Med. 1979; 90:348.

196. Bjornsson TD et al: Interaction of clofibrate with warfarin I. Effect of clofibrate on the disposition of the optical enantiomorphs of warfarin. J Pharmacokinetics Biopharm. 1977; 5:495.

197. Pond SM et al: The effects of allopurinol and clofibrate on the elimination of coumarin anticoagulants in man. Aust N Z J Med. 1975; 5:324.

198. Schrogie JJ et al: The anticoagulant response to bishydroxycoumarin II. The effect of D-thyroxine, clofibrate and norethandrolone. Clin Pharmacol Ther. 1967; 8:70.

199. Rothstein E: Warfarin effect enhanced by disulfiram (Antabuse). JAMA. 1972; 221:1052.

200. O'Reilly RA: Interactions of sodium warfarin and disulfiram (Antabuse) in man. Ann Intern Med. 1973; 78:73.

201. O'Reilly RA: Dynamic interaction between disulfiram and separated enantiomorphs of racemic warfarin. Clin Pharmacol Ther. 1981; 29:332.

202. Koch-Weser J: Potentiation by glucagon of the hypoprothrombinemic action of warfarin. Ann Intern Med. 1970; 72:331.

203. Kazmier FJ: A significant interaction between metronidazole and warfarin. Mayo Clin Proc. 1976; 51:782.

204. Aggler PM et al: Potentiation of anticoagulant effect of warfarin by phenylbutazone. N Engl J Med. 1967; 276:496.

205. Schary WL et al: Warfarin-phenylbutazone interactions in man: A long term multiple dose study. Res Commun Chem Pathol Pharmacol. 1975; 10:663.

206. Gallus A et al: Sulphinpyrazone and warfarin: A probable drug interaction. Lancet. 1980; 1:535.

207. Jamil A et al: Interaction between sulphinpyrazone and warfarin. Chest. 1981; 79:375.

208. Davis et al: Possible interaction of sulphinpyrazone with coumarins. N Engl J Med. 1978; 299:953.

209. O'Reilly RA et al: Racemic warfarin and trimethoprim-sulfamethoxazole interaction in humans. Ann Intern Med. 1979; 91:34.

210. O'Reilly RA: Stereoselective interaction of TMP/SMX with the separated enantiomorphs of racemic warfarin in man. N Engl J Med. 1980; 302:33.

211. Sioris LJ et al: Potentiation of warfarin anticoagulation by sulfisoxazole. Arch Intern Med. 1980; 140:546.

212. Lumholtz B et al: Sulfamethizole-induced inhibition of diphenylhydantoin, tolbutamide, and warfarin metabolism. Clin Pharmacol Ther. 1978; 17:731.

213. Medical News: Possible interaction occurs with aspirin and two drugs. JAMA. 1970; 214:39.

214. Quick AJ et al: Influence of acetylsalicylic acid and salicylamide on the coagulation of blood. J Pharmacol Exper Ther. 1960; 128:95.

215. Weiss HJ: Platelet physiology and abnormalities of platelet function. N Engl J Med. 1975; 293:580.

216. Weiss HJ: Antiplatelet drugs—A new pharmacologic approach to the prevention of thrombosis. Am Heart J. 1976; 92:86.

217. Fausa O: Salicylate-induced hypoprothrombinemia. Acta Med Scand. 1970; 188:403.

218. O'Reilly RA et al: Impact of aspirin and chlorthalidone on the pharmacodynamics of oral anticoagulant drugs in man. Ann NY Acad Sci. 1971; 179:173.

219. Vagenakis AG et al: Enhancement of warfarin-induced hypoprothrombinemia by thyrotoxicosis. Hopkins Med J. 1972; 131:69.

220. Vessel ES et al: Impairment of drug metabolism in man by allopurinal and nortriptyline. N Engl J Med. 1970; 283:1484.

221. Rawlins MD et al: Influence of allopurinol on drug metabolism in man. Br J Pharmacol. 1973; 48:693.

222. Edwards MS et al: Decreased anticoagulant tolerance with oxymetholone. Lancet. 1971; 2:221.

223. Husted S et al: Increased sensitivity to phenprocoumon during methyltestosterone therapy. Eur J Clin Pharmacol. 1976; 10:209.

224. Sellers EM et al: Potentiation of warfarin-induced hypoprothrombinemia by chloral hydrate. N Engl J Med. 1970; 283:827.

225. Griner PF et al: Chloral hydrate and warfarin interaction: clinical significance? Ann Intern Med. 1971; 74:540.

226. Sellers EM et al: Kinetics and clinical importance of displacement of warfarin from albumin by acidic drugs. Ann NY Acad Sci. 1971; 179:213.

227. Boston Collaborative Drug Surveillance Program: Interaction between chloral hydrate and warfarin. N Engl J Med. 1972; 286:53.

228. Udall JA: Clinical implications of warfarin interactions with five sedatives. Am J Cardiol. 1975; 35:67.

229. Udall JA: Warfarin-chloral hydrate interaction, pharmacological activity and clinical significance. Ann Intern Med. 1974; 81:341.

230. Sellers EM et al: Enhancement of warfarin-induced hypoprothrombinemia by triclofos. Clin Pharmacol Ther. 1972; 13:912.

231. Nappi JM: Warfarin and phenytoin interaction. Ann Intern Med. 1979; 90:852.

232. Koch-Weser J: Hemorrhagic reactions and drug interactions in 500 warfarin treated patients (abstract). Clin Pharmacol Ther. 1973; 14:139.

233. Vessell ES et al: Failure of indomethacin and warfarin to interact in normal human volunteers. J Clin Pharmacol. 1975; 15:486.

234. Self TH et al: Possible interaction of indomethacin and warfarin. Drug Intell Clin Pharm. 1978; 12:580.

235. Breckenridge A et al: Dose-dependent enzyme induction. Clin Pharmacol Ther. 1973; 14:514.

236. Robinson DS et al: Interaction of commonly prescribed drugs and warfarin. Ann Intern Med. 1970; 72:853.

237. Antlitz AM et al: Effect of butabarbital on orally administered anticoagulants. Curr Ther Res. 1968; 10:70.

238. Johansson SA: Apparent resistance to oral anticoagulant therapy and influence of hypnotics on some coagulation factors. Act Med Scand. 1968; 184:297.

239. Levy G: Pharmacokinetic analysis of the effect of barbiturate on the anticoagulant action of warfarin in man. Clin Pharmacol Ther. 1970; 11:372.

240. Corn M: Effect of phenobarbital and glutethimide on biological half-life of warfarin. Thromb Diath Haemorrh. 1966; 16:606.

241. MacDonald MG et al: Clinical observations of possible barbiturate interference with anticoagulation. JAMA. 1968; 204:97.

242. MacDonald MG et al: The effects of phenobarbital, chloral betaine, and glutethimide administration on warfarin plasma levels and hypoprothrombinemic responses in man. Clin Pharmacol Ther. 1969; 10:80.

243. Kendall AG et al: Warfarin-carbamazepine interaction. Ann Intern Med. 1981; 94:280.

244. Hansen IM et al: Carbamazepine-induced acceleration of diphenylhydantoin and warfarin metabolism in man. Clin Pharmacol Ther. 1971; 12:539.

245. O'Reilly RA: Interaction of sodium warfarin and rifampin studies in man. Ann Intern Med. 1974; 81:337.

246. O'Reilly RA: Interaction of chronic daily warfarin therapy and rifampin. Ann Intern Med. 1978; 83:506.

247. Romankiewics JA et al: Rifampin and warfarin: A drug interaction. Ann Intern Med. 1975; 82:224.

248. Robinson DS, Benjamin DM et al: Interaction of warfarin and nonsystemic gastrointestinal drugs. Clin Pharmacol Ther. 1971; 12:491.

249. Jahnchen E et al: Enhanced elimination of warfarin during treatment with cholestyramine. Br J Clin Pharmacol. 1978; 5:437.

250. Meinertz T et al: Interruption of the enterohepatic circulation of phenprocoumon by cholestyramine. Clin Pharmacol Ther. 1977; 21:731.

251. O'Reilly RA: Lack of effect of mealtime table wine on the hypoprothrombinemia of oral anticoagulants. Am J Med Sci. 1979; 277:189.

252. Mielke CH et al: Effects of zomepirac on hemostasis in healthy adults and on platelet function in vitro. J Clin Pharmacol. 1980; 20–409.

253. Serlin MJ et al: Interaction between diflunisal and warfarin. Clin Pharmacol Ther. 1980; 28:493.

254. Penner JA et al: Lack of interaction between ibuprofen and warfarin. Curr Ther Res. 1975; 18:862.

255. O'Brien JR: Effect of anti-inflammatory agents on platelets. Lancet. 1968; 1:894.

256. Carter SA: Potential effect of sulindac on response of prothrombin-time to oral anticoagulants. Lancet. 1979; 2:698.

257. Loftin JP et al: Interaction between sulindac and warfarin: Different results in normal subjects and in an unusual patient with a potassium-losing renal tubular defect. J Clin Pharmacol. 1979; 19:733.

258. Slattery JT et al: Effect of naproxen on the kinetics of elimination and anticoagulant activity of a single dose of warfarin. Clin Pharmacol Ther. 1979; 25:51.

259. Jain A et al: Effect of naproxen on the steady-state serum concentration and anticoagulant activity of warfarin. Clin Pharmacol Ther. 1979; 25:61.

260. Brogden RN et al: Diclofenac sodium: A review of its pharmacological properties and therapeutic use in rheumatic diseases and pain of varying origin. Drugs. 1980; 20:24.

261. Savitsky JP et al: Fenbufen-warfarin interaction in healthy volunteers. Clin Pharmacol Ther. 1980; 27:284.

262. Kelly JG et al: Clinical pharmacokinetics of oral anticoagulants. Clin Pharmacokinetics. 1979; 4:1.

263. O'Reilly RA: Stereoselective interaction of sulphinpyrazone with racemic warfarin and its separated enantiomorphs in man. Circulation. 1982; 65:202.

264. Hull R et al: Adjusted subcutaneous heparin versus warfarin sodium in the long-term treatment of venous thrombosis. N Engl J Med. 1982; 306:189.

Chapter 16

Respiratory Diseases

H. William Kelly

The major function of the respiratory system, in conjunction with the cardiovascular system, is to provide adequate oxygen to body tissues. The respiratory tract transports oxygen (O_2) from the environment to the blood and carbon dioxide (CO_2) from the blood to the environment. The lung's primary function is to exchange gas, although it also filters toxic materials, metabolizes compounds, and protects the body from environmental microorganisms. Diseases of the respiratory tract may interfere with gas exchange through alteration of *ventilation* or *diffusion*. Ventilation refers to the mechanics by which air enters and leaves the alveoli, while diffusion refers to the passage of O_2 and CO_2 across the alveolar walls. This chapter concentrates on the therapy of the more common upper and lower respiratory tract diseases as well as the drug-induced pulmonary diseases. More detailed reviews of the basic physiology and pathophysiology of respiratory tract diseases have been presented elsewhere (1–3).

PULMONARY FUNCTION TESTS

Spirometry. The spirometer (Fig. 1) is used to measure lung volumes and flow rates. As the patient breathes, he displaces the bell, and the pen deflection reflects the volume of air entering or exiting the lung. The *tidal volume* is the volume of gas inspired or expired during normal breathing. The volume during maximal inspiration and

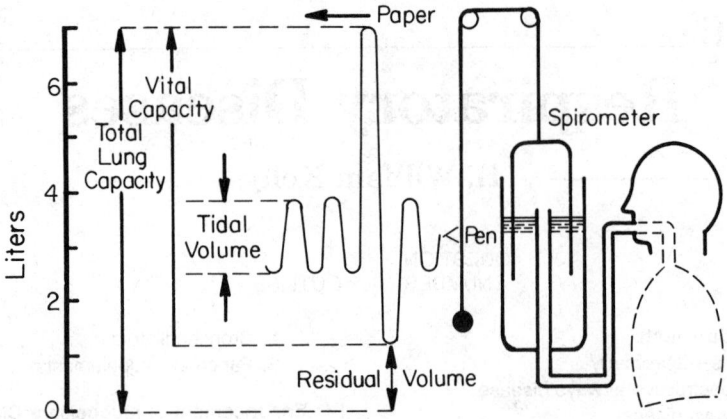

Figure 1. Spirometric Graphs During Quiet Breathing and Maximal Breathing.

expiration is defined as the *vital capacity (VC)*. The *residual volume (RV)* is the volume of air left in the lung after maximal expiration. The volume of gas left after a normal expiration is the *functional residual capacity (FRC)*. *Total lung capacity (TLC)* is the vital capacity plus the residual volume. Patients with obstructive pulmonary disease tend to have a decreased VC, an increased RV, and an increased or normal TLC, while patients with classical restrictive pulmonary disease have a decrease in all lung volumes (1). However, patients may have mixed lesion diseases, in which case simple changes in lung volumes are unlikely to occur until the disease has advanced considerably.

Forced expiration maneuvers amplify the ventilation abnormalities produced by disease. The most useful simple clinical test for ventilation dysfunction is the forced expiration volume. This is measured by having the patient exhale as forcefully and completely as possible after maximal inspiration into a spirometer. This is often done in a spirometer which measures flow and volume (Fig. 2), and measurements are made from the resulting flow/volume curve. The *forced expiratory volume in the first second (FEV₁)* and the total volume expired or *forced vital capacity (FVC)* are the most commonly used measurements because they are the most reproducible. Normally, the FEV_1 is 80% of the FVC and is often reported as the FEV_1/FVC ratio. Figure 3 depicts typical flow/volume curves for obstructive and restrictive lung disease. Obstructive diseases such as asthma, bronchitis, and emphysema pro-

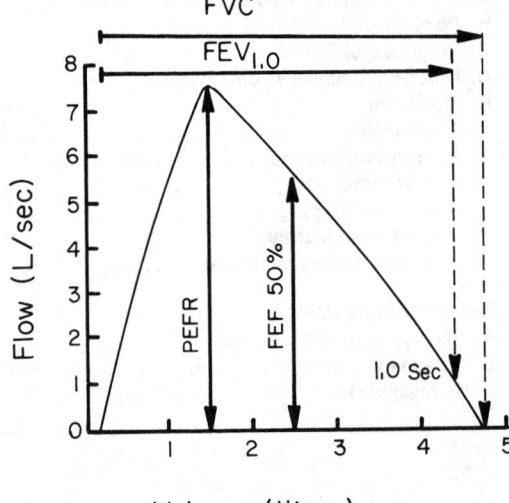

Figure 2. Flow/Volume Curve Resulting from A Forced Expiratory Maneuver.

duce a decrease in the FEV_1 and FEV_1/FVC ratio. Restrictive diseases depress both the FEV_1 and FVC so that the FEV_1/FVC ratio may be normal or even greater than normal (2,3).

The *peak expiratory flow rate (PEFR)* is the maximal flow which can be produced during the forced expiration. The PEFR is easy to measure and is therefore commonly used in emergency rooms and clinics to quickly assess the effectiveness of bronchodilators in the treatment of acute asthma attacks. The changes in PEFR generally

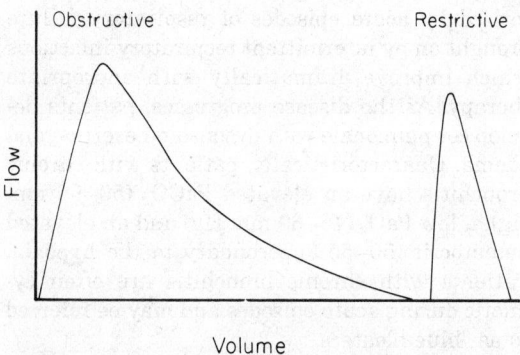

Figure 3. A Flow/Volume Curve with Typical Patterns for Obstructive and Restrictive Disease.

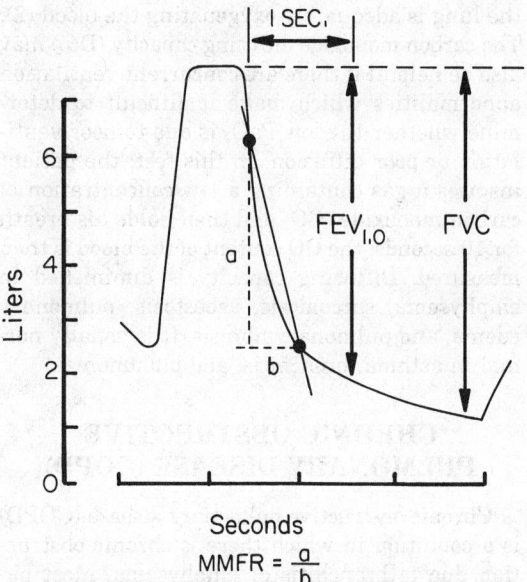

Figure 4. Volume/Time Curve Resulting from A Forced Expiratory Maneuver.

parallel those of the FEV_1; however, the PEFR is a less reproducible measure than the FEV_1. The *maximal midexpiratory flow rate (MMFR or MMEF)* is the flow rate measured over the middle half of expiration. The MMFR is measured on the effort-independent portion of the forced expiratory volume curve or that portion of flow which is only dependent on the elastic recoil of the lung (Fig. 4). The expiratory flow at 50% vital capacity (FEF 50%) is an equivalent measurement taken from a flow/volume curve (Fig. 2). These are more sensitive measures of air flow resistance in the small airways (eg, those less than 2.0 mm in diameter) (2).

Obstructive versus Restrictive Airway Disease. In simplest terms, obstructive disease limits airflow during expiration and restrictive disease limits airflow during inspiration. Restrictive disease results from a loss of elasticity and a consequent inability to expand the lung; therefore, a typical flow volume curve shows markedly depressed volumes with increased flow rates (when corrected for the volume). In obstructive diseases such as chronic bronchitis (characterized by increased mucous in the bronchial lumen), emphysema (characterized by airway collapse), or asthma (characterized by bronchospasm), maximal expiration begins at high lung volumes and the flow rates are depressed. The markedly depressed flows at low lung volumes give the characteristic scooped out appearance of the obstructive flow/volume curve (Fig. 3). Because the MMFR is the most sensitive test of small airways disease, some of the earliest changes in chronic obstructive pulmonary disease may be detected with this measurement.

Reversible Airway Obstruction. Spirometry is often used to diagnose bronchospasm or reversible airways disease, which is most commonly seen in asthma; however, obstruction from bronchiolar wall edema and excess mucous may also be "reversible." Significant clinical reversibility is defined as a 15–20% improvement in FEV_1 or PEFR following a challenge with a bronchodilator (4). Bronchospasm can also be measured by spirometry before and after an inhalation challenge of histamine or methacholine which will produce a 15–20% decrease in FEV_1 in asthmatics (5).

Limitations of Spirometry. Since the FEV_1 and the PEFR are both highly effort-dependent, complete patient cooperation is required for reliable results. This limits the utility of spirometric tests in severely ill or very young patients. The FEV_1 and PEFR are also relatively insensitive to small airway changes, and early mucous plugging and bronchospasm in small bronchioles may not be detectable. Although the MMFR is a more sensitive test of airway obstruction, it is also much more variable, requiring larger changes (30–40%) to be clinically significant.

Evaluation of Diffusion Capacity. Arterial blood gases (PaO_2, $PaCO_2$, and pH) are the best laboratory tests for determining whether or not the lung is adequately oxygenating the blood (2). The carbon monoxide diffusing capacity (Dco) may also be helpful if there are concurrent ventilation abnormalities which make it difficult to determine whether the low PaO_2 is due to poor ventilation or poor diffusion. In this test, the patient inspires a gas containing a low concentration of carbon monoxide (CO) and then holds his breath for 10 seconds; the CO content of the blood is then measured. Diffusing capacity is diminished in emphysema, sarcoidosis, asbestosis, pulmonary edema, and pulmonary fibrosis. It is usually normal in asthma, bronchitis, and pneumonias.

CHRONIC OBSTRUCTIVE PULMONARY DISEASE (COPD)

Chronic obstructive pulmonary disease (COPD) is a condition in which there is chronic obstruction due to bronchitis or emphysema. Most patients with COPD present with characteristics of both diseases, although in many there is a predominance of either emphysema or bronchitis. See Table 1.

Chronic bronchitis is a condition characterized by excessive mucous production and can be diagnosed on the basis of the patient's history. Airways obstruction in this condition is caused by inflammation and edema of the bronchioles as well as mucous plugs. The patient is generally obese and has a long history of cigarette smoking; there is a cough productive of sputum at least three months of the year. The disease is charac-

terized by acute episodes of respiratory failure brought on by intermittent respiratory infections which improve dramatically with appropriate therapy. As the disease progresses, patients develop cor pulmonale with dyspnea on exertion and edema. Characteristically, patients with chronic bronchitis have an elevated $PaCO_2$ (50–60 mm Hg), a low PaO_2 (45–60 mm Hg) and an elevated hematocrit (50–55%) secondary to the hypoxia. Patients with chronic bronchitis are often cyanotic during acute episodes and may be referred to as "blue bloaters."

Emphysema, like bronchitis, is characterized by a long smoking history with chronic obstruction resulting in a decreased FEV_1, FVC, and MMFR. However, the underlying pathology differs in that the obstruction is due to alveolar tissue destruction and scarring which decrease the elastic recoil and cause a loss of tissue tractional support; this leads to bronchiolar collapse during expiration. In contrast to patients with chronic bronchitis, patients with emphysema are thin and give a long history of dyspnea with minimal cough that is only slightly productive of sputum. Further, recurrent respiratory infections and cor pulmonale are not usually associated with the disease process. The patient has obvious difficulty breathing and uses accessory muscles vigorously to help him breathe. There is an increased respiratory rate, often with grunting on inspiration and followed by prolonged expiration through pursed lips. The arterial blood gases and hematocrit are generally slightly abnormal or within

Table 1.

CLINICAL PATTERNS OF CHRONIC BRONCHITIS AND EMPHYSEMA

Characteristic	Chronic Bronchitis	Emphysema
Synonyms	Blue Bloater	Pink-Puffer
Age of onset	45–65	55–75
Cigarette smoking	+	+
Major symptom	chronic cough	dyspnea
Cor pulmonale	present	absent
Body type	obese	thin
Sputum	copious	scanty
Pulmonary functions		
FEV_1	↓	↓
FVC	↓	↓
Residual volume	↑	↑ ↑
Total lung capacity	normal, ↓	↑ ↑
Diffusing capacity	normal	↓

normal limits and for this reason these individuals may be referred to as "pink puffers."

The primary theoretical importance of differentiating between these two causes of COPD is that while emphysema is an irreversible process which may only be treated by minimizing insults and preventing its progression, chronic bronchitis is a reversible, treatable condition. In actuality, most patients present with features of both conditions and treatment differs little regardless of the diagnosis.

Cigarette smoking is clearly the most important factor in the pathogenesis of chronic obstructive pulmonary disease (6,7). Increases in bronchial reactivity and significant obstruction in small airways can be demonstrated in smokers without clinical symptomatology and in children and other non-smokers chronically exposed to the cigarette smoke of others (8,10). Air pollution is another predisposing factor to COPD.

The role of recurrent respiratory tract infections in the pathogenesis of chronic bronchitis is much less clear. In a critical review of the literature, Tager found no conclusive evidence to support the role of infection as a causative factor in COPD (11). A number of studies have demonstrated an increased colonization of the sputum of chronic bronchitics with bacteria and mycoplasmas. While a number of these investigations have been able to demonstrate an increase in antibody titers against these bacteria during acute exacerbations, a clearcut pathogenic role in the progression of the disease has not been defined. Studies evaluating the prophylactic administration of antibiotics effective against these bacteria have also failed to demonstrate a pathogenic role for these bacteria in that there was no decrease in the number of acute exacerbations with moderate disease. Also, the progressive rate of decline in FEV_1 was not significantly different between the treated and untreated groups (11).

Although recurrent infections do not appear to be the cause of the mucous hypersecretion, there is evidence that increased mucous secretion does predispose the patient to increased infection (11). Further clinical examples of this phenomenon would be the increased number of bacterial respiratory infections in patients with cystic fibrosis, bronchiectasis, and Kartagener's syndrome (immotile cilia), diseases characterized by either increased mucous secretion or decreased mucociliary clearance.

The prognosis for patients with COPD is highly variable and depends principally upon the severity of obstruction. In general, 50% of patients live five years or more following the onset of clinical disability. The disease progresses insidiously with intermittent, acute exacerbations; the two most common causes of death are cor pulmonale and respiratory failure.

1. L.Y. is an overweight, 55-year-old female bus driver who presents with a chief complaint of breathlessness, dyspnea, and an increasing cough productive of purulent sputum over the past three days. Five days prior to this episode, the patient developed signs and symptoms of an upper respiratory tract infection and began taking tetracycline 250 mg qid, aspirin 650 mg every four hours for her fever and headache, and Contac, one capsule as needed for her stuffiness.

The past medical history reveals that the patient was diagnosed as having chronic bronchitis four years previously. At that time she had a two pack per day history of smoking for 30 years and was advised to stop smoking. The patient also gave a history of frequent chest infections since childhood. There has been an increasing frequency and severity of these infections over the past five years, some resulting in hospitalization. The patient has had a chronic productive cough for the past 10 years.

Physical examination revealed a slightly cyanotic, obese female who was tachycardic and tachypneic. She exhibited three to four word breathlessness and pursed her lips during expiration. Her chest was hyperinflated and resonant to percussion and there were rales and rhonchi on auscultation. She had 2 + pretibial edema and a temperature of 38° C.

Laboratory tests were reported as follows: WBC 10,000/mm³, pH 7.38, PaO_2 48 mm Hg, $PaCO_2$ 50 mm Hg. Pulmonary function tests included the following: FEV_1 0.7 L (34% of predicted), FVC 1.5 L, MMFR 25% of predicted.

The patient was diagnosed as having acute respiratory insufficiency secondary to an acute exacerbation of chronic bronchitis. She was begun on amoxicillin 500 mg orally every six hours, aminophylline 0.5 mg/kg/hr IV following a loading dose of 6 mg/kg, inhaled me-

taproterenol (0.3 ml of a 50 mg/ml solution diluted in 2.5 cc of normal saline and administered by a compressed air nebulizer every four hours), and methylprednisolone 0.5 mg/kg every six hours intravenously. The patient was also placed on low flow oxygen (approximately 24%) by nasal cannula.

Was the diagnosis of chronic bronchitis consistent with the patient's history and physical examination?

Although L.Y. has some symptoms consistent with emphysema such as tachypnea, a resonant chest and a prolonged expiratory phase with pursed lips, most of her signs, symptoms and past medical history are consistent with chronic bronchitis. These include her long history of smoking, recurrent respiratory infections, and a productive cough. Her shortness of breath, rales, and edema are consistent with cor pulmonale, which is more common in patients with chronic bronchitis; her abnormal blood gases are also consistent with chronic bronchitis.

2. Why was the patient placed on amoxicillin?

Although chronic prophylaxis with antibiotics is of no therapeutic benefit, few practitioners would argue with the intermittent use of antibiotics to treat acute exacerbations in chronic bronchitis; data to support this practice, however, are weak. Tager found that of the six double-blind studies using a placebo control, only two demonstrated a statistically significant advantage for the use of antibiotics in treating acute exacerbations (11). Most studies compare one antibiotic with another without a placebo control. The bacteria most commonly isolated from the sputum of chronic bronchitics are *Hemophilus influenzae* and *Diplococcus pneumoniae* (11). *Mycoplasma pneumoniae* and viruses have also been implicated in these acute exacerbations. Amoxicillin or ampicillin 500 mg every six hours, tetracycline 250-500 mg every six hours or co-trimoxazole (Bactrim DS) one tablet every twelve hours are the most frequent regimens used. All appear to be equally effective.

3. Comment on the use of bronchodilators and corticosteroids in L.Y. Is this patient's airways obstruction reversible?

Reversibility usually refers to obstruction caused by bronchospasm; however, airways obstruction caused by mucous plugs and bronchiolar inflammation with edema is also reversible.

Many chronic bronchitics will also have hypertrophy of bronchial smooth muscle and hyperreactive airways (12). A recent study of ten patients with irreversible airflow obstruction demonstrated improved pulmonary mechanics with therapeutic doses of *theophylline* (13). Theophylline has also been shown to increase alveolar ventilation and improve right ventricular performance in COPD patients without significantly changing lung mechanics (14,15). Because of these findings, many investigators feel a trial of bronchodilators with careful monitoring is indicated in chronic bronchitics who are in acute respiratory failure. Ambulatory patients should be given bronchodilators chronically only if they have had a documented response to a challenge with bronchodilators.

The role of *corticosteroids* in chronic bronchitis is less clear. In an excellent review of the literature, Sahn found that of 17 studies only six demonstrated a beneficial effect of corticosteroids in the treatment of bronchitis (16). However, because individual patients had a beneficial response Sahn recommended that any patient with COPD with worsening symptoms be given an objectively monitored, finite trial of corticosteroids. A more recent double-blind placebo-controlled trial in 44 chronic bronchitis patients with acute respiratory insufficiency demonstrated that 0.5 mg/kg methylprednisolone every six hours significantly improved pulmonary mechanics in the first 72 hours (17).

4. Was the administration of oxygen appropriate in L.Y.? How should it be administered? What are the dangers of oxygen therapy?

Patients such as L.Y. with hypercapnic hypoxemia should be given controlled, low dose oxygen therapy (inspired oxygen concentration of 24%) if the PaO_2 values are less than 50 mm Hg (19). Serial arterial blood gas measurements should be used to monitor improvement of the hypoxemia and hypercapnea in L.Y. Improvement in physical signs such as cyanosis, tachycardia, and mental status are also useful monitoring parameters.

The administration of oxygen to COPD patients with acute respiratory insufficiency, such as L.Y., may cause progressive acidosis and stupor or coma secondary to carbon dioxide narcosis. This is caused by decreasing the hypoxic respiratory drive in patients whose hypercapnic stimulation to respiration has been blunted from chronic carbon dioxide retention. Bone et al found that the PaO_2 and pH were more sensitive predictors of patients who would develop carbon dioxide narcosis than the degree of hypercapnia (23). In their series, patients who developed narcosis had an average PaO_2 of 41 ± 9 mm Hg and a pH of 7.27 ± 0.04 versus an average PaO_2 of 55 ± 10 mm Hg and a pH of 7.36 ± 0.07 (P < 0.0001) in those who did not develop narcosis. The $PaCO_2$ was not significantly different in the two groups. L.Y.'s PaO_2 of 48 mm Hg and pH of 7.38 indicate that she is not at high risk for carbon dioxide narcosis using these criteria. Nevertheless, the arterial pH and $PaCO_2$ must be monitored closely.

Dried secretions with decreased tracheal clearance of mucous and tracheitis may be caused by the administration of oxygen which is inadequately humidified. These symptoms have also been described in six normal subjects who were administered 90–95% oxygen for six hours (19).

Oxygen toxicity of the lung usually occurs at oxygen concentrations greater than 40%, although no absolutely safe concentration has been established (19). Inspired oxygen concentrations (FiO_2) of between 50 and 100% carry a significant risk of toxicity. The duration required to produce the toxicity seems to be inversely proportional to the concentration. Pathologically, oxygen toxicity consists of atelectasis, edema, alveolar hemorrhage, inflammation, fibrin deposition, ciliated cell damage, and hyalinization of alveolar membranes (20,21). In premature infants, oxygen therapy carries the additional risk of inducing blindness by causing retrolental fibroplasia (22). These patients may also develop bronchopulmonary dysplasia, a chronic obstructive pulmonary disease of infancy.

5. What are the benefits of chronic home oxygen therapy? Should this patient receive chronic oxygen therapy?

The goal of chronic home oxygen therapy in patients with severe COPD is to improve their general well-being and prolong their lives. Levin initially demonstrated an improvement in the general well-being of such patients receiving continuous low flow oxygen therapy (24). Since then, numerous studies have demonstrated improvements in exercise tolerance and neurophysiological parameters such as memory (25–27). In 1970, Neff reported that continuous home oxygen therapy could extend the life of patients with severe

COPD (28), and preliminary data from a large controlled study by the Medical Research Council of Great Britain have also demonstrated a decrease in mortality in patients using low flow O_2 (1–3 liters/min) 15 hours a day (29). Chronic O_2 therapy improves life span by decreasing pulmonary vascular resistance and reversing polycythemia; this prevents cor pulmonale, a leading cause of morbidity and mortality in these patients (27,29).

The substantial cost of home oxygen therapy and the possible risk of further lung damage have resulted in the establishment of guidelines for placing patients on home oxygen therapy. The patient should have a PaO_2 below 50–55 mm Hg at rest, measured several times during a stable period while breathing room air. Patients with a daytime PaO_2 consistently above 55 mm Hg who have clinical signs of significant chronic tissue hypoxemia such as polycythemia, cor pulmonale, pulmonary hypertension, and profound dyspnea and hypoxemia with exercise and patients with significant nocturnal hypoxemia should also receive chronic oxygen therapy (27). Although L.Y. fills many of the criteria for home oxygen therapy at this time, she is in acute exacerbation and will have to be evaluated following stabilization.

6. If L.Y. is started on home oxygen therapy, how many hours during the day should it be administered? Describe the best method for its administration.

Because of evidence of toxicity from 24-hour oxygen therapy and studies indicating improvement with as little as 15 hours of therapy, a large cooperative study group was formed to compare 12-hour versus 24-hour home oxygen therapy (29,30). The Nocturnal Oxygen Therapy Trial Group (NOTTG) reported results of therapy in 203 patients who were followed for at least one year. Entry criteria included resting hypoxemia ($PaO_2 \leq 55$ mm Hg) or a $PaO_2 \leq 59$ mm Hg together with edema, a hematocrit $\geq 55\%$, cor pulmonale on ECG, or an FEV_1/FVC ratio of less than 70% after treatment with a bronchodilator. The results showed an overall mortality in the 12-hour nocturnal group which was 1.94 times greater than that of the 24-hour continuous group (p = 0.01) (31). Therefore oxygen should be administered at least 12–15 hours daily and possibly 24 hours/day.

The usual method of administering oxygen is through a nasal cannula in a range of 1 to 4 liters

Table 2. (32)

EXPECTED FiO$_2$ FROM VARIOUS DEVICES

Device	Flow Rate (L/min)	FiO$_2$(%)
Simple Mask	3–4	28–30
	5–6	35–42
	7–8	44–54
	>8	55–60
Rebreathing Mask	5	60
	7	70
	10	99
Nasal Cannula	1	24
	2	28
	3	32
	4	36

per minute (27). This method delivers fractional levels of inspired oxygen (FiO$_2$) which improve the resting PaO$_2$ to 60–80 mm Hg. This should be titrated to the individual to relieve exertional dyspnea and other signs of hypoxia. Table 2 lists the different methods of administering O$_2$ and the expected FiO$_2$ from each method. The nasal cannula is preferred by most patients, while the masks provide greater humidification.

CYSTIC FIBROSIS

Cystic fibrosis (CF) is the most common lethal genetic disease of Caucasians and occurs with a frequency of 1:1500 to 1:2500 (33). It is an autosomal recessive trait with the heterozygous carrier occurring in 1 of 20 persons in a Caucasian population. The basic defect of CF is unknown, but it is characterized clinically by the secretion of thick, tenacious mucous in the exocrine glands which causes obstruction. Sites of obstruction include the lung airways, paranasal sinuses, pancreas, small intestine, uterine cervix, and male genital tract (34). The two most significant clinical problems in CF are malabsorption secondary to obstruction of the pancreas and a lack of digestive enzymes and chronic lung disease secondary to recurrent infections. The pulmonary disease in CF is obstructive in nature, resembling chronic bronchitis, with mucous plugging, chronic infection, bronchiectasis, and fibrosis. It accounts for 95% of the mortality in these patients (34).

7. **R.S., a 17-year-old male with a history of cystic fibrosis, presents with a chief complaint of increased tiredness over the last week and three days of increased cough and sputum production. The sputum has also changed color and has been blood tinged during the last day. The patient's past medical history is significant for his cystic fibrosis and numerous hospitalizations in the past for pneumonia. Current medications include Pancrease, three capsules with meals and one or two with snacks; sustained-release theophylline 500 mg every 12 hours; metaproterenol metered dose inhaler, two puffs qid before postural drainage; Aquasol E and multiple vitamin supplementation.**

On physical examination, the patient presents as a thin, pale young man in mild respiratory distress with a constant productive cough. The patient is admitted and begun on the following regimen: tobramycin 2.5 mg/kg/ dose every six hours, ticarcillin 50 mg/kg/dose every four hours, and nafcillin 30 mg/kg/dose every four hours, all by intravenous infusion; probenecid 40 mg/kg/day orally in four divided doses; and theophylline and metaproterenol. Chest physical therapy (CPT) and postural drainage every six hours are continued.

Why was this particular antibiotic regimen selected for this patient?

The pathogens most commonly isolated from the sputum of CF patients are *Staphylococcus aureus, Pseudomonas aeruginosa,* and *Hemophilus influenzae* (35,36). Many patients become chronically colonized with pseudomonas which become extremely difficult to eradicate. CF patients are frequently placed on an antibiotic regimen which covers staphylococcus and pseudomonas at the first subtle signs of infection. These are exhibited in this patient by increased fatigue, increased cough and sputum production, and by the changes in the consistency and color of his sputum. Improved patient survival in CF may be attributed in large part to improved antimicrobial therapy.

Initial therapy of acute exacerbations often consists of an aminoglycoside (gentamicin or tobramycin) plus carbenicillin or ticarcillin with or without an anti-staphylococcal penicillin such as nafcillin. This regimen covers the most common etiologic organisms.

8. **Why were such high doses of antibiotics**

ordered for R.S.? Are aerosolized antibiotics useful?

There are several reasons why higher doses are used in CF patients. The aminoglycoside and penicillin antibiotics penetrate bronchial secretions poorly (37,38). This commonly results in antimicrobial sputum levels which are less than the minimum inhibitory concentration (MIC) for the infecting organisms in CF patients (39,40). Also, an increase in the renal clearance of penicillins has been observed in CF patients, resulting in more frequent dosing and the addition of probenecid to their regimens (41,42). The renal clearance of amikacin (43) and the volume of distribution and total plasma clearance of gentamicin (142) and tobramycin (143) are significantly increased for patients with CF. Since nomograms or guidelines for aminoglycoside dosing have been derived from populations which did not include subjects with CF, such generalized approaches to dosing must not be used for CF patients. Because CF patients have unique dosing requirements, routine monitoring of aminoglycoside serum concentrations are essential in these patients. Because of their malabsorption problems, CF patients also have a greater than normal lean body mass to surface area ratio which increases their distribution volumes of aminoglycosides if calculated on a weight basis (44). A number of clinical studies have demonstrated the need for higher mg/kg doses in CF patients to achieve comparable peak serum aminoglycoside levels when compared to non-CF patients (43,45,46). This is often corrected by basing the dose on body surface area. This patient's tobramycin dose of 2.5 mg/kg every six hours is appropriate (143). Subsequent doses should be adjusted according to serum concentrations.

Some cystic fibrosis treatment centers advocate using aerosolized antibiotics to overcome the difficulty in achieving adequate antibiotic sputum levels. At present there are no convincing data to support this practice. At least two small clinical studies have demonstrated no increased benefit from the addition of aerosolized antibiotics to the regimen of CF patients treated with adequate systemic therapy (45,47).

9. What is the indication for bronchodilators in R.S.?

The use of bronchodilators in the treatment of CF is controversial. Mellis and Levison demonstrated bronchial hyperactivity in CF patients which correlated with the severity of their lung disease (48). Clinical studies have variably demonstrated worsening or improvement in pulmonary function following the administration of bronchodilators depending on the measurement technique (49,50). Beta-2-adrenergic agents demonstrably increase mucociliary transport in CF patients (51). The routine use of bronchodilators in all CF patients is not recommended, but bronchodilators are warranted in patients with concomitant asthma or documented reversible bronchospasm. Also, a trial of bronchodilators with close monitoring and follow-up of pulmonary function tests and clinical well-being may be warranted in patients with severe pulmonary disease.

10. This patient is receiving Pancrease as a pancreatic enzyme replacement. What are the goals of therapy and how does Pancrease differ from other enzyme preparations?

The goals of pancreatic enzyme therapy in children with CF are to reduce steatorrhea and establish adequate nutrition for growth. Pancreatic enzyme products are produced from dessicated beef or pork pancrease. The preparations available include a powder, tablets, capsules, and enteric coated tablets. Since much of the enzyme activity of these preparations is destroyed by the acidic environment of the stomach, very high doses have been recommended (52). To minimize this problem, enteric coated tablets have been formulated, but they are usually less effective than uncoated preparations (52). Recently, antacids and/or cimetidine have been added to the enzyme regimens with improved therapeutic results (53). This patient is receiving Pancrease which is a capsule containing enteric coated microspheres of enzyme. This dosage form appears to be more efficacious than other enzyme replacements and combination therapy with antacids or cimetidine is unnecessary (53,54). The dose required is three tablets with each meal as opposed to 12 tablets of other enzyme products. The ingestion of so many tablets or powders with each meal has been particularly onerous to patients, and it is our experience that Pancrease is the most palatable of the products currently available.

11. What is the purpose of the chest physical therapy (CPT) and postural drainage in this patient's therapy?

The lung's primary defense against irritants and infectious agents is the mucociliary transport system. Patients with CF not only have excess mucous secretion but an impairment of cilia function (55). This impaired ciliary function contributes to recurrent pulmonary infections.

The purpose of CPT and postural drainage in this patient is to improve his mucociliary clearance. Chest physical therapy by mechanical vibrator or manual clapping of the thorax produces vibrations which loosen mucous in the bronchiolar lumens. Postural drainage then utilizes gravity flow to help remove the loose secretions. Although CPT and postural drainage are commonly prescribed for patients with CF and chronic bronchitis, the efficacy of this form of therapy remains controversial (59). Graham demonstrated that CPT was of no benefit in the treatment of patients with acute pneumonia (60). In patients with COPD, the data are less clear. While some studies have demonstrated an increased sputum production and some improvement in lung volumes following CPT, others have shown no benefit and potentially harmful hypoxemia during CPT in patients with acute exacerbations of chronic bronchitis (59, 61–64). Oldenburg recently demonstrated that no effect of postural drainage could be detected if cough was suppressed and that chest physiotherapy did not show any better effect than cough alone (65).

In older patients with CF, good exercise programs are often as beneficial as complicated programs of routine CPT with postural drainage. In conclusion, the use of physiotherapy in CF and other disease states needs further controlled evaluation to document its benefit. Therefore, when considering its use, the possible risks and cost to benefit ratios should be considered. As with any form of therapy, careful objective and subjective follow-up evaluation of the patient is an essential part of therapy.

12. On the second day of hospitalization, R.S. is begun on N-acetylcysteine by inhalation, 4 cc of a 10% solution every 6 hours just prior to CPT and postural drainage. Is N-acetylcysteine an effective mucolytic agent? What other mucolytic agents are available? Should this patient be placed on mucolytic therapy chronically?

Mucolytic agents such as glycerin and propylene glycol decrease the viscosity of mucous by increasing its water content through hygroscopic activity; others break down the mucous glycoprotein. N-acetylcysteine (Mucomyst) contains free sulfhydryl groups which interact with and break the mucoprotein disulfide bonds. Dornase (Dornovac) and trypsin (Tryptar) are proteolytic enzymes which break down the proteins in mucous. Alevaire, a mixture of sodium bicarbonate and tyloxapol, a surfactant, and plain sodium bicarbonate are used to decrease the adhesiveness of mucoid secretions to the respiratory epithelium.

The administration of *bland aerosols* such as normal saline, hypotonic saline, or hypertonic saline have been used extensively in combination with chest physiotherapy, postural drainage, and percussion to enhance mucociliary clearance and improve pulmonary function in patients. A current review by Wanner on the use of bland aerosols concluded that except for the induction of cough by hypertonic saline and the induction of bronchospasm in asthmatics, there are no conclusive data demonstrating benefit from bland aerosol therapy in cystic fibrosis or chronic bronchitis (57). Nocturnal mist tent therapy in cystic fibrosis has no demonstrated benefit (57,58).

There is no question that *N-acetylcysteine* and *pancreatic dornase* are effective mucolytics *in vitro* in that they both significantly decrease sputum viscosity (56,57). The detergent Alevaire produces the same effect as water or normal saline. In patients with chronic bronchitis and cystic fibrosis, the results with a 10% and 20% inhalation of N-acetylcysteine have been inconclusive. While a number of studies have demonstrated an increased amount of sputum with a decreased viscosity 30–60 minutes following the inhalation of N-acetylcysteine and pancreatic dornase, long-term studies have all failed to demonstrate any positive effect of these agents (34, 55–57). In contrast, the direct instillation of 10% N-acetylcysteine has been life-saving in patients with acute bronchial mucous impaction and has demonstrated efficacy in opening atelectatic portions of the lung (56,57,66). Acutely, enzymes and N-acetylcysteine cause irritation and bronchospasm and should therefore be administered with isoproterenol in patients with hyperactive airways.

13. Are there other pharmacologic means to improve mucociliary clearance in R.S.? What agents could further depress the mucociliary clearance in this patient?

Pharmacologic agents can improve mucociliary transport by decreasing mucous viscosity or by increasing ciliary beating. *Beta-2-adrenergic agents* increase mucociliary transport by stimulating mucous production and ciliary beat frequency (34,55). *Cholinergic agents* increase transport by stimulating ciliary function and mucous production, but their clinical use is limited because they also stimulate bronchospasm. *Methylxanthines* stimulate ciliary function and mucous production, thus increasing mucociliary transport in animal models (55).

Expectorant drugs such as guaifenisin (Robitussin), ammonium chloride, sodium citrate, terpin hydrate, and ipecac increase mucous secretion by causing gastric irritation. Subemetic doses initiate reflex stimulation of the vagal efferent nerves supplying the bronchial glands. Ziment calls this the gastropulmonary mucokinetic vagal reflex (56). Iodides such as potassium iodide (SSKI) are thought to have a direct stimulating effect on the bronchial glands as well as a mucolytic and an indirect vagal effect. Although there are no objective data to support this contention, many clinicians consider iodides to be the most effective of the expectorant drugs.

A number of well-controlled, double-blind studies have failed to show any expectorant effect for guaifenisin over placebo in doses up to 400 mg (twice the recommended dosage) four times daily (55,56,67). There has been a similar lack of evidence for terpin hydrate, ammonium chloride, and ipecac at the usual recommended dosages. Dosages high enough to produce an effect with these agents, such as 2400 mg per day of guaifenisin, also produce significant gastrointestinal upset (56). Iodides have also failed to demonstrate a consistent expectorant effect but have demonstrated considerable toxicity when taken chronically in cystic fibrosis and chronic bronchitis (34,55,56,68). Chronic iodide therapy has caused acne, induced goiter and hypothyroidism, and is associated with severe hypersensitivity reactions (56,69).

In conclusion, many of the current methods for increasing mucociliary clearance are of questionable benefit. When considering either drugs or physiotherapy, the possible risks and cost to benefit ratios should be considered. Careful objective and subjective follow-up of the patient is an essential part of therapy.

Agents which impair mucociliary transport include chronic cigarette smoking, viral respiratory tract infections, low inspired humidity, general anesthesia, anticholinergics, and narcotic analgesics (55).

COMMON COLD

14. J.G., a 38-year-old female, requests a medication to treat her cold. She complains of a headache, sore throat, malaise, cough, congestion, and some rhinitis. The patient's history reveals that she has hypertension which is well controlled with hydralazine, propranolol, and hydrochlorthiazide; she has no drug allergies or history of chronic lung disease. What further information would be helpful in deciding how to treat this patient? Would an antibiotic be useful in this patient?

The etiologic agent for the "common cold" is a virus. The rhinoviruses are the most common causative agents, while the echoviruses, adenoviruses, coxsackie viruses, and parainfluenza viruses are also known etiologic agents. The signs and symptoms of a viral cold include a sore throat, cough, rhinitis, headache, and slight fever; they are non-specific and could be presenting symptoms of potentially more serious problems. A brief history by the practitioner can readily detect situations which require a more extensive work-up. First, one should determine if the patient's symptoms are those she usually associates with a cold and whether or not other family members have similar symptoms. Does the patient have a chronic lung disease or significant cardiovascular disease beyond the hypertension for which she is taking medication? How long has she had the symptoms? A chronic cough may be the first sign of chronic bronchitis, or the only presenting symptom of asthma. If the patient is producing mucopurulent sputum in large quantities, she may have a bacterial bronchitis or pneumonia. Rhinitis may be a sign of allergic hay fever, sinusitis (particularly if purulent), or vasomotor rhinitis. Chronic nasal stuffiness may also be a sign of decongestant abuse, or nasal polyps. Headache may also be a sign of bacterial sinus infection particularly if the patient has point tenderness over a sinus area. A sore throat could be streptococcal pharyngitis. A viral flu often mimics the common cold but usually will present with more severe constitutional symptoms. In infants and young children, many common viral illnesses, chicken pox, measles, and rubella initially present with "cold-like" symptoms. This patient presents with minimal symptomatology and a negative history of chronic lung disease; therefore, antibiotics are not indicated.

15. The patient's cough is non-productive and irritating, and she would like an antitussive agent. How should her cough and cold be treated?

The common cold is a self-limiting illness which has a course of 5–7 days; therefore, any treatment regimen should be of short duration. Treatment is symptomatic and as such should be tailored to meet the needs of the patient. For more extensive reviews of the available products, the reader should refer to other resources (70,71). In providing symptomatic therapy for the common cold, the practitioner should use the opportunity for patient education. The patient should be made aware that a cough is a protective, beneficial mechanism for clearing excess secretions and that the most effective oral expectorant is adequate fluid intake. Cough suppressants will not stop the cough completely, but should decrease the cough and suppress severe paroxysms which prevent adequate rest at night. Codeine 5–10 mg, detromethorphan 15–30 mg, and noscapine 15–30 mg, given four to six times daily, appear to be equally effective as cough suppressants (70,71). [The dose of codeine for children should not exceed 1 mg/kg/day (72).] If the patient has an irritative nonproductive cough, the use of syrups (honey and lemon juice with whiskey) or cough drops which provide a soothing demulcent effect may be adequate (70,73). For more severe sore throats, lozenges containing a local anesthetic agent such as benzocaine may provide more relief (71,73).

16. The patient would like a decongestant. Which non-prescription decongestant would be the most appropriate for this patient?

The available decongestants are alpha-adrenergic stimulants which cause vasoconstriction. The oral decongestants with proven efficacy include pseudoephedrine (Sudafed), 60 mg four times daily, phenylpropanolamine 25–50 mg three times daily, and phenylephrine 10 mg every four hours (71). Phenylephrine is a direct alpha agonist while pseudoephedrine and phenylpropanolamine work indirectly through the release of endogenous norepinephrine. Phenylephrine is erratically absorbed and is not recommended for oral use. Oral decongestants are not selective for the nasal vasculature and will cause systemic vasoconstriction. When taken in the recommended dosage, they do not significantly increase blood pressure; however, it is generally best to avoid these preparations in patients with a history of hypertension (such as J.G.) or cardiac arrhythmias (70,71). Therefore, a topical decongestant would be more appropriate for this patient. Phenylephrine 0.25–0.5% (Neo-Synephrine), Naphazoline 0.05% (Privine), Oxymetazoline 0.05% (Afrin), and Xylometazoline 0.1% (Sinex-L.A.) are all effective. Phenylephrine has a short duration of action and must be used every 1–2 hours. Naphazoline causes significant burning and irritation locally, as well as central depression and is not recommended. Oxymetazoline and xylometazoline are long-lasting with a duration of 8–12 hours and require less frequent dosing; they are the topical decongestants of choice.

Topical nasal decongestants should not be used for more than 3–5 days since prolonged use is associated with rebound congestion and dependence. The newer, long-acting decongestants have the same potential for abuse and rebound congestion as phenylephrine (Neo-synephrine). Antihistamines which are commonly included in nonprescription cold preparations dry secretions through their anticholinergic effect and have no place in the therapy of viral colds.

DRUG-INDUCED PULMONARY DISEASES

Drug-induced pulmonary dysfunction mimics the entire spectrum of pathologic conditions of the respiratory system: apnea can be induced by narcotics, asthma can be caused by aspirin, and infection can be induced by immunosuppressants. The following table focuses on primary drug-induced pulmonary diseases. A number of drugs which have significant adverse effects on pulmonary function through their central nervous system depressant effects (e.g., barbiturates and narcotics) are not included. The table is organized by pathophysiologic state induced by the agents. For more extensive information, the reader should refer to several excellent reviews (91–97).

Table 3.

DRUG-INDUCED PULMONARY DISEASES

Condition, Drugs, Frequency, Mechanism	Clinical Remarks
Pulmonary Edema	
Heroin Common. Due to an outpouring of edema fluid into the alveoli. The mechanism of the increased capillary permeability is unknown (91–93,98–101).	The syndrome is associated with a mortality rate of approximately 10%. It usually occurs after IV administration but has been reported to follow nasal administration ("snorting"). Patients usually present in coma with depressed respiration or marked respiratory distress. Dyspnea, tachypnea, hypotension, cyanosis, tachycardia, and severe hypoxemia are common. It does not appear to be dose related although it may often follow an overdose. Symptoms occur within 2 hours following administration and usually clear in 1–2 days. X-ray clearing occurs in 2–5 days; however, significant decreases in pulmonary function such as FVC, dynamic compliance and diffusing capacity take much longer to improve. Treatment consists of naloxone (Narcan), respiratory support and oxygen therapy. Secondary bacterial and aspiration pneumonias are frequent complications.
Methadone (Dolophine) Common with overdose. The mechanism is the same as for heroin (91–93,98,102,103).	Occurs following oral administration as much as 6 hours after the dose. Symptoms and treatment are the same as for heroin. May take longer to improve due to a longer duration of action relative to heroin.
Propoxyphene (Darvon) Uncommon. Mechanism thought to be the same as heroin and methadone, but may also be related to postictal pulmonary edema.	Propoxyphene is structurally similar to methadone. Has occurred exclusively following overdose situations. Treatment is the same as for heroin-induced edema.
Ethchlorvynol (Placidyl) Uncommon. Increased alveolar capillary permeability. Noncardiogenic (98,105–107).	It appears to be a dose dependent reaction which occurs more frequently with intravenous administration. Pulmonary edema has been reported with oral administration in fatal overdose; however, this occurred with as little as 450 mg following IV administration. Much higher lung tissue levels of the drug are reached during IV administration. Patients present with dyspnea and dry cough which occur within an hour following injection. The X-ray picture is typical of pulmonary edema. Symptoms clear rapidly. Treatment is symptomatic.
Chlordiazepoxide (Librium) Rare. Noncardiogenic. Mechanism unknown (108).	One reported case following injection of the contents of capsule. Has not been reported with parenteral preparation.
Salicylate Uncommon. Noncardiogenic, increased vascular permeability to fluid and protein (98,109–111).	Has been reported with overdoses as well as patients with "therapeutic" anti-inflammatory levels treated for acute rheumatic fever. In non-overdose situations, symptoms typically appear 2 to 8 days following the initiation of therapy. Patients improve on withdrawal of salicylates.

Table 3. (continued)

DRUG-INDUCED PULMONARY DISEASES

Condition, Drugs, Frequency, Mechanism	Clinical Remarks
Dextran 40 (Rheomacrodex) Rare. Mechanism unknown, probably increased capillary permeability. Noncardiogenic (112).	One case report in which symptoms occurred 4 days into therapy.
Hydrochlorothiazide (Hydrodiuril) Uncommon. Mechanism unknown. Noncardiogenic, non-immunologic (98,113–115).	Symptoms occur within an hour following oral administration of a single dose and rapidly subside within 24 hours. X-ray clears within 2–6 days and diffusing capacity may take a month to return to normal. Most patients have had previous history of thiazide exposure with mild reaction; however, it has occurred with a first exposure. Has never been reported with any other thiazide diuretic.
Phenylbutazone (Butazolidin) Rare. Cardiogenic from sodium retention (93,97).	Reported in elderly patients with pre-existing heart disease. Avoid in patients who should be sodium restricted.
Epinephrine (Adrenalin) Rare. Mechanism unknown (93,97).	Occurs due to accidental overdose during anesthesia.
Intravenous fluids particularly electrolyte solutions. Common. Mechanism is cardiovascular fluid overload (97,116).	Commonly occurs in shock and cardiac failure. Careful monitoring of central venous pressure will prevent. Most comon cause of iatrogenic pulmonary edema. Patients who develop adult respiratory distress syndrome from shock are particularly susceptible. These patients should be treated with positive end expiratory pressure (PEEP) to prevent leakage.

Pulmonary Fibrosis

Busulfan (Myleran) Common. Exact mechanism is unknown but is believed to be due to chemical alveolitis with proliferation of granular pneumocytes and fibrosis of alveolar walls (91–95).	Insidious in onset. Symptoms usually occur 3 to 4 years after therapy is initiated. It presents as a dry hacking cough, tachypnea, cyanosis dyspnea, and low grade fever. X-ray shows diffuse interstitial and intra-alveolary infiltrates. Differential diagnosis includes opportunistic infection, leukemic infiltration, and radiation fibrosis. Pulmonary function tests are typical of restrictive lung disease with a diffusion defect. Clinical course is one of progression with no reversibility. High dose corticosteroids have been tried with little apparent benefit.
Cyclophosphamide (Cytoxan) Rare. Mechanism unknown, thought to be the same as busulfan (91–93,95,117–119).	The clinical picture and pulmonary function is the same as busulfan lung. It follows continuous low dose therapy and has occurred in children 4–6 years after the drug has been discontinued. Rapidly progressive.
Chlorambucil (Leukeran) Rare. Mechanism unknown but probably the same as busulfan and cyclophosphamide which are also alkylating agents (95,120,121).	Typically occurs after 2 years of daily therapy. Symptoms and histology same as busulfan lung.
Other alkylating agents: Melphalan (Alkeran), Uracil Mustard. Rare. Mechanism same as for busulfan and cyclophosphamide (95).	All the alkylating agents except nitrogen mustard and thiotepa have been associated with the syndrome. Except for busulfan, it appears to be a rare complication but it may represent an inherent toxicity of this group of drugs. Caution should be used when these agents are given with other drugs associated with fibrosis.

Table 3. (continued)

DRUG-INDUCED PULMONARY DISEASES

Condition, Drugs, Frequency, Mechanism	Clinical Remarks
Bleomycin (Blenoxane) Common. The overall incidence is estimated at 11%. Mechanism is direct cytotoxic injury to the lung epithelium probably due to free-radical generation following binding of drug to DNA. It is the dose limiting toxicity of the drug with a 10% death rate in patients receiving >550 mg (94,95,119,122–124).	The clinical presentation is characterized by non-productive cough, dyspnea with occasional fever, dry basilar rales and skin pigmentation. Onset is 4 to 10 weeks after beginning therapy. The lung disease is restrictive with a severe diffusion defect. Older patients (60–70 years) appear to be more susceptible. The toxicity is potentiated by radiation given either concomitantly or sequentially, high oxygen concentrations, and possibly adriamycin. The disease is usually insidiously progressive and irreversible. Total dose is restricted to 450 mg or less. Routine monitoring of pulmonary function tests has been of questionable value. Steroid therapy has been reported to be beneficial in some cases.
Mitomycin Uncommon. Mechanism is unknown (95,119,125).	The clinical presentation is like bleomycin; however, the relative dosages were low with a cumulative dose of as little as 40 mg/m^2. The toxicity appears 3–6 months following initiation of treatment and may occur following the second course. High oxygen tension appears to potentiate the toxicity. Postoperative patients should be ventilated with an FiO_2 of 30% or less. Corticosteroids have been reported to improve some patients but others have died of respiratory insufficiency despite steroid therapy.
Methotrexate Uncommon. It appears to be an allergic reaction with fibrosis; noncaseating granuloma formation with lymphocytic infiltrates (91,92,94,95,119).	The mean onset of toxicity occurs 12–200 days after administration. There is no correlation with dose and 65% of the patients will have peripheral eosinophilia. It has been reported after oral, intravenous, and intrathecal use. Symptoms include dry cough, dyspnea, cyanosis. High dose prednisone will induce a rapid remission with radiographic clearing. Appears to be completely reversible.
BCNU (Carmustine) Uncommon. The mechanism is unknown. It appears to be a dose related toxicity (95,119,126,127).	It has occurred after cumulative doses of 580 mg/m^2 to 2,100 mg/m^2 with a duration of therapy from 6 months to 3 years. It presents as a typical restrictive fibrosis with an insidious cough, dyspnea and hypoxemia with a diffusion defect. Steroid therapy has not been effective in altering the course. It frequently has been a rapidly fatal disease. One case associated with semustine, an experimental nitrosourea, has also been reported.
6-Mercaptopurine (Purinethol) Rare. Mechanism unknown (95,117).	
Nitrofurantoin (Macrodantin) Rare. Mechanism unknown (91–94,128,129).	Pulmonary fibrosis from nitrofurantoin occurs with chronic administration usually after 6 months to 6 years of therapy. It is much more rare than the acute syndrome (see below). The clinical pattern consists of a dry cough, exertional dyspnea, and fever with a restrictive pattern on pulmonary function testing. The x-ray is consistent with diffuse interstitial fibrosis and the patients exhibit a diffusing defect. Most cases have been reversible following discontinuation of the drug and institution of steroid therapy. It appears to occur most frequently in postmenopausal women.
Radiation—Cobalt irradiation in Hodgkins and breast carcinoma Common. Two types: Acute hypersensitivity—not dose dependent; chronic—related to total dose (>6000 rads) and total area irradiated (94,130).	The acute form is fulminating occasionally with effusions. The chronic form presents with insidious cough and dyspnea. Clinical presentation is warmth and tightness of chest, dry cough, fever, rales, and occasional friction rubs. Radiographic changes begin at the hilum and spread peripherally. Occasionally responds to steroids although steroids do not prevent late fibrosis. Incidence has significantly decreased with shielding.

Table 3. (continued)

DRUG-INDUCED PULMONARY DISEASES

Condition, Drugs, Frequency, Mechanism	Clinical Remarks
Oxygen Frequent. A related reaction which occurs at increasing frequency as FiO_2 goes over 50%. Toxicity is caused by the formation of superoxide anion (O_2^-), a highly reactive cytotoxic free radical. This can oxidate sulfhydryl enzymes, inactivate DNA, and result in lipid peroxidation of cellular membranes (20, 21,131,132).	Clinical pathology is extensive and is generally regarded in two stages: the acute or exudative stage and chronic proliferative stage. The acute phase consists of perivascular peribronchiolar, interstitial and alveolar edema, and alveolar hemorrhage with necrosis of the pulmonary endothelium. Phase two consists of exudate resorption, alveolar thickening and collagen and elastin deposition in the interstitium of alveolar walls. The patient may have irreversible emphysematous and fibrotic changes. The clinical picture may be obstructive, restrictive, or a mixture of the two. Bronchopulmonary dysplasia (BPD) is a chronic obstructive pulmonary disease produced in premature infants who require O_2 and ventilatory support for the treatment of infant respiratory distress syndrome. As neonatal intensive care units are saving the lives of progressively more premature infants, the incidence of BPD is increasing. Although the relative role of positive pressure ventilation in the production of BPD is important, the high O_2 requirements of these babies play a significant role in the pathogenesis of this disease.
Paraquat (Chevron Ortho Spot Weed and Grass Killer) Common. Annually, more than 120 deaths are reported. Mortality following ingestion is from 33 to 50%. Mechanism is due to O_2 toxicity by superoxide free radical production (21, 91,94,133,134).	Toxicity can appear after oral doses as low as 15 to 20 cc. It presents as progressive dyspnea with radiographic evidence of pulmonary edema which may appear several days after ingestion. It became popular because foreign governments used paraquat to exfoliate illicit marijuana fields. However, paraquat is readily inactivated by exposure to sunlight and is destroyed by burning. Therefore, it is unlikely that any significant toxicity would occur from smoking a marijuana cigarette which had been exposed. All reported fatal cases have been from oral ingestion. Therapy is supportive, although the enzyme superoxide dimutase has been shown to improve outcome in animals by preventing formation of (O_2^-)ions. A high FiO_2 in patients requiring ventilatory support will hasten their demise.
Methysergide (Sansert) Common. A dose and duration related side effect. Part of the chronic fibrosis that it causes. Mechanism is unknown (91–93,97).	The fibrosis is a pleuropulmonary fibrosis as opposed to the interstitial fibrosis produced by other agents. Methysergide is the only drug that will produce a chronic pleural effusion as well. Onset is insidious with the patient having taken the drug at least 6 months. Symptoms include acute pleuritic pain or progressive dyspnea with x-ray changes showing pleural fibrosis. Involvement may be unilateral or bilateral. The syndrome is usually completely reversible upon discontinuation of the drug.
Gold (Myochrysine) Uncommon. Mechanism is unknown; however, it does not appear to be immunologically mediated (135–137).	Clinical symptoms usually occur after 300 to 400 mg total dose has been given. Symptoms include dyspnea and a nonproductive cough. X-ray is compatible with diffuse interstitial fibrosis and histology is the same as for other drug-induced pulmonary fibroses. Pulmonary function tests show a restrictive pattern with a diffusion abnormality. Symptoms resolve with discontinuation of the drug. Steroids have no therapeutic benefit.
Penicillamine (Cuprimine) Rare. Mechanism is unknown (138).	Only one reported case in the literature. Symptoms occurred after 12 months of therapy. Symptoms and pulmonary function tests were consistent with interstitial fibrosis.
Pindolol Rare. Mechanism is unknown (139).	Pindolol is a beta blocker which is structurally similar to practolol, a drug well known as a cause of fibrotic disease. Practolol has been removed from the market in the United Kingdom. This is the first reported case with pindolol.

Table 3. (continued)

DRUG-INDUCED PULMONARY DISEASES

Condition, Drugs, Frequency, Mechanism	Clinical Remarks
Ganglionic blocking agents (hexamethonium, mecamylamine, pentolinium) Rare. Mechanism unknown (91,93,97).	These drugs are rarely used so this reaction is of historical interest. Patients present with classical pulmonary fibrosis a few months to a year following initiation of therapy. Of interest is that hexamethonium is structurally similar to busulfan.

Pulmonary Infiltrates With Eosinophilia (Loeffler's Syndrome)

Nitrofurantoin Common. Mechanism is unknown (91–94,97,129).	Onset of symptoms occurs 2 hours to 10 days following drug administration. Symptoms include fever, chills, cyanosis, dyspnea, may resemble pulmonary edema or an acute asthma attack. X-ray shows diffuse alveolar infiltrates with occasional small pleural effusions. Eosinophilia occurs in one-third of the patients. Symptoms regress within 24–48 hours of stopping the drug.
Para-aminosalicylic (PAS) acid Common. Probably an allergic reaction (91,92,94,97).	This reaction is becoming much less common with the decreased use of PAS in the treatment of tuberculosis. Eosinophils may be as high as 26%. Rechallenge usually reproduces the reaction in 2 days. Sputum does not demonstrate eosinophilia. Classical symptoms of high fever leukocytosis, eosinophilia, cough, and dyspnea occur with all the agents in this section. Treatment of choice is discontinuation of the offending agent.
Penicillin Rare. An allergic reaction (91,92,94,97).	
Sulfonamides Rare, allergic reaction (91–94,97).	Has even been reported with sulfonamide vaginal cream. Other sulfa like drugs will cross react and cause the syndrome such as sulfasalazine and the sulfonylurea, chlorpropamide.
Procarbazine (Matulane) Rare. Possibly an allergic reaction (93,95).	Will improve with steroid therapy. May progress to fibrosis.
Pituitary snuff Rare. Allergic reaction (91–93,96).	More commonly produces asthma attacks but has caused a number of cases of allergic alveolitis.
Imipramine (Tofranil) Rare. Possible allergy (93,97).	Treatment of choice is to discontinue drug.
Cromolyn sodium (Intal) Rare. Allergy (93,97,140).	Cromolyn has also been associated with a chronic allergic granulomatous disease of the lung.
Mephenesin Rare. Probably allergy (93,97).	See Imipramine, above.

Pulmonary Hypertension

Magnesium trisilicate (talc) Common only in drug abusers. Arteritis and angiothrombosis of the pulmonary vasculature is part of a foreign body reaction (91,92,94,97,141).	The reaction is caused by any inert substance injected into the veins. Talc is a common filler for many oral drugs which may be taken intravenously by drug addicts. Cotton fibers have also been implicated. The reaction was common in "blue velvet" abusers. Talc was an inert filler in tripelennamine tablets (an antihistamine) one of the constituents of a "blue velvet" injection. Corn starch from dissolved tablets has also been implicated in granuloma formation and pulmonary hypertension. The reaction has also been reported after the intravenous use of alpha sympathomimetics from nasal inhalers.

References

1. West JB: *Respiratory Physiology—The Essentials.* The Williams and Wilkins Co., Baltimore, 1974.
2. West JB: *Pulmonary Pathophysiology—The Essentials.* The Williams and Wilkins Co., Baltimore, 1977.
3. Comroe et al: *The Lung—Clinical Physiology and Pulmonary Function Tests.* 2nd edition, Year Book Medical Publishers, Inc., Chicago, 1977.
4. Costello JF: Asthma. In *Diseases of the Chest,* edited by Henshaw HC and Murray JF, WB Saunders, Philadelphia, 1980, p 525.
5. Chai H et al: Standardization of bronchial inhalation challenge procedures. J Allergy Clin Immunol. 1975; 56:323.
6. Mitchell RS: Chronic airways obstruction. In *Textbook of Pulmonary Disease,* 2nd edition, Gerald L. Baum, Little, Brown and Company, Boston, 1974, p 579.
7. Anderson DO et al: Role of tobacco smoking in the causation of chronic respiratory disease. N Engl J Med. 1962; 267:787.
8. Gerrard JW et al: Increased nonspecific bronchial reactivity in cigarette smokers with normal lung function. Am Rev Respir Dis. 1980; 122:577.
9. Yarnell JWG et al: Respiratory illness, maternal smoking habit and lung function in children. Br J Dis Chest. 1979; 73:230.
10. White JR et al: Small-airways dysfunction in nonsmokers chronically exposed to tobacco smoke. N Engl J Med. 1980; 302:720.
11. Tager I et al: Role of infection in chronic bronchitis. N Engl J Med. 1975; 292:563.
12. Snider GL: Control of bronchospasm in patients with chronic obstructive pulmonary diseases. Chest. 1978; 73:927.
13. Eaton ML et al: Efficacy of theophylline in "irreversible" airflow obstruction. Ann Intern Med. 1980; 92:758.
14. Burki NK: Resting ventilatory pattern, mouth occlusion pressure, and the effects of aminophylline in asthma and chronic airways obstruction. Chest. 1979; 76:629.
15. Matthay RA et al: Effects of aminophylline upon right and left ventricular performance in chronic obstructive pulmonary disease. Am J Med. 1978; 65:903.
16. Sahn SA: Corticosteroids in chronic bronchitis and pulmonary emphysema. Chest. 1978; 73:389.
17. Albert RK et al: Controlled clinical trial of methylprednisolone in patients with chronic bronchitis and acute respiratory insufficiency. Ann Intern Med. 1980; 92:753.
18. Sackner MA et al: Pulmonary effects of oxygen breathing; a 6-hour study in normal men. Ann Intern Med. 1975; 82:40.
19. Snider GL et al: Oxygen therapy; oxygen therapy in medical patients hospitalized outside of the intensive care unit. Am Rev Respir Dis. 1980; 122(2):29.
20. Deneke SM et al: Normobaric oxygen toxicity of the lung. N Engl J Med. 1980; 303:76.
21. Frank L et al: Oxygen toxicity. Am J Med. 1980; 69:117.
22. Bland RD: Special considerations in oxygen therapy for infants and children. Am Rev Respir Dis. 1980; 122(2):45.
23. Bone RC et al: Controlled oxygen administration in acute respiratory failure in chronic obstructive pulmonary disease. Am J Med. 1978; 65:896.
24. Levin BE et al: The role of longterm continuous oxygen administration in patients with chronic airway obstruction with hypoxemia. Ann Intern Med. 1967; 66:639.
25. Block AJ et al: Chronic oxygen therapy. Treatment of chronic obstructive pulmonary disease at sea level. Chest. 1974; 65:279.
26. Bradley BL et al: Oxygen-assisted exercise in chronic obstructive lung disease. Am Rev Respir Dis. 1978; 118:239.
27. Flick MR et al: Chronic oxygen therapy. Med Clin North Am. 1977; 61:1397.
28. Neff TA et al: Long-term continuous oxygen therapy in chronic airway obstruction. Ann Intern Med. 1970; 72:621.
29. Fenley DC et al: Nocturnal hypoxemia and long-term domiciliary oxygen therapy in "blue and bloated" bronchitics. Physiopathologic correlations. Chest. 1980; 77:305.
30. Petty TL et al: Continuous oxygen in chronic airway obstruction (observations on possible oxygen toxicity and survival). Ann Intern Med. 1971; 75:361.
31. NOTTG: Continuous or nocturnal oxygen therapy in hypoxemic chronic obstructive lung disease. A clinical trial. Ann Intern Med. 1980; 93:391.
32. Ziment I: Respiratory gases. In *Respiratory Pharmacology and Therapeutics,* by I. Ziment, W. B. Saunders, Philadelphia, 1978, p 442.
33. Bowman BH et al: Current concepts in genetics—cystic fibrosis. N Engl J Med. 1976; 294:937.
34. Wood RE et al: State of the art: Cystic Fibrosis. Am Rev Respir Dis. 1976; 113:833.
35. May JR et al: Bacterial infection in cystic fibrosis. Arch Dis Child. 1972; 47:908.
36. Mearns MB et al: Bacterial flora in respiratory tract in patients with cystic fibrosis. 1950–1970. Arch Dis Child. 1972; 47:902.
37. Pennington JE et al: Concentrations of gentamicin and carbenicillin in bronchial secretions. J Infect Dis. 1973; 128:63.
38. Pennington JE et al: Tobramycin in bronchial secretions. Antimicrob Agents Chemother. 1973; 4:299.
39. Marks MI et al: Carbenicillin and gentamicin: Pharmacologic studies in patients with cystic fibrosis and pseudomonas pulmonary infections. J Pediatr. 1971; 79:822.
40. Saggers BA et al: In vivo penetration of antibiotics into sputum in cystic fibrosis. Arch Dis Child. 1968; 43:404.
41. Jusko WJ et al: Enhanced renal excretion of dicloxacillin in patients with cystic fibrosis. Pediatrics. 1975; 56:1038.
42. Yaffe SJ et al: Pharmacokinetics of methicillin in patients with cystic fibrosis. J Infect Dis. 1977; 135:828.
43. Vogelstein B et al: The pharmacokinetics of amikacin in children. J Pediatr. 1977; 91:333.
44. Zaske DE: Counter point discussion—aminoglycosides. In *Applied Pharmacokinetics,* edited by WE Evans, JJ Schentag, and WJ Jusko, Applied Therapeutics, Inc., San Francisco, 1980, p 210.
45. Hoff GE et al: Tobramycin treatment of pseudomonas aeruginosa infections in cystic fibrosis. Scand J Infect Dis. 1974; 6:333.

46. Lau WK et al: Amikacin therapy of exacerbations of pseudomonas aeruginosa infections in patients with cystic fibrosis. Pediatrics. 1977; 60:372.

47. Huang NN et al: Carbenicillin in patients with cystic fibrosis: clinical pharmacology and therapeutic evaluation. J Pediatr. 1971; 78:338.

48. Mellis CM et al: Bronchial reactivity in cystic fibrosis. Pediatrics. 1978; 61:446.

49. Larsen GL et al: A comparative study of inhaled atropine sulfate and isoproterenol hydrochloride in cystic fibrosis. Am Rev Respir Dis. 1979; 119:399.

50. Shapiro GG et al: The paradoxical effect of adrenergic and methylxanthine drugs in cystic fibrosis. Pediatrics. 1976; 58:740.

51. Wood RE et al: Tracheal mucociliary transport in patients with cystic fibrosis and its stimulation by terbutaline. Am Rev Respir Dis. 1975; 111:733.

52. Graham DY: Enzyme replacement therapy of exocrine pancreatic insufficiency in man. N Engl J Med. 1977; 296:1314.

53. Regan PT et al: Comparative effects of antacids, cimetidine and enteric coating on the therapeutic response to oral enzymes in severe pancreatic insufficiency. N Engl J Med. 1977; 297:854.

54. Graham DY: An enteric-coated pancreatic enzyme preparation that works. Digestive Dis Scie. 1979; 24:906.

55. Wanner A: Clinical aspects of mucociliary transport. Am Rev Respir Dis. 1977; 116:73.

56. Editor: Pathophysiology and pharmacology of sputum. In *Respiratory Pharmacology and Therapeutics,* edited by I Ziment, WB Saunders Co., Philadelphia, 1978, p 41.

57. Wanner A et al: Clinical indications for and effects of bland, mucolytic, and antimicrobial aerosols. Am Rev Respir Dis. 1980; 122:79.

58. Bureau MA et al: Late effect of nocturnal mist tent therapy related to the severity of airway obstruction in children with cystic fibrosis. Pediatrics. 1978; 61:842.

59. Menkes H et al: Physical therapy: rationale for physical therapy. Am Rev Respir Dis. 1980; 122:127.

60. Graham WGB et al: Efficacy of chest physiotherapy and intermittent positive-pressure breathing in the resolution of pneumonia. N Engl J Med. 1978; 299:624.

61. Newton DAG et al: Effect of physiotherapy on pulmonary function, a laboratory study. Lancet. 1978; 2:228.

62. Bateman JRM et al: Regional lung clearance of excessive bronchial secretions during chest physiotherapy in patients with stable chronic airways obstruction. Lancet. 1979; 1:294.

63. Connors AE et al: Chest physical therapy, the immediate effect on oxygenation in acutely ill patients. Chest. 1980; 78:559.

64. Newton DAG et al: Physiotherapy and intermittent positive-pressure ventilation of chronic bronchitis. Br Med J. 1978; 2:1525.

65. Oldenburg FA et al: Effects of postural drainage, exercise, and cough on mucus clearance in chronic bronchitis. Am Rev Respir Dis. 1979; 120:739.

66. Donaldson JC et al: Acetylcysteine for life-threatening acute bronchial obstruction. Ann Intern Med. 1978; 88:656.

67. Hirsch SR et al: The expectorant effect of glyceryl guaiacolate in patients with chronic bronchitis. Chest. 1973; 63:9.

68. Fallsers CJ et al: Controlled study of iodotherapy for childhood asthma. J Allergy Clin Immunol. 1966; 38:183.

69. Committee on Drugs of the American Academy of Pediatrics. Adverse reactions to iodide therapy of asthma and other pulmonary diseases. Pediatrics. 1976; 57:272.

70. Ziment I: Medications for coughs and colds. In *Respiratory Pharmacology and Therapeutics,* by I Ziment, WB Saunders, Philadelphia, 1978, p 282.

71. Cormier JF et al: Cold and allergy products. In *Handbook of Non Prescription Drugs,* 6th Edition, by American Pharmaceutical Association, Washington, D. C., 1979, p 73.

72. Committee on Drugs: Use of codeine and dextromethorphan-containing cough syrups in pediatrics. Pediatrics. 1978; 62:118.

73. Bickerman H: Clinical pharmacology of antitussive drugs. Clin Pharmacol Ther. 1962; 3:353.

74. Calvert JC: Cough: differential diagnosis and treatment. Drug Intell Clin Pharm. 1976; 10:640.

75. Anon: Vitamin C and the common cold. Med Let Drugs Ther. 1974; 16:85.

76. Lucey JF: The xanthine treatment of apnea of prematurity. Pediatrics. 1975; 55:584.

77. Kattwinkel J: Neonatal apnea: pathogenesis and therapy. J Pediatr. 1977; 90:342.

78. Kuzemko JA et al: Apnoeic attacks in the newborn treated with aminophylline. Arch Dis Child. 1973; 48:404.

79. Shannon DC et al: Prevention of apnea and bradycardia in low-birthweight infants. Pediatrics. 1975; 55:589.

80. Uauy R et al: Treatment of severe apnea in prematures with orally administered theophylline. Pediatrics. 1975; 55:595.

81. Myers TF et al: Low-dose theophylline therapy in idiopathic apnea of prematurity. J Pediatr. 1980; 96:99.

82. Gerhardt T et al: Effect of aminophylline on respiratory center activity and metabolic rate in premature infants with idiopathic apnea. Pediatrics. 1979; 63:537.

83. Gerhardt T et al: Aminophylline therapy for idiopathic apnea in premature infants: effects on lung function. Pediatrics. 1978; 62:801.

84. Aranda JV et al: Pharmacokinetic aspects of theophylline in premature newborns. N Engl J Med. 1976; 295:413.

85. Giacoia G et al: Theophylline pharmacokinetics in premature infants with apnea. J Pediatr. 1976; 89:829.

86. Grygiel JJ et al: Effect of age on patterns of theophylline metabolism. Clin Pharmacol Ther. 1980; 28:456.

87. Brazier JL et al: Plasma xanthine levels in low birthweight infants treated or not treated with theophylline. Arch Dis Child. 1979; 54:194.

88. Boutroy MJ et al: Methylation of theophylline to caffeine in premature infants. Lancet. 1979; 1:830.

89. Aranda JV et al: Pharmacokinetic profile of caffeine in the premature newborn infant with apnea. J Pediatr. 1979; 94:663.

90. Somani SM et al: Caffeine and theophylline: serum/CSF correlation in premature infants. J Pediatr. 1980; 96:1091.

91. Rosenow EC: The spectrum of drug induced pulmonary disease. Ann Intern Med. 1972; 77:977.

92. Whitcomb ME: Drug-induced lung disease. Chest. 1973; 63:418.

93. Martin DW et al: Drug-induced lung disease: the price of progress. Calif Med. 1973; 119:48.

94. Lippmann M: Pulmonary reactions to drugs. Med Clin North Am. 1977; 61:1353.

95. Weiss RB: Cytotoxic drug-induced pulmonary disease: update 1980. Am J Med. 1980; 68:259.

96. Editor: Respiratory Manifestations. In *Clinical Problems with Drugs,* edited by LE Cluff, GJ Caranasos, and RB Stewart, WB Saunders, Philadelphia, 1975, p 142.

97. Brewis RAL: Respiratory disorders. In *Textbook of Adverse Drug Reactions,* edited by DM Davies, Oxford University Press, New York, 1977, p 103.

98. Shanies HM: Noncardiogenic pulmonary edema. Med Clin North Am. 1977; 61:1319.

99. Steinberg AD et al: The clinical spectrum of heroin pulmonary edema. Arch Intern Med. 1968; 122:122.

100. Duberstein JL et al: A clinical study of an epidemic of heroin intoxication and heroin-induced pulmonary edema. Am J Med. 1971; 51:704.

101. Frand UI et al: Heroin-induced pulmonary edema: sequential studies of pulmonary function. Ann Intern Med. 1972; 77:29.

102. Frand UI et al: Methadone-induced pulmonary edema. Ann Intern Med. 1972; 76:975.

103. Aronow R et al: Childhood poisoning: an unfortunate consequence of methadone availability. JAMA. 1972; 219:321.

104. Bogartz LJ et al: Pulmonary edema associated with propoxyphene intoxication. JAMA. 1971; 215:259.

105. Glauser FL et al: Ethchlorvynol (Placydyl)-induced pulmonary edema. Ann Intern Med. 1976; 84:46.

106. Self TH et al: Intravenous ethchlorvynol-induced pulmonary edema. Drug Intell Clin Pharm. 1979; 13:96.

107. Glauser FL et al: Pulmonary tissue concentrations of ethchlorvynol after intravenous injection. Am Rev Respir Dis. 1977; 115:83.

108. Richman S et al: Acute pulmonary edema associated with librium abuse. Radiology. 1972; 103:57.

109. Davis PR et al: Pulmonary edema and salicylate intoxication. Ann Intern Med. 1974; 80:553.

110. Bowers RE et al: Salicylate pulmonary edema: the mechanism in sheep and review of the clinical literature. Am Rev Respir Dis. 1977; 115:261.

111. Alexander WD et al: Disadvantageous effects of salicylate in rheumatic fever. Lancet. 1962; 1:768.

112. Kaplan AI et al: Dextran 40: another cause of drug-induced noncardiogenic pulmonary edema. Chest. 1975; 68:376.

113. Steinberg AD: Pulmonary edema following ingestion of hydrochlorothiazide. JAMA. 1968; 204:825.

114. Beaudry C et al: Severe allergic pneumonitis from hydrochlorothiazide. Ann Intern Med. 1973; 78:251.

115. Bell RT et al: Hydrochlorothiazide-induced pulmonary edema, report of a case and review of the literature. Arch Intern Med. 1979; 139:817.

116. Venus B et al: Treatment of the adult respiratory distress syndrome with continuous positive airway pressure. Chest. 1979; 76:257.

117. Sostman HD et al: Cytotoxic drug-induced lung disease. Am J Med. 1977; 62:608.

118. Alvarado CS et al: Late-onset pulmonary fibrosis and chest deformity in two children treated with cyclophosphamide. J Pediatr. 1978; 92:443.

119. Willson JKV: Pulmonary toxicity of antineoplastic drugs. Cancer Treat Rep. 1978; 62:2003.

120. Godard P et al: Interstitial pneumonia and chlorambucil. Chest. 1979; 76:471.

121. Cole SR et al: Pulmonary disease with chlorambucil therapy. Cancer. 1978; 41:455.

122. Holoye PY et al: Bleomycin hypersensitivity pneumonitis. Ann Intern Med. 1978; 88:47.

123. Brown WG et al: Reversibility of severe bleomycin-induced pneumonitis. JAMA. 1978; 239:2012.

124. Lewis BM et al: Routine pulmonary function tests during bleomycin therapy, tests may be ineffective and potentially misleading. JAMA. 1980; 243:347.

125. Buzdar AV et al: Pulmonary toxicity of mitomycin. Cancer. 1980; 45:236.

126. Durrant JR et al: Pulmonary toxicity associated with bischloroethyl-nitrosourea (BCNU). Ann Intern Med. 1979; 90:191.

127. Crittenden D et al: Pulmonary fibrosis after prolonged therapy with 1,3-bis-z-chloroethyl-1-nitrosourea. Chest. 1977; 72:372.

128. Rosenow EC et al: Chronic nitrofurantoin pulmonary reaction. N Engl J Med. 1968; 279:1258.

129. Simonson W et al: Nitrofurantoin pneumonitis. Drug Intell Clin Pharm. 1977; 11:654.

130. Stone D et al: Fatal pulmonary insufficiency due to radiation effect upon the lung. Am J Med. 1956; 21:211.

131. Frank L et al: The lung and oxygen toxicity. Arch Intern Med. 1979; 139:347.

132. Northway WH et al: Workshop on bronchopulmonary dysplasia. J Pediatr. 1979; 85(2):815.

133. Copland GM et al: Fatal pulmonary intra-alveolar fibrosis after paraquat ingestion. N Engl J Med. 1974; 291:290.

134. Fairshter RD et al: Paraquat poisoning. Am J Med. 1975; 59:751.

135. Winterbauer RH et al: Diffuse pulmonary injury associated with gold treatment. N Engl J Med. 1976; 294:919.

136. Terho EO et al: Pulmonary damage associated with gold therapy, a report of two cases. Scan J Respir Dis. 1979; 60:345.

137. Weaver LT et al: Lung changes after gold salts. Br J Dis Chest. 1978; 72:247.

138. Eastmond CJ: Diffuse alveolitis a complication of penicillamine treatment for rheumatoid arthritis. Br Med J. 1976; 1:1506.

139. Musk AW et al: Pindolol and pulmonary fibrosis. Br Med J. 1979; 2:581.

140. Lobel H et al: Pulmonary infiltrates with eosinophilia in an asthmatic patient treated with disodium cromoglycate. Lancet. 1972; 2:1032.

141. Robertson CH: Pulmonary hypertension and foreign body granulomas in IV drug abusers. Am J Med. 1976; 61:557.

142. Kearns GL et al: Dosing implications of altered gentamicin disposition in patients with cystic fibrosis. J Pediatr. 1982; 100:312.

143. Kelly HW et al: Pharmacokinetics of tobramycin in cystic fibrosis. J Pediatr. 1982; 100:318.

Chapter 17

Asthma

Donald L. Uden and Gary D. Smith

Asthma is defined by the American Thoracic Society as a disease which is characterized by increased responsiveness of the trachea and bronchi to various stimuli and manifested by widespread narrowing of the airways; the disease changes in severity either spontaneously or as a result of treatment (1). This extensive narrowing of the airways is secondary to bronchoconstriction and mucosal edema with increased mucous production. The bronchoconstriction results from contraction of smooth muscle which surrounds the bronchiole. The mucosal edema and increased mucous production result from inflammation of lung tissue. These actions cause both narrowing and physical obstruction of the bronchial tubes.

Symptoms. Wheezing, coughing, and dyspnea are the major symptoms associated with asthma and are of variable duration and severity (2–4).

These symptoms frequently are precipitated by upper respiratory tract infections (viral and bacterial), exercise, irritants (allergic, chemical, and physical), psychological problems, or climate (4–13). Therefore, when wheezing and coughing accompany respiratory difficulty, a diagnosis of asthma should be considered, especially when these problems develop in association with an upper respiratory tract infection in a pediatric patient.

Diagnosis. The diagnosis of asthma should be based on a good patient history which details the nature of symptoms, precipitating or aggravating factors, and the profile of the typical asthma attack. Pulmonary function testing which documents the reversibility of airway obstruction is of value when establishing the diagnosis of asthma (15). An increase of pulmonary function of 15–

20% over baseline after bronchodilator administration indicates reversibility of the airway obstruction (16,17). Significant improvement of pulmonary function after bronchodilator therapy indicates that a reversible component exists; however, lung function may still not be optimized (15). The absence of this optimal reversibility may indicate that excessive inflammation and edema are present and warrants treatment with corticosteroids. The most useful pulmonary function tests to evaluate airway response are the forced vital capacity (FVC), forced expiratory volume in one second (FEV_1), and forced mid-expiratory flow (FEF_{25-75}). Of these, the FEF_{25-75} is the least effort-dependent and provides the most accurate information about small airway obstruction (17). The FVC, FEV_1, and the FEF_{25-75} are decreased in asthma, although the FVC is sometimes normal.

Treatment Goals. The goal of therapy is to prevent emergency physician visits, minimize interference with sleep and physical activity, and to promptly relieve symptoms when they occur (14). Pharmacologic approaches to treatment should be directed at reversing either the bronchoconstriction and/or the pulmonary inflammatory response of mucosal edema and increased mucous production. Beta-adrenergic agonists, anticholinergics, corticosteroids, theophylline, and cromolyn sodium are useful agents for the management of asthma.

Pathophysiology and Mechanisms of Drug Action. An asthmatic attack can be initiated by mast cells whose membranes have been altered by antigen, infection, exercise, stress, or climate. These injured cell membranes permit influx of calcium into the mast cells which subsequently release vasoactive mediators such as histamine, slow reacting substance of anaphylaxis (SRS-A), and eosinophil chemotactic factor (ECF-A). These vasoactive mediators then cause bronchiole smooth muscle contraction and tissue edema (18).

Cyclic adenosine monophosphate (cAMP) inhibits the influx of calcium through the altered membranes of mast cells, and cyclic guanosine monophosphate (cGMP) enhances this calcium influx (19). Cyclic AMP is formed from the con-

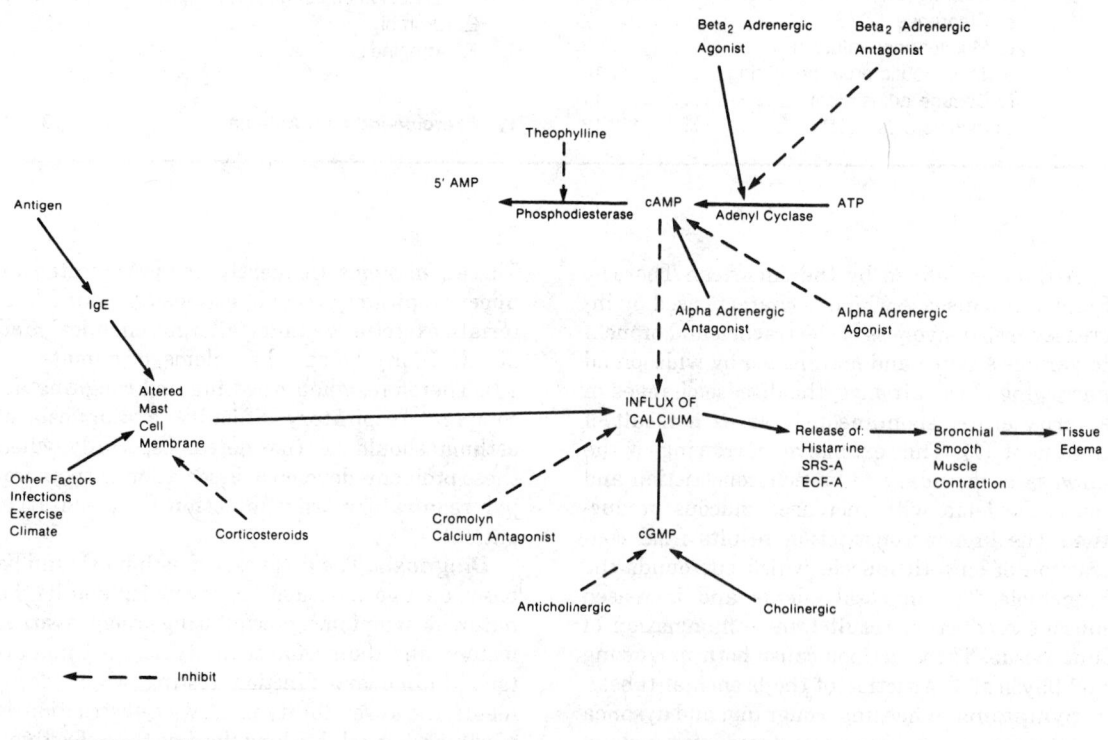

Figure 1. Pathophysiology of an Asthmatic Attack

version of adenosine triphosphate (ATP) in the cell; this conversion is enhanced by beta-adrenergic agonists and alpha-adrenergic antagonists. It is inhibited by beta-adrenergic antagonists and alpha-adrenergic agonists. The cAMP is metabolized to 5'AMP by the enzyme phosphodiesterase, and its degradation can be prevented by inhibition of phosphodiesterase with theophylline. However, the direct inhibitory effect of theophylline on phosphodiesterase does not occur at clinically achievable serum concentrations; therefore theophylline may affect a prostaglandin which regulates phosphodiesterase (20). Theophylline also might increase cAMP by blocking the release of histamine from the mast cell (21,22). *In vitro*, theophylline and beta-adrenergic agonists synergistically inhibit histamine release, but whether this synergy occurs clinically is uncertain (21).

Drugs, such as cromolyn sodium, also may inhibit the influx of calcium into mast cells (23,24). Cromolyn sodium stabilizes the mast cell membrane, and thereby prevents the release of the vasoactive mediators. It does not block the effects of these mediators once released and does not dilate the bronchioles. Corticosteroids can stabilize cell membranes, prevent the release of vasoactive substances, and even protect the cells from the vasoactive effects of these mediators (25). The precise anti-asthmatic mechanism of action of corticosteroids is unknown, but their anti-inflammatory effects decrease the amount of fluid leakage into bronchioles and minimize production of mucous and edema.

ACUTE ASTHMA

1. **A six-year-old cyanotic male, weighing 30 kg, presents to the emergency room with a history of chronic asthma and complaints of dyspnea, wheezing, and coughing. These symptoms began three days ago and were associated with the onset of a cold-like illness. This present illness has resulted in missed school days, limitation of activity, and night awakenings due to cough and chest tightness. What presenting subjective or objective data are consistent with acute asthma in this patient?**

Asthma occurs in approximately 2% of the general population and is the most common chronic disease of childhood. Symptoms generally occur during the first five years of life in 65% of patients and are responsible for significant morbidity and many missed days of school (2). Thus, the age of this patient and the interruption of his daily routine are consistent with the usual pattern of asthma. Likewise, the association of exacerbations of asthma with upper respiratory tract infections such as this patient's cold is common. The symptoms of dyspnea, wheezing, and coughing also are consistent with asthma. Finally, this patient's cyanosis is a result of inadequate oxygenation secondary to deterioration of his asthma.

Laboratory Evaluation

2. **What initial laboratory information should be obtained to evaluate the severity of this asthmatic attack?**

Initial laboratory evaluations should include arterial blood gas (ABG) determination and a chest x-ray (26–28). Blood gas determinations may have to be repeated as often as every 15 minutes if the patient is in respiratory failure or if respiratory failure seems imminent (26). Acute respiratory failure can be defined, in the absence of metabolic alkalosis, as an arterial O_2 (P_aO_2) of less than 55–60 mm Hg or an arterial CO_2 (P_aCO_2) greater than 45–50 mm Hg at sea level (29). The chest x-ray should provide information as to the presence of a pneumothorax, atelectasis, or a pulmonary infection (26).

Therapy

3. **The patient's ABG results show a P_aO_2 of 65, P_aCO_2 of 32, and pH of 7.35. No infiltrates are present on chest x-ray and pulmonary infection is highly unlikely despite the finding of air trapping on the chest x-ray. The ABG results are not compatible with acute respiratory failure, although the clinical assessment based on subjective and objective data is that of acute asthma. What therapeutic intervention would be of the highest priority at this time?**

Oxygen administration by nasal cannula or ventilation mask is highly appropriate for this cyanotic 6-year-old patient (26–28). The oxygen should be humidified to prevent further drying of the airways. The fraction of the inspired oxygen delivered is determined by the results of ABG; and oxygen in a concentration of 22% would be reasonable for this patient at this time.

Administration of fluids also is important. Rapid respiratory rates and the work of breathing may increase fluid loss, and hydration is essential to the clearing of dried mucous plugs.

4. Sympathomimetics. In addition to oxygen, sympathomimetic therapy with epinephrine or terbutaline should be included into the therapeutic plan for this patient. What would be an appropriate dose for this patient and how quickly should he be expected to respond to this sympathomimetic therapy?

Both drugs significantly improve pulmonary function when doses of 0.01 mg/kg (0.5 mg maximum dose) are used (30,31). Asthma symptoms abate within 15–20 minutes after the dose is administered. If the patient's symptoms do not improve or reoccur after the previous dose, the dose may be repeated twice at 20–30 minute intervals. Both are equivalent with respect to onset of action and side effects when tested in patients with acute asthma symptoms (32–35).

5. Theophylline with Sympathomimetics. The patient received 0.3 ml (0.3 mg) of subcutaneous terbutaline with minimal change in his clinical status. Would additional bronchodilator therapy with theophylline be indicated?

Concurrent administration of sympathomimetic drugs such as epinephrine, isoproterenol, ephedrine, isoetharine, metaproterenol, and terbutaline with theophylline raises the question of "Can one achieve a greater degree of bronchodilation with theophylline and a sympathomimetic drug in combination than with either drug alone?" According to Powell and Jackson (36) this question has no definitive answer because studies have not compared dose-response curves which have achieved maximal bronchodilation with theophylline, a sympathomimetic, and a combination of the two. Nevertheless, in this clinical situation, theophylline should be administered because some studies suggest that the combination of beta-adrenergic agonists produces greater bronchodilation than either drug alone (37,38). Moreover, these drugs seem to have different mechanisms of action, and this patient does not seem to be responding to terbutaline alone.

Prior to the administration of theophylline, a careful medication history must be obtained to determine if the patient has taken theophylline in the previous 24 hours. This history will also help to detect other medications which may influence the clearance of theophylline.

6. Theophylline Volume of Distribution. When calculating the loading dose of theophylline, does the volume of distribution (Vd) of theophylline need to be adjusted for this patient?

The reported values for the volume of distribution (Vd) of theophylline range from 0.3–0.7 L/kg (39,43–45) and average approximately 0.45 L/kg (450 ml/kg) for adults and children (44). This Vd for theophylline seems to remain relatively constant from infancy to adulthood and even in the presence of diseases such as congestive heart failure (46) or severe liver disease (47). Therefore, adjustments for changes in the Vd for this patient are unnecessary.

7. Theophylline Clearance. What clinical situations can affect the clearance of theophylline?

The metabolic clearance of theophylline is dependent upon age, concurrent disease states, drug therapy, diet, and smoking habits (see Table 1). The mean half-life of theophylline in premature infants with apnea ranges from 20–30 hours and in children (1–17 years of age) with nonacute asthma from 3–4 hours. The half-life then increases to about 7–8 hours in non-smoking, healthy, adults (48,49,51).

Disease states which decrease theophylline clearance are hepatic cirrhosis, acute respiratory infections, pulmonary edema, and cor pulmonale. Prolonged fever and hypoxia may also be associated with decreased theophylline clearance (46, 47,55,56).

Drugs which may decrease theophylline clearance include erythromycin, troleandomycin, cimetidine, propranolol, metoprolol, trivalent influenza vaccine, and thiabendazole.

The macrolide antibiotics, erythromycin and troleandomycin, appear to substantially reduce theophylline clearance. Despite some conflicting reports (57–61,66) and subsequent confusion regarding the status of this drug interaction, the preponderance of recent evidence indicates that this interaction is of clinical significance. Increases in theophylline serum concentrations and signs of theophylline toxicity have been noted when erythromycin was administered to patients previously stabilized on theophylline (57–61,66). Furthermore, serum theophylline levels decrease when erythromycin is discontinued. As a result, some clinicians routinely decrease theophylline doses by 25% when erythromycin therapy is to be initiated. In contrast, others simply prefer to add the erythromycin while closely monitoring patients for signs of theophylline toxicity rather than altering two variables which may affect the steady-state of theophylline.

Cimetidine also can predictably decrease theophylline clearance by as much as 43–49% (62–65). Since cimetidine probably begins to reduce theophylline elimination as soon as therapeutic serum levels of cimetidine are achieved, a new steady-state serum theophylline level will be observed by the second day of cimetidine therapy (109).

Propranolol and metoprolol in rapid metabolizers can inhibit the metabolism of theophylline, but this drug interaction requires more study before a clinical perspective can be derived. Preliminary results also indicate that influenza vaccine is associated with considerable increases (as much as 122%) in serum theophylline concentrations (108). Elevated theophylline levels and signs of theophylline toxicity also were noted in one patient who received thiabendazole, but confirmation of this supposed drug interaction is needed.

Diet also may affect the clearance of theophylline. Dietary intake of charcoal broiled foods and high protein diets are associated with increased theophylline elimination, while high carbohydrate diets decrease elimination (70–73).

Smoking of tobacco or marijuana cigarettes also seems to affect the clearance of theophylline. Nicotine and polycyclic hydrocarbons may increase theophylline clearance because of hepatic microsomal enzyme induction (67–69).

8. *Theophylline Loading Dose.* According to this patient's mother, he has not received theophylline or any medications in the 24 hours prior to admission to the emergency room. What would be a reasonable initial dose of theophylline for this patient?

Since no theophylline had been ingested in the previous 24 hours, a loading dose should be administered to rapidly achieve the desired therapeutic serum concentration of 10–20 mcg/ml which effectively minimizes asthma symptoms. Theophylline serum concentrations greater than 10 mcg/ml inhibit exercise-induced bronchospasms, and serum concentrations above 15 mcg/ml have an even more profound effect. The bronchodilator effects of theophylline increase in proportion to the logarithm of the serum concentration over a range of 5 to 20 mcg/ml (39–43).

A loading dose of theophylline can be calculated as follows: Loading dose (L.D.) = Desired serum concentration (Cp) × volume of distribution (Vd) × patient weight.

The units of measure for the loading dose are in milligrams; the desired serum concentration in mcg/ml; the volume of distribution in ml/kg; and the patient weight in kilograms.

Loading doses will result in variable peak serum theophylline concentrations because of intersubject variability in volumes of distribution. For this reason, the loading dose should be calculated to achieve a mean serum concentration near the lower end of the therapeutic range (i.e., 10 to 15 mcg/ml). Furthermore, ideal body weight should be used in calculations because theophylline does not readily enter adipose tissue.

If the desired serum concentration of theophylline for this patient is 15 mcg/ml, the initial dose of theophylline for this patient can be calculated by use of the above equation as follows:

$$
\begin{aligned}
\text{L.D.} &= (\text{Cp})(\text{Vd})(\text{Patient weight}) \\
&= (15 \text{ mcg/ml})(450 \text{ ml/kg})(30 \text{ kg}) \\
&= 202.5 \text{ mg of theophylline}
\end{aligned}
$$

Since theophylline can be administered intravenously only as aminophylline (80% theophylline), the loading dose of aminophylline must be corrected as follows:

$$
\frac{202.5 \text{ mg theophylline}}{0.8} = 253 \text{ mg of aminophylline}
$$

9. *Theophylline Maintenance Infusion.* Based upon the above calculations, 250 mg of aminophylline was administered to this patient intravenously over 15 minutes. If a continuous intravenous infusion of aminophylline is started, what infusion rate would maintain therapeutic concentrations of theophylline in this patient?

The optimal method to maintain serum theophylline concentrations, once a therapeutic level is attained with a loading dose, is by a continuous intravenous infusion at a rate that matches the elimination rate at the desired serum concentration. Unfortunately, the rate at which theophylline is eliminated varies among individuals, resulting in a wide range of dosage requirements for continued therapy (110). See Table 1. Nevertheless, rates of infusion which will result in an average serum theophylline concentration of 10 mcg/ml have been derived from mean pharmacokinetic data appropriate for patients of various ages and clinical conditions (Table 2). Since the daily dose of theophylline which is needed to provide therapeutic concentrations for this particular patient is unknown, it would be reasonable to

Table 1.

FACTORS ASSOCIATED WITH VARIATION IN THEOPHYLLINE ELIMINATION (110).

Factors	Age Mean ± S.D. (years)	No. of Patients	Clearance Mean ± S.D. (ml/min/kg)	Half-Life Mean ± S.D. (hours)	Reference
AGE					
Premature Neonates					
with Apnea	7.5 ± 4.4 days	6	0.29 ± 0.1	30 ± 6.5	48
	41 ± 12 days	8	0.64 ± 0.3	20 ± 5.3	52
Infants					
under 6 mos.	12 ± 4 weeks	8	Incomplete data	14 ± 4	54
	18 ± 2 weeks	3	0.8 ± 0.1	6.9 ± 1	111
6 to 11 mos.	34 ± 10 weeks	4	2.0 ± 0.5	4.6 ± 1.2	111
	34 ± 7 weeks	5	Incomplete data	3.7 ± 1	112
Young children					
1–4 years	2.5 ± 0.9	10	1.7 ± 0.6	3.4 ± 1.1	49
Older children					
4–12 years	9.4 ± 3	17	1.5 ± 0.4	Not measured	136
13–15 years	14 ± 0.8	6	0.8 ± 0.2	Not measured	136
6–17 years	10.7 ± 2.6	30	1.4 ± 0.6	3.7 ± 1.1	44
Adults					
—otherwise healthy nonsmoking asthmatics	31 ± 10	16	0.65 ± 0.19	8.7 ± 2.2	45
—healthy non-smoking volunteers	22–35[a]	19	0.86 ± 0.35	8.1 ± 2.4	69
—healthy non-smoking volunteers	20–32(25.5)[b]	15	0.67 ± 0.13	8.2 ± 1.2	132
Elderly					
—nonsmokers with normal cardiac, liver and renal function	67 ± 5.7	9	0.59 ± 0.07	7.4 ± 1.1	146
ABNORMAL PHYSIOLOGY					
Fever					
—associated with acute viral upper respiratory tract illness	9–15[a]	6 (During illness)	Not measured	7.0 ± 3.0	56
		(1 month later)	Not measured	4.1 ± 2.4	
Cor pulmonale	64[a]	8	0.48 ± 0.2	Not measured	147
Acute pulmonary edema	71 ± 10	9	0.33(0.067-2.35)[d]	19(3.1-82)[d]	46
Hepatic cirrhosis	52 ± 8.2	9	0.43(0.13-3.3)[d]	14.1(7.1-59.1)[d]	47
	56 ± 4	8	0.21(0.1-0.6)[d]	32(10.4-56)[d]	148

administer theophylline at an infusion rate of 0.85 mg/kg/hour according to this table. Therefore, this patient should receive about 32 mg of aminophylline per hour by constant IV infusion (theophylline dose divided by 0.8 to correct for the aminophylline salt and multiplied by this patient's weight of 30 kg). Because no one constant infusion rate can reliably yield both optimum benefit and safety for all patients, this initial infusion rate may need to be adjusted. Adjustments should be based upon measurements of serum theophylline if this drug is to be continued at full therapeutic doses for more than 12 to 24 hours.

In this particular situation, monitoring serum theophylline concentrations would be especially appropriate because this patient's loading dose of theophylline was aimed at achieving a serum concentration of 15 mcg/ml.

10. A constant IV infusion of aminophylline at 35 mg/hour is ordered for this patient. When should serum samples be obtained to monitor theophylline concentrations?

A serum sample should be assayed to determine the serum theophylline concentration 15 to 30 minutes after the administration of the load-

Table 1. (continued)

FACTORS ASSOCIATED WITH VARIATION IN THEOPHYLLINE ELIMINATION

Factors	Age Mean ± S.D. (years)	No. of Patients	Clearance Mean ± S.D. (ml/min/kg)	Half-Life Mean ± S.D. (hours)	Reference
SMOKING HISTORY					
Marijuana alone	20–25[a]	7	1.2 ± 0.5	4.3 ± 1.2	69
Marijuana and cigarettes	19–27[a]	7	1.5 ± 0.4	4.3 ± 1	69
Cigarettes	33[c]	10	Not measured	4.1 ± 1	158
Cigarettes (heavy smokers)	22–31(27)[b]	7	1.05 ± 0.32	5.4 ± 1	132
Ex-cigarette smokers (for at least 2 years)	22–39(28)[b]	6	0.85 ± 0.2	6.4 ± 1	132
CONCURRENT DRUGS					
Triacetyloleandomycin (TAO)	39 ± 15	8 (Before)	0.70 ± 0.14	Not measured	66
		(After)	0.34 ± 0.05	Not measured	
Erythromycin base	23 ± 2.2	8 (Before)	0.82 ± 0.17	6.7 ± 0.19	108
		(After)	0.60 ± 0.11	8.3 ± 1.8	
Phenobarbital	23–32(27)[b]	6 (Before)	0.75 ± 0.35	Not measured	159
		(After 1 mo.)	1.0 ± 0.5	Not measured	
ABERRANT DIETS					
Low carbohydrate—high protein	22–29[a]	6 (Before)	e	8.1 ± 2.4	161
		(After 2 wks.)		5.2 ± 1	
Charcoal-broiled beef	22–32[a]	8 (Before)	e	6.0 ± 1	162
		(After 7 days of Diet)		4.7 ± 0.4	

[a] Age range. Individual ages were not reported.
[b] Age range and mean. Standard deviation was not reported.
[c] Mean age. Individual data not reported.
[d] Median and range. Mean and standard deviations were not meaningful because of large range of values.
[e] Calculation on weight basis not reported.

Table 2.

CONTINUOUS THEOPHYLLINE DOSAGE FOR
ACUTELY ILL PATIENTS FOLLOWING
AN INITIAL LOADING DOSE (110)

Patient age/Clinical condition	infusion rate* (mg/kg/hr)
Neonates	0.13
Infants 2–6 months	0.4
Infants 6–11 months	0.7
Children 1–9 years of age	0.8
Children over 9 and otherwise healthy adults who smoke.	0.6
Otherwise healthy non-smoking adults	0.4
Cardiac decompensation, cor pulmonale, and liver dysfunction	0.2

*These are guidelines for initial infusion rates of theophylline (aminophylline = theophylline/0.80) to achieve a target serum concentration of 10 μg/ml (7.5 μg/ml for neonates). Final dosage requirements may be higher or lower and should be guided by serum theophylline measurement. Use ideal body weight for obese patients.

ing dose of this drug or at the beginning of the IV infusion. Another serum sample should be obtained 6 to 8 hours later to determine whether the theophylline serum concentration is within the desired therapeutic range. Empirical adjustments of the infusion rate followed by repeat serum measurements can then maintain serum concentrations at the desired level. Thereafter, it would be prudent to monitor serum theophylline concentrations every 24 hours during the infusion. More frequent determinations of serum theophylline concentrations may be necessary if the patient's symptoms deteriorate or if symptoms of theophylline toxicity occur.

11. The serum theophylline concentration 15 minutes after the loading dose was 14 mcg/ml and eight hours later it was 11 mcg/ml. The patient's overall clinical condition seems to have improved; however, the wheezing is still prominent. How should his dose of theophylline be adjusted to provide additional relief of his symptoms?

The patient's clinical condition has slightly improved; however, the serum theophylline concentration appears to be decreasing. This decrease in the serum concentration of theophylline is not surprising because the loading dose of theophylline was supposed to produce a serum concentration of approximately 15 mcg/ml while the rate of intravenous infusion was based upon calculations to provide a concentration of about 10 mcg/ml. Therefore, it would be reasonable to "fine tune" this patient's dose of theophylline by increasing the total daily dose by 10%. Table 3 provides guidelines for the adjustments of theophylline doses based upon serum theophylline concentrations.

12. Corticosteroids. This patient has received terbutaline subcutaneously and theophylline by intravenous infusion after an initial loading dose. Would the addition of corticosteroids to this therapy be of benefit to this patient?

An acute exacerbation of asthma is associated with pulmonary inflammatory changes which result in edema and increased mucous production in the lung. Therefore, it would seem reasonable to add corticosteroids to the treatment plan of patients who are suffering from an acute asthmatic attack. Corticosteroids, perhaps as a result of anti-inflammatory effects, can decrease morbidity and hypoxemia and improve the response of patients to bronchodilators (83–86). Corticosteroids are the only anti-asthmatic agents that can effectively reverse the airway obstruction which has become poorly responsive to bronchodilators.

This patient's exacerbation of asthma is severe enough to require hospitalization and does not seem to be responding to bronchodilator therapy. In patients such as this, corticosteroids are exceedingly important and should not be withheld.

13. What should be the dose of corticosteroid for this patient?

The initial dosage and the maintenance dosage of corticosteroids for the acute management of severe asthma are controversial. There is even a lack of consensus as to the best choice of a corticosteroid preparation and the preferred route of administration. In essence, empirical choices and empirical doses abound. Fortunately, these empirical regimens usually are all successful provided that doses are large enough to decrease pulmonary inflammation, edema, and mucous production. Most clinicians recommend doses of 4 to 8 mg/kg of hydrocortisone (or its equivalent) every 4 to 6 hours (25,27,28). Some clinicians advocate much larger doses because the potential benefits seem to outweigh the adverse risks when the course of treatment is so brief.

Hydrocortisone or methylprednisolone are usually considered to be the corticosteroids of choice when administered intravenously, although there is no evidence to suggest that other intravenous corticosteroids are either inferior or superior. Methylprednisolone may be preferred when very large corticosteroid doses are used because of its relative lack of mineralocorticoid effects.

This patient is only six years of age and anti-inflammatory doses of 1 or 2 mg/kg of methylprednisolone every 4 to 6 hours seem reasonable. Therapy should be continued until the patient has been asymptomatic for 24 hours. Long-term corticosteroid therapy is unwarranted in this pediatric patient at this time.

Table 3.

DOSE ADJUSTMENT FOLLOWING SERUM THEOPHYLLINE CONCENTRATION MEASUREMENT (53,110)

Peak Theophylline Concentration (μg/ml)	Approximate Adjustment in Total Daily Dose*	Comment
<5	100% increase	If patient is asymptomatic, consider trial off drug, repeat measurement of serum concentration after dose adjustment.
5–7.9	50% increase	
8–9.9	20% increase	Even if patient is transiently asymptomatic at this level, an increased serum concentration may better prevent symptoms when the airways are stressed by vigorous exertion, allergen exposure, or a viral respiratory infection.
10–13.9	Cautions 10% increased if clinically indicated	If patient is asymptomatic, no increase is necessary; if bronchodilator responsive symptoms persist, increase cautiously as indicated.
14–19.9	None	If "breakthrough" in asthmatic symptoms occurs at the end of dosing interval, change to slow-release product and repeat serum theophylline measurements.
	Occasional intolerance requires a 10% decrease.	If side effects occur, decrease total daily dose as indicated.
20–24.9	10% decrease	Even if side effects are absent.
25–29.9	25% decrease	Even if apparent side effects are absent, omit next dose and decrease total daily dose as indicated; repeat measurement of serum concentration after adjustment.
30–34.9	33% decrease	
≥35	50% decrease	Omit next two doses, decrease as indicated, and repeat measurement of serum theophylline concentration after adjustment.

*To avoid toxicity:

(1) Assure that the sample represents a peak concentration obtained at steady state (e.g. no missed or extra doses with close approximation of prescribed dosing intervals during previous 48 hours).

(2) Use reliable laboratory; if result appears questionable, repeat determination if not initally performed in duplicate.

(3) The increase of 50% or 100% should be made in 25% increments at two-day intervals to further assure safety and tolerance. The serum concentration may increase disproportionate to dosage increase as the therapeutic range is entered.[34,35]

CHRONIC ASTHMA

Theophylline

14. A constant IV infusion of aminophylline at 1.3 mg/kg/hour has resulted in a steady state theophylline concentration of 14 mcg/ml in this patient. The asthma symptoms have decreased significantly and oral therapy is to be initiated. What would be an appropriate oral dose of theophylline for this patient?

Once the appropriate daily theophylline dose is established and the patient's condition improved, subsequent theophylline can be administered orally by dividing the same total daily dose into the intervals appropriate for the absorption characteristics of the chosen oral preparation. If a slow release theophylline product is chosen, patients should be dosed every 8 to 12 hours. For a rapid release product, the dosage should be given every 6 hours. In this patient the 24 hour theophylline dose is:

1.3 mg/kg/hr × 30 kg × 24 hours/day × 0.8 (aminophylline is 80% theophylline) = 748.8 mg per day of theophylline.

15. *Serum Concentrations.* When should serum concentrations of theophylline be measured when this patient is switched to oral theophylline therapy?

Blood samples obtained for guidance of long-term theophylline therapy are of value only when steady-state conditions are present. A serum measurement is valid only if no doses have been missed in the previous 48 hours, no extra doses have been taken, the interval between doses has been approximately equal, and no erythromycin or other factors which could potentially alter theophylline clearance transiently are present (110).

Because of the short half-life of theophylline in pediatric patients, trough concentrations tend to be substantially lower than peak concentrations, and therapy based on trough concentrations without consideration of corresponding peak concentrations will lead to problems. Therefore, we feel that theophylline dosage adjustments are best guided by peak serum concentrations, because both the efficacy and toxicity of theophylline correlate well with peak concentrations. When utilizing peak concentrations, care must be taken to avoid error due to delayed absorption; see the chapter entitled Clinical Pharmacokinetics. For rapid release products such as solutions and plain uncoated tablets, the serum theophylline concentration should peak about two hours after dosing (53). For slow release products such as Slo-Phyllin Gyrocaps, Theo-dur, or Sustaire, the peak serum theophylline concentration should be expected about four hours after the dose. Nevertheless, serum samples can be obtained three to seven hours after the morning dose to approximate the peak concentration in most patients who receive Theo-dur (110).

16. Once this patient has been stabilized on oral theophylline, how often should his serum concentration of theophylline be monitored?

Following the establishment of a dosage regimen that maintains theophylline serum concentrations within the therapeutic range, measurements of theophylline levels only need to be obtained once a year in adults because clearance and dosage usually are stable. This patient, however, is only six years of age and periods of rapid growth may significantly alter weight-adjusted dosages. Therefore, repeat measurements of serum theophylline concentrations may be needed every six months. Changes in factors which affect the clearance of theophylline would, of course, necessitate more frequent serum monitoring (110).

17. *Theophylline Product Formulation.* Would a plain theophylline formulation or a sustained released theophylline preparation be best for this patient?

Plain uncoated tablets of theophylline are rapidly absorbed and are most appropriate for the acute management of asthma. However, slow-release formulations of theophylline are more appropriate for the treatment of chronic asthma because those preparations produce minimal peak to trough fluctuations (90). Although some slow-release theophylline products are incompletely and erratically absorbed, others such as Theo-dur have reliable absorption characteristics (Table 4). Therefore, a sustained-release theophylline preparation would be preferred for the chronic management of this patient's asthma especially because children tend to eliminate theophylline more rapidly than adults. Furthermore, slow-release formulations of medications permit dosing at times other than during school hours and thereby alleviate some of the potential psychological stresses

Table 4.

SLOW RELEASE THEOPHYLLINE AND
PERCENT SERUM FLUCTUATIONS (90)

| Product | t½ = 3.7 hr | | t½ = 8.2 hr |
	q 8 hr	q 12 hr	q 12 hr
Slophyllin Gyrocap	61%	225%	69%
Elixophylline - SR	59%	131%	49%
Quibron T-SR	33%	128%	46%
Theolair SR	57%	149%	53%
Theo-dur (200 mg or 300 mg)	17%	38%	16%
Theo-dur (100 mg)	31%	87%	34%
Constant - T	51%	153%	54%
Theovent	63%	168%	58%
Somophyllin CRT	50%	130%	47%
Labid	108%	247%	73%

Above are some widely used slow-released theophylline products and the predicted percent fluctuations in an average child and adult (t½ = 3.7 hr and 8.2 hr, respectively) if continuously dosed every 8 or 12 hours. Calculated to maintain a mean serum concentration of 15 mcg/ml.

which might be associated with medication taking in the presence of peers at school.

18. *Initiation of Theophylline in Ambulatory Patients.* **A 25-year-old, 45 kg patient had asthma as a child. Her asthmatic attacks diminished during her adolescence and responded reasonably well to non-prescription inhaler therapy. She now complains of chronic night cough and shortness of breath associated with activity. A decision has been made to treat this patient's asthma with theophylline. What would be a reasonable initial dose of theophylline for this ambulatory patient and what would be a reasonable plan for optimizing the theophylline dosage for chronic therapy?**

The initial theophylline dose should be 400 mg/day or 16 mg/kg/day, whichever is less. The dose can then be increased by approximately 25% increments *if tolerated* at three day intervals to the average dose for the appropriate age group (see Figure 2). A serum sample should be obtained to monitor the peak serum theophylline concentration if all doses have been taken as scheduled for the past 48 hours. The theophylline dose can then be adjusted based upon the results of the theophylline serum concentration according to Table 3. Therefore, this particular 45-kg patient should receive 400 mg of theophylline each day in divided doses initially. The daily theophylline dose may be increased if tolerated to 500 mg according to Figure 2 and the patient should be scheduled for another clinic visit in order to obtain a serum theophylline concentration and to otherwise evaluate therapy.

19. *Theophylline Salts.* **This patient's physician prefers Choledyl over plain theophylline tablets. What would be an appropriate initial daily dose of Choledyl for the patient in the previous question?**

Theophylline salts and derivatives, such as theophylline ethylenediamine (Aminophylline), oxtriphylline (Choledyl), and theophylline sodium glycinate (Theofort) are not equivalent on a weight basis. The actual theophylline content of these preparations must be known in order to properly calculate or estimate doses for a patient (see Table 5). In this particular instance, only 64% of a 100 mg tablet of Choledyl consists of active theophylline. Therefore, the daily theophylline dose for this patient should be divided by 0.64. It has been determined that this patient should receive 400 mg/day of theophylline initially. Thus, a comparable dose of Choledyl would be approximately 625 mg/day. Unfortunately, Choledyl tablets are available as coated 100 mg or 200 mg tablets and it would be difficult for this patient to take 1.5 tablets four times daily. As an alternative, 1.5 teaspoonsful of the 100 mg/5 ml Choledyl elixir would provide the needed flexibility for this patient's initial daily dose. Other alternatives would be the use of a theophylline preparation other than Choledyl or administration of the Choledyl daily dose other than in four equally divided doses.

20. *Theophylline Toxicity.* **What symptoms are commonly associated with high serum levels of theophylline?**

Symptoms associated with excessive serum theophylline concentrations are related to the gastrointestinal (GI) tract, central nervous system, and cardiovascular system. These symptoms

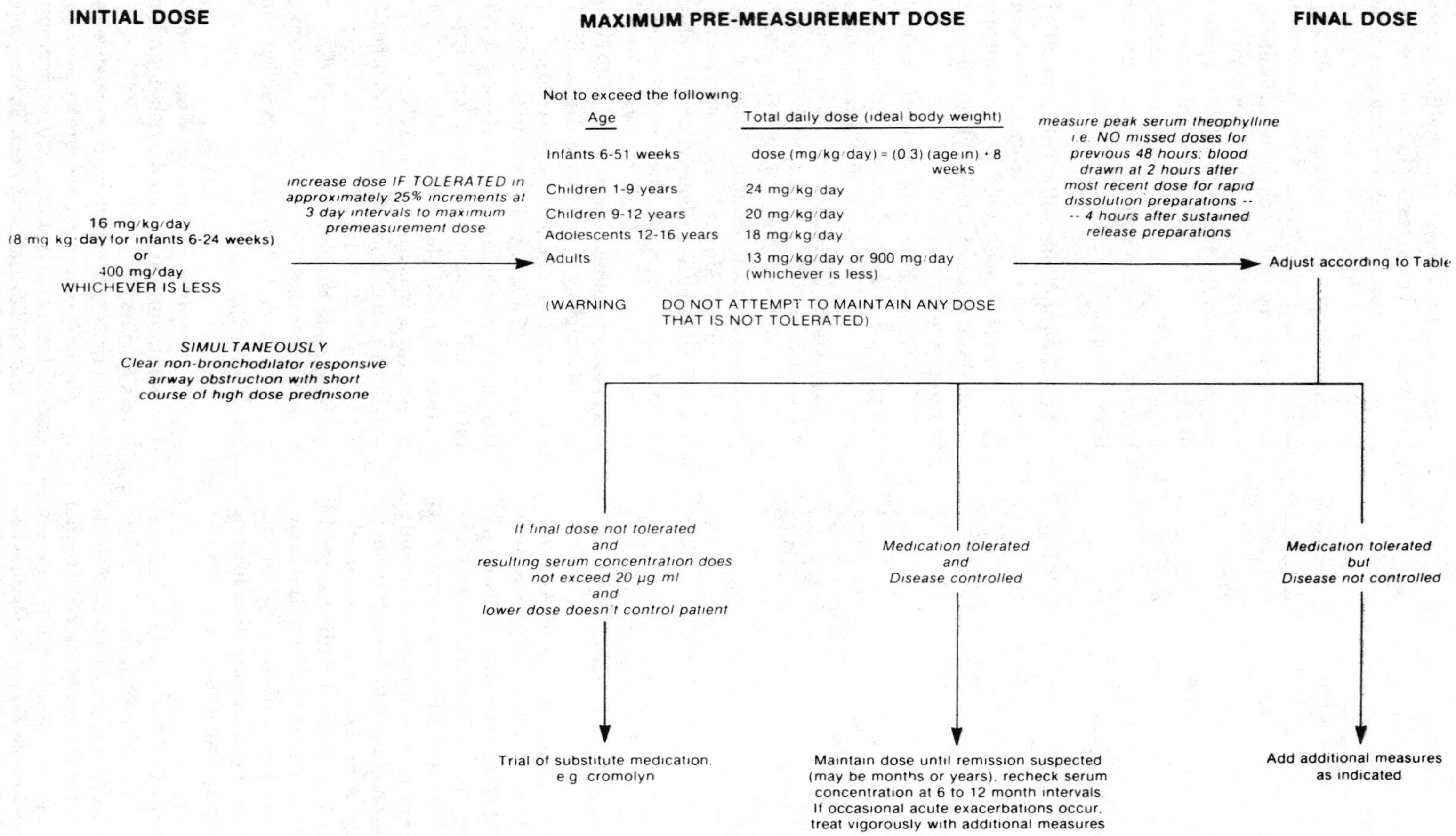

INITIAL DOSE   MAXIMUM PRE-MEASUREMENT DOSE   FINAL DOSE

Not to exceed the following:

Age	Total daily dose (ideal body weight)
Infants 6-51 weeks	dose (mg/kg·day) = (0.3) (age in) + 8
	weeks
Children 1-9 years	24 mg/kg·day
Children 9-12 years	20 mg/kg·day
Adolescents 12-16 years	18 mg/kg·day
Adults	13 mg/kg·day or 900 mg/day
	(whichever is less)

(WARNING   DO NOT ATTEMPT TO MAINTAIN ANY DOSE
             THAT IS NOT TOLERATED)

increase dose IF TOLERATED in
approximately 25% increments at
3 day intervals to maximum
premeasurement dose

16 mg/kg·day
(8 mg/kg·day for infants 6-24 weeks)
or
400 mg/day
WHICHEVER IS LESS

SIMULTANEOUSLY
Clear non-bronchodilator responsive
airway obstruction with short
course of high dose prednisone

measure peak serum theophylline
i.e. NO missed doses for
previous 48 hours; blood
drawn at 2 hours after
most recent dose for rapid
dissolution preparations --
-- 4 hours after sustained
release preparations

Adjust according to Table

If final dose not tolerated
and
resulting serum concentration does
not exceed 20 µg/ml
and
lower dose doesn't control patient

Trial of substitute medication.
e.g. cromolyn

Medication tolerated
and
Disease controlled

Maintain dose until remission suspected
(may be months or years). recheck serum
concentration at 6 to 12 month intervals.
If occasional acute exacerbations occur.
treat vigorously with additional measures

Medication tolerated
but
Disease not controlled

Add additional measures
as indicated

Figure 2. Guide to Theophylline Therapy (53,110)

Table 5.

PERCENTAGE OF ANHYDROUS THEOPHYLLINE
AND THE EQUIVALENT DOSE OF VARIOUS
THEOPHYLLINE SALTS

Salt	% Theophylline	Equivalent Dosage (mg)
Theophylline anhydrous	100%	100 mg
Theophylline monohydrate	91	110
Aminophylline anhydrous	86	116
Aminophylline dihydrate	79	127
Theophylline monoethanolamine	75	133
Oxtriphylline (choline theophylline)	64	156
Theophylline sodium glycinate	49	200
Theophylline calcium salicylate	48	208

include nausea, vomiting, diarrhea, abdominal discomfort, irritability, headaches, insomnia, seizures, and cardiac arrhythmias (138–140). GI symptoms may not precede the occurrence of seizures (138,140). Therefore, it is important not to ignore any symptoms associated with theophylline toxicity. If these symptoms are present, a serum theophylline level should be obtained, and the dose adjusted, if necessary, according to Table 3.

21. How should accidental overdosages of oral theophylline be managed medically?

Ingestion of an oral theophylline dose which may result in signs of theophylline toxicity requires immediate treatment with syrup of ipecac, followed by activated charcoal after emesis (141). Monitoring of serum theophylline concentrations is imperative. Many patients with very high serum theophylline concentrations survive without any aftereffects; however, death or permanent brain damage are common when seizures occur. Prompt reduction of theophylline concentrations can prevent seizures. Therefore, charcoal hemoperfusion

may be indicated clinically when the serum theophylline concentration is greater than 60 mcg/ml because this procedure can rapidly remove theophylline (142–145). The risks of the charcoal hemoperfusion procedure probably are not warranted when the serum theophylline concentration is less than 40 mcg/ml, and the benefits versus risk ratio must be carefully balanced by the clinical status of the patient when serum theophylline concentrations are between 40–60 mcg/ml. Peritoneal dialysis is not adequate for the management of theophylline poisoning (110,142). Hemodialysis, however, may be a reasonable alternative to charcoal hemoperfusion in medical facilities which do not have the capability to initiate charcoal hemoperfusion (163).

Ephedrine

22. A 15-year-old asthmatic patient has been treated with Quibron-T/SR 300 mg twice a day. Despite a steady state peak serum theophylline concentration of 16 mcg/ml, she is continuing to experience brief episodes of bronchospasm three to four times a week. Although additional bronchodilator therapy with a beta-adrenergic agent may be desirable, why would ephedrine be the least desirable agent?

Seven beta-adrenergic agonists are available for clinical use (Table 6); of these, only ephedrine, metaproterenol, terbutaline, and albuterol are available in an oral dosage form. Metaproterenol, terbutaline, and albuterol selectively stimulate the beta$_2$-adrenergic receptors in the bronchi to a greater extent than the beta$_1$-adrenergic receptors in the heart. In contrast, ephedrine possesses both weak alpha-adrenergic as well as beta$_1$-and beta$_2$-adrenergic activity. Moreover, ephedrine mediates its weak bronchodilator effects indirectly through the release of norepinephrine. When compared to these other agents, ephedrine has a shorter duration of action, a lower peak effect, and more adverse effects (102–106). Furthermore, ephedrine adds little to the bronchodilation which is achievable with therapeutic doses of theophylline, and the combination of these two drugs produces synergistic toxicity (106).

Aerosolized Sympathomimetics

23. A 45-year-old man has been treated in emergency medical facilities for acute asth-

Table 6.

SYMPATHOMIMETIC BRONCHODILATORS

Drug	Route	Approximate Duration Effect	Pediatric Dose	Adult Dose	Availability
Epinephine	SQ	0.5–3 hr	.01 mg/kg (0.5 max)	0.1mg/kg (0.5 max)	IV,SQ
Ephedrine	PO	3–5 hr	3–6mg/kg/day	100–150mg/day	PO
Isoproterenol	MDI	1½–2 hr	NA	NA	MDI,NEB,IV,SL
Isoetharine	MDI	1½–2 hr	NA	NA	MDI,NEB
Metaproterenol	PO	3–4 hr	2mg/kg/day	40–80mg/day	PO,MDI,NEB
	MDI	4–6 hr	2–8 inhalations/ day	2–8 inhalations/ day	
Terbutaline	PO	4–6 hr	0.23mg/kg/day	7.5–15mg/day	PO,SQ,IV,NEB,MDI
	SQ	0.5–6.0 hr	.01mg/kg (0.5mg max. dose)	0.1mg/kg (0.5mg max. dose)	
	MDI	6–8 hr	2–8 inhalations/ day	2–8 inhalations/ day	
Albuterol	MDI	6–8 hr	2–8 inhalations/ day	2–8 inhalations/ day	MDI,PO
	PO	4–6 hr	NA	8–16mg/day	

matic attacks three times in the past six months. On each occasion his wheezing and dyspnea completely cleared following two subcutaneous injections of terbutaline. Should this patient be given a prescription for an oral or an aerosolized sympathomimetic drug for use at the onset of his symptoms?

Patients with intermittent asthma should be treated initially with an inhaled beta$_2$-agonist. Beta-adrenergic drugs when administered by inhalation have a more rapid onset of action and a longer duration of action than when administered orally (114,115). Inhalation of these sympathomimetic drugs also induces significant bronchodilation with only minimal adverse effects. Thus, the administration of beta-adrenergic drugs by inhalation should be preferred over oral administration for the management of this patient's infrequent acute attacks.

24. Which beta-adrenergic bronchodilator would be most appropriate for this patient?

Albuterol, metaproterenol, isoetharine, and isoproterenol currently are available for inhalation in the USA. Of these drugs, albuterol has the longest duration of action and the least side effects (116,117). Although individual patients vary in their response to different bronchodilators, 0.2 mg of albuterol has been shown to be more effective and longer-lasting than 1.5 mg of metaproterenol or 1.0 mg of isoproterenol (118). Furthermore, adverse effects with albuterol are less common than with either isoproterenol or metaproterenol at equal bronchodilatory doses. Since the clinical usefulness of the beta$_2$-adrenergic bronchodilator, albuterol, is well established, it would seem to be the most appropriate inhaler for managing the infrequent acute asthmatic attacks of this patient. Nevertheless, the efficacy and degree of selectivity of available agents are probably clinically indistinguishable when used in appropriate dosages by inhalation.

Albuterol is also known as salbutamol in Europe where it has been widely utilized for the management of patients with asthma for many years.

25. Aerosol Instructions. What instructions should this 45-year-old patient receive concerning the proper usage of his inhaler?

The pharmacological benefits from pressurized metered-dose aerosol inhalers are dependent upon achievement of an adequate concentration of the inhaled medication at appropriate bronchial receptors. Variables such as the rate and depth of inhalation, length of time that the breath is held after inhalation, and placement of the inhaler mouthpiece into the mouth can affect the bronchial concentration of inhaled medications. Therefore, patients must understand and be able to properly use these inhaler devices. Although manufacturer's instruction sheets are dispensed along with the inhaler, the effectiveness of this method of patient instruction has not been adequately evaluated (119).

Physicians, pharmacists, and nurses give little or no advice to hospitalized patients commencing bronchodilator inhaler therapy (120) and these practitioners sometimes are unsure themselves how to use bronchodilator aerosols. It is not surprising that surveys of the clinical use of pressurized aerosols indicate that 14–75% of patients used their inhalers incorrectly (121–123). These surveys, unfortunately, failed to accurately define the criteria used to determine correct technique and, as a result, interpretations or extrapolations from these surveys are suspect.

It would seem wise to supplement the manufacturers' printed instructions with a demonstration of proper techniques in the use of these inhalation devices. There is adequate evidence that medication counseling can significantly improve patient adherence to prescribed therapeutic regimens. Furthermore, one particular study has demonstrated that the manufacturer's printed instruction does not appear to be sufficient by itself to teach patients how to use their inhalers; however, supplemental verbal instruction followed by a practice session using an empty inhaler significantly increased the correct use of the inhaler (119).

Individualized patient counseling in lieu of the manufacturer's printed instructions may also be appropriate if patients can be provided with continual follow-up instructions. In this situation, patients should be informed if verbal instructions are different than the manufacturer's printed instructions. Individualized patient counseling can take advantage of recent studies which evaluate how aerosolized medications can best be administered. However, the potential for confusion should not be underestimated if printed instructions are different from verbal instructions.

If the particular situation is conducive to individualized patient counseling, the following information should be supplied to the patient. This adult patient should be instructed to *shake the canister well* immediately before each use and to remove the cap. The amount of medication reaching bronchial receptors can be increased if the metered-dose inhaler is held approximately two inches from an open mouth, or if the medication is inhaled through a four-inch paper tube spacer which is placed on the end of the actuator (127–131). The patient should *tilt* his *head back slightly* to form as straight a channel as possible to maximize the depth of airway penetration by the drug. The next step is to *breathe out fully but normally*. The dose of the drug will be more uniformly distributed in the lungs when inhaled after a normal exhalation (133–135). The patient should then *breathe in deeply and slowly* over 4–5 seconds while simultaneously depressing fully the top of the metal canister. A fourteen-fold higher concentration of the drug will be deposited in the lung after a slow 4–5 second inhalation (0.5 L/second) as compared to a fast 1–2 second inhalation (2.0 L/second) because more drug reaches the small airways instead of impacting on the large airways (133,135). Likewise, the depth of inhalation also enhances the amount of drug retained by the lung. The patient should then *hold his breath* for about 5–10 seconds after inhalation to prevent exhaling particles of drug which would normally deposit in the lung due to gravitational effects. If another inhalation has been prescribed, the patient should allow five to ten minutes for the first inhaled dose to take effect and then he should repeat the entire above procedure. Afterwards, the *inhaler should be cleaned thoroughly*. The patient should remove the metal canister and wash the plastic case and cap by rinsing thoroughly in warm running water at least once a day. After thoroughly drying the plastic case and cap, the metal canister should be put back into the case with a twisting motion, and the cap should be put back on.

In addition to these instructions concerning administration techniques, the patient also should be warned not to increase the number or the frequency of inhalations without specific authorization from his physician. The patient should also consult with his physician if his symptoms worsen. Finally, the medication should not be stored near heat or an open flame because the contents of the inhaler are under pressure.

Corticosteroids

26. An 11-year-old male with chronic asthma has been treated with albuterol by

inhalation and Theo-dur 400 mg twice a day. Over the past two months he has experienced three exacerbations of his asthma symptoms, but he has been able to avoid hospitalization because he responded in each of these occasions to short "bursts" of prednisone (20 mg bid × 5 days). In each instance, his coughing and wheezing would clear by the fourth to fifth day of therapy and would gradually return about 10–14 days after discontinuation of this corticosteroid. Should this patient receive chronic corticosteroid therapy?

The repeated use of short courses of prednisone in the past 8 weeks indicates a probable need for maintenance corticosteroid therapy. However, all therapeutic interventions should be evaluated before exposing this actively growing 11-year-old patient to the growth-suppressant and other adverse effects of long-term corticosteroids. If after determining that this patient would not benefit from additional theophylline or beta$_2$-adrenergic medications, and if the precipitating events of these recent asthmatic attacks cannot be prevented, then chronic corticosteroid therapy can be initiated after assessing the risks for this patient.

The adverse effects of corticosteroids are significant (see chapter entitled Disorders of the Adrenals) and must not be regarded lightly in this situation. Therefore, all efforts must be made to minimize these adverse effects. The initial corticosteroid doses should always be reduced after asthma symptoms are controlled to the lowest possible dose that is still compatible with continued control. Alternate-day corticosteroid therapy has been used extensively to treat asthmatics and has been associated with considerably less risk than daily corticosteroid therapy. Prednisone given in single doses on alternate mornings may well be reasonable for this patient. Moreover, growth has been shown to be unaffected by prednisone doses of 30 to 60 mg every other day in children with nephrotic syndrome or ulcerative colitis (200). If these data can be extrapolated to asthmatic children, then comparable corticosteroid doses should not adversely affect the growth of this child. Although alternate-day steroid therapy is preferable to daily therapy, aerosol corticosteroid therapy also minimizes adverse systemic effects and appears to offer clinical results comparable to alternate-day therapy (151–155).

27. *Oral versus Aerosol Corticosteroids.* **The decision has been made to continue this** patient's theophylline and albuterol and to begin chronic corticosteroid therapy. Would alternate-day prednisone or would aerosolized beclomethasone be preferred?

At this time, there is not a definitive answer to this question and the decision must be based on subjective assessment and clinical judgment. Both alternate-day prednisone and inhaled beclomethasone dipropionate have advantages over daily prednisone therapy in terms of adrenal suppression and other systemic effects. Similar suppression of the hypothalamic-pituitary-adrenal function was noted when 400 to 800 mcg per day of beclomethasone dipropionate were compared to 20 to 40 mg of alternate-day prednisone in children with chronic asthma (156). The adrenal suppression in this study may have been due to the relatively large doses of the aerosol preparation as this adverse effect is, in general, dose dependent (150). Although large doses of beclomethasone by inhalation may be associated with suppression of plasma cortisol and inhibition of metarapone stimulation, inhaled beclomethasone generally has not been associated with clinical hypercorticism. Hypercorticism can occur clinically with alternate-day prednisone therapy. Therefore, it would seem that aerosol beclomethasone would be preferred for this patient at this time (155).

28. *Beclomethasone Aerosol Dosage.* **What would be an appropriate dose of beclomethasone for this patient initially?**

The effectiveness of beclomethasone dipropionate is clearly dose related, as 1600 mcg/day is more effective than 800 mcg/day, and 400 mcg/day is more effective than 200 mcg/day (149–151). The usual adult dose of beclomethasone initially is two 50 mcg inhalations three or four times daily. However, initial dosages of beclomethasone are highly variable. The usual mean beclomethasone dose for adults is about 400–600 mcg/day. A "mean" dose by definition implies that half of the patients require more than 400–600 mcg/day and that half of the patients require less. Therefore, different clinical situations and different patients may dictate the need for either a larger or a smaller dose than the "mean" dose. Some clinicians prefer to initiate therapy in adults with 600–800 mcg/day and to gradually decrease the dose until the minimum effective dose is determined for a given patient. This approach suggests that if a patient is in sufficient need of beclomethasone, a larger dose is preferred initially in hopes of preventing hospitalization and/or short "bursts" of systemic corticosteroid therapy. On the other hand, an initial beclomethasone dose of 300–400 mcg/day may be more appropriate if a patient has just finished a short "burst" of oral prednisone. The usual dosage for children more than six years of age is one or two inhalations three or four times a day. Therefore, it would be reasonable for this 11-year-old patient to initiate therapy with two inhalations (100 mcg) four times daily. This dose should be re-evaluated subsequently. Several weeks may pass before the full benefits from this medication are achieved, but a single aerosol dose of beclomethasone produces noticeable benefits in two hours and peak effects in about eight hours (155).

29. *Patient Instructions.* What instructions should this patient and his parents receive concerning proper usage of beclomethasone dipropionate?

This patient should inhale his beclomethasone aerosol using the same techniques that he uses with his albuterol inhaler (see Question 25). In addition, he should gargle or drink fluids immediately after using his beclomethasone to remove residual corticosteroids from the oral cavity. Such action will decrease the probability of developing oral candidiasis (160,164).

The patient also must be informed that this medication, unlike his albuterol, must be used continuously on a daily basis, even when he is asymptomatic. Beclomethasone by aerosol is not intended to treat acute asthmatic attacks and is contraindicated until the acute episode has subsided because the inhaled powder further aggravates already hyperactive airways. Furthermore, the aerosol may not effectively reach occluded airways during the acute attack, and instead of receiving additional corticosteroid, because of the associated stress, the patient receives less or none. These patients should be given a reserve supply of oral prednisone and instructions to begin corticosteroid therapy because deaths have occurred under these circumstances (155,157). This patient's parents should be encouraged to seek medical advice for him at the first sign of an acute exacerbation of asthma.

30. This patient's mother claims that her son seems to experience decreasing benefits from the beclomethasone as the canister becomes empty. What might be a reasonable explanation which could account for this observation?

When the beclomethasone aerosol is activated, the canister is designed to deliver approximately 50 mcg of drug for each inhalation. However, reliance on the delivery of a metered 50 mcg dose cannot be assured beyond 200 inhalations, and usage of the canister until empty is not recommended (157). Since this patient has been needing two inhalations of the beclomethasone every eight hours, he should need a refill every 33 days (200 inhalations divided by six inhalations per day). It would also be useful to inform the patient or his parents of the estimated refill date and to encourage the maintenance of a daily asthma diary. Finally, the patient should also be reminded to shake the canister well just prior to use because beclomethasone dipropionate aerosol is a suspension (157).

31. This 11-year-old patient continues to experience periodic episodes of asthma symptoms. His peak serum theophylline concentration is 16 mcg/ml on Theo-dur 400 mg twice a day, and he continues to use albuterol and beclomethasone by inhalation. Although this patient receives continual positive reinforcement and instruction on proper inhaler use (Questions 25,29,30), he periodically rebels, as a typical adolescent, and uses his inhalers haphazardly. What would be a reasonable therapeutic approach to the management of this problem?

The majority of patients are unable to benefit from inhaler-dispensed medications primarily because they are unable or unwilling to operate these devices appropriately. Although careful and continuous instruction of patients in the proper techniques of using inhalers can alleviate this problem, many young children simply are not candidates for this type of treatment. This patient has needed three short "bursts" of prednisone over a span of about eight weeks prior to his use of beclomethasone (see Question 26) and probably needs to receive predictable doses of corticosteroids. If this patient is reluctant or unable to properly use his inhaler device, oral corticosteroid therapy may be needed. Alternate-day prednisone would be preferred over daily prednisone because it is associated with considerably less risk (see Disorders of the Adrenals chapter).

In pediatric patients, the dose of prednisone (or its equivalent) is about 1.0–2.0 mg/kg every other day (4). Many other dosage recommendations are available but none have been proven to be superior to any other. In essence, the initial corticosteroid doses should be large enough to control asthma symptoms and subsequent doses should be gradually reduced to the lowest dose which can control these symptoms. One alternate-day dosage regimen which has been recommended for children and adults is as follows (99): prednisone 10 mg every other day for children less than 1 year of age, 20 mg for ages 1–3, 30 mg for ages 3-12, and 40 mg for ages 12 and older.

Cromolyn

32. A 9-year-old patient has experienced asthmatic symptoms three to four days of the week throughout the school year for the past four years, and has a history of allergy to animal dander. He has been unable to tolerate the gastrointestinal effects of theophylline even though peak serum concentrations have never been higher than 8 to 10 mcg/ml; and terbutaline 2.5 mg three times daily caused a coarse hand tremor which interfered with his writing ability at school. Why should this patient be given a trial of cromolyn?

Theophylline is more effective than cromolyn in preventing asthmatic symptoms, is more convenient to administer, requires less frequent administration when sustained release formulations are used, and is less expensive. However, this patient has been unable to tolerate theophylline even when peak theophylline serum concentrations were well below 20 mcg/ml. Any patient with chronic perennial asthma who cannot tolerate theophylline or beta-adrenergic therapy should receive a trial of cromolyn sodium (Intal). Although cromolyn has no bronchodilating or anti-asthmatic effects and is not appropriate for treatment of acute asthmatic symptoms, it is clearly of value in the prophylactic management of asthma.

Cromolyn is effective in 52–89% of patients with asthma (167–172). It may be even more effective in young patients or in those with allergy-mediated asthma. Therefore, this 9-year-old patient with a four-year history of allergy-mediated asthma may respond remarkably well to this drug.

33. If this patient's asthmatic symptoms are not related to a known allergen, would cromolyn sodium still be effective?

Cromolyn blocks the release of the chemical mediators (eg, histamine, serotonin, and slow reacting substance of anaphylaxis) of IgE-mediated hypersensitivity reactions. It appears to do this by acting on the surface of mast cells to stabilize the cell membrane and to protect it from the effects of antigen-antibody reactions that would otherwise release these mediators of bronchospasm. It does not interfere directly with the antigen-antibody interaction, nor does it oppose the action of the mediators once they are released (99). At the cellular level, the actual mechanism of cromolyn's action still is unclear. Currently, it is thought that cromolyn prevents the influx of calcium into mast cells, thereby inhibiting calcium-dependent, antigen-induced mediator release (100). Since cromolyn inhibits allergen-induced release of mediators from mast cells, it could be inferred that its major use would be in allergy-mediated asthma.

Cromolyn additionally blocks nonimmunological stimulation of mediator release from mast cells. The ability of this drug to protect susceptible individuals from asthmatic attacks provoked by phospholipase A, dextran, polymyxin-B, hyperventilation, air, exercise, and aspirin also suggests that cromolyn has nonspecific mast cell membrane stabilizing effects (175–180). Since allergic factors alone do not accurately predict a favorable response to cromolyn, patients without a demonstrable allergen should not be deprived of a trial of cromolyn just because this drug gives the appearance of being primarily effective in allergy-mediated asthma.

34. What is the mechanism by which cromolyn capsules are administered?

Cromolyn is administered as a powder by inhalation. It is commercially available in gelatin capsules which contain 20 mg of the drug and an equal amount of lactose. The drug particles of cromolyn are 2 to 6 microns in size and are too fine to flow well in an airstream. Therefore, lactose particles which are much larger in size are blended in with the cromolyn to improve the airflow properties of the mixture. The gelatin capsule which contains this powder blend is inserted into a special Spinhaler device that punctures the capsule. When the patient inhales through the Spinhaler mouthpiece, a plastic propeller-like rotor is activated and the powder blend enters the respiratory tract in the form of a finely particulate aerosol. The small cromolyn particles reach the peripheral airways and the large lactose particles deposit in the oropharynx and the trachea (101).

35. What instructions should this patient and his parents receive concerning proper use of the cromolyn Spinhaler?

The inhalation techniques for administration of cromolyn are not as complicated as those which are required for the sympathomimetic metered-dose inhalers (see Question 25). Nevertheless, proper inhalation technique is associated with a better therapeutic response (181). The patient should be taught according to the manufacturer's instructions which accompany the commercially available product and the patient should demonstrate his technique subsequently. The patient also should be reminded to take several inhalations in order to extract as much of the powder from a single capsule as possible. If inhalation of this powered aerosol causes bronchial irritation or wheezing, subsequent administrations of cromolyn should be preceded by a prophylactic puff of a beta$_2$-adrenergic aerosolized bronchodilator. Finally and most importantly, the patient must understand that cromolyn is not indicated for the treatment of an acute attack of asthma or for status asthmaticus, and that cromolyn inhalations must be temporarily discontinued should an acute attack develop.

36. This patient was started on a dosage regimen of one 20 mg cromolyn capsule to be inhaled four times a day at spaced intervals. When should patients begin to respond to cromolyn and how much time is usually needed before judging the efficacy of this therapy?

The time of onset of effectiveness of cromolyn differs, and depends on the type of chronic asthma which is being treated. Predictable seasonal asthma often responds to cromolyn in 4 to 14 days, and the concomitant use of bronchodilators can be reduced in about three to six weeks. For perennial and unresponsive asthma a few months may elapse before the optimal benefits from cromolyn are realized (167). Generally, most patients respond to cromolyn within four weeks (174). If patients continue to experience significant

symptoms after four weeks of cromolyn, alternative therapy should be considered, although some clinicians might increase the dose before abandoning this drug (107). Adverse effects to cromolyn generally are not dose-related and for the most part are related to irritation of the inhaled powder (187,188).

37. If this patient is unable to use the Spinhaler effectively, how else might the cromolyn be administered?

Some children may have difficulty inhaling cromolyn from the Spinhaler. For these children, a 20 mg capsule can be dissolved in 2 ml of normal saline or water and nebulized by a face mask (189).

Atropine

38. What is the role of atropine in the medical management of asthma?

The clinical disease of asthma is currently thought to reflect not only the effects of bronchospasm but also of inflammation and epithelial damage. The effects of epithelial damage are mediated by the vagus, and the role of cholinergic receptors in asthma may be of considerable importance (81,82). Therefore, anticholinergic drugs such as atropine can be used to manage asthmatic symptoms. Previously, anticholinergic drugs were thought to be contraindicated in asthmatics because of the anticholinergic drying effect on bronchial mucous. However, this drying effect does not seem to be significant when atropine is administered by inhalation. Thus, atropine aerosol could be a major addition to the pharmacological armamentarium useful in the management of asthma, especially if asthmatics with a significant cholinergic component to their asthma can be identified. Much research is being conducted in this area and aerosolized atropine may play an increasingly large role in asthma management in the not too distant future (180,70–75). At present, inhaled anticholineric drugs such as atropine or ipratropium bromide (76–80) should be given a trial in those patients who do not adequately respond to more traditional therapy.

EXERCISE-INDUCED ASTHMA

39. A 10-year-old female experiences asthmatic attacks after short periods of exercise

which seldom last more than six minutes. These bronchospastic attacks are severe enough to prevent this fifth grade child from participating in school, church, or social activities which require physical exertion. Is this the typical pulmonary response to exercise of asthmatics?

Approximately 75–93% of asthmatics will develop bronchospasm with sufficient exercise (7–13), and the severity of the bronchospasm is dependent upon the duration, intensity and type of physical exercise (190–192). The asthmatic patient generally experiences bronchodilation about 2–3 minutes after the start of exercise, and bronchoconstriction after about 6 minutes of exercise. The bronchoconstriction may force termination of the exercise; however, if exercising continues in spite of the bronchospasm, the asthma symptoms may end. Supposedly, the bronchodilation is a result of an initial sympathetic surge from the exercise and the bronchoconstriction a result of the release of chemical mediators such as histamine or SRS-A. When these chemical mediators are depleted from their storage sites, the asthma symptoms terminate despite continuation of the exercise activity (193,194). The stimuli which provoke the release of chemical mediators are unknown, but hyperpnea, hypocapnia, lactic acidosis, air temperature, and humidity may play a role (194).

40. What pharmacological interventions are effective in the management of exercise-induced asthma?

Theophylline, beta-adrenergic agonists, or cromolyn (11,14–25,88–93,180,195–199) can prevent the occurrence of exercise-induced asthma more effectively than anticholinergics or corticosteroids (25–28,93–97,180) in the majority of patients. Theophylline and cromolyn are preferable for the exercise-induced asthma (EIA) of patients with chronic perennial asthma. Theophylline is especially effective in preventing EIA when theophylline serum concentrations are within the acceptable therapeutic range. Although cromolyn is as effective as theophylline in preventing EIA (180), it is not a bronchodilator and must be administered immediately prior to physical exercise for optimal effects. Furthermore, the cromolyn only will protect the patient from EIA for about 1–2 hours (98).

For patients who experience asthmatic symptoms only when exercising, the inhaled beta-adrenergic drugs such as metaproterenol or albuterol are preferred (180,195–198). These agents are beta$_2$-adrenergic specific, have a rapid onset of action, are convenient to administer, and have minimal side effects. Oral beta-adrenergic medications are not advocated because their peak action occurs about 90 minutes after a dose and the exercise activity must be properly synchronized (197–199).

References

1. American Thoracic Society: Committee on diagnostic standards for non-tuberculosis respiratory disease: Definition and classification of chronic bronchitis, asthma, and pulmonary emphysema. Am Rev Resp Dis. 1962; 85:762.

2. National Institute of Allergy and Infectious Diseases Task Force Report: Asthma and the other allergic diseases. Washington, D.C., U.S. Government Printing Office: 1979;1–20. (NIH Publication no 79-387).

3. Corrao WM et al: Chronic cough as the sole presenting manifestation of bronchial asthma. N Engl J Med. 1979; 300:633.

4. Leffert F: The management of chronic asthma. J Pediatr. 1980; 97:875.

5. McIntosh K et al: The association of viral and bacterial respiratory infections with exacerbations of wheezing in young asthmatic children. J Pediatr. 1973; 82:578.

6. Minor TE et al: Viruses as precipitants of asthma attacks in children. JAMA. 1974; 227:292.

7. Jones RS et al: The place of physical exercise and bronchodilator drugs in the assessment of the asthmatic child. Arch Dis Child. 1963; 38:539.

8. Sly RM: Exercise related changes in airway obstruction: Frequency and clinical correlates in asthmatic children. Ann Allergy. 1970; 28:1.

9. Silverman M et al: Standardization of exercise tests in asthmatic children. Arch Dis Child. 1972; 47:882.

10. Bierman CD et al: Incidence of exercise induced asthma in children. Pediatrics. 1975; 56:847.

11. Anderson SD et al: Inhaled and oral salbutamol in exercise induced asthma. Am Rev Respir Dis. 1976; 114:493.

12. Kattan M et al: The response to exercise in normal and asthmatic children. J Pediatr. 1978; 92:718.

13. Godfrey S et al: Problems of exercise induced asthma. J Allergy Clin Immunol. 1973; 52:199.

14. Ekwo E et al: Evaluation of a program for the pharmacologic management of children with asthma. J Allergy Clin Immunol. 1978; 61:240.

15. McFadden ER et al: Acute bronchial asthma. Relations between clinical and physiologic manifestations. N Engl J Med. 1973; 288:221.

16. Rupple G: Testing regimens, before and after bronchodilator studies. In *Manual of Pulmonary Function Testing,* CV Mosby Co, 1975, p 69.

17. Ayer LN et al: A guide to the interpretation of pulmonary function tests. Pamphlet, Pfizer Pharm, New York, New York, 1978.

18. Middleton E: Antiasthmatic drug therapy and calcium ions. Review of pathogenesis and role of calcium. J Pharm Sci. 1980; 69:243.

19. Brisson GR et al: The stimulus secretion coupling of glucose-induced release: VII. A proposed site of action for adenosine 3'5' cyclic monophosphate. J Clin Invest. 1972; 51:232.

20. Horrobin DF et al: Methylxanthine phosphodiesterase inhibitors behave as prostaglandin antagonists in a perfused rat mesenteric artery preparation. Prostaglandins. 1977; 13:33.

21. Lichtenstein LM et al: Histamine release in vitro: Inhibition by catecholamines and methylxanthines. Science. 1968; 161:902.

22. Assen ESK et al: Inhibition by sympathomimetic amines of histamine release induced by antigen in passively sensitized human lung. Nature. 1969; 224:1028.

23. Kerr JW et al: Effect of receptor blocking drugs and disodium cromoglycate on histamine hypersensitivity in bronchial asthma. Br Med J. 1970; 2:139.

24. Johnson HG et al: Prevention of calcium ionophore-induced release of histamine in rat mast cells by disodium cromoglycate. J Immunol. 1975; 114:514.

25. Morris H: Pharmacology of corticosteroids in asthma. In *Allergy: Principles and Practice,* edited by E Middleton, CE Reed, and EF Ellis, St. Louis, 1978, p 464.

26. Leffert F: The management of acute severe asthma. J Pediatr. 1980; 96:1.

27. Fireman P: Status asthmaticus in children. In *Allergy: Principles and Practice,* edited by E Middleton, CE Reed, and EF Ellis, St. Louis, 1978, p 780.

28. Petty T: Status asthmaticus in adults. In *Allergy: Principles and Practice,* edited by E Middleton, CE Reed, and EF Ellis, St. Louis, 1978, p 771.

29. The respiratory system: Acute respiratory failure. In *Critical Care Manual,* edited by RF Wilson, UpJohn, p 4.

30. Davis WJ et al: Terbutaline in the treatment of acute asthma in childhood. Chest. 1977; 72:614.

31. Pang LM et al: Terbutaline in the treatment of status asthmaticus. Chest. 1977; 72:469.

32. Sly MR et al: Comparison of subcutaneous terbutaline with epinephrine in the treatment of asthma in children. J Allergy Clin Immunol. 1977; 59:128.

33. Smith PR et al: A comparative study of subcutaneously administered terbutaline and epinephrine in the treatment of acute bronchial asthma. Chest. 1977; 71:129.

34. Glass P et al: Evaluation of a new beta$_2$-adrenergic receptor stimulant, terbutaline, in bronchial asthma. I. Subcutaneous comparison with epinephrine. Curr Ther Res. 1973; 15:141.

35. Simons FER et al: Dose response of subcutaneous terbutaline and epinephrine in children with asthma. Am J Dis Child. 1981; 135:214.

36. Powell JR et al: Theophylline: Counterpoint discussion. In *Applied Pharmacokinetics: Principles of Therapeutic Drug Monitoring,* 1st ed, edited by WE Evans, JJ Schentag, and WJ Jusko, Applied Therapeutics, Inc., San Francisco, 1980.

37. Wolfe J et al: Bronchodilator effects of terbutaline and aminophylline alone and in combination in asthmatic patients. N Engl J Med. 1978; 298:363.

38. Smith J et al: Theophylline and aerosolized terbutaline in the treatment of bronchial asthma. Chest. 1980; 78:816.

39. Jenne J et al: Pharmacokinetics of theophylline application to adjustment of the clinical dose of aminophylline. Clin Pharmacol Ther. 1972; 13:349.

40. Weinberger M et al: Evaluation of oral bronchodilator therapy. J Pediatr. 1974; 84:421.

41. Weinberger M et al: Interaction of ephedrine and theophylline. Clin Pharmacol Ther. 1975; 17:585.

42. Hambleton G et al: Comparison of cromoglycate (cromolyn) and theophylline in controlling symptoms of chronic asthma. Lancet. 1977; 1:381.

43. Mitenko P et al: Rational intravenous doses of theophylline. N Engl J Med. 1973; 289:600.

44. Ellis E et al: Pharmacokinetics of theophylline in children with asthma. Pediatrics. 1976; 58:542.

45. Hendeles L et al: Disposition of theophylline after a single intravenous infusion of aminophylline. Am Rev Resp Dis. 1978; 118:97.

46. Piafsky KM et al: Theophylline kinetics in acute pulmonary edema. Clin Pharmacol Ther. 1977; 21:310.

47. Piafsky KM et al: Theophylline disposition in patients with hepatic cirrhosis. N Engl J Med. 1977; 296:1495.

48. Aranda JV et al: Pharmacokinetic aspects of theophylline in premature newborns. N Engl J Med. 1976; 295:413.

49. Loughnan P et al: Pharmacokinetic analysis of the disposition of intravenous theophylline in young children. J Pediatr. 1976; 88:874.

50. Weinberger M et al: Intravenous aminophylline dosage use of serum theophylline measurement for guidance. JAMA. 1976; 235:2110.

51. Zaske D et al: Oral aminophylline therapy. Increased dosage requirement in children. JAMA. 1977; 237:1453.

52. Giacoia G et al: Theophylline pharmacokinetics in premature infants with apnea. J Pediatr. 1976; 89:829

53. Hendeles L et al: Guide to oral theophylline therapy for treatment of chronic asthma. Am J Dis Child. 1978; 132:876.

54. Nassif EG et al: Theophylline disposition in infancy. Presented at American Academy of Pediatrics Annual Meeting, San Francisco, 1979.

55. Vozeh S et al: Changes in theophylline clearances during acute illness. JAMA. 1978; 240:1882.

56. Chang KC et al: Altered theophylline pharmacokinetics during acute respiratory viral illness. Lancet. 1978; 1:1132.

57. Cummins LH et al: Erythromycin's effect on theophylline blood levels. Pediatrics. 1977; 59:144.

58. Kozak PP et al: Administration of erythromycin to patients on theophylline. J Allergy Clin Immunol. 1977; 16:149.

59. Laforce C et al: Effect of erythromycin on theophylline clearance in asthmatic children. J Pediatr. 1981; 99:153.

60. Zarowitz BJ et al: Effect of erythromycin base on theophylline kinetics. Clin Pharmacol Ther. 1981; 29:601.

61. Prince RA et al: Effect of erythromycin on theophylline kinetics. J Allergy Clin Immunol. 1981; 68:427.

62. Roberts R et al: Cimetidine impairs the elimination of theophylline and antipyrine. Gastroenterology. 1981; 81:19.

63. Jackson JE et al: Cimetidine decreases theophylline clearance. Am Rev Respir Dis. 1981; 123:615.

64. Campbell MA et al: Cimetidine decreases theophylline clearance. Ann Intern Med. 1981; 95:68.

65. Weinberger M et al: Decreased theophylline clearance due to cimetidine. N Engl J Med. 1981; 304:672.

66. Weinberger M et al: Inhibition of theophylline clearance by troleandomycin. J Allergy Clin Immunol. 1977; 59:228.

67. Hunt S et al: Effects of smoking on theophylline disposition. Clin Pharmacol Ther. 1976; 19:546.

68. Jusko WJ et al: Role of tobacco smoking in pharmacokinetics. J Pharmacokinetic Biopharm. 1978; 6:7.

69. Jusko WJ et al: Enhanced biotransformation of theophylline in marijuana and tobacco smokers. Clin Pharmacol Ther. 1978; 24:406.

70. Tinkelman DG et al: Inhibition of exercise-induced bronchospasm by atropine. Am Rev Respir Dis. 1976; 114:87.

71. Itkin IH et al: The role of atropine as a mediator blocker of induced bronchial obstruction. J Allergy Clin Immunol. 1970; 45:178.

72. Yu DYC et al: Inhibition of antigen-induced bronchoconstriction by atropine in asthmatic patients. J Appl Physiol. 1972; 32:823.

73. Cavanaugh MJ et al: Inhaled atropine sulfate: Dose response characteristics. Am Rev Respir Dis. 1976; 114:517.

74. Brady RE et al: The value of atropine in the documentation of reversible airway obstruction. Ann Allergy. 1979; 42:211.

75. Hemstreet MP: Atropine nebulization—Simple and safe. Ann Allergy. 1980; 44:138.

76. Storms WW et al: Aerosol SCH 1000—An anticholinergic bronchodilator. Am Rev Respir Dis. 1975; 111:419.

77. Gross NJ: SCH 1000: A new anticholinergic bronchodilator. Am Rev Respir Dis. 1975; 112:823.

78. Poppius H et al: Comparative trial of a new anticholinergic bronchodilator, SCH 1000, and salbutamol in chronic bronchitis. Br Med J. 1973; 4:134.

79. Petrie GR et al: Comparison of aerosol ipratropium bromide and salbutamol in chronic bronchitis and asthma. Br Med J. 1975; 1:430.

80. Ruffin RE et al: A comparison of the bronchodilator activity of SCH 1000 and salbutamol. J Allergy Clin Immunol. 1977; 59:136.

81. Vincent NJ et al: Factors influencing pulmonary resistance. J Appl Physiol. 1970; 29:236.

82. Gold WM et al: Role of vagus nerves in experimental asthma in allergic dogs. J Appl Physiol. 1972; 33:719.

83. Pierson WE et al: A double-blind trial of corticosteroid therapy in status asthmaticus. Pediatrics. 1974; 54:282.

84. Ellul-Micalef R et al: Effect of intravenous prednisolone in asthmatics with diminished adrenergic responsiveness. Lancet. 1975; 2:1269.

85. Arnaud A et al: Treatment of acute asthma. Effect of intravenous corticosteroids and beta$_2$-adrenergic agonists. Lung. 1979; 156:43.

86. Loren ML et al: Corticosteroids in the treatment of acute exacerbations of asthma. Ann Allergy. 1980; 45:67.

87. Harfi H et al: Treatment of status asthmaticus in children with high doses and conventional doses of methylprednisolone. Pediatrics. 1978; 61:829.

88. Collins JV et al: Intravenous corticosteroids in treatment of acute bronchial asthma. Lancet. 1970; 2:1047.

89. Ahrens R et al: The clinical pharmacology of drugs used in the treatment of asthma. In Pediatric Pharmacology, edited by S Yaffe, New York, NY, 1981; Chapter 15:p 268.

90. Weinberger M et al: Relationship of formulation and dosing interval to fluctuation of serum theophylline concentration in children with chronic asthma. J Pediatr. 1981; 99:145.

91. Streck W et al: Pituitary adrenal recovery following short-term suppression with corticosteroids. Am J Med. 1979; 66:910.

92. Wood DW et al: Intravenous isoproterenol in the management of respiratory failure in childhood status asthmaticus. J Allergy Clin Immunol. 1972; 50:75.

93. Klaustermeyer WB et al: Intravenous isoproterenol: Rationale for bronchial asthma. J Allergy Clin Immunol. 1975; 55:325.

94. Thiringer G et al: Comparison of infused and inhaled terbutaline in patients with asthma. Scand J Respir Dis. 1976; 57:17.

95. Williams SJ et al: Comparison of inhaled and intravenous terbutaline in acute severe asthma. Thorax. 1981; 36:629.

96. May CS et al: Intravenous infusion of salbutamol in the treatment of asthma. Br J Clin Pharmacol. 1975; 2:503.

97. Bloomfield P et al: Comparison of salbutamol given intravenously and by intermittent positive-pressure breathing in life-threatening asthma. Br Med J. 1979; 1:848.

98. Hambleton G et al: Comparison of IV salbutamol with IV aminophylline in the treatment of severe acute asthma in childhood. Arch Dis Child. 1979; 54:391.

99. Weinberger M et al: Clinical pharmacology of drugs used for asthma. Ped Clin N Amer. 1981; 28:47.

100. Foreman JC et al: Cromoglycolate and other antiallergic drugs: A possible mechanism of action. Br Med J. 1976; 1:820.

101. Ziment I: Cromolyn sodium. In Respiratory Pharmacology and Therapeutics, 1st ed., WB Saunders Company, Philadelphia, 1978.

102. Kennedy MCS et al: Oral sympathomimetic amines in treatment of asthma. Br Med J. 1963; 2:1506.

103. Chervinsky P et al: Metaproterenol tablets: Their duration of effect by comparison with ephedrine. Curr Ther Res. 1975; 17:507.

104. Geumei A et al: Evaluation of a new oral B$_2$ adrenoreceptor stimulant bronchodilator, terbutaline. Pharmacol. 1975; 13:201.

105. Tashkin DP et al: Double blind comparison of acute bronchial and cardiovascular effects of oral terbutaline and ephedrine. Chest. 1975; 68:155.

106. Weinberger MM et al: Evaluation of oral bronchodilator therapy in asthmatic children. J Pediatr. 1974; 84:421.

107. Bernstein LI et al: Therapy with cromolyn sodium. Ann Intern Med. 1978; 89:228.

108. Hansten PD: Erythromycin and theophylline. Drug Interactions Newsletter. 1981; 1:5.

109. Hansten PD: Cimetidine interactions. Drug Interactions Newsletter. 1981; 1:43.

110. Hendeles L et al: Theophylline. In *Applied Pharmacokinetics: Principles of Therapeutic Drug Monitoring*, edited by WE Evans, JJ Schentag, WJ Jusko, Applied Therapeutics, Inc., 1980, San Francisco.

111. Rosen JP et al: Theophylline pharmacokinetics in the young infant. Pediatrics. 1979; 64:248.

112. Simons FER et al: Pharmacokinetics in infancy. J Clin Pharmacol. 1978; 18:472.

113. Svedmyr N et al: Drugs in the treatment of asthma. Pharm Ther. 1978; 3:397.

114. Shim C et al: Bronchial response to oral versus aerosol metaproterenol in asthma. Ann Intern Med. 1980; 93:428.

115. Dulfano MJ et al: The bronchodilator effects of terbutaline: Route of administration and patterns of response. Ann Allergy. 1976; 37:357.

116. Choo-Kang YFJ et al: Controlled comparison of the bronchodilator effects of three B-adrenergic stimulant drugs administered by inhalation to patient with asthma. Br Med J. 1969; 2:287.

117. Murray AB et al: The effects of pressurized isoproterenol and salbutamol in asthmatic children. Pediatrics. 1974; 54:746.

118. Anon: Albuterol. Med Lett Drugs Ther. 1981; 23:81.

119. Roberts RJ et al: A comparison of various types of patient instruction in the proper administration of metered inhalers. Drug Intell Clin Pharm. 1982; 16:53.

120. Cope CA et al: Counseling patients with chronic obstructive lung disease in the use of bronchodilator aerosols. Drug Intell Clin Pharm. 1982; 16:65.

121. Epstein SW et al: Survey of the clinical use of pressurized aerosol inhalers. Canadian Med J. 1979; 120:813.

122. Orehek J et al: Patient error in use of bronchodilator metered aerosols. Br Med J. 1976; 1:76.

123. Paterson IC et al: Use of pressurized aerosols by asthmatic patients. Br Med J. 1976; 1:76.

124. Harper TB et al: Techniques of administration of metered-dose aerosolized drugs in asthmatic children. Am J Dis Child. 1981; 135:218.

125. Davies DS: Pharmacokinetics of inhaled substances. Postgrad Med J. 1975; 51(Suppl 7):69.

126. Newman SP et al: Deposition of pressurized aerosols in the human respiratory tract. Thorax. 1981; 36:52.

127. Connolly CK: Method of using pressurized aerosols. Br Med J. 1975; 5:21.

128. Moren F: Drug deposition of pressurized inhalation aerosols I. Influence of actuator tube design. Int J Pharm. 1978; 1:205.

129. Bloomfield P et al: A tube spacer to improve inhalation of drugs from pressurized aerosols. Br Med J. 1979; 2:1479.

130. Gomm SA et al: Effect of an extension tube on the bronchodilator efficacy of terbutaline delivered from a metered dose inhaler. Thorax. 1980; 35:552.

131. Ellul-Micalef R et al: Use of a special inhaler attachment in asthmatic children. Thorax. 1980; 35:620.

132. Powell JR et al: The influence of cigarette smoking and sex on theophylline disposition. Am Rev Resp Dis. 1977; 116:17.

133. Newman SP et al: Simple instructions for using pressurized aerosol bronchodilators. J Royal Soc Med. 1980; 73:776.

134. Riley DJ et al: Enhanced responses to aerosolized bronchodilator therapy in asthma using respiratory maneuvers. Chest. 1979; 76:501.

135. Newhouse MT et al: Deposition and fate of aerosolized drugs. Chest. 1978; 73:936.

136. Ginchansky E et al: Relationship of theophylline clearance to oral dosage in children with chronic asthma. J Pediatr. 1977; 91:655.

137. Macfarlane JT et al: Irregularities in the use of regular aerosol inhalers. Thorax. 1980; 35:477.

138. Zwillich C et al: Theophylline-induced seizure in adults. Ann Intern Med. 1975; 82:784.

139. Jacobs M et al: Clinical experience with theophylline. Relationship between dosage, serum conc., and toxicity. JAMA. 1976; 235:1983.

140. Hendeles L et al: Frequent toxicity from IV aminophylline infusions in critically ill patients. Drug Intell Clin Pharm. 1977; 11:12.

141. Stinek C et al: Inhibition of theophylline absorption by activated charcoal. J Pediatr. 1979; 2:314.

142. Weinberger M et al: Role of dialysis in the management and prevention of theophylline toxicity. Dev Pharmacol Ther. 1980; 1:26.

143. Ehler S et al: Massive theophylline overdose, rapid elimination by charcoal hemoperfusion. JAMA. 1978; 240:474.

144. Lawyer C et al: Treatment of theophylline neurotoxicity with resin hemoperfusion. Ann Intern Med. 1978; 88:516.

145. Russo ME: Management of theophylline intoxication with charcoal-column hemoperfusion. N Engl J Med. 1979; 300:24.

146. Nielsen-Kudsk F et al: Pharmacokinetics of theophylline in ten elderly patients. Acta Pharmacol Toxicol. 1978; 42:226.

147. Vicuna N et al: Impaired theophylline clearance in patient with cor pulmonale. Br J Clin Pharmacol. 1979; 7:33.

148. Mangione A et al: Pharmacokinetics of theophylline in hepatic disease. Chest. 1978; 73:616.

149. Spitzer SA et al: Beclomethasone dipropionate and chronic asthma. Chest. 1976; 70:38.

150. Klein R et al: Treatment of chronic childhood asthma with beclomethasone dipropionate aerosol: I. A double-blind crossover trial in nonsteroid-dependent patients. Pediatrics. 1977; 60:7.

151. Toogood JH et al: A graded dose assessment of the efficacy of beclomethasone dipropionate aerosol for severe chronic asthma. J Allergy Clin Immunol. 1977; 59:298.

152. Webb DR: Beclomethasone in steroid-dependent asthma; effective therapy and recovery of hypothalamo-pituitary-adrenal function. JAMA. 1977; 238:1508.

153. Godfrey S et al: A three and five year follow up of the use of the aerosol steroid, beclomethasone dipropionate, in childhood asthma. J Allergy Clin Immunol. 1978; 62:335.

154. McCoy RJ et al: Beclomethasone dipropionate in twice daily treatment of asthma. Aust Fam Physician. 1980; 9:721.

155. Williams MH Jr: Beclomethasone dipropionate. Ann Intern Med. 1981; 95:464.

156. Wyatt R et al: Effects of inhaled beclomethasone dipropionate and alternate-day prednisone on pituitary-adrenal function in children with chronic asthma. N Engl J Med. 1978; 299:1387.

157. Fischer RG et al: Beclomethasone dipropionate aerosol: patient consultation recommendations. Drug Intell Clin Pharm. 1979; 13:767.

158. Jenne J et al: Decreased theophylline half-life in cigarette smokers. Life Sci. 1975; 17:195.

159. Landay RA et al: Effect of phenobarbital on theophylline disposition. J Allergy Clin Immunol. 1978; 62:27.

160. Pingleton WW et al: Oropharyngeal candidiasis in patients treated with triamcinolone acetonide aerosol. J Allergy Clin Immunol. 1977; 4:254.

161. Kappas A et al: Influence of dietary protein and carbohydrate on antipyrine and theophylline metabolism in man. Clin Pharmacol Ther. 1976; 20:643.

162. Kappas A et al: Effect of charcoal-broiled beef on antipyrine and theophylline metabolism. Clin Pharmacol Ther. 1978; 23:445.

163. Anderson JR et al: Effects of hemodialysis on theophylline kinetics. J Allergy Clin Immunol. 1982; 69:137 (Supplement—January).

164. Chervinsky P et al: Incidence of oral candidiasis during therapy with triamcinolone acetonide aerosol. Ann Allergy. 1979; 43:80.

165. Slavin RG et al: Multicenter study of flunisolide aerosol in adult patients with steroid-dependent asthma. J Allergy Clin Immunol. 1980; 66:379.

166. Vlasses P et al: Adrenocortical function after chronic inhalation of fluocortinbutyl and beclomethasone dipropionate. Clin Pharmacol Ther. 1981; 29:643.

167. Hyde JS et al: Short- and long-term prophylaxis with cromolyn sodium in chronic asthma. Chest. 1973; 63:875.

168. Berman BA et al: Cromolyn sodium in the treatment of children with severe perennial asthma. Pediatrics. 1975; 55:621.

169. Crisp J et al: Cromolyn sodium therapy for chronic perennial asthma. JAMA. 1974; 229:787.

170. Smith JM et al: Clinical trial of disodium cromoglycate in treatment of asthma in children. Br Med J. 1968; 2:340.

171. Friday GA et al: Cromolyn therapy for severe asthma in children. J Pediatr. 1973; 83:299.

172. Mascia AV et al: Clinical experience with long term cromolyn sodium administration in 53 asthmatic children. Ann Allergy. 1976; 37:1.

173. Gaddie J et al: The effect of disodium cromoglycate on pulmonary function in asthma. Br J Dis Chest. 1972; 66:254.

174. Bernstein IL et al: A controlled study of cromolyn sodium sponsored by the Drug Committee of the American Academy of Allergy. J Allergy Clin Immunol. 1972; 50:235.

175. Marshall R: Protective effect of disodium cromoglycate on rat peritoneal mast cells. Thorax. 1972; 27:38.

176. Orr TSC et al: Disodium cromoglycate, an inhibitor of mast cell degranulation and histamine release induced by phospholipase A. Nature. 1969; 233:197.

177. Orr TSC et al: The effect of disodium cromoglycate on the release of histamine and degranulation of rat mast cells induced by compound 48/80. Life Sci. 1971; 10:805.

178. Breslin ABX et al: Effect of sodium cromoglycate on asthmatic reactions to environmental temperature changes. Clin Allergy. 1975; 5:325.

179. Clarke PS: Effect of disodium cromoglycate on exacerbations produced by hyperventilation. Br Med J. 1971; 1:317.

180. Godfrey S et al: Inhibition of exercise-induced asthma by different pharmacological pathways. Thorax. 1976; 31:137.

181. Smith JM et al: Observations on the safety of disodium cromoglycate in long-term use in children. Clin Allergy. 1972; 2:143.

182. Silverman M et al: Use of serial exercise tests to assess the efficacy and duration of action of drugs for asthma. Thorax. 1973; 28:574.

183. Silverman M et al: Time course of effect of disodium cromoglycate on exercise-induced asthma. Arch Dis Child. 1972; 47:419.

184. Berman BA et al: Cromolyn sodium in the treatment of children with severe perennial asthma. Pediatrics. 1975; 55:621.

185. Chai H et al: Steroid sparing effects of disodium cromoglycate (DSC) in children with severe chronic asthma. Proceedings of the VII International Congress of Allergology. Excerpta Med. 1970; 232:385.

186. Hiller EJ et al: Betamethasone-17-valerate aerosol and disodium cromoglycate in severe childhood asthma. Br J Dis Chest. 1975; 69:103.

187. Sheffer AL et al: Immunologic components of hypersensitivity reactions to cromolyn sodium. N Engl J Med. 1975; 293:1220.

188. Settipane GA et al: Adverse reactions to cromolyn. JAMA. 1979; 241:811.

189. Hiller EJ et al: Nebulized sodium cromoglycate in young asthmatic children. Arch Dis Child. 1977; 52:875.

190. Burr ML et al: Peak expiratory flow rates before and after exercise in school children. Arch Dis Child. 1974; 49:923.

191. Haynes RL et al: An assessment of the pulmonary response to exercise in asthma and an analysis of the factors influencing it. Am Rev Respir Dis. 1976; 114:739.

192. Eggleston PA et al: A standardized method of evaluating exercise induced asthma. J Allergy Clin Immunol. 1976; 58:414.

193. Godfrey S: Exercise-induced asthma. Allergy. 1978; 33:229.

194. Edmunds AT et al: The refractory period after exercise induced asthma: its duration and relation to the severity of exercise. Am Rev Respir Dis. 1978; 117:247.

195. Bakran I et al: Aminophylline vs salbutamol in exercise induced asthma. Int J Clin Pharmacol Ther Tox. 1980; 18:442.

196. Anderson SD et al: Inhaled and oral bronchodilator therapy in exercise induced asthma. Aust NZ J Med. 1975; 5:544.

197. Morse JLC et al: The effects of terbutaline in exercise induced asthma. Am Rev Respir Dis. 1976; 113:89.

198. Francis PWJ et al: Oral and inhaled salbutamol in the prevention of exercise induced bronchospasm. Pediatrics. 1980; 66:103.

199. Pollock et al: Relationship of serum theophylline concentration to inhibition of exercise induced bronchospasm and comparison with cromolyn. Pediatrics. 1977; 60:840.

200. Sadeghi-Nejad A et al: Adrenal function, growth, and insulin in patients treated with corticoids on alternate days. Pediatrics. 1969; 43:277.

Chapter 18

Upper Gastrointestinal Diseases

Donald M. Moran, William A. Watson, and John Russo, Jr.

Gastric and duodenal ulcer, or peptic ulcer disease (PUD), Zollinger-Ellison syndrome (ZE), and gastroesophageal reflux disease (GRD) are upper gastrointestinal disorders sharing a common abnormality: too much acid and pepsin activity for the degree of local tissue resistance. Hydrolytic and proteolytic digestion of the exposed mucosa occur followed by inflammation, necrosis, and ulceration. Gastric hypersecretion appears to be the primary causative event at one end of the disease spectrum. This is supported by the finding that 93% of patients afflicted with ZE develop peptic ulcer disease (1). At the opposite end of the spectrum, acid secretion plays a lesser role and mucosal resistance becomes more important. Gastric ulcer, for example, is a disease typified by a reduced basal and stimulated acid output. Some acid is required, however, since PUD rarely develops in patients with achlorhydria. Therapy for these disorders is directed at correction of the apparent imbalance between acid and pepsin activity and mucosal resistance. Success of therapy is measured in terms of symptom control, ulcer healing and the prevention of complications secondary to the disease or its treatment. (2)

PEPTIC ULCER DISEASE

Although all ulcerating lesions of the gastroduodenal area have traditionally been labelled as peptic ulcers, these lesions differ in anatomical location, etiology, clinical presentation and genetic relationships.

Peptic ulcer disease (PUD) is characteristic to man and occurs in 10%–15% of the population. Prior to 1900, gastric ulcers occurred more commonly than duodenal ulcers and both were more common in women. Today, both trends have reversed throughout the world except in Japan where gastric ulcer is still more common. Gastric ulcers are two to three and a half times more prevalent in males, and males have up to ten times more duodenal ulcers than females. The incidence of gastric ulcers seems to increase with age. Ulcers occur most commonly between the ages of 20 and 50 years.

Pathophysiology. The traditional acid-peptic theory remains valid for the *duodenal ulcer*. Patients with these ulcers have higher "average" outputs of hydrochloric acid than do ulcer-free persons. The word average is important since nearly half of the persons with duodenal ulcer have normal acid secretion. While some persons with duodenal ulcers may secrete more acid, their ulcers will heal spontaneously with little or no therapeutic intervention, and this healing is not accompanied by a decrease in gastric acid output. Several theories have been proposed to explain the complex interrelationship between acid secretion and duodenal ulcer. For example, the person with duodenal ulcer may have an abnormally high "vagal tone"; excessive humoral (gastrin) stimulation of acid; impaired inhibition of gastric secretion; or a greater capacity to secrete acid. Unfortunately, all of these theories evolve entirely around acid secretion, and it is important to realize that peptic activity may have an equally important role in duodenal ulcer pathogenesis.

Although some patients with *gastric ulcer* are hypersecretors of acid, most secrete either normal or less than normal amounts. Therefore, it is probably reasonable to focus more attention on mucosal resistance than on acid and pepsin in this type of ulcer. Gastric ulcer may result from poor gastric emptying which leads to stasis of the gastric contents. This is followed by gastritis which lowers mucosal resistance to minimal amounts of acid and pepsin. The gastric mucosa has the capacity to prevent the penetration of normal concentrations of acid; however, when acid concentrations are increased, the mucosal barrier is broken and hydrogen ions penetrate the stomach wall resulting in mucosal damage. Pyloric sphincter dysfunction may also contribute to the pathogenesis of gastric ulcers by allowing reflux of duodenal contents into the stomach. The resultant bile, bile salts, and urea reaching the stomach will cause a break in the gastric mucosa even at low concentrations of acid, permitting the back-diffusion of hydrogen ions. The acid damage to mucosa and acid-pepsin lead to ulceration. However, this sequence of events is only theoretical, and the true cause of gastric ulcer remains to be established.

Clinical Presentation. Clinically, ulcer patients complain of recurrent episodes of abdominal pain over a period of several years. The pain may be nonspecific but is usually described as a gnawing or burning in the epigastric region, reaching maximum intensity just prior to meals. The pain is readily relieved by food, antacid, or vomiting. Although the pain may awaken the patient from his sleep, it is unusual to experience pain on awakening in the morning. About 10%

of persons with PUD will present with complications: hematemesis, GI bleeding, perforation, or obstruction. Peptic ulcer is a chronic disease, and is characterized by remission and exacerbation of symptoms over 20–30 years.

Management of PUD

1. *Comparison of Cimetidine and Antacids.* A.G., a 39-year-old woman, is hospitalized following a two-day history of postprandial vomiting and the passage of loose, tarry stools. She was in her normal state of health until two months ago when she first noticed the onset of intermittent, burning epigastric pain. The pain was localized to just below the xiphoid process, did not radiate, and was readily relieved by the administration of antacid. Her present medications include warfarin 5 mg po daily for recurrent deep venous thrombosis and multiple antacid preparations as needed for epigastric pain. The antacids have become progressively less effective for relief of this complaint. She smokes one pack per day. An upper GI series demonstrated a duodenal ulcer.

In the hospital she is treated with IV fluids; cimetidine (Tagamet), 300 mg q6h IV; and an aluminum-magnesium (Al/Mg) hydroxide antacid, 30 ml as needed for stomach pain. An upper GI series reveals the presence of an ulcer crater in the duodenum. Once stabilized, A.G. is discharged on cimetidine, 300 mg qid and antacids as needed for eight weeks and is advised to avoid any foods which she associates with ulcer pain. Why was cimetidine used as the primary therapeutic agent in this patient? Is cimetidine more effective than antacids?

Cimetidine reduces gastric acidity by blocking histamine at H_2 receptors on parietal cells in the stomach. Parietal cells mediate gastric acid secretion, and during cimetidine therapy both nocturnal and basal acid secretion are reduced (146). Cimetidine was selected as the primary agent for the treatment of A.G.'s peptic ulcer disease because she had a history of unsatisfactory results with antacid therapy. However, it is questionable whether A.G. had an adequate trial of antacid therapy in view of the fact that she was taking these agents on an "as needed" basis. The dose and form (liquid vs tablet) of antacid she was tak-

ing are also unknown. Cimetidine should not be viewed as a more potent therapeutic agent but as an alternative to antacids. A review of the literature indicates that both modes of therapy are associated with ulcer healing.

Studies conducted outside the United States show that cimetidine is superior to placebo in the promotion of duodenal ulcer healing (9–12). After 4–6 weeks of therapy, healing was demonstrated in approximately 85% of the cimetidine-treated patients; this compared to a healing rate of approximately 35% in the placebo groups. An American study also demonstrated an improved rate of healing in cimetidine-treated patients as compared to a control group, but the differences were not statistically significant at six weeks (13). This study did not demonstrate that cimetidine was ineffective; however, it did demonstrate a high rate of healing with placebo therapy. In this study, placebo was defined as 15 ml of an Al/Mg hydroxide preparation taken as needed for the relief of ulcer pain. Aluminum hydroxide was substituted if diarrhea occurred. Only antacid tablets were permitted in the other studies. The suspension formulation, considered superior to the tablets because of its greater surface area and ease of mixing with gastric contents, may have been responsible for the apparent efficacy of this "placebo."

Although studied less extensively, similar healing rates are reported in gastric ulcer patients treated with cimetidine or antacid. Table 1 summarizes Freston's (14) findings that antacid intake in gastric ulcer patients can heal ulcers as well as cimetidine if taken in sufficient amounts. Studies designed to assess cimetidine's efficacy have changed many long-held beliefs with regard to the role of antacids in PUD therapy. As late as 1976 they were recommended only to decrease gastric acidity and alleviate symptoms (15).

It is clear from the findings of the studies cited that much remains to be resolved regarding the pathophysiology and treatment of peptic ulcer disease. For example, one study of duodenal ulcer patients showed endoscopically proven healing rates in untreated populations which were comparable to those seen in cimetidine-treated patients (16). Another demonstrated that antacid tablets, which have been assumed to be inferior to liquid antacid preparations, were as effective as antacid suspensions administered by the same regimen (17).

Table 1.

DIFFERENCES BETWEEN ANTACIDS
ADMINISTERED IN VARYING DOSAGES
AND CIMETIDINE IN THE HEALING OF
GASTRIC ULCERS (14)

Mean Antacids Consumed (mEq/day)	Difference in % of Healed Ulcers
4	30
14	32
279	19
345	-2

2. *Life Style and Diet.* Will a change in A.G.'s life-style or diet enhance healing of her peptic ulcer?

Numerous empiric recommendations are made to patients with PUD. For example, many patients are encouraged to avoid stress; however, prevention or relief of stress has not been proven to enhance ulcer healing. Further, it is not known whether stress plays a role in the development of new ulcers or brings attention to existing ulcers. Major life style changes have not been proven to decrease the likelihood of recurrent ulcers or their complications. Similarly, sedatives, tranquilizers or mood elevating drugs are not indicated in the management of PUD and should be administered only if another co-existing condition requires them (18). A.G.'s smoking will inhibit duodenal ulcer healing and should be discouraged (17,19).

The cornerstone of PUD therapy has been dietary restriction, but specific recommendations vary greatly and lack scientific support. There is no evidence that a bland diet will enhance healing or prevent recurrence. The prophylactic restriction of spices, acid fruit juices or "rough" foods is of no proven value (20,21). If this patient feels that particular foods are causing discomfort, they should be avoided. Arbitrary and rigid restriction of foods or other substances will only serve as a source of frustration and distract her from complying with other aspects of therapy.

3. *Monitoring Parameters.* Is pain relief a reliable monitoring parameter for assessing ulcer healing?

Symptom control is an unreliable parameter to use to determine the presence of PUD or to assess whether or not an ulcer has healed (22). The immediate clinical response to therapy is usually good and symptomatic improvement occurs following a variety of therapeutic regimens including diet, rest, antacids, psychotherapy, reassurance or a change in environment (19–21). Table 2 shows the results of one study which compared antacid and placebo therapy. Freedom from ulcer pain was a poor predictor of ulcer healing, and a healed ulcer did not ensure symptomatic relief. Despite this, symptom control is one goal of therapy and it is important even in the absence of objective evidence of healing. Therefore, antacids, anticholinergic agents, diet or any other form of treatment which provides subjective pain relief should be used as needed to relieve pain unless they are contraindicated for other reasons. However, because symptomatic relief correlates poorly with healing, all patients who become asymptomatic should be counseled to finish their course of therapy.

4. Should endoscopy be utilized as a routine monitoring parameter to assess the success of A.G.'s ulcer treatment?

Endoscopy of the gastrointestinal (GI) tract is an uncomfortable procedure but is safe and indicated for all patients with *gastric* ulcers. It should be accompanied by a biopsy and brush cytology to rule out malignancy. A.G. has a duodenal ulcer, which is generally responsive to therapy and is not commonly associated with malignancy. Therefore, routine endoscopy is unnecessary unless A.G. continues to experience symptoms similar to those which led to her hospitalization.

Table 2.

EVALUATION OF PEPTIC ULCER SYMPTOMS
AS A PREDICTOR OF HEALING DURING
DUODENAL ULCER THERAPY (19)

	Aluminum/ Magnesium Antacid 30 ml 7 Times Daily	Inert Placebo Prn
Endoscopic Healing at 4 weeks	78%	45%
Asymptomatic at 4 weeks	69%	63%

Endoscopy is also useful when a discrepancy exists between symptoms and other diagnostic tests, or for patients with a history of frequent recurrent peptic ulcer disease. In the latter group, it is useful to confirm healing before maintenance therapy is initiated.

Cimetidine

5. *Dosing.* Is cimetidine 300 mg qid for eight weeks an appropriate course of therapy for A.G.? When should she take her medication?

Initial PUD therapy has been conducted with doses ranging from 0.8 to 1.6 gm per day. In the United States, 300 mg four times daily is commonly used. In most other countries, 200 mg three times daily and 400 mg at bedtime is prescribed. Both regimens are arbitrary and equally effective. The initial course of therapy lasts six to eight weeks (27).

The bioavailability of oral tablets ranges from 60 to 70% (28). While no difference in bioavailability is noted when a 200 mg dose is given with a meal or during fasting (29), decreased bioavailability occurs when cimetidine is given with antacids. However, this doesn't influence the period of time that plasma concentrations are above the suggested therapeutic levels and is not a clinically significant interaction (30). Cimetidine should be taken during or just after meals, to permit optimal acid inhibition in the interdigestive period (31). This utilizes the combined buffering activity of the food, antacids, and cimetidine.

6. *Long-Term Therapy.* Will further drug treatment be necessary after A.G. completes an eight-week course of therapy?

Cimetidine heals ulcers but does not cure PUD. Once discontinued, 60–80% of patients experience a recurrence in six months (22–24). However, early case reports of rapid and severe recurrence following the discontinuation of cimetidine do not appear to reflect the normal course of events (22,25). Predictors of recurrence have been difficult to define. Ulcer recurrence is not affected by the duration of therapy, and further studies are needed to confirm a reported inverse correlation with the daily dose of cimetidine and a direct correlation with the duration of illness (22,24).

Low-dose maintenance therapy with cimetidine (400 mg hs or 400 mg bid plus antacids taken as needed for pain) lowers the recurrence rate to between 15 and 30%. The expense and potential risk of toxicity with chronic therapy precludes routine cimetidine maintenance for all ulcer patients. Currently, it should be reserved for those patients who have a history of frequent recurrences following endoscopically confirmed healing (26). A.G. does not fit this criterion.

7. *Oral Anticoagulant Interaction.* Will A.G.'s anticoagulant therapy be affected by cimetidine therapy?

Cimetidine potentiates the effects of anticoagulants by decreasing the rate of drug metabolism (32,33). Soft-tissue and urinary tract bleeding occurred in a patient previously stabilized on warfarin seven days after cimetidine therapy was initiated. This patient's prothrombin time (PT) rose from 27 to 83 seconds; the control value was 11 seconds (32). This has been confirmed in studies of other patients stabilized on anticoagulants including phenindione and nicoumalone. Cimetidine therapy increased the PT a mean of 12.6 seconds (range 5 to 23.4). In normal subjects, cimetidine causes a reversible but significant increase in PT and plasma warfarin concentrations (33). A.G. should be carefully monitored in the first two weeks of cimetidine therapy. The dose of anticoagulant will probably need to be decreased.

8. *Other Interactions.* Does cimetidine affect the metabolism of other drugs?

Cimetidine decreases the hepatic metabolism of many other drugs including diazepam (34), chlordiazepoxide (35), antipyrine (36), phenytoin (208), theophylline (208) and others. This effect can be observed after 30 hours of pretreatment (34). It is not presently understood whether cimetidine or one of its metabolites is responsible (34), but cimetidine may competitively bind to some portion of the cytochrome P-450 system (37). Cimetidine does not appear to interfere with glucuronidation (38). Cimetidine reduces the clearance of propranolol through competitive inhibition of hepatic microsomal enzymes and the reduction of hepatic blood flow. This effect may enhance propranolol-induced bradycardia (39). Cimetidine drug interactions have recently been reviewed (208).

9. *Side Effects.* What side effects may occur during cimetidine administration?

Cimetidine-associated *gynecomastia* and *gal-*

actorrhea have been reported with an overall incidence of less than 1.4 cases per 100,000 patients (40–43). These effects most commonly occur after more than four months of cimetidine use (40,42), are unrelated to elevated cimetidine levels (40), and are usually not bothersome enough to require discontinuation of the drug (41). Both gynecomastia and galactorrhea are readily reversible following discontinuation of cimetidine therapy. The mechanism by which cimetidine induces these effects is uncertain, but it may be related to serum prolactin levels which are elevated in patients with galactorrhea (42) and 15–60 minutes after an IV dose of cimetidine (44). However, patients on chronic cimetidine therapy do not demonstrate an elevation in serum prolactin concentrations (40–42,45). The weak antiandrogenic effects of cimetidine currently offer the best explanation for the development of gynecomastia and galactorrhea (46).

Cimetidine also suppresses spermatogenesis and increases plasma testosterone concentrations (47, 48). Impotence has also been reported (49).

Although cimetidine has no detectable effect on serum immunoreactive parathyroid hormone (iPTH) in euparathyroid patients (50–52), in patients with primary hyperparathyroidism (51), and hyperparathyroidism secondary to chronic renal failure (52), serum iPTH levels are decreased. However, serum ionized calcium, phosphorous or magnesium concentrations are unaffected. The mechanism is unknown, but it has been suggested to be a direct, dose-related effect on the parathyroid gland, which is slowly reversible upon discontinuation of cimetidine (52). Other cimetidine side effects are discussed in Questions 10 & 11.

10. Five weeks after initiation of cimetidine therapy A.G.'s son returns from the Peace Corps. He has a positive intradermal skin test for tuberculosis. A.G. requests an intradermal TB test. Can cimetidine therapy affect the results of her TB test?

Six weeks of cimetidine therapy have been associated with an augmented, delayed hypersensitivity response to intradermal antigen skin testing (53,54). This effect is likely to be related to the H_2 histamine antagonizing effect of cimetidine, since it appears that H_2 receptors are found on some lymphocytes and these may modulate the inflammatory reaction (53,55). A.G. should wait until cimetidine therapy is completed before undergoing skin testing.

11. How significant are the renal, dermatologic, gastrointestinal and other side effects reported during cimetidine administration?

With its widespread use, it is not surprising that a large number of complications have been associated with cimetidine, including cholestatic jaundice in children (56), a hypersensitivity-type hepatitis (57), drug fever (58), Stevens-Johnson syndrome (59), exfoliative dermatitis (60), severe diarrhea (61), erosive gastritis (62), and interstitial nephritis (63). Many of these reports require further evaluation before a cause-effect relationship can be established.

Cimetidine's effect on creatinine clearance has been specifically evaluated. The slight decrease in creatinine clearance is probably secondary to competition between cimetidine and creatinine for renal tubular secretion and has little clinical significance (64).

The development of H_2-receptor antagonists has also led to identification of H_2-receptors in most organ systems (65), thus accounting for the wide variety of reported side effects, including mental status changes, attributed to cimetidine. McGuigan's comprehensive review provides further discussion of the adverse effects of cimetidine (66). Cimetidine-induced mental status changes are discussed further in the chapter on Acute Stress Erosions.

Antacids

Schwartz's dictum, "no acid—no ulcer," has provided the longstanding basis for antacid therapy in PUD. Raising the intragastric pH from 1.0 to 3.5 eliminates 99% of the hydrogen ion in gastric juice and inhibits the proteolytic activity of secreted pepsin, hence attenuating two factors known to overwhelm gastric mucosal resistance (67–69). The usefulness of antacids in achieving this end, however, has in the past been controversial (70).

Although elevation of the gastric pH to 3.5 is a reasonable if arbitrary goal, maintaining the pH at this level throughout the day is difficult (71). Early studies which examined the effect of antacids on gastric pH were conducted in fasting subjects or in subjects receiving concurrent milk feedings. These situations are not representative of the actual clinical population and the findings cannot be extrapolated to all PUD patients (72–76). Acid neutralization was shown to be of short duration (20–40 minutes), and this was attributed to rapid gastric emptying of the antacid or enhanced acid secretion.

Investigators have since described standard methods for assessing antacid potency *in vitro* which correlate well with *in vivo* activity (77,78). Utilizing these techniques, the acid neutralizing capacity of some antacids has been shown to vary 30-fold (79,80) prompting the recommendation that antacids be dosed on the basis of milliequivalents of neutralizing capacity rather than as a specific number of tablets or an arbitrary volume. For instance, a 5-fold reduction in gastric acidity for two hours in a duodenal ulcer patient would require more than 150 mEq of antacid in most patients (78). As Table 3 indicates, this amount var-

Table 3.

COMPARISON OF ALUMINUM-MAGNESIUM
HYDROXIDE CONTAINING ANTACIDS

	Dose to Neutralize 152 mEq Acid (ml)	Sodium Content (mEq) of Ulcer Regimen*
Delcid	18	12.1
Maalox Therapeutic Concentrate	27	2.1
Mylanta II	30	2.5
Gelusil II	32	2.9
Simeco	35	14.7–29.4
Aludrox	54	3.6
Maalox	56	8.5
Maalox Plus	56	8.5
Mylanta	61	2.5
Gelusil	66	3.2
Riopan	69	<2.9
Riopan Plus	72	<9.7
Kolantyl	72	9.7

*Based on neutralizing dose given seven times daily.
Adapted from Dutro MP et al: N Engl J Med. 1980; 302:967.

ies from 18–72 ml depending on the antacid selected.

Fordtran and Collyns (81) found that 4 gm of calcium carbonate given one hour after a meal reduced gastric acidity to 38% of the control value for four hours. Doubling the dose increased both the degree and duration of neutralization. A dose of 15 ml of Al/Mg gel had comparable effects. Deering and Malagelada (82) measured the amount of acid delivered to the duodenum after a meal in ulcer patients given cimetidine or Al/Mg hydroxide gel. Cimetidine reduced the four-hour postprandial delivery of titratable acid and hydrogen ion by 63% and 86% respectively. Al/Mg hydroxide, 30 ml given one and three hours after a meal, lowered the titratable acidity and hydrogen ion concentration by 47% and 74% respectively. The fall in acid delivered to the duodenum was concluded to be comparable for both regimens, although more fluctuation would be expected with the antacid. Therefore, antacids reduce gastric acidity if taken in sufficient amounts. Complete around-the-clock neutralization of all intragastric acid, however, resulting in a pH of 7 is not achieved, nor is this necessary to achieve healing of the ulcer.

12. *Antacid Selection and Dosing.* K.R., a 54-year-old male with a chief complaint of epigastric pain, is found by endoscopy to have a duodenal ulcer. A decision is made to treat him with antacids. Which antacid should be used? What dose should he be given? How often? What should the duration of therapy be?

Duodenal ulcer patients such as K.R. require large amounts of antacid to achieve adequate buffering. Effective doses are approximately 150 mEq of neutralizing capacity, which can be achieved with approximately two tablespoonfuls of the more concentrated aluminum-magnesium hydroxide antacids such as Delcid, Maalox Therapeutic Concentrate, Gelusil II and Mylanta II (see Tables 3 & 4) (78). The aluminum-magnesium hydroxide antacids are the most commonly used products because the aluminum hydroxide, which is constipating, balances the diarrheal effects of the magnesium hydroxide. The selection of the specific antacid should be based upon the patient's taste preference and cost.

Two tablespoonfuls of antacid should be ingested one and three hours after meals and at bedtime for a period of six weeks. This regimen is based upon the results of studies using similar antacid regimens. With this regimen, healing rates were greater in antacid-treated patients than placebo-treated patients (19) and similar to patients treated with cimetidine 800 mg/day and 1200 mg/day (83). A duration of six to eight weeks is based upon the finding that 50% of duodenal ulcers heal completely in six weeks.

To promote compliance away from home, it may be necessary to recommend that patients carry a chewable tablet preparation with them. The cost of therapy with tablet antacids is generally comparable to that with liquid antacids, although a very large number of tablets must be consumed to reach the targeted neutralizing capacity (84). Table 4 shows that between 9 and 32 Al/Mg tablets would have to be taken as a single dose, depending on the product, to adequately buffer intragastric acid.

13. *Antacid-Induced Diarrhea and Constipation.* **Two days after K.R. begins his antacid regimen, he complains of severe diarrhea (six stools in one night). Could this be secondary to his antacid? What can be done? What other gastrointestinal problems should be anticipated in association with antacid therapy?**

Although aluminum-magnesium hydroxide antacids are formulated to minimize diarrhea secondary to the magnesium salt or constipation secondary to the aluminum salt, individual patients commonly experience gastrointestinal side effects. Diarrhea seems to occur more commonly and is a troublesome side effect which may discourage compliance and pose a risk for fluid and electrolyte imbalances (85). In these instances aluminum hydroxide, a less potent antacid, is incorporated into the antacid regimen to counteract the laxative effect of magnesium hydroxide, a potent neutralizing substance. To regulate bowel function, Morrissey and Barreras (67) recommend that four to eight doses per day of the Al/Mg preparation be supplemented with four to eight doses of a non-magnesium preparation such as aluminum hydroxide gel. The patient can be given the option of alternating the intake of the magnesium or non-magnesium product as needed to control diarrhea or constipation. Diphenoxylate (Lomotil) or other antidiarrheals are unnecessary.

Patients taking aluminum hydroxide antacids alone or in excessive amounts relative to their Al/Mg hydroxide antacids can develop constipation. K.R. should be instructed to seek medical attention if constipation develops and persists in the face of abdominal pain, distention, vomiting or fever. High doses of antacids in liquid or tablet form can lead to intestinal obstruction (86,87). Hemodialysis and renal transplant patients, in particular, appear to be at high risk for fecal impaction while using aluminum hydroxide preparations (88). Calcium-containing antacids have long been suspected of possessing a constipating action as well, but this has never been supported with objective evidence (89).

Table 4.

NEUTRALIZING CAPACITY OF
AL/MG TABLET ANTACIDS

Antacid	Acid Neutralizing (mEq/Tablet) Capacity	Number of Tablets Containing 150 mEq
Camalox	16.7	9
Mylanta II	11.0	14
Riopan Plus	10.0	15
Gelusil II	8.2	19
Maalox Plus	5.7	27
Digel	4.7	32

Adapted from Drake D et al: Ann Intern Med. 1981; 94:215.

14. *Electrolyte Content of Antacids.* **J.R. is a 48-year-old male with essential hypertension who has been counseled regularly about the importance of compliance with his diuretic prescription and low-calorie, low-salt diet; however, his weight and blood pressure continue to rise. Last month he began taking two tablets of Alka-Seltzer Antacid after meals for relief of a "sour stomach." Two days ago, his stomach pain worsened and relief can now be obtained only if he induces vomiting of his meals. He looks pale and sullen and complains of feeling dizzy. Is the electrolyte content of this preparation or alternative antacids of clinical concern?**

Alka-Seltzer Antacid contains 1 gm sodium bicarbonate and 0.3 gm potassium bicarbonate per effervescent tablet. Although this is a potent, fast-acting antacid preparation, probably best suited for relief of occasional episodes of heartburn, chronic use should be discouraged (67). Two grams of sodium bicarbonate contain 24 mEq sodium and 24 mEq bicarbonate; both are readily absorbed and predispose patients to metabolic complications (67). Daily absorption of 21 mEq of sodium, existing as a contaminant in one antacid preparation, led to fluid retention in patients with cirrhosis and labile congestive heart failure (90). Additionally, a link between salt intake and hypertension probably exists (91). Increasing the sodium intake from 9 mEq to 240 mEq daily in a small group of salt-sensitive hypertensive patients led to an 18% increase in mean arterial blood pressure, along with weight gain (92). To imply that antacid therapy will surely predispose to a hemodynamic imbalance, however, is misleading. Table 3 demonstrates that many currently formulated Al/Mg hydroxide antacids are remarkably low in sodium content and should not contribute significantly to a patient's daily sodium intake. The dangers of sodium loading secondary to antacid use today are probably overstated for most patients.

Excess bicarbonate ion which is absorbed after ingestion of two to four teaspoonfuls of sodium bicarbonate is normally compensated for by an increased renal excretion of bicarbonate (93). At larger doses, or in patients with renal insufficiency, the excretory capacity for bicarbonate can be exceeded, in which case serious metabolic alkalosis follows. The daily intake of sodium bicarbonate should not exceed 200 mEq in patients under 60 years of age or 100 mEq in patients over 60 years of age (94).

Since J.R. has reported the onset of epigastric pain relieved by vomiting, medical evaluation is strongly recommended. His symptoms suggest something more than just indigestion, perhaps gastric outlet obstruction (95). With vomiting, hydrogen and chloride are lost and this can result in a metabolic alkalosis (95). The additional exogenous administration of bicarbonate in the form of Alka-Seltzer Antacid could precipitate a dangerous degree of alkalosis; its use should therefore be strongly discouraged.

15. *Milk-Alkali Syndrome.* D.J. is a 30-year-old female who presents to the Emergency Room complaining of nausea, vomiting, lethargy, and diarrhea of three days duration.

Blood chemistries reveal the following: calcium 12.5 mg/dl (9.0–11.0 mg/dl), phosphorus 4.8 mg/dl (3.0–4.5 mg/dl), carbon dioxide content 35 mEq/L (24–30 mEq/L), potassium 2.8 mEq/L (3.8–5.2 mEq/L), BUN 30 mg/dl (7–18 mg/dl), and creatinine 2.0 mg/dl (0.7–1.2 mg/dl). The patient admits to having taken four tablets of Titralac (420 mg CaCo₃/tablet) every day for the past three days to relieve her "queasy" stomach. The intern who examines her suspects the milk-alkali syndrome caused by antacid use as her most likely diagnosis. What is the milk-alkali syndrome?

The term *milk-alkali syndrome* describes the metabolic complications and symptoms which arise from a high calcium intake combined with any factor which produces an alkalosis (96,97). Although rarely seen by gastroenterologists today, the syndrome was previously described in ulcer patients for whom a milk and alkali regimen had been prescribed (around-the-clock administration of sodium bicarbonate, calcium carbonate, magnesium carbonate, and bismuth oxycarbonate). In the early, reversible stages, patients complain of anorexia, nausea, and weakness (98,99). Additionally, they may demonstrate hypercalcemia, hyperphosphatemia, azotemia, and alkalosis. Progression of the syndrome into its chronic and irreversible stage is characterized by florid renal failure and metastatic calcification of soft tissues (98,100). D.J.'s symptoms and laboratory values are consistent with early milk-alkali syndrome.

The syndrome was first believed to be a complication in 1% of 3,000 ulcer patients (101) given 2 to 4 gm of calcium carbonate hourly, but systematic studies performed later demonstrated it can occur in up to 25% of patients receiving 30–40 gm of the antacid daily (102,103). Clinical features of hypercalcemia or alkalosis usually developed within three days of therapy, and creatinine clearance values fell an average of 19% from control values 3, 5, and 7 days after treatment. The patients in one study (103) were also receiving an anticholinergic drug, but the role it may have played in affecting calcium absorption or the patient's symptomatic complaints was not delineated.

It is unlikely that the daily ingestion of four tablets of Titralac could have precipitated milk-alkali syndrome in D.J. Although 16% of an orally administered dose of calcium carbonate is systemically absorbed, the hypercalcemia which results from the single ingestion of 1 to 12 gm of the antacid is only transient, lasting several hours (104). In fact, 20 gm of calcium carbonate has been administered daily for 18–30 days to normal individuals without apparent adverse effects (105). The increased absorption of calcium was accompanied by a compensatory rise in urinary calcium excretion. The propriety of prescribing doses on the order of 20 to 40 gm daily, however, must be questioned. The relationship between hypercalciuria and renal calculi (106), as well as the relationship between hypercalciuria and calcium carbonate ingestion implies that excess ingestion of calcium could lead to calcium nephropathy (103,107). Silica calculi have been documented in the renal tract of some antacid users (108,109). If an organic basis exists for antacid therapy in this patient, a non-calcium preparation should be recommended. Her current presentation, however, will require further work-up. A thorough drug history should be elicited to help rule out vitamin D intoxication or inappropriate diuretic use. It should also be remembered that hyperparathyroidism, sarcoidosis, or malignant tumor could similarly explain D.J.'s clinical findings.

16. *Acid Rebound.* What is the role of calcium carbonate in PUD treatment? Does it produce acid rebound?

Calcium carbonate is a potent and rapid acting antacid. Two grams readily brings 100 ml of 0.1 N hydrochloric acid to a pH above 6, and four grams given one hour after eating will reduce gastric acidity to 38% of the control value four hours after the meal (67,81). Enthusiasm over calcium carbonate's use has waned, however, because electrolyte and renal disturbances are associated with its use and its clinical efficacy in healing peptic ulcers has been questioned.

One controlled study suggests that intensive calcium carbonate therapy delays pain relief and peptic ulcer healing (110); another (111) found two-hourly calcium carbonate dosing to be more effective than placebo in healing gastric ulcer, but not duodenal ulcer. This discrepancy in response (gastric vs duodenal) might be explained by the association between calcium carbonate use and gastric hypersecretion or acid rebound (112,113). Calcium carbonate is the only antacid shown to produce this effect in humans (114–117). Eight grams of calcium carbonate induced gastric hypersecretion for up to 5.5 hours after ingestion in 24 chronic duodenal ulcer patients (114). This effect was not reproduced with the administration

of 30–60 ml of Al/Mg hydroxide or 4–8 gm of sodium bicarbonate. In another study, Barreras (115) gave four equivalent neutralizing doses of calcium carbonate, sodium bicarbonate and magnesium hydroxide hourly to 20 fasting duodenal ulcer patients. The average rate of acid secretion observed in association with calcium carbonate was double that found in the basal state or with other antacids. The mechanism for this phenomenon is not clear. It occurs in fasting and nonfasting subjects and is seen with all calcium salts (89). Hypercalcemia may be one mechanism by which increased acid secretion occurs, but the concentration of serum calcium correlates poorly with acid output (118,120). Gastrin stimulation has been postulated as another mechanism, and studies have demonstrated that a small but statistically significant rise in serum gastrin following the administration of 0.5 to 2.0 gm of calcium carbonate parallels a stimulated acid secretion in fasting subjects both with and without duodenal ulcer (120,121). This response was not duplicated with the administration of intravenous calcium gluconate, although instillation of calcium carbonate into the small intestine will provoke acid hypersecretion (118,121). Contact between calcium and the antrum is not an apparent requirement for acid stimulation to occur. Under clinical conditions, the effect of hypersecretion on gastric acidity is initiated by the buffering capacity of the antacid remaining in the stomach, or by a second meal or dose of antacid (85). Vigorous calcium carbonate therapy, therefore, probably results in sustained but buffered gastric hypersecretion. Whether this affects the natural history of the disease by expanding the parietal cell mass or enhancing nocturnal gastric acidity remains to be clarified (85).

In light of the discrepancies about its clinical efficacy, the phenomenon of acid rebound, and the potential toxicity of this drug, the use of calcium carbonate is not recommended for the treatment of peptic ulcer disease.

17. *Antacid-Digoxin Interaction.* A.L. is a 65-year-old arthritic man with worsening congestive heart failure. His medications include aspirin 3.9 gm daily, furosemide (Lasix) 20 mg every morning, and Mylanta II 30 ml prn stomach upset. The patient will be started on digoxin. Will antacids affect the bioavailability of this drug?

The pharmacokinetics of digoxin are altered by

concurrent administration of antacids, but correlation with an alteration in therapeutic effect is not established. Binnion (118) reported that the 8-hour serum area under the curve measured for digoxin was decreased in three subjects given Al/Mg antacid (Maalox) compared to eight control subjects. Statistical analysis and measurement of urinary excretion were not performed. Brown and Juhl (119) found that 60 ml of aluminum hydroxide, magnesium hydroxide, and magnesium trisilicate gels given with 0.75 mg of digoxin acutely lowered the area under the curve by 9 to 13% in 10 normal subjects. Measurement of the effect on steady-state concentrations was not performed. The mechanism for this interference is unclear and cannot be entirely related to physical adsorption or alterations in gut transit time. Until the significance of this interaction is known, proper spacing of the dosages should be advised when antacids and digitalis glycosides are taken concurrently.

18. *Other Antacid-Drug Interactions.* Are there other antacid-drug interactions which should be anticipated in A.L.? What other drugs interact with antacids?

Antacids affect the absorption, dissolution, adsorption, chelation, ionization, gastric emptying, and urinary excretion of many drugs (120). In the context of A.L., the arthritic patient, data exist to show that concomitant administration of Al/Mg hydroxide with *aspirin* can cause a significant reduction in serum salicylate concentration, whereas the converse (discontinuation of antacid administration) can gradually increase serum salicylate to a potentially toxic concentration (121–123). The mechanism is attributable to an antacid-induced increase in urinary pH which consequently increases the renal elimination of salicylate (124,125). Additional evidence demonstrates that antacids can accelerate the rate of aspirin's absorption from the stomach (120,121). If salicylates and antacids are to be given concurrently for chronic arthritic therapy, dosage adjustment should be based on regular monitoring of the serum concentration and therapeutic response. (Also see the chapter entitled Rheumatic Diseases.)

Two other interactions of known clinical significance do exist. The *tetracyclines* are poorly absorbed when given with antacids due to chelation of polyvalent cations by the antibiotic (120,126). An earlier report (127) that a high intragastric pH also retards the absorption of tetracycline has recently been refuted (128,129), thus vindicating cimetidine as one therapeutic alternative when acid reduction and tetracycline therapy must occur concomitantly. Staggering the administration of antibiotic and antacid by several hours is another alternative.

Cardiac arrythmia, elevated serum quinidine levels, and prolongation of intraventricular conduction have been reported following administration of absorbable and nonabsorbable antacids to patients stabilized on *quinidine* (130,131). As quinidine is a weak base which undergoes some renal elimination, alkalinization of the urine could enhance tubular reabsorption of the drug and its pharmacologic effect. Monitoring of serum quinidine levels is recommended when regular administration of antacids is begun.

Antacid Formulation Additives

19. *Simethicone.* After a lunch of corned beef, cabbage and draft beer, P.U. returns to work feeling "bloated." His secretary gives him a tablet of Mylicon (simethicone 40 mg) to chew for relief. What is simethicone? Is it likely to be effective in this situation?

Simethicone is a chemically inert gastric defoaming agent (132). It lowers surface tension, causing small gas bubbles to coalesce into a form that can be more easily eliminated through belching or passing flatus (133). Simethicone has been reported to be valuable in reducing the incidence of postoperative ileus (134,135) and in treating excessive intestinal gas and bloating (136). One placebo-controlled trial demonstrated 50 mg of simethicone to be effective in relieving the symptoms of functional upper gastrointestinal disorders (137). Data collected from another group imply that 40 to 80 mg of the drug administered orally prior to endoscopy is a simple way of insuring adequate visualization of the GI mucosa during endoscopic examination (138). Conversely, Souranta et al (139) state that it does not reduce the amount of gas in the gastrointestinal tract as viewed by abdominal radiography and, therefore, is not a useful adjunct in preparing the patient for radiologic exam. They explain the discrepancy between clinical relief of symptoms and radiologic findings as perhaps attributable to simethicone's ability to accelerate the transit of intestinal gas without affecting total volume.

Since simethicone has no acid-neutralizing capabilities (131,136), its incorporation into many antacid products is peripheral to the management of peptic ulcer. The manufacturers state that simethicone is added for relief of gas-related complaints, although statistics on the incidence of such symptoms in patients with peptic ulcer disease are not available. In the case of P.U., the occasional use of simethicone is probably safe, inexpensive, and possibly beneficial. Future dietary discretion, however, should be reinforced as an alternative to the use of over-the-counter drug products.

20. *Oxethazaine*. D.B. is a 42-year-old male who was discharged from the hospital following a diagnosis of benign gastric ulcer. The patient needs an antacid for relief of epigastric pain, but his insurance does not reimburse him for over-the-counter medications. To circumvent this problem, Oxaine M (Al/Mg hydroxide and oxethazaine) 5 ml po 15 minutes before meals and at bedtime is prescribed. What is oxethazaine?

Oxethazaine is a local anesthetic which resembles lidocaine but is chemically stable in an acid pH (140). It is incorporated into an antacid mixture to manage pain due to peptic ulcer, esophagitis, and gastritis. Early clinical studies seemed to uphold the product's marketing claims that oxethazaine and aluminum hydroxide in combination were more effective than aluminum hydroxide alone in the relief of pain and in providing acid neutralization to duodenal ulcer, but the number of patients involved was small and the methodology employed was not entirely objective (141,142). Oxethazaine was believed to inhibit the antral release of gastrin through a local action on mucosal nerve tracts (143,144), thereby reducing gastric secretion. This hypothesis has since been refuted by immunoreactive gastrin studies performed in 30 normal and PUD patients (145). The combination of oxethazaine and aluminum hydroxide did not hinder gastrin release in either the basal or food-stimulated state, possibly because oxethazaine was adsorbed and inactivated by the antacid. The pharmacologic effect of this product, if any, is probably due to the acid neutralizing capacity of the antacid alone.

Anticholinergic Drugs

21. *Indications*. D.M. is a 65-year-old male accountant whose chief complaint is inter-

mittent, gnawing epigastric pain which is relieved by food. The pain awakens him frequently at approximately 1:00–2:00 a.m. and he obtains relief with baking soda. This pain has been occurring off and on for the past six years. However, during the past two months the pain has become intense and frequent. He is currently taking L-dopa (Dopar) for Parkinson's Disease. An upper GI series is performed and shows a duodenal ulcer. He is treated with cimetidine 300 mg and 15 mg propantheline (Probanthine) hs.

What is the role of anticholinergic drugs in the treatment of PUD? Will the addition of such an agent to cimetidine lead to greater suppression of gastric acid secretion?

There is insufficient evidence to support the use of anticholinergic drugs as first-line agents in the treatment of PUD. Competitive antagonism of acetylcholine by anticholinergic drugs reduces acid secretion by 25–30% (146). In contrast, both nocturnal and basal acid secretion are reduced by 90–95% for 5–7 hours following a 300 mg dose of cimetidine, and meal-stimulated acid secretion is inhibited by about 70% for more than three hours (146).

The use of anticholinergic agents has been complicated by the long-held notion that they must be administered at near-toxic doses to adequately suppress gastric acid secretion (147–148). This is unnecessary. A single 15 mg dose of propantheline is equivalent to the optimal effective dose (averaging 48 mg) in suppressing gastric acid secretion for three hours after administration to duodenal ulcer patients (149).

Anticholinergics should be used as adjuncts to antacid and cimetidine therapy. Their ability to control the circadian pattern of gastric acid secretion should be utilized in patients with persistent nocturnal pain (150,151). Anisotropine methylbromide (Valpin) 80 mg administered at 8:00 p.m. suppresses nighttime gastric acid secretion and symptoms without significant side effects (152).

Propantheline tablets 15 mg have additive suppressive effects on acid secretion when combined with cimetidine. This combination may be of value in patients resistant to cimetidine alone (149).

22. *Anticholinergic Interactions*. D.M. is taking L-dopa for Parkinson's Disease. Will his propantheline therapy affect his re-

sponse to L-dopa? How do anticholinergic drugs affect the disposition of other drugs?

Although the stomach is not an important site of absorption for most drugs, including L-dopa, the rate of gastric emptying can alter drug absorption from the small intestine. Clinically significant interactions can occur between anticholinergic agents and other drugs, but their significance depends on the dose, the particular anticholinergic drug administered, and the effect that delayed gastric emptying has on the drug in question. For example, concurrent administration with drugs exhibiting anticholinergic properties of their own, such as tricyclic antidepressants, is likely to accentuate those properties. Delayed gastric emptying can reduce the bioavailability of drugs like *L-dopa* and *penicillin G,* which are degraded during prolonged contact with stomach acid. *Phenothiazine* bioavailability is also reduced due to delayed gastric emptying and possibly increased intestinal metabolism. *Acetaminophen* (Tylenol) exhibits delayed absorption but equal bioavailability when administered with high doses of propantheline. Other drugs show indirect evidence of increased bioavailability during anticholinergic therapy. There is increased urinary tract recovery of nitrofurantoin (Macrodantin) and more frequent extrapyramidal reactions associated with methotrimeprazine (Levoprome) use (153,154). Drug interactions with anticholinergics should be approached with an understanding of their adjunctive role in PUD therapy.

23. *Side Effects.* **What is the risk of precipitating an attack of narrow-angle glaucoma following the administration of an anticholinergic agent to D.M.? Are there situations in which anticholinergic agents are contraindicated? What side effects should be expected with their use?**

Acute attacks of narrow-angle glaucoma occur when the pupil dilates and outflow of aqueous fluid is obstructed. Blurred vision, halos and pain progressing to blindness may occur, requiring rapid medical and possibly surgical treatment (155).

The topical administration of anticholinergic agents in a heterogenous North American population, not screened for glaucoma, may induce an attack in 1 per 4,000 persons over 30 years of age and in 1 per 100 persons more than 40 years old. The systemic administration of atropine may produce an attack, but since the quantity of drug reaching the eye is less, the intensity of its action

would also be less. Anisotropine methylbromide (Valpin), dicyclomine (Bentyl), or methixene HCl (Tremonil), have little or no effect on the pupil and, therefore, a minimal tendency to induce glaucoma (155).

Patients with a history of narrow-angle glaucoma should definitely not receive anticholinergic agents; those with open-angle glaucoma have a relative contraindication to the use of these agents. Since anticholinergic agents are primarily used for symptom control in patients with PUD and other effective agents are available for pain management, anticholinergic agents should be avoided in patients with glaucoma. If anticholinergic agents must be used, concurrent treatment with ocular pilocarine will maintain the intraocular pressure within normal limits (156,157).

Other conditions in which anticholinergic agents are contraindicated include reflux esophagitis due to increased gastroesophageal regurgitation, which is characterized by pain which may be confused with ischemic heart pain; pyloric stenosis, where delayed gastric emptying may accentuate symptoms of obstruction; and prostatic hypertrophy, since urinary retention may be a complication of anticholinergic drugs (158,159). Other side effects include dry mouth, blurred vision, impotence and increased heart rate.

Surgical Management

24. *Indications.* **A.J. has been purchasing a variety of antacid products weekly for more than six months. He complains of typical ulcer pain which has not changed during this time and has not noticed any blood loss or other signs of progressing disease. He believes he has an ulcer but is afraid to seek medical care because he fears surgery. Is he likely to need surgical treatment of his PUD?**

Surgical treatment is required in about 15% of all duodenal ulcer patients at some point in their disease. Indications include hemorrhage, perforation, obstruction, or PUD which is resistant to medical management (intractable ulcer) (160).

Various procedures are used, but all aim to cure PUD through a reduction in gastric acid secretion. Elective surgery provides satisfactory to excellent results in about 90% of cases. Indications for surgery in gastric ulcer patients are similar to those for PUD patients (160); in addition, surgery is indicated if the gastric ulcer is found to be malignant.

Based on his relatively mild, nonprogressive symptoms, A.J. would not be a candidate for surgery unless he had a malignant gastric ulcer. He should seek medical attention for diagnosis and therapeutic recommendations.

25. *Drug Therapy for Complications.* Unfortunately, A.J.'s PUD was complicated by worsening symptoms, obstruction, and perforation, which required partial gastrectomy. What drug therapy problems should be anticipated when monitoring him as a postgastrectomy patient?

Anemia. Half of the patients with a partial gastrectomy will become anemic after 20 years, although few will be symptomatic. Sixty percent of these will be iron deficient as a result of reduced intake, poor absorption, and occult blood loss. In 30%, vitamin B_{12} deficiency occurs due to reduction in the concentration of intrinsic factor in gastric juice. Total gastrectomy is associated with a complete loss of intrinsic factor. Folate deficiency is the least common cause of anemia and is unlikely to occur alone.

Monthly B_{12} injections are mandatory for patients who have undergone total gastrectomy and highly recommended in patients such as A.J. who have had a partial gastrectomy. The need for chronic iron and folate therapy is less well defined, but treatment may be deferred since long-term follow-up will be required in these patients (161).

Osteomalacia. Osteomalacia is a potential postgastrectomy complication due to vitamin D deficiency in patients who restrict their intake of fatty foods due to postprandial discomfort. Malabsorption is not a problem except in the presence of steatorrhea (162).

Diminished Drug Bioavailability. An association between gastrectomy and tuberculosis stimulated an evaluation of the bioavailability of antitubercular agents following this procedure (165). The absorption of p-aminosalicylic acid (P.A.S.), isoniazid (INH), and rifampin (Rifadin) are unaffected (153,164). Antrectomy with gastroduodenostomy does not affect ethambutol (Myambutol) absorption; however, if a selective vagotomy to control postgastrectomy syndromes is performed, there is a significant reduction in ethambutol bioavailability (165). Similar findings made with sulfisoxazole (Gantrisin) and quinidine point to the significant changes that

modifications from surgical procedures can have on drug bioavailability (165).

The use of bethanechol (Urecholine) to control delayed gastric emptying following gastrectomy has met limited success but early reports with metoclopromide (Reglan) are promising, and increased use of this drug in the future may affect drug bioavailability in these patients (166).

Drug and Disease-Induced Ulcers

26. J.G. is a 52-year-old patient taking at least eight aspirin tablets daily for rheumatoid arthritis over the past five years. He noted frequent burning and gnawing epigastric pain during the past two months. Endoscopy revealed small lesions in the prepyloric area. Could J.G.'s aspirin usage be the cause of his PUD? If so, how should his rheumatoid arthritis be treated? What other drugs are ulcerogenic?

Many drugs have been associated with the formation of erosions or ulceration of the esophagus, stomach, or small bowel; aspirin and potassium chloride tablets are most solidly implicated. Aspirin ingestion could be associated with J.G.'s ulcer. Utilization of enteric coated aspirin and treatment of the ulcer will probably lessen J.G.'s chance for a drug-related ulcer. Newer nonsteroidal antiinflammatory agents require further evaluation of their ulcerogenic potential (167–169). The reader is referred to the chapter entitled Rheumatic Diseases for a further discussion of the ulcerogenesis of nonsteroidal antiinflammatory agents. The ulcerogenicity of corticosteroids is poorly defined (170). Agents such as reserpine, coffee, and cigarettes are not associated with an increased frequency of peptic ulceration. Table 5 summarizes data concerning drug-induced erosion and ulceration.

27. What is the effect of underlying disease on the development of ulcers? What is the added effect of drug therapy for that disease?

Available data suggest that ulcers do not occur more frequently in patients with rheumatic diseases or Crohn's disease than in the general population (171). A recent study, however, concluded that patients receiving aspirin for their rheumatic disease were more likely to develop ulcers during their course of therapy. Gastric ulcers were

Table 5.

EFFECTS OF DRUGS ON THE
GASTROINTESTINAL TRACT

Agent	PUD	Erosion/ Gastritis
Corticosteroids	no	no
Aspirin	yes	yes
Indomethacin	no	yes
Phenylbutazone/ Oxyphenbutazone	no	yes
Ibuprofen	no	yes[a]
Naproxen	no	yes[a]
Sulindac	no	yes[a]
Cigarettes (nicotine)	no[b]	no
Coffee (caffeine)	no[b]	no[c]
Alcohol	no[b]	yes[d]
Reserpine	no	no
Potassium Chloride	no	yes

[a]May be a dose-response relationship (167,168).
[b]Association has been noted; no cause-effect relationship established (172).
[c]Not tested (171).
[d]Produces acute gastritis; controversy over whether it can produce chronic disease (173).

found in 17% of patients with presentations similar to J.G.'s; this compares to a 2% incidence of gastric ulcers in the general population. Also, the aspirin preparation used influenced the incidence of ulceration. Regular and buffered aspirin users had incidence of 23% and 31% respectively; this compared with a 6% incidence in users of enteric coated aspirin (169).

The prevalence of peptic ulceration varies in different chronic liver diseases. It is more common in hepatitis B-associated chronic liver disease, alcoholic liver disease and primary biliary cirrhosis and less common in hepatitis B antigen-negative chronic active hepatitis when compared to the general population. Corticosteroid therapy does not alter these findings (174).

New Drugs

28. What new drugs and therapeutic approaches may be used in the future medical treatment of PUD?

The role of conventional acid reducing therapy in managing PUD is being challenged by the development of a wide range of new drugs. Table 6 lists the various "new" remedies which have been used to treat peptic ulcer disease. These include antipepsins, antigastrins, drugs enhancing mucosal resistance and gastric motility, as well as agents affecting corticohypothalamic pathways. Their impact on the natural history of PUD, however, is still unclear, and carefully controlled studies of many of these agents are lacking.

Sucralfate. Under the broad category of cytoprotective compounds, sucralfate, a sulfated disaccharide which is structurally related to heparin but has no anticoagulant effects, has recently been made available for general use under the trade name Carafate. Once in solution it becomes a highly polar anion which preferentially adheres to the ulcer and protects it from further exposure to acid, pepsin and bile. Sucralfate also directly inhibits bile and pepsin activity and blocks back-diffusion of gastric acid and pepsin. (175)

Sucralfate, one gram administered one half hour before meals and at bedtime, is superior to placebo and comparable to cimetidine in healing gastric and duodenal ulcers after four to twelve weeks of therapy (176,177). The rate of ulcer recurrence one year after completion of an eight-week course is also comparable to that seen with cimetidine (176).

Probably because of its minimal absorption, adverse reactions have been minor (4.7%) and primarily related to gastrointestinal complaints. They include constipation (2.2%), diarrhea, nausea, gastric discomfort, dry mouth, rash, pruritus, back pain, dizziness, sleepiness and vertigo (175).

Antacids may be used as required for pain relief during sucralfate therapy. However, a certain level of acidity is required for its activation and neither antacids nor meals should be taken less than one-half hour before or sooner than one hour after administration. For this reason, it can not be assumed that combined cimetidine-sucralfate or high dose antacid-sucralfate therapeutic regimens will be superior to drug treatment with single agents.

Carbenoxolone. Other cytoprotective agents

have generated much interest. Carbenoxolone sodium, a derivative of licorice root, has potential value in the management of both gastric and duodenal ulcer (27). It lengthens the life-span of gastric epithelial cells; increases the production, secretion and viscosity of gastric mucus; and minimizes back diffusion of hydrogen ions in the presence of bile (140). Hypertension, edema and hypokalemia secondary to its mineralocorticoid side actions may limit its use in some patients.

Prostaglandins. Drugs with antisecretory and cytoprotective action include prostaglandins of the E and A type (178). In humans, PGE_2 given orally for two weeks to 10 patients with gastric ulcer was associated with greater healing than placebo (179). Experiments performed with 15-methyl PGE_2 and 16,16-dimethyl PGE_2 show the same trend in both gastric and duodenal ulcer (178). Additionally, prostaglandins may be useful in preventing gastrointestinal erosions caused by nonsteroidal antiinflammatory agents (179).

Bismuth Salts. The colloidal bismuth salts are classified as mucosal protectants (140). At an acidic pH, they chelate with protein and amino acids produced by necrotic ulcer tissue, thus insulating it from further peptic digestion (180). Impressive results have been obtained in the treatment of duodenal and gastric ulcers. Few side effects are reported.

H$_2$ Receptor Blockers. Agents aimed at altering the intragastric acid-pepsin balance include a new generation of H_2 receptor blockers which are more potent and have a longer duration of action than cimetidine. Ranitidine is a new histamine H_2-receptor antagonist which decreases gastric acidity by the same mechanism of action as cimetidine. It is well tolerated, with side effects largely confined to skin rash, headache, and dizziness. In the treatment of duodenal ulcer and benign gastric ulcer disease, ranitidine is as effective as cimetidine. Patients who are unresponsive to or intolerant of the high cimetidine doses often required to control Zollinger-Ellison syndrome have also been successfully treated with ranitidine. Hepatic drug metabolism does not appear to be influenced, and no clinically significant drug interactions have been reported. Its twice daily dosing schedule may be valuable in maintaining patient compliance, although this remains to be demonstrated.

Trimipramine, a tricyclic antidepressant, and **pirenzepine** are also antisecretory compounds,

although their mechanism of action is believed to be independent of cholinergic or histamine mediated pathways (181,182). Preliminary studies suggest that they are valuable in providing symptomatic relief from peptic ulcer, although objective data clearly defining their role does not exist.

Sulpiride. Sulpiride is another central nervous system acting drug with antidepressant and antisecretory properties. Classified as a hypothalamic neuroleptic, the drug is believed to inhibit the cephalic phase of acid and gastrin secretion as well as stimulate antral tone and increase gastric mucosal blood flow (17,27). Lam et al (17) investigated the efficacy of the drug in 101 duodenal ulcer patients and found the combination of antacid tablets and sulpiride to be more effective than placebo in healing ulcers. Sulpiride alone did not appear to be more efficacious than placebo. This contrasts the findings of two French

Table 6.

CLASSIFICATION OF NEWER DRUGS
FOR THE TREATMENT
OF PEPTIC ULCER DISEASE

Drugs Affecting Mucosal Resistance
Cytoprotectives
　　Carbenoxolone Sodium
　　Sucralfate
　　Geranyl Farnesylacetate
　　Methyl Prostaglandins
Ulcer Insulators
　　Colloidal Bismuth Salts

Drugs Affecting Acid-Pepsin Activity
Acid Inhibitors
　　H_2- Receptor Antagonists
　　　(e.g., Cimetidine, Ranitidine, Tiotidine)
　　Pirenzipine
　　Trimipramine
Antipepsins
　　Carageenin
　　Amylopectin
Antigastrins
　　Proglumide

Drugs Acting on Cortico Hypothalamic Pathways
　　Sulpiride

Drugs Affecting Gastric Emptying
　　Metoclopramide

Adapted from Marks IN: Drugs. 1980; 20:283.

groups who found sulpiride to be effective in the management of chronic peptic ulceration and prophylaxis of acute stress ulceration (140). Enthusiasm for the drug was, at one time, high because of its purported psychotropic properties. Sulpiride was believed to be particularly well suited for the treatment of peptic ulceration in which psychosomatic overtones were marked. Again, evidence to support this is absent.

ZOLLINGER-ELLISON SYNDROME

The Zollinger-Ellison Syndrome (ZE) is characterized by single or multiple non-beta islet cell adenomas of the pancreas which release large quantities of gastrin into the plasma. This results in a 10–20 fold increase in the amount of acid secreted and a high incidence of ulcers. Diagnosis is based on elevated serum gastrin levels and on an enormously elevated "basal" secretion of HCl that is minimally stimulated following the administration of histamine. (3) A patient with ZE usually presents with epigastric pain beginning 30 minutes to 3 hours after a meal. Unlike peptic ulcer disease, which is characterized by remissions and exacerbations, ZE patients experience pain that is likely to be more persistent, progressive and less responsive to food or antacids. Patients may also present with diarrhea secondary to the gastric hypersecretion and hypercalcemia related to concurrent hyperparathyroidism. Other comparisons between PUD and ZE are displayed in Table 7.

29. Cimetidine Treatment for ZE. B.G. is a 45-year-old man who presents with severe abdominal pain. About six months ago he noted the onset of intermittent epigastric burning pain relieved with food or antacids.

For the past six months the pain has become much more severe and the frequency of the pain has increased to the point of being almost continuous. In the past three months, the patient has noted the onset of loose, frequent stools (approximately 8–10 per day) and he has lost 25 lbs over the past six months. His stool is positive for occult blood. Basal acid secretion, the Histalog stimulation test, and serum gastrin levels are consistent with ZE. What is the role of cimetidine therapy in this patient's treatment? Will cimetidine eliminate the need for surgery?

The primary goal in the treatment of gastrin-producing islet cell tumors has been the complete control of hormonally-induced gastric hypersecretion or surgical removal of the tumor. Prior to the availability of cimetidine, total gastrectomy was the only sure method of controlling ulcer diathesis in a majority of patients and was considered a life-saving procedure. Recent postoperative follow-up studies dispute this and indicate that the most important factors affecting survival are the resectability and extent of the tumor, not the type of gastric operation performed. Cimetidine produces a "chemical gastrectomy" and, like the surgically-performed gastrectomy, is indicated for the prophylactic treatment of the clinical consequences of gastrinomas such as epigastric pain, ulcers, diarrhea, steatorrhea, gastrointestinal bleeding or perforation. Because cimetidine does not affect tumor growth, surgical resection of the tumor is still necessary (183,184). However, because these tumors may be multiple and small, complete resection may be impossible.

30. When should B.G. be started on cimetidine? What doses should be used?
Cimetidine usually provides immediate symp-

Table 7.

COMPARISON OF PUD AND ZE

Parameter	Duodenal Ulcer	Gastric Ulcer	Zollinger-Ellison Syndrome
Prevalence	10%	2.5%	uncommon
Average age of onset	4th decade	6th decade	20–50 years
Location	duodenal bulb (95%)	lesser curvature within 6 cm of the pylorus 60%	1st portion of duodenum 75%
Male:female	2:1	3:1–4:1	3:2

tomatic relief and should be started as soon as the diagnosis is confirmed by secretin challenge (183). Although as little as 800 mg daily has been used, it is reasonable to start B.G. on a dose of 300 mg four times daily and titrate the dose as necessary to control symptoms (185). Doses up to 600 mg qid have been required in some cases. Preoperative treatment will provide time for nutritional support and stabilization of the patient, making him a better operative risk. It will also provide time to complete endocrine studies and decide on the most appropriate surgical procedures; hyperparathyroidism is reported in 25% of these patients and other endocrine tumors have been found as well (183).

If B.G. has a total gastrectomy, cimetidine can be discontinued immediately postoperatively. Otherwise, it will be required for life or until a total gastrectomy is performed (183).

31. B.G. is to be discharged on cimetidine. What are the risks and benefits of this "chemical gastrectomy"?

The major benefits of cimetidine therapy are symptom control and avoidance of a total surgical gastrectomy with its attendant nutritional consequences (see Question 25). Probably more than 80% of such patients remain below ideal weight and many are severe nutritional cripples. The major reason for weight loss is reduced intake associated with postprandial distress known as the postgastrectomy or "dumping" syndrome (186).

Long-term cimetidine treatment is not without risks. In most patients, noncompliance is followed by a rapid return of symptoms (184). However, the ZE syndrome is cyclic and patients may stop taking their medication without apparent problems only to suffer complications such as gastrointestinal bleeding or gastric outlet obstruction during an exacerbation (183). A vagotomy can facilitate postoperative cimetidine therapy; however, as the disease progresses, higher and more frequent doses may be needed for symptom control. Eventually, cimetidine may become ineffective, forcing a total gastrectomy when the patient is a poorer surgical risk due to advanced age (183,185,187,188). Long-term side effects of cimetidine may force the patient into a similar situation.

32. Other Drugs for ZE. Are other drugs useful in the treatment of Zollinger-Ellison syndrome?

Antacid and anticholinergic agents have been unsuccessful when used alone to control symptoms. They may be combined with cimetidine if high doses of the latter fail to control symptoms satisfactorily. Anticholinergics would be contraindicated in B.G. because he has a partial gastric outlet obstruction and esophagitis. Evaluations of streptozotocin and chlorozotocin are now underway (193).

GASTROESOPHAGEAL REFLUX DISEASE

Gastroesophageal reflux disease (GRD) refers to a clinical syndrome produced by the reflux of gastric or duodenal contents into the esophagus (4). Heartburn, the most common clinical manifestation, typically appears after a meal and is frequently aggravated by physical strain, bending over, or the recumbent position (5). Regurgitation, dysphagia, and hemorrhage are other symptomatic complaints, but their expression may portend the presence of more severe anatomic involvement including esophagitis, esophageal stricture, esophageal ulceration, pulmonary fibrosis or infection. Patients most severely affected by the disease seem to have an impaired ability to clear the esophagus of refluxed fluid by swallowing (5).

GRD and *hiatus hernia* are not synonymous. At one time it was believed that herniation of the stomach into the mediastinum (hiatus hernia) predisposed or caused reflux, but correlation between symptoms and radiographic evidence of herniation has been poor (6,7). It is currently thought that reflux is primarily the result of a weakened lower esophageal sphincter, a muscular, high pressure zone located between the stomach and esophagus that serves as an anti-reflux barrier (8). Compromise of this sphincter by mechanical, hormonal, neural, or pharmacologic means may allow gastric contents to flow back into the esophagus.

33. Predisposing Factors. J.N. is a 20-year-old prima gravida female who is 30-weeks pregnant. She presents to the clinic with a two-week history of substernal burning which awakens her at night and leaves a sour taste in her mouth. A rim of caked antacid encircles her lips; she attributes this to the usage of Gaviscon tablets. She smokes 1½ packs of

low tar cigarettes daily and usually drinks a glass of wine before retiring at night. Her obstetrician examines her and concludes she is probably experiencing mild GRD. What are this patient's predisposing risk factors for reflux?

The tone of the lower esophageal sphincter is modulated by a number of excitatory and inhibitory control mechanisms. Nerve tracts, secreted hormones, and a host of pharmacologic agents including the xanthines, sympathomimetics, cholinergics, and dopaminergics have been shown to affect the sphincter's function (8). Progesterone, for example, causes a significant reduction in sphincter pressure, perhaps explaining why heartburn is a frequent complaint during pregnancy. Nicotine relaxes the sphincter and alcohol reduces both sphincter pressure and peristaltic contraction in the distal esophagus.

Eating or drinking prior to retiring at night additionally serve to fill the stomach with material that can then later be refluxed into the esophagus. Dietary indiscretion in the form of fatty foods also tends to decrease lower esophageal sphincter pressure and delay gastric emptying, both of which may worsen reflux disease. The increased intragastric and intra-abdominal pressure that occur secondary to weight gain may also serve to compromise the gastroesophageal sphincter gradient.

34. Treatment. What are the therapeutic approaches to the treatment of GRD? What would you recommend for J.N.?

Therapy for patients with gastroesophageal reflux is directed towards reduction of the reflux by physical methods, by strengthening the sphincter muscle pharmacologically, or by altering the quantity or character of the gastric content available for reflux (5). As a first step, dietary adjustments, including decreased fat ingestion, avoidance of nicotine and alcohol, and restriction of other specific foods that incite symptoms (eg, chocolate, citrus juices) may help to reduce the number of reflux episodes (190). Simple elevation of the head of the patient's bed at night is an often effective, though overlooked, way to protect the esophagus from nocturnal reflux. If these measures do not afford adequate relief, J.N. should receive a trial of antacids or alginate. For intermittent attacks, antacids are probably the safest and most convenient mode of treatment, al-

though their efficacy in severe esophagitis is dubious. A controlled trial performed in patients with GRD of at least two year's duration showed that 30 ml of an antacid given one hour after meals and at bedtime provided symptomatic relief in 17% of patients followed for three years or longer (191). The antacid was ineffective in patients with severe reflux symptoms, gross esophagitis at endoscopy, and severe sphincter incompetence. More recently, studies examining the efficacy of cimetidine in GRD have suggested that the H_2-blockers could supplement or even replace antacids in the treatment of reflux esophagitis (192–195). Subjects were given cimetidine 300 to 400 mg after meals and at bedtime or placebo for four to eight weeks. Cimetidine caused a significant decrease in symptom frequency and in esophageal acid sensitivity when tested with an acid infusion (194). Objective improvement of esophagitis as determined by esophagoscopy and histology, however, has not been demonstrated unequivocally. (Also see Question 36.)

As a last step in medical therapy, increasing lower esophageal sphincter pressure pharmacologically with the cholinergic drug, bethanechol or the dopamine antagonist, metoclopramide might offer an advantage not afforded by previously discussed measures. Thanik and colleagues (196) found that 25 mg of bethanechol given four times daily for four weeks with antacid therapy decreased the symptoms of esophagitis and resulted in more complete endoscopic healing of erosions and ulcerations than antacid therapy alone. Metoclopramide stimulates smooth muscle of the upper GI tract, thereby increasing lower esophageal sphincter tone and stimulating gastric emptying. One controlled study has found it effective in providing symptomatic relief from reflux, though endoscopic and histologic findings were not reported (197).

When medical therapy does not control the manifestations of reflux, then surgery should be considered. A number of anti-reflux procedures are available, each with their own proponents, but all are aimed at strengthening the integrity of the lower esophageal sphincter. One controlled clinical trial has shown that surgery is a particularly rational and effective form of management (191), offering significant relief to 73% of the patients studied.

In light of the abrupt onset of symptoms in this patient, measures aimed at curtailing consumption of cigarettes, wine, and fat-rich foods might prove beneficial until her child has been delivered.

35. What is Gaviscon?

Gaviscon is an antacid preparation containing alginic acid, sodium alginate, sodium bicarbonate, magnesium trisilicate and aluminum hydroxide. After the tablet is chewed, it forms a viscous foam that floats on top of the liquid surface within the stomach and acts as a barrier to reflux. The product has been shown to decrease the number of reflux episodes by a nongravitational mechanism independent of the lower esophageal sphincter, and it decreases the percentage of time during which the esophageal pH is in the acid range (198,199). Symptomatic relief of heartburn and regurgitation are also obtained with the drug's use (200–202), but until controlled studies are performed documenting that Gaviscon can uniformly prevent or help heal the chronic complications of gastroesophageal reflux, it should be viewed as a palliative therapeutic measure.

36. Should J.N. receive cimetidine during pregnancy or while she is breast feeding?

Cimetidine has not been found teratogenic in animal studies (203); however, no data exist in humans. Transient hepatic impairment was noted in a newborn whose mother received cimetidine 1.2 gm/daily for the last month prior to delivery (204). A higher incidence of clinically important jaundice was also noted in a trial of single-dose cimetidine prior to caesarean section, with jaundice occurring in 5 out of 20 infants whose mothers received cimetidine versus 2 of 20 in the control group (206). The potential for hepatic impairment due to maternal cimetidine therapy requires further evaluation.

Two studies of single-dose therapy before caesarean section have not resulted in effects on infant parameters which the authors could attribute to cimetidine. Cimetidine is detectable in umbilical cord blood, at a lower concentration than maternal venous blood, after a single dose (205, 206).

Presently, alternative therapy, such as antacids, should be utilized in the pregnant patient. In the patient who does receive cimetidine before delivery, the infant should be closely observed for signs of hepatic impairment.

Cimetidine does appear in breast milk, equilibrating slowly with plasma. After chronic dosing, milk cimetidine concentrations are much higher than plasma concentrations. Up to 6 mg of drug may be ingested by an infant consuming a liter of breast milk per day (207). Although this is a very small dose, breast feeding while on cimetidine is not advisable until more is understood about its pharmacologic effects on newborns.

References

1. Isenberg J et al: Pathogenesis of peptic ulcer. In *Gastrointestinal Disease*, 2nd ed, edited by MH Sleisinger and JS Fordtran, W.B. Saunders Co., Philadelphia, 1978, p 792.

2. Spiro HM: Moynihan's Disease? The diagnosis of duodenal ulcer. N Engl J Med. 1974; 291:567.

3. McGuigan JE: The Zollinger-Ellison syndrome. In *Gastrointestinal Disease*, 2nd ed, edited by MH Sleisinger and JS Fordtran, W.B. Saunders Co., Philadelphia, 1978, p 860.

4. Cohen S et al: The pathophysiology and treatment of gastroesophageal reflux disease. Arch Intern Med. 1978; 138:1398.

5. Pope CE: Gastroesophageal reflux disease. In *Gastrointestinal Disease*, 2nd ed, edited by MH Sleisinger and JS Fordtran, W.B. Saunders Co., Philadelphia, 1978, p 541.

6. Cohen S et al: Does hiatus hernia affect competence of the lower esophageal sphincter. N Eng J Med. 1971; 284:1053.

7. Stilson W et al: Hiatal hernia and gastroesophageal reflux. Radiology. 1969; 93:1323.

8. Fox S et al: Control of lower esophageal sphincter pressure and acid reflux. Clin Gastroenterol. 1979; 8:37.

9. Bank S et al: Histamine H_2-receptor antagonists in the treatment of duodenal ulcers. S Afr Med J. 1976; 50:1781.

10. Blackwood WS et al: Cimetidine in duodenal ulcer: Controlled trial. Lancet. 1976; 2:174.

11. Bodemar G et al: Cimetidine in the treatment of active duodenal and prepyloric ulcers. Lancet. 1976; 2:161.

12. Hetzel DJ et al: Cimetidine treatment of duodenal ulcer: Short term clinical trial and maintenance study. Gastroenterology. 1978; 74:389.

13. Binder HJ et al: Cimetidine in the treatment of duodenal ulcer: A multicenter double-blind study. Gastroenterology. 1978; 74:380.

14. Freston JW: Cimetidine in the treatment of gastric ulcer: Review and commentary. Gastroenterology. 1978; 74:426.

15. Grossman MI et al: A new look at peptic ulcer. Ann Intern Med. 1976; 84:57.

16. Collen MR et al: Cimetidine vs. placebo in duodenal ulcer therapy: a six-week, controlled, double-blind investigation without any antacid therapy. Dig Dis Sci. 1980; 25:744.

17. Lam SK et al: Treatment of duodenal ulcer with antacid and sulpiride: a double-blind controlled study. Gastroenterology. 1979; 76:315.

18. Ingelfinger FJ: Let the ulcer patient enjoy his food. In *Controversy in Internal Medicine,* edited by FJ Ingelfinger, AS Relman, and M Finland, W.B. Saunders Co., Philadelphia, 1966, p 171.

19. Peterson WL et al: Healing of duodenal ulcer with an antacid regimen. N Engl J Med. 1977; 297:341.

20. Sturdevant RAL et al: Duodenal ulcer. In *Gastrointestinal Disease,* 2nd ed, edited by MH Sleisinger and JS Fordtran, W.B. Saunders Co., Philadelphia, 1978, p 840.

21. Buchman E et al: Unrestricted diet in the treatment of duodenal ulcer. Gastroenterology. 1969; 56:1016.

22. Dronfield MW et al: Controlled trial of maintenance cimetidine treatment in healed duodenal ulcer: short and long term effects. Gut. 1979; 20:526.

23. Gray GR et al: Long term cimetidine in the management of severe duodenal ulcer dyspepsia. Gastroenterology. 1978; 74:397.

24. Bardham KD et al: Double-blind comparison of cimetidine and placebo in the maintenance of healing of chronic duodenal ulceration. Gut. 1979; 20:158.

25. Wallace WA et al: Perforation of chronic peptic ulcers after cimetidine. Br Med J. 1977; 2:865.

26. Ippoliti A et al: The pharmacology of peptic ulcer. Clin Gastroenterol. 1979; 8:53.

27. Marks IN: Current therapy in peptic ulcer. Drugs. 1980; 20:283.

28. Walkenstein SS et al: Bioavailability of cimetidine in man. Gastroenterology. 1978; 74:360.

29. Bodemar G et al: The absorption of cimetidine before and during maintenance treatment with cimetidine and the influence of a meal on the absorption of cimetidine—studies in patients with peptic ulcer disease. Br J Clin Pharmacol. 1979; 7:23.

30. Bodemar G et al: Diminished absorption of cimetidine caused by antacids. Lancet. 1979; 1:444.

31. Spence RW et al: Influence of a meal on the absorption of cimetidine. Digestion. 1976; 14:127.

32. Silver BA et al: Cimetidine potentiation of the hypoprothrombinemic effect of warfarin. Ann Intern Med. 1979; 90:348.

33. Serline MJ et al: Cimetidine: interaction with oral anticoagulants in man. Lancet. 1979; 2:317.

34. Klotz U et al: Delayed clearance of diazepam due to cimetidine. N Engl J Med. 1980; 302:1012.

35. Desmond PV et al: Cimetidine impairs elimination of chlordiazepoxide in man. Ann Intern Med. 1980; 93:266.

36. Puuronen J et al: Effect of cimetidine on microsomal drug metabolism in man. Eur J Clin Pharmacol. 1980; 18:185.

37. Rendic S et al: Interaction of cimetidine with liver microsomes. Xenobiotica. 1979; 9:555.

38. Klotz U et al: Effect of cimetidine on the clearance of benzodiazepines. N Engl J Med. 1980; 303:754.

39. Feely J et al: Reduction of liver blood flow and propranolol metabolism by cimetidine. N Engl J Med. 1981; 304:692.

40. Spence RW et al: Gynaecomastia associated with cimetidine. Gut. 1979; 20:154.

41. Delle Fase GF et al: Gynaecomastia with cimetidine. Lancet. 1977; 1:1319.

42. Bateson MC et al: Galactorrhea with cimetidine. Lancet. 1977; 2:247.

43. Davis TG et al: Evaluation of a worldwide spontaneous reporting system with cimetidine. JAMA. 1980; 243:1912.

44. Daubresse JC et al: Plasma-prolactin and cimetidine. Lancet. 1978; 1:99.

45. Spiegel AM et al: Serum-prolactin in patients receiving chronic oral cimetidine. Lancet. 1978; 1:881.

46. Winters SJ et al: Cimetidine is an antiandrogen in the rat. Gastroenterology. 1975; 76:504.

47. Van Thiel DH et al: Hypothalamic-pituitary-gonadal dysfunction in men using cimetidine. N Engl J Med. 1979; 300:1012.

48. White MC et al: Endocrine function after cimetidine. N Engl J Med. 1979; 301:502.

49. Wolfe M: Impotence on cimetidine therapy. N Engl J Med. 1979; 300:94.

50. Ljunghall S et al: Serum concentrations of parathyroid hormone in euparathyroid subjects during cimetidine therapy. N Engl J Med. 1980; 303:1178.

51. Palmer FJ et al: Cimetidine and hyperparathyroidism. N Engl J Med. 1980; 302:692.

52. Jacob AI et al: Reduction by cimetidine of serum parathyroid hormone levels in uremic patients. N Engl J Med. 1980; 302:671.

53. Avella J et al: Effect of histamine H_2-receptor antagonists on delayed hypersensitivity. Lancet. 1978; 1:624.

54. Jones FGC: Cimetidine and the delayed hypersensitivity response. Lancet. 1978; 1:80.

55. Plaut M et al: Modulation of inflammation by histamine receptor-bearing cells. In *Histamine Receptors,* edited by TO Yellin, SP Medical and Scientific Books, New York, 1979, p 351.

56. Lilly JR et al: Cimetidine cholestatic jaundice in children. J Surg Res. 1978; 24:384.

57. Lorenzini I et al: Cimetidine-induced hepatitis. Dig Dis Sci. 1981; 26:275.

58. McLoughlin JC et al: Cimetidine fever. Lancet. 1978; 1:499.

59. Ahmed AH et al: Stevens-Johnson syndrome during treatment with cimetidine. Lancet. 1978; 2:433.

60. Yontis PL et al: Cimetidine-induced exfoliative dermatitis. Dig Dis Sci. 1980; 25:73.

61. Field R et al: Diarrhea from cimetidine. N Engl J Med. 1978; 299:262.

62. Webster J et al: Erosive gastritis and duodenitis during continuous cimetidine treatment. Br Med J. 1978; 1:20.

63. Davis TG et al: Evaluation of a worldwide spontaneous reporting system with cimetidine. JAMA. 1980; 243:1912.

64. Dubb JW et al: Effect of cimetidine on renal function in normal man. Clin Pharmacol Ther. 1978; 24:76.

65. Yellin TO (editor): *Histamine Receptors,* SP Medical and Scientific Books, New York, 1979.

66. McGuigan JE: A consideration of the adverse effects of cimetidine. Gastroenterology. 1981; 80:181.

67. Morrissey JF et al: Antacid therapy. N Engl J Med. 1974; 290:550.

68. Piper DW et al: PH stability and activity curves of pepsin with special reference to their clinical importance. Gut. 1964; 5:506.

69. Goldberg HI et al: Role of acid and pepsin in acute experimental esophagitis. Gastroenterology. 1969; 56:228.

70. Morris T et al: Progress report. Antacids and peptic ulcer—a reappraisal. Gut. 1979; 20:538.

71. Littman A et al: Antacids and anticholinergic drugs. Ann Intern Med. 1975; 82:544.

72. Tomenius J et al: Continuously recorded pH of gastric and duodenal contents in situ with the evaluation of the efficacy of some antacids in vivo. Acta Med Scand. 1960; 166:25.

73. Grossman MI: Duration of action of antacids. Clin Res. 1960; 8:125.

74. Kirsner JB et al: Effects of various antacids on hydrogen-ion concentration of gastric contents. Am J Digest Dis. 1940; 7:85.

75. Kirsner JB: Further study of effect of various antacids on hydrogen-ion concentration of gastric contents. Am J Dig Dis. 1941; 8:53.

76. Price AV et al: Alkali requirement for continuous neutralization of gastric contents in gastric and duodenal ulcer. Clin Sci. 1956; 15:285.

77. Piper DW et al: An evaluation of antacids in vitro. Gut. 1964; 5:585.

78. Fordtran JS et al: In vivo and in vitro evaluation of liquid antacids. N Engl J Med. 1973; 288:923.

79. Jones B et al: Which antacid? An assessment of liquid antacids. Practitioner. 1977; 219:559.

80. Barry RE et al: Sodium content and neutralizing capacity of some commonly used antacids. Br Med J. 1978; 1:413.

81. Fordtran JS et al: Antacid pharmacology in duodenal ulcer. Effects of antacids on postcibal gastric acidity and peptic activity. N Engl J Med. 1966; 274:922.

82. Deering TB et al: Comparison of an H_2 receptor antagonist and a neutralizing antacid on postprandial acid delivery into the duodenum in patients with duodenal ulcer. Gastroenterology. 1977; 73:11.

83. Ippoliti AF et al: Cimetidine versus intensive antacid therapy for duodenal ulcer: a multicenter trial. Gastroenterology. 1978; 74:393.

84. Drake D et al: Neutralizing capacity and cost effectiveness of antacids. Ann Intern Med. 1981; 94:215.

85. Peterson WL et al: Reduction of gastric acidity. In Gastrointestinal Disease, 2nd ed, edited by MH Sleisinger and JS Fordtran, W.B. Saunders Co., Philadelphia, 1978, p 891.

86. Potyk D: Intestinal obstruction from impacted antacid tablets. N Engl J Med. 1970; 283;134.

87. Brettschneider L et al: Intestinal obstruction due to antacid gels. Complication of medical therapy for gastrointestinal bleeding. Gastroenterology. 1965; 49:291.

88. Welch JP et al: Management of antacid impactions in hemodialysis and renal transplant patients. Am J Surg. 1980; 139:561.

89. Clemens JD et al: Calcium carbonate and constipation: A historical review of medical mythopoeia. Gastroenterology. 1977; 72:957.

90. Rimer DG et al: Sodium content of antacids. JAMA. 1960; 173:995.

91. Dahl LK: Salt and hypertension. Am J Clin Nutr. 1972; 25:231.

92. Kawasaki T et al: The effect of high-sodium and low-sodium intakes on blood pressure and other related variables in human subjects with idiopathic hypertension. Am J Med. 1978; 64:193.

93. Green FW et al: Pharmacology and clinical use of antacids. Am J Hosp Pharm. 1975; 32:425.

94. 21 CFR Part 331, Code of Federal Regulations—Food and Drug Administration, Chapter 1, title 21, part 331: Antacid products for over-the-counter (OTC) human use.

95. Walker CO: Complications of peptic ulcer disease and indications for surgery. In Gastrointestinal Disease, 2nd ed, edited by MH Sleisinger and JS Fordtran, W.B. Saunders Co., Philadelphia, 1978, p 914.

96. Petersen WL et al: Reduction of gastric acidity. In Gastrointestinal Disease, 2nd ed, edited by MH Sleisinger and JS Fordtran, W.B. Saunders Co., Philadelphia, 1978, p 891.

97. Texter EC et al: The milk-alkali syndrome. Amer J Dig Dis. 1966; 11:913.

98. Sanderson PH: Alkalosis: a medical muddle. J R Coll Physicians Lond. 1978; 12:201.

99. Cope CL: Base changes in the alkalosis produced by the treatment of gastric ulcer with alkalies. Clin Sci. 1936; 2:287.

100. Burnett CH et al: Hypercalcemia without hypercalciuria or hypophosphatemia, calcinosis and renal insufficiency. N Engl J Med. 1949; 240:787.

101. Wenger J et al: The milk-alkali syndrome. Hypercalcemia, alkalosis and azotemia following calcium carbonate therapy of peptic ulcer. Gastroenterology. 1975; 33:745.

102. McMillan DE et al: The milk-alkali syndrome: a study of the acute disease with comments on the development of the chronic condition. Medicine. 1965; 44:485.

103. Stiel JN et al: Hypercalcemia in patients with peptic ulceration receiving large doses of calcium carbonate. Gastroenterology. 1967; 53:900.

104. Ivanovich P et al: The absorption of calcium carbonate. Ann Intern Med. 1967; 66:917.

105. Clarkson EM et al: The effect of a high intake of calcium carbonate in normal subjects and patients with chronic renal failure. Clin Sci. 1966; 30:425.

106. Hodgkinson A et al: The urinary excretion of calcium and inorganic phosphate in 344 patients with calcium stone of renal origin. Br J Surg. 1958; 46:10.

107. Vincent PC et al: The effect of large doses of calcium carbonate on serum and urinary calcium. Amer J Dig Dis. 1966; 11:286.

108. Herman JR et al: New type of urinary calculus caused by antacid therapy. JAMA. 1960; 174:1206.

109. Joekes AM et al: Multiple renal silica calculi. Br Med J. 1973; 1:146.

110. Baume PE et al: Failure of potent antacid therapy to hasten healing in chronic gastric ulcers. Australas Ann Med. 1969; 18:113.

111. Hollander D et al: Antacids vs placebos in peptic ulcer therapy. A controlled double-blind investigation. JAMA. 1973; 226:1181.

112. Breuhaus HC et al: Nocturnal gastric secretion in normal and duodenal ulcer patients on various forms of therapy. Gastroenterology. 1950; 16:172.

113. Barreras RF: Calcium and gastric secretion. Gastroenterology. 1973; 64:1168.

114. Fordtran JS: Acid rebound. N Engl J Med. 1968; 279:200.

115. Barreras RF: Acid secretion after calcium carbonate in patients with duodenal ulcer. N Engl J Med. 1970; 282:1402.

116. Levant JA et al: Stimulation of gastric secretion and gastrin release by single oral doses of calcium carbonate in man. N Engl J Med. 1973; 289:555.

117. Behar J et al: Calcium stimulation of gastrin and gastric acid secretion: effect of small doses of calcium carbonate. Gut. 1977; 18:442.

118. Binnion PF: Absorption of different commercial preparations of digoxin in the normal human subject, and the influences of an antacid, antidiarrhoeal and ion-exchange agents. In *Symposium on Digitalis,* edited by O. Storstein, Glydenidal Norsk Forlag, Oslo, 1973, p 216.

119. Brown DD et al: Decreased bioavailability of digoxin due to antacids and kaolin-pectin. N Engl J Med. 1976; 295:1034.

120. Hurwitz A: Antacid therapy and drug kinetics. Clin Pharmacokinetics. 1977; 2:269.

121. Levy G et al: Decreased serum salicylate concentrations in children with rheumatic fever treated with antacid. N Engl J Med. 1975; 293:323.

122. Hansten PD et al: Effect of antacid and ascorbic acid on serum salicylate concentration. J Clin Pharmacol. 1980; 20:326.

123. Smith PK et al: Studies on the pharmacology of salicylates. J Pharmacol. 1946; 87:237.

124. Levy G et al: Urine pH and salicylate therapy. JAMA. 1971; 217:81.

125. Gibaldi M et al: Effect of antacids on pH of urine. Clin Pharmacol Ther. 1974; 16:520.

126. Kunin G et al: Clinical pharmacology of the tetracycline antibiotics. Clin Pharmacol Ther. 1961; 2:51.

127. Barr WH et al: Decrease of tetracycline absorption in man by sodium bicarbonate. Clin Pharmacol Ther. 1971; 12:779.

128. Kramer PA et al: Tetracycline absorption in elderly patients with achlorhydria. Clin Pharmacol Ther. 1978; 23:467.

129. Garty M et al: Effect of cimetidine and antacids on gastrointestinal absorption of tetracycline. Clin Pharmacol Ther. 1980; 28:203.

130. Zinn MB: Quinidine intoxication from alkali ingestion. Texas Medicine. 1970; 66:64.

131. Gerhardt RE et al: Quinidine excretion in aciduria and alkalinuria. Ann Intern Med. 71:927, 1969.

132. Kimura KK et al: Therapeutic use of methyl polysiloxane. Curr Ther Res. 1964; 6:202.

133. Rider JA et al: Use of silicone in the treatment of intestinal gas and bloating. JAMA. 1960; 174:2052.

134. Roberts M et al: Methyl-polysiloxane in postoperative gas pains. JAMA. 1963; 183:595.

135. Danhof IE et al: Accelerated transit of intestinal gas with simethicone. Obstet Gynecol. 1974; 44:148.

136. Pellegrino PC et al: Management of gastroenteric gas syndromes. Am J Gastroenterol. 1961; 36:450.

137. Bernstein JE et al: A double-blind trial of simethicone in functional disease of the upper gastrointestinal tract. J Clin Pharmacol. 1974; 14:617.

138. McDonald GB et al: Pre-endoscopic use of oral simethicone. Gastrointest Endoscopy. 1978; 24:283.

139. Suoranta H et al: The value of simethicone in abdominal preparation. Radiology. 1979; 133:307.

140. Bank S et al: Evaluation of new drugs for peptic ulcer. Clin Gastroenterol. 1973; 2:379.

141. Pontes JF et al: Double-blind comparison of an oxethazaine-antacid combination against the antacid alone in the treatment of duodenal ulcer pain. Curr Ther Res. 1975; 18:315.

142. Novaes CC et al: A comparison of the acid neutralizing effects of a combination of antacid plus oxethazaine compared to antacid alone in duodenal ulcer patients. Curr Ther Res. 1975; 18:125.

143. Posey EL et al: Inhibition of food stimulated gastrin release by a topical anesthetic. Amer J Dig Dis. 1969; 14:787.

144. Posey EL et al: Inhibition of acetylcholine-stimulated gastrin release by the topical anesthetic, oxethazaine. Amer J Gastroenterol. 1971; 55:54.

145. Taggart GJ et al: The effect of mucaine on gastrin release in man. Aust NZ J Med. 1978; 8:397.

146. Finkelstein W et al: Cimetidine. N Engl J Med. 1978; 299:992.

147. Ivey K: Anticholinergics: do they work in peptic ulcer? Gastroenterology. 1975; 68:154.

148. Sun DCH et al: Optimal effective dose of anticholinergic drug in peptic ulcer therapy. Arch Intern Med. 1956; 97:442.

149. Feldman M et al: Effect of low-dose propantheline on food stimulated gastric acid secretion. N Engl J Med. 1977; 297:1427.

150. Moore JG et al: Circadian rhythm of gastric acid secretion in man. Nature. 1970; 266:1261.

151. Freston JW et al: A double-blind evaluation of the nocturnal antisecretory effects of anisotropine methylbromide in man. Dose response and duration of action studies. J Clin Pharmacol. 1977; 17:29.

152. Bowers JH et al: Effect of nighttime anisotropine methylbromide on duodenal ulcer healing and pain: a double-blind controlled trial. J Clin Pharmacol. 1978; 18:365.

153. Nimmo WS: Drugs, diseases and altered gastric emptying. Clin Pharmacokinetics. 1976; 1:189.

154. Hansten PD: *Drug Interactions,* 4th ed., Lea and Febiger, Philadelphia, 1979.

155. Grant WM: Ocular complications of drugs. JAMA. 1969; 207:2089.

156. Hiatt RL et al: Systemically administered anticholinergic drugs and intraocular pressure. Arch Opthal. 1970; 84:735.

157. Lazenby GW et al: Anticholinergic medication in open-angle glaucoma. Arch Opthal. 1970; 84:719.

158. Piper DW et al: Medical management of peptic ulcer. With reference to anti-ulcer agents in other gastrointestinal diseases. Drugs. 1972; 3:366.

159. Bettarello A et al: Effect of autonomic drugs on gastroesophageal reflux. Gastroenterology. 1960; 39:340.

160. Way LW: Stomach and duodenum. In *Current Surgical Diagnosis and Treatment,* 4th ed, Lange Medical Publications, Los Altos, CA, 1979, p 465.

161. After Gastrectomy. Lancet. 1976; 2:891.

162. Gertner JM et al: 25-Hydroxycholecalciferol absorption in steatorrhea and postgastrectomy osteomalacia. Br Med J. 1977; 1:1310.

163. Steiger Z et al: Pulmonary tuberculosis after gastric resection. Am J Surg. 1976; 131:668.

164. Hagelund CHH et al: Absorption of rifampicin in gastrectomized patients: effect of meals. Scand J Resp Dis. 1977; 58:241.

165. Venho VMK et al: Effect of gastric surgery on gastrointestinal drug absorption in man. Scand J Gastroenterol. 1975; 10:43.

166. Davidson ED et al: Use of metoclopramide in patients with delayed gastric emptying following gastric surgery. Ann Surg. 1977; 43:40.

167. Lanza FL et al: The effects of ibuprofen, indomethacin, aspirin, naproxen, and placebo on the gastric mucosa of normal volunteers. Dig Dis Sci. 1979; 24:823.

168. Caruso I et al: Gastropic evaluation of antiinflammatory agents. Br Med J. 1980; 1:75.

169. Silvoso GR et al: Incidence of gastric lesions in patients with rheumatic diseases on chronic aspirin therapy. Ann Intern Med. 1979; 91:517.

170. Conn HO et al: Nonassociation of adrenocorticosteroid therapy and peptic ulcer. N Engl J Med. 1976; 294:473.

171. Cooke AR: Drug damage to the gastroduodenum. In *Gastrointestinal Disease*, 2nd ed., edited by MH Sleisinger and JS Fordtran, W.B. Saunders Co., Philadelphia, 1978, p 807.

172. Friedman GD et al: Cigarettes, alcohol, coffee and peptic ulcer. N Engl J Med. 1974; 290:469.

173. Wolff G: Does alcohol cause chronic gastritis? Scand J Gastroenterol. 1970; 5:289.

174. Kirk AP et al: Peptic ulceration in patients with chronic liver disease. Dig Dis Sci. 1980; 24:756.

175. McGraw BF et al: Sucralfate. Drug Intel Clin Pharmacy. 1981; 15:578.

176. Marks IN et al: Ulcer healing and relapse rates after initial treatment with cimetidine or sucralfate. J Clin Gastroenterol. 1981; 3(Suppl 2):163.

177. Martin F et al: Comparison of the healing capacities of sucralfate and cimetidine in the short-term treatment of duodenal ulcer: A double-blind randomized trial. Gastroenterology. 1982; 82:401.

178. Robert A: Prostaglandins and digestive diseases. In *Advances in Prostaglandin and Thromboxane Research*, edited by B Samuelsson, PW Ramwell and R Paoletti, Raven Press, New York, 1980, p 1533.

179. Fung WP et al: Effect of prostaglandin E_2 on the healing of gastric ulcers: a double-blind endoscopic trial. Aust NZ J Med. 1976; 6:121.

180. Brogden RN et al: Tri-potassium Di-citrato Bismuthate: a report of its pharmacological properties and therapeutic efficacy in peptic ulcer. Drugs. 1976; 12:401.

181. Abrahamsson H et al: Pharmacological and clinical aspects of some drugs used in peptic ulcer treatment. Scand J Gastroenterol. 1979; 14(Suppl 55):117.

182. Wetterhus S et al: Experience with trimipramine in the treatment of peptic ulcer. Scand J Gastroenterol. 1979; 14(Suppl 55):124.

183. Zollinger RM et al: Primary peptic ulcerations of the jejunum associated with islet cell tumors: twenty-five-year appraisal. Ann Surg. 1980; 192:422.

184. McCarthy DM: Report on the United States experience with cimetidine in Zollinger-Ellison syndrome and other hypersecretory states. Gastroenterology. 1978; 74:453.

185. Lamers CBH et al: Long term treatment with histamine H_2-receptor antagonists in Zollinger-Ellison syndrome. Am J Gastroenterol. 1978; 70:286.

186. Randal HT: Alterations in gastrointestinal tract function following surgery. Surg Clin North Am. 1958; 38:585.

187. Richardson CT et al: Effect of vagotomy in Zollinger-Ellison syndrome. Gastroenterology. 1979; 77:682.

188. Groorke JF et al: Zollinger-Ellison syndrome unresponsive to cimetidine. Am J Gastroenterol. 1979; 72:168.

189. Southwest Oncology Group Protocol 7935: Chemotherapy of functioning and nonfunctioning islet cell carcinoma, Phase II. Ronald Bukowski, M.D., Study Coordinator.

190. Castell DO: Medical therapy of reflux esophagitis. Ann Intern Med. 1980; 93:926.

191. Behar J et al: Medical and surgical management of reflux esophagitis. N Engl J Med. 1975; 293:263.

192. McCluskie RA et al: Cimetidine in the treatment of oesophagitis. In Cimetidine: Second International Symposium on Histamine H_2-Receptor Antagonists, edited by WL Burland and MA Simkins, Royal College of Physicians, London, 1976. *Excerpta Medica,* 1977, p 287.

193. Wesdorp E et al: Oral cimetidine in reflux esophagitis: a double-blind controlled trial. Gastroenterology. 1978; 74:821.

194. Behar J et al: Cimetidine in the treatment of gastroesophageal reflux. Gastroenterology. 1978; 74:441.

195. Powell-Jackson P et al: Effect of cimetidine in the symptomatic gastroesophageal reflux. Lancet. 1978; 2:1068.

196. Thanik KO et al: Reflux esophagitis: effect of oral bethanechol on symptoms and endoscopic findings. Ann Intern Med. 1980; 93:805.

197. McCallum RW et al: A controlled trial of metoclopramide in symptomatic gastroesophageal reflux. N Engl J Med. 1977; 296:354.

198. Malmud LS et al: The mode of action of alginic acid compound in the reduction of gastroesophageal reflux. J Nucl Med. 1979; 20:1023.

199. Stanciu C et al: Alginate/antacid in the reduction of gastroesophageal reflux. Lancet. 1974; 1:109.

200. Graham DY et al: Symptomatic reflux esophagitis: a double-blind controlled comparison of antacids and alginate. Curr Ther Res. 1977; 22:653.

201. Barnardo DE et al: A double-blind controlled trial of Gaviscon in patients with symptomatic gastro-oesophageal reflux. Curr Med Res Opin. 1975; 3:388.

202. Beeley M et al: Medical treatment of symptomatic hiatus hernia with low density compounds. Curr Med Res Opin. 1972; 1:63.

203. Leslie GB et al: A toxicological profile of cimetidine. In Burland WL, Simkins MA (Editors), *Cimetidine: Proceedings of the Second International Symposium on Histamine H_2-Receptor Antagonists,* Oxford, Excerpta Medica, 1977, p 30.

204. Glade G et al: Cimetidine in pregnancy. Am J Dis Child. 1980; 134:87.

205. Howe JP et al: Effect of cimetidine in reducing intragastric acidity in patients undergoing elective caesarean section. In Torsoli A, Lucchelli PE, Brimblecombe RW (Editors), H_2-*Antagonists,* Oxford, Excerpta Medica, 1980, pp 174–184.

206. Wilson J: Effect of intravenous cimetidine on intragastric pH at caesarean section. In Torsoli A, Lucchelli PE, Brimblecombe RW (Editors), *H₂-Antagonists,* Oxford, Excerpta Medica, 1980, pp 185–190.

207. Somogyi A et al: Cimetidine excretion into breast milk. Br J Clin Pharmac. 1979; 7:627.

208. Hansten PD: Cimetidine interactions. Drug Interactions Newsletter, 1981; 1:43.

Chapter 19

Acute Stress Erosions

William A. Watson and John Russo, Jr.

Erosions of the gastric mucosa caused by physical stress are called acute stress erosions (ASE's) and are an important therapeutic consideration in critically ill patients. ASE's commonly occur following major thermal injuries, head trauma, sepsis, hypotension, extensive trauma, multiple organ system disease, and during the postoperative period of major surgical procedures (1,2). Recent reports suggest that the incidence of ASE's is 84–100% following these events.

It is important to diagnose and treat ASE's early because they may rapidly progress from the relatively benign foci of pallor and hyperemia which develop within 24 hours of an injury to acute ulcers complicated by hemorrhage and perforation 2–18 days later (3–5). Although subclinical bleeding (Hemoccult positive gastric contents) is common, the overall incidence of significant bleeding is less than 10%. The latter is probably secondary to the progressive erosion of the lesion into the submucosal layer of the gastrointestinal lining where there is a higher concentration of arteries (1,6,7). Under these conditions, the mortality is close to 50% (8). Identified risk factors are listed in Table 1.

The diagnosis of ASE is difficult since symptoms rarely occur before complications are evident. In one study, bleeding was the first presenting sign in 50% of patients; 25% of the patients presented with massive hemorrhage (9). Hematemesis and melena are seen with equal frequency (8). Endoscopy is the preferred method of locating and differentiating ASE's from other lesions, but angiography may be useful when the site of bleeding is not identified by endoscopy. Barium examinations are not generally useful in detecting stress ulcers (10,11).

ASE's are generally located in the proximal portion of the stomach; however, other sites have been identified (1). Patients with severe head injury may develop lesions in the esophagus, stomach, and duodenum (8,12). Duodenal and gastroduodenal lesions and a higher incidence of perforation are linked to major thermal injury (3,9). Silen and Skillman (11) suggest that the lower incidence of antral and duodenal lesions in the acutely ill patient may be related to a lack of aggressive evaluation of those areas of the gastrointestinal tract.

Although many theories regarding the pathogenesis of ASE's have been proposed, the majority of evidence supports the role of three factors: acid secretion; mucosal integrity; and gastric mucosal blood flow (13,14).

The presence of acid is critical to the development of ASE's (3,16,17). The rate of acid secretion

Table 1.

RISK FACTORS FOR COMPLICATIONS
OF ACUTE STRESS EROSIONS (2,5,10,18,21)

Hypotension	Acute clinical deterioration
Sepsis	Jaundice
Respiratory insufficiency	Four or more organ system injuries
Renal failure	Hyperalimentation
Coma Peritonitis	Major operative procedures

varies in different clinical conditions as well as at different times during the course of disease. For example, patients who have undergone neurosurgery are hypersecretors of gastric acid (15). In contrast, acid secretion is decreased immediately following traumatic injury, but is increased 3–5 days thereafter or when hypotension is corrected (4).

When the integrity of the gastric mucosal barrier is decreased, more acid diffuses from the lumen of the stomach into the mucosa. ASE and its complications arise from this back diffusion (18,19).

Decreased gastric mucosal blood flow is most likely the major factor underlying the development of ASE's (4,8,15,19). The gastric mucosa contains no glycogen and is unable to use anaerobic glycolysis efficiently as an alternative source of energy; it is therefore particularly vulnerable to ischemia (8). Ischemia of the gastric mucosa produces a severe energy deficit which ultimately results in a breakdown of normal mucosal defenses and cellular necrosis (20).

1. W.J., a 25-year-old male, is transferred to a regional burn treatment center eight hours after sustaining a 50% total body surface area burn. W.J. is confused and unable to provide any medical history. Appropriate burn resuscitation is undertaken. Should ASE treatment be started immediately?

Two therapeutic options face the clinician treating a patient at risk for ASE: withhold treatment until complications develop or initiate prophylactic therapy immediately. Less than 10% of patients at risk for ASE develop complications; however, once significant hemorrhage or perforation occurs, the mortality rate is 50% or greater

(6,8). Therefore, treatment should not be withheld from high risk patients. Prophylaxis has been successful in patients with major thermal injury (22), severe head injury (12), and other critically ill patients (23). Successful management of any of the underlying conditions listed in Table 1 is also critical to the prevention of ASE complications.

2. What is the goal of prophylaxis?

As McElwee and associates (24) have demonstrated, prophylaxis is designed to limit gastric lesions to erythema and to prevent their progression to erosions and ulcerations which could result in hemorrhage or perforation. Because abolishment of all lesions does not appear to be possible, prophylaxis is directed at the prevention of complications.

Intraluminal buffering is presently the prophylactic technique of choice (1,8,11). It is effective and can be easily monitored through pH determinations of gastric contents (22,23,25,26). Cimetidine has also been used in this regard and may have the added beneficial effect of maintaining gastric mucosal blood flow during hypotension (27). Other potentially useful agents include carbenoxolone, prostaglandins, and corticosteroids (1). Since these agents do not alter the intraluminal pH, it is more difficult to monitor their effects.

3. How much intraluminal buffering is necessary for successful prophylaxis?

There is no agreement with regard to the pH that should be maintained for the prophylactic treatment of ASE patients. Some investigators have used a pH of 3.5 as the lower limit on the grounds that pepsin activity is minimal at this pH. Others have attempted to maintain the gastric pH at a level of 4, 5 or 7. (Table 2 summarizes the efficacy data from investigators studying the prophylactic treatment of ASE's). *In vitro* evaluation of the effects of pH on coagulation indicates that aberrations occur at a pH of less than 6.8 (30). This may explain the subclinical bleeding observed in most patients with ASE's (7) and supports those investigators who use a higher pH as a therapeutic goal. A lower limit of pH 5 is used at many institutions.

4. Which agents are useful in raising intraluminal pH and how should prophylaxis be initiated?

Table 2.

RESULTS OF CLINICAL TRIALS: THEIR pH GOAL AND EFFICACY

Reference Number	pH Goal	Maximum pH Attained	Efficacy* (percent)
2	3.5	not listed	antacids (titrated dose) — 37/37 (100%) cimetidine (max. 400 mg every 4 hours) — 31/38 (82%)
12	not defined	approximately 4.2	control — 6/24 (25%) cimetidine (300 mg every 4 hours) — 21/26 (81%)
22	7.0	not listed	control — 17/24 — (71%) antacids (titrated dose) — 23/24 (97%)
23	3.5	"usually 7 to 8" greater than 5 in all but 2 cases	control 37/49 — (76%) antacids (dose titrated) 49/51 — (96%)
24	5.0	not listed	antacids (dose titrated) — 14/14 (100%) cimetidine (400 mg every 4 hours) — 13/13 (100%)
28	4.0	not listed	antacids (dose titrated) pH — 35/37 (95%) bleeders — 35/37 (95%) cimetidine (up to 300 mg every 3 hours) pH — 27/40 (68%) bleeders — 37/40 (93%)

*Efficacy is defined as the ability to prevent gastroduodenal hemorrhage.

Any form of therapy which increases the intraluminal pH above 5 appears to be useful in the prophylactic treatment of ASE. Antacids (2,23,24,28), cimetidine (12,24,28,31,32), and antacids with nutritional supplements (26) are all clinically efficacious.

Prophylactic therapy should be initiated as soon as possible following injury, and it has been suggested that treatment prior to major surgery may be beneficial (33).

Antacids and cimetidine, alone or in combination, are acceptable. Both are approximately equivalent with regard to side effects; however, ease of administration favors cimetidine. Regardless of the regimen used, successful prophylaxis requires routine gastric pH monitoring with dosing adjustment made as needed to maintain gastric pH at the desired level. No correlation has been found between plasma cimetidine concentrations and intraluminal pH (34,35). Figure 1 provides dosing guidelines for therapy designed to maintain gastric pH above 5.

5. How is prophylaxis monitored?

Intraluminal pH and evidence of bleeding are equally important parameters. Two means of determining pH are available: aspiration of intraluminal contents through a nasogastric (NG) tube and intraluminal pH probes. These probes are expensive and are used primarily for research purposes (36,37).

When intraluminal contents are directly examined via aspiration, it is important that the sample be representative of total gastric contents. The NG tube must be placed in the dependent portion of the stomach, as pH varies in different areas (37). The total gastric contents can be aspirated and thoroughly mixed before the pH is determined, although this may be cumbersome and impractical. Most commonly, hourly samples are evaluated. When this method is used, it is important to avoid testing the residual fluid volume in the NG tube and to test the actual gastric contents.

The patient should also be evaluated for signs

ALGORITHM FOR THE TREATMENT OF ACUTE STRESS EROSIONS

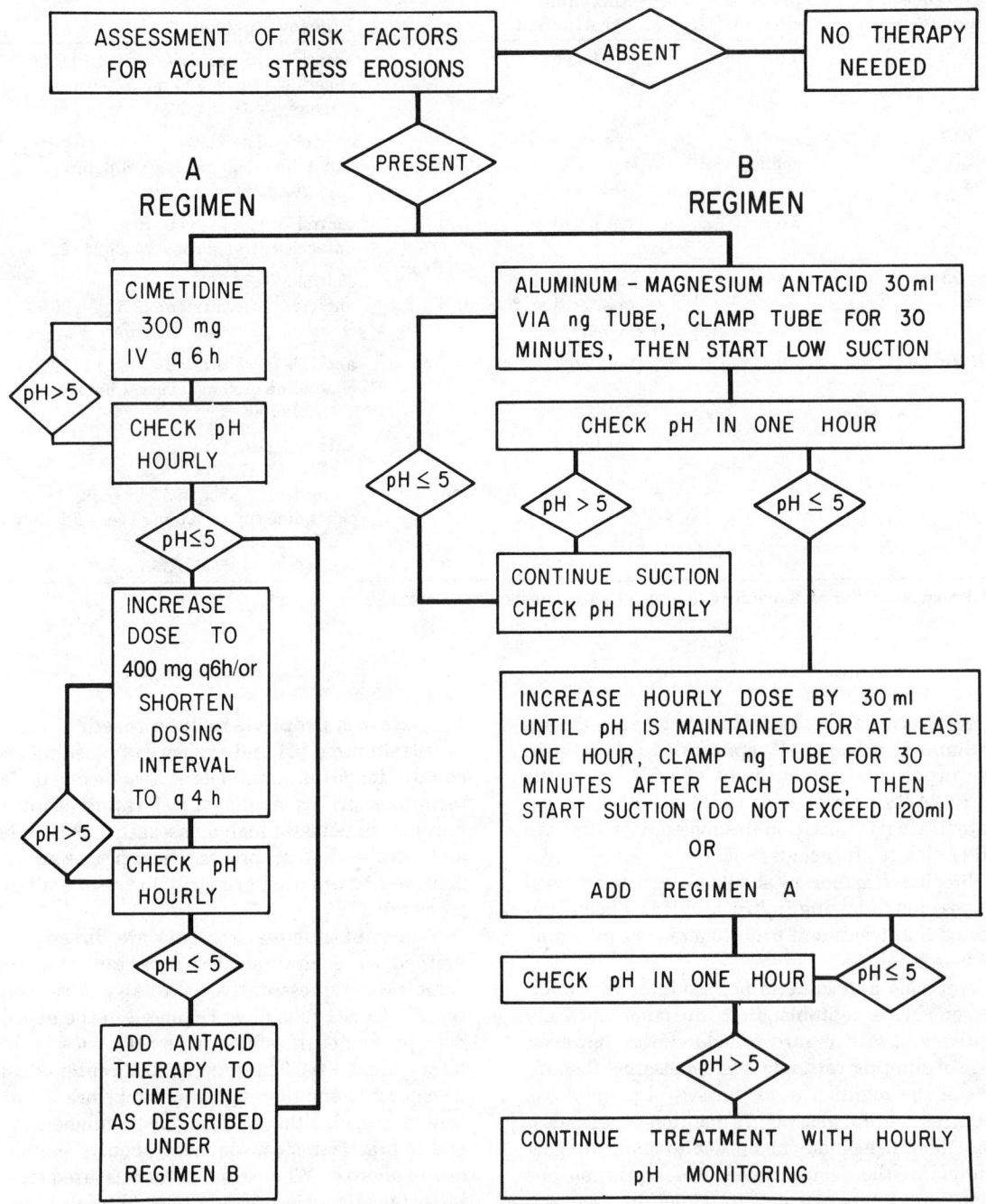

Figure 1. Treatment of Acute Stress Erosion. The clinician has the option of initiating treatment with either Regimen A or B and combining the regimens to achieve optimal pH control. Once control is achieved therapy should continue until risk factors for ASE and its complications have been corrected.

of bleeding from ASE's. Stool and NG aspirates should be routinely checked for blood, utilizing both visual, bedside or laboratory analysis. The pH of blood in the gastric aspirate is 6.5 or greater; therefore, visual examination of the gastric aspirate is important to rule out the presence of blood as a source of a falsely elevated pH. Systemic signs of bleeding, such as hypotension, tachycardia, oliguria, and a decreasing hematocrit should also be evaluated.

6. The day after W.J. is admitted to the burn treatment center, his family arrives. His wife indicates that he has been treated for a duodenal ulcer for the last three months and has been taking antacids seven times a day. Does the presence of an active or healed peptic ulcer alter the prophylactic therapy of ASE's?

There is no information available concerning the significance of a previous history of peptic ulcer disease in patients like W.J. One would expect that the presence of active ulcers might increase the risk of hemorrhage or perforation. As with other patients, aggressive prophylactic therapy should be initiated and repeatedly positive aspirates should be actively investigated.

7. After four days of successful prophylaxis with IV cimetidine, W.J. pulled all of his IV lines out. A crushed cimetidine tablet was administered through the NG tube. One hour later the aspirate was positive for occult blood. Do oral cimetidine tablets affect tests for occult blood?

When cimetidine tablets are administered, a false positive test for occult blood in nasogastric aspirate can be obtained using the Hemoccult method (38). A dye, FDC Blue Lake No. 2, has been identified as the cause of the reaction, not cimetidine (39). This dye's effect on stool testing has not been evaluated.

Since this result was found within four hours of administration, a false positive reaction may be the problem. However, major gastrointestinal bleeding begins two days after the initial insult; therefore, if a positive reaction persists when intravenous cimetidine is resumed, actual gastrointestinal bleeding must be ruled out.

8. A.F. is a 20-year-old male who is transferred to the trauma center from a local community hospital. Approximately one week prior to admission A.F. sustained abdominal and head trauma secondary to a motor vehicle accident. As a result of his injuries he developed several complications including sepsis and acute renal failure. On admission, he is obtunded and febrile. Medications include cimetidine 300 mg intravenously every 6 hours and antacids as needed to maintain the gastric pH above 5. Cimetidine is discontinued because "it causes mental status changes complicating assessment of the patient's neurological status." A magnesium-aluminum antacid is ordered hourly and as needed to control gastric acidity. Could cimetidine be the cause of this patient's obtundation? If so, how can it be ruled out?

There is an association between cimetidine and changes in mental status. Restlessness and confusion are usually the first signs, progressing to disorientation, agitation, hallucinations, focal twitching, unresponsiveness, apneic spells and seizures. It is usually seen within 24 to 48 hours of therapy, and the elderly as well as patients with renal and/or hepatic dysfunction are at greatest risk (40).

Mental status changes may be a result of cimetidine's effect on H_2-receptors in the central nervous system (41). Both H_1 and H_2 histamine receptors are present in the central nervous system (CNS); however, it is difficult to separate their actions. Presently, cimetidine's specific role remains obscure (42,43), but it does penetrate the blood brain barrier. CNS levels of 0.4 mcg/ml or more and trough serum levels of 1.25 mcg/ml or more correlate with mental status changes (40,41). The frequency of this effect has been reported to be as high as 17%; however, in the general population it is probably closer to the 7.3 reported cases per 100,000 patients treated (44).

When mental status changes occur, they should reverse within 2–3 days following discontinuation of the cimetidine. If serum cimetidine levels are available, it is also possible to individualize the dosing regimen to reverse and minimize mental deterioration (40). This may be accomplished by decreasing the dose and/or increasing the dosing interval to maintain therapeutic concentrations while avoiding toxic levels. Physostigmine has been used to reverse the mental changes caused by cimetidine; however, its use is not recommended because it too has nonspecific central nervous system activity and toxicity (45,46).

When evaluating cimetidine-induced mental

status changes, it should also be determined if the patient is currently receiving diazepam or chlordiazepoxide therapy since cimetidine can potentiate the sedative effects of these agents (47,48). See the Upper Gastrointestinal Diseases chapter for further discussion of cimetidine drug interactions.

9. Does the dose of cimetidine need to be adjusted in patients such as A.F. with impaired renal function?

Cimetidine dosage adjustments for patients with impaired renal function are listed in Table 3. These and other published recommendations are based on stable patient populations without consideration for concurrent hepatic dysfunction which further impairs drug clearance (49–55). In critically ill patients, these recommendations cannot be expected to guarantee adequate pH control or eliminate the possibility of cimetidine-associated mental status changes.

The need for a post-hemodialysis dose has been the subject of considerable confusion (51,52,54). Notwithstanding its substantial dialyzability, the amount of cimetidine removed by four hours of hemodialysis constitutes only 8–14% of the administered dose; therefore, major dosing adjustments are not required following dialysis (51). Similarly, peritoneal dialysis removes only a small fraction of the administered dose (50).

10. What are the adverse effects of antacid therapy in critically ill patients?

Magnesium excretion declines with advancing renal failure; the diseased kidney is unable to maintain magnesium homeostasis at glomerular filtration rates of less than 10 to 30 ml/min (55,56). Although cases of hypermagnesemia in acute renal failure are reported in the absence of exogenous

magnesium intake, symptomatic *hypermagnesemia* usually occurs in patients also receiving enemas, intravenous fluids or antacids which contain magnesium. The oral administration of as little as 180 ml/day of a magnesium containing antacid for three days has resulted in symptomatic hypermagnesemia (57).

As serum levels rise from 3 to 15 mEq/L, symptoms progress from a tendency to hypotension to drowsiness, weakness, respiratory depression, loss of deep tendon reflexes, coma, prolonged QT interval and cardiac arrest (58).

In the absence of serum magnesium levels, hypermagnesemia should be suspected in symptomatic patients particularly if their anion gap is low. It should also be considered in a septic patient with lactic acidosis whose anion gap is normal since magnesium can act as an "unmeasured cation" (59). Both peritoneal and hemodialysis can be used to control hypermagnesemia (58).

Aggressive aluminum hydroxide antacid therapy may also cause *hypophosphatemia* secondary to the formation of insoluble aluminum phosphate complexes in the gut which are then excreted in the feces. Magnesium may also contribute to phosphate depletion with serum phosphate levels falling below 1 mg/dl. Consequences of phosphate depletion include impaired oxygen release from erythrocytes; depressed chemotactic, phagocytic and bactericidal activity of granulocytes; elevated calcium levels when assessed in light of the serum albumin concentration; and mental status changes (60). This can be prevented by adjusting the phosphorus content of parenteral fluids.

Medication *bezoars* due to antacids, especially those with aluminum hydroxide gel, are also a consideration. Obstruction secondary to bezoars may result in severe complications (61).

Clearly, all therapeutic options for stress ulcers place the patient at risk of mental status changes and other side effects. Therapy should be undertaken with an appreciation for these potential complications so that appropriate monitoring and adjustments in drug therapy can be made as needed.

11. Are there any interactions between antacids and constant suction through a nasogastric tube that should be considered?

Decreased gastrointestinal motility predisposes patients to pulmonary aspiration of the intestinal contents, and the removal of gastric con-

Table 3.

CIMETIDINE DOSAGE ADJUSTMENT foR RENAL DYSFUNCTION

Cl_{cr} (ml/min)	0–20	20–40	>40
Cimetidine/ 6 hours	150 mg	225 mg	300 mg
Alternate schedule	300 mg/ 12 hrs	300 mg/ 8 hrs	300 mg/ 6 hrs

Modified from Luk GD et al: Ann Intern Med. 1979; 90:991

tents with continuous nasogastric suction minimizes this problem (11,62). When antacid therapy is utilized, suction must be interrupted for approximately 30 minutes after each dose to permit the antacids to mix with gastric contents. This procedure increases the risk of aspiration. Cimetidine does not require clamping of the NG tube. Its use will reduce the number of antacid doses required and thus the frequency of clamping the NG tube. It also decreases the volume of gastric secretion (63).

12. After five days of successful prophylactic therapy, A.F. develops an abdominal abscess and his gastric pH falls to 2.5. Therapy with increased doses of cimetidine and antacid therapy have no effect on pH. Is there a relationship between the development of sepsis and ineffective intraluminal buffering?

Two prospective studies have identified an association between the failure of ASE prophylaxis and the inability to increase intraluminal pH with antacids and cimetidine during sepsis (21,28). In more than half of the patients, a failure in pH control occurred before or within 48 hours of the onset of sepsis (28). If failure of pH control occurs after initial success, sepsis should be considered as a potential cause.

13. B.M., a 56-year-old female with metastatic cancer, is admitted to the surgical intensive care unit post-operatively. She was previously treated with radiotherapy, and has a WBC of 2000/mm^3 as well as a sick-sinus syndrome. What considerations for prophylactic therapy of ASE's are required in a patient with this history?

Since a previous H$_2$-receptor antagonist was linked with agranulocytosis, cimetidine's effects on bone-marrow have been scrutinized. It was initially considered safe because it lacked the thiourea moiety which was suspected to be the problem with metiamide; furthermore, it was safely used in a patient with metiamide-induced agranulocytosis (65). More recently, several reports of cimetidine-associated granulocytopenia, leukopenia, and thrombocytopenia have been published (66–73). These effects have been observed 1–49 days following the initiation of cimetidine therapy and may be caused by both bone-marrow suppression and increased peripheral cellular destruction. Present incidence data show 2.3 cases of decreased blood cell count per 100,000 treated patients (44).

Patients with prior marrow suppressive therapy such as B.M. and features of immunoallergic disease appear to be at risk for developing this complication (70,74). Freston suggests there is no reason to conclude that cimetidine causes suppression of blood cell counts in patients with uncomplicated acid-peptic disease based upon current data (75). Alternatives to cimetidine should be considered in B.M. until this problem has been more accurately defined. If no alternative is available, blood cell counts should be monitored and cimetidine discontinued if suppression is noted.

Cimetidine-associated sinus bradycardia has been reported and supported by rechallenge (76). It appears that digoxin and procedures that produce histamine release may predispose patients to the effects of cimetidine on the myocardium (77) since cimetidine has no effect on heart rate or sinus node function in unmedicated patients (78).

References

1. Moody FG: Acute stress erosions and ulceration. In *Gastrointestinal Diseases*, 2nd ed, edited by MH Sleisenger and JS Fordtran, W.B. Saunders, Philadelphia, 1978, p 826.

2. Priebe JH et al: Antacid versus cimetidine in preventing acute gastrointestinal bleeding. N Engl J Med. 1980; 302:426.

3. Czaja AJ et al: Acute gastric disease after cutaneous thermal injury. Arch Surg. 1975; 110:600.

4. Lucas CE et al: Natural history and surgical dilemma of "stress" gastric bleeding. Arch Surg. 1971; 102:266.

5. Skillman JJ et al: Respiratory failure, hypotension, sepsis, and jaundice—a clinical syndrome associated with lethal hemorrhage from acute stress ulceration of the stomach. Am J Surg. 1969; 117:523.

6. Menguy R: The prophylaxis of stress ulceration. N Engl J Med. 1980; 302:461.

7. Skillman JJ et al: Stress ulcers. Lancet. 1972; 2:1303.

8. Moody FG et al: Stress ulcers: their pathogenesis, diagnosis, and treatment. Surg Clin North Am. 1976; 56:1469.

9. Moncrief JA et al: Curling's ulcer. J Trauma. 1964; 4:481.

10. Czaja AJ et al: Acute duodenitis and duodenal ulceration after burns—clinical and pathological characteristics. JAMA 1975; 232:621.

11. Silen W et al: Gastrointestinal responses to injury and infection. Surg Clin North Am. 1976; 56:945.

12. Halloran LG et al: Prevention of acute gastrointestinal complications after severe head injury: a controlled trial of cimetidine prophylaxis. Am J Surg. 1980; 139:44.

13. O'Neill JA et al: Studies related to the pathogenesis of Curling's ulcer. J Trauma. 1967; 7:275.

14. Chernov MS et al: Stress ulcer: a preventable disease. J Trauma. 1972; 12:831.

15. Skillman JJ et al: The gastric mucosal barrier: clinical and experimental studies in critically ill and normal man, and in the rabbit. Ann Surg. 1970; 172:564.

16. Rosenthal A et al: Gastrin levels and gastric acidity in the pathogenesis of acute gastroduodenal disease after burns. Surg Gynecol Obstet 1977; 144:232.

17. Robbins R et al: Studies of gastric secretion in stressed patients. Ann Surg. 1972; 175:555.

18. Gordon MJ et al: Divergent nature of gastric mucosal permeability and gastric acid secretion in sick patients with general surgical and neurosurgical disease. Ann Surg. 1973; 178:285.

19. Silen W et al: Stress ulcer, acute erosive gastritis and the gastric mucosal barrier. Advances Intern Med. 1974; 19:195.

20. Menguy R et al: Gastric mucosal energy metabolism and "stress ulceration." Ann Surg. 1974; 180:538.

21. Martin LF et al: Failure of cimetidine prophylaxis in the critically ill. Arch Surg 1979; 114:492.

22. McAlhany JC et al: Antacid control of complications from acute gastroduodenal disease after burns. J Trauma. 1976; 16:645.

23. Hastings PR et al: Antacid titration in the prevention of acute gastrointestinal bleeding: a controlled, randomized trial in 100 critically ill patients. N Engl J Med. 1978; 298:1041.

24. McElwee HP et al: Cimetidine affords protection equal to antacids in prevention of stress ulceration following thermal injury. Surgery. 1979; 86:620.

25. Watson LC et al: Prevention of upper gastrointestinal hemorrhage in 582 burned children. Am J Surg. 1976; 132:790.

26. Solem LD et al: Antacid therapy and nutritional supplementation in the prevention of Curling's ulcer. Surg Gynecol Obstet. 1979; 148:367.

27. Levine BA et al: Cimetidine prevents reduction in gastric mucosal blood flow during shock. Surgery. 1978; 84:113.

28. Martin LF et al: Failure of gastric pH control by antacids or cimetidine in the critically ill: a valid sign of sepsis. Surgery. 1980; 88:59.

29. Hollander F: What is pH? Gastroenterology. 1945; 4:497.

30. Green FW et al: Effect of acid and pepsin on blood coagulation and platelet aggregation. Gastroenterology. 1978; 74:38.

31. Jones RH et al: Cimetidine: prophylaxis against upper gastrointestinal haemorrhage after renal transplantation. Br Med J. 1978; 2:398.

32. Macdougall BRD et al: H$_2$-receptor antagonists and antacids in the prevention of acute gastrointestinal haemorrhage in fulminant hepatic failure. Lancet. 1977; 1:617.

33. Levine BA et al: The role of cimetidine in the prevention of stress induced gastric mucosal injury. Surg Gynecol Obstet. 1979; 148:399.

34. Kohler TR et al: Cimetidine pharmacokinetics in trauma patients. Surg Forum. 1979; 30:12.

35. Cohen IA et al: Relationship between cimetidine plasma levels and gastric acidity in acutely ill patients. Am J Hosp Pharm. 1980; 37:375.

36. Herrmann V et al: Evaluation of intragastric pH in acutely ill patients. Arch Surg. 1979; 114:511.

37. Abasov IT et al: Application of intragastric pH-metry for diagnostic and therapeutic control of gastric diseases. Am J Gastroenterology. 1977; 67:229.

38. Norfleit RG et al: False-positive "Hemoccult" reaction with cimetidine. N Engl J Med. 1980; 302:467.

39. Schentag JJ: False-positive "Hemoccult" reaction with cimetidine. N Engl J Med. 1980; 303:110.

40. Kimelblatt BJ et al: Dose and serum concentration relationships in cimetidine-associated mental confusion. Gastroenterology. 1980; 78:791.

41. Schentag JJ et al: Pharmacokinetic and clinical studies in patients with cimetidine-associated mental confusion. Lancet. 1979; 1:177.

42. Stayavivad J et al: Iontophoretic studies of histamine and histamine antagonists in the feline vestibular. Eur J Pharmacol. 1977; 41:17.

43. Sastry HSR et al: Depression of rat cerebral cortical neurones by H$_1$ and H$_2$ histamine receptor agonists. Eur J Pharmacol. 1976; 38:269.

44. Davis TG et al: Evaluation of a worldwide spontaneous reporting system with cimetidine. JAMA. 1980; 243:1912.

45. Mogeinicki SR et al: Physostigmine reversal of cimetidine-induced mental confusion. JAMA. 1979; 241:826.

46. Callaham M: Tricyclic antidepressant overdose. JACEP. 1979; 8:413.

47. Klotz V et al: Delayed clearance of diazepam due to cimetidine. N Engl J Med. 1980; 302:1012.

48. Desmond PV et al: Cimetidine impairs elimination of chlordiazepoxide (Librium) in man. Ann Intern Med. 1980; 93:266.

49. Luk GD et al: Cimetidine and impaired renal function. Ann Intern Med. 1979; 90:991.

50. Vaziri ND et al: Peritoneal dialysis clearance of cimetidine. Am J Gastroenterology. 1979; 71:572.

51. Vaziri ND et al: Hemodialysis clearance of cimetidine. Arch Intern Med. 1978; 138:1685.

52. Ma KW et al: Effects of renal failure on blood levels of cimetidine. Gastroenterology. 1978; 74:473.

53. Larsson R et al: Oral absorption of cimetidine and its clearance in patients with renal failure. Eur J Clin Pharmacol. 1979; 15:153.

54. Canavan JSF et al: Cimetidine clearance in renal failure. In Cimetidine: Proceedings of the Second International Symposium on Histamine H$_2$-Receptor Antagonists, edited by WD Burland and MA Simkins. Amsterdam—Oxford, Excerpta Medica, 1977, p 75.

55. Robinson RR et al: Renal factors responsible for the hypermagnesemia of renal disease. J Lab Clin Med. 1959; 53:572.

56. Stelle TH et al: The contribution of the chronically diseased kidney to magnesium homeostasis in man. J Lab Clin Med. 1968; 71:455.

57. Randall RE, Jr et al: Hypermagnesemia in renal failure: etiology and toxic manifestations. Ann Intern Med. 1964; 61:73.

58. Mordes JP et al: Excess magnesium. Pharmacol Rev. 1978; 29:273.

59. Emmett M et al: Hypermagnesemia and hypotension. Ann Intern Med. 1976; 84:340.

60. Knochel JP: The pathophysiology and clinical characteristics of severe hypophosphatemia. Arch Intern Med. 1977; 137:203.

61. Korenman MD et al: Intestinal obstruction from medication bezoars. JAMA. 1978; 240:54.

62. LeFrock JL et al: Aspiration pneumonia: a ten-year review. Am Surg. 1979; 45:305.

63. Finkelstein W et al: Cimetidine. N Engl J Med. 1978; 299:992.

64. Feldman EJ et al: Effects of metiamide on gastric acid hypersecretion, steatorrhea and bone-marrow function in a patient with systemic mastocytosis. N Engl J Med. 1976; 295:1178.

65. Fleischer D et al: Cimetidine therapy in a patient with metiamide-induced agranulocytosis. N Engl J Med. 1977; 296:342.

66. Chang HK et al: Bone-marrow suppression associated with cimetidine. Ann Intern Med. 1979; 91:580.

67. Lopez-Loque A et al: Cimetidine and bone-marrow toxicity. Lancet. 1978; 1:444.

68. Druart F et al: Association of cimetidine and bone-marrow suppression in man. Dig Dis Sci. 1979; 24:730.

69. Collen MJ: Cimetidine-associated thrombocytopenia and leukopenia. West J Med. 1980; 132:257.

70. Posnett DN et al: Cimetidine-induced neutropenia: a possible dose-related phenomenon. Arch Intern Med. 1979; 139:584.

71. Isaacs AJ: Cimetidine and thrombocytopenia. Br Med J. 1980; 6210:294.

72. Ufberg IH et al: Transient neutropenia in a patient receiving cimetidine. Gastroenterology. 1977; 73:635.

73. Byron JW: Mechanism for histamine H_2-receptor induced cell-cycle changes in the bone marrow stem cell. Agents Action. 1977; 7:209.

74. Pariente EA et al: Cimetidine-induced bone marrow suppression. Dig Dis Sci. 1980; 25:396.

75. Freston JW: Cimetidine and granulocytopenia. Ann Intern Med. 1979; 90:264.

76. Ligumsky M et al: Cimetidine and arrhythmia suppression. Ann Intern Med. 1978; 89:1008.

77. Levi R et al: Histamine-drug-disease interactions and cardiac function. In *Histamine Receptors*, edited by TO Yellin, SP Medical and Scientific Books, New York, 1979, p 99.

78. Engel TR et al: Histamine$_2$ receptor antagonism by cimetidine and sinus-node function. N Engl J Med. 1979; 301:591.

Chapter 20

Inflammatory Bowel Disease

George E. Dukes, Jr.

Inflammatory bowel disease is a generic classification for a group of non-specific, idiopathic inflammatory disorders of the gastrointestinal tract. By convention, inflammatory bowel disease is divided into two major disorders: ulcerative colitis and Crohn's disease (granulomatous enteritis). Both ulcerative colitis and Crohn's disease frequently affect a similar group of patients (Table 1), run a course characterized by exacerbations and remissions, tend to be chronic in nature, have similar extra-intestinal manifestations (Table 2) and may be associated with a positive family history of inflammatory bowel disease (1,2). While there are many similarities in the natural

Table 1.

POPULATION CHARACTERISTICS OF PATIENTS AT
HIGH RISK FOR DEVELOPING INFLAMMATORY
BOWEL DISEASE (6,9)

1. No sexual predilection.

2. Third to sixth decades of life.

3. Ethnic predilection for western (northern European,
   Anglo-Saxon, or northeastern European) greater than
   Oriental populations.

4. Urban greater than rural dwellers.

5. Caucasian.

6. Jews living in Europe and North America.

7. Occurs in familial clusters.

Table 2.

EXTRA-INTESTINAL COMPLICATIONS OF
ULCERATIVE COLITIS AND CROHN'S DISEASE
(1,4,5,10–12)

Manifestation	Ulcerative Colitis	Crohn's Disease
Arthritis/arthralgia	25%	33%
Erythema nodosum/ pyoderma gangrenosum	4%	5%
Abnormal liver function tests	50%	30%
Iritis/uveitis	5%	4%
Ankylosing spondylityis	15%	10%
Growth retardation	18%	13%

history and clinical features of these diseases, they differ extensively in their pathophysiology, anatomic distribution and clinical course (Table 3) (1,3–6).

When considering inflammatory bowel disease therapy, one must appreciate that the etiology of the disease is unknown and, therefore, precludes definitive therapy. Additionally, specific therapy will depend on the anatomical location of the disease. The major therapeutic goals should be to: induce remission, prevent relapse, and symptomatically control the clinical manifestations of the disease and its intestinal and extra-intestinal complications. This chapter will concentrate on the first two goals. Symptomatic treatment is covered in other chapters of this text.

ULCERATIVE COLITIS

1. *Pathophysiology and Clinical Presentation.* C.M. is a 25-year-old white female college student who has had episodic watery diarrhea and colicky abdominal pain, relieved by defecation, for the past nine months. Eight weeks prior to admission, the diarrhea increased to 3–5 semi-formed stools daily. The frequency of the stools gradually increased to 5–10 times per day one week ago. At this time, the patient noted bright red blood in the stools. Stool frequency has now increased to 10–15 per day and the volume of each stool is estimated to be only "one-half

cupful". She feels a great urgency to defecate even though the volume is small. She has not traveled outside the United States and has not taken any antibiotics recently.

The patient complained of anorexia and a ten pound weight loss over the past two months. For the past four months she has had intermittent swelling, warmth and tenderness of the left knee which is unassociated with trauma. She denied any difficulties with her eyes or skin rashes. A review of other body systems and social and family history were noncontributory.

She appears to be a slightly anxious and tired young female of normal body habitus. Her temperature is 101°F and her pulse rate is 100 and regular. Physical examination is normal except for evidence of acute arthritis of the left knee and tenderness of the left lower abdomen to palpation.

Stool examination shows a watery effluent that contains numerous red and white cells with no trophozoites. Stool cultures and an amebiasis indirect hemagglutination test are negative. Her hematocrit is 39% with a hemoglobin of 9 gm/dl; the WBC is 15,000/mm^3 with 82% PMNs; the erythrocyte sedimentation rate is 70 seconds (normal = <20mm/hr, Westergren); serum albumin is 2.4 gm/dl (3.5–5.0 gm/dl). Other pertinent laboratory values include an alkaline phosphatase of 210μ (normal = 30–110μ), an SGOT of 55μ (normal =

Table 3.

PATHOPHYSIOLOGIC DIFFERENCES BETWEEN ULCERATIVE
COLITIS AND CROHN'S DISEASE (1,3–6,13,14)

Characteristic	Ulcerative Colitis	Crohn's Disease
1. Incidence	6.4/100,000/year	5.5/100,000/year
2. Anatomical location	colon and rectum	mouth to anus
3. Distribution	continuous, diffuse, mucosal	segmental, focal, transmural
4. Bowel wall	shortened, loss of haustral markings, generally not thickened	rigid, thick, edematous and fibrotic
5. Gross rectal bleeding	common	infrequent
6. Crypt abscesses	common	less frequent
7. Fissuring with sinus formation	absent	common
8. Noncaseating granulomas	absent	common
9. Strictures	absent	common
10. Abdominal mass	infrequent	common
11. Abdominal pain	infrequent	common
12. Toxic megacolon	occasional	rare
13. Bowel carcinoma	greatly increased	slightly increased

10–40μ) and a serum potassium of 3.1 mEq/L (3.5–5.0 mEq/L).

Sigmoidoscopy gave evidence of a granular, edematous and friable mucosa with ulcerations extending from the anus to approximately 20 cm. A barium enema shows confluent disease extending from the rectum to transverse colon.

Which symptoms, signs and laboratory data are consistent with ulcerative colitis? Describe the pathophysiologic basis for C.M.'s clinical presentation.

Ulcerative colitis is an inflammation of the mucosal layer of the colon and rectum (4). Characteristically, the inflammation does not extend beyond the submucosa, and transmural ulcers are rare. Upon examination, the mucosa appears erythematous and is very friable. C.M. presents with the classical clinical symptoms of ulcerative colitis: chronic diarrhea, rectal bleeding and abdominal pain (15). The diarrhea is secondary to the decreased colonic absorption of water and electrolytes and to diminished colonic segmental contractions which normally serve to decrease bowel content flow. A good indication of the severity of the patient's disease is the volume of stool passed per day (4). As the severity of the disease increases, incontinence and nocturnal diarrhea commonly occur. In addition to the diarrhea, the malabsorption of water and electrolytes will cause dehydration, weight loss (as observed in C.M.), and electrolyte disturbances.

C.M.'s rectal bleeding is secondary to colonic mucosal erosions and occurs in essentially all patients with ulcerative colitis (1). Generally, bright red blood mixed in the stools indicates a colonic origin, whereas blood streaking of the stools indicates an anal or rectal origin. The anemia associated with ulcerative colitis is generally secondary to this rectal bleeding. It presents as a hemorrhagic or iron deficiency anemia depending upon the acuteness of the bleeding. C.M.'s hypoalbuminemia is also exacerbated by chronic colonic bleeding (4).

C.M.'s abdominal pain and cramping are caused by spasm of the irritated and inflamed colon. This abdominal pain, often called tenesmus, is commonly associated with urgency to defecate. As illustrated by C.M., the pain is usually relieved with defecation even though the stool volume may be small.

The patient's other signs and symptoms demonstrate that ulcerative colitis is a systemic disease and not just a disease of the gastrointestinal tract. Her nonspecific symptoms include anorexia, fatigue, weight loss, anxiety and tachycardia and may become profound in severe ulcerative colitis (4). The arthritis and elevated liver enzymes (alkaline phosphatase and SGOT) in this patient are indicative of the extra-intestinal manifestations that occur in ulcerative colitis (Table 2) (11). The fever, leukocytosis and increased sedimentation rate are also systemic manifestations of an inflammatory disease.

Remission Induction

2. What agents can be used to induce disease remission in this patient? What evidence is there to support your choice? By what mechanism do these agents exert their beneficial effects?

Corticosteroids. Corticosteroids are widely accepted as the most effective agents for the induction of remission of acute exacerbations of ulcerative colitis (7,8,16–18). This beneficial effect of corticosteroids was first demonstrated by Truelove and Witts in 1955 (19). In this comparative trial of cortisone and placebo, the cortisone was more effective in the induction of disease remission in all patients than was placebo, but the response rate decreased with increasing severity of the disease and was greater among patients with a first attack of the disease. Subsequent controlled trials with prednisone (20–23), prednisolone (24,25) and hydrocortisone (20,26–29) have confirmed the beneficial effects of corticosteroids in inducing remissions in these patients.

Even though corticosteroids are effective inducers of disease remission in patients with acute ulcerative colitis, they probably do not alter the underlying disease process (17). Their beneficial effect is thought to be exerted through their non-specific anti-inflammatory properties (16).

Sulfasalazine. Sulfasalazine has also been shown to induce remission in patients with acute exacerbations of ulcerative colitis (30,31). Dick and colleagues (31) demonstrated that 45% of their acute ulcerative colitis patients obtained remission from their disease after three weeks of sulfasalazine therapy. Sulfasalazine is commonly used as the initial therapeutic agent for inducing remission in mild attacks of ulcerative colitis because it is effective and safe relative to the corticosteroids (8,16). However, in a controlled trial, sulfasalazine was significantly less effective than corticosteroids in inducing remission after two weeks of treatment (76% with steroids, 52% with sulfasalazine) (32). The combination of sulfasalazine and corticosteroids is also used for remission induction in acute ulcerative colitis even though adequate controlled trials are not available to recommend this form of concomitant therapy (17,18).

3. Corticosteroids are available for administration by various routes: parenterally, topically, and orally. Which route of administration should be utilized for C.M.'s corticosteroid therapy?

Parenteral corticosteroids and hospitalization are mandatory for patients such as C.M. with severe acute ulcerative colitis to prevent its potentially dangerous progression (4,15,16,18). Recent studies have shown that the absorption and efficacy of oral corticosteroids are decreased in this type of patient (33). Truelove and Jewell (34) defined the patient population requiring parenteral corticosteroids as those having greater than six bloody stools per day, fever greater than 99.5°F, heart rate greater than 90 beats per minute, anemia, increased erythrocyte sedimentation rate and abdominal tenderness. C.M. meets these criteria and should receive corticosteroids by this route.

The question of which corticosteroid is best used parenterally in ulcerative colitis has been addressed extensively. Adrenal corticotrophic hormone (ACTH), which stimulates the endogenous release of corticosteroids, has been advocated as the parenteral agent of choice in this disease (17). Two recent controlled trials comparing the efficacy of ACTH to parenteral hydrocortisone have demonstrated no overall advantage of either agent; hydrocortisone, however, was superior in patients previously treated with corticosteroids (35,36). Since hydrocortisone has significant mineralocorticoid effects which may exacerbate electrolyte imbalances already induced by the ulcerative colitis, a synthetic corticosteroid with high anti-inflammatory and low mineralocorticoid properties, such as prednisone or methylprednisolone, should be used (15,18).

Parenteral corticosteroid therapy for ulcerative colitis should be designed to achieve a rapid therapeutic response. This may be attained with a high initial dose followed by a gradual dosage reduction to minimize development of corticosteroid adverse reactions (15). The initial dose, as well as the rate of a subsequent dosage reduction, should be individualized based on the severity of the patient's signs, symptoms, and disease course. Up to 75% of patients with severe ulcerative colitis will respond to corticosteroid doses equivalent to 160 mg prednisone daily; the majority respond to 60–80 mg prednisone or its equivalent per day (23).

4. When is the oral route of corticosteroid administration indicated in ulcerative colitis? What are the most appropriate dosages?

Oral corticosteroids are effective for the treatment of mild to moderate acute ulcerative colitis and may be substituted for parenteral corticosteroids once a satisfactory initial response has been achieved (8,16,18). As with parenteral corticosteroids, the dose should be individualized to the patient's disease course and symptomatology. In a controlled trial, 40 mg of prednisone daily was significantly more efficacious than 20 mg daily in controlling ambulatory patients with moderately severe acute ulcerative colitis (21). Sixty mg of prednisone daily had no additional therapeutic value but did cause more side effects. Additionally, a single 40 mg morning dose of prednisone was as effective and more convenient than an equivalent divided dose (10 mg qid). Furthermore, this dosage schedule was less toxic and less likely to cause adrenal suppression (22,37). Therefore, the initial dose of corticosteroid for a patient with moderately severe acute ulcerative colitis is 40 mg of prednisone or its equivalent administered once daily in the morning.

Oral corticosteroids should induce remission within two to four weeks, at which time an attempt should be made to gradually withdraw the drug (18). The total corticosteroid treatment course should last only four to eight weeks (16). If remission does not occur, the patient may require parenteral corticosteroids and hospitalization.

5. When are topical corticosteroids indicated in the management of acute ulcerative colitis? How do they exert their beneficial effect? What are the limitations for use of each topical corticosteroid dosage form in the treatment of this disease?

Topically administered corticosteroids, in the form of suppositories, foams and retention enemas, are effective in the management of acute mild ulcerative colitis which is limited to the distal colon and rectum (20,24–29,38–43). But, to justify the use of such a difficult and socially unacceptable route of administration, a clear-cut advantage of either increased efficacy or decreased side effects over other administration routes for these agents must be demonstrated.

Theoretically, corticosteroids administered via this topical route would provide a high concentration of drug to the diseased mucosal area, exerting a local anti-inflammatory effect while averting systemic side effects. Unfortunately, several well-designed investigations have established that variable but significant systemic absorption (up to 90%) and adrenal suppression does occur from the topical administration of corticosteroids to the rectum and distal colon (28, 29,44,45). Therefore, the beneficial effects produced by topical use of these agents may accrue from systemic as well as local effects. The relatively low incidence of corticosteroid side effects associated with topical administration, may be due to the low doses utilized and to the infrequent administration (1–2 times daily) needed to control mild acute ulcerative colitis (16). When prednisolone is given in equivalent doses orally and rectally, the incidence of side effects and therapeutic effects are similar (16).

If corticosteroids are to be utilized topically for the management of mild acute ulcerative colitis, the corticosteroid of choice would be the one with the lowest absorptive characteristics (44). Unfortunately, there is no comparative trial of the absorption characteristics of all corticosteroids available for administration by this route. The evidence available indicates that, of the hydrocortisone salts, the acetate is absorbed the least (28). Also, betamethasone valerate has been shown to cause less adrenal suppression than therapeutically equivalent doses of prednisolone-21-phosphate (43).

Since corticosteroid topical therapy of ulcerative colitis depends in theory on drug contact with the affected mucosa, the anatomical location of the disease and the distribution characteristics of the dosage form must be considered in the selection of the proper dosage form. For instance, if the disease is limited to the distal portion of the rectum (proctitis), corticosteroid *suppositories*, which have a very limited area of distribution and have been shown to be more effective than placebo suppositories, should be used (24). Two suppositories daily for four to six weeks is generally sufficient to induce disease remission in patients with mild acute proctitis (8).

Retention enemas of corticosteroids which will allow distribution of the drug to a much greater colonic area than the suppository dosage form can be utilized in patients with more extensive disease. Retention enemas can distribute corticosteroids proximal to the hepatic flexture (46), although the extent of drug distribution varies among patients (47). The enema volume can be individualized to the extent of the patient's disease by adding barium to the estimated enema volume needed and following its distribution by x-ray (47).

Corticosteroid retention enemas are best utilized at bedtime when the patient is inactive and better able to retain the medication for a prolonged period of time (15). Ideally, the enema should be instilled as a bolus, with the patient in the supine position. The patient should alternate positions every 20 minutes from supine to left decubitus to right decubitus to prone to promote maximal topical coverage (4). If the patient cannot retain the initial volume, it can be decreased and slowly dripped in over 20–30 minutes (16). Alternatively, foam preparations of corticosteroids have been advocated as a dosage form that is easier for patients to retain, although the extent to which the foam distributes proximally is unknown (39,40). If the patient cannot retain the enema, despite these measures, an alternate route of corticosteroid administration will have to be utilized.

6. What particular corticosteroid side effects are of importance in patients with ulcerative colitis specifically, and inflammatory bowel disease in general?

Corticosteroid side effects and precautions for use often limit the therapeutic effectiveness of these agents and should never be overlooked (49);

these are covered in detail elsewhere in this text (See Chapter on Disorders of the Adrenals). Certain glucocorticoid side effects are of particular importance in patients with inflammatory bowel disease in that they may mimic, mask or intensify symptoms or complications of this disease. For instance, it is well documented that corticosteroids cause cutaneous atrophy (50). Patients with ulcerative colitis are predisposed to intestinal wall perforation and drug-induced cutaneous atrophy will only intensify this predisposition. In addition, the symptoms of one of the major complications of intestinal perforation, peritonitis, may be masked by the use of corticosteroids. Drug-induced cutaneous atrophy and the decreased wound healing associated with corticosteroid use may contribute to operative morbidity and mortality in patients with inflammatory bowel disease (51), although this has been disputed (52). Other corticosteroid side effects that may be secondary to either the drug and/or the inflammatory bowel disease include retardation of growth and development in prepubertal patients; osteoporosis with secondary pathologic fractures and spinal column decompression; and hypokalemic alkalosis (49).

Maintenance of Remission

7. C.M.'s symptoms decreased significantly after an initial course of parenteral corticosteroids. She was successfully changed to 40 mg of oral prednisone once daily without recurrence of her disease symptoms. What drug regimen should be used to maintain a disease remission in this ulcerative colitis patient?

Oral *sulfasalazine* significantly reduces the incidence of relapse in ulcerative colitis patients who are in remission (31,53–55). In a double-blind controlled trial, 70% of patients taking 2 gm of sulfasalazine daily by mouth maintained disease remission, whereas only 21% of those receiving placebo were symptom-free after one year (54). This study was subsequently confirmed in patients for up to three years using sigmoidoscopic and biopsy abnormalities as relapse criteria (54). One investigation showed that as the dose of sulfasalazine was increased, both the prophylactic efficacy and the incidence of side effects of the drug increased (55). A two gram dose appeared to provide optimal balance between adverse and beneficial effects in these patients. Therefore, two grams is the recommended prophylactic dose, although the dose should be individualized if adverse effects appear or beneficial effects are not achieved (16).

Oral and topical corticosteroids are ineffective in preventing relapse of ulcerative colitis once remission has occurred (26,56,57). Studies have shown that 100 mg hydrocortisone hemisuccinate twice weekly by retention enema (26), 50 mg oral cortisone twice daily (56) or 15 mg oral prednisone daily (57) cause significant side effects and fail to maintain previously induced disease remission in ulcerative colitis patients.

On the basis of the above, C.M.'s prednisone should be gradually tapered and discontinued over a one to two-month period. Concomitantly, sulfasalazine (2 gm daily) should be initiated as prophylaxis against disease relapse. Prophylactic therapy should be continued indefinitely unless intolerable side effects develop (16,18).

8. By what mechanism does sulfasalazine maintain disease remission in patients with ulcerative colitis? Describe its absorption and elimination.

Sulfasalazine exerts an anti-inflammatory therapeutic effect through a complex series of events. Structurally, sulfasalazine is a combination of a sulfonamide antibiotic, sulfapyridine, in an azo linkage with 5-aminosalicylic acid. Following oral administration, 20–30% of the parent compound is absorbed in the proximal small intestine (58,59). The absorbed sulfasalazine is not metabolized *in vivo*; 25–50% of the absorbed drug is excreted unchanged in the bile and the remainder is excreted by the kidneys (59). Ultimately, 75–85% of the oral dose reaches the colon where diazo bond cleavage by bacterial azo-reductases produces sulfapyridine and 5-aminosalicylic acid (58,60–63). It appears that the ability to split the azo linkage is inherent in the majority of bacterial species normally found in the human intestine (60). The liberated sulfapyridine is readily absorbed and metabolized in liver by acetylation, hydroxylation and glucuronidation before it is excreted in the urine as the metabolite or free drug (64). Since the acetylation rate of sulfapyridine is genetically determined (65,66), its half-life of elimination is dependent on the patient's acetylation phenotype and varies between 5–13 hours (67).

The 5-aminosalicylate liberated in the colon is poorly absorbed (68), although a small portion can be recovered in the urine in the acetylated form (69). This is in contrast to orally administered 5-aminosalicylic acid which is well absorbed proximally in the gastrointestinal tract (16). Factors that alter the normal absorption and metabolism of sulfasalazine and therefore increase the amount of unaltered sulfasalazine excreted in the feces and decrease the amount of liberated sulfapyridine and 5-aminosalicylic acid include a rapid intestinal transit time (69,70), a sterile colon (60–63), and surgical removal of the colon (63).

Recent evidence indicates that the beneficial activity of sulfasalazine is due to the local effects of 5-aminosalicylic acid, not the sulfapyridine component (68,71,72). In two double-blind controlled trials, both 5-aminosalicylate and sulfasalazine were significantly more effective than sulfapyridine in the treatment of patients with inflammatory bowel diseases (68,71). In another study, 5-aminosalicylate was significantly more effective than sulfapyridine or placebo in preventing disease relapses in ulcerative colitis patients (72). Furthermore, 5-aminosalicylic acid and sulfasalazine inhibit prostaglandin synthetase activity, whereas sulfapyridine does not (73–75). It is well known that prostaglandins play a significant role in the inflammatory process (76). Patients with acute untreated ulcerative colitis have high levels of prostaglandins in the stool, colonic venous blood and urine (74,75,77–79), as well as increased prostaglandin synthetase activity in rectal mucosal biopsy specimens (80). Therefore, prostaglandins probably contribute to the pathogenesis of ulcerative colitis.

On the basis of this evidence, sulfasalazine most likely serves as a carrier molecule which delivers the active moiety, 5-aminosalicylic acid, to the diseased colonic mucosa in relatively high concentrations. There, 5-aminosalicylic acid inhibits prostaglandin synthesis locally and supresses inflammation.

9. What are the adverse effects of sulfasalazine which must be monitored in C.M? What are their etiologies? How can they be minimized?

Sulfasalazine adverse effects occur frequently (21%–88% of patients) (66,81). They can cause significant morbidity and often limit the drug's clinical usefulness. These adverse effects appear to be of two types: dose-related or idiosyncratic. See Table 4.

The majority of sulfasalazine adverse reactions are dose-related (81) and occur more frequently when the dose is four or more grams per day (32,55,66,81). These adverse effects correlate

Table 4.

SULFASALAZINE ADVERSE EFFECTS

	Reference
I. Dose-Related Reactions	
A. *General*	
Nausea, vomiting, anorexia headache, fever, arthralgias	55, 66, 81
B. *Hematologic*	
Heinz body anemia	81, 83, 84, 85
G-6-PD deficiency hemolytic anemia	85, 86, 87, 88
Reticulocytosis	16, 55, 87
Leukopenia	17
Megaloblastic anemia	89, 90
C. *Others*	
Cyanosis	53, 81
Male infertility	91, 92, 93
Neonatal kernicterus	94
II. Idiosyncratic Reactions	
A. *Hematologic*	
Agranulocytosis	95
Autoimmune hemolytic anemia	85, 87, 88, 96
B. *Dermatologic*	
Skin rash	81, 97, 98, 99
Toxic epidermal necrolysis	100
Exfoliative dermatitis	16, 81
C. *Pulmonary*	
Bronchospasm, infiltrates, eosinophilia, fibrosing alveolitis	101, 102, 103
D. *Gastrointestinal*	
Hepatotoxicity	97, 98, 99, 104, 105, 106
Pancreatitis	107
E. *Other*	
Lupus-like syndrome	108
Raynaud's phenomenon	109
Nephrotic syndrome	97
Paresthesias	110

more specifically to serum concentrations of sulfapyridine which exceed 50 mcg/ml (55,66,68,81). Since sulfapyridine is acetylated (65,66), genetically-determined slow acetylators (60% of the population) (82) experience a higher incidence of the "dose-related" adverse effects than fast acetylators (55,66,70,81).

Generally, sulfasalazine dose-related adverse effects occur early in the course of therapy. It is important to note that the concurrent use of corticosteroids may mask certain adverse effects of sulfasalazine (eg, malaise, arthralgia, rash, fever, etc.) and these will become apparent once the corticosteroids are withdrawn (17).

Dose-related sulfasalazine adverse effects can be minimized by initiating the patient on a low dose (0.5 gm daily) and gradually increasing the amount to tolerated therapeutic levels of 2–4 gm per day (17,53,55,81). If dose-related reactions do occur, the drug should be discontinued until the symptoms subside; then, sulfasalazine should be reinstituted at a lower dosage. Although enteric-coated sulfasalazine tablets are available, they offer no demonstrated advantage and because they are also more expensive, their use is unjustified.

Idiosyncratic reactions to sulfasalazine are rare, but they cause significantly more morbidity and mortality. Since many of these reactions are similar to the sensitivity reactions associated with the sulfonamide derivatives, they are thought to be secondary to the sulfapyridine component of the parent compound (4). The severe sequelae associated with these reactions may be minimized through vigilance for the occurrence of these reactions, avoidance of the use of sulfasalazine in patients with documented sensitivity reactions to sulfonamides, and prompt withdrawal of sulfasalazine at the first indication that such a reaction is occurring.

10. What drugs can interact with C.M.'s sulfasalazine therapy?

Since bacterial cleavage of sulfasalazine's diazo bond is necessary to liberate its active moiety, 5-aminosalicylic acid, concomitant therapy with antibiotics could theoretically diminish this activity (64). Liberated sulfapyridine itself will suppress some bacterial species in patients with inflammatory bowel disease (111); however, a significant drug interaction does not occur because most *E. coli* are resistant to this sulfonamide derivative (112). Since the majority of intestinal bacteria have the ability to split the azo linkage of sulfasalazine (60), the clinical significance of an antibiotic-sulfasalazine interaction is probably minimal.

Therapeutic serum levels of sulfapyridine are produced following the administration of sulfasalazine (58,60–63); therefore, drugs which interact with sulfonamides, in general, must be used cautiously in patients taking sulfasalazine. The majority of sulfapyridine interactions occur as a result of competitive protein binding with other highly bound agents—for example, the coumarin anticoagulants (113), oral hypoglycemic agents (114) and bilirubin (94).

The concomitant administration of ferrous sulfate and sulfasalazine results in reduced sulfasalazine serum levels (115). This is probably secondary to iron-salicylate chelation in the gastrointestinal tract resulting in decreased absorption of the sulfasalazine. Although it has not been demonstrated, this chelation should also decrease the absorption of iron that is often prescribed for patients with anemia secondary to the inflammatory bowel disease. This phenomenon can be minimized by maximizing the interval between the administration of the individual agents.

Other sulfasalazine drug interactions include interference with folic acid absorption (89,90) and decreased serum digoxin levels (116).

11. What additional drugs have been or are used to either induce or maintain disease remission in patients with ulcerative colitis? What is their demonstrated efficacy?

Immunosuppressive agents such as azathioprine (117–119), 6-mercaptopurine (120,121), 6-thioguanine, busulphan, nitrogen mustards and cyclophosphamide have been used to treat ulcerative colitis patients (122). Of these agents, only azathioprine has been studied sufficiently. Although initial clinical observations were favorable, subsequent double-blind trials indicate that these agents are ineffective in most cases of ulcerative colitis. In a controlled double-blind study, 2.5 mg/kg/day of azathioprine added to a standard corticosteroid regimen had a negligible effect on inducing remission of an acute ulcerative colitis attack (117). These investigators continued the trial for one year to determine the effect of azathioprine on the rate of relapse of ulcerative colitis. Although not significant, there was a favorable trend for azathioprine in those patients

treated after a relapse of colitis. This contrasts to a trial of azathioprine versus sulfasalazine in maintaining patients in disease remission which showed no difference in efficacy, although no placebo control was used (118). One additional study demonstrated that even though azathioprine had no effect on the overall clinical course of the ulcerative colitis, it did permit a significant reduction of the corticosteroid dose in steroid-dependent patients (119). In summary, azathioprine may have a limited effect in maintaining remission of ulcerative colitis; however, serious adverse-effects (eg, leukopenia, thrombocytopenia, alopecia, liver damage, etc.) occur in almost all patients and this offsets its limited value (123).

Cromolyn sodium (disodium cromoglycerate), which inhibits the release of inflammatory substances from sensitized mast cells, has been used to alter the clinical course of ulcerative colitis (124–129). In an initial trial, topically applied cromolyn sodium was more effective than placebo in preventing acute attacks of ulcerative colitis (124). This trial was supported to some extent by Mani and colleagues (125) who studied cromolyn sodium in patients taking sulfasalazine to maintain remission of the ulcerative colitis. Although the relapse rate was unchanged, there were significant improvements in the patients' sense of well being, and in the sigmoidoscopic and rectal biopsy appearances in the cromolyn sodium group. Conversely, recent studies have shown that this drug is no better than placebo when given by mouth to patients with chronic active ulcerative colitis (126); furthermore, it was statistically less effective than sulfasalazine in maintaining remission of the disease (127–129). Additional studies are needed to define the role of cromolyn sodium in the treatment of ulcerative colitis.

Toxic Megacolon

12. One year has passed since C.M. last had an acute attack of ulcerative colitis. She has been taking sulfasalazine 1 gm tid only. She now presents with a fever of 104°F, a heart rate of 110 beats per minute, abdominal pain, weakness, and a sudden decrease in frequency of bowel movements. Physical examination discloses abdominal distention with non-localized rebound tenderness, tympany, and an absence of bowel sounds. Ab-

normal laboratory values include a leuko-cytosis of 15,000 WBC/mm³ and a serum potassium of 3.0 mEq/L. A plain x-ray of the abdomen shows the transverse colon to be dilated to 9 cm. What is the most probable cause of C.M.'s symptoms? What are poten-tial sequelae of this complication of inflam-matory bowel disease? What drugs ought to be avoided in this patient? What medical therapeutic modalities ought to be con-sidered?

C.M.'s signs and symptoms are consistent with an acute dilation of the colon associated with sys-temic toxemia. This complication of ulcerative co-litis, commonly referred to as toxic megacolon, is reported to occur in 1.6–13% of patients with this disease (14,130). Toxic megacolon is also a com-plication of Crohn's colitis and ileocolitis (131–133).

Toxic megacolon represents the most life-threatening complication of inflammatory bowel disease and has an overall mortality rate of up to 30% (134). Signs and symptoms present in C.M. which are consistent with toxic megacolon in-clude prostration, a fever greater than 101.5°F, tachycardia, electrolyte imbalance, abdominal pain and tenderness, leukocytosis, dilation of the colon to a diameter greater than 6 cm, and signs of diminished colonic peristalsis as evidenced by de-creased stool frequency and the absence of bowel sounds. Other signs which are consistent with this diagnosis but which are not illustrated by C.M. include dehydration, anemia, and hypoalbumi-nemia (4,135).

C.M. is hypokalemic; this decreases the mus-cular tone and predisposes her to the develop-ment of toxic megacolon. Other factors which pre-dispose patients with inflammatory bowel disease to toxic megacolon include antispasmodics such as the opiates or anticholinergic agents (134, 136,137); irritant cathartics such as castor oil; barium enemas (135,138); and hypoproteinemia which produces bowel wall edema.

Colonic perforation followed by peritonitis and hemorrhage are the major complications of toxic megacolon (135). C.M.'s condition should be con-sidered a medical emergency.

General supportive measures are used to ar-rest the necrotic process taking place in the colon (4,135). C.M.'s bowel should be put to rest. Noth-ing should be taken by mouth and nasogastric suction should be initiated to prevent passage of swallowed air and fluid into the colon. Fluid and electrolyte imbalances must be corrected. In C.M.'s case, the hypokalemia which predisposes her to toxic megacolon should be corrected as quickly as possible. She should also be given adequate nu-tritional support, including total parenteral nu-trition if a prolonged course is anticipated. High doses of corticosteroids should be initiated. C.M. is not currently taking steroids, but if she were, the dose would need to be increased to prevent adrenal insufficiency. A blood sample should be sent for culture and sensitivity and C.M. should be initiated on empiric antibiotic therapy since she exhibits signs and symptoms of systemic bac-teremia (leukocytosis, fever, prostration). There must be antibiotic coverage for anaerobes since these bacteria occur in large numbers in the colon (eg, clindamycin). Other measures which may be appropriate in other patients with toxic megaco-lon would include discontinuance of any drugs (opiates, anticholinergic agents) which might be predisposing the patient to this condition and blood transfusions to correct any existing anemia or hy-poalbuminemia. C.M. must be monitored care-fully for signs of improvement or persistent dil-atation, perforation, peritonitis and hemorrhage.

Surgical Management

13. C.M. has been treated as described above for three days. Nevertheless, her ab-dominal plain x-rays indicate no diminution in the caliber of the distended bowel, her temperature continues to spike to 103°F with negative blood cultures, and the abdomen re-mains distended and silent. Fluid and elec-trolyte imbalances have been restored. How should the patient be managed at this point?

Within the first 72 hours of therapy and ob-servation, the need for corrective surgery will be determined (4,135). There are three general pat-terns of response: improvement, status quo or de-terioration (135).

Those who improve with medical therapy dem-onstrate decreased colonic distention, a return of bowel sounds and a decreased pulse and temper-ature. Medical management should be continued in these patients as long as they continue to show a progressive beneficial response. Unfortunately, only 6–30% of toxic megacolon patients respond satisfactorily to medical therapy. (134–135).

C.M.'s course is illustrative of the majority of toxic megacolon patients who show fluctuating degrees of response to medical management. These patients may appear to respond initially with decreased tachycardia and fever, but become toxic again in 2–3 days. Despite signs of improvement, there is little or no change in bowel sounds or colonic size. Perforation of the colon may occur in as many as 50% of these individuals (4) unless they are surgically managed (subtotal colectomy and ileostomy) (134,135). Several studies have demonstrated that early surgery will reduce the overall mortality rate in patients such as C.M. (140–142).

Some patients with toxic megacolon deteriorate despite medical therapy. In these individuals, any of the following constitutes a surgical emergency (135): free perforation or peritonitis; severe, localized tenderness usually over the left quadrant; septic shock; and massive hemorrhage. Even with immediate surgery, mortality will be 50% in this group (134).

14. What factors are considered in determining whether surgery is indicated for a patient with ulcerative colitis? What are the indications for surgery in ulcerative colitis patients besides unresponsive toxic megacolon as described above?

Of the various therapeutic modalities available for the management of ulcerative colitis, surgery is the most definitive form of therapy in that it is curative in most instances (4,143). Since the lesion of ulcerative colitis is generally localized and continuous, colectomy will remove the primary focus of the disease. It will also eliminate both the extra-intestinal and local complications of ulcerative colitis in most patients. Unfortunately, the operative mortality for an elective colectomy with ileostomy is at least 2% (141). Additionally, patients may require further surgery for anastomotic leaks, intraperitoneal abscesses, adhesions, obstruction, stomal ileitis and mechanical problems associated with the ileostomy (4). Patient acceptability of ileostomies is also poor and major psychological adjustments are required of the patients and their families (144,145). Patients must be given support and educated with regard to the care of their ileostomies; this includes the prevention and management of common skin problems as well as control of odor and leakage of the effluent (145,146). Therefore, even though ulcerative colitis can be cured by surgery, it is indicated only after all reasonable non-operative forms of therapy have been exhausted.

Surgery is indicated in the treatment of ulcerative colitis when the patient fails to respond to medical management acutely or chronically; develops uncontrollable drug-related complications; becomes incapacitated from the disease or its drug therapy; fails to grow and develop at a normal rate; or develops carcinoma of the rectum or colon (4,8,17,147). Additionally, patients who have had universal colitis for more than ten years or who demonstrate premalignant changes on rectal biopsy are surgically managed as a prophylactic measure against colonic carcinoma (149–151).

CROHN'S DISEASE

15. *Pathophysiology and Clinical Presentation.* J.P. is a 30-year-old white male who was entirely well until 18 months ago when he developed crampy right lower quadrant abdominal pain associated with an increased frequency of semi-formed stools (4–5 per day). The pain was episodic at first, exacerbated by meals and somewhat relieved by defecation. During this period of time, the patient experienced anorexia and a 15-pound weight loss. He denied any changes in vision, joint pains, or the appearance of skin rashes. He has not traveled out of the United States or taken antibiotics recently.

Physical examination was essentially normal except for a temperature of 99.5°F and soft, loose, watery stools that were streaked with fat and guaiac positive. There was tenderness of the abdomen upon palpation of the right lower quadrant. Pertinent laboratory values included a hematocrit of 38%, hemoglobin of 9 gm/dl, WBC of 14,000/mm³, and an erythrocyte sedimentation rate of 60 seconds (normal <20 mm/hr, Westergren).

Sigmoidoscopy and rectal biopsy were negative. Stool cultures were negative, as was the examination for signs of trophozoites. A barium enema showed an edematous ileocecal valve and a terminal ileum which had a nodular irregularity of the mucosa.

Which of J.P.'s symptoms, signs and laboratory data are consistent with Crohn's disease? Describe the pathophysiologic basis for this patient's clinical presentation.

Crohn's disease is a granulomatous inflammatory process which may involve any portion of the digestive tract from the mouth to the anus (1,5,6,152,153). Unlike ulcerative colitis, the inflammation is characteristically transmural and this leads to deep ulcerations, adhesions which connect loops of bowel to one another or the peritoneum, and fistula formation (5,11). The inflammatory process is typically patchy with diseased bowel separated by lengths of normal bowel. The majority of patients (55%) have disease involving the colon and terminal ileum (ileocolitis); an additional 14% have disease which is confined to the terminal ileum (terminal ileitis), 3% have involvement of other areas in the small intestine and 15% have disease which is restricted to the colon (153). The location of the disease within the gastrointestinal tract is a partial determinant of the patient's clinical presentation as well as disease complications (153,154).

J.P., like the vast majority of patients with Crohn's disease, presents with the classical triad of abdominal pain, diarrhea, and weight loss (1). He also complains of the most frequent symptom, right lower quadrant abdominal pain, which is secondary to an indolent inflammatory process in the ileocecal area (5). Diarrhea is also a characteristic symptom; however, in contrast to ulcerative colitis, the stools are usually partly formed and there is generally no gross blood visible. If the disease is limited to the colon, the diarrhea may be of the same quality and quantity as that associated with ulcerative colitis. If the disease is limited to the ileum, as it appears to be with J.P., the diarrhea is generally moderate, with four to six stools daily. Also, if there is significant ileal involvement, bile salt malabsorption will occur resulting in steatorrhea. Weight loss may be pronounced in patients with long-standing Crohn's disease (1); this is due to anorexia and malabsorption secondary to fistula formation which bypasses large sections of the small bowel, the blind loop syndrome, and bile salt malabsorption.

Another common symptom of Crohn's disease exhibited by J.P. is a low grade fever which rarely exceeds 102°F unless disease complications (eg, infection, intra-abdominal abscess or fistula formation) occur (5). Fever may be the earliest and only manifestation of this disease.

Rectal bleeding occurs in patients with Crohn's disease, particularly those with colonic involvement, although it is not as common as that associated with ulcerative colitis (153,154). Slow blood loss may occur in patients with disease limited to the small intestine and this may cause positive guaiac feces and eventually iron-deficiency anemia. This is illustrated by J.P. Massive hemorrhage is usually a late complication of Crohn's disease and generally is due to transmural ulceration and subsequent erosion into a major blood vessel.

J.P.'s leukocytosis and increased erythrocyte sedimentation rate demonstrate that, like ulcerative colitis, Crohn's disease is a systemic disease. Extra-intestinal manifestations such as arthritis, liver disease, and skin rash occur in Crohn's disease with the same frequency as ulcerative colitis (Table 2) (1,11).

Most patients with Crohn's disease have recurrent, symptomatic episodes of pain and diarrhea with gradual progression of their disease to shorter and shorter asymptomatic periods (5). Although the clinical course is generally progressive, 10% of the patients will remain essentially asymptomatic after a few acute episodes (152). Other patients may only manifest a slight fever for years until a late complication of the disease such as fistula formation develops. Alternatively, Crohn's disease may be rapidly progressive (153).

Remission Induction

16. What agents can be utilized to induce a remission of J.P.'s Crohn's disease? What evidence is there to support the use of these agents?

Since the clinical course of Crohn's disease varies so tremendously among patients (152,154), the management of this disease must be individualized to the patient's condition (5). The anatomical location of the disease is also an important determinant of therapy (155). Unfortunately, the latter has only recently been recognized as an important consideration in the determination of therapy. The majority of investigations evaluating the treatment of acute symptomatic Crohn's disease have ignored this factor, and are therefore difficult to assess.

Corticosteroids. Corticosteroids are the most widely used therapeutic agents for the treatment of active, symptomatic Crohn's disease (156). Initial uncontrolled reports of the use of these agents to induce disease remission were encouraging (156–158). Subsequently, three large retrospective studies confirmed that 50–90% of patients treated with corticosteroids improved as manifested by an increased appetite; decreased fever, pain and diarrhea; increased sense of well-being; increased hematocrit and decreased erythrocyte sedimentation rate (160–162). These studies also demonstrated that clinical improvement did not necessarily correlate with improvement in roentgenogram results and that the beneficial effects appeared to be short-term. The only double-blind, controlled trial of corticosteroid treatment of acute symptomatic Crohn's disease has been the National Cooperative Crohn's Disease Study (NCCDS) which reported its findings in 1979 (155). The results indicate that a dose of 0.25–0.75 mg/kg/day of prednisone adjusted to the severity of the patient's disease, was significantly superior to placebo in inducing remission during a four-month trial period (60% with prednisone; 30% with placebo). When the anatomical location of the disease was considered, prednisone was significantly more effective than placebo in patients with involvement of the ileum alone or ileum and colon than when the disease was confined to the colon.

Sulfasalazine. Sulfasalazine is also widely recommended and utilized in treating mildly symptomatic Crohn's disease patients (17,18), although there are only two controlled trials on which to base this use (155,163). In both of these investigations sulfasalazine was significantly superior to placebo in the induction of Crohn's disease remission. The NCCDS found that although sulfasalazine was more effective than placebo, it was less effective when compared to prednisone (155). In addition, these investigators demonstrated that the beneficial effect of sulfasalazine was confined to patients with disease involving the colon or the colon and ileum; sulfasalazine was not effective in patients with small bowel disease (155). This is not unexpected since colonic bacterial metabolism of sulfasalazine is necessary to release the active moiety, 5-aminosalicylic acid (see Question 8) (68,71,72).

There are other relevant observations concerning the use of sulfasalazine and corticosteroids in inducing remission of Crohn's disease. Previously untreated patients respond better to sulfasalazine than placebo or prednisone, and patients who are unresponsive to prednisone are unlikely to be responsive to sulfasalazine (155). The combination of prednisone and sulfasalazine is no more effective than prednisone therapy alone and the total dose of prednisone needed to control the disease symptoms is not decreased with the addition of sulfasalazine (164). Additionally, extra-intestinal manifestations of Crohn's disease do not significantly improve with corticosteroid or sulfasalazine therapy (155).

Based on this information, the drug therapy recommendations for remission induction in Crohn's disease patients are as follows:

1. For patients with disease confined to the colon, prescribe sulfasalazine.

2. For patients with disease confined to the small bowel (such as J.P.) prescribe prednisone.

3. Previously untreated patients with disease of the ileum and colon should receive sulfasalazine. If there is no response within four months, the patient should be switched to prednisone.

Remission Maintenance

17. After four weeks of prednisone (40 mg daily), J.P. experienced fewer symptoms of Crohn's disease: 1–2 well-formed stools per day, increased appetite and weight, decreased abdominal pain and tenderness, and normal body temperatures. Should the prednisone be discontinued? What agents are effective in maintaining remission of symptoms in patients with Crohn's disease?

Once prednisone has induced remission of active symptomatic Crohn's disease, attempts should be made to slowly reduce the dose (18). The NCCDS demonstrated that the incidence of relapse was the same whether corticosteroids were continued or discontinued in patients with quiescent Crohn's disease (155). This study confirms retrospective observations (160–162) and several controlled trials (165–168) which show that continued corticosteroid therapy in this group of patients is ineffective in preventing relapse and may be associated with increased mortality and need for surgical intervention.

The NCCDS also demonstrated that the continued use of sulfasalazine in patients with asymptomatic Crohn's disease was not significantly more effective in preventing recurrence of symptoms than placebo during a two-year period (155). These findings are in agreement with earlier observations and conclusions from controlled trials (163,166,169,170).

In summary, J.P. should not be maintained on any drugs during the remission phase since long-term prophylactic therapy with sulfasalazine or corticosteroids is ineffective in preventing relapse of active symptomatic Crohn's disease. Additionally, the problems that arise from long-term therapy with these drugs may be qualitatively and quantitatively greater than no therapy in such patients (155,171).

Chronic Symptomatic Crohn's Disease

18. Five weeks after starting to taper J.P.'s prednisone dosage (currently taking 10 mg per day), the patient complains of increased diarrhea (3–4 watery stools per day), fevers of 100°F, and increased abdominal pain. What is your recommendation?

In the majority of patients who have been treated with corticosteroids to induce remission of active symptomatic Crohn's disease, reduction of the corticosteroid dosage will result in exacerbation of disease symptoms (18). In the NCCDS, only 40% of patients receiving remission induction with prednisone could be withdrawn completely from the drug (155). Furthermore, 30% of those patients experienced at least one flare-up of symptoms before they were withdrawn completely. The addition of sulfasalazine does not facilitate prednisone withdrawal (164).

A significant portion of patients with Crohn's disease experience mild symptoms chronically (5,153) and up to 50% of Crohn's disease patients will require continued low-dose corticosteroid treatment (5–15 mg of prednisone per day) to suppress these symptoms (16,172). Withdrawal of corticosteroids in this group of patients results in significant clinical deterioration (155).

In patients who require continued corticosteroid therapy to suppress symptoms of Crohn's disease, concomitant immunosuppressive therapy significantly reduces the corticosteroid dosage requirement (173–175). Of the immunosuppressive agents tested in this situation, azathioprine has been suggested as the agent of choice (18). The possible steroid-sparing effect of immunosuppressive agents must be weighed against their potentially severe adverse effects (eg, bone marrow suppression and increased incidence of malignancy) (171,176,177). In J.P.'s case, the prednisone dose should first be increased to a level that suppresses his symptoms. This should be followed by repeated attempts to withdraw the drug. If

these attempts are unsuccessful, J.P. may require chronic corticosteroid suppressive therapy; the addition of azathioprine for its corticosteroid-sparing effect is also a possible consideration.

19. What additional drugs have been or are used to either induce or maintain remission in patients with Crohn's disease? What is their demonstrated efficacy?

Immunosuppressive agents, with azathioprine being the most widely studied, have been utilized to induce and maintain remission in patients with Crohn's disease (123). The NCCDS has shown that azathioprine is no more effective than placebo in inducing remission; the anatomical distribution of the disease was not a factor in this lack of response (155). Although this conclusion supports the results of several controlled trials (178,179), there is at least one controlled study which found azathioprine to be effective (175). The use of immunosuppressives for the maintenance of remission in patients with Crohn's disease is controversial (123). The NCCDS showed that azathioprine alone, in a dose of 1 mg/kg/day, was no more effective than placebo in preventing disease relapse (155). This is in agreement with a trial by Watson (180), but contradicts the conclusions of Willoughby (173) and O'Donoghue (176) who found that larger doses of azathioprine, 2 mg/kg/day, may maintain disease remission. Because the risk of toxicity from these agents is great and because an azathioprine-responsive group of patients cannot be predicted, additional investigations into immunosuppressive maintenance therapy of quiescent Crohn's disease are warranted before routine use can be justified.

Investigations into other forms of drug therapy of Crohn's disease have recently produced some interesting findings. *Metronidazole,* in preliminary studies, has been shown to be effective in the treatment of patients with Crohn's disease confined to the colon or perianal area, but not in patients with ileocolitis or ileitis (181,182). Larger controlled studies are necessary to define its role in the treatment of Crohn's disease. It has also been suggested that nonspecific immunostimulant agents such as levamisole and BCG vaccine may have a beneficial effect in Crohn's disease (183); however, there is little evidence at present to indicate that these agents are efficacious in this disease state (184,185).

Surgical Management

20. After six years of remission, J.P. is hospitalized for an acute exacerbation of right lower quadrant pain associated with abdominal distention, lack of bowel movements, and vomiting over the last 24 hours. Roentgenographic studies indicate partial small bowel obstruction at the terminal ileum. Surgery revealed that the mucosa of the terminal 40 cm of the ileum was inflamed and thickened. In all, 50 cm of the terminal ileum was removed along with the ascending colon to the hepatic flexure. The remaining small bowel was anastomosed directly to the transverse colon. What factors are considered in determining whether surgery is indicated in Crohn's disease? What are the indications for surgery in Crohn's disease?

Since medical therapy of Crohn's disease is often inadequate, 78% of all patients with this disease will undergo surgery within 20 years of symptom onset (186). In contrast to ulcerative colitis, however, surgical removal of the involved bowel in Crohn's disease is not a definitive form of therapy (5,143). Crohn's disease can recur even after extensive resections. Various investigations have determined that cumulative recurrence rates after surgery for this disease are as high as 80%, depending on the surgical procedure and disease location (154,187,188). Therefore, multiple operations, and all their attendant risks, are often necessary over the life span of the Crohn's disease patient (143). Depending on the amount and site of the bowel removed during surgery, specific malabsorption syndromes can occur (eg, vitamin B_{12} malabsorption with removal of the terminal ileum) (5). If an ileostomy is part of the surgical procedure, the patient will have to undergo significant psychosocial adjustments (see Question 14). Therefore, surgery is indicated only for specific complications which are unresponsive to alternate forms of therapy and should be postponed whenever possible.

Generally accepted indications for surgical intervention in patients with Crohn's disease include (17,143,147,148,153) failure of medical management; incapacitation due to the disease or its drug therapy; retarded growth and development; intestinal obstruction; fistula formation; abscess formation; toxic megacolon; perforation and hemorrhage; and carcinoma.

References

1. Farmer RG: Clinical features and nature history of inflammatory bowel disease. Med Clin North Am. 1980; 64:1103.
2. Farmer RG et al: Studies of family history among patients with inflammatory bowel disease. Clin Gastro. 1980; 9:271.
3. Huizenga KA: Symptoms, signs and pathophysiology of bowel complications of chronic ulcerative colitis and Crohn's colitis. In *Inflammatory Bowel Disease,* edited by JB Kirsner and RG Shorter, Lea and Febiger, Philadelphia, 1975, p 109.
4. Cello JP et al: Ulcerative colitis. In *Gastrointestinal Disease,* 2nd ed, edited by MH Sleisenger and JS Fordtran, Saunders, Philadelphia, 1978, p 1597.
5. Donaldson RM: Crohn's disease of the small bowel. In *Gastrointestinal Disease,* 2nd ed, edited by MH Sleisenger and JS Fordtran, Saunders, Philadelphia, 1978, p 1052.
6. Cello JP et al: Crohn's disease of the colon. In *Gastrointestinal Disease,* 2nd ed, edited by MH Sleisenger and JS Fordtran, Saunders, Philadelphia, 1978, p 1658.
7. Northfield TC: Ulcerative colitis and Crohn's colitis: differential diagnosis and treatment. Drugs. 1977; 14:198.
8. Jacknowitz AI: Ulcerative colitis and its treatment. Am J Hosp Pharm. 1980; 37:1635.
9. Mendeloff AI: The epidemiology of inflammatory bowel disease. Clin Gastro. 1980; 9:259.
10. Rankin GB et al: National Cooperative Crohn's Disease Study: Extra intestinal manifestations and perianal complications. Gastroenterology. 1979; 77:914.
11. Smith JN et al: Complications and extraintestinal problems in inflammatory bowel disease. Med Clin North Am. 1980; 64:1161.
12. Kern F: Extraintestinal complications of chronic ulcerative and Crohn's disease of the colon. In *Inflammatory Bowel Disease,* edited by JB Kirsner and RG Shorter, Lea and Febiger, Philadelphia, 1975, p 127.
13. Brahme F et al: Crohn's disease in a defined population. Gastroenterology. 1975; 69:342.
14. Edwards FC et al: The course and prognosis of ulcerative colitis III. Complications. Gut. 1964; 5:1.
15. Rosenbert IH et al: Gastrointestinal disorders. In *Clinical Pharmacology,* 2nd ed, edited by K Melmon and H Morrelli, Macmillan, New York, 1978, p 432.
16. Lennard-Jones JE et al: Drug treatment of inflammatory bowel disease. Clin Gastro. 1979; 8:187.

17. Korelitz BI: Therapy of inflammatory bowel disease, including use of immunosuppressive agents. Clin Gastro. 1980; 9:331.

18. Singleton JW: Medical therapy of inflammatory bowel disease. Med Clin North Am. 1980; 64:1117.

19. Truelove SC et al: Cortisone in ulcerative colitis. Br Med J. 1955; 2:1041.

20. Lennard-Jones JE et al: Assessment of prednisone, salazopyrin and topical hydrocortisone hemisuccinate used as out-patient treatment for ulcerative colitis. Gut. 1960; 1:217.

21. Baron JH et al: Out-patient treatment of ulcerative colitis: comparison between three doses of oral prednisone. Br Med J. 1962; 2:441.

22. Powell-Tuck J et al: A comparison of oral prednisone given as single or multiple daily doses for active proctocolitis. Scand J Gastroenterol. 1978; 13:833.

23. Kristensen M et al: High dose prednisone treatment in severe ulcerative colitis. Scand J Gastroenterol. 1974; 9:177.

24. Lennard-Jones JE et al: A double-blind controlled trial of prednisolone-21-phosphate suppositories in treatment of idiopathic proctitis. Gut. 1962; 3:207.

25. Matts SGF: Local treatment of ulcerative colitis with prednisolone-21-phosphate enemas. Lancet. 1960; 1:517.

26. Truelove SC: Treatment of ulcerative colitis with local hydrocortisone hemisuccinate sodium. A report on a controlled therapeutic trial. Br Med J. 1958; 2:1072.

27. Watkinson G: Treatment of ulcerative colitis with topical hydrocortisone hemisuccinate sodium. A controlled trial employing restricted sequential analysis. Br Med J. 1958; 2:1077.

28. Farmer RG et al: Treatment of ulcerative colitis with hydrocortisone enemas—comparison of absorption and clinical response. Am J Gastroenterol. 1970; 54:229.

29. Farmer RG et al: Treatment of ulcerative colitis with hydrocortisone enemas. Dis Colon Rectum. 1970; 13:355.

30. Baron JH et al: Sulphasalazine and salicylazosulfadimidine in ulcerative colitis. Lancet. 1962; 1:1094.

31. Dick AP et al: Controlled trial of sulphasalazine in treatment of ulcerative colitis. Gut. 1964; 5:437.

32. Truelove SC et al: Comparison of corticosteroid and sulphasalazine therapy in ulcerative colitis. Br Med J. 1962; 2:1708.

33. Elliott PR et al: Prednisone absorption in acute colitis. Gut. 1980; 21:49.

34. Truelove SC et al: Intensive intravenous regimen for severe attacks of ulcerative colitis. Lancet. 1974; 1:1067.

35. Kaplan HP et al: A controlled evaluation of intravenous adrenocorticotropic hormone and hydrocortisone in the treatment of acute colitis. Gastroenterology. 1975; 69:91.

36. Powell-Tuck J et al: A controlled comparison of corticotropin and hydrocortisone in the treatment of severe proctocolitis. Scand J Gastroenterol. 1977; 12:971.

37. Myles AB et al: Single daily dose corticosteroid treatment. Effect on adrenal function and therapeutic efficacy in various diseases. Ann Rheumatic Dis. 1971; 30:149.

38. Brown EH et al: Topical steroid therapy for ulcerative colitis: report of 50 cases. Am J Gastroenterol. 1961; 36:343.

39. Scherl ND et al: Adjunctive use of a steroid rectal foam in the treatment of ulcerative colitis. Dis Colon Rectum. 1973; 16:149.

40. Ruddell WSJ et al: Treatment of distal ulcerative colitis (proctosigmoiditis) in relapse: comparison of hydrocortisone enemas and rectal hydrocortisone foam. Gut. 1980; 21:885.

41. Misiewicz JJ et al: Comparison of oral and rectal steroids in the treatment of proctocolitis. Proc Royal Soc Med. 1964; 57:561.

42. Matts SGF: Betamethasone enema in ulcerative colitis. Gut. 1962; 3:312.

43. Multicentre Trial: Betamethasone 17-valerate and prednisone 21-phosphate retention enemas in proctocolitis. Br Med J. 1971; 3:84.

44. Powell-Tuck J: Plasma prednisolone levels after administration of prednisolone-21-phosphate as a retention enema in colitis. Br Med J. 1976; 1:193.

45. Lima JJ et al: Bioavailability of hydrocortisone retention enemas in normal subjects. Am J Gastroenterol. 1980; 73:232.

46. Lennard-Jones JE: Medical management of ulcerative colitis. Can J Surg. 1974; 17:420.

47. Swarbrick ET et al: Enema volume as an important factor in successful topical corticosteroid treatment of colitis. Proc Royal Soc Med. 1974; 67:753.

48. Clark ML: A local foam aerosol in ulcerative colitis. Practitioner. 1977; 219:103.

49. Haynes RC et al: Adrenocorticotropic hormone; adrenocortical steroids and their synthetic analogs; inhibitors of adrenocortical steroid biosynthesis. In *The Pharmacological Basis of Therapeutics,* 6th ed, edited by AG Gilman, LS Goodman and A Gilman, Macmillan, New York, 1980, p 1466.

50. Colomb D: Cutaneous manifestations in long-term general corticotherapy. Study of 100 cases. Presse Med. 1971; 79:1011.

51. Knudsen L et al: Early complications in patients previously treated with corticosteroids. Scand J Gastroenterol. 1976; 11(Suppl 3):123.

52. Jalon KN et al: Influence of corticosteroids in the results of surgical treatment for ulcerative colitis. N Engl J Med. 1971; 282:588.

53. Misiewicz JJ et al: Controlled trial of sulphasalazine in maintenance therapy for ulcerative colitis. Lancet. 1965; 1:185.

54. Dissanayake AS et al: A controlled therapeutic trial of long term maintenance treatment of ulcerative colitis with sulphasalazine (salaxopyrin). Gut. 1973; 14:923.

55. Azad Khan AK et al: Optimal dose of sulphasalazine for the maintenance treatment of ulcerative colitis. Gut. 1980; 21:232.

56. Truelove SC et al: Cortisone and corticotrophin in ulcerative colitis. Br Med J. 1959; 1:387.

57. Lennard-Jones JE et al: Prednisone as a maintenance treatment for ulcerative colitis in remission. Lancet. 1965; 1:188.

58. Schroder H et al: Absorption, metabolism, and excretion of salicylazo-sulfapyridine in man. Clin Pharmacol Ther. 1972; 13:506.

59. Das KM et al: Small bowel absorption of sulfasalazine and its hepatic metabolism in human beings, cats, and rats. Gastroenterology. 1979; 77:280.

60. Peppercorn MA et al: The role of bacteria in the metabolism of salicylazosulfapyridine. J Pharmacol Exper Ther. 1972; 181:555.

61. Peppercorn MA et al: Distribution studies of salicylazosulfapyridine and its metabolites. Gastroenterology. 1973; 64:240.

62. Schroder H et al: Azo reduction of salicyl-azo-sulfapyridine by germ-free and conventional rats. Xenobiotica. 1973; 3:225.

63. Das EM: The role of the colon in the metabolism of salicylazosulfapyridine. Scand J Gastroenterol. 1974; 9:137.

64. Goldman P et al: Sulfasalaxzine. N Engl J Med. 1975; 293:20.

65. Evans DAP et al: Human acetylation polymorphism. J Lab Clin Med. 1964; 63:394.

66. Schroder H et al: Acetylator phenotype and adverse effects of sulphasalazine in healthy subjects. Gut. 1972; 13:278.

67. Das KM et al: Clinical pharmacokinetics of sulfasalazine. Clin Pharmacokinetics. 1976; 1:406.

68. Klotz U et al: Therapeutic efficacy of sulfasalazine and its metabolites in patients with ulcerative colitis and Crohn's disease. N Engl J Med. 1980; 303:1499.

69. van Hees PAM et al: Influence of intestinal transit time on azo-reduction of salicylazosulfapyridine (salazopyrin). Gut. 1979; 20:300.

70. Azad Khan AK et al: Circulating levels of sulfasalazine and its metabolites and their relation to the clinical efficacy of the drug in ulcerative colitis. Gut. 1980; 21:706.

71. Azad Khan AK et al: An experiment to determine the active therapeutic moiety of sulphasalazine. Lancet. 1977; 2:892.

72. van Hees PAM et al: Effect of sulfapyridine, 5-aminosalicylic acid and placebo in patients with idiopathic proctitis: a study to determine the active therapeutic moiety of sulphasalazine. Gut. 1980; 21:632.

73. Butt AA et al: Effects on prostaglandin biosynthesis of drugs affecting gastrointestinal function. Gut. 1974; 15:344.

74. Gould SR et al: Production of prostaglandins in ulcerative colitis and their inhibition by sulphasalazine. Gut. 1976; 17:828.

75. Sharon P et al: Role of prostaglandins in ulcerative colitis. Enhanced production during active disease and inhibition by sulfasalazine. Gastroenterology. 1978; 75:638.

76. Ferreira SH et al: Prostaglandins and signs and symptoms of inflammation. In Prostaglandin Synthetase Inhibitors, edited by HJ Robinson and JR Vane, Ravin Press, New York, 1974, p 175.

77. Gould SR: Increased prostaglandin production in ulcerative colitis. Lancet. 1975; 2:98.

78. Gould SR: Assay of prostaglandin-like substances in faeces and their measurement in ulcerative colitis. Prostaglandins. 1976; 11:489.

79. Rampton DS et al: Rectal mucosal prostaglandin E_2 release and its relation to disease activity, electrical potential difference, and treatment in ulcerative colitis. Gut. 1980; 21:591.

80. Harris DW et al: Determination of prostaglandin synthetase activity in rectal biopsy material and its significance in colonic disease. Gut. 1978; 19:875.

81. Das KM et al: Adverse reactions during salicylazosulfapyridine therapy and the relation with drug metabolism and acetylator phenotype. N Engl J Med. 1973; 289:491.

82. Evans DAP: An improved and simplified method of detecting the acetylator phenotype. J Med Genet. 1969; 6:405.

83. Spriggs AI et al: Heinz-body anaemia due to salicylazosulphapyridine. Lancet. 1958; 1:1039.

84. Bottiger LE et al: The occurrence of Heinz bodies during azulfidine treatment of ulcerative colitis. Gastroenterol Basel. 1963; 100:33.

85. Gabor P: Hemolytic anemia as adverse reaction to salicylazosulfapyridine (letter). N Engl J Med. 1973; 289:1372.

86. Cohen SM et al: Ulcerative colitis and erythrocyte G-6-PD deficiency. JAMA. 1968; 205:116.

87. Goodacre RL et al: Hemolytic anemia in patients receiving sulfasalazine. Digestion. 1978; 17:503.

88. van Hees PAM et al: Hemolysis during salicylazosulfapyridine therapy. Am J Gastroenterol. 1979; 70:501.

89. Franklin JL et al: Impaired folic acid absorption in inflammatory bowel disease; effects of salicylazosulfapyridine (Azulfidine). Gastroenterology. 1973; 64:517.

90. Schneider RE et al: Megaloblastic anemia associated with sulphasalazine treatment. Br Med J. 1977; 2:1638.

91. Levi AJ et al: Male infertility due to sulphasalazine. Lancet. 1979; 2:276.

92. Toth A: Reversible toxic effect of salicylazosulfapyridine on seman quality. Fertil Steril. 1979; 31:538.

93. Traub AI et al: Male infertility due to sulphasalazine. Lancet. 1979; 2:639.

94. Hensleigh PA et al: Maternal absorption and placental transfer of sulfasalazine. Amer J Obstet Gynec. 1977; 127:443.

95. Jamsnidi K et al: Azulfidine agranulocytosis with bone marrow megakaryocytosis and plasmacytosis. Minn Med. 1972; 55:545.

96. Fishman FL et al: Non-oxidative hemolysis due to salicylazosulfapyridine: evidence for an immune mechanism. Gastroenterology. 1973; 64:A441.

97. Chester AC et al: Hypersensitivity to salicylazosulfapyridine: renal and hepatic toxic reactions. Arch Intern Med. 1978; 138:1138.

98. Mihas AA et al: Sulfasalazine toxic reactions: hepatitis, fever and skin rash with hypocomplementemia and immune complexes. JAMA. 1978; 239:2590.

99. Sotolongo RP et al: Hypersensitivity reaction to sulfasalazine with severe hepatotoxicity. Gastroenterology. 1978; 75:95.

100. Strom J: Toxic epidermal necrolysis (Lyell's syndrome): a report on four cases with three deaths. Scand J Infect Dis. 1969; 1:209.

101. Jones GR et al: Sulphasalazine induced lung disease. Thorax. 1972; 27:713.

102. Davies D et al: Fibrosing alveolitis and treatment with salicylazosulfapyridine. Gut. 1974; 15:185.

103. Tydd TF et al: Sulphasalazine lung. Med J Aust. 1976; 1:570.

104. Sotolongo RP et al: Azulfidine (sulfasalazine) induced hepatic injury. Am J Dig Dis. 1978; 23:956.

105. Callen JP et al: Granulomatous hepatitis associated with salicylazosulfapyridine therapy. South Med J. 1978; 71:1159.

106. Gully RM et al: Hepatotoxicity of salicylazosulfapyridine. Am J Gastroenterol. 1979; 72:561.

107. Block MB et al: Pancreatitis as an adverse reaction to salicylazosulfapyridine. N Engl J Med. 1970; 282:380.

108. Griffiths ID et al: Sulfasalazine-induced lupus syndrome in ulcerative colitis. Br Med J. 1977; 4:1188.

109. Reid J et al: Raynaud's phenomenon induced by sulphasalazine. Postgrad Med J. 1980; 56:106.

110. Wallace IW et al: Neurotoxicity associated with a reaction to sulphasalazine. Practitioner. 1970; 204:850.

111. West B et al: Effects of sulphasalazine (salazopyrin) on faecal flora in patients with inflammatory bowel disease. Gut. 1974; 15:960.

112. Cooke EM et al: Properties of strains of Escherichia coli carried in different phases of ulcerative colitis. Gut. 1974; 15:143.

113. Hansten PD: *Drug Interactions,* 4th ed., Lea and Febiger, Philadelphia, 1979, p 57.

114. Ibid, p 103.

115. Das KM et al: Effect of iron and calcium on salicylazosulphapyridine metabolism. Scot Med J. 1973; 18:45.

116. Juhl RP et al: Effects of sulfasalazine on digoxin bioavailability. Clin Pharmacol Ther. 1976; 20:387.

117. Jewell DP et al: Azathioprine in ulcerative colitis. Final report on a controlled clinical trial. Br Med J. 1974; 4:627.

118. Caprilli R et al: A double-blind comparison of the effectiveness of azathioprine and sulfasalazine in idiopathic proctocolitis—preliminary report. Am J Dig Dis. 1975; 20:115.

119. Rosenberg JL et al: A controlled trial of azathioprine in the management of chronic ulcerative colitis. Gastroenterology. 1975; 69:96.

120. Korelitz BI et al: Long-term immunosuppressive therapy of ulcerative colitis. Am J Dig Dis. 1973; 18:317.

121. Korelitz BI et al: Long-term observation of children with ulcerative colitis treated with an immunosuppressive drug (6-mercaptopurine). Gastroenterology. 1977; 72:A60.

122. Bean RHD: Treatment of ulcerative colitis with antimetabolites. Br Med J. 1966; 1:1081.

123. Sachar AB et al: Immunotherapy in inflammatory bowel disease. Med Clin North Amer. 1978; 62:173.

124. Heatly RV et al: Disodium cromoglycate in the treatment of chronic proctitis. Gut. 1975; 16:559.

125. Mani V et al: Treatment of ulcerative colitis with oral disodium cromoglycate: a double-blind controlled trial. Lancet. 1976; 1:439.

126. Buckell NA et al: Controlled trial of disodium cromoglycate in chronic persistent ulcerative colitis. Gut. 1978; 19:1140.

127. Langman MJS et al: Disodium cromoglycate maintenance treatment of ulcerative colitis. Acta Allergologica. 1977; 13:76.

128. Dronfield MW et al: Comparative trial of sulfasalazine and oral sodium cromoglycate in the maintenance of remission in ulcerative colitis. Gut. 1978; 19:1136.

129. Willoughby CP et al: Comparison of disodium cromoglycate and sulphasalazine as maintenance therapy for ulcerative colitis. Lancet. 1979; 1:119.

130. Jalan KN et al: An experience of ulcerative colitis: I. Toxic dilation in 55 cases. Gastroenterology. 1969; 57:68.

131. Farmer RG et al: Clinical patterns in Crohn's disease: a statistical study of 615 cases. Gastroenterology. 1975; 68:627.

132. Greenstein AJ et al: Crohn's disease of the colon. III. Toxic dilatation of the colon in Crohn's colitis. Am J Gastroenterol. 1975; 63:117.

133. Grieco MB et al: Toxic megacolon complicating Crohn's colitis. Ann Surg. 1980; 191:75.

134. Binder SC et al: Toxic megacolon in ulcerative colitis. Gastroenterology. 1974; 66:909.

135. Fazio VW: Toxic megacolon in ulcerative colitis and Crohn's colitis. Clin Gastroenterol. 1980; 9:389.

136. Garrett JM et al: Colonic mortality in ulcerative colitis after opiate administration. Gastroenterology. 1967; 53:43.

137. Smith FW et al: Fulminant ulcerative colitis with toxic dilatation of the colon: medical and surgical management of eleven cases with observations regarding etiology. Gastroenterology. 1962; 24:233.

138. Goldberg H et al: The barium enema and toxic megacolon: cause-effect relationship? Gastroenterology. 1975; 68:617.

139. Cohn EM et al: Ulcerative colitis with hypopotassemia. Gastroenterology. 1956; 30:950.

140. Goligher JC et al: Surgical treatment of severe attacks of ulcerative colitis, with special reference to the advantages of early operation. Br Med J. 1970; 4:703.

141. Ritchie JK: Results of surgery for inflammatory bowel disease: a further survey of one hospital region. Br Med J. 1974; 1:264.

142. Binder SC et al: Emergency and urgent operations for ulcerative colitis. Arch Surg. 1975; 110:284.

143. Glotzer DJ: Operation in inflammatory bowel disease: indications and type. Clin Gastroenterol. 1980; 9:371.

144. Corbett JJ: The ostomy patient: surgical and physiological implications. US Pharm. 1980; 5:41.

145. Phillips SF: Life with an ileostomy. In *Gastrointestinal Disease,* 2nd ed, edited by MH Sleisenger and JS Fordtran, Saunders, Philadelphia, 1978, p 1653.

146. Steiner JF: The ostomy patient: pharmaceutical aspects. US Pharm. 1980; 5:53.

147. Kirsner JB: Current medical and surgical opinions on important therapeutic issues in inflammatory bowel disease. Am J Surg. 1980; 140:391.

148. Gryboski J et al: Inflammatory bowel disease in children. Med Clin North Amer. 1980; 64:1185.

149. Morson BC et al: Rectal biopsy as an aid to cancer control in ulcerative colitis. Gut. 1967; 8:423.

150. Fuson JA et al: Endoscopic surveillance for cancer in chronic ulcerative colitis. Am J Gastroenterol. 1980; 73:120.

151. Butt JH et al: A practical approach to the risk of cancer in inflammatory bowel disease. Med Clin North Amer. 1980; 64:1203.

152. Hellers G: Crohn's disease in Stockholm County, 1955 to 1974. A study of epidemiology, results of surgical treatment and long term prognosis. Scand J Gastroenterol (Suppl). 1979; 490:1.

153. Merkhjian HS et al: Clinical features and natural history of Crohn's disease. Gastroenterology. 1979; 77:898.

154. Farmer RG et al: Clinical patterns in Crohn's disease: a statistical study of 615 cases. Gastroenterology. 1975; 68:627.

155. Summers RW et al: National Cooperative Crohn's Disease Study: results of drug treatment. Gastroenterology. 1979; 77:847.

156. Singleton JW: Corticosteroids for Crohn's disease. Ann Intern Med. 1979; 90:983.

157. Gray SJ et al: Treatment of ulcerative colitis and regional enteritis with ACTH. Arch Intern Med. 1951; 87:646.

158. Stanley MM et al: The use of corticotrophin (ACTH) in the treatment of chronic regional enteritis. Med Clin North Am. 1951; 35:1255.

159. Sauer WG et al: Experiences with the use of corticotrophin in regional enteritis. Gastroenterology. 1952; 22:550.

160. Jones JH et al: Corticosteroids and corticotrophin in the treatment of Crohn's disease. Gut. 1966; 7:181.

161. Sparberg N et al: Long-term corticosteroid therapy for regional enteritis: an analysis of 58 courses in 54 patients. Am J Dig Dis. 1966; 865.

162. Cooke WT et al: Corticosteroid or corticotrophin therapy in Crohn's disease (regional enteritis). Gut. 1970; 11:921.

163. Anthonisen P et al: The clinical effect of salazosulphapyridine (Salazopyrin [R]) in Crohn's disease. Scand J Gastroenterol. 1974; 9:549.

164. Singleton JW et al: A trial of sulfasalazine as adjunctive therapy in Crohn's disease. Gastroenterology. 1979; 77:887.

165. Lefton HB et al: Ileorectal anastomosis for Crohn's disease of the colon. Gastroenterology. 1975; 69:612.

166. Bergman L et al: Postoperative treatment with corticosteroids and salazosulphapyridine (Salazopyrin [R]) after radical resection for Crohn's disease. Scand J Gastroenterol. 1976; 11:651.

167. Rhodes J et al: Effect of low dose steroids on clinical relapse in Crohn's disease. Gut. 1978; 19:606.

168. Smith RC et al: Low-dose steroids and clinical relapse in Crohn's disease: a controlled trial. Gut. 1978; 19:606.

169. Baron JH et al: Sulphasalazine in asymptomatic Crohn's disease: a multicentre trial. Gut. 1977; 18:69.

170. Wenckert A et al: The long-term prophylactic effect of salazosulphapyridine (Salazopyrin [R]) in primarily resected patients with Crohn's disease. A controlled double-blind trial. Scand J Gastroenterol. 1978; 13:161.

171. Singleton JW et al: National Cooperative Crohn's Disease Study: adverse reaction to study drugs. Gastroenterology. 1979; 77:870.

172. Kaufman S et al: A prospective study of the course of Crohn's disease. Dig Dis Sci. 1979; 24:269.

173. Willoughby JMT et al: Controlled trial of azathioprine in Crohn's disease. Lancet. 1971; 2:944.

174. Rosenberg JL et al: A controlled trial of azathioprine in Crohn's disease. Amer J Dig Dis. 1975; 20:721.

175. Present DH et al: Treatment of Crohn's disease with 6-mercaptopurine: a long-term randomized double-blind study. N Engl J Med. 1980; 302:981.

176. O'Donoghue DP et al: Double-blind withdrawal trial of azathioprine as maintenance treatment for Crohn's disease. Lancet. 1978; 2:955.

177. Kinlen LJ et al: Collaborative United Kingdom—Australian study of cancer in patients treated with immunosuppressive drugs. Br Med J. 1979; 2:1461.

178. Rhodes J et al: Controlled trial of azathioprine in Crohn's disease. Lancet. 1971; 2:1273.

179. Klein M et al: Treatment of Crohn's disease with azathioprine: a controlled evaluation. Gastroenterology. 1974; 66:916.

180. Watson WC et al: Azathioprine in the management of Crohn's disease: a randomized crossover study. Gastroenterology. 1974; 66:796.

181. Blichfeldt P et al: Metronidazole for Crohn's disease: a double-blind crossover clinical trial. Scand J Gastroenterol. 1978; 13:123.

182. Bernstein LH et al: Healing of perineal Crohn's disease with metronidazole. Gastroenterology. 1980; 79:357.

183. Segal AW et al: Levamisole in the treatment of Crohn's disease. Lancet. 1977; 2:382.

184. Wesdorp E et al: Levamisole in Crohn's disease: a double-blind controlled trial. Gut. 1977; 18:A971.

185. Burnham WR et al: Oral BCG vaccine in Crohn's disease. Gut. 1979; 20:229.

186. Mekhjian HS et al: National Cooperative Crohn's Disease Study: factors determining recurrence of Crohn's disease after surgery. Gastroenterology. 1979; 77:907.

187. de Dombal FT: Recurrent Crohn's disease. Can J Surg. 1974; 17:408.

188. Allan R et al: Crohn's disease involving the colon: an audit of clinical management. Gastroenterology 1977; 73:723.

Chapter 21

Pancreatitis

John Russo, Jr. and Kelly D. Mutchie

Pancreatitis is a common, complex disease of the pancreas characterized by a broad spectrum of symptoms and often, multiple organ involvement. Although the terms "acute" and "chronic" are used when referring to these patients, it has not been established that acute and chronic pancreatitis are etiologically linked. At present, it is most useful to view acute and chronic pancreatitis as two disease states. Acute pancreatitis is characterized by attacks of severe, steady and boring upper abdominal pain usually radiating to the back, chest or lower abdomen with patients occasionally obtaining relief by sitting with the trunk flexed, knees drawn up and arms folded across the abdomen. Such attacks may occur once or repeatedly and are frequently accompanied by nausea and vomiting. Chronic pancreatitis may initially present in the same way or begin insidiously with mild bouts of abdominal pain. The major difference between these conditions is that pancreatic function returns to normal in the acute form, whereas permanent damage to the pancreas occurs as a consequence of the chronic form. This eventually impairs pancreatic function resulting in malabsorption, steatorrhea, azotorrhea and frank diabetes. The most sucessful approach to the treatment of either disease is to identify and eliminate the etiologic factor. If this is not possible, therapy is directed toward symptomatic relief and treatment of the complications.

ACUTE PANCREATITIS

Drug-Induced Pancreatitis

1. A.C. is a 20-year-old, moderately obese woman who was well until eight months ago when she experienced her first bout of abdominal pain followed by three more episodes occurring at one to four-week inter-

vals. Each episode lasted for two to three days without further symptoms. Oral cholecystography was negative following her fourth attack and a low fat diet was prescribed. She has been noncompliant with the diet and now presents to the emergency room with complaints of severe abdominal pain radiating to the left shoulder. Her abdomen is tender and resistant to palpation and bowel sounds are diminished. Intravenous cholangiography is normal. Family history is positive for diabetes mellitus and atherosclerosis. WBC is 20,000/mm³ with 79% polys and 10% bands, serum is lactescent, glucose 200 mg/dl, SGOT 35 mU/ml (8–35), LDH 100 mU/ml (54–134), serum amylase 350 u/dl (60–180), serum calcium 8.5 mg/dl (8.5–10.5). Current medications include a combined estrogen-progestogen oral contraceptive for the past nine months, chlordiazepoxide (Librium) taken as needed for five years, and "pain pills" as needed to control her abdominal pain. She limits consumption of alcoholic beverages to white wine in small amounts. The diagnosis of acute pancreatitis is made and treated with nasogastric (NG) suction, IV fluid therapy and meperidine (Demerol) 75–100 mg IV every 3 hours as needed for pain. What might be the cause of A.C.'s pancreatitis?

Ethanol. Successful management requires recognition and elimination of the cause of the disease. Sixty to 80% of patients with pancreatitis have either cholelithiasis or a history of alcohol abuse (1). A.C.'s diagnostic work up is negative for the former and her history of ethanol ingestion does not fit the typical pattern. Most patients with alcohol-induced pancreatitis have had a history of alcohol abuse for at least two years and usually five to ten years elapse before the onset of symptoms. The type of alcoholic beverage consumed is not important but the daily consumption of approximately 150 ml appears to be directly toxic to the pancreas. This results in increased protein secretion, intraductal plug formation (2), and the appearance of free proteolytic activity (chymotrypsin) despite the presence of adequate levels of trypsin inhibitor. Normal pancreatic secretions show no free proteolytic activity (3). Other potential etiologic factors are listed in Table 1.

Estrogen. Many findings in A.C.'s history are consistent with estrogen-induced pancreatitis.

Table 1.

FACTORS ASSOCIATED WITH THE DEVELOPMENT OF PANCREATITIS

Biliary Tract Disease	Heredity
Alcoholism	Hyperlipoproteinemia (Type 1 & 5)
Peptic Ulcer Disease	
Trauma	Infection
Surgery	Hypercalcemia
Vascular Diseases	Drugs (see Table 2)

Typically symptoms occur within three months of the start of estrogen therapy; in A.C.'s case, the initial symptoms occurred one month after she had started her birth control pills. Also, obese individuals with a family history of diabetes mellitus and atherosclerosis such as A.C. appear to be predisposed to this problem. Finally, A.C.'s serum was lactescent which is consistent with the hypertriglyceridemia associated with estrogen-induced pancreatitis. Other findings which would further support an estrogen-induced pancreatitis include: a diabetic glucose tolerance curve, lipemia retinalis, and Type IV or V serum lipid patterns. The precise mechanism of this drug-induced disease is unknown but it appears to be associated with estrogen-mediated hypertriglyceridemia. If her pancreatitis is estrogen-induced, discontinuation of the drug should lead to resolution of symptoms within two weeks as well as a gradual decrease in the triglycerides (4–6).

2. What other drugs should be considered when ruling out drug-induced pancreatitis?

More than thirty agents are implicated in the induction of pancreatitis (7,8); however, a realistic approach to this question necessitates conducting a medication history, with agents in Table 2 being foremost in the evaluation.

Azathioprine. Azathioprine-induced pancreatitis appears to be a hypersensitivity reaction. It typically occurs within three weeks of starting therapy, improves within 24 hours of discontinuing the drug and is exacerbated upon rechallenge with a single dose (9–11).

Tetracycline. Pancreatitis is a feature of a clinical syndrome known as "tetracycline-induced fatty liver of pregnancy." Risk factors include high daily doses (3.6–6 gm) of tetracycline, pregnancy and impaired renal function. Tetracycline should be discontinued in patients with pancreatitis under the conditions described above since the course of the disease is severe and some fatalities have been reported (12).

Diuretics and Sulfa Drugs. Supporting evidence for other forms of drug-induced pancreatitis is weak. Case reports, animal data demonstrating inflammatory and necrotic changes after chronic treatment and elevated serum amylase levels following administration form the basis for *benzothiadiazine*-induced pancreatitis (7,8,13). *Furosemide* (7,8) and *sulfa drugs* such as sulfamethizole (Urobiotic) and salicylazosulfapyridine (Azulfidine) have less clinical supporting evidence (although rechallenge has been undertaken in some cases). The structural similarity of these drugs to *thiazides* is often used to support the case for thiazide-induced pancreatitis (8). Isolated cases of acute pancreatitis associated with structurally unrelated diuretics such as ethacrynic acid (Edecrin) and chlorthalidone (Hygroton) have been reported (7,8). Spironolactone (Aldactone) has not been implicated in the induction of pancreatitis.

L-asparaginase. Pancreatitis secondary to *L-asparaginase* is reported in approximately 7% of patients during and four to ten weeks after treatment. L-asparaginase, through its hydrolysis to L-aspartic acid deprives rapidly proliferating leukemic cells of L-asparagine thus interfering with intracellular protein synthesis. Organs with high rates of protein synthesis such as the pancreas are vulnerable to this effect. Young females, older than nine years, may be at greater risk than males since serum estrogens, which prolong and potentiate L-asparaginase activity, begin to rise in women at this time (14).

Calcium. Hypercalcemia (> 11 mg/dl) secondary to a wide variety of causes including vitamin D administration, hyperalimentation, calcium infusion tests, hemodialysis and hyperparathyroidism may precipitate pancreatitis (8).

Treatment

3. Is A.C.'s current therapy sufficient? Is there any way of predicting whether A.C. will develop severe or lethal complications of her acute pancreatitis?

At this point, A.C. is being treated appropriately with a combination of intravenous fluids, nasogastric suction, and analgesics.

Intravenous fluid replacement is the cornerstone of treatment of acute pancreatitis. The inflamed pancreas and retroperitoneal bed can serve as a massive third space reservoir for body fluids and as a result, large amounts of intravenous fluid and colloid may be required to maintain intravascular volume and blood pressure (see chapter on *Fluid and Electrolyte Disorders* for discussion of monitoring techniques).

Nasogastric (NG) suction and the maintenance of a fasting state minimizes the release of gastrin and acid into the duodenum which can stimulate pancreatic secretion. The goal of therapy is to "rest" the pancreas since the secretion of enzyme rich fluids can intensify inflammation of the organ. The nasogastric tube should be utilized as described in the chapter on *Acute Stress Erosions.* Recently, benefits of continuous gastric suction have been questioned in two reports demonstrating no differences in complications and mortality rates between groups with and without NG suction (21,22). Milder cases may not require this treatment but it should be instituted in patients with ileus or severe disease.

Further recommendations for the therapy of pancreatitis have been hampered by an inability to recognize those patients who are at particular

Table 2.

DRUGS ASSOCIATED WITH PANCREATITIS

Azathioprine (Imuran)

Calcium (hypercalcemia)

Chlorothiazide (Diuril) and Hydrochlorothiazide (Esidrix)

Chlorthalidone (Hygroton)

Corticosteroids

Estrogens: oral contraceptives, conjugated estrogens (Premarin), diethylstilbesterol, chlorotrianisene (Tace)

Ethacrynic acid (Edecrin)

Ethanol

Furosemide (Lasix)

L-asparaginase

Sulfonamides

Tetracycline (Achromycin)

risk for complications or death early in the disease process. Table 3 lists early signs associated with the development of severe and lethal complications of pancreatitis. Ranson and colleagues (15,16) found that patients who exhibited three or more of these within 48 hours of admission were at high risk for the development of serious complications or death from their pancreatitis. Eventually, these criteria may be used to assess the efficacy of more aggressive therapeutic modalities. Until then, these prognostic signs should be used to monitor the course of disease and to guide further treatment decisions.

Of note is that serum amylase is not listed in Table 3. Serum amylase is elevated in 90% of cases of pancreatitis within eight hours of onset and is strongly suggestive of its diagnosis when values exceed 200 Somogyi units; however, the degree to which it is raised correlates poorly with the severity of the condition. In fact, it may be normal in as many as one-third of patients with pancreatic abcess (17).

On the basis of the criteria listed in Table 3, A.C.'s prognosis looks favorable at this time. She exhibits only one of the unfavorable prognostic indicators.

4. What drugs have been used to minimize pancreatic secretions?

Antacids and *cimetidine* have been used in addition to nasogastric suction to further minimize pancreatic secretions and as prophylaxis against stress ulcers. Cimetidine does not appear to have any specific effects that alter the course of acute pancreatitis (20).

Anticholinergic drugs have been widely prescribed for this purpose without demonstrated efficacy (23). Experimental work suggests that atropine inhibits enzyme secretion to a greater extent than it inhibits synthesis resulting in a 70 to 80% increase in tissue enzyme content. If pancreatitis is caused or perpetuated by escape of proteases from damaged acinar cells, the use of drugs which cause enzyme accumulation in the pancreas seems inadvisable (24). Further, anticholinergic side effects such as urinary retention, tachycardia, ileus, and excessive dryness of the mouth could further complicate evaluation of the patient's fluid therapy; thus, their use is discouraged.

Other agents including acetazolamide (Diamox) (25), vasopressin (Pitressin) (26) and glucagon (27) also lack clinical evidence of efficacy in the management of acute pancreatitis.

5. Aprotinin (Trasylol) has been discussed for many years as a potential breakthrough in the search for an agent which directly inhibits proteolytic enzymes. What is its current status?

Aprotinin shortens the course of experimentally-induced pancreatitis but the results of clinical trials are conflicting (27–29). This may be due to the timing of the first injection, dosing, or the heterogenicity of the patient populations studied. Until these questions are answered, the indications for aprotinin in the treatment of acute pancreatitis will remain undefined.

6. A.C. is receiving meperidine for pain relief. Are other analgesics superior to this drug

Table 3.
ELEVEN EARLY FINDINGS WHICH CORRELATE WITH SEVERE ILLNESS AND DEATH (15,16)*

On Admission	During the Initial 48 Hours
Age > 55 years	Hematocrit fall > 10 percentage points
Blood glucose level > 200 mg%	BUN rise > 5 mg%
White blood cell count > 16,000/ml^3	Lowest serum calcium < 8 mg%
SGOT > 250 Fraenkel units%	Lowest PaO$_2$ < 60 mm Hg
LDH > 350 IU/l	Base deficit > 4 mEq/l
	Estimated fluid sequestration > 6 liters

*In patients with more than three positive prognostic signs, there is a high risk of serious illness or death. The risk is small in those with less than three early signs.

in the management of pain associated with acute pancreatitis?

Pain secondary to pancreatic inflammation or exudation can be severe and its alleviation may require the use of potent analgesics. Studies reporting superiority of any agent base their findings on post cholecystectomy patients with T-tube drainage of the biliary tract (see Fig. 1 in the chapter on Acute Cholecystitis), *not* patients with acute pancreatitis (30,31). It is assumed that narcotic-induced duct pressure changes in this stable population accurately reflect changes in the pancreatic duct pressures in patients with pancreatitis and that increases in pressure correlate with the severity of pain. The traditional use of meperidine as the drug of choice in pancreatitis is based on data generated from these studies and on the theoretical advantages of its chemical structure. Originally, the drug was intended to combine the chemical features of atropine and papaverine and was to be used as a smooth muscle relaxant (32). In fact, meperidine produces spasm of the duodenal wall surrounding the sphincter of Oddi, and the difference between its effect and an equianalgesic dose of morphine has not been shown to be statistically or clinically different (30,32). A recent study of pentazocine (Talwin) suffers from similar deficiencies in study design (31).

Since there is little or no evidence to indicate that any analgesic harms a patient with pancreatitis, the primary basis for drug selection should be analgesic efficacy.

Parenteral meperidine (50–100 mg) or morphine (5–15 mg) should be initiated *following* completion of the patient's initial work-up since these agents can increase serum amylase levels substantially and may thereby potentially confuse the diagnosis. The patient's analgesic response to the narcotics and the total dose administered over 24 hours should be monitored. There must also be constant evaluation of the patient's respiratory rate, especially if the narcotics are administered intravenously (also see chapter on Pain). The clinician should be aware that increased pain may be the first sign of complications such as a pancreatic pseudocyst.

Complications

7. What are the complications of acute pancreatitis which should be anticipated in A.C.?

Complications of acute pancreatitis may involve many organ systems and include cardiovascular failure, respiratory failure, renal failure, coagulation changes, neuropsychiatric changes and others (1). Three complications deserve specific attention.

First, uncomplicated acute pancreatitis is a sterile inflammatory process but *infections* such as pancreatic abscesses occur in 3 to 9% of patients. Persistence of fever, ileus and tenderness and anorexia beyond three days or deterioration one to four weeks after initial improvement should alert the clinician to the possibility of abscess formation (33). Patients with postsurgical pancreatitis and those displaying more than three of the early prognostic signs listed in Table 3 are also at increased risk of abscess formation (34). Antibiotics should be initiated prior to surgical drainage of the abscess. *E. coli* and klebsiella account for almost 50% of organisms cultured from these abscesses. *B. fragilis*, pseudomonas and staphylococci are also isolated frequently (35). An aminoglycoside plus clindamycin (Cleocin) or another agent to cover anaerobes should be started preoperatively and continued pending cultures and sensitivity results. Appropriate changes can be made at that time.

Nutritional depletion in patients with acute pancreatitis is documented (36) and this may inhibit healing, increase the risk of infectious complications and make the patient a poorer operative risk (37). This can be minimized through adequate nutritional support. In mild cases, oral feedings may be resumed once all signs of pancreatic inflammation have resolved; reactivation of pancreatitis and abscess formation have been observed in patients fed too soon (34). To minimize potential insults to the pancreas, elemental diets which stimulate pancreatic secretions less than standard diets are used to initiate oral feedings (38). Patients with severe disease and who are not likely to tolerate oral feedings should be treated with intravenous hyperalimentation as soon as practical but within 48 hours of admission. This may be supplemented with intrajejunal feedings as a preliminary step to oral alimentation when bowel function returns as evidenced by active peristaltic sounds (38).

Hypocalcemia is another complication of pancreatitis and is the best recognized objective index of its severity. Indications for treatment include a serum calcium below 8 mg/dl or clinical evidence of hypocalcemia such as numbness of the fingers; tingling and burning of the extremities, lips and tongue; muscle cramps; or a positive Trousseau test or Chvostek's sign (17,39). Calcium gluconate (10 ml of a 10% solution) should be administered by intravenous infusion over six to eight hours and then adjusted as needed to maintain a normal serum calcium level. Since depressed magnesium levels inhibit the response of the parathyroid gland to hypocalcemia, it may be necessary to administer 6 gm $MgSO_4$ IV daily for three to five days to replace total body stores of magnesium in patients who are hypomagnesemic (40). Patients in alcohol withdrawal are particularly susceptible to this problem. Patients with creatinine clearance values less than 30 ml/min must be treated more conservatively to avoid magnesium toxicity (41).

CHRONIC PANCREATITIS

8. T.C. is a 43-year-old man with recurrent abdominal pain of eight years duration. The pain is mid-epigastric and typically occurs after eating or long drinking episodes. He began drinking 22 years ago. Over the last two years, the pain has been related less to meals and alcohol ingestion and has been more persistent, often lasting several days at a time. Three years ago, he began passing bulky, foul-smelling stools containing oily, floating material. He has lost 30 pounds over the past two years. There was tenderness to deep palpation in the mid-epigastrium but the remainder of the physical examination was unremarkable. The fasting blood sugar was 200 mg/dl and microscopic examination of the stool revealed numerous fat globules and undigested meat fibers. Small bowel x-ray revealed a malabsorption pattern and a secretin test was positive for pancreatic insufficiency. This patient's most distressing problem is chronic pain. Other than narcotic analgesics, what can be done to alleviate this complaint?

Persistent pain with minor fluctuations is one of the most difficult therapeutic problems in the management of chronic pancreatitis. Possible causes include; distension, chronic pancreatic or perineural inflammation, and pressure from one or more pseudocysts. Ductal obstruction secondary to stones or strictures may cause pain which begins promptly after meals and lasts several

hours; at times, it may cause nausea and vomiting. Other causes of abdominal pain to be ruled out include penetrating duodenal ulcer, cholecystitis and malingering in an effort to obtain more narcotic analgesics. In addition to total abstinence from alcohol, which may or may not result in clinical improvement at this stage of the disease, two other approaches may be beneficial. First, the patient should be instructed to avoid large meals rich in fat and protein. A liquid elemental diet may also be tried to control pain and maintain nutrition. Second, cimetidine may be beneficial alone or in combination with antacids and anticholinergic agents to minimize delivery of gastric acid into the duodenum (42).

9. T.C.'s fasting glucose level is 200 mg/dl. Should he be treated with insulin?

The development of glucose intolerance is a more common complication of chronic pancreatitis than is steatorrhea. This is probably related to the fact that experimentally, greater than 70% of the pancreas must be resected before the diabetic state is induced, while steatorrhea does not occur until the enzyme output is less than 10% of normal. Fortunately, elevations in blood glucose levels are usually well tolerated and uncomplicated by diabetic ketoacidosis or the chronic sequelae of diabetes such as diabetic retinopathy and nephropathy.

Attempting to regulate this patient's blood glucose level may be a hazardous undertaking. The diabetic state in chronic pancreatitis is extremely brittle. Basal glucagon and insulin levels may be normal but there is deficient glucagon and insulin reserve. Therefore, if exogenously administered insulin causes hypoglycemia, the deficiency in glucagon reserve will prevent restoration of serum glucose to normal (43). This can be life threatening, particularly in an alcoholic who is likely to be noncompliant with diet as well as many other aspects of diabetic therapy.

10. Why is T.C. passing bulky stools that contain oily, floating material?

Steatorrhea (excessive loss of fat in the feces) and azotorrhea (excessive loss of nitrogen in the feces) are frequently encountered in patients such as T.C. with chronic pancreatitis and are associated with a 90% reduction in the pancreatic secretion of lipase and trypsin (44). Lipase secretion appears to be reduced more rapidly than trypsin; therefore, steatorrhea is usually the initial finding (47). Pancreatic insufficiency secondary to chronic pancreatitis can have an insidious or rapid onset depending upon the cause of the pancreatitis (45–48). Patients with alcohol-induced chronic pancreatitis such as T.C. typically have the condition for several years before symptoms of gastric pain and diarrhea appear. In contrast, patients with carcinoma of the pancreas typically have a more rapid onset of pancreatic insufficiency. Steatorrhea can be minimized by prescribing exogenous pancreatic enzymes for the patient.

11. Compare the commercially available pancreatic enzymes with regard to enzyme potency, formulation, dose and efficacy.

There are many commercially available pancreatic enzyme preparations (Table 4). *In vitro* tests of commercial pancreatic supplements demonstrate a wide variation in enzyme potency (50–52) and it has been shown that the *in vivo* potency correlates with the enzyme activity measured *in vitro*. Therefore, a high potency product should be selected to minimize the need for large numbers of pills. Many products are manufac-

tured with an enteric coating which theoretically allows the tablet to pass through the low pH of the stomach without significant inactivation of the enzymes. However, evidence suggests that many of the enteric-coated tablets may decrease the *in vivo* potency of the enzymes due to reduced bioavailability (52). Recently, a microencapsulated enteric preparation (Pancrease) has been shown to be effective in the therapy of malabsorption due to pancreatic insufficiency (53,54); a second microencapsulated product, Cotazym-S, is also available. In general, these capsules appear to be as effective in the treatment of chronic alcoholic pancreatitis as standard tablets (53,54) and in some patients, fewer capsules may be required to achieve the same response as larger doses of the standard tablets. Furthermore, in one study, five of six patients preferred the microspheres over the enzyme preparations they had used previously because there was no bloating, cramping or abdominal discomfort associated with their use (53).

The enzyme tablets (Cotazym, Viokase, Ilozyme) and the enteric-coated microsphere cap-

Table 4.

COMPARISON OF ENZYME ACTIVITIES PRESENT IN COMMERCIAL
PANCREATIC ENZYME PREPARATIONS

Preparation	Manufacturer	Type	Lipase	Enzyme Activity (U/Unit)	
				Trypsin	Amylase
Ilozyme	Warren-Teed	Tablet	3,600	3,444	329,600
Ku-zyme Hp	Kremers-Urban	Capsule	2,330	3,082	594,048
Festal	Hoechst-Roussel	Enteric	2,073	488	219,200
Cotazym	Organon	Capsule	2,014	2,797	499,200
Viokase	Viobin	Tablet	1,636	1,828	277,333
Ro-Bile	Rowell	Enteric	539	661	68,000
Entozyme	A H Robins	Enteric	495	668	39,000
Enzapan	Norgine	Enteric	297	381	29,100
Phazyme	Reed-Carnick	Enteric	210	620	15,800
Ku-Zyme	Kremers-Urban	Capsule	170	25	37,700
Digolase	Boyle	Capsule	44	143	16,850
Arco-Lase	Arco	Tablet	29	106	19,000
Kanulase	Dorsey	Tablet	11	590	517
Zypan	Standard Process	Tablet	10	296	441

Modified from Graham (52): Refer to reference for explanation of units.

sules (Pancrease and Cotazym-S) are the most commonly used products in the United States (Table 5). Viokase is also available as a powder (one teaspoonful is equivalent to seven Viokase tablets) and Cotazym is available as a granule (one packet is equivalent to two Cotazyme capsules). Most preparations are derived primarily from hog and beef pancreas, but Viokase, derived only from beef pancreas is available on special order for patients allergic to pork.

12. How should T.C.'s enzymes be dosed? What factors can alter his response? What are reasonable therapeutic endpoints?

The lower limit of lipase activity necessary for efficient lipolysis is approximately 8,000 units per hour (approximately 10% of the lower limit of normal output as measured in healthy subjects)(49). Therefore, 32,000 units of lipase (8,000 units per hour for four postprandial hours) would be necessary to provide minimal lipolytic activity if all the pancreatic enzyme reached the duodenum in an active form (49). This is equivalent to six to eight Viokase tablets per meal. Administration of the enzymes hourly does not improve their effectiveness (55).

Complete elimination of the steatorrhea is usually not accomplished by enzyme replacement therapy (49) and the response varies from patient to patient. The failure of the oral enzyme preparations to completely abolish steatorrhea is related to several factors which limit the quantity of enzyme reaching the duodenum: differing enzyme potency of the commercial products; inac-

tivation of the enzymes in the acidic environment of the gastrointestinal tract; and the dietary fat intake. These factors are responsible for the large dose requirements for enzymes in pancreatic insufficiency. Nevertheless, there should be a substantial reduction in the number and quantity of fat in the stools a few days following the initiation of enzyme therapy. The ultimate goal of therapy is to improve digestion and to supply adequate caloric absorption to produce weight gain and to minimize excessive diarrhea and steatorrhea.

13. Once T.C. is initiated on enzyme therapy what side effects should be anticipated?

Pancreatic enzymes appear to be relatively free from side effects but allergic reactions characterized by watery eyes and sneezing have been reported in patients as well as family members who have been exposed to the product. This is particularly associated with the powder dosage form. As noted earlier, if this reaction is related to an allergy to the hog enzyme, Viokase prepared from beef pancreas is available on special request.

Dose-related hyperuricosuria and hyperuricemia have been observed in cystic fibrosis patients taking more than 6.5 gm/day of pancreatic extract (64,65). This is most likely related to the high purine content of the enzymes.

14. If T.C. fails to respond to Viokase, is he more likely to respond to the microencapsulated form?

Regan et al (54) compared the effectiveness of a microencapsulated preparation (Pancrease) with

Table 5.

PANCREATIC ENZYMES (Manufacturers' Information)

Preparation	Source	Dosage Form	Enzyme Activity per Unit Dosage (N.F. Units)		
			Lipase	Protease	Amylase
Cotazym	Hog Pancreas	Capsules	8,000	30,000	30,000
		Packets U/pkt	16,000	60,000	60,000
*Viokase	Hog Pancreas	Tablets	6,500	32,000	48,000
		Powder: 1 tsp	45,000	225,000	337,500
Ilozyme	Hog Pancreas	Tablets	9,600	40,000	40,000
Pancrease	Hog Pancreas	Capsules (microspheres)	4,000	25,000	20,000
Cotazym-S	Hog Pancreas	Capsules (microspheres)	5,000	20,000	20,000

*Also available as beef source

a standard enzyme tablet (Viokase) in six patients with alcohol-induced pancreatitis, such as T.C. The mean reduction of steatorrhea was similar in both groups; however, in two of the six patients receiving Pancrease, steatorrhea was completely abolished. Both of these had supranormal acid output in that the intragastric pH never rose above 5.5.

This study suggests that the enteric-coated preparations may be more beneficial in patients with increased gastric secretion. Pancrease is an enteric coated preparation with a pH-dependent polymer that maintains its integrity at low pH but becomes unstable as the pH increases above 5. Therefore, Pancrease appears to be most effective in patients who have very acidic conditions in the upper intestine in which the pH is maintained below 4 (54). Pancrease (4–6 capsules with meals) would be an alternative to Viokase for T.C., especially if the patient demonstrates a highly acidic condition in the upper intestine. Pancrease, therefore, may eliminate the need for cimetidine administration in some patients.

15. Three weeks following the initiation of enzymes, T.C. still has excessive steatorrhea and has not gained weight. What methods can be used to improve delivery of active enzymes to the duodenum?

Orally administered pancreatic enzymes are rapidly inactivated by acid; this inactivation can be further increased by the proteolytic action of pepsin (57). Therefore, the addition of antacids or bicarbonate to increase the pH in the stomach and duodenum have been suggested to decrease inactivation of the enzyme. Evidence to support the concomitant use of antacids, however, is minimal. In fact, Regan, et al (54) demonstrated that antacids failed to enhance the effect of oral enzyme therapy on fat malabsorption.

Cimetidine, an H_2-receptor antagonist that decreases gastric acid secretion and increases gastric pH, has been used in conjunction with pancreatic enzymes in adults and children (54,58,59). These investigations have demonstrated that cimetidine significantly increases the efficiency of pancreatic enzymes. Cimetidine appears to have a low incidence of toxicity during short-term use, but more studies are needed to evaluate its prolonged use.

The acid secretory capacity of the stomach of patients with pancreatic insufficiency can vary, thus influencing the amount of enzymes required. For example, patients with alcohol-induced pancreatic insufficiency may have an impaired gastric secretory capacity (60–62), while the gastric secretion in patients with non-alcoholic chronic pancreatitis may be normal or greater than normal (62). Generally, patients with chronic pancreatitis have a significantly higher gastric pH during the early postprandial period and a significantly lower pH in the last postprandial period compared to healthy individuals (55). Since T.C. has not demonstrated a dramatic reduction in steatorrhea in response to enzyme replacement, cimetidine, 300 mg one-half hour before meals should be prescribed to reduce and possibly abolish the steatorrhea.

References

1. Ranson JHC: Acute pancreatitis. Cur Prob Surg. 1979; 16:1.
2. Sarles H: Chronic calcifying pancreatitis—chronic alcoholic pancreatitis. Gastroenterology. 1974; 66:604.
3. Renner IG et al: Profiles of pure pancreatic secretions in patients with acute pancreatitis: the possible role of proteolytic enzymes in pathogenesis. Gastroenterology. 1978; 75:1090.
4. Bank S et al: Case Reports: Hyperlipaemic pancreatitis and the pill. Postgrad Med J. 1970; 46:576.
5. Davidoff F et al: Marked hyperlipidemia and pancreatitis associated with oral contraceptive therapy. N Engl J Med. 1973; 289:552.
6. Glueck CJ et al: Estrogen-induced pancreatitis in patients with previously covert familial type V hyperlipoproteinemia. Metabolism. 1972; 21:657.
7. Nakashima Y et al: Drug-induced acute pancreatitis. Surg Gyn Obstet. 1977; 145:105.
8. Mallory A et al: Drug-induced pancreatitis: a critical review. Gastroenterology. 1980; 78:813.
9. Nogueira JR et al: Acute pancreatitis as a complication of Imuran therapy in regional enteritis. Gastroenterology. 1972; 62:1040.
10. Paloyan D et al: Azathioprine-associated acute pancreatitis. Am J Dig Dis. 1977; 22:839.
11. Huizenga KA et al: Pancreatitis: a specific complication of azathioprine treatment of Crohn's Disease. Gastroenterology. 1976; 70:895.
12. Kucers A et al: The Use of Antibiotics. 2nd ed. JB Lippincott Co, Phila, 1975, p 399.
13. Bourke JB et al: Drug-associated primary acute pancreatitis. Lancet. 1978; 1:706.

14. Weetman RM et al: Latent onset of clinical pancreatitis in children receiving L-asparaginase therapy. Cancer. 1974; 34:780.

15. Ranson JHC et al: Prognostic signs and nonoperative peritoneal lavage in acute pancreatitis. Surg Gyn Obstet. 1976; 143:209.

16. Ranson JHC et al: Statistical methods for quantifying the severity of clinical acute pancreatitis. J Surg Res. 1977; 22:79.

17. Jacobs ML et al: Acute pancreatitis: analysis of factors influencing survival. Ann Surg. 1977; 185:43.

18. Warshaw AJ: The kidney and changes in amylase clearance. Gastroenterology. 1976; 71:702.

19. Levitt MD et al: Is the Cam/Ccr ratio of value for the diagnosis of pancreatitis? Gastroenterology. 1978; 75:118.

20. Meshkinpour H et al: Cimetidine in the treatment of acute alcoholic pancreatitis: a randomized, double-blind study. Gastroenterology. 1979; 77:687.

21. Levant JA et al: Nasogastric suction in the treatment of alcoholic pancreatitis: a controlled study. JAMA. 1974; 229:51.

22. Switz DM: Acute alcoholic pancreatitis: effect of clinical presentation and therapies on outcome at a V.A. hospital (abstract). Ann Intern Med. 1973; 78:816.

23. Cameron JL et al: Evaluation of atropine in acute pancreatitis. Surg Gyn Obstet. 1979; 148:206.

24. Soergel KH: Medical treatment of acute pancreatitis: what is the evidence? Gastroenterology. 1978; 74:620.

25. Anderson MC et al: Use of carbonic anhydrase inhibitor in the treatment of pancreatitis. Am J Dig Dis. 1966; 11:367.

26. Pissiotis CA et al: Effect of vasopressin on pancreatic blood flow in acute hemorrhagic pancreatitis. Am J Surg. 1972; 123:203.

27. Welbourn RB et al: Death from acute pancreatitis. Lancet. 1977; 2:632.

28. Trapnell JE et al: A controlled trial in the treatment of acute pancreatitis. Br J Surg. 1974; 61:177.

29. Imrie CW et al: A single-center doubleblind trial of Trasylol therapy in primary acute pancreatitis. Br J Surg. 1978; 65:337.

30. Kjellgren K: The influence of morphine and pethidine in combination with levallorphan on biliary duct pressure after cholecystectomy. Brit J Anaesth. 1960; 2:32.

31. Economou G et al: A cross-over comparison of the effect of morphine, pethidine, pentazocine and phenazocine on biliary pressure. Gut. 1971; 12:218.

32. Gaensler EA et al: A comparative study of the action of Demerol and opium alkaloids in relation to biliary spasm. Surgery. 1948; 23:211.

33. Warshaw AL: Pancreatic abscesses. N Engl J Med. 1972; 287:1234.

34. Ransom JHC et al: Prevention, diagnosis and treatment of pancreatic abscess. Surgery. 1977; 82:99.

35. Holden JE et al: Pancreatic abscess following acute pancreatitis. Arch Surg. 1976; 111:858.

36. Blackburn GL et al: New approaches to the management of severe acute pancreatitis. Am J Surg. 1976; 131:114.

37. Dionigi R et al: Nutrition and infection. J Parent & Ent Nut. 1979; 3:62.

38. Feller JH et al: Changing methods in the treatment of severe pancreatitis. Am J Surg. 1974; 127:196.

39. Ranson JHC et al: Prognostic signs and the role of operative management in acute pancreatitis. Surg Gynecol Obstet. 1974; 139:69.

40. Flink EB: Therapy of magnesium deficiency. NY Acad Med. 1969; 162:901.

41. Mordes JP et al: Excess magnesium. Pharmacol Rev. 1978; 29:273.

42. Banks PA: Treatment of chronic pancreatitis. In *Pancreatitis*, Plenum Medical Book Co., New York, 1979, p 209.

43. Banks PA: Clinical features of chronic pancreatitis. In *Pancreatitis*, Plenum Medical Book Co., New York, 1979, p 189.

44. DiMagno EP et al: Relations between pancreatic enzyme outputs and malabsorption in severe pancreatic insufficiency. N Engl J Med. 1973; 288:813.

45. Howard JM et al: The etiology of pancreatitis: a review of clinical experience. Ann Surg. 1960; 152:135.

46. Sarles H et al: Observations on 205 confirmed cases of acute pancreatitis, recurring pancreatitis, and chronic pancreatitis. Gut. 1965; 6:545.

47. DiMagno EP et al: Relationship between alcoholism and pancreatic insufficiency. Ann NY Acad Sci. 1975; 252:200.

48. DiMagno EP et al: The relationships between pancreatic ductal obstruction and pancreatic secretion in man. Mayo Clin Proc. 1979; 54:157.

49. DiMagno EP et al: Medical treatment of pancreatic insufficiency. Mayo Clin Proc. 1979; 54:435.

50. Giulian BB et al: Treatment of pancreatic exocrine insufficiency: in vitro lipolytic activities of pancreatic lipase and fifteen commercial pancreatic supplements. Ann Surg. 1967; 165:564.

51. Pairent FW et al: Pancreatic exocrine insufficiency: the enzyme content of commercial pancreatic supplements. Arch Surg. 1975; 110:739.

52. Graham DY: Enzyme replacement therapy of exocrine pancreatic insufficiency in man: relation between in-vitro enzyme activities and in-vivo potency in commercial pancreatic extracts. N Engl J Med. 1977; 296:1314.

53. Graham DY: An enteric-coated pancreatic enzyme preparation that works. Dig Dis Sci. 1979; 24:906.

54. Regan PT et al: Comparative effects of antacids, cimetidine and enteric coating on the therapeutic response to oral enzymes in severe pancreatic insufficiency. N Engl J Med. 1977; 297:854.

55. DiMagno EP et al: Fate of orally ingested enzymes in pancreatic insufficiency: comparison of two dosage schedules. N Engl J Med. 1977; 296:1318.

56. French AB et al: Effect of pancreatic replacement therapy on metabolic balance in adolescent fibrocystic disease. J Lab Clin Med. 1967; 70:1005.

57. Heizer WD et al: Gastric inactivation of pancreatic supplements. Bull Johns Hopk Hosp. 1965; 116:261.

58. Regan PT et al: Rationale for the use of cimetidine in pancreatic insufficiency. Mayo Clin Proc. 1978; 53:79.

59. Cox KL et al: The effect of cimetidine on maldigestion in cystic fibrosis. J Pediatr. 1979; 94:488.

60. Kravety RE et al: Gastric secretion in chronic pancreatitis. Ann Intern Med. 1969; 63:776.

61. Chey WY et al: Gastric secretion in patients with chronic pancreatitis and in chronic alcoholics. Arch Intern Med. 1968; 122:399.

62. Bunk S et al: Gastric acid secretion in pancreatic disease. Gastroenterology. 1966; 51:649.
63. Hill D: Pancreatic extract lung sensitivity. Med J Austr. 1975; 2:533.
64. Stapleton FB et al: Hyperuricosuria due to high-dose pancreatic extract therapy in cystic fibrosis. N Engl J Med. 1976; 295:246.
65. Nousia-Arvanitakis S et al: Therapeutic approach to pancreatic extract-induced hyperuricosuria in cystic fibrosis. J Pediatr. 1977; 90:302.

Chapter 22

Acute Cholecystitis

John Russo, Jr.

The gallbladder is a distensible outpouching of the extrahepatic biliary duct system which stores, concentrates, and discharges micellar bile complexes into the duodenum during periods of digestion. The location of the gall bladder and other important structures of the bile duct system are shown in Figure 1.

A prolonged imbalance between the cholesterol, phospholipid, and conjugated bile acid components of bile will lead to gallstone formation within the gallbladder. These calculi become clinically significant when forced into the cystic duct by gallbladder contractions which occur in response to cholecystokinin release following a meal. Lodgement or passage of calculi through the cystic duct and common bile duct is usually accompanied by the sudden onset of severe mid-epigastric or right upper quadrant pain which may last 1–3 hours. Attacks of biliary "colic" occur at unpredictable intervals at any time of the day or night and are often accompanied by nausea.

In cases of prolonged obstruction, inflammation of the gallbladder ensues (acute cholecystitis). Bacterial infection of the gallbladder and its contents occurs in 75% of patients with obstruction of the cystic duct. Acute cholecystitis is accompanied by a low grade fever, an increased white count with a shift to the left, and right upper quadrant tenderness. The serum bilirubin and alkaline phosphatase may be moderately elevated, and the serum transaminase levels may be increased. Frank jaundice and chills are unusual.

The abdominal pain can be more generalized than that observed in biliary colic.

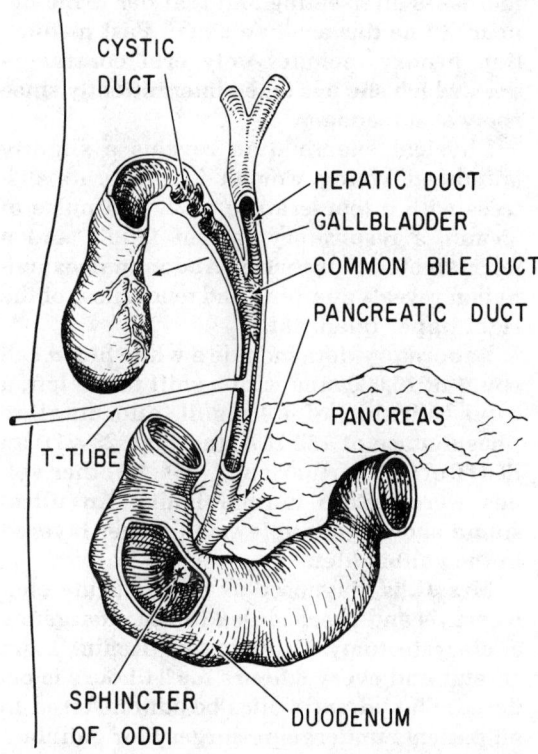

Figure 1. Anatomic relationship between the gallbladder, pancreas and duodenum with placement of a T-tube drain.

Acute cholecystitis is corrected surgically, but the role of antibiotic therapy in the prevention of postoperative infections is important, and often controversial. The therapeutic principles applied when assessing the need for antibiotics and initiating appropriate therapy are applicable to all surgical procedures where prophylactic antibiotic therapy is being considered.

1. *Antibiotic Therapy.* **Mrs. C. is a 24-year-old woman with a chief complaint of nausea and sharp cramping epigastric pain radiating to the right subscapular region which has lasted for three days. She experienced her first episode of epigastric pain three years prior to admission following the birth of her first child; that episode lasted one hour and subsided spontaneously. She is now three months postpartum with her third child and has experienced more frequent painful episodes; each lasts approximately 12 hours and is accompanied by nausea and occasional vomiting. Recently she has noted that the pain increases after eating and that her urine appears to be darker than usual. Past medication history includes only oral contraceptives which she has taken intermittently since she was a teenager.**

Physical examination reveals a slightly jaundiced young woman in moderate distress with a temperature of 38°C, a pulse of 95/min, a respiratory rate of 17/min and a normal blood pressure. Abdominal examination reveals guarding and tenderness of the right upper quadrant.

Laboratory data include a white blood cell count of 16,000/mm³ with a shift to the left, a total bilirubin of 4.3 mg/dl, and alkaline phosphatase of 152 IU/L (normal: 23–71), an SGOT of 96 IU/L (normal: 7–26). All other values were within normal limits. An ultrasound showed multiple small stones layered in the gallbladder.

Mrs. C. is diagnosed as having acute cholecystitis and is scheduled for an emergency cholecystectomy. Cephalothin (Keflin) 1 gm IV stat and every 6 hours for 24 hours is ordered. Should antibiotics be administered to all patients undergoing surgery for gallbladder disease?

In young, otherwise healthy patients cholecystectomy carries little risk of infection. In fact, the postoperative infection rate is less than 2% in two-thirds of all patients with gallbladder disease (1,2). Surgical procedures are considered "clean" when the risk of postoperative infection is this low, and prophylactic antibiotic therapy is unjustified (3,4). Patients with decreased resistance, valvular heart disease or other cardiac abnormalities are possible exceptions (4,5). However, Mrs. C. is at risk for postoperative infection, as discussed in Question 2.

2. Is it possible to identify patients at high risk for postoperative infection? Why is prophylactic antibiotic therapy appropriate for this patient?

Infection of the bile with enteric organisms (bile sepsis) is the major risk factor for postoperative infectious complications. It is present in approximately one-third of cholecystectomy cases, and these patients are 40 times more likely to experience postoperative infections than those whose bile cultures are negative (1). One approach to this problem is to aspirate and gram-stain gallbladder bile intraoperatively. Antibiotics can then be administered prior to gallbladder excision if bacteria are identified. Advocates of this technique state that it permits administration of more specific antibiotics and limits unnecessary patient exposure (6). This is the only method by which all patients with bile sepsis can be guaranteed coverage, but it is time consuming and may require additional personnel to carry out the microscopic evaluation.

Alternatively, it is possible to assess risk factors for bile sepsis and to use antibiotics in those patients who are at risk. Table 1 lists four risk factors associated with bile sepsis more than 50% of the time.

Mrs. C. has two risk factors: jaundice and the need for emergency surgery. She does not meet the age criteria even if we lower it to 60 years as

Table 1.

RISK FACTORS FOR BILE SEPSIS
IN CHOLECYSTITIS (1,6)

Factors	Positive Cultures (%)
Age greater than 70 years	54–72
Jaundice at surgery	65–90
Emergency surgery	60–100
Choledocholithiasis	58–63

one group has done (7). Preoperatively, it is not possible to predict with certainty if she has choledocholithiasis (calculi in the common bile duct). Its incidence is reportedly between 2.5% and 25% of patients with acute cholecystitis; the greatest frequency is reported when the diagnosis is made solely by clinical criteria, while lower rates occur when histopathologic findings are analyzed (8–10). Jaundice is an unreliable marker for choledocholithiasis and may reflect other causes of obstruction, including compression of the common bile duct by an acutely inflamed gallbladder, pancreatitis, hepatitis, or choledochal sphincter spasm. Laboratory studies, such as serum bilirubin, alkaline phosphatase levels, and intravenous cholangiography are also unreliable. Intraoperative cholangiography is the diagnostic method of choice, and if positive, antibiotics should be administered prior to cholecystectomy with common bile duct exploration (8,9).

3. To what extent will prophylactic antibiotic therapy reduce the risk of postoperative infection in Mrs. C.?

Postoperative wound infections (in biliary surgery) occur in 27% of high risk patients (2) and in 11% of all cholecystitis patients regardless of the presence of risk factors or infected bile (12). The appropriate use of antibiotics as an adjunct to optimal surgical technique reduces this complication to 4% in the former group and 2% in the latter group, an infection rate similar to that found in "clean" surgical procedures. Similar findings are reported for septicemia (11), but not in the prevention of abscess formation. The potential consequences of septicemia require no further elaboration. However, wound infections can progress to septicemia or cellulitis and can double the postoperative stay, thereby significantly increasing hospitalization expenses (13).

4. Evaluate the choice of antibiotic therapy for Mrs. C.

The choice of antibiotic depends upon the organisms responsible for bile sepsis. Table 2 provides a representative list of organisms cultured from bile of 215 patients and is likely to be representative of findings in most institutions. E. coli predominates with gram-negative aerobes found in over 70% of infected bile. A cephalosporin, such as cephalothin which was prescribed for Mrs. C., will provide adequate coverage for a majority of

these strains as well as staphylococci. More complete coverage requires combination therapy such as an aminoglycoside plus ampicillin. Both reduce the incidence of wound infections (11,12), but the specific choice of agents depends on the organisms commonly isolated and their antibiotic sensitivity at a particular institution.

The time of administration is critical if optimal results are to be achieved. Antibiotics must not only be able to kill or suppress the invading bacteria but act before biochemical lesions have occurred (eg, within three hours of contamination) (14). To accomplish this, antibiotics are started one to two hours preoperatively and administered for no longer than 24 to 48 hours as illustrated by Mrs. C.'s orders (15). Antibiotic therapy initiated post-surgically is ineffective (12), and initiating therapy earlier or prolonging it beyond 48 hours has not been shown to improve results (16–18). Despite this, a recent study indicates that prolongation of prophylactic antibiotic therapy is common and may account for 20 to 25% of all antimicrobial drug therapy in hospitals (19). This area of therapeutics should be a target for cost containment by all clinicians.

5. Is it important to achieve high antibiotic bile concentrations?

It is widely assumed that high bile concentrations of an antibiotic are essential to the successful therapy of patients with biliary sepsis. Studies measuring these levels in patients with T-tube drains as shown in Figure 1 demonstrate that the bile levels for many antibiotics greatly exceed the corresponding serum levels (20–22). This tech-

Table 2.

MICROORGANISMS ISOLATED FROM THE BILE
IN 215 CHOLECYSTECTOMY PATIENTS

Escherichia coli	48 %
Streptococci (including enterococci 10% and anaerobic streptococci 16%)	33 %
Klebsiella	22 %
Staphylococci	7 %
Enterobacter	7 %
Clostridia	3.7%
Bacteroides fragilis	3.7%
Pseudomonas	2.3%

Modified from Jarvinen H et al: Ann Clin Res. 1978; 10:247.

nique has been criticized because T-tubes promote free drainage of bile, reflecting normal physiology. They do not provide any indication of antibiotic bile levels found during acute cholecystitis (6). Table 3 shows that the pathology associated with high risk cholecystitis patients has a dramatic effect. Following the administration of ampicillin, 500 mg within two hours of surgery, simultaneous serum, common bile duct bile and gallbladder bile were obtained. Patients at low risk for bile sepsis (no obstruction) attained bile concentrations of ampicillin at least twice those found in serum. Cystic duct obstruction resulted in subtherapeutic ampicillin levels in the gallbladder bile, and common bile duct obstruction was associated with undetectable antibiotic levels in the bile (23).

It appears that adequate bile concentrations of antibiotics are not attainable in cholecystitis when there is obstruction to bile flow (11,24). The success of prophylactic antibiotic therapy must be dependent upon the achievement of therapeutic tissue levels and this is related to the serum level, not the bile level attained (11,24,25).

6. *Drug-Induced Cholecystitis.* **Mrs. C.'s history associates her gallbladder disease with pregnancy. Does such an association exist, and could the use of oral contraceptives contribute to her condition?**

Yes. Multiparity appears to predispose women to gallbladder disease, and there is evidence that exogenously administered estrogens also increase this risk, possibly by elevating bile cholesterol levels (26,27). The Coronary Drug Project found that men taking 2.5 or 5 mg conjugated estrogens daily were at increased risk for cholecystitis (28), and the Boston Collaborative Drug Surveillance Program reported similar findings in women below the age of 35 taking oral contraceptives (29).

Although not applicable in this patient, similar findings are reported during chronic thiazide and clofibrate therapy (28,30).

7. *Medical Therapy for Gallstones.* **Mr. C. recently read that it is possible to dissolve gallstones and wishes to know if a drug can be used to treat his wife, thereby avoiding any risks associated with surgery.**

Numerous reports on gallstone dissolution with chenodeoxycholic acid (CDC) have attracted great interest, and unless significant adverse effects from this drug are reported, many patients in the United States will soon have this drug available as a therapeutic option. Its mechanism of action is not completely understood, but biliary excretion of cholesterol is lower when CDC constitutes the main bile acid secreted; this may be due to diminished cholesterol synthesis.

Clinical trials report total dissolution of stones in 12–20% of patients following one to three years of therapy. Part of this modest response may be due to noncompliance, subtherapeutic doses (10–15 mg/kg body weight per day is recommended), use of the drug to dissolve large stones (>2 cm in diameter) which respond poorly, and perhaps treatment of stones composed of pigments which, unlike cholesterol stones, are unaffected by CDC. Diarrhea, a dose-dependent side effect of CDC, and a recurrence rate of 30% once therapy is discontinued also make this a less attractive alternative than it would initially appear. CDC is also contraindicated in women of childbearing age and patients with known or suspected disease of the liver parenchyma.

If these limitations are evaluated in an average patient population, it is estimated that 18–20% would qualify for therapy and that less than half could expect complete dissolution after one to three years. Although CDC will not dramati-

Table 3.

EFFECT OF DUCT OBSTRUCTION ON AMPICILLIN LEVELS

Cholelithiasis	Ampicillin Concentration (mcg/ml)		
	Serum	Common Bile Duct Bile	Gallbladder Bile
No Obstruction	6.2 ± 0.46	22.3 ± 3.78	13.1 ± 2.69
Cystic Duct Obstruction	5.8 ± 0.88	12.9 ± 2.88	1.45 ± 0.80
Common Bile Duct Obstruction	6.8 ± 1.09	—	—

Modified from Mortimer PR et al: Brit Med J. 1969; 3:88.

cally reduce the number of cholecystectomies performed, it will probably be of value in patients who are at high risk for surgery and those who have small radiolucent stones and a functioning gallbladder (31).

References

1. Chetlin SH et al: Biliary bacteremia. Arch Surg. 1971; 102:303.
2. Chetlin SH et al: Preoperative antibiotics in biliary surgery. Arch Surg. 1973; 107:319.
3. Cruse PJE et al: A five-year prospective study of 23,649 surgical wounds. Arch Surg. 1973; 107:206.
4. MacLean LD: Prophylactic antibiotic therapy in surgery. Can J Surg. 1975; 18:243.
5. Kaplan EL et al: Prevention of bacterial endocarditis. Circulation. 1977; 56:139A.
6. Keighley MRB et al: Antibiotic treatment of biliary sepsis. Surg Clin North Am. 1975; 55:1379.
7. Kune GA et al: Are antibiotics necessary in acute cholecystitis. Med J Aust. 1975; 2:627.
8. Pitluk HC et al: Choledocholithiasis associated with acute cholecystitis. Arch Surg. 1979; 114:887.
9. Cheung LY et al: Jaundice in patients with acute cholecystitis: its validity as an indication for common bile duct exploration. Am J Surg. 1975; 130:746.
10. Watkin DFL et al: Jaundice in acute cholecystitis. Br J Surg. 1971; 58:570.
11. Keighley MBR et al: Antibiotics in biliary disease: the relative importance of antibiotic concentrations in the bile and serum. Gut. 1976; 17:495.
12. Stone HH et al: Antibiotic prophylaxis in gastric, biliary and colonic surgery. Ann Surg. 1976; 184:443.
13. Green JW et al: Postoperative wound infection: a controlled study of the increased duration of hospital stay and direct cost of hospitalization. Ann Surg. 1977; 185:264.
14. Burke JF: Preoperative antibiotics. Surg Clin North Am. 1963; 43:665.
15. Hurley DL et al: Perioperative prophylactic antibiotics in abdominal surgery: a review of recent progress. Surg Clin North Am. 1979; 59:919.
16. Ledger WJ et al: Guidelines for antibiotic prophylaxis in gynecology. Am J Obstet Gynecol. 1975; 121:1038.
17. Conte JE Jr et al: Antibiotic prophylaxis and cardiac surgery: a prospective double-blind comparison of single-dose versus multiple-dose regimens. Ann Intern Med. 1972; 76:943.
18. Goldmann DA et al: Cephalothin prophylaxis in cardiac valve surgery: a prospective, double-blind comparison of two-day and six-day regimens. J Thorac Cardiovasc Surg. 1977; 73:470.
19. Shapiro M et al: Use of antimicrobial drugs in general hospitals: patterns of prophylaxis. N Engl J Med. 1979; 301:351.
20. Furesz S et al: Experimental data for the use of Rifamycin S.V. in biliary infections: in vitro activity against various pathogenic bacteria and bile concentrations in man. Chemotherapia. 1963; 7:365.
21. Hammond JB et al: Factors affecting the absorption and biliary excretion of erythromycin and two of its derivatives in humans. Clin Pharmacol Exper Ther. 1960; 3:308.
22. Turner FP: Fatal *Clostridium welchii* septicaemia following cholecystectomy. Am J Surg. 1956; 144:1008.
23. Mortimer PR et al: Ampicillin levels in human bile in the presence of biliary tract disease. Br Med J. 1969; 3:88.
24. Jarvinen H et al: Antibiotics in acute cholecystitis. Ann Clin Res. 1978; 10:247.
25. Waterman NG et al: Antibiotic concentrations in hepatic interstitial and wound fluid. Surg Gynecol Obstet. 1976; 142:235.
26. Bennion L J et al: Effects of oral contraceptives on the gallbladder bile of normal women. N Engl J Med. 1976; 294:189.
27. Pertsemlidis D et al: Effects of clofibrate and of an estrogen-progestin combination on fasting biliary lipids and cholic acid kinetics in man. Gastroenterology. 1974; 66:565.
28. The Coronary Drug Project Research Group: Gallbladder disease as a side effect of drugs influencing lipid metabolism. N Engl J Med. 1977; 296:1185.
29. Boston Collaborative Drug Surveillance Program: Oral contraceptives and venous thromboembolic disease, surgically confirmed gallbladder disease and breast tumours. Lancet. 1973; 1:1399.
30. Rosenberg L et al: Thiazides and acute cholecystitis. N Engl J Med. 1980; 303:546.
31. Schersten T: Medical treatment of gallstones: clinical evaluation of the indication. Scand J Gastroent. 1978; 13:129.

Chapter 23

Congenital Biliary Atresia

Kelly D. Mutchie and John A. Bosso

Congenital biliary atresia, which results in obstructive or cholestatic jaundice in infancy, is the pathologic closure of a major portion or segment of the extrahepatic biliary tree. Its etiology and pathogenesis are unclear (1). Intrahepatic biliary atresia or hypoplasia, which accounts for less than 10% of cases of obstructive jaundice, will not be discussed.

The incidence of biliary atresia is approximately 1 in 25,000 live births. Jaundice and hepatomegaly always occur but may not be detected for several weeks after birth. In surgically unrepaired cases, the prognosis is hopeless and death due to hepatic failure usually occurs by the end of the second year of life (2). This condition may be surgically corrected by the original or a variation of the Kasai procedure or portoenterostomy shown in Figure 1 (3–5). Successful biliary drainage is accomplished in a high percentage of patients when this procedure is performed in the first 60 days of life. Nevertheless, bile flow may not reach adequate levels for 6 to 12 months postoperatively (5). Progressive intrahepatic disease invariably occurs and few patients survive beyond 5 to 10 years of age, although some long-term survivors have been reported (2).

Patients who have had successful operations present the clinician with a number of chronic management problems including recurrent cholangitis, osteomalacia and osteoporosis, nutritional deficiencies and failure to thrive, portal hypertension, and psycho-social problems.

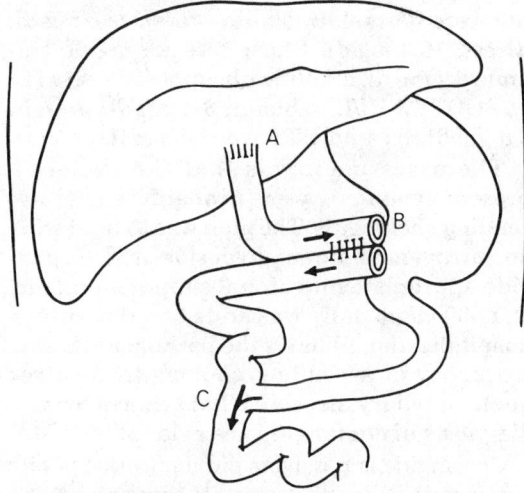

Figure 1. Schematic illustration of operation for patients with biliary atresia. Arrows indicate direction of intestinal and bile flow. Adapted from Barkin (reference 5) by permission from Journal of Pediatrics.

1. K.M. is a 10-month-old, white male who is admitted with a chief complaint of lethargy and fever for two days. The diagnosis of biliary atresia was made at 2 weeks of age and a Kasai procedure was performed when he was six weeks old which resulted in a decrease in serum bilirubin over a four-month period. In the interim, the patient has had

two hospitalizations for ascending cholangitis, which have been treated with intravenous antibiotics. The patient has no documented allergies. He is presently taking phenobarbital, 30 mg daily at bedtime and trimethoprim/sulfamethoxazole (Bactrim) one teaspoonful every 12 hours.

Physical examination revealed an acutely ill, markedly jaundiced, responsive, alert infant. Vital signs: temperature 40°C, pulse 140/min, respiratory rate 48/min, weight 9.8 kg (25th percentile for height and weight). Eyes had marked scleral icterus. The liver was palpated 4 cm below the right costal margin.

Admitting laboratory values were as follows: white cell count 11,000 leukocytes/mm^3 (15% bands, 38% segmented neutrophils, 40% lymphocytes, and 7% monocytes), hemoglobin 13.7 gm/dl, and hematocrit 40.6%. Serum sodium, potassium, chloride, and bicarbonate were normal. Bilirubin—total: 12.0 mg/dl, direct: 10.0 mg/dl. Phosphate 1.9 mg/dl, calcium 8.7 mg/dl, alkaline phosphatase 1214 IU/L, SGOT 73 IU/L, albumin 3.2 gm/dl, protein 6.3 gm/dl. PT and PTT were normal.

The assessment was that the patient's present symptoms were probably due to ascending cholangitis. The plan was to treat with an intravenous aminoglycoside and to provide appropiate nutritional support. Vitamin D, 1,000 IU po daily was added on day two of hospitalization. What is the pathogenesis and frequency of ascending cholangitis as a sequela of biliary atresia? What criteria for the diagnosis of cholangitis are evident in K.M.?

Cholangitis is a universal complication of biliary atresia following successful hepatic portoenterostomy. Although the pathogenesis remains unclear, evidence supports the role of an ascending infection. Hitch and co-workers demonstrated that bacterial colonization occurs during the first postoperative month in these patients (6). Bilirubin clearance correlates directly with the number of different bacteria and bacterial count, and cholangitis appears to be more common in patients with good bilirubin excretory function (5–7). The onset is variable, but the first episode generally occurs in the first six to nine months following surgery. Barkin et al (5) reported that all patients in their study population with successful bile drainage had at least one and as many as seven attacks of cholangitis during the first post-

operative year. The average number of episodes was 4.8 per patient during the first year, and 2.5 episodes per patient during the second year.

The diagnosis of cholangitis is based on clinical signs and laboratory data. A high fever associated with an elevation in white blood cell count is usually present as illustrated by K.M. Serum bilirubin levels also increase, but often not for 24 to 36 hours after the onset of symptoms. In K.M., the elevated serum bilirubin is accompanied by jaundice and scleral icterus.

2. Was it appropriate to initiate aminoglycoside therapy in K.M.? What is the role of prophylactic antibiotic therapy in K.M.?

Acute cases of cholangitis should be treated with a 10-day course of intravenous aminoglycosides (5). If this therapy is initiated immediately, a rapid response generally occurs followed by a return of the serum bilirubin levels to normal.

Hitch et al (6) evaluated the effect of several antibiotics on the colonization of the bilioenteric conduit and found that none, except trimethoprim/sulfamethoxazole, which is excreted into the bile, affected the number of different types of bacteria or the bacterial count. Despite these results, the authors' clinical impression was that aminoglycosides were most effective in the treatment of acute cholangitis. This was explained by the fact that biliary concentrations of antibiotics do not necessarily correlate with tissue antibiotic concentrations. This assumption correlates well with canine studies in which gentamicin is relatively concentrated in both hepatic and other soft tissue even though it is barely detectable in bile fluids (8).

Because the majority of episodes of cholangitis appear during the first postoperative year, many clinicians recommend prophylactic long-term antibiotic therapy during this period. Kobayashi et al (7) evaluated the effect of prophylactic ampicillin therapy on the incidence of cholangitis. The duration of therapy was 10–14 months and 18% of the patients who received long-term antibiotic therapy developed cholangitis. In contrast, 59% of patients receiving no antibiotic therapy developed this complication. The use of prophylactic antibiotics seems reasonable, although this practice is based upon limited clinical data. The choice of trimethoprim/sulfamethoxazole in this patient also appears to be rational based upon its effects on the bacterial colonization of the bilioenteric conduit (6).

3. What is the rationale for the use of phenobarbital in K.M.?

Phenobarbital is often administered to patients with biliary atresia in an attempt to stimulate bile excretion (5). Stiehl et al (9) demonstrated that phenobarbital stimulated bile secretion and biliary excretion of bile salts in two children with intrahepatic cholestasis. Other studies have demonstrated that phenobarbital induces those microsomal processes concerned with drug, steroid, and bilirubin metabolism (10). As with prophylactic antibiotics, data supporting the therapeutic efficacy of phenobarbital in biliary atresia are incomplete. However, since cholangitis during the first postoperative year is most likely due to ascending infection which may be facilitated by intrahepatic cholestasis, these agents may be of some benefit.

4. K.M.'s height and weight are in the 25th percentile. What is the most probable explanation for this observation?

Adequate nutrition and growth are important concerns in patients with biliary atresia, because they are unable to efficiently digest fat and as a result develop a malabsorption syndrome characterized by steatorrhea, vitamin D and vitamin K deficiency, and growth retardation (11,12). Patients such as K.M. who have undergone successful portoenterostomies can be expected to achieve normal bile outputs approximately one year following surgery (5). Until adequate bile flow is achieved, however, they will require nutritional support and vitamin supplementation.

Medium chain triglycerides (MCT) provide a source of absorbable fat which permits growth (11,12). MCT's are contained in some infant formulas and may be added to others (see the Pediatric Therapy chapter).

Supplementation of vitamin K, a fat soluble vitamin, may be required if malabsorption of that vitamin occurs to the extent that a prolonged prothrombin time is observed. This results from a decreased synthesis of the vitamin K-dependent clotting factors.

Supplementation of vitamin D may also be required as discussed in Question 5. The degree of vitamin D absorption is related to the severity of biliary obstruction and therefore to the degree of steatorrhea.

5. Radiographic studies performed on the second hospital day revealed decreased bone density. What is the most likely explanation for this finding as well as his abnormal serum phosphate, calcium, and alkaline phosphatase levels?

K.M.'s abnormal bone x-ray, his high alkaline phosphatase and his low serum calcium and phosphate are consistent with the diagnosis of rickets, a disease characterized by bone demineralization.

This complication of biliary atresia is caused primarily by the malabsorption of vitamin D (cholecalciferol) (13,14) and perhaps by the impaired hydroxylation and activation of vitamin D by the liver (13). The latter mechanism is controversial, however (14). Phenobarbital therapy may also increase the catabolism of vitamin D to inactive metabolites and thereby predispose the patient to this complication (15–17). Rickets is observed in virtually all patients with biliary atresia and the diagnosis is made at a mean age of 10.6 months (5).

Several preparations of vitamin D are available, and many have been used in the prevention and treatment of rickets with varying degrees of success. Vitamin D_2 (ergocalciferol) is the biologically inactive form of vitamin D which must be hydroxylated by the liver and then the kidney to an active form. It is an oil soluble vitamin which requires the presence of bile acids to be completely absorbed. It is not surprising that the response of patients with biliary atresia to oral vitamin D_2 is variable and unpredictable. Kooh et al report three cases of children with biliary atresia on daily doses ranging from 400 U to 10,000 U of vitamin D_2 who developed hypocalcemia, hypophosphatemia, and bone demineralization. All responded in 3–4 weeks on 3000 IU weekly of intravenous vitamin D_2 (14).

Nevertheless, the extent of malabsorption often is not complete in these children and can be overridden by pharmacological doses of vitamin D_2. Whereas 400 IU is the usual daily nutritional requirement for vitamin D_2, doses of 1000–2000 IU daily as prescribed for K.M. are common; doses of 4000–10,000 IU daily may be required in frankly rachitic children.

The therapeutic response to vitamin D therapy will be exhibited by an increase in serum phosphate and serum calcium. The onset of response is generally within 2–10 days and normalization can be expected 3–4 weeks following the onset of therapy. The complete healing of bony lesions may take somewhat longer (18). Hypercalcemia is the major complication of vitamin D therapy.

    If K.M. is unresponsive to conventional modes of therapy, 25-hydroxy vitamin D$_3$, (calcediol, Calderol) 4–5 mcg/kg/day orally or 1,25-dihydroxy vitamin D$_3$ (calcitriol, Rocaltrol) 0.2 mcg/kg/day parenterally may be used (18,19).

References

1. Haas JE: Bile duct and liver pathology in biliary atresia. World J Surg. 1978; 2:561.
2. Kasai M et al: Technique and results of operative management of biliary atresia. World J Surg. 1978; 2:571.
3. Kasai M et al: Surgical treatment of biliary atresia. J Pediatr Surg. 1968; 3:665.
4. Lilly JR and Hitch DC: Postoperative ascending cholangitis following portoenterostomy for biliary atresia: measures for control. World J Surg. 1978; 2:581.
5. Barkin RM et al: Biliary atresia and the Kasai operation: continuing care. J Pediatr. 1980; 96:1015.
6. Hitch DC et al: Identification, quantification, and significance of bacterial growth within the biliary tract after Kasai's operation. J Pediatr Surg. 1978; 13:563.
7. Kobayashi A et al: Congenital biliary atresia. Am J Dis Child. 1976; 130:830.
8. Waterman NG et al: Antibiotic concentration in hepatic interstitial and wound fluid. Surg Gynecol Obstet. 1976; 142:235.
9. Stiehl A et al: The effects of phenobarbital on bile salts and bilirubin in patients with intrahepatic and extrahepatic cholestasis. N Engl J Med. 1972; 286:858.
10. Thaler MM et al: Phenobarbital-induced changes in NADPH-cytochrome C reductase and smooth endoplasmic reticulum in human liver. J Pediatr. 1972; 80:302.
11. Silverberg M et al: Nutritional requirements of infants and children with liver disease. Am J Clin Nutr. 1980; 23:604.
12. Weber A et al: The malabsorption associated with chronic liver disease in children. Pediatrics. 1972; 50:73.
13. Daum F et al: 25-hydroxycholecalciferol in the management of rickets associated with extrahepatic biliary atresia. J Pediatr. 1976; 88:1041.
14. Kooh SW et al: Pathogenesis of rickets in chronic hepatobiliary disease in children. J Pediatr. 1979; 94:870.
15. Heubi JE et al: 1, 25-dihydroxyvitamin D$_3$ in childhood hepatic osteodystrophy. J Pediatr. 1979; 94:977.
16. Jubiz W et al: Plasma 1, 25-dihydroxyvitamin D levels in patients receiving anticonvulsant drugs. J Clin Endocrinol Metab. 1977; 44:617.
17. Hahn TJ et al: Serum 25-hydroxycalciferol levels and bone mass in children on chronic anticonvulsant therapy. N Engl J Med. 1975; 292:550.
18. Tsang RC: Rickets. In *Current Pediatric Therapy,* 9th ed, edited by SS Gellis and BM Kagan, WB Saunders Company, Philadelphia, 1980, p 336.
19. Glorieux FH et al: Bone response to phosphate salts, ergocalciferol, and calcitrol in hypophosphatemic vitamin D rickets. N Engl J Med. 1980; 303:1023.

Chapter 24

Alcoholic Cirrhosis

Joseph P. Gee and Lucia K. Jim

Cirrhosis can best be defined as a chronic disease of the liver in which diffuse hepatic parenchymal cell destruction has led to the active formation of connective tissue and nodular regeneration with resultant disorganization of the normal lobular architecture (1). The classification of cirrhosis is still undergoing evolution; a confusing array of nomenclature and inconsistent criteria are found in current literature (2). LaMont has classified cirrhosis into the following categories: Laennec's, postnecrotic, biliary (primary or secondary), hemochromatosis, cardiac or congestive, or rare and nonspecific cirrhosis (3). The most prevalent type of cirrhosis in the United States and Western Europe is Laennec's cirrhosis, and alcoholism is the most common cause (2,4–6). The incidence of cirrhosis among chronic alcoholics is 10–20% (3). Other contributing factors such as malnutrition and genetic factors have also been suggested (7,8). Other major types of cirrhosis seen in the United States are postnecrotic and biliary cirrhosis (4).

Pathogenesis. The pathogenesis of alcoholic cirrhosis is not completely understood. Alcohol alone causes fatty infiltration and ultrastructural changes in the livers of animals and alcoholic and non-alcoholic man. Diet supplementation does not prevent alcohol-induced lesions in man, but diet deficiency has been shown in animal studies to potentiate the injurious effect of alcohol. The major biochemical alteration, an increase in the NADH:NAD ratio, is produced by the oxidation of alcohol and results in hyperlipidemia, fatty liver, ketosis, hypoglycemia, hyperlactacidemia, and other abnormalities in the microsomal enzyme system. Electron microscopic study of fatty liver produced experimentally by the administration of alcohol reveals changes in the mitochondria and rough endoplasmic reticulum comparable to those seen in patients with alcoholic hepatitis, suggesting that fatty liver may represent the precursor of alcoholic hepatitis. Since only a limited number of alcoholics develop hepatitis, and all of these don't progress to cirrhosis, factors other than alcohol (ie, genetic predisposition, other hepatotoxins) could contribute to the pathogenesis of cirrhosis (6). The latter point is further supported by the observation that some cases of alcoholic hepatitis do not progress to cirrhosis in spite of continued excessive drinking and others progress to cirrhosis despite documented abstinence (11,12). Cirrhosis is probably the result of fibrosis secondary to hepatocyte inflammation and necrosis. However, the interrelationships between fatty liver, alcoholic hepatitis, and cirrhosis have yet to be elucidated.

Clinical Features. Cirrhosis may be asymptomatic for a variable length of time or may appear in an active, symptomatic phase in which alcoholic hepatitis is most often noted as the primary lesion. The most common subjective complaints, which are nonspecific for hepatocellular injuries, include anorexia, nausea, abdominal discomfort, weakness, weight loss, easy fatigability, and malaise. Hepatosplenomegaly, jaundice, ascites, and peripheral edema are usually found on physical examination. Spider angiomas and palmar erythema are common signs of liver disease.

Portal Hypertension. Many signs and symptoms of advanced liver cirrhosis are related to complications secondary to the development of portal hypertension. The portal vein collects blood from the splanchnic area, which includes the abdominal portion of the digestive tract, the pancreas, and the spleen, and transports the blood to the liver (Fig. 1). At the liver hilum, the portal vein separates into a right and a left branch. Portal venous blood passes through a capillary system in the splanchnic viscera and leads to the hepatic sinusoids. Portal venous blood differs from most other venous blood in being: under slightly higher pressure in order to overcome the resistance of the hepatic sinusoids, higher in oxygen content because of the relatively high blood flow through the splanchnic area, and containing many nutrients and bacterial waste products from the digestive tract that are being routed to the liver. Normal portal venous pressure is about 5 to 10 mm Hg (13). In advanced cirrhosis, blood flow can be blocked by fibrous regenerative nodules. These nodules compress and distort the hepatic veins, leading to increased portal venous pressure (14). Proliferation of endothelial and sinusoidal cells might also significantly increase portal pressure in alcoholic hepatitis (15). Other causes for increased resistance to portal venous flow include extrahepatic vein thrombosis, schistosomiasis, and post-hepatic venous obstruction (eg, Budd-Chiari syndrome, metastatic liver tumor). If such increase in portal venous pressure persists, normal lymph and blood flow are interfered with, followed by development of collateral blood vessels and intrahepatic shunts (13). The natural sites for the development of collateral circulation are the low pressure veins and venules in the submucosa of the esophagus, rectum, anterior abdominal wall, splenic vein, and parietal peritoneum. Thus, portal hypertension is often accompanied by splenic enlargement, esophageal and gastric varices, abdominal collaterals, ascites, hemorrhoids, and symptoms related to the shunting of venous blood away from the liver. Splenomegaly is commonly associated with hematologic disorders (eg, thrombocytopenia, low grade hemolytic anemia, and neutropenia) (16). Ruptured esophageal varices, however, are the most common life-threatening complications of portal hypertension (13,17,18). Other major complications related to advanced cirrhosis include hepatic encephalopathy and renal failure (19,20).

Laboratory Findings. Laboratory evaluation does not measure the functional capacity of the liver but only gives a rough qualitative estimate of the liver dysfunction. Conventional biochemical liver tests include the serum transaminases (SGOT, SGPT), alkaline phosphatase, and serum bilirubin. The serum transminases are enzymes which are released from the normal turnover of liver cells. A persistent elevation of serum transaminases represents increased leakage from injured hepatocytes rather than from dead cells and thus does not correlate quantitatively with the liver dysfunction due to hepatocellular necrosis (2). In the presence of jaundice, an elevation of serum alkaline phosphatase greater than three times the normal value of 2–5 units (Bodansky) usually indicates obstruction rather than hepatocellular necrosis. A low activity of serum alkaline phosphatase is diagnostically more useful to rule out obstruction, since mild elevation of the enzyme is normally found in adolescents undergoing rapid growth and pregnant women in the third trimester. Elevations up to 30–50% above the upper limits of normal may not be unusual in geriatric patients, because alkaline phosphatase levels usually increase with increasing age (2). Isolation of the hepatic isoenzyme of elevated alkaline phosphatase or concurrent elevation of gamma glutamyl transpeptidase are suggestive of hepatic origin. In cirrhosis, alkaline phosphatase levels may be affected not only by the liver disease but also by the secondary effect of the disease on bone metabolism (2). An elevation of total bilirubin concentration is not a sensitive indicator of either biliary obstruction or hepatocellular injury. Elevation of unconjugated bilirubin may imply mild or early hepatocyte injury even though the total bilirubin remains normal.

Serum albumin is not usually regarded as part of liver function tests. Although serum albumin is synthesized by the hepatic parenchymal cells, changes in albumin concentration are non-specific and insensitive to liver disease and have little

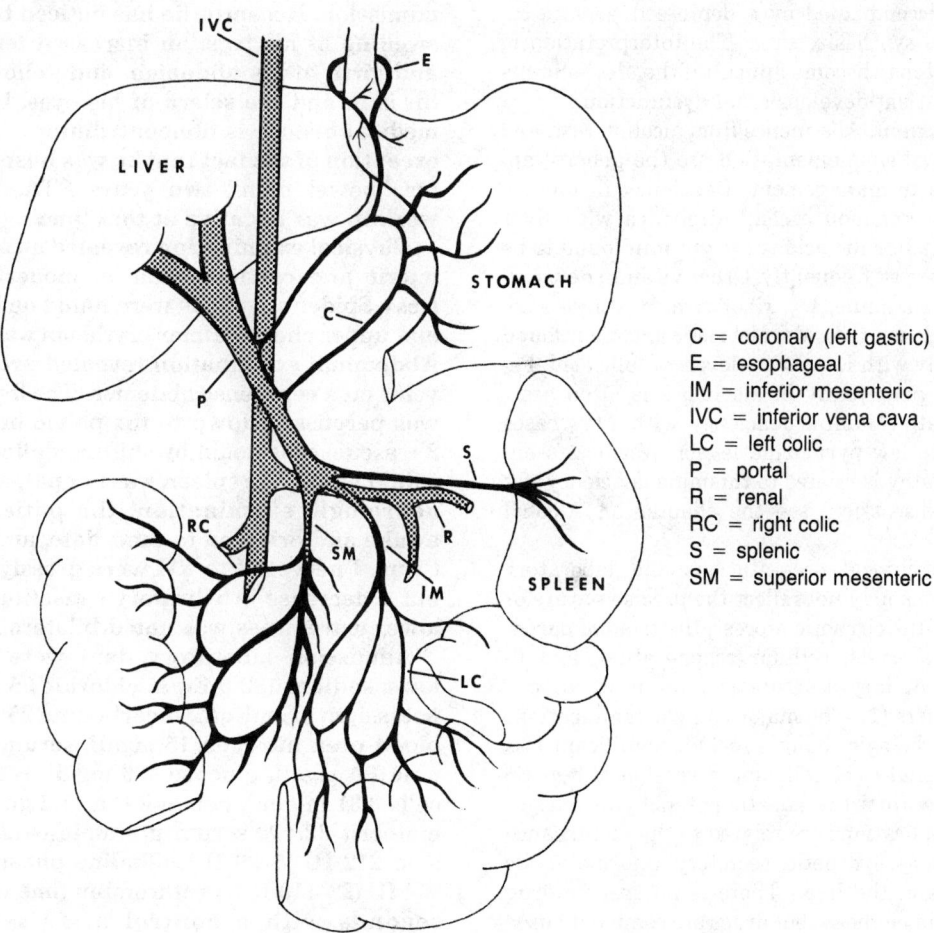

C = coronary (left gastric)
E = esophageal
IM = inferior mesenteric
IVC = inferior vena cava
LC = left colic
P = portal
R = renal
RC = right colic
S = splenic
SM = superior mesenteric

Figure 1. Schematic Diagram of Portal Venous System

value in the differential diagnosis of liver diseases. However, a low serum albumin (<3 gm/dl) that is unresponsive to therapy indicates an unfavorable prognosis.

Prolongation of prothrombin time due to chronic obstructive jaundice, celiac disease, and hypovitaminosis K usually can be improved within 24 hours after a 10 mg dose of vitamin K. This response does not occur with diffuse hepatocellular disease and thus may be of some diagnostic value (21,22). A prolonged prothrombin time which is unresponsive to parenteral vitamin K often indicates an imminent development of fulminant hepatic failure and is a poor prognostic sign in chronic hepatocellular disease (22).

Blood urea nitrogen (BUN) below 5 mg/dl is characteristic of alcoholic cirrhosis and is uncommon in patients with other forms of cirrhosis (2). The low BUN is attributed to inadequate protein intake accompanied by a depressed hepatic capacity to synthesize urea. The interpretation of the BUN may become difficult if the alcoholic cirrhotic patient develops renal dysfunction.

Treatment. Abstinence from alcohol, rest, and nutritional supplementation are the general approaches to management. Deficiency in dietary intake is common among alcoholics with liver disease (23). Folic acid is the vitamin found to be deficient most frequently. Other vitamin deficiencies are thiamine, B_{12}, riboflavin, nicotinic acid, and pyridoxine (24). Megaloblastic anemia is found commonly with low serum levels of folic acid. Peripheral neuropathy in alcoholics is often associated with thiamine deficiency, with a few cases related to low pyridoxine levels. Wernicke's encephalopathy is related to thiamine deficiency (for further discussion, see the chapter on Alcohol Abuse).

While clinical presentations and laboratory evaluations may not reflect the precise nature or extent of the cirrhotic process, the triad of parenchymal necrosis, cellular regeneration, and fibrotic nodullary scarring is present in all cirrhotic livers (1). The major clinical ramifications of the pathologic changes include significant loss of functional liver cells and diversion of hepatic blood flow from the hepatic parenchyma. Resultant complications are related to the disturbance of the many synthetic, secretory, and metabolic functions of the liver. There is no specific drug therapy for cirrhosis, but drugs are commonly used to treat secondary complications of cirrhosis.

Therefore, this chapter will emphasize the secondary complications of cirrhosis and their management.

ASCITES

1. R.W. is a 54-year-old male with a two-week history of nausea, vomiting, and lower abdominal cramps without diarrhea. Despite chronic anorexia, he has managed to eat about two meals a day and drink a fifth of vodka per day for the past two years. During this time he experienced a reported 30 pound weight loss. He began drinking nine years prior to admission (PTA) when his wife became an invalid secondary to a brain tumor. His alcohol consumption increased from one pint to a fifth daily two years prior to this admission. Recently, he has noticed bilateral swelling of his legs, an increased tenseness and girth of his abdomen, and yellowing of his skin and the sclera of his eyes. His past medical history is noncontributory with the exception of the fact that he was hospitalized for "bowel pain" two years PTA. The GI workup was negative at that time.

Physical examination revealed an afebrile, icteric and cachetic male in moderate distress. Spider angiomas were found on his face and upper chest. Palmar erythema was noted. Abdominal examination revealed prominent veins on a very tense abdomen. The liver edge was percussed down to the pelvic brim and 2+ ascites was noted by shifting dullness and a fluid wave. The spleen was not palpable. On neurologic examination, the patient was awake and oriented to time, date, and place. Cranial nerves II to XII were grossly intact, but a decrease in vibratory sensation of the lower extremities was noted bilaterally.

Admission laboratory data were as follows: sodium 132 mEq/L, chloride 95 mEq/L, potassium 3.8 mEq/L, bicarbonate 25 mEq/L, blood urea nitrogen 15 mg/dl, serum creatinine 1.4 mg/dl, glucose 136 mg/dl, red blood cells 3.31 m/mm³, hemoglobin 11.2 gm/dl, hematocrit 32.4%, serum glutamic oxaloacetic acid 212 IU (5–29 IU), alkaline phosphatase 954 IU (22–110 IU), prothrombin time was 13.5 seconds with a control of 12 seconds, total:direct bilirubin was 18.8 mg/dl:10.7 mg/

dl, albumin was 2.3 gm/dl, and stool guaiac was positive.

The impression on admission was alcoholic cirrhosis, ascites, and heme positive stools.

Why did R.W. present with cachexia and a history of weight loss despite eating two meals daily?

Alcoholics are known to have poor dietary habits. Deficiency in dietary protein is one of the reasons for the common history of weight loss obtained from alcoholic cirrhotic patients. One study showed an average weight gain of 3.1 kg over a 3-week period after 56 alcoholic patients were reinstated to a normal diet (25). In addition, chronic alcohol consumption often contributes to the depletion of liver glycogen stores. Furthermore, hepatic gluconeogenesis is inhibited, possibly due to increases in the NADH:NAD ratio caused by alcohol metabolism (26).

Demand for glucose as a source of energy leads to mobilization of amino acid from the muscles. This results in muscle wasting in the cirrhotic patient (24). Interestingly, high protein diet is not necessary to maintain a positive nitrogen balance in the cirrhotic patient. A normal protein intake of 35 to 50 gm per day is sufficient to keep cirrhotic patients in protein equilibrium or positive nitrogen balance (27).

2. What subjective and objective evidence are compatible with alcoholic cirrhosis in this patient?

R.W.'s presentation of a long history of alcohol abuse, cachexia, hypoalbuminemia, jaundice, and his admission laboratory data are all consistent with advanced cirrhosis. The presence of ascites and prominent abdominal veins are suggestive of portal hypertension. His compromised coagulation system, evidenced by the prolonged prothrombin time, indicates possible hepatocellular dysfunction. Liver biopsy is usually required to confirm the presence and severity of cirrhosis; however, in view of R.W.'s prolonged prothrombin time, the risk of a biopsy must be considered. The presence of a normal BUN and an elevated direct or conjugated serum bilirubin is suggestive of some remaining hepatic parenchymal function. Therefore, the suspicion of alcoholic cirrhosis in R.W.'s case is supported primarily by his long history of alcoholism; nonspecific complaints of nausea, abdominal cramps, anorexia, and jaundice; the presence of hepatomegaly and ascites; hypoalbuminemia; and elevation of liver enzymes.

The severity of cirrhosis may be assessed by noting the liver's ammonia capturing function (ie, BUN), conjugatory function (ie, direct serum bilirubin), responsiveness of the prolonged prothrombin time to vitamin K therapy, and presence of other complications of parenchymal failure (ie, encephalopathy, portal hypertension, esophageal varices). The marked elevation of alkaline phosphatase and conjugated serum bilirubin in R.W.'s case may indicate extrahepatic cholestasis, a phenomenon reported in some patients with alcoholic liver injuries (28,29). More comprehensive reviews of the biochemical evaluation of liver diseases can be found elsewhere (22,30).

3. *Causes of Ascites*. What physiological mechanisms predispose this patient to fluid accumulation in the peritoneal cavity?

Accumulation of fluid in the peritoneal cavity, medically referred to as ascites, is most frequently anteceded by cirrhosis. At present, three theories are postulated to explain the accumulation of ascitic fluid. The classical theory is that formation of ascites results from a combination of increased hydrostatic pressure and decreased plasma oncotic pressure (31,32). In cirrhotic patients, the hepatic outflow is blocked and eventually results in back pressure which leads to portal hypertension and increased splanchnic blood volume, as is evident by R.W.'s prominent abdominal veins (13,33). Ascites may be produced by exudation of fluid from the splanchnic capillary bed and the liver surface when the drainage capacity of the lymphatic system is exceeded. In addition, R.W.'s hypoalbuminemia (2.3 gm/dl), due to impaired albumin synthesis in the liver, favors the formation of ascites (34). As fluid exudation continues, the arterial perfusion of vital organs is transiently reduced because of plasma volume contraction. Reduced blood flow to the kidneys and abnormal hepatic hemodynamics activate the renin-angiotensin-aldosterone system (35,36). Increased aldosterone enhances the distal tubular reabsorption of sodium and water, thus expanding the total blood volume. However, this circulatory compensation can also aggravate the portal hypertension, increase the splanchnic blood volume, and establish a vicious cycle.

Lieberman proposed the "overflow" theory which suggests that ascites accumulate only after the plasma volume expands from renal retention of sodium and water (37). Excess fluid then "overflows" into the peritoneal cavity from the congested portal system.

An alternative proposal is the "lymph imbalance" theory (38). Visceral edema from lymph imbalance is suggested as the primary stimulus to retention of salt and water by the kidney. Subsequent expansion of the extracellular fluid volume further leads to increases in visceral lymph production which eventually exceeds lymph return and results in ascites.

Regardless of whether the kidney initiates or secondarily causes ascites, it avidly reabsorbs sodium and water. Thus, treatment of ascites is mainly directed at the removal of excess sodium and water.

4. Goals of Therapy. What are the therapeutic goals in the management of this patient's ascites?

The goals of therapy for R.W.'s ascites are to mobilize ascitic and edema fluid and to prevent major complications including hepatorenal syndrome, variceal bleeding, bacterial peritonitis, hernias, pleural effusions, and respiratory disorders (31). Treatment of ascites in this patient should be undertaken cautiously and gradually, since acid-base imbalance, hypokalemia, or intravascular volume depletion caused by overly aggressive therapy may lead to compromised renal function, hepatic encephalopathy and death. Medical management of ascites involves bed rest, restriction of sodium and water intake, and utilization of diuretics to effect salt and water loss (31,32,39–41).

5. The 24-hour urinary electrolytes for R.W. were reported to be: sodium 10 mEq/L and potassium 28 mEq/L. The medical intern suggested that R.W. be placed on sodium and water restriction. Do you agree?

Sodium restriction and bed rest will result in diuresis in many patients with cirrhosis and ascites; the degree of success depends on the duration of the restriction (39,42,43). Restriction to 20 mEq of sodium per day is common, and less than 10 mEq/day may be required (40,41). Patients with normal or increased urinary sodium excretion (>10 mEq/L) are most likely to respond to this type of conservative treatment (39). Since this patient has a urinary sodium of 10 mEq/L which indicates a borderline renal capacity to excrete free water, he

may benefit from sodium restriction. Water restriction as part of the initial treatment should probably be avoided in this patient whose serum sodium concentration was within normal limits (132 mEq/L). Water and sodium restriction should be reserved for patients whose poor renal capacity to excrete free water results in excessive water retention and dilutional hyponatremia (<130 mEq/L) (32–39). Patients with low urinary sodium excretion (<10 mEq/L), but normal or near normal free water clearance and normal renal function, appear to benefit from the addition of diuretics (39). Patients with reduced 24-hour urinary excretion of sodium as well as diminished glomerular filtration rate and free water clearance are commonly resistant to medical treatment and have a poor prognosis (39).

6. Diuretic Therapy. R.W. was placed on 500 mg sodium restriction after initial evaluation. Spironolactone 100 mg/day was ordered to induce diuresis. Is spironolactone a rational choice in the treatment of ascites? Can other potassium-sparing diuretics be used?

In general, most cirrhotic patients have high circulating levels of aldosterone. The fluid loss into the peritoneal cavity causes a contraction of the intravascular volume which decreases renal perfusion and leads to activation of the renin-angiotensin-aldosterone system (31,32). Hepatic shunting also serves to increase aldosterone production by similarly decreasing renal blood flow. In addition, aldosterone is substantially metabolized by the liver, and hepatic dysfunction prolongs the biologic half-life and action of aldosterone (44). Aldosterone acts on the distal renal tubule to enhance sodium retention and potassium loss, and the ideal diuretic is one with anti-aldosterone and potassium sparing effects. Therefore spironolactone, an aldosterone antagonist, is a rational choice in R.W. when more conservative measures fail to mobilize fluid overload (32,43,45). A starting dose of 100 mg/day is reasonable in treating most patients with ascites (40,45,46). If the patient's response is unsatisfactory, the dosage should be increased slowly (every two to four days) because of the long half-life of spironolactone. Triamterene (Dyrenium), a potassium sparing diuretic without anti-aldosterone activity, can be used as an effective alternative to spironolactone if intolerable side effects occur with spironolactone (eg, gynecomastia) (39,41).

7. What laboratory parameters should be monitored to ensure the therapeutic effectiveness of spironolactone therapy for this patient?

The 24-hour urinary sodium to potassium (Na:K) ratio can be used to define the need for increasing doses of spironolactone (45,47). Patients with low baseline urinary Na:K ratio (less than one,) which indicates high intrinsic mineralocorticoid (ie, aldosterone) activity, may require anywhere from 200 to 1000 mg/day of spironolactone alone (45,48). Because this patient's urinary Na:K ratio is less than one, spironolactone 200 mg/day may be a better starting dose. Generally, if there is still no response following reversal of the urinary Na:K ratio or if diuresis remains insufficient after four or more days of increasingly larger doses of spironolactone, a thiazide (eg, hydrochlorothiazide 50 mg/day), metolazone (5 mg/day), or furosemide (20 mg/day) can be added on a continuous or intermittent basis (40,45,49). Doses of the adjunctive diuretics may be doubled after two or more days if necessary.

**8. *Complications of Diuretic Therapy.*
Spironolactone 200 mg/day was ordered as recommended. Three days later, R.W.'s urinary sodium and potassium levels were 48 mEq/L and 30 mEq/L, respectively. Fluid intake was 1400 ml and urinary output was 750 ml. The medical intern wants to add furosemide to the diuretic therapy because of insufficient diuresis. What potential complications due to diuretic therapy should be watched for in this patient? Suggest guidelines to minimize these complications.**

The most common complications to monitor for in this patient are hypokalemia, hyponatremia, metabolic alkalosis, encephalopathy, and azotemia (43,50). Azotemia usually results from overdiuresis with subsequent compromise of intravascular volume and decreased renal perfusion. With salt restriction alone, patients with ascites can mobilize only about 300 ml of ascitic fluid daily. Patients with both edema and ascites can mobilize up to 800 ml of nonascitic fluid and no more than 300 ml of ascitic fluid per 24-hour period (51). Although diuretic agents enhance fluid mobilization, they result in maximal loss of 930 ml of ascitic fluid as compared to 4.7 liters of nonascitic fluid (51). Thus, the fluid loss during diuresis is chiefly at the expense of nonascitic fluid which may result in plasma volume contraction

and decreased renal perfusion. To avoid overdiuresis, it is best to limit maximal daily fluid loss to <300 ml per day for patients with ascites alone and ≤1 liter per day for those with both ascites and edema (51,52). Since this patient presented with both edema and ascites, a fluid loss of up to one liter/day would be reasonable. Gradual diuresis avoids diuretic-induced depletion of extracellular fluid volume by permitting ascitic fluid to equilibrate with the plasma volume. By using these guidelines, untoward effects from diuretic therapy, which may occur in as many as 75% of diuretic-treated cirrhotic patients with ascites, can be minimized (43,50).

Hypokalemic hypochloremic alkalosis and hyponatremia are the other frequently encountered abnormalities (43,53,54). Many cirrhotics initially have a deficit in total body potassium and are predisposed to this metabolic abnormality. Hypokalemic alkalosis can generally be corrected with adequate potassium chloride supplementation. Since this patient has some degree of renal impairment (serum creatinine 1.4 mg/dl) and is being given spironolactone, his serum potassium level should be monitored closely. His potassium chloride dosage should then be adjusted accordingly to avoid hyperkalemia. Hyponatremia, if present, can usually be corrected by temporary withdrawal of diuretics.

Disorientation and asterixis are signs of encephalopathy and demand immediate discontinuation of diuretics if present. Increases in either serum creatinine (>0.5 mg/dl) or BUN (> 10 mg/dl) from baseline also necessitate cessation of diuretics for a few days to allow volume expansion through fluid equilibration because of the grave prognosis of hepatorenal syndrome (40,41,55–57).

9. *Paracentesis.* Furosemide 40 mg po bid was given and subsequently increased to 160 mg bid without major improvement in diuresis. Laboratory data revealed that R.W.'s serum creatinine had increased to 3.2 mg/dl and BUN to 45 mg/dl. Serum electrolytes were potassium 3.1 mEq/L, sodium 130 mEq/L, chloride 88 mEq/L, and bicarbonate 32 mEq/L. R.W. became progressively short of breath. Paracentesis was performed. Why? What are the limitations and complications of this procedure?

Paracentesis is a procedure for tapping the abdominal cavity for the removal of ascitic fluid. It is usually performed for diagnostic purposes, but it is also used therapeutically in patients with refractory ascites not responsive to diuretic therapy and causing compromised respiratory and cardiac functions, as in this case (3,32,59). Removal of as little as one liter of fluid may provide considerable relief from the respiratory distress that occurs with massive ascites. Usually there is rapid reaccumulation of ascites after paracentesis due to transudation of fluid from the interstitial and plasma compartments into the peritoneal cavity (51); therefore, paracentesis is not a definitive treatment for ascites. The major complications of too vigorous paracentesis include hypotension, hemoconcentration, shock, oliguria, encephalopathy, and hepatorenal syndrome (52,56). Other potential complications of paracentesis are hemorrhage, perforation of the abdominal viscera, infection, and protein depletion.

10. *Alternative Therapy.* **What other modes of therapy are available for the management of intractable ascites? How would these alternatives be applied in this patient?**

Intractable ascites is uncommon and is difficult to treat. Alternative regimens include albumin infusion and reinfusion of the ascitic fluid into the systemic circulation by a peritoneovenous (LeVeen) shunt. Elevation of decreased serum albumin levels has been shown to promote diuresis in cirrhotic patients with ascites and edema (60,61). However, the effects of albumin infusion are seldom long-lasting, and variceal hemorrhage may be precipitated (62). In view of this patient's rising BUN and creatinine levels and the grave prognosis of hepatorenal syndrome, peritoneovenous shunt would be a better choice.

Peritoneovenous shunt, which is surgically implanted, consists of a valve implanted in the abdominal wall, an intra-abdominal cannula, and an outflow tube tunneled subcutaneously from the valve to a neck or a shoulder vein to empty into the superior vena cava (63). This procedure is contraindicated in the presence of peritonitis, esophageal varices, recurrent coma, coagulopathy, significant cardiac failure, and acute alcoholic hepatitis. In view of this patient's elevated prothrombin time, extra measures must be taken prior to surgery, ie, administration of vitamin K and fresh frozen plasma. Resistant ascites has been successfully treated with LeVeen shunt, and reversal of the usually fatal hepatorenal syndrome has also been reported (64–67). However, the basic hepatic abnormalities remain unchanged, and

whether the overall survival rate is improved remains to be established (68). Pulmonary edema frequently occurs after peritoneovenous shunt from the increased volume of fluid returning to the heart. Intravenous furosemide is usually administered during the first two to three days after operation to augment diuresis (68). Other possible complications of peritoneovenous shunt include consumption coagulopathy, fever, wound infection, septicemia, and gastrointestinal bleeding (69–71).

ESOPHAGEAL VARICES

11. A 55-year-old, pale-looking female with known primary biliary cirrhosis was admitted for a chief complaint of hematemesis. The patient has a history of recurrent upper gastrointestinal bleeding and documented esophageal varices but no history of angina pectoris or myocardial infarction. On examination, blood pressure was 78/40 mm Hg, pulse rate was 110 beats/min and respiration rate was 22/min. Skin was cold. Chest and cardiac examinations were within normal limits. Abdominal examination revealed ascites and a palpable spleen. Bowel sounds were normal. Laboratory values included hemoglobin 7 gm/dl, hematocrit 22%, albumin 3.0 gm/dl, serum glutamic oxaloacetic transaminase 160 IU (5–29 IU), serum glutamic pyruvic transaminase 250 IU (4–33 IU), alkaline phosphatase 40 IU (22–110 IU), and creatinine 2.0 mg/dl. The prothrombin time was 18 seconds with a control of 12 seconds. Serum electrolytes were all within normal limits. Electrocardiogram revealed sinus tachycardia.

What treatment endeavors are of the highest priority in managing this patient's hematemesis?

The goals of therapy are to stop or slow down blood loss and to treat hypovolemic shock if it develops. Initial treatment consists of cold saline irrigation of the stomach via a nasogastric tube to induce local vasoconstriction and intravenous administraton of Lactated Ringers or normal saline solution to maintain blood pressure. Whole blood is transfused if there are signs of hypovolemia or if the blood loss is severe.

Hypovolemic symptoms in this patient include pallor, cold and clammy skin, rapid pulse, and systolic blood pressure less than 80 mm Hg. Fresh blood is preferable because of its hemostatic properties and should constitute one-third or one-fourth of the total number of units administered if possible (33,72). If the prothrombin time is greater than 15 seconds, as in this case, intravenous or oral vitamin K administration is recommended. The patient should be monitored for electrolyte and metabolic abnormalities (eg, potassium, sodium, bicarbonate), hypoxia (eg, pO_2, pH), and decreased urinary output. Behavioral changes, mental confusion, asterixis, and other signs of hepatic encephalopathy should be closely watched for. Evacuation of retained gastric blood with magnesium sulfate or lactulose is essential to prevent ammonia production and hepatic encephalopathy. Sterilization of gut flora with neomycin is also helpful.

12. Three units of whole blood and one unit of fresh frozen plasma were transfused initially. The stomach was lavaged with iced saline and the gastric aspirate from the nasogastric tube continued to be strongly positive for blood. Vitamin K (Aqua-Mephyton) 20 mg was administered by slow IV push. Four hours later, her bleeding still persisted. What other therapeutic interventions can be used to control her bleeding esophageal varices?

In general, if the bleeding persists after lavage and blood replacement, emergency endoscopy can be extremely useful to rule out other causes of upper GI bleeding. Fiberoptic esophagoscopy is considered highly accurate in locating esophageal varices (73–75). If necessary, selective angiography may be utilized (13,72). Once the diagnosis of esophageal or gastric varices is made, one of two treatment modalities may be chosen. The Sengstaken-Blakemore tube may permit effective *balloon tamponade* of esophageal varices and stop the bleeding (76,77). However, complications are many and include pneumonitis, aspiration, esophageal ulceration or rupture, and asphyxia (13,78). Alternatively, intravenous or intra-arterial *vasopressin infusion* may be used. Intravenous vasopressin can be initiated with a constant infusion pump at 0.2 U/min and later increased to 0.4 U/min if the bleeding does not stop. The maximal dose recommended is 0.9 U/min.

Vasopressin is a potent stimulator of smooth muscle, particularly those of capillaries and arterioles. Its mechanism of action is postulated to be through vasoconstriction of the mesenteric arteriolar bed. This decreases blood flow into the portal system and results in reduction of collateral flow into the esophageal varices (79,80).

13. *Administration of Vasopressin.* Should the route of administration for vasopressin be intra-arterial or intravenous?

Earlier studies found that intravenous bolus injections of vasopressin significantly reduced the portal pressure and controlled bleeding from esophageal varices (81–84). However, most patients required multiple doses of vasopressin (84). In an attempt to reduce systemic adverse effects of vasopressin, superior mesenteric arterial (SMA) infusion of vasopressin was utilized to stop bleeding from esophageal varices (85). Although SMA vasopressin infusion was successful, the incidence of side effects remained high (86–93). Subsequently, a more sustained reduction of portal venous pressure was observed after continuous IV infusion of vasopressin than after an IV bolus (94,95). The infusion also caused less abdominal cramping, substernal discomfort, and cardiac arrhythmias. When intravenous infusion of vasopressin was compared to SMA infusion, hemostatic control occurred in 64% of the intravenous group and 50% of the SMA group, although the difference was not statistically significant (96). However, complications were more frequent in the SMA group (i.e., catheter complications and cardiac arrhythmias). Furthermore, the intravenous route is easier to use and does not require angiographic placement of the catheter, thus allowing prompt institution of therapy. In summary, intravenous infusion appears to be as efficacious as SMA infusion, although some refractory patients may respond to the SMA and not the intravenous route (97–99).

14. What would be an appropriate initial infusion rate of vasopressin for this patient and what guidelines should be followed for subsequent adjustment?

Starting doses for intravenous infusion range from 0.2 to 0.4 U/min, increasing to 0.9 U/min if necessary (95–97,100). Larger doses (1.2–1.5 U/min) do not control hemorrhage in patients who are unresponsive to lower doses (97). Intra-arterial infusions were given at 0.1 to 0.5 U/min (96–98). Since many of the side effects are dose related, the lowest effective dose should be used whenever possible. When the bleeding is controlled, it is customary to taper the vasopressin dose over 24–48 hours (89,95,96,101), but there is no evidence that tapering the dose decreases the incidence of rebleeding or side effects (100).

15. *Complications of Vasopressin Therapy.* During the intravenous vasopressin infusion in this patient, blanching of the skin near the injection site and abdominal cramps are noted. Are these symptoms related to vasopressin therapy? What other subjective and objective data need to be monitored in this patient to minimize the toxicities associated with vasopressin?

Skin blanching and abdominal cramps are common side effects of vasopressin. Other minor complications include mild hypertension, fecal incontinence, benign arrhythmias, phlebitis, and hematoma at the infusion site (102).

Complications from vasopressin therapy are related to its vasoconstrictive and its antidiuretic hormonal effects as well as to the catheter placement procedure. Fatal complications have been reported (97,103). Major complications occurred at a rate of 9% in the SMA group and 6.3% in the intravenous group in one study (104). Minor complications occurred in 29% of the SMA group and 38% of the intravenous group. Reported major complications are cardiac and respiratory arrest; ventricular arrhythmias; angina and myocardial infarction; reduced cardiac output and acute cardiac failure (97,101,103–107); infections: spontaneous bacterial peritonitis and sepsis (97,101,104,108); vascular: local arterial bleeding, venous and arterial thrombosis; hepatic, gastric, intestinal and splenic infarcts; gangrene (109–113); and systemic: water intoxication and electrolyte imbalance (87,110,111,114).

16. *Alternative Therapy.* If vasopressin therapy fails to control the bleeding esophageal varices in this patient, what are other therapeutic alternatives?

Surgical management of bleeding esophageal varices is aimed at reducing the portal venous pressure. Portacaval anastomosis has been reported to decrease the frequency of hemorrhage and increase long-term survival (17,18,115–117). However, hepatic encephalopathy may be observed in a high percentage (11–31.5%) of patients depending on the patient's preoperative condition (18,115,117–119) Details of portacaval

shunts and other types of operative procedures are reviewed elsewhere (13,117).

Injection sclerotherapy for esophageal varices with ethanolamine oleate has recently received much attention (120–124). This procedure involves insertion of a rigid esophagoscope to visualize actively bleeding esophageal varices and injection of a sclerosing agent into each varix to induce immediate hemostasis. Terblanche accomplished a 92% control rate with a single injection and a satisfactory outcome in 72% of admissions (122,123). The 25-month mortality rate of 41% compares favorably with other conservative and emergency surgical measures for control of bleeding esophageal varices. However, since the underlying portal hypertension is not affected, the therapeutic role of injection sclerotherapy remains to be defined.

Unfortunately, even if the bleeding is effectively controlled by vasopressin, the mortality rate associated with bleeding esophageal varices does not improve significantly (17,125,126). On the other hand, surgical portal systemic shunts following temporary control of hemorrhage with vasopressin have been reported to improve the long-term survival rate of these patients (17,18). Thus, if this patient is a suitable surgical candidate, perhaps a portacaval shunt should be considered when the acute bleeding episode subsides.

17. *Precautions to Minimize Recurrence.* This patient subsequently recovered from her acute episode of varix bleeding. How should she be counseled as to activities, alcohol, diet, and non-prescription medications prior to her discharge from the hospital?

Patient education should emphasize the importance of abstinence from alcohol. Information and referral to available community services should be given to the patient and family. It would be best for the patient to avoid salicylates and other medications that could irritate gastric and esophageal mucosa (eg, salicylamide, indomethacin). To prevent worsening of portal hypertension and ascites, the patient should adhere to the prescribed low salt diet and avoid medications that are high in sodium content (eg Alka-Seltzer, Soda Mint). Avoidance of certain activities that increase the chance of bleeding must be emphasized. Heavy lifting, vomiting, coughing, sneezing, ingestion of a large meal, and stool straining due to constipation all can increase intra-abdominal pressure and should be minimized. Prophylactic use of antacids and stool softeners which prevent mucosal irritation and constipation, respectively, can be employed.

HEPATIC ENCEPHALOPATHY

Hepatic coma or encephalopathy is a metabolic disorder of the CNS which occurs in patients with either advanced cirrhosis or fulminant hepatic failure with or without spontaneous or surgically induced portal-systemic shunting of blood (127). The clinical features usually include altered mental state, fetor hepaticus, asterixis, and a slow EEG pattern (127,128). During the early phase of the encephalopathy the altered mental state may present as a slight derangement of judgment or personality or change of mood. Drowsiness and confusion become more prominent as the encephalopathy progresses. Finally, unresponsiveness to arousal and deep coma ensue. Fetor hepaticus, a peculiar sweetish, musty odor in the breath, is considered to be pathognomonic of hepatic encephalopathy. This pungent odor of the breath is believed to be due to circulating mercaptans (128). Asterixis, or flapping tremor, is the most characteristic neurologic abnormality in hepatic encephalopathy. It can be demonstrated by having the patient hyperextend his wrist with the forearms outstretched and fingers separated. Asterixis is not specific for hepatic encephalopathy; it may also be present in uremia, hypokalemia, heart failure, respiratory failure, and sedative overdose (129). Although a slowing wave frequency on the EEG may occur in other severe metabolic disturbances such as hypoglycemia, uremia, and CO_2 retention, the EEG abnormality that occurs with liver disease is almost always indicative of impending hepatic coma (127,130).

In most cases hepatic encephalopathy is fully reversible without leaving structural lesions or residual sequelae, thus suggesting that hepatic encephalopathy is a metabolic/neurophysiologic disorder rather than an organic disorder. Many causes have been suggested, including ammonia, fatty acids, mercaptans, and weak neurotransmitters, but none of these has been incriminated as the single cause in all cases. The pathogenesis of hepatic encephalopathy is postulated to be multifactorial and includes increased susceptibility to various "toxins" (eg, altered permeability

of the blood-brain barrier), perhaps because of the absence of some protective substances normally produced by the healthy liver. No crucial protective substance has yet been identified, but an increase in blood-brain transport has been demonstrated (131). Of the many implicated toxins, ammonia is accepted as the primary toxin because plasma concentration of ammonia is greatly elevated in 90% of the patients with hepatic encephalopathy (127). Fatty acids and mercaptans may potentiate the toxic effects of ammonia by inhibiting its detoxification (132).

Changes in plasma amino acids have been associated with hepatic coma (133,134). An increase in phenylalanine, tyrosine, and methionine and a decrease in branched chain amino acids have been observed in hepatic encephalopathic patients. These changes in plasma amino acids might result in depletion of some true neurotransmitters and accumulation of weak neurotransmitters, thus altering normal cerebral function (133,134). The exact mechanism(s) of the plasma amino acid changes in the induction of coma is not clear, but evidence to support the importance of such changes in hepatic encephalopathy is accumulating (133). Furthermore, improvement of the mental status of hepatic encephalopathic patients has been associated with normalization of the plasma amino acid profile (135). Presently, active research is directed toward the formulation of intravenous amino acid preparations for the treatment of hepatic coma (133–135).

Although the precise etiology of hepatic encephalopathy is still unknown, certain biochemical and physiologic changes help delineate factors which may contribute to the genesis of neuropsychiatric symptoms (136). Portal-systemic shunting, whether a consequence of cirrhosis or surgical decompression of portal hypertension, remains the primary predisposing factor to hepatic coma. The shunted blood bypasses the liver's normal process of nitrogen detoxification, thus predisposing the patient to hepatic encephalopathy.

Of all the toxins suspected to cause coma, ammonia and certain amino acids are the most frequently studied and are generally held responsible. Other precipitating factors (see Table 1) increase the serum ammonia or produce excessive somnolence in patients with impending hepatic coma. Excess nitrogen load and metabolic or electrolyte abnormalities may increase ammonia levels (127,137,138).

18. R.C. is a 57-year-old male who was admitted to the hospital because of nausea, vomiting, and abdominal pain. He had a long history of alcohol abuse with multiple hospital admissions for alcoholic gastritis and alcohol withdrawal. Physical examination revealed a very cachetic male. His mentation was cloudy, but he was responsive to name and place. Tense ascites and edema were noted. The liver was percussed at 9 cm below the right costal margin. The spleen was not palpated and no active bowel sounds were heard. Laboratory results on admission included sodium 132 mEq/L, potassium 3.7 mEq/ L, chloride 98 mEq/L, bicarbonate 27 mEq/L, blood urea nitrogen 24 mg/dl, serum creatinine 1.4 mg/dl, hemoglobin 9.2 gm/dl, hematocrit 24.1%, serum glutamic oxaloacetic transaminase 520 IU (5–29 IU), alkaline phosphatase 218 IU (22–110 IU), lactic dehydrogenase 305 IU (82–226 IU), and total bilirubin 3.5 mg/dl; prothrombin time was 22 seconds with a control of 12 seconds.

A 60 gm protein, 2000 Kcal diet was ordered. Lasix 40 mg bid was ordered in an attempt to reduce the edema and ascites. Morphine sulfate and prochlorperazine were ordered for his abdominal pain and nausea, respectively. Two days after admission, R.C. had an episode of hematemesis. He became mentally confused and at times nonrespon-

Table 1.

FACTORS WHICH MAY PRECIPITATE
HEPATIC ENCEPHALOPATHY

Cause	Therapeutic Considerations
I. Excess nitrogen load	

A. Gastrointestinal bleeding
    1. esophageal varices
    2. hemorrhoid
    3. peptic ulcer
	A. Avoid gastric irritants; correct hypoprothrombinemia with vitamin K; give stool softener to prevent variceal bleeding from straining; evacuate blood in bowel with lactulose or magnesium citrate.

B. Excess dietary protein	B. Limit protein intake to 1 gm/kg; avoid protein with high ammoniagenic potential.

C. Azotemia
    1. diuretic-induced hypovolemia
    2. uremia of renal failure
    3. excessive enterohepatic circulation of BUN
	C. Avoid over-diuresis; use neomycin or lactulose prophylactically to decrease gut ammonia genesis from urea.

D. Infection - tissue catabolism	D. Treat infection with appropriate antibiotics.
E. Constipation - increased ammonia genesis due to increased gut transit time	E. Use stool softener and laxatives prophylactically.
II. Metabolic and electrolyte abnormalities	

A. Hypokalemia
    1. diuretic-induced
    2. dietary deficiency
    3. excessive diarrhea
    4. hyperaldosteronism
	A. Avoid over-diuresis; KCl replacement; control diarrhea; spironolactone therapy for ascites.

B. Alkalosis
    1. hypokalemia-induced
    2. excessive nausea & vomiting
	B. Correct hypokalemia; HCl infusion (150 ml HCl/L H_2O 0.5–2L in 24 hr) if needed; antiemetic therapy.

III. Drug-induced CNS depression	
A. Sedatives	A. Avoid long acting sedatives; use non-metabolized sedatives (ie, oxazepam).
B. Tranquilizers	B. Avoid phenothiazines because of association with hepatotoxicity.
C. Narcotic analgesics	C. Avoid hypoxia from respiratory depression.

sive to verbal command. A nasogastric tube was inserted and produced coffee ground material upon continuous suctioning. Iced saline lavage was performed until the aspirate became clear. The next morning the patient was still in a confused mental state and showed prominent asterixis. Fetor hepaticus was noted in his breath. An EEG showed slowing wave frequency. Other laboratory data included hemoglobin 7.4 gm/dl, hematocrit 21.2%, serum potassium 3.1 mEq/L, serum creatinine 1.4 mg/dl, blood urea nitrogen 36 mg/dl, prothrombin time 22 seconds, and stool guaiac was 4+ positive. Impending hepatic coma and upper GI bleeding were added to the problem list.

Identify the probable precipitating causes of hepatic encephalopathy in this case.

The most apparent cause which precipitated the encephalopathy in R.C. was the sudden onset of upper gastrointestinal bleeding, a frequent complication of advanced cirrhosis. Gastrointestinal hemorrhage provides excess protein for ammonia genesis by the gut flora. The degradation of blood protein in the gut results in absorption of large amounts of ammonia and possibly other toxins into the portal system. Other important contributory factors in this case are diuretic-induced hypovolemia (blood urea nitrogen: serum creatinine>20), hypokalemia (potassium <3.1 mEq/L), azotemia (blood urea nitrogen>36 mg/dl), and potential for the development of systemic alkalosis (eg, hypokalemia, continuous nasogastric suction). Overzealous diuretic therapy enhances hepatic encephalopathy by inducing prerenal azotemia, and more importantly, by promoting hypokalemia and metabolic alkalosis. Hypokalemia increases the concentration of ammonia in renal venous blood (139). Alkalosis, frequently associated with hypokalemia, promotes diffusion of nonionic ammonia and other amines into the central nervous system. The associated intracellular acidosis "traps" the ammonia by converting it back to ammonium ion (NH_4^+) (136). Another possible contributory factor to R.C.'s encephalopathy may be the sedating effect of morphine sulfate and prochlorperazine.

19. What are other precipitating causes of hepatic encephalopathy?

Besides gastrointestinal hemorrhage and certain electrolyte abnormalities, excessive dietary protein, tissue catabolism from severe infections, and constipation can also contribute to excess nitrogen load in the genesis of hepatic coma (see Table 1).

Sedating drugs also may be hazardous in patients with cirrhosis. Drugs that have frequently been associated with hepatic encephalopathy are: opiates (eg, morphine, methadone, meperidine, codeine), sedatives (eg, benzodiazepines, barbiturates, chloral hydrate, paraldehyde), and tranquilizers (eg, phenothiazines) (140). Encephalopathy precipitated by most drugs can be explained by increased CNS sensitivity and a decrease in hepatic clearance and subsequent accumulation. In addition, the effects of morphine (141), chlorpromazine (142,143), and diazepam (144) may be increased in liver disease because of decreased plasma protein binding.

20. *Treatment.* What steps should be taken to manage R.C.'s hepatic encephalopathy?

After identifying and removing precipitating causes of hepatic coma, therapeutic management is aimed primarily at reducing the amount of ammonia or nitrogenous products in the circulatory system. All protein intake should be stopped completely at the onset of encephalopathy. Dietary protein can then be gradually increased at 10–20 gm/day every two to five days depending on the clinical response. Vegetable protein may be better tolerated than animal protein (145), because vegetable protein contains less methionine and aromatic amino acids which are less ammoniagenic (127).

Keto-analogues, the nitrogen-free structural analogs of the corresponding essential amino acids, can be given intravenously or orally to offset hyperammonemia and poor nitrogen balance (146). Preliminary studies show minor improvement in nitrogen balance but noticeable improvement of neuropsychiatric symptoms and decline in plasma glutamine and blood ammonia levels (147).

Bowel sterilization also is an important adjunctive therapy in the management of hepatic encephalopathy. The two agents most commonly used for this purpose are neomycin, a nonabsorbable antibiotic, and lactulose, a nonutilizable disaccharide.

21. How are neomycin and lactulose used in hepatic encephalopathy? Which agent would be more appropriate for this patient?

Neomycin, in doses of one to two grams orally four times daily, or as a 1% solution given as a retention enema for 20–60 minutes four times daily, is effective in reducing plasma ammonia levels presumably by decreasing the urease-producing and other bacteria in the gut lumen. Approximately 1–3% of a dose of neomycin is absorbed and may cause oto- and nephro-toxicity, especially in patients with renal failure (148,149). Routine monitoring of serum creatinine, urine protein, and creatinine clearance is advisable for patients receiving high doses or prolonged therapy. Neomycin therapy may also produce a reversible malabsorption syndrome (150) which not only suppresses the absorption of fat, nitrogen, carotene, iron, vitamin B_{12}, xylose, and glucose, but also decreases the absorption of various drugs such as digoxin, penicillin, and vitamin K (151–153).

Lactulose is also efficacious in the treatment of hepatic encephalopathy (154,155). This disaccharide is broken down by gut bacteria to form lactic, acetic, and formic acids which acidify the colon from its normal pH of 7 to a pH of 5 in addition to producing an osmotic diarrhea (156). The proposed mechanisms of action are: acidification of the colon reduces the absorption of non-ionized ammonia and favors the growth of weak ammonia-producing bacteria like Lactobacillus acidophilus over proteolytic ammonia producers such as E. coli; and the osmotic diarrhea decreases the intestinal transit time available for ammonia production and absorption (127,156,157). Lactulose also may reduce ammonia concentration by serving as a bacterial substrate for either increasing bacterial assimilation of ammonia or reducing deamination of nitrogenous compounds (158). Lactulose syrup (67 gm/100 ml) has been used successfully in both acute and chronic hepatic encephalopathy. In the acute situation, initial doses of 30 to 45 ml are given three times daily and titrated to the production of three soft stools per day. When the oral route of administration is undesirable, as in the treatment of comatose patients, a rectal retention enema of 300 ml of lactulose in 700 ml of tap water or equal parts of normal saline and lactulose can be given for one hour. The beneficial clinical effect of lactulose enema occurs within 12 hours, as compared to 24 to 48 hours for oral lactulose (159,160). With chronic administration of lactulose 50–150 ml in three divided daily doses, patients are afforded better dietary protein tolerance (161,162). Besides monitoring the colonic pH with pHydrion

indicator paper, caution should be taken not to induce excessive diarrhea which may lead to dehydration and hypokalemia, both of which have been associated with exacerbations of hepatic encephalopathy (see Question 8). Although lactulose is generally well tolerated, 20% of patients may complain of gaseous distention, flatulence or belching (156,157). The excessive sweetness of the syrup can be reduced by diluting it with fruit juice, carbonated beverages or water.

Clinical trials comparing lactulose and neomycin reveal similar effectiveness for both agents in the treatment of hepatic encephalopathy (154,155). Occasionally, a patient who does not respond to one will respond to the other (156,162,163). In the treatment of an acute exacerbation, neomycin may produce a faster response than lactulose (164); however, there does not seem to be a consensus on this matter (165). In view of R.C.'s decreased renal function (serum creatinine 1.4 mg/dl), the 1–3% absorption of neomycin may result in accumulation and thereby increase the risk of oto- and nephrotoxicity. The interference of vitamin K absorption by neomycin may further impair the patient's already compromised coagulation status (prothrombin time 22 seconds). Therefore, lactulose may be more suitable than neomycin for R.C., especially when used for prolonged therapy. To hasten the onset of response, lactulose can be given as an initial loading dose of 30–40 ml every hour until catharsis occurs. If the patient does not have a gag reflex, lactulose enema may elicit a response within 20 minutes to an hour (159).

22. Would the combined use of neomycin and lactulose have any additive beneficial effect for this patient?

There is some evidence that the combination of lactulose and neomycin may be more effective than either drug alone (166). However, the concomitant use of lactulose and neomycin remains a controversial issue. Theoretically, sterilization of gut flora by neomycin would significantly impair the bacterial degradation of lactulose to its organic acid metabolites which are required for colonic acidification. In a study of nine patients with hepatic encephalopathy, the combined use of lactulose and neomycin reduced fasting ammonia to half the levels achieved by the use of either agent alone (167). The explanation for the additive effect of the two drugs is not clear, but the observation suggests that degradation of lactulose may not be essential for reduction of ammonia level (127). Other circumstantial evidence in support of such a theory includes: clinical response to lactulose enema can occur within 20–60 minutes, a time too short for any significant bacterial degradation to take place (159); the concentration of ammonia in a fecal incubation system with lactulose was lower than that of a lactic-acetic acid mixture (159); and undegraded lactulose has a low pH of 3.8 and thus may acidify the intestine without bacterial conversion to the organic acids (158). Furthermore, neomycin may not totally prevent the bacterial degradation of lactulose. One study suggests that one-third to one-half of cirrhotic patients can degrade lactulose in the presence of therapeutic doses of neomycin (168). Perhaps some strains of *Lactobacillus acidophilus* are resistant to neomycin (168), or perhaps neomycin therapy does not sterilize the gastrointestinal tract completely (168–170). Lactulose should be tried first, and if satisfactory results do not occur, neomycin alone should be given a trial (171). If both agents fail when used singly, the two agents can then be tried together. A stool pH below 6 reflects the synergistic effect of the two agents. When combination therapy fails to reduce the stool pH below 6, *Lactobacillus acidophilus* (Enpac, Lactinex) may be given orally as a capsule or rectally as an enema to ensure degradation of lactulose in the presence of neomycin (168). While combination use of lactulose and neomycin has been shown to have additive beneficial effects and both drugs to be equally effective, lactulose alone may be more desirable for long term use, since it has less toxic side effects than neomycin.

23. *Alternative Therapy.* What alternative treatments have been tried in patients with chronic encephalopathy which is resistant to conventional therapy?

For patients with chronic encephalopathy who have become resistant to protein restriction and lactulose or neomycin, total *colectomy* or colonic bypass may eliminate the source of ammonia or other nitrogenous toxins. However, the long-term survival rate has not been demonstrated to be significantly different from patients who are treated medically (127). Therefore, the indication for colonic bypass is still limited.

Levodopa and *bromocriptine* have been tried experimentally for the treatment of refractory chronic hepatic encephalopathy. The pharmacological basis for this treatment modality is the false neurotransmitter theory, believed by some to explain the pathogenesis of hepatic encephalopathy. The false neurotransmitter theory is based on the observation that amino acid precursors such as phenylethanolamine or octopamine appear to accumulate in the CNS as the severity of hepatic encephalopathy increases (172). These beta-hydroxylated phenylethylamines are false neurochemical transmitters. Normally they are metabolized by the monoamine oxidase system in the liver and excreted readily in the urine. In cirrhotic patients, with shunting of hepatic blood flow and impaired metabolic function of the hepatocytes, these false neurotransmitters accumulate and displace the active neurotransmitters, norepinephrine and dopamine. Administration of a large quantity of levodopa, a precursor of dopamine and norepinephrine, would theoretically reverse the effect of these false neurotransmitters. Indeed, early clinical trials reported striking improvement of abnormal EEG recordings and temporary improvement of sensorium in hepatic coma patients who received up to 5 gm of levodopa (172–174). The arousal began as early as 15 minutes after levodopa was administered. Unfortunately, therapy had to be withdrawn from most patients because of concern for gastric bleeding and excessive nausea and vomiting. In a more recent controlled trial in 75 cirrhotic patients, there was no significant difference between patients treated with levodopa, levodopa with carbidopa, or placebo; levodopa was concluded to be ineffective in the treatment of hepatic encephalopathy (175).

Bromocriptine, a dopaminergic agonist, has also been studied; one study showed no beneficial effect while another reported some improvement (176,177). Thus, the exact role of bromocriptine in hepatic coma awaits more extensive study.

References

1. Conn HO: Cirrhosis. In *Diseases of the Liver*, 4th ed, edited by L Schiff, JB Lippincott, Philadelphia, 1975, p 833.
2. Galambos JT: *Cirrhosis*, edited by LH Smith Jr, WB Saunders, Philadelphia, 1979.
3. LaMont JT: Cirrhosis. In *Harrison's Principles of Internal Medicine*, edited by KJ Isselbacher, RD Adams et al, 9th ed, McGraw-Hill, New York, 1980, p 1473.
4. Robbins SL et al: The hepatobiliary system and the pancreas. In *Basic Pathology*, 4th ed, edited by SL Robbins and M Angell, WB Saunders Company, Philadelphia, 1972, p 441.
5. Popper H et al: The social impact of liver diseases. N Engl J Med. 1969; 281:1455.
6. Lieber CS: Liver adaptation and injury in alcoholism. N Engl J Med. 1973; 288:356.
7. Brunt PW: Alcohol and the liver. Gut. 1971; 12:222.
8. Sherlock S: Causes and effects of acute liver damage. Scand J Gastroenterology. 1970; 6:187S.
9. Klatskin G: Alcohol and its relation to liver damage. Gastroenterology. 1961; 41:443.
10. Masse L et al: Trends in mortality from cirrhosis of the liver, 1950–1971. World Health Statistics Report. 1976; 29:40.
11. Brunt PW et al: Studies in alcoholic liver disease in Britain. I. Clinical and pathological patterns related to natural history. Gut. 1974; 15:52.
12. Galambos JT: Natural history of alcoholic hepatitis III. Histological changes. Gastroenterology. 1972; 63:1026.
13. Reynolds TB: Portal Hypertension. In *Diseases of the Liver*, 4th ed, edited by L Schiff, JB Lippincott, Philadelphia, 1975, p 330.
14. Kelty RH et al: The relation of the regenerated hepatic nodule to the vascular bed in cirrhosis. Mayo Clin Proc. 1950; 25:17.
15. Leevy CM et al: Mesenchymal-cell proliferation in liver disease of the alcoholic. JAMA. 1964; 187:598.
16. ten Hove W et al: Hepatic circulation and portal hypertension. Postgrad Med. 1973; 53:135.
17. Orloff MJ et al: The complications of cirrhosis of the liver. Ann Intern Med. 1967; 66:165.
18. Orloff MJ et al: Long-term results of emergency portacaval shunt for bleeding esophageal varices in unselected patients with alcoholic cirrhosis. Ann Surg. 1980; 192:325.
19. Lesesne HR et al: Alcoholic liver disease. Postgrad Med. 1973; 53:101.
20. Galambos JT: Alcoholic hepatitis: its therapy and prognosis. Prog Liver Dis. 1972; 4:567.
21. Curtis SJ: A guide to the practical use of liver function tests. Hospital Medicine. 1974; 10:51.
22. Rosoff L et al: Biochemical tests for hepatobiliary disease. Surg Clin North Am. 1977; 57:257.
23. Leevy CM et al: B-complex vitamins in liver disease of the alcoholic. Am J Clin Nutr. 1965; 16:339.
24. Mezey E: Liver disease and nutrition. Gastroenterology. 1978; 74:770.
25. Mezey E et al: Metabolic impairment and recovery time in acute ethanol intoxication. J Nerv Ment Dis. 1971; 153:445.
26. Forsander OA: Influence of the metabolism of ethanol on the lactate/pyruvate ratio of rat-liver slices. Biochem J. 1966; 98:244.
27. Gabuzda GJ et al: Metabolism of dietary protein in hepatic cirrhosis. Nutritional and clinical considerations. Am J Clin Nutr. 1970; 23:479.
28. Phillips GB et al: Liver disease of the chronic alcoholic simulating extrahepatic biliary obstruction. Gastroenterology. 1957; 33:236.
29. McGill DB: Steatosis, cholestasis, and alkaline phosphatase in alcoholic liver disease. Am J Dig Dis. 1978; 23:1057.
30. Scheife RT: Serum enzyme levels. Hosp Pharm. 1974; 9:394.
31. Conn HO: The rational management of ascites. Prog Liver Dis. 1972; 4:269.
32. Summerskill WHJ et al: Ascites. In *Diseases of the Liver*, 4th ed, edited by L Schiff, JB Lippincott, Philadelphia, 1975, p 424.
33. Resnick RH: Portal hypertension. Med Clin North Am. 1975; 59:945.
34. Zimon DS et al: Albumin to ascites: Demonstration of a direct pathway bypassing the systemic circulation. J Clin Invest. 1969; 48:2074.
35. Wong PY et al: Studies on the renin-angiotensin-aldosterone system in patients with cirrhosis and ascites: Effect of saline and albumin infusion. Gastroenterology. 1979; 77:1171.
36. Bosch J et al: Hepatic hemodynamics and the renin-angiotensin-aldosterone system in cirrhosis. Gastroenterology. 1980; 78:92.
37. Lieberman FL et al: The relationship of plasma volume, portal hypertension, ascites, and renal sodium retention in cirrhosis: The overflow theory of ascites formation. Ann NY Acad Sci. 1970; 170:202.
38. Witte CL et al: Lymph imbalance in the genesis and perpetuation of the ascites syndrome in hepatic cirrhosis. Gastroenterology. 1980; 78:1059.
39. Arroyo V et al: A rational approach to the treatment of ascites. Postgrad Med J. 1975; 51:558.
40. Frakes JT: Physiologic considerations in the medical management of ascites. Arch Intern Med. 1980; 140:620.
41. Mitchell K et al: Management of the patient with ascites. Drugs. 1980; 19:383.
42. Davidson CS: Cirrhosis of the liver treated with prolonged sodium restrictions. JAMA. 1955; 159:1257.
43. Gregory PB et al: Complications of diuresis in the alcoholic patient with ascites: a controlled trial. Gastroenterology. 1977; 73:534.
44. Sadee W et al: Pharmacokinetics of spironolactone, canrenone and canrenoate-K in humans. J Pharmacol Exper Ther. 1973; 185:686.
45. Eggert RC: Spironolactone diuresis in patients with cirrhosis and ascites. Br Med J. 1970; 4:401.
46. Hoyumpa AM Jr: A guide to treatment of ascites. Drug Ther. 1979; 4:33.
47. Alexander WD et al: The urinary sodium: potassium ratio and response to diuretics in resistant oedema. Postgrad Med J. 1977; 53:117.

48. Campra JL et al: Effectiveness of high-dose spironolactone therapy in patients with chronic liver disease and relatively refractory ascites. Am J Dig Dis. 1978; 23:1025.

49. Hillenbrand P et al: Use of metolazone in the treatment of ascites due to liver disease. Br Med J. 1971; 4:266.

50. Sherlock S et al: Complications of diuretic therapy in hepatic cirrhosis. Lancet. 1966; 1:1049.

51. Shear L et al: Compartmentalization of ascites and edema in patients with hepatic cirrhosis. N Engl J Med. 1970; 282:1391.

52. Gabuzda GJ: Cirrhosis, ascites, and edema. Gastroenterology. 1970; 58:546.

53. Vesin P: Potassium metabolism and diuretics administration in liver cirrhosis. Postgrad Med J. 1975; 51:545.

54. Gabuzda GJ et al: Relation of potassium depletion to renal ammonium metabolism and hepatic coma. Medicine. 1966; 45:481.

55. Shear L et al: Renal failure in patients with cirrhosis of the liver. Am J Med. 1965; 39:184.

56. Metz RJ et al: The hepatorenal syndrome. Surg Gynecol Obstet. 1976; 143:297.

57. Wong PY et al: The hepatorenal syndrome. Gastroenterology. 1979; 77:1326.

58. Shear L: Ascites: Pathogenesis and treatment. Postgrad Med. 1973; 53:165.

59. Guazzi M et al: Negative influence of ascites on the cardiac function of cirrhotic patients. Am J Med. 1975; 59:165.

60. Dykes PW: A study of the effects of albumin infusion in patients with cirrhosis of the liver. Quart J Med. 1961; 30:297.

61. Wilkinson P et al: The effect of repeated albumin infusions in patients with cirrhosis. Lancet. 1962; 2:1125.

62. Boyer JL et al: Effect of plasma volume expansion on portal hypertension. N Engl J Med. 1966; 275:750.

63. LeVeen HH et al: Peritoneovenous shunting for ascites. Ann Surg. 1974; 80:580.

64. Wapnick S et al: LeVeen continuous peritoneal-jugular shunt: improvement of renal function in ascitic patients. JAMA. 1977; 237:131.

65. Fullen WD: Hepatorenal syndrome: reversal by peritoneovenous shunt. Surgery. 1977; 82:337.

66. Berkowitz HD et al: Improved renal function and inhibition of renin and aldosterone secretion following peritoneovenous (LeVeen) shunt. Surgery. 1978; 84:120.

67. Blendis LM et al: The renal and hemodynamic effects of the peritoneovenous shunt for intractable hepatic ascites. Gastroenterology. 1979; 77:250.

68. Stanley MM: Treatment of intractable ascites in patients with alcoholic cirrhosis by peritoneovenous shunting (LeVeen). Med Clin North Am. 1979; 63:523.

69. Lerner RG et al: Disseminated intravascular coagulation complication of LeVeen peritoneovenous shunts. JAMA. 1978; 240:2064.

70. Dupas JL et al: Superior vena cava thrombosis as a complication of peritoneovenous shunt. Gastroenterology. 1978; 75:899.

71. Markey W et al: Hemorrhage from esophageal varices after placement of the LeVeen shunt. Gastroenterology. 1979; 77:341.

72. Malt RA: Control of massive upper gastrointestinal hemorrhage. N Engl J Med. 1972; 286:1043.

73. Conn HO et al: Observer variation in the endoscopic diagnosis of esophageal varices. N Engl J Med. 1965; 272:830.

74. Conn HO et al: Fiberoptic and conventional esophagoscopy in the diagnosis of esophageal varices. Gastroenterology. 1967; 52:810.

75. Yajko RD et al: Current management of upper gastrointestinal bleeding. Ann Surg. 1975; 181:474.

76. Pitcher JL: Safety and effectiveness of the modified Sengstaken-Blakemore tube: a prospective study. Gastroenterology. 1971; 61:291.

77. Bauer JJ et al: The use of the Sengstaken-Blakemore tube for immediate control of bleeding esophageal varices. Ann Surg. 1974; 179:273.

78. Merigan TC et al: Gastrointestinal bleeding with cirrhosis. N Engl J Med. 1960; 263:579.

79. Nusbaum M et al: Pharmacologic control of portal hypertension. Surg. 1967; 62:299.

80. Conn HO et al: Hepatic arterial escape from vasopressin-induced vasoconstriction: an angiographic investigation. Am J Roentgenol. 1973; 119:102.

81. Kehne JH et al: The use of surgical pituitrin in the control of esophageal varix bleeding. Surg. 1956; 39:917.

82. Schwartz SI et al: The use of intravenous pituitrin in treatment of bleeding esophageal varices. Surg. 1959; 45:72.

83. Merigan T: Effect of intravenously administered posterior pituitary extract on hemorrhage from bleeding esophageal varices. N Engl J Med. 1962; 266:134.

84. Conn HO et al: Multiple infusions of posterior pituitary extract in the treatment of bleeding esophageal varices. Ann Intern Med. 1962; 57:804.

85. Nusbaum M et al: Control of portal hypertension by selective mesenteric arterial drug infusion. Arch Surg. 1968; 97:1005.

86. Murray-Lyon IM et al: Treatment of bleeding oesophageal varices by infusion of vasopressin into the superior mesenteric artery. Gut. 1973; 14:59.

87. Nusbaum M et al: Control of portal hypertension. Arch Surg. 1974; 108:342.

88. Millette B et al: Portal and systemic effects of selective infusion of vasopressin into the superior mesenteric artery in cirrhotic patients. Gastroenterology. 1975; 69:6.

89. Conn HO et al: Intraarterial vasopressin in the treatment of upper gastrointestinal hemorrhage; a prospective, controlled clinical trial. Gastroenterology. 1975; 68:211.

90. Palmer FJ et al: Arterial vasoconstrictor therapy for bleeding oesophageal varices. Med J Aust. 1976; 1:143.

91. Kaufman SL et al: Control of variceal bleeding by superior mesenteric artery vasopressin infusion. Am J Roentgenol. 1977; 128:567.

92. Getzen LC et al: Survival following infusion of Pitressin into the superior mesenteric artery to control bleeding esophageal varices in cirrhotic patients. Ann Surg. 1978; 187:337.

93. Sherman LM et al: Selective intra-arterial vasopressin. Ann Surg. 1979; 189:298.

94. Thomford N et al: Intravenous vasopressin in patients with portal hypertension; advantage of continuous infusion. J Surg Res. 1975; 18:113.

95. Rigberg LA et al: Continuous low dose peripheral vein Pitressin infusion in the control of variceal bleeding. Am J Gastroenterology. 1977; 68:481.

96. Johnson WC et al: Control of bleeding varices by vasopressin. Ann Surg. 1977; 186:369.

97. Chojkier M et al: A controlled comparison of continuous intraarterial and intravenous infusions of vasopressin in hemorrhage from esophageal varices. Gastroenterology. 1979; 77:540.

98. Chojkier M et al: Intraarterial vs. intravenous vasopressin in the treatment of massive upper gastrointestinal hemorrhage. Gastroenterology. 1978; 75:958.

99. Davis GB et al: Advantage of intraarterial over intravenous vasopressin infusion in gastrointestinal hemorrhage. Am J Roentgenol. 1977; 128:733.

100. Chojkier M et al: Reply-vasopressin infusion. Gastroenterology. 1980; 78:420.

101. Conn HO et al: Selective intraarterial vasopressin in the treatment of upper gastrointestinal hemorrhage. Gastroenterology. 1972; 63:634.

102. Bouillon R et al: Miscellaneous hormones and prostaglandins. In *Side Effects of Drugs,* Annual 4, edited by MNG Dukes, Excerpta Medica, Amsterdam—Oxford, 1980, p 311.

103. Slotnik IL et al: Cardiac accidents following vasopressin injection (Pitressin). JAMA. 1951; 146:1126.

104. Greenfield AJ et al: Vasopressin in control of gastrointestinal hemorrhage: complications of selective intraarterial vs. systemic infusions. Gastroenterology. 1979; 76:1144.

105. Beller BM et al: Pitressin-induced myocardial injury and depression in a young woman. Am J Med. 1971; 51:675.

106. Sirinek KR et al: Isoproterenol in offsetting adverse effects of vasopressin in cirrhotic patients. Am J Surg. 1975; 129:130.

107. Alves M et al: Gastric infarction. A complication of selective vasopressin infusion. Dig Dis Sci. 1979; 24:409.

108. Mallory A et al: Selective intra-arterial vasopressin infusion for upper gastrointestinal tract hemorrhage. Arch Surg. 1980; 115:30.

109. Mogan GR et al: Infected gangrene. A serious complication of peripheral vasopressin administration. Am J Gastroenterology. 1980; 73:426.

110. Marubbio AT: Antidiuretic hormone effect of Pitressin during continuous Pitressin administration. Gastroenterology. 1972; 62:1103.

111. Marubbio AT et al: Control of variceal bleeding by superior mesenteric artery Pitressin perfusions—complications and indications. Dig Dis. 1973; 18:539.

112. Berardi RS: Vascular complications of superior mesenteric artery infusion with Pitressin in treatment of bleeding esophageal varices. Am J Surg. 1974; 127:757.

113. Greenwald RA et al: Local gangrene: a complication of peripheral Pitressin therapy for bleeding esophageal varices. Gastroenterology. 1978; 74:744.

114. McSwain GR et al: Antidiuretic hormone effect of vasopressin therapy for gastrointestinal hemorrhage. South Med J. 1979; 72:895.

115. Grace ND et al: The present status of shunts for portal hypertension in cirrhosis. Gastroenterology. 1966; 50:684.

116. Hourigan K et al: Elective end-to-side portacaval shunt: results in 64 cases. Br Med J. 1971; 4:473.

117. Schwartz SI: Liver. In *Principles of Surgery,* 3rd ed, edited by SI Schwartz, GT Shires, et al, McGraw-Hill, New York, 1979, p 1269.

118. Reynolds TB et al: Clinical comparison of end-to-side and side-to-side portacaval shunt. N Engl J Med. 1966; 274:706.

119. Mikkelsen WP: Therapeutic portacaval shunt. Arch Surg. 1974; 108:302.

120. Raschke E et al: Management of hemorrhage from esophageal varices using the esophagoscopic sclerosing method. Ann Surg. 1973; 177:99.

121. Shields R: Injection sclerotherapy for oesophageal varices. Lancet. 1979; 2:365.

122. Terblanche J et al: A prospective evaluation of injection sclerotherapy in the treatment of acute bleeding from esophageal varices. Surg. 1979; 85:239.

123. Terblanche J et al: A prospective controlled trial of sclerotherapy in the long term management of patients after esophageal variceal bleeding. Surg Gynecol Obstet. 1979; 148:323.

124. Jones RS: Sclerotherapy of bleeding esophageal varices. Gastroenterology. 1979; 77:596.

125. Garceau AJ et al: The natural history of cirrhosis. I. Survival with esophageal varices. N Engl J Med. 1963; 268:469.

126. Orloff MJ: Emergency portacaval shunt: a comparative study of shunt, varix ligation and non-surgical treatment of bleeding esophageal varices in unselected patients with cirrhosis. Ann Surg. 1967; 166:456.

127. Hoyumpa AM Jr et al: Hepatic encephalopathy. Gastroenterology. 1979; 76:184.

128. Schenker S et al: Hepatic encephalopathy: current status. Gastroenterology. 1974; 66:121.

129. Conn HO: Asterixis in non-hepatic disorders. Am J Med. 1960; 29:647.

130. Parsons-Smith BG et al: The electroencephalograph in liver disease. Lancet. 1957; 2:867.

131. James JH et al: Hyperammonemia, plasma amino acid imbalance, and blood brain aminoacid transport: a unified theory of portal systemic encephalopathy. Lancet. 1979; 2:772.

132. Zieve L et al: Synergism between mercaptans and ammonia or fatty acids in the production of coma: a possible role of mercaptans in the pathogenesis of hepatic coma. J Lab Clin Med. 1974; 83:16.

133. Fischer JE et al: The role of plasma amino acids in hepatic encephalopathy. Surgery. 1975; 78:276.

134. Fischer JE et al: The effect of normalization of plasma amino acids on hepatic encephalopathy in man. Surgery. 1976; 80:77.

135. Smith AR et al: Alterations in plasma and CSF amino acids, amines and metabolites in hepatic coma. Ann Surg. 1978; 187:343.

136. Zieve L: Pathogenesis of hepatic coma. Arch Intern Med. 1966; 118:211.

137. Maddrey WC et al: Chronic hepatic encephalopathy. Med Clin North Am. 1975; 59:937.

138. Fischer JE et al: Pathogenesis and therapy of hepatic coma. Prog Liver Dis. 1976; 5:363.

139. Shear L et al: Potassium deficiency and endogenous ammonia overload from kidney. Am J Clin Nutr. 1970; 23:614.

140. Breen KJ: Hepatic coma: present concepts of pathogenesis and therapy. Prog Liver Dis. 1972; 4:301.

141. Laidlaw J et al: Morphine tolerance with hepatic cirrhosis. Gastroenterology 1961; 40:389.

142. Read AE et al: Effects of chlorpromazine in patients with hepatic disease. Br Med J 1969; 3:497.

143. Maxwell JD et al: Plasma disappearance and cerebral effects of chlorpromazine in cirrhotics. Clin Sci. 1972; 43:143.

144. Branch RA et al: Intravenous administration of diazepam in patients with chronic liver disease. Gut. 1976; 17:975.

145. Greenberger NJ et al: Effects of vegetable and animal protein diets in chronic hepatic encephalopathy. Am J Dig Dis. 1977; 22:845.

146. Maddrey WC et al: Effects of keto-analogues of essential amino acids in portalsystemic encephalopathy. Gastroenterology. 1976; 71:190.

147. Maddrey WC et al: Arginine and ornithine salts of branched-chain ketoacids in portal-systemic encephalopathy (abstr). Clin Res. 1978; 26:322A.

148. Poth EJ et al: Neomycin, a new intestinal antiseptic. Texas Rep Biol Med. 1970; 8:353.

149. Breen KJ et al: Neomycin absorption in man: studies of oral and enema administration and effect of intestinal ulceration. Ann Intern Med. 1972; 76:211.

150. Longstreth GF et al: Drug-induced malabsorption. Mayo Clin Proc. 1975; 50:284.

151. Lindenbaum J et al: Inhibition of digoxin absorption by neomycin. Gastroenterology. 1976; 71:399.

152. Cheng SH et al: Effect of orally administered neomycin on the absorption of penicillin V. N Engl J Med. 1962; 267:1296.

153. Faloon WW: Metabolic effects of non-absorbable antibacterial agents. Am J Clin Nutr. 1970; 23:645.

154. Conn HO et al: Comparison of lactulose and neomycin in the treatment of chronic portal-systemic encephalopathy. Gastroenterology. 1977; 72:573.

155. Atterbury CE et al: Neomycin-sorbitol and lactulose in the treatment of acute portal systemic encephalopathy. A controlled, double-blind clinical trial. Digestive Dis. 1978; 23:398.

156. Avery GS et al: Lactulose: A review of its therapeutic and pharmacological properties with particular reference to ammonia metabolism and its mode of action in portal systemic encephalopathy. Drugs 1972; 4:7.

157. Romankiewicz JA: Medical management of hepatic encephalopathy. U.S. Pharmacist. 1978; 3:H-6.

158. Vince A et al: Effect of lactulose on ammonia production in a fecal incubation system. Gastroenterology. 1978; 74:544.

159. Kersh ES et al: Lactulose enemas. Ann Intern Med. 1973; 78:81.

160. Bircher J et al: Treatment of chronic portal systemic encephalopathy with lactulose. Lancet 1966; 2:890.

161. Elkington SG et al: Lactulose in the treatment of chronic portal-systemic encephalopathy. N Engl J Med. 1969; 281:408.

162. Bircher J et al: Treatment of chronic portal-systemic encephalopathy with lactulose. Am J Med. 1971; 51:148.

163. Zeegen R et al: Some observations on effects of treatment with lactulose on patients with chronic hepatic encephalopathy. Quart J Med. 1970; 39:245.

164. Simmons F et al: Controlled clinical trial of lactulose in hepatic encephalopathy. Gastroenterology. 1970; 59:827.

165. Fessel JM et al: Lactulose in treatment of acute hepatic encephalopathy. Am J Med Sci. 1973; 266:103.

166. Conn HO: Interaction of lactulose and neomycin. Drugs. 1972; 4:4.

167. Pirotte J et al: Comparative study of basal arterial ammonemia and of orally-induced hyperammonemia in chronic portal systemic encephalopathy, treated with neomycin, lactulose, and an association of neomycin and lactulose. Digestion. 1974; 10:435.

168. Read AE et al: Lactobacilli acidophilus (Enpac) in treatment of hepatic encephalopathy. Br Med J. 1966; 1:1267.

169. Loh WP et al: Fecal flora of man after oral administration of chlortetracycline or oxytetracycline. Arch Intern Med. 1955; 95:74.

170. Weinstein L et al: Effect of paromomycin on bacterial flora of human intestine: studies of total numbers and specific components. JAMA. 1961; 178:891.

171. Conn HO et al: Lactulose and neomycin: combined therapy. In *Hepatic Coma Syndromes and Lactulose,* Williams & Wilkins, Baltimore, 1979; p 340.

172. Fischer JE et al: Treatment of hepatic coma and hepatorenal syndrome. Am J Surg. 1972; 123:222.

173. Parkes JD et al: Levodopa in hepatic coma. Lancet. 1970; 2:1341.

174. Stefanini M et al: Levodopa in hepatic failure. JAMA. 1972; 220:1247.

175. Michel H et al: Treatment of cirrhotic hepatic encephalopathy with L-dopa. A controlled trial. Gastroenterology. 1980; 79:207.

176. Uribe M et al: Treatment of chronic portal systemic encephalopathy with bromocriptine. Gastroenterology. 1979; 76:1347.

177. Morgan MY et al: Successful use of bromocriptine in the treatment of chronic hepatic encephalopathy. Gastroenterology. 1980; 78:663.

Chapter 25

Viral Hepatitis

Joseph P. Gee and Lucia K. Jim

Hepatitis, or inflammation of the liver, may be caused by various factors such as viruses, bacteria, or chemicals. Viral hepatitis is a systemic infection which predominantly affects the liver. Viral hepatitis is caused by at least three distinct etiologic agents—hepatitis A virus (HAV), hepatitis B virus (HBV), and hepatitis non-A non-B virus(es) (1). Hepatocellular disease produced by other viruses, such as the Epstein-Barr virus and cytomegalovirus, is considered separate from viral hepatitis, because hepatic inflammation is less clinically prominent than other systemic manifestations.

Although hepatitis A and B viruses produce clinically similar diseases in man, the two forms can be distinguished by their antigenic properties. The third type, non-A non-B virus(es), has yet to be definitively described. Because it is not detected by the routine antigenic screening employed by blood banks, non-A non-B virus causes about 90% of post-transfusion hepatitis (2–4).

There are approximately 53,000 clinically recognized cases of viral hepatitis reported in the United States each year (5). About 55% reportedly are caused by hepatitis A, 30% are caused by hepatitis B, and the remaining 15% are unspecified as to type.

Hepatitis A

Other names for hepatitis A include infectious hepatitis, short-incubation hepatitis, and MS-1 hepatitis. Symptoms of infection with hepatitis A are usually acute in onset, and infections occur primarily in children and young adults. The incubation period is 15 to 50 days (mean: 25 to 28 days).

Serology. Hepatitis A virus (HAV) is only transiently detectable in the serum and is usually of very low titer; however, antibodies to the hepatitis A virus can be monitored serologically. The serum concentration of anti-hepatitis A antibodies (anti-HA) begins to increase about two weeks after patients have become infectious. Maximal serum concentrations of these antibodies are reached in several months and may be detectable for about ten years. The presence of anti-HA is associated with immunity from subsequent HAV infection (6).

Although 18% to 80% of adults in the United States have positive anti-HA serum (7), the frequency of adults with positive anti-HA serum can be as high as 90–100% in certain hyperendemic areas of the world (8). However, less than 5% of individuals with anti-HA serum have a history of clinical hepatitis. These studies suggest that HAV infection is common, usually mild, and self-limiting.

Clinical Presentation. The symptoms of hepatitis A infection are generally abrupt in onset and frequently include fever, malaise, anorexia, myalgia, headache, nausea, and abdominal discomfort. Scleral icterus is uncommon, but it may occur one to two weeks after the onset of prodromal symptoms. Hepatitis A infection tends to be benign and self-limited when compared with hepatitis B and non-A non-B hepatitis. Furthermore, hepatitis A infections do not appear to produce a chronic carrier state, chronic liver disease, or cirrhosis. With the exception of some elderly patients, those infected with hepatitis A virus

rarely develop fulminant hepatitis. The fatality rate from hepatitis A infection is about 0.01%.

Routes of Transmission. Direct personal contact is the main route of transmission of hepatitis A, and the fecal-oral route is most often involved. The feces of patients with hepatitis A remain infectious for about two weeks before and about two weeks after the onset of symptoms (9). Accordingly, hepatitis A occurs in epidemic form, especially in areas where sanitation is poor. Contaminated water, uncooked shellfish, and other foods also play a role in the spread of hepatitis A virus. Although one report suggested that hepatitis A can be contracted in a hemodialysis unit, parenteral transmission is extremely rare (10).

Hepatitis B

Hepatitis B is also known as serum hepatitis, long-incubation hepatitis, MS-2 hepatitis, hepatitis B surface antigen (HBsAg)-positive hepatitis, and Australia antigen-positive hepatitis. Unlike hepatitis A, symptoms of infection due to hepatitis B can be either acute or insidious in onset, infections occur in all age groups, and the virus has a longer incubation period (range: 45 to 180 days).

Serology. The hepatitis B virus (HBV) is a 42-nm double shelled virus, originally known as the Dane particle. It consists of an inner nucleocapsid core designated as the *hepatitis B core antigen (HBcAg)* and an outer lipoprotein coat termed the *hepatitis B surface antigen (HBsAg)* (11). A third serologic marker of HBV, called the *"e" antigen (HBeAg),* is associated with the intact virus and high serum levels of hepatitis B viral-specific DNA-polymerase activity (11,12).

HBsAg first appears in serum three to 11 weeks after inoculation and is the first manifestation of HBV infection. HBsAg often persists throughout the clinical illness and disappears one to 13 weeks after appearance of the laboratory abnormalities. Persistence of HBsAg beyond 13 weeks occurs infrequently (4%) and is commonly associated with chronic hepatitis (13). *Specific antibodies to HBsAg (anti-HBs)* develop several weeks to months after clearance of HBsAg from the serum. Development of anti-HBs signals recovery from hepatitis B, absence of infectivity, and protection from future HBV infection.

Free HBcAg is not found in serum and can only be detected by concentrating and disrupting circulating Dane particles (6,11). *Antibody to hepatitis core antigen (anti-HBc)* is detected 12 to 20 weeks after exposure to HBV. Anti-HBc has been identified in all cases of acute HBV infection and carrier states and is present in 98% of HBsAg-positive serum samples (14). Although only 1% of HBsAg-negative donors are positive for anti-HBc, transfused blood from these donors is infectious (14).

HBeAg is a soluble protein found only in HBsAg-positive serum. HBeAg appears during the incubation period, within one week after detection of HBsAg and before biochemical abnormality. Since HBeAg is regularly associated with signs of active viral replication, "e" antigen is an important index of infectivity (11).

Clinical Presentation. The clinical presentation of acute hepatitis B is similar to that of hepatitis A with a few exceptions. The onset of symptoms due to infection with hepatitis B is usually insidious, with fatigue, anorexia and other gastrointestinal complaints, and is often followed by jaundice. Arthralgias, urticaria, and a serum-sickness-like prodrome may occur in 10–20% of patients with hepatitis B but rarely in those with hepatitis A. Fever is usually absent. The duration of the clinical course is frequently longer for hepatitis B than for hepatitis A. The fatality rate is low but is significantly increased by age and underlying debilitating states (15,16).

Routes of Transmission. Transmission of hepatitis B virus is most often by parenteral inoculation of virus-containing material. Hepatitis B can also be spread by intimate physical contact or transmitted from HBsAg-positive mothers to their fetuses or neonates (6). HBsAg has been detected from tears, sneeze droplets, saliva, breast milk, urine, semen, menstrual blood, and vaginal secretions of hepatitis B patients; however, the infectivity of these secretions is not yet known (17).

1. *Acute Viral Hepatitis.* M.E., a 20-year-old student nurse, was seen in the clinic with chief complaints of tiredness, loss of appetite, vomiting, itching, and joint pain. Several weeks prior to this clinic visit, she began feeling increasingly fatigued and began losing her appetite. One day prior to this visit she noticed dark urine. Three months ago she and her husband spent three weeks in India. After returning from the trip, she did a one-month clerkship rotation on the oncology ward. She takes no medications and does not consume alcohol.

Physical examination revealed a well nourished female in moderate distress. Her temperature was 98°F. Her sclerae were markedly icteric, her skin appeared jaundiced, and there were scratch marks on both arms. Her abdomen was full with right upper quadrant tenderness, the liver was slightly enlarged, and the spleen was not enlarged. No shifting dullness was appreciated.

Laboratory studies revealed: Serum glutamic oxaloacetic transaminase 920 IU/L (6–18), serum glutamic pyruvic transaminase 1500 IU/L (3–26), alkaline phosphatase 110 IU/L (21–91), total bilirubin 10 mg/dl (1.0) and direct bilirubin 8.5 mg/dl (0.4), prothrombin time 12 seconds, and positive test for serum HBsAg.

What clinical features of viral hepatitis are illustrated by this patient?

Assuming that alcohol and drugs can be ruled out because of their negative history of intake, the patient's history of travel abroad and close contact with immunosuppressed patients is suggestive of either hepatitis A or hepatitis B infection. Her presenting symptoms and signs of fatigue, anorexia, vomiting, pruritus, dark urine, scleral icterus, and elevated liver function test results are compatible with a diagnosis of acute viral hepatitis. The absence of ascites and her normal prothrombin time denote a good prognosis.

Viral hepatitis usually begins with the onset of vague symptoms. In hepatitis A, abrupt onset of fatigue, headache, anorexia, and vomiting may be the first manifestations of the disease. Right upper quadrant abdominal fullness and tenderness may be present as in this case. A flu-like syndrome including fever, myalgia, pharyngitis and coryza may be described but was absent in M.E. These presenting symptoms may eventually subside in a large percentage of patients and the hepatitis remains unnoticed. A few patients will go on to develop clinical jaundice 2 to 14 days after the onset of symptoms. Dark urine and light stools due to bilirubinemia usually precede jaundice by 1 to 5 days. Transient pruritus may occur at this stage. When the disease is acquired parenterally (ie, hepatitis B) the symptoms are similar to those of hepatitis A but, as was the case with M.E., the onset is more insidious and fever is usually absent. The serum sickness-like prodrome of skin eruption, urticaria, polyarthralgia, and arthritis, which are thought to be caused by circulating immune complexes, occurs more frequently in hepatitis B patients. M.E.'s complaints of joint pain and itching may be part of the serum sickness-like prodrome of hepatitis B. Once jaundice appears, the clinical features of hepatitis A and B are essentially identical.

With the onset of jaundice, the prodromal symptoms usually subside. The post-icteric recovery phase varies from 2 to 12 weeks. It is usually more prolonged in acute hepatitis B, and complete clinical and biochemical recovery requires 3 to 4 months in most cases.

2. Why is hepatitis B viral infection the most likely cause of this patient's acute hepatitis?

Hepatitis A virus is a potential cause since she has recently traveled to a densely populated country. However, the incubation period in this case was longer than that usually reported for hepatitis A. Serologic testing for anti-HA is of little diagnostic value because of its delayed appearance after an acute infection and its presence in a high percentage of adults in the United States (7). Hepatitis B viral infection is also a potential cause of her acute hepatitis because she was in close contact with immunosuppressed oncology patients who were likely to be HBsAg-positive carriers. Her work as a nurse required handling of contaminated needles, blood, and other body fluids which may have further exposed her to potential contamination. The more convincing evidence includes the incubation period of about seven weeks, which coincides with that of hepatitis B, and the positive HBsAg in her serum, which confirmed acute hepatitis B infection.

3. *Treatment.* Outline a rational treatment plan for M.E.'s presumed hepatitis B infection.

It may be desirable to hospitalize M.E. to ensure fluid and food intake because of her prolonged anorexia and vomiting and in order to perform a more complete diagnostic work-up. Hydroxyzine 50 mg or prochlorperazine 10 mg orally or IM every four to six hours can be used to treat her vomiting. *The management of acute viral hepatitis is nonspecific.* Hospitalization may be required for proper diagnosis, for clinically severe illness, and for elderly patients because of the high mortality rate in this group. Previously healthy persons with hepatitis B generally recover completely and may be treated on an outpatient basis with close monitoring of liver function tests and clinical signs and symptoms.

Measures should be taken to minimize spread of the hepatitis virus. Thorough hand washing with soap and water is probably the most effective means of prevention. Patients with hepatitis B often transmit infection to close contacts, especially sexual partners. Persons who have acute hepatitis B or are asymptomatic HBsAg carriers should have separate razors, toothbrushes, washcloths, and other personal items. Blood-contaminated bandages, sanitary napkins, or other objects should be discarded in waterproof plastic bags. Samples of blood and other body fluids should be properly labeled with precautions. Those who handle contaminated items should wear disposable gloves and wash their hands thoroughly afterwards. Instruments, utensils, and surfaces must be cleansed and sterilized or disinfected.

Bed rest is recommended initially, but prolonged bed rest beyond the duration of clinical disease is unnecessary. Patients who feel well may be allowed to ambulate as tolerated (16,18). In addition to the subjective improvement of symptoms, declining serum transaminase levels may be used as a guide to ambulation.

4. *Immunoglubins.* Would immune serum (gamma) globulin (ISG) or hepatitis B immune globulins (HBIG) be of any benefit in the management of this patient's hepatitis B viral infection? How do these products differ?

Gamma immunoglobulins for intramuscular administration are sterile protein solutions that contain antibodies derived from pooled human plasma. The concentrations of anti-HA and anti-HBs in *immune serum globulin (ISG)* vary depending on donor exposure to the type of viral hepatitis. In the U.S., all lots of ISG contain quantities of anti-HA sufficient for protection against hepatitis A virus. ISG manufactured after 1977 has regularly contained detectable anti-HBs titers in the range of 1:100 and can reasonably be expected to provide some passive immunization against hepatitis B virus. Immunoglobulins prepared from donor pools pre-selected for the presence of anti-HBs generally have much higher titers of anti-HBs (>1:100,000) than standard ISG and are designated as *hepatitis B immune globulins (HBIG).* It appears that this product can minimize symptoms or prevent infection entirely if given within 7 days after exposure to hepatitis B virus (20,22–24). The protection lasts for about four months (24). Neither product would be of any value for patient M.E., since she already has active viral hepatitis; she will subsequently aquire active immunity for hepatitis B virus.

5. Under what circumstances would the use of immune serum globulin (ISG) or hepatitis immune globulin (HBIG) be indicated? (Also see previous question.) What doses are used?

Hepatitis A. In the event of hepatitis A exposure, 0.02 ml/kg given intramuscularly early in the incubation period will prevent symptoms and jaundice (21). Subclinical infection with serum transaminase elevation followed by immunity probably occurs in these individuals. ISG offers greatest prophylactic value if administered within one to two weeks of exposure to hepatitis A virus; its prophylactic value decreases with increased elapsed time after exposure. ISG is ineffective if given more than two weeks after exposure and in the treatment of active disease. Routine administration of ISG is indicated for household or institutional contacts who are at substantial risk of being infected with hepatitis A virus, or foodhandlers exposed to the virus who may be involved in its spread. ISG is not required for casual contacts. ISG prophylaxis is also recommended for travelers to tropical or developing countries; an intramuscular dose of 0.02 ml/kg is given prior to travel of less than 3 months duration. For longer travel, a dose of 0.05 ml/kg can be given every 4 to 6 months (16).

Hepatitis B. The major indication for the use of HBIG is after a single exposure to a relatively large inoculum of hepatitis B virus. At present, the U.S. Public Health Service recommends HBIG for post-exposure prophylaxis of patients or staff accidentally exposed to blood known to contain HBsAg and for neonates whose mothers had acute hepatitis B in the third trimester of pregnancy or who are HBsAg-positive at the time of delivery (20). The recommended dose for acute exposure is 0.06 ml/kg intramuscularly within 24 hours. This dose should be repeated one month later. For neonates, the dose of HBIG is 0.5 ml IM as a single dose as soon as possible after delivery but not later than 24 hours. The same dose (0.5 ml) should be repeated 3 months and 6 months later (20).

HBIG is not recommended for pre-exposure prophylaxis of hepatitis B (20). Passive immunization is not routinely recommended for patients and staff of hemodialysis units. Precautions such as serologic screening of patients and staff, segregation of carriers, and environmental hygiene should be encouraged. In selected circumstances where hepatitis B virus is endemic, ISG is as effective as HBIG for pre-exposure prophylaxis. The recommended dose of ISG is 0.05–0.07 ml/kg IM and is repeated at four-month intervals for as long as the risk of hepatitis B virus transmission persists. Patients receiving passive immunization should be checked for the presence of anti-HBs before each injection; in those found positive, prophylaxis can be discontinued due to presumed acquisition of active immunity.

6. *Pruritus.* M.E. complained of itching when she first came to the clinic. Her skin on both arms revealed scratch marks. What is the most likely cause of her pruritus and how should it be treated?

The exact cause of the pruritus which accompanies hepatitis or obstructive biliary diseases is unknown. It is currently believed that high blood levels of bile salts result in deposition in the subcutaneous tissues and thereby cause pruritus. Bile salts are the final products of cholesterol degradation. In man, the liver synthesizes only about 800 mg of bile acids per day. However, about 25 gm of bile salts are secreted into the biliary tree daily and are reabsorbed from the small bowel (biliary enterohepatic recycling) (25). Generally, pruritus associated with acute viral hepatitis is mild and requires no treatment. Whereas that of primary biliary cirrhosis is often intense and requires medical attention.

Treatment of pruritus is nonspecific and symptomatic. Topical dressings of Burow's solution or phenolated calamine lotion can be applied for temporary relief of itching. Antihistamines such as hydroxyzine can be given at a dose of 25–50 mg orally every six hours for relief of pruritus and for sedation (26,27).

Cholestyramine, an anion exchange resin which decreases the enterohepatic recycling of bile salts, can be used effectively to decrease pruritus if other more conservative measures fail (ie, topical dressings and antihistamines).

If pruritus is severe, the patient's nails should be cut short and kept clean to decrease excoriation and infection. Wearing cotton mittens may help, particularly if the patient scratches during sleep.

7. After a trial of hydroxyzine, calamine lotion, and oatmeal baths with minimal relief of pruritus, cholestyramine was ordered for M.E. How does cholestyramine exert its therapeutic effect?

Cholestyramine (Cuemid, Questran) is an insoluble quarternary ammonium anion exchange resin that disrupts biliary enterohepatic recycling by firmly binding bile salts in the bowel; the bile salts are then excreted in the feces. Therefore, cholestyramine decreases itching by reducing bile acids in the serum and, ultimately, those deposited in dermal tissues. The efficacy of cholestyramine depends upon the ability of the bile salts to reach the duodenum where the exchange takes place. Patients with complete biliary obstruction will therefore not respond to cholestyramine.

Cholestyramine is administered orally. The recommended adult dosage is 4 gm three or four times daily with meals. It should be mixed with fruit juices or soups because of its offensive pungent odor and should be allowed to stand in the selected vehicle for one to two minutes prior to stirring so that it will absorb moisture and disperse evenly. It usually takes one to three weeks for dramatic relief of itching to occur (25,33–34); however, some relief may occur within the first week (33).

8. After M.E. was started on cholestyramine 4 gm orally qid, she complained of abdominal cramps. Is this a common side effect of cholestyramine? What other potential untoward reactions or drug interactions should one monitor for?

Toxicity resulting from cholestyramine is negligible, although large doses may induce steatorrhea and hypoprothrombinemia. Gastrointestinal symptoms are common and may include nausea, abdominal cramping, diarrhea, or constipation. If the abdominal cramps become unbearable for M.E., reducing the cholestyramine dose to 4 gm tid may alleviate her symptoms.

By increasing the fecal excretion of bile salts, cholestyramine interferes with fat and fat-soluble vitamin absorption. Patients receiving long-term resin therapy should also receive water-soluble formulations of vitamin A, D, and K or IM injections of these vitamins. Although not pertinent to this patient, decreased absorption of drugs such as digoxin and warfarin by co-administration of cholestyramine can be significant. Patients who are taking these drugs should be advised to take them as far apart from their cholestyramine doses as possible to minimize this drug interaction (35,36).

Transfusion Hepatitis

Human blood products occasionally transmit hepatitis. Specific blood products can be classified as high risk, average risk, or safe. The actual risk of infection following transfusion depends on the donor population, the number of units transfused, and the susceptibility of the recipient to viral hepatitis (37). Since routine screening of blood donors for HBsAg takes place, most cases of transfusion-associated hepatitis is that of the non-A non-B type. The remaining few cases are caused by hepatitis B virus that was not detected at the time of donation; hepatitis A virus is an extremely rare cause of transfusion hepatitis (38,39).

In general, the risk of hepatitis following transfusion of pooled blood (blood derived from large numbers of donors) or of blood obtained from commercial (paid) donors is greater than the risk following transfusion of blood from volunteer donors (40). Average risk preparations include whole blood and its components, such as plasma and red cells, that are prepared without pooling. High risk derivatives are those that are pooled and cannot be sterilized (eg, fibrinogen and clotting factor concentrates). Safe products are those that have been sterilized by heating for ten hours at 60°C or prepared by ethanol fractionation. Albumin, thrombin, fibrinolysin, and the immune serum globulins are considered risk-free.

9. *Risk of Transfusion Hepatitis.* N.P. is a 62-year-old man with polycystic kidney disease who has been on hemodialysis for the past eleven years. He was admitted with a hemoglobin of 7 gm/dl (normal: 13–18 gm/dl) and a chief complaint of dyspnea on exertion. Two units of whole blood were ordered. Why should N.P. be screened for viral hepatitis?

N.P. should be routinely screened for the presence of HBsAg in his serum because he probably requires blood transfusion on a chronic basis and the risk of hepatitis increases with the total number of units transfused. His immune system is probably suppressed and thus he is a likely candidate for becoming an asymptomatic HBsAg-positive carrier. If the result for HBsAg is positive, he should be treated as potentially infectious and appropriate precautions should be employed (see Question 3).

10. Why are ISG or HBIG not indicated for N.P. as prophylaxis against hepatitis B and non-A non-B post-transfusion hepatitis?

The routine use of ISG to prevent post-transfusion hepatitis B in N.P. is probably not warranted since the blood banks routinely screen for HBsAg. Because of its cost and its questionable efficacy, passive immunization is not recommended for patients and staff of hemodialysis units except in selected areas where HBV is endemic (20). (Also see Question 5.)

Approximately 90% of post-transfusion hepatitis is now related to non-A non-B virus(es). Although data from studies of the effect of ISG and HBIG prophylaxis on the incidence of and morbidity and mortality from transfusion-associated hepatitis have suggested that ISG and HBIG may be effective in reducing transfusion-associated non-A non-B hepatitis, especially the icteric variety (41–44), additional studies are needed to verify these findings. The efficacy of ISG and HBIG in preventing or attenuating non-A non-B hepatitis in other epidemiologic settings must be better defined before routine prophylactic use of immunoglobulins can be recommended.

Sequelae of Hepatitis B Viral Infection

Approximately 10% of hepatitis B viral infections develop into a chronic carrier state in which HBsAg remains detectable in the serum from several years to the patient's lifetime (1). The carrier state can be totally asymptomatic or it may present as active liver disease (ie, chronic hepatitis). Immunosuppressed patients who contracted hepatitis B viral infection at an early age are especially predisposed to the development of chronic liver disease. Cellular immune response is important in terminating the infection and in the genesis of autoimmunity. The absence of competent T-cell function would favor the development of the chronic carrier state and promote chronic liver damage (45). Characteristically, chronic carriers with no anti-HBs and high titers of anti-HBc and HBeAg are at high risk of developing active liver disease and transmitting the infection to others (1).

Chronic hepatitis can be differentiated morphologically into chronic persistent and chronic active hepatitis (6). *Chronic persistent hepatitis (CPH),* a continuing inflammatory reaction in the liver, is almost always benign and self-limited.

Thus, no therapy is required. *Chronic active hepatitis (CAH)* is associated with more severely deranged liver functions and multilobular necrosis on liver biopsy. Unlike CPH, the syndrome of CAH is progressive and may lead to cirrhosis or fulminant hepatic failure.

Steroid Treatment of CAH. Chronic active hepatitis may be caused by hepatotoxic drugs and autoimmune (lupoid) reactions in addition to hepatitis B and possibly non-A non-B virus(es). The autoimmune form of CAH, which affects predominantly women and usually presents with positive LE cells, smooth muscle antibodies and antinuclear antibodies, is usually responsive to steroid therapy (46). The Mayo Clinic studies suggest that CAH patients with HBsAg-negative serum and severe symptomatic disease may benefit from steroid therapy (47,48). More recent studies (49,50) revealed that steroid therapy not only is ineffective in HBsAg-positive CAH but may have deleterious consequences, because the immunosuppressive effect of steroids may potentiate hepatitis B viral replication in these HBsAg-positive chronic infections (51). The results of these studies seem to suggest that the absence of HBsAg in the serum is crucial for the beneficial and safe use of steroids in CAH. Nevertheless, two previous studies suggested that steroid therapy may be ineffective in the treatment of CAH of viral origin whether it is HBsAg-positive or -negative (52,53); conclusive evidence may not be available until non-A non-B agents can be identified by serologic testing.

11. *Chronic Active Hepatitis.* J.R. is a 25-year-old Navy veteran who was admitted to the VA medical center for liver biopsy. His previous medical record revealed that J.R. first developed acute viral hepatitis 4 years ago, shortly after entering boot camp for military training. Since then, J.R. complained of persistent fatigue, anorexia, diarrhea and stomach upset. He was seen at the VA medical center one year ago for evaluative studies. Liver biopsy at that time was consistent with "mild piecemeal necrosis." His persistent fatigue and elevated SGOT prompted this admission for re-biopsy and consideration of steroid therapy. Current laboratory data included: WBC 1,500/mm^3 (4,300–10,800/mm^3), platelets 75,000/mm^3 (150,000–350,000/mm^3), alkaline phosphatase 93 IU/L (20–48 IU/L),

serum glutamic oxaloacetic transaminase 418 IU/L (6–18 IU/L), and serum globulins 6 gm/dl (2.3–3.5 gm/dl). Serum HBsAg was negative. The biopsy report was consistent with progressive multilobular necrosis, thus confirming the diagnosis of CAH. Steroid therapy was initiated.

Why was steroid therapy indicated for J.R.?

Steroid therapy is indicated in this case because J.R.'s laboratory and biopsy results are consistent with the subset of CAH patients who may derive beneficial effects from steroid therapy. The criteria for therapy for CAH based on the Mayo Clinic studies include symptoms for at least 10 weeks, sustained SGOT elevations 10 times greater than normal, or 5 times greater than normal with concurrent doubling of serum globulins, and liver biopsies showing at least piecemeal necrosis or multilobular necrosis (55,56). Since J.R. presented with HBsAg-negative CAH and meets all four of the Mayo Clinic criteria for treatment, steroid therapy may be given a trial.

12. Assuming that drug therapy is deemed justified in J.R.'s condition, what drug regimens are available for the treatment of CAH? Which regimen is more appropriate for J.R.?

Two treatment regimens appear to be equally effective in the management of severe CAH. Both high-dose prednisone with a tapering schedule and a lower dose of prednisone combined with a fixed dose of azathioprine have been demonstrated to be effective in controlling the inflammatory manifestations of the disease. Both regimens result in a greater than 60% remission rate after three years of therapy, and the relapse rate with both is about 20% (48). Because the frequency of drug-induced side effects is less with the combination regimen than with prednisone alone (10% versus 44%), the combination schedule is preferred for patients in whom azathioprine is not contraindicated by pretreatment cytopenia (48,56,57).

The dosage of the two treatment regimens has varied among different authors. Summerskill et al, of the Mayo Clinic, recommend that prednisone alone should be initiated at 60 mg daily for one week, 40 mg daily for the next week, then 30 mg for the following two weeks, and then maintained at 20 mg daily. When the patient goes into remission, the maintenance dose is slowly tapered over the next six weeks and discontinued. The initial schedule is repeated if the patient relapses. In patients where the risk of steroid side effects is high (eg, osteoporosis, diabetes, hypertension, secondary infections, and acne problems), prednisone at one-half of the scheduled daily dose can be used in combination with azathioprine 50 mg daily (48,58). Treatment with azathioprine alone at a dosage of 100–200 mg daily has been attempted, but the results are inferior to those obtained with corticosteroids. Furthermore, drug toxicity from azathioprine, including hepatotoxicity, nausea, emesis, rash, and cytopenia, may mask the manifestation of the liver disease itself. At a low dose of 50 mg daily, however, these toxicities are reported in less than 10% of patients (56). In the case of J.R., his current thrombocytopenia (platelet count 75,000/mm^3) and low WBC (1,500/mm^3) can be considered contraindications to the use of azathioprine; therefore, he should be treated with prednisone alone.

13. *Antiviral Agents.* If J.R.'s serum had been HBsAg-positive, steroid treatment would not have been considered. Are antiviral drugs effective in the treatment of chronic hepatitis B infections?

Because of the possible deleterious effects of steroid therapy on HBsAg-positive chronic active hepatitis (49–51), several antiviral agents, including interferons, ribavirin, and adenine arabinoside, have been extensively evaluated for the treatment of HBsAg-positive chronic hepatitis B viral infections. The goal in treating thse HBsAg-positive patients is to eradicate the virus. Unfortunately, none of the antiviral agents studied have achieved this goal, although transient inhibition of viral replication has been demonstrated.

Interferons are small glycoproteins produced by virally infected cells. Interferons can induce non-infected animal cells to synthesize a protein capable of inhibiting the production of virally coded protein (59). Two antigenically distinguishable interferons from humans have been described: one produced in leukocytes and the other in fibroblasts (12). The observation that patients with hepatitis B viral infection have low levels of circulating interferons led to the hypothesis that decreased interferon production might be responsible for failure of the host to eliminate the virus (60). Clinical trials of leukocyte-derived interferon in patients with HBsAg-positive CAH demonstrated suppression of Dane particle production during the period of treatment (61,62). In a majority of the patients, Dane particles were again demonstrated once therapy was ceased. Fibroblast-derived interferon appears to produce more unpredictable results than leukocyte-derived interferon (63). Thus, limited studies with interferons have been encouraging, but the high cost of production and limited availability of interferons has confined their use to experimental situations. An interferon inducer (polyriboinosinic polyribocytidylic acid) has also been demonstrated to have similar effectiveness in animals, but this agent is too toxic for clinical use (64).

Ribavirin (virazole), a nucleotide analog which inhibits viral DNA synthesis in vitro, was found to have no significant effect on DNA polymerase, HBsAg concentration, or liver function in a short-term trial with six HBsAg-positive patients (65).

Adenine arabinoside (ARA-A, vidarabine), a potent inhibitor of viral DNA synthesis, was demonstrated to be effective in decreasing DNA polymerase and HBsAg concentrations during treatment of HBsAg-positive CAH patients (66,67). In the study by Chadwick et al, two 5-day courses of ARA-A 10mg/kg/day produced a consistent but transient fall in HBV-specific DNA polymerase activity. A further increase in dose to 20 mg/kg/day similarly produced only a transient effect (66). Permanent inhibition of DNA polymerase was seen only in one female patient treated by Pollard et al, and this is the only patient in whom HBsAg fell to zero during treatment (67). Due to the low solubility of the drug, it must be given as continuous intravenous infusion in large volumes of fluid. The long-term side effects have not been well established.

Chloroquine and *quinacrine* have been shown to inhibit hepatitis B viral DNA polymerase in vitro (68). The adjunctive use of these drugs with interferons or other antiviral agents has been suggested. However, one preliminary trial of chloroquine 200 mg daily following an intravenous course of ARA-A did not maintain the suppression of HBV DNA polymerase (69).

References

1. Seto DS: Viral hepatitis. Pediatr Clin North Am. 1979; 26:305.

2. Alter HJ et al: The emerging pattern of post-transfusion hepatitis. Am J Med Sci. 1975; 270:329.

3. Purcell RH et al: Non-A, non-B hepatitis. Yale J Biol Med. 1977; 49:243.

4. Aach RD et al: Post-transfusion hepatitis: current perspectives. Ann Intern Med. 1980; 92:539.

5. Centers for Disease Control: Reported morbidity and mortality in the United States, 1978. Morbid Mortal Weekly Rep. 1979; 27:3.

6. Reed JS et al: Viral hepatitis: epidemiologic, serologic and clinical manifestations. DM. 1979; 25:1.

7. Szmuness W et al: Distribution of antibody to hepatitis A antigen in urban adults. N Engl J Med. 1976; 295:755.

8. Szmuness W et al: The prevalence of antibody to hepatitis A antigen in various parts of the world. Am J Epidemiol. 1977; 106:392.

9. Dienstag JL et al: Fecal shedding of hepatitis A antigen. Lancet. 1975; 1:765.

10. Szmuness W et al: Hepatitis type A and hemodialysis: a seroepidemiologic study in 15 U.S. centers. Ann Intern Med. 1977; 87:8.

11. Czaja AJ: Serologic markers of hepatitis A and B in acute and chronic liver disease. Mayo Clin Proc. 1979; 54:721.

12. Zuckerman AJ: Human viral hepatitis. Pharmacol Ther. 1980; 10:1.

13. Nielsen JO et al: Incidence and meaning of persistence of Australia antigen in patients with acute viral hepatitis: development of chronic hepatitis. N Engl J Med. 1971; 285:1157.

14. Hoofnagle JH et al: Antibody to hepatitis B core antigen: a sensitive indicator of hepatitis B virus replication. N Engl J Med. 1974; 290:1336.

15. Mistilis SP et al: Management of chronic hepatitis, Part one: Diagnosis. Med J Aust. 1980; 1:152.

16. Dienstag JL et al: Acute viral hepatitis. In *Harrison's Principles of Internal Medicine,* 9th ed, edited by KJ Isselbacher et al., McGraw-Hill, New York, 1980, p 1459.

17. Gitnick GL et al: The liver and the antigens of hepatitis B. Ann Intern Med. 1976; 85:488.

18. Greenberg H et al: Hepatitis A. In *Infectious Diseases,* 2nd ed, edited by PD Hoeprich, Harper & Row, Hagerstown, Maryland, 1977, p 604.

19. Bryan JA: Viral hepatitis. 2. Prevention and control. Postgrad Med. 1980; 68:81.

20. Centers for Disease Control: Recommendation of the Immunization Practices Advisory Committee (ACIP): Immune globulin for protection against viral hepatitis. Atlanta: Centers for Disease Control. 1981; 30(No. 34):423.

21. Public Health Service Advisory Committee on Immunization Practices: Immune serum globulin for protection against viral hepatitis. Ann Intern Med. 1972; 77:427.

22. Redeker AG et al: Hepatitis B immune globulin as a prophylactic measure for spouses exposed to acute type B hepatitis. N Engl J Med. 1975; 293:1055.

23. Prince AM et al: Hepatitis B "immune" globulin: effectiveness in prevention of dialysis-associated hepatitis. N Engl J Med. 1975; 293:1063.

24. Grady GF et al: Hepatitis B immune globulin—prevention of hepatitis from accidental exposure among medical personnel. N Engl J Med. 1975; 293:1067.

25. Van Itallie TB et al: The treatment of pruritus and hy-
    percholesteremia of primary biliary cirrhosis with
    cholestyramine. N Engl J Med. 1961; 265:469.

26. Anon.: Atarax (hydroxyzine) for itching. Med Letter Drugs
    Ther. 1980; 22:4.

27. Harvey RP et al: A controlled trial of therapy in chronic
    urticaria. (Abstr) J Allergy Clin Immunol. 1980; 65:190.

28. Kaiser HB: Cimetidine in chronic urticaria. Lancet. 1980;
    2:206.

29. Aymard JP et al: Cimetidine for pruritus in Hodgkin's
    disease. Br Med J. 1980; 1:151.

30. Harrison AR et al: Pruritus, cimetidine and polycy-
    themia. N Engl J Med. 1979; 300:433.

31. Trolle D: Decrease of total serum bilirubin concentration
    in newborn infants after phenobarbitone treatment.
    Lancet. 1968; 2:705.

32. Stiehl A et al: The effects of phenobarbital on bile salts
    and bilirubin in patients with intrahepatic and extra-
    hepatic cholestasis. N Engl J Med. 1972; 286:858.

33. Datta DV et al: Treatment of pruritus of obstructive
    jaundice with cholestyramine. Br Med J. 1963; 1:216.

34. Schaffner F: Cholestyramine, a boon to some who itch.
    Gastroenterology. 1964; 46:67.

35. Brown DD et al: Decreased bioavailability of digoxin due
    to hypocholesterolemic interventions. Circulation. 1978;
    58:164.

36. Robinson DS et al: Interaction of warfarin and nonsys-
    temic gastrointestinal drugs. Clin Pharmacol Ther. 1971;
    12:491.

37. Goldfield M: Some epidemiologic studies of transfusion-
    associated hepatitis. In *Transmissible Disease and Blood
    Transfusion*, edited by TJ Greenwalt, and GA Jamieson,
    Grune & Stratton, New York, 1974, p 141.

38. Feinstone S et al: Transfusion associated hepatitis not
    due to A or B viruses. N Engl J Med. 1975; 292:767.

39. Chircu LV et al: Post-transfusion hepatitis: antigen/
    antibody systems correlated with non-A, non-B hepati-
    tis. J Med Virology. 1980; 6:147.

40. Barker JF et al: Viral hepatitis B: Detection and pro-
    phylaxis. In *Transmissible Disease and Blood Transfu-
    sion*, edited by TJ Greenwalt and GA Jamieson, Grune
    & Stratton, New York, 1974, p 81.

41. Knodell RG et al: Efficacy of prophylactic gamma-glob-
    ulin in preventing non-A non-B post-transfusion hepa-
    titis. Lancet. 1976; 1:577.

42. Knodell RG et al: Development of chronic liver disease
    after acute non-A non-B post-transfusion hepatitis: role
    of λ globulin prophylaxis in its prevention. Gastroenter-
    ology. 1977; 72:902.

43. Seeff LB et al: A randomized, double blind controlled
    trial of the efficacy of immune serum globulin for the
    prevention of post-transfusion hepatitis: a Veterans
    Administration Cooperative Study. Gastroenterology.
    1977; 72:111.

44. Seeff LB et al: Immunoprophylaxis of viral hepatitis.
    Gastroenterology. 1979; 77:161.

45. Eddleston ALWF et al: Inadequate antibody response to
    HBAg or suppressor T-cell defect in active chronic hep-
    atitis. Lancet. 1974; 2:1543.

46. Wright EC et al: Treatment of chronic active hepatitis:
    an analysis of three controlled trials. Gastroenterology.
    1977; 73:1422.

47. Czaja AJ et al: Corticosteroid treated chronic active hep-
    atitis in remission: uncertain prognosis of chronic per-
    sistent hepatitis. N Engl J Med. 1981; 304:5.

48. Summerskill WHJ et al: Prednisone for chronic active
    liver disease: Dose titration, standard dose, and combi-
    nation with azathioprine compared. Gut. 1975; 16:876.

49. De Groote J et al: Long-term follow-up of chronic active
    hepatitis of moderate severity. Gut. 1978; 19:510.

50. Lam KC et al: Deleterious effect of prednisolone in HBsAg-
    positive chronic active hepatitis. N Engl J Med. 1981;
    304:380.

51. Scullard GH et al: The effect of immunosuppressive ther-
    apy on hepatitis B viral infection in patients with chronic
    hepatitis. Gastroenterology. 1979; 77:A40 (abstr).

52. Gregory PB et al: Steroid therapy in severe viral hepa-
    titis: a double-blind, randomized trial of methyl-pred-
    nisolone versus placebo. N Engl J Med. 1976; 294:681.

53. Ware A et al: Controlled trial of corticosteroid therapy
    in severe acute viral hepatitis. Gastroenterology. 1978;
    75:992 (abstr).

54. Redeker AG: Treatment of chronic active hepatitis, good
    news and bad news. N Engl J Med. 1981; 304:420.

55. Czaja AJ et al: Chronic hepatitis: To treat or not to treat?
    Med Clin North Am. 1978; 62:71.

56. Czaja AJ: Current problems in the diagnosis and man-
    agement of chronic active hepatitis. Mayo Clin Proc. 1981;
    56:311.

57. Uribe M et al: Steroid side effects during therapy of chronic
    active liver diseases (CALD): What to expect, (abstr).
    Gastroenterology. 1976; 71:932.

58. Soloway RD et al: Chronic active liver disease: classifi-
    cation and treatment. Postgrad Med. 1973; 53:88.

59. Thomas HC et al: Immunological and anti-viral therapy
    of chronic hepatitis B virus infection. Clin Gastroenter-
    ology. 1980; 9:85.

60. Tolentino P et al: Decreased interferon response by lym-
    phocytes from children with chronic hepatitis. J Infect
    Dis. 1975; 132:459.

61. Greenberg HB et al: Human leukocyte interferon and
    hepatitis B virus infection. N Engl J Med. 1976; 295:517.

62. Merigan TC et al: Antiviral therapy. In *Viral Hepatitis*,
    edited by GH Vigas, SN Cohen and R Schmid, Franklin
    Institute Press, Philadelphia, 1978.

63. Weimar W et al: Fibroblast interferon in HBs antigen
    positive chronic active hepatitis. Lancet. 1977; 2:1282.

64. Purcell RH et al: Modification of chronic hepatitis B vi-
    rus infection in chimpanzees by administration of an in-
    terferon inducer. Lancet. 1976; 2:757.

65. Jain S et al: Trial of ribavarin for the treatment of HBsAg
    positive chronic liver disease. J Antimicrob Chemother.
    1978; 4:369.

66. Chadwick RG et al: HBs antigen positive chronic liver
    disease: inhibition of DNA polymerase activity by vi-
    darabine. Br Med J. 1978; 2:531.

67. Pollard RB et al: The effect of vidarabine on chronic hep-
    atitis B virus infection. JAMA. 1978; 239:1648.

68. Hirschman SZ et al: Inhibition of hepatitis B DNA po-
    lymerase by intercalating agents. Nature. 1978; 271:681.

69. Thomas HC: Immunostimulant in treatment of HBs an-
    tigen positive chronic active liver disease. In *Immune
    Reactions in Liver Disease*, edited by ALWF Eddleston,
    JCP Weber and R Williams, Tunbridge Wells: Pitman
    Medical, 1979, p 281.

Chapter 26

Adverse Effects of Drugs on the Liver

Lucia K. Jim

In general, adverse drug effects on the liver represent only a small segment of the total spectrum of hepatic diseases. Drug-induced jaundice occurs in less than 5% of icteric patients admitted to general hospitals (1,2), but the relative incidence might be higher in elderly patients (3) and in patients who receive psychoactive or antituberculous drugs (4,5). Drugs, however, play a much more important role in hepatic necrosis and account for 20–30% of the cases of fulminant hepatic failure (6,7).

Classification

Drug-induced hepatic injury can be classified according to the morphology of the injury, the presumed mechanism, and the circumstances of drug-induced damage. Drug-induced hepatic injury can be characterized as either acute or chronic. Acute hepatic injury produced by drugs can be cytotoxic, cholestatic, or a mixed presentation of both. Cytotoxic hepatic injury can be due to necrosis, steatosis, or a combination thereof.

Hepatic Necrosis. Hepatic necrosis leads to hepatocellular jaundice and a viral hepatitis-like syndrome. In this situation, laboratory values for serum transaminases are often elevated from 10 to 200 times the upper limit of normal, and values for alkaline phosphatases are usually modestly increased to no more than three times normal values (8). Hepatic necrosis often results in fulminant hepatic failure and fatalities range from 10 to 50% (9).

Steatosis. Drug-induced acute steatosis, such as that caused by parenteral tetracycline, usually manifests as mild jaundice and moderately elevated concentrations of serum transaminase (9,10).

Cholestasis. Drug-induced cholestatic injury often resembles extrahepatic obstructive jaundice (8,11). In this instance, pruritus and jaundice are the main manifestations. Transaminase levels are only moderately elevated in most cases. Alkaline phosphatase levels are usually elevated more than three-fold in cholestasis associated with erythromycin estolate or chlorpromazine, but are lower in cholestasis provoked by anabolic and contraceptive steroids (12). The mortality rate for cholestatic injury is much lower than that for cytotoxic damage and is believed to be less than 1% (9).

Mixed forms of jaundice with cytotoxic and cholestatic features can be caused by para-aminosalicylic acid, sulfonamides, and phenylbutazone (9,11,13). The mortality rate of the mixed form seems to depend on the extent of cytotoxic injury.

Chronic Active Hepatitis. Chronic active hepatitis (CAH) is a syndrome which has only been recognized in the last two decades. It may progress during the course of drug therapy and may eventually result in post-necrotic cirrhosis. This syndrome of CAH can also be caused by hepatitis B virus, "non-A, non-B" viruses, or by an "autoimmune" (or lupoid) mechanism. Drugs associated with CAH include oxyphenisatin, methyldopa, nitrofurantoin, isoniazid, dantrolene, sulfonamides, perhexiline maleate, propylthiouracil, acetaminophen, and probably chlorpromazine and halothane (9,14–17). The clinical picture of drug-induced CAH is a mixture of characteristic features of both acute and chronic hepatic injury. Patients may first present with features of acute hepatocellular injury or clinical evidence of cirrhosis. Physical examinations often reveal a firm enlarged liver, splenomegaly, and spider angiomas with or without ascites. Jaundice, anorexia, and fatigue are common. Arthralgias or "arthritis" may occur. Serum transaminases are usually moderately elevated; hyperglobulinemia and hypoalbuminemia are characteristic; and antinuclear antibodies may be found in the serum (16–20). Recognition that drug-induced CAH can present as an "autoimmune" type picture is extremely important because withdrawal of the responsible drug may lead to marked improvement and eventually complete resolution of the disease.

Other Forms. Other forms of chronic hepatic disease are: steatosis and fatty cirrhosis in some patients after prolonged administration of methotrexate (21); peliosis hepatis, benign and malignant hepatic tumors which develop in recipients of contraceptive and anabolic steroids (22–25);

Budd-Chiari syndrome caused by hepatic vein occlusion resulting from the thrombogenic effect of the contraceptive steroids (26,27); and hepatic granulomas with or without other evidence of hepatic injury produced by phenylbutazone (28), chlorpropamide (29), allopurinol (30), and others (8,14).

In general, prognosis of drug-induced hepatotoxicity is good when the offending agent is withdrawn, but this is affected to a significant degree by the type of liver injury (9). The more cytotoxic the injury, the more likely is hepatic failure and death; the more cholestatic the injury, the better the prognosis.

Mechanisms of Hepatic Injury

The two major mechanisms by which drugs induce hepatic injury are *intrinsic hepatotoxicity* and *idiosyncracy* (see Table 1). Intrinsic hepatotoxins (eg, chloroform) have the inherent property of predictably injuring the liver. Idiosyncratic or unpredictable hepatotoxins (eg, halothane) cause hepatic damage only in a small number of uniquely susceptible individuals. The major differences between these two types of hepatotoxins are listed in Table 2.

Intrinsic. Intrinsic hepatotoxins can be subdivided into direct and indirect toxins. Direct intrinsic hepatotoxins (eg, carbon tetrachloride) destroy hepatocytes by a physiochemical attack. There are no known direct hepatotoxins that are used as therapeutic agents (9,17). Indirect hepatotoxins are the antimetabolites and related compounds which produce structural changes of the hepatocyte by competitive inhibition of essential metabolites or by interference with selective metabolic or secretory processes of the hepatocyte. These changes can be cytotoxic or cholestatic. Indirect intrinsic hepatotoxins that produce cytotoxic changes are tetracycline, mechlorethamine, alcohol, acetaminophen, and 5-mercaptopurine (9,11). Indirect intrinsic cholestatic hepatotoxins, such as several C-17 alkylated anabolic and contraceptive steroids (31,32), produce jaundice and hepatic dysfunction by specific interference with mechanisms for excretion of bile or uptake of its constituents from the blood.

Idiosyncracy. Hepatic injury due to host idiosyncracy can be caused by hypersensitivity reactions or by other mechanisms such as an aberrant metabolic pathway for the drug in the susceptible patient. Idiosyncratic hepatic injuries also may be cytotoxic, cholestatic, or mixed (9,11). The liver injury may be tentatively attributed to hypersensitivity when it develops after a "sensitization" period of one to five weeks, and is accompanied by systemic characteristics of rash, fever, and eosinophilia (8). These hallmarks of hypersensitivity suggest that the hepatic injury is due to drug allergy, especially when such findings are supported by a prompt recurrence of the syndrome in response to a challenge dose of the drug. Examples of drugs causing allergic hepatic dysfunctions are methyldopa, phenytoin, para-aminosalicyclic acid, chlorpromazine, erythromycin estolate, and halothane (8,12). Idiosyncratic hepatic injury also can be caused by toxic metabolites (33–35). The idiosyncratic or unpredictable hepatic injury which results from a metabolic aberration rather than hypersensitivity usually develops after variable latent periods of one week to 12 months or longer, and usually is not accompanied by fever, rash, eosinophilia, or by histological findings of eosinophilic or granulomatous inflammation in the liver. In addition, reproduction of the hepatic injury requires administration of the drug for a period of days or weeks, rather than for only one or two doses, presumably to allow for accumulation of toxic metabolites. For example, the idiosyncratic jaundice provoked by isoniazid and iproniazid is the result of the hepatotoxic metabolites of these agents (33,35).

The classification of the mechanism of hepatic injury by an individual drug into intrinsic predictable hepatotoxicity or unpredictable idiosyncracy can sometimes be impossible and in many

Table 1.

MECHANISMS OF DRUG-INDUCED HEPATOTOXICITY

Classification	Lesion	Incidence
I. Intrinsic Hepatotoxicity		
1. Direct hepatotoxins	Necrosis & Steatosis	High
2. Indirect hepatotoxins		
a. Cytotoxic	Steatosis or Necrosis	High
b. Cholestatic	Bile casts	High
II. Host Idiosyncracy		
1. Hypersensitivity	Cytotoxic or Cholestatic	Low
2. Metabolic abnormality	Cytotoxic or Cholestatic	Low

Table 2.

CHARACTERISTICS OF INTRINSIC VS
IDIOSYNCRATIC HEPATOTOXINS

Intrinsic	Idiosyncratic
1. A distinctive histologic pattern is observed for any given drug.	1. Variable histologic pattern of lesions.
2. Dose dependent hepatotoxicity.	2. Dose independent hepatotoxicity.
3. Elicited in all individuals.	3. Only a small fraction of exposed individuals affected.
4. Reproducible in experimental animals.	4. Cannot be reproduced in experimental animals.
5. Predictable appearance of lesions and usually a brief latent period following exposure.	5. Appearance of lesions bears no temporal relationship to the institution of drug therapy.
6. No extrahepatic manifestations of hypersensitivity.	6. Lesions often accompanied by extrahepatic manifestations of hypersensitivity (eg, fever, rash, and eosinophilia).

instances both major types of mechanisms may have a role.

1. Evaluation of Possible Drug-Induced Liver Disease. A 72-year-old woman with a 12-year history of non-insulin dependent diabetes is admitted with chief complaints of generalized weakness, loss of appetite, a mild rash over the chest and thighs, and increasing itchiness. The patient also noted dark urine, light-colored stools, and yellow pigmentation of the skin. Her past medical history includes diabetes controlled by diet until one month ago, and hypertension treated with hydrochlorothiazide (HCTZ) and methyldopa for the past four years. One month ago she was started on chlorpropamide 500 mg daily when her fasting blood glucose was found to be 390 mg/dl. There is no history of fever, abdominal pain, fatty food intolerance, alcoholism, exposure to hepatitis virus, or blood transfusion.

On admission, the patient appears weak and icteric. Other significant findings include a macular rash on the upper chest wall and a slightly tender but normal sized liver. Vital signs are all within normal limits. Laboratory findings show serum glutamic oxaloacetic transaminase (SGOT) 370 units/ml, serum glutamic pyruvic transaminase (SGPT) 740 units/ml, lactic dehydrogenase (LDH) 384 IU/ml, alkaline phosphatase 587 IU, bilirubin ratio of total:direct (T:D) 5.1 mg/dl:4.9mg/dl, and albumin 4.1 gm/dl. All other chemistry data are within normal limits. A complete blood count (CBC) and differential count are normal. Tests for antinuclear antibody (ANA) and hepatitis B antigen (HB-Ag) are both negative. Ultrasound shows a normal biliary tract system, with no obstruction in the bile ducts, gallbladder, or near the head of the pancreas.

The patient is placed on a 1200-calorie a day with no added salt diet and lente insulin 20 units daily. All other drugs are discontinued. Cholestyramine (Questran) 4 gm three times daily is started for itching. By the fifth day of hospitalization, her laboratory values are SGOT 85 units/ml, SGPT 214 units/ml, alkaline phosphatase 288 IU, and bilirubin T:D 2.5 mg/dl:1.7 mg/dl. Her blood glucose is gradually controlled with increasing doses of lente insulin. Her blood pressure increased

to 190/105 mm Hg and HCTZ 50 mg twice daily is re-started. Two days later, her blood pressure is 160/90 mm Hg. Her lente insulin dose has been increased to 35 units daily and a fasting blood glucose of 190 mg/dl is noted. What signs and symptoms are suggestive of hepatitis in this patient?

Weakness, anorexia, dark urine, light-colored stools, icterus, pruritus, hyperbilirubinemia, and elevated alkaline phosphatase levels suggest cholestatic jaundice. The slightly tender liver and the highly elevated SGOT and SGPT levels suggest hepatocellular damage. The clinical presentation of this patient is consistent with that of a mixed cholestatic-cytotoxic hepatic injury.

2. How can the potential etiology of drug-induced hepatitis be determined, and what was the most likely etiology in this patient?

Drug-induced hepatic injury should be suspected in every patient with jaundice. Negative history of fever, abdominal pain, and fatty food intolerance rules out gall bladder disease in this patient. She has no history of alcoholism, exposure to hepatitis virus, or blood transfusion. In addition, negative ultrasound studies rule out the possibility of extrahepatic obstructive jaundice. The presence of macular rash together with a rapid decline of serum transaminase, alkaline phosphatase, and bilirubin levels toward normal when all drugs are withdrawn supports the assessment of drug-induced hepatitis in this patient.

There are three possible causes for this patient's drug-induced hepatitis, namely, chlorpropamide, HCTZ and methyldopa. HCTZ is not a likely candidate since hypersensitive cholestatic jaundice is very rarely associated with thiazide diuretics, and this patient has taken the drug for four years. Methyldopa has been reported to cause acute hepatocellular injury, chronic active hepatitis, and, rarely, cholestatic jaundice. However, most cases of methyldopa-induced hepatic injury occur within the first three months of exposure (9). Thus, methyldopa is probably not the causative agent in this patient. Chlorpropamide, on the other hand, has been reported to cause a mixed cholestatic-cytotoxic injury. Onset of the injury is usually within two to six weeks of sulfonylurea therapy. The incidence of hepatotoxic effects due to chlorpropamide is about 0.5% (9,36). Rash, fever and eosinophilia are described in some patients prior to, or concomitant with, the appearance of jaundice (36,37), although fever and eosinophilia are absent in this patient. In view of this patient's recent history of chlorpropamide intake and the physical and laboratory findings, chlorpropamide seems to be the most probable cause. However, the possibility of methyldopa-induced hepatic injury cannot be ruled out without a liver biopsy and an undesireable rechallenge test with methyldopa.

To determine the etiology of drug-induced hepatic injury, a detailed drug history should be obtained for all patients with jaundice. Special attention should be paid to the duration of exposure to a specific drug and its relationship to the onset of symptoms. A history of taking nonprescription drugs such as laxatives and vitamins, birth control pills, and illicit drugs should be sought. Predisposing factors to drug-induced hepatitis, if any, should be noted. These factors vary with the agent involved and can include nutritional status, alcoholism, and pre-existent liver or kidney disease, previous history of exposure, gestation in females, sex, and age.

The presumptive diagnosis of drug-induced hepatic injury requires a history of exposure to a drug, awareness of the characteristic syndrome produced by various agents and a search for supportive evidence. If the liver injury is accompanied by fever, rash and eosinophilia, the likelihood of drug-induced disease increases. However, lack of these features does not exclude the possibility of drug-induced disease (9,11). Differentiation of drug-induced hepatocellular injury from viral hepatitis involves evaluation of the epidemiologic circumstances, serologic studies to exclude virus B hepatitis (eg, HB-Ag), and determination of whether a history of receiving blood transfusions or injection with a contaminated syringe exists. Distinction of drug-induced cholestatic jaundice from extrahepatic obstructive jaundice often requires radiographic or ultrasonic studies. If liver biopsy reveals cholestasis with an eosinophil-rich portal inflammation, drugs become a likely etiology.

3. Should this patient be given a challenge dose of chlorpropamide to confirm the etiology of her drug-induced hepatitis?

Confirmation of the etiology may be obtained by giving a rechallenge dose of the incriminated drug. Recurrence of hepatic dysfunction or hyperbilirubinemia after a test dose offers valuable support for the diagnosis. Failure to develop abnormalities, however, does not preclude drug-induced dysfunction because only 40 to 60% of patients show a recurrence of hepatic injury after a test dose (9). Furthermore, some drugs will produce the hepatic injury only after an extended period (1 to 12 weeks) of readministration. Testing for the effect of a challenge dose can be potentially dangerous if the drug is known to cause hepatocellular injury, whereas rechallenge is considered safe if the drug usually leads to cholestasis alone. Therefore, risk must be weighed against benefit before giving a challenge dose of an incriminated drug to a patient.

Rechallenge of this patient with chlorpropamide is potentially dangerous because of her clinical picture of hepatocellular injury. Since alternative agents (ie, insulin) can be used to manage her diabetes, giving a test dose of the offending drug is not warranted.

4. *Treatment.* How should drug-induced hepatic injuries be treated?

Once the diagnosis has been made, the presumed offending drug should be withdrawn. In this case, all medications taken prior to admission were discontinued. The management of drug-induced jaundice is similar to the treatment of other hepatic diseases. Treatment usually includes a diet high in carbohydrate, moderately high in protein, and adequate in calories, (eg, 2000–3000 calories/day). However, a lower caloric diet is prescribed for this patient because of her diabetes. Treatment of jaundice is mainly supportive. If itching is severe, the use of cholestyramine to enhance the rate of bile acid excretion may alleviate the symptoms. If possible, the use of chlorpropamide, and perhaps methyldopa, should be avoided in future therapy for this patient and appropriate alternative drugs be used instead.

If present, ascites, esophageal variceal bleeding, and other complications are treated accordingly. The use of large doses of glucocorticoids (eg, 1000 mg hydrocortisone daily) in acute hepatic failure is largely empirical and awaits evaluation in future studies (9,17).

Drugs Reported to Cause Clinically Significant Hepatic Dysfunction

There are many reports of drug-related hepatitis in the literature. Most of these are reports of single cases involving one drug. Many reports of adverse drug effects on the liver are difficult to evaluate because: a) biopsy studies are not reported or adequate descriptions and illustrations for proper morphologic classification are lacking; b) some patients received several potentially hepatotoxic drugs concurrently; c) certain patients had pre-existing hepatic diseases that were not drug related; and d) very few patients had been rechallenged with the drug. Furthermore, hepatic drug effects that occurred early after exposure may differ in character from those that occur later (eg, chlorpromazine). In addition, certain drugs may cause various types of morphologic responses via different mechanisms (ie, hepatotoxic vs idiosyncratic). In an attempt to summarize and facilitate discussion of the vast amount of information on this subject, only drugs that have been implicated in causing significant liver dysfunction are listed in Table 3. The hepatotoxicity of acetaminophen and antituberculous agents (eg,

isoniazid) are covered in Poisoning and Tuberculosis chapters, respectively, and will not be presented here. Oxyphenisatin, a laxative compound, has been reported to cause many cases of acute and chronic hepatic disease and has been banned from this country since the early 1970's. For more details on oxyphenisatin-induced hepatic injury, other references can be consulted (38–43).

A discussion of the types of morphologic findings and presumed mechanism of toxicity for each drug is included. References are listed so that more detailed information may be obtained if desired. In the section entitled "Clinical Remarks," prominent clinical features such as clinical presentation, dose and duration of therapy associated with the adverse effect, pertinent laboratory data, and prognosis are summarized.

Table 3.

DRUG-INDUCED HEPATOTOXICITY

Drug: a) Incidence, b) Morphology, and c) Mechanism	Clinical Remarks
Allopurinol a) rare b) submassive or massive necrosis cholestatic or granulomatous hepatitis c) hypersensitivity (30,44–48)	Onset of symptoms varies from 7 days to 6 weeks. Mild to moderate increases in alkaline phosphatase and SGOT have been reported in most cases. Several instances of generalized hypersensitivity and severe hepatitis have been described. Rarely, death may result from hepatic failure.
Androgenic steroids a) high incidence of hepatic dysfunction; low incidence of cholestatic jaundice b) cholestasis with minor or no portal inflammation; dilation of sinusoids; peliosis hepatis; adenoma and carcinoma? c) indirect intrinsic hepatotoxin (22,23,31,49–60)	Only anabolic steroids with an alkyl group in the C-17 position have been incriminated in causing hepatic dysfunction and jaundice. Testosterone and 19-nortestosterone and their esters do not exhibit adverse effects on the liver. Although a majority of recipients of therapeutic doses of the C-17 anabolic steroids promptly develop impairment of BSP excretion, only very few patients develop jaundice. Cholestatic jaundice usually develops in patients taking the drug for one or more months. The rate of development and the severity of hepatic dysfunction are dose-dependent. The larger the daily dose, the more likely is the development of jaundice. However, the development of jaundice among recipients of therapeutic doses apparently also depends on individual susceptibility. Furthermore, pre-existing liver disease enhances the hepatic dysfunction caused by the steroid. Jaundice may be preceded by nonspecific symptoms such as malaise, mild anorexia, and nausea. Pruritus may be present in about 10% of patients. Serum transaminase levels are usually less than 100 IU. Values for alkaline phosphatase are normal or modestly elevated in most patients. Serum bilirubin levels can be very high (> 30 mg/dl).

Table 3. (continued)

DRUG-INDUCED HEPATOTOXICITY

Drug: a) Incidence, b) Morphology, and c) Mechanism	Clinical Remarks
	The main effect of the anabolic steroid appears to be at the canalicular level, producing a selective interference with excretion of conjugated bilirubin. Prognosis is good for patients with steroid-induced jaundice or hepatic dysfunction. Recovery is prompt for anicteric patients with dysfunction but may take weeks to months for those with jaundice after the drug is stopped.
	Methyltestosterone has been implicated in rare instances of primary biliary cirrhosis. Rarely, anabolic steroids have led to peliosis hepatis. Peliosis hepatis is a vascular lesion that may rupture and lead to hemoperitoneum in some patients. Death has been reported in patients with necrosis associated with peliosis hepatis. Hepatic adenoma and carcinoma have also been ascribed to the taking of anabolic steroids, but the association remains to be confirmed by future studies.
Aspirin and other salicylates a) high b) focal hepatic necrosis c) intrinsic hepatotoxicity (61–70)	Can affect up to 50% of patients with high salicylate blood levels. Most patients who have developed hepatic injury have had levels >25 mg/dl, although a few instances have been noted at levels as low as 10 mg/dl. The injury is manifested by increased serum transaminases (10 to 40-fold) and is reversible upon withdrawal of the drug. Bilirubin levels are normal or moderately elevated. Patients with juvenile arthritis, systemic lupus erythematosis, and rheumatic fever seem to be more vulnerable.
Azathioprine a) rare b) cholestasis; minor hepato-cellular injury c) idiosyncracy (71–79)	Only a few isolated instances of jaundice have been attributed to azathioprine. While azathioprine has been used in the treatment of chronic active hepatitis, worsening of the hepatic disease may also occur.
Carmustine (BCNU) a) dose related b) necrosis c) intrinsic hepatotoxin (80–84)	Nitrosoureas apparently act as alkylating agents and have been found to produce hepatic injury in experimental animals and in up to 25% of patients taking therapeutic doses of BCNU. The hepatic injury produced by BCNU has ranged from reversible jaundice and abnormal levels of SGOT to severe hepatic necrosis.
Chlorpromazine (CPZ) a) 0.5 to 1% b) cholestasis; scattered focal areas of necrosis c) hypersensitivity (4,85–97)	The effect of age, sex, race, or other factors on vulnerability to CPZ jaundice has not been established. In approximately 80% of the cases, icterus develops between one to four weeks of CPZ treatment. In rare instances, jaundice has developed after the first dose. Prodromal symptoms consist of fever, itching, abdominal pain, anorexia and nausea. Skin rash is only observed in about 5% of reported cases. CPZ jaundice often resembles extra-hepatic obstructive jaundice. Severe pruritus is common and may be the first evidence of hepatic injury in some patients. Serum alkaline phosphatase and cholesterol levels are often markedly

Table 3. (continued)

DRUG-INDUCED HEPATOTOXICITY

Drug: a) Incidence, b) Morphology, and c) Mechanism	**Clinical Remarks**
	elevated. Serum transaminase levels are increased slightly to moderately in almost all patients. Eosinophilia has been noted in 60 to 80% of cases reported. The outlook for CPZ jaundice is good. Cholestatic jaundice associated with CPZ often resolves within 8 weeks but occasionally may last up to one year or longer. Some of the patients with prolonged cholestasis have developed a syndrome resembling that of primary biliary cirrhosis. The clinical syndrome is characterized by itching, xanthoma, hepatomegaly, and splenomegaly. Although it has been suggested that this syndrome is frequently benign and reversible, two cases of irreversible cirrhosis and fatality due to CPZ have been described.
	Other phenothiazines have also been reported to cause cholestatic jaundice, but no reliable estimate of the incidence is available. Since there is a potential for cross-sensitivity between chlorpromazine and other phenothiazines, it is best to avoid using any agent in this class for patients who have had CPZ jaundice.
Chlorpropamide a) 0.5% b) mixed cholestatic-cytotoxic injury c) hypersensitivity hepatotoxicity? (29,36,37,98–104)	Host factors that modify the susceptibility to hepatic injury are unknown. Onset of jaundice is usually between 2 to 6 weeks of chlorpropamide therapy. The initial symptoms are anorexia, nausea and vomiting. Soon thereafter dark urine, jaundice, and clay-colored stools appear. Pruritus and hepatomegaly are common. Fever, rash, and eosinophilia occur frequently but not in all cases. Because of an apparent dose-dependent relationship it has been suggested that direct hepatotoxicity of chlorpropamide may be responsible for some cases of jaundice. Values for serum liver enzymes and bilirubin are consistent with the picture of cholestatic jaundice with a minor component of hepatocellular damage. Complete recovery generally occurs within one to three months after chlorpropamide is stopped. Patients who have recovered from chlorpropamide jaundice apparently do not relapse when given tolbutamide. Other sulfonylureas in clinical use (ie, acetohexamide, tolbutamide, and tolazamide) have also been reported to cause jaundice, but the incidence appears to be very low.
Contraceptive steroids a) dose related b) A. cholestasis (32,105–118) B. adenoma, peliosis hepatis (23,119–127) C. Budd-Chiari syndrome (26,27) D. Carcinoma? (25,128,129)	A. Estrogens have been found to selectively interfere with BSP and bilirubin excretion by the liver. The importance of structural specificity of the estrogen molecule in causing hepatic dysfunction has been established. The phenolic character of ring A and the addition of an alkyl group at the C-17 position of the estrogen molecule seem to be responsible for the injury. Progesterone has little or no demonstrable adverse effect on hepatic function by itself but may enhance the hepatic injury produced by the estrogens if given together. The incidence of jaundice appears to be very low and is estimated to be 1 per 10,000 recipients in most countries and 1 per 4000 recipients in Sweden. Hepatic dysfunction occurs much more frequently and may be as high as 40 to 50% of patients taking these

Table 3. (continued)

DRUG-INDUCED HEPATOTOXICITY

Drug: a) Incidence, b) Morphology, and c) Mechanism	**Clinical Remarks**
c) indirect hepatotoxin; genetic predisposition?	agents. Postmenopausal women appear to be more susceptible to hepatic dysfunction induced by estrogen than younger women. Certain ethnic groups (Swedes, Chileans) seem to be more prone to develop anicteric dysfunction than others. Up to 50% of patients who develop jaundice while taking contraceptive steroids have a previous history of jaundice or itching during pregnancy. Onset of the jaundice is usually during the first six months of therapy and often in the first cycle. Jaundice is preceded by nonspecific symptoms including malaise, anorexia, nausea, and pruritus. Splenomegaly is not seen, and hepatomegaly is infrequent. Bilirubin levels are moderately elevated in most cases ($\geq$10 mg/dl) but values higher than 20 mg/dl have been described. Other biochemical features resemble the jaundice produced by the C-17 alkylated anabolic steroids. Prognosis of the cholestatic jaundice is good. In most individuals the clinical syndrome resolves completely within one month. B. Hepatic adenoma was a very rare tumor before the widespread use of contraceptive steroids. Since then, the increase in incidence of adenoma seems to have paralleled the increased use of oral contraceptives. Women taking the contraceptive steroids for periods greater than five years appear to be at higher risk of developing an adenoma than those who have taken the preparation for less than three years. One-third to one-half of patients found to have adenoma remains asymptomatic. Approximately one-third may present with a painful, tender mass. The remaining one-fourth to one-third of reported patients often presents with a sudden life-threatening intra-abdominal hemorrhage secondary to rupture of the adenoma. Prognosis is good if resection of the adenoma can be accomplished prior to rupture. For patients with hemoperitoneum, the outlook is fair if the diagnosis is made promptly and the tumor resected. Otherwise, death may result from hemorrhagic shock, coagulation abnormalities, and related complications. Peliosis hepatis is a rare complication from contraceptive steroids and often occurs along with the adenoma. C. Budd-Chiari syndrome is characterized by acute or subacute development of abdominal pain, hepatomegaly, portal hypertension, ascites, edema, and moderate jaundice. This syndrome is caused by thrombosis and subsequent occlusion of the hepatic veins. Although this complication is very rare, an extremely high mortality rate clearly makes it an important consideration in the use of estrogens. D. A few cases of hepatic carcinoma have recently been ascribed to the use of contraceptive steroids, but the cause-effect relationship awaits confirmation.

Table 3. (continued)

DRUG-INDUCED HEPATOTOXICITY

Drug: a) Incidence, b) Morphology, and c) Mechanism	Clinical Remarks
Dantrolene a) Hypertransaminasemia 　– without jaundice – 1.2% 　– overt hepatic injury – 0.4% b) chronic active hepatitis-like; submassive and massive necrosis c) idiosyncracy; 　toxic metabolites 　(130–133)	The incidence and severity of the hepatic injury appear to be related to the duration of therapy and to the age of the patient. Clinical onset of hepatic injury has been delayed for at least 45 days after starting the drug in almost all cases. In a study of 1044 patients, all fatalities have occurred in patients over 30 years of age and after at least 2 months of therapy. Females have a higher fatality rate than males, although there appears to be no significant difference in the incidence of hepatic injury between sexes. The development and the severity of hepatic injury seem to be dose-related. Doses above 300 mg/day are more likely to produce hepatic injury than smaller doses, and doses of 200 mg/day or less rarely lead to liver damage.
Erythromycin estolate a) 2 % b) cholestasis; mixed cholestatic-cytotoxic injury c) hypersensitivity 　(134–145)	With the exception of two cases of hepatotoxicity (326,327) associated with erythromycin ethylsuccinate, the estolate salt is the only form of erythromycin reported to cause hepatic injury. Onset of symptoms is usually between the tenth and twentieth day of exposure. Abdominal pain occurs in approximately 75% of the cases. Icterus may precede or accompany GI complaints such as anorexia, nausea, and vomiting. Fever is mild and rash is often absent. Eosinophilia occurs frequently. Serum bilirubin values are generally below 5 mg/dl. SGOT and alkaline phosphatase levels are consistent with the picture of cholestatic jaundice. Response to a challenge dose in patients who have had a previous reaction to estolate is usually prompt. The hepatic injury is reversible and jaundice often subsides within two to five weeks after the drug is stopped.
Fluphenazine a) rare b) cholestasis c) hypersensitivity 　(146)	See chlorpromazine
Glucocorticoids a) dose related b) steatosis c) hepatotoxicity 　(147–149)	Hepatic steatosis secondary to glucocorticoids is usually of little clinical consequence. However, occasionally this may lead to fat embolism in the vascular bed of major organs (eg, lung) resulting in tissue damage and fatality.
Haloperidol a) low	The incidence has been estimated to be between 0.2 to 3% of recipients. Most reported cases of jaundice appear to be cholestatic.

Table 3. (continued)

DRUG-INDUCED HEPATOTOXICITY

Drug: a) Incidence, b) Morphology, and c) Mechanism	**Clinical Remarks**
b) cholestasis	
c) hypersensitivity (150–151)	

Halothane

a) infrequent

b) centrizonal necrosis; steatosis; massive necrosis

c) hypersensitivity; metabolic idiosyncracy? (152–167)

The incidence and severity appear to be greater in females and enhanced by obesity. Susceptibility is particularly enhanced by previous exposure to halothane, especially if the interval between the exposures is less than 3 months. Irradiation may also increase susceptibility to halothane hepatitis. Jaundice is rare in children and young adults under 30 years of age. The clinical syndrome of halothane-induced liver disease often consists of a history of unexplained delayed fever postoperatively (>3 days) after halothane anesthesia. There is usually a latent period of 5 to 14 days between the anesthetic episode and the appearance of hepatic injury, but it may appear as early as one day after the operation in patients who have had multiple prior exposures to halothane. Fever with or without chills, aching, anorexia, nausea, and abdominal distress precede jaundice in 75% of the patients. Once jaundice has appeared, other manifestations of serious hepatocellular damage often develop rapidly. Coagulation abnormalities, ascites, renal insufficiency, gastrointestinal bleeding, and encephalopathy may follow. Values for serum transaminases are markedly elevated ($\geq$3000 IU) whereas alkaline phosphatase is only modestly increased. Eosinophilia has been observed in 20 to 50% of reported cases. Rash is uncommon. The mortality rate for halothane hepatitis ranges from 14 to 67%. An average fatality rate of 40% was reported in a review of 404 cases.

6-mercaptopurine (6-MP)

a) dose related

b) cholestasis with fatty hepatic necrosis

c) indirect intrinsic hepatotoxin (168–173)

Liver injury with jaundice has been reported in 6 to 40% of leukemic patients treated with 6-MP. Adults appear to be more susceptible to the hepatic injury than children. Onset of overt hepatic injury is usually within one to two months of receiving the drug. Jaundice commonly appears as the first sign, followed by pruritus. Blood transaminase values are generally below 250 IU. Alkaline phosphatase values are moderately to markedly elevated. Doses in excess of 2.5 mg/kg are more likely to cause hepatic injury. Prognosis depends on the degree of cytotoxic injury.

Methimazole

a) rare

b) cholestasis

c) hypersensitivity (174–177)

Onset of the syndrome is usually during the first four weeks of therapy but may be as late as three months. Rash, fever, lymphadenopathy, and agranulocytosis may occur in various combinations. The cholestatic jaundice associated with methimazole is reversible. Death appears to have been the result of concomitant agranulocytosis and bone marrow depression rather than the hepatic injury.

Table 3. (continued)

DRUG-INDUCED HEPATOTOXICITY

Drug: a) Incidence, b) Morphology, and c) Mechanism	**Clinical Remarks**
Methoxyflurane a) rare b) similar findings as in halothane hepatitis c) hypersensitivity; metabolic aberration? (178–181)	The clinical syndrome and hepatic lesions from methoxyflurane are very similar to those observed in halothane hepatitis. Halothane and methoxyflurane appear to cross react in patients with a history of halothane hepatitis.
Methotrexate (MTX) a) dose related b) steatosis; necrosis; fibrosis; cirrhosis c) indirect intrinsic hepatotoxin (21,182–195)	MTX frequently produces biochemical evidence of hepatic injury, and occasionally gives rise to overt clinical signs of liver disease. Fatty liver, fibrosis, or cirrhosis has been reported in over 100 cases of psoriatic patients treated with MTX. Treatment of leukemia, choriocarcinoma, rheumatoid arthritis, and other diseases with MTX has also led to hepatic injury. It has been suggested that the likelihood of hepatic injury is directly related to the duration of therapy and inversely related to the length of the interval between doses. Other risk factors may include alcoholism and perhaps severity of psoriasis. Biochemical changes provide insensitive reflections of MTX-induced hepatic injury. Mildly elevated SGOT and SGPT and slightly abnormal values for BSP excretion are usually observed for one to two days after a dose of MTX. However, cirrhosis may develop insidiously without marked elevation of liver enzyme levels. Prognosis depends on the severity of the hepatic injury at the time of its diagnosis. Some patients may have developed cirrhosis and the associated complications by the time MTX-induced injury is recognized. Some of these patients may progress to hepatic failure and death. Early recognition of this syndrome can decrease irreversible hepatic damage and improve long-term survival. Preventive measures include giving large intermittent rather than small daily doses of MTX, monitoring serum enzyme values and BSP excretion test regularly (on a monthly basis), and performing liver biopsy at regular intervals (6 to 12 months).
Methyldopa a) low b) cytotoxic injury; subacute or bridging necrosis; rare cholestasis; chronic active hepatitis c) hypersensitivity; toxic metabolite? (16,18,33,196–206)	Incidence of methyldopa-induced hepatic injury is difficult to estimate. Elevated serum transaminase levels and impaired hepatic function have been reported in an incidence as low as 1% and as high as 27%. In some patients the serum enzyme levels have returned to normal despite continued therapy with methyldopa. Cholestasis is a very rare presentation of methyldopa-induced hepatic disease and is reversible upon cessation of the drug. The incidence of severe cytotoxic injury is estimated to be less than 0.1% of recipients. Patients reported to have methyldopa hepatitis are often older than 35 years of age and predominantly female. Acute hepatic injury has appeared within four weeks of therapy in 50% of the patients reported and within four to twelve weeks in 25% of the

Table 3. (continued)

DRUG-INDUCED HEPATOTOXICITY

Drug: a) Incidence, b) Morphology, and c) Mechanism	**Clinical Remarks**
	cases. Others may have a latent period for up to one year. The syndrome of methyldopa-induced hepatic injury resembles acute viral hepatitis. There has usually been a prodromal period of fever, chills, malaise, anorexia, nausea, vomiting, occasional right upper quadrant tenderness, and pruritus. Jaundice, dark urine, and hepatomegaly usually follow in severe cases. Rash, lymphadenopathy, and arthralgia have been rare. Biochemical features resemble those of cytotoxic injury. Eosinophilia has been rare among patients with acute hepatic injury. The fatality rate from acute hepatic injury is estimated to be 10%. For those patients who survive, withdrawal of the drug results in rapid recovery in most cases.
	Chronic active hepatitis induced by methyldopa resembles "autoimmune" type CAH. Biopsy of the liver has revealed confluent areas of lobular collapse, intense inflammatory response in the portal and periportal areas, and, in some cases, evidence of cirrhosis. Positive Coombs test, LE factor, antinuclear and anti-smooth muscle antibodies may be observed. Clinical presentation may be a mixture of acute and chronic hepatitis. In some patients, hepatosplenomegaly and spider angiomas may develop when the syndrome is first recognized.
	To prevent irreversible liver injury or death, it is advisable to monitor liver enzyme tests regularly during the first three months of therapy, particularly in females. Periodic checks for the first three years may also be indicated.
Mithramycin a) dose related b) necrosis c) intrinsic hepatotoxin (207–210)	Biochemical evidence of hepatic injury has been found in 25 to 100% of recipients of "full" oncotherapeutic doses. Values for SGOT and SGPT may be as high as 1000 IU. Hepatocellular jaundice may occur. Hepatotoxicity appears to be lower in the doses used to treat Paget's disease and hypercalcemia. An alternate-day regimen used to treat carcinomatosis also seems to have an acceptable level of hepatotoxicity.
Monoamine oxidase inhibitors (iproniazid, isocarboxazid, phenelzine) a) low b) hepatocellular damage c) metabolic idiosyncracy (211–216)	Iproniazid, the first antidepressant to produce hepatic injury, was withdrawn from the market because of many reported cases of fulminant hepatic failure. Severe hepatitis has been encountered in patients given phenelzine for periods of 18 days to five months. The clinical features and the histologic findings in the liver are indistinguishable from those of severe viral hepatitis. The reported mortality rate is about 15%. Tranylcypromine, a non-hydrazine MAO inhibitor, rarely causes jaundice.

Table 3. (continued)

DRUG-INDUCED HEPATOTOXICITY

Drug: a) Incidence, b) Morphology, and c) Mechanism	**Clinical Remarks**
Nitrofurantoin a) rare b) cholestasis; mixed cholestatic-cytotoxic injury; chronic active hepatitis c) hypersensitivity (19,20,217–223)	The onset of the symptoms of hepatic injury is usually abrupt with fever and eosinophilia in over half of the patients. Approximately two-thirds of the patients have had previous exposure to nitrofurantoin. The latent period prior to the development of symptoms ranges from two days to five months. Jaundice has been recognized in almost all cases reported. The prognosis of acute jaundice induced by nitrofurantoin is good. Biochemical abnormalities and jaundice are generally reversible when the drug is stopped. Chronic active hepatitis of the "lupoid" type is rare and may be accompanied by pulmonary lesions.
Oxacillin a) low b) anicteric hepatic dysfunction; rare cases of cholestatic jaundice reported c) hypersensitivity? idiosyncracy? (224–231)	Oxacillin has been associated with rare cholestatic jaundice and numerous cases of anicteric hepatic dysfunction. Liver transaminase levels can be as high as 1000 IU in some cases. Alkaline phosphatase levels are only modestly elevated and serum bilirubin remains normal in most patients. Eosinophilia accompanies only about 25% of the cases. Upon cessation of oxacillin, liver enzyme values generally return to normal within two weeks. Apparently there is no cross hepatotoxicity between oxacillin and other penicillins. Nafcillin or penicillin G can often be substituted without recurrence of liver injury.
Penicillin a) very rare b) necrosis; granuloma; "lupoid" hepatitis c) hypersensitivity (232–243)	Only several cases of hepatic dysfunction have been associated with penicillin G. Almost all cases reported were associated with systemic hypersensitivity reactions such as urticaria, rash, anaphylactic shock, systemic granulomatous response, serum sickness, or exfoliative dermatitis. Carbenicillin, ampicillin, and amoxicillin have also been reported to lead to elevated transaminase levels.
Phenindione a) <0.5% b) mixed cholestatic-cytotoxic c) hypersensitivity (244–251)	Overt hepatic injury induced by phenindione is always associated with generalized allergic reactions. The onset is usually during the third or fourth week of drug administration. The hepatic injury appears to be of the mixed cytotoxic and cholestatic type. Values for serum transaminases are usually below 500 IU. Alkaline phosphatase levels have been moderately to markedly elevated. As a rule, hepatitis subsides following withdrawal of phenindione. The case fatality rate of patients with phenindione jaundice is reported to be 10% and is probably the result of severe generalized hypersensitivity rather than that of hepatic failure.
Phenylbutazone a) 0.25% b) local or diffuse parenchymal necrosis with or without cholestasis	Onset of illness often occurs within four to six weeks of therapy but occasionally can occur after 12 months of therapy. Hypersensitivity has been postulated to be responsible for the hepatic injury produced by phenylbutazone due to the accompanying sys-

Table 3. (continued)

DRUG-INDUCED HEPATOTOXICITY

Drug: a) Incidence, b) Morphology, and c) Mechanism	Clinical Remarks
c) hypersensitivity; intrinsic toxicity? (28,252–256)	temic manifestations. However, allergic symptoms are found in only 50% of the cases reported in the literature. Since an apparent relationship between dose and toxicity was observed more frequently in the early years of administering high doses of phenylbutazone, it has been suggested that intrinsic toxicity of the drug may also play a role. The clinical characteristics include fever, rash, arthralgia, nausea, vomiting, and abdominal pain which may precede or accompany the jaundice. Approximately two-thirds of reported cases have had cytotoxic injury with or without cholestasis and steatosis. In about 30% of patients, cholestasis with little or no parenchymal injury has been observed. Granuloma may also be found in a few cases. A fatality rate of 12% has been reported in patients with hepatic necrosis. Patients with cholestasis and granulomatous lesion generally recover, although the lesion may take up to four months to resolve.
Phenytoin (DPH) a) low; <1% b) cytotoxic injury with varying degrees of cholestasis; necrosis c) hypersensitivity (257–268)	Children seem to be less vulnerable to hepatic injury from phenytoin. Almost 80% of reported cases involve adults over 20 years of age. Symptoms generally occur after one to five weeks of therapy. Fever, rash, lymphadenopathy, and eosinophilia appear in almost all patients. Jaundice then follows. Leukocytosis with lymphocytosis and atypical lymphocytes is common. The syndrome resembles that of serum sickness. Biochemical features are similar to those of severe viral hepatitis. Values for SGOT and SGPT are very high (range 200–2000 IU). Serum alkaline phosphatase level is modestly elevated. The prognosis of this syndrome is grave; case fatality rate is estimated to be 40%. Presumably, this high mortality rate is due partly to accompanying severe hypersensitivity reactions (eg, exfoliative dermatitis) and partly to resulting hepatic failure.
Prochlorperazine a) rare b) cholestasis c) hypersensitivity (269–271)	See chlorpromazine
Propylthiouracil (PTU) a) rare b) hepatocellular injury; chronic active hepatitis; cholestasis c) hypersensitivity (272–277)	Signs and symptoms of hepatocellular damage usually appear within two to four weeks after initiation of the drug. Two cases of chronic active hepatitis and one case of cholestatic jaundice secondary to PTU have been described. Fatal cases of PTU-induced jaundice have been due to hepatic necrosis or to accompanying agranulocytosis.

Table 3. (continued)

DRUG-INDUCED HEPATOTOXICITY

Drug: a) Incidence, b) Morphology, and c) Mechanism	**Clinical Remarks**
Quinidine a) rare b) mixed hepatocellular injury; granulomata c) hypersensitivity (278–283)	Mild hepatic injury induced by quinidine most commonly occurs within 6 to 12 days of initiation of treatment. Quinidine-induced hepatitis is usually heralded by fever in association with elevated SGOT, SGPT, LDH and alkaline phosphatase levels. Jaundice has not been reported. Discontinuation of the drug usually results in rapid resolution of fever and laboratory abnormalities. Upon re-challenge with a single dose of quinidine, most patients have promptly developed fever and elevations of serum transaminases, supporting hypersensitivity as a mechanism.
Sulfonamides a) 0.5–1% b) mainly cytotoxic injury; mixed-hepatocellular injury; subacute hepatic necrosis with cirrhosis; chronic active hepatitis c) hypersensitivity; mild hepatotoxicity (284–291)	Clinical presentation of hepatic injury often occurs within 5 to 14 days, but occasionally presents as late as several months. About 25% of the patients with hepatic dysfunction have had prior exposures to sulfonamides. The reaction is characterized by fever, rash, and signs of visceral and bone marrow injury. The clinical and morphologic features of such reactions resemble those of serum sickness. Acute hepatitis occurs in about 0.6% of patients undergoing sulfanilamide therapy and less frequently in individuals who receive other sulfonamide derivatives. Usually, the onset of symptoms is sudden, with fever, anorexia, nausea, vomiting, and sometimes rash. Jaundice appears on the third to sixth day after the onset of fever, but may be delayed for as long as two weeks. Dark urine and acholic stools are frequent, and hepatomegaly may be noted. Prognosis depends on the extent of cytotoxic injury. Case fatality rate is reportedly above 10%. Patients who survive generally recover slowly over a period of several weeks to months.
Tetracyclines a) low b) microvesicular fat droplets in hepatocytes; massive steatosis c) intrinsic hepatotoxicity (10,292–302)	Chlortetracycline, oxytetracycline, and tetracycline have been reported to produce hepatic steatosis. The development of clinically significant fatty liver appears to depend on the presence of high blood levels of the drug. Large doses (>1.5 gm/day) of tetracycline, especially when given intravenously to pregnant women or individuals with renal disease, may give rise to severe hepatic injury. Clinical manifestations usually appear 4–10 days after initiation of tetracycline therapy. Early symptoms include nausea, vomiting, and abdominal pain. Mild jaundice then follows. Hemorrhagic complications, azotemia, syncope, hypotension, shock, and coma may develop subsequently. The mortality rate from this syndrome is approximately 80%. This serious untoward reaction can be avoided by using safer alternative antibiotics whenever possible or by keeping the intravenous dose of tetracycline below 1 gm/day.
Thioridazine a) low b) cholestasis	See chlorpromazine

Table 3. (continued)

DRUG-INDUCED HEPATOTOXICITY

Drug: a) Incidence, b) Morphology, and c) Mechanism	Clinical Remarks
c) hypersensitivity (303,304)	
Tricyclic antidepressants (amitriptyline, imipramine, desipramine) a) rare to infrequent b) cholestasis; hepatic necrosis c) hypersensitivity plus slight toxicity (305–311)	Most of the reported cases have been cholestatic. Jaundice usually appears between the seventh and 110th day of treatment. Biochemical and histologic features are usually those of mild cholestasis. Severe hepatic necrosis and death have been reported rarely.
Trifluoperazine a) rare b) cholestasis c) hypersensitivity (312,313)	See chlorpromazine
Valproic acid a) unknown b) steatosis; focal or massive necrosis c) intrinsic hepatotoxicity? (314–320)	Hepatotoxicity produced by valproic acid has only been recognized recently. Liver injury has been described as elevation of serum transaminases, hypofibrinogenemia, and a Reye's-like syndrome. Over fourteen cases of fatal hepatic necrosis have thus far been associated with valproic acid. Therefore, it is essential to monitor serum enzyme levels regularly when a patient is placed on the drug.
Vitamin A a) dose related b) fatty liver; nonspecific hepatocellular degeneration; fibrosis; cirrhosis c) intrinsic hepatotoxin (321–325)	Chronic vitamin A intoxication results from intake of large amounts (>40,000 IU daily) of the vitamin for months to years. Systemic manifestations of the syndrome include anorexia, weight loss, fatigability, mild fever, pallor, and night sweats. Pruritus, dry skin, hair loss, as well as pain and tenderness of bone are characteristics. Hepatomegaly and splenomegaly have been reported in about half of the cases. Jaundice is rare. Ascites, portal hypertension, and other clinical signs of cirrhosis have been observed in a few reported cases. Laboratory studies may reveal anemia, leukopenia, increased sedimentation rate, and proteinuria. Hepatic injury may be evidenced by impaired BSP excretion, elevated levels of alkaline phosphatase and SGOT, hypoalbuminemia, and hypoprothrombinemia. The prognosis of patients with impaired hepatic function and hepatomegaly is usually good if the vitamin A intake is discontinued. However, once ascites and portal hypertension are present, the syndrome may persist even after cessation of the vitamin. Current restrictions in the vitamin A content of nonprescription preparations may limit the likelihood of overdose.

References

1. Bjorneboe M et al: Infective hepatitis and toxic jaundice in a municipal hospital during a five-year period. Acta Med Scand. 1967; 182:491.

2. Koff RS et al: Profile of hyperbilirubinemia in three hospital populations. Clin Res. 1970; 18:680.

3. Eastwood HOH: Causes of jaundice in the elderly: a survey of diagnosis and investigation. Geront Clin. 1971; 13:69.

4. Graham GS: Chlorpromazine jaundice in a general hospital. Br Med J. 1957; 2:1080.

5. Shimano K: Drug-induced hepatic injury with special reference to antitubercular agents. Acta Hepatol Japan. 1965; 6 suppl:74.

6. Ritt DJ et al: Acute hepatic necrosis with stupor or coma: An analysis of thirty-one patients. Med. 1969; 48:151.

7. Caravati CM et al: Acute massive hepatic necrosis with fatal hepatic failure. Am J Dig Dis. 1971; 16:803.

8. Zimmerman HJ: Drug-induced liver disease. Drugs. 1978; 16:25.

9. Zimmerman HJ: *Hepatotoxicity: Adverse Effects of Drugs and Other Chemicals on the Liver.* Appleton-Century Crofts, New York, 1978.

10. Peters RL et al: Tetracycline-induced fatty liver in nonpregnant patients. Am J Surg. 1967; 113:622.

11. Klatskin G: Toxic and drug-induced hepatitis. In *Diseases of the Liver,* 4th ed, edited by L Schiff, JB Lippincott, Philadelphia, 1975, p 604.

12. Zimmerman HJ: Liver disease caused by medicinal agents. Med Clin North Am. 1975; 59:897.

13. Simpson DG et al: Hypersensitivity to para-aminosalicylic acid. Am J Med. 1960; 29:297.

14. Zimmerman HJ: Drug-induced chronic hepatic disease. Med Clin North Am. 1979; 63:567.

15. Maddrey WC et al: Drug-induced chronic hepatitis and cirrhosis. Prog Liver Dis. 1979; 6:595.

16. Maddrey WC et al: Drug-induced chronic liver disease. Gastroenterology. 1977; 72:1348.

17. Maddrey WC: Drug-related acute and chronic hepatitis. Clin Gastroenterol. 1980; 9:213.

18. Rodman JS et al: Methyldopa hepatitis. A report of six cases and review of the literature. Am J Med. 1976; 60:941.

19. Black M et al: Nitrofurantoin-induced chronic active hepatitis. Ann Intern Med. 1980; 92:62.

20. Sharp JR et al: Chronic active hepatitis and severe hepatic necrosis associated with nitrofurantoin. Ann Intern Med. 1980; 92:14.

21. Dahl MGC et al: Methotrexate hepatotoxicity in psoriasis—comparison of different dose regimens. Br Med J. 1972; 1:654.

22. Johnson LF et al: Association of androgenic-anabolic steroid therapy with development of hepatocellular carcinoma. Lancet. 1972; 2:1273.

23. Bagheri SA et al: Peliosis hepatis associated with androgenic-anabolic steroid therapy: A severe form of hepatic injury. Ann Intern Med. 1974; 81:610.

24. Baker AL et al: Liver adenoma associated with oral contraceptive pill administration. Digestive Dis. 1978; 23:53s.

25. Ham JM et al: Hepatocellular carcinoma possibly induced by oral contraceptives. Digestive Dis. 1978; 23:38s.

26. Sterup K et al: Budd-Chiari syndrome after taking oral contraceptives. Br Med J. 1967; 4:660.

27. Hoyumpa AM Jr et al: Budd-Chiari syndrome in women taking oral contraceptives. Am J Med. 1971; 50:137.

28. Ishak KG et al: Granulomas and cholestatic hepatocellular injury associated with phenylbutazone. Report of two cases. Am J Dig Dis. 1977; 22:611.

29. Rigberg LA et al: Chlorpropamide-induced granulomas. JAMA. 1976; 235:409.

30. Simmons F et al: Granulomatous hepatitis in a patient receiving allopurinol. Gastroenterology. 1972; 62:101.

31. Kory RC et al: Six-month evaluation of anabolic drug, norethandrolone in underweight persons. II. Bromsulfalein (BSP) retention and liver function. Am J Med. 1959; 26:243.

32. Kottra LL et al: Estrogen pharmacology. III. Effect of estradiol on plasma disappearance rate of sulfobromophthalein in man. Arch Intern Med. 1966; 117:373.

33. Mitchell JR et al: Metabolic activation of drugs to toxic substances. Gastroenterology. 1975; 68:392.

34. Mitchell JR et al: Metabolic activation: Biochemical basis for many drug-induced liver injuries. Prog Liver Dis. 1976; 5:259.

35. Dybing E: Activation of α-methyldopa, paracetamol and furosemide by human liver microsomes. Acta Pharmacol Et Toxicol. 1977; 41:89.

36. Reichel J et al: Intrahepatic cholestasis following administration of chlorpropamide. Am J Med. 1960; 28:654.

37. Hamff LH et al: The effect of tolbutamide and chlorpropamide on patients exhibiting jaundice as a result of previous chlorpropamide therapy. Ann NY Acad Sci. 1959; 74:820.

38. Reynolds TB: Recurring jaundice associated with ingestion of a laxative "Dialose Plus." Gastroenterology. 1969; 56:418.

39. McHardy G et al: Jaundice and oxyphenisatin. JAMA. 1970; 211:83.

40. Reynolds TB et al: Chronic active and lupoid hepatitis caused by a laxative, oxyphenisatin. N Engl J Med. 1971; 285:813.

41. Fischer MG et al: Recurrent jaundice induced by oxyphenisatin. Am J Gastroenterology. 1972; 58:58.

42. Gjone R et al: Liver disease associated with a "non-constipatory" iron preparation. Lancet. 1973; 1:421.

43. Dietrichson O et al: The incidence of oxyphenisatin-induced liver damage in chronic non-alcoholic liver disease. A controlled investigation. Scand J Gastroenterology. 1974; 9:473.

44. Kantor G: Toxic epidermal necrolysis, azotemia and death after allopurinol therapy. JAMA. 1970; 212:478.

45. Young J et al: Severe allopurinol hypersensitivity. Arch Intern Med. 1974; 134:553.

46. Esperitu CR et al: Allopurinol-induced granulomatous hepatitis. Am J Dig Dis. 1976; 21:804.

47. Boyer TD et al: Allopurinol hypersensitivity and liver damage. Western J Med. 1977; 126:143.

48. Butler RC et al: Acute massive hepatic necrosis in a patient receiving allopurinol. JAMA. 1977; 237:473.

49. Foss GL et al: Oral methyltestosterone and jaundice. Br Med J. 1959; 1:259.

50. Schaffner F et al: Cholestasis produced by the administration of norethandrolone. Am J Med. 1959; 26:249.

51. Schaffner F et al: Changes in bile canaliculi produced by norethandrolone: Electron microscopic study of human and rat liver. J Lab Clin Med. 1960; 56:623.

52. Marquardt GH et al: Effect of anabolic steroids on liver function tests and creatine excretion. JAMA. 1961; 175:851.

53. Wilder EM: Death due to liver failure following the use of methandrostenolone. Can Med Assoc J. 1962; 87:768.

54. Gilbert EF et al: Intrahepatic cholestasis with fatal termination following norethandrolone therapy. JAMA. 1963; 185:538.

55. deLorimier AA et al: Methyltestosterone, related steroids, and liver function. Arch Intern Med. 1965; 116:289.

56. Ticktin HE et al: Effects of a synthetic anabolic agent on hepatic function. Am J Med Sci. 1966; 251:674.

57. Glober GA et al: Biliary cirrhosis following the administration of methyltestosterone. JAMA. 1968; 204:170.

58. Editorial: Liver tumors and steroid hormones. Lancet. 1973; 2:1481.

59. Gordon GG et al: Effect of chronic alcohol use on hepatic testosterone 5α-A-Ring reductase in the baboon and the human being. Gastroenterology. 1979; 77:110.

60. Nadell J et al: Peliosis hepatis. Twelve cases associated with oral androgen therapy. Arch Pathol Lab Med. 1977; 101:405.

61. Russell AS et al: Serum transaminase during salicylate therapy. Br Med J. 1971; 2:428.

62. Athreya BH et al: Aspirin-induced abnormalities of liver function. Am J Dis Child. 1973; 126:638.

63. Rich RR et al: Salicylate hepatotoxicity in patients with juvenile rheumatoid arthritis. Arthritis Rheum. 1973; 16:1.

64. Seaman WE et al: Aspirin-induced hepatotoxicity in patients with systemic lupus erythematosus. Ann Intern Med. 1974; 80:1.

65. Wolfe JD et al: Aspirin hepatitis. Ann Intern Med. 1974; 80:74.

66. Sillanpaa M et al: Acute liver failure and encephalopathy (Reye's syndrome?) during salicylate therapy. Acta Paediatr Scand. 1975; 64:877.

67. Barone R et al: Salicylate-induced hepatic injury. Arthritis Rheum. 1976; 19:964.

68. Miller JJ et al: Correlations between transaminase concentrations and serum salicylate concentration in juvenile rheumatoid arthritis. Arthritis Rheum. 1976; 19:115.

69. Seaman WE et al: The effect of aspirin on liver tests in patients with rheumatoid arthritis or systemic lupus erythematosus and in normal volunteers. Arthritis Rheum. 1976; 19:155.

70. O'Gorman T et al: Salicylate hepatitis. Gastroenterology. 1977; 72:726.

71. Mackay IR et al: Treatment of chronic active hepatitis and lupoid hepatitis with 6-mercaptopurine and azathioprine. Lancet. 1964; 1:899.

72. Corley CC Jr et al: Azathioprine therapy of "autoimmune" diseases. Am J Med. 1966; 41:404.

73. Sparberg M et al: Intrahepatic cholestasis due to azathioprine. Gastroenterology. 1969; 57:439.

74. Torisu M et al: Immunosuppression, liver injury, and hepatitis in renal, hepatic and cardiac homograft recipients: with particular reference to the Australia Antigen. Ann Surg. 1971; 174:620.

75. Malekzadeh MH et al: Hepatic dysfunction after renal transplantation in children. J Pediatr. 1972; 81:279.

76. Zardy A et al: Irreversible liver damage after azathioprine. JAMA. 1972; 222:690.

77. Briggs WA et al: Hepatitis affecting hemodialysis and transplant patients. Arch Intern Med. 1973; 132:21.

78. Rashid A et al: Liver disease in kidney transplant patients receiving azathioprine. Arch Intern Med. 1973; 132:29.

79. Ware AJ et al: Spectrum of liver disease in renal transplant recipients. Gastroenterology. 1975; 68:755.

80. DeVita VT et al: Clinical trials with 1,3-bis(2-chloroethyl)-1-nitrosourea, NSC-409962. Cancer Res. 1965; 25:1876.

81. Moertel CG et al: Therapy of advanced gastrointestinal cancer with 1,3-bis(2-chloroethyl)-1-nitrosourea (BCNU). Clin Pharmacol Ther. 1968; 9:652.

82. Thompson GR et al: The hepatotoxicity of 1,3-bis(2-chloroethyl)-1-nitrosourea (BCNU) in rats. J Pharmacol Exper Ther. 1969; 166:104.

83. Walker MD et al: BCNU (1,3-bis-(2-chloroethyl)-1-nitrosourea; NSC-409962) in the treatment of malignant brain tumor. Cancer Chemother Reports. 1970; 54:263.

84. Lessner HE et al: Toxicity study of BCNU (NSC-409962) given orally. Cancer Chemother Reports. 1974; 58:407.

85. Kelsey JR et al: Chlorpromazine jaundice. Gastroenterology. 1955; 29:865.

86. Stein AA et al: Hepatic pathology in jaundice due to chlorpromazine. JAMA. 1956; 161:508.

87. Hollister LE: Allergy to chlorpromazine manifested by jaundice. Am J Med. 1957; 23:870.

88. Waitzkin L: Hepatic dysfunction during promazine therapy. N Engl J Med. 1957; 257:276.

89. Schneider EM et al: Chlorpromazine jaundice: The effect of continued chlorpromazine ingestion in the presence of chlorpromazine jaundice. South Med J. 1958; 51:287.

90. Zelman S: Liver cell necrosis in chlorpromazine jaundice (allergic cholangitis): A serial study of 26 needle biopsy specimens in nine patients. Am J Med. 1959; 27:708.

91. Herron G et al: Jaundice secondary to promazine and an analysis of possible cross sensitivities between phenothiazine derivatives. Gastroenterology. 1960; 38:87.

92. Read AE et al: Chronic chlorpromazine jaundice with particular reference to its relationship to primary biliary cirrhosis. Am J Med. 1961; 31:249.

93. Kohn NN et al: Xanthomatous biliary cirrhosis following chlorpromazine. Am J Med. 1961; 31:665.

94. Walker CD et al: Biliary cirrhosis induced by chlorpromazine. Gastroenterology. 1966; 51:253.

95. Bolton BH: Prolonged chlorpromazine jaundice. Am J Gastroenterology. 1967; 48:497.

96. Ishak KG et al: Hepatic injury associated with the phenothiazines: Clinicopathologic and follow-up study of 36 patients. Arch Path. 1972; 93:283.

97. Russel RI et al: Active chronic hepatitis after chlorpromazine ingestion. Br Med J. 1973; 1:655.

98. Knick B: Clinical and experimental studies with chlorpropamide in diabetes mellitus, in normal individuals, and in nondiabetics with hepatic disease. Ann NY Acad Sci. 1958–1959; 74:858.

99. Brown G et al: Hepatic damage during chlorpropamide therapy. JAMA. 1959; 170:2085.

100. Haunz EA et al: Liver function in chlorpropamide therapy. Five-year clinical study of 181 patients. JAMA. 1964; 188:237.

101. Goldstein MJ et al: Jaundice in a patient receiving acetohexamide. N Engl J Med. 1966; 275:97.

102. Baird RW et al: Cholestatic jaundice from tolbutamide. Ann Intern Med. 1960; 53:194.

103. Gregory DH et al: Chronic cholestasis following prolonged tolbutamide administration. Arch Path. 1967; 84:194.

104. Van Thiel DH et al: Tolazamide hepatotoxicity. Gastroenterology. 1974; 67:506.

105. Eisalo A et al: Hepatic impairment during the intake of contraceptive pills. Clinical trial with postmenopausal women. Br Med J. 1964; 2:426.

106. Mueller MN et al: Estrogen pharmacology. I. The influence of estradiol and estriol on hepatic disposal of sulfobromophthalein. J Clin Invest. 1964; 43:1905.

107. Boake WC et al: Intrahepatic cholestatic jaundice of pregnancy followed by Enovid-induced cholestatic jaundice. Ann Intern Med. 1965; 63:302.

108. Larsson-Cohn U et al: Jaundice during treatment with oral contraceptive agents. Report of two cases. JAMA. 1965; 193:84.

109. Stoll AB et al: Liver damage from oral contraceptives. Br Med J. 1966; 1:960.

110. Ockner RK et al: Hepatic effects of oral contraceptives. N Engl J Med. 1967; 276:331.

111. Larsson-Cohn U et al: Liver ultrastructure and function in icteric and non-icteric women using oral contraceptive agents. Acta Med Scand. 1967; 181:257.

112. Roman P et al: The liver toxicity of oral contraceptives, a critical review of the literature. Med J Aust. 1968; 2:682.

113. Urban E et al: Liver dysfunction with mestranol but not with norethynodrel in a patient with Enovid-induced jaundice. Ann Intern Med. 1968; 68:598.

114. Sabel GH et al: Biliary stasis after mestranol-norethindrone ingestion. Obstet Gynecol. 1968; 31:375.

115. Metreau J et al: Oral contraceptives and the liver. Digestion. 1972; 7:318.

116. Drill VA: Benign cholestatic jaundice of pregnancy and benign cholestatic jaundice from oral contraceptives. Am J Obstet Gynecol. 1974; 119:165.

117. Haemmerli HU: Jaundice during pregnancy. In Diseases of the Liver, 4th ed, edited by L Schiff, JP Lippincott, Philadelphia, 1975, p 1336.

118. Kern F et al: Effect of estrogens on the liver. Gastroenterology. 1978; 75:512.

119. Berg JW et al: Hepatomas and oral contraceptives. Lancet. 1974; 2:349.

120. Antoniades K et al: Hemoperitoneum from liver cell adenoma in a patient on oral contraceptives. Surg. 1975; 77:137.

121. Frederick WC et al: Spontaneous rupture of the liver in patients using contraceptive pills. Arch Surg. 1974; 108:93.

122. Ameriks JA et al: Hepatic cell adenomas, spontaneous liver rupture, and oral contraceptives. Arch Surg. 1975; 110:548.

123. Ishak KG et al: Benign tumors of the liver. Med Clin North Am. 1975; 59:995.

124. Edmondson HA et al: Liver cell adenomas associated with the use of oral contraceptives. N Engl J Med. 1976; 294:470.

125. Klatskin G: Hepatic tumors: Possible relationship to use of oral contraceptives. Gastroenterology. 1977; 73:386.

126. Omer FB et al: Focal nodular hyperplasia of the liver and contraceptive steroids. Acta Hepato-Gastroenterol. 1978; 25:319.

127. Poulsen H et al: Liver disease with periportal sinusoidal dilatation. Digestion. 1973; 8:441.

128. Davis M et al: Histological evidence of carcinoma in a hepatic tumor associated with oral contraceptives. Br Med J. 1975; 4:496.

129. Hoch-Ligeti C: Angiosarcoma of the liver associated with diethylstilbestrol. JAMA. 1978; 240:1510.

130. Ogburn RM et al: Hepatitis associated with dantrolene sodium. Ann Intern Med. 1976; 84:53.

131. Schneider R et al: Dantrolene hepatitis. JAMA. 1976; 235:1590.

132. Utili R et al: Dantrolene-associated hepatic injury. Gastroenterology. 1977; 72:610.

133. Donegan JH et al: Massive hepatic necrosis associated with dantrolene therapy. Digestive Dis. 1978; 23 Suppl:48s.

134. Kohlstaedt KG: Propionyl erythromycin ester lauryl sulfate and jaundice. JAMA. 1961; 178:89.

135. Johnson DF et al: Allergic hepatitis caused by propionyl erythromycin ester of lauryl sulfate. N Engl J Med. 1961; 265:1200.

136. Havens WP: Cholestatic jaundice in patients treated with erythromycin estolate. JAMA. 1962; 180:30.

137. Gilbert FJ: Cholestatic hepatitis caused by esters of erythromycin and oleandomycin. JAMA. 1962; 182:1048.

138. Robinson MM: Demonstration by "challenge" of hepatic dysfunction associated with propionyl erythromycin ester lauryl sulfate. Antibiotic Chemother. 1962; 12:147.

139. Brown AR: Two cases of untoward reaction after "Ilosone." Br Med J. 1963; 2:913.

140. Fischer HW et al: Mimicry of acute cholecystitis by erythromycin estolate reactions. Report of 2 cases. Am J Med Sci. 1964; 247:283.

141. McKenzie I et al: Two cases of jaundice following "Ilosone." Med J Aust. 1966; 1:349.

142. Braun P: Hepatotoxicity of erythromycin. J Infect Dis. 1969; 119:300.

143. Rogers RS: Abdominal distress and erythromycin estolate. Lancet. 1972; 2:1198.

144. Oliver LE et al: "Biliary colic" and Ilosone. Med J Aust. 1973; 1:1148.

145. Lloyd-Still JD et al: Erythromycin estolate hepatotoxicity. Am J Dis Child. 1978; 132:320.

146. Walters GM et al: Jaundice following administration of fluphenazine dihydrochloride. Am J Psychiatry. 1963; 120:81.

147. Steinberg H et al: Hepatomegaly with fatty infiltration secondary to cortisone therapy. Case report. Gastroenterology. 1952; 21:304.

148. Hill RB Jr: Fatal fat embolism from steroid-induced fatty liver. N Engl J Med. 1961; 165:318.

149. Jones JP et al: Systemic fat embolism after renal homo-transplantation and treatment with corticosteroids. N Engl J Med. 1965; 273:1453.

150. Gerle B et al: Clinical observations of the side effects of haloperidol. Acta Psychiat Scand. 1964; 40:65.

151. Crane GE et al: A review of clinical literature on halo-peridol. Int J Neuropsychiat. 1967; 3:Suppl 5111.

152. Lindenbaum J et al: Hepatic necrosis associated with halothane anesthesia. N Engl J Med. 1963; 268:525.

153. Herber R et al: Liver necrosis following anesthesia. Arch Intern Med. 1965; 115:266.

154. Cooperative study: Subcommittee on the national halothane study of the committee on anesthesia, NAS-NRC summary of the national halothane study. JAMA. 1966; 197:775.

155. Little DM Jr: Effects of halothane on liver function. In Clinical Anesthesia: Halothane, edited by NM Greene, FA Davis, Philadelphia, 1968, p 85.

156. Peters RL et al: Hepatic necrosis associated with halothane anesthesia. Am J Med. 1969; 47:748.

157. Klion FM et al: Hepatitis after exposure to halothane. Ann Intern Med. 1969; 71:467.

158. Hughes M et al: Recurrent hepatitis in patients receiving multiple halothane anesthetics for radium treatment of carcinoma of the cervix uteri. Gastroenterology. 1970; 58:790.

159. Carney FMT et al: Halothane hepatitis: A critical review. Anesth Analgesia. 1972; 51:135.

160. Byrd BF et al: Serious sequelae of general anesthesia. Ann Surg. 1972; 175:673.

161. Paull A et al: Halothane hepatitis—A report of five cases. Med J Aust. 1974; 1:954.

162. Inman WHW et al: Jaundice after repeated exposure to halothane: An analysis of reports to the Committee on Safety of Medicine. Br Med J. 1974; 1:5010.

163. Trowell J et al: Controlled trial of repeated halothane anesthetics in patients with carcinoma of the uterine cervix treated with radium. Lancet. 1975; 1:821.

164. Moult P et al: Halothane-related hepatitis. Quart J Med. 1975; 44:99.

165. Bottinger LE et al: Halothane-induced liver damage: An analysis of the material reported to the Swedish Adverse Drug Reaction Committee, 1966–1973. Acta Anesth Scand. 1976; 20:40.

166. Schlipper W et al: Recurrent hepatitis following halothane exposures. Am J Med. 1978; 65:25.

167. Kline MM: Enflurane-associated hepatitis. Gastroenterology. 1980; 79:126.

168. Farber S: Summary of experience with 6-mercaptopurine. Ann NY Acad Sci. 1954; 60:412.

169. Frei E III et al: A comparative study of two regimens of combination chemotherapy in acute leukemia. Blood. 1958; 13:1126.

170. Clark PA et al: Toxic complications of treatment with 6-mercaptopurine. Two cases with hepatic necrosis and intestinal ulceration. Br Med J. 1960; 1:393.

171. Acute leukemia group B: Studies of sequential and combination anti-metabolite therapy in acute leukemia: 6-mercaptopurine and methotrexate. Blood. 1961; 18:431.

172. Einhorn M et al: Hepatotoxicity of mercaptopurine. JAMA. 1964; 188:802.

173. Shorey J et al: Hepatotoxicity of mercaptopurine. Arch Intern Med. 1968; 122:54.

174. Specht NW et al: Death due to agranulocytosis induced by methimazole therapy. JAMA. 1952; 149:1010.

175. Rosenbaum H et al: Agranulocytosis and toxic hepatitis from methimazole. JAMA. 1953; 152:27.

176. Martinez-Lopez JL et al: Drug-induced hepatic injury during methimazole therapy. Gastroenterology. 1962; 43:84.

177. Fischer MG et al: Methimazole-induced jaundice. JAMA. 1973; 223:1028.

178. Crandall WB et al: Nephrotoxicity associated with methoxyflurane. Anesthesiology. 1966; 27:591.

179. Judson JA et al: Possible cross-sensitivity between halothane and methoxyflurane. Anesthesiology. 1971; 35:527.

180. Halpren BA et al: Interstitial fibrosis and chronic renal failure following methoxyflurane anesthesia. JAMA. 1973; 223:1239.

181. Joshi PH et al: The syndrome of methoxyflurane-associated hepatitis. Ann Intern Med. 1974; 80:395.

182. Hutter RVP et al: Hepatic fibrosis in children with acute leukemia: A complication of therapy. Cancer. 1960; 13:288.

183. Hersh EM et al: Hepatotoxic effects of methotrexate. Cancer. 1966; 19:600.

184. Coe RD et al: Cirrhosis associated with methotrexate. Treatment of psoriasis. JAMA. 1968; 206;1515.

185. Muller SA et al: Cirrhosis caused by methotrexate in the treatment of psoriasis. Arch Dermatol. 1969; 100:523.

186. McDonald CJ et al: Parenteral methotrexate in psoriasis. A report on the efficacy and toxicity of long-term intermittent treatment. Arch Dermatol. 1969; 100:655.

187. Vogler WR: Treatment of rheumatoid arthritis with amethopterin. Clin Res. 1970; 18:46.

188. Goldstein DP: Five years' experience with the prevention of trophoblastic tumors by the prophylactic use of chemotherapy in patients with molar pregnancy. Clin Obstet Gynecol. 1970; 13:945.

189. Moojin RO et al: Monitoring methotrexate therapy in psoriasis. Arch Dermatol. 1970; 101:646.

190. Dubin HV et al: Liver disease associated with methotrexate treatment of psoriatic patients. Arch Dermatol. 1970; 102:498.

191. Weinstein G: Evaluation of possible chronic hepatotoxicity from methotrexate for psoriasis. Arch Dermatol. 1970; 102:613.

192. Editorial: Psoriasis, methotrexate, and cirrhosis. JAMA. 1970; 212:314.

193. Filip DJ et al: Pulmonary and hepatic complications of methotrexate therapy of psoriasis. JAMA. 1971; 216:881.

194. Almeyda J et al: Structural and functional abnormalities of the liver in psoriasis before and during methotrexate therapy. Br J Dermatol. 1972; 87:623.

195. Podurgiel BJ et al: Liver injury associated with methotrexate therapy for psoriasis. Mayo Clin Proc. 1973; 48:787.

196. Elkington SG et al: Hepatic injury caused by L-alpha-methyldopa. Circulation. 1969; 40:589.

197. Tysell JE Jr et al: Hepatitis induced by methyldopa (Aldomet). Report of a case and a review of the literature. Am J Dig Dis. 1971; 16:849.

198. Eliastam M et al: Hepatitis, arthritis and lupus cell phenomena caused by methyldopa. Am J Dig Dis. 1971; 16:1014.

199. Hoyumpa AM Jr et al: Methyldopa hepatitis: Report of three cases. Am J Dig Dis. 1973; 18:213.

200. Brouillard RP et al: Methyldopa associated hepatitis. JAMA. 1973; 224:904.

201. Rehman OU et al: Methyldopa-induced submassive hepatic necrosis. JAMA. 1973; 224:1390.

202. Goldstein GB et al: Drug-induced active chronic hepatitis. Am J Dig Dis. 1973; 18:177.

203. Schweitzer IL et al: Acute submassive hepatic necrosis due to methyldopa. Gastroenterology. 1974; 66:1203.

204. Toghill PJ et al: Methyldopa liver damage. Br Med J. 1974; 3:545.

205. Maddrey WC et al: Severe hepatitis from methyldopa. Gastroenterology. 1975; 68:351.

206. Cacace LG et al: Alpha-methyldopa (Aldomet) hepatitis. Drug Intell Clin Pharm. 1976; 10:144.

207. Ansfield FJ: Clinical studies with mithramycin. Oncology. 1969; 23:283.

208. Kennedy BJ: Mithramycin therapy in advanced testicular neoplasms. Cancer. 1970; 26:755.

209. Foley JF et al: The treatment of metastatic testicular tumors. J Urol. 1972; 108:439.

210. Ryan WG: Mithramycin in Paget's disease of bone. Lancet. 1973; 1:1319.

211. Felix A et al: Iproniazid hepatitis. Report of five cases and review of pertinent literature. Arch Intern Med. 1959; 104:72.

212. Rosenblum LE et al: Hepatocellular jaundice as a complication of iproniazid therapy. Arch Intern Med. 1960; 105:583.

213. Benack RT et al: Jaundice associated with isocarboxazid therapy. N Engl J Med. 1961; 264:294.

214. Knight JA: Drug-induced hepatic injury: Marplan hepatitis. Am J Psychiatry. 1961; 118:73.

215. Griffith GC et al: Jaundice and hepatitis in patients who have received hydrazine-base monamine oxidase inhibitors. Am J Med Sci. 1962; 244:592.

216. Bandt C et al: Liver injury associated with tranylcypromine therapy. JAMA. 1964; 188:752.

217. Cook GC et al: Jaundice and its relation to therapeutic agents. Lancet. 1965; 1:175.

218. Jokela S: Liver disease due to nitrofurantoin. Gastroenterology. 1967; 53:306.

219. Adverse effects of drugs commonly used in the treatment of urinary tract infection. A report from the Australian Drug Evaluation Committee. Med J Aust. 1972; 1:435.

220. Goldstein LI et al: Hepatic injury associated with nitrofurantoin therapy. Am J Dig Dis. 1974; 19:987.

221. Klemola H et al: Anicteric liver damage during nitrofurantoin medication. Scand J Gastroenterology. 1975; 10:501.

222. Engel JJ et al: Cholestatic hepatitis after administration of furan derivatives. Arch Intern Med. 1975; 135:733.

223. Selroos O et al: Lupus-like syndrome associated with pulmonary reaction to nitrofurantoin: Report of three cases. Acta Med Scand. 1975; 197:125.

224. Klein I et al: Oxacillin-associated hepatitis. Am J Med Sci. 1963; 245:399.

225. Pas AT et al: Cholestatic hepatitis following the administration of sodium oxacillin. JAMA. 1965; 191:138.

226. Dismukes WE: Oxacillin-induced hepatic dysfunction. JAMA. 1973; 226:861.

227. Olans RN et al: Reversible oxacillin hepatotoxicity. J Pediatr. 1976; 89:835.

228. Pollock AA et al: Hepatitis associated with high dose oxacillin therapy. Arch Intern Med. 1978; 138:915.

229. Bruckstein AH et al: Oxacillin hepatitis. Am J Med. 1978; 64:519.

230. Onorato IM et al: Hepatitis from intravenous high dose oxacillin therapy. Ann Intern Med. 1978; 89:497.

231. Taylor C et al: Oxacillin and hepatitis. Ann Intern Med. 1979; 90:857.

232. Waugh D: Myocarditis, arteritis and focal hepatic, splenic and renal granulomas apparently due to penicillin sensitivity. Am J Pathol. 1952; 28:437.

233. Ross S et al: Alpha-amino-benzyl-penicillin—new broad spectrum antibiotic: Preliminary clinical and laboratory observations. JAMA. 1962; 182:238.

234. Murphy ES et al: Shock, liver necrosis, and death after penicillin injection. Arch Pathol. 1962; 73:13.

235. Valdivia-Barriga V et al: Generalized hypersensitivity with hepatitis and jaundice after the use of penicillin and streptomycin. Gastroenterology. 1963; 45:114.

236. Girard JP et al: Lupoid hepatitis following administration of penicillin. Helvetica Medica Acta. 1967; 34:23.

237. Neu HC et al: Carbenicillin: Clinical and laboratory experience with a parenterally administered penicillin for treatment of pseudomonas infections. Ann Intern Med. 1969; 71:903.

238. Bodey GP et al: Carbenicillin therapy for pseudomonas infections. JAMA. 1971; 218:62.

239. Davies GE et al: Drug-induced immunological effects on the liver. Br J Anaesth. 1972; 44:941.

240. Kosmidis J et al: Amoxicillin—pharmacology, bacteriology, and clinical studies. Br J Clin Pract. 1972; 26:341.

241. Goldstein LI et al: Hepatic injury associated with penicillin therapy. Arch Pathol. 1974; 98:114.

242. McArthur JE et al: Stevens-Johnson syndrome with hepatitis following therapy with ampicillin and cephalexin. NZ Med J. 1975; 81:390.

243. Wilson FM et al: Anicteric carbenicillin hepatitis: Eight episodes in four patients. JAMA. 1975; 232:818.

244. East EN et al: Severe sensitivity reaction (hepatitis, dermatitis, and pyrexia) attributable to phenylindanedione. Can Med Assoc J. 1957; 77:1028.

245. Jones NL: Hepatitis due to phenindione sensitivity. Br Med J. 1960; 2:504.

246. Brooks RH et al: Dermatitis, hepatitis and nephritis due to phenindione (phenylindanedione). Ann Intern Med. 1960; 52:706.

247. Portal RW et al: Phenindione hepatitis complicating anticoagulant therapy. Br Med J. 1961; 2:1318.

248. Perkins J: Phenindione sensitivity. Lancet. 1962; 1:127.

249. Garnet ES et al: A fatal case of phenindione sensitivity. Br Med J. 1962; 2:1023.

250. Perkins J: Phenindione jaundice. Lancet. 1962; 1:125.

251. Mohamed SD: Sensitivity reaction to phenindione with urticaria, hepatitis, and pancytopenia. Br Med J. 1965; 2:1475.

252. Kuzell WC et al: Phenylbutazone. Further clinical evaluation. Arch Intern Med. 1953; 92:603.

253. Fisher JH: Fatal phenylbutazone hepatitis. Can Med Assoc J. 1960; 83:1211.

254. Juul J: Acute poisoning with butazolidine (phenylbutazone). Acta Pediatr Scand. 1965; 54:503.

255. Ecker JA: Phenylbutazone hepatitis. Am J Gastroenterology. 1965; 43:23.

256. Fowler PD et al: Phenylbutazone and hepatitis. Rheumatol Rehabil. 1975; 14:71.

257. Gropper AL: Diphenylhydantoin sensitivity: Report of a fatal case with hepatitis and exfoliative dermatitis. N Engl J Med. 1956; 254:522.

258. Siegel S et al: Diphenylhydantoin (dilantin) hypersensitivity with infectious mononucleosis-like syndrome and jaundice. J Allergy. 1961; 32:447.

259. Bajoghli M: Generalized lymphadenopathy and hepatosplenomegaly induced by diphenylhydantoin. Pediatrics. 1961; 28:943.

260. Braverman IM et al: Dilantin-induced serum sickness: Case report and inquiry into its mechanisms. Am J Med. 1963; 35:418.

261. Harinasuta U et al: Diphenylhydantoin sodium hepatitis. JAMA. 1968; 203:1015.

262. Pezzimenti JF et al: Anicteric hepatitis induced by diphenylhydantoin. Arch Intern Med. 1970; 125:118.

263. Dhar GJ et al: Diphenylhydantoin-induced hepatic necrosis. Postgrad Med. 1974; 56:128.

264. Kleckner HB et al: Severe hypersensitivity to diphenylhydantoin with circulating antibodies to the drug. Ann Intern Med. 1975; 83:522.

265. Lee TJ et al: Diphenylhydantoin-induced hepatic necrosis. Gastroenterology. 1976; 70:422.

266. Campbell CB et al: Cholestatic liver disease associated with diphenylhydantoin therapy. Am J Dig Dis. 1977; 22:255.

267. Parker WA et al: Phenytoin hepatotoxicity: A case report and review. Neurology. 1979; 29:175.

268. Koren JF et al: Phenytoin hypersensitivity reaction: Hepatic necrosis. Drug Intell Clin Pharm. 1980; 14:252.

269. Mechanic RC et al: Chlorpromazine-type cholangitis. Report of a case occurring after the administration of prochlorperazine. N Engl J Med. 1958; 259:778.

270. Solomon FA et al: Jaundice due to prochlorperazine (Compazine). Am J Med. 1959; 27:840.

271. McFarland RB: Fatal drug reaction associated with prochlorperazine (Compazine). Am J Clin Path. 1963; 40:284.

272. Amerbein JA et al: Granulocytopenia, lupus-like syndrome, and other complications of propylthiouracil therapy. J Pediatr. 1970; 74:54.

273. Parker LN: Hepatitis and propylthiouracil. Ann Intern Med. 1975; 82:228.

274. Fedotin MS et al: Liver disease caused by propylthiouracil. Arch Intern Med. 1975; 135:319.

275. Eisen MJ: Fulminant hepatitis during treatment with propylthiouracil. N Engl J Med. 1963; 249:814.

276. Mihas AA et al: Fulminant hepatitis and lymphocyte sensitization due to propylthiouracil. Gastroenterology. 1976; 70:770.

277. Colwell AR Jr et al: Propylthiouracil-induced agranulocytosis, toxic hepatitis, and death. JAMA. 1952; 148:639.

278. Deisseroth A et al: Quinidine-induced liver disease. Ann Intern Med. 1972; 77:595.

279. Chajek T et al: Quinidine-induced granulomatous hepatitis. Ann Intern Med. 1974; 81:774.

280. Handler SD et al: Quinidine hepatitis. Arch Intern Med. 1975; 135:871.

281. Koch MJ et al: Quinidine toxicity: A report of a case and a review of the literature. Gastroenterology. 1976; 70:1136.

282. Djur JR: Quinidine hepatotoxicity. JAMA. 1976; 235:908.

283. Geltner D et al: Quinidine hypersensitivity and liver involvement. A survey of 32 patients. Gastroenterology. 1976; 70:650.

284. Garvin CF: Toxic hepatitis due to sulfanilamide. JAMA. 1938; 111:2283.

285. Cline EW: Acute yellow atrophy of the liver following sulfanilamide medication. JAMA. 1938; 111:2384.

286. Longcope WT: Serum sickness and analogous reactions from certain drugs, particularly the sulfonamides. Med. 1943; 22:251.

287. Chaikin NW et al: Acute hepatitis; clinical observations in 63 cases. Am J Dig Dis. 1945; 12:151.

288. Dujovne CA et al: Sulfonamide hepatic injury. N Engl J Med. 1967; 277:785.

289. Tisdale WA: Focal hepatitis, fever, and skin rash following therapy with sulfamethoxypyridazine, a long-acting sulfonamide. N Engl J Med. 1958; 258:687.

290. Tonder M et al: Sulfonamide-induced chronic liver disease. Scand J Gastroenterology. 1974; 9:93.

291. Sotolongo RP et al: Hypersensitivity reaction to sulfasalazine with severe hepatotoxicity. Gastroenterology. 1978; 75:95.

292. Schultz JC et al: Fatal liver disease after intravenous administration of tetracycline in high dosage. N Engl J Med. 1963; 269:999.

293. Briggs RC: Tetracycline and liver disease. N Engl J Med. 1963; 269:1386.

294. Gough GS et al: Additional case of fatal liver disease with tetracycline therapy. N Engl J Med. 1964; 270:157.

295. Dowling HF et al: Hepatic reactions to tetracycline. JAMA. 1964; 188:307.

296. Whalley PJ et al: Tetracycline toxicity in pregnancy. JAMA. 1964; 189:357.

297. Horwitz ST et al: Fatal liver disease during pregnancy associated with tetracycline therapy. Obstet Gynecol. 1964; 23:826.

298. Kunelis CT et al: Fatty liver of pregnancy and its relationship to tetracycline therapy. Am J Med. 1965; 38:359.

299. Davis JS et al: Tetracycline toxicity. Am J Obstet Gynecol. 1966; 95:523.

300. Hansen CH et al: Impaired secretion of triglycerides by the liver: A cause of tetracycline-induced fatty liver. Proc Soc Exp Biol Med. 1968; 128:143.

301. Robinson MJ et al: Tetracycline-associated fatty liver in the male. Am J Dig Dis. 1970; 15:857.

302. Hoyumpa AM Jr et al: Fatty liver: Biochemical and clinical considerations. Am J Dig Dis. 1975; 20:1142.

303. Reinhart MJ et al: Suggestive evidence of hepatotoxicity concomitant with thioridazine hydrochloride use. JAMA. 1966; 197:767.

304. Barancik M et al: Thioridazine-induced cholestasis. JAMA. 1967; 200:69.

305. Malitz S et al: Preliminary evaluation of Tofranil in a combined in-patient and out-patient setting. Can Psychiat Assoc J. 1959; Suppl 4:152.

306. Cunningham ML: Acute hepatic necrosis following treatment with amitriptyline and diazepam. Br J Psychiatry. 1965; 111:1107.

307. Biagi RW et al: Intrahepatic obstructive jaundice from amitriptyline. Br J Psychiatry. 1967; 113:1113.

308. Horst DA et al: Prolonged cholestasis and progressive hepatic fibrosis following imipramine therapy. Gastroenterology. 1980; 79:550.

309. Powell WJ et al: Lethal hepatic necrosis after therapy with imipramine and desipramine. JAMA. 1968; 206:642.

310. Short MH et al: Cholestatic jaundice during imipramine therapy. JAMA. 1968; 206:1791.

311. Yon J et al: Hepatitis caused by amitriptyline therapy. JAMA. 1975; 232:833.

312. Kohn N et al: Cholestatic hepatitis associated with trifluoperazine. N Engl J Med. 1961; 264:549.

313. Margulies AI et al: Jaundice associated with the administration of trifluoperazine. Can Med Assoc J. 1968; 98:1063.

314. Sodium valproate: A new anticonvulsant. Med Let Drugs Ther. 1977; 19:93.

315. Willmore LJ et al: Effect of valproic acid on hepatic function. Neurology. 1978; 28:961.

316. Donat JF et al: Valproic acid and fatal hepatitis. Neurology. 1979; 29:273.

317. Sussman NM et al: A direct hepatotoxic effect of valproic acid. JAMA. 1979. 242:1173.

318. Suchy FJ et al: Acute hepatic failure associated with the use of sodium valproate. N Engl J Med. 1979; 300:962.

319. Gerber N et al: Reye-like syndrome associated with valproic acid therapy. J Pediatr. 1979; 95:142.

320. Young RSK et al: Fatal Reye-like syndrome associated with valproic acid. Ann Neurol. 1980; 7:389.

321. Stimson WH: Vitamin A intoxication in adults: Report of a case with a summary of the literature. N Engl J Med. 1961; 265:369.

322. Rubin E et al: Hepatic injury in chronic hypervitaminosis A. Am J Dis Child. 1970; 119:132.

323. Muenter MD et al: Chronic vitamin A intoxication in adults. Am J Med. 1971; 50:129.

324. Muenter MD: Hypervitaminosis A. Ann Intern Med. 1974; 80:105.

325. Russell RM et al: Hepatic injury from chronic hypervitaminosis A resulting in portal-hypertension and ascites. N Engl J Med. 1974; 291:435.

326. Viteri AL et al: Erythromycin ethylsuccinate-induced cholestasis. Gastroenterology. 1979; 76:1007.

327. Greenlaw CW et al: Hepatotoxicity possibly associated with erythromycin ethylsuccinate. Drug Intell Clin Pharm. 1979; 13:236.

Chapter 27

Kidney Diseases

John G. Gambertoglio, Richard J. Mangini, and Daniel C. Robinson

There is an ever-increasing number of patients with renal disease. In good part this is due to the use of chronic dialysis and renal transplantation for those who would otherwise die from end-stage renal failure.

The clinical features, pathogenesis, and treatment of some of the more commonly encountered forms of renal disease are described in this chapter. These are acute and chronic renal failure, diabetes insipidus, and the syndrome of inappropriate antidiuretic hormone secretion. In addition, some commonly used drugs which have been associated with nephrotoxic effects are also reviewed.

In order to assess drug therapy, it is necessary to have a basic understanding of the disease process. This chapter discusses the important aspects of renal disease, but emphasis is placed on drugs and drug therapy.

ACUTE RENAL FAILURE

Acute renal failure (ARF) can be defined as a sudden decline in renal function, accompanied by an accumulation of nitrogenous waste products normally excreted by the kidney. It is caused by a process within the kidney itself and is not reversed by correction of extrarenal factors, ie, pre-renal and post-renal causes of azotemia. Urine volume may vary over a wide range in ARF. A urine volume less than 50 ml per day constitutes *anuria.* If the urine volume is less than 400 ml but greater than 50 ml per day, it is described as *oliguria.* However, the urine volume may be much higher, exceeding one liter or more. This is referred to as *nonoliguric* or *high-output acute renal failure.* A cursory examination of daily input and output is, therefore, inadequate for monitoring patients who are receiving potentially nephrotoxic drugs. It has been demonstrated that up to 50% of drug-induced ARF cases are nonoliguric (1). Commonly, the term *acute tubular necrosis (ATN),* which describes a histopathological change within the kidneys, is used; however, patients with ARF frequently do not exhibit evidence of tubular necrosis. In fact, histological changes within the kidney do not correlate very well with the functional capacity of the kidney. Therefore, the terms acute tubular necrosis and acute renal failure are not synonymous (2–4).

There are a number of causes of acute renal failure. These may be classified into three major categories. The first are diseases affecting the glomerulus and small blood vessels of the kidney. Examples of these include: systemic lupus erythematosus, infective endocarditis, acute post streptococcal glomerulonephritis, malignant hypertension, pregnancy, and drug-induced vasculitis. The second category includes disorders that result in ischemia to the kidney: severe trauma, major hemorrhage, crush injury, intra-operative ischemia, transfusion reactions, and sepsis. The last major category is renal failure caused by nephrotoxins. Among these are the following chemicals or drugs: heavy metals and their compounds, organic solvents, glycols, pesticides, radio-contrast media, and antibiotics. Finally, approximately 20% of the cases of ARF are termed idiopathic because no identifiable cause exists (2–5).

Pre-renal azotemia may be defined as a decline in creatinine clearance or glomerular filtration rate (GFR) caused by an event which decreases renal perfusion pressure or causes severe renal vasoconstriction. The most common etiology is hypovolemia which decreases renal blood flow and produces renal ischemia. The hypovolemia may be secondary to blood loss or excessive fluid losses from the gastrointestinal tract or from severe burns. The overuse of diuretics can also cause pre-renal azotemia, especially if patients are on sodium-restricted diets. Vasodilatation of peripheral blood vessels secondary to antihypertensive drugs or septicemia can decrease renal perfusion. Other causes of pre-renal azotemia include decreased cardiac output secondary to impaired cardiac function (eg, myocardial infarction), congestive heart failure, obstruction of the renal vasculature by emboli, and increased renal vascular resistance due to surgery and anesthesia. In most instances pre-renal failure is readily reversible when the extra-renal factors are corrected. However, should the pre-renal cause be prolonged for an extended period, irreversible damage to the kidneys could result (2,3).

Post-renal azotemia is simply an accumulation of waste products which is caused by an obstruction along the urinary tract. Obstruction of the ureters may be caused by stones, blood clots, uric acid and sulfonamide crystals, and papillary necrosis from analgesic abuse. Tumors and retroperitoneal fibrosis (methysergide therapy) may also cause obstruction by impinging on or surrounding the ureters. Carcinoma, infection of the bladder, prostatic hypertrophy and ganglionic blockers may lead to bladder neck obstruction along the urethra. The finding of anuria (no urine excretion) or alternating anuria and polyuria (large urine volume) in a patient with decreased renal function is very suggestive of obstruction. Removal of the obstruction, when possible, will reverse the renal failure (2,3).

The clinical course of the patient who develops acute renal failure not associated with pre-renal or post-renal azotemia is dependent on the severity of the renal injury. Oliguria starts within a few hours of the insult and progresses over the next 24 to 48 hours. With certain nephrotoxic chemicals, however, the onset of oliguria may be delayed for several days. Once established, oliguria may last from one day to six weeks, the average being 7 to 12 days. The nonoliguric form of acute renal failure is generally associated with a lesser degree of renal injury and a better overall prognosis.

Following the oliguric phase of acute renal failure, urine volume progressively increases. This signals the return of renal function. On the average, the blood urea nitrogen (BUN) becomes normal within approximately 15 to 20 days after the onset of diuresis. The recovery phase, during which the clinical signs and symptoms of uremia subside, may take two or three months. Most patients are well enough to resume normal activities by this time. Testing may reveal subclinical defects in renal function, such as impaired concentrating ability, which may persist for up to one year. In others, a permanent reduction in glomerular filtration rate (GFR) which is not clinically important may exist (2–5).

Diagnosis

1. M.B., a 38-year-old, 82 kg male, was admitted to the hospital because of persistent nausea, vomiting, and diarrhea that is thought to be due to a viral infection. He has a history of hypertension and has been treated with sodium restriction, hydrochlorothiazide, and methyldopa. Admission orders included bedrest, the encouragement of oral fluids, hydrochlorothiazide 50 mg bid, and methyldopa 250 mg tid. On day two the patient's blood pressure was 70/30 mm Hg with a rapid pulse and a urine volume of less than 10 ml/hr. Dry mucous membranes and decreased skin turgor were noticed on physical exami-

nation. Serum electrolytes at this time were sodium 147 mEq/L (132–145 mEq/L), potassium 7 mEq/L (3.5–4.7 mEq/L), chloride 110 mEq/L (95–108 mEq/L) and CO_2 content 19 mEq/L (24–32 mEq/L). The serum creatinine was 4.0 mg/dl and the BUN was 60 mg/dl. The plasma osmolality was 310 mOsm/kg. Examination of the urine revealed the following: sodium 7 mEq/L, potassium 25 mEq/L, urea 900 mg/dl, creatinine 70 mg/dl, and osmolality 800 mOsm/kg.

Based on M.B.'s admission diagnosis and history, what factors were most likely responsible for his low blood pressure on day two of his hospitalization?

M.B.'s admission orders included oral fluids, hydrochlorothiazide, and methyldopa. In view of his history of nausea, vomiting, and diarrhea, a careful physical examination on admission may have revealed a low blood pressure and tachycardia. His antihypertensive therapy should have been withheld until correction of his fluid balance was attained. Replacement of his fluid deficit requires intravenous administration of fluids since oral fluids would not be well tolerated in a patient with presumed viral enteritis.

2. What is the nature of M.B.'s renal problem? How can it be determined whether it is acute renal failure, pre-renal azotemia, or post-renal azotemia?

Since pre-renal and post-renal azotemia are usually readily reversible, precipitating causes must first be considered. If these are excluded as an explanation of the patient's renal failure, then the diagnosis of acute renal failure must be considered.

M.B. exhibits a number of physical findings which suggest volume depletion as a cause of pre-renal azotemia. These include dry mucous membranes, decreased skin turgor, and orthostatic hypotension with increased pulse rate. The physical examination did not reveal any findings suggestive of post-renal azotemia. Such an examination would include percussion of the abdomen for an enlarged bladder, palpation for kidney enlargement, and a pelvic examination in females for cervical malignancy or a rectal examination in males for an enlarged prostate in order to rule out obstruction. In addition, excretion urography and bladder catheterization may be needed.

Specific laboratory tests are very helpful in distinguishing the cause of azotemia. In general, one can differentiate pre-renal failure from acute renal failure by examination of the urine. In a patient with pre-renal azotemia who is otherwise normal, tubular function is intact and the kidney responds normally to a decrease in renal perfusion or volume depletion. Therefore, if oliguria is due to pre-renal factors, the urine should be highly concentrated, the urinary sodium concentration should be decreased, and the urine urea and creatinine concentrations should be increased as evidenced in M.B. Generally, patients in acute or intra-renal failure do not have intact tubular function and will not be able to conserve sodium and water normally.

Table 1 compares the usual urinary findings in pre-renal azotemia and acute renal failure. M.B.'s urinary findings further substantiate a diagnosis of pre-renal azotemia as opposed to acute renal failure. In addition to these findings, his plasma urea to creatinine ratio is greater than 10 to 1 which is also suggestive of pre-renal azotemia. Urine composition is not very useful in distinguishing post-renal failure from acute renal failure, since in certain types of obstruction it may be similar to that of pre-renal azotemia or acute renal failure (2–4).

3. M.B. was taking hydrochlorothiazide when his urinary indices were evaluated. What effect would this be expected to have?

Since diuretics uniformly increase the renal

excretion of sodium, they may cause misleading results in diagnostic tests which depend on urine sodium concentration. Increases in urine sodium are more consistent with acute renal failure than with pre-renal azotemia (See Table 1). The low urine sodium seen in M.B. despite the influence of hydrochlorothiazide is highly suggestive of a pre-renal etiology (2,5,6).

4. Are there other factors which may cause misinterpretation of the urinary indices?

The urine of older patients and those with chronic renal disease may not be concentrated despite the presence of pre-renal azotemia. Also, the urinary sodium of some patients with non-oliguric acute renal failure may be less than 20 mEq/L (2).

Management

5. Now that a diagnosis of pre-renal azotemia has been established, how should M.B. be managed?

Every effort should be made to correct any contributing factors. In the case of M.B. it is imperative that the fluid imbalances associated with dehydration and hypovolemia be corrected as soon as possible to prevent progressive ischemic renal injury. An estimate of the total fluid deficit can be obtained by examining the plasma osmolality. Since osmotic activity is equal in all body fluids except the renal medulla, any increase in plasma osmolality will represent a decrease in total body water (See chapter on Fluid and Electrolyte Disorders). For example, in the adult male total body water (TBW) represents approximately 60% of total body weight. For M.B. this would be 82 kg $\times$ 0.60 = 49.2 kg or 49.2 liters.

$$\text{corrected TBW} = \frac{49.2 \text{ L} \times 285 \text{ mOsm/kg (normal)}}{310 \text{ mOsm/kg (patient)}}$$

$$= 45.2 \text{ L}$$

$$\text{fluid deficit} = 49.2 - 45.2$$

One method of replacing this fluid would be to give 45% of the deficit over the initial 8 hours, 25% over the next 16 hours and 30% over the next 24 hours. Urine output must be assessed continuously once rehydration has begun. If output does not increase significantly during the first one to two hours, the possibilities of either an incorrect diagnosis or ischemic renal injury must be con-

Table 1.

URINARY FINDINGS IN PRE-RENAL AZOTEMIA AND ACUTE RENAL FAILURE

	Pre-renal azotemia	Acute renal failure
urine sodium concentration (mEq/L)	<20	>40
urine osmolality (mOsm/kg)	>500	<400
urine/plasma creatinine	>40	<20
renal failure index: $\frac{U(Na)}{U/P(Creat.)}$	<1	>2
urine sediment	normal	granular casts cellular debris

Adapted from Schrier RW and Conger JD, 1980 (2)

sidered. Potassium should not be included in the initial intravenous solutions until an assessment of renal potassium excretion can be made.

6. Assuming that volume expansion failed to restore M.B.'s renal function, what further measures might be taken? How are appropriate drugs used, and what complications may accompany their use?

In patients whose renal function remains impaired once hypovolemia has been corrected, improvement in cardiac function or replacement of glucocorticoid hormones may correct the oliguria if heart failure or adrenal insufficiency exist (5).

It has been demonstrated that drugs which increase urine excretion may prevent the development of acute renal failure following pre-renal azotemia and may convert oliguric to non-oliguric renal failure. This latter effect is important in view of recent evidence that mortality is lower in non-oliguric than in oliguric renal failure (26% versus 50%) (1,7). Mannitol and potent diuretics such as furosemide and ethacrynic acid are commonly used to increase urine flow. The success of these maneuvers depends largely upon their early administration after the onset of oliguria and adequate replacement of urinary water and electrolytes to prevent further volume depletion.

Osmotic Diuretics. Mannitol is a nondiffusable hexahydric sugar. Following intravenous administration, it distributes within the plasma and interstitial spaces but does not enter cells (8,9). Dosage recommendations are quite variable, but, in general, 10 to 25 gm of mannitol are infused intravenously over 5 to 10 minutes. Urine output is then measured, and if it is not greater than 40 ml/hour over a one to three hour period, a repeat dose may be given. Should the patient fail to respond to a second challenge, no further mannitol should be administered. If there is an adequate response (greater than 30 ml/hour), then mannitol should be continued, either by a continuous infusion or by repeated injection, in order to maintain a high rate of urinary flow (approximately 100 ml/hour). This is continued until the patient is able to sustain a sufficient urine output on his own. Within a 24-hour period, no more than 100 gm of mannitol should be administered unless the urinary flow rate exceeds 100 ml/hour (5).

Complications in the use of mannitol include excessive intravascular volume expansion, hyponatremia, fluid overload, pulmonary edema, congestive heart failure, and hypertension. Since mannitol is entirely excreted unchanged in the urine, patients with pre-existing renal failure can potentially accumulate the drug. Another consideration is that mannitol is available as a 25% supersaturated solution which commonly crystallizes. This can be avoided by heating the solution or using the less concentrated 20% solution.

Loop Diuretics. Furosemide and ethacrynic acid represent useful alternatives in patients with congestive heart failure, excessive hydration, or chronic renal failure, where mannitol is contraindicated. Furosemide is used more frequently since it is less ototoxic and more conveniently prepared and administered than ethacrynic acid (10,11). However, in terms of diuretic potency they are essentially equivalent. Nierenberg (12) has reviewed 17 studies in which furosemide or ethacrynic acid were administered in treating acute renal failure. There was no consistency with regard to dose. In the only randomized, controlled study, established acute renal failure was treated with 3 mg/kg of furosemide followed every four hours by equal doses if diuresis was maintained between 20 and 100 ml/hour. If urine flow remained below 20 ml/hour, a 6 mg/kg dose was given. Patients were given 1.5 mg/kg every four hours if urine flow was between 100 and 150 ml/hour. Only 10 of 33 patients treated with furosemide had a diuretic response. There was no significant difference between the control and treatment groups with respect to duration of oliguria, number of dialyses, or the mean period of renal insufficiency (13). Other controlled, nonrandomized studies suggest that large doses of furosemide will shorten the duration of oliguria and shorten the time to achieve a daily urine output of 1500 ml. The requirement for dialysis may also be modestly decreased (12).

Once pre-renal azotemia is ruled out with appropriate urinary indices, a trial dose of furosemide, 1.5 mg/kg, may be given. If no response is obtained in four hours, the initial dose may be doubled. There is no advantage to be gained from giving further furosemide challenges in the absence of a response, since in such cases acute renal failure is probably well established (4).

7. How should M.B. be managed with respect to fluids, electrolytes, and nutrition once a diagnosis of acute renal failure has been established?

Therapy at this point can be divided into conservative management and dialysis. The aim of therapy is to limit the intake of all substances requiring renal excretion.

Fluid. A fluid intake of 400 ml plus measured volume losses (urine, GI drainage, etc.) is considered average in a 70 kg man. With excessive tissue catabolism, as in traumatic injury or sepsis, there is an increased endogenous liberation of fluid, making daily requirements smaller. In contrast, profuse sweating or diarrhea would increase fluid requirements. The patient should be weighed daily as a simple check on overall fluid balance (5,21).

Electrolytes. Since the kidneys are no longer able to concentrate or dilute urine during acute renal failure, regulation of solute balance and hence osmolality is dependent upon the net osmotic intake. The serum sodium concentration will usually remain normal if sodium intake is maintained between 30 and 60 mEq per day. Hyponatremia, if present, usually represents serum dilution from excess body water, and management requires further fluid restriction. Within days of the onset of acute renal failure, serum phosphorus tends to rise and serum calcium falls. The use of oral phosphate-binding antacids will minimize both of these problems. If hypocalcemia is manifested by latent tetany, calcium gluconate (30 ml of a 10% solution) may be administered slowly. Caution must be exercised when correcting acidosis with the administration of alkalinizing solutions since the abrupt lowering of ionized calcium may cause tetany (5,21). See the section on Chronic Renal Failure for further discussion of electrolyte abnormalities.

Nutrition. The reduction or prevention of protein catabolism is necessary if accumulation of the nitrogenous metabolites responsible for uremic symptoms is to be prevented. During the stress associated with acute renal failure, energy demands can be met by the use of hypertonic glucose (37 to 47%). Glucose administration also elevates serum insulin levels, causing reduced muscle protein breakdown and improved protein synthesis. Although protein-free diets were once advocated, it is now recognized that diets composed of high-quality protein (0.5 to 0.6 gm/kg per day) may decrease azotemia and improve clinical status (5,22,23). Thus the management of M.B. requires careful monitoring of fluid losses, daily weights, regulation of solute intake, the use of phosphate-binding antacids, and a diet containing high-quality protein. See the chapter on Pa-

renteral Nutrition for specific nutritional recommendations.

8. *Trauma-Induced Renal Failure.* J.A. is a 44-year-old male who sustained multiple injuries from an automobile accident. On examination in the emergency room he was semiconscious with severe hypotension. Crush injuries were noted on his lower extremities. How does the management of a trauma patient such as this differ from the management of the patient described in Question 1?

Depending on the degree of muscle damage incurred, variable amounts of myoglobin are released into the circulation. Large amounts of filtered myoglobin may precipitate and cause a sludging in renal tubules which promotes renal failure. Myoglobinuria produces a red-brown urine which tests positive when treated with routine indicators such as orthotolidine, benzidine, and guaiac. More sophisticated laboratory procedures are necessary to distinguish hemoglobinuria and hematuria from myoglobinuria (14). Examination of the BUN to serum creatinine ratio may reveal a value less than the normal of 10:1 because creatinine phosphate released from damaged muscle causes a relatively more rapid rise in the serum creatinine. Other indicators of damaged muscle include elevated creatine phosphokinase (CPK) and serum glutamic oxaloacetic transaminase (SGOT). Treatment of myoglobinuria is directed at increasing renal blood flow with mannitol and maintaining myoglobin solubility with sodium bicarbonate. This "trauma cocktail" consists of a liter of 5% dextrose from which 200 ml have been removed. Two ampules of sodium bicarbonate (100 mEq) and two ampules of mannitol (25 gm) are then added. One liter is given at a rate of 250 ml/hr. If urine output is adequate at the end of four hours, the solution is continued at a rate which will replace hourly urine losses. If no response is seen at four hours, it is assumed that renal parenchymal damage is present and further trials will be of no benefit (15).

9. *Furosemide-Induced Ototoxicity.* S.D. is a 25-year-old, 60 kg woman who developed septic shock five days after an uncomplicated cesarean section. Despite the administration of fluids, oliguria developed over the

next 12 hours. Acute tubular necrosis was diagnosed by an analysis of urine (many darkly pigmented granular casts) and a renal failure index (see Table 1) greater than 5. Two rapid intravenous boluses of furosemide, 120 mg followed by 360 mg several hours later, were given unsuccessfully in an attempt to increase urine flow. Minutes after the second dose, the patient noted the sudden onset of bilateral deafness and could hear only shouted commands (adapted from reference 12).

What factors contributed to the development of furosemide ototoxicity in this patient? How might it have been prevented?

Furosemide induced ototoxicity is an uncommon finding, occurring in less than 0.2% of patients receiving less than 80 mg (12,16,17). It is significant that all reported cases of ototoxicity have occurred in patients with impaired renal function. Doses greater than 100 mg are, however, seldom given for conditions other than acute renal failure. The coadministration of furosemide with other potentially ototoxic drugs such as aminoglycosides may potentiate this toxicity, although this has not been proven.

Hearing loss appears to be most closely related to the rate of furosemide administration. The rate at which S.D. received her furosemide is not known. However, infusions of large doses at 25 mg per minute produced acute reversible hearing loss in 50 to 60% of those patients studied (18). Doses given at 15 mg per minute were noted to produce only "minor hearing losses which the subjects were not aware of" (19). The manufacturer's recommendations are conflicting in that the text refers to the administration of 80 mg of IV furosemide over 1 to 2 minutes; however, specific recommendations on infusion suggest that large doses be given no faster than 4 mg per minute (20). In our experience, infusions given at 15 mg per minute are well tolerated without clinical sequelae. Thus, S.D. should have received her doses over 8 and 24 minutes respectively.

CHRONIC RENAL FAILURE

Chronic renal failure may be defined as a progressive deterioration in renal function as evidenced by a rise in BUN and serum creatinine, a decline in creatinine clearance, and the development of uremic symptoms.

The term *uremia* refers to the symptom complex associated with severe renal functional impairment. It may take months, or even years, to reach what is termed end-stage renal failure. The downhill progression of renal function depends on the primary cause of the renal failure, the frequency of relapsing episodes of acute renal failure, and on the occurrence of complications which accompany renal failure (24–28).

The causes of chronic renal failure are multiple and include glomerulonephritis, pyelonephritis, and polycystic renal disease. Some systemic diseases leading to chronic renal failure are diabetes mellitus, amyloidosis, lupus erythematosus, hypertension, polyarteritis nodosa, tuberculosis, sickle-cell anemia, and multiple myeloma (29). A number of agents can cause interstitial nephritis which represents a potentially preventable or reversible form of chronic renal failure. These include drugs, hyperuricemia, oxalate deposition, and heavy metals (24).

In general, kidney damage which leads to chronic renal failure is irreversible. However, there are cases in which renal function that is already compromised may become further reduced over a period of days to months because of reversible pre-renal or post-renal factors. These reversible factors must be sought and corrected to prevent further deterioration of the patient's renal function and to restore it to pre-existing levels. These factors include obstructive uropathy, urinary tract infection, or any cause of acute renal failure which diminishes renal perfusion. Drugs can also cause reversible renal toxicity. Examples include diuretic-induced hypovolemia, decreased renal perfusion secondary to antihypertensives, and nephrotoxic antibiotics such as cephaloridine, methicillin, amphotericin, and the aminoglycosides. Obstruction can also occur secondary to crystalluria induced by sulfonamides, uricosurics, or radiocontrast dyes (24–28).

The major complications of chronic renal failure are listed in Table 2. Some of these are discussed in more detail in the cases which follow.

Anemia

10. M.S. is a 49-year-old female with chronic renal failure secondary to a long history of diabetes and hypertension. She was admitted to the hospital with a chief complaint of severe abdominal pain, nausea, and vomit-

ing. An upper gastrointestinal series revealed a small peptic ulcer. She also complains of arthritic type pain in her knees and

Table 2.

COMPLICATIONS OF CHRONIC RENAL FAILURE

Hematological	anemia
Hemostasis defects	bleeding
Metabolic	carbohydrate intolerance
	hyperuricemia
Endocrine	abnormalities in calcium
	and phosphorus
	hyperparathyroidism
	renal osteodystrophy
	sexual dysfunction
	infertility
Cardiovascular	hypertension
	congestive heart failure
	pericarditis
	atherosclerosis
Gastrointestinal	anorexia
	nausea
	vomiting
	G.I. bleeding
	ulcers
Neurological	headache
	lethargy
	muscular irritability and
	cramps
	asterixis
	paresthesias
	motor weakness
	seizures
	coma
Dermatological	pallor
	hyperpigmentation
	ecchymosis
	pruritus
	uremic frost
	calcium deposition
Fluid/Electrolyte	sodium and potassium
	imbalance
	acidosis
	extracellular fluid imbalance
Psychological	depression
	anxiety
	psychosis
Infection	increased susceptibility
	hepatitis

hands for which she has been treating herself with aspirin. Because the aspirin frequently caused her gastrointestinal irritation, she has been taking Maalox with each dose. On physical examination she appeared pale and in moderate distress from her abdominal pain. Her blood pressure was 170/100 mm Hg, her heart rate was 70/minute, and her respiratory rate was 14/minute. Ophthalmologic examination revealed arteriolar narrowing without exudates. Heart and chest examination were within normal limits. Her extremities revealed characteristic arthritic changes. No spleen or liver enlargement were noted. X-ray showed bony deformities secondary to arthritis and density changes consistent with renal osteodystrophy. She stopped taking all medications two days prior to admission because of increasing GI symptoms.

Laboratory data included the following: Sodium 143 mEq/L (normal 132–145), potassium 5.8 mEq/L (normal 3.5–4.7), chloride 110 mEq/L (normal 95–108), CO_2 Content 18 mEq/L (normal 24–32), calcium 7.5 mg/dl (normal 8.4–10.4), phosphorus 5.4 mg/dl (normal 2.5–5), magnesium 4.3 mg/dl (normal 1.4–2.6), uric acid 12 mg/dl (normal 1.5–6.6 for females), hemoglobin 8 gm/dl (normal 11.5–15.5 for females), hematocrit 24% (normal 35–46 for females), platelet count 74,000/cu mm (normal 150,000–450,000), glucose, fasting 200 mg/dl (normal 60–120), serum creatinine 6.0 mg/dl (normal less than 1.4), blood urea nitrogen 80 mg/dl (normal 5–25), creatinine clearance 15 ml/min (normal 108 ± 20 for females).

Her present medications include: hydrochlorothiazide 50 mg bid, methyldopa 500 mg qid, maalox 30 cc prn, NPH insulin 10 units q AM, aspirin 600 mg prn.

What are the characteristics and etiology of the anemia seen in M.S.?

Patients with chronic renal failure inevitably develop anemia, and the occurrence of pallor and fatigue are the earliest clinical signs. The anemia first becomes evident when the serum creatinine exceeds 3 mg/dl and worsens progressively as renal function declines (30,31).

The anemia of chronic renal failure will usually stabilize at a hematocrit of approximately 20 to 25% in the absence of other associated anemias. The anemia is characteristically normochromic and normocytic in nature unless a concomitant iron or folate deficiency exists. Uremic anemia is generally well tolerated except in elderly patients or those with angina pectoris, cerebral ischemia, or congestive heart failure. Our patient appears to tolerate her anemia well since there is no evidence of tachycardia, tachypnea, or heart enlargement suggestive of failure. The increased tolerance to uremic anemia is in part due to increased RBC adenosine triphosphate (ATP), 2,3-diphosphoglycerate (2,3-DPG), and metabolic acidosis which lowers oxygen's affinity for hemoglobin, allowing for greater tissue oxygenation (31,32).

A number of factors have been demonstrated to contribute to the anemia of chronic renal failure. Reduced erythrocyte production appears to be the most significant etiologic factor. Due to progressive damage to kidney tissue, erythropoietin production, an endocrine product of the kidney, is diminished (31,33). As a result, red blood cell formation in the marrow is reduced and anemia occurs. However, the fact that anephric patients can respond, though inefficiently, to hemorrhage or hypoxia with a reticulocytosis demonstrates that total hormonal control of erythropoiesis may not lie within the kidney. In fact, extrarenal production through a hepatic erythropoietin globulin has been described (34). However, this non-renal source is minimal, since anephric patients usually cannot stimulate erythropoiesis as well as patients with remnant kidneys (31).

Inhibitors of erythropoiesis may also exist in the plasma of patients with chronic renal failure. These substances may inhibit the production of erythropoietin, the bone marrow response to erythropoietin, and/or the synthesis of heme. The existence of these substances is confirmed by the observation that dialyzed patients who have no increase in blood erythropoietin levels display improvement in erythropoiesis. This, as well as other evidence, indicates that there may be a dialyzable erythroid depressant factor in renal failure (31,34,35).

The red blood cell lifespan is reduced to 30 to 60% of normal in chronic renal failure patients. The hemolysis is generally mild, and is due to the abnormal chemical environment of uremia. The exact nature of these hemolytic factors in uremic plasma is unknown, and the hemolysis is not uniformly reversed with dialysis. Other causes contributing to or aggravating the hemolysis are

malignant hypertension, hypersplenism, and dialysis fluid that has been contaminated with copper, nitrates, or chloramine. In addition, use of a hypotonic dialysate may lead to a fatal hemolytic episode (31). Yawata et al (36), found that 50% of uremic patients have a uremic plasma factor which inhibits the RBC hexose monophosphate shunt's ability to generate NADPH, thereby reducing the RBC's ability to handle oxidative stress. Hence, survival is reduced. Some patients may need to be screened for red-cell hexose monophosphate shunt deficiency since drugs known to cause glucose-6-phosphate dehydrogenase hemolytic anemia may produce the same reaction in these patients.

Blood loss is a frequent contributing factor to the anemia of chronic renal disease (31). Because of the impaired hemostasis of uremia, gastrointestinal tract and intradermal bleeding are frequent. M.S. has a peptic ulcer and a history of aspirin ingestion; both factors can be responsible for some G.I. blood loss. Although a stool guaiac was not performed in M.S. most uremic patients will have a positive test. In addition, dialysis patients have an obligate blood loss that is related to the techniques and complications inherent in dialysis. It has been estimated that blood loss approximates 75 ml per dialysis treatment or 22 units of whole blood per year (37). Patients on hemodialysis are given heparin during the procedure and occasionally receive warfarin or antiplatelet drugs to prevent clotting. Thus, bleeding may occur from the administration of these drugs.

Iron deficiency may develop secondary to blood loss. The diagnosis of iron deficiency anemia by laboratory parameters is difficult since serum iron is typically low in chronic renal failure. Serum ferritin, which reflects bone marrow stores of iron, may be the best objective measure of deficiency. A low serum ferritin is consistent with iron deficiency; however, a normal or high value does not rule out iron deficiency since marrow iron is often high as a result of impaired incorporation of iron into hemoglobin. Treatment is, therefore, often based on a careful history and evidence of chronic blood loss.

In a study of patients on maintenance hemodialysis who were iron deficient as evidenced by a low serum ferritin, a greater erythropoietic response was seen with oral iron sulfate than with parenteral iron dextran. Oral iron supplementation represents the treatment of choice in most patients (38).

Folic acid deficiency as evidenced by low folate levels and macrocytosis is not uncommon in renal failure (39–42). However, a recent study by Paine et al (43), noted subnormal serum folate levels in only 10% of chronic renal failure patients who were not on dialysis, and none had a megaloblastic anemia. Nevertheless, folate deficiency occurs most frequently in patients on dialysis since folic acid is readily removed by dialysis (44).

Pyridoxine (Vitamin B_6) deficiency has been observed in both chronic renal failure and hemodialysis patients. It is mentioned here because of the marked similarities between this deficiency and the symptoms of uremia, which include skin hyperpigmentation and peripheral neuropathy. Higher requirements are necessary for patients taking isoniazid, hydralazine, oral contraceptives, thyroid hormones, and levodopa (45,46).

11. How should M.S.'s anemia be treated?

Treatment of the anemia of chronic renal failure includes a variety of approaches. Initially, it is important to correct any iron deficiency with oral ferrous sulfate, 300 mg three times daily, or parenteral iron in patients who show evidence of gastrointestinal intolerance or noncompliance. Based on M.S.'s history of aspirin use and peptic ulcer disease, parenteral iron replacement should be utilized. Folic acid is usually administered orally at a dose of 1 mg per day. Pyridoxine is given daily in the form of a multivitamin which contains from 1 to 5 mg per tablet. In addition to vitamin and mineral supplements, adequate oral nutrition is very important (41,45). Also see chapter on Anemias.

Although dialysis does not fully correct the anemia, it has been shown that regular dialysis will improve erythrokinetics and may be essential in the management of uremic anemia (34,47). At the initiation of hemodialysis, the hematocrit frequently falls and then progressively increases over the next 6 to 12 months. The effect of dialysis on erythropoiesis rarely restores the hematocrit to normal, but can raise it to the low thirties (31).

Blood transfusions are avoided, if possible, in patients with chronic renal failure because there is a risk of hepatitis, iron overload, and further suppression of erythropoiesis. Transfusions may,

however, be required in certain patients to restore oxygen carrying capacity and alleviate the symptoms of anemia. Recent evidence indicates that blood transfusions given to dialysis patients can increase graft survival following renal transplantation (24,28).

12. Are androgens effective in the treatment of the anemia of chronic renal failure?

Androgens can increase erythropoiesis in many chronic renal failure patients. They act by directly or indirectly raising erythropoietin levels, thereby increasing RBC production. Various clinical trials have been conducted using a number of androgenic compounds at different dosages. The interpretation of many of these studies is complicated because most are not controlled and patients were sometimes iron and vitamin deficient, given blood transfusions, or not treated for sufficient periods of time. Thus, direct comparison of the data to determine which androgen is the most suitable or the most potent is extremely difficult.

The most commonly used androgens include the orally administered 17-alpha-alkylated products, oxymetholone, fluoxymesterone, and methyltestosterone, or parenterally administered testosterone enanthate or nandrolone decanoate. Male patients usually require larger amounts of a given androgen than females to elicit a similar hematologic response. Anephric patients generally do not respond as well to androgen therapy as do patients with intact kidneys; therefore, nephrectomized patients may, therefore, require a higher dose of androgen. The maximum response from androgen therapy may not be observed for three or more months.

Side effects reported from the use of androgens in chronic renal failure patients on dialysis include: virilization, weight gain, muscle soreness, abnormal hair growth, priapism, acne, and swelling and hematoma at injection sites. Some of these effects are particularly disturbing to female patients, such as M.S., who sometimes refuse androgen therapy. Nandrolone decanoate is preferred in females since it has a high anabolic: androgenic ratio and produces fewer undesirable masculinizing effects (30). Hepatic dysfunction with hepatomegaly and abnormal liver function tests may occur. The orally administered 17-alpha-alkylated compounds are generally considered more hepatotoxic than the others and have been associated with the development of hepatocellular carcinoma (48). Despite these effects, androgens are useful to dialysis patients in improving their anemia and in reducing symptoms and may reduce the number of blood transfusions they require.

Doses. Nandrolone decanoate (Decadurabolin) 100–200 mg is commonly administered intramuscularly at weekly intervals. Alternative therapy includes oral administration of fluoxymesterone (Halotestin) in doses of 30 mg/day for males and 10 mg/day for females (35,49–54).

Other methods that have been used in treating the anemia of chronic renal failure include splenectomy, histidine supplementation and even the administration of exogenous erythropoietin (27,31).

Hemostatic Defects

13. M.S. (Question 10) was noted to have thrombocytopenia. Describe the quantitative and qualitative defects of platelets associated with uremia.

Uremia is frequently complicated by excessive bleeding as evidenced by ecchymosis, purpura, low-grade gastrointestinal bleeding, epistaxis, and less commonly, profuse gastrointestinal hemorrhage.

Estimates of moderate to severe hemorrhage vary from 12 to 63% of patients depending on the study (55). Capillary fragility and a decrease in plasma coagulation factors have been excluded by most investigators as major causes of uremic bleeding. A quantitative deficiency of platelets has been suggested as a cause for the bleeding tendency in uremics since thrombocytopenia (less than 150,000/mm^3) has been reported in up to 53% of renal failure patients. However, values of less than 50,000/mm^3 are rarely seen (55), and it is generally agreed that thrombocytopenia is not a significant causative factor of uremic bleeding. Platelet lifespan has also been shown to be normal. A functional platelet defect in uremic platelets has been demonstrated although its exact nature is unknown. Earlier reports suggested an inhibition or deficiency of platelet factor 3 (56,57); however, the prolonged bleeding times observed in uremics cannot totally be accounted for on this basis. The possibility of defects in platelet adhesion and ADP-induced aggregation have also been considered. Apparently, abnormalities of several platelet functions lead to the overall platelet defect (57,58).

A specific uremic toxin responsible for defective platelet function has not been identified. However, guanidinosuccinic acid, phenol, and phenolic acids are toxins known to accumulate in uremia which have been shown to produce qualitative platelet defects. Whatever the specific toxin, the platelet abnormalities of uremia can be corrected and normal hemostasis maintained with frequent hemodialysis or peritoneal dialysis. Whenever bleeding occurs, thorough dialysis is the treatment of choice (58).

A regular dialysis program and avoidance of antiplatelet drugs can substantially reduce the occurrence of uremic bleeding. The aspirin taken by M.S. is a very potent inhibitor of platelet aggregation and its use should be avoided whenever possible in uremic patients. A list of drugs which have clinically important antiplatelet activity is provided in Table 3.

Calcium and Vitamin D Metabolism

14. Describe the mechanisms responsible for the hyperphosphatemia and hypocalcemia observed in M.S.

Hypocalcemia associated with hyperphosphatemia, hyperparathyroidism, and vitamin D resistance are frequent problems of chronic renal failure which may lead to the secondary complication of renal osteodystrophy. Pathologic studies indicate that 55 to 80% of patients dying of chronic renal failure have renal osteodystrophy (61). This major cause of disability refers to one or more of the following disorders: osteomalacia, osteitis fibrosa cystica, osteosclerosis, or osteoporosis associated with chronic renal failure.

No single mechanism has yet been identified as being responsible for the diverse forms of bone disease seen. Hyperparathyroidism, which is seen

Table 3.

DRUGS WITH ANTIPLATELET ACTIVITY

acetylsalicylic acid	indomethacin
carbenicillin	oxyphenbutazone
dextran	penicillin G
dipyridamole	phenylbutazone
hydroxychloroquine	sulfinpyrazone

(59,60)

at all stages of renal impairment, is certainly responsible for the development of osteitis fibrosa cystica. Phosphate retention plays a major role in the development of secondary hyperparathyroidism. For each decrement in renal function there is a transient and possibly undetectable rise in serum phosphorus. This slight hyperphosphatemia results in a decrease in ionized calcium which stimulates the release of parathyroid hormone (PTH) (see Fig. 1). An increase in PTH tends to bring serum calcium levels toward normal by increasing tubular phosphate excretion. Normalization of serum phosphate promotes the renal conversion of 25-hydroxycholecalciferol (25-HCC) to 1,25-dihydroxycholecalciferol (1,25-DHCC), thus enhancing intestinal calcium absorption and bone mobilization. At glomerular filtration rates of less than 30 ml per minute the loss of nephrons and persistent hyperphosphatemia reduce the synthesis of 1,25-DHCC. Low circulating 1,25-DHCC results in bone resistance to PTH and calcium malabsorption (62).

15. How should M.S.'s renal osteodystrophy and calcium and phosphate abnormalities be managed?

The objectives of management for osteodystrophy associated with chronic renal failure are to: a) keep serum calcium and phosphorus levels near normal, b) suppress PTH secretion, and c) restore normal skeletal development. The degree of renal impairment largely determines the therapy selected (63).

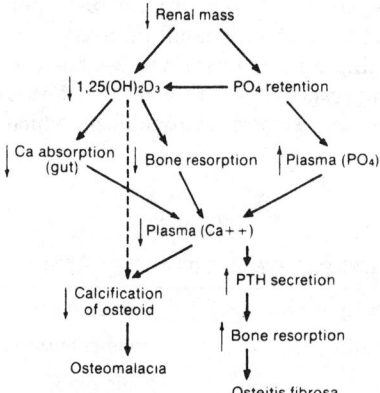

Figure 1. Pathogenesis of secondary hyperparathyroidism and osteodystrophy (osteitis fibrosa plus osteomalacia) in chronic renal insufficiency. Adapted from Kidney International (reference 166) with permission.

Phosphate-Binding Gels. During the early stages of renal impairment, dietary phosphorus could be reduced through restriction of meat, milk, legumes, and carbonated beverages. Since this may be difficult, phosphate-binding gels may be incorporated. A comparison of available phosphate-binding antacids is given in Table 4. When 15 to 30 ml of aluminum carbonate (Basaljel) or aluminum hydroxide (Amphojel) are administered with or immediately following meals and at bedtime, dietary phosphate and phosphate contained in gastrointestinal secretions form an insoluble complex which is excreted in the stool. Aluminum hydroxide capsules (Alucaps) may be substituted if the antacid gels are poorly tolerated. Up to 3 or 4 capsules may be administered with meals (45). Serum phosphorus levels should be measured to permit adjustment of antacids and prevent the development of severe hypophosphatemia.

Oral Calcium. Oral calcium supplementation may be necessary because the intestinal absorption of calcium is impaired in renal failure and because uremic patients who consume few dairy products ingest insufficient amounts of calcium. Since calcium is absorbed by passive ionic diffusion as well as under the influence of vitamin D (64–67), oral supplementation may normalize serum calcium without the addition of vitamin D therapy. A total calcium intake of 1 to 1.5 gm should be provided by supplementing dietary calcium with calcium gluconate (9% Ca), calcium carbonate (40% Ca), or calcium lactate (13% Ca). Oral calcium should not be initiated until serum phosphorous levels are below 5.5 to 6.0 mg/dl. A calcium–phosphate product greater than 70 must be avoided because soft tissue calcification may occur (63,65). Calcific deposits may occur in the heart, lung, skeletal muscle, blood vessel walls, and periarticular tissue (66).

Vitamin D. If the above regimens have not been successful in maintaining a normal serum calcium or PTH level, then a trial of vitamin D is warranted. Vitamin D is available as ergocalciferol (vitamin D_2), cholecalciferol (vitamin D_3), 25-hydroxycholecaliferol (25-HCC), 1,25-dihydroxycholecalciferol (1,25-DHCC, calcitriol), and the synthetic dihydrotachysterol (DHT). The response to vitamins D_2 and D_3 can vary substantially depending on the degree of renal failure and the ability of the kidney to convert these vitamins to the biologically active 1,25-DHCC. Vitamin D_2 doses of 4,000–200,000 IU/day (0.1 mg–

Table 4.

PHOSPHATE BINDING CAPACITY OF
SELECTED ANTACIDS

Product	Contents	Phosphate Binding Capacity	Elemental Aluminum Content (gm/30 ml)
Amphojel	Aluminum hydroxide	+2	0.636
Basaljel	Aluminum carbonate	+4	0.87
Phosphaljel	Aluminum phosphate	0	
Gelusil	Aluminum & magnesium hydroxide	+3	
Maalox	Aluminum & magnesium hydroxide	+3	0.716
Mylanta	Aluminum & magnesium hydroxide & simethicone	+2	
Riopan	Aluminum-magnesium hydroxide complex	+1	0.276
Titralac	Calcium carbonate & glycine	0	0

Adapted from Bailey (47).

5 mg) may be required to produce improvement in skeletal disease (63). The potential for vitamin D intoxication and sustained hypercalcemia which may require weeks for resolution is a major hazard associated with pharmacologic doses of vitamin D. In contrast, a physiologic dose of 1,25-DHCC (0.5–2.0 mcg/day) produces an initial response within days. Furthermore, because 1,25-DHCC has a short half-life, hypercalcemia can be corrected rapidly should intoxication occur (62,63,68). Serum calcium levels are used to modify the dose of 1,25-DHCC. If the serum calcium does not increase by 0.5 mg/dl 4 to 6 weeks after 1,25-DHCC has been initiated, the dose should be increased by 0.25–0.5 mcg/day. This approach may be continued until serum calcium reaches the normal range. Frequent calcium determinations are needed to detect hypercalcemia which may occur with prolonged therapy (69). DHT (0.2 to 1 mg/day) was the only agent available for the management of vitamin D-resistant renal osteodystrophy until the recent introduction of 1,25-DHCC and 25-HCC. It shares the advantages of a short half-life and rapid onset of action (70). However, like the newer 1-alpha-hydroxycholecalciferol (1-HCC) it must undergo hepatic 25-hydroxylation before it becomes active. Patients with severe hepatic disease or those receiving phenobarbital or phenytoin, which impair 25-hydroxylation, may have an impaired response to DHT or 1-HCC (68,71,72).

There are several reports in the literature which warn about the use of vitamin D congeners in non-dialyzed patients such as M.S. In a study of non-dialyzed patients with moderate to advanced renal disease, a deterioration in renal function was noted in patients taking 1-HCC (5.5% per month decrease in creatinine clearance during treatment compared to a decrease of 1.7% per month prior to and 2.5% per month after treatment). Similar changes have also been noted with 1,25 DHCC and DHT (70,73,74). Others have not witnessed this change in renal function or have attributed it to transient or sustained hypercalcemia which may cause renal damage secondary to an elevated calcium-phosphate product and subsequent deposition of calcium salts in renal tissue. Caution must be exercised to avoid hypercalcemia by administering the lowest effective dose and obtaining frequent calcium determinations (69,75). Despite many advances in the management of renal osteodystrophy, bone disease will not improve in 20–30% of patients because of unidentifiable factors which may be of importance in its pathogenesis (76).

Gastrointestinal Complications

16. M.S.'s (Question 10) chief complaint includes severe abdominal pain, nausea, and vomiting. Could these be related to her chronic renal failure?

There is a high incidence of gastric acid hypersecretion and duodenal ulcer secondary to elevated serum gastrin levels in uremics. Gastrin levels are inversely related to renal function, probably because its renal degradation is reduced (77). The saliva of uremics contains a high concentration of urea which undergoes transformation to ammonia through the action of salivary urease. The ammonia which is swallowed produces an erosive gastritis leading to further GI discomfort. Gastric ammonia is then absorbed and converted back to urea in the liver, thus completing the cycle (78). Physical examination may reveal a malodorous breath characteristic of ammonia which is often associated with nausea, vomiting, and loss of appetite. Gastric acid hypersecretion is treated with antacids or cimetidine. Hypersecretion should, however, be documented since serum gastrin levels may be elevated without a subsequent rise in gastric acid secretion (77). Lowering serum urea concentrations by dialysis may be the only way to control the local production of ammonia.

Patients with GI symptoms should also be carefully questioned about their use of drugs which are irritating to the GI tract.

17. *Complications of Antacid Therapy.* A.C. was seen in the nephrology clinic with complaints of generalized muscle weakness and depression. His chronic renal failure has been treated conservatively over the past four years. The only recent change in therapy was a substitution of Amphogel for AlternaGel because of increased palatability. He maintained his previous dose of 30 ml before meals and at bedtime. How might this change in therapy be related to his current symptoms? What other antacid-induced problems should be monitored in chronic renal failure patients?

Aluminum-containing Antacids. Amphogel and AlternaGel are both antacids which contain aluminum hydroxide. They contain 64 mg/ml and 120 mg/ml aluminum hydroxide respectively and therefore differ greatly in their phosphate binding capacity. By maintaining the same volume of antacid, A.C. has doubled the amount of phosphate binders he receives. The use of aluminum-containing antacids can cause excessive *phosphate depletion* if serum phosphorus is not carefully followed. The complications resulting from hypophosphatemia include: hypercalcemia, hypercalciuria, osteomalacia and fractures, and defects in erythrocyte, leukocyte, and platelet function related to decreased adenosine triphosphate and 2,3-DPG. The symptoms of phosphate depletion include generalized muscle weakness, malaise, tremors, absence of deep tendon reflexes, bone pain, mental depression, convulsions, and even coma. The complications of hypophosphatemia are generally reversible upon phosphate replacement (79–82).

Long-term administration of aluminum may not in itself be without toxicity. Aluminum antacids are supposedly nonabsorbable, and aluminum does not appear to accumulate in normal subjects after repeated doses of aluminum compounds (83). Nevertheless, significant *elevations in serum* and *tissue aluminum* have been noted in renal failure patients receiving aluminum hydroxide. Berlyne et al (84,85) have described a syndrome of aluminum toxicity in uremic rats consisting of periorbital bleeding, lethargy, anorexia, and death. Elevated plasma levels of aluminum and deposition of aluminum in numerous organs including the brain, liver, heart, muscle, and especially bone were found. Berlyne et al recommend that the use of aluminum salts be curtailed in renal failure patients because of the possibility of aluminum toxicity. However, their failure to measure phosphate levels as well as their administration of parenteral and soluble oral salts of aluminum make their conclusions difficult to evaluate (86). In fact, Thurston et al (87) found that even though small amounts of aluminum are absorbed and deposited in bone, no toxicity related to aluminum itself could be demonstrated in uremic rats. They did show, however, that in normal rats growth-stunting, secondary to aluminum antacid therapy, was related to phosphate depletion. It is thought that some of the toxicity related to aluminum antacid treatment is related to phosphate depletion and can be prevented by avoidance of hypophosphatemia.

Alfrey et al (88) also demonstrated elevated levels of aluminum in muscle, bone, and brain tissue in dialyzed patients who were receiving aluminum antacid therapy. They suggest a relationship between the excess aluminum levels and the development of a fatal neurologic syndrome referred to as the dialysis encephalopathy syndrome. Additional studies are needed to further define this complication.

Magnesium-containing Antacids. Antacids containing magnesium should be used cautiously, if at all, in renal failure patients. Significant amounts of magnesium from antacids and cathartics can be absorbed from the gastrointestinal tract. Since magnesium levels within the body are controlled by glomerular filtration and distal tubular reabsorption, a lowering of the glomerular filtration rate below 20 ml/min results in a reduced clearance of magnesium (63,89–92). If a patient with this degree of renal failure or worse is presented with a magnesium load, *magnesium intoxication* may develop. The occurrence of magnesium toxicity in renal failure patients, secondary to antacid or cathartic therapy, is well documented (89,93,94). Ingestion of 150 to 300 ml per day of magnesium-containing products can result in rapid intoxication in these patients (95). Moderate amounts of magnesium-containing antacids can be used if the patient is on regular dialysis (eg, hemodialysis for four hours, three times a week) and avoids ingestion of large quantities of magnesium. However, if the patient has severe renal dysfunction that does not yet require dialysis or is on irregular maintenance dialysis, magnesium compounds should be avoided (63).

Hypermagnesemia is evidenced clinically by central nervous system signs of lethargy, weakness, hyporeflexia, and hypotension. Electrocardiographic abnormalities can be noted at serum concentrations of 8 mEq/L, while complete heart block, coma, and respiratory depression usually occur at higher blood levels.

Treatment for hypermagnesemia consists of administration of parenteral calcium salts (5 to 10 mEq) if severe symptoms of intoxication such as respiratory depression or cardiac arrhythmias are present. Unfortunately, calcium injections are not uniformly effective (89,96). If kidney function is adequate, intravenous furosemide and saline administration can be used to enhance renal magnesium excretion. Dialysis against a bath containing little (1.5 mEq/L) or no magnesium can substantially reduce magnesium levels within four to six hours (89,96). In addition, all magnesium-containing preparations should be discontinued.

Calcium-containing Antacids. Antacids containing calcium should also be used with caution because of the possibility of developing the milk-alkali syndrome, hypercalcemia, nephrocalcinosis, and/or worsening renal function (97,98). Calcium carbonate also has been associated with a rebound increase in gastric acid secretion (99). The significance of this in patients with renal failure is not yet determined. However, this problem is of concern since calcium preparations seem to be effective acid-neutralizing agents, and patients with renal failure frequently receive calcium salts for calcium replacement therapy.

Constipation and fecal impaction are also associated with calcium and aluminum antacids. In fact, intestinal obstruction may even result from the development of solid concretions of antacid in the intestine, especially in patients with renal failure (100). Such obstructions have resulted in rectal-vaginal fistula formation and may require surgical intervention and removal.

Potassium Balance

18. M.S. (described in Question 10) is hyperkalemic (serum potassium 5.8 mEq/L). Describe the mechanisms by which potassium imbalance occurs in chronic renal failure.

Most of the daily load of potassium, approximately 100 mEq, is removed from the body by the kidney. Gastrointestinal losses account for only minimal amounts of potassium elimination.

Potassium is normally filtered at the glomerulus and undergoes nearly complete reabsorption throughout the renal tubule. The potassium excreted in the urine is chiefly the result of distal tubular secretion. A variety of factors affect this distal secretion of potassium, including aldosterone, sodium load presented to the distal reabsorptive site, hydrogen ion secretion, the amount of unreabsorbable anions, urinary flow-rate, diuretics, and potassium intake (101–103).

Serum potassium levels are relatively well-maintained within normal limits in patients with chronic renal failure. With a creatinine clearance greater than 5 ml per minute, the development of hyperkalemia is rare without an endogenous or exogenous load of potassium. This balance is maintained despite a decreasing nephron population and an overall drop in glomerular filtration. The remaining nephron population undergoes adaptive hypertrophy to enhance the distal tubular secretion of potassium per nephron, which is mediated by elevated levels of aldosterone. Increased gastrointestinal secretion and fecal losses may account for up to 50% of the daily potassium losses in patients with severe renal insufficiency (24,101,104).

Episodic *hyperkalemia* can develop in a patient with chronic renal failure under several conditions. Excess potassium loads may result from exogenous sources such as increased dietary intake or drugs (105). Endogenous sources of potassium include cellular destruction, as for example in the hemolysis of red blood cells, rhabdomyolysis, and catabolic states. Metabolic or respiratory acidosis may cause a redistribution of intracellular potassium to the extracellular space. For each 0.1 unit change in blood pH, there is a corresponding opposite change of 0.6 mEq/L in the serum potassium level (24). Potassium-sparing diuretics such as spironolactone or triamterene should be avoided in the presence of renal failure since they decrease tubular secretion of potassium, and their use has been associated with fatal hyperkalemia (106,107). Diabetic patients with normal renal function may develop hyperkalemia from the administration of these diuretics (101). Some diabetic patients with only mild degrees of renal failure may also develop hyperkalemia as a result of low plasma renin levels and subsequently lowered aldosterone levels (24,101).

Paradoxically, *hypokalemia* can occur in chronic renal failure patients. The potassium deficiency can be due to inadequate dietary intake or excessive gastrointestinal (GI) losses. This is related to the anorexia, nausea, vomiting, and diarrhea which accompany the GI irritation that occurs in the uremic patient. Protracted vomiting may lead to hypokalemia through induction of a hypochloremic alkalosis and through loss of potassium-rich fluids. Furthermore, hypovolemia and other conditions may induce hyperaldosteronism which will enhance urinary losses of potassium (24,101). Other causes of hypokalemia include glucocorticoid therapy, Cushing's syndrome, licorice abuse, laxative abuse, excessive diuretic therapy, and renal tubular acidosis (101,104). Also see the chapters on Fluid and Electrolyte Disorders and Congestive Heart Failure.

19. Is treatment of M.S.'s potassium indicated? How should severe hyperkalemia be managed?

Treatment of hyperkalemia depends upon the serum level of potassium as well as the presence or absence of symptoms and electrocardiographic (ECG) changes. Manifestations of hyperkalemia include weakness, confusion, and muscular or respiratory paralysis. Early ECG changes include peaked T waves, followed by a decreased R wave amplitude, widened QRS complex, and a prolonged P-R interval. This may progress to complete heart block with absent P waves, and finally a sine wave. Ventricular arrhythmias or cardiac arrest may ensue if no effort to lower serum potassium is initiated. Hyperkalemic ECG changes are uncommon at potassium levels of less than 7 mEq/L but occur regularly at levels above 8 mEq/L.

Since M.S. has a mild potassium elevation of 5.8 mEq/L, no specific treatment is required. Generally, no treatment is necessary if potassium is less than 6.5 mEq/L and there are no ECG changes. If potassium levels rise above 6.5 mEq/L, especially with neuromuscular symptoms or changes in the ECG, treatment should be instituted.

Treatment of hyperkalemia consists of three basic modalities. The first is calcium administration to counteract the effects of excess potassium on the heart. Second, glucose or alkali therapy lowers serum potassium by shifting it from extracellular to intracellular fluid compartments. Thirdly, exchange resins or dialysis are used to remove potassium from the body.

Calcium. In the presence of life-threatening arrhythmias, 5 to 10 ml of a 10% calcium gluconate solution may be given intravenously over 2 minutes to antagonize the cardiac toxicity of hyperkalemia. The injection may be repeated in 5 minutes; continuous monitoring of the ECG is mandatory. The cardiac response to an injection of calcium begins within 5 minutes and lasts from 1 to 2 hours. Since administration of calcium does not lower the serum potassium, other modes of treatment must also be instituted. Patients receiving digitalis should be given calcium cautiously.

Bicarbonate. Additional emergency treatment consists of *sodium bicarbonate* 50 mEq injected intravenously over 5 minutes. This may be repeated every 10 to 15 minutes as needed to reverse ECG abnormalities. Sodium bicarbonate is used because the alkaline systemic pH it produces favors the shift of potassium intracellularly, and the sodium load enhances distal tubular potassium secretion. It should be used cautiously in patients with congestive heart failure.

Glucose plus Insulin. Glucose and insulin infusions also shift potassium intracellularly. One unit of insulin for every 2 grams of glucose is administered. Two to three hundred ml of a 20% glucose solution containing 20 to 30 units of regular insulin are infused over 30 to 60 minutes. This should produce a 1 to 2 mEq/L reduction of serum potassium for approximately 12 to 24 hours. The glucose-insulin infusion can then be continued at a slower rate and titrated against the serum potassium level. Sodium bicarbonate may be added to the solution containing glucose and insulin. The onset of effect is less than 30 minutes with either alkali or glucose-insulin therapy. The volume of fluid administered is a consideration in oliguric patients or those with heart failure or hypertension.

Cation Exchange Resins. Cation exchange resins also lower serum potassium and maintain low potassium levels. Rectal retention enemas containing 50 gm of sodium polystyrene sulfonate (Kayexalate) suspended in 50 ml of 70% sorbitol and 100 ml of tap water can reduce serum potassium levels by 0.5 to 2.0 mEq/L, 30 to 90 minutes after a single dose. The enema should be retained for at least 30 to 60 minutes and may be repeated as needed thereafter. The sorbitol is used to prevent fecal impactions.

On a chronic basis, oral Kayexalate may be given in a dose of 15 to 20 grams three to four times daily. The dose should be suspended in 20 ml of 70% sorbitol with water added if necessary. The onset of action when given orally ranges from 2 to 12 hours, somewhat longer than when given rectally. The oral route of administration may be preferred by some patients despite some nausea. Semi-diarrhea should be induced with sorbitol before the administration of oral Kayexalate to prevent constipation and fecal impaction. Since this resin exchanges sodium for potassium, consideration must be given to patients with heart failure or elevated blood pressure. Although the oral administration of Kayexalate is often considered unpalatable, it should not be mixed with citrus juices or solutions containing high concentrations of potassium as this will render the resin ineffective.

Dialysis. Hemodialysis and peritoneal dialysis are also effective means of lowering serum potassium, but the results take several hours, making these methods relatively slow. Thus, they should not be used as the primary mode of treatment in emergency situations (4,24,101,103,104, 108–112).

Hyperuricemia

20. Why is M.S.'s serum uric acid elevated (Question 10)? How does chronic renal failure affect uric acid disposition? Does M.S.'s serum uric acid of 12 mg/dl require treatment? What treatments are utilized?

Chronic renal failure is associated with hyperuricemia that is due to reduced excretion of uric acid by the kidneys. Uric acid is normally freely filtered at the glomerulus; only a small fraction of protein-bound urate is not filtered. Up to 98% of the filtered urate load is reabsorbed by the proximal tubules and then secreted distal to the site of reabsorption. It is now believed that uric acid undergoes another reabsorptive process in the latter portion of the proximal tubule after it is secreted. The small fraction of filtered uric acid (6–10%) which finally appears in the urine results from the secreted uric acid that escapes proximal tubular reabsorption. The final reabsorption process is believed to protect the nephron from excessive concentrations of uric acid, and therefore from uric acid stones (113).

As kidney function decreases and the nephron population is reduced, the fractional excretion of filtered urate increases. This means that as the tubular reabsorptive and secretory capacity diminishes with renal failure, there is an increase in the fractional amount of glomerularly filtered urate which escapes reabsorption. Therefore, as renal function decreases, glomerular filtration takes over a greater proportion of the renal excretion of uric acid. In the anuric patient, gastrointestinal secretion provides the only means of urate excretion from the body (113–115).

The degree of hyperuricemia correlates with the severity of renal dysfunction. Serum urate levels are usually maintained within normal limits until the creatinine clearance drops below 30 ml/min, at which point serum urate levels begin to rise. Urate levels may rise well above 20 mg/dl with severe renal failure (114,115).

Excessive urate levels may give rise to three complications: gouty attacks and arthritis; uric acid stones; and urate deposition nephropathy. For unknown reasons gouty attacks and arthritis are not likely to occur in renal failure despite the presence of excessive urate levels. Rarely is urate-lowering therapy begun to prevent gouty attacks in these patients (116). Only if a patient has had a previous gouty history should gouty attacks be expected. The occurrence of slowly progressive renal disease due to gout alone is controversial. Even though this common association exists, the evidence suggests that hyperuricemia is more a result of chronic renal failure than a cause of chronic renal failure. Berger and Yu (117), in a long-term follow-up study of 524 gouty patients, found little evidence that deterioration in renal function occurred more rapidly in their subjects than in a non-gouty population matched for age. They added that the presence of renal urate deposits correlated poorly with renal function (118). Treatment is therefore aimed at those patients with a history of gouty attacks and those with evidence of urate stones. Since M.S. has a negative history, treatment is not indicated.

The conservative management of urate stones, in patients with adequate renal function, consists of liberal fluid intake to reduce the concentration of urinary uric acid, and urinary alkalinization to maintain a urinary pH of 6.0–6.5. A pH greater than 6.5 is not desirable because of possible calcium phosphate crystallization (119,120). Allopurinol may be added if fluid and alkalinization have failed. Uricosuric drugs are ineffective in lowering urate levels if the creatinine clearance is less than 30 ml/min, since tubular function is diminished (114,115,120). There is also the possibility that uricosurics could give rise to a greater incidence of stone formation because of the increased excretion of uric acid.

Allopurinol can be started at 200 to 300 mg per day, usually as a single dose (120–123). Since allopurinol and oxypurinol (a major active metabolite) are both cleared renally, accumulation occurs with decreased renal function (124). Therefore it is necessary to titrate the dose in renal failure. A fair number of patients may be adequately controlled on a smaller dose. Since gouty attacks are uncommon in these patients, prophylactic colchicine is not necessary. Its toxicity, which may be greater in renal failure (125,126), is thereby avoided.

In patients with chronic, irreversible renal failure who have creatinine clearances less than 5 to 10 ml/min, urate-lowering therapy should be questioned as there is essentially no renal function left to save. Invariably most of these patients will come to dialysis which may obviate the need for drug therapy since uric acid is partially dialyzable.

Hyperglycemia

21. M.S. has an elevated fasting glucose. Is this common in chronic renal failure? What mechanisms are involved, and what are the implications for treatment?

Although approximately 70% of uremic patients have varying degrees of "uremic diabetes" manifested by an abnormal glucose tolerance test and elevated fasting insulin levels, fasting blood sugars are generally normal. Peripheral insensitivity to circulating insulin is a well established mechanism of carbohydrate intolerance in uremic patients. This insensitivity has been attributed to several physiologic conditions and chemical substances present in renal failure. These include acidosis, total body potassium deficiency, and elevated growth hormone, urea and guanidinosuccinic acid (77,127–131). However, no one factor has been proven to be conclusively responsible.

Other mechanisms for uremic diabetes include defects in insulin secretion and insulin metabolism (77,128). Uremic diabetes rarely requires treatment since marked symptomatic hyperglycemia and ketoacidosis are rare. However, abnormalities of carbohydrate metabolism in uremics can be partially normalized within several weeks following initiation of hemodialysis (128,131). The exact mechanism by which this is accomplished is unknown.

It is well known that the kidney, as well as the liver, is important in the degradation of insulin within the body (77,130,132,133). Thirty to forty percent of the insulin reaching the kidneys is cleared by this organ. Insulin is normally filtered by the glomerulus; it then undergoes nearly complete proximal tubular reabsorption and catabolism, with less than 2% of the filtered load appearing in the urine. Patients with mild to moderate renal failure have reduced renal degradation of insulin, but they still manage to catabolize a significant amount (132,134). However, in patients with severe renal disease, the insulin half-life may be slightly prolonged and the amount of insulin renally degraded is reduced (77,130–132,135). Insulin requirements of diabetic patients may be decreased in severe renal failure because of altered insulin kinetics. Marked insulin sensitivity with fatal hypoglycemia has been reported in these patients (77,133,136).

M.S. has a history of diabetes and exhibits an elevated fasting glucose as part of her disease process. Control of her diabetes with only 10 units of NPH insulin prior to her acute illness exemplifies the increased sensitivity to insulin in chronic renal failure.

Hypertension

22. When M.S. was admitted to the hospital (Question 10), her blood pressure was 170/100 mm Hg. What is the relationship between hypertension and chronic renal failure? How should hypertension be treated in patients with chronic renal failure?

The kidney plays a major role in the control of blood pressure by regulating extracellular fluid volume and through the renin-angiotensin system (137–139). Hypertension is known to induce renal failure by damaging the renal vasculature. As a consequence, the impaired renal perfusion leads to increased renin secretion which further aggravates the hypertension and worsens renal failure. A vicious cycle is thus established, and in many cases it is unclear which came first, the hypertension or the renal failure (140). In an individual with chronic renal failure, it is often difficult to establish if the hypertension is associated predominantly with volume expansion or high renin levels. However, the primary cause of the hypertension in most of these patients is extracellular volume expansion. This volume overload exists because the kidney is no longer able to excrete fluids efficiently (140–142).

Since elevated blood pressure results in kidney damage, aggressive antihypertensive therapy can improve renal function and long-term survival (143–145). Therefore, the aim of antihypertensive treatment in chronic renal failure patients is to prevent further renal damage. When treating hypertensive patients with renal failure, drugs which cause excessive venous pooling and thus have a substantial orthostatic component (eg, guanethidine) should be avoided. An acute drop in blood pressure can further reduce or even eliminate any remaining renal function. The treatment of hypertension in patients with renal failure is thus complicated by the fact that either too high or too low a blood pressure may have a detrimental effect on residual kidney function. Hence,

antihypertensive drugs which minimally reduce or have no effect on renal blood flow are commonly used (eg, methyldopa, hydralazine). Despite the use of these drugs, patients may still develop elevations in their BUN and serum creatinine at the initiation of therapy. These are caused by reduced renal perfusion secondary to lowered blood pressure. Therapy should be continued, as the elevations are transient and should not be taken as a sign of worsening renal function unless severe hypotension is present (144).

23. M.S.'s hypertension has been treated with hydrochlorothiazide. How should her diuretic therapy be modified in view of her renal function?

Diuretics are relatively mild antihypertensive agents and act primarily by reducing extracellular fluid volume. In patients with renal failure not requiring dialysis, diuretics are the most common treatment modality. Because the effectiveness of thiazides as diuretics is reduced when the creatinine clearance is less than 20–30 ml/min, furosemide is usually the preferred agent. The ability of furosemide to maintain urine flow in patients with renal failure has been adequately demonstrated (146–150). Because diuretics increase renin release, a better response is observed in patients classified as low-renin hypertensives. Less diuretic-induced renin stimulation occurs in these patients compared to normal or high renin producers (151). Because M.S.'s creatinine clearance is only 15 ml/min, she should be given furosemide instead of hydrochlorothiazide at an initial dose of 40 mg daily or 20 mg twice daily.

24. If M.S.'s hypertension is not controlled with diuretics, what other agents or methods of blood pressure reduction could be used?

Antihypertensive therapy at this point would include the addition of methyldopa, propranolol, prazosin or clonidine. Each of these drugs is capable of lowering renin release without compromising renal blood flow (152–156). Hydralazine in combination with either clonidine, methyldopa, or propranolol can be used for further blood pressure control without a significant risk of developing reflex tachycardia. Minoxidil in combination with propranolol and furosemide is effective in the control of hypertension in chronic renal failure patients refractory to other therapy. Thus, it represents the treatment of choice in refractory hypertension and is effective regardless of the degree of renal failure. Minoxidil is not used initially because of the weight gain and edema which invariably occur in non-dialyzed patients. Hypertrichosis is another drawback to its use (157–159).

In patients with severe acute hypertension and renal failure, the direct-acting vasodilators diazoxide (160) or nitroprusside (161) are frequently used. The control of hypertension with diazoxide has been shown to be a critical factor in improving renal function in patients with chronic renal failure (160). The continued administration of nitroprusside to patients with renal failure can lead to accumulation of the toxic metabolite thiocyanate (162–163). Neither diazoxide, nitroprusside, minoxidil, or hydralazine adversely affect renal blood flow, and all are potent stimulators of renin release (140).

Reserpine and guanethidine are rarely used in the patient with renal failure because of frequent side effects. Additionally, guanethidine adversely affects renal blood flow.

Hemodialysis is extremely effective in reducing extracellular fluid volume and lowering blood pressure (140,147,164). Since volume expansion is the major cause of hypertension in chronic renal failure patients, hemodialysis is effective in controlling blood pressure in the majority of cases (137,147). When hemodialysis is initiated, antihypertensive medications may be given in lower doses or even discontinued in some patients. However, in a minority of patients whose hypertension is primarily related to elevated renin levels, the response to dialysis is usually not significant (140).

Bilateral nephrectomy has been used to control blood pressure when antihypertensive drug treatment and dialysis have failed. This procedure eliminates the source of the excessive renin production and controls the patient's hypertension (165).

In summary, aggressive antihypertensive therapy should be initiated in renal failure patients with hypertension. The aim of such therapy is to improve the patient's renal function if possible and to prevent further organ damage and complications of hypertension. Antihypertensive drug administration is clearly the most important therapeutic approach. However, dialysis or nephrectomy may also be necessary.

DIABETES INSIPIDUS

Diabetes insipidus is a disorder of water metabolism caused by a relative deficiency of the antidiuretic hormone, arginine vasopressin (AVP).

The normal production and secretion of AVP as well as the proper functioning of the hypothalamic thirst center are essential for the maintenance of extracellular fluid osmolality and water balance (see Fig. 2). AVP is manufactured in the supraoptic and paraventricular nucleus of the hypothalamus and is then tranported via the neurohypophyseal tract to the posterior pituitary where it is stored for release into the general circulation. The major physiologic factor which controls day-to-day AVP production and release is plasma osmolality. Elevations in plasma osmolality, sensed by hypothalamic osmoreceptors, result in an increased AVP production and secretion. A decrease in plasma osmolality has the opposite effect. AVP generation is secondarily controlled by volume depletion, which is mediated through vagal nerve impulses from arterial and venous baroreceptors as well as through cardiopulmonary stretch receptors. Pain, emotion, stress, temperature, and drugs can also influence the synthesis and secretion of AVP. Once

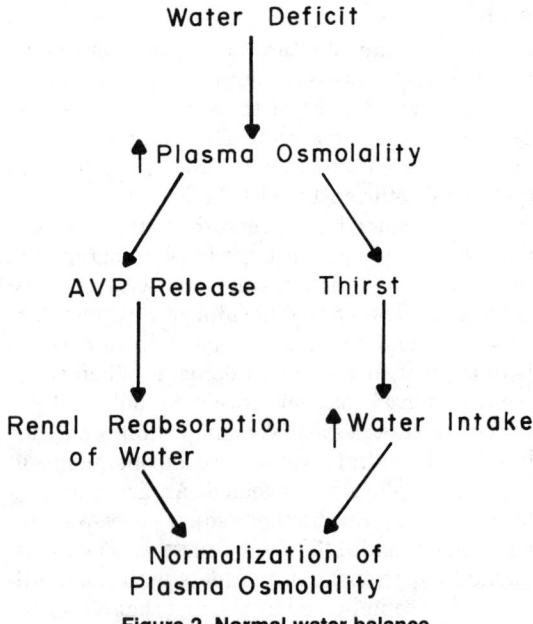

Figure 2. Normal water balance.

Table 5.

MAJOR CAUSES
OF NEUROGENIC DIABETES INSIPIDUS

Primary (idiopathic/familial)
Head Trauma (accidental/neurosurgical)
Malignancy (primary/metastatic)

in the circulation, AVP is transported to the kidney where it binds to renal tubular cell membranes and activates adenyl cyclase, which in turn generates cyclic-AMP. The end result of this biochemical reaction is an increase in the permeability of the renal collecting tubules to water. This leads to an increase in water reabsorption and a lowering of plasma osmolality.

Diabetes insipidus usually results from a partial or complete deficiency in the production and secretion of AVP from the neurohypophysis. The major causes of neurogenic diabetes insipidus can be found in Table 5. AVP deficiency can be permanent such as with the congenital form of the disease or transient as is frequently the case following accidental or neurosurgically-induced diabetes insipidus.

There is also a rare congenital form of this disease called nephrogenic diabetes insipidus. In these patients there are more than sufficient levels of circulating AVP. However, the renal tubules are totally or partially insensitive to the action of the hormone from birth. Polyuric syndromes unresponsive to vasopressin are also associated with a number of clinical conditions including certain forms of chronic renal disease. Several drugs (lithium, demeclocycline, and methoxyflurane) can also produce a nephrogenic state in patients treated with these agents (167–177).

25. *Diabetes Insipidus.* J.J. is a 14-year-old male admitted to the hospital for partial hypophysectomy to reduce an expanding pituitary tumor. The post-operative course was uncomplicated until immediately after surgery when the patient complained about voiding copious amounts of urine (polyuria) and thirst (polydipsia). Blood and urine chemistries were normal. Urine specific gravity was 1.003. Polyuria abated after 24 hours, only to reappear on the fourth post-operative day with the patient voiding 12 liters per day of urine with a specific gravity of 1.002. Because of the possibility of post-operative diabetes insipidus, the patient underwent a 14-hour water deprivation test. Baseline plasma and urinary osmolality (Posm and Uosm) were 295 mOsm/kg and 179 mOsm/kg respectively. Weight was 58.7 kg. During the 14 hours of water deprivation, the patient's weight fell to 56.2 kg. Posm gradually rose to a high of 322 mOsm/kg by 14 hours. Despite fluid deprivation and rising Posm, the patient failed to concentrate his urine (Uosm = 185 mOsm/kg). After the 14 hours the patient was administered 5 units of pitressin tannate in oil intramuscularly. Uosm promptly rose to 950 mOsm/kg and urine volume fell dramatically to a rate of less than 40 ml/hr. Over the next 5 days the patient was maintained on intermittent injections (5 U) of aqueous vasopressin. Since the patient's condition did not remit during the period of hospitalization, consideration was given to the long-term management of this patient. Vasopressin analogs, chlorpropamide, and diuretics were therapeutic alternatives considered. The patient was eventually discharged on desmopressin acetate (DDAVP) at a dose of 10 mcg intranasally prn. At the 2-week follow-up the patient still required DDAVP 10 mcg every 14 to 18 hours. However, he was able to taper the use of DDAVP over the next three months and was finally able to discontinue its use.

What features in this case are consistent with a diagnosis of diabetes insipidus?

Continuous production of inappropriately large volumes of hypotonic urine (Uosm < 200 mOsm/kg; specific gravity < 1.005) is indicative of diabetes insipidus. J.J. also complained of intense thirst (polydipsia), another classic symptom. To distinguish diabetes insipidus from other polyuric syndromes, J.J. underwent two diagnostic procedures. The first was a water deprivation test to determine if the patient had the ability to concentrate urine. When dehydrated, a normal person will respond by concentrating urine (Uosm > 800 mOsm/kg) while maintaining plasma osmolality at approximately 285 mOsm/kg. J.J. had an obvious inability to concentrate urine as evidenced by the production of an inappropriately dilute urine (Uosm = 185 mOsm/kg) in the face of an elevated plasma osmolality (Posm = 322 mOsm/kg). It should be noted that patients with a partial AVP deficiency may be able to produce mildly hypertonic urines.

Next, the patient was administered a test dose of pitressin (vasopressin) which allows the clinician to distinguish between neurogenic and nephrogenic forms of diabetes insipidus. Since J.J. responded to pitressin by producing a concentrated urine, the diagnosis of neurogenic diabetes insipidus secondary to surgical trauma was made (167–177).

26. What was the rationale behind the use of the various vasopressin analogs in this patient?

Treatment of diabetes insipidus is not an emergency situation. In fact, as long as patients have an intact thirst mechanism and an adequate fluid supply, they are not in immediate danger of fluid and electrolyte imbalance. Treatment is initiated nonetheless, not only to relieve the inconvenience of polydipsia and polyuria, but also to avoid rapid dehydration in a situation of involuntary water deprivation (eg, head injury, unconsciousness). Treatment consists of vasopressin, synthetic vasopressin analogs, thiazide diuretics, and a variety of non-hormonal drugs which can produce antidiuresis.

Vasopressin and its synthetic analogs are the principal treatment of neurogenic diabetes insipidus, which is J.J.'s diagnosis. These agents are ineffective in treating the nephrogenic variant of this clinical condition. Two preparations of vasopressin and two synthetic analogs of vasopressin are currently available for general use. (See Table 6.)

Table 6.

VASOPRESSIN PREPARATIONS AND ANALOGS AVAILABLE FOR GENERAL USE

Vasopressin
   (Pittressin synthetic)—aqueous solution 20 U/cc
   (Pittressin tannate in oil)—5 U/cc

Lysine vasopressin (Diapid)—2 U/spray

Desmopressin acetate (DDAVP)—0.1 mg/ml

Aqueous pitressin provides short amelioration of polyuria and therefore requires repeated administration every 3 to 4 hours as indicated by urine output (> 150 to 200 ml/hour). The initial dose of aqueous vasopressin is 5 units intramuscularly or subcutaneously; however, smaller amounts may be used. The dose may be increased to 20 units or more if control with smaller doses is inadequate. Because of this preparation's short duration of action, it is used primarily for diagnostic purposes and for titration of patients during the early stages of diabetes insipidus when the severity and duration of the disease are not yet determined. This was the reason for the use of aqueous pitressin in J.J.

Besides its use as a diagnostic agent, *pitressin tannate in oil* has long been the treatment of choice for treating prolonged episodes or chronic diabetes insipidus because of its 24- to 72-hour duration of action. Following a test dose of 1.5 to 2.5 units, a maintenance dose of 2.5 to 5.0 units is administered intramuscularly as needed; this is determined by urinary output. The drug is preferably administered at night. In administering the tannate in oil preparation, it is important to remember that it is a suspension requiring thorough agitation before use. Ignorance of this fact has been the cause of a number of "vasopressin-resistant" cases of diabetes insipidus. Despite the fact that water intoxication is most likely to occur with this preparation, it is recommended over the aqueous solution for maintenance therapy. Because of the availability of newer synthetic vasopressin analogs, the tannate in oil preparation was not used in this patient.

Although considered but not used in this patient, *lysine vasopressin* (Diapid), available as a nasal spray, is more acceptable for many patients than the tannate in oil vasopressin. This preparation is dosed every 3 to 6 hours as required to control polyuria. It is conveniently administered, and water intoxication is rare. The local, systemic, and pulmonary allergic reactions commonly associated with the older, still available, posterior pituitary snuff powder have practically been eliminated. The dose is one to two sprays in one or both nostrils (to a total of four sprays), four times a day initially. If polyuria is not controlled, it is recommended that the dosing frequency be decreased rather than increasing the amount of drug per dose, since excessive amounts will be lost by swallowing. Overnight control may be difficult due to this preparation's short duration of action.

A new synthetic vasopressin analog, *desmopressin acetate (DDAVP)* has recently been released in the United States. This agent has become the agent of choice for most clinicians treating cases of chronic neurogenic diabetes insipidus. DDAVP, like lysine vasopressin, offers the convenience of intranasal administration. However, DDAVP's longer duration of action of 8 to 20 hours (average, 12 hours) allows more satisfactory control of symptoms with one or two inhalations of 2.5 to 20 mcg/day. Dosing every 8 hours may be required in some patients. The drug is administered intranasally by use of a calibrated plastic tube whereby the patient blows the solution into the nasal cavity where it is absorbed. The pharmacist who dispenses this medication should make sure that the patient has been instructed in the proper technique for administering this drug.

Adverse reactions to this medication are minimal with headache, nausea, and nasal congestion/rhinitis being the most common. Unlike vasopressin, DDAVP has no significant vasopressor or oxytocic effects at therapeutic doses. No significant hypersensitivity reactions have been reported. J.J. suffered no adverse effects from DDAVP.

Because of the convenience of administration and lack of side effects, particularly hyponatremia, DDAVP was chosen for J.J.

J.J. should be monitored for electrolyte changes caused by excessive or insufficient vasopressin. Intake of hypertonic fluids should be avoided since an increased sodium load increases urine volume. Urine output, urine osmolality, serum osmolality, and specific gravity should be monitored closely during the patient's hospitalization in order to determine the proper dose of vasopressin or its analogs. At home, J.J. should be instructed to follow symptoms of polyuria and polydipsia in order to determine the proper time to administer his medications. Since hypokalemia, hypercalcemia, and hypercalciuria can cause resistance to vasopressin, these electrolyte abnormalities should be avoided (167,171,172,175,177).

27. Although they were not used in this patient, diuretics (particularly thiazide-type diuretics) were considered as therapeutic alternatives. What place do diuretics have in the treatment of diabetes insipidus? How do they paradoxically decrease urine volume?

Diuretics, particularly thiazide-type diuretics, have been used in the treatment of diabetes insipidus because of their paradoxical ability to reduce urine volume by 30 to 50%. Although patients excrete a smaller quantity of a less hypotonic urine, the urine does not become hypertonic. The usual dose of hydrochlorothiazide is 50 to 100 mg a day or an equivalent dose of another thiazide. Furosemide has also been successfully used to reduce urine volume in these patients. Although diuretics are limited to an adjuvant role in the treatment of neurogenic diabetes insipidus, they are the only drug therapy available for patients with nephrogenic diabetes insipidus.

The principal mechanism by which the chronic administration of diuretics reduces urine volume is by inducing a mild sodium deficit and volume contraction which results in an increased proximal tubular reabsorption of sodium and water. The reduction in the solute and fluid load presented to the ascending loop of Henle and the cortical diluting segment impairs the generation of free water, thereby decreasing urine volume. A low sodium diet enhances, while a high sodium diet blunts the antidiuresis. In addition to the above mechanism, thiazides impair the generation of free water by their ability to block sodium reabsorption in the cortical diluting segment of the nephron (167,169,175).

28. Because of the limited action of thiazide diuretics in the treatment of neurogenic diabetes insipidus, consideration was given to the use of other non-hormonal oral preparations, such as chlorpropamide, to treat J.J.'s diabetes insipidus. What are the roles of drugs such as chlorpropamide, carbamazepine, and clofibrate in the treatment of patients with neurogenic diabetes insipidus?

As with vasopressin, *chlorpropamide* is effective only in the treatment of neurogenic diabetes insipidus. Chlorpropamide appears to act by augmenting the action of AVP on the distal tubule of the nephron. An additional central mode of action has also been reported. Chlorpropamide's ability to produce antidiuresis and a hypertonic urine depends on residual pituitary function and the dose of chlorpropamide.

The usual dose of chlorpropamide for treating diabetes insipidus is 125 to 250 mg/day. Doses as high as 500 mg/day have been used when satisfactory control is not achieved; however, the incidence of hypoglycemia at this dose prohibits the use of chlorpropamide in many patients. The addition of a thiazide diuretic such as hydrochlorothiazide to chlorpropamide therapy is an effective alternative to increasing the dose of chlorpropamide to 500 mg/day. The addition of thiazides potentiates the action of chlorpropamide by their ability to decrease free water clearance and reduce urine volume by 30 to 50%. In addition, the ability of thiazides to impair insulin release tends to blunt the hypoglycemic action of chlorpropamide. Although not selected for use in J.J., chlorpropamide's effectiveness and ease of treatment have made it a popular choice for the treatment of patients with partial deficiencies in the production and secretion of AVP.

Prompt reversal of clinical signs and symptoms of vasopressin-sensitive diabetes insipidus has also been reported in a majority of patients treated with 400 to 800 mg/day of *carbamazepine.* Current evidence indicates that carbamazepine achieves its antidiuresis by either enhanced synthesis or release of AVP. As with chlorpropamide, the effects of carbamazepine appear to be dose-related. Additionally, the combination of carbamazepine and chlorpropamide has been used to treat diabetes insipidus. The combination offers equal effectiveness, while allowing dosage reduction and a decrease in the toxicity of each agent.

The antidiuretic effect of *clofibrate,* a lipid lowering agent, has been successfully utilized to treat patients with diabetes insipidus. In doses of 1.5 to 2.25 gm/day, clofibrate has been shown to cause a striking decrease in urine volume within 24 hours in a majority of treated patients with neurogenic diabetes insipidus. Response depends on residual neurohypophyseal function and the dose of clofibrate. The mechanism appears to be one of enhanced release of AVP. Clofibrate has been used in combination with other agents, such as chlorpropamide, with synergistic effects.

Acetaminophen has also been reported to improve polyuria and water balance in patients with neurogenic diabetes insipidus (169,171,172,175).

DILUTIONAL HYPONATREMIA

29. E.T. is a 62-year-old woman who was admitted to the hospital with the chief com-

plaint of increasing dizziness, fatigue, and confusion over a three week period. The patient was in good health with the exception of a 5-year history of congestive heart failure and mild hypertension controlled with 0.125 mg/day of digoxin and 50 mg/day of hydrochlorothiazide and a 2-year history of adult onset diabetes mellitus treated at present with 250 mg/day of chlorpropamide which was recently added to dietary controls. On admission, plasma and urine chemistries were taken. Of note, serum sodium was 113 mEq/L, serum chloride was 87 mEq/L, and the BUN was 4 mg/dl. Plasma osmolality was 240 mOsm/kg, while urine osmolality was 415 mOsm/kg. Urine sodium concentration was 54 mEq/L. Except for an altered mental status, the patient had no obvious abnormalities on physical examination; no evidence of dehydration was present.

Based on clinical symptoms and laboratory data, the presumptive diagnosis of dilutional hyponatremia secondary to chlorpropamide was made. Chlorpropamide and hydrochlorothiazide were discontinued, and the patient was placed on water restriction. Serum sodium rose to 119 mEq/L within 24 hours and by the end of the third hospital day the serum sodium had risen to 135 mEq/L with complete clearing of neurological symptoms. Water restriction was discontinued. Hydrochlorothiazide was resumed, but chlorpropamide was replaced with acetohexamide. The patient was discharged after five days and has not suffered any electrolyte imbalances since.

How was the diagnosis of dilutional hyponatremia made in this patient?

The diagnosis of dilutional hyponatremia is based on five criteria, all of which were fulfilled by E.T. First, hyponatremia (serum sodium = 113 mEq/L) and hypoosmolality of the plasma (Posm = 240 mOsm/kg) caused by excessive water retention were both present. Second, renal sodium wasting (urinary sodium = 54 mEq/L) existed despite the presence of hyponatremia. This phenomenon is related to volume expansion which increases GFR and sodium diuresis. The third criteria is the formation of a less than maximally dilute urine in the face of plasma hypotonicity. E.T. had an inappropriately concentrated urine (Uosm = 415 mOsm/Kg) for her plasma osmolality of 240 mOsm/Kg. Fourth, the absence of dehydration, and finally, normal renal and adrenal function. In fact, these patients tend to have lower than normal BUN's as illustrated by E.T. (BUN = 4 mg/dl) (168,172,176).

Because the development of dilutional hyponatremia coincided with the initiation of chlorpropamide treatment in E.T., chlorpropamide was considered to be the most likely cause.

30. What role did chlorpropamide play in the development of dilutional hyponatremia in this patient? What other conditions did the patient have which may have predisposed her to the development of this complication? Why was she switched from chlorpropamide to another sulfonylurea, acetohexamide?

Chlorpropamide possesses an antidiuretic action which has been demonstrated in water-loaded normal subjects, patients with diabetes mellitus and those with neurogenic diabetes insipidus. Chlorpropamide acts mainly by enhancing the action of AVP on the renal collecting ducts, although there is evidence that chlorpropamide stimulates AVP release as well. The antidiuretic action of chlorpropamide has been shown to be additive with that of thiazide diuretics (as was the case in E.T.) and carbamazepine.

In some patients, the antidiuretic action of chlorpropamide can cause significant water retention resulting in a dilutional hyponatremic state indistinguishable from the syndrome of inappropriate secretion of antidiuretic hormone (SIADH). This side effect has been frequently reported to complicate chlorpropamide treatment. In one study of diabetic patients treated with chlorpropamide, dilutional hyponatremia occurred in 4% of the patients. Current evidence suggests that chlorpropamide-induced hyponatremia is most common in patients with an underlying tendency to retain water, such as those with congestive heart failure. Congestive heart failure may have contributed to the development of hyponatremia in E.T.

Tolbutamide has also been shown to have antidiuretic properties. There are several case reports which implicate tolbutamide as a cause of dilutional hyponatremia, although the incidence appears to be considerably less than that reported for chlorpropamide. Conversely, tolazamide and acetohexamide have been shown to have a diuretic action in water-loaded subjects. This was the reason why E.T. was switched to acetohexamide after the hyponatremic episode with chlorpropamide (171,172,176).

31. What other drugs have been reported to cause a dilutional hyponatremic state resembling SIADH (syndrome of inappropriate antidiuretic hormone)?

Besides chlorpropamide and tolbutamide, a number of other drugs have been reported to cause a dilutional hyponatremic state resembling SIADH. The antidiuretic action of carbamazepine is well documented, and this effect has been used therapeutically in the treatment of neurogenic diabetes insipidus. Carbamazepine has no intrinsic AVP activity, but apparently it induces water retention by increasing AVP release, as evidenced by reports of elevated AVP levels following treatment with carbamazepine. Carbamazepine antidiuresis is additive with that of chlorpropamide and is blocked by phenytoin. Dilutional hyponatremia has been described as a complication of carbamazepine treatment in patients with seizure disorders, trigeminal neuralgia, and psychogenic polydipsia. The risk of developing dilutional hyponatremia appears to be correlated with the dose and serum level of carbamazepine.

Clofibrate, a hypolipidemic agent, has significant antidiuretic properties in patients with neurogenic diabetes insipidus and in normal subjects. However, dilutional hyponatremia has only been reported in a psychogenic water drinker receiving 6 to 8 gm/day of clofibrate.

Impaired water excretion secondary to cyclophosphamide has been documented. Impaired water load excretion has been reported in 17 of 19 cancer patients receiving 50 mg/kg of cyclophosphamide. Signs of hyponatremia, hypoosmolality, and inappropriately concentrated urine appeared within 4 to 12 hours following the dose. The effect lasted up to 20 hours. The course of events can be related in time to the excretion of active metabolites in the urine. Impaired water excretion could not be attributed to the patients' clinical conditions. A case of hyponatremia following a 3 gm dose of cyclophosphamide has been reported in a patient with oat cell carcinoma. Hyponatremia persisted for ten days. Drug-induced SIADH or the release of an AVP substance were suggested as possible mechanisms in this patient. Impaired water excretion due to cyclophosphamide may be an important consideration during treatment with this drug, since patients are usually instructed to increase fluid intake to prevent hemorrhagic cystitis. Therefore patients must be monitored for signs of water intoxication, especially when receiving large doses of cyclophosphamide.

Diuretic-induced hyponatremia may be caused by excessive saluresis or by impairing the excretion of a water load. In the former, the patient suffers from a deficit of total body water and an even larger deficit of total body sodium (hypovolemic hyponatremia). In the latter, the deficit in total body sodium is associated with an excess of total body water (dilutional hyponatremia). Dilutional hyponatremia secondary to diuretics is indistinguishable from SIADH except that hypokalemia and metabolic alkalosis are usually present and sodium levels return to normal within several days after stopping diuretics. Elevated AVP levels have been demonstrated, although thiazides can impair free water excretion in the absence of elevated AVP because of their ability to prevent sodium reabsorption in the cortical diluting segment of the nephron.

SIADH secretion has been described with *vincristine* treatment in both adults and children. Water intoxication usually occurs one to two weeks after initiation of vincristine treatment. Other manifestations of vincristine neurotoxicity are invariably present as well. An abnormal secretion of AVP from the neurohypophysis has been suggested as a possible mechanism, based on reports of elevated AVP levels in some patients. Enhanced neurohypophyseal secretion of AVP may be related to a disruptive effect of vincristine on the microtubules of the neurohypophysis. The incidence of vincristine SIADH is not known, but there is evidence to suggest that this is a dose-related phenomenon. Several cases of dilutional hyponatremia have also been reported following high-dose vinblastine treatment.

Other drugs reported to cause dilutional hyponatremia include amitriptyline, fluphenazine, phenformin, and thiothixene. Oxytocin, a hormone used to induce labor, has weak AVP activity and can produce dilutional hyponatremia when administered in large doses to water-loaded patients. Surgical patients exposed to pre-operative barbiturates, general anesthesia, and/or intraoperative narcotic agents can release excessive amounts of AVP, manifested by impaired water excretion, and on rare occasion produce hyponatremia (171,172,176).

32. What is the appropriate treatment of a patient presenting with dilutional hyponatremia? Was E.T. (Question 29) properly treated?

The treatment of dilutional hyponatremia depends upon the clinical status of the patient. Correction of hyponatremia is the first concern. Patients should be placed on water restriction regardless of the etiology of dilutional hyponatremia. Administration of 500 to 1000 ml/day of fluid induces a negative free water balance and encourages renal tubular reabsorption of sodium in most patients. In patients with severe symptomatic hyponatremia, more aggressive therapy may be indicated. Negative free water balance with rapid correction of hyponatremia can be achieved by the intravenous administration of furosemide (1 mg/kg) with concomitant hourly replacement of urinary sodium losses with hypertonic saline. Potassium, magnesium, and other electrolyte losses produced by furosemide need to be replaced. Infusion of hypertonic saline (3 to 5%) alone has been used to produce rapid but temporary correction of hyponatremia. However, since sodium loads are rapidly excreted by these patients, plasma sodium levels are only transiently increased. Because of the danger of circulatory overload, this treatment modality is rarely indicated.

Removal or correction of the cause of hyponatremia is also a primary concern. Patients with drug-induced water intoxication usually respond to discontinuation of the offending agent. In other patients where hyponatremia is due to inappropriate secretion of antidiuretic hormone as the result of some underlying pathological process, surgical or medical correction of the problem will be necessary. In those patients where the disease state cannot be reversed, administration of *lithium carbonate* or *demeclocycline* has been shown to be useful for the treatment of chronic forms of SIADH. Both of these drugs function by inhibiting the action of AVP on the collecting ducts of the kidney, thereby creating a functional diabetes insipidus. *Phenytoin,* which blocks AVP release, has been shown to improve impaired water balance in patients with SIADH. However, this effect is usually transient and therefore not useful for chronic treatment in many patients with SIADH. Because of a lower incidence of toxicity, demeclocycline is preferred by most clinicians for the treatment of chronic SIADH (168,172,176).

Because symptoms of hyponatremia developed over a several week period, aggressive therapy was not indicated for E.T. She was placed on simple water restriction (500 ml/day) and the offending agent, chlorpropamide, was withdrawn. Hydrochlorothiazide was also withdrawn because of its antidiuretic properties in this situation.

ADVERSE EFFECTS OF DRUGS ON THE KIDNEY

Many drugs used in the treatment of a wide variety of medical conditions can induce significant adverse effects upon the kidney. Nephropathy due to some agents is suggested by isolated case reports, while that due to others is clearly documented by laboratory investigation and clinical studies. The potential for and frequency of renal damage due to a particular drug depends primarily upon the drug's mechanism and site of nephrotoxicity. However, the exact incidence of nephrotoxicity due to any drug is difficult to predict and can be influenced by a number of factors including concurrent administration of other nephrotoxic agents, preexisting renal disease, and other underlying disease states.

Drug nephrotoxicity may occur at a number of sites (see Fig. 3). These include the renal vasculature, the glomerulus, the renal tubule (both proximal and distal), the collecting ducts, the interstitium, the pelvicalyceal system, and the ureters.

Several mechanisms exist whereby drug-induced renal damage may develop. First, a parent drug or metabolite may exert a direct toxic effect

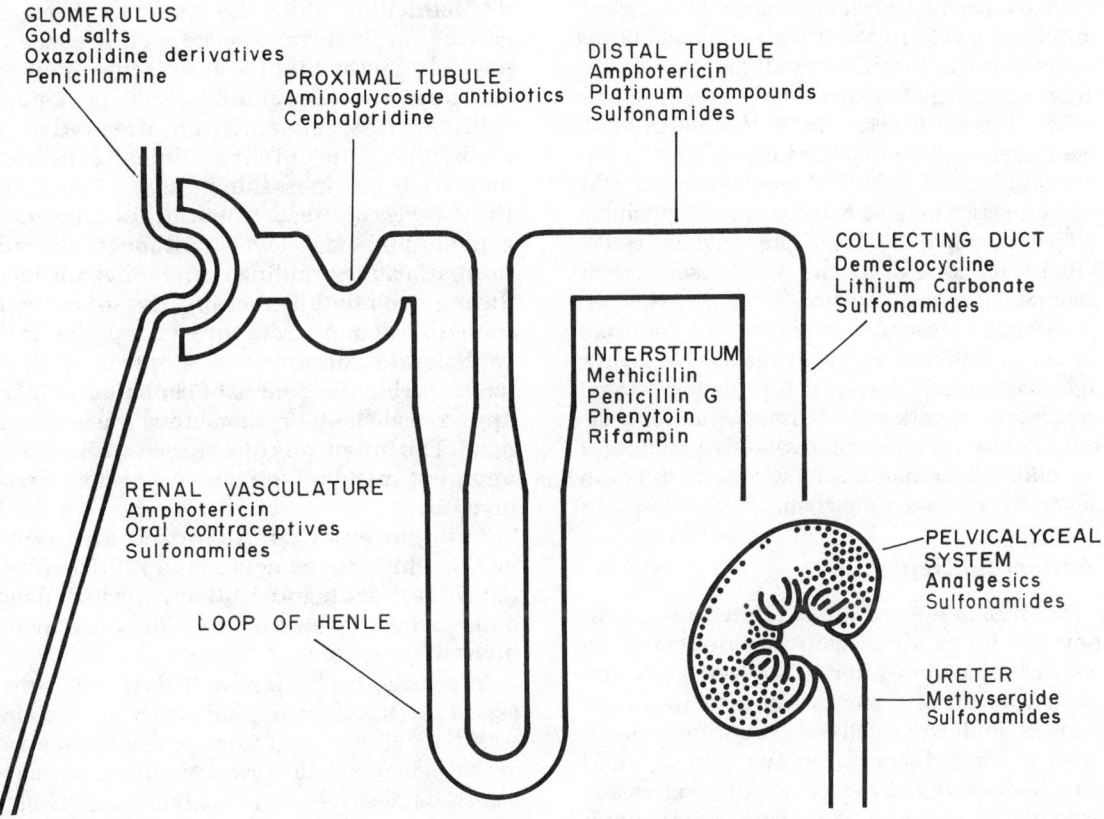

Figure 3. Possible sites of drug nephrotoxicity.

on renal cells (protoplasmic toxin). Tubular cell damage and necrosis are usually the result of a directly nephrotoxic drug. In addition, a drug can indirectly cause kidney damage by creating a condition within the patient which can potentially lead to deterioration in renal function (eg, hypertension induced by oral contraceptive agents). A drug may also act as an immunogen and elicit an immune reaction whereby the renal vasculature (vasculitis), glomerulus (glomulonephritis), or tubules and interstitium (tubulointerstitial disease) may be damaged. The immune reaction to a drug is due to antibody formation in response to either a drug antigen or a drug hapten-protein which combine to form a complete antigen. The formed antigen-antibody complex, either circulating or tissue bound, can elicit an inflammatory response with resultant renal tissue damage. An additional mechanism by which drugs can cause kidney damage is mechanical obstruction of the tubules, collecting ducts, or ureters (obstructive nephropathy). This may result from a) a parent compound or metabolite exceeding its solubility in the urine and precipitating out of solution, forming crystals and stones, b) a drug increasing the excretion of a poorly soluble material, or c) a drug creating a condition in which the ureters may be impinged upon (eg, retroperitoneal fibrosis). A further mechanism whereby renal function may be reduced is a drug-induced decrease in renal blood flow (pre-renal azotemia). Finally, for some drugs the mechanism of their nephrotoxicity is not known.

Although a complete discussion of the nephrotoxic potential of all the available therapeutic agents is beyond the scope of this chapter, several nephrotoxic agents will be discussed in some detail in order to provide representative samples of the different mechanisms by which the drug can adversely alter renal function.

Methicillin Nephritis

33. B.S. is a 4-week-old premature infant boy (1.8 kg at birth) who was delivered by caesarian section after a 32-week gestation period because of increasing toxemia in the mother. Following delivery, the infant developed a Staphylococcal aureus osteomyelitis which showed x-ray evidence of progressive osseous changes in the distal tibial metaphysis and first metatarsal despite a 10-day course of methicillin at a dose of 300 mg/kg/day.

The infant (weight 2.3 kg) was transferred to a university hospital for evaluation and treatment of osteomyelitis of the right leg. On admission, physical examination showed an active, alert baby in no apparent distress. Physical findings were unremarkable except for osteomyelitis involving the right ankle, distal tibia, knee, and part of the great toe. Admission laboratory data were unremarkable except for a WBC of 14,200/mm^3 with 22% eosinophils. Temperature was 38°C (rectal). Urine, blood, and aspirate cultures were taken on admission and were all subsequently reported as negative. The infant was maintained on 300 mg/kg/day of methicillin until the fourth hospital day at which time hematuria (4+), pyuria (too many to count), and mild proteinuria (1+) were noted on urinalysis. At the time, WBC was 11,900/mm^3 with 17% eosinophils. Serum creatinine was 0.4 mg/dl. Methicillin, which the infant had been receiving for 22 days, was stopped because of possible methicillin-induced acute interstitial nephritis. Cephalothin, 300 mg/kg/day initially, was chosen as an alternative to methicillin. The infant's clinical condition improved, but increasing doses of cephalothin were required to maintain adequate cephalothin cidal levels. Although the abnormal urinary findings gradually subsided during cephalothin therapy, the infant continued to demonstrate an eosinophilia until cephalothin therapy was stopped 32 days later. During the course of cephalothin therapy, a transient erythematous rash developed. The infant was discharged without any apparent residual effects from the osteomyelitis.

This patient was diagnosed as having methicillin-induced acute interstitial nephritis. What is acute interstitial nephritis? What other drugs besides methicillin cause acute interstitial nephritis?

Interstitial nephritis is a distinct histopathological pattern of renal tissue injury in which interstitial cellular infiltration and inflammation of the kidney are the primary finding on renal biopsy. Because histologic and functional tubular changes are invariably present as well, the term tubulointerstitial disease has been introduced to describe this lesion. Renal tubular cell damage and other tubular structural abnormalities are usually adjacent to or surrounded by interstitial cellular inflammation. In the acute form of interstitial nephritis, interstitial edema is generally present, while fibrosis is absent. The glomeruli are normal.

Presently, drugs and bacterial infections (particularly pyelonephritis) are considered to be the two main causes of acute interstitial nephritis. Although a number of drugs have been implicated as causing this form of nephrotoxicity (see Table 7), acute interstitial nephritis is most often described following the administration of penicillin analogs, primarily methicillin.

Over 100 cases of acute interstitial nephritis secondary to methicillin have been reported. Available data indicate that toxicity is immunologically mediated. Both the humoral and cell-mediated components of the immune system have been implicated in the clinicopathogenesis of methicillin nephritis (178–193).

34. Since B.S. did not have a renal biopsy, how was the diagnosis of methicillin nephritis made? Was it based on the patient's clinical findings, and if so what are the clinical manifestations which characterize methicillin nephritis?

The presumptive diagnosis of methicillin nephritis in B.S. was based on his urinalysis and white blood cell differential. Clinical manifestations of methicillin-induced nephritis usually become evident within the first four weeks (average 15 days) following initiation of the drug (186). Toxicity appears to be immunologically mediated and is not dose dependent, although the incidence reportedly increases with a duration of treatment greater than ten days. Onset of toxicity is evidenced by the presence of a systemic immune reaction characterized by eosinophilia (79%), fever (87%) and rash (24%) which is usually maculopapular or morbilliform in nature. Allergic manifestations may antedate or occur concurrently with urinary abnormalities which are present in over 90% of patients with methicillin nephritis. Microscopic to gross hematuria (97%), mild to moderate proteinuria (94%), and sterile pyuria (93%) are the principal abnormal urinary findings, all of which were found in B.S. Eosinophils can be demonstrated by Wright stain of the urine of patients with methicillin nephritis, although this was not done in this patient. In one patient series, eosinophiluria averaging more than 33% was present in each of nine patients with methicillin nephritis (189). Some authors consider eosinophiluria to be of considerable value in the diagnosis of methicillin and other drug-induced causes of acute interstitial nephritis.

Deterioration of renal function is a potential sequela of methicillin nephritis (179,186,188). Renal impairment ranges from minor elevations in the blood urea nitrogen and/or serum creatinine to oliguric or anuric renal failure requiring hemodialysis. Renal failure appears to be more common in adults and occurs in over 60% of patients 16-years or older; in children this complication only occurs about 10% of the time (186). As noted in B.S., renal function did not deteriorate despite the presence of an abnormal urinalysis.

Table 7.

DRUGS REPORTED TO CAUSE
ACUTE INTERSTITIAL NEPHRITIS

Allopurinol

Azathioprine

Cephalosporins
  Cephalexin
  Cephaloridine
  Cephalothin

Cimetidine

Ethambutol

Non-steroidal antiinflammatory drugs

Para aminosalicylic acid

Penicillins
  Ampicillin
  Carbenicillin
  Methicillin
  Nafcillin
  Oxacillin
  Penicillin G

Phenindione

Phenobarbital

Phenytoin

Rifampin

Sulfonamides (including co-trimoxazole)

Thiazide diuretics

(188,192)

Less commonly reported complications include impaired renal concentrating ability and systemic acidosis (186). Cogan et al (191) recently described a patient with methicillin nephritis who had evidence of renal sodium wasting, hyperchloremic acidosis, and hyperkalemia in addition to renal insufficiency. In some patients, hematuria may be associated with dysuria. This finding may indicate the presence of hemorrhagic cystitis, a recently reported complication of methicillin therapy. Hemorrhagic cystitis can develop concurrently with acute interstitial nephritis (184, 185).

35. Methicillin was withdrawn from B.S. Is this proper management for acute interstitial nephritis? Since this is an allergic reaction, are corticosteroids indicated?

Drug discontinuation is the proper management for methicillin-induced interstitial nephritis. Although drug toxicity may transiently worsen, improvement usually occurs within 48 hours. Complete reversal of the allergic and renal manifestations of methicillin nephritis generally requires several days to four to five weeks. In patients with severe renal dysfunction, the course of renal failure can be prolonged; several months, and in some cases more than a year, may be required for renal function to return to pre-methicillin levels. Permanent impairment of renal function has been described but is rare (179, 186,188).

There is anecdotal evidence to suggest that corticosteroids have a beneficial effect in the treatment of renal failure secondary to methicillin. In one series of 14 patients with methicillin nephritis, retrospective evaluation indicated that treatment with prednisone resulted in a rapid return to near normal renal function, while renal dysfunction persisted in those patients who did not receive steroids (189). Despite the apparent success of some with steroid treatment, others still question its value in methicillin nephritis. In regards to B.S., steroids would not have been indicated since renal function did not deteriorate (186).

Methicillin should not be readministered since evidence of toxicity can rapidly reappear.

36. Cephalothin was substituted for methicillin in B.S. Could another penicillin analog have been used instead of cephalothin?

Since current evidence indicates that methicillin nephritis is the result of an immune reaction, it raises the question of which alternative antibiotic can be administered with the least risk of cross-antigenicity. Immune responses among penicillin analogs are heterogenous, thus explaining conflicting reports of their ability to exacerbate methicillin-induced interstitial nephritis (188). In one patient who had developed interstitial nephritis during combined methicillin-penicillin treatment, the inadvertent administration of 4 grams of ampicillin resulted in a prompt rise in eosinophils and a reappearance of renal dysfunction (180). Because of the likelihood of cross-antigenicity, most authorities recommend avoidance of any penicillin derivative in patients who have developed methicillin nephritis. In this patient, other penicillin analogs were considered but were not chosen based on the recommendation of the Clinical Pharmacology consultant.

Although allergic cross-reactivity has been demonstrated between penicillin analogs and cephalosporin derivatives, its existence is not extensive. However, since recurrence of nephritis has been reported following the substitution of methicillin with a cephalosporin, such substitution should be initiated with caution. It is interesting to note that B.S.'s eosinophilia persisted following the substitution of cephalothin for methicillin, although the abnormal urinary sediment cleared. Vancomycin or clindamycin may be useful alternative antibiotics for Staphylococcal infections since they have not been shown to cause acute interstitial nephritis (186,188).

37. What is the incidence of nephritis caused by methicillin? Is it greater than that caused by penicillin analogs, particularly nafcillin?

Scattered case reports of methicillin nephritis first appeared in the 1960's and early 1970's. Although the actual incidence of methicillin nephritis was difficult to determine from these case reports, it was considered to be rare. However, evidence from subsequent retrospective and prospective studies in both children and adults suggest that the incidence of methicillin nephritis has been underestimated, especially when patients are treated for periods of ten days or more. The incidence of this complication has been placed at 10 to 20% by these more recent studies (182–

184,186,187,190). As for B.S., this was the fifth child on the pediatric service diagnosed to have methicillin nephritis in an eight-week period.

Interstitial nephritis has also been attributed to other penicillin analogs, particularly penicillin and ampicillin. Although the exact incidence is not known, the risk appears to be considerably less than with methicillin (188,191).

On rare occasions, nephritis has been reported to occur during treatment with nafcillin (188,193). However, none of the case reports described in the literature clearly implicate nafcillin as a cause of interstitial nephritis. Data from a study comparing the incidence of adverse reactions due to methicillin or nafcillin in 70 adult patients with Staphylococcal aureus endocarditis have been reported (190). Forty-one patients received 12 gm/day or more of methicillin for 8 to 52 days, while 29 received 12 gm/day of nafcillin for 6 to 67 days. The clinical and bacteriologic response to the two different antibiotics was comparable. However, drug reactions (fever, rash, urinary sediment abnormalities, hematologic toxicity) occurred in 16 of 41 (39%) of the methicillin-treated patients but in only four of 29 (14%) of the nafcillin-treated patients. Of these patients, five receiving methicillin (12%) developed hematuria, two with biopsy-documented acute interstitial nephritis, while none of the nafcillin-treated patients had any evidence of renal or urinary tract abnormalities. Furthermore, in a recent prospective analysis of 210 patients administered nafcillin, no clinically evident cases of acute interstitial nephritis due to nafcillin were found (194).

Based on the available evidence, use of methicillin on the pediatric service was discontinued, and nafcillin was used in its place. During a six month follow-up, no cases of interstitial nephritis were reported.

Aminoglycoside Nephrotoxicity

38. J.R. is a 61-year-old, 77.2 kg female who was admitted for induction chemotherapy for acute myelogenous leukemia with daunomycin, cytosine arabinoside, and 6-thioguanine. The patient did well until the tenth hospital day when she spiked a fever to 39.5° C (see Fig. 4). Her WBC had fallen from an admission value of 14,750/mm^3 to 1100/mm^3. Blood cultures were taken and the patient was started on gentamicin 5 mg/kg/day, cephalothin 12 gm/day, and carbenicillin 30 gm/day, all administered intravenously. Renal function tests and urinalysis were normal at this time. Despite repeatedly negative blood cultures, the patient remained febrile with temperatures ranging between 39.2° and 40.1° C. Peak and trough gentamicin levels ranged between 6.5 and 8.4 mcg/ml and 1.8 and 2.4 mcg/ml respectively. No dosage adjustment was made. The patient's WBC reached a nadir of 700/mm^3 on the fourteenth day. An abnormal urinary sediment, consisting of 1+ protein, 4–5 WBC/HPF, and some renal tubular cells and granular casts, was also noted on this day. Urinary specific gravity was 1.004. The following day, serum creatinine was reported to be 1.7 mg/dl. Urine volume was 2,250 ml/24 hr. The dose of gentamicin was reduced to 4 mg/kg/day. Because of a falling serum potassium (2.8 mEq/L from 4.5 mEq/L), potassium supplementation was initiated. As noted in Fig. 4, her serum creatinine continued to rise. The gentamicin dose was further reduced to 3 mg/kg/day on the nineteenth hospital day. The dose of carbenicillin was also reduced to 20 gm/day. The gentamicin was finally discontinued because of its probable nephrotoxic effects when her serum creatinine reached 5.0 mg/dl on the twenty-second hospital day. The serum creatinine peaked at 5.8 mg/dl on the twenty-third day. Despite failing renal function, urine output remained above 500 ml/24 hr. All antibiotics were withdrawn on the twenty-sixth day when the patient defervesced. Renal function steadily improved over the next two weeks, with renal function tests returning to near baseline by that time. Potassium requirements also fell after antibiotics were discontinued.

What is the usual course of gentamicin-induced nephrotoxicity? Did J.R. present with a typical course?

Renal toxicity due to gentamicin is a potential complication of this drug. The incidence of gentamicin nephrotoxicity is generally considered to be between 5 and 10%, although estimates ranging from less than 2% to higher than 50% (depending on the criteria used to determine nephrotoxicity) have been reported.

J.R. typifies the usual course of gentamicin-induced nephrotoxicity: a gradual, modest rise in serum creatinine which promptly reverses on discontinuation of gentamicin. Evidence of toxicity generally appears within the first two weeks of treatment. In this patient the first sign of toxicity, an abnormal urinary sediment, occurred after four days. Proteinuria, which is the major finding, is generally mild in cases of gentamicin nephrotoxicity. This was the situation in J.R. whose proteinuria never exceeded 1+ during the period of rising serum creatinine. White blood cells and cylindruria are also a common finding, while red blood cells are not. Renal concentrating ability may also be impaired. (Urinary specific gravity was 1.004 in J.R.) Abnormal urinary sediment usually precedes the development of markedly impaired renal function, as exemplified by this case.

Renal failure is usually non-oliguric in nature. Characteristically, J.R. maintained a urinary output of >500 ml/24 hr, despite a serum creatinine in excess of 5 mg/dl. It should be realized, however, that oliguric or anuric renal failure occasionally does occur. Its onset may be rapid and its course prolonged, requiring dialysis in some cases.

A complex metabolic disorder apparently related to renal tubular dysfunction has been reported as an uncommon but troublesome complication of treatment with gentamicin and other aminoglycoside antibiotics. This syndrome may occur in the absence of declining renal function and has been reported most frequently in patients undergoing chemotherapy (particularly adriamycin) who are receiving large doses of aminoglycosides. The syndrome is characterized by

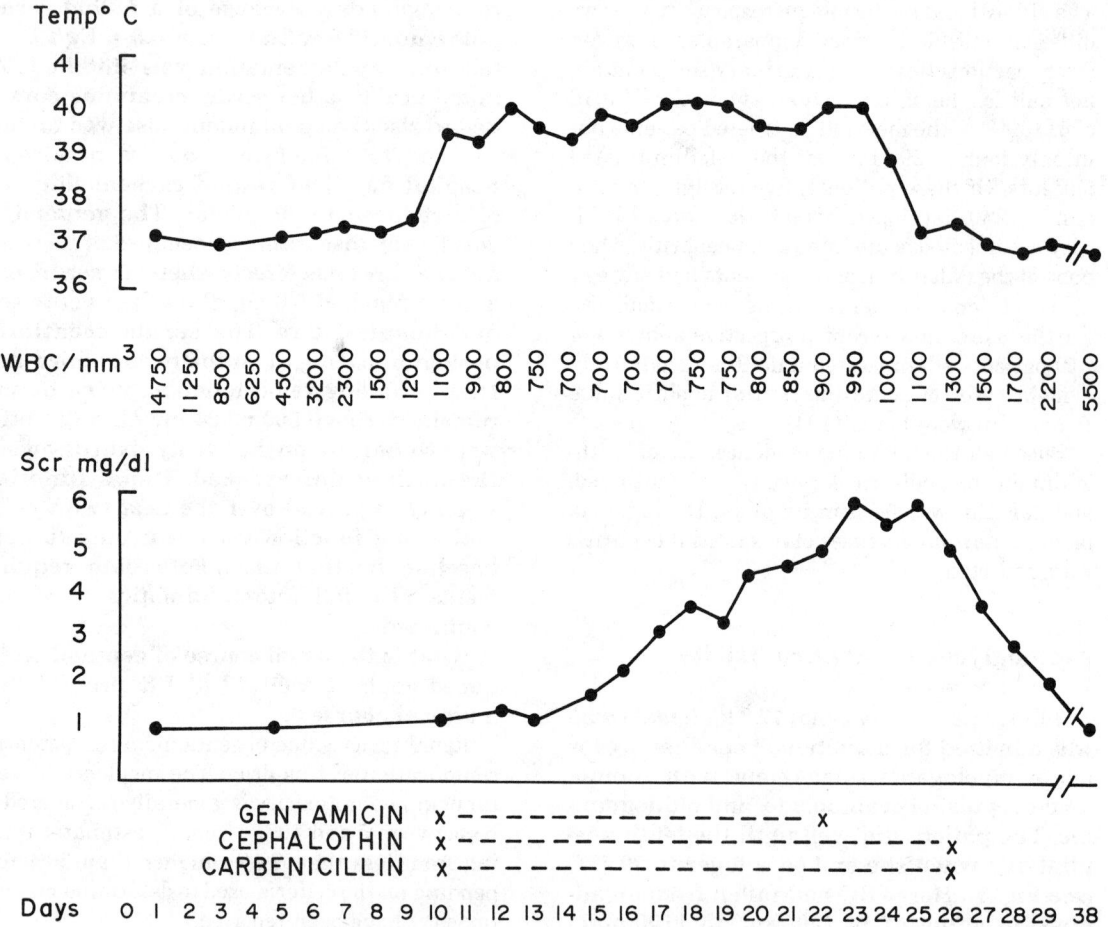

Figure 4. Patient data, aminoglycoside nephrotoxicity.

hypomagnesemia, hypocalcemia, and hypokalemia secondary to renal electrolyte wasting. Low circulating parathyroid hormone levels have been reported despite the presence of hypocalcemia. Excessive urinary loss of phosphate, sodium, and uric acid may also be seen. Electrolyte wasting, requiring replacement in most cases, may persist for two to eight weeks even after withdrawal. J.R.'s hypokalemia is probably due to carbenicillin, not gentamicin, since she has no other electrolyte abnormalities (195–198).

39. What is the mechanism of gentamicin-induced renal failure? Are there any characteristics peculiar to J.R. or her treatment which could have increased the risk of nephrotoxicity secondary to gentamicin?

Gentamicin and other aminoglycoside antibiotics appear to exert a direct nephrotoxic effect on renal tubular epithelial cells which results in cellular vacuolization with variable degrees of degeneration and necrotic changes. Although the exact cellular mechanism is not clear, it is well established that gentamicin accumulates in the renal cortex and that there is a correlation between the cortical concentration of gentamicin and the risk of nephrotoxicity (197,198).

A number of factors have been reported to potentiate gentamicin nephrotoxicity (See Table 8), although not all have been definitively shown to alter risk in human subjects (197,198).

Of particular interest is the presence of two reported risk factors in J.R.: high trough levels and concomitant administration of cephalothin.

Table 8.

FACTORS WHICH MAY INCREASE THE RISK OF GENTAMICIN NEPHROTOXICITY

Age

Concomitant administration of cephalothin

Concomitant administration of loop diuretics

Excessive serum gentamicin levels
  Peak levels > 12 mcg/ml
  Trough levels > 2 mcg/ml

Hypotension/hypovolemia

Preexisting renal dysfunction

Prolonged duration of therapy (> 10 days)

Recent exposure to aminoglycoside antibiotics

The relationship between high trough levels and nephrotoxicity was reported in a study of more than 80 patients in which it was observed that patients who experienced a decline in renal function while receiving gentamicin all had trough levels of 2 mcg/ml or more. Conversely, those patients with levels less than 2 mcg/ml suffered no deterioration in renal function. Although a clear cut cause and effect relationship was not established, avoidance of high trough levels appears prudent (199).

As with gentamicin and other aminoglycosides, proximal tubular damage is a potential toxic effect of cephalosporin antibiotics. Animal data and clinical experiments indicate that cephaloridine is the most nephrotoxic cephalosporin. This is related to the excessive concentrations of cephaloridine which accumulate in proximal tubular cells due to this drug's characteristic inability to readily diffuse across the luminal membrane (200). The nephrotoxic potential of other cephalosporins is considered to be substantially less or nonexistent as compared to cephaloridine. Cases of cephalothin-induced renal damage as evidenced by mild proteinuria, a rise in serum creatinine and/or BUN, and oliguric renal failure have been reported but only after administration of large doses for prolonged periods of time (200).

With respect to the combination of gentamicin and cephalothin, a possible adverse interaction is suspected. Although there are animal data and some clinical evidence to the contrary, several controlled studies indicate that the incidence of renal dysfunction is substantially higher in patients receiving an antibiotic regimen containing both gentamicin and cephalothin than in patients administered regimens without this combination. This effect of cephalothin appears to extend to other aminoglycosides as well. Whether other cephalosporins potentiate gentamicin nephrotoxicity is not presently known (198,200,201).

In retrospect, the concomitant administration of cephalothin and gentamicin and the presence of high trough levels were considered to have been contributing factors in the renal toxicity experienced by this patient.

40. Is there any validity to the claim that other aminoglycoside agents would have been less nephrotoxic than gentamicin in this patient?

Aminoglycoside antibiotics differ in their nephrotoxic potential. All aminoglycoside antibiotics accumulate in the renal cortex to varying degrees, and although there is a correlation between an individual aminoglycoside's cortical concentration and its risk of nephrotoxicity, no such correlation exists among the various aminoglycoside agents.

Clearly, neomycin is the most nephrotoxic aminoglycoside. Because of this high risk potential, neomycin is not administered parenterally. In fact, cases of acute renal failure have been reported following local irrigation with neomycin solutions or oral administration of the drug. Conversely, streptomycin is the least nephrotoxic aminoglycoside. Netilmicin, an experimental aminoglycoside, is considered to have a relatively low nephrotoxic risk potential, while gentamicin, kanamycin, amikacin, and tobramycin appear to have an intermediate risk potential. Although differences in the incidence and degree of renal damage exist in experimental models, clinically the risk of nephrotoxicity with gentamicin, amikacin, tobramycin, and kanamycin has been considered to be somewhat comparable. However, recent data have been reported which suggest that tobramycin (which has essentially the same therapeutic indications as gentamicin) may in fact be less nephrotoxic than gentamicin. In one controlled study, nephrotoxicity (defined as a rise in serum creatinine of 0.5 mg/dl or more) developed in 19 of 72 (26%) patients receiving gentamicin but in only 9 of 74 (12%) patients receiving tobramycin. The severity of renal dysfunction did not differ. Further controlled studies are necessary to confirm these findings (197,198,202).

Amphotericin Nephrotoxicity

41. L.A. is a 19-year-old male from the central valley of California who was transferred to the university hospital with a pleural effusion, an enlarging right lower lobe infiltrate, and bulging fissures. The patient was febrile to 40.1°C; admission white count was 30,000/mm^3. All bacterial cultures to date were negative. The patient's condition had deteriorated despite antibiotic treatment at the local hospital. An open lung and pleural biopsy were performed. Microscopic examination suggested coccidioidomycosis, and it

was decided that amphotericin B should be started. Baseline renal function studies showed a serum creatinine of 0.8 mg/dl, a creatinine clearance of 115 ml/min, and a normal urinalysis. A 1 mg test dose of amphotericin was well tolerated. The dose was then progressively increased to 60 mg/day (1 mg/kg) over one week. Amphotericin was administered with 25 mg of hydrocortisone and 500 units of heparin in 500 ml of D5W. A 25 gm dose of mannitol was also administered along with each dose of amphotericin. The patient's condition improved rapidly once amphotericin was initiated. The patient's course was predictably complicated by amphotericin-induced renal dysfunction. On the tenth day, urinalysis demonstrated 2–3 casts/HPF (cylindruria), 2–3 WBC/HPF, and the presence of tubular epithelial cells. Serum creatinine was reported to be 1.2 mg/dl. Over the next three weeks cylindruria persisted and serum creatinine progressively rose. On the eighteenth day the patient was started on potassium gluconate because of a falling serum potassium (2.9 mEq/L). By the twentieth day the potassium requirements were fixed at 100 mEq/day. On the twenty-seventh day urinalysis showed 10–15 casts/HPF, urinary specific gravity was 1.003, and urinary pH was 6.7. Serum creatinine had risen to 3.1 mg/dl, and creatinine clearance was 37 ml/min. Because of the patient's worsening renal function, amphotericin was withheld pending improvement in renal function. After 72 hours serum creatinine fell to 2.4 mg/dl. At this time amphotericin was reinstituted at a dose of 60 mg every other day. With this dosage regimen the patient continued to improve while his renal function stabilized. The patient completed a six week course of therapy at which time the serum creatinine was 2.8 mg/dl and creatinine clearance was 48 ml/min. The patient had received a total dose of 1800 mg. Renal function improved steadily following completion of amphotericin therapy. Within two weeks the patient's serum creatinine had fallen to 1.7 mg/dl. He was also able to discontinue potassium supplements. At the two-month follow-up, serum creatinine was 1.1 mg/dl.

By what mechanism does renal impairment due to amphotericin B occur? What is

the typical clinical presentation? Comment on the management of this patient.

As was the case in L.A., nephrotoxicity is the major dose-limiting factor of treatment with amphotericin B. Functionally, toxicity is characterized by a reduction in GFR, a rise in serum creatinine, and renal tubular dysfunction.

A wide range of renal histopathologic changes due to amphotericin have been described. These include vacuolization of smooth muscle cells in the media of the arterioles and arteries of the kidney, thickening and/or fragmentation of the glomerular basement membranes, focal or diffuse tubular degeneration and atrophy, and nephrocalcinosis of both the proximal and distal convoluted tubules. Although a reduction in renal blood flow with resultant cortical ischemia is considered by many to be the primary mechanism of amphotericin nephrotoxicity, the contribution of direct tubule cell toxicity and that of calcium deposition cannot be overlooked.

A rise in serum creatinine occurs in over 80% of patients who receive amphotericin. Impaired renal function may be mild and self-limited or progressive as was the situation with L.A. whose serum creatinine rose steadily over a three-week period. This rise in serum creatinine was accompanied by the presence of cylindruria in the urine. Cylindruria is a common finding in the urine of patients with amphotericin-induced renal damage. Amphotericin was withheld in L.A. in accord with the generally accepted recommendation that amphotericin be withheld for 24 to 48 hours when the serum creatinine reaches 2.5 to 3.0 mg/dl in order to allow renal function to improve. Amphotericin should then be reinstituted at one-half the original dose and increased gradually.

Distal renal tubular acidosis is another potential adverse effect of amphotericin on the kidney. It is believed to be the result of a direct toxic effect of the drug on tubular epithelial cells. The syndrome is characterized by excessive excretion of bicarbonate and potassium in the urine, defective citrate excretion, and impaired renal concentrating ability. Potassium wasting due to amphotericin was the most likely cause of L.A.'s hypokalemia. The potassium deficit can be substantial in some patients, and supplemental requirements of 100 to 200 mEq of potassium a day may be required. L.A. required 100 mEq/day. Potassium was administered to this patient in the form of potassium gluconate instead of the chloride salt because distal renal tubular acidosis results in the unusual metabolic imbalance of hypokalemic acidosis. These patients also have an impaired ability to excrete an acid load, although metabolic acidosis usually does not occur. Nephrocalcinosis secondary to a persistently alkaline urine may also occur.

Particular attention should be given not only to renal function but also to electrolyte and acid-base balance in patients who are receiving amphotericin (203–207).

42. Are the nephrotoxic effects of amphotericin always reversible?

Tubular dysfunction and renal insufficiency are usually reversible upon withdrawal of amphotericin. This was the case with L.A.; renal function had returned to near normal two weeks after completion of his amphotericin therapy and was essentially normal at the end of two months. However, in some cases reversal upon withdrawal of amphotericin may be prolonged, and on occasion renal function does not return to baseline values. The correlation between the degree and persistence of renal insufficiency as related to total dose of amphotericin is disputed. However, total doses of more than 4 grams should be used with caution since there is some evidence to suggest a greater incidence of permanent renal damage at this dosage level (203–207).

43. Why was mannitol administered to L.A.?

Several possible methods have been suggested for reducing amphotericin nephrotoxicity. These include alternate day administration of amphotericin and infusion of mannitol just prior to the administration of amphotericin. Prophylactic administration of alkali has also been proposed to prevent the development of renal tubular acidosis. In this patient, alternate day administration of amphotericin was used following the temporary withdrawal of the drug due to worsening renal function.

It has been reported in animal experiments and uncontrolled clinical trials that the osmotic diuretic, mannitol, prevents the rise in serum creatinine which normally accompanies amphotericin administration. However, in the only controlled study, mannitol infusions not only proved to be ineffective, but renal biopsy samples indicated that patients receiving the combination of amphotericin and mannitol had more severe renal arteriolar vacuolization. Based on these data, it would appear that mannitol should not be used for the prevention of amphotericin nephrotoxicity.

As for the other modalities, their success is based on uncontrolled clinical trials and therefore must await further controlled trials before a definite conclusion about their usefulness can be made (206).

Lithium Nephrotoxicity

44. J.B. is a 49-year-old male who was placed on lithium carbonate 900 mg/day eight years ago after a hospitalization for manic illness. The patient has been maintained on this regimen since that time, although several subsequent manic episodes required a temporary increase in the lithium dose. The patient's lithium levels have usually fallen within the range of 0.5 to 1.2 mEq/L, although on two separate occasions levels of 2.8 and 2.2 mEq/L were recorded in association with episodes of acute lithium intoxication apparently related to restriction of sodium intake. Besides these two episodes of lithium intoxication, the patient has a six-year history of polyuria (5 to 7 liters/day) secondary to lithium. The patient, who is presently free of any manic symptoms, is now being admitted to the university hospital for evaluation of abnormal renal function. Admission renal function tests were serum creatinine 2.8 mg/dl, BUN 28 mg/dl (values 2 years previously were 1.1 mg/dl and 13 mg/dl, respectively). Urinary sediment results were as follows: trace protein, 0–2 WBC/HPF, 0–2 RBC/HPF, and no casts. On urinalysis, the patient's urine had a specific gravity of 1.003 with a urine osmolality of 188 mOsm/kg. A renal biopsy showed evidence of nonspecific histologic changes. Interstitial fibrosis, tubular atrophy, and glomerular sclerosis were most pronounced. Because of a possible association with lithium treatment, the Nephrology and Clinical Pharmacology Departments were contacted for consultation as to the possible effects of lithium on the kidney. Based on recommendations by both departments, lithium was discontinued and the patient was placed on another antipsychotic medication.

What are the adverse effects of lithium on the kidney which were illustrated in this patient?

This patient illustrates the important functional and histological abnormalities associated with the chronic use of lithium. The best known adverse effect of lithium on the kidney is decreased renal concentrating ability and polyuria. J.B. was obviously experiencing this as a side effect as evidenced by his history of polyuria of 5 to 7 liters/day and his low urinary specific gravity and osmolality. Lithium-induced disturbances in water clearance are caused by resistance to the action of antidiuretic hormone (vasopressin). Lithium-induced polyuria can be seen during the first several weeks following the initiation of treatment, although as was the case in this patient, it may appear as a late complication of long-term lithium administration. Although the potential for serious alteration in water balance exists, for many patients polyuria is only a minor inconvenience while for others it is a troublesome problem which threatens patient compliance. In some patients, a reduction in dose may be necessary in an attempt to reduce the degree of polyuria. Concurrent administration of thiazide-type diuretics has been shown to be useful in reducing lithium dosage requirements while improving the degree of polyuria. This treatment modality was considered at one time for J.B., but he refused to take any additional medications. Discontinuation of lithium may be required in an occasional patient. Although normal urinary concentrating ability usually returns within several weeks, there are an increasing number of reports of persistent polyuria following lithium withdrawal, suggesting the possibility of permanent renal damage in some patients. In this patient, polyuria improved following withdrawal of lithium; however, a urine output of 3 to 4 liters/day persisted for six months after lithium was discontinued. The patient was lost to follow-up at that time.

Aside from the effects of lithium on the renal concentrating ability of the kidney, permanent renal damage secondary to chronic histologic changes, such as that found in our patient, have been recently described in patients receiving long-term treatment with lithium salts. In one study of 14 patients with acute lithium intoxication and/or nephrogenic diabetes insipidus, renal biopsy specimens demonstrated a significant degree of focal nephron atrophy associated with interstitial fibrosis in 13 of the patients (208). Glomerular sclerosis was also present in most of the patients. These nonspecific changes were significantly more common in lithium-treated psychiatric patients as compared to a control sample of non-psychiatric patients. All patients had received lithium for a year or more. An inverse correlation was reported between creatinine clearance and the degree of chronic histologic changes on renal biopsy.

In a subsequent investigation of 110 patients treated with lithium for six months or more, 18 (26%) had clinical evidence of renal disease which was attributed to lithium (209). In 14 patients biopsy documentation of chronic interstitial nephritis with fibrosis was found. Renal concentrating ability was markedly impaired in all 18 patients, and polyuria was present in 15. However, only minor changes in the glomerular filtration rates were found. Impairment of renal concentrating ability was correlated to both the duration of lithium treatment and the degree of tubular damage.

Because of methodological deficiencies in the design of these two studies, the incidence of these chronic lesions and their association to high dose and/or prolonged use of lithium is disputed. The possibility of permanent renal damage secondary to lithium has spurred a number of investigators to examine patients on long-term lithium with regard to renal function and histologic changes. Although other instances of chronic lesions similar to those described above have been reported, most authorities consider that if these lesions are in fact related to lithium administration, their occurrence is not common. Even if they are present, serious renal dysfunction appears to be rare.

Despite the apparent infrequency of chronic renal lesions associated with lithium treatment, lithium was considered the most likely cause of impaired renal function in J.B. As mentioned above, discontinuation of lithium resulted in improvement in his polyuria; however, renal function tests had not improved at the time the patient was lost to follow-up.

Finally, there are several reports of nephrotic syndrome developing during treatment with lithium salts. In two cases, renal biopsy provided evidence of minimal change or lipoid nephrosis. Proteinuria resolved in both cases upon withdrawal of lithium and reappeared in one patient who was rechallenged with lithium. This patient had neither clinical (excessive proteinuria) nor biopsy evidence of minimal change nephrosis (208–214).

Analgesic Nephropathy

45. H.G. is a 47-year-old female who was admitted to the hospital for treatment of acute renal failure. The patient, who appeared older than her stated age, was in apparent distress, complaining of severe lower back pain which was not substantially relieved by a 50 mg intramuscular dose of meperidine administered in the emergency room.

Laboratory data reported on admission were: serum creatinine 12 mg/dl, BUN 145 mg/dl, serum potassium 5.7 mEq/L, serum bicarbonate 15 mEq/L; urinalysis: RBC's > 25/HPF, WBC's 10–15/HPF, and protein 1+; urine output was < 20 ml/hr. Blood pressure was 160/110 mm Hg.

Past medical history was significant for analgesic abuse which began at the age of 23. At that time the patient began taking various analgesic remedies including APC tablets (aspirin, phenacetin, and caffeine) on a regular basis (three to six tablets a day) for headaches and for dysmenorrhea. At the age of 26, the patient was treated medically for a gastric ulcer, and the ulcer subsequently required surgical intervention when she was 28. The patient has taken antacids on an irregular basis since that time. Iron supplements were also required for iron deficiency anemia secondary to excessive gastrointestinal blood loss. The patient was instructed to avoid aspirin. Analgesic abuse was not considered. At the age of 31, the patient saw her local physician for various somatic complaints which included chronic headache, weakness, malaise, sleeplessness, and nocturia. All laboratory tests at that time were normal. The physician prescribed a tranquilizer. Because the patient was dissatisfied with her medical care, she sought other physicians who in turn prescribed a variety of analgesics, sleep medications, and tranquilizers. At age 38, during a physical exam required for employment, the patient was noted to have an abnormal urinalysis: 4–5 WBC/HPF, 2–3 RBC/HPF, trace protein, specific gravity 1.004. Urine cultures were negative.

Serum creatinine was found to be 1.5 mg/dl. The patient was referred to a nephrologist who performed additional tests. She was found to have significantly impaired renal concentrating ability. Creatinine clearance was 68 ml/min. An intravenous urogram was performed and showed changes consistent with renal papillary necrosis. Strongly suspecting analgesic nephropathy, the nephrologist questioned the patient thoroughly, after which she admitted to excessive analgesic use. It was estimated that the patient had ingested in excess of 4 kg of phenacetin and 6 kg of aspirin since age 23. The patient was advised to discontinue the use of all analgesic agents.

Despite these warnings, the patient continued taking over-the-counter analgesics (Empirin Compound, Excedrin, Tylenol, Bufferin) and her renal function continued to decline. Serum creatinine was 4.3 mg/dl two months prior to admission. After her last physician visit two weeks prior to admission, the patient was treated with ampicillin for a urinary tract infection.

Based on the patient's past medical history and present clinical condition, a presumptive diagnosis of acute oliguric renal failure secondary to obstruction, probably due to a sloughed papilla, was made. The presence of a urinary tract infection may have exacerbated the situation.

Dialysis was instituted, electrolyte abnormalities were corrected, and blood pressure was controlled. However, surgical intervention was required to remove the obstruction. Following surgery, renal function improved; serum creatinine was 4.6 mg/dl at the time of discharge 18 days later. Because of this episode, the patient stated she would discontinue all analgesic agents. The patient was followed in nephrology clinic, and at her last visit nine months after hospitalization, her serum creatinine was 3.2 mg/dl.

What is analgesic nephropathy and which analgesics were the most likely cause in this case?

Analgesic nephropathy is a form of renal disease characterized by renal papillary necrosis and chronic interstitial nephritis caused by the chronic consumption of various analgesic preparations.

The earliest histologic change which has been demonstrated in these patients is partial or complete papillary necrosis; interstitial nephritis occurs secondary to processes which begin in the deeper zones of the medulla. Renal cortical tissue is not involved in the early stages of renal damage. It has not been established whether the initiating event in the development of papillary necrosis is ischemia or a direct toxic effect of analgesics.

The identity of the analgesics involved in the pathogenesis of these renal lesions remains controversial. Phenacetin has long been considered the principal causative agent in analgesic nephropathy. However, in experimental animal models phenacetin and its metabolite, acetaminophen, when given alone are considered less nephrotoxic than aspirin alone. In addition, combinations of analgesics such as aspirin plus phenacetin when given in either high doses for a short period of time or lower doses over a prolonged period of time produce a relatively higher incidence of papillary necrosis than single agents. Dehydration apparently increases the medullary concentration of these agents and thereby substantially increases the incidence of papillary necrosis. To summarize, in experimental animal models the relative ability to produce papillary necrosis is as follows: aspirin + phenacetin > aspirin alone > phenacetin or acetaminophen alone.

Although renal papillary necrosis has been reported after long-term ingestion of single agents such as aspirin, acetaminophen, and other nonsteroidal antiinflammatory drugs including indomethacin and phenylbutazone, analgesic nephropathy due to single agents is uncommon. The majority of cases have been reported in patients ingesting combination products, especially those containing phenacetin. Such was the case with H.G. who primarily abused aspirin, phenacetin, and caffeine tablets. The association between phenacetin and cases of analgesic nephropathy led to the withdrawal of phenacetin from the market in several countries. While withdrawal of phenacetin in some countries has been associated with a reduction in the death rates from analgesic nephropathy (Denmark, Sweden, Canada), in other countries no such reduction has been shown (Switzerland, Australia).

Most authorities consider patients who ingest

excessive quantities of analgesic combination products to be at the greatest risk of developing analgesic nephropathy (215–231).

46. How was the initial diagnosis of analgesic nephropathy made in H.G.? Is this patient fairly typical of patients with analgesic nephropathy?

Although analgesic nephropathy was once considered rare in this country, rising awareness of this problem has led to its identification in an increasing number of patients. Analgesic nephropathy has been estimated to be the cause of 20% of all cases of chronic interstitial nephritis and 7% of all cases of chronic renal failure in the U.S. This patient demonstrates several characteristics of this syndrome. Patients who present with analgesic nephropathy are predominately middle-aged women with a history of headaches and other various somatic complaints (eg, weakness, malaise). H.G. was 38 years old with a 15-year history of headaches at the time of diagnosis. Psychiatric disturbances and addictive habits such as smoking, alcoholism, use of psychotropic drugs, and laxative abuse are frequently present. Gastrointestinal symptoms occur in approximately half of patients who abuse analgesics, particularly those who abuse aspirin-containing preparations. Anemia is also present in a high proportion of patients with analgesic nephropathy. Anemia may be due to chronic renal failure and/or aspirin-induced gastrointestinal blood loss. Methemoglobinemia and sulfhemoglobinemia may also develop in patients who abuse phenacetin-containing combinations. The latter was not present despite H.G.'s use of phenacetin. An increased incidence of atherosclerosis and ischemic heart disease has been found. Premature aging (present in this patient) has been emphasized by several authorities as a feature of analgesic nephropathy.

Any patient who has a history of ingesting 1 gm/day of an analgesic for one or more years or has ingested a total of 2 to 3 kg should be considered at risk for the development or presence of analgesic nephropathy. At the time the diagnosis of analgesic nephropathy was made in H.G., her total intake far exceeded these minimum values. Denial of analgesic intake, as occurred with this patient, is a problem that makes diagnosis difficult. It should be emphasized that the risks of lower doses of analgesics on renal structure have not been adequately investigated.

Renal impairment is insidious in onset. Renal tubular dysfunction (impaired concentrating ability, defective renal acidification, sodium wasting), mild proteinuria, microscopic hematuria, sterile pyuria, and azotemia usually occur during the course of the disease. A reduced concentrating ability is frequently the earliest sign of renal damage. Renal involvement commonly progresses to end stage renal failure with continued analgesic abuse.

The diagnosis of partial or complete papillary necrosis can be made from an intravenous urogram. This was done in this patient. A normal urogram does not rule out papillary necrosis, since it may represent an early stage of papillary necrosis not detectable by urogram or papillary necrosis in situ. Serial urograms may be beneficial. If radiographic data are inconclusive, renal biopsy may be necessary to demonstrate chronic interstitial nephritis. Because of H.G.'s history of analgesic abuse, clinical features, and radiologic evidence, renal biopsy was not considered necessary for the diagnosis.

Sloughed papillary tissue can cause obstruction and acute renal failure, as exemplified by H.G. and is clinically evident by renal colic and macroscopic hematuria. Infectious pyelonephritis is commonly superimposed and may further compromise renal function (215–231).

47. How should patients with analgesic nephropathy be managed? Should H.G. have been managed any differently than she was?

The reversibility and prognosis of analgesic nephropathy are related to the severity of renal damage at the time of diagnosis and to whether or not the patient refrains from further analgesic use. This latter point must be emphasized to patients with analgesic nephropathy since present evidence indicates that renal function stabilizes or often improves when analgesic abuse is stopped. Control of blood pressure, urinary tract infection, and early treatment of obstructive uropathy (as was done in H.G.) are essential for preserving residual renal function. This patient's renal function probably would have normalized if she had refrained from analgesic use when the problem was initially diagnosed. Her renal function did improve once she stopped taking analgesic medications after her episode of acute renal failure, although renal function did not return to normal. The patient's prognosis is probably fair if she continues to abstain from analgesic use. The appearance of persistent heavy proteinuria (not present in this patient) indicates glomerular damage and carries a poor prognosis (221,223,225).

The occurrence of persistent hematuria, particularly after the withdrawal of analgesic preparations, should alert the physician to the possibility of transitional cell carcinoma of the lower urinary tract. Since 1965, over 100 cases of uroepithelial tumors of the renal pelvis have been reported following prolonged and/or excessive analgesic intake. Multiple uroepithelial tumors involving the ureters and bladder have been described as well. Malignancy usually occurs after years of analgesic abuse and may even occur following cessation of analgesic use and in the absence of active papillary necrosis (232). The possibility that such a malignancy could eventually develop in this patient must be considered in her long-term management. Patients with analgesic nephropathy are reportedly eight times more likely to develop transitional cell carcinoma of the urinary tract than the general population. Overall prognosis for these patients is generally poor with a less than 40% five-year survival rate (232). Current evidence implicates phenacetin, or more specifically, its N-hydroxylated metabolite, as a probable carcinogenic factor (232).

Gold Nephropathy

48. R.M. is a 62-year-old woman who was evaluated by her local physician in 1976 because of complaints of joint stiffness and soreness. The patient was diagnosed to have rheumatoid arthritis (ESR 65 mm/hr; positive rheumatoid factor). Routine urinalysis was normal at this time. Therapeutic doses of aspirin were prescribed with a good initial response. However, in 1978, because of progression of her disease, prednisone was started with the maintenance dose fixed at 12.5 mg/day. Urinalysis and renal function tests were normal at this time. Over the next two years the patient required increasing doses of prednisone to control her symptoms. Finally, in February of 1980, the patient was referred to the University Rheumatology Clinic for evaluation of her disease. It was decided that in addition to her prednisone she should be started on gold therapy. Pertinent laboratory values at the time were ESR

55 mm/hr, serum creatinine 1.0 mg/dl, BUN 9 mg/dl, and normal urinalysis. The patient was to be followed by her local physician with periodic visits to the clinic. Sodium thiomalate (Myochrysine) was started at 25 mg initially, followed by 50 mg weekly. With this regimen the patient's condition improved. After six months the patient's gold dose was decreased to 50 mg twice a month and after another three months was decreased to 50 mg a month. During the first nine months of treatment, urinalyses were unremarkable except for transient proteinuria which occurred at the beginning of treatment. Increasing proteinuria was noted by the patient's local physician starting in December of 1980. Proteinuria reached a high of 3+ in March of 1981. The patient's urine was not tested again until her clinic visit in May. At this time the patient was found to have 3+ ankle edema. Urinalysis showed 4+ proteinuria, 1+ hematuria, and 1–2 RBC casts/HPF. Serum albumin was 2.7 mg/dl. The 24-hour albumin excretion was 6.5 gm. Serum creatinine was 1.1 mg/dl and BUN was 15 mg/dl. Serum cholesterol was 355 mg/dl. A renal biopsy was performed and showed membranous glomerulonephritis on light microscopy. Immunofluorescent staining was positive for IgG. Gold inclusions were also found in proximal tubular cells but not in the glomerulus. Based on the working diagnosis of gold-induced nephrotic syndrome, gold salts were discontinued. Within seven weeks proteinuria improved, with 24-hour albumin excretion being less than 300 mg/day. Gold salts were readministered at this time because of worsening symptoms. Within two months proteinuria recurred (750 to 1100 mg/24 hr). Gold salts were withdrawn and the patient was maintained on higher doses of prednisone. Consideration was given to starting penicillamine at a future date.

49. What characteristics did R.M. display which led to the diagnosis of gold-induced nephrotic syndrome? Was this patient's toxicity related to the dose of gold salts? What is proper management of patients with gold-induced nephrotoxicity?

The appearance of persistent proteinuria, and less frequently, microscopic hematuria, is usually the first clinical indication of renal toxicity. This can occur at any time during treatment. As was the case in R.M., proteinuria may become so severe that the nephrotic syndrome develops. The nephrotic syndrome can be defined by the presence of proteinuria of > 3.5 gm/day, hypoalbuminemia < 3.0 mg%, hypercholesterolemia, and edema. All four criteria were met by this patient.

Pathologically, the nephrotic syndrome caused by gold salts is due to immune-complex membranous glomerulonephritis. This was demonstrated in this patient's renal biopsy. Subendothelial deposits of an unidentified immunogen as well as IgG and other immunoglobulins have been reported by investigators using immunofluorescent techniques. IgG was identified in this patient's biopsy sample. Deposits of gold in tubular epithelial cells are also a commonly reported biopsy finding (present in our patient). Although this suggests an additional direct toxic effect of gold on the kidney, the overall contribution of these gold deposits to nephrotoxicity is not clear. Overall, the development of gold nephropathy cannot be consistently related to dose, duration of treatment or blood levels of gold.

Proteinuria usually clears within several weeks or months. In persistent cases, steroid treatment may be beneficial. On occasion, azotemia and chronic renal failure may develop, especially in patients in whom gold salts are continued in the face of the nephrotic syndrome. It is generally recommended that gold salts be withheld until the urinary sediment clears if a patient develops persistent proteinuria or microscopic hematuria; gold salts can subsequently be reinstituted at a lower dose. The local physician in this patient's case may not have been fully aware of the nephrotoxic potential of gold salts and therefore continued gold in the presence of persistent proteinuria. It wasn't until the patient was seen in the Rheumatology Clinic that the diagnosis was made and gold salts discontinued. Although it is often recommended that gold salts not be readministered once the nephrotic syndrome has developed, this was done in R.M. with fairly rapid reappearance of proteinuria. Gold salts were not administered again (233–240). Also see the chapter on Rheumatic Diseases.

It should be noted that penicillamine, which is being considered for further use in this patient, has been reported to cause nephrotic syndrome secondary to immune-complex membranous glomerulonephritis. It is not known whether the development of nephrotic syndrome while on gold salts enhances the risk of penicillamine-induced glomerulonephritis.

Oral Contraceptive Nephrotoxicity

50. S.B. is a 37-year-old, moderately obese (85 kg) female who presented to her local physician with a 6-month history of severe frontal headaches (for which the patient took various headache remedies) and a 3-week history of increasing shortness of breath, dyspnea on exertion, and persistent nausea and vomiting. Blood pressure at this time was 220/140 mm Hg. Hypertensive retinopathy (papillary edema, hemorrhagic exudates) was present. Urinalysis revealed 4+ proteinuria. The patient was on no medication at this time except for a mestranol-norethindrone oral contraceptive combination product which had been started 8 months previously, after her third pregnancy and delivery. The patient's pregnancy had been complicated by persistent edema and mild to moderate hypertension during the final three months.

The patient was admitted to the hospital for treatment of malignant hypertension apparently due to her oral contraceptive medication. Admission blood pressure was 230/150 mm Hg. Serum creatinine was 6.4 mg/dl, and BUN was 75 mg/dl. An intravenous pyelogram showed no evidence of impaired blood flow to either kidney. Her oral contraceptive medication was discontinued, and parenteral antihypertensives (diazoxide, hydralazine, and furosemide) were administered. Blood pressure was brought under control by the third hospital day, at which time the patient was switched to oral antihypertensive agents (methyldopa and furosemide). Despite control of blood pressure, renal insufficiency persisted, and the patient was discharged after 12 days with a serum creatinine of 2.4 mg/dl and a creatinine clearance of 45 ml/min. The patient's renal function had not improved at a follow-up visit 7 months after discharge. The patient is presently using an alternate form of birth control.

Hypertension is a well known side effect of oral contraceptives. Was S.B. at any greater

risk of developing hypertension; should she have been monitored more closely?

This case points out the need for early detection of oral contraceptive-induced hypertension. Although the increase in blood pressure is frequently minor, marked increases may be seen. The development of malignant hypertension, which occurred in S.B., is always a potential hazard. Blood pressure should be monitored regularly, especially during the initial months of treatment. This was not done in this patient who was at increased risk because of her age, weight problem, and history of hypertension during pregnancy. Patients should also be instructed to report symptoms such as headache, persistent nausea or emesis which are possible indicators of hypertension. If this patient had been properly monitored, it is possible she may not have developed renal failure (241,242).

The development of hypertensive arteriolar nephrosclerosis is a potential sequela of malignant hypertension. Azotemia, acute oliguric renal failure and, in some cases, end-stage renal failure requiring nephrectomy may result. Hemolytic anemia secondary to microangiopathy, did not occur in S.B., but is frequently present. Withdrawal of the offending agent and control of blood pressure are imperative to preserve renal function. Although blood pressure was controlled in this patient, some degree of irreversible renal damage apparently had already taken place (243–246).

Oral contraceptives can also induce renal failure secondary to renal vein thrombosis. This is a rare but serious complication of oral contraceptive therapy. The severity and rapidity of onset of renal impairment depends primarily on the location of the thrombus and the degree of occlusion. The patient may present acutely with sudden onset of lower back pain. Evidence of renal damage may range from an abnormal urinalysis (proteinuria/hematuria) to severe azotemic renal failure or, in chronic cases, nephrotic syndrome. Renovascular hypertension may also develop. Although this patient did present with some features of renal vein thrombosis (proteinuria, azotemia), the lack of changes characteristic of renal vein thrombosis on the pyelogram tend to rule out this diagnosis (247,248).

References

1. Anderson RJ et al: Nonoliguric acute renal failure. N Engl J Med. 1977; 296:1134.
2. Schrier RW et al: Acute renal failure. In *Renal and Electrolyte Disorders,* 2nd ed, edited by RW Schrier, Little, Brown and Company, Boston, 1980, p 375.
3. Cronin RE et al: Acute renal failure: diagnosis, pathogenesis, and management. Hosp Med. 1976; 12:26.
4. Levinsky NG et al: Acute renal failure. In *The Kidney,* edited by BM Brenner and FC Rector, WB Saunders Company, Phil., 1976, p 806.
5. Franklin SS et al: Acute renal failure. In *Clinical Disorders of Fluid and Electrolyte Metabolism,* 3rd ed, edited by MH Maxwell and CR Kleeman, McGraw-Hill Book Co., New York, 1980, p 745.
6. Valtin H (ed): Diuretics. In *Renal Dysfunction: Mechanisms Involved in Fluid and Solute Imbalance,* Little, Brown and Company, Boston, 1979, p 167.
7. Schrier RW: Acute renal failure. Kidney International. 1979; 15:205.
8. Barry KG et al: Oliguric renal failure: evaluation and therapy by the intravenous infusion of mannitol. JAMA. 1962; 179:510.
9. Silverberg DS et al: The use of mannitol in oliguric renal failure. Med Clin North Am. 1966; 50:1159.
10. Miller RR et al (eds): *Drug Effects in Hospitalized Patients,* John Wiley and Sons, New York, 1976, p 86.
11. Meriwether WD et al: Deafness following a standard intravenous dose of ethacrynic acid. JAMA. 1971; 216:795.
12. Nierenberg DW: Furosemide and ethacrynic acid in acute tubular necrosis. West J Med. 1980; 133:163.
13. Kleinknecht D et al: Furosemide in acute oliguric renal failure—a controlled trial. Nephron. 1976; 17:51.
14. Bradley GM et al: Examination of the urine. In *Todd-Sanford Clinical Diagnosis by Laboratory Methods,* 15th ed, edited by I Davidsohn and J Henry, WB Saunders Company, Phil., 1974, p 41.
15. Humphreys MH et al: Acute renal failure in trauma patients. West J Med. 1975; 123:148.
16. Naranjo CA et al: Furosemide-induced adverse drug reactions during hospitalization. Am J Hosp Pharm. 1978; 35:794.
17. Greenblatt DJ et al: Clinical toxicity of furosemide in hospitalized patients. Am Heart J. 1977; 94:6.
18. Wigand ME et al: Ototoxic side effects of high doses of furosemide in patients with uremia. Postgrad Med J. 1971(suppl); 47:54.
19. Cooperman LB et al: Toxicity of ethacrynic acid and furosemide. Am Heart J. 1973; 85:831.
20. Anonymous: Lasix: package insert. Hoeschst-Roussel Pharmaceuticals Inc. 1979.
21. Stein JH et al: Acute renal failure: clinical aspects and pathophysiology. Contr Nephrol. 1978; 14:118.
22. Kopple JD: Total parenteral nutrition and parenteral fluid therapy. In *Clinical Disorders of Fluid and Electrolyte Metabolism,* 3rd ed, edited by M Maxwell and C Kleeman, McGraw-Hill, New York, 1980, p 413.

23. Blackburn GL et al: Criteria for choosing amino acid therapy in acute renal failure. Am J Clin Nutr. 1978; 31:1841.

24. Alfrey AC: Chronic renal failure: manifestations and pathogenesis. In *Renal and Electrolyte Disorders,* 2nd ed, edited by RW Schrier, Little, Brown and Company, Boston, 1980, p 409.

25. Crowe LR et al: Diagnosis and management of chronic renal insufficiency. Hosp Med. 1976; 12:6.

26. Merrill JP et al: Uremia. N Engl J Med. 1970; 282:953 and 1014.

27. Schonfeld PY et al: A general description of the uremic state. In *The Kidney,* edited by BM Brenner and FC Rector, WB Saunders, Phil., 1976, p 1423.

28. Walser M: The conservative management of the uremic patient. In *The Kidney,* edited by BM Brenner and FC Rector, WB Saunders, Phil., 1976, p 1613.

29. Valtin H: Chronic renal failure: adaptation of balances. In *Renal Dysfunction: Mechanisms Involved in Fluid and Solute Imbalance,* Little, Brown and Company, Boston, 1979, p 257.

30. Fried W: Hematologic complications of chronic renal failure. Med Clin North Am. 1978; 62:1363.

31. Eschbach JW et al: The hematologic consequences of renal failure. In *The Kidney,* edited by BM Brenner and FC Rector, WB Saunders, Phil. 1976, p 1522.

32. Lichtman MA et al: Erythrocyte glycolysis, 2,3-diphosphoglycerate and adenosine triphosphate concentration in uremic subjects: relationships to extracellular phosphate concentration. J Lab Clin Med. 1970; 76:267.

33. Ersley AJ: Renal biogenesis of erythropoietin. Am J Med. 1975; 58:25.

34. Koch KM et al: Anemia of the regular hemodialysis patient and its treatment. Nephron. 1974; 12:405.

35. Shahidi NT: Androgens and erythropoiesis. N Engl J Med. 1973; 289:72.

36. Yawata Y et al: Abnormal red cell metabolism causing hemolysis in uremia: a defect potentiated by tap water hemodialysis. Ann Intern Med. 1973; 79:362.

37. Parker PA et al: Therapy of iron deficiency anemia in patients on maintenance dialysis. Nephron. 1979; 23:181.

38. Gokal R et al: Iron metabolism in hemodialysis patients. Quarterly J Med (New Series). 1979; 48:369.

39. Hampers CL et al: Megaloblastic hematopoiesis in uremia and in patients on long-term hemodialysis. N Engl J Med. 1967; 276:551.

40. Hines JD et al: Abnormal folate binding proteins in azotemic patients. Blood. 1973; 42:997.

41. Kopple JD et al: Vitamin nutrition in patients undergoing maintenance hemodialysis. Kidney International. 1975; 7:S-79.

42. Whitehead VM: Hemostasis of folic acid in patients undergoing maintenance hemodialysis. N Engl J Med. 1968; 279:970.

43. Paine CJ et al: Folic acid binding proteins and folate balance in uremia. Arch Intern Med. 1976; 136:756.

44. Skoutakis VA et al: Folic acid dosage for chronic hemodialysis patients. Clin Pharmacol Ther. 1975; 18:200.

45. Holliday MA et al: Nutritional management of chronic renal disease. Med Clin North Am. 1979; 63:945.

46. Grangrande A et al: Management of dialysis anemia: effective or ineffective. In *Dialysis Review,* edited by AM Davison, JB Lippincott Company, Phil., 1978, p 144.

47. Bailey GL (ed): *Hemodialysis, Principles and Practice,* Academic Press, New York, 1972.

48. Johnson FL et al: Association of androgenic-anabolic steroid therapy with development of hepatocellular carcinoma. Lancet. 1972; 2:1273.

49. Alexander MR: Use of androgens in chronic renal failure patients on maintenance hemodialysis. Am J Hosp Pharm. 1976; 33:242.

50. DeGowin RL et al: Erythropoiesis and erythropoietin in patients with chronic renal failure treated with hemodialysis and testosterone. Ann Intern Med. 1970; 72:913.

51. Doane BD et al: Response of uremic patients to nandrolone decanoate. Arch Intern Med. 1975; 135:972.

52. Eschbach JW et al: Improvement in the anemia of chronic renal failure with fluoxymesterone. Ann Intern Med. 1973; 78:527.

53. Fried W et al: The hematologic effect of androgen in uremic patients: study of packed cell volume and erythropoietin responses. Ann Intern Med. 1973; 79:823.

54. Hendler ED et al: Controlled study of androgen therapy in anemia of patients on hemodialysis. N Engl J Med. 1974; 291:1046.

55. Rabiner SF: Bleeding in uremia. Med Clin North Am. 1972; 56:221.

56. Hutton RA: Hemostatic mechanism in uremia. Am J Clin Path. 1968; 21:406.

57. Weiss HJ: Bleeding disorders due to abnormal platelet function. Med Clin North Am. 1973; 57:517.

58. Merrill JP: Uremia. N Engl J Med. 1970; 282:953.

59. Mustard JF et al: Platelets, thrombosis, and drugs. Drugs. 1975; 9:19.

60. Weiss HJ: Platelet physiology and abnormalities of platelet function. N Engl J Med. 1975; 293:580.

61. Rasmussen H: Parathyroid hormone, calcitonin, and the calciferols. In *Textbook of Endocrinology,* edited by RH Williams, WB Saunders Company, Phil., 1974, p 758.

62. Jacobs MD: Vitamin D deficient states—pathophysiology and treatment. West J Med. 1979; 131:305.

63. Coburn JW et al: Altered divalent ion metabolism in renal disease and renal osteodystrophy. In *Clinical Disorders of Fluid and Electrolyte Metabolism,* 3rd ed, edited by M Maxwell and C Kleeman, McGraw-Hill, New York, 1980, p 1209.

64. Coburn JW et al: Intestinal absorption of calcium and the effect of renal insufficiency. Kidney International. 1973; 4:96.

65. Hanley DA et al: Secondary hyperparathyroidism in chronic renal failure. Med Clin North Am. 1978; 62:1319.

66. Contiguglia SR et al: The nature of soft tissue calcification in uremia. Kidney International. 1973; 4:229.

67. Avioli LV et al: Renal osteodystrophies. In *The Kidney,* edited by BM Brenner and FC Rector, WB Saunders Company, Phil., 1976, p 1542.

68. Favus MJ: Vitamin D physiology and some clinical aspects of the vitamin D endocrine system. Med Clin North Am. 1978; 62:1291.

69. Massry SG: Requirements of vitamin D metabolites in patients with renal disease. Am J Clin Nutr. 1980; 33:1530.

70. Teredesai P et al: Therapy of renal osteodystrophy with dihydrotachysterol in nondialyzed patients. Clin Nephr. 1980; 13:31.

71. Pierides AM et al: Barbiturate and anticonvulsant treatment in relation to osteomalacia with hemodialysis and renal transplantation. Br Med J. 1976; 1:190.

72. Pierides AM et al: 1-a-hydroxycholecalciferol in hemodialysis renal osteodystrophy. Adverse effects of anticonvulsant therapy. Clin Nephr. 1976; 5:189.

73. Nielsen HE et al: 1-a-hydroxyvitamin D₃ treatment of non-dialyzed patients with chronic renal failure. Effects on bone mineral, metabolism, and kidney function. Clin Nephr. 1980; 13:103.

74. Christiansen C et al: Decreased renal function in association with administration of 1,25-dihydroxyvitamin D₃ to patients with stable advanced renal failure. Contr Nephr. 1980; 18:139.

75. Healy MD et al: Effects of long-term therapy with calcitriol in patients with moderate renal failure. Arch Intern Med. 1980; 140:1030.

76. Norman AW et al: Recent advances in the endocrinology of vitamin D and implications for renal failure. Contr Nephr. 1978; 14:190.

77. Feldman HA et al: Endocrinology and metabolism in uremia and dialysis: a clinical review. Medicine. 1975; 54:345.

78. Depner TA et al: Chronic renal failure. In Strauss and Welt's Diseases of the Kidney, 3rd ed, edited by LE Earley and CW Gottschalk, Little, Brown and Company, Boston, 1979, p 211.

79. Abrams EE et al: Case reports: antacid induction of phosphate depletion syndrome in renal failure. West J Med. 1974; 120:157.

80. Bloom WL et al: Osteomalacia with pseudofractures caused by the ingestion of aluminum hydroxide. JAMA. 1960; 174:181.

81. Boelens PA et al: Hypophosphatemia with muscle weakness due to antacids and hemodialysis. Am J Dis Child. 1970; 120:350.

82. Knochel JP: Hypophosphatemia. West J Med. 1981; 134:15.

83. Poole JW et al: Investigation of aluminum blood levels in man after oral administration of an aluminum-containing complex, potassium glucaldrate. J Pharm Sci. 1965; 54:651.

84. Berlyne GM et al: Aluminum toxicity in rats. Lancet. 1972; 1:564.

85. Berlyne GM: Aluminum toxicity. Lancet. 1972; 2:47.

86. Bailey RR: Aluminum toxicity in rats and man. Lancet 1972; 2:276.

87. Thurston H et al: Aluminum retention and toxicity in chronic renal failure. Lancet. 1972; 1:881.

88. Alfrey AC et al: The dialysis encephalopathy syndrome. Possible aluminum intoxication. N Engl J Med. 1976; 294:184.

89. Alfrey AC: Disorders of magnesium metabolism. In Renal and Electrolyte Disorders, 2nd ed, edited by RW Schrier, Little, Brown and Company, 1980, p 299.

90. Randall RE Jr et al: Hypermagnesemia in renal failure: etiology and toxic manifestations. Ann Intern Med. 1964; 61:73.

91. Wacker WEC et al: Magnesium metabolism. N Engl J Med. 1968; 278:712.

92. Wacker WEC et al: Magnesium metabolism. N Engl J Med. 1968; 278:772.

93. Ditzier JW: Epsom-salts poisoning and a review of magnesium ion physiology. Anesthesiology. 1970; 32:378.

94. Mansouri K et al: Zinc, copper, magnesium and calcium in dialyzed and non-dialyzed uremic patients. Arch Intern Med. 1970; 125:88.

95. Bailey GL et al: Pharmacodynamics in renal failure. In Hemodialysis: Principles & Practice, edited by GL Bailey, Academic Press, New York, 1972, p 117.

96. Parfitt AM et al: Clinical disorders of calcium, phosphorus, and magnesium metabolism. In Clinical Disorders of Fluid and Electrolyte Metabolism, 3rd ed, edited by MH Maxwell and CR Kleeman, McGraw-Hill Company, New York, 1980, p 947.

97. David DS et al: Hypercalcemia after renal transplantation. N Engl J Med. 1973; 289:398.

98. Randall RE et al: The milk-alkali syndrome. Arch Intern Med. 1961; 107:63.

99. Levant JA et al: Stimulation of gastric secretion and gastrin release by single oral doses of calcium carbonate in man. N Engl J Med. 1973; 289:555.

100. Townsend CM Jr. et al: Intestinal obstruction from medication bezoar in patients with renal failure. N Engl J Med. 1973; 288:1058.

101. Gabow PA et al: Disorders of potassium metabolism. In Renal and Electrolyte Disorders, 2nd ed, edited by RW Schrier, Little, Brown and Company, Boston, 1980, p 183.

102. Schwartz WB: Potassium and the kidney. N Engl J Med. 1955; 253:601.

103. Whang R: Hyperkalemia: diagnosis and treatment. Am J Med Sci. 1976; 272:19.

104. Schultze RG et al: Potassium: physiology and pathophysiology. In Clinical Disorders of Fluid and Electrolyte Metabolism, 3rd ed, edited by MH Maxwell and CR Kleeman, McGraw-Hill Company, New York, 1980, p 113.

105. Pearson RE et al: Potassium content of selected medicines, foods and salt substitutes. Hosp Pharm. 1971; 6:6.

106. Cohen AB: Hyperkalemic effects of triamterene. Ann Intern Med. 1966; 65:521.

107. Herman E et al: Fatal hyperkalemic paralysis associated with spironolactone. Arch Neurol. 1966; 15:74.

108. Berlyne GM: Dangers of kayexalate in the treatment of hyperkalemia in renal failure. Lancet 1966; 1:167.

109. Cacioppo PL et al: Orange juice treated with exchange resin. N Engl J Med. 1972; 287:361.

110. Chamberlain MJ: Emergency treatment of hyperkalemia. Lancet. 1964; 1:464.

111. Levy N et al: Citrus juice treated with exchange resins. N Engl J Med. 1973; 289:753.

112. Rovner DR: Use of pharmacologic agents in the treatment of hypokalemia and hyperkalemia. Rational Drug Therapy. 1972; 6:1.

113. Rieselbach RE et al: Influence of the kidney upon urate homeostasis in health and disease. Am J Med. 1974; 56:665.

114. Smyth CJ: Diagnosis and treatment of gout. In Arthritis and Allied Conditions, 8th ed, edited by JL Hollander, Lea & Febiger, Phil, 1972, p 1112.

115. Wyngaarden JB: The etiology and pathogenesis of gout. In Arthritis and Allied Conditions, 8th ed, edited by JL Hollander, Lea & Febiger, Phil, 1972, p 1071.

116. Fessel WF et al: Correlates and consequences of asymptomatic hyperuricemia. Arch Intern Med. 1973; 132:44.

117. Berger L: Renal function in gout: IV. An analysis of 524 gouty subjects including long-term follow-up studies. Am J Med. 1975; 59:605.

118. Lassiter WE: Uric acid and the kidney. In Strauss and Welt's Diseases of the Kidney, 3rd ed, edited by LE Earley and CW Gottschalk, Little, Brown and Company, Boston, 1979, p 1217.

119. Smith LH: Urolithiasis. In Strauss and Welt's Diseases of the Kidney, 3rd ed, edited by LE Earley and CW Gottschalk, Little, Brown and Company, Boston, 1979, p 893.

120. Pyrah LN: Uric acid calculi. In Renal Calculus, Springer-Verlag, New York, 1979, p 320.

121. Symposium: Gout with renal complications. Ann Rheum Dis. 1966; 25:668.

122. Yu TF: Milestones in the treatment of gout. Am J Med. 1974; 56:676.

123. Wilson JD et al: Allopurinol in the treatment of uremic patients with gout. Ann Rheum Dis. 1967; 26:136.

124. Elion GB et al: Renal clearance of oxypurinol, the chief metabolite of allopurinol. Am J Med. 1968; 45:69.

125. Wallace SL et al: Plasma levels of colchicine after oral administration of a single dose. Metabolism. 1973; 22:749.

126. Wallace SL et al: Colchicine plasma levels: implications as to pharmacology and mechanism of action. Am J Med. 1970; 48:443.

127. Bagdade JD: Disorders of carbohydrate and lipid metabolism in uremia. Nephron. 1975; 14:153.

128. DeFronzo RA et al: Carbohydrate metabolism in uremia, a review. Medicine. 1973; 52:469.

129. Horton DS et al: Carbohydrate metabolism in uremia. Ann Intern Med. 1968; 68:63.

130. Rabkin R et al: Effect of renal disease on renal uptake and excretion of insulin in man. N Engl J Med. 1970; 282:182.

131. Knochel JP et al: The pathophysiology of uremia. In *The Kidney*, edited by BM Brenner and FC Rector, WB Saunders Company, Philadelphia, 1976, p 1448.

132. Corvilain J et al: Labeled insulin catabolism in chronic renal failure and in the anephric state. Diabetes. 1971; 20:467.

133. Rubinstein AH et al: Role of the kidney in insulin metabolism and excretion. Diabetes. 1968; 17:161.

134. Fuss M et al: I^{125}-insulin metabolism in chronic renal failure treated by renal transplantation. Kidney International. 1974; 5:372.

135. Navalesi R et al: Insulin metabolism in chronic uremia and in the anephric state: effect of the dialytic treatment. J Clin Endocrinol Metab. 1975; 40:70.

136. Greenblatt DJ: Insulin sensitivity in renal failure. N Y State J Med. 1974; 74:1040.

137. Del Greco F et al: Hypertension of chronic renal failure: role of sodium and the renal pressor system. Kidney International. 1975; 7:S176.

138. Kincaid-Smith P et al: Hypertension and the kidney. Kidney International. 1975; 8:S151.

139. Weidmann P et al: Hypertension in terminal renal failure. Kidney International. 1976; 9:294.

140. McDonald KM et al: The kidney in hypertension. In *Renal and Electrolyte Disorders*, 2nd ed, edited by RW Schrier, Little, Brown and Company, Boston, 1980, p 345.

141. Davies DL et al: Abnormal relation between exchangeable sodium and the reninangiotensin system in malignant hypertension and in hypertension with chronic renal failure. Lancet. 1973; 1:683.

142. Vertes V et al: Hypertension in end-stage renal disease. N Engl J Med. 1969; 280:978.

143. Mroczek WJ et al: The value of aggressive therapy in the hypertensive patient with azotemia. Circulation. 1969; 40:893.

144. Woods JW et al: Management of malignant hypertension complicated by renal insufficiency. N Engl J Med. 1967; 277:57.

145. Woods JW et al: Management of malignant hypertension complicated by renal insufficiency, a follow-up study. N Engl J Med. 1974; 291:10.

146. Sulliven JF et al: Use of furosemide in the oliguria of acute and chronic renal failure. Postgrad Med J. 1971; 47:S26.

147. Lazarus JM et al: Hypertension in chronic renal failure: treatment with hemodialysis and nephrectomy. Arch Intern Med. 1974; 133:1059.

148. Muth RG: Diuretic properties of furosemide in renal disease. Ann Intern Med. 1968; 69:249.

149. Rastogi SP et al: High-dose furosemide in the treatment of hypertension in chronic renal insufficiency and of terminal renal failure. Postgrad Med J. 1971; 47:S45.

150. Ulvila JM et al: Blood pressure in chronic renal failure: effect of sodium intake and furosemide. JAMA. 1972; 220:233.

151. Vaughan ED Jr et al: The volume factor in low and normal renin essential hypertension. Its treatment with either spironolactone or chlorthalidone. In *Hypertension Manual*, edited by JH Laragh, New York, Yorke Medical Books, 1973, p 851.

152. Buhler FR et al: Propranolol inhibition of renin secretion: a specific approach to diagnosis and treatment of renin-dependent hypertensive diseases. N Engl J Med. 1972; 287:1209.

153. Pettinger WA: Clonidine, a new antihypertensive drug. N Engl J Med. 1975; 193:1179.

154. Guerrero IM: Treatment of hypertension complicated with renal failure. In *Arterial Hypertension*, edited by M Velasco, Excerpta Medica, Amsterdam, 1980, p 298.

155. Brogden RN et al: Prazosin: a review of its pharmacologic properties and therapeutic efficacy in hypertension. Drugs. 1977; 14:163.

156. Harter HR et al: Effects of prazosin in the control of blood pressure in hypertensive dialysis patients. J Cardiovascular Pharmacol. 1979; 1:S43.

157. Pettinger WA et al: Minoxidil—an alternative to nephrectomy for refractory hypertension. N Engl J Med. 1973; 289:167.

158. Javier R et al: Long-term treatment with minoxidil in patients with severe renal failure. J Cardiovascular Pharmacol. 1980; 2:S149.

159. Davidson RC et al: Cardiovascular manifestations of renal failure. In *Strauss and Welt's Diseases of the Kidney*, 3rd ed, edited by LE Earley and CW Gottschalk, Little, Brown and Company, Boston, 1979, p 263.

160. Mathew TH et al: The use of diazoxide in hypertensive crises. Drugs. 1971; 2:73.

161. Ahearn DJ et al: Treatment of malignant hypertension with sodium nitroprusside. Arch Intern Med. 1974; 133:187.

162. Cacace L et al: Treatment of hypertensive emergencies with sodium nitroprusside. Drug Intell Clin Pharm. 1970; 4:187.

163. Koch-Weser J: Hypertensive emergencies. N Engl J Med. 1974; 290:211.

164. Hull AR et al: The control of hypertension in patients undergoing regular maintenance hemodialysis. Kidney International. 1975; 7:S184.

165. Lazarus JM et al: Urgent bilateral nephrectomy for severe hypertension. Ann Intern Med. 1972; 76:733.

166. Goldsmith RS et al: Effects of calcium and phosphorous on patients maintained on dialysis. Kidney International. 1975; 7:S118.

167. Coggins CH et al: Diabetes insipidus. Am J Med. 1967; 42:807.

168. Bartter FC et al: The syndrome of inappropriate secretion of antidiuretic hormone. Am J Med. 1967; 42:790.

169. Nawar T et al: Non-hormonal drugs for the treatment of diabetes insipidus. Can Med Assoc J. 1972; 107:1225.

170. Hayes RM: Antidiuretic hormone. N Engl J Med. 1976; 295:659.

171. Miller M et al: Drug-induced states of impaired water excretion. Kidney International. 1976; 10:96.

172. Moses AM et al: Pathophysiology and pharmacologic alterations in the release and action of ADH. Metabolism. 1976; 25:697.

173. Singer I et al: Drug-induced states of nephrogenic diabetes insipidus. N Engl J Med. 1976; 294:507.

174. Weitzman RE et al: The clinical physiology of water metabolism: Part I. West J Med. 1979; 131:373.

175. Weitzman RE et al: The clinical physiology of water metabolism: Part II. West J Med. 1979; 131:486.

176. Weitzman RE et al: The clinical physiology of water metabolism: Part III. West J Med. 1980; 132:16.

177. Cohen JJ et al: Neurogenic diabetes insipidus. Kidney International. 1979; 15:572.

178. Schrier RW et al: Nephropathy associated with penicillin and homologues. Ann Intern Med. 1966; 64:116.

179. Baldwin DS et al: Renal failure and interstitial nephritis due to penicillin and methicillin. N Engl J Med. 1963; 279:1245.

180. Gilbert DN et al: Interstitial nephritis due to methicillin, penicillin and ampicillin. Ann Allergy. 1970; 28:378.

181. Border WA et al: Antitubular basement membrane antibodies in methicillin-associated interstitial nephritis. N Engl J Med. 1974; 291:381.

182. Sanjad SA et al: Nephropathy, an underestimated complication of methicillin therapy. Pediatr. 1974; 84:873.

183. Ooi BS et al: Acute interstitial nephritis. Am J Med. 1975; 59:614.

184. Yow MD et al: A ten-year assessment of methicillin-associated side effects. Pediatrics. 1976; 58:329.

185. Bracis R et al: Methicillin hemorrhagic cystitis. Antimicrob Agents Chemother. 1977; 12:438.

186. Ditlove J et al: Methicillin nephritis. Medicine. 1977; 56:483.

187. Nolan CM et al: Nephropathy associated with methicillin therapy: Prevalence and determinants in patients with staphylococcal bacteremia. Arch Intern Med. 1977; 137:997.

188. Appel GB et al: The nephrotoxicity of antimicrobial agents. N Engl J Med. 1977; 296:663.

189. Galpin JE et al: Acute interstitial nephritis due to methicillin. Am J Med. 1978; 65:756.

190. Kancir LM et al: Adverse reactions to methicillin and nafcillin during treatment of serious staphylococcal aureus infections. Arch Intern Med. 1978; 138:909.

191. Cogan MC et al: Sodium wasting, acidosis and hyperkalemia induced by methicillin interstitial nephritis. Am J Med. 1978; 64:500.

192. Van Ypersele de Strihou C: Oliguric interstitial nephritis. Kidney International. 1979; 16:751.

193. Bodendorfen TW: Nafcillin-induced interstitial nephritis. JAMA. 1980; 244:2609.

194. Barriere SL et al: Absence of nafcillin-associated nephritis. West J Med. 1980; 133:472.

195. Bar RS et al: Hypomagnesemic hypocalcemia secondary to renal magnesium wasting—a possible consequence of high dose gentamicin therapy. Ann Intern Med. 1975; 82:646.

196. Hypocalcemia with hypoparathyroidism and renal tubular dysfunction associated with aminoglycoside therapy. Cancer. 1977; 39:1410.

197. Cronin RE: Aminoglycoside nephrotoxicity: pathogenesis and prevention. Clin Nephr. 1979; 11:251.

198. Kaloyanides GJ et al: Aminoglycoside nephrotoxicity. Kidney International. 1980; 18:571.

199. Dahlgren JG et al: Gentamicin blood levels: a guide to nephrotoxicity. Antimicro Agents Chemotherapy. 1975; 8:58.

200. Barza M: The nephrotoxicity of cephalosporins: an overview. J Infect Dis. 1978; 137:S60.

201. Mannion JG et al: Cephalosporin-aminoglycoside synergistic nephrotoxicity: fact or fiction? Drug Intell Clin Pharm. 1981; 15:248.

202. Smith CR et al: Double-blind comparison of the nephrotoxicity and auditory toxicity of gentamicin and tobramycin. N Eng J Med. 1980; 302:1106.

203. Lovine G et al: Nephrotoxicity of amphotericin B. Arch Intern Med. 1963; 112:92.

204. Butler WT et al: Nephrotoxicity of amphotericin B: early and late effects in 81 patients. Ann Intern Med. 1964; 61:175.

205. Utz JP et al: Amphotericin B toxicity. Ann Intern Med. 1964; 61:334.

206. Burgess JL et al: Nephrotoxicity of amphotericin B, with emphasis on changes in tubular function. Am J Med. 1972; 53:77.

207. Maddux MS et al: A review of complications of amphotericin B therapy. Drug Intell Clin Pharm. 1980; 14:177.

208. Hestbech J et al: Chronic renal lesions following long-term treatment with lithium. Kidney International. 1977; 12:205.

209. Hansen HE et al: Chronic interstitial nephropathy in patients on long-term lithium treatment. Quarterly J Med. 1979; 48:577.

210. Neu C et al: Renal damage associated with long-term use of lithium carbonate. J Clin Psychiat. 1979; 40:460.

211. Jenner FA: Lithium and the question of kidney damage. Arch Gen Psychiatry. 1979; 36:888.

212. Hwang S et al: Long-term maintenance lithium therapy and possible irreversible renal damage. J Clin Psychiatry. 1980; 41:11.

213. Myers JB et al: Effects of lithium on the kidney. Kidney International. 1980; 18:601.

214. Singer I: Lithium and the kidney. Kidney International. 1981; 19:374.

215. Steward JH et al: Analgesic abuse and kidney disease. Aust N Z J Med. 1976; 6:498.

216. Gloor FJ: Changing concepts in pathogenesis and morphology of analgesic nephropathy as seen in Europe. Kidney International. 1978; 13:27.

217. Burry A: Pathology of analgesic nephropathy: Australian experience. Kidney International. 1978; 13:34.

218. Dubach UC et al: Epidemiological study in Switzerland. Kidney International. 1978; 13:41.

219. Murray RM: Genesis of analgesic nephropathy in the United Kingdom. Kidney International. 1978; 13:50.

220. Gault MN et al: Analgesic nephropathy in Canada: Clinical management and outcome. Kidney International. 1978; 13:58.

221. Murray TG et al: Analgesic-associated nephropathy in the USA: Epidemiologic, clinical and pathogenetic features. Kidney International. 1978; 13:64.

222. Stewart JH: Analgesic abuse and renal failure in Australia. Kidney International. 1978; 13:72.

223. Nanra RS et al: Analgesic nephropathy: Etiology, clinical syndrome and clinicopathologic correlations in Australia. Kidney International. 1978; 13:79.

224. Lindvall N: Radiological changes of renal papillary necrosis. Kidney International. 1978; 13:93.

225. Nanra RS et al: Clinical and pathological aspects of analgesic nephropathy. Br J Clin Pharmacol. 1980; 10:3598.

226. Duggin GS: Mechanisms in development of analgesic nephrology. Kidney International. 1980; 18:553.

227. Holland EA: Experimental renal papillary necrosis. Kidney International. 1978; 13:5.

228. Shelly JH: Pharmacological mechanisms of analgesic nephropathy. Kidney International. 1978; 13:15.

229. Abel JA: Analgesic nephropathy: A review of the literature 1967–1970. Clin Pharmacol Ther. 1971; 12:583.

230. Shelley JM: Phenacetin through the looking glass. Clin Pharmacol Ther. 1967; 3:427.

231. Kindcaid-Smith P: Analgesic abuse and the kidney. Kidney International. 1980; 17:250.

232. Dengtsson U et al: Malignancies of the urinary tract and their relation to analgesic abuse. Kidney International. 1978; 13:107.

233. Vaamonde CA et al: The nephrotic syndrome as a complication of gold therapy. Arthritis Rheum. 1970; 13:826.

234. Silverberg DS et al: Gold nephropathy. Arthritis Rheum. 1970; 13:812.

235. Katz A et al: Gold nephropathy. Arch Pathol. 1973; 96:133.

236. Tornroth T et al: Gold nephropathy prototype of membranous glomerulonephritis. Am J Pathol. 1974; 75:573.

237. Tornroth T et al: The development and resolution of glomerular basement changes associated with subepithelial immune deposits. Am J Pathol. 1975; 79:219.

238. Yarom R et al: Nephrotoxic effect of parenteral and intra-articular gold. Arch Pathol. 1975; 99:36.

239. Watanabe I et al: Gold nephropathy. Arch Pathol Lab. 1976; 100:632.

240. Husseri FE et al: Gold nephropathy in juvenile rheumatoid arthritis. Am J Dis Child. 1979; 133:50.

241. Laragh JH: Oral contraceptive-induced hypertension—nine years later. Am J Obstet Gynecol. 1976; 126:141.

242. Dalen JE et al: Oral contraceptives and cardiovascular disease. Am Heart J. 1981; 101:626.

243. Zacherle BJ et al: Irreversible renal failure secondary to hypertension induced by oral contraceptives. Ann Intern Med. 1972; 77:83.

244. Dunn FG et al: Malignant hypertension associated with use of oral contraceptives. Br Heart J. 1975; 37:336.

245. Schoolwerth AC et al: Nephrosclerosis postpartum and in women taking oral contraceptives. Arch Intern Med. 1976; 136:178.

246. Jackson B et al: The hemolytic uremic syndrome and oral contraceptives. Aust N Z J Med. 1976; 6:530.

247. Slick GL et al: Hypertension, renal vein thrombosis and renal failure. Clin Nephrol. 1975; 3:70.

248. Delin K et al: Multiple arterial occlusions and hypertension probably caused by an oral contraceptive. Clin Nephrol. 1976; 6:453.

Chapter 28

Fluid and Electrolyte Disorders

Lawrence J. Hak and Cynthia B. Dunham

The internal environment of the body is maintained primarily by renal mechanisms which regulate fluid and electrolyte balance and by cell membranes which maintain the intracellular electrolyte composition. Cell membranes are normally impermeable to anions and either actively retain or extrude cations (1–4). Most all membranes are permeable to both sodium and potassium which diffuse passively down concentration gradients. Therefore, in order to maintain an intracellular sodium concentration of 10 mEq/L with an extracellular concentration of 140 mEq/L, sodium must be actively extruded from the intracellular fluid (ICF) (5); the reverse is true for potassium. This process is accomplished through the Na^+-K^+-ATPase system located on the cell membrane (6).

The solute concentration of body fluids varies within a usual range of 280 to 295 milliosmoles per kilogram of water (mOsm/kg H_2O) (4). Particles in solution create osmotic gradients which induce water movement across semipermeable membranes from areas of lower particle concentration to those of higher concentration. When the particle concentration on each side of the membrane is the same, water movement will cease. Since all cell membranes are freely permeable to water (7), addition of solute to one body compartment will cause the movement of water between compartments to eliminate osmotic gradients (8). Thus, the osmolality of the ICF and the extracellular fluid (ECF) will always be equal, although their solute compositions are markedly different (2–4).

Estimation of Osmolality

For univalent ions, 1 mEq = 1 mOsm. Sodium represents over 90% of the ECF cations (9), and each cation is accompanied by an anion. Therefore, plasma osmolality (P_{Osm}) is primarily a function of sodium and its accompanying anions. It may be estimated using the following equation (4,10,11):

$$P_{Osm} = 2\ Na^+(mEq/L) + \frac{BUN\ (mg/dl)}{2.8} \qquad (Eq.\ 1)$$
$$+ \frac{Glucose\ (mg/dl)}{18}$$

For example, to calculate the plasma osmolality of a patient with a serum Na of 142 mEq/L, a BUN of 26 mg/dl, and a glucose of 85 mg/dl:

$$P_{Osm} = 2\ (142) + \frac{26}{2.8} + \frac{85}{18}$$
$$= 298\ mOsm/kg\ H_2O$$

Since urea, like water, is freely permeable to most cell membranes, it will not affect fluid shifts between compartments and therefore is not considered in calculating the effective osmolality (E_{Osm}) (2,12); thus:

$$E_{Osm} = 2\ (Na^+) + \frac{Glucose}{18} \qquad (Eq.\ 2)$$

From the above equation, it can be seen that glucose and urea contribute very little to plasma osmolality. Therefore, with the exception of patients with hyperglycemia, the effective osmolality of body fluids can be estimated simply by multiplying the serum sodium by two.

Equivalent Weights

Electrolytes in solution combine according to their electrical charges (ionic valence) rather than according to their molecular or atomic weights. The standard of reference for electrical equivalence is one atomic weight of hydrogen; thus, an equivalent weight of any ion is that amount which will replace or combine with one atomic weight or one gram of hydrogen.

The equivalent weight of a substance (ie, the weight of one electrochemical equivalent) may be calculated by dividing the gram atomic or formula weight by the ionic valence. The milliequivalent weight is then equal to the equivalent weight divided by 1000 (1,13).

The principles of equivalence are illustrated below. Following are common formulae and mEq weights which are used (1,13):

$$Eq\ Wt = \frac{gram\ atomic\ or\ formula\ weight}{valence} \qquad (Eq.\ 3)$$
$$mEq = \frac{Eq\ weight\ (gm)}{1000} \qquad (Eq.\ 4)$$
$$mEq/L = \frac{mg/100\ ml}{atomic\ weight} \times valence \times 10 \qquad (Eq.\ 5)$$

The following problems illustrate application of the above principles.

Problem 1. It is recommended that a patient receive a diet restricted to 2 grams/day of sodium. How many mEq/day of sodium does this represent?

Table 1.
MILLIEQUIVALENT WEIGHT OF COMMON SUBSTANCES

Substance	Weight (gm)
Na^+	0.023
K^+	0.039
Ca^{++}	0.020
Mg^{++}	0.012
Cl^-	0.0355
HCO_3^-	0.061
NaCl	0.0585
KCl	0.0746
$NaHCO_3$	0.084

mEq wt of sodium = 0.023 grams

$$mEq = \frac{Wt \text{ of substance}}{mEq \text{ wt}}$$

$$= \frac{2 \text{ gm}}{0.023 \text{ gm/mEq}} \qquad (Eq. 4)$$

$$= 86.9 \text{ mEq } Na^+$$

Problem 2. How many mEq/L of NaCl are present in a solution of 0.9% NaCl (normal saline)?

$$mEq/L = \frac{mg/100 \text{ ml}}{formula \text{ wt}} \times valence \times 10$$

$$= \frac{900 \times 1 \times 10}{58.5} \qquad (Eq. 5)$$

$$= 154 \text{ mEq/L of } Na^+$$
$$\text{and } 154 \text{ mEq/L of } Cl^-$$

Problem 3. How many mEq of calcium are contained in a liter of solution which contains 10 mg/100 ml of $CaCl_2 \cdot 2H_2O$?

$$mEq/L = \frac{mg/100 \text{ ml} \times 10 \times valence}{formula \text{ wt}}$$

$$= \frac{(10) \times (10) \times (2)}{147} \qquad (Eq. 5)$$

$$= 1.36 \text{ mEq/L}$$

In referring to normal plasma electrolyte concentrations, milliequivalents are generally used for substances which are highly ionized in plasma, for example, sodium, potassium, chloride, and bicarbonate. Calcium is usually reported in mg/dl rather than mEq/L. Calcium is approximately 40% bound to proteins and 10% complexed with citrate, phosphate, etc., while about 50% exists in the ionized form (14). Since bound calcium is not ionized, it is not electrochemically equivalent. Most plasma assay procedures for calcium measure both the bound and the ionized forms; therefore, the laboratory reports calcium as mg/dl.

Similarly, inorganic phosphate is found in serum in two forms: $H_2PO_4^-$ and $HPO_4^=$, the relative proportions of each being dependent on pH. Because it is not possible to provide a single valence for phosphate, the total phosphorus is measured and reported as mg/dl rather than mEq/L (15).

Body Water Distribution

Normally, total body water (TBW) in males represents approximately 60% of body weight. In females TBW is approximately 50% of body weight. These percentages vary according to the relative amount of fat present (16). In a 75 kg male, TBW is approximately 45 liters. This fluid is distributed into two compartments. Two-thirds (30 liters) is intracellular fluid (ICF) and one-third is extracellular fluid (ECF). The ECF is further subdivided with approximately 75% (11.25 L) in the interstitial space and 25% (3.75 L) in the intravascular space (3,16). Since body water is held within compartments by osmotically active substances, it follows that two-thirds of the body's osmotically active substances are found in the ICF with the remaining one-third in the ECF. Since the quantity of osmotically active substances in the ICF is relatively fixed, the ICF volume is determined by water balance. Salts of sodium comprise greater than 90% of the osmotically active substances of the ECF; therefore, ECF volume is controlled by sodium balance (3,4). With this in mind, it is possible to estimate the changes that would occur in body fluid compartments if 2 liters of normal saline or 3 liters of D5W were administered to a 75 kg male.

Because Na^+ and Cl^- ions are confined to the ECF compartment and saline is isosmotic with normal body fluids, the entire two liters of solution will remain in the ECF and total body os-molality will not change.

$$\boxed{\begin{array}{c|c} ECF & ICF \\ \hline 15\ L & 30L \end{array}}_{45L} \quad + \quad 3L\ D5W \quad = \quad \boxed{\begin{array}{c|c} ECF & ICF \\ \hline 16\ L & 32L \end{array}}_{48L}$$

As glucose solutions are administered, endo-geneous insulin secretion will cause the glucose to enter the intracellular space where it will either be metabolized or stored as glycogen. In either case, the number of osmotically active particles in the intracellular compartment will not change significantly because of the addition of glucose particles. The net volume changes in body fluid compartments will be the same as if free water were administered. Thus, since two-thirds of the body's osmotically active substances are in the intracelluar compartment and one-third in the extracellular compartment, two liters of water will enter the intracelluar compartment, one liter will remain in the extracellular compartment and to-tal body osmolality will decrease.

Fluid Requirements

The minimum daily water requirement is ap-proximately 1300 ml, while approximately 2300 ml are needed for usual body function. These water requirements (in ml) may be broken down as follows:

	Minimal (ml)	Usual (ml)
Insensible Loss		
Respiration	500	500
Sweat	500	500
Urine	500	1500
Water production	1500	2500
from catabolism	−200	−200
	1300	2300

To prevent azotemia, a minimum urine output of 500 ml/day is necessary. Maximal renal effi-ciency occurs with a urine output of about 1500 ml/day.

Increased water loss through the skin occurs with elevations of body or environmental tem-perature which increase maintenance water re-quirements. Fever increases insensible water loss by 10–15% for each Centigrade degree rise in

temperature (17–19). Rises in environmental temperature result in variable water loss as sweat; as much as 16 L/day may be lost (20).

Supplemental fluids will also be required when there are excess gastrointestinal (GI) losses or when there is "third-spacing" of body fluids. GI losses may be increased by vomiting, nasogastric suction, diarrhea, or drainage of large fluid vol-umes from ileostomies, colostomies or enterocu-taneous fistulae. Such losses will require both fluid and electrolyte replacement (Table 2). "Third-spacing" represents the abnormal sequestration of body fluids in a space which generally does not contain substantial volumes of fluid. Conditions associated with third space loss include perito-nitis, burns, intestinal obstruction and ascites (9).

Hyperosmolality

1. A 26-year-old male diabetic presents to clinic complaining of polyuria, polydipsia and 3+ to 4+ glycosuria which he states began shortly after he developed symptoms of a "cold." Routine laboratory data revealed: Na 130 mEq/L, K 4.0 mEq/L, Cl 101 mEq/L, CO_2 24 mEq/L, BUN 26 mg/dl, creatinine 0.9 mg/dl, and glucose 500 mg/dl. How has this pa-tient's hyperglycemia altered his fluid and electrolyte balance?

Plasma osmolality in this patient would be es-timated to be 297 mOsm/kg H_2O which is high:

$$P_{Osm} = 2\ (130) + \frac{500}{18} + \frac{26}{2.8} \qquad (Eq.\ 1)$$

$$= 260 + 27.7 + 9.2$$

$$\cong 297\ mOsm/kg\ H_2O$$

As P_{Osm} increases, the following changes take place. Osmoreceptors in the thirst center, sensing

Table 2.

SODIUM AND POTASSIUM CONTENT OF BODY FLUIDS

Body Fluid	Sodium (mEq/L)	Potassium (mEq/L)
Gastric	40–80	5–15
Pancreatic	130–150	0–10
Small bowel	80–140	0–10
Diarrhea	120–140	15–20
Sweat	40–80	0–5

Adapted from Anderson RJ et al (reference 9).

an increase in body fluid osmolality, stimulate thirst and cause an increased oral intake of fluid (21). The osmoreceptors in the supraoptic nuclei of the hypothalamus send stimuli to the posterior pituitary causing the release of antidiuretic hormone (ADH) which promotes water reabsorption in the distal tubule and collecting duct of the nephron (22–24). However, as the serum glucose rises above the renal threshold for glucose reabsorption, an osmotic diuresis occurs preventing maximal ADH-stimulated water reabsorption (25). As the osmotic diuresis increases tubular fluid volume, the tubular fluid concentration of sodium will be less than that of the tubular epithelial cells and peritubular spaces so that sodium will passively diffuse back into the tubular fluid causing a natriuresis (25). Ultimately, deficits of both total body sodium and water will occur.

2. How has the patient's hyperglycemia affected his serum sodium concentration? How will correction of the patient's hyperglycemia influence serum sodium?

This example represents a situation in which the primary disturbance leading to hyponatremia is an abnormal distribution of water between the ICF and ECF compartments. The high glucose concentration in the plasma creates an osmotic gradient, favoring the movement of water from the intracelluar to the extracelular compartment. The increased extracellular water results in dilution of the serum sodium leading to hyponatremia (26). If total body water content does not change, for each rise of 100 mg/dl in plasma glucose concentration above normal, serum sodium concentration declines by approximately 1.6 mEq/L (27). Therefore, correction of this patient's hyperglycemia should result in a rise in the serum sodium concentration to approximately 136 mEq/L.

Hyponatremia has also been reported with mannitol administration as a result of the same mechanism by which glucose promotes shifts of water to the ECF (4,25,28).

3. How should his fluid and electrolyte imbalances be corrected?

Insulin should be administered to enhance the uptake and utilization of glucose by cells and to alleviate hyperosmolality. Intravenous 0.9% or 0.45% sodium chloride (NaCl) is required initially to replace salt and water which have been lost through osmotic diuresis. This is particularly important if the patient is exhibiting signs and symptoms consistent with dehydration (poor skin turgor, increased pulse rate, and postural hypotension). Eventually, 0.45% NaCl or dextrose 5% and 0.45% NaCl will be required to completely restore normal fluid balance.

Hyponatremia

4. A 55-year-old female was found on routine laboratory studies to have a serum sodium of 130 mEq/L. What conclusions can one draw from this patient's serum sodium? What factors may cause a false hyponatremia?

Hyponatremia is defined as a serum sodium concentration of less than 135 mEq/L; although the serum sodium is a useful estimate of P_{Osm}, it is not a reflection of total body sodium.

The ultimate choice of therapy for hyponatremia depends upon an accurate assessment of ECF as well as total body sodium since hyponatremia can occur in the presence of a normal, expanded, or contracted ECF volume. It is therefore necessary to determine whether total body sodium and water are normal, increased or decreased. This assessment is made by analysis of the clinical setting in which the hyponatremia occurs, urinary sodium concentration and osmolality, and physical assessment parameters.

Prior to an extensive workup of the patient with hyponatremia, factitious causes should be excluded. The reported value for serum sodium may not reflect the true ECF sodium concentration in patients with hyperlipemia or hyperproteinemia. In the presence of hyperlipemia, the sodium concentration of plasma water may be normal but the lipids reduce the quantity of water per unit volume of plasma resulting in a pseudohyponatremia (10,26). Hyponatremia has also been reported in patients with multiple myeloma with hyperproteinemia (29). In this situation, hyponatremia appears to occur secondary to high concentrations of paraproteins which have a net positive charge. These positively charged proteins have a "displacing" effect on sodium (29). In both of these cases, measured plasma osmolality is normal.

Dilutional hyponatremia caused by hyperglycemia must also be excluded as a cause of hyponatremia.

5. *Syndrome of Inappropriate ADH*. A.B. is a 56-year-old white female with oat cell

carcinoma of the lung, admitted for radiation therapy. Physical examination is unremarkable with the exception of a 2.5 kg weight gain since her last clinic visit. No edema is present. Laboratory findings are remarkable only for a serum sodium of 124 mEq/L and a chloride of 90 mEq/L. All other laboratory values are normal, including glucose and triglycerides. Urinalysis revealed a urine sodium concentration of 90 mEq/L and an osmolality of 650 mOsm/kg H_2O. She is on no medications and has received no chemotherapy. What is the etiology of this patient's hyponatremia? How should it be treated?

Hyponatremia in patients such as A.B. occurs as a result of excessive antidiuretic hormone (ADH) activity leading to increased total body water (30–32). ADH activity may be increased as a result of certain tumors (30,32–34), pneumonia and tuberculosis (32), psychosis (35), or drugs (Table 3) which increase ADH activity by increasing its secretion or potentiating its renal effects (36–45).

In these patients, total body sodium content may be normal or slightly decreased. This is explained by a decrease in proximal tubular sodium reabsorption secondary to the slight ECF volume expansion that occurs with ADH-induced water retention. Although significant water retention may occur, there are few clinical signs of volume excess since only ⅓ of the retained water remains in the ECF. Edema is rarely present if hyponatremia is solely attributable to ADH effects. Urine sodium concentration will be high and urine osmolality will be inappropriately high for the level of serum osmolality.

The primary form of therapy for hyponatremia due to increased ADH activity is restriction of free water. Although the absolute level of restriction may be variable, it must be of a magnitude great enough to effect a net negative daily fluid balance. Restriction of water intake to a level approximating daily urine output should result in a net fluid loss equaling daily insensible water loss, which should lead to a slow return of the serum sodium toward normal. If possible, the cause of the increased ADH activity should be removed (ie, removal of offending drugs, treatment of tumor or infection, etc.).

In patients with chronic hyponatremia due to tumors or other noncorrectable primary causes of the syndrome of inappropriate ADH (SIADH), de-

meclocycline may be used (46–49). At doses of 600–1200 mg/day, demeclocycline produces a reversible dose-related nephrogenic diabetes insipidus, thus inhibiting the response to ADH at the collecting duct. The advantage of this therapy is primarily one of comfort to the patient, in that it attenuates the need for severe restriction of fluid intake. Its use should be limited to patients who are able to drink normally so that excessive volume depletion can be avoided. It should not be used in patients with renal insufficiency, and patients on long-term therapy should be warned of its photosensitizing effects.

6. Hyponatremia in Congestive Heart Failure. W.H is a 62-year-old white male with a four-year history of congestive heart failure (CHF), admitted with a two-week history of increasing shortness of breath and dyspnea on exertion. Physical examination was significant for rales in the lungs bilaterally, the presence of an S_3 gallop, and 4+ pitting edema to the knees in both extremities. Serum electrolytes were as follows: Na 124 mEq/L, K 3.3 mEq/L, Cl 90 mEq/L, CO_2 33 mEq/L, BUN 30 mg/dl, and serum creatinine 1.2 mg/dl. Urinalysis showed a sodium concentration of 10 mEq/liter and an osmolality of 600 mOsm/kg H_2O. What is the cause of hyponatremia in this patient? In what other situations can hyponatremia present with clinical signs of sodium and water excess? How should the hyponatremia be managed?

This patient illustrates the classic presentation of hyponatremia resulting from CHF (50). In CHF, cardiac output is decreased, resulting in decreased renal perfusion. This "apparent" volume deficit results in increased proximal tubular sodium and water reabsorption and activation of the renin-angiotensin-aldosterone system (51). Diminished cardiac return activates volume receptors in the left atrium (22,52) to stimulate the secretion of ADH (53–55). The net effect is an increase in total body sodium and water content, with water retained in excess of sodium.

The avid retention of sodium and water by the kidney results in a low urine sodium concentration. Urine osmolality is high due to decreased urine flow in the collecting duct and increased water reabsorption due to ADH activity. The presence of edema denotes total body sodium excess.

Two other situations in which hyponatremia occurs with increased total body salt and water content are cirrhosis and nephrotic syndrome (26). Again, there is renal salt and water retention due to a decrease in "effective" intravascular volume. As in CHF, urine sodium concentration is low and osmolality is high.

Hyponatremia which occurs in the setting of an expanded ECF volume and an increase in total body sodium may also be seen in patients with acute or chronic renal insufficiency when sodium and water intake exceed the excretory ability of the kidneys. In contrast to patients with CHF, cirrhosis or nephrosis, urine sodium concentration may be high with an isotonic urine.

Therapy for hyponatremia with increased ECF volume is restriction of salt and water intake combined with therapy directed toward correction of the underlying disorder. In patients with CHF, such as W.H., an attempt should be made to improve cardiac output which will increase renal perfusion and increase sodium delivery to distal diluting sites through the use of digitalis, afterload reduction and diuretic therapy.

7. Hyponatremia With Dehydration. S.D. is a 47-year-old male admitted with a three-day history of profuse diarrhea, nausea and vomiting due to viral gastroenteritis. He has been unable to eat any solids although he has managed to drink some Coca-Cola. Physical examination is remarkable for dry mucous membranes, absence of axillary sweat, a resting tachycardia of 110 beats/minute and a standing blood pressure of 90/50. Urinalysis showed a sodium concentration of 10 mEq/liter and an osmolality of 850 mOsm/kg H₂O. Serum sodium is 124 mEq/L, the BUN is 40 mg/dl, and the creatinine is 1.0 mg/dl. What is the etiology of this patient's hyponatremia? How should it be treated?

Hyponatremia with true total body sodium depletion can occur in individuals with excessive renal sodium losses secondary to diuretic use (36,56), interstitial renal disease, or mineralocorticoid deficiency, or in those such as S.D. with GI losses from vomiting or diarrhea (9,10,26). See Table 2.

Initially, sodium loss causes a decrease in ECF volume. Resultant homeostatic mechanisms involve increased proximal tubular sodium and water reabsorption, secretion of aldosterone and

ADH as well as a concomitant increase in thirst. In response to the thirst stimulus, salt poor fluids are often ingested, with ⅔ of this solute free water entering the ICF and ⅓ remaining in the ECF. The portion remaining in the ECF worsens the hyponatremia without sufficiently restoring intravascular volume, while the elevated ADH prevents the kidney from producing a dilute urine despite the presence of hyponatremia and hyposmolality. A similar picture of hyponatremia is often produced iatrogenically in the hospitalized patient whose GI or urinary losses of sodium and water are replaced with sodium-free solutions such as 5% dextrose in water.

In true salt depletion hyponatremia with ECF volume contraction, therapy should consist of isotonic saline solution until volume deficits are repaired. The urine output, urine and serum electrolytes, and intravascular volume status should be monitored.

8. Treatment of Symptomatic Hyponatremia. A 40-year-old male released 5 days ago from the hospital with newly diagnosed small cell carcinoma of the lung, was brought to the emergency room just after having a grand mal seizure. He was unresponsive on arrival. History is significant for the fact that the patient was ingesting large quantities of juices and soft drinks until the day prior to his seizure at which time he became confused and somewhat somnolent. His admission laboratory values were: Na 110 mEq/L, K 3.2 mEq/L, Cl 86 mEq/L, HCO₃ 24 mEq/L, BUN 5 mg/dl, Creatinine 1.0 mg/dl. His weight was 60 kg, which was not different from his usual weight. No edema was present. What symptoms in this patient are consistent with hyponatremia? How should this patient's hyponatremia be treated?

The symptoms of hyponatremia depend on the etiology of the low sodium, the magnitude of the decrease, and the acuteness with which it occurs (10,57,58).

Whether hyponatremia is the result of salt depletion or is dilutional, the net effect is a decrease in effective extracellular osmotically active substances and a relative overhydration of the intracellular space. This produces symptoms of weakness, nausea, difficulty in concentration, headache and somnolence (10,57,58). In severe cases, as described above, seizures may occur (58).

Symptomatic hyponatremia is a medical emergency and in clinical practice is managed with hypertonic (3% or 5%) saline (59). The amount of sodium necessary to raise the serum sodium to 140 mEq/L can be estimated using the following formula (59):

$$(140 - \text{patient's Na})(\text{total body water} = \text{mEq Na in liters})$$

$$(\text{Eq. 6})$$

Assuming that total body water in the above patient is 36 liters (0.6 × 60 kg), his sodium deficit will be 1080 mEq: (140 − 110)×(36). Half the estimated deficit may be replaced over the first 8 hours. Treatment is continued until the serum sodium is 130 mEq/L or until neurologic symptoms improve. The remainder of his deficit may be replaced slowly over several days. Sufficient fluid and sodium to replace insensible water loss and urine output should also be provided. An alternative therapy which may successfully produce a negative water balance is the use of 0.9% NaCl and furosemide. Furosemide is given to induce a diuresis, and hourly urine losses of sodium are replaced with 0.9% NaCl (60).

POTASSIUM

The potassium content of a normal 70 kg male is approximately 3500 mEq, over 98% of which is located intracellularly (61). A very small portion (50 mEq) of total body potassium is present in the ECF under normal conditions; the ECF potassium concentration ranges between 3.5–5.0 mEq/L (62). Of the potassium present in the ICF, the greatest part is found in skeletal muscle (63,64).

For adults, the usual daily dietary intake of potassium ranges from 50–150 mEq (63). The daily loss of potassium is roughly equivalent to daily potassium intake, permitting the maintenance of total body potassium stores within narrow limits. Normally, more than 90% of the potassium ingested is excreted in the urine; only small amounts are lost in the sweat and feces (65,66). The kidneys will increase potassium excretion in response to augmented intake, but in states of total body potassium deficits, the kidney is unable to totally avoid potassium excretion and urinary losses range from 5–10 mEq/day (64). In addition to daily intake, the retention or elimination of potassium by the kidneys is influenced by a number of other factors including sodium intake, aldosterone, flow rate of tubular fluid in the distal nephron, ammonia metabolism, and systemic acid-base status (67,68,69).

Clinical Manifestations of Hypokalemia and Hyperkalemia. One of the major functions of potassium is maintenance of the excitatory properties of neuromuscular tissue. The resting membrane potential of cells is a function of and varies directly with the ratio of intracellular to extracellular potassium concentration (70,71). Since the normal intracellular potassium concentration is approximately 140 mEq/L and the extracellular concentration is approximately 3.5 mEq/L, it is evident that small alterations in intracellular potassium concentration do not significantly affect the ratio or the resting membrane potential. However, small alterations of extracellular potassium significantly affect the ratio and in turn the resting membrane potential.

Rapid or pronounced changes in extracellular potassium concentration would have the following consequences (70,72,73). In *hypokalemia,* the ratio of intracellular to extracellular potassium concentration increases. This increases the resting membrane potential so that a greater than normal stimulus is required to obtain an action potential. Clinically, neuromuscular dysfunction including weakness and paralysis may be observed. Cardiac abnormalities including defects in cardiac conduction and predisposition to atrial and ventricular ectopy may be seen (74,75). Gastrointestinal dysfunction with decreased bowel motility and gastric atony (76) may be observed, and, if severe enough, hypokalemia may result in respiratory muscle paralysis (77).

Hyperkalemia, on the other hand, decreases the ratio of intracellular to extracellular potassium concentration, resulting in a decreased resting membrane potential and an enhanced state of excitability. Effects on cardiac conduction may be life-threatening. Enhanced conduction is seen with mild hyperkalemia, while more pronounced or extremely rapid elevations of the serum potassium induce rapid depression of cardiac conduction which may lead to ventricular tachyarrhythmias or asystole (78–80). If the alteration in extracellular potassium concentration occurs slowly so that equilibration between intracellular and extracellular potassium concentration occurs, the ratio does not change significantly, and excitability disturbances may not be observed (81).

This may explain why patients with chronic renal failure and end stage renal disease tolerate modestly elevated serum potassium levels without clinical signs or symptoms.

Potassium also plays an important role in carbohydrate and protein metabolism and in enzymatic reactions (66). Physiologic concentrations of intracellular potassium are required for glycogen synthesis in liver and in skeletal muscle. Small reductions in intracellular potassium concentrations result in significant reductions in protein synthesis (82). Many enzyme systems (82–85) require potassium, including ATPase which hydrolyzes ATP for release of energy for numerous metabolic processes (86,87). Insulin secretion is blunted in hypokalemia (88–90), and the diuretic-induced hyperglycemia noted in latent diabetics may be ameliorated by potassium repletion (89–92).

Hypokalemia

9. An 18-year-old female comes to the emergency room with a four-day history of anorexia, nausea and vomiting which she attributes to the "stomach flu". Physical examination reveals poor skin turgor and dry mucous membranes. Laboratory values are as follows: Na 134 mEq/L, K 3.0 mEq/L, Cl 90 mEq/L, CO_2 32 mEq/L, BUN 24 mg/dl, and creatinine 0.8 mg/dl. Discuss the possible etiologies for this patient's hypokalemia.

Potassium depletion occurs in situations where potassium loss exceeds intake, and commonly occurs with vomiting, nasogastric suction or diarrhea (93). See Table 2. The hypokalemia that occurs with vomiting or nasogastric suction is multifactorial. Potassium content of gastric fluid ranges from 5 to 15 mEq/liter (9,93), thus accounting for a portion of the loss. However, the major contributing factor is renal potassium wasting. When HCl is lost from the body, metabolic alkalosis occurs and large amounts of bicarbonate are presented to the distal nephron. This increases potassium secretion into the tubular fluid and loss in the urine (77,93). This urinary potassium loss is augmented by an increase in aldosterone secretion stimulated by volume depletion (51).

The metabolic alkalosis observed in this patient may also cause transcellular redistribution of potassium into the ICF compartment, lowering the serum potassium concentration by approximately 0.6 mEq/L for each 0.1 unit change in pH (66,93).

Although fecal potassium content is low and losses by this route are usually minimal, potassium losses in the stool may increase greatly in the presence of diarrhea (94). An obvious cause of hypokalemia which is often overlooked occurs in patients who take nothing by mouth as is the case with this patient. This also occurs in hospitalized patients if sufficient potassium is not induced in intravenous fluids to replace urinary or other losses.

There are other causes of hypokalemia which are not illustrated by this patient. Hypokalemia may be seen in chronic alcoholics, or in severe starvation states where potassium intake is so markedly reduced that renal excretion exceeds intake (64). Also, if such patients receive sufficient quantities of glucose and/or amino acids to increase the intracellular potassium stores but only receive enough potassium to replace urinary losses, total body potassium deficits and hypokalemia will ensue (95). Additionally, administration of large glucose loads or insulin will acutely decrease the serum potassium by promoting its movement into intracellular spaces (61).

Hypokalemia secondary to urinary potassium loss occurs in patients with renal tubular acidosis (96–99) and mineralocorticoid excess, including primary (100,101) and secondary (93) hyperaldosteronism, in individuals who ingest excessive amounts of licorice (102), and in primary magnesium deficiency (103). Drugs may also cause hypokalemia by a variety of mechanisms (104–127). Also see Table 3 and Question 10.

10. T.J. is a 20-year-old white male with acute lymphocytic leukemia (ALL) in relapse, currently undergoing therapy with high dose cytosine arabinoside (ARA-C) and L-asparaginase. His hospital course has been complicated by severe, prolonged neutropenia, gram-negative sepsis and pulmonary aspergillosis. Current antimicrobial therapy consists of:

> **Carbenicillin 5 gm IV q4h**
> **Tobramycin 100 mg IV q8h**
> **Septra DS 1 tablet po bid**
> **Nystatin oral suspension 600,000**
> **units q4h swish and swallow**
> **Amphotericin B 35 mg IV qd**

He has also experienced marked hypokalemia requiring administration of large

amounts of potassium chloride to maintain the serum potassium in the low normal range. Currently, the serum potassium is stable at 3.5 mEq/L on a regimen of: potassium chloride 40 mEq po tid, spironolactone 100 mg po bid, and potassium chloride 30 mEq/L of D5 ½ NS at a "keep vein open" rate. What are potential drug-related cause of hypokalemia in this patient? Discuss the mechanisms by which drugs cause hypokalemia.

A number of drugs are known to cause hypokalemia; thus, the possibility of a drug-induced etiology should always be considered in the patient who becomes hypokalemic (104–127) (Table 3).

T.J. is receiving several *antibiotics* which have been associated with increased renal potassium loss and hypokalemia. Hypokalemia can occur with the use of carbenicillin and penicillin in large doses (107–112). Carbenicillin acts as a nonreabsorbable anion and increases electrical negativity in the tubular lumen (111). As a result, hydrogen and potassium are secreted into the tubule to maintain electrical neutrality. Amphotericin B causes a defect in distal tubular function which makes the tubules passively permeable to a number of electrolytes including potassium (113–115). Significant hypokalemia may occur requiring large potassium supplementation in patients receiving this drug. Aminoglycosides have been reported to cause hypokalemia by increasing renal loss, although the mechanism is not entirely clear (116,117). Therefore, tobramycin must also be considered as a potential cause of hypokalemia in T.J.

Other drugs which cause hypokalemia which are not illustrated by this patient include the diuretics and laxatives. Hypokalemia is a commonly quoted complication of *diuretic therapy* with furosemide, ethacrynic acid, thiazides, and metolazone, although there is disagreement in the literature as to its true incidence and clinical significance (128,129). The proposed mechanism for diuretic-induced hypokalemia is increased delivery of sodium to the distal tubular sites for sodium-potassium exchange (126,127). Extracellular fluid volume contraction with alkalosis resulting in secondary hyperaldosteronism may in large part be responsible for renal potassium wasting from diuretics (128). Although routine potassium supplementation is commonly prescribed for patients receiving diuretics, the extent

Table 3.

DRUG-RELATED DISORDERS OF FLUID AND ELECTROLYTES

HYPONATREMIA	HYPERKALEMIA
Sodium Depletion	arginine hydrochloride
diuretics	indomethacin,
Increased ECF OAS	prostaglandin
mannitol	inhibitors
Increased ADH activity	penicillin G potassium
acetaminophen	potassium supplements
barbiturates	salt substitutes
carbamazepine	spironolactone
chlorpropamide	succinylcholine
clofibrate	triamterene
morphine, opiates	
nicotine	HYPOPHOSPHATEMIA
vinca alkaloids	aluminum carbonate
	aluminum, magnesium
HYPOKALEMIA	hydroxides
aminoglycosides	diuretics
amphotericin B	
antibiotic-associated	HYPERCALCEMIA
pseudomembranous	calcium
colitis	lithium
carbenicillin, penicillin	tamoxifen
diuretics (except	thiazides
spironolactone,	vitamin A
triamterene)	vitamin D
laxatives	
mineralocorticoids	HYPOMAGNESEMIA
	diuretics
HYPERMAGNESEMIA	gentamicin
magnesium-containing	
antacids	
milk of magnesia	

of renal potassium wasting and the need for potassium supplementation seem to differ greatly depending on the setting in which the diuretic is used (128). Significant potassium depletion seems less likely in the hypertensive patient treated with diuretics in comparison to the patient with edema, where such factors as dietary sodium restriction, secondary hyperaldosteronism, and acid-base status may influence the extent and significance of the potassium loss (128,129).

Laxative abuse is a common setting in which hypokalemia occurs. Laxative-induced hypokalemia has been reported secondary to magnesium or phosphate containing cathartics as well as phenolphthalein, bisacodyl, castor oil, cascara and other stimulant laxatives (118–124). High rates

(15 to 55 mEq/L) of potassium loss in stool occur, and the subsequent laxative-induced volume depletion produces a state of hyperaldosteronism which further augments potassium excretion. Laxative abuse should be suspected in patients in whom no apparent cause for hypokalemia can be identified.

Other situations in which drugs may be implicated as a cause for hypokalemia include antibiotic-associated pseudomembranous colitis (104) and the use of ACTH, mineralocorticoids, and glucocorticoid preparations with mineralocorticoid activity (93). For a discussion of the treatment of hypokalemia, see chapter on Congestive Heart Failure.

Hyperkalemia

11. *Etiology.* **J.R., a 50-year-old black male with a long history of insulin dependent diabetes mellitus, hypertension, and chronic renal insufficiency, is admitted with a chief complaint of weakness, increasing somnolence and lower extremity swelling. He was last discharged from the hospital six months earlier following admission for severe fluid overload which required therapy with large doses of diuretics. He was successfully diuresed with furosemide and discharged from the hospital on the following medications: Methyldopa 500 mg bid, furosemide 120 mg bid, Extra Strength Basaljel 15 ml tid pc, Shohl's Solution 10 ml tid and NPH Insulin 15 units sc q am. He was prescribed a 40 gram protein, chronic renal failure diet with potassium restriction and was also fluid restricted. At the time of discharge all electrolytes were normal. Creatinine clearance (Cl_{Cr}) at that time was 10 ml/minute with a BUN of 74 mg/dl and a creatinine of 9.4 mg/dl. He states that he had done well since that time, complying with diet and medications, until about two weeks prior to admission when he began experiencing some lower extremity swelling. At the local emergency room he was given a prescription for Aldactone 100 mg po qd, which he began taking at that time. He experienced no improvement in the lower extremity swelling, but noted increasing weakness and was admitted with the complaints previously described. Electrolytes on admission included Na 135 mEq/L, K 6.5 mEq/L,**

Cl 111 mEq/L, CO_2 13 mEq/L, BUN 100 mg/dl, creatinine 15 mg/dl, and glucose 456 mg/dl. An electrocardiogram revealed peaked T waves. A 24-hour urine collection revealed a Cl_{Cr} of 6 ml/minute. What are the causes of hyperkalemia? What are possible etiologies of hyperkalemia in the above patient?

As discussed below, a number of factors may have contributed to the development of hyperkalemia in J.R. Renal function has declined to a point where adaptive changes in excretion may be inadequate to maintain a normal potassium balance. In addition, renal potassium excretion may have been impaired by the use of spironolactone. Potassium shifts from the intracellular space to the extracellular space may also have occurred secondary to acidosis and hyperglycemia.

In any patient who presents with hyperkalemia, it is helpful to determine whether the elevation in serum potassium is due to a redistribution of potassium between the ICF and ECF, an increase in the total body potassium, or a spurious lab value.

Causes of *spurious elevations* of the serum potassium should be considered. *In vitro* release of potassium due to hemolysis of red cells is a common cause of artifactual hyperkalemia (64). Diseases associated with marked thrombocytosis or leukocytosis may result in an elevated serum potassium due to leakage of potassium from these cells (130–133). Prior exercise or trauma to tissue in the area from which the blood sample is obtained may falsely elevate the serum potassium (134). Blood samples obtained near intravenous potassium infusion sites may also misleadingly imply hyperkalemia.

A number of factors may influence the redistribution of potassium from the ICF to the ECF causing hyperkalemia. *Systemic acidosis* may cause an elevation of the serum potassium due to a shift of intracellular potassium to the extracellular compartment. For each decrease in the plasma pH of 0.1 unit there is an increase in the serum potassium of 0.6 mEq/L (66,93). The mechanism by which these changes in serum potassium occur with changes in pH is unclear. Early reports suggest an exchange of hydrogen ion for potassium across cell membranes (135). More recent evidence indicates that serum bicarbonate modulates serum potassium levels (136). Others suggest that although acidosis due to mineral acids is associated with hyperkalemia, acidosis secondary to organic acids such as lactic acid may not (137,138).

Redistribution of potassium with hyperkalemia may be seen with severe *digitalis toxicity* which interferes with Na^+-K^+-ATPase function (139,140). *Depolarizing agents* such as succinylcholine cause release of potassium from muscle cells by altering membrane permeability and may produce life-threatening hyperkalemia, particularly in patients who have renal failure and/or preexisting hyperkalemia (141,142). *Hyperglycemia* may cause hyperkalemia through an osmotic effect causing fluid containing potassium to shift to the ECF space. *Insulin deficiency* may also play a role in hyperglycemia-induced hyperkalemia (138). Finally, infusions of *arginine hydrochloride* may result in hyperkalemia due to an intracellular exchange of arginine, a cationic amino acid, for potassium (143).

Hyperkalemia commonly occurs in patients with *renal insufficiency*; however, it is usually not seen in non-oliguric patients until the Cl_{Cr} is less than 5 ml/minute. This potassium balance is maintained through adaptive changes in renal and gastrointestinal potassium excretion (144–147). As the nephron mass is reduced, distal tubular secretion of potassium is increased. In addition, fecal potassium excretion is increased through a net increase in colonic potassium secretion (147). However, certain factors may interfere with or override this adaptation and precipitate hyperkalemia in the patient with impaired renal function.

In the setting of renal insufficiency, large or sudden increases in the potassium load, from either endogenous or exogenous sources, can lead to hyperkalemia. The endogenous potassium load may be increased as a result of hemolysis, tissue destruction or necrosis, or severe catabolic states. This is often the case in acute renal failure due to trauma or severe injury. In these settings, the potassium is released at a rate that exceeds the excretory capabilities of the kidneys. Sources of exogenous potassium include dietary intake of high potassium foods, oral or parenteral administration of potassium salts, salt substitutes which may contain up to 60 mEq of potassium per teaspoonful, potassium penicillin G, clay-eating, and transfusion of stored bank blood.

Drugs such as *spironolactone* or *triamterene* that interfere with distal tubular potassium secretion may impair its renal excretion. Thus, they should be avoided in patients with renal insuffi-

ciency. It is also important to be aware that these potassium sparing diuretics can produce hyperkalemia in patients with normal renal function if administered in conjunction with large doses of potassium supplements or salt substitutes.

Hypoaldosteronism is associated with a decrease in renal potassium excretion and may lead to hyperkalemia. A syndrome consisting of hyperkalemia with hypoaldosteronism, most likely resulting from low renin secretion, has been reported (148,149). This syndrome of "hyporeninemic hypoaldosteronism" has been most frequently described in patients with diabetic renal disease or chronic renal failure due to tubulointerstitial disease (149). A similar reversible syndrome has been reported in association with the use of *indomethacin* and other prostaglandin inhibitors (148,150). Inhibition of renal prostaglandin synthesis may suppress renin secretion in susceptible individuals and lead to the development of hyperkalemia.

12. *Treatment.* A.D., a 15-year-old previously healthy male, was brought unconscious to the emergency room following a crush injury sustained when a tractor which he was driving overturned, pinning him for several hours. Following preliminary evaluation, he was transferred to the intensive care unit. Vital signs on admission included: BP 100/60 mm Hg, P 110/min, Temp 38.6°C, Resp 30/min. Evidence of extensive trauma to the abdomen and lower extremities was present with extensive bleeding into soft tissue. Bowel sounds were absent and the abdomen was markedly distended. A nasogastric tube was placed and a large amount of guaiac positive material was aspirated. Urine sediment, electrolytes and osmolality were consistent with acute renal failure. Other laboratory data included: Na 138 mEq/L, K 6.8 mEq/L, Cl 100, CO_2 10 mEq/L, BUN 40 mg/dl, creatinine 2.2 mg/dl, glucose 120 mg/dl, hematocrit 31, WBC 18,600 with marked left shift. Arterial blood gas values were as follows: pO_2 89; pCO_2 28; pH 7.23. Chest x-ray showed multiple rib fractures, a flat plate of the abdomen revealed an ileus pattern and an electrocardiogram revealed tall peaked T waves, a prolonged PR interval, and widened QRS complexes. In the emergency room he received 50 mEq of sodium bicarbonate, 50 ml of 50% dextrose and 10 ml of 10% calcium gluconate intravenously. Fifty grams of Kayexalate in 70% sorbitol was administered as a retention enema. The repeat serum potassium 4 hours later was 7.1 mEq/L. Sodium bicarbonate, 50% glucose and calcium gluconate were again administered, with an additional 50 grams of Kayexalate as a retention enema. Because the serum potassium 2 hours later had fallen only to 6.5 mEq/L, acute hemodialysis was performed against a dialysate bath containing no potassium. This patient presents with a number of abnormal ECG findings. Discuss the ECG changes which may be caused by elevation of the serum potassium.

Hyperkalemia causes a number of characteristic abnormalities in cardiac conduction which, if present, influence the decision to treat the hyperkalemia and the aggressiveness with which the treatment is carried out. The earliest change seen in the electrocardiogram (ECG) is peaking or "tenting" of T waves, which correlates generally with a potassium level of 5.9–6.5 mEq/liter. Shortening of the QT interval may also be seen. As the serum potassium exceeds 6.5 mEq/liter, flattening of P waves, prolongation of the PR interval and widening of QRS complexes may be seen. At a serum potassium greater than 8 mEq/liter, a sine wave pattern consistent with marked depression of cardiac conduction and with the potential of life threatening arrythmias or asystole develops (80,151).

13. Emergency treatment of this patient's hyperkalemia included Kayexalate, calcium, sodium bicarbonate, and ultimately hemodialysis. What was the rationale for their use? What other modes of therapy are available for the emergency treatment of hyperkalemia?

The emergency treatment of hyperkalemia may include measures designed to antagonize the membrane effects of potassium, shift potassium from the extracellular to the intracellular compartment, or reduce the total body potassium content by increasing its removal from the body (152–157).

Calcium should be administered initially to reverse life-threatening ECG changes. Calcium salts antagonize the cardiac toxicity of potassium (155). The intravenous infusion of 10 to 30 ml of a 10% solution of calcium gluconate (4.5 mEq Ca^{++} per 10 ml) over 3 to 4 minutes may reverse cardiac conduction abnormalities within several min-

utes; this effect of calcium is transient. Calcium does not alter the serum potassium level, and serves only as a temporizing measure until therapy designed to produce cellular potassium shifts or to increase potassium removal takes effect. Caution should be exercised in digitalized patients, as calcium potentiates the effects of the cardiac glycosides and may produce digitalis toxicity.

The intravenous administration of *glucose and insulin* may be the most effective mode of emergency treatment of hyperkalemia. Any number of combinations of glucose-insulin in varying amounts have been suggested. Administration of 50 grams of glucose plus 10 units of regular insulin should decrease the serum potassium within 15 to 30 minutes as potassium moves intracellularly with glucose and is stored with glycogen (152).

Two issues should be addressed when glucose and insulin are used to treat hyperkalemia in patients such as A.D. who have renal failure. First, caution should be exercised against the injudicious use of large doses of insulin along with the glucose. Severe, sustained hypoglycemia may occur as a result of the prolonged half-life of insulin in renal failure (159). Secondly, it should be emphasized that glucose and insulin have no effect on total body potassium content; they merely shift potassium intracellularly. Hyperkalemia in most patients with renal failure is largely due to increased total body potassium content. Thus, glucose and insulin (or glucose alone) should be used in conjunction with measures to reduce the total body potassium content in these patients.

Sodium bicarbonate will also shift potassium into cells. It has been shown to be of particular value in rapidly lowering the serum potassium in patients like A.D. who are also acidotic (158), although it may also be effective in patients with a normal arterial pH. Recent studies have demonstrated that the intracellular shift of potassium with bicarbonate administration occurs even when there is no change in pH (136). Sodium bicarbonate in a dose of 50 mEq should be administered over several minutes and may be repeated as necessary. Like glucose and insulin, this therapy has no effect on total body potassium content and should not be substituted for measures which decrease potassium load when hyperkalemia is due to total body potassium excess. Because of its sodium content, repeated administration of sodium bicarbonate may result in ECF volume expansion and fluid overload as well as hypernatremia, particularly in the setting of renal insufficiency.

Excess potassium can be removed from the body through the use of the cation exchange resin *sodium polystyrene sulfonate (Kayexalate)*. Administered orally or as a retention enema, Kayexalate exchanges sodium for potassium in the gastrointestinal tract (156,157). Although somewhat slower in onset than other modalities used to treat hyperkalemia, Kayexalate readily and effectively lowers total body potassium content. Each gram of the resin will bind approximately 1 mEq of potassium and release 2–3 mEq of sodium if sufficient time is allowed for maximal exchange. With rectal administration, Kayexalate should be retained for at least 30 minutes. When given orally, it should be administered with sorbitol to prevent constipation due to Kayexalate, and to induce diarrhea which will also increase fecal potassium excretion. Continued administration of large amounts of Kayexalate in patients with renal failure can cause ECF volume expansion, CHF and pulmonary edema if its contribution to the patient's sodium intake is overlooked (157).

Although an effective measure for reducing total body potassium content, dialysis is seldom required for the emergency treatment of hyperkalemia due to the effectiveness of the cation exchange resins. However, dialysis may be required in situations which preclude the use of the gastrointestinal tract, or in patients (illustrated by A.D.) who have a sustained, high release of tissue potassium and have renal failure. Peritoneal dialysis, which can remove up to 15 mEq/hour of potassium, is less effective than hemodialysis, which can remove up to 50 mEq/hour (64).

PHOSPHORUS

The normal adult body contains between 500 and 700 grams (approximately 20,000 mmoles) of phosphorus, of which 80–85% is found in bone (160–162). The remainder is primarily found in the intracellular space, with about 9% in skeletal muscle. Only about 0.05% is found in the extracellular space (162).

The dietary intake of phosphorus varies greatly due to its abundance in all naturally occurring foods, but approximates 1 gram daily (161). Approximately 90% of the phosphorus absorbed in the gastrointestinal tract is excreted by the kidneys; the remaining 10% is excreted in the feces (161,162). Renal excretion is regulated by glomerular filtration and tubular reabsorption, in part under the influence of parathyroid hormone (PTH) (161).

Intracellular stores of organic phosphorus are incorporated into ribonucleic acids, cell membrane phospholipids and phosphorylated adenine and guanine nucleotides and play an important role in intermediary metabolism (160,161). A small fraction is present in the form of inorganic phosphorus for the synthesis of ATP. The creation of the high energy phosphate bond is associated with the origins of life, for without this means of energy transfer, cellular growth and reproduction would not be possible. Phosphorus is also important in the regulation of glycolysis, in the delivery of oxygen to tissues through regulation of 2, 3-diphosphoglycerate (2,3-DPG), and in the excretion of fixed acids by the kidney where it functions as an important urinary buffer (161).

Normal serum levels of inorganic phosphorus vary with age. The normal range in adults is 2.7–4.5 mg/dl; it is 4.0–7.1 mg/dl in children (161). As with all electrolytes, the serum level of phosphorus is not indicative of body stores or of phosphorus balance. For example, severely depleted alcoholics may develop rhabdomyolysis from extremely low intracellular concentrations of phosphorus (161). As cellular destruction occurs, intracellular phosphorus is released and the serum phosphorus may rise to normal or even elevated levels while stores remain depleted (162,163). Alternatively, refeeding of severely malnourished patients drives phosphorus intracellularly as cellular anabolism is promoted, resulting in depression of serum levels at a time when body stores remain unchanged or are increasing (161).

Hypophosphatemia

14. *Etiology.* W.S. is a 42-year-old, 63 kg male with a 20-year history of diabetes and chronic alcoholism who was admitted to the hospital after experiencing four days of diarrhea, vomiting and severe epigastric pain. His history is significant for multiple hospitalizations for acute pancreatitis, and malnutrition with a 30 to 40 pound weight loss in the past two years.

On admission, W.S. complained of severe abdominal pain and appeared icteric. Vital signs were stable. Pertinent laboratory find-

ings included: Na 133 mEq/L, K 3.9 mEq/L, Cl 100 mEq/L, CO_2 30 mEq/L, BUN 30 mg/dl, creatinine 1.4 mg/dl, glucose 365 mg/dl, Ca 8.3 mg/dl, albumin 2.2 gm/dl, phosphorus 3.0 mg/dl, and amylase 900. A nasogastric tube (NG) was placed and guaiac positive material was aspirated. He was placed on NG suction and Amphogel alternating with Gelusil was begun.

The diagnosis of acute pancreatitis and pancreatic pseudocyst was made and total parenteral nutrition (TPN) was begun by central vein. Three days later, W.S. became irritable, was noted to be intermittently confused and complained of diffuse muscle weakness. Laboratory studies revealed normal Ca, Mg, K and glucose levels, but the serum phosphorus was 0.8 mg/dl. Describe clinical situations in which hypophosphatemia may occur. What is the etiology of hypophosphatemia in this patient?

Clinical hypophosphatemia occurs as a result of any one or combination of three basic mechanisms: decreased GI absorption or increased GI loss, increased renal excretion, and intracellular shifts (160–162). Moderate hypophosphatemia is defined as a serum phosphorus level of 2.0–2.5 mg/dl and may or may not be accompanied by clinical signs and symptoms. With severe hypophosphatemia, defined as a serum phosphorus less than 1 mg/dl, clinical manifestations are commonly present.

Because food is abundant in phosphorus, dietary deficiences are rare. Notable exceptions include patients with severe starvation, prolonged vomiting, malabsorption states (160), or the hospitalized patient who is not eating but is receiving intravenous dextrose or parenteral nutritional solutions containing inadequate phosphorus supplementation (160–162; 164–171). In such patients, the administration of glucose stimulates insulin secretion which in turn facilitates the passage of glucose and phosphorus into cells (172,173). In severe depletion states, profound hypophosphatemia may develop, possibly as a result of the entry of much of the administered glucose into skeletal muscle where large quantities of phosphorus are utilized (174).

Severe hypophosphatemia from ingestion of large quantities of phosphate binding antacids, such as aluminum hydroxide, aluminum carbonate or magnesium hydroxide, has been reported in patients with normal renal function (175–178) as well as in those with renal failure (179–181).

With the extensive use of phosphate binding agents, particularly in patients with end stage renal disease receiving chronic dialysis, the potential for development of hypophosphatemia should be kept in mind, especially in those patients whose dietary intake may be low on the basis of anorexia. Excessive phosphorus losses may occur in patients on dialysis or who are taking diuretics as well as in patients with systemic acidosis, renal tubular defects and hyperparathyroidism (160–162).

Severe or profound hypophosphatemia is most commonly seen in severe alcoholics (160,161, 163,182–184); in patients with diabetic ketoacidosis (DKA) (160–162,185), severe respiratory alkalosis (160–162,186,187), or the nutritional recovery syndrome (160–162,188); following the initiation of TPN therapy (160–162;164–171) and in the recovery period following major burns (161,162). All of these situations are associated with large intracellular phosphorus shifts. In some of these situations, the severe depression of the serum phosphorus occurs during the treatment period. In diabetic ketoacidosis, for example, acidosis promotes intracellular organic substrate metabolism with release of phosphate into the ECF, while glucosuria, ketonuria and osmotic diuresis augment phosphate excretion. This produces a normal serum phosphorus in the face of intracellular depletion. With insulin therapy, volume repletion and correction of acidosis, intracellular shifts occur and profound hypophosphatemia may develop (160–162, 185).

The etiology of hypophosphatemia in W.S. is multifactorial. With malnutrition and alcoholism both increasing the likelihood for preexisting phosphate depletion, TPN therapy caused intracellular phosphate shifts. There was apparently inadequate phosphate supplementation to meet the needs of anabolism. Increased gastrointestinal losses caused by phosphate binding antacids in combination with these factors resulted in the development of symptomatic hypophosphatemia.

15. *Signs and Symptoms.* How do the findings of weakness, irritability and confusion in W.S. relate to the serum phosphorus level of 0.8 mg/dl? What are other biochemical and clinical manifestations of hypophosphatemia?

Since intracellular phosphorus is required for almost every metabolic process, major alterations in cellular metabolism are expected to occur. Mild symptoms such as muscle weakness, malaise, paresthesias and irritability may be present at serum levels less than 2 mg/dl. At levels less than 1 mg/dl, significant alterations in hematologic and neuromuscular function are observed.

The central nervous system (CNS) effects of hypophosphatemia resemble metabolic encephalopathy (161,170) with irritability, weakness, numbness, paresthesias, confusion, obtundation, seizures and coma (161,167,170,171). The pathophysiology of these findings is unclear, but may involve decreased glucose utilization by the brain secondary to reduction in inorganic phosphate or CNS hypoxia resulting from decreased erythrocyte 2,3-DPG (161).

Musculoskeletal abnormalities such as bone pain, pseudofractures, weakness or paralysis, myopathy and rhabdomyolysis have been attributed to hypophosphatemia (160–162;178,180,181). If severe enough, paralysis of respiratory muscles and respiratory failure can occur (189). Myocardial contractility may be depressed and can result in the development of congestive cardiomyopathy and heart failure (177,190).

With severe depletion of erythrocyte inorganic phosphate, glycolysis is suppressed, limiting the production of 2,3-DPG and ATP. Reduced levels of these substances increase the affinity of hemoglobin for oxygen and decrease oxygen delivery to tissues (161,191–194). Impaired tissue oxygen delivery has been implicated as a cause for the persistent coma seen in some patients undergoing treatment for diabetic ketoacidosis (192–194). It has been suggested that decreased erythrocyte 2,3-DPG may be involved in the hepatic dysfunction and coma seen in alcoholics through creation of a relative hypoxia to liver and CNS tissue (160,161).

Hemolysis associated with hypophosphatemia is rare. It is usually seen only at serum phosphorus levels below 0.2–0.5 mg/dl, and is then usually accompanied by other stress such as sepsis or severe acidosis (161,195).

Impaired granulocyte function has been demonstrated in hypophosphatemia (191,196). Depression of chemotactic, phagocytic and bactericidal activity of granulocytes has been reported in hypophosphatemic dogs which reversed following phosphate repletion (196).

16. *Treatment.* Could the development of hypophosphatemia have been avoided in W.S.?

As with any electrolyte abnormality, identification of patients at risk for the development of hypophosphatemia and prevention with appropriate phosphorus supplementation is the best therapy. In the case of W.S., hypophosphatemia should have been anticipated and could probably have been avoided with appropriate supplementation in the TPN solution. In patients with normal renal function receiving TPN, hypophosphatemia can usually be prevented with the administration of 10–15 mmoles of phosphorus as sodium or potassium phosphate for each 1000 kcal the patient receives (15,197). Renal failure patients receiving TPN are usually hyperphosphatemic at the outset of therapy and probably should not be given phosphorus initially unless the serum level is low or normal. If the patient's metabolic requirements are met, intracellular movement of phosphorus may normalize serum levels within two to five days. At this point, the addition of 5–10 mmoles of phosphorus per 1000 kcal will usually prevent hypophosphatemia.

Hypophosphatemia during the treatment of diabetic ketoacidosis can be avoided if part of the potassium replacement is provided as potassium phosphate (15,185). Lentz et al (15) suggest administration of approximately 20 mEq/L of potassium replacement as the phosphate salt. As most commercially available parenteral solutions of potassium phosphate contain 3 mmoles of phosphorus and 4.4 mEq of potassium per ml, this recommendation provides approximately 14 mmoles of phosphorus/liter.

Although the best management is certainly prevention, the development of hypophosphatemia requires implementation of definitive therapy. The choice of therapy is dictated by the clinical setting, the phosphorus level and the presence or absence of symptoms.

17. Is W.S. a good candidate for oral phosphate replacement?

Oral supplementation is a desirable form of therapy for mild hypophosphatemia in patients who can tolerate oral intake (15,160–162). Doses of 1 to 2 grams of elemental phosphorus per day (30 to 60 mmoles) may be given in three or four divided doses. A number of oral preparations are available (Table 4). An unpleasant side effect of some oral phosphate replacement solutions is diarrhea. Although it can be minimized by diluting the dose in water, it creates the potential for unreliable gastrointestinal (GI) absorption. With the life-threatening complications that may accompany severe hypophosphatemia, a more reliable form of therapy is necessary. Because of the extremely low phosphorus level, the presence of symptoms and the inability to use the GI tract, parenteral rather than oral phosphate replacement would be the preferred therapy for W.S.

18. Outline therapeutic guidelines for the treatment of severe hypophosphatemia.

Patients such as W.S. who have severe hypophosphatemia and/or are unable to tolerate oral therapy should be treated parenterally. Since it is not possible to predict either the magnitude of the phosphorus deficit or the degree of elevation of the serum phosphorus following a given replacement dose (15), the goal of therapy is to select a dose that will raise the phosphorus from dangerously low levels but will not produce toxicity.

Based on analysis of available data concerning phosphorus balance, Lentz et al (15) suggest that an initial phosphorus dose of 0.08 to 0.16 mmoles/kg as sodium or potassium phosphate be infused over six hours, followed by close monitoring of serum levels. A 25–50% higher initial dose is suggested if symptoms are present; however, to avoid complications, the dose should not exceed 0.24 mmoles/kg. The goal of this regimen is to raise the phosphorus to a safe level without producing toxic effects such as hyperphosphatemia, hypocalcemia, and metastatic calcification (15,-198–200).

An alternative treatment regimen for severe hypophosphatemia has been recently proposed. Vannetta et al (201) suggest the following regimen for treatment of severe hypophosphatemia in normokalemic adults with normal renal function: administration of 9 mmoles of phosphorus as potassium phosphate in half normal saline as a continuous intravenous infusion during a 12-hour period, repeating the dose at 12-hour intervals until the serum phosphorus exceeds 1 mg/dl.

A number of treatment plans would be acceptable for the treatment of hypophosphatemia in W.S. First, it is important to verify that the TPN solution is providing the recommended 15 mmoles of phosphorus per 1000 kcal. If he is indeed receiving this amount of phosphorus, the likelihood exists, in this severely depleted patient in whom glucose is providing a continued stimulus for in-tracellular movement of phosphorus, that an additional 10 to 15 mmoles of phosphorus should raise the serum level to within a safe range and would be unlikely to cause any toxicity. It is impossible to predict how much phosphorus will ultimately be required to maintain the serum phosphorus within the normal range. It is important to obtain serum phosphorus determinations on a daily basis until the serum phosphorus stabilizes, keeping in mind that additional supplementation may be necessary.

Caution should always be observed when intravenous or oral phosphate therapy is attempted in the patient with renal insufficiency and serum phosphorus levels must be closely monitored. Similar caution should be exercised in the patient with hypercalcemia. In addition, the sodium and potassium load incurred with phosphate replacement should always be considered, particularly in the patient with congestive heart failure, renal insufficiency, or other disease states in which sodium and potassium metabolism are altered. See Table 4 for sodium and potassium content of phosphate replacement products.

CALCIUM

The total body calcium content varies according to the size of the skeleton and the density of bone; more than 99% of body calcium is found in the skeleton (202). The remaining calcium is distributed between intracellular and extracellular compartments, and the concentration in these two compartments is similar (203).

In normal persons the serum calcium is maintained within a narrow range of 8.5 to 10.5 mg/100 ml. This concentration reflects a dynamic equilibrium between bound and unbound calcium in the serum (14). Approximately 40% of the calcium present in the serum is bound to proteins, primarily albumin. Approximately 10% is present in the form of complexes with citrate, phosphate, etc., otherwise known as the diffusible fraction. The free or ionized calcium constitutes the remaining 50% of the serum calcium (14, 204,205). This ionized form is the physiologically active form and it is this ionized calcium concentration which is rigidly maintained within a narrow range by very sensitive homeostatic mechanisms. Hormonal regulation of the serum calcium concentration involves a complex interplay be-

Table 4.

PHOSPHORUS REPLACEMENT SOLUTIONS

PREPARATION	PHOSPHATE (mmoles/ml)	SODIUM (mEq/ml)	POTASSIUM (mEq/ml)
Cow's milk	0.029	0.025	0.035
Fleet's Phospho-Soda	4.1	4.8	—
Neutra-Phos	*0.107	*0.095	*0.095
	(8.1 mmoles/250 mg)	(7.1 mEq/250 mg)	(7.1 mEq/250 mg)
Neutra-Phos K	*0.107	—	*0.190
	(8.1 mmoles/250 mg)		(14.2 mEq/250 mg)
Potassium phosphate injection	3	—	4.4
Sodium phosphate injection	3	4.0	—

Table adapted from: Lentz et al (reference 15).
*Concentration present when prepared according to instructions of manufacturer (contents of one 250 mg capsule dissolved in 75 ml water).

tween the effects of parathyroid hormone, calcitonin and Vitamin D on the skeleton, kidney and gastrointestinal tract (206).

Since a large proportion of the calcium present in the serum is bound to albumin, changes in the serum albumin may affect the total serum calcium level even though the physiologically active ionized form may be normal. For each decrease in serum albumin concentration of 1.0 gm/dl, the total serum calcium decreases by approximately 0.8 mg/dl. Therefore, accurate interpretation of the serum calcium is dependent on the concomitant measurement of the serum albumin (14).

The amount of calcium absorbed in the gastrointestinal tract is dependent on dietary calcium intake and the efficiency of intestinal absorption. Although intestinal calcium absorption is primarily an active process regulated by 1,25-dihydroxycholecalciferol, intestinal absorption of calcium can occur by passive diffusion. Quantities of calcium greater than 2 gm/day are required for passive calcium absorption to occur (207,208). At the usual dietary calcium intake of 400–800 mg/day passive absorption is negligible and Vitamin D stimulated active transport of calcium is required to maintain calcium balance (209–211). GI absorption ranges from 5–50% of intake, with the higher percent absorption ocurring in individuals with low dietary calcium intake (202). Obligatory daily losses average 100 mg in the urine and 150 mg in the feces. These losses are independent of dietary intake.

The role of calcium in normal body functions has been reviewed (212). In addition to its key role in normal bone structure, calcium acts to help maintain cellular membrane excitability, nerve tissue excitability, and contractility of skeletal, smooth and cardiac muscle. It functions as a co-factor in the activation of various enzyme systems, including those of the pancreas; it is necessary for appropriate function of the coagulation system; and it also affects the secretory activity of endocrine and exocrine glands.

Hypercalcemia

19. *Etiology.* **L.C., a 54-year-old white female, was admitted to the hospital in a coma. She was in her usual state of good health until two years prior to admission when biopsy of a breast mass revealed adenocarcinoma. Initial therapy consisted of radical mastectomy with node dissection, radiation therapy and chemotherapy. Despite multiple courses of treatment, the disease progressed with widespread metastases to the liver and bone. According to her family, her severe bone pain was well-controlled with narcotic analgesics and she was generally well until approximately two weeks prior to admission when she began complaining of easy fatigability, diffuse muscle weakness and anorexia. At this time she confined herself to bed and refused all food intake except for small amounts of fluids. Approximately one week prior to admission, she began experiencing episodes of intermittent disorientation and confusion which progressed until the evening of admis-**

sion when she was found by her daughter to be unarousable. Medications on admission included: tamoxifen 10 mg po bid, hydrochlorothiazide 50 mg po qd, Brompton's Cocktail 15–30 ml q3h prn pain, DOSS 100 mg tid, MOM 30 ml po prn. On admission to the hospital, she was responsive only to painful stimuli. Vital signs were: BP 130/80 supine, dropping to 100/70 with 30° elevation of the head of the bed; pulse 90/min, respirations 20/min. Physical examination revealed diffuse hyporeflexia; the skin was dry with poor turgor, mucous membranes were dry and axillary sweat was absent. Her weight was 50 kg which was 3.5 kg lower than that recorded at her last clinic visit one month prior to admission. Laboratory data were as follows: Na 144 mEq/L, K 4.0 mEq/L, Cl 100 mEq/L, CO_2 30 mEq/L, BUN 40 mg/dl, creatinine 2.8 mg/dl, glucose 130 mg/dl, calcium 14.8 mg/dl, phosphorus 3.2 mg/dl, and albumin 2.8 gm/dl. Electrocardiogram revealed shortening of the QT interval. Discuss the causes of hypercalcemia. What are the possible etiologies for hypercalcemia in this patient?

Causes of hypercalcemia may be divided into two groups: those related to increased resorption from bone and those related to increased intestinal absorption. Malignancy and hyperparathyroidism are the two most common causes of hypercalcemia (14).

Hypercalcemia can occur as a common consequence of almost any malignancy, but is especially common with breast cancer, squamous cell carcinoma of the lung, multiple myeloma and certain renal carcinomas (14,213,214). A number of mechanisms may be involved, including tumor production of polypeptides with PTH-like activity (215–216), production of prostaglandins which cause bone resorption (217–222), production of factors that stimulate osteoclast activity (osteoclast activating factors; OAF) (223) and direct bone resorption due to skeletal metastases (14,214).

Primary or secondary hyperparathyroidism is a common cause of hypercalcemia (14,224,225). Primary hyperparathyroidism occurs as a result of parathyroid adenomas, hyperplasia and malignancy (14) and may be asymptomatic or characterized by fatigue, nervous irritability and other nonspecific somatic complaints. Secondary hyperparathyroidism is most commonly seen in patients with acute or chronic renal failure (226, 227).

In addition to hyperparathyroidism and malignancy, hypercalcemia is also associated with sarcoidosis and other granulomatous diseases, Paget's Disease of the bone, milk-alkali syndrome, hyperthyroidism, immobilization, and recovery from acute renal failure secondary to rhabdomyolysis (14). Drugs known to cause hypercalcemia include the thiazide diuretics (228–231), Vitamin D (232), Vitamin A (233), tamoxifen (234), lithium (235) and calcium supplements (236). In addition, volume depletion and dehydration can result in decreased urinary calcium excretion and aggravate hypercalcemia.

The primary underlying cause for hypercalcemia in this patient is malignancy with skeletal metastases causing bone resorption. It may also be aggravated by immobilization and volume contraction. Possible drug-related etiologies in this patient include the thiazide diuretic and tamoxifen.

20. What are the signs and symptoms of hypercalcemia? How are they manifested in L.C.?

Essentially, every organ system may be affected by hypercalcemia. Multiple psychiatric disturbances may occur, with the symptoms often proportional to the degree of hypercalcemia and the rate at which it develops, although this is not always the case. Tiredness, lethargy, apathy and depression or agitation, nervousness and insomnia may occur. The electroencephalogram may show diffuse slow activity. Neurotic behavior, psychomotor retardation, agitated depression and paranoia have all been reported to occur with hypercalcemia, and are reversible as the calcium level returns to normal. Headaches and generalized muscle weakness are also common (237–240).

Gastrointestinal manifestations include anorexia, nausea, vomiting, and constipation or diarrhea (241). Increased gastric acid and pepsin secretion occur, which may explain the increased incidence of peptic ulcer disease in conditions associated with hypercalcemia (242).

A number of cardiac arrhythmias may occur during hypercalcemia (14,243). ECG changes which may occur include shortening of the QT interval, prolongation of the PR interval and broadening of T waves. The inotropic effect of the digitalis glycosides is potentiated by hypercalcemia and their toxicity may be enhanced. Thus, digitalis should be used cautiously in hypercalcemic patients.

Hypercalcemia affects both the glomerular filtration and tubular function of the kidney (244–246). Renal blood flow and glomerular filtration rate are reduced and have been attributed to the vasoconstrictive effects of calcium on the renal vasculature. The polyuria and secondary polydipsia seen with hypercalcemia are a result of inhibition of the adenyl cyclase-cyclic AMP system which is responsible for mediation of the effects of ADH on the collecting duct; this causes a defect in water conservation and concentrating ability. Calcium also inhibits solute transport in the loop of Henle which may lower medullary tonicity and contribute to the renal concentrating defects. Most of the functional abnormalities are corrected with normalization of the serum calcium. If allowed to persist, however, hypercalcemia can lead to renal calcium deposition and chronic renal insufficiency.

Acute hypercalcemia may result in hypertension which reverses as the serum calcium level returns to normal (247,248). Chronic hypercalcemia may also be accompanied by hypertension. It has been estimated that over 70% of patients with chronic primary hyperparathyroidism and up to 35% of those with hypercalcemia of any etiology are hypertensive (247). Normal renal function may be a prerequisite for normotension once serum calcium levels are returned to normal in hyperparathyroidism (247). In severe or chronic hypercalcemia, volume depletion may occur preventing the development of hypertension.

Signs and symptoms in L.C. which are consistent with hypercalcemia include fatigue, muscle weakness, anorexia, dehydration and the electrocardiographic abnormalities.

21. What modes of therapy are available to manage L.C.'s hypercalcemia? Discuss these in order of their use.

As with most electrolyte disorders, treatment of hypercalcemia should be primarily aimed at correction of the underlying cause. However, when patients such as L.C. present with symptomatic hypercalcemia, immediate therapy to lower the serum calcium level is required.

Fluid Replacement. Since hypercalcemia is usually accompanied by vomiting and polyuria, and almost all patients present with dehydration (206), initial therapy should consist of intravenous normal saline in sufficient quantity to rehydrate the patient and increase urine output to at least 100 ml/hour.

Saline and Furosemide. Once urine output reaches 100 ml/hour, intravenous furosemide may be given at doses of 80 to 100 mg every one to two hours (249). Since calcium reabsorption in the nephron appears to be linked to sodium reabsorption (250), the natriuretic effect of furosemide in consort with the saline-induced diuresis increases urinary calcium excretion. Hourly urine volume should be measured as well as periodic urinary potassium and magnesium to assess the extent of their losses and to determine the need for intravenous replacement. As might be expected, if the volume of intravenous saline replacement is insufficient to replace urinary loss, the reduction in ECF volume and the resultant increase in tubular reabsorption of sodium and calcium will ultimately negate the desired calciuretic effects. This therapy is best carried out with a central venous catheter in place for monitoring of fluids (206). This therapy must be administered cautiously to patients with such underlying diseases as congestive heart failure or renal insufficiency.

Mithramycin, an antibiotic that has antitumor activity especially in the treatment of embryonal cell carcinoma of the testis has recently become a mainstay in the therapy of malignant hypercalcemia (253–255). Although the exact mechanism of action of mithramycin is unknown, it has been proposed that it acts through inhibition of RNA synthesis (253). PTH directly stimulates bone resorption possibly by initiating the development of osteoclast differentiation (256), a process which is related to an increased synthesis of RNA within the osteoclast (253). Thus, it is likely that mithramycin exerts its activity by inhibiting the effect of PTH on the osteoclast. Also, small doses of mithramycin have been shown to block the hypercalcemic action of pharmacologic doses of vitamin D (257).

Cumulative doses of mithramycin, like those used in tumor therapy, are quite toxic and may cause fever, nausea, vomiting, and dermatitis (253). Hemorrhage resulting from vascular damage, thrombocytopenia, altered platelet function, and depression of factors II, V, VII and X (258) may occur in over 50% of the patients (253). Hepatic dysfunction occurs regularly and is associated with elevated levels of SGOT, SGPT and LDH; the morphologic finding is usually central lobular necrosis (253). [Severe renal damage, although less frequent, does occur with cumulative doses;

mild renal damage with proteinuria, is common (253).]

Although serious toxicity limits the use of mithramycin as a tumor agent, the doses used to treat hypercalcemia (25 to 150 mcg/kg/week) are well tolerated (254,259). The drug may be administered by IV bolus or by IV infusion over 24 hours. Gradual decreases in serum calcium levels occur usually within 48 hours after its administration. The duration of the effect is variable and repeated doses may be required every 3 to 7 days.

Calcitonin is an agent which rapidly lowers serum calcium through inhibition of bone resorption (264). With an onset of action of several hours and relative freedom from toxicity, calcitonin is attractive for acute management of symptomatic hypercalcemia (264–268), particularly in patients with renal or hepatic disease. The most promising use for calcitonin is in hypercalcemia associated with malignancy (264,268). Results of therapy in other hypercalcemic states is less impressive. At this time, calcitonin is not a first-line agent for acute management of hypercalcemia of malignancy, but in situations where other therapies may be contraindicated, it should be strongly considered as an alternative. Chronic therapy with calcitonin is limited by development of resistance to the hypocalcemic effect within several days, although one study suggests that the simultaneous use of glucocorticoids may inhibit this escape phenomenon (268).

Glucocorticoids are widely used in the therapy of hypercalcemia although the exact mechanism by which they lower serum calcium remains unknown. Most patients like L.C. with breast cancer as well as those with sarcoidosis, myeloma, lymphoma or leukemia will respond to prednisone 40 to 60 mg daily (251); this is in part due to the antitumor effect of the steroids (213, 214,252). These agents also exert an anti-vitamin D effect which may decrease both bone resorption and gastrointestinal absorption of calcium (252).

Prostaglandin Inhibitors. The use of indomethacin in doses of 75 to 150 mg/day or aspirin in doses of 1.8 to 4.8 grams/day may be effective in treatment of hypercalcemia of malignancy associated with increased prostaglandin production (220–222). These agents presumably inhibit prostaglandin cyclooxygenase and thus interfere with prostaglandin synthesis (221). A therapeutic response is more likely to occur in patients who have certain solid tumors which are not complicated by bone metastases, whose urinary excretion of PGE-M, a urinary metabolite of the E prostaglandins, is increased, and whose PTH levels are not elevated. The presence of skeletal metastases results in a blunted or partial response to therapy. If PGE-M excretion is not elevated, regardless of whether or not bone metastases are present, patients are unlikely to respond to this therapy. L.C. has bone metastases and is therefore less likely to respond to therapy with these agents.

Phosphates. Although inorganic phosphates lower serum calcium when administered orally or by IV infusion, the mechanisms by which they do so is unclear since the renal excretion of calcium actually decreases during therapy (260,261). Several investigators (260–262) propose precipitation of $CaHPO_4$ as the mechanism, while others (263) believe phosphate administration promotes bone formation. The available evidence supports the theory that calcium is removed from the blood and deposited as a phosphate precipitate in soft tissue and bone. Although clinical complications generally do not occur, hypotension and acute renal failure have been associated with the rapid administration of intravenous phosphate solution (198).

22. E.M. is a 50-year-old female with the diagnosis of primary hyperparathyroidism who at this time refuses surgery. Although she has been relatively asymptomatic, she consistently has serum calcium levels ranging between 11.5 and 12.5 mg/100 ml. What measures should be used to control this patient's hypercalcemia?

When surgery is not feasible, adequate salt and water intake must be assured to prevent dehydration, which will decrease the renal excretion of calcium and accentuate the hypercalcemia by decreasing the extracellular volume. Agents which may cause hypercalcemia should be avoided (see Table 3). Also, careful use of digitalis glycosides is necessary to prevent calcium potentiated digitalis toxicity. Immobilization of the patient should be minimized as this accelerates bone resorption. Restriction of calcium in the diet is usually of no benefit since most of the calcium is being resorbed from the bones; however, milk products which contain vitamin D should not be taken. If these measures are unsuccessful, oral phosphates should be added to the regimen in a dosage of 1 to 3 grams of elemental phosphorus per 24 hours. Antacid preparations should not be taken concomitantly as these agents bind phosphate in the gut.

Hypocalcemia

23. When it is observed, what are the signs and symptoms of hypocalcemia?

The major manifestation of hypocalcemia is tetany. Earliest symptoms are numbness of the fingers and tingling or burning in the extremities. As hypocalcemia progresses, muscle cramps may occur followed by visible muscle spasms of the extremities. In several cases generalized convulsions are observed (241).

A widened S-T segment is seen on electrocardiogram, and impaired cardiac contractility can ultimately lead to cardiac enlargement and heart failure (151,241). Thinning and loss of body hair usually occurs with chronic hypocalcemia. In addition, the skin becomes dry and keratotic, resembing eczema.

Hypocalcemia occurs in malabsorptive states and in primary and secondary hypoparathyroid states. Also see chapter on Kidney Diseases for a discussion of the treatment of hypocalcemia associated with chronic renal failure. Acute shifts of ionized calcium onto protein which may follow rapid correction of acidosis may also be associated with the symptomatology described above.

MAGNESIUM

Hypermagnesemia

24. F.C. is a 36-year-old black male with end stage renal failure (Cl_{Cr} 4 ml/min) who is currently being managed by diet and drug therapy while awaiting admission into a chronic hemodialysis program. His regimen includes a 40 gm protein diet, calcium carbonate 1 gram po tid, aluminum carbonate gel (Basaljel Extra Strength) 15 ml tid pc, multivitamins 1 qd, and Shohl's Solution 10 ml tid. He was brought to the emergency room where he appeared to be uremic, with drowsiness and a clouded sensorium. Initial laboratory values were Na 139 mEq/L, K 4.2 mEq/L, Cl 102 mEq/L, CO_2 18 mEq/L, BUN 74 mg/dl, Cr 12.5 mg/dl, and glucose 89 mg/dl. An

electrocardiogram (ECG) revealed a prolonged P-R interval and a broadened QRS complex. On questioning the patient and his family, it was concluded that adherence to both diet and prescribed drug regimens was excellent; however, the patient had been constipated for the past two weeks and had been taking milk of magnesia several times a day for the past week. A serum magnesium level was drawn and found to be 7.2 mEq/L. How does the kidney handle magnesium normally and in renal failure? What is the etiology of F.C.'s hypermagnesemia?

The major pathway for magnesium excretion is renal, with regulation of renal excretion controlled by both filtration and reabsorption. Of approximately 1800 mg/day of magnesium filtered at the glomerulus, only 3–5% is lost in the urine. Active magnesium reabsorption occurs throughout the nephron (269–272). With advancing renal failure, magnesium excretion generally declines.

Generally, the serum magnesium concentration in a patient with chronic renal failure such as F.C. is normal or only slightly elevated as long as magnesium containing compounds are not ingested (269,273). However, as illustrated by this case, the use of magnesium containing laxatives or antacids by patients with renal insufficiency can rapidly result in the development of severe hypermagnesemia (273,274).

25. What are the signs and symptoms of hypermagnesemia? Are this patient's neurologic and ECG findings consistent with hypermagnesemia? How should he be treated?

Signs and symptoms of hypermagnesemia occur secondary to its effects on the cardiovascular and neurologic systems. Common cardiovascular effects of hypermagnesemia include hypotension and abnormal cardiac conduction with ECG changes. Increased P-R interval, increased QRS complex, prolonged QT interval, decreased P-wave voltage and peaking of T waves have all been reported. At very high concentrations, heart block or asystole may occur. Effects on the nervous system include mental status changes, hyporeflexia, respiratory paralysis and coma. Early clinical findings may include nausea, vomiting and hypotension, thus making the diagnosis in patients such as the one described above difficult to distinguish from uremia (269). Thus, this patient's clouded sensorium and ECG findings are consistent with hypermagnesemia.

The management of symptomatic hypermagnesemia includes discontinuation of magnesium-containing compounds and administration of calcium to reverse the toxic effects of magnesium. Calcium (5–10 mEq) will usually reverse the respiratory depression and heart block due to hypermagnesemia (270). Peritoneal or hemodialysis against a dialysate bath low in magnesium are also effective in reducing elevated magnesium concentrations (269,273,274).

Hypomagnesemia

26. A 35-year-old male was admitted to the hospital after a generalized convulsion. He has had regional enteritis for the past 10 years requiring surgery on two occasions for removal of diseased bowel. The most recent surgery was four weeks prior to his seizure. Since that surgery he has had continual diarrhea and food intake has been poor. On admission he was confused and had multiple focal seizures. His serum calcium was 7.5 mg/dl. Intravenous administration of calcium returned his serum calcium level to normal; however, his state of consciousness did not improve and he experienced another seizure. At this time his serum magnesium level was 0.9 mEq/L and intravenous administration of magnesium was begun. By the next day, his CNS symptoms had cleared, his neuromuscular irritability had disappeared and his appetite was improved. What is the etiology of this patient's hypomagnesemia? Are the clinical findings consistent with those of hypomagnesemia?

Magnesium deficiency with hypomagnesemia may occur due to decreased intake or absorption of magnesium, or excessive urinary, fecal or other GI losses of magnesium (275–280). Malabsorption syndromes, extensive intestinal resection, starvation, and protein calorie malnutrition are associated with decreased intake or absorption of magnesium. Excessive magnesium may also be lost through prolonged nasogastric suction, laxative overuse, severe diarrhea and intestinal fistulae. With the long history of regional enteritis, recent surgical resection of diseased bowel and the four-week history of anorexia and persistent diarrhea, a low magnesium intake as well as impaired absorption are likely explanations for this patient's hypomagnesemia. Excessive urinary

magnesium losses may be seen with diuretic therapy, chronic alcoholism, hyperaldosteronism, hypercalcemia, diabetes with acidosis, hyperthyroidism, leukemia with lysozymuria and gentamicin toxicity.

The clinical manifestations of hypomagnesemia are primarily neuromuscular, including weakness, muscle fasciculations with tremor, occasional tetany, and hyperreflexia. CNS changes may include anxiety, delirium or psychosis as well as seizures. Associated laboratory findings may include hypocalcemia, hypokalemia or hypophosphatemia.

27. Parenteral magnesium replacement is indicated in this patient due to the severity of symptoms and because adequate GI absorption of magnesium is unlikely. Outline possible treatment plans for magnesium replacement. What precautions are necessary when administering parenteral magnesium?

Therapy for hypomagnesemia is in large part empiric since estimation of the magnesium deficit is difficult. Consequently, a number of dosing schedules have been suggested (270,276,277,281). Flink (281) suggests the following plan for parenteral therapy in patients with normal renal function:

Intramuscular route (50% $MgSO_4$): On day 1 give 2 grams (16.3 mEq Mg^{++}) every 2 hours for three doses and then every 4 hours for four doses. On day 2 give 1 gram (8.1 mEq Mg^{++}) every 4 hours for six doses. On days 3 to 5 give 1 gram (8.1 mEq Mg^{++}) every 6 hours. The total magnesium dose is 32 grams (260 mEq Mg^{++}).

Intravenous administration (50% $MgSO_4$): On day 1 give 6 grams (49 mEq Mg^{++}) in 1000 ml solution containing glucose over 3 hours. Follow with 5 grams (40 mEq Mg^{++}) in each of two one-liter solutions to be administered through the day. On days 2–5 give 6 grams (49 mEq Mg^{++}) distributed equally in the total intravenous fluids of the day.

Alternatively, Massry and Seelig (270) suggest that significant magnesium depletion may be associated with a magnesium deficit of 1 to 2 mEq/kg. The amount required to correct this deficit will be about twice this amount because approximately 50% of the administered dose is lost in the urine. They recommend that 40–50% of the calculated deficit be administered by the IM or IV route in the first 24 hours and that the remainder be administered over the next two to four days.

Whatever regimen is chosen, a reduced dose may be required in patients with renal insufficiency and serial magnesium determinations must be monitored closely. If magnesium is adminis-tered intravenously, rapid infusion should be avoided to prevent acute hypermagnesemia with hypotension and respiratory depression. Massry and Seelig (270) suggest that 50 mEq of magnesium be infused over 4–6 hours; further they recommend against exceeding 100 mEq over 12 hours.

References

1. Hays RM: Dynamics of body water and electrolytes. In *Clinical Disorders of Fluid and Electrolyte Metabolism,* 3rd ed, edited by M Maxwell and C Kleeman, McGraw-Hill, New York, 1980, p 1.
2. Carroll HJ et al: Electrolyte physiology and body composition, Chapter 1. In *Water, Electrolyte, and Acid-Base Metabolism,* Lippincott, Philadelphia, 1978, p 1.
3. McCurdy DK: Hyperosmolar hyperglycemic nonketotic diabetic coma. Med Clin North Am. 1970; 54:683.
4. Feig PU et al: The hypertonic state. N Engl J Med. 1977; 297:1444.
5. Leaf A: Cell swelling. A factor in ischemic tissue injury. Circulation. 1973; 48:455.
6. Katz AL et al: Physiologic role of sodium-potassium-activated adenosine triphosphatase in the transport of cations across biologic membranes. N Engl J Med. 1968; 278:253.
7. Edelman IS: Exchange of water between blood and tissues, characteristics of deuterium oxide equilibration in body water. Am J Physiol. 1952; 171:279.
8. Leaf A et al: The mechanism of the osmotic adjustment of body cells as determined in vivo by the volume of distribution of a large water load. J Clin Invest. 1954; 33:1261.
9. Anderson RJ et al: Sodium Depletion States, Chapter 7. In *Sodium and Water Homeostasis,* edited by B Brenner and J Stein, Churchill Livingstone, New York, 1978, p 154.
10. Fuisz RE: Hyponatremia. Medicine. 1963; 42:149.
11. Berl T et al: Water metabolism and the hypo-osmolar syndromes. In *Sodium and Water Homeostasis,* edited by B Brenner and J Stein, Churchill Livingstone, New York, 1978, p 1.
12. Goldberg M: Hyponatremia. Med Clin North Am. 1981; 65:251.
13. Shroeder R: The meaning of milliequivalents. Minnesota Pharmacist. 1969; 10:10.
14. Lee DBN et al: The pathophysiology and clinical aspects of hypercalcemic disorders (Medical Progress). West J Med. 1978; 129:278.
15. Lentz RD et al: Treatment of severe hypophosphatemia. Ann Intern Med. 1978; 89:941.
16. Edelman IS et al: Anatomy of body water and electrolytes. Am J Med. 1959; 27:256.
17. Keitel HG: The prevention and treatment of fluid balance disorders in specific diseases. In *The Pathophysiology and Treatment of Body Fluid Disturbances,* Appleton-Century-Croft, New York, 1962, p 145.
18. Weil WB et al: Fluid balance. In *Fluid and Electrolyte Metabolism in Infants and Children. A Unified Approach,* Grune and Stratton, New York, 1977, p 29.
19. Goldberger E: General principles of water and electrolyte therapy. In *A Primer of Water, Electrolyte and Acid-Base Syndromes,* 6th ed, Lea and Febiger, Philadelphia, 1980, p 367.
20. Carroll HJ et al: Deficits of salt and water involving renal and nonrenal exchange, Chapter 3. In *Water, Electrolyte and Acid-Base Metabolism,* Lippincott, Philadelphia, 1980, p 73.
21. Wolf AV: Amometric analysis of thirst in man and dog. Am J Physiol. 1950; 161:75.
22. Hays RM: Antidiuretic hormone. N Engl J Med. 1972; 295:659.
23. Leaf A et al: The normal antidiuretic mechanism in man and dog: Its regulation by extracellular fluid tonicity. J Clin Invest. 1952; 31:54.
24. Verney EB: Croonian lecture: The antidiuretic hormone and the factors which determine its release. Proc R Soc Lond. 1947; 135:25.
25. Gennari FJ et al: Osmotic diuresis. N Engl J Med. 1974; 291:714.
26. DeFronzo RA et al: Pathophysiologic approach to hyponatremia. Arch Intern Med. 1980; 140:897.
27. Katz MA: Hyperglycemia-induced hyponatremia—calculation of expected serum sodium depression. N Engl J Med. 1973; 289:843.
28. Nissenson AR et al: Mannitol. West J Med. 1979; 131:277.
29. Frick PG et al: Hyponatremia associated with hyperproteinema in multiple myeloma. Helv Med Acta. 1966; 33:317.
30. Martinez-Maldonado M: Inappropriate antidiuretic hormone secretion of unknown origin. Kidney Int. 1980; 17:554.
31. Newsome HH: Vasopressin: Deficiency, excess and the syndrome of inappropriate antidiuretic hormone secretion. Nephron. 1979; 23:125.
32. Cooke CR et al: The syndrome of inappropriate antidiuretic hormone secretion (SIADH): Pathophysiologic mechanisms in solute and volume regulation. Medicine. 1979; 58:240.
33. Takacs FJ: Fluid and electrolyte problems in patients with advanced carcinoma. Med Clin North Am. 1974; 59:449.
34. Glassock RJ et al: Kidney and electrolyte disturbances in neoplastic diseases. Contr Nephrol. 1977; 7:2.

35. Dubovsky SL et al: Syndrome of inappropriate secretion of antidiuretic hormone with exacerbated psychosis. Ann Intern Med. 1973; 79:551.

36. Moses AM et al: Drug-induced dilutional hyponatremia. N Engl J Med. 1974; 290:1234.

37. deBodo RC et al: The antidiuretic action of barbiturates (phenobarbital, amytal, pentobarbital) and the mechanism involved in this action. J Pharmacol Exper Ther. 1944; 82:74.

38. Moses AM et al: Clofibrate-induced antidiuresis. J Clin Invest. 1973; 52:535.

39. deBodo RC: The antidiuretic action of morphine and its mechanism. J Pharmacol Exper Ther. 1944; 82:74.

40. Moses AM et al: Mechanism of chlorpropamide induced antidiuresis in man: Evidence for release of ADH and enhancement of peripheral action. Metabolism. 1973; 22:59.

41. Robertson GL et al: Vincristine neurotoxicity and abnormal secretion of antidiuretic hormone. Arch Intern Med. 1973; 132:720.

42. Cadnapaphornchai P et al: Mechanism of the effect of nicotine on renal water excretion. Am J Physiol. 1974; 227:1216.

43. Kimura T et al: Mechanism of carbamazepine (Tegretol)-induced antidiuresis: Evidence for release of antidiuretic hormone and impaired excretion of a water load. J Clin Endocrinol Metab. 1974; 38:356.

44. deFronzo RA et al: Water intoxication in man after cyclophosphomide therapy: Time course and relation to drug activation. Ann Intern Med. 1973; 78:861.

45. Miller M et al: Drug-induced states of impaired water excretion. Kidney Int. 1976; 10:90.

46. deTroyer A: Demeclocycline: Treatment for syndrome of inappropriate antidiuretic hormone secretion. JAMA. 1977; 237:2723.

47. deTroyer A et al: Correction of antidiuresis by demeclocycline. N Engl J Med. 1975; 293:915.

48. Cherrill DA et al: Demeclocycline treatment in the syndrome of inappropriate antidiuretic hormone secretion. Ann Intern Med. 1975; 83:654.

49. Forrest JN et al: Superiority of demeclocycline over lithium in the treatment of chronic syndrome of inappropriate secretion of antidiuretic hormone. N Engl J Med. 1978; 298:173.

50. Weston RE et al: The pathogenesis and treatment of hyponatremia in congestive heart failure. Am J Med. 1958; 29:558.

51. Humes HD et al: The kidney in congestive heart failure. In Sodium and Water Homeostasis, edited by B Brenner and J Stein, Churchill Livingstone, New York, 1978, p 51.

52. Gupta PD et al: Responses of atrial and aortic baroreceptors to nonhypotensive hemorrhage and to transfusion. Am J Physiol. 1966; 211:1429.

53. Gupta PD et al: Role of atrial afferents in the tachycardia and increased antidiuretic hormone levels of moderate hemorrhage. Fed Proc. 1966; 25:571.

54. Leaf A et al: An antidiuretic mechanism not regulated by extracellular fluid tonicity. J Clin Invest. 1952; 31:60.

55. Share L et al: Cardiovascular receptors and blood titer of antidiuretic hormone. Am J Physiol. 1962; 203:425.

56. Fichman MP et al: Diuretic-induced hyponatremia. Ann Intern Med. 1971; 75:853.

57. Arieff AI et al: Neurologic manifestations and morbidity of hyponatremia: Correlation with brain water and electrolytes. Medicine. 1976; 55:121.

58. Arieff AI et al: Effects on the central nervous system of hypernatremic and hyponatremic states. Kidney Int. 1976; 10:104.

59. Covey CM et al: Disorders of sodium and water metabolism and their effects on the central nervous system. In Sodium and Water Homeostasis, edited by B Brenner and J Stein, Churchill Livingstone, New York, 1978; p 212.

60. Hantman O et al: Rapid correction of hyponatremia in the syndrome of inappropriate secretion of antidiuretic hormone. Ann Intern Med. 1973; 78:870.

61. Scribner BH et al: Symposium: water and electrolytes interpretation of the serum potassium concentration. Metabolism. 1956; 5:468.

62. Scully RE et al (eds): Normal Reference Laboratory Values. N Engl J Med. 1980; 302:37.

63. Woodbury DM: Physiology of body fluids. In Physiology and Biophysics II. Circulation, Respiration and Fluid Balance, 20th ed, edited by T Ruch and H Patton, WB Saunders, Philadelphia, 1974, p 450.

64. Kliger AS: Disorders of Potassium Balance. In Acid Base and Potassium Homeostasis, edited by B Brenner and J Stein, Churchill Livingstone, New York, 1978, p 168.

65. Carroll HJ et al: Disturbances in potassium metabolism. In Water Electrolyte and Acid-Base Metabolism, Lippincott, Philadelphia, 1978, p 178.

66. Welt LG et al: The consequences of potassium depletion. J Chron Dis. 1960; 11:213.

67. Suki WN: Disposition and regulation of body potassium: An overview. Am J Med Sci. 1976; 272:31.

68. Schultze RG: Recent advances in the physiology and pathophysiology of potassium excretion. Arch Intern Med. 1973; 131:885.

69. Gennari FJ et al: Role of the kidney in potassium homeostasis. Kidney Int. 1975; 8:1.

70. Williams JA et al: Effects of nephrectomy and KCl on transmembrane potentials, intracellular electrolytes, and cell pH of rat muscle and liver in vivo. J Physiol. 1971; 212:117.

71. Eckel RE et al: Membrane potentials in K-deficient muscle. Am J Physiol. 1963; 205:307.

72. Grob D et al: Potassium movement in normal subjects, effects on muscle function. Am J Med. 1957; 23:340.

73. Grob D et al: Potassium movement in patients with familial periodic paralysis. Relationship to the defect in muscle function. Am J Med. 1957; 23:356.

74. Schwartz WB et al: The electrocardiogram in potassium depletion. Its relation to the total potassium deficit and the serum concentration. Am J Med. 1954; 16:395.

75. Davidson S et al: Ectopic beats and atrioventricular conduction disturbances in patients with hypopotassemia. Arch Intern Med. 1967; 120:280.

76. Schultze RG et al: Potassium: physiology and pathophysiology. In Clinical Disorders of Fluid and Electrolyte Metabolism, 3rd edition, edited by M Maxwell and C Kleeman, McGraw-Hill, New York, 1980, p 113.

77. Cohen JJ: Disorders of potassium balance. Hospital Practice. 1979; 119.

78. Fisch C: Relation of electrolyte disturbances to cardiac arrhythmias. Circulation. 1973; 47:408.

79. Fisch C et al: Potassium and the monophasic action potential, electrocardiogram, conduction and arrhythmias. Progr Cardiovasc Dis. 1966; 8:387.

80. Ettinger PO et al: Hyperkalemia, cardiac conduction and the EKG: A review. Am Heart J. 1974; 88:360.

81. Newmark SR et al: Hyperkalemia and hypokalemia. JAMA. 1975; 231:631.

82. Muntwyler E et al: Muscle electrolyte composition and balances of nitrogen and potassium in potassium-deficient rats. Am J Physiol. 1953; 174:283.

83. Pitts BJR: The relationship of the K-activated phosphatase to the Na, K-ATPase. Ann NY Acad Sci. 1974; 242:293.

84. Tobin T et al: Studies on the two phosphoenzyme conformation of Na-K-ATPase. Ann NY Acad Sci. 1974; 242:120.

85. Wilde WS: Potassium. In *Mineral Metabolism,* Vol. II, edited by Comor and Bronner, Academic Press, New York, 1962, p 73.

86. Epstein FH et al: Role of sodium, potassium-ATPase in renal function. Ann NY Acad Sci. 1974; 242:519.

87. Knox WH et al: Mechanism of action of aldosterone with particular reference to Na-K-ATPase. Ann NY Acad Sci. 1974; 242:471.

88. Rowe JW et al: Effect of experimental potassium deficiency on glucose and insulin metabolism. Metabolism. 1980; 29:498.

89. Chowdhury FR et al: Chlorthalidone-induced hypokalemia and abnormal carbohydrate metabolism. Horm Metab Res. 1970; 2:13.

90. Gorden P: Glucose intolerance with hypokalemia-failure of short-term potassium depletion in normal subjects to reproduce the glucose and insulin abnormalities of clinical hypokalemia. Diabetes. 1973; 22:544.

91. Rapoport MI et al: Thiazide-induced glucose intolerance treated with potassium. Arch Intern Med. 1964; 113:405.

92. Wolf FW et al: Further observations concerning the hyperglycemic activity of benzothiadiazines. Diabetes. 1964; 13:115.

93. Nardone DA et al: Mechanisms in hypokalemia: Clinical correlation. Medicine. 1978; 57:435.

94. Fordtran JS et al: Water and electrolyte movement in the intestine. Gastroenterology. 1966; 50:263.

95. Dudrick SJ et al: Parenteral hyperalimentation, metabolic problems and solutions. Ann Surg. 1972; 176:259.

96. Sebastian A et al: Renal potassium wasting in renal tubular acidosis (RTA). J Clin Invest. 1971; 50:667.

97. Mudge GH: Clinical patterns of tubular dysfunction. Am J Med. 1958; 24:785.

98. Makler RF et al: Potassium-losing renal disease. Quart J Med. 1956; 25:21.

99. Burnett CH et al: An analysis of some features of renal tubular dysfunction. Arch Intern Med. 1958; 102:881.

100. Conn JW: Primary aldosteronism, a new clinical syndrome. J Lab Clin Med. 1955; 45:3.

101. Relman AS et al: Electrolyte balance and acid-base metabolism in primary aldosteronism. J Clin Invest. 1957; 36:923.

102. Tourtellotte CR et al: Hypokalemia, muscle weakness, and myoglobinuria due to licorice ingestion. West J Med. 1970; 113:51.

103. Gitelman HJ et al: A new familial disorder characterized by hypokalemia and hypomagnesemia. Trans Assoc Am Phys. 1966; 79:221.

104. Lawson DH et al: Severe hypokalemia in hospitalized patients. Arch Intern Med. 1979; 139:978.

105. Chesney RW: Drug-induced hypokalemia. Am J Dis Child. 1976; 130:1055.

106. Danilevicus Z: Another form of iatrogenic hypokalemia. JAMA. 1976; 236:2657.

107. Cabizuka SV et al: Carbenicillin associated hypokalemic alkalosis. JAMA. 1976; 236:956.

108. Funada H et al: Hypokalemia during massive treatment with carbenicillin. Chemotherapy. 1976; 24:1527.

109. Stapleton FB et al: Hypokalemia associated with antibiotic treatment. Am J Dis Child. 1976; 130:1104.

110. Brunner FP et al: Hypokalemia, metabolic alkalosis and hypernatremia due to "massive" sodium penicillin therapy. Br Med J. 1968; 4:550.

111. Lipner HI et al: The behavior of carbenicillin as a non-reabsorbable anion. J Lab Clin Med. 1975; 86:183.

112. Klatersky J et al: Carbenicillin and hypokalemia. Ann Intern Med. 1973; 78:774.

113. Burgess JL et al: Nephrotoxicity of amphotericin B, with emphasis on changes in tubular function. Am J Med. 1972; 53:77.

114. McCurdy DK et al: Renal tubular acidosis due to amphotericin B. N Engl J Med. 1968; 278:124.

115. Drutz DJ et al: Hypokalemic rhabdomyolysis and myoglobinuria following amphotericin B therapy. JAMA. 1970; 211:824.

116. Schwartz JH et al: Fanconi syndrome with cephalothin and gentamicin therapy. Cancer. 1978; 41:769.

117. Cronin RE: Aminoglycoside nephrotoxicity: pathogenesis and prevention. Clin Neph. 1979; 11:251.

118. Oster JR et al: Laxative abuse syndrome. Am J Gastroenterology. 1980; 74:451.

119. Morris AI et al: Surreptitious laxative abuse. Gastroenterology. 1979; 77:780.

120. LaRusso NR et al: Surreptitious laxative ingestion. Mayo Clin Proc. 1975; 50:706.

121. Heizer WD et al: Protein-losing gastroenteropathy and malabsorption associated with factitious diarrhea. Ann Intern Med. 1968; 68:839.

122. Kramer P et al: Factitious diarrhea induced by phenolphthalien. Arch Intern Med. 1964; 114:634.

123. Gassain VV et al: Surreptitious laxation and hypokalemia. Ann Intern Med. 1972; 76:671.

124. Fleming BJ et al: Laxative-induced hypokalemia, sodium depletion and hyperreninemia. Ann Intern Med. 1975; 83:60.

125. Puschett JB: Comparative study on the effects of metolazone and other diuretics on potassium excretion. Clin Pharmacol Ther. 1974; 15:397.

126. Morgan T et al: A study by continuous microperfusion of water and electrolyte movements in the loop of Henle and distal tubule of the rat. Nephron. 1969; 6:388.

127. Malnic G et al: Micropuncture study of distal tubular potassium and sodium transport in rat nephron. Am J Physiol. 1971; 221:1192.

128. Kassirer JP et al: Diuretics and potassium metabolism: A reassessment of the need, effectiveness and safety of potassium therapy. Kidney Int. 1977; 11:505.

129. Morgan TO: Potassium replacement; supplements or potassium-sparing diuretics? Drugs. 1979; 18:218.

130. Hartmann RC et al: Studies on thrombocytosis: I. Hyperkalemia due to release of potassium from platelets during clotting. J Clin Invest. 1958; 37:699.

131. Salomon J: Spurious hypoglycemia and hyperkalemia in myelomonocytic leukemia. Am J Med Sci. 1974; 267:359.

132. Bellevue R et al: Pseudo-hyperkalemia and extreme leukocytosis. J Lab Clin Med. 1975; 85:660.

133. Hartmann RC et al: The relationship of platelets to the serum potassium concentration. J Clin Invest. 1955; 34:938.

134. Skinner SL: Cause of erroneous potassium levels. Lancet. 1961; 1:478.

135. Scribner BH et al: The effect of acute respiratory acidosis on the internal equilibrium of potassium. J Clin Invest. 1955; 34:1276.

136. Fraley DS et al: Correction of hyperkalemia by bicarbonate despite constant blood pH. Kidney Int. 1977; 12:354.

137. Orringer CE et al: Natural history of lactic acidosis after grand-mal seizures. N Engl J Med. 1977; 297:796.

138. Cox M: Potassium homeostasis. Med Clin North Am. 1981; 65:363.

139. Bismuth C et al: Hyperkalemia in acute digitalis poisoning. Prognostic significance and therapeutic implications. Clin Toxicol. 1973; 6:153.

140. Smith TW et al: Suicidal and accidental digoxin ingestion. Report of five cases with serum digoxin level correlations. Circulation. 1971; 44:29.

141. Weintraub HD et al: Changes in plasma potassium concentration after depolarizing blockers in anesthetized man. Br J Anesth. 1969; 41:1048.

142. Walton JD et al: Suxamethonium hyperkalemia in uremic neuropathy. Anaesthesia. 1973; 28:666.

143. Hertz P et al: Arginine-induced hyperkalemia in renal failure patients. Arch Intern Med. 1972; 130:778.

144. Silva P et al: Adaptation to potassium. Kidney Int. 1977; 11:466.

145. Van Ypersele de Strinou C: Potassium homeostasis in renal failure. Kidney Int. 1977; 11:491.

146. Cox M et al: The defense against hyperkalemia: the roles of insulin and aldosterone. N Engl J Med. 1978; 299:525.

147. Bastl C et al: Increased large intestinal secretion of potassium in renal insufficiency. Kidney Int. 1977; 12:9.

148. deFronzo RA: Hyperkalemia and hyporeninemic hypoaldosteronism. Kidney Int. 1980; 17:118.

149. Schambelan M et al: Prevalence, pathogenesis, and functional significance of aldosterone deficiency in hyperkalemic patients with renal insufficiency. Kidney Int. 1980; 17:89.

150. Tan SY et al: Indomethacin-induced prostaglandin inhibition with hyperkalemia. A reversible cause of hyporeninemic hypoaldosteronism. Ann Intern Med. 1979; 90:783.

151. Surawicz B: Relationship between electrocardiogram and electrolytes. Am Heart J. 1967; 73:814.

152. Merrill JP et al: Clinical recognition and therapy of acute potassium intoxication. Ann Intern Med. 1950; 33:797.

153. Whang R: Hyperkalemia: diagnosis and treatment. Am J Med Sci. 1976; 272:19.

154. Kunis CL et al: The emergency treatment of hyperkalemia. Med Clin North Am. 1981; 65:165.

155. Kass RS: Multiple effects of calcium antagonists on plateau currents in cardiac Purkinje fibers. J Gen Physiol. 1975; 66:169.

156. Scherr L et al: Management of hyperkalemia with a cation exchange resin. N Engl J Med. 1961; 264:115.

157. Berlyne GM et al: Dangers of Resonium A in the treatment of hyperkalemia in renal failure. Lancet. 1966; 167.

158. Schwartz KC et al: Severe acidosis and hyperpotassemia treated with sodium bicarbonate infusion. Circulation. 1959; 19:215.

159. Rubenstein AH et al: Role of the kidney in insulin metabolism and excretion. Diabetes. 1968; 17:161.

160. Fitzgerald F: Clinical hypophosphatemia. Ann Rev Med. 1978; 29:177.

161. Knochel JP: The pathophysiology and clinical characteristics of hypophosphatemia. Arch Intern Med. 1977; 137:203.

162. Kreusser W et al: The phosphate-depletion syndrome. Contr Nephrol. 1978; 14:162.

163. Knochel JP: Hypophosphatemia in the alcoholic. Arch Intern Med. 1980; 140:613.

164. Sheldon GF et al: Complications of nutritional support. Crit Care Med. 1980; 8:35.

165. Dudrick SJ: Parenteral hyperalimentation: metabolic problems and solutions. Ann Surg. 1972; 176:259.

166. Allen TR et al: Hypophosphatemia occurring in patients receiving total parenteral hyperalimentation. Fed Proc. 1971; 30:580.

167. Prins JC et al: Hyperalimentation, hypophosphatemia and coma. Lancet. 1973; 1:1253.

168. Sheldon GF et al: Phosphate depletion and repletion: relation to parenteral nutrition and oxygen transport. Ann Surg. 1975; 182:683.

169. Tovey SJ et al: Hypophosphatemia and phosphorus requirements during intravenous nutrition. Postgrad Med J. 1977; 53:289.

170. Silvis SE et al: Paresthesias, weakness, seizures, and hypophosphatemia in patients receiving hyperalimentation. Gastroenterology. 1972; 62:513.

171. Furlan AJ et al: Acute areflexic paralysis. Association with hyperalimentation and hypophosphatemia. Arch Neurol. 1975; 32:706.

172. Annino JS et al: The effect of eating on some of the clinically important chemical constituents of the blood. Am J Clin Path. 1959; 31:155.

173. Forsham PH et al: Changes in inorganic serum phosphorus during intravenous glucose tolerance test as an adjunct to diagnosis of early diabetes mellitus. Proc Am Diabetes Assoc. 1950; 9:101.

174. Corredor DG et al: Enhanced postglucose hypophosphatemia during starvation therapy of obesity. Metabolism. 1969; 18:754.

175. Bloom WL et al: Osteomalacia with pseudofractures caused by the ingestion of aluminum hydroxide. JAMA. 1960; 174:1327.

176. Ansari A: Antacid-induced phosphorus depletion and repletion. Minn Med. 1970; 53:837.

177. Darsee JR et al: Reversible severe congestive cardiomyopathy in 3 cases of hypophosphatemia. Ann Intern Med. 1978; 89:867.

178. Lotz M et al: Evidence for a phosphorus-depletion syndrome in man. N Engl J Med. 1968; 278:409.

179. Lichtman MA et al: Erythrocyte adenosine triphosphate depletion during hypophosphatemia in a uremic subject. N Engl J Med. 1969; 280:240.
180. Boelens PA et al: Hypophosphatemia with muscle weakness due to antacids and hemodialysis. Am J Dis Child. 1970; 120:350.
181. Abrams DE et al: Antacid induction of phosphate depletion syndrome in renal failure. West J Med. 1974; 120:157.
182. Ryback RS et al: Clinical relationships between serum phosphorus and other blood chemistry values in alcoholics. Arch Intern Med. 1980; 140:673.
183. Flink EB: Mineral metabolism in alcoholism. In *The Biology of Alcoholism: Biochemistry,* edited by B Kissin and H Gegleiter, Plenum Press, New York, 1971, Vol. 1.
184. Stein JH et al: Hypophosphatemia in acute alcoholism. Am J Med Sci. 1966; 252:78.
185. Kreisberg RA: Diabetic ketoacidosis: New concepts and trends in pathogenesis and treatment. Ann Intern Med. 1978; 88:681.
186. Okel BB et al: Prolonged hyperventilation in man: Associated electrolyte changes and subjective symptoms. Ann Intern Med. 1961; 108:757.
187. Mostellar ME et al: The effects of alkalosis on plasma concentration and urinary excretion of inorganic phosphate. J Clin Invest. 1964; 43:138.
188. Schnitker MA et al: A clinical study of malnutrition in Japanese prisoners of war. Ann Intern Med. 1951; 35:69.
189. Newman JF et al: Acute respiratory failure associated with hypophosphatemia. N Engl J Med. 1977; 296:1101.
190. O'Connor LR et al: The effect of hypophosphatemia on myocardial performance in man. N Engl J Med. 1977; 297:901.
191. Lichtman MA: Hypoalimentation during hyperalimentation. N Engl J Med. 1974; 290:1432.
192. Ditzel J: Effect of plasma inorganic phosphate on tissue oxygenation during recovery from diabetic ketoacidosis. From International Symposium on Oxygen Transport to Tissue. In *Adv Exper Med Biol,* edited by H Dicher and D Bruley, Plenum, New York, 1973, 37A:163.
193. Ditzel J: Importance of plasma inorganic phosphate on tissue oxygenation during recovery from diabetic ketoacidosis. Horm Metab Res. 1973; 5:471.
194. Ditzel J: Impaired oxygen release caused by alterations of the metabolism in the erythrocytes in diabetes. Lancet. 1972; 1:721.
195. Jacob HS et al: Acute hemolytic anemia with rigid red cells in hypophosphatemia. N Engl J Med. 1971; 285:1446.
196. Craddock PR et al: Acquired phagocyte dysfunction. A complication of the hypophosphatemia of parenteral hyperalimentation. N Engl J Med. 1974; 290:1403.
197. Turco SJ et al: Methods of ordering and use of intravenous phosphate. Hospital Pharmacy. 1975; 10:320.
198. Shackney S et al: Precipitous fall in serum calcium, hypotension and acute renal failure after intravenous phosphate therapy of hypercalcemia. Ann Intern Med. 1967; 66:906.
199. Winter RJ et al: Diabetic ketoacidosis induction of hypocalcemia and hypomagnesemia by phosphate therapy. Am J Med. 1979; 67:897.
200. Zipf WB et al: Hypocalcemia, hypomagnesemia and transient hypoparathyroidism during therapy with potassium phosphate in diabetic ketoacidosis. Diabetes Care. 1979; 2:265.
201. Vannatta JB et al: Efficacy of intravenous phosphorus therapy in the severely hypophosphatemic patient. Arch Intern Med. 1981; 141:885.
202. Lutwak L et al: Current concepts of bone metabolism. Ann Intern Med. 1974; 80:630.
203. Epstein FH: Calcium and the kidney. Am J Med. 1968; 45:700.
204. Walser M: Ion association VI. Interactions between calcium, magnesium, inorganic phosphate and citrated protein in normal human plasma. J Clin Invest. 1961; 40:723.
205. Moore EW: Ionized calcium in normal serum, ultrafiltrates and whole blood determined by ion-exchange electrodes. J Clin Invest. 1970; 49:318.
206. Singer FR et al: Hypercalcemia and hypocalcemia. Clin Neph. 1977; 7:154.
207. Clarkson EM et al: The effect of high intake of calcium carbonate in normal subjects and patients with chronic renal failure. Clin Sci. 1966; 30:415.
208. Meyrier A et al: The influence of high calcium carbonate intake on bone disease in patients undergoing hemodialysis. Kidney Int. 1973; 4:146.
209. Brickman AS et al: 1, 25 dihydroxyvitamin D-3 in normal man and patients with renal failure. Ann Intern Med. 1974; 80:161.
210. DeLuca HF: Vitamin D endocrinology. Ann Intern Med. 1976; 85:367.
211. Norman AW: 1, 25-Dihydroxy-vitamin D-3: A kidney-produced steroid hormone essential to calcium homeostasis. Am J Med. 1974; 57:21.
212. Carroll HJ et al: Disturbances in calcium, phosphate and magnesium metabolism. In *Water, Electrolyte and Acid-Base Metabolism—Diagnosis and Management,* Lippincott, Philadelphia, 1978, p 306.
213. Muggia FM et al: Hypercalcemia associated with neoplastic disease. Ann Intern Med. 1970; 73:281.
214. Mazzaferri EL et al: Treatment of hypercalcemia associated with malignancy. Seminars in Oncology. 1978; 5:141.
215. Riggs BL et al: Immunologic differentiation of primary hyperparathyroidism from hyperparathyroidism due to nonparathyroid cancer. J Clin Invest. 1971; 50:2079.
216. Sherwood LM et al: Production of parathyroid hormone by nonparathyroid tumors. J Clin Endocrinol Metab. 1967; 27:140.
217. Klein DC et al: Prostaglandins: Stimulation of bone resorption in tissue culture. Endocrinology. 1970; 86:1436.
218. Tashjian AH Jr et al: Prostaglandins, calcium, metabolism and cancer. Fed Proc. 1974; 33:81.
219. Tashjian AH: Prostaglandins, hypercalcemia and cancer. N Engl J Med. 1975; 293:1317.
220. Seyberth HW et al: Prostaglandins as mediators of hypercalcemia associated with certain types of cancer. N Engl J Med. 1975; 293:1278.
221. Seyberth HW et al: Prostaglandins and hypercalcemic states. Ann Rev Med. 1978; 29:23.
222. Brereton HD et al: Indomethacin-responsive hypercalcemia in a patient with renal-cell adenocarcinoma. N Engl J Med. 1974; 291:83.
223. Mundy GR et al: Bone-resorbing activity in supernatants from lymphoid cell lines. N Engl J Med. 1974; 290:867.

224. Boonstra CE et al: Hyperparathyroidism detected by routine serum calcium analysis—Prevalence in a clinic population. Ann Intern Med. 1965; 63:468.

225. Christensson T et al: Prevalence of hypercalcemia in a health screening in Stockholm. ACTA Med Scand. 1976; 200:131.

226. Massry SG et al: Secondary hyperparathyroidism in chronic renal failure. Arch Intern Med. 1969; 124:431.

227. Massry SG et al: Divalent ion metabolism in patients with acute renal failure—Studies on the mechanism of hypocalcemia. Kidney Int. 1974; 5:437.

228. Stote R et al: Hydrochlorothiazide effects on serum calcium and immunoreactive parathyroid hormone concentrations. Ann Intern Med. 1972; 77:587.

229. Brickman AS et al: Changes in serum and urinary calcium during treatment with hydrochlorothiazide: Studies on mechanisms. J Clin Invest. 1972; 51:945.

230. Breslau N et al: The role of volume contraction in the hypocalcuiric action of chlorothiazide. Kidney Int. 1976; 10:164.

231. Popovtzer MM et al: The acute effect of chlorthiazide on serum ionized calcium: evidence for a parathyroid hormone-dependent mechanism. J Clin Invest. 1975; 55:1295.

232. Chaplin H et al: Vitamin D intoxication. Am J Med Sci. 1971; 221:369.

233. Frame B et al: Hypercalcemia and skeletal effects in chronic hypervitaminosis A. Ann Intern Med. 1974; 80:44.

234. O'Connell TX: Hypercalcemia induced by tamoxifen. Am J Surg. 1981; 14:277.

235. Christensson TAT: Lithium, hypercalcemia and hyperparathyroidism. Lancet. 1976; 2:144.

236. McMillan DF et al: The milk-alkali syndrome: a study of the acute disorder with comments on the development of the chronic condition. Medicine. 1965; 44:485.

237. Lehrer GM et al: Neuropsychiatric presentation of hypercalcemia. J Mt Sinai Hospital, New York, 1960; 27:10.

238. Henson RA: The neurological aspects of hypercalcemia: With special reference to primary hyperparathyroidism. J Roy Coll Surg London. 1966; 1:41.

239. Schott GD: Hypercalcemic stupor as a presentation of lymphosarcoma. J Neurol Neurosurg Psychiatry. 1975; 38:382.

240. Moure JMB: The electroencephalogram in hypercalcemia. Arch Neurol. 1967; 17:34.

241. Weiner M et al: Signs and symptoms of electrolyte disorders. Yale J Biol Med. 1970; 43:76.

242. Wilder WT et al: Peptic ulcer in primary hyperparathyroidism. Ann Intern Med. 1960; 105:536.

243. Voss DM et al: Cardiac manifestations of hyperparathyroidism with presentation of previously unreported arrhythmia. Am Heart J. 1967; 73:235.

244. Thier SO: Renal insufficiency and hypercalcemia. Kidney Int. 1978; 14:194.

245. Ritz E et al: The kidney in disorders of calcium metabolism. Contr Nephrol. 1977; 7:114.

246. Benabe JE et al: Hypercalcemic nephropathy. Arch Intern Med. 1978; 138:777.

247. Blum M et al: Reversible hypertension caused by the hypercalcemia of hyperparathyroidism, Vitamin D toxicity, and calcium infusion. JAMA. 1977; 237:262.

248. Massry SG et al: Blood calcium levels and hypertension. Contr Nephrol. 1977; 8:117.

249. Suki WN et al: Acute treatment of hypercalcemia with furosemide. N Engl J Med. 1970; 283:836.

250. Martinez-malonado M et al: Diuretics in nonedematous states. Physiological basis for clinical use. Arch Intern Med. 1973; 131:797.

251. Lazor MZ et al: Mechanism of adrenalsteroid reversal of hypercalcemia in multiple myeloma. N Engl J Med. 1964; 270:749.

252. Chopra D et al: Hypercalcemia and malignant disease. Med Clin North Am. 1975; 59:441.

253. Kennedy BJ: Metabolic and toxic effects of mithramycin during tumor therapy. Am J Med. 1970; 49:494.

254. Slayton RE et al: New approach to the treatment of hypercalcemia. The effect of short term treatment with mithramycin. Clin Pharmacol Ther. 1971; 12:833.

255. Singer FR et al: Mithramycin treatment of intractable hypercalcemia due to parathyroid carcinoma. N Engl J Med. 1970; 283:634.

256. Ryan WG et al: Effects of mithramycin on Paget's disease of bone. Ann Intern Med. 1969; 70:549.

257. Parsons V et al: Effect of mithramycin on calcium and hydroxyproline metabolism in patients with malignant disease. Br Med J. 1967; 1:474.

258. Monto RW et al: Observations on the mechanism of hemorrhagic toxicity in mithramycin (NSC-24559) therapy. Cancer Res. 1969; 29:697.

259. Edwards CRW: Mithramycin treatment of malignant hypercalcemia. Br Med J. 1968; 3:167.

260. Goldsmith RS et al: Inorganic phosphate treatment of hypercalcemia of diverse etiologies. N Engl J Med. 1966; 274:1.

261. Hebert LA et al: Studies of the mechanism by which phosphate infusion lowers serum calcium concentration. J Clin Invest. 1966; 45:1886.

262. Massry SG et al: Inorganic phosphate treatment of hypercalcemia. Arch Intern Med. 1968; 121:307.

263. Carrol E et al: Stimulation of bone formation by inorganic phosphate and inhibition of bone resorption by thyrocalcitonin. J Clin Invest. 1967; 46:1043.

264. Austin LA et al: Calcitonin: Physiology and pathophysiology. N Engl J Med. 1981; 304:269.

265. Wisneski LA et al: Salmon calcitonin in hypercalcemia. Clin Pharmacol Ther. 1978; 24:219.

266. Nilsson O et al: Salmon calcitonin in the acute treatment of moderate and severe hypercalcemia in man. ACTA Med Scan. 1978; 204:249.

267. Sjoberg HE et al: Acute treatment with calcitonin in primary hyperparathyroidism and severe hypercalcemia of other origin. ACTA Chir Scand. 1975; 141:90.

268. Binstock ML et al: Effect of calcitonin and glucocorticoids in combination on the hypercalcemia of malignancy. Ann Intern Med. 1980; 93:269.

269. Mordes JP et al: Excess magnesium. Pharmacol Rev. 1978; 29:273.

270. Massry SG: The clinical pathophysiology of magnesium. Contr Nephrol. 1978; 14:64.

271. Massry SG et al: Hypomagnesemia and hypermagnesemia. Clin Neph. 1977; 7:147.

272. Barker ES et al: Studies on renal excretion of magnesium in man. J Clin Invest. 1959; 38:1733.

273. Randall RE et al: Hypermagnesemia in renal failure. Etiology and toxic manifestations. Ann Intern Med. 1964; 61:73.

274. Alfrey AC et al: Hypermagnesemia after renal homotransplantation. Ann Intern Med. 1970; 73:367.

275. Wacker WEC et al: Magnesium metabolism. N Engl J Med. 1968; 278:772.

276. Flink EB et al: Magnesium deficiency after prolonged parenteral fluid administration and after chronic alcoholism, complicated by delerium tremens. J Lab Clin Med. 1954; 43:169.

277. Hanna S et al: The syndrome of magnesium deficiency in man. Lancet. 1960; 2:172.

278. Dunn MJ et al: Magnesium depletion in normal man. Metabolism. 1966; 15:884.

279. Fitzgerald MG: Experimental study of magnesium deficiency in man. Clin Sci. 1956; 15:635.

280. Gitelman HJ et al: Magnesium deficiency. Ann Rev Med. 1969; 20:233.

281. Flink EB: Therapy of magnesium deficiency. Ann New York Acad Sci. 1969; 162:901.

Chapter 29

Acid-Base Disorders

Thomas J. Cali

Normal Acid-Based Metabolism

Normal metabolism results in the production of approximately 20,000 mMol of carbonic acid and 80 mMol of nonvolatile acids daily. The lungs, the kidneys, bicarbonate and other buffer systems maintain the concentration of hydrogen ion in the extracellular fluid at an almost constant level. Arterial blood pH varies from 7.38 to 7.42 in a healthy person; venous blood and interstitial fluid pH vary between 7.33 and 7.37 (1) and intracellular pH is generally believed to vary from 4.5 to 7.4 depending upon the rate of metabolism and local tissue blood flow (2).

The pH can be calculated from the following equation:

$$pH = pK + \log \left[\frac{HCO_3^-}{H_2CO_3} \right]$$

$$= 6.1 + \log \left[\frac{HCO_3^-}{(0.03)(pCO_2)} \right] \quad \text{(Eq. 1)}$$

An important concept illustrated by this equation (the Henderson-Hasselbalch equation) is that it is the ratio of HCO_3^- to H_2CO_3, not their absolute concentrations, that determines the pH. It therefore follows that if both the HCO_3^- and pCO_2 are increased or decreased proportionately, the ratio remains fixed and the pH is not affected.

The serum bicarbonate is primarily regulated by the kidneys, while the pCO_2 is under pulmonary control. Thus, the compensatory actions of these organ systems preserve the ratio of HCO_3^- to pCO_2. Changes in the ratio resulting from increased or decreased HCO_3^- are metabolic disturbances, while changes in the ratio caused by increased or decreased pCO_2 are respiratory disturbances.

Acidosis causes central nervous system (CNS) depression, which may lead to coma or death (3), while alkalosis causes CNS excitation and is likely to result in a convulsive disorder or tetany. Arterial pH can vary from 6.8 to 7.7 and still be compatible with life.

Acid-base disturbances cannot be assessed on the basis of a serum bicarbonate or respiratory rate alone. To illustrate, an elevated serum bicarbonate is consistent with both metabolic alkalosis and chronic respiratory acidosis; similarly, hyperventilation is consistent with both respiratory alkalosis and metabolic acidosis. Therefore, the patient's laboratory studies, signs, and symptoms cannot be assessed without considering his or her medical history.

Laboratory Tests

A thorough understanding of the following laboratory tests is essential for assessment of acid-base balance.

CO_2 Content (Normal 24–30 mM/L); CO_2 Combining Power; Serum bicarbonate (Normal 23–28 mEq/L). Ninety-five percent of the value obtained as CO_2 *content* is HCO_3^-. If a CO_2 content is 20 mM/L, the corresponding HCO_3^- level is 19 mEq/L in venous blood. The *CO_2 combining power* is a measure of HCO_3^- in the plasma after equilibration of plasma with an atmosphere having a pCO_2 of 40 mm Hg. *Bicarbonate* reported with blood gases represents the actual HCO_3^- concentration in arterial blood as calculated from the Henderson-Hasselbalch equation. Bicarbonate ion changes in the same direction as CO_2 content in acid-base disorders. The CO_2 content is the most commonly used test (4).

Arterial pH (Normal 7.38–7.42). Arterial pH is the pH which is determined immediately after arterial blood is collected in a glass, heparinized syringe. Arterial pH is essential in determining the severity of a disorder and in monitoring the therapy of mixed disorders (4).

Arterial pCO_2 (Normal 35–45 mm Hg). The pCO_2 measures the partial pressure of carbon dioxide in arterial blood. It indicates the level of respiratory acid and its contribution to total hydrogen ion activity. An increase in pCO_2 is consistent with respiratory acidosis, while a decrease in pCO_2 is consistent with respiratory alkalosis (4).

Serum Chloride (Normal 96–106 mEq/L). The serum chloride level may indicate acid re-

tention or base excretion by the kidney. Hypochloremia may increase proximal tubular reabsorption of bicarbonate, leading to metabolic alkalosis. Hyperchloremia may reflect the addition of hydrogen ion with chloride ion in the extracellular fluid (ECF) and is consistent with metabolic acidosis (4).

Arterial pO_2 (normal 80–90 mm Hg). Acidosis shifts the oxygen-hemoglobin dissociation curve downward and to the right, decreasing oxygen-hemoglobin binding and increasing tissue delivery of oxygen (5). Alkalosis has the opposite effect. An acidotic patient with a pO_2 of 70 mm Hg could be oxygenating tissues appropriately.

Anion Gap. The principle of electroneutrality dictates that the sum of all positive charges in the extracellular fluid (ECF) be exactly neutralized by an equal number of negative charges. The serum sodium and potassium account for 95% of all cations present in the ECF. Chloride and bicarbonate represent the anionic components but account for only 85% of ECF anions. Therefore, the sum of the measured anions does not fully equal the sum of the measured cations. This difference, measured in mEq/L, is termed the anion gap. Under normal conditions the unmeasured anions, representing anionic protein, sulfates, phosphates, and anionic groups of organic ions, total approximately 12–14 mEq/L (6,7).

$$\begin{matrix} \text{Anion} \\ \text{Gap} \end{matrix} = \left(\begin{matrix} \text{Serum} \\ Na^+ \end{matrix} + \begin{matrix} \text{Serum} \\ K^+ \end{matrix} \right) - \left(\begin{matrix} \text{Serum} \\ Cl^- \end{matrix} + \begin{matrix} \text{Serum} \\ HCO_3^- \end{matrix} \right)$$
$$(Eq.\ 2)$$

Since the serum concentration of potassium is relatively low, the above formula can be shortened:

$$\begin{matrix} \text{Anion} \\ \text{Gap} \end{matrix} = \left(\begin{matrix} \text{Serum} \\ Na^+ \end{matrix} \right) - \left(\begin{matrix} \text{Serum} \\ Cl^- \end{matrix} + \begin{matrix} \text{Serum} \\ HCO_3^- \end{matrix} \right)$$
$$= 12\text{–}14\ mEq/L$$
$$(Eq.\ 3)$$

Metabolic Acidosis

An elevated anion gap gives the clinician a clue to the etiology of a metabolic acidosis. An anion gap above 30 mEq/L is usually indicative of an identifiable organic anion acidosis such as lactic acidosis or ketoacidosis (8), or of ingestion of substances such as ethylene glycol, methanol, or salicylates. Small elevations in the anion gap (to 15–16 mEq/L) are occasionally seen in patients with respiratory alkalosis. True elevations in the anion gap always indicate acidosis of metabolic origin. The effect of other primary acid-base abnormalities on the anion gap is not consistent or predictable.

Metabolic acidosis characterized by an increased chloride level and a normal anion gap is commonly referred to as hyperchloremic metabolic acidosis. There are three major causes: an excessive acid load, large losses of alkaline body fluids, and diminished acid excretion by the kidneys. See Table 1. Rapid volume expansion with intravenous fluids can also cause a mild metabolic acidosis through dilution of plasma bicarbonate (6,9).

Metabolic Alkalosis

Loss of acid from the body is by far the most common cause of metabolic alkalosis. This occurs when there are excessive losses of upper gastrointestinal fluid (eg, vomiting and naso-gastric suction) and when hydrogen ion excretion (or bicarbonate reabsorption) by the kidneys is increased. Rarely, alkali therapy will cause a metabolic alkalosis (7,10).

Table 2 lists the common causes of metabolic acidosis (except hyperchloremic), metabolic alkalosis, respiratory acidosis, and respiratory alkalosis.

Table 1.

COMMON CAUSES OF HYPERCHLOREMIC METABOLIC ACIDOSIS

I. **Excess Acid Load**
  A. Hyperalimentation (see chapter on Parenteral Nutrition)
  B. Acidifying Agents
    1. Ammonium chloride
    2. Arginine HCl
    3. Lysine HCl

II. **Large Losses of Alkaline Body Fluids**
  A. Diarrhea, ileostomy, colostomy
  B. Excessive cathartic use
  C. Pancreatic fistula

III. **Decreased Renal Excretion of Acid**
  A. Renal tubular acidosis (see chapter on Kidney Diseases)
  B. Carbonic anhydrase inhibitors
    1. Acetazolamide
    2. Sulfamylon
  C. Uremia (occasionally)

Diagnosis

The four primary acid-base disorders affect pH, hydrogen ion concentration, pCO_2 and HCO_3^- in the following way:

	pH	(H^+)	pCO_2	HCO_3^-
Metabolic acidosis	↓	↑	↓	↓
Metabolic alkalosis	↑	↓	↑	↑
Respiratory acidosis	↓	↑	↑	↑
Respiratory alkalosis	↑	↓	↓	↓

Note: Dotted arrows indicate compensatory changes.

When evaluating laboratory data, clinicians must remember that they are treating a patient and not abnormal laboratory values. Patients must always be evaluated clinically, and if laboratory data are inconsistent with the overall clinical picture, other confirmatory tests should be performed. Laboratory data concerning acid-base balance can be especially misleading in patients with two ongoing primary disturbances. A highly abnormal CO_2 (greater than 40 mM/L) with a relatively normal pH may be manifested in the presence of concurrent metabolic alkalosis and respiratory acidosis, and does not reflect a medical emergency. These two disorders tend to move CO_2 in the same direction, but pH in opposite directions as follows:

$$\text{Metabolic alkalosis} = \uparrow CO_2 \text{ content}, \uparrow pH$$
$$\text{Respiratory acidosis} = \uparrow CO_2 \text{ content}, \downarrow pH$$

On the other hand, concurrent metabolic acidosis and respiratory acidosis could result in an extremely low pH (less than 7.0) and a relatively normal CO_2 content due to off-setting effects:

$$\text{Metabolic acidosis} = \downarrow CO_2 \text{ content}, \downarrow pH$$
$$\text{Respiratory acidosis} = \uparrow CO_2 \text{ content}, \downarrow pH$$

The relatively normal CO_2 content in this situation is grossly misleading, as the pH may be so depressed as to be considered a medical emergency. Since CO_2 content is usually among the first laboratory data received, the above distinction is essential.

Table 2.

COMMON CAUSES OF ACID-BASE DISORDERS

Metabolic Acidosis[1]	*Metabolic Alkalosis*
(Increased anion gap)	Nasogastric suction
Renal failure	Vomiting
Diabetic ketoacidosis	Chloruretic diuretics
Alcoholic ketoacidosis	Glucocorticoids
Starvation ketosis	Cushings disease
Lactic acidosis	Chloride restriction
Substance ingestion	Alkali therapy
Salicylate	Antacid use
Ethylene glycol	
Methanol	
Paraldehyde	
Respiratory Acidosis	*Respiratory Alkalosis*
CNS depression	Psychogenic hyperventilation
Obstructive lung disease	Gram negative sepsis
Mechanical hypoventilation	Salicylate intoxication
Status asthmaticus	Mechanical overventilation
Pneumothorax	Pneumonia
Abdominal distention	High altitude

[1] The causes of metabolic acidosis listed here are accompanied by an increase in the anion gap. Table 1 lists causes of metabolic acidosis which are associated with a normal anion gap (hyperchloremic metabolic acidosis).

HYPERCHLOREMIC METABOLIC ACIDOSIS

1. *Acetazolamide-Induced.* R.G., a 54-year-old male, is being seen in the ophthalmology clinic. Three days prior to this visit, therapy was begun with acetazolamide sustained release capsules for chronic open angle glaucoma. The patient has returned to clinic complaining of shortness of breath, polyuria and polydipsia.

Laboratory studies reveal the following: Sodium 136 mEq/L, Potassium 6.1 mEq/L, Chloride 108 mEq/L, CO_2 Content 15 mM/L, pO_2 96 mm Hg, pCO_2 36 mm Hg, and pH 7.22. Assess this patient's acid-base disorder.

The low CO_2 content and pH are both consistent with metabolic acidosis and the low pCO_2 (increased respiratory rate) is consistent with respiratory alkalosis or compensated metabolic acidosis. The normal unmeasured anion concentration and high serum chloride level, together with the history and evidence above, indicate that the patient has metabolic acidosis with respiratory compensation secondary to acetazolamide therapy.

2. How does acetazolamide induce metabolic acidosis?

The formation of carbonic acid from carbon dioxide and water is catalyzed by carbonic anhydrase (CA) in the cells of the proximal tubules. Following the dissociation of carbonic acid to hydrogen ion and bicarbonate, the hydrogen ion is secreted (in exchange for sodium) into the tubule, and the bicarbonate is reabsorbed (with sodium) into the blood stream. Acetazolamide inhibits CA, thereby decreasing the generation, and ultimately the secretion, of acid and the reabsorption of sodium. A mild metabolic acidosis results.

3. What treatment is indicated for this patient? Would sodium bicarbonate be indicated on an acute basis?

Acetazolamide produces a natriuresis and diuresis by decreasing the intracellular generation of hydrogen ion which is normally exchanged for tubular sodium. This effect will diminish in 7 to 10 days as CA activity increases; therefore, the patient should be instructed to continue therapy and maintain adequate hydration.

Sodium bicarbonate would not be indicated, nor would it be effective in an acute situation. Normally, filtered bicarbonate is buffered and completely resorbed in the proximal tubule. However, since acetazolamide decreases proximal tubular hydrogen ion availability, any additional bicarbonate filtered by the glomerulus would be excreted in the urine and would have no permanent systemic effect.

4. The patient was placed on sodium bicarbonate, 650 mg four times daily and was given a three month's supply. Is the patient at risk of developing metabolic alkalosis from chronic ingestion of oral sodium bicarbonate? How is bicarbonate normally handled by the body?

Normally, the maximum tubular reabsorption (Tm) for bicarbonate is 25 mEq/L, and any excess bicarbonate is eliminated in the urine. Therefore, alkalosis rarely occurs secondary to exogenous bicarbonate ingestion unless the Tm for this anion is increased.

Examples of factors which increase the Tm include chloride or potassium depletion and situations which increase sodium reabsorption. In the latter instance, sodium is exchanged for hydrogen ion, thereby generating excess bicarbonate which must be reabsorbed. Volume contraction and the administration of glucocorticoids are other examples of factors which increase sodium and, indirectly, bicarbonate reabsorption (11–13).

5. Why is R.G.'s serum potassium elevated?

Up to 50% of the hydrogen ion is buffered by intracellular organic anions and protein. In acidosis, excess hydrogen ion moves intracellularly; to maintain electroneutrality, sodium and potassium are displaced into the extracellular fluid compartment. Therefore, hyperkalemia is commonly observed in acidotic individuals. Clinicians use a general rule of thumb that for every 0.1 unit pH change from the normal value of 7.4 one can expect a reciprocal change in the serum potassium value of 0.6 mEq/L (7,14).

6. *Spironolactone-Induced.* B.K., a 50-year-old male with documented alcoholic cirrhosis, is admitted to the hospital for a prolonged prothrombin time, a guaiac-positive stool, and anemia (hemoglobin 11.5 gm/dl). His weight is 3 kg less than it was during a previous admission 6 months ago, and he currently receives spironolactone 50 mg four times daily. Renal function is unchanged.

Laboratory studies reveal the following: Sodium 131 mEq/L, Potassium 5.8 mEq/L, Chloride 112 mEq/L, CO_2 Content 12 mM/L, pO_2 90 mm Hg, pCO_2 32 mm Hg, and pH 7.26. Assess this patient's acid-base status.

The pH, low CO_2, and elevated serum potassium are consistent with metabolic acidosis. The decreased pCO_2 may indicate primary respiratory alkalosis or compensation for metabolic acidosis. The normal unmeasured anion concentration and elevated serum chloride concentration, considered with the history and previous information, indicate that the patient has compensated metabolic acidosis. The elevated serum potassium concentration is evidence possibly implicating spironolactone as the etiology of the acidosis.

7. How does spironolactone induce metabolic acidosis?

Spironolactone causes metabolic acidosis through several mechanisms. Spironolactone directly antagonizes aldosterone's ability to increase distal tubular hydrogen ion secretion, resulting in retention of hydrogen ion (17,18). Spironolactone antagonizes the ability of aldosterone to affect distal tubular potassium secretion (19), resulting in hyperkalemia (20), as in this patient. Elevations in serum potassium have been observed to impair renal ammonia production and excretion (21), thereby impairing urinary acidification and thus contributing to the acidosis.

8. What treatment is indicated for this patient?

Gabow and associates (22) reported six patients with hyperchloremic metabolic acidosis induced by spironolactone. Mean serum bicarbonate concentration decreased by approximately 7 mEq/L. Discontinuation of the spironolactone resulted in a spontaneous reversal in the serum bicarbonate depression. While patients may occasionally require supplementation with alkali, drug discontinuation should sufficiently restore the plasma bicarbonate concentration, reversing the acidosis. Drug discontinuation should also normalize the serum potassium concentration providing no other source for hyperkalemia is present.

METABOLIC ACIDOSIS WITH ANION GAP

9. A 60-year-old, 65 kg alcoholic male presented with complaints of vomiting and shortness of breath for the preceding 10–12 hours. These symptoms followed a prolonged drinking binge and a period of abstinence from food. He was admitted with the diagnosis of possible metabolic acidosis secondary to alcohol abuse. In the emergency room, he was alert with a supine blood pressure of 130/85, a pulse of 80/min and a respiratory rate (RR) of 32/min. He became progressively less responsive.

Laboratory studies revealed: Sodium 139 mEq/L, Potassium 5.1 mEq/L, Chloride 106 mEq/L, Bicarbonate 4 mEq/L, pH 7.0, pCO$_2$ - 14 mm Hg, CO$_2$ content 3 mM/L, BUN 72 mg/dl and Glucose 86 mg/dl. A urinalysis revealed a pH of 5.0 and the presence of ketones. There were no salicylates or crystals. The serum lactate concentration was dramatically elevated.

Assess this patient's acid-base status and comment on the possible causes.

This patient has a severe metabolic acidosis (pH 7.0; HCO$_3^-$ 4 mEq/L; CO$_2$ content 3 mM/L; urine pH 5.0) with a large anion gap [139 −(106 + 4) = 29 mEq/L] and respiratory compensation (RR 32/min; pCO$_2$ 14 mm Hg). The various causes of metabolic acidosis with an increased anion gap are listed in Table 2. In this case, food abstinence and appreciable alcohol intake apparently resulted in the accumulation of excessive amounts of nonvolatile acids, thus explaining the presence of urinary ketones and increased serum lactate. Except for his normal glucose level, these find-

ings could be consistent with diabetic ketoacidosis, a common cause of metabolic acidosis (23). Other drugs and conditions which result in lactic acidosis (25) include: shock—all types (29,31), diabetes mellitus (23,32), phenformin (24–27,33–35), leukemia (36), glycogen storage disease (37), ethanol (38,39), exercise (40,41), epinephrine (42), and severe anemia (43).

10. Should this patient's acidosis be treated? What are the goals of therapy, and what are the dangers of correcting the acidosis too rapidly?

This patient's acidosis is severe (pH < 7.1) and deserves immediate therapy. When the serum bicarbonate falls to 5 mEq/L or less, the situation is very serious, since at this level maximum respiratory compensation (pCO$_2$ = 15 mm Hg) has occurred, and small changes in the bicarbonate will result in large changes in the pH. The goal of therapy is to increase the pH to greater than 7.2 or to increase the bicarbonate by 4–6 mEq/L over 6–12 hours. The bicarbonate may then be increased to a level of approximately 15 mEq/L over the next 24 hours. Blood gases should be monitored every 2–3 hours to assess the patient's response to therapy (44).

11. How should this patient be treated?

Sodium bicarbonate is generally considered the agent of choice since it provides a direct source of bicarbonate ion.

Clinicians have used the following formula to estimate the initial doses of sodium bicarbonate. It is based upon the premise that the volume of distribution (Vd) for bicarbonate is approximately 50% of body weight.

$$\text{Bicarbonate Dose (mEq)} = 0.5 \times \text{Body Weight (Kg)} \times \text{Desired Increase in Serum HCO}_3^- \text{(mEq/L)} \quad \text{(Eq. 4)}$$

Assuming the initial goal of therapy is to increase the serum bicarbonate by 6 mEq/L, the dose for this patient can be calculated as follows:

$$\text{Bicarbonate Dose (mEq)} = 0.5 \times 65 \times 6 \text{ mEq/L} = 195 \text{ mEq}$$

Rapid and full correction of the acidosis is unnecessary and may be dangerous for the following reasons. Compensatory hyperventilation may persist 36–48 hours after acidosis has been corrected, placing the patient in jeopardy of a respiratory alkalosis. Second, the methods for determining the doses of the alkalinizing agents are, at best, estimates and these agents may in themselves produce a metabolic alkalosis. Rapid correction has also been said to aggravate cerebrospinal fluid acidosis, resulting in deterioration in the condition of such patients (45). Severe hypokalemia can occur, because potassium is redistributed from extracellular to the intracellular spaces. Finally, tetany resulting from rapid shifts of free, ionized calcium onto serum protein can occur when there is an acute increase in pH (44). It should also be kept in mind that since many of the agents used to treat metabolic acidosis are sodium salts, volume overload and pulmonary edema are potential complications of therapy. Therefore, patients are initially treated empirically with approximately one-half the calculated dose of bicarbonate.

12. Four hours after the sodium bicarbonate was administered, repeat arterial blood gases revealed that the patient's bicarbonate was only 7 mEq/L. The patient was judged to be "alkali resistant." What are some causes of bicarbonate resistance?

Patients may require higher than predicted doses of bicarbonate when there is a high rate of production of endogenous acid (eg, lactic acidosis or ketoacidosis) and when there are large, continuous losses of bicarbonate (eg, severe diarrhea).

In some patients, large amounts of hydrogen ion are sequestered intracellularly. In these individuals, large amounts of bicarbonate move into the cells and the volume of distribution is increased. This Vd apparently diminishes as the acidosis is corrected (46).

Although clinically untested, Garella (55) recommends that an initial dose of bicarbonate be based upon a Vd equal to 100% of body weight if the HCO_3^- is less than 5 mEq/L. This method should be used very cautiously if the acidosis is produced by an anion such as lactate, which can eventually be metabolized to bicarbonate. This patient ultimately responded well to an additional 89 mEq of bicarbonate.

13. What other agents and methods are available for the treatment of metabolic acidosis? What are their advantages and disadvantages?

First, every effort should be made to identify and correct the underlying etiology of the metabolic acidosis (eg, shock, diabetic ketoacidosis, diarrhea). However, when metabolic acidosis is severe or if it persists, consideration should be given to the use of alkalinizing agents. As pointed out above, sodium bicarbonate is generally considered the agent of choice. Other treatments include the following.

Sodium Lactate and Sodium Acetate. Sodium lactate and sodium acetate are used to treat metabolic acidosis because they are metabolized to bicarbonate; however, since their effectiveness depends on their conversion to bicarbonate, sodium bicarbonate remains the agent of choice. Sodium lactate should not be used to treat lactic acidosis, because lactate metabolism is impaired in these individuals and bicarbonate is not likely to be generated.

THAM. THAM (Tris-hydroxymethyl-amino methane), or tromethamine, buffers hydrogen ion and generates bicarbonate. Although THAM lowers the pCO_2, it depresses ventilation and can aggravate hypoxia in patients with chronic obstructive pulmonary disease (10). THAM is highly alkaline, and administration may result in local vascular spasm, pain, phlebitis or thrombosis (47). There are two theoretical advantages of THAM over bicarbonate. First, in a patient who will not tolerate a sodium load THAM may expand ECF volume less than sodium bicarbonate (47). Secondly, THAM may penetrate cells more rapidly than sodium bicarbonate (48). This latter effect is probably unnecessary, actually may be detrimental (49), and is unproven. Since THAM has no proven advantage over bicarbonate and has additional side effects, sodium bicarbonate is still preferred.

Methylene Blue. Methylene blue (tetramethylthionine chloride) can function as a hydrogen ion donor:acceptor. Theoretically, it could benefit metabolic acidosis by generating NAD from $NADH_2$ (52). However, the clinical use of methylene blue has been limited, and results have not been dramatic.

Dialysis. Dialysis is of particular value if the metabolic acidosis is caused by a dialyzable substance. Additionally, dialysis may be useful to maintain the desired fluid balance in a patient who is unable to accommodate the sodium load which accompanies sodium bicarbonate administration.

METABOLIC ALKALOSIS

14. Thiazide-Induced. M.S. is a 63-year-old, 104 lb female with a long history of hypertension and congestive heart failure. For the past six months, she has been bothered by dependent edema despite intermittent therapy with digoxin and hydrochlorothiazide 50 mg every other day. On admission, supine BP was 160/80 mm Hg, pulse was 88/min and regular, respiratory rate was 28/min and temperature was normal. Physical examination revealed neck vein distension at 45°, cardiomegaly, and an S_3 gallop. A liver edge was palpated 3 cm below the left costal margin, and she had bilateral thigh and ankle edema.

She was treated with bedrest, salt restriction, digoxin 0.25 mg daily and furosemide 80 mg twice daily. By the next morning she had lost six pounds and her supine blood pressure was 105/60 mm Hg. Her laboratory values were as follows:

	On Admission	Hospital Day 2
Sodium	137 mEq/L	135 mEq/L
Potassium	3.6 mEq/L	2.9 mEq/L
Chloride	98 mEq/L	90 mEq/l
CO_2 content	28 mM/L	33 mM/L
pH	—	7.50
pCO_2	—	42 mm Hg
Urine pH	6.4	5.2
BUN	31 mg/dl	48 mg/dl
Creatinine	1.0 mg/dl	1.1 mg/dl

Assess the patient's acid-base status on hospital day two. What is the etiology of this patient's acid-base imbalance?

The elevated CO_2 content, low serum chloride and increased pH are all consistent with a metabolic alkalosis. The normal pCO_2 is further indication that the alkalosis is of metabolic, not respiratory origin.

The alkalosis in this patient is almost certainly an effect of over-diuresis as indicated by the weight loss, decreased blood pressure, elevated BUN, decreased chloride, and decreased potassium.

Diuretics may produce alkalosis by several mechanisms. First, diuretic-induced hypochloremia causes a greater proportion of sodium to be reabsorbed in exchange for hydrogen ion; thus, the proximal tubular reclamation of bicarbonate is increased. Secondly, if a patient is made hypokalemic by diuretics, a greater portion of so-

dium will be reabsorbed in exchange for hydrogen ion (rather than potassium) in the distal segment of the tubule. Finally, extracellular fluid contraction in itself can produce metabolic alkalosis.

Although metabolic alkalosis is usually associated with both chloride and potassium deficits, chloride depletion is the critical factor in most cases of metabolic alkalosis. In the presence of metabolic alkalosis and profound hypochloremia, reabsorption of filtered chloride is almost complete, and a urinary chloride determination will demonstrate virtually no chloride in the urine (ie, less than approximately 10 mEq/L). If more than 10 mEq/L of chloride is found in the urine in the absence of diuretics, it is likely that the potassium deficiency is contributing to the alkalosis (56).

15. Why is this patient's urine acidic?

Healthy individuals with an average dietary intake excrete urine that is acidic. In acidosis, the urinary pH falls as renal excretion of acid increases. In acute metabolic alkalosis, the renal transport maximum (Tm) for bicarbonate is exceeded and urine becomes alkaline. If metabolic alkalosis is chronic, urinary pH may be normal. Patients with acute metabolic alkalosis and hypokalemia reabsorb bicarbonate ion in the distal and proximal tubule, perpetuating the alkalosis and producing paradoxical aciduria (4).

16. Besides discontinuing or adjusting the diuretic therapy, how should this patient be managed? How should correction of the acid-base imbalance be monitored?

In general, metabolic alkalosis should be managed by correcting the underlying cause. Any fluid deficits (57) and ion disturbances which are present should also be corrected.

Hypochloremia must be corrected, since a significant portion of sodium which is filtered by the kidney will be reabsorbed through cation (K^+ and H^+) exchange as long as there is a chloride deficit. This can be accomplished by replacing fluid losses with sodium chloride, and to some extent by correcting the potassium deficit with potassium chloride. As chloride is replaced, the patient will undergo a bicarbonate diuresis and the alkalosis will be corrected (58,59). Fluids should be replaced cautiously in this patient since she was admitted in congestive heart failure and has a history of hypertension.

If therapy is appropriate, serial laboratory values should reflect an increasing serum potassium as well as an increasing serum chloride. The CO_2 content should be decreasing at this time. The urine chloride should be monitored to determine the adequacy of chloride replacement (7); urine chloride concentrations of 60–100 mEq/L are indicative of ECF chloride repletion. Serial blood gases should be monitored if necessary. Other important parameters to monitor in this patient include her weight, blood pressure and signs and symptoms of congestive heart failure.

17. What agents are available for the management of more severe forms of metabolic alkalosis? How is their dosage determined?

In the rare cases when alkalosis is severe (eg, characterized by tetany associated with convulsions or severe respiratory depression), an acid such as arginine monohydrochloride, ammonium chloride, or dilute (0.1N–0.2N) hydrochloric acid may need to be administered (60,61). However, ammonium chloride is limited by its CNS toxicity, and dilute hydrochloric acid must generally be administered through a central vein. Arginine monohydrochloride has been shown to cause hyperkalemia (62) and hyperglycemia (63).

Since bicarbonate has an apparent volume of distribution approximately equal to 50% of total body weight (9), the required dose of acid can be approximated according to the following formula:

$$\frac{\text{Dose}}{\text{(in mEq)}} = \frac{(0.5)(\text{Weight in kg})}{(\text{Bicarbonate Decrement Desired})} \quad \text{(Eq. 5)}$$

For example, if the serum bicarbonate level in a 70 kg patient is 39 mEq/L and one wishes to decrease this to 29 mEq/L, the calculation is:

$$\text{Acid required (mEq)} = (0.5)\,(70)\,(10)$$
$$= 350 \text{ mEq}$$

If this amount of acid (arginine monohydrochloride) is added to infusions of sodium and potassium chloride, the serum bicarbonate should decrease to 29 mEq/L in approximately 12–24 hours.

18. How is injectable hydrochloric acid solution prepared?

Distilled water for injection can be used to dilute a concentrated hydrochloric acid solution to 0.2 N. This solution is filtered through the glass portion of a millipore filter. An equal volume of 10% dextrose solution or enough sodium chloride to produce physiologic saline solution should be added, yielding either 0.1N HCl in Dextrose 5% or 0.1N HCl in 0.9% NaCl (64). These solutions can be determined to be sterile by culture prior to administration.

RESPIRATORY ACIDOSIS

19. An elderly male is admitted to a hospital with chronic obstructive pulmonary disease (COPD) and increasing pulmonary failure. Laboratory data on admission include:

Venous		Arterial	
Sodium	138 mEq/L	pH	7.33
Potassium	5.0 mEq/L	pCO_2	68 mm Hg
Chloride	98 mEq/L	pO_2	60 mm Hg
Bicarbonate	35 mEq/L		

Assess this patient's acid-base disorder. What are some common causes of this disorder, and what are the body's normal compensatory mechanisms?

The patient's history and blood gases (acidic pH, hypoxia, and hypercapnea) are consistent with chronic respiratory acidosis. The markedly elevated serum bicarbonate level could be consistent with a primary metabolic alkalosis but most likely represents the presence of compensatory metabolic alkalosis in this patient. Since it takes several days for maximal renal compensation to occur in response to hypercapnea, acute respiratory acidosis is accompanied by a rather small elevation in serum bicarbonate. If serum bicarbonate levels are greater than 30 mEq/L, as in this situation, a superimposed metabolic alkalosis should be suspected (65,10). Acutely, hemoglobin and tissue buffers are responsible for defending the body against excessive hydrogen ion concentrations.

Any drug or condition which produces hypoventilation can cause respiratory acidosis. Examples of these include central nervous system depressant drugs, generalized pulmonary diseases, disorders affecting the respiratory muscles, diseases of the central nervous system, and extreme obesity (7,10,65). Also see Table 2.

20. After treatment with mechanical ventilation, the following data were reported by the laboratory:

Venous		Arterial	
Sodium	138 mEq/L	pH	7.50
Potassium	4.8 mEq/L	pCO_2	45 mm Hg
Chloride	95 mEq/L	pO_2	95 mm Hg
Bicarbonate	35 mEq/L		

Assess the patient's current acid-base abnormality. How should his treatment be altered?

The mechanical respirator has corrected the respiratory acidosis as evidenced by the normal pO_2 and pCO_2. However, since it takes several days for renal compensatory mechanisms to return to normal, this therapy has placed the patient in uncompensated metabolic alkalosis. Although the patient is unable to correct this metabolic imbalance by hypoventilation because he is on a respirator, bicarbonate diuresis will eventually occur.

The patient's respirator should be adjusted to a slower rate to maintain the pCO_2 greater than 45 mm Hg, while at the same time avoiding a hypoxic level that would compromise respiratory function. The CO_2 content should be monitored, and as a bicarbonate diuresis begins, the patient's ventilation can be increased in keeping with the objectives of his pulmonary disease therapy.

Generally, the goal of therapy is to correct the underlying disorder and improve ventilation; immediate restoration of a normal pH is unnecessary and may result in complications, as illustrated in the above case. It should also be emphasized that the production of alkalosis is particularly undesirable in patients with chronic pulmonary disease because it depresses respiratory drive (10,65).

RESPIRATORY ALKALOSIS

21. **A 28-year-old female was admitted to the labor room of University Hospital. Physical examination revealed a pregnant woman who was having 60 second contractions every three to four minutes. Her cervix was dilated to 7 cm and the head of the fetus was engaged. She was under full control using the La Maze breathing technique. Several hours later her contractions became much stronger and recurred every 30–60 seconds. She complained of numbness and tingling around her lips, lightheadedness, and cramping in her calves. She was panting and blowing to control her labor pains and to keep herself from "bearing down."**

Assess this patient's acid-base status. What other conditions are associated with this particular acid-base imbalance? What changes in laboratory values would be expected? How should she be treated?

This patient has all the signs and symptoms (perioral paresthesia, lightheadedness, muscle cramps) of acute respiratory alkalosis which was caused by voluntary hyperventilation. The pathogenesis of these symptoms is unclear but is probably related to changes in cerebral circulation and ionic calcium levels which occur in alkalosis. Generally, any condition that stimulates respiration increases the elimination of carbon dioxide and can potentially produce respiratory alkalosis (7,10,65). These include mechanically assisted ventilation, central nervous system disease involving the medullary respiratory center, any hypoxic condition (eg, anemia, residence in high altitudes, pulmonary embolism), cirrhosis, hypermetabolic conditions (eg, hyperthyroidism, fever, gram negative sepsis), salicylate intoxication, and psychogenic hyperventilation.

When there is an acute drop in the pCO_2, bicarbonate is consumed to make carbonic acid which is converted to CO_2 and expired. The low pCO_2 value increases the bicarbonate to pCO_2 ratio (see Eq. 1), resulting in a respiratory alkalosis. Thus, acute respiratory alkalosis is characterized by an elevated pH, a decreased pCO_2, and a modest decrease in the serum bicarbonate. Even when the pCO_2 decreases acutely from 40 mm Hg to 15 mm Hg, the accompanying drop in serum bicarbonate only amounts to 7–8 mEq/L. A serum bicarbonate which is less than 15 mEq/L suggests the presence of a concurrent metabolic acidosis (65).

The treatment of respiratory alkalosis is directed at correction of the underlying problem. In this case, for example, the patient should simply be instructed to take some deep breaths and to breathe a bit more slowly. Psychogenic hyperventilators can be instructed to place a bag over their nose and mouth and rebreathe the carbon dioxide. It is rarely necessary to administer respiratory suppressants or 5% carbon dioxide (10,65). The morbidity and mortality associated with respiratory alkalosis has been correlated with pCO_2 values, as illustrated by the summary results of a retrospective study of 114 patients with respiratory alkalosis (66). Shock and sepsis occurred more frequently in Group 1 patients.

	pCO$_2$	Mortality
Group 1	15 mm Hg	88%
Group 2	20–25 mm Hg	77%
Group 3	25–30 mm Hg	73%
Group 4	35–45 mm Hg	29% (p<.001)

MIXED ACID-BASE DISORDERS

22. A one and one-half-year-old child is admitted to the emergency room with a history of salicylate ingestion. The following laboratory studies were obtained: Sodium 140 mEq/L, Potassium 5.0 mEq/L, Chloride 95 mEq/L, CO$_2$ Content 10 mEq/L, pH 7.30, pCO$_2$ 20 mm Hg, and Bicarbonate 9.5 mEq/L.

A diagnosis of metabolic acidosis and respiratory alkalosis was made, and the patient was placed on a mechanical respirator. Several hours later the pCO$_2$ was 45 mm Hg and the pH was 6.95. Assess the patient's acid-base disorder at this time.

Initially the patient had metabolic acidosis and respiratory alkalosis with a relatively normal pH. Improved ventilation removed the respiratory alkalosis leaving pure uncompensated metabolic acidosis with a pH of 6.95 and placed the patient in grave danger. See chapter on Poisonings for further information on the treatment of salicylate intoxication.

23. What general principle of the treatment of mixed disorders does this case illustrate? Name some other clinical situations where mixed acid-base disorders frequently occur.

Generally, the same principles used to treat primary disorders may also be applied to the therapy of mixed acid-base disorders. However, if mixed disorders exert the same effect on pH, a medical emergency generally exists, and therapy must be vigorous. On the other hand, if the mixed disorders exert opposite effects on pH (as in this case), overzealous therapy may produce an uncompensated disorder and thereby create a medical emergency.

Concurrent metabolic and respiratory acidosis occur following a cardiac arrest (67) and must be treated vigorously with sodium bicarbonate. Respiratory acidosis and metabolic alkalosis occur in patients with chronic obstructive pulmonary disease, and concurrent metabolic acidosis and respiratory alkalosis occur in patients who are intoxicated with salicylates or those with the hepatorenal syndrome or septic shock.

References

1. Guyton AC: *Textbook of Medical Physiology,* 5th edition, Philadelphia, WB Saunders Company, 1976.

2. Carter NW: Intracellular pH. Kidney Internat. 1972; 1:341.

3. Relman AS: Metabolic consequences of acid-base disorders. Kidney Internat. 1972; 1:347.

4. Fleischer WR: Laboratory assessment of acid-base imbalance. Geriatrics. 1974; 29:96.

5. Davenport HW: *The ABC of Acid-Base Chemistry,* Sixth Edition, The University of Chicago Press, 1974.

6. Emmett ME et al: Clinical use of the anion gap. Medicine. 1977; 56:38.

7. McCurdy DM: Mixed metabolic and respiratory acid-base disturbances: Diagnosis and treatment. Chest. 1972; 62 (suppl):35S.

8. Gabow PA et al: Diagnostic importance of an increased serum anion gap. N Engl J Med. 1980; 303:854.

9. Beeson PB et al: *Textbook of Medicine,* 14th edition, Philadelphia, WB Saunders Company, 1975.

10. Makoff DL: Acid-base metabolism in *Clinical Disorders of Fluid and Electrolyte Metabolism,* 2nd ed., edited by Maxwell MH, Kleeman CR, New York, McGraw-Hill Book Co., 1972, pp 297.

11. Pitts RF: Control of renal production of ammonia. Kidney Internat. 1972; 1:297.

12. Pitts RF: *Physiology of the Kidney and Body Fluids,* 3rd edition, Chicago Yearbook Medical Publishers, Inc. 1974.

13. Rastegar A et al: Physiologic consequences and bodily adaptations to hypercapnia and hypocapnia. Chest. 1972; 62 (suppl):28S.

14. Costrini NV and Thomson WM (eds): *Manual of Medical Therapeutics,* Ed 22. Little, Brown and Co., Boston 1977.

15. Knochel JP et al: The role of aldosterone in renal physiology. Arch Intern Med. 1973; 131:876.

16. Ludens JH et al: Aldosterone stimulation of acidification of urine by isolated urinary bladder of the Columbian toad. Am J Physiol. 1974; 226:1321.

17. Szylman P et al: Role of hyperkalemia in the metabolic acidosis of isolated hypoaldosteronism. N Engl J Med. 1976; 294:361.

18. Perez GO et al: Renal acidosis and renal potassium handling in selective hypoaldosteronism. Am J Med. 1974; 57:809.

19. Liddle GW: Aldosterone antagonist. Arch Intern Med. 1958; 102:998.

20. Greenblatt DJ et al: Adverse reactions to spironolactone. JAMA. 1973; 225:40.

21. Tannen RL: Relationship of renal ammonia production and potassium homeostasis. Kidney Internat. 1977; 11:453.

22. Gabow PA et al: Spironolactone-induced hyperchloremic acidosis in cirrhosis. Ann Intern Med. 1979; 90:338.

23. Felig P: Diabetic ketoacidosis. N Engl J Med. 1974; 290:1360.

24. Conlay LA: Phenformin and lactic acidosis. JAMA. 1976; 235:1575.

25. Olivia PB: Lactic acidosis. Am J Med. 1970; 48:209.

26. Brach BB et al: A review of deaths due to suspected lactic acidosis at a large metropolitan hospital. South Med J. 1975; 68:202.

27. Anon: Phenformin: New labeling and possible removal from market. FDA Drug Bull. 1977; 7:6.

28. Cady LD Jr et al: Quantitation of severity of critical illness with special reference to blood lactate. Crit Care Med. 1973; 1:75.

29. Peretz DL et al: Lactic acidosis: a clinically significant aspect of shock. Can Med Assoc J. 1964; 90:673.

30. Hopkins RW et al: Hemodynamic aspects of hemorrhagic and septic shock. JAMA. 1965; 191:731.

31. Maclean LD et al: Patterns of septic shock in man—A detailed study of 56 patients. Ann Surg. 1967; 166:543.

32. Daughaday WH et al: Lactic acidosis as a cause of non-ketotic acidosis in diabetic patients. N Engl J Med. 1967; 267:1010.

33. Milisci RE et al: Phenformin-induced lactic acidosis. Am J Med Sci. 1973; 265:447.

34. Steiner DF et al: Respiratory inhibition and hypoglycemia by biguanides and decamethylenediguanide. Biochem et Biophys Acta. 1958; 30:329.

35. Walker RS et al: Mode of action and side effects of phenformin hydrochloride. Br Med J. 1960; 2:1567.

36. Field M et al: Lactic acidosis in acute leukemia. Clin Res. 1963; 11:193.

37. Howell RR et al: Glucose-6-phosphatase deficiency glycogen storage disease. Pediatrics. 1962; 29:553.

38. Seligson D et al: Some metabolic effects of ethanol in humans. Clin Res Proc. 1953; 1:86.

39. Sullivan JF et al: Renal excretion of lactate and magnesium in alcoholism. Am J Clin Nutr. 1966; 18:231.

40. Bruce RA et al: Anaerobic metabolic response to acute maximal exercise in male athletes. Am Heart J. 1964; 67:643.

41. Turrell ES et al: The acid-base equilibrium of the blood in exercise. Am J Physiol. 1942; 137:742.

42. Greene NM: Effect of epinephrine on lactate, pyruvate and excess lactate production in normal human subjects. J Lab Clin Med. 1961; 58:682.

43. Siebert DJ et al: Assessment of tissue anoxemia in chronic anemia by the arterial lactate pyruvate ratio and excess lactate formation. J Lab Clin Med. 1967; 69:177.

44. Kassirer JP: Serious acid-base disorders. N Engl J Med. 1974; 291:773.

45. Plum F et al: Acid-base balance of cisternal and lumbar cerebrospinal fluid in hospital patients. N Engl J Med. 1973; 289:1346.

46. Relman AS et al: Profound acidosis resulting from excessive ammonium chloride in previously healthy subjects: a study of two cases. N Engl J Med. 1961; 265:848.

47. Bleich HL et al: Tris buffer (THAM)—an appraisal of its physiologic effects and clinical usefulness. N Engl J Med. 1966; 274:782.

48. Robin ED et al: Intracellular acid-base relations and intracellular buffers. Ann NY Acad Sci. 1961; 92:539.

49. Adler S et al: Intracellular acid-base regulation. II. The response of muscle cells to changes in CO_2 tension of extracellular bicarbonate concentration. J Clin Invest. 1965; 44:8.

50. Waters WC III et al: Spontaneous lactic acidosis. Am J Med. 1963; 35:781.

51. Ewy GA et al: Lactic acidosis associated with phenformin therapy and localized tissue hypoxia. Ann Intern Med. 1963; 59:878.

52. Tranquada RE et al: Methylene blue in the treatment of lactic acidosis. Clin Res. 1963; 11:230.

53. Huckabee WE: Lactic acidosis. Am J Cardiol. 1963; 12:663.

54. Taradash MR et al: Vasodilator therapy of idiopathic lactic acidosis. N Engl J Med. 1975; 293:468.

55. Garella S et al: Severity of metabolic acidosis as a determinant of bicarbonate requirements. N Engl J Med. 1973; 289:121.

56. Garella S et al: Saline-resistant metabolic alkalosis or "chloride-wasting nephropathy." Ann Intern Med. 1970; 73:31.

57. Earley LE et al: Sodium metabolism. N Engl J Med. 1969; 281:72.

58. Cohen JJ: Correction of metabolic alkalosis by the kidney after isometric expansion of extracellular fluid. J Clin Invest. 1968; 47:1181.

59. Cohen JJ: Selective chloride retention in repair of metabolic alkalosis without increasing filtered load. Amer J Physiol. 1970; 218:165.

60. Harken AH et al: Hydrochloric acid in the correction of metabolic alkalosis. Arch Surg. 1975; 110:819.

61. Williams SE: Hydrogen ion infusion for treating severe metabolic alkalosis. Br Med J. 1976; 5/15:1189.

62. Hertz P et al: Arginine induced hyperkalemia in renal failure patients. Arch Intern Med. 1972; 130:778.

63. Felig P et al: The glycemic responses to arginine in man. Diabetes. 1972; 21:308.

64. Harken A et al: Hydrochloric acid in the correction of metabolic alkalosis. Arch Surg. 1975; 110:819.

65. Brackett NC Jr et al: Acid-base response to chronic hypercapnia in man. N Engl J Med. 1969; 280:124.

66. Mazzara JT et al: Extreme hypocapnia in the critically ill patient. Am J Med. 1974; 56:450.

67. Bishop RL et al: Sodium bicarbonate administration during cardiac arrest. JAMA. 1976; 235:506.

68. Hill JB: Salicylate intoxication. N Engl J Med. 1973; 288:1110.

69. Albert MS: Quantitative displacement of acid-base equilibrium in metabolic acidosis. Ann Intern Med. 1967; 66:312.

Chapter 30

Parenteral Nutrition

Gail W. McSweeney

Good nutrition is necessary for normal growth and development as well as cell function and regeneration. Until recently, it was impossible to provide adequate nourishment to individuals with special nutritional requirements or those persons who were unable to ingest, absorb or metabolize usual foods. There were many attempts to solve

this dilemma, but it was not until the 1960's that specialized nutritional support became feasible (1,2). At that time, the food components needed by the body were identified and quantified, and the development of technology to separate and recombine these components for specific patient needs followed. The delivery systems used to supply these specialized nutritional products enterally or parenterally also became available. It is now possible to supply all known nutrients individually or in combination. The aim of this therapy is to maintain normal nutritional status; meet the special needs of specific patient groups such as pregnant women and children; and to supply extra or special nutrients to correct deficits or heal injuries.

The use of specialized nutritional support should only be considered if all attempts at normal alimentation and supplementation have failed. These products may be equivalent to normal foods, but they are not superior to them.

Malnutrition

The two major types of malnutrition observed clinically are marasmus and kwashiorkor. These differ in the magnitude with which they affect the visceral protein mass, which is made up of the plasma proteins (albumin, globulins, transferrin, transport proteins), immunoglobulins, clotting factors, red and white blood cells, and lymphocytes. Although these proteins account for only 5% of the body mass, they play a critical role in the maintenance of homeostasis and host defense. These proteins have short half-lives in contrast to other body components and are particularly susceptible to acute changes in nutritional status. Without them, circulating plasma volume, hematologic integrity, and defense against injury and infection are impossible to maintain, and patients succumb to cardiovascular collapse, infection, or exsanguination. They are also unable to withstand the insults of injury, major surgery, or cancer chemotherapy (12–14).

Marasmus. Marasmus is protein-calorie malnutrition which usually results from chronic semi-starvation in the absence of stress. The patient appears thin or cachectic, but the visceral protein mass is generally intact. In this form of malnutrition, the patient has efficiently mobilized peripheral fat and protein stores for energy and cell regeneration. Only in extreme circumstances will homeostatic mechanisms fail.

Kwashiorkor. Kwashiorkor is a disease caused by protein deficiency; it most commonly occurs in two situations. In the first, the patient's diet is deficient in or devoid of protein but contains sufficient calories to supply energy for biochemical functions. However, because the body is unable to recapture 0.5–0.7 gm/kg of protein from cell

turnover each day, the nitrogen building blocks needed to regenerate the visceral protein mass are eventually depleted. The peripheral fat stores are often intact because adequate calories have been ingested, and the patient does not appear malnourished. He may even be slightly puffy from the edema caused by low plasma albumin levels.

Kwashiorkor also occurs in patients who are stressed as a result of infection, burns, trauma, or disease. In this situation, the hormones released in response to stress prevent the mobilization and utilization of fat as a source of energy. As a consequence, the visceral protein mass is used as a primary source of energy for normal metabolic processes. The hormones involved in this process are the catecholamines, cortisol, glucagon, and insulin. The catecholamines, cortisol and glucagon all stimulate gluconeogenesis, a process which utilizes amino acids from visceral proteins. Fat is not utilized as an energy source in this setting because it cannot be converted to glucose by the body. Insulin, which is released in response to the increased glucose, inhibits lipolysis and stimulates the conversion of glucose to fat. Hyperglycemia and elevated urea levels (a by-product of gluconeogenesis) are common consequences of this hormonal milieu (16–20).

Because the visceral protein mass is small, significant protein depletion can occur rapidly. When this happens, vascular integrity, wound healing, immunocompetence, and oxygen-carrying capacity decline and the patient succumbs despite pharmacologic or surgical intervention (15).

It is common to see both types of malnutrition superimposed on one another, particularly in hospitalized patients. From a therapeutic standpoint, it is more appropriate to view these conditions as metabolic processes rather than as states-of-being. For example, a patient who is septic will be in a kwashiorkor mode, inefficiently using current body energy stores and any nutritional supplements; when this stress is alleviated and recovery begins, the patient's metabolic set will be that of the efficient marasmic.

Nutritional Assessment

An assessment of the type and degree of malnutrition is essential before one can determine the need for nutritional support, the goals of nutritional therapy, and the patient's prognosis. This process involves assessing the status of the patient's peripheral fat, peripheral protein, and visceral protein mass. The patient's values are compared to standard values for "normals" to estimate the degree of depletion. The degree of catabolism or the rate at which metabolism is progressing is also estimated.

Peripheral Fat. The triceps skin fold (TSF) thickness is a direct caliper measurement of the mid upper arm fat and is used to estimate peripheral fat stores. The standard TSF thickness values are 12.5 mm for men and 16.5 mm for women.

Peripheral Protein. There are several measures of peripheral protein. The arm muscle circumference (AMC) is a direct measurement of mid upper arm muscle stores and, like the triceps skin fold thickness, is compared to standard values. AMC standards for men and women are 25.3 cm and 23.2 cm, respectively.

Creatinine is a by-product of muscle metabolism and is elaborated at a constant rate depending upon the peripheral protein mass. The amount excreted in a 24-hour period can be determined by measuring the creatinine in an accurate 24-hour urine collection. The patient's value is compared to the norm for men (23 mg/kg) and women (18 mg/kg).

Visceral Protein. The status of the visceral protein mass is based upon direct laboratory measures of the proteins which comprise this compartment. In interpreting the results of these values, it is important to keep in mind that many factors other than nutritional status, such as liver disease and cancer, can independently produce abnormal values. Albumin, an important plasma protein, has a large volume of distribution and a long half-life (20 days); therefore it is an insensitive measurement of the current visceral protein mass (24). In contrast, transferrin (which has a half-life of seven days) rises and falls more rapidly in response to depletion and more accurately reflects the condition of the visceral protein mass (25). The total iron binding capacity can be used to approximate transferrin levels. The total peripheral lymphocyte count and immunologic status (as determined by response to skin tests) may also be used to assess the visceral protein mass, but the specificity and sensitivity of these determinations are under debate (26).

Catabolism. The rate of protein loss (catabolism) can be estimated from the amount of urea eliminated in a 24-hour urine collection. Before any interpretation of catabolism is made, 4 grams of nitrogen should be added to the urine nitrogen value to account for non-urea nitrogen in sweat, urine, and feces. Any nitrogen loss which exceeds the usual turnover of 0.08–0.11 grams of nitrogen per kilogram (of existing weight) is considered abnormal. Unfortunately, it is impossible to determine the compartment (visceral or peripheral protein) in which catabolism is primarily occurring (21–23).

Vitamins and Minerals. A careful diet and weight history is indispensible to the determination of specific vitamin and mineral deficiencies. It will also enable the clinician to estimate how rapidly the nutritional deficits have developed and will provide an indication of whether the patient is likely to be in a marasmic or kwashiorkor nutritional status.

Overall Evaluation. When the nutritional measurements discussed above are less than 80% of normal, a patient is considered to be moderately malnourished; patients whose values are less than 60% of normal are considered to be severely malnourished. If the nutritional deficits are in the visceral or central protein mass, the patient is at much greater risk for developing severe and life-threatening complications. Also, the degree of abnormality in each of the tests differs when the patient is in a marasmic or kwashiorkor mode (see Tables 1 and 2). An evaluation of stress as well as these tests will help the clinician determine whether the patient has marasmus or kwashiorkor and to establish the therapeutic goals accordingly.

Indications

When it becomes apparent that a patient will be unable to meet his nutritional requirements, the duration of this problem should be estimated. If this time will exceed five days or if the patient is currently malnourished, nutritional support should be considered (3). It is much easier to maintain the body cell mass or to repair small deficits than to replete a seriously ill patient (4–7). Although malnutrition occurs most commonly in patients with gastrointestinal problems, it can occur in any population. Moderate to severe malnutrition has been demonstrated in up to 20% of hospitalized patients (8–11).

Methods of Providing Nutritional Support

Repair of nutritional deficits or maintenance of the body cell mass can be achieved through

Table 1.

DISTRIBUTION OF THE BODY CELL MASS IN A 70 KG NON-OBESE MAN

Cell Mass	Body Weight (%)	Protein Mass (%)	Caloric Reserves	Assessment Parameters
Peripheral Fat	25	—	160,000 kcal	Triceps skin fold thickness
Peripheral Protein	35	~36	30,000 kcal	Arm muscle circumference Creatinine excretion index Urine urea nitrogen
Visceral and Plasma Proteins	5	~14	—	Albumin, Total Protein, Transferrin, Retinol Binding Protein, Clotting Factors, Immunoglobulins
Bone, Skin	10	~50	—	—
Extracellular Fluid	25	—	—	—

Table 2.

COMPARATIVE ASSESSMENTS OF MARASMUS AND KWASHIORKOR

Parameter	Marasmus	Kwashiorkor
Weight/Height Ratio	↓	nl, ↓ ; or ↑
Triceps Skin-fold Thickness	↓	nl
Arm Muscle Circumference	↓	nl
Albumin	nl or ↓	↓
Transferrin	nl or ↓	↓
Immunologic Function	nl or ↓	↓

administration of nutrients into the gastrointestinal tract (enteral) or into the venous system (parenteral). Intravenous nutrition should be considered only when enteral support is impossible. Examples of situations when the gastrointestinal tract cannot be used are post-duodenal complete obstruction, ileus, high output fistulas, and total malabsorption. Inability to chew, swallow or absorb complex foodstuffs are not contraindications to enteral nutrition.

Enteral Nutrition. A variety of enteral products are available commercially and can be given to patients lacking some or all digestive ability. The protein and calorie components are pre-digested and only sufficient absorptive surface area (approximately 3 feet of functioning jejunum) is absolutely required for enteral support to be fea-

sible. Table 3 lists the classes of enteral products available and their uses.

The method of administration of enteral products is variable. They can be eaten or drunk by the patient or infused by feeding tube into the stomach, duodenum, or jejunum. Tubes inserted into these portions of the gastrointestinal tract through the skin are used for patients with proximal obstructions (such as esophageal carcinoma or gastric outlet obstruction) or patients with depressed gag reflexes or altered states of consciousness in whom aspiration of stomach contents is a significant risk (107–115).

Parenteral Nutrition. Parenteral nutrition is indicated only when use of the gastrointestinal tract is impossible or the absorptive ability is insufficient to meet nutritional requirements.

Table 3.

PRODUCTS FOR ENTERAL NUTRITION

Class	Characteristics	Uses
Chemically Defined (eg, Vivonex, Precision LR, Travasorb, Vital, Vipep)	fiber-free, low fat; require little, if any, digestion	short bowel, fistulas, pancreatitis, jejunal feeding
Lactose-Free (eg, Ensure, Isocal, Osmolite)	fiber-free, lactose-free; require fat and protein digestion	lactose intolerance, duodenal feeding with intact digestive and absorptive ability
Milk or Meat Base (eg, Meritine, Formula 2, Compleat B)	complex protein, fat and carbohydrate diets; require complete digestion	oral or gastric feeding with intact digestive and absorptive ability

Table 4.

PRODUCTS FOR PARENTERAL NUTRITION

Nutrient Class	Products	Concentrations Available
Free l-amino acids Balanced (essential and non-essential)	Aminosyn, FreAmine, Travasol	3, 3.5, 5, 5.5, 7, and 10%
Essential	Aminosyn RF, Nephramine	5.1%
Dextrose	—	10–70% in 10% increments
Fat	Intralipid, Liposyn, Travamulsion	10 and 20%

The products for parenteral administration of nutrients are amino acid solutions, dextrose solutions, and fat emulsions. Electrolyte, vitamin, and mineral preparations to make the regimen nutritionally complete are also available. The balanced amino acid solutions are mixtures of essential and non-essential individual l-amino acids; d-amino acids are not readily utilized by the body. Although the products, listed in Table 4, differ slightly in their composition, they can be considered therapeutically equivalent in most instances. Their biologic value, or ability to supply the amounts and types of amino acids needed for protein maintenance and anabolism, is very high, and they contain approximately 40% essential amino acids.

Goals of Therapy

The goals and outcomes of nutritional therapy are quite different in kwashiorkor and marasmic individuals. In the former, the primary defect is in the utilization, not the availability, of nutrients. Therefore, the primary goal of nutritional therapy in a stressed patient is to reduce and minimize catabolism of the visceral protein mass. Infusion of excessive quantities of calories and protein will not achieve a faster rate of anabolism than the hormonal milieu can support and may instead result in hyperglycemia, fat accumulation, and azotemia. It may only be possible to reduce the rate of catabolism in these patients until the stress causing the metabolic inefficiency is removed.

In contrast, patients in a marasmic mode should become anabolic with adequate nutritional repletion. These patients are able to use nutrients efficiently because their hormonal environment is not deranged. If catabolism continues in spite of therapy, the patient's nutritional status should be reassessed to assure that his requirements are being met.

1. *Nutritional Assessment.* J.G., a 20-year-old male with a six-month history of ulcerative colitis, is admitted with a chief complaint of massive bloody diarrhea for three days, weakness, and a 30-pound weight loss over the past two months. During these two months, he has experienced nausea, vomiting, some anorexia, and 4–5 diarrheal stools each day. His usual well-balanced diet has been maintained, but the amount of food consumed has been greatly reduced due to recurrent nausea and vomiting.

On physical examination, J.G. was found to be a thin (180 cm; 56 kg), pale, white male with no acute distress who exhibited slight guarding over his left lower quadrant. His temperature was 36.5° C, his respiratory rate was 15/min, his pulse was 120/min, and his blood pressure (lying) was 110/65 mm Hg with no orthostatic changes. Relevant laboratory data included the following: sodium 140 mEq/L; potassium 3.6 mEq/L; chloride 105 mEq/L; bicarbonate 20 mEq/L; albumin 4.2 gm/dl; total protein 7.3 gm/dl; prothrombin time 11.5 seconds; partial thromboplastin time 33 seconds, blood urea nitrogen 12.0 gm/dl; creatinine 0.7 gm/dl; hemoglobin 10 gm/dl; hematocrit 32%; total iron binding capacity 225 mcg/dl (nl: 250–400 mcg/dl); 24-hour creatinine excretion 1150 mg; 24-hour urinary urea nitrogen 15 gm.

The patient's arm muscle circumference is 17.9 cm and his triceps skin fold thickness is 8.5 mm. Gastrointestinal evaluation reveals that J.G. has a complete colonic obstruction, probably due to the inflammatory process, and he is placed on nothing by mouth. Assess J.G.'s nutritional status, and determine whether total parenteral nutrition is indicated.

There are several indications that J.G.'s visceral protein mass is not significantly depleted. His serum albumin and protein levels are within normal limits, and the TIBC or serum transferrin is within 90% of normal. The prothrombin time is also normal, indicating that clotting factors are not significantly depleted. The red blood cells, which make up a portion of the visceral protein mass, are low but this can be explained by his bloody diarrhea and chronic disease process. The low hemoglobin and hematocrit should be evaluated further to determine the etiology of his anemia. (See the chapter on Anemias for a complete discussion of this problem.)

There is substantial evidence, however, that J.G.'s peripheral fat and peripheral muscle mass are decreased and that he is moderately malnourished. His triceps skin fold thickness of 8.5 mm is 68% (8.5 mm/12.5 mm) of normal and his arm muscle circumference of 17.9 cm is 71% (17.9 cm/25.3 cm) of normal. Furthermore, his 24-hour creatinine excretion of 1150 mg is approximately 70% of normal if one considers that his ideal body weight is 71 kg and that his normal output should be 1640 mg (71 kg × 23 mg/kg ideal weight). This information, together with his 30-pound weight loss and his dietary history which indicates that he has been eating a well-balanced diet in smaller amounts, is consistent with marasmus.

J.G.'s 24-hour urinary urea nitrogen output of 15 gm is approximately twice normal for his weight, indicating that he is catabolic and could easily progress to a more severe state of malnutrition before he is able to eat normally. This evaluation plus the fact that he may require surgery, which will produce another major drain on his metabolic reserves and place him in a kwashiorkor mode of malnutrition, make him a candidate for immediate protein and calorie repletion therapy.

Because enteral nutrition is contraindicated in the presence of a complete obstruction, total parenteral nutrition is indicated to replete his current nutritional deficits and to prevent further deterioration of his metabolic status.

2. *Calculation of Nutritional Requirements.* Estimate J.G.'s fluid, caloric, protein, electrolyte, and vitamin requirements for his total parenteral nutrition solution.

Water, Dextrose, Protein. Table 5 lists the requirements for parenteral nutrition fluids for well-nourished patients who will require maintenance therapy only because they are unable to take or absorb nutrients for a prolonged period of time and for patients such as J.G. who are malnourished and in various states of stress. For the purpose of estimating J.G.'s initial 24-hour requirements, one can assume that with the exacerbation of his ulcerative colitis he is in a state of moderate stress. Also, calculations are based upon J.G.'s *existing* rather than ideal body weight to avoid the complications associated with excessive protein and glucose supplementation. For J.G., the approximate fluid, calorie, and protein requirements are 2220 ml, 2240 kcal, and 67 gm, respectively:

Fluids
(cc/24 hr) = 1500 cc + (20 cc/kg)(36 kg)
= 2220 cc

Non-protein
Calories = (40 kcal/kg)(56 kg)
= 2240 kcal

Protein (gm) = (1.2 gm/kg)(56 kg)
= 67 gm

Electrolytes. The quantities of electrolytes which should be added to the total parenteral nutrition (TPN) solution are determined by several factors: the patient's existing electrolyte imbalances; the existence of abnormal sources of electrolyte loss such as diarrhea, nasogastric suction, fistulas, or ostomy outputs; extraordinary requirements for intracellular electrolytes which are needed for effective anabolism.

J.G. is currently hypokalemic and slightly hyperchloremic secondary to diarrheal fluid losses; therefore, his TPN fluids will have to be tailored to replete his total body potassium stores and minimize his hyperchloremia. This may be accomplished by providing a portion of his potassium replacement with potassium phosphate or acetate salts. At the present time, J.G. does not have any abnormal source of potassium loss. He has not been placed on nasogastric suction and his diarrhea has subsided. Should he develop an exogenous source of potassium loss, the fluid and ions from that source would be quantified and added to the TPN regimen.

Table 5.

BASIC NUTRITIONAL REQUIREMENTS PER 24 HOURS

Water	1500 cc (first 20 kg) + 20 cc/kg thereafter	
Non-Protein calories	maintenance	35 kcal/kg
	moderate stress	40 kcal/kg
	severe stress 45 kcal/kg. These patients are often inefficient in their handling of nutrients. Watch for signs of overfeeding (cholestasis, fatty liver) and/or azotemia.	
Protein	maintenance	0.5–1 gm/kg
	moderate stress	1–1.2 gm/kg
	severe stress	1.2–1.5 gm/kg
Electrolytes (patients with normal laboratory values)		
	Na	3–5 mEq/100cc.
	K	2 mEq/100cc + 20 mEq/1000 non-protein calories
	PO_4	0.1–0.2 mM/kg + 10 mM/1000 non-protein calories
	Cl	2/3 of the Na requirement
	Mg	0.1 mEq/kg + 8 mEq/1000 non-protein calories
	Ca	0.2–0.4 mEq/kg
	Ac	will be added as needed to balance
Vitamins and Minerals		
	Multivitamin preparation	Amount to meet the Recommended Daily Allowance (RDA) or to correct deficiencies
	Folic acid	1 mg
	Zinc	5 mg + 15 mg/L abnormal small bowel losses
	Copper	2 mg
	B_{12}	100–1000 mcg given at the initiation of therapy

Ions involved in glucose utilization or those which occupy intracellular space will be needed in quantities which exceed normal replacement values. These include potassium, magnesium, and phosphate (39,40). Potassium is essential for the transport of glucose across cell membranes and is also the major cation within the cell. Consequently, three to four times the usual replacement amount is needed by a patient manufacturing new body cell mass.

The major extracellular ions, sodium, chloride, and calcium, will be needed in the usual replacement quantities because vascular volume is not significantly altered by the anabolic process.

Vitamins. Vitamins must be present in sufficient quantities for metabolic processes to proceed normally. The B complex vitamins serve as co-enzymes in absorptive and metabolic processes as well as in the transfer of energy from protein, fats and, particularly, carbohydrates to cells and its storage as ATP. They also catalyze the formation of nucleic acids, genes, hormones, enzymes, structural proteins, cell membranes, prostaglandins, and myelin sheaths. The B vitamins are water-soluble molecules and, with the exception of vitamin B-12, are not stored to a great extent by the body.

Vitamin C, another water-soluble vitamin, is required for collagen synthesis. This is essential for capillary synthesis and stability, wound healing, and maintenance of the integument (41).

The precise actions of the fat-soluble vitamins are not completely understood, but it is known that their functions are highly specialized and specific. Vitamin A is essential for vision, the production of mucus-secreting epithelial cells, bone growth and development, and spermatogenesis. Vitamin D is partially responsible for calcium and phosphate homeostasis and bone calcification. Vitamin K is required for prothrombin generation and the conversion of fibrin to fibrinogen. The role of vitamin E is unknown, but it may be instrumental in the protection of some subcellular components, such as mitochondria and lysosomes, from destruction by peroxidases (42).

The recommended daily allowances for vitamins are listed in Table 6. Depending on the patient's status, these amounts may be sufficient, but a therapeutic formula may be indicated in patients with deficits. Significant deficiencies of folic acid, vitamin C, and the B complex vitamins have been observed in hospitalized patients (9, 11,43).

Table 6.

GUIDELINES OF THE AMERICAN MEDICAL ASSOCIATION/NUTRITION ADVISORY GROUP FOR PARENTERAL MULTIVITAMINS IN ADULTS AND CHILDREN (AGED 11 AND ABOVE)

Vitamin	Daily Requirement
A	3300 IU
D	200 IU
C	100 mg.
Folic acid	400 mcg
Niacin	40 mg
Riboflavin	3.6 mg
Thiamine	3 mg
Pyridoxine	4 mg
Vitamin B_{12}	5 mcg
Pantothenic acid	15 mg
Biotin	60 mcg

3. *Formulation.* **Describe how a solution which would meet J.G.'s calculated nutritional requirements could be manufactured from the available commercial preparations. Are there any formulation problems which should be anticipated?**

Amino acid and dextrose solutions are available in a wide variety of concentrations, as noted in Table 4. The products selected for use must be able to be combined with all additives to a final volume of 2200 cc, the amount of fluid needed to meet J.G.'s requirement.

The electrolyte and vitamin preparations are available in differing concentrations, so it is best to calculate the volume they will contribute to the final solution first. J.G.'s 24-hour requirement for these (refer to Table 5) is as follows:

Na .... 66 mEq (30 mEq/L)
K .... 88 mEq (40 mEq/L)
P .... 28 mM (13 mM/L)
Cl .... 32 mEq (15 mEq/L)
Mg .... 21 mEq (10 mEq/L)
Ca .... 15 mEq (7 mEq/L)
Zn .... 5 mg
Cu .... 2 mg
Folic Acid .... 1 mg
Multivitamin Injection .. 5 cc.

The amount of chloride to be given is slightly less than maintenance to correct the patient's slight hyperchloremia. It is usual practice to add the vitamin and mineral additives to only one liter per day.

These additive requirements correspond to the following volumes when the identified stock solutions are used, assuming Travasol 8.5% will be the amino acid base in this example. Travasol 8.5% contains Cl 35 mEq/L and Acetate 54 mEq/L as some amino acids can only be solubilized as salts.

NaHPO₄ 4 mEq Na- 3 mM P/cc .... 4.3 cc
KCl 2 mEq of each/cc .... 1.4 cc
Ca Gluconate 0.45 mEq Ca/cc ...... 15.5 cc
MgSO₄ 0.5 mEq Mg/cc .... 10 cc
NaAc 2 mEq of each/cc .... 6.4 cc
KAc 2 mEq of each/cc .... 18.6 cc

This volume is 56 cc and the final concentration of acetate in the solution (needed to balance the cations) will be 69 mEq. The amino acid stock solution will be Travasol 8.5% and the dextrose stock solution 70%. Their contribution to the solution will be 950 cc. This corresponds to 350 cc of the amino acid solution and 430 cc of the 70% dextrose. The remaining 164 cc needed to reach the final volume of one liter will be supplied by Sterile Water for Injection, USP. Infusion of 2.2 liters of this 30% dextrose—3% amino acid solution with additives per 24 hours will meet J.G.'s nutritional needs.

When preparing J.G's solution, it is important to realize that high concentrations of calcium and phosphate may precipitate. There are several variables which determine the solubility of calcium and phosphate in these solutions: calcium and phosphate concentrations; amino acid concentration; pH; temperature; and time. Solubility is prolonged if the pH of the solution is below 6.0 and the ambient temperature is below 75°F. Often, precipitation is not immediate and can occur during the infusion, particularly in the IV catheter. In general, no more than 10 mEq of calcium should be added to any solution containing phosphate. Further, if the amino acid concentration is less than 2.5%, particular attention should be paid to the temperature and infusion period. In many cases, it may be best to add the ions individually to alternating solutions (44,118).

4. Subclavian vs Peripheral Administration. Should the solution described above be infused through a peripheral vein or a subclavian catheter? Under what circumstances may the peripheral route be used?

The solution prescribed for J.G. is extremely hypertonic and cannot be infused peripherally. Solutions administered through the subclavian vein are immediately diluted by large volumes of blood so that irritation of the intima is negligible or absent. The greatest risks associated with the subclavian route are the complications which can occur at the time of catheter insertion: pneumothorax, hemothorax, subclavian artery catheterization, and tearing of the vein. However, in the hands of an experienced practitioner, the incidence of these is less than 1%. In J.G.'s case, the risk of the procedure is minimal compared to the risks and complications associated with continued malnutrition (27).

Administration of nutritional solutions through peripheral veins are appropriate if caloric needs are small, if they can be partially met by oral alimentation, or nutritional therapy will only be required for a short duration of time. J.G. meets none of these criteria. The solutions which are commonly used for peripheral alimentation, such as 10% dextrose—2.75% amino acids plus electrolytes, are very hypertonic (1100–1400mOsm/ L) and frequently cause thrombosis and phlebitis. Since J.G. may require parenteral nutrition for weeks to months, it is likely that peripheral venous access would be exhausted before his nutritional needs could be met. Furthermore, the volume of fluid which would be required to meet his metabolic needs with 10% dextrose solutions and fat emulsions may produce volume overload (119).

5. Rate of Administration; Hyperglycemia. Following placement of a subclavian catheter, J.G.'s parenteral nutrition fluid is ordered to run at a rate of 100 ml/hr. The following day his urine glucose levels are noted to be more than 2% and his urine output is greater than his parenteral intake. Explain. How can this be minimized?

J.G. does not have a history of diabetes mellitus, making this an unlikely explanation for his glycosuria. A serum glucose determination would undoubtedly reveal hyperglycemia, as his renal threshold for glucose has been exceeded in the presence of normal kidney function. Metabolic adaptation to large intravenous glucose loads is usually necessary, and the initial infusion rate of TPN solutions should be 40–50 cc/hour in an adult.

Insulin secretion, particularly in debilitated and stressed patients, takes time to equilibrate to the demand. The best way to minimize J.G.'s glycosuria is to reduce the infusion rate to 50 cc/hour. It can be increased over 24–48 hours to his final infusion rate of 90 cc/hour while blood and urine glucose determinations are made to evaluate his tolerance to the glucose load.

Insulin administration is not the treatment for hyperglycemia in non-diabetic patients. Patients without islet cell defects will adjust quickly to glucose infusions; the problem is not inability to manufacture or secrete insulin, but rather a delayed response to stimulation. Administration of exogenous insulin may cause hypoglycemia.

Some very stressed patients will never adjust to large glucose loads. Again, insulin is not the best treatment. Stress causes the release of catecholamines and glucagon which, in combination with other metabolic responses to injury, cause a physiologic insulin resistance (probably at the receptor site) with resultant hyperglycemia. There is also probably a decreased rate of intracellular glucose oxidation. Again, the problem is not lack of endogenous insulin. Giving insulin to the patient may correct the hyperglycemia, but the oxidation rate will not be affected and intracellular fat accumulations can result (see Question 6 on complications of therapy) (2,13,16,18,19,40,45). Therefore, the infusion rate must be adjusted to the patient's ability to metabolize the glucose load.

In diabetic or pancreatectomized patients, insulin administration is necessary. This can be accomplished by subcutaneous injection of regular insulin or by addition of regular insulin to the TPN solution. Blood and urine sugars should be monitored every 6–8 hours to ensure adequate therapy. The amount of insulin added to glass or plastic containers and administered through plastic IV tubing will not be the amount that reaches the patient. Approximately 40–50% will adhere to the delivery system. Because the exact availability cannot be determined, the insulin dose should be titrated slowly (116,117).

6. Complications from Overfeeding. On the third day of hospitalization, it is decided to schedule J.G. for surgery on the tenth hospital day if his obstruction does not resolve. In anticipation of this surgery, it is decided to increase J.G.'s calories to 5000 and his 24-hour protein intake to 150 gm to ensure repletion of his deficits by that date. Is this pos-

sible? What problems may be encountered with this therapy?

Anabolism is not a mass action process and supplementation of nutrients beyond the requirements will not accelerate biochemical processes. Glucose oxidation occurs at a rate of 0.5 gm/kg/hr in an adult. The maximum amount of nitrogen which can be converted to protein is 6–10 gm/day in a relatively stable, marasmic patient such as J.G.; in a stressed individual, it is usually less. Albumin synthesis by the liver occurs at a normal rate of 200 mg/kg/day; under ideal circumstances, this rate may be doubled. Since the normal amount of total body albumin is 5 gm/kg (350 gm/70 kg) and albumin is distributed throughout total body water, it is unlikely that even at maximal synthetic rates (28 gm/70 kg/day) that the serum albumin levels will be affected dramatically over a short period of time.

Overfeeding, as in this case, can cause significant metabolic complications. Excess amino acids are transformed to glucose through gluconeogenesis. If the amount of glucose generated exceeds the body's oxidative capacity, it will be converted (as will excess infused glucose) to fat or hyperglycemia will result. Urea is a by-product of amino acid metabolism. If excessive amounts are produced, dehydration may result through the obligate water loss which occurs when urea is eliminated renally. Further, if the renal capacity for the elimination of urea is exceeded, azotemia will occur. Other signs of overfeeding include: elevation in liver enzyme concentrations with a cholestatic pattern due to fatty infiltration of hepatocytes, hepatomegaly, an increase in the urine output and urine urea content and, possibly, azotemia (36). The arterial pCO_2 may also increase because 8 moles of CO_2 are produced for each mole of oxygen consumed when glucose is converted to fat. If the amount of carbon dioxide produced exceeds the lung's capacity to remove it, the arterial pCO_2 increases. These problems can be alleviated by reducing the amount of calories and nitrogen in the nutritional solution (37,38).

7. Other Complications. What other complications of TPN therapy should be anticipated in J.G.? How should these be monitored and prevented?

Sepsis. Sepsis can occur at any time in a patient receiving fluid through a subclavian catheter. Several factors predispose these patients to sepsis. The tip of the catheter lying in the vena cava is constantly bathed in a dextrose solution which provides a nidus for bacterial or fungal growth. Further, TPN patients are often on drugs, such as steroids, antibiotics, and cancer chemotherapeutic agents, which impair host defenses. It is important to note that the infusate is rarely the source of infection since the solutions are too hypertonic to support bacterial growth; however, some yeasts and fungi can survive (122).

To prevent sepsis, scrupulous aseptic technique must be observed during catheter insertion, dressing changes, and manipulation of the infusion tubing. No other solutions should be piggybacked into the line, and all TPN solutions should be prepared with strict adherence to aseptic technique.

The manifestations of sepsis or an infected catheter tip include fever, chills, and leukocytosis; however, a change in glucose tolerance in a previously stabilized patient may be the only sign (45). The subclavian line should be removed only if no other source of infection can be found or if it is obvious that it is the source of infection.

Hyperchloremic Metabolic Acidosis. Hyperchloremic metabolic acidosis can arise from the generation of HCl from the metabolism of arginine and lysine (46,47) or from the addition of too much chloride ion to the solution. This problem can be remedied through substitution of the acetate salt (which is metabolized to bicarbonate) for the chloride salts of sodium and potassium. Bicarbonate itself should not be added to TPN solutions because it produces pH changes with attendant compatibility and CO_2 production problems.

Hyperammonemia. Hyperammonemia is most often observed in neonates, but can occur in adults with massive hepatic decompensation. The inability to convert ammonia to urea may be due to insufficient numbers of hepatocytes. It may also be due to deficiencies in arginine, ornithine, or aspartic acid, which are involved in urea formation from ammonia. Intravenous arginine may be administered to counteract this problem, but metabolic acidosis may result from its use. Signs and symptoms of acidosis should be corrected if they occur (48,49,108).

Anemia. Anemia is commonly observed in patients ill enough to require parenteral nutrition, but its specific etiology should be determined and corrected if possible. Occasionally, vitamin B-12 and iron may be required since the base parenteral nutrition solutions and vitamin preparations do not contain these nutrients.

8. *Monitoring of TPN Therapy.* **How can one assess whether J.G.'s nutritional therapy is adequate?**

The parameters which should be monitored while patients are on parenteral nutrition are listed in Table 7.

The adequacy of the electrolyte content of the TPN fluid is easily monitored through daily measurement of the serum sodium, potassium, chloride, and bicarbonate for the first 3–5 days and three times weekly thereafter. Calcium, phosphate, and magnesium levels should be measured weekly. Electrolyte abnormalities are the most common complications of total parenteral nutrition therapy; however, imbalances are entirely preventable if the patient is carefully monitored. The frequency of the electrolyte measurements should be increased if J.G. develops any medical problem which may produce abnormal shifts or losses of electrolytes such as diarrhea, vomiting, renal dysfunction, or peritonitis.

It will be more difficult to determine if J.G.'s caloric and nitrogen intake are adequate. Accurate measurements of J.G.'s fluid intake and urine output will enable the clinician to determine if he is urinating excessively secondary to glucosuria or increased amounts of urea in the urine. Glucosuria may be an indication of too much glucose, inadequate glucose utilization (secondary to stress or pancreatic insufficiency), or too much nitrogen (gluconeogenesis). An excessive amount of urea in the urine relative to J.G.'s nitrogen intake would indicate continued catabolism. This may be due to inadequate amounts of nitrogen, stress (due to inefficiency of utilization in the kwashiorkor mode), or to inadequate amounts of non-protein calories, electrolytes, or vitamins which are required for anabolism.

In addition to the nitrogen balance studies which are assessed through the measurement of urine urea (see Table 7), nitrogen retention can also be monitored through improvement in the serum albumin and TIBC. As mentioned previously, these values are not likely to change quickly even at maximum anabolic rates, so weekly measurements should be sufficient.

Weight gain is another indication of anabolism. However, any gain in weight in excess of 2 pounds weekly is probably secondary to fat or fluids. The maximum weight gain which can be

Table 7.

MONITORING PROTOCOL FOR
TOTAL PARENTERAL NUTRITION

1. **Baseline Studies:** Complete blood count (CBC), platelet count, Prothrombin time, SMA-6, SMA-12, Mg

2. **Daily Studies During Stabilization (initial 3–5 days):** Urine glucose and ketones q 8 hours, SMA-6, blood glucose, accurate records of intake and output, and body weight.

3. **Routine Studies After Initial Stabilization**
   a. Daily: Intake and output, body weight, urine glucose and ketones
   b. Three Times Weekly: SMA-6
   c. Weekly: CBC, SMA-12, Mg, prothrombin time

Nitrogen Balance: Most patients should have a nitrogen balance determination after they have achieved stabilization on a nutritional regimen that is calculated to meet their protein and calorie requirements. Nitrogen balance studies are also indicated after significant adjustments in the protein and glucose contents of TPN solution or major changes in the activity or metabolic status of the patient.

Approximately 90% of the nitrogen lost/day is excreted in the urine. Urea nitrogen constitutes 70% of total nitrogen excreted in the urine. An estimate of total nitrogen excretion/day can be obtained as follows: send an aliquot of 24 hr urine collection for urine urea nitrogen (same as BUN assay). Convert to grams of N lost/day and add 4. The additional 4 gm is a constant that reasonably estimates daily nitrogen loss as ammonia, uric acid, creatinine, amino acids, etc.

N_{bal} = Nitrogen Intake/24 hours −
Nitrogen Loss/24 hours

N_{bal} = Amino Acid Nitrogen (16% of protein) in gm −
(Urine Urea Nitrogen in gm + 4 gm)

In adults, TPN therapy can stimulate at most about 4–10 grams of positive N_2 balance or 1/3 lb of protoplasmic weight gain per day. Maximal protoplasmic weight gain per week is about 2 lbs. Greater weight gain than this represents fat or fluid.

attributed to positive nitrogen balance is one-third pound per day.

If J.G. remains catabolic, the adequacy of his repletion and stress status should be re-evalu-

ated. Because he is currently in a stable, marasmic mode, his catabolic status should gradually reverse itself; if this does not occur, additional protein and calories may be indicated. The clinical goal should be to achieve a positive nitrogen balance of 4–10 gm/day. However, if J.G.'s clinical status deteriorates or he enters a kwashiorkor mode, this goal may not be achievable.

9. *Renal Failure.* **On day 14 of J.G.'s hospital stay, he is operated on for his colonic obstruction. Two days later, he develops acute renal failure. What complications related to his parenteral nutrition therapy must be anticipated? What changes will be required?**

There are three potential complications which may arise as a result of this therapy in a patient in renal failure. These are volume overload, electrolyte imbalances (hyperkalemia, hyperchloremia, etc), and exacerbation of uremia through ureagenesis.

Exacerbation of uremia is the primary problem which needs to be anticipated in these patients since urea is a by-product of amino acid metabolism. Solutions which contain only essential amino acids are commercially available for use in patients such as J.G. with renal failure. Theoretically, if sufficient calories are supplied along with these essential amino acids, the liver can recapture the urea nitrogen and manufacture non-essential amino acids. This has not been conclusively demonstrated, making the use of these special solutions controversial. Some believe that the fall in blood urea nitrogen levels associated with the use of these products is simply related to a suppression of gluconeogenesis (which promotes protein breakdown and the mobilization and metabolism of amino acids) by glucose infusions or to the administration of smaller quantities of amino acids. Therefore, this author recommends balanced solutions containing essential and non-essential amino acids which can be utilized directly by J.G. without prior transamination by the liver (50–52,120).

It is unlikely that J.G. will be able to tolerate his current volume of TPN. This problem can be minimized by administering a more concentrated solution and supplementing a smaller volume with fats to provide an adequate caloric intake. In some patients it may become impossible to meet all nutritional requirements under these circumstances. For J.G., one liter of 35% dextrose and 5% amino acid solution with 500 cc of a 20% fat solution will provide 50 gm of nitrogen and 2200 kcal. Also see Questions 14–18 for an expanded discussion of fat therapy. The most concentrated base fluids which are commercially available are a 70% dextrose and a 10% amino acid solution.

Hyperkalemia, as well as other electrolyte imbalances, is another potential problem in patients with renal failure. If the patient's azotemia is severe enough to warrant dialysis therapy, electrolyte imbalances may be managed this way. If the patient is not on dialysis, daily potassium levels must be measured and the electrolyte content of the parenteral nutrition fluids must be adjusted accordingly. As discussed earlier, large quantities of potassium are required for effective utilization of glucose.

10. Discontinuation of Parenteral Nutrition. Three weeks postoperatively, J.G.'s renal and gastrointestinal problems resolve. How can he best be returned to oral feedings?

Long-term insult to and disuse of the gastrointestinal tract produces atony and an alteration of normal secretory functions. Therefore, the return of J.G. to oral alimentation must be gradual and should begin with small quantities of easily digestible foods; a clinical dietitian should be central to this process. Intravenous nutrition should be continued until the patient is able to support himself nutritionally with oral feedings; the amount infused is reduced as oral intake increases to ensure good nutrition during the transition period (113).

11. Liver Disease. A patient with severe liver disease and malnutrition requires parenteral nutrition. What special problems must be anticipated in such a patient?

Unfortunately, this situation can present an insoluble nutritional problem. The liver is responsible for the manufacture of the visceral protein mass and if there are insufficient numbers of functioning hepatocytes to accomplish visceral protein repletion, malnutrition becomes irreversible. Patients with severe liver disease have particular difficulty metabolizing phenylalanine, methionine, and tryptophan; this results in elevated levels of these amino acids and an imbalance of the plasma amino acids. This is important because these amino acids may be involved in the development of encephalopathy through the generation of false neurotransmitters. These amino acids are precursors of epinephrine, norepinephrine, and dopamine. Therefore, high levels of these protein building blocks may produce derangements in the metabolic pathways in which these hormones are synthesized and function. Another postulate for the development of encephalopathy in these patients is hyperammonemia. See Question 7 on complications of therapy.

The nutrition of patients with severe liver disease should be initiated with 20 gm of amino acids daily. If this is not tolerated, the patient may be terminally decompensated. If the patient's sensorium is not affected, the amount of nitrogen should be increased gradually until signs of protein overload (such as encephalopathy) appear or the patient's nutritional needs are met. There are no commercially available intravenous amino acid solutions which lack phenylalanine, methionine, and tryptophan. However, even if there were, it is unknown whether effective anabolism could proceed without these amino acids (53–55).

12. Pediatric Patients. M.W. is a 20-day-old, 4.2 kg infant who was born with a congenital omphalocele (evisceration of the stomach, one-third of the liver and portions of the intestine). On the day of delivery, the infant was taken to surgery where closure of the omphalocele was performed with placement of a Dacron graft over the abdominal cavity. Two days later the patient developed signs of necrotizing enterocolitis, and parenteral nutrition was considered. How will therapy in this and other pediatric patients differ from that of the adult?

The nutritional requirements for pediatric patients receiving parenteral nutrition are summarized in Table 8. The primary difference between TPN in these patients compared to adults is in the amounts of protein and energy required for maintenance and growth of the body mass. For patients weighing less than 10 kg like M.W., 100–125 kcal/kg (as opposed to 35 kcal/kg for an adult) and 2–2.5 gm/kg of protein are required for maintenance, and 10–20% more amino acids and calories are required for growth and development. Infants and children can oxidize glucose for calories faster than adults; this process can approach a rate of 1.5 gm glucose/kg/hour. Unfortunately, premature infants have difficulty handling calories because their metabolic processes are underdeveloped. The introduction of fat emulsions as an alternative energy source has

Table 8.

BASIC REQUIREMENTS FOR
PEDIATRIC PATIENTS (PER 24 HOURS)

Water	100 cc/kg for first 10 kg
	50 cc/kg for next 10 kg
	20 cc/kg thereafter
Protein	2.0–2.5 gm/kg
Non-protein Calories	100–125 kcal/kg for first 10 kg
	50–60 kcal/kg for next 10 kg
	20–25 kcal/kg thereafter
Na	2–4 mEq/kg/day
K	1–4 mEq/kg/day
Cl	3–5 mEq/kg/day
Mg	0.5–1.0 mEq/kg/day
Ca	1.0–3.0 mEq/kg/day
PO_4	0.5–1.0 mM/kg/day
MVI	0.25–0.5 cc/kg
Folic acid	25–50 mcg/kg
Zinc	40–100 mcg/kg
Copper	20 mcg/kg
B-12	10 mcg/kg

eased this problem somewhat, but these children have impaired fat metabolism as well.

The most common problem encountered in the administration of parenteral nutrition to this age group is the delivery of sufficient amounts of nutrients in a fluid volume which the child can tolerate. This is particularly a problem in sick and premature infants who often have accompanying pulmonary, cardiac, and renal problems which impair their ability to tolerate volume loads. Because of these special metabolic characteristics, all infants and children receiving total parenteral nutrition should initially be monitored several times daily to assess the assimilation of nutrients and tolerance to the volume load. Adjustments should be made in the nutrition therapy accordingly (56–59).

13. Recommend a solution for M.W. How should the solution be initiated and evaluated?

As long as M.W.'s renal, cardiac, and pulmonary status remain stable, his fluid requirement will be 420 cc/day, his caloric requirement will be 420–525 kcal/day, and his protein requirement will be 8–10 gm/day. This corresponds to a solution of 35% dextrose and 2.5% amino acids with appropriate electrolyte, vitamin, and mineral additives infused at a rate of 18 cc/hr. This therapy should be instituted very slowly (beginning with a rate as low as 5 cc/hr) and his response should be followed closely. If M.W.'s ability to oxidize glucose is impaired and hyperglycemia results, then up to 60% of his total caloric requirement can be substituted with a fat emulsion (see section on fat emulsion therapy). The adequacy of his repletion should be evaluated as previously described for J.G. in Questions 6–8. He should be particularly monitored for hyperammonemia and metabolic acidosis, as infants are susceptible to these complications of total parenteral nutrition (36, 46,48,49,121).

FAT EMULSIONS

Intravenous fat emulsions have been available commercially as an adjunct to nutritional support since 1974. The emulsions are stabilized and maintained by egg yolk phospholipids to a mean particle size of 0.13 microns, a size which is within the range of naturally occurring chylomicrons (60). Numerous investigators have demonstrated that these fat particles are cleared from the blood in the same manner and rate as fat absorbed from the gastrointestinal tract (61,62). Once they enter the bloodstream, chylomicrons are rapidly covered by an apoprotein released from lipoproteins. At this point, lipoprotein lipase from the capillary endothelium acts on the fat to form free fatty acids (FFA's) for energy (63). If the generated FFA's exceed the body's current needs, they will be re-esterified and stored in adipose cells. This reaction occurs in the presence of alpha-glycerophosphate, a glycogen derivative (64).

Because fat particles have no tonicity of their own, glycerol is added to render the emulsions isotonic (300 mOsm/L). This property makes it possible to manufacture emulsions with varying and high caloric concentrations which are not hypertonic (65).

Products. There are three commercially available products (Intralipid, Liposyn, and Travamulsion) and their composition is listed in Table 9. Travamulsion and Intralipid contain soybean oil and Liposyn contains safflower oil. Both

Table 9.

FAT EMULSIONS 10%

COMPOSITION OF AVAILABLE PREPARATIONS

	Intralipid	Liposyn	Travamulsion
Fatty Acid (by percent):			
Linoleic	54	77	56
Linolenic	8	—	6
Oleic	26	13	23
Palmitic	9	7	11
Stearic	—	2.5	—
Egg phospholipids	1.2	1.2	1.2
Osmolality	280 mOsm/L	300 mOsm/L	270 mOsm/L
pH	5.5–9	8.3	5.5–9
Glycerol	2.25%	2.25%	2.25%

product types contain egg yolk phospholipid as an emulsifying agent and glycerol and are available in 10% and 20% concentrations. The 10% concentration provides 1.1 kcal/cc and the 20% concentration provides 2.0 kcal/cc.

For adults and normal pediatric patients, either product type can be used for essential fatty acid or caloric replacement. Liposyn, the safflower oil emulsion, has a slightly higher concentration of linoleic acid, but the dose of this EFA required can easily be met with either product type. The primary difference between these two product types is in their linolenic acid content which is higher in the soybean oil emulsions. Linolenic acid is found in high concentrations in nerve tissue. Because nerve tissue does not regenerate and is completely developed at term, the linolenic content is only relevant to premature infants. Although the absolute need for this fatty acid has not been established, soybean oil may be the preferred product in this population (81).

Indications. The first and primary indication for fat emulsions is in the prevention or treatment of essential fatty acid deficiency (EFAD). Man requires linoleic acid for cell membrane synthesis and stabilization, but is incapable of synthesizing it. A deficiency of linoleic acid is characterized clinically by a scaly skin, sparse hair growth or alopecia areata, poor wound healing, and thrombocytopenia. Body fat stores contain approximately 10% linoleate.

The second indication for fat emulsions is the provision of non-protein calories for patients receiving parenteral nutrition whose caloric requirements cannot be met by glucose. This may be related to an inability to effectively metabolize and assimilate glucose or to volume restriction.

14. *Essential Fatty Acid Deficiency.* B.R. is a 39-year-old, 70 kg male who was in his usual state of good health until he was involved in a motor vehicle accident three days ago. He sustained compound fractures of both legs and internal injuries which required splenectomy and correction of a small bowel perforation. A central venous catheter was inserted and B.R. was initiated on parenteral nutrition solutions which provided 75 grams of amino acids and 2500 non-protein calories daily. Why is B.R. currently a candidate for fat therapy?

The appearance of essential fatty acid deficiency varies depending upon the previous existence of poor nutrition, the efficiency of fatty acid mobilization from existing stores, and the requirement for fatty acid for new cell synthesis (67–69). No absolute rate of endogenous utilization or replacement requirements can be calculated. A non-injured patient with chronically poor nutrition may not develop signs of fatty acid deficiency for several months, depending on the quantity of fat stores. In contrast, a severely injured patient such as B.R. may become deficient quickly because increased amounts of linoleate will be required for new cell synthesis. Also, hormone imbalances associated with injury and high glucose levels may impair normal mobilization of the patient's own fatty acid stores (70,71). For these reasons, B.R. is a candidate for fat emulsion therapy now.

15. How can the presence of essential fatty acid deficiency (EFAD) be detected in B.R.?

Fatty acid deficiency cannot be detected by assessing derangements in cell membrane lipid layers directly. Instead, this disorder is diagnosed indirectly through the measurement of plasma fatty acid ratios. The essential fatty acid, linoleic acid, belongs to a family of long-chain, unsaturated fatty acids with a double bond six carbons from the terminal carbon (n-6). Oleic acid, a nonessential fatty acid, belongs to a family with a double bond nine carbons from the terminal carbon (n-9). The body preferentially metabolizes fatty acids in the n-6 group, and if these are not available, the n-9 fatty acids will be in greater abundance relative to the n-6 fatty acids. The biochemical test used to determine fatty acid deficiency is called a triene:tetraene (n-9:n-6) ratio. A ratio of less than 0.4 is considered normal; if the ratio is greater than 0.4, it is assumed that insufficient linoleic acid is available for metabolism and that a deficiency state exists (72). This test is also used to determine the adequacy of fat emulsion therapy.

16. *Requirements and Administration.* How much fat emulsion should B.R. receive and how should it be administered?

Between two and eight percent of the caloric requirements as *linoleic acid* is generally adequate to prevent and treat essential fatty acid deficiency (73,74). Because B.R. has been severely injured, his need for essential fatty acids (EFA's) will be high as he generates new cells. For this reason, 8% of his non-protein caloric requirements should be provided in the form of linoleic acid. One should note that the concentration of this EFA in the two product types differs considerably. Triene:tetraene ratios should be obtained two or three times weekly and the amount of infused fat adjusted to keep the ratio below 0.4. Under no circumstances should the non-protein caloric contribution of fat exceed 60%, since sufficient glucose must be provided to maximize anabolism.

All three fat emulsion products are isotonic and can be administered through central or peripheral venous lines. No other substances should be added to fat emulsion products because any agent which alters the pH or the emulsion's characteristics can cause particle coalescence or cracking of the emulsion (75). Piggyback administration with dextrose-amino acid solutions is permissible as long as the contact time between the two is brief. Also, there should be no in-line filtration since fat particles are too large to pass through the membrane. For the first 30 minutes the emulsion should be infused at a rate of 1 ml/min; if no adverse reactions occur, the rate may be increased.

17. *Complications and Side Effects.* What are the risks and side effects of fat emulsion therapy? Are there any contraindications to its use?

Because both emulsions are stabilized by egg yolk phospholipids, a history of severe egg allergy precludes their use. Patients with alterations in reticuloendothelial system function, such as those with respiratory distress syndrome, may accumulate fat in their lungs, resulting in compromised gas exchange (64,76). A history of hyperlipidemia is not a contraindication to the use of fat emulsions, but clearance of lipid from the blood should be monitored closely in patients with this disorder by measurement of serum triglycerides. B.R. should be evaluated for a history of egg allergy and hyperlipidemia prior to the initiation of fat emulsion therapy.

Acute reactions to fat emulsion therapy are generally mild and transient and do not require discontinuation of therapy. These include fever (3%), chills, shivering, vomiting, and chest pain.

Delayed reactions to fat emulsion therapy include thrombocytopenia, hepatomegaly, and splenomegaly. Transient elevation in liver function tests occur, but the actual effect on hepatic function is difficult to assess since prolonged infusions of protein and carbohydrate also induce structural changes in the liver. B.R. should have liver function tests weekly while he is receiving fat therapy (80).

When fat comprises more than 60% of the non-protein calories over a prolonged period of time, a syndrome of overloading can occur. This is characterized clinically by focal seizures, fever, leukocytosis, and shock (79).

18. *Peripheral Administration as Source of Calories.* Three weeks after TPN is insti-

tuted, B.R. develops a mediastinal infection which necessitates the removal of his central venous catheter. Because there is a threat of pulmonary edema, B.R.'s fluids are limited to three liters daily. Phlebitis precludes the administration of solutions more concentrated than 10% glucose. How can B.R.'s caloric needs be met peripherally?

Fat emulsions are widely used as a calorie source and their high caloric density makes them ideal for patients who have no central venous access or whose calories must be delivered in the smallest possible volume. The 20% emulsions have the caloric density of 58.8% dextrose and because they are isotonic, they can be given through a peripheral vein.

Ideally, B.R.'s parenteral nutrition should provide 1.2–1.5 grams of protein per kg per day or 84–105 grams. It should also provide 40 kcal/kg or 2800 non-protein calories. Since no more than 60% of these calories can be provided as fat and B.R. is limited to 3 liters daily, it will be impossible to meet his caloric needs. The best that can be done is to administer approximately 2.5 liters of a 10% dextrose—4% amino acid solution (1000 calories and 100 gm protein) daily and 500 cc of 20% fat emulsion (1000 calories). This combination provides his total protein requirement but only 2000 of his 2800 calorie requirement; however, the contribution of fat is less than 60%.

The fat emulsion should be infused slowly so that B.R.'s ability to metabolize the fat will not be exceeded. B.R. should also be free of a fat emulsion therapy for at least four hours daily for the first few days of therapy. His serum should be checked at the end of this period for lipid clearance. Once tolerance has been established, the fat emulsion can be infused over 24 hours.

TRACE ELEMENTS

Trace elements are those which occur in amounts which are less than 0.01% of the body mass. Their presence is required in minute amounts for enzyme activity, synthesis and stabilization of proteins and nucleic acids, mitochondrial energy generation, membrane transport, nerve conduction, and muscle contraction.

The gastrointestinal absorption of all trace metals is regulated by the mucosa through complexation with ligand proteins secreted by the pancreas. A ligand is a group, molecule, or ion that forms a complex with a central metallic atom.

Metals generally occur in foods as organo-complexes, but they are absorbed individually with ligands (83–86). In patients who are unable to ingest or absorb a normal diet, trace metals may have to be given intravenously. Their activity is entirely physiologic, and administration of amounts in excess of those needed for biochemical processes may produce adverse effects (87).

Elements which are essential include zinc, copper, iron, iodine, and cobalt (as vitamin B-12). Evidence which supports the essentiality of chromium, manganese, and selenium is accumulating. Iron and cobalt (as vitamin B-12) are discussed in detail in the Anemias chapter and a discussion of iodine can be found in the chapter entitled Thyroid Diseases.

Zinc. Zinc stores in the adult vary from 1–2 grams. The major route of excretion is through secretion into the duodenum and jejunum with reabsorption in the mid-jejunum. Only minute amounts are lost in the urine (88,89). The major repositories for this metal are in skeletal muscle, skin, bone, and the pancreas. The role of zinc at these sites is probably related to its enzymatic activity since it is a component of DNA polymerase. Mitosis necessary for cellular proliferation in wound healing, maintenance of the integument, and replacement of cells lining the gastrointestinal tract is facilitated by this metalloenzyme. Additionally, zinc is required for synthesis and mobilization from the liver of retinol binding protein, the carrier of vitamin A (90,91). This fat-soluble vitamin is necessary for the synthesis of collagen fibrils and fibers. Zinc requirements can usually be met with a dose of 40 mcg/kg/day.

The signs of zinc deficiency vary but the major symptoms include bullous, vesicular, or acrodermatitis-like lesions around body orifices or extremities; alopecia; poor wound healing; glucose intolerance secondary to impaired insulin synthesis and release (97); hypogeusia (decreased taste perception); hyposmia (decreased sense of smell) (98); diarrhea; and growth retardation in children (92–96).

Copper. The human adult has a store of 100–150 mg of copper. It is found chiefly in the liver and in the blood bound to ceruloplasmin. The major route of copper excretion is through the bile; reabsorption occurs in the duodenum and proximal jejunum (99). A dose of 20 mcg/kg/day will replace losses.

This metal has two major roles in the body. Copper, bound to ceruloplasmin, aids in the mobilization of iron and its conversion to the ferric form necessary for hemoglobin synthesis. Therefore, severe deficiency results in a microcytic anemia, even in the presence of adequate total body iron. Administration of copper should be considered in patients with a microcytic anemia unresponsive to iron therapy (98). Copper is also a component of a metalloenzyme involved in collagen cross-linking, lysyl oxidase. Vitamin C is necessary for the hydroxylation of proline and lysine to procollagen, and copper is a component of the ascorbic acid oxidase enzyme as well (91). The signs of copper depletion include microcytic anemia, neutropenia, and poor wound healing (100,101).

Chromium, Manganese, Selenium. Chromium, manganese and selenium deficiency states have been described in patients who have had no oral intake for several years. Body stores of these metals are unknown.

Manganese is needed for mitochondrial energy generation as a component of the metallo-enzyme, pyruvate carboxylase. It may also have a role in DNA and RNA synthesis. The signs of deficiency include hypocholesterolemia and ataxia. Replacement is achieved with 0.4 to 2 mg per day in the adult (91).

Chromium is part of the nicotinic acid-amino acid complex called "glucose tolerance factor." It potentiates the activity of insulin at the receptor site, and the signs of deficiency are glucose intolerance and elevated free fatty acid levels. Replacement can be achieved with the oral administration of 20 mcg/day in the adult (102).

Selenium is found in glutathione peroxidase in the red blood cell. A replacement dose has not been determined and there is no available parenteral product (103,104).

19. L.M. is a 35-year-old female with a three-week history of profuse diarrhea which is occasionally bloody and has occurred as often as twelve times per day. She has a five-year history of Crohn's disease but no other significant medical problems. Two years ago, L.M. had a 12 cm ileal resection. Pertinent findings on admission include a dry, cool skin, patchy alopecia, vesicular lesions around the nose and mouth, orthostatic changes, and a 20-lb weight loss in three weeks.

Laboratory findings were as follows: Sodium 132 mEq/L, Potassium 2.5 mEq/L, Chloride 105 mEq/L, Bicarbonate 20 mEq/L, Al-

bumin 3.2 gm/dl (3.5–5), Serum Zn 89 mcg/dl (95–105), Hemoglobin 12 gm/dl, Hematocrit 37%, MCV 95 microns^3, and MCHC 28 gm/dl (31–35). Colonoscopic findings included granulomatous changes in the ileum and cecum consistent with Crohn's disease.

Assess L.M.'s overall clinical status. How should she be managed?

L.M.'s most acute problems are hypovolemia, dehydration, and hypokalemia. These should be corrected with intravenous normal saline and potassium chloride since gastrointestinal absorption of fluid and electrolytes may not be reliable in the presence of her Crohn's disease (refer to the chapter on Fluid and Electrolyte Disorders for guidelines).

Vigorous nutritional support should be instituted. L.M. has had a rapid and significant weight loss, and her low plasma albumin level suggests a serious reduction in visceral protein. Crohn's disease is characterized by a transmural lesion of the bowel and the risk of perforation is quite high. Exacerbations may last for months in spite of drug therapy, and malabsorption can be almost complete due to intestinal hypermotility. For these reasons, L.M. will require central intravenous nutrition rather than an enteral formula.

20. Evaluate L.M.'s zinc status and balance.

L.M.'s history of diarrhea and the presence of skin lesions and alopecia indicate she is probably deficient in zinc. The low serum zinc level is a less reliable indicator of total body zinc depletion because 98% of the element is located intracellularly (92,93). Since albumin is the primary transport protein for zinc, hypoalbuminemia (as in this patient) may give the appearance of a deficiency in a patient with normal stores (13). It has been demonstrated by several investigators that serum zinc does not correlate well with intracellular concentrations or signs of depletion. Clinical findings and zinc balances are the most reliable parameters to follow (95,96).

Zinc is a trace element which is primarily excreted by the gastrointestinal tract (97) and L.M. has had prolonged, unusual losses via this route. The small bowel secretes zinc and losses beyond the normal turnover of 40 mcg/kg/day correlate well with stool volume (88,89). Patients with a history of vomiting or nasogastric suction will not lose unusual quantities of this metal. Wolman et al have quantitated zinc losses in stool (97). In patients with an intact small bowel, 17 mg/L stool will be excreted. In those with major resections of small bowel, 12 mg/L of stool will be lost. L.M.'s previous ileal resection was not a major loss of absorptive surface for zinc as the metal is reabsorbed in the jejunum.

21. Estimate a replacement dose of zinc for L.M. How should it be administered?

In calculating a replacement dose of zinc for L.M. several factors should be kept in mind: normal zinc turnover (40 mcg/kg/day); any continuing diarrhea (17 mg/L); and current deficits. She has had a three-week history of diarrhea but has not had a major small bowel resection which could alter her reabsorption of zinc.

L.M. should be weighed to determine her maintenance need and then questioned about the volume of the diarrhea she has been experiencing to estimate her current deficit. Any continuing abnormal stool losses should be quantified daily.

Adverse reactions to trace metals given intravenously have not been reported. Physico-chemical incompatibility has also not been reported and there does not appear to be a problem with the addition of zinc to TPN solutions. The daily dose would be a total of L.M.'s daily maintenance requirement, continuing losses, and the portion of the initial deficit required to normalize the body stores within 7–10 days. In the interim, L.M. should be watched closely for glucose intolerance, which is associated with profound zinc deficiency.

The chloride or sulfate salts of zinc are available from various manufacturers. Because individual requirements vary depending on age, sex, and clinical condition, the Nutrition Advisory Group of the American Medical Association recommends replacement with individual metals rather than with combination products (87).

Zinc is available orally as the sulfate salt. The dosage form is a 220 mg capsule and is appropriate for patients with adequate duodeno-jejunal surface area and gastrointestinal transit times. Metals are actively transported across the mucosa, so the amount absorbed is a function of the body's need. Although the bioavailability of the product is good, L.M. should not receive an oral preparation because her current gastrointestinal transit time is greatly reduced.

22. Are there any other trace elements which may have to be replaced in L.M.?

With the history of bloody diarrhea and the presence of a low hematocrit, L.M. may have low iron stores. Since her red blood cell indices do not currently reflect a microcytic anemia, a peripheral smear, and serum iron and a TIBC would be helpful in establishing the specific diagnosis for the anemia. The amount of terminal ileum resected was minimal and has not predisposed this patient to folic acid and B_{12} deficiency. Intravenous iron therapy is probably not indicated at this time because a hypersensitivity reaction is a risk and oral iron therapy can be given, if indicated, when the patient begins taking foods by mouth. Folic acid and B-12 can be given safely by the intravenous route in depleted patients.

Normal copper turnover through bile losses is 20 mcg/kg/day. Recapture in the small bowel is very efficient, so only patients losing large amounts of bile are at risk of developing a deficiency. L.M. does not fit these criteria and probably does not require copper replacement above the usual turnover amounts (101).

Because L.M. has not been without oral intake for an extended period, administration of other metals is probably not required.

23. Parenteral nutrition is ordered for L.M. and 1 gm of zinc sulfate is ordered to be added to the first liter. This is done to immediately correct her total body zinc deficit. What are the risks of trace metal overdose in this situation?

Toxicity has not been described in association with the intravenous administration of physiologic amounts of the available trace metal products. However, tubular necrosis was reported in a patient who received 7.4 gm of zinc over a 60-hour period (105–106). Because quantitative toxicity data are not available and because L.M.'s deficiency is not life threatening, it is more reasonable to replace her total body deficit over a 7–10 day period.

24. Which trace metals are currently available commercially?

Zinc, copper, chromium, and manganese are available for intravenous use from various manufacturers as the chloride or sulfate salts. Each product varies in concentration, but none exceeds 5 mg/cc. Zinc sulfate is the only trace element which is available in an oral form as a single entity. Copper, manganese, chromium, and zinc are found in varying amounts in many oral vitamin and mineral products.

References

1. Dudrick SJ et al: Long-term parenteral nutrition with growth, development and positive nitrogen balance. Surgery. 1968; 64:134.

2. Dudrick SJ et al: Principles and practice of parenteral nutrition. Gastroenterology. 1971; 61:901.

3. Goodgame JT: A critical assessement of the indications for total parenteral nutrition. Surg Gynecol Obstet. 1980; 151:433.

4. Rich AJ et al: Ketosis and nitrogen excretion in under-nourished surgical patients. J Parenteral Enteral Nutr. 1979; 3:350.

5. Abbott WE et al: Effect of starvation, infection and injury on the metabolic processes and body composition. NY Acad Sci Ann. 1963; 110:941.

6. Moore FD et al: Surgical injury: Body composition, protein metabolism and neuroendocrinology. In: Ballinger WF (ed), *Manual of Surgical Nutrition*, WB Saunders, Philadelphia, 1975; p 169.

7. Cuthbertson DP: The metabolic response to injury and its nutritional implications: retrospect and prospect. J Parenteral Enteral Nutr. 1979; 3:108.

8. Bistrian B et al: Protein status of general surgical patients. JAMA. 1974; 230:858.

9. Bistrian B et al: Prevalence of malnutrition in general medical patients. JAMA. 1976; 235:1567.

10. Willcutts H: Nutritional assessment of 1000 surgical patients in an affluent community hospital, abstracted. J Parenteral Enteral Nutr. 1977; 1:4.

11. Weinsier RL et al: Hospital malnutrition: a prospective evaluation of general medical patients during the course of hospitalization. Am J Clin Nutr. 1979; 32:418.

12. Cuthbertson DP et al: Note on the effect of injury on the levels of plasma proteins. Br J Exp Path. 1935; 16:471.

13. Wilmore DW: Hormonal responses and their effect on metabolism. Surg Clin North Am. 1976; 56:999.

14. Jeejeebhoy KN et al: The comparative effects of nutritional and hormonal factors in the synthesis of albumin, fibrinogen and transferrin. In: Ciba Foundation Symposium, *Protein Turnover*, Associated Science Publishers, Amsterdam, 1973.

15. Clowes GHA et al: Energy metabolism in sepsis; treatment based on different patterns in shock and high output stage. Ann Surg. 1974; 179:684.

16. Wilmore DW et al: Catecholamines: mediators of the hypermetabolic response to thermal injury. Ann Surg. 1974; 180:653.

17. Moore FD et al: La maladie port-operatoire: is there order in variety? The six stimulus-response sequences. Surg Clin North Amer. 1976; 56:803.

18. Meguid MM et al: Hormone-substrate interrelationships following trauma. Arch Surg. 1974; 109:776.

19. Alberti KGMM et al: Relative role of the various hormones in mediating the metabolic response to injury. J Parenteral Enteral Nutr. 1980; 4:141.

20. Clowes GHA et al: Energy metabolism and proteolysis in traumatized and septic man. Surg Clin North Amer. 1976; 56:1169.

21. Blackburn GL et al: Nutritional and metabolic assessment of the hospitalized patient. J Parenteral Enteral Nutr. 1977; 1:11.

22. Blackburn GL et al: Nutritional assessment of the hospitalized patient. Med Clin North Amer. 1979; 63:1103.

23. MacKenzie T et al: Clinical assessment of nutritional status using nitrogen balance. Fed Proc. 1974; 33:683.

24. Forse RA et al: Serum albumin and nutritional status. J Parenteral Enteral Nutr. 1980; 4:450.

25. Smith M et al: Transferrin as a measure of the efficiency of parenteral and enteral nutrition. J Parenteral Enteral Nutr. 1979; 1:9.

26. Bistrian B et al: Cellular immunity in adult marasmus. Arch Intern Med. 1977; 137:1408.

27. Johnson C et al: Parenteral hyperalimentation. Drug Intell Clin Pharm. 1975; 9:493.

28. Brennan MF et al: Glycerol: major contributor to the short term protein sparing effect of fat emulsions. Ann Surg. 1975; 182:386.

29. Cahill GF et al: Hormone-fuel interrelationships during fasting. J Clin Invest. 1966; 45:1751.

30. Loomis WF et al: Reversible inhibition of the coupling between phosphorylation and oxidation. J Biol Chem. 1975; 250:290.

31. Lipman F: Mechanism of peptide bond formation. Fed Proc. 1949; 8:597.

32. O'Connell RC et al: Nitrogen conservation in starvation: graded responses in intravenous glucose. J Clin Endocrinol Metab. 1974; 39:555.

33. Rothschild MA et al: Albumin synthesis. N Engl J Med. 1972; 286:749.

34. MacFayden BV et al: Clinical and biochemical changes in liver function during intravenous hyperalimentation. J Parenteral Enteral Nutr. 1979; 3:438.

35. Lindor KD et al: Liver function values in adults receiving total parenteral nutrition. JAMA. 1978; 241:984.

36. Sondheimer JM et al: Cholestatic tendencies in premature infants on and off total parenteral nutrition. Pediatrics. 1978; 62:984.

37. Askanazi J et al: Influence of total parenteral nutrition on fuel utilization in injury and sepsis. Ann Surg. 1980; 191:40.

38. Askanazi J et al: Respiratory changes induced by large glucose loads in total parenteral nutrition. JAMA. 1980; 243:1444.

39. Manery JF et al: The distribution of electrolytes in mammalian tissues. J Biol Chem. 1939; 127:657.

40. Moore FD et al: Energy and maintenance of the body cell mass. J Parenteral Enteral Nutr. 1980; 4:228.

41. Sebrell WH et al: *The Vitamins*, ed. 2, vol. 1–7. Academic Press, New York, 1978.

42. DeLuca HF: (ed.), *The Fat-Soluble Vitamins*, vol. 2, In: *The Handbook of Lipid Research*, Plenum Press, New York, 1978.

43. Hill GL et al: Malnutrition in surgical patients. An unrecognized problem. Lancet. 1977; 1:689.

44. Hull RL: Physicochemical considerations in intravenous hyperalimentation. Am J Hosp Pharm. 1974; 31:236.

45. Dahn M et al: The sepsis-glucose intolerance riddle: a hormonal explanation. Surgery. 1979; 86:423.

46. Chan JC et al: pH and titratable acidity of amino acid mixtures used in hyperalimentation. JAMA. 1972; 220:1119.

47. Chan JC et al: Hyperalimentation with amino acids and casein hydrolysate solutions: mechanisms of acidosis. JAMA. 1972; 220:1700.

48. Heird WC et al: Total parenteral nutrition: the state of the art. J Pediatr. 1975; 86:2.

49. Heird WC et al: Hyperammonemia resulting from intravenous alimentation using a mixture of synthetic L amino acids, a preliminary report. J Pediatr. 1972; 81:162.

50. Motil KJ et al: Complications of essential amino acid hyperalimentation in children with acute renal failure. J Parenteral Enteral Nutr. 1980; 4:32.

51. Kopple JD et al: Nitrogen balance and plasma amino acid levels in uremic patients fed an essential amino acid diet. Am J Clin Nutr. 1974; 27:806.

52. Abel RM et al: Intravenous essential amino acids and hypertonic dextrose in patients with acute renal failure. Am J Surg. 1972; 123:631.

53. Striebel JP et al: Parenteral nutrition and coma therapy with amino acids in hepatic failure. J Parenteral Enteral Nutr. 1979; 3:240.

54. Rosen HM et al: Plasma amino acid patterns in hepatic encephalopathy of differing etiology. Gastroenterology. 1977; 72:483.

55. Fischer JE et al: False neurotransmitters and hepatic failure. Lancet. 1971; 2:75.

56. Kerner JA et al: Parenteral alimentation. Semin Perinatol. 1979; 32:417.

57. Dweck HS et al: Glucose intolerance in infants of very low birth weight. Pediatrics. 1974; 53:189.

58. Cohen IT et al: Peripheral total parenteral nutrition employing a lipid emulsion (Intralipid): complications encountered in pediatric patients. J Pediatr Surg. 1977; 12:837.

59. Conners RH et al: Pediatric total parenteral nutrition; efficacy and toxicity of a new fat emulsion. J Parenteral Enteral Nutr. 1980; 4:384.

60. Schoefl GI: The ultrastructure of chylomicra and of the particles in an artificial fat emulsion. Proc R Soc Lond (Biol). 1968; 169:147.

61. Hallberg D: Elimination of exogenous lipids from the blood stream. An experimental methodological and clinical study in dog and man. Acta Physiol Scand. 1965; 65 (suppl 254): 1.

62. Rossner S et al: Elimination of parenterally administered fat. Studies on removal sites for Intralipid in normo- and hyperlipemic subjects. Acta Chir Scand Suppl. 1976; 466:56.

63. Erkelens DW et al: Availability of apoprotein CII in relation to the maximal removal capacity for an infused triglyceride emulsion in man. Metabolism. 1979; 28:495.

64. Shennan AT et al: The effects of gestational age on intralipid tolerance in newborn infants. Pediatrics. 1977; 91:134.

65. Wretlind A: Development of fat emulsions. J Parenteral Enteral Nutr. 1981; 5:230.

66. Bivins BA et al: Parenteral safflower oil emulsion. Ann Surg. 1980; 191:307.

67. Blackburn GL: Evaluation of safflower oil in the prevention biochemical changes of essential fatty acid deficiency in adult hospital patients receiving TPN. Liposyn Research Conference Proceedings, Abbott Laboratories, North Chicago, 1979.

68. Crawford MA: Essential fatty acid requirements in infancy. Am J Clin Nutr. 1978; 31:2181.

69. Bistrian B et al: Low plasma cortisol and hematologic abnormalities associated with essential fatty acid deficiency in man. J Parenteral Enteral Nutr. 1981; 5:141.

70. Stern TP et al: Essential fatty acid deficiency in patients receiving simultaneous parenteral and oral nutrition. J Parenteral Enteral Nutr. 1980; 4:343.

71. Wolfram G et al: Factors influencing essential fatty acid requirement in TPN. J Parenteral Enteral Nutr. 1978; 2:634.

72. Holman RT: Essential fatty acid deficiency. In: *Progress in the Chemistry of Fats and Other Lipids*, 9, part 2. Pergamon Press, Oxford, 1968; p 329.

73. O'Neill JA et al: Essential fatty acid deficiency in surgical patients. Ann Surg. 1977; 185:535.

74. Hallberg D et al: Experimental and clinical studies with fat emulsion for intravenous nutrition. Nutr Dieta. 1966; 8:245.

75. Black CD et al: Stability of intravenous fat emulsions. Arch Surg. 1980; 115:891.

76. Friedman Z et al: Effect of parenteral fat emulsion of the pulmonary and reticuloendothelial system in the newborn infant. Pediatrics. 1978; 61:694.

77. Shenkin A et al: Parenteral nutrition. World Rev Nutr Dietet. 1978; 28:1.

78. Bierman EL et al: Transport and metabolism of triglycerides and fatty acids. In: *Fat Emulsions in Parenteral Nutrition.* American Medical Association, Chicago, 1977.

79. Belin RP et al: Fat overload with 10% soybean oil emulsion. Arch Surg. 1976; 111:1391.

80. Sasaki H et al: Toxicity testing of fat emulsions II. Ultrastructure changes in the liver following administration of a new intravenous fat emulsion (Intralipid). Am J Clin Nutr. 1965; 16:37.

81. Tinoco ET et al: Linolenic acid deficiency. Lipids. 1979; 14:166.

82. Schroeder HA et al: Trace element analysis in clinical chemistry. Clin Chem. 1971; 17:461.

83. O'Dell B: Dietary factors that affect biological availability of trace elements. Ann NY Acad. 1972; 199:70.

84. Askari A et al: Zinc, copper and parenteral nutrition in cancer. J Parenteral Enteral Nutr. 1980; 4:561.

85. Ulmer D: Trace elements. N Engl J Med. 1977; 297:318.

86. Evans GW: Zinc absorption and transport. D Oberleas (ed.) *Trace Elements in Human Health and Disease*, vol 2, Academic Press, New York, 1976; p 186.

87. Anon: Guidelines for essential trace elements. Preparations for parenteral use. JAMA. 1979; 241:2051.

88. Matseshe JW et al: Recovery of dietary iron and zinc from the proximal intestine of healthy man: studies of different meals and supplements. Am J Clin Nutr. 1980; 33:1946.

89. Sandstrom B et al: Zinc absorption from composite meals. II. Influence of the main protein source. Am J Clin Nutr. 1980; 33:1778.

90. Solomon MW et al: The interaction of Vitamin A and zinc: implications for human nutrition. Am J Clin Nutr. 1979; 33:2031.

91. Burch R et al: Newer aspects of the roles of zinc, manganese and copper in human nutrition. Clin Chem. 1975; 21:501.

92. Solomon NW: On the assessment of trace mineral nutrition in patients on total parenteral nutrition. Nutr Suppl Serv. 1981; 1:13.

93. Kay RG et al: A syndrome of acute zinc deficiency during total parenteral nutrition in man. Ann Surg. 1976; 183:331.

94. Canfield WK et al: Plasma zinc values in children recovering from protein-calorie malnutrition. J Pediatr. 1980; 97:87.

95. Latimer JS et al: Clinical zinc deficiency during zinc supplemented total parenteral nutrition. J Pediatr. 1980; 97:434.

96. Lowry SF et al: Abnormalities of zinc and copper during total parenteral nutrition. Ann Surg. 1979; 189:120.

97. Wolman SL et al: Zinc in total parenteral nutrition. Requirements and metabolic effects. Gastroenterology. 1979; 76:458.

98. Casper RC et al: An evaluation of trace metals, vitamins and taste functions in anorexia nervosa. Am J Clin Nutr. 1980; 33:1801.

99. Sternlieb L: Copper and the liver. Gastroenterology. 1979; 78:1615.

100. Hull R: Use of trace elements in total parenteral nutrition. Am J Hosp Pharm. 1974; 31:759.

101. Taper JL et al: Effects of zinc uptake on copper balance in adult females. Am J Clin Nutr. 1980; 33:1077.

102. Jeejeebhoy KN et al: Chromium deficiency, glucose intolerance and neuropathy reversed by chromium supplementation in patient receiving long term parenteral nutrition. Am J Clin Nutr. 1977; 30:531.

103. Van Rij AM et at: Selenium and total parenteral nutrition. J Parenteral Enteral Nutr. 1979; 3:235.

104. Van Rij AM et al: Selenium supplementation in total parenteral nutrition. J Parenteral Enteral Nutr. 1981; 5:120.

105. Geoyer G: Acute intravenous zinc poisoning. Br Med J. May 28, 1979; p 1390.

106. Bogden JD et al: Elevated plasma zinc concentration in renal dialysis patients. Am J Clin Nutr, 1980; 33:1088.

107. Heymsfield SB et al: Enteral hyperalimentation: an alternative to central venous hyperalimentation. Ann Int Med. 1979; 90:63.

108. Page CP et al: Safe, cost effective postoperative nutrition. Defined formula diet via needle-catheter jejunostomy. Am J Surg. 1979; 138:939.

109. Heitkemper ME et al: Rate and volume of intermittent enteral feeding. J Parenteral Enteral Nutr. 1981; 5:125.

110. Silk DB et al: Use of a peptide rather than free amino acid nitrogen source in chemically defined "elemental" diets. J Parenteral Enteral Nutr. 1980; 4:548.

110. Sleisenger MH et al: Protein digestion and absorption. N Engl J Med. 1979; 300:659.

111. Hoover HC et al: Nutritional benefits of immediate postoperative feeding of an elemental diet. Am J Surg. 1980; 139:153.

112. Moss G: Maintenance of gastrointestinal function after bowel surgery and immediate enteral full nutrition. II. Clinical experience, with objective demonstration of intestinal absorption and motility. J Parenteral Enteral Nutr. 1981; 5:215.

113. Shin CS et al: Early morphologic changes in the intestine following massive resection of the small intestine and parenteral nutrition therapy. Surg Gyn Obstet. 1980; 151:246.

114. Keith RG: Effect of a low fat elemental diet on pancreatic secretion during pancreatitis. Surg Gyn Obstet. 1980; 151:337.

115. Bondy RA et al: Comparison of two commercial low residue diets and a low residue diet of common foods. J Parenteral Enteral Nutr. 1979; 3:226.

116. Wingert TD et al: Insulin absorption to an air-eliminating in-line filter. Am J Hosp Pharm. 1981; 38:382.

117. Weber SS et al: Availability of insulin from parenteral nutrient solutions. Am J Hosp Pharm. 1977; 34:353.

118. Eggert LD et al: Calcium and phosphate compatibility in parenteral nutrition solutions for neonates. Am J Hosp Pharm. 1982; 39:49.

119. Gazitua R et al: Factors determining peripheral vein tolerance to amino acid infusions. Arch Surg. 1979; 114:897.

120. Mirtallo JM et al: A comparison of essential and general amino acid infusions in the nutritional support of patients with compromised renal function. J Parenteral Enteral Nutr. 1982; 6:109.

121. Seashore JH et al: Hyperammonemia during total parenteral nutrition in children. J Parenteral Enteral Nutr. 1982; 6:114.

122. Wilkinson WR et al: Growth of microorganisms in parenteral nutritional fluids. Drug Intell Clin Pharm. 1973; 7:226.

Chapter 31

Hyperlipidemias

— Ralph H. Raasch —

Metabolism and Classification of Lipoproteins

Hyperlipidemia or hyperlipoproteinemia are terms used to describe an increased plasma lipid concentration of cholesterol and/or triglyceride. The terms are often used synonymously since lipids are not freely soluble and are carried by proteins in the circulation. Lipoproteins have been classified based upon their electrophoretic and ultracentrifugation characteristics (1).

There are five classes of lipoprotein based upon ultracentrifugation or density characteristics: chylomicrons, very low density lipoproteins (VLDL), intermediate density lipoproteins (IDL), low density lipoproteins (LDL), and high density lipoproteins (HDL). The corresponding electrophoretic mobility and major lipid constituents of these lipoproteins are summarized in Table 1 (2,3).

Elevation of the serum cholesterol, triglyceride, or both, occurs secondary to increases in the various lipoproteins. A system of phenotyping lipoprotein elevations has been established depending upon which lipoprotein is increased. These lipoprotein phenotypes and the general ranges of elevation of plasma cholesterol and triglyceride are summarized in Table 2 (4).

Dietary fat is hydrolyzed in the small intestine into the major breakdown products, fatty acids and monoglycerides. These are then incorporated by the absorptive cells of the gut into chylomicrons, the large, triglyceride-rich lipoproteins. The chylomicrons are secreted into the lymphatic system and eventually reach the plasma. Triglyceride may also be synthesized in the liver from free fatty acids, glucose, or acetate. This "endogenous" triglyceride is combined with phospholipid, unesterified cholesterol, and protein and secreted into hepatic venous blood as VLDL.

Triglyceride in chylomicrons and VLDL is transported to adipose tissue and muscle for storage and utilization. The activity of lipoprotein lipase, which catalyzes triglyceride uptake by adipose tissue and skeletal muscle, is enhanced by insulin secretion during and after meals. With the loss of triglyceride to adipose tissue and muscle, a lipoprotein of intermediate density (IDL) remains in the plasma. This lipoprotein has also

Table 1.

CLASSIFICATION AND COMPOSITION OF PLASMA LIPOPROTEINS

Lipoprotein Class	Density (gm/ml)	Electrophoretic Mobility	Major Lipid Constituents
Chylomicrons	< 0.95	Origin	Dietary triglyceride
VLDL	0.95–1.006	Prebeta	Endogenous triglyceride
IDL	1.006–1.019	Slow prebeta or broad beta	Cholesterol ester, triglycerides
LDL	1.019–1.063	Beta	Cholesterol ester
HDL	1.063–1.210	Alpha	Cholesterol ester

Table 2.

CLASSIFICATION OF HYPERLIPOPROTEINEMIA

Lipoprotein Phenotype	Lipoprotein Elevated	Plasma Cholesterol	Plasma Triglyceride
TYPE I	Chylomicrons	< 300 mg%	> 1000 mg%
TYPE IIa	LDL	> 240 mg%	< 160 mg%
TYPE IIb	VLDL, LDL	> 240 mg%	> 160 mg%
TYPE III	IDL	> 240 mg%	> 160 mg%
TYPE IV	VLDL	< 300 mg%	160–1000 mg%
TYPE V	VLDL, Chylomicrons	< 240 mg%	> 1000 mg%

been called a remnant particle. The remnant appears to be taken up quickly by the liver where it is converted to the cholesterol-rich LDL. The liver removes further triglyceride as well as some cholesterol and surface proteins in converting the remnant to LDL.

Extrahepatic tissues remove LDL from the plasma and use the lipoprotein as the chief cholesterol source for membrane synthesis. An LDL surface protein, apoprotein B, appears to be specifically bound to the cell surface of extrahepatic tissue. The LDL is then absorbed by the cell in an endocytotic vesicle, and the cholesterol ester is hydrolyzed to unesterified cholesterol which is used in membrane synthesis. A feedback system regulates LDL uptake by the cell so that the presence of intracellular free cholesterol inhibits further uptake of LDL as well as endogenous cholesterol synthesis.

High-density lipoproteins (HDL) are synthesized in the liver and primarily contain phospholipids and apoproteins. The lipid-poor HDL carry phospholipid and unesterified cholesterol from the surface of chylomicrons and VLDL as the triglyceride cores of these lipoproteins are being metabolized; the liver then removes cholesterol from HDL. HDL may also enhance the release of free cholesterol from extrahepatic tissues. Hence, HDL transports cholesterol from cells to the liver for excretion (1,2,5).

Diagnosis

There are two major diagnostic procedures used to place patients into specific lipoprotein phenotypes. The first is to measure a serum triglyceride and serum cholesterol concentration. The second is to place the patient's plasma sample in the refrigerator for twelve hours and observe its appearance.

Plasma triglycerides should be measured at least 10–12 hours after the ingestion of a meal, since the dietary triglycerides carried by the chylomicrons will not be completely metabolized for that period of time. In contrast to the triglyceride concentration, serum cholesterol levels are not greatly altered by the cholesterol or triglyceride content of meals (5).

The appearance of the plasma differs following refrigeration depending upon the specific type of lipoprotein which is elevated. For example, in patients with hyperchylomicronemia, a creamy layer will appear at the top of the sample. In contrast, an increase in VLDL will produce uniform turbidity of the plasma. Other lipoprotein phenotypes produce clear plasmas or a combination of a turbid plasma with a creamy supernatant. Table 3 summarizes the appearances of refrigerated plasma for each of the lipoprotein phenotypes. Since it may not be possible to distinguish between types IIb, III, and IV on the basis of appearance alone, it is important to use the serum triglyceride and cholesterol levels in conjunction to place the patient into the correct phenotypic group. This step is critical to the selection of therapy (1,6).

Hyperlipidemia secondary to various diseases generally resolves if the primary disease is treated appropriately. Increased serum cholesterol and LDL levels occur in hypothyroidism, nephrotic syndrome, and following an excessive and sustained intake of cholesterol and saturated fats (7–9). Hypercholesterolemia can also be caused by the commonly-used thiazide diuretics (10); how-ever, this increase is generally minimal (10%) and can be prevented by a low cholesterol diet.

Hypertriglyceridemia and increased levels of VLDL are associated with obesity and can occur in patients with chronic renal failure, hypothyroidism, and diabetes mellitus (11–14). Chronic alcohol ingestion and therapy with estrogens, oral contraceptives, or glucocorticoids may also be responsible for elevated triglyceride levels (15–17).

The pathological consequences of hyperlipidemia are an increased incidence of atherosclerosis and an increased risk of coronary heart disease. The bulk of evidence indicates that there is a positive correlation between dietary fat intake, serum cholesterol concentrations and the incidence of atherosclerosis and coronary heart disease in middle-aged men (18–22). Occasional studies and reviews question this correlation engendering debate regarding the importance of a low cholesterol diet in the treatment of coronary heart disease (23,24). A positive correlation between hypertriglyceridemia and coronary heart disease is much weaker than that between elevated cholesterol levels and heart disease (25). Other risk factors for coronary heart disease include age, sex, hypertension, diabetes, and smoking.

As indicated in Table 1, most serum cholesterol is found in LDL and HDL. However, in most early studies that assessed cholesterol levels and coronary heart disease, the cholesterol was not separated into LDL- and HDL-cholesterol. Two-thirds of serum cholesterol is usually carried in LDL, and there is a close correlation between total cholesterol and LDL-cholesterol. The importance of differentiating LDL-cholesterol from HDL-cholesterol is that there is a strong correlation between HDL-cholesterol levels and the *absence* of coronary heart disease (26). Women, middle-aged men who exercise, and non-smokers have higher HDL-cholesterol than comparable male smokers who do not regularly exercise. Obesity and diabetes are associated with lower-than-average HDL-cholesterol levels as well (27–30). Interestingly, alcohol ingestion is associated with increased HDL-cholesterol levels, although this does not necessarily mean coronary heart disease is reduced by alcohol intake (31,32).

Based upon these considerations, the goals of therapy are to lower the serum cholesterol (preferably LDL-cholesterol) and triglyceride concentrations, and perhaps raise HDL-cholesterol levels, in hopes that a decrease in the incidence of cardiovascular death might result (33). A variety

Table 3.

PLASMA APPEARANCE IN HYPERLIPOPROTEINEMIA

Lipoprotein Phenotype	Appearance, 12 hours at 4°C
I	Creamy supernatant with clear infranatant
IIa	Clear
IIb	Uniform turbidity
III	Uniform turbidity; creamy supernatant may also be present
IV	Uniform turbidity
V	Creamy supernatant with turbid infranatant

Table 4.

SUMMARY OF SELECTED DRUGS USED IN HYPERLIPIDEMIA

Drug	Effect on Serum Lipids	Primary Indication	Mechanism	Dosage	Side Effects
Sitosterol (34–36)	Decreases cholesterol 10–15% with diet	Mild Type IIa	Decreases cholesterol absorption	3 gm daily	Nausea, diarrhea.
Probucol (37–39)	Decreases cholesterol 12–25% with diet	Mild Type IIa	Decreases cholesterol synthesis; increases excretion of bile acids	500 mg bid with meals	Increased triglyceride, diarrhea, flatulence (ventricular fibrillation reported in dogs, not in man).
Dextrothyroxine (40,41)	Decreases cholesterol 10–20% with diet	Mild Type IIa	Increases cholesterol catabolism	4–8 mg daily	Angina, tachycardia.
Clofibrate (42–45)	Decreases triglyceride and cholesterol 5–10% with diet	Types III, IV, V	Decreases free fatty acids; increases biliary, fecal cholesterol; decreases VLDL synthesis	1 gm bid	Gallstones, nausea, myositis, hepatomegaly.
Niacin (43,46–48)	Decreases triglyceride and cholesterol 10–20% with diet	Types II, III, IV, V	Decreases hepatic production of triglycerides and VLDL	0.25 gm tid increased to 2.5 gm tid with meals	Flushing, urticaria, anorexia, hyperglycemia, peptic ulceration, jaundice, hyperuricemia.
Cholestyramine (49–52)	Decreases cholesterol 20–40% with diet	Type IIa and IIb	Increases bile salt formation from cholesterol; increases LDL catabolism	4 gm tid ac initially, 4 gm qid (ac&hs) maintenance	Constipation, flatulence, nausea, heartburn. Increased triglyceride levels.
Colestipol (53–55)	Decreases cholesterol 16–40% with diet	Type IIa and IIb	Increases bile salt formation from cholesterol	15–30 gm per day, given bid to qid	Constipation, nausea, flatulence, increased triglyceride levels.

of dietary and drug regimens are available for use. However, certain drugs are more effective than others in specific hyperlipidemias. The drugs used to treat hyperlipidemias are summarized in Table 4.

HYPERCHOLESTEROLEMIA

1. C.R. is a 45-year-old, 75 kg male who has noticed the appearance, over the past several months, of intermittent chest pain which is worsened by exercise and relieved by rest. He is a moderately active business-man who smokes 1–2 packs of cigarettes per day and drinks alcoholic beverages several times per week. Physical examination is re-markable for small nodular swellings on both elbows. His father died at age 62 as a result of a myocardial infarction, and his mother is alive at age 65 but suffers from mild diabetes mellitus. Pertinent laboratory data obtained after an overnight fast include: fasting plasma glucose 105 mg/dl (normal 65–115 mg/dl), serum albumin 4.5 gm/dl (normal 3.5–5.0 gm/dl), total protein 7.5 gm/dl (normal 6.5–8.3 gm/dl), serum thyroxine 7.5 mcg/dl (normal 4.5–11.5 mcg/dl), resin T_3 uptake 43% (normal 35–45%), serum cholesterol 360 mg/dl (normal 130–230 mg/dl), serum triglyceride 140 mg/dl (normal < 160 mg/dl), and trace urine protein. A plasma sample left in the refrigerator over-night appears clear. Other laboratory data are within normal limits. He takes no medi-cations with the exception of over-the-counter analgesics for occasional headaches. How should C.R.'s hyperlipidemia be classified?

Several considerations should be made when classifying elevated lipid levels into the lipopro-tein phenotypes. First, since C.R. had blood drawn for lipid determination after an overnight fast, it is unlikely that the concentrations obtained were influenced by a recent meal. Since serum choles-terol levels are not raised by a previous meal, this is only a serious consideration when serum tri-glyceride levels are elevated. Secondly, there is no evidence that C.R. has a secondary hypercho-lesterolemia due to hypothyroidism or nephrotic syndrome since his thyroid function tests and plasma and urine proteins are normal. However, there is the possibility that large intakes of di-etary cholesterol may be increasing his serum cholesterol concentration (56).

After ruling out the above possibilities, the elevated serum cholesterol, the normal serum tri-glyceride, and the clear refrigerated plasma sam-ple are consistent with Type IIa hyperlipoprotein-emia. If a serum electrophoresis were done (not routinely suggested), it is likely that an increased amount of LDL would be observed.

In the absence of evidence for a secondary hy-percholesterolemia in C.R., a primary or genetic hypercholesterolemia should be considered. Pri-mary disease occurs secondary to an alteration in a single gene (monogenic familial hypercholes-terolemia), or several genes (polygenic hypercho-lesterolemia, familial combined hyperlipidemia). Familial hypercholesterolemia is inherited as an autosomal dominant disorder which affects the extrahepatic cellular receptor for LDL. As a re-sult, endogenous cholesterol synthesis is not sup-pressed by the cellular uptake of LDL-choles-terol, and hypercholesterolemia occurs. The heterozygous patient has approximately 50% nor-mal and 50% abnormal LDL-receptors, resulting in a serum cholesterol level two to three times normal. In the rare homozygous patient, LDL-receptors are nearly absent, causing severe hy-percholesterolemia (>600 mg/dl). A family dis-tribution of hypercholesterolemia consistent with an autosomal dominant disorder (50% of first-degree relatives) and the presence of tendon xan-thomas, xanthelasmas, and arcus corneae are ob-served in familial hypercholesterolemia (5,57). The small nodular swellings on C.R.'s elbows are pos-sibly tendon xanthomas. As is often the case, an insufficient knowledge of the cholesterol levels of relatives exists here, but C.R.'s father died of car-diovascular disease. It is very possible that C.R. has a monogenic familial hypercholesterolemia.

The polygenic hyperlipidemias account for the elevated cholesterol levels in 5% of the general population. The precise etiology is unknown, but the hypercholesterolemia is probably related to multiple genetic and environmental factors. Pa-tients with the polygenic disorder usually do not present with physical signs of increased choles-terol (xanthomas, etc.), and no more than 10% of first-degree relatives are affected. Because C.R. does have physical signs of increased cholesterol excess, it is unlikely that his hypercholesterole-mia is of the polygenic type (57).

2. Will treating and lowering the total serum cholesterol concentration reduce C.R.'s chance of suffering from severe coronary

**heart disease? How can the serum choles-
terol level be lowered?**

Several studies indicate that a statistically
significant reduction of non-fatal myocardial infarction occurs with a 10% lowering of serum cholesterol, but a significant reduction in total mortality rate has not been observed.

Even though vegetarian diets or low cholesterol, low saturated fat diets decrease serum cholesterol levels (58,59), they do not significantly
reduce the incidence of coronary heart disease
compared to the normal, unmodified diet. However, within the population studied, there is a
nonstatistical association between a low cholesterol diet and decreased incidence of coronary heart
disease (60–63).

The addition of various cholesterol-lowering
drugs such as clofibrate or niacin to dietary treatment has not been demonstrated to significantly
lower overall mortality when compared to diet
plus placebo. However, lowering cholesterol levels with these drugs does appear to significantly
reduce the incidence of non-fatal myocardial infarction. An unexpected finding of one of these
studies (64) was an increase in deaths from all
causes in the patient groups receiving clofibrate
compared to patients receiving placebo (43,64–
67).

Based upon the available information, it would
appear reasonable to lower C.R.'s serum cholesterol in an attempt to reduce his chances of suffering a non-fatal myocardial infarction. Clofibrate should be avoided.

**3. What are reasonable treatment goals for
C.R. in terms of desired cholesterol or triglyceride concentrations? How often should
these concentrations be assessed?**

The goal of therapy for C.R. is to lower the
serum cholesterol levels to 230 mg/dl or less without raising the triglyceride concentration. Four
weeks is usually sufficient for any form of dietary
or drug therapy to produce a maximal effect on
plasma lipid concentrations. Therefore, fasting
lipid levels should initially be assessed at monthly
intervals and the treatment regimen changed if
necessary. Once the therapeutic goal has been
achieved, levels can be reassessed every three to
six months (33).

**4. What dietary modifications should be
made to treat C.R.'s hyperlipidemia? Is dietary management sufficient for C.R.?**

Dietary modification is the initial therapy of
choice for C.R.'s hypercholesterolemia. Restriction of dietary cholesterol to less than 300 mg per
day (equivalent to 1½ eggs), reduction in dietary
saturated fat to 10% of total caloric intake, and
increasing unsaturated fat intake to 15–20% of
total caloric intake are the general recommendations for reducing serum cholesterol (68). A diet
of this type involves the use of fish, shellfish,
poultry, and veal rather than beef, lamb, ham, or
pork, and substitutes vegetable oils for animal
fat. Serum cholesterol levels may decrease by 10–
15% when this diet is followed by hypercholesterolemic patients for at least twelve weeks; however, this diet therapy may not always reduce
cholesterol levels significantly (38,69). Advice from
a dietitian can be very helpful in devising a diet
that the patient will follow.

If C.R. responds like the average patient to dietary therapy, with a 10% reduction in his serum
cholesterol concentration (to 320 mg/dl), he would
still have significant hypercholesterolemia.
Therefore, dietary therapy alone is not likely to
reduce serum cholesterol adequately, and drug
therapy in addition to diet appears necessary in
this case. Because C.R. has signs of atherosclerotic disease (angina-like chest pain), a family
history of heart disease, and he smokes, the use
of drugs in addition to diet is indicated (33).

**5. What would be the most rational drug
therapy for C.R.?**

Table 4 lists the drugs which alter serum lipid
and lipoprotein levels. When combined with dietary therapy, the total reduction in cholesterol
concentration averages 10–15% with beta-sitosterol (70) and up to 20–40% with cholestyramine
or colestipol (49,50,53). (See Table 4.) The cholesterol-lowering capability of the other agents indicated for Type IIa hyperlipoproteinemia is generally between these percentages.

At this point, a brief consideration of the potential toxic effects of these drugs in C.R. should
be made. Dextrothyroxine was associated with an
increase in mortality rate in patients with angina
pectoris in the Coronary Drug Project (41). C.R.'s
chest pain is consistent with angina, so dextrothyroxine should be avoided if possible. Niacin in
the necessary dosage of 1–2.5 gm tid consistently
causes flushing of the skin which may persist with
continued treatment (71). Although not officially
approved for hypercholesterolemia, neomycin can

reduce cholesterol by 20% when combined with diet (72); however, its potential for severe toxicity with long-term use makes it unacceptable for use as an initial agent (73–75). This reluctance to use neomycin more frequently has been criticized (76).

Because the magnitude of serum cholesterol reduction is generally greatest with the bile salt binding resins (cholestyramine, colestipol), they are the most rational drugs to use in C.R. However, a reasonable argument can be made for the use of probucol because it is easily administered compared to the resins, and this may improve compliance. Both cholestyramine and colestipol bind bile salts, interrupting their enterohepatic circulation. This in turn stimulates an increased bile salt formation from cholesterol (51,55). Cholestyramine has also been shown to increase the catabolism of LDL via a mechanism involving the binding of LDL to cellular receptors (52). Both drugs given in adequate dosage are equally effective in lowering serum cholesterol and LDL (77). Since colestipol is odorless and tasteless compared to cholestyramine, colestipol would be the bile salt binding resin of choice initially. However, colestipol may be slightly more expensive than cholestyramine.

6. What information should be given to C.R. regarding his bile acid sequestrant therapy?

Both colestipol and cholestyramine are available in dry powder form and must be hydrated before ingestion. This can be done by adding the powder to at least 120 ml water (for cholestyramine, the powder should be placed on the surface to allow hydration without clumping), soups, or fruit preparations with high fluid content.

Colestipol should be taken before meals (dosage is usually 10 gm, or 2 packets bid). Twice daily dosing is usually as effective as administration three or four times a day and is more likely to result in compliance (78). These resins occasionally cause bloating and constipation which can be controlled by a stool softener or by the addition of bran to the diet (54). The medication should not be taken dry (79).

7. If C.R. responds to the colestipol and diet therapy, it is likely that he will be maintained on this regimen indefinitely. What complications of chronic colestipol therapy should be anticipated?

In addition to decreasing the serum cholesterol

and LDL-cholesterol, bile salt sequestrants also increase VLDL-triglyceride and HDL-triglyceride. However, this effect on the triglyceride level is usually transient and of greatest magnitude in patients whose serum triglyceride levels are elevated prior to therapy (54,77,80). Therefore, bile salt sequestrant therapy in patients with Type IIb hyperlipidemia (increased serum cholesterol and triglyceride) may induce severe hypertriglyceridemia. Since C.R. has normal triglycerides, this potential adverse effect is unlikely to be significant.

Chronic bile salt sequestrant therapy may alter the absorption of nutrients and other drugs. Serum folate levels may be reduced in children, but serum concentrations of vitamins A, E, D, and K do not change significantly (81). Reports of vitamin K deficiency in adults (hypoprothrombinemia) due to cholestyramine have appeared (82), but bleeding as a complication is probably only significant when there is concurrent liver disease (83). Because C.R. is on an adequate diet to help control his hypercholesterolemia, it is unlikely that he will develop nutrient deficiencies due to colestipol or cholestyramine unless he develops liver disease. In children, periodic folate levels should be monitored and folate supplementation should be given (1 mg/day) if necessary (84).

Cholestyramine and colestipol have been reported to alter the absorption or enterohepatic circulation of warfarin (85), digitoxin (86), chlorothiazide (87), thyroxine (88), and iron (89), resulting in decreased absorption and increased fecal excretion of these drugs. No consistent effect on serum digoxin levels has been observed (90), and blood levels of clofibrate have been unaltered by the concurrent ingestion of colestipol (93). In general, other drugs should be taken at least one hour before or four hours after cholestyramine or colestipol administration to reduce the risk of an interaction. If an oral medication is prescribed for C.R., this recommendation should be made.

8. After a six-month trial of diet and colestipol, C.R.'s cholesterol level is 270 mg/dl and his fasting triglyceride level has increased to 210 mg/dl despite close adherence to therapy. How should he be managed at this point?

Several studies have demonstrated that the addition of a second lipid-lowering drug to diet and cholestyramine or colestipol therapy can further reduce serum cholesterol. The addition of clofibrate caused a total cholesterol reduction of 28% compared to a range of 16–25% with diet-colestipol alone. Niacin, however, caused a total reduction of cholesterol from 45–47% when added to a diet plus colestipol regimen (54,91). When cholestyramine was added to a diet plus probucol regimen, the average decrease in serum cholesterol was raised from 7.7% to 18.2% (92). Niacin and clofibrate will also decrease the elevated serum triglyceride levels caused by bile salt sequestrant therapy (54).

Because cholesterol is lowered to the greatest extent by the addition of niacin, a combined regimen of diet, colestipol and niacin is the most appropriate management at this point. The colestipol dosage can be maximized to 30 gm per day (10 gm tid or 15 gm bid) and niacin can be initiated at a dose of 250–300 mg tid with meals. The niacin dose can be increased every two to four weeks as tolerated until a usual total daily dose of 6–8 gm is reached (54,91).

9. Common side effects associated with niacin therapy include cutaneous flushing and increases in liver function tests (aspartate aminotransferase, alkaline phosphatase). What measures can be taken to minimize these side effects?

Niacin-induced cutaneous flushing is caused by prostaglandin release (94); therefore, prostaglandin synthetase inhibitors have been used to reduce this side effect. Small doses of aspirin (from 120–300 mg) taken one-half hour before niacin ingestion have been noted to cause a marked diminution in flushing (54,91).

Increases in liver function tests are associated with the rate at which the daily niacin dose is increased as well as the total daily dose. Increases in aspartate aminotransferase and alkaline phosphatase were noted when daily doses of niacin were increased by more than 2.5 gm per month. For example, abnormal liver function tests occurred if dose was increased from 1 gm tid to 2 gm tid (daily dose increase >2.5 gm) in less than one month (54). A total daily dose of greater than 6.0–7.5 gm/day for prolonged periods also increases the risk of hepatotoxicity (54,91).

Other side effects of niacin therapy, such as hyperglycemia and hyperuricemia, should be assessed with appropriate laboratory tests every three to six months.

HYPERTRIGLYCERIDEMIA

10. S.L. is a 54-year-old, 65 kg female who was in good health until diabetes was diagnosed six months ago. When the diagnosis was made, she weighed 75 kg and her initial treatment regimen was with diet. Insulin therapy was added three months after diagnosis. She is 5 feet, 2 inches tall.

Laboratory data noted in her initial workup included the following: fasting plasma glucose 350 mg/dl (normal < 115 mg/dl), urine glucose 1–2%, serum albumin 4.0 gm/dl (normal 3.5–5.0 gm/dl), serum cholesterol 160 mg/dl (normal 130–230 mg/dl), serum triglyceride 650 mg/dl (normal < 160 mg/dl). Serum electrolytes, BUN, creatinine, and thyroid function tests were within normal limits. On follow-up examination, the fasting plasma glucose had fallen to 140 mg/dl as a result of treatment, but several subsequent fasting triglyceride levels remained elevated at 300 mg/dl. A refrigerated plasma sample was turbid.

Her medication history is negative for estrogen, corticosteroid, oral contraceptive, or thyroid replacement therapy. Treatment to lower the triglyceride level is under consideration. What are the effects of obesity and diabetes on S.L.'s serum triglyceride levels?

Elevated serum triglyceride levels can be caused by increased levels of VLDL, chylomicrons, or a combination of the two. As discussed previously, triglycerides are normally elevated postprandially secondary to increased chylomicron levels. Increased levels of VLDL most commonly account for a clinical picture characterized by moderately elevated fasting triglyceride levels in the presence of normal cholesterol levels (Type IV). The turbid appearance of S.L.'s refrigerated plasma without a creamy top layer indicates that her plasma triglyceride levels are elevated secondary to an elevated VLDL. This is generally related to a genetic predisposition for the overproduction of triglyceride-rich VLDL by the liver. Overproduction is also stimulated by high carbohydrate diets, obesity, hyperinsulinism, estrogens, and excessive alcohol consumption (5,95,96). A genetically determined decreased catabolism of VLDL (decreased lipoprotein lipase activity) may also account for an elevated triglyceride level. Decreased catabolism may also be present in diabetics who are insulin deficient, since insulin enhances the activity of lipoprotein lipase (5). Other causes of decreased catabolism include hypothyroidism, azotemia, and nephrotic syndrome (12, 13,97).

S.L.'s obesity and adult onset diabetes are associated with hyperinsulinemia and are contributing factors to her hypertriglyceridemia. The fact that her triglycerides have remained elevated despite diabetic control and weight reduction indicates that she has familial or endogenous hypertriglyceridemia (Type IV) (15). Individuals with endogenous hypertriglyceridemia and diabetes will continue to have moderately elevated triglycerides (200–500 mg/dl) following diabetic treatment and control. Familial hypertriglyceridemia is not associated with an increased risk of diabetes; these two genetic disorders appear to be independent of one another (98).

11. Should S.L. be treated for her elevated triglyceride level?

Many investigators have claimed that elevated triglyceride levels contribute to an increased risk of coronary artery disease (99–101). However, the results of their studies have been questioned on the basis of poor methodology or lack of statistical adjustment for other risk factors in coronary artery disease. When the incidence of coronary artery disease is adjusted for other risk factors such as serum cholesterol, systolic blood pressure, cigarette smoking, and age, there is no statistically significant association between hypertriglyceridemia and coronary artery disease (25).

Because a direct link between hypertriglyceridemia and coronary artery disease is lacking, one could question whether treatment of an apparently healthy person with hypertriglyceridemia is rational. However, there is a reduced risk of coronary artery disease in individuals with elevated levels of HDL-cholesterol, and these are low in individuals such as S.L. with Type IV hyperlipidemia (102). There are many investigators now studying the treatment of Type IV hyperlipidemia to determine whether a reduction in the serum triglyceride is associated with an increased HDL-cholesterol and a concomitant decrease in coronary artery disease.

12. What is the effect of dietary treatment for Type IV hyperlipidemia on HDL-cholesterol levels?

Dietary therapy for Type IV hyperlipidemia is designed to achieve ideal body weight and to avoid excessive carbohydrate and alcohol intake. No more than 45% of the total caloric intake should be provided as carbohydrate, and equivalent amounts of polyunsaturated and saturated fat should be provided (103). S.L. should attempt to reduce her weight to approximately 50 kg.

The above dietary therapy may cause a reduction in plasma triglyceride by more than 50% (98,104). However, even though there is an inverse correlation between elevated plasma triglyceride and decreased HDL-cholesterol in untreated Type IV hyperlipidemia (102), dietary treatment that effectively lowers plasma triglyceride does not raise HDL-cholesterol (104). Theoretically, therefore, dietary therapy is unlikely to change the risk of coronary artery disease.

Since moderate alcohol consumption elevates HDL-cholesterol levels (31,32), it is questionable whether S.L. should eliminate alcohol from her diet. The elimination of alcohol from the diet will only result in lowered triglyceride levels if the patient consumes more than 8% of her calories as alcohol. Therefore, after a period of weight loss, alcohol may be allowed as long as it does not exceed 3–5% of her total caloric intake; this may raise the HDL-cholesterol concentrations (104).

13. Should S.L. be given clofibrate in addition to diet to further lower her plasma triglycerides and perhaps raise her HDL-cholesterol levels? What are the indications for clofibrate therapy?

Clofibrate (1 gm bid) may lower the serum triglyceride by as much as 40% over a period of 6 weeks in diabetics (106) and patients with Type IV hyperlipidemia (105) who are already on diet therapy. An increase in HDL-cholesterol is associated with this fall in triglycerides, but the absolute levels are still significantly lower than those found in normal controls (105). Unfortunately, this rise in HDL-cholesterol is apparently transient, because HDL-cholesterol levels return to baseline levels six months following the initiation of clofibrate (104).

Current studies do not strongly support the addition of clofibrate to diet in the treatment of Type IV hyperlipidemia. A lowering of triglyceride levels associated with an increase in HDL-cholesterol and a reduction in the risk of coronary artery disease has not been demonstrated. Since clofibrate therapy is also associated with some risk (43,44,64,107,108), its routine use in the treatment of Type IV hyperlipidemia cannot be advocated at this time.

In contrast, clofibrate is effective in lowering elevated triglyceride levels and elevating low HDL-cholesterol levels associated with chronic renal failure (109). Therapy is associated with relatively little toxicity as long as the dose of clofibrate is reduced to 1–1.5 gm weekly in divided doses (110). In this form of secondary hypertriglyceridemia, clofibrate increases lipoprotein lipase activity and thereby increases the clearance of triglyceride from circulating VLDL. Further investigation is necessary to determine whether these changes in lipoprotein levels will reduce the rate of mortality from cardiovascular disease in chronic renal failure patients on dialysis.

Clofibrate is also very effective in reversing the symptoms and clinical signs associated with the uncommon Type III hyperlipidemia (elevated IDL). HDL-cholesterol rises significantly secondary to clofibrate therapy in this type of disease (42). However, whether the increase in HDL-cholesterol reduces the consequences of the premature atherosclerosis associated with Type III hyperlipidemia remains to be determined.

References

1. Havel RJ: Classification of the hyperlipidemias. Ann Rev Med. 1977; 28:195.
2. Jackson RL et al: Lipoproteins and lipid transport: structural and functional concepts. In *Hyperlipidemia Diagnosis and Therapy*, edited by BM Rifkind and RI Levy, Grune & Stratton, New York, 1977; p 1.
3. Simons LA and Gibson JC: Lipids: *A Clinician's Guide*, University Park Press, Baltimore, 1980; p 1.
4. Ibid, p 53.
5. Brunzell JD et al: Pathophysiology of lipoprotein transport. Metabolism. 1978; 27:1109.
6. Yeshurun D et al: Drug treatment of hyperlipidemia. Am J Med. 1976; 60:379.
7. Mishkel MA et al: Hypothyroidism, an important cause of reversible hyperlipidemia. Clin Chem Acta. 1977; 74:139.
8. Spritz N et al: Effects of dietary fats on plasma lipids and lipoproteins: an hypothesis for the lipid-lowering effect of unsaturated fatty acids. J Clin Invest. 1969; 48:78.
9. Ibels LS et al: Studies in the nature and causes of hyperlipidemia in uremia, maintenance dialysis and renal transplantation. Quarterly J Med. 1975; 44:601.
10. Grimm RH et al: Effects of thiazide diuretics on plasma lipids and lipoproteins in mildly hypertensive patients. Ann Intern Med. 1981; 94:7.
11. Olefsky JM et al: Decreased insulin binding to adipocytes and circulating monocytes from obese subjects. J Clin Invest. 1976; 57:1165.
12. Bagdade JD et al: Hypertriglyceridemia: a metabolic consequence of chronic renal failure. N Engl J Med. 1968; 279:181.
13. Pykalisto OJ et al: Reversal of decreased human adipose tissue lipoprotein lipase and hypertriglyceridemia after treatment of hypothyroidism. J Clin Endocrinol Metab. 1976; 43:549.
14. Pykalisto OJ et al: Determinants of human adipose tissue lipoprotein lipase. Effect of diabetes and obesity on basal and diet-induced activity. J Clin Invest. 1975; 56:1108.
15. Lieber CS: Effects of ethanol upon lipid metabolism. Lipids. 1974; 9:103.
16. Hazzard WR et al: Estrogens and triglyceride transport: increased endogenous production as the mechanism for the hypertriglyceridemia of oral contraceptive therapy, in *Endocrinology*, Proc IV Int Cong of Endocrinology, Excerpta Medica, Amsterdam, 1973, p 1006.
17. El-Shaboury AM et al: Hyperlipidemia in asthmatic patients receiving long-term steroid therapy. Br Med J. 1973; 2:85.
18. Shekelle RB et al: Diet, serum cholesterol, and death from coronary heart disease. N Engl J Med. 1981; 304:65.
19. Mohley RW: The role of dietary fat and cholesterol in atherosclerosis and lipoprotein metabolism. West J Med. 1981; 134:34.
20. Gofman JW et al: Evaluation of serum lipoproteins and cholesterol measurements as predictors of clinical complications of atherosclerosis. Circulation. 1956; 14:691.
21. Kannel WB et al: Serum cholesterol, lipoproteins and the risk of coronary heart disease: the Framingham study. Ann Intern Med. 1971; 74:1.
22. Stamler J: Dietary and serum lipids in the multifactorial etiology of atherosclerosis. Arch Surg. 1978; 113:21.
23. Nichols AB et al: Independence of serum lipid levels and dietary habits: the Tecumseh study. JAMA. 1976; 236:1948.
24. Mann GV: Diet-heart: end of an era. N Engl J Med. 1977; 297:644.
25. Hulley SB et al: Epidemiology as a guide to clinical decisions. The association between triglyceride and coronary heart disease. N Engl J Med. 1980; 302:1383.
26. Gordon T et al: High density lipoprotein as a protective factor against coronary heart disease. Am J Med. 1977; 62:707.
27. Castelli WP et al: HDL cholesterol and other lipids in coronary heart disease: the Cooperative Lipoprotein Phenotyping study. Circulation. 1977; 55:767.
28. Hartung GH et al: Relation of diet to high-density-lipoprotein cholesterol in middle-aged marathon runners, joggers, and inactive men. N Engl J Med. 1980; 302:357.
29. Hulley SB et al: Plasma high-density lipoprotein cholesterol level: influence of risk factor intervention. JAMA. 1977; 238:2269.
30. Miller GJ et al: Plasma-high-density-lipoprotein concentration and development of ischemic heart disease. Lancet. 1975; 1:16.
31. Castelli WP et al: Alcohol and blood lipids. Lancet. 1977; 2:153.

32. Devenyi P et al: Alcohol and high-density lipoproteins. Can Med Assoc J. 1980; 123:981.

33. Steinberg D et al: Management of hyperlipidemia. Arch Surg. 1978; 113:55.

34. Lees AM et al: Plant sterols as cholesterol-lowering agents: clinical trials in patients with hypercholesterolemia and studies of sterol balance. Atherosclerosis. 1977; 28:325.

35. Farquhar JW et al: Response of serum lipids and lipoproteins of man to beta-sitosterol and safflower oil—a long-term study. Circulation. 1958; 17:890.

36. Kudchodkar BJ et al: Effects of plant sterols on cholesterol metabolism in man. Atherosclerosis. 1976; 23:239.

37. Brown HB et al: The additive effect of probucol on diet in hyperlipidemia. Clin Pharmacol Ther. 1974; 16:44.

38. LeLorier J et al: Diet and probucol in lowering cholesterol concentrations. Arch Intern Med. 1977; 137:1429.

39. Marshall FN et al: Sensitization to epinephrine-induced ventricular fibrillation produced by probucol in dogs. Toxicol Appl Pharmacol. 1973; 24:594.

40. Schwandt P et al: The effect of d-thyroxine on lipoprotein lipids and apolipoproteins in primary type IIa hyperlipoproteinemia. Atherosclerosis. 1980; 35:301.

41. Coronary Drug Project Research Group: Findings leading to further modification of its protocol with respect to dextrothyroxine. JAMA. 1972; 220:996.

42. Falko JM et al: Type III hyperlipoproteinemia. Rise in high-density lipoprotein levels in response to therapy. Am J Med. 1979; 66:303.

43. The Coronary Drug Project Research Group: Clofibrate and niacin in coronary heart disease. JAMA. 1975; 231:360.

44. Coronary Drug Project: Gallbladder disease as a side effect of drugs influencing lipid metabolism. N Engl J Med. 1977; 296:1185.

45. Angelin B et al: Biliary lipid composition during treatment with different hypolipidemic drugs. Eur J Clin Invest. 1979; 9:185.

46. Carlson LA et al: The effect of nicotinic acid on plasma lipids in patients with hyperlipoproteinemia during the first week of treatment. J Atherosclerosis Res. 1968; 8:667.

47. Christensen NA et al: Nicotinic acid treatment of hypercholesterolemia: comparison of plain and sustained-action preparations and report of two cases of jaundice. JAMA. 1961; 177:546.

48. Molnar GD et al: The effect of nicotinic acid in diabetes mellitus. Metabolism. 1964; 13:181.

49. Howard RP et al: Effect of cholestyramine administration on serum lipids and on nitrogen balance in familial hypercholesterolemia. J Lab Clin Med. 1966; 68:12.

50. Weisweiler P et al: The effect of cholestyramine on lipoprotein lipids in patients with primary type IIa hyperlipoproteinemia. Atherosclerosis. 1979; 33:295.

51. Moore RB et al: Effect of cholestyramine on the fecal excretion of intravenously administered cholesterol-4-14C and its degradation products in a hypercholesterolemic patient. J Clin Invest. 1968; 47:1664.

52. Shepart J et al: Cholestyramine promotes receptor-mediated low-density lipoprotein catabolism. N Engl J Med. 1980; 302:1219.

53. Goodman DS et al: The effects of colestipol resin and colestipol plus clofibrate on the turnover of plasma cholesterol in man. J Clin Invest. 1973; 52:2646.

54. Kane JP et al: Normalization of low-density-lipoprotein levels in heterozygous familial hypercholesterolemia with a combined drug regimen. N Engl J Med. 1981; 304:251.

55. Miller NE et al: Effects of colestipol, a new bile-acid-sequestering resin, on cholesterol metabolism in man. J Lab Clin Med. 1973; 82:876.

56. Kritchevsky D: Food products and hyperlipidemia. Arch Surg. 1978; 113:52.

57. Motulsky AG: The genetic hyperlipidemias. N Engl J Med. 1976; 294:823.

58. Sacks FM et al: Plasma lipids and lipoproteins in vegetarians and controls. N Engl J Med. 1975; 292:1148.

59. Glueck CJ et al: Dietary fat and atherosclerosis. Am J Clin Nutr. 1979; 32:2703.

60. Davis CE et al: Clinical trials of lipid lowering and coronary artery disease prevention. In *Hyperlipidemia Diagnosis and Therapy,* edited by BM Rifkind and RI Levy, Grune & Stratton, New York, 1977, p 79.

61. Miettinen M et al: Effect of cholesterol-lowering diet on mortality from coronary heart-disease and other causes. Lancet. 1972; 2:835.

62. Leren P: The effect of plasma cholesterol-lowering diet in male survivors of myocardial infarction: a controlled trial. Acta Med Scand. [Suppl] 1966; 466:5.

63. Frantz ID et al: The Minnesota coronary survey: effect of diet on cardiovascular events and deaths. Circulation. 1975; 51–52:Suppl 2:II.

64. Committee of Principal Investigators: A co-operative trial in the primary prevention of ischemic heart disease using clofibrate. Br Heart J. 1978; 40:1069.

65. Rosenhamer G et al: Effect of combined clofibrate-nicotinic acid treatment in ischemic heart disease. Atherosclerosis. 1980; 37:129.

66. Committee of Principal Investigators: W.H.O. cooperative trial on primary prevention of ischemic heart disease using clofibrate to lower serum cholesterol: mortality follow-up. Lancet. 1980; 2:379.

67. The Coronary Drug Project Research Group. Influence of adherence to treatment and response of cholesterol on mortality in the coronary drug project. N Engl J Med. 1980; 303:1038.

68. National Heart, Lung, and Blood Institute: *The Dietary Management of Hyperlipoproteinemia,* DHEW Publication No. (NIH) 78-110, 1978, p 13.

69. Wilson WS et al: Serial lipid and lipoprotein responses to the American Heart Association fat-controlled diet. Am J Med. 1971; 51:491.

70. Joyner C et al: The effect of sitosterol administration upon the serum cholesterol level and lipoprotein pattern. Am J Med Sci. 1955; 230:636.

71. Martz BL: Drug management of hypercholesterolemia. Am Heart J. 1979; 97:389.

72. Miettinen TA: Effects of neomycin alone and in combination with cholestyramine on serum cholesterol and fecal steroids in hypercholesterolemic subjects. J Clin Invest. 1979; 64:1485.

73. Breen KJ et al: Neomycin absorption in man: studies of oral and enema administration and effect of intestinal ulceration. Ann Intern Med. 1972; 76:211.

74. Jacobsen ED et al: Malabsorptive syndrome induced by neomycin: morphologic alterations in the jejunal mucosa. J Lab Clin Med. 1960; 56:245.

75. Hvidt S et al: Malabsorption induced by small doses of neomycin sulfate. Acta Med Scand. 1963; 173:699.

76. Samuel P: Treatment of hypercholesterolemia with neomycin—a time for reappraisal. N Engl J Med. 1979; 301:595.

77. Glueck CJ et al: Colestipol and cholestyramine resin: comparative effects in familial Type II hyperlipoproteinemia. JAMA. 1972; 222:676.

78. Gundersen K et al: Cholesterol—lowering effect of colestipol hydrochloride given twice daily in hypercholesterolemic patients. Atherosclerosis. 1976; 25:303.

79. Cohen MI et al: Intestinal obstruction associated with cholestyramine therapy. N Engl J Med. 1969; 280:1285.

80. Witztum JL et al: Bile sequestrant therapy alters the compositions of low-density and high-density lipoproteins. Metabolism. 1979; 28:221.

81. West RJ et al: The effect of cholestyramine on intestinal absorption. Gut. 1975; 16:93.

82. Gross L et al: Hypoprothrombinemia and hemorrhage associated with cholestyramine therapy. Ann Intern Med. 1970; 72:95.

83. Bressler R et al: Treatment of hypercholesterolemia and hypertriglyceridemia by anion exchange resin. South Med J. 1966; 59:1097.

84. Lees AM et al: Agents used to treat hyperlipidemia and atherosclerosis. In *Handbook of Drug Therapy,* edited by RR Miller and DJ Greenblatt, Elsevier, New York, 1979, p 707.

85. Jahnchen E et al: Enhanced elimination of warfarin during treatment with cholestyramine. Br J Clin Pharmacol. 1978; 5:437.

86. Caldwell JH et al: Interruption of the enterohepatic circulation of digitoxin by cholestyramine. J Clin Invest. 1971; 50:2638.

87. Kauffman RE et al: Effect of colestipol on gastrointestinal absorption of chlorothiazide in man. Clin Pharmacol Ther. 1973; 14:886.

88. Northcutt RC et al: The influence of cholestyramine on thyroxine absorption. JAMA. 1969; 208:1857.

89. Thomas FB et al: Inhibition of the intestinal absorption of inorganic and hemoglobin iron by cholestyramine. J Lab Clin Med. 1971; 78:70.

90. Hall WH et al: Effect of cholestyramine on digoxin absorption and excretion in man. Am J Cardiol. 1977; 39:213.

91. Illingworth DR et al: Colestipol plus nicotinic acid in treatment of heterozygous familial hypercholesterolemia. Lancet. 1981; 1:296.

92. Boyden TW et al: Synergistic effects of probucol and cholestyramine to lower serum cholesterol. J Clin Pharmacol. 1981; 21:48.

93. DeSante KA et al: The effect of colestipol hydrochloride on the bioavailability and pharmacokinetics of clofibrate. J Clin Pharmacol. 1979; 19:721.

94. Svedmyr N et al: Influence of indomethacin on flush induced by nicotinic acid in man. Acta Pharmacol Toxicol. 1977; 41:397.

95. Olefsky JM et al: Reappraisal of the role of insulin in hypertriglyceridemia. Am J Med. 1974; 57:551.

96. Brunzell JD et al: Plasma triglyceride and insulin levels in familial hypertriglyceridemia. Ann Intern Med. 1977; 87:198.

97. Kekki M et al: Plasma triglyceride metabolism in the adult nephrotic syndrome. Eur J Clin Invest. 1971; 1:345.

98. Brunzell JD et al: Evidence for diabetes mellitus and genetic forms of hypertriglyceridemia as independent entities. Metabolism. 1975; 24:1115.

99. Castelli WP et al: HDL cholesterol and other lipids in coronary heart disease. Circulation. 1977; 55:767.

100. Goldstein JL et al: Hyperlipidemia in coronary heart disease. I. Lipid levels in 500 survivors of myocardial infarction. J Clin Invest. 1973; 52:1533.

101. Carlson LA et al: Ischemic heart-disease in relation to fasting values of plasma triglycerides and cholesterol. Lancet. 1972; 1:865.

102. Schaeffer EJ et al: Plasma-triglycerides in regulation of H.D.L.—cholesterol levels. Lancet. 1978; 2:391.

103. National Heart, Lung, and Blood Institute: *The Dietary Management of Hyperlipoproteinemia,* DHEW Publication No. (NIH) 78-110, 1978, p 47.

104. Witztum JL et al: Normalization of triglycerides in Type IV hyperlipoproteinemia fails to correct low levels of high-density-lipoprotein cholesterol. N Engl J Med. 1980; 303:907.

105. Brook JG et al: The concentration of high density lipoprotein in patients with Type IV hyperlipoproteinemia and the effect of clofibrate. Atherosclerosis. 1980; 36:461.

106. Calvert GD et al: The effects of clofibrate on plasma glucose, lipoproteins, fibrinogen, and other biochemical and haematological variables in patients with mature onset diabetes mellitus. Eur J Clin Pharmacol. 1980; 17:355.

107. Pierides AM et al: Clofibrate-induced muscle damage in patients with chronic renal failure. Lancet. 1975; 2:1279.

108. Cumming A: Acute renal failure and interstitial nephritis after clofibrate treatment. Br Med J. 1980; 281:1529.

109. Goldberg AP et al: Increase in lipoprotein lipase during clofibrate treatment of hypertriglyceridemia in patients on hemodialysis. N Engl J Med. 1979; 301:1073.

110. Goldberg AP et al: Control of clofibrate toxicity in uremic hypertriglyceridemia. Clin Pharmacol Ther. 1977; 21:317.

Chapter 32

Surgical Antibiotic Prophylaxis

B. Joseph Guglielmo

Surgical antibiotic prophylaxis has long been a topic of great controversy. Although there is extensive literature on the prevention of surgical infections with antimicrobials, few of the published studies have been adequately designed. Chodak and Plaut reviewed the English language literature from 1960–1976 on the subject. Trials in genitourinary and cardiovascular surgery were not included. Of 131 studies, only 24 were considered well-designed, valuable studies (1).

Despite the lack of good information, the use of prophylactic antibiotics in surgery is extensive and often inappropriate (2,3).

Classification of Surgical Wounds

In 1964, the Ad Hoc Committee of the Committee on Trauma of the National Research Council formulated a standard classification of surgical wounds according to the following criteria (4):

Clean. The gastrointestinal, respiratory, and urinary tract are not entered, no inflammation is encountered, and no break in aseptic technique occurs. One large prospective study observed that of 36,383 clean wounds, only 624 later became infected (1.7%) (5).

Clean-Contaminated. The gastrointestinal or respiratory tract is entered without significant spillage or mechanical drainage. Included in this category are procedures involving entry into the vagina, the uninfected biliary tract, or genitourinary tract. The previously mentioned prospective study observed that 664 of 7,335 wounds (8.8%) became infected (5).

Contaminated. Acute inflammation (without pus formation) is encountered; there is a major break in sterile technique or gross spillage from the gastrointestinal tract occurs. Incisions into infected biliary or urinary tracts are also included in this category. Of 2,613 contaminated wounds studied prospectively, 458 (17.5%) became infected (5).

663

Dirty. Perforated, viscous wounds with the presence of pus or wounds from a dirty source (e.g., trauma) are included. The definition implies the presence of organisms in ordinarily sterile tissue before the operation and an active infectious process. In this category, 660 of 1,586 wounds (41.6%) were found to be infected (5).

Risk Factors

The decision to use antibiotic prophylaxis should be based on many variables. The risk of surgical infection must be compared to the risks, costs, and ecologic impact of antibiotic usage. One major prospective study observed a 5.4% incidence of antibiotic-induced side effects in 7,765 consecutive patient admissions, 2,877 of whom received antibiotics (6).

Another important determinant is the health of the patient. Malnutrition, immunosuppressive therapy, and chronic illnesses may predispose the individual to postoperative infection. These variables may empirically necessitate the use of prophylactic antibiotics.

Since the wound infection rate for "clean" surgery is relatively low, the financial and ecologic impact most likely exceeds the benefits derived from antibiotic prophylaxis. The exception to this would be such cases where an infection is likely to be of catastrophic consequence. Examples would include procedures involving insertion of prosthetic material such as artificial joints, vascular grafts, and cardiac valves.

"Clean-contaminated" procedures involve the presence of abundant resident flora, where minor spillage is difficult to avoid even with the most careful technique. Much of the controversy regarding the use of antibiotic prophylaxis is associated with this category.

In "contaminated" and "dirty" operations, organisms are already present in ordinarily sterile sites, and the use of antimicrobial agents represents therapy rather than prophylaxis.

Antibiotic Choice and Timing

The agent chosen should have activity against most, but not necessarily all, of the major microbes likely to be encountered. Additionally, the drug(s) should be relatively nontoxic and, if possible, inexpensive.

The classic work of Burke (7) and Alexander (8) clearly demonstrates the need for a therapeutic antibiotic concentration in the blood stream and vulnerable tissue at the time of wound contamination. Antibiotic administration given postoperatively cannot be considered adequate prophylaxis, since the incidence of infectious complications associated with such administration is equal to that in patients who receive no antibiotics (9).

1. *Colorectal Surgery.* **G.B. is a 50-year-old woman who was admitted one day before elective colorectal surgery. A diagnosis of carcinoma of the large bowel was made recently, and surgical resection is the planned treatment.**

Physical examination revealed a cachectic woman with a history of 9 kg weight loss over the previous three months (current weight 60 kg). Increased frequency of bowel movements and chronic fatigue were also noted by the patient. Except for the gastrointestinal system, all organ systems were normal.

Laboratory data included: hemoglobin 10.4 gm/dl, hematocrit 29.7%, white blood cell count 8500/mm³, blood urea nitrogen 28 mg/dl, serum creatinine 2.3 mg/dl, carcinoembryonic antigen was elevated, and the stool guaiac was positive. Vital signs were within normal limits. She was taking no medications and had no history of allergies.

The following orders were written on the day before surgery:

1) **Clear liquid diet**
2) **Supplemental IV fluids as needed**
3) **Magnesium sulfate 50% 30 ml po at 10:00 AM and 2:00 PM**
4) **Neomycin sulfate 1.0 gm and erythromycin 1.0 gm po at 1:00 PM, 2:00 PM, and 11:00 PM**

Comment on the appropriateness of the antibiotic prophylaxis selected for this patient.

Fecal flora, a mixture of aerobic and anaerobic bacteria, reside in the distal ileum, colon, and rectum. The most common pathogens encountered after colorectal surgery are *Escherichia coli* and *Bacteroides fragilis;* however, enterococcus, other aerobic coliforms, and anaerobes also commonly cause infection (10,11). The colon harbors as many as 10^{13} bacteria per cubic milliliter. This large concentration of bacteria at least partially explains why surgery involving the large bowel has always been associated with a high prevalence of postoperative infection.

Combinations of "nonabsorbable" antibiotics effective against gram-negative enteric aerobes (neomycin, kanamycin, phthalylsulfathiazole) in combination with antimicrobials effective against anaerobes (tetracyclines, erythromycin, metronidazole) have consistently been shown to be highly effective in the prevention of infection in colorectal surgery (12–19).

Parenterally, cephaloridine (20), lincomycin (21), gentamicin plus lincomycin or metronidazole (10), and metronidazole alone (22) have all been shown to decrease postoperative infection.

Of the above regimens, perhaps the most established in the United States is the neomycin-erythromycin bowel preparation first studied by Clarke and colleagues. Utilizing neomycin 1.0 gm plus erythromycin 1.0 gm at 1:00 PM, 2:00 PM, and 11:00 PM on the preoperative day, a 9% (5/56) rate of postoperative sepsis was observed compared to 43% (26/60) in the control group (15).

When oral neomycin, kanamycin, or phthalylsulfathiazole are used without the addition of an antibiotic with adequate anaerobic coverage, the incidence of postoperative sepsis is 40–50%. However, when tetracycline, erythromycin, or metronidazole are added to the above, the sepsis rate decreases to 8–13% (18,19,23).

Thus, the above combination of an oral erythromycin-neomycin bowel preparation is a rational and well-established choice for antibiotic prophylaxis in this patient (see Table 1).

2. The surgical resident decides to discontinue the neomycin-erythromycin order. Instead, he orders cefamandole 1.0 gm IV to be administered on call to the operating room, then every 6 hours for 48 hours. He claims intravenous antibiotics are as effective as oral antibiotics and that cephalosporins are relatively safe drugs. Is this change a rational alternative to the neomycin-erythromycin bowel preparation? Are parenteral antibiotics effective as prophylaxis for bowel surgery?

Two investigations have compared cephalothin to oral antibiotic bowel preparations (24,25). In one study, septic complications occurred in 39% of patients receiving cephalothin without oral neomycin-erythromycin; however, those receiving the oral bowel preparation, with or without cephalothin, had only a 6% infection rate (25). This high rate of sepsis with cephalothin alone is similar to the postoperative sepsis rate observed in patients who received no preoperative antibiotics (12,

14–17). Cefamandole, one of the newer cephalosporins, appears to offer no therapeutic advantages when compared with cephalothin in elective colonic surgery (26). Cephaloridine, however, has been shown to compare favorably with the neomycin-erythromycin oral preparation (27).

Intravenous metronidazole given immediately prior to surgery and repeated in 8 and 16 hours has been shown to be as effective as oral metronidazole given for two days preoperatively (28). Keighley compared the effects of an oral regimen of metronidazole and kanamycin to a parenteral regimen of the same two drugs. The oral metronidazole was discontinued 36 hours preoperatively and the oral kanamycin was discontinued 12 hours before the operation. The parenteral preparations were given immediately before and after surgery. The rate of infection was significantly greater in patients receiving the oral regimen, despite the fact that the concentration of bacteria in the gut of the parenteral group far exceeded that of the oral group. This study supports the suggestion that it is blood and tissue levels rather than colonic antibiotic concentrations that are critical in the prevention of infection (29). However, the efficacy of non-absorbable antibiotics has been documented by many well-designed studies, showing clearly that high intraluminal concentrations of antibiotic are important (12,14–16). Thus, while investigations have shown certain parenteral regimens to be as effective as oral antibiotic bowel preparations, the use of cefamandole or cephalothin as sole preoperative antibiotic prophylaxis in colorectal surgery is unjustified. In cases of emergency colorectal surgery, a combination of IV aminoglycoside, clindamycin and perhaps penicillin should be the treatment of choice, based on their efficacy in the treatment of abdominal infection.

3. The resident agrees to the use of the oral neomycin-erythromycin bowel preparation in this patient; however, he also orders intravenous clindamycin and gentamicin to supplement neomycin and erythromycin. Does this regimen offer any advantage over neomycin-erythromycin alone in this patient? Would other parenteral antibiotics in combination with neomycin-erythromycin offer any advantage?

Because the neomycin-erythromycin bowel preparation is very effective against *E. coli* and *B. fragilis* and the rate of infection with its use is relatively low, one might speculate that documentation of a further decrease in the rate of sepsis would require study with great numbers of patients. Perioperative gentamicin and clindamycin added to the oral neomycin-erythromycin preparation produces no observable decrease in infection rate (30). However, the addition of intravenous cefazolin to the same oral bowel preparation has been observed to produce a significant decrease in wound infection (9). It is likely that the high prevalence of wound infection due to *Staphylococcus aureus* in this study accounted for the reduction of wound sepsis in the cefazolin-treated group. Thus, there are conflicting data regarding the efficacy of parenteral antibiotics when used in combination with oral agents. While intravenous clindamycin and gentamicin do not appear to significantly further reduce postoperative sepsis, in colorectal surgery cefazolin has been shown to be useful when *S. aureus* is a common pathogen.

4. *Duration of Prophylaxis.* Immediately after G.B.'s colorectal surgery, the following antibiotics are ordered: clindamycin 600 mg

IV every 6 hours for seven days and gentamicin 80 mg IV every 8 hours for seven days. How long after surgery should prophylactic antibiotics be continued?

It has been observed in many investigations that a short course of antibiotic prophylaxis is as effective as a longer course in the prevention of postoperative infection. Stone and associates have shown that five days of postoperative antibiotics are no better than perioperative therapy alone in the prophylaxis of elective gastric, biliary and colonic surgery (31). Other investigators have observed similar results in colorectal surgery (32), biliary surgery (33), vaginal hysterectomy (34,35), cesarean section (36), and "clean" procedures such as cardiothoracic surgery (37,38) and total hip arthroplasty (39).

Therefore, there is no need to continue prophylactic antibiotics for longer than 24 to 48 hours after surgery.

5. *Antibiotic-Associated Pseudomembranous Colitis.* Because of postoperative fever and a mild leukocytosis (11,500/mm³), G.B.'s clindamycin and gentamicin were continued. On

Table 1.

Suggested Antibiotic Regimens for Surgical Prophylaxis

Surgery	Antibiotic Prophylaxis
Colorectal	Neomycin 1.0 gm and erythromycin 1.0 gm at 1 p.m., 2 p.m, 11 p.m. on the preoperative day (See Question 1)
Gastroduodenal	Cephalosporin[1] for high risk patients (See Question 6)
Biliary	Cephalosporin[1] for high risk patients (See Question 7)
Vaginal Hysterectomy	Cephalosporin[1] or ampicillin[2] (See Question 8)
Abdominal Hysterectomy	Cephalosporin[1] (conflicting data on efficacy, see Question 9)
Cesarean section	Cephalosporin[1] or ampicillin[2] for high risk patients (See Question 10)
Orthopedic	Cephalosporin[1] or penicillinase-resistant penicillin[3] (See Question 11 for specific procedures)
Cardiac	Cephalosporin[1] or penicillinase-resistant penicillin[3] In cases involving placement of prosthetic material, antibiotics may be continued until all "lines" are removed (See Question 12)
Vascular	Cephalosporin[1] or penicillinase-resistant penicillin[3] (See Question 13 for specific procedures)

1. Cefazolin 500 mg to 1.0 gm IV at induction of anesthesia, then postoperatively every 6–8 hrs × 24 hrs. Cephalothin 1.0 to 2.0 gm IV as above then postoperatively every 4–6 hrs × 24 hrs.

2. Ampicillin 1.0 gm IV at induction of anesthesia, then postoperatively every 6 hrs × 24 hrs.

3. Nafcillin or oxacillin or methicillin 1.0 gm IV at induction of anesthesia, then postoperatively every 6 hrs × 24 hrs.

the sixth day of therapy, she complains of abdominal cramping and diarrhea. Her temperature is 38.5° C and her leukocyte count has increased to 24,700/mm³. Sigmoidoscopy shows greenish-yellow raised lesions on the mucosal surface consistent with pseudomembranous colitis. *Clostridia difficile* toxin titers from stool are pending. The diagnosis is antibiotic-associated pseudomembranous colitis. Her antibiotic therapy is discontinued. What is pseudomembranous colitis, and how should it be treated?

Pseudomembranous colitis is a severe and sometimes lethal consequence of antibiotic use. One etiology appears to be an exotoxin produced by *Clostridia difficile* overgrowth in the bowel (47). The classic presentation is acute onset of moderate watery diarrhea, abdominal cramping, fever, and leukocytosis. Sigmoidoscopy reveals discrete yellow plaque-like lesions on the mucosal surface. While the above signs and symptoms usually begin after four to nine days of antibiotic therapy, some cases occur up to three weeks after discontinuation of antibiotic therapy (40–42). Clindamycin (43), lincomycin, and ampicillin have been the most commonly implicated antibiotics, although tetracyclines, cephalosporins (45), and trimethoprim-sulfamethoxazole (46) have been implicated as well.

Treatment is directed against the offending organism, *Cl. difficile,* and its exotoxin. The most commonly used treatment is oral vancomycin 125 to 500 mg three to four times daily for seven to fourteen days (48–50). The minimum inhibitory concentration (MIC) for vancomycin is 0.5 to 16 mcg/ml. Since vancomycin is poorly absorbed, fecal concentrations of 700 to 3000 mcg/gm are produced; these concentrations are many times higher than the required MIC (48,49). Metronidazole is also highly effective against anaerobes such as *Cl. difficile* and has been shown to be effective in the treatment of pseudomembranous colitis (51). Cholestyramine resin, which apparently binds the bacterial exotoxin, has also proven to be useful in this disease (52).

Fever and abdominal cramping should resolve within 48–72 hours after the initiation of proper therapy; resolution of the diarrhea requires four to fourteen days (43). Although relapses after vancomycin therapy have been reported, they do not appear to be due to the emergence of resistant strains. *Cl. difficile* strains isolated from these patients have been sensitive to vancomycin MIC's of 2 mcg/ml or less, and these patients have responded to retreatment with vancomycin or cholestyramine (53).

6. *Gastroduodenal Surgery.* R.B. is a 43-year-old male who is admitted to the general surgery service for a chronic duodenal ulcer. His medical history reveals no other medical problems or previous operative procedures. He is scheduled for surgery tomorrow morning. Are prophylactic antibiotics indicated for this patient? Are they necessary for other gastroduodenal surgical procedures?

Bacterial flora are infrequent in the normal or hypersecretory stomach, because gastric acid rapidly kills swallowed organisms. Conditions involving low acid output, such as gastric cancer and gastric ulcers, might be expected to be associated with higher bacterial counts and resultant infection rate. Confirming this hypothesis, one study reported a 6% prevalence of infection in pyloroplasty and vagotomy, 13.4% in gastric ulcer surgery, 17.2% in procedures for gastric carcinoma, and 25% when intraluminal blood was found during the operation (5). Other investigators have made similar observations (54).

The most common infecting organisms in gastroduodenal surgery are *Streptococci viridans, Escherichia coli,* and anaerobes. Like the normal stomach, the normal duodenum, jejunum, and upper ileum harbor low concentrations of resident bacterial flora. However, the distal two to three feet contain fecal flora whose concentration increases as the ileocecal valve is approached. With obstruction, the small bowel rapidly becomes populated with high concentrations of fecal organisms, and surgical intervention requires prophylactic treatment with antibiotics.

Patients with duodenal ulcer (such as R.B.) are at low risk for infection as a result of gastroduodenal procedures (55). However, patients with pyloric stenosis, gastric ulcer, or gastric carcinoma are at relatively high risk, and the benefits of prophylactic antibiotics for gastroduodenal procedures in these patients have been clearly demonstrated (55). (See Table 1.)

7. *Biliary Tract Surgery.* M.R. is a 70-year-old woman with acute cholecystitis who is scheduled for surgery. Is antibiotic prophylaxis indicated? If so, what antibiotics would be appropriate?

Surgical procedures involving sterile bile result in very low infection rates; however, certain risk factors for bacterbilia and resultant infection have been identified. In a retrospective study of 1,421 cases of biliary tract surgery, 33% of all bile cultures were positive for bacteria at surgery, and positive biliary culture was associated with postoperative infection forty times more frequently than negative culture (56). Risk factors that were identified as being associated with positive bile cultures were acute cholecystitis, common duct stones with or without jaundice, and age greater than 70 years. *E. coli* was the organism most often isolated in these patients. Subsequently, the same authors prospectively studied antibiotic prophylaxis in these high risk patients, and those who received antibiotic prophylaxis (with cephaloridine) had a lower infection rate than the patients who served as controls (57). Postoperative sepsis was most often associated with *Escherichia coli, Klebsiella pneumoniae,* and *Staphylococcus aureus.* Enterococcus and anaerobes were isolated to a lesser extent. Thus, an antibiotic regimen effective against the three major organisms would most likely offer optimal protection.

In addition to the cephalosporins (9,33,57), trimethoprim-sulfamethoxazole (59) and gentamicin (58) have been shown to be effective in prophylaxis in biliary tract surgery. Penetration of the prophylactic antibiotic into the bile does not appear to be essential (60).

Since this patient is 70 years old and presents with acute cholecystitis, she is at risk for having bacteria in her bile, and a short course of perioperative cephalosporins or trimethoprim-sulfamethoxazole is justified. (See Table 1.) It should be noted that some practitioners utilize antibiotic prophylaxis for all surgery involving the biliary tract, since the intraoperative cholangiogram may occasionally demonstrate an unexpected stone in the common bile duct (9).

8. *Vaginal Hysterectomy.* L.T. is a 46-year-old woman with a recent history of abnormal uterine bleeding and vaginal discharge. Vaginal biopsy is positive for squamous cell carcinoma. There is no evidence of invasive disease; the cancer localized to the intraepithelial layer of the cervix. The diagnosis is carcinoma *in situ,* and she is scheduled for vaginal hysterectomy. Recommend an appropriate prophylactic antibiotic regimen for this patient.

As with colorectal surgery, the primary pathogens in obstetric and gynecologic surgery involve fecal flora. The most common infecting bacteria are *E. coli,* the enterococcus, and anaerobes, with other Enterobacteriaceae being less frequently isolated (31, 61–75). Several studies have shown a clear benefit from the use of antibiotic prophylaxis in vaginal hysterectomies. Most of the studies involve cephalosporins such as cephaloridine (34,61–64), cephradine (35), cephalothin (65), cefazolin (66–68), and cefoxitin (69–70). However, penicillins (71–74), tetracyclines (71), aminoglycosides (72), and cotrimoxazole (trimethoprim-sulfamethoxazole) (75) have also been used successfully as prophylaxis in vaginal hysterectomies.

Since infections in the operative site are often difficult to assess, postoperative complications in these studies are commonly described in terms of "febrile morbidity." This classification usually refers to a temperature of $> 38°$ C on two separate occasions at least 6 hours apart, excluding the first 24 hours. Fever from noninfectious causes (eg, drug-related, atelectasis, etc.) may often be included in this classification. Furthermore, many of the investigations include bacteriuria as well as other miscellaneous infections in their statistical analysis. Nevertheless, based on the rate of pelvic and wound infection, the benefit of antibiotics is still obvious. Thus, a course of perioperative cephalosporins would be a reasonable choice for prophylaxis in this patient. (See Table 1.)

9. *Abdominal Hysterectomy.* Would the decision to use antibiotic prophylaxis be the same if the above individual required an abdominal hysterectomy rather than surgery by the vaginal route?

The benefit of antibiotic prophylaxis in abdominal surgery is not as obvious as with vaginal hysterectomy. While some studies show dramatic decreases in postoperative pelvic and wound infection (65,66,68,76–78), others do not show a clear benefit (73,74,79,80).

The discrepancy between studies can be at least partially explained by the inherently lower rate of infection associated with abdominal hysterectomy. Since the surgical incision with the abdominal operation is in a "clean" or noncontaminated area, the risk of infection is lower than with vaginal hysterectomy. Thus, the benefits of antibiotic prophylaxis are less clearly apparent. Reported infection rates in abdominal hysterectomy without antibiotics range from 9 to 40% (65,66 68,73,74,76–79) (see Question 8 for assessment of postoperative infection). Antibiotic prophylaxis for abdominal hysterectomy is controversial, and it appears that it is not warranted except in hospitals with high infection rates for this procedure. (See Table 1.)

10. *Cesarean Section.* **G.J. is a 27-year-old woman who is admitted to the obstetrics unit at the local hospital. She is now at term in her first pregnancy and has been in excellent health. The last few visits with her obstetrician have documented that the baby is breeched; thus she must undergo cesarean section. Are antibiotics effective in decreasing postoperative infection in cesarean section? Should they be recommended in the above individual?**

The use of prophylactic antibiotics for cesarean section is also controversial. As with vaginal and abdominal hysterectomy, the use of the parameter "febrile morbidity" complicates evaluation of the benefit of antibiotic prophylaxis (see Question 8). Many studies document a decreased rate of endometritis with prophylactic antibiotics. However, the incidence of serious wound infection and septicemia is generally low; most studies report a rate of < 5%. The addition of prophylactic antibiotics has only variably been shown to decrease the rate of these more serious infections (81–91).

Certain risk factors may predispose patients to infection. A retrospective study determined four factors that identify the patient most likely to develop febrile morbidity: use of general anesthesia, obesity (> 30 pounds over pregravid desirable weight), low hematocrit (< 30%), and labor prior to delivery (92). Another prospective study identified various risk factors associated with postoperative endometritis. Duration of labor, number of vaginal examinations, and number of rectal examinations were all definite risk factors. Parity, rupture of the membranes, and skill of the operator also were significantly correlated to the rate of postoperative endometritis (93). Others have arrived at similar conclusions, observing that only women in labor had a significant decrease in the rate of endometritis when antibiotics were administered. There was no endometritis in those patients who had no labor prior to their cesarean sections (85).

If antibiotics are considered necessary in high risk cesarean section patients, ampicillin or cephalosporins are appropriate choices. Because the passage of antibiotics to the fetus is a potential problem, some investigators have elected to give the antibiotic after cord clamping (87,88) or immediately postoperatively (89). Gordon et al found no difference in infection rate between giving ampicillin preoperatively and administering the drug after clamping the umbilical cord (88). If antibiotics are to be used, a short course of therapy is as effective as a full five-day course in reducing postoperative infection (36). (See Table 1.)

11. *Orthopedic Surgery. Second Generation Cephalosporins.* **S.N. is a 57-year-old woman with rheumatoid arthritis and degenerative joint disease. She has been admitted for insertion of a prosthesis in her left hip (total hip arthroplasty). The following orders are written on the day before surgery: Cefamandole 2 gm IM on call to the operating room; repeat 2 gm IV intraoperatively, then 1 gm IV every 6 hours until drainage tubes are removed. Is antibiotic prophylaxis warranted? Is the use of cefamandole justified for prophylaxis of total hip arthroplasty rather than a first-generation cephalosporin such as cefazolin or cephalothin?**

Although the rate of infection in bone surgery without prosthetic material is low (103,104), the value of prophylactic antibiotics in total hip arthroplasty has been clearly demonstrated (102). Furthermore, because of the catastrophic consequences of postoperative infection in this setting, antimicrobial prophylaxis is generally recommended (105,106). The organisms most likely to cause postoperative infection after total hip replacement are staphylococci, both *S. aureus* and *S. epidermidis* (105,106). These organisms are susceptible to penicillinase-resistant antibiotics such as nafcillin, cephalosporins, and vancomycin. Those isolates of staphylococci which are resistant to beta-lactam compounds remain susceptible to vancomycin, and infections caused by these resistant isolates must be treated with this agent. Fortunately, the vast majority of staphylococci are sensitive to the penicillins and cephalosporins.

Antibiotic selection is based on several factors: high level of antibacterial activity, adequate tissue penetration, clinical experience with the agent, and relative cost. Many orthopedic surgeons in the United States utilize cephalosporins for prophylaxis (2). This is partly because the cephalosporins have better gram-negative activity than the penicillinase-resistant penicillins. However, the most important considerations in this particular case are the relative anti-staphylococcal activity and relative cost of cefamandole compared to a parenteral first-generation cephalosporin. Cefoxitin, the other available second-generation cephalosporin, is distinctly inferior to first-generation agents or cefamandole against gram-positive organisms (107). Several studies have compared the *in vitro* activity of cefamandole to older cephalosporins. In general, the activity of these agents against *S. aureus* is comparable (108–111). Most isolates are susceptible to 0.5 mcg/ml or less. Cephalothin and cephapirin are perhaps slightly more active than cefamandole against these isolates, but this difference is not clinically significant. *Staphylococcus epidermidis* is more resistant to cephalosporins. Minimal inhibitory concentrations for 90% of isolates are on the order of 1–2 mcg/ml. However, some strains may have MIC values as high as 8–16 mcg/ml (110). In conclusion, the differences between cefamandole and older cephalosporins with regard to anti-staphylococcal activity are minimal. Generally, a few more percent of staphylococcal isolates are susceptible to cefamandole at a concentration of 8–16 mcg/ml. However, because these higher concentrations of drug are difficult to achieve in tissues, especially bone these differences are also of questionable clinical significance (112).

Also of importance is the lack of published data documenting the effectiveness of cefamandole in this situation. Although it is reasonable to expect that cefamandole would be effective, far more clinical experience has been gained with older agents. It is also theoretically possible that infection following use of a broader spectrum agent such as cefamandole would be caused by more resistant gram-negative organisms and would therefore be more difficult to treat. Finally, on a per gram basis, cefamandole is approximately twice as expensive as cefazolin or cephalothin and nearly three times as expensive as cephapirin. Consideration must be given to the amount of money spent on more expensive prophylaxis for a questionable increase in efficacy. On the other hand, an argument can be made that the prevention of even one or two infections of hip prostheses would save enough money and patient morbidity in the long term so as to outweigh any increased

drug costs. Only large-scale controlled clinical trials cananswer these questions, and for the time being each clinician must analyze susceptibility and cost data in their institutions to reach a decision. (See Table 1).

12. *Cardiac Surgery.* **L.G., a 28-year-old male with a history of rheumatic heart disease, has a 12-year history of a murmur consistent with mild mitral stenosis and mitral regurgitation. Over the last four months his murmur has become much more prominent. Additionally, he has developed severe dyspnea with light physical activity and 3+ pitting edema over both lower legs. Physical examination is notable for coarse rales and an S_3 gallop. For the past six weeks he has been maintained on digoxin, furosemide, and hydralazine without significant relief of his shortness of breath. After consultation with a cardiothoracic surgeon, mitral valve replacement is recommended. Is antibiotic prophylaxis necessary in cardiac surgery? What antibiotic regimens are appropriate?**

Operative procedures involving the heart are classified as "clean" procedures with a low rate of infection. However, the devastating effects of prosthetic valve endocarditis and mediastinitis mandate the use of prophylactic antibiotics in this surgical setting. It is well documented that *Staphylococcus aureus, Staphylococcus epidermidis,* and diptheroids sp. are the most likely infecting agents. Thus, antibiotic therapy should be directed against these potential pathogens. Cephalosporins and semisynthetic anti-staphylococcal penicillins are the most commonly used antibiotics, and the length of prophylaxis varies from one dose to as long as one week postoperatively (37, 94–98). The most devastating infection in cardiac surgery, endocarditis, occurs with much greater frequency in cases involving the placement of prosthetic material. In aorta-coronary bypass grafts, this complication is rare or non-existent. Thus, it is important to note the types of cardiac surgery performed in each study. Additionally, since the infection rate is so low, an extremely large study group is necessary to prove the benefit of a specific regimen.

The value of knowing the sensitivity patterns at the specific hospital where the surgery is performed is illustrated by Myerowitz and colleagues. A significant decrease in serious infections (endocarditis, sepsis) was observed in patients receiving cephalothin when compared to methicillin. The main isolated pathogen was coagulase-negative staphylococci resistant to methicillin and sensitive to cephalothin (96).

Goldmann et al have shown that a two-day regimen is as effective as a six-day regimen in preventing postoperative infection (95). On the basis of a small series of patients undergoing cardiac surgery, Conte et al suggest that a single preoperative dose may be sufficient antibiotic prophylaxis (37). However, since it is well known that infections such as UTI's, pneumonia, and transient bacteremia can produce endocarditis, some clinicians prefer continuing antibiotics until all "lines" are removed after surgery involving valve replacement or the insertion of prosthetic material. A review by Everett and Hirschmann lists such procedures as nasotracheal intubation and suctioning, urethral catheterization, and the presence of intravascular lines as being responsible for bacteremia (99). However, the lack of endocarditis in Goldmann's series of 200 patients who received two days of treatment (95) suggests that continued antibiotic use is unnecessary. These patients averaged 2.2 days with endotracheal tube, 5.3 days with Foley catheter, 14.1 days with pacemaker, 7.0 days with CVP catheter, 5.4 days with peripheral IV catheter, 2.6 days with arterial line, and 3.7 days with pulmonary artery catheter (95).

While a case can be made for continuing antibiotics in valve replacement and surgery involving prosthetic material, it is difficult to justify the continuation of long-term antibiotics in aorta-coronary bypass grafts. However, the recent investigation by Fong et al suggests short-term antibiotics will decrease sternal wound infections in coronary bypass surgery (98). Since resultant mediastinitis is a strong possibility in patients with deep sternal wound infections, short-course prophylaxis is justifiable in this setting.

Therefore, prophylaxis is necessary in patients such as L.G. who will undergo a valve replacement procedure possibly involving placement of prosthetic material. The use of antibiotics in coronary artery bypass graft is more controversial; however, the risk of mediastinitis suggests that their use may be beneficial in this setting. The antimicrobial agent used in L.G.'s case should have good activity against staphylococci, but the choice of drug depends on resistance patterns at the hospital. Cephalosporins or nafcillin/methicillin ap-

pear to be good choices. While length of therapy should be short in aorta-coronary bypass surgery, length of prophylaxis in procedures involving cardiac valve replacement and other prosthetic material is less clear.

13. Vascular Surgery. Like orthopedic and cardiac surgery, most vascular surgeries are classified as "clean." What evidence supports the use of prophylactic antibiotics in vascular surgery?

Two studies to date attempt to define the role of antibiotics in prevention of postoperative infection in vascular surgery. Kaiser et al conclusively showed that perioperative cefazolin significantly decreased the rate of wound infection in 462 patients undergoing surgery of the abdominal aorta and lower extremity vasculature. Four vascular graft infections were observed, all in the control group. Cefazolin-sensitive, coagulase-positive staphylococci were the most common pathogens in this investigation (100). The results of Pitt et al suggest that the instillation of cephradine at the wound site is as effective as systemic drug in decreasing groin wound infection (101).

As is the case with cardiac surgery, any vascular surgery involving placement of prosthetic material should include antibiotic prophylaxis. Abdominal and lower extremity vascular surgery, with or without prosthesis, should also include prophylactic antibiotics. (See Table 1.)

Third Generation Cephalosporins

14. Postoperative Complications. L.G. (Question 11) is given cefazolin for perioperative prophylaxis of his mitral valve replacement. The cefazolin is discontinued on the third postoperative day when the intra-arterial lines and endotracheal tube are removed. However, on the eighth postoperative day he suffers a cardiac arrest. He is successfully resuscitated, reintubated, and returned to the coronary care unit. The following day the patient becomes febrile to 40°C. Physical examination reveals rales, rhonchi, and dullness to percussion in the right lung. Chest x-ray reveals infiltrates in the right middle and lower lobes. Gram-stain of suctioned material from the patient's endotracheal tube reveals sheets of polymorphonuclear leukocytes and many gram-negative

Table 2.

COMPARISON OF CEPHALOSPORINS

Name	Antibacterial Spectrum	Half-Life (hrs) (Normal Renal Function)	Half-Life (hrs) (Anuria)	Primary Route of Elimination	Adverse Effects	Comments
Cephalothin/ Cephapirin	Streptococci, staphylococci, E. coli, Proteus mirabilis, some Klebsiella. Enterococci are resistant to all cephalosporins.	0.5	3–4	Renal/Metabolism	Hypersensitivity reactions, Coombs' positivity; phlebitis and pain on IV or IM administration; pseudomembranous colitis is rare.	Prototype agent for first generation cephalosporins; cephapirin is virtually identical; both are metabolized to less active desacetyl derivative.
Cephradine/ Cephalexin	Same as cephalothin, but most organisms are less susceptible.	0.8	8–15	Renal	Same as cephalothin.	Cephradine is also available as parenteral product; sodium content of parenteral form is high (7 mEq Na$^+$/gm)
Cefazolin	Same as cephalothin.	1.4–2.2	18–36	Renal	Same as cephalothin.	Protein binding of 85–90%; small volume of distribution and slow clearance result in high, prolonged serum levels.
Cefadroxil	Same as cephalothin, with slightly better activity against gram-negative bacilli.	1.5	20–24	Renal	Same as cephalothin.	Oral agent with longer half-life is dosed twice daily.
Cefaclor	Same as cephalothin; increased activity against H. influenzae.	0.7	1.5–2.0	Renal/Biliary	Same as cephalothin.	Alternative agent for treatment of otitis media.
Cefamandole	Better activity against some gram-negative bacilli including H. influenzae and indole-positive Proteus.	0.9–1.5	15–20	Renal	Same as cephalothin.	Certain isolates, including enterobacter and ampicillin-resistant H. influenzae, may become resistant during therapy.
Cefoxitin	Better activity against many Enterobacteriaceae including Serratia, Klebsiella, and Proteus. Good activity against Bacteroides.	0.7	13–22	Renal	Same as cephalothin.	Useful with or without an aminoglycoside, in intraabdominal infections or as a sole agent in pelvic infections.

Agent	Spectrum of Activity			Route of Elimination	Adverse Effects	Comments
Cefotaxime	Excellent activity against most Enterobacteriaceae; some *Serratia* and most *P. aeruginosa* are resistant; anaerobic activity comparable to cefazolin or cefamandole. Gram-positive activity comparable to cefamandole.	0.8–1.4	3–4	Renal/Metabolism	Same as cephalothin; superinfection with resistant organisms (eg, enterococci, *Pseudomonas*) may occur.	Third generation agents are broad enough in spectrum to warrant their use as sole agents in initial therapy of serious bacterial infection. Addition of aminoglycoside or antipseudomonal penicillin is warranted if *Serratia* or *Pseudomonas* are likely pathogens.
Moxalactam	Poor gram-positive activity; activity against Enterobacteriaceae and *Pseudomonas* is comparable to cefotaxime; anaerobic activity comparable to or slightly better than cefoxitin.	2.0–3.0	20–24	Renal	Same as cefotaxime; hypoprothrombinemia presumably due to eradication of gut flora has been reported; alcohol intolerance has been noted in a few patients (see Question 14).	This agent and cefotaxime appear to penetrate meninges in quantities sufficient to treat gram-negative bacillary meningitis; poor activity of moxalactam and others against *Listeria*, enterococci and other streptococci make them poor choices as sole agents for neonatal meningitis.
Cefoperazone	Activity against gram-positive organisms and Enterobacteriaceae is not as good as cefotaxime; good activity against *Pseudomonas*; anaerobic activity is comparable to cefazolin or cefamandole.	2.0	2.0	Biliary	Same as cefotaxime; alcohol intolerance has also been noted (see Question 14).	Small volume of distribution, slow renal clearance result in high prolonged serum levels; as with moxalactam, can be dosed every 8–12 hours.

bacilli of a single morphology. What infecting organisms are most likely? What initial antibiotic therapy should be instituted? Comment on the appropriateness and potential toxicities of third generation cephalosporins (eg, cefotaxime, moxalactam, cefoperazone) in this patient.

The presence of gram-negative bacilli in the patient's endotracheal secretions may reflect only colonization of the upper portions of the bronchial tree. However, the large numbers of neutrophils combined with the presence of an apparently single type of gram-negative organism and the patient's clinical history and physical examination make the likelihood of parenchymal infection of the lung very high (113,114).

The organisms most likely to produce this infection have been altered by the duration of this patient's hospitalization. Enteric gram-negative bacilli colonize the pharynx and upper airways of patients within a few days of hospitalization (114). Aspiration of pharyngeal secretions during the cardiac arrest and inoculation of the bronchi and lower airways during intubation are the likely factors in the pathogenesis of the infection (113). Organisms producing infection in this setting vary according to institutional flora. These include *Klebsiella, Enterobacter, Serratia, Acinetobacter,* and *Pseudomonas aeruginosa* (113,114). Initial therapy of this infection must provide coverage for these organisms.

Generally, therapy consists of an aminoglycoside with or without the addition of an extended spectrum penicillin such as carbenicillin or ticarcillin. The added penicillin provides some coverage for aminoglycoside-resistant organisms and synergy in combination with the penicillins against many of the possible organisms, especially *Pseudomonas aeruginosa.* Alternatively, a first or second generation cephalosporin could be combined with the aminoglycosides, but synergy against some of the possible organisms, particularly *Pseudomonas,* is lacking (113).

Available third generation cephalosporins, cefotaxime, moxalactam, and cefoperazone are active against most, if not all, of the possible pathogens in this case. Cefotaxime and moxalactam are significantly more active than older cephalosporins against the Enterobacteriaceae (115–118) and *Hemophilus influenzae* (119,120). Although they possess some activity against *Serratia marcescens* and *Pseudomonas aeruginosa,*

many isolates are resistant. Cefoperazone is somewhat less active against the Enterobacteriaceae than either cefotaxime or moxalactam but has good activity against *Pseudomonas* (117,120). Additionally, these agents are frequently active against aminoglycoside-resistant and cephalothin-resistant isolates (121,122).

Open clinical trials of third generation cephalosporins have demonstrated their efficacy in the management of gram-negative pneumonia (123–126). Clinical failures and the development of resistance have been noted with the use of cefotaxime and moxalactam in the management of pneumonia due to *Pseudomonas aeruginosa* (127). More clinical experience is needed with cefoperazone and other third generation agents in this infection before they can be routinely recommended.

Adverse Effects. A distinct advantage of the available third generation cephalosporins is their relative lack of toxicity. To date, no reports of oto- or nephrotoxicity have been published. It is not known whether combinations of these agents with aminoglycosides would result in enhanced nephrotoxicity. Renal function should be carefully monitored in this patient who suffered a hypotensive episode during the cardiac arrest. Adverse reactions reported thus far for these agents include those noted for other cephalosporins such as phlebitis, hypersensitivity reactions, transient elevations of liver enzymes, and minor hematological abnormalities. A few, more unusual reactions have been noted with moxalactam and cefoperazone and deserve comment. Several cephalosporins, including the two just mentioned, possess a methyltetrazol moiety on the "3" position of the cephalosporin nucleus. This is chemically similar to disulfiram, and in alcohol-fed animals, methyltetrazol can produce significant increases in acetaldehyde levels (*Personal Communication:* J. Wold, Lilly Research Laboratories). Cases of a *disulfiram-like reaction* in patients treated with either moxalactam or cefoperazone who subsequently received alcohol have been reported (127–131). Cefamandole also has this moiety as part of its structure but this reaction has not been reported. *Hypoprothrombinemia*, with bleeding episodes, has been reported with moxalactam given in large doses to neutropenic cancer patients (131). This is presumably due to eradication of gastrointestinal flora which synthesize vitamin K. There are probably other factors involved including predisposing underlying conditions such as carcinoma and thrombocytopenia. Nonetheless, the hypoprothrombinemia was rapidly reversed with administration of phytonadione.

Colonization and superinfection with resistant pathogens has been described for third generation cephalosporins. Of particular concern are superinfections with enterococci (132) and *Pseudomonas aeruginosa*. Infections with these pathogens in an already debilitated host are very difficult to treat and are frequently fatal.

It is unlikely that these reactions would arise in our patient since he has no significant underlying conditions, but careful monitoring of his vital signs, physical examination, and culture data are crucial. Given this information and the clinical circumstances, it seems that the appropriate initial therapy for this patient should include an aminoglycoside to provide full gram-negative coverage. A second agent, either an extended spectrum penicillin or a third generation cephalosporin, would provide synergy and broaden coverage. Once the organism is identified and susceptibility tests performed, more specific therapy can be selected. If the organism is susceptible to a first or second generation cephalosporin (eg, Klebsiella), then that may be appropriate sole therapy for this infection. If the organism is found to be *Enterobacter, Serratia* or *Pseudomonas*, a third generation agent either alone or combined with an aminoglycoside would be appropriate therapy.

Parenchymal pulmonary infections are difficult to treat, and large doses of these agents would be necessary. Cefotaxime should be given in doses of 1–1.5 gm every 4–6 hours. Moxalactam and cefoperazone are eliminated more slowly and can be given every 8 to 12 hours (eg, 2–3 gm q 8–12 hr).

In conclusion, if the organisms producing nosocomial infection in a given institution are found to be highly susceptible to third generation cephalosporins, then these agents may be used alone in the initial therapy of serious gram-negative infection. If this information is not available, it seems prudent, at this time, to include an aminoglycoside in the initial regimen until culture and sensitivity results are available.

References

1. Chodak GW et al: Use of systemic antibiotics for prophylaxis in surgery. Arch Surg. 1977; 112:326.

2. Shapiro M et al: Use of antimicrobial drugs in general hospitals. Patterns of prophylaxis. N Engl J Med. 1979; 301:351.

3. Castle M et al: Antibiotic use at Duke University Medical Center. JAMA. 1977; 237:2819.

4. Ad Hoc Committee of the Committee on Trauma, Division of Medical Sciences, National Academy of Sciences-National Research Council: Postoperative wound infections: the influence of ultraviolet irradiation of the operating room and various other factors. Ann Surg. 1964; 160 (Suppl 2):23.

5. Cruse P: Infection surveillance: identifying the problems and the high risk patient. South Med J. 1977; 70(Suppl):4.

6. Caldwell JR et al: Adverse reactions to antimicrobial agents. JAMA. 1974; 230:77.

7. Burke JF: Effective period of preventive antibiotic action in experimental incisions and dermal lesions. Surgery. 1961; 50:161.

8. Alexander JW et al: Penicillin prophylaxis of experimental staphylococcal wound infections. Surg Gynecol Obstet. 1965; 120:243.

9. Stone HH et al: Antibiotic prophylaxis in gastric, biliary and colonic surgery. Ann Surg. 1976; 184:443.

10. Feathers RS et al: Prophylactic systemic antibiotics in colorectal surgery. Lancet. 1977; ii:4.

11. Arabi Y et al: Influence of bowel preparation and antimicrobials on colonic microflora. Br J Surg. 1978; 65:555.

12. Washington JA et al: Effect of preoperative antibiotic regimen on development of infection after intestinal surgery: prospective, randomized, double-blind study. Ann Surg. 1974; 180:567.

13. Jorgenson SJ et al: Prophylactic treatment with bacitracin-neomycin and tetracycline in surgery of colon and rectum. Acta Chir Scand. 1974; 140:491.

14. Goldring J et al: Prophylactic oral antimicrobial agents in elective colonic surgery. A controlled trial. Lancet. 1975; ii:997.

15. Clarke JS et al: Preoperative oral antibiotics reduce septic complications of colon operations: results of prospective, randomized, double-blind clinical study. Ann Surg. 1977; 186:251.

16. Matheson DM et al: Randomized multicentre trial of oral bowel preparation and antimicrobials for elective colorectal operations. Br J Surg. 1978; 65:597.

17. Höjer H et al: Systemic prophylaxis with doxycycline in surgery of the colon and rectum. Ann Surg. 1978; 187:362.

18. Taylor SA et al: The use of metronidazole in the preparation of the bowel for surgery. Br J Surg. 1979; 66:191.

19. Wapnick S et al: Reduction of postoperative infection in elective colon surgery with preoperative administration of kanamycin and erythromycin. Surgery. 1979; 85:317.

20. Polk HC et al: Postoperative wound infection: a prospective study of determinant factors and prevention. Surgery. 1969; 66:97.

21. Keighley MRB et al: Prophylaxis against anaerobic sepsis in bowel surgery. Br J Surg. 1976; 63:538.

22. Eykyn SJ et al: Prophylactic perioperative intravenous metronidazole in elective colorectal surgery. Lancet. 1979; ii:761.

23. Rosenberg IL et al: Preparation of the intestine in patients undergoing major large bowel surgery, mainly for neoplasms of the colon and rectum. Br J Surg. 1971; 58:266.

24. Burton JGW et al: A trial of cephalothin sodium in colon surgery to prevent wound infection. Arch Surg. 1977; 112:1169.

25. Condon RE et al: Preoperative prophylactic cephalothin fails to control septic complications of colorectal operations: results of controlled clinical trial. Am J Surg. 1979; 137:68.

26. Slama TG et al: Comparative efficacy of prophylactic cephalothin and cefamandole for elective colon surgery. Am J Surg. 1979; 137:593.

27. Lewis RT et al: Antibiotics in surgery of the colon. Can J Surg. 1978; 21:339.

28. Dion YM et al: The influence of oral versus parenteral preoperative metronidazole on sepsis following colon surgery. Ann Surg. 1980; 192:221.

29. Keighley MRB et al: Comparison between systemic and oral antimicrobial prophylaxis in colorectal surgery. Lancet. 1979; i:894.

30. Barber MS et al: Parenteral antibiotics in elective colon surgery? A prospective, controlled clinical study. Surgery. 1979; 86:23.

31. Stone HH et al: Prophylactic and preventive antibiotic therapy. Timing, duration and economics. Ann Surg. 1979; 189:691.

32. Higgins AF et al: Single and multiple dose cotrimoxazole and metronidazole in colorectal surgery. Br J Surg. 1980; 67:90.

33. Strachan CJL et al: Prophylactic use of cephazolin against wound sepsis after cholecystectomy. Br Med J. 1977; i:1254.

34. Ledger WJ et al: Guidelines for antibiotic prophylaxis in gynecology. Am J Obstet Gynecol. 1975; 121:1038.

35. Mendleson J et al: Effect of single and multidose cephradine prophylaxis on infectious morbidity of vaginal hysterectomy. Obstet Gynecol. 1979; 53:31.

36. D'Angelo LJ et al: Short versus long-course prophylactic antibiotic treatment in cesarean section patients. Obstet Gynecol. 1980; 55:583.

37. Conte JE et al: Antibiotic prophylaxis and cardiac surgery. A prospective double-blind comparison of single-dose versus multiple-dose regimens. Ann Intern Med. 1972; 76:943.

38. Goldmann DA et al: Cephalothin prophylaxis in cardiac valve surgery. A prospective, double-blind comparison of two-day and six-day regimens. J Thorac Cardiovasc Surg. 1977; 73:470.

39. Pollard JP et al: Antibiotic prophylaxis in total hip replacement. Br Med J. 1979; i:707.

40. Gorbach SL et al: Pseudomembranous colitis: A review of its diverse forms. J Infect Dis. 1977; 135 (Suppl):S 89.

41. Totten M et al: Clinical and pathological spectrum of antibiotic associated colitis. Am J Gastroenterol. 1978; 69:311.

42. Cammerer RC et al: Clinical spectrum of pseudomembranous colitis. JAMA. 1976; 235:2502.

43. Tedesco FJ: Clindamycin and colitis: a review. J Infect Dis. 1977; 135 (Suppl):S 95.

44. Christie D: Ampicillin associated colitis. J Pediatr. 1975; 87:657.

45. Tures JF et al: Cephalosporin-associated pseudomembranous colitis. JAMA. 1976; 236:948.

46. Cameron A et al: Pseudomembranous colitis and cotrimoxazole. Br Med J. 1977; i:1321.

47. Bartlett JG et al: Antibiotic-associated pseudomembranous colitis due to toxin-producing clostridia. N Engl J Med. 1978; 298:531.

48. Keighley MRB et al: Randomized controlled trial of vancomycin for pseudomembranous colitis and postoperative diarrhea. Br Med J. 1978; ii:1667.

49. Tedesco F et al: Oral vancomycin for antibiotic-associated pseudomembranous colitis. Lancet. 1978; ii:226.

50. Modigliani R et al: Vancomycin for antibiotic-induced colitis. Lancet. 1978; i:97.

51. Dinh HT: Treatment of antibiotic-induced colitis by metronidazole. Lancet. 1978; i:338.

52. Burbige EJ et al: Pseudomembranous colitis. Association with antibiotics and therapy with cholestyramine. JAMA. 1975; 231:1157.

53. George WL et al: Relapse of pseudomembranous colitis after vancomycin therapy. N Engl J Med. 1979; 301:414.

54. Gatehouse D et al: Prediction of wound sepsis following gastric operations. Br J Surg. 1979; 65:551.

55. Lewis RT et al: Discriminate use of antibiotic prophylaxis in gastroduodenal surgery. Am J Surg. 1979; 138:640.

56. Chetlin SH et al: Biliary bacteremia. Arch Surg. 1971; 102:303.

57. Chetlin SH et al: Preoperative antibiotics in biliary surgery. Arch Surg. 1973; 107:319.

58. Keighley MRB et al: A controlled trial of parenteral prophylactic gentamicin therapy in biliary surgery. Br J Surg. 1975; 62:275.

59. Morran C et al: Prophylactic co-trimoxazole in biliary surgery. Br Med J. 1978; ii:462.

60. Keighley MRB et al: Antibiotics in biliary disease: the relative importance of antibiotic concentrations in the bile and serum. Gut. 1976; 17:495.

61. Ledger WJ et al: Prophylactic cephaloridine in the prevention of postoperative pelvic infections in premenopausal women undergoing vaginal hysterectomy. Am J Obstet Gynecol. 1973; 115:766.

62. Breedon JT et al: Low dose prophylactic antibiotics in vaginal hysterectomy. Obstet Gynecol. 1974; 43:379.

63. Ohm MJ et al: The effect of antibiotic prophylaxis on patients undergoing vaginal operations. Am J Obstet Gynecol. 1975; 123:590.

64. Forney JP et al: Impact of cephalosporin prophylaxis on conization-vaginal hysterectomy morbidity. Am J Obstet Gynecol. 1976; 125:100.

65. Allen JL et al: Use of a prophylactic antibiotic in elective major gynologic operations. Obstet Gynecol. 1972; 39:218.

66. Swartz WH et al: T-tube suction drainage and/or prophylactic antibiotics. A randomized study of 451 hysterectomies. Obstet Gynecol. 1976; 47:665.

67. Lett WJ et al: Prophylactic antibiotics for women undergoing vaginal hysterectomy. J Reprod Med. 1977; 19:51.

68. Jennings RH: Prophylactic antibiotics in vaginal and abdominal hysterectomy. South Med J. 1978; 71:251.

69. Mickal A et al: Cefoxitin sodium: double-blind vaginal hysterectomy prophylaxis in premenopausal patients. Obstet Gynecol. 1980; 56:222.

70. Hemsell DL et al: Cefoxitin for prophylaxis in premenopausal women undergoing vaginal hysterectomy. Obstet Gynecol. 1980; 56:629.

71. Bolling DR et al: Prophylactic antibiotics for vaginal hysterectomies. Obstet Gynecol. 1973; 41:689.

72. Harralson JD et al: The effect of prophylactic antibiotics on pelvic infection following vaginal hysterectomy. Am J Obstet Gynecol. 1974; 120:1046.

73. Roberts JM et al: Low-dose carbenicillin prophylaxis for vaginal and abdominal hysterectomy. Obstet Gynecol. 1978; 52:83.

74. Grossman JH et al: Prophylactic antibiotics in gynecologic surgery. Obstet Gynecol. 1979; 53:537.

75. Mathews DD et al: A double-blind trial of single-dose chemoprophylaxis with co-trimoxazole during vaginal hysterectomy and repair. Br J Obstet Gynaecol. 1979; 86:737.

76. Holman JF et al: Perioperative antibiotics in major elective gynecologic surgery. South Med J. 1978; 71:417–420.

77. Mathew DD et al: A randomized controlled trial of a short course of cephaloridine in the prevention of infection after abdominal hysterectomy. Br J Obstet Gynaecol. 1978; 85:381–385.

78. Karhunen M et al: Single dose of tinidazole in prophylaxis of infections following hysterectomy. Br J Obstet Gynaecol. 1980; 87:70.

79. Mathews DD et al: A double-blind trial of single-dose chemoprophylaxis with cotrimoxazole during total abdominal hysterectomy. Br J Obstet Gynaecol. 1977; 84:894.

80. Ohm MJ et al: The effect of antibiotic prophylaxis on patients undergoing total abdominal hysterectomy. I. Effect on morbidity. Am J Obstet Gynecol. 1976; 125:442.

81. Gibbs RS et al: Prophylactic antibiotics in cesarean section: a double blind study. Am J Obstet Gynecol. 1972; 114:1048.

82. Morrison JC et al: The use of prophylactic antibiotics in patients undergoing cesarean section. Surg Gynecol Obstet. 1973; 136:425.

83. Gibbs RS et al: A follow-up study on prophylactic antibiotics in cesarean section. Am J Obstet Gynecol. 1973; 117:419.

84. Moro M et al: Prophylactic antibiotics in cesarean section. Obstet Gynecol. 1974; 44:688.

85. Rothbard MJ et al: Prophylactic antibiotics in cesarean section. Obstet Gynecol. 1975; 45:421.

86. Kreutner AK et al: Perioperative antibiotic prophylaxis in cesarean section. Obstet Gynecol. 1978; 52:279.

87. Wong R et al: Prophylactic use of cefazolin in monitored obstetric patients undergoing cesarean section. Obstet Gynecol. 1978; 51:407.

88. Gordon HR et al: Prophylactic cesarean section antibiotics: maternal and neonatal morbidity before or after cord clamping. Obstet Gynecol. 1979; 53:151.

89. Iskovitz J et al: The effect of prophylactic antibiotics on febrile morbidity following cesarean section. Obstet Gynecol. 1979; 53:162.

90. Phelan JP et al: Prophylactic antibiotics in cesarean section: a double-blind study of cefazolin. Am J Obstet Gynecol. 1979; 133:474.

91. Gall SA: The efficacy of prophylactic antibiotics in cesarean section. Am J Obstet Gynecol. 1979; 134:506.

92. Green SL et al: Risk factors associated with post cesarean section febrile morbidity. Obstet Gynecol. 1980; 56:269.

93. Rehu M et al: Risk factors for febrile morbidity associated with cesarean section. Obstet Gynecol. 1980; 56:269.

94. Goodman JS et al: Infection after cardiovascular surgery. N Engl J Med. 1968; 278:117.

95. Goldmann DA et al: Cephalothin prophylaxis in cardiac valve surgery. A prospective, double-blind comparison of two-day and six-day regimens. J Thorac Cardiovasc Surg. 1977; 73:470.

96. Myerowitz PD et al: Antibiotic prophylaxis for open heart surgery. J Thorac Cardiovasc Surg. 1977; 73:625.

97. Pien FD et al: Comparative study of prophylactic antibiotics in cardiac surgery. Clindamycin versus cephalothin. J Thorac Cardiovasc Surg. 1979; 77:908.

98. Fong IW et al: The value of prophylactic antibiotics in aorta-coronary bypass operations. A double-blind randomized study. J Thorac Cardiovasc Surg. 1979; 78:908.

99. Everett ED et al: Transient bacteremia and endocarditis prophylaxis. A review. Medicine. 1977; 56:61.

100. Kaiser AB et al: Antibiotic prophylaxis in vascular surgery. Ann Surg. 1978; 188:283.

101. Pitt HA et al: Prophylactic antibiotics in vascular surgery: topical, systemic, or both? Ann Surg. 1980; 192:356.

102. Ericson C et al: Cloxacillin in the prophylaxis of postoperative infections of the hip. J Bone Joint Surg. 1973; 55A:808.

103. Boyd RJ et al: A double-blind clinical trial of prophylactic antibiotics in hip fractures. J Bone Joint Surg. 1973; 55A:1251.

104. Pavel A et al: Prophylactic antibiotics in clean orthopaedic surgery. J Bone Joint Surg. 1974; 56A:777.

105. DiPiro JT et al: Antimicrobial prophylaxis in surgery: Parts 1 & 2. Am J Hosp Pharm. 1981; 38:320,487.

106. Hirschmann JV et al: Antimicrobial prophylaxis: A critique of recent trials. Rev Infect Dis. 1980; 2:1.

107. Eickhoff TC et al: In vitro comparison of cefoxitin, cefamandole, cephalexin, and cephalothin. Antimicrob Agents Chemother. 1976; 9:994.

108. Eykyn S et al: Antibacterial activity of cefamandole, a new cephalosporin antibiotic, compared with cephalothin, cephaloridine and cephalexin. Antimicrob Agents Chemother. 1973; 3:657.

109. Bodey GP et al: In vitro studies of cefamandole. Antimicrob Agents Chemother. 1976; 9:452.

110. Eykyn S et al: Antibacterial activity of cefuroxime, a new cephalosporin, compared with that of cephaloridine, cephalothin and cefamandole. Antimicrob Agents Chemother. 1976; 9:690.

111. Washington JA: Differences between cephalothin and newer parenterally absorbed cephalosporins in vitro: A justification for separate disks. J Infect Dis. 1978; 137(suppl):S32.

112. Schurman DJ et al: Cefazolin concentrations in bone and synovial fluid. J Bone Joint Surg. 1978; 60-A:359.

113. Reyes MP: The aerobic gram-negative bacillary pneumonias. Med Clin North Am. 1980; 64:363.

114. Eickhoff TC: Pulmonary infections in surgical patients. Surg Clin North Am. 1980; 60:175.

115. Neu HC et al: Antibacterial activity of a new l-oxa cephalosporin compared with that of other beta-lactam compounds. Antimicrob Agents Chemother. 1979; 16:141.

116. Jorgensen JH et al: In vitro activities of moxalactam and cefotaxime against aerobic gram-negative bacilli. Antimicrob Agents Chemother. 1980; 17:937.

117. Kurtz TO et al: Comparative in vitro activity of moxalactam, cefotaxime, cefoperazone, piperacillin and aminoglycosides against gram-negative bacilli. Antimicrob Agents Chemother. 1980; 18:645.

118. Barry AL et al: In vitro evaluation of LY127935(6059S) compared with cefotaxime, eight other beta-lactams and two aminoglycosides. J Antimicrob Chemother. 1980; 6:775.

119. Jorgensen JH et al: In vitro activities of cefotaxime and moxalactam against Hemophilus influenzae. Antimicrob Agents Chemother. 1980; 17:516.

120. Baker CN et al: In vitro antimicrobial activity of cefoperazone, cefotaxime moxalactam, azlocillin, mezlocillin, and other beta-lactam antibiotics against Neisseria gonorrhoeae and Hemophilus influenzae, including beta-lactamase producing strains. Antimicrob Agents Chemother. 1980; 17:757.

121. Hall WH et al: Comparative activities of the oxa-beta-lactam LY127935, cefotaxime, cefoperazone, cefamandole, and ticarcillin against multiple resistant gram-negative bacilli. Antimicrob Agents Chemother. 1980; 17:273.

122. Verbist L: Comparison of in vitro activities of eight beta-lactamase-stable cephalosporins against beta-lactamase-producing gram-negative bacilli. Antimicrob Agents Chemother. 1981; 19:407.

123. Dudley MN et al: Microbiology, pharmacology, and clinical use. Clin Pharm. 1982 In press.

124. Tofte RW et al: Moxalactam therapy for a wide spectrum of bacterial infections in adults. Antimicrob Agents Chemother. 1981; 19:740.

125. Lentino JR et al: Therapy of lower respiratory tract infections with moxalactam. Antimicrob Agents Chemother. 1981; 19:801.

126. Livingston WK et al: Clinical evaluation of moxalactam. Antimicrob Agents Chemother. 1981; 20:88.

127. Platt R et al: Moxalactam therapy of infections caused by cephalothin-resistant bacteria: influence of serum inhibitory activity on clinical response and acquisition of antibiotic resistance during therapy. Antimicrob Agents Chemother. 1981; 20:351.

128. Neu HC et al: Interaction between moxalactam and alcohol. Lancet. 1980; 1:1422.

129. Foster TS et al: Disulfiram-like reaction associated with a parenteral cephalosporin. Am J Hosp Pharm. 1980; 37:858.

130. McMahon FG: Disulfiram-like reaction to a cephalosporin. JAMA. 1980; 243:2397.

131. Fainstein V et al: Moxalactam and ticarcillin or tobramycin for the treatment of neutropenia cancer patients. Abst #317. Proc. 21st Intersci Conference Antimicrob Agents Chemother, Chicago, Ill. Nov. 4–6, 1981.

132. Yu VL: Enterococcal superinfection and colonization after therapy with moxalactam, a new broad spectrum antibiotic. Ann Intern Med. 1981; 94:784.

Chapter 33

Tuberculosis

Earl S. Ward and Lloyd Y. Young

Tuberculosis is a bacterial infection caused by the organism *Mycobacterium tuberculosis.* In humans, the lung is the most common site of infection, although numerous other areas (meninges, bones, joints, peritoneum, genitourinary tract, skin) may also become infected (1). If unrecognized or left untreated, the infection *may* progress to clinical disease and lead to necrosis and cavitation of the patient's lung. In addition, a person with cavitary tuberculosis is a health hazard to those with whom he is in close contact, since the organism can be transmitted to others (2).

Mycobacterium tuberculosis is an aerobic bacillus that stains acid-fast (Ziehl-Neelsen method or fluorescence technique) and is therefore sometimes referred to as an acid-fast bacillus (AFB). It thrives in organs of relatively high oxygen tension such as the apices of the lung, the renal parenchyma, the growing ends of the bones, and the cerebral cortex (2).

Tubercle bacilli are transmitted by aerosolized droplets expectorated from a person with pulmonary tuberculosis. These droplets are small enough (less than 10 microns) to remain airborne for a considerable period of time. Transmission of these particles can be blocked by adequate room ventilation, ultraviolet light, and by chemotherapy of the source case (3–9). Tubercle bacilli are not transmitted on objects such as dishes, clothing, or bedding (9). Family household contacts and those in institutions (hospitals, nursing homes, prison) sharing an enclosed environment with a source case are at a major risk for infection (10,11).

The droplet nuclei containing tubercle bacilli enter the lungs where their small size allows them to reach the respiratory bronchioles and alveoli where they may establish infection. This initial infection usually occurs in the lower segment(s) of the lung. Persons that have been previously infected with tubercle bacilli are protected from reinfection by a specific immunity mediated by T lymphocytes. In the non-immune (susceptible) host, the bacilli multiply initially unopposed by normal host defense mechanisms. The tubercle bacilli that are taken into the macrophage during phagocytosis may remain viable for extended periods of time. These organisms may enter the lymphatic system and disseminate to other organs of the body. After a period of three to ten weeks, a specific T lymphocyte-mediated immune response should develop and prevent further multiplication of these bacilli. The T lymphocytes

cause release of lysosomal enzymes from macrophages which destroy some bacilli but also damage host tissues. The result of this immune response is tissue healing with granuloma formation. The bacilli contained in the granuloma may survive and remain dormant for many years. For unknown reasons, these granulomas may break down in later years leading to either pulmonary or extrapulmonary clinical disease (2,12–16). Today, most cases of tuberculosis result from a reactivation (break down of a granuloma) of a previous infection, rather than a new infection (2).

A clear distinction should be made between infection and clinical disease. *Infection* with tuberculosis refers to harboring the bacilli within the body with no x-ray changes, negative bacteriologic studies, and no clinical symptoms. Infection is suspected when the tuberculin skin test (PPD-Mantoux) is greater than 10 mm. *Clinical disease* (Tuberculosis) results when a lack of host defense mechanisms allow infection to progress to one or more organs and produce clinical symptoms, x-ray changes, or positive bacteriologic studies. The definite diagnosis of tuberculosis is dependent on the isolation of *M. tuberculosis* from the sputum, spinal fluid, urine, or tissue biopsy (1,14). It takes 6 to 8 weeks for this culture to become positive. The risk of developing clinical disease within five years after infection is 5 to 15% if left untreated. The highest risk occurs in the first one to two years following infection (17). Many persons harbor the bacilli for a lifetime but remain at risk of developing clinical disease at any time.

Certain risk factors such as diabetes mellitus, silicosis, gastrectomy, crowded living conditions, alcohol abuse, chronic renal failure, hematologic disease, reticuloendothelial disease, and corticosteroid use increase the chances of developing clinical tuberculosis (2,13).

There has been a dramatic decline in the incidence of tuberculosis since 1900 largely due to effective chemotherapy and early recognition of source cases. In 1980, 27,749 cases of tuberculosis (case rate 12.3 per 100,000) were reported in the United States. This represents an increase in cases of 0.3% from the number of cases reported in 1979. This is only the second time since 1953 that an increase in the number of cases reported has occurred (18). The major reason for this increase is the high incidence of tuberculosis among Southeast Asian refugees admitted to this country. The incidence of tuberculosis is estimated to be 40 times higher in this group than in the general U.S. population (19). The overall incidence of tuberculosis is higher in the southern half of the U.S. and in major cities. The poor, the elderly, and non-caucasians also exhibit a higher incidence.

With the recognition that tuberculosis can be effectively treated with outpatient drug therapy, the responsibility of treatment has shifted from the sanatorium to the community hospital, private physician, and health department (20–22). The need for early recognition and treatment necessitates that all practitioners become familiar with the tuberculosis disease process and the principles of treatment.

1. M.W., a 40-year-old female, is admitted to the hospital with a two-month history of cough which has recently become productive, fatigue, night sweats, and a five pound weight loss. Other medical problems include diabetes mellitus which is controlled with 10 units of NPH insulin daily.

Physical examination and chest x-ray were essentially normal. A PPD skin test and sputum collections for culture and sensitivity and for acid-fast bacilli (AFB) were ordered as part of this patient's diagnostic workup. Initial laboratory tests were within normal limits.

The result of the PPD skin test, read at 48 hours, was a palpable induration of 14 mm. Her sputum smear was positive for AFB, and additional sputum cultures for *M. tuberculosis* were ordered to confirm a diagnosis of active disease.

What subjective findings does this patient have that are consistent with tuberculosis?

This patient's history of cough, which gradually became productive, fatigue, and night sweats are all consistent with the classic symptoms of tuberculosis (2,14,28). The cough is usually nonproductive in the early stages and later becomes productive. The sputum may contain blood (hemoptysis) in the later stages in patients with advanced cavitary disease. Other symptoms include anorexia which may result in weight loss, fever, pleuritic pain, and general malaise. Many patients with pulmonary tuberculosis (active disease) have no acute symptoms, and cases are often found following routine chest x-rays for another illness. Since symptoms often occur in persons with pre-existing pulmonary disease or pneu-

monia, they are often not attributed to tuberculosis.

Misdiagnosis. A report from a private urban hospital showed that over a one year span almost 50% of the cases of active tuberculosis were misdiagnosed (29). More than one-third of their patients with active tuberculosis had no sweats, chills, or malaise, and fewer than 50% had fever. Cough was evident in 80% of these patients, but only 25% had hemoptysis. Although dullness over the apices of the lungs and post-tussive rales are expected in tuberculosis, fewer than one-third of the above patients showed any abnormal pulmonary signs upon physical examination. As a result of the lack of clinical symptoms, tuberculosis was not suspected in 44% of the cases from another institution, nor was it diagnosed in up to 95% of cases in some other reports. A subsequent report by Greenbaum et al showed that 50% of patients in a teaching hospital with pulmonary tuberculosis, confirmed by isolation of *M. tuberculosis,* were misdiagnosed at the time of their admission (30).

2. *PPD Skin Test.* What is the PPD skin test and how should the results be interpreted in this patient?

The *PPD skin test* (Mantoux test) is a diagnostic tool used for the detection of infection with *M. tuberculosis.* The abbreviation PPD refers to the purified protein derivative of *M. tuberculosis* which is prepared from a culture of tubercle bacilli. The skin test (intermediate-strength PPD) is performed by injecting 0.1 ml of solution containing 5 tuberculin units (TU) intracutaneously into the volar or dorsal portion of the forearm (23). The solution, stabilized with Tween 80, should be administered immediately after its withdrawal from the vial (14,24).

In the presence of mycobacterial infection, a delayed hypersensitivity reaction to the tubercle bacillus or to its components develops in the host. Upon re-exposure to the tuberculin antigen (PPD skin test), the host's immune system responds with a characteristic inflammatory reaction at the site of exposure. This reaction usually will develop within 2 to 10 weeks after infection (16).

This patient's reaction is positive (14 mm). A palpable induration of greater than 10 mm diameter, 48–72 hours after administration is considered to be a positive reaction; a reading of 5–

9 mm is considered doubtful; and 0–4 mm is interpreted as a negative reaction (14). The average reaction in the presence of *M. tuberculosis* infection is 16 mm ± 8 mm (23). This measurement is not based upon the erythematous zone, but rather on the palpable induration which represents a localized thickening of the skin due to edema and accumulation of sensitized lymphocytes (2). A reaction of 5 mm or more may be significant when testing a close contact of a person with tuberculosis (14). If less than a 10 mm reaction is considered positive, a larger percentage of these reactions may be due to cross-reacting mycobacteria other than *M. tuberculosis.*

This patient's positive reaction to PPD (5 TU) does not imply clinical disease. It merely signifies that she may have been infected previously with *M. tuberculosis* or possibly an atypical "cross-reacting" mycobacterium which are present in areas such as the southeastern United States (23). However, since her clinical symptoms are consistent with tuberculosis, and she has a positive skin test response and a positive sputum smear, a diagnosis of active disease can be made. To confirm this diagnosis, *M. tuberculosis* must be isolated from the sputum.

3. Would a negative tuberculin skin test have eliminated the possibility of infection with *M. tuberculosis* in this patient?

A negative skin test may be the result of technical error but most frequently occurs in individuals who have had no prior infection with *M. tuberculosis* or who have only recently been infected, or who are anergic.

Anergy or decreased ability to respond to antigens may be due to severe debility, old age, high fever, sarcoidosis, corticosteroids, immunosuppressive drugs, hematological disease, reticuloendothelial disease, overwhelming disseminated (miliary) tuberculosis, recent virus infection, or vaccination. The nutritional status of the patient is also of concern, since the number of positive skin tests in patients with tuberculosis infection increases with the correction of malnutrition (25,26).

A "false-negative" reaction may occur in 15–20% of persons infected with *M. tuberculosis* (2). In a study by Nash et al, 25% of patients with active pulmonary tuberculosis failed to respond to (5 TU) PPD (27).

Therefore, a negative response to 5 TU in this patient would not have excluded tuberculosis infection.

The use of 250 TU strength of PPD (second-strength PPD) for persons not responding to 5 TU is not recommended, because these results cannot be interpreted using the American Thoracic Society Guidelines (14).

4. *Treatment.* How should treatment be initiated in this patient pending the results of the sputum culture and sensitivity?

Effective treatment of tuberculosis requires a period of intensive drug therapy with at least two bactericidal drugs. This patient, with uncomplicated pulmonary tuberculosis, should be started on isoniazid (INH) 300 mg and rifampin 600 mg in a single daily dose. This initial phase of treatment should last two to three months. This combination of INH-rifampin sterilizes the lesions and sputum faster than the standard three drug regimen of INH, streptomycin, and ethambutol (31). There is no additional benefit obtained from adding either ethambutol or streptomycin to this initial INH – rifampin combination except in cases of extrapulmonary tuberculosis or when primary drug resistance is suspected (32–35). The dosage of rifampin is extremely important when using this two drug regimen. Doses of rifampin less than 600 mg a day in combination with INH are associated with decreased effectiveness, and dosages of less than 9 mg/kg/day may not be effective in treating pulmonary tuberculosis (36).

This patient, who is also a diabetic, should also be placed on pyridoxine 10 mg/day, since she may be at a higher risk of developing peripheral neuropathy (see Question 14) (37).

She should cease to be infectious about two to four weeks after initiation of chemotherapy at which time the number of organisms in her sputum should be significantly reduced (3–8). If there are no complications from her drug therapy or disease, she may be released from the hospital as soon as her symptoms resolve. Most patients with uncomplicated pulmonary tuberculosis do not require hospitalization (4,58,59).

5. Why is multiple drug therapy indicated for the treatment of active disease?

Multiple drug therapy is needed to prevent the development of resistance strains of bacilli and to sterilize the sputum and lesions as quickly as possible. The drugs available for the treatment of tuberculosis vary in their ability to accomplish these tasks (see Table 1) (38).

The drugs that are effective against tubercle bacilli can be divided into two groups: primary and secondary (see Table 2). The foundation of treatment should be with primary drugs such as isoniazid and rifampin. Both INH and rifampin are bactericidal against the fast growing extracellular bacilli in the lung cavity. Rifampin also has activity against intracellular organisms that are usually dormant but undergo periods of active growth (slow multipliers) (38,39). This ability to penetrate and destroy the slow-growing, persistent intracellular organisms makes rifampin extremely valuable in short-course chemotherapy regimens.

The secondary drugs streptomycin, ethambutol, and pyrazinamide are generally less effective or more toxic than the primary agents. They are primarily used in combination with INH – rifampin when drug-resistant organisms are suspected or to treat extrapulmonary tuberculosis infections. Streptomycin is active against the fast multiplying extracellular organisms and is very effective when given daily for two months followed by two to three times a week administration (40). Streptomycin must be given intramuscularly which is painful and may decrease patient compliance. Also, like all aminoglycosides, streptomycin can cause ototoxicity and/or renal toxicity. Ethambutol is bacteriostatic and is moderately effective against the fast growing bacilli. It

has very little sterilizing activity and is used primarily in the prevention of drug-resistant organisms (38,41). Pyrazinamide is effective against intracellular bacilli whose growth is partially inhibited by the acidic environment within the macrophage. It is very effective in sterilizing the lesions and appears to be most active in the first two months of treatment (38,41–44). Pyrazinamide appears to be an essential drug if the duration of treatment is to be less than 9 months.

The other drugs used in the treatment of tuberculosis, capreomycin, kanamycin, cycloserine, ethionamide, and aminosalicylic acid are usually reserved for cases involving drug-resistant organisms, drug toxicity, or patient intolerance to the other agents.

6. Six weeks later the sputum cultures from M.W. were found to be positive for *M. tuberculosis* and subsequently shown to be sensitive to the current drug regimen of INH and rifampin. What drug regimen would be appropriate for continued therapy in this patient and how long should treatment be maintained?

For years, the standard treatment of tuberculosis was INH 300 mg daily with ethambutol 15 to 25 mg/kg/day for a period of 18 to 24 months. Streptomycin 1 gm per day intramuscularly (IM) was used for the first two months to prevent development of INH-resistant organisms (2). A recent study demonstrated that daily INH and rifampin for 20 weeks followed by daily INH and ethambutol until the sputum is negative for one year is very effective (36). Successful treatment of uncomplicated tuberculosis is possible in 12 to 18 months of treatment providing that INH and rifampin are used for the first 20 weeks. If drugs other than INH and rifampin are used in the initial phase, treatment must be continued 18 to 24 months (56,57). Subsequent reports indicate that in regimens containing INH and rifampin, the duration of therapy may be successfully shortened to 9–12 months (45–47).

The British Thoracic and Tuberculosis Association has reported successful results utilizing treatment regimens of INH and rifampin with either streptomycin or ethambutol daily for two months, followed by INH and rifampin for 4 to 10 months (45).

In addition, two reports indicate successful results with the continuation phase given once or

Table 1.

GRADING OF ANTIBACTERIAL DRUGS

Activity	Prevention of Drug Resistance	Sterilizing Activity
High	Isoniazid	Rifampin
	Rifampin	Pyrazinamide
	Streptomycin	Isoniazid
	Ethambutol	Streptomycin
	Thiacetazone	Ethambutol
Low	Pyrazinamide	Thiacetazone

Reprinted with permission from Mitchison DA: Basic mechanisms of chemotherapy. Chest. 1979; 76 (Suppl):771.

Table 2.

SUMMARY OF ANTITUBERCULAR DRUGS

Drug	Daily Dose	Twice-weekly Dose	Peak Blood Levels	Primary Toxicities	Dosage Adjustment In Renal Impairment	Comments
PRIMARY DRUGS						
Isoniazid (INH)	Adults: 5–10 mg/kg (max 300 mg) Children: 10 mg/kg (max 300 mg)	15 mg/kg	2–5 mcg/ml	Peripheral neuropathy; hepatic dysfunction; skin rashes; fever; arthralgia, SLE syndrome.	No	Neuropathy preventable by pyridoxine 10 mg. Increases serum levels of phenytoin.
Rifampin (RIF)	Adults: 600 mg Children: 10–15 mg/kg (max 600 mg)	600 mg 15 mg/kg (max 600 mg)	8 mcg/ml	Hepatic dysfunction; thrombocytopenia; renal failure; "flu-like" syndrome; cutaneous reactions.	No	Red discoloration of body secretions (perspiration, saliva, urine). Induces hepatic metabolism of warfarin, corticosteroids, diazepam, quinidine, digoxin, and oral contraceptives.
SECONDARY DRUGS						
Ethambutol (EMB)	15–25 mg/kg	50 mg/kg	2–5 mcg/ml	Retrobulbar neuritis; peripheral neuritis; headache; skin rashes.	Yes	Routine vision tests of questionable value. 50% excreted unchanged in urine.
Streptomycin (SM)	Adults: 1 gm IM Children: 20–40 mg/kg		20–40 mcg/ml	Vestibular and/or auditory dysfunction of 8th nerve; renal dysfunction; skin rashes; neuromuscular blockade.	Yes	Audiometric and neurological examinations recommended. 60–80% excreted unchanged in urine.
Pyrazinamide (PZA)	25–35 mg/kg (max 3 gm)	50 mg/kg (max 3 gm)	60 mcg/ml	Hepatitis (3–6%); hyperuricemia; fever; skin rashes; arthralgia; hemolytic anemia.	Yes	SGOT monthly. Hyperuricemia. Nearly 100% excreted in urine.

MISCELLANEOUS DRUGS

Drug	Dose				Remarks
Capreomycin (CPM)	1 gm	30–35 mcg/ml	(See SM)	Yes	(See SM)
Kanamycin (KM)	Adults: 10 mg/kg Children: 15 mg/kg	15–30 mcg/ml	Auditory dysfunction primarily. (See also SM)	Yes	(See SM)
Cycloserine (CS)	15 mg/kg	10 mcg/ml	CNS toxicity (psychosis and convulsions); headache; tremor; fever; skin rashes.	Yes	Contraindicated in epileptic patients. Some toxicity preventable by pyridoxine. 65% excreted unchanged in urine.
Ethionamide (ETA)	15 mg/kg	20 mcg/ml	GI irritation (50%); hepatitis (esp. diabetics); gynecomastia; impotence; postural hypotension; difficulty in diabetic management.	No	Must be given with meals or antacids. SGOT monthly.
Aminosalicylic Acid (PAS)	200–300 mg/kg	7–8 mcg/ml	GI upset (10%); anemia in G6PD deficient patients; skin rashes; fever; hepatitis; hypothyroidism.	Yes	Must be taken with meals or antacids. 100% excreted into urine. False positive reaction with Clinitest. May increase levels of INH.

twice a week (46,47). One of these reports demonstrated the effectiveness of one month of INH 300 mg and rifampin 600 mg daily, followed by INH 900 mg and rifampin 600 mg twice a week for eight additional months (47). Three months after beginning therapy, 95% of all patients studied had a negative sputum culture.

Attempts to shorten the duration of therapy to less than nine months have been less successful with relapse rates of greater than 5%, a rate considered unacceptable in the United States (32, 35,44,48–51). Since decreasing the duration of chemotherapy can be advantageous in the treatment of tuberculosis, the American Thoracic Society (ATS) and the Centers for Disease Control (CDC) recently issued guidelines (see Table 3) for short-course chemotherapy in the United States (52–54).

There are two options for the continuation phase of treatment in this patient. Treatment may be continued either daily (self-administered) or twice-weekly (supervised). Daily therapy would consist of INH 300 mg and rifampin 600 mg in a single dose. Twice-weekly therapy would consist of INH 15 mg/kg and rifampin 600 mg given in a single dose. Because she is a diabetic, this patient should be treated until the sputum cultures have remained negative for 12 months (36). The ATS/CDC recommends that therapy not be shortened to 9 months until the effectiveness of treatment is known in this group of patients. Because therapy will be extended in this patient, twice-weekly supervised administration is recommended. This approach would require fewer doses of rifampin and should result in substantial cost savings (55). Pyridoxine 10 mg/day should be continued.

7. Monitoring of Therapy. What subjective and objective findings should be monitored for in this patient to ensure effective therapy wth minimal side effects?

Subjective. This patient should be questioned about the occurrence of adverse reactions secondary to INH and rifampin (see Table 2). Specifically, she should be asked about gastrointestinal complaints of anorexia, nausea, or vomiting which may be an indication of possible hepatitis. Since she is a diabetic and is at greater risk for development of peripheral neuropathy, she should be questioned about numbness and tingling in her extremities. However, isoniazid peripheral neuropathy should not be a problem in this patient since she is being maintained on pyridoxine 10

Table 3.

GUIDELINES FOR SHORT-COURSE TUBERCULOSIS CHEMOTHERAPY (52–54)

1. A "core" of isoniazid and rifampin must be used for a minimum of 9 months. This is an acceptable regimen for patients with uncomplicated pulmonary tuberculosis. Therapy should not be shortened in patients with drug-resistant, extrapulmonary tuberculosis, or in patients with other medical conditions such as diabetes, silicosis, and immunosuppressive diseases. In addition, patients being treated with immunosuppressive drugs should not be placed on shortened therapy.

2. The initial phase of treatment usually does not require hospitalization unless symptoms are severe or the patient is a public health hazard.

3. Treatment should be initiated in adults with isoniazid 300 mg and rifampin 600 mg daily. Ethambutol 15 mg/kg daily should be added if the patient has emigrated from an area of high drug resistance, has a history of prior drug treatment for TB, or if the patient is living in an area of high drug resistance. Ethambutol should be continued until drug susceptibility studies show susceptibility to both INH and rifampin. Resistance to either drug will require a change in the chemotherapy and the duration of treatment.

4. The initial phase of treatment should last for 2 weeks to 2 months. Treatment may be continued either daily (self-given) or changed to twice-weekly (supervised). In the twice-weekly regimen, patients should receive INH 15 mg/kg and rifampin 600 mg in one dose. Patients receiving rifampin intermittently should be observed for side effects such as thrombocytopenia (purpura, petechiae, hematuria) or the "flu syndrome".

5. Treatment must be continued a minimum of 9 months and in some cases longer, until the sputum culture has been negative for at least 6 months. Over 90% of patients become sputum negative within 3 months of initiation of therapy. If compliance is questionable or if there is evidence of disseminated disease or complicating medical conditions, treatment should be extended to longer than 6 months after the sputum has become negative.

6. Patients should be monitored for 12 months after completion of therapy.

mg daily. She should also be examined for and questioned about petechiae, bruises, or hematuria, since thrombocytopenia is more common with twice-weekly rifampin.

Objective. A pre-treatment hematocrit, white blood cell count, platelet count, BUN, SGOT, and bilirubin should be determined. Since the patient is over 35 years of age and therefore at increased risk of developing INH and/or rifampin hepatotoxicity, her serum transaminase levels should be monitored monthly at least initially (see Questions 9 and 10). Most INH and rifampin hepatotoxicity occurs within the first four months of therapy (60,61).

Sputum cultures and smears for acid-fast bacilli should be done every one to two weeks initially and then monthly after the sputum cultures become negative (2). With appropriate therapy, sputum smears should be negative in about six to eight weeks. The sputum cultures take longer than the smear to become negative, but are usually negative within three to five months (10).

Intensive follow-up is usually not required after the successful completion of chemotherapy (57). However, since most relapses occur during the first six months after the treatment is completed, it would be advisable to obtain sputum specimens (if possible) at 3, 6, and 12 months. Relapse is usually due to incomplete eradication of organisms rather than the development of drug-resistant organisms (57). Chest x-rays should be done only if there are signs and symptoms suggestive of a recurrence of active disease (54).

8. Preventative Treatment. M.W.'s 51-year-old husband is skin tested with 5 TU strength PPD to determine if he is infected with *M. tuberculosis*. He has a 10 mm reaction to the skin test which is classified as "positive." He does not have any clinical symptoms or x-ray findings suggestive of tuberculosis at this time. Is he at risk of developing active disease? What are the current recommendations for using isoniazid preventive therapy, and should he be treated?

This man is at greater risk of developing active disease, because he is a household contact of a patient with active disease. During the first year after infection, the risk of developing active disease is 2.5%. However, this risk increases to 5% if upon initial evaluation the household contact has a tuberculin positive skin test (62).

Preventive therapy of tuberculosis with isoniazid decreases the bacterial population in those taking the drug. Therefore, INH preventive therapy is not really prophylactic therapy but in ac-

tuality reflects treatment of an infection. Such therapy reduces future morbidity from tuberculosis in the groups at high risk of developing active disease. Persons treated with INH who have not received prior chemotherapy for tuberculosis had a 60% reduction in bacteriologically proven disease over a seven year period when compared to persons receiving a placebo (63). Benefits from preventive therapy usually outweigh the risks of iatrogenic drug reactions, because every person with a positive PPD skin test reaction is at risk of developing clinical disease throughout his or her lifetime.

The American Thoracic Society and the Centers for Disease Control have balanced the risks of developing active tuberculosis against the risk of INH toxicity and have jointly established the following guidelines and priorities for determining who should receive preventive therapy (62):

a. Household members or close associates of persons with newly diagnosed tuberculosis. This group has a high risk of developing active disease.

b. Positive tuberculin reactors with findings on chest x-ray consistent with non-progressive disease who have not received adequate prior treatment with INH. The risk of disease reactivation in these individuals is between 1.0 and 4.5% per year.

c. Newly infected individuals (those who have had a skin test conversion within the last two years). A converter is a person that has a 6 mm increase in induration from less than 10 mm to greater than 10 mm. These individuals have a 5% risk of developing active disease the first year after infection.

An increase in reaction size may not represent a skin test conversion but may be due to a "booster effect." (See Question 11). The booster effect occurs with increasing frequency in persons over the age of fifty and must be considered when determining whether a positive skin test conversion actually represents a new infection.

d. Positive tuberculin reactors with the following special clinical situations may require INH preventive therapy:

(i) prolonged therapy with glucocorticoids, (ii) immunosuppressive therapy, (iii) leukemia, Hodgkin's disease, or other hematologic or reticuloendothelial disease, (iv) diabetes mellitus, (v) silicosis, and (vi) postgastrectomy patients.

e. Other positive tuberculin skin test reactors not included in a. through d. should be considered on a case by case basis as to the advisability of preventive therapy. Age is an important factor in the equation of benefits of therapy. Tuberculin reactors who are over 35 years of age are not to be routinely treated with INH, because the risk of INH hepatitis in this age group outweighs the potential benefits of therapy. (See Questions 9 and 10). These individuals, however, should receive preventive therapy if other risk factors, outlined above, are present. INH preventive therapy is mandatory for children under six years of age. In a study of urban school children, 3,000 PPD skin test converters were treated with INH and compared prospectively with 1,200 untreated children (66). The incidence of tuberculosis in the untreated group was 60 times that of the treated children.

This man should be placed on isoniazid 300 mg/day given as a single daily dose for 12 months. Even though he has a higher chance of developing liver damage (2.3%) because of his age, he is at a high risk of developing clinical disease. Based on the preceding discussion, it would seem that the benefits of preventive treatment outweigh the possible risks of hepatitis. He should be educated and questioned frequently about the clinical symptoms of hepatitis which are often associated with gastrointestinal complaints. Pretreatment serum transaminase and bilirubin determinations should be made to rule out pre-existing liver disease. The need for monthly or routine monitoring of those laboratory values is controversial and will be discussed thoroughly in Question 9.

9. INH Hepatitis. After two months of INH preventive therapy, the man described in the previous question was found to have an elevated SGOT, 130 mU/ml (Normal: 7–40 mU/ml). Should isoniazid be discontinued in this patient to prevent liver damage secondary to INH?

Approximately 10 to 20% of INH recipients may have elevated liver enzymes upon routine laboratory evaluation (67,68). Most patients with mild subclinical hepatic damage do not progress to overt hepatitis and recover completely even while continuing INH therapy (69). However, continuation of INH in the presence of clinical symptoms can result in severe hepatocellular toxicity which is associated with a higher fatality rate than when INH is discontinued immediately (69,70).

There is some doubt as to whether biochemical monitoring of liver function is of value in the detection of liver toxicity secondary to INH. The ATS/CDC do not recommend routine liver function tests unless there are symptoms suggestive of hepatitis (62). However, in a recent study involving 1000 patients receiving INH, 47 out of 64 patients, with SGOT levels elevated to the point where the drug should have been discontinued, did not have signs or symptoms of hepatitis (60). Another investigator reported that subclinical hepatic injury occurs early in treatment with INH and is reversible if detected early with routine liver function tests at least during the first three months (71). Hepatic injury is most common in the first three months of treatment (69). For these reasons, patients receiving INH preventive therapy should probably receive monthly liver function tests (60,77). Other experts suggest that only those persons at high risk of developing hepatitis (eg, daily alcohol consumers, persons over 35, those taking other hepatotoxic drugs, and those with liver disease) receive routine liver function tests (15). INH should be temporarily discontinued if the SGOT level exceeds 3 to 5 times the normal value (60,72).

Since this man's SGOT is three times the upper range of the normal value and he is over 35 years old, INH should be temporarily discontinued until the levels return to normal (68). At that time INH should be resumed at a lower dosage and the laboratory tests rechecked. If the SGOT increases again, the drug should be discontinued. In addition to laboratory monitoring, the patient should be reminded of the importance of reporting any gastrointestinal symptoms which might suggest hepatitis. INH hepatitis is often associated with gastrointestinal symptoms (55% of patients) such as nausea, anorexia, vomiting, and abdominal discomfort. Some patients (35%) complain of a viral-like illness, and others are asymptomatic until the onset of jaundice (10%). Other patients have had hepatomegaly (33%), hyperbilirubinemia (25%), and prolonged prothrombin times (35%) (69).

10. What are the proposed causes of INH hepatitis? Does the 51-year-old man de-

scribed in Question 8 have an increased risk of developing INH hepatitis?

Isoniazid-induced hepatitis has been characterized as being clinically, biochemically, and histologically indistinguishable from viral hepatitis (69). Viral hepatitis, however, primarily affects young adults, while INH hepatitis occurs most frequently in older patients (17). The development of INH hepatitis has been linked to several factors including acetylator status, aging, and daily alcohol consumption.

People who are rapid acetylators were believed to have a greater risk of developing INH hepatitis than slow acetylators. Rapid acetylators of INH form monoacetylhydrazine, a compound which can cause liver damage, more rapidly than slow acetylators (67,73,74). However, rapid acetylators would also eliminate this compound at a faster rate, which should equalize the risk of toxicity between slow and fast acetylators (75). One study demonstrated a different incidence of hepatitis between Asian males and females who were both fast acetylators. This study suggests that hepatitis is probably due to factors other than acetylator phenotype (76). Thus, it appears that acetylator status may not be a major factor in the development of INH hepatitis.

Age and concurrent daily alcohol ingestion are probably more significant factors in the development of INH hepatitis (62,76). Progressive liver damage is rare in individuals less than 20 years of age. It occurs in approximately 0.3% of individuals between the ages of 20–34 years; in up to 1.2% of those between the ages of 35–49 years; and in up to 2.3% of persons 50 years of age or older (62).

This 51-year-old man has an increased risk of developing hepatitis secondary to isoniazid. He should be monitored closely according to the guidelines in Question 9.

11. Skin Test Booster Phenomenon. A 50-year-old male hospital employee receiving his annual tuberculin skin test (PPD-Mantoux) had an 8 mm reaction. Since this was a 5 mm increase from the previous year, it was decided to re-test him in one week. The result of the repeat skin test was 14 mm. He denies exposure to persons with clinical tuberculosis. What is the significance of this reaction, and should this man be placed on INH preventive therapy?

Some persons experience a marked increase in the size of a tuberculin skin test reaction which may not be due to *M. tuberculosis* infection (78). This reaction, or "booster" phenomenon, is not fully understood but may be due to a remote tuberculosis infection or a sensitivity to non-tuberculosis mycobacteria. The tuberculin skin test itself can act as a stimulus to cause an increase in reaction size when repeat tests are performed every one to two years. The incidence of this reaction appears to increase with age and can occur as soon as one week after a previous test (79,80).

Since serial tuberculin testing is recommended for hospital employees, it becomes important to distinguish a possible booster reaction from a recent infection with *M. tuberculosis* (20,81–83). Persons who exhibit an increase of 6 mm from less than 10 mm to greater than 10 mm may be mistaken for recent converters and given INH preventive therapy unnecessarily. To determine if a reaction is due to boosting, a second identical skin test should be administered one week after the first. The results of this test should be read in 48 to 72 hours. If the repeat test is positive (greater than 10 mm), the reaction should be classified as a booster reaction and should not be treated with INH. If the repeat test is less than 10 mm but changes to positive (with a 6 mm increase) after one year, the person should be classified as a recent converter and managed according to the recommendations in Question 8 (79).

The increase in reaction size in this man is probably due to the booster effect. Since he is over 35-years-old, he would not be a candidate for INH preventive therapy. When tested in the future, 14 mm should be considered as his baseline value (81).

12. Drug-Resistant Organisms. A 29-year-old Asian male was skin tested with 5 TU strength PPD because his sister, with whom he lives, developed active tuberculosis. The sensitivity report, from her sputum culture, documented organisms resistant to INH. His skin test is positive (14 mm), but his chest x-ray and sputum smears for acid-fast bacilli are negative. What is the incidence of primary infections with drug-resistant organisms? Should this man receive INH preventive therapy?

Primary drug resistance is defined as infection with bacteria which are resistant to drugs in persons who have not received these drugs previously. The overall primary resistance rate for drugs used in the treatment of tuberculosis is 7.1% with the highest incidence of drug-resistant bacilli reported in Harlingen, Texas (15.1%). The resistance rates to antitubercular medications vary among racial and ethnic groups with Asians and Hispanics having the highest rate of resistance. Their rates are 12.7% and 12.6% respectively, compared to the combined rate of 5.6% for other race/ethnic groups. Resistance rates are highest for INH (4.1%) and streptomycin (3.9%). Resistance rates for rifampin, ethambutol, and other drugs studied are less than 1%, as shown in Table 4. Younger patients have higher resistance rates (12.1% among those 0–10 years of age) than older patients (3.2% among those more than 90-years-old) (84,85).

Tubercle bacilli that are resistant to the usual drugs can be transmitted to persons who have never received chemotherapy. The Centers for Disease Control reported a multiple case community outbreak of drug-resistant tuberculosis in Mississippi (86,87). Containment of a tuberculosis outbreak such as this requires not only aggressive treatment of active cases, but also prevention of future cases in tuberculin positive reactors. There is no clinical evidence to determine whether INH is effective in the treatment or prevention of drug-resistant tuberculosis, and there is no evidence to indicate the efficacy of other antitubercular drugs in the prevention of tuberculosis.

There are three approaches that should be considered in this case (87). The first approach is to use INH as preventive therapy. INH has been reported to be effective in the prevention of disease despite *in vitro* resistance (86,88,89). However, INH has sometimes failed to prevent tuberculosis when INH-resistant organisms were present (90). The second approach would be to use rifampin alone or in combination with INH or ethambutol (2,90–92). Since rifampin has not been clinically evaluated as a single preventive drug, the addition of a second drug might be more acceptable. The combination of INH–rifampin would probably be more effective but may not be cost justified unless 50% or more of the cases in a given area are infected with organisms that are resistant to INH (93). The third approach would be to administer no drugs and follow the patient closely for 3 to 5 years. Koplan et al found, by a decision analysis technique, a two- to seven-fold increase in the number of cases of tuberculosis using the third approach when compared to the first two approaches (93). This increase makes the last approach the least acceptable.

The man in this case is in close contact with a relative who has clinical tuberculosis and is therefore a candidate for preventive therapy. He

Table 4.

PRIMARY RESISTANCE TO ANTITUBERCULOSIS DRUGS IN THE UNITED STATES

Drugs	Race/ethnic group													
	Caucasian (N = 3,050)		Black (N = 2,712)		Asian (N = 355)		Hispanic (N = 1,229)		Am. Ind. (N = 162)		Other (N = 39)		Total (N = 7,547)	
	No.	%	No.	%	No.	%	No.	%	No.	%	No.	%	No.	%
Streptomycin	82	2.7	84	3.1	27	7.6	94	7.6	5	3.1	2	5.1	294	3.9
Isoniazid	84	2.8	90	3.3	30	8.5	98	8.0	6	3.7	1	2.6	309	4.1
Para-amino-salicylic acid	15	0.5	28	1.0	7	2.0	10	0.8	2	1.2	0	0.0	62	0.8
Rifampin	4	0.1	7	0.3	0	0.0	4	0.3	0	0.0	0	0.0	15	0.2
Ethambutol	6	0.2	7	0.3	1	0.3	9	0.7	0	0.0	0	0.0	23	0.3
Cycloserine	2	0.1	3	0.1	0	0.0	4	0.3	0	0.0	0	0.0	9	0.1
Ethionamide	13	0.4	19	0.7	7	2.0	19	1.5	2	1.2	0	0.0	60	0.8
Kanamycin	1	0.0	2	0.1	1	0.3	3	0.2	0	0.0	0	0.0	7	0.1
Capreomycin	4	0.1	2	0.1	1	0.3	3	0.2	0	0.9	0	0.0	10	0.1
Overall resistance rate to ≥ 1 drug	158	5.2	164	6.0	45	12.7	155	12.6	9	5.6	3	7.7	534	7.1

Reprinted from Center for Disease Control: Primary resistance to antituberculosis drugs—United States. Morbid Mortal Weekly Rep. 1980; 29:345.

should be placed on INH 300 mg a day. Since his sister has documented INH-resistant organisms, it might be advantageous to add rifampin 600 mg daily to the INH regimen.

This man should be monitored closely to ensure prompt detection of active disease and early institution of appropriate therapy. Other close associates of his sister should be contacted and skin tested with 5 TU strength PPD. Positive tuberculin reactors should be managed according to the current recommendations outlined in Question 8. Negative reactors should be re-tested in approximately three months.

13. *BCG Vaccine.* A 25-year-old female refugee from Cambodia was given a routine physical examination upon entering this country. As part of this examination, she received a tuberculin skin test with 5 TU strength PPD. The result of this test was positive with an induration of 12 mm. She denied previous treatment for tuberculosis, but remembered receiving a tuberculosis vaccine (BCG) several years ago. What is BCG vaccine? Does this positive skin test indicate infection with *M. tuberculosis*?

BCG (Bacillus of Calmette and Guerin) is a human vaccine derived from a strain of bovine mycobacterium. It is used in many foreign countries with a high incidence of tuberculosis to prevent the disease in persons who are tuberculin negative (no immunity to tuberculosis infection). There are many different BCG vaccines available worldwide, and all of them differ with respect to immunogenicity, efficacy, and reactogenicity (23). These factors may account for the varied degrees of protection afforded by the vaccine. In trials conducted in the United States, the protective effect derived from BCG vaccine ranged from 0 to 80% (94,95).

Prior vaccination with BCG usually results in a positive tuberculin skin test. It is impossible to differentiate between a positive skin test due to BCG and that due to infection with *M. tuberculosis* (96). Therefore, she should be treated as having a positive tuberculin skin test and managed according to the guidelines outlined in Question 8. The possibility of organisms that are resistant to INH should also be considered. (See Question 12).

Adverse reactions to the BCG vaccine vary according to the type, dosage, and age of the vaccine. Osteomyelitis, prolonged ulceration at the vaccination site, lupoid reactions, lymphadenitis, disseminated BCG infection, and death have all been reported (94,98).

BCG vaccine is not recommended for use in the routine prophylaxis of tuberculosis in the United States. The risk of exposure to tuberculosis in this country is relatively low, and other methods of control (eg, treatment of high risk groups) are usually adequate (97). BCG vaccine should only be used in persons who are tuberculin negative who are repeatedly exposed to highly infectious, untreated patients with active disease (tuberculosis) (96,97).

14. *INH Adverse Effects.* C.W., a 50 kg, 35-year-old female, is being treated for active disease with INH 900 mg and rifampin 900 mg twice a week. Is 900 mg of INH twice-weekly an appropriate dose for a 50 kg patient? What side effects, other than hepatotoxicity, might occur in this patient receiving INH?

According to the Guidelines for Short-Course Chemotherapy (Table 3), this patient should be receiving 750 mg (15 mg/kg) rather than 900 mg of INH. This higher dosage *may* result in a greater chance for the development of INH side effects and should be reduced.

Isoniazid may rarely cause a direct dose-dependent peripheral neuropathy when dosages of 5 mg/kg/day are used. However, as many as 20% of patients may experience this problem when doses exceed 6 mg/kg/day (37,99). This peripheral neuropathy is a result of competitive inhibition of pyridoxine in neural enzyme systems. Clinically, the patient usually experiences a numbness or tingling in the feet or hands. This problem can be prevented by the concurrent administration of pyridoxine 10 mg daily. This side effect is most common in alcoholic, diabetic, and malnourished patients who should always receive pyridoxine (37). Other patients probably do not need pyridoxine unless they are receiving more than 6 mg/kg/day of INH.

Convulsions, responsive to large parenteral doses of pyridoxine (100 to 200 mg/day), have also been reported in patients with no history of a previous seizure disorder who were receiving large doses of INH (100).

Allergic reactions consisting of arthralgia, skin rash, swelling of the tongue, and fever can also occur (37,102). Isoniazid has also been associated with arthritic symptoms (103), lupus erythematosus (104), and in as many as 50% of patients, an increased prevalence of antinuclear antibodies.

Other reactions that may occur with INH are dry mouth, epigastric distress, central nervous system stimulation and depression, psychoses, hemolytic anemia, pyridoxine-responsive anemia, agranulocytosis, acne, and pellagra (37,40, 99,101,101A).

In addition to the above mentioned adverse reactions, there is a clinically significant drug interaction between INH and phenytoin. INH inhibits the hepatic metabolism of phenytoin which can result in an increased blood level. Patients receiving these two drugs should be observed for signs of phenytoin toxicity such as nystagmus, ataxia, or drowsiness. They should also receive periodic serum level monitoring of phenytoin so that the dosage may be adjusted if necessary (105). INH also inhibits the metabolism of diazepam, but rifampin has the opposite effect on diazepam metabolism and INH–rifampin combination therapy stimulates the metabolism of diazepam (122a).

15. *Rifampin Adverse Effects.* **One month after beginning her twice-weekly (supervised) therapy, the patient in Question 14 developed a flu-like syndrome. Laboratory data were normal except for a slightly decreased platelet count. Could this patient's flu-like syndrome be related to her drug therapy? What other adverse reactions should be monitored for in a patient receiving rifampin?**

A flu-like syndrome has been reported with intermittent administration of rifampin. This syndrome is rarely seen with usual doses of 600 mg twice-weekly, but the incidence increases with dosages of greater than 900 mg. This also appears to be true if the dosage interval is increased to one week or longer (36,106–108). Unless the symptoms are severe, discontinuation of the drug is unnecessary (105). It would be advisable to decrease the dosage of rifampin to 600 mg in this patient and change to daily therapy until the symptoms subside. Twice-weekly therapy may then be resumed as long as the dosage of rifampin is not increased above 600 mg.

The platelet count should be monitored closely, since thrombocytopenia is also reported to occur more frequently with the intermittent administration of rifampin (109,110). The proposed mechanism for the development of this thrombocytopenia is that anti-rifampin antibodies are adsorbed onto platelets, resulting in damage to the platelet (105). The reduction in dosage and change to daily therapy should prevent a further decrease in the platelet count. However, if the platelets continue to decrease, rifampin should be discontinued immediately.

In addition to these side effects which occur more frequently with intermittent administration of higher dosage rifampin, 3 to 4% of patients taking normal doses may experience adverse reactions (36,109). The most common of these reactions are nausea, vomiting, fever, and rash (37).

Rifampin, like isoniazid, may also cause elevated liver enzymes and possibly hepatotoxicity. Older patients, alcoholics, and those with preexisting liver disease may be more susceptible to the development of hepatotoxicity (111). However, a recent study showed no significant difference in adverse reactions between alcoholic and nonalcoholic patients. Therefore, the use of rifampin and isoniazid is not contraindicated in alcoholic patients (112). Active hepatitis would be the primary contraindication to the usage of INH–rifampin combination therapy (57). If the SGOT increases 3 to 5 times above normal, both INH and rifampin should be discontinued temporarily until the laboratory values return to normal. The INH should then be resumed at a lower dosage, gradually increasing up to 300 mg a day. Rifampin may be restarted at a lower dosage, gradually increasing up to 600 mg or ethambutol 15 mg/kg/day may be substituted. If rifampin is discontinued, therapy must be extended to at least 18 to 24 months. Serum transaminase levels should probably be determined weekly during the first month after resuming therapy. Thereafter, monthly determinations should be adequate.

Acute renal failure has also occurred with rifampin (113,116). This reaction may occur with both intermittent or daily administration and may last as long as 12 months (117). The reaction is probably due to a hypersensitivity reaction involving rifampin antibodies (107). Rifampin should be discontinued until renal function returns to normal. However, both rifampin and isoniazid may be given in normal dosages to patients with preexisting renal failure (118,119).

Other reactions to rifampin include the hepatorenal syndrome, hemolysis, leukopenia, and anemia (37). The development of these reactions would require discontinuation of the drug. Another problem associated with rifampin is due to its chemical makeup. It is an orange-red crystalline powder which is distributed widely to body fluids and may discolor saliva, tears, urine, and sweat. Patients using rifampin should be cautioned not to use soft contact lenses because of possible discoloration.

Rifampin is also a potent enzyme inducer. It has been reported to increase the metabolism of corticosteroids, oral contraceptives, quinidine, diazepam, warfarin, and digoxin (37,120–122b). It may be necessary to increase the dosage of these drugs while the patient is receiving rifampin. Women who are taking rifampin should use an alternative birth control method.

16. Steroids; Drug-Resistant Organisms. A 25-year-old Hispanic female is admitted to the hospital with cough, hemoptysis, and fever. She has a positive PPD skin test and her sputum is positive for acid-fast bacilli. She has been receiving prednisone 20 mg daily for one month following an acute exacerbation of asthma. She is also receiving a sustained release theophylline preparation (200 mg every 12 hours). Her serum theophylline level is 12 mcg/ml. What effects do steroids have on the development of tuberculosis? How should this patient be treated?

Steroids interfere with monocyte-macrophage mobility and function which may result in an increased risk of tuberculosis and a depression of tuberculin reactivity (123). Persons infected with tuberculosis who are receiving steroids are at a greater risk for developing clinical tuberculosis (2). Even though steroids may depress skin reactivity to tuberculin, masking TB, it is possible to have a positive reaction to PPD (124).

Patients who are from areas of high drug resistance should be treated initially as if they had INH-resistant organisms. Since this Hispanic patient has an 8% chance of primary resistance to INH (see Table 4), treatment should be initiated with three or four drugs until the results of sputum culture and sensitivity are determined (85). The Center for Disease Control (CDC) recommends the addition of ethambutol 15 mg/kg/daily to the INH-rifampin combination (see Question 4). An alternative would be to add both streptomycin and pyrazinamide to the INH-rifampin regimen (55). The combination of streptomycin

and pyrazinamide is bactericidal against both extracellular and intracellular tubercule bacilli as long as neither drug is withdrawn (125).

If drug susceptibility studies confirm INH-resistant organisms, the drug regimen should be revised and the duration of treatment extended to longer than nine months (52,54,126). The isoniazid, rifampin and ethambutol regimen could be continued for 12 to 18 months or until the sputum remains negative for one year. The alternative regimen consisting of INH, rifampin, streptomycin, and pyrazinamide given twice-weekly for nine months has proven to be effective in recent trials (125). However, more study is needed to determine the toxicity and efficacy of this regimen. If either rifampin or INH is discontinued, therapy should be continued at least 18 to 24 months (2).

If the tubercle bacilli are not resistant to INH or rifampin, the patient should be treated according to the short-course chemotherapy guidelines outlined in Table 3.

This patient may also require an adjustment in her prednisone dosage, since rifampin may increase its metabolism and thus diminish the steroid's effectiveness (37,105,122).

17. Ethambutol Adverse Effects. A 65-year-old female was placed on INH 300 mg/day, rifampin 600 mg/day, and ethambutol 1200 mg/day for initial treatment of tuberculosis (active disease). Two months after the initiation of therapy, she began having blurred vision. A routine eye examination and visual field test resulted in diagnosis of optic neuritis. There was no evidence of glaucoma, cataracts, or retinal damage. Laboratory tests were within normal limits except for an elevated serum uric acid (9.7 mg/dl) and an elevated serum creatinine (1.4 mg/dl). There were no symptoms of joint pain associated with the elevated serum uric acid and no past history of gout. Her calculated creatinine clearance (ClCr) based on her weight of 60 kg was 50 ml/minute. Could the visual problem be related to her medications?

This patient's decrease in visual acuity is compatible with ethambutol-induced optic neuritis. This condition is characterized by central scotomas, loss of green color vision, or less commonly as a peripheral vision defect. The intensity of these ocular effects is related to the duration of continued therapy after the first noted appearance of decreased visual acuity (37). The optic neuritis is dose related and is extremely rare. It is reported to occur in less than 2% of those persons receiving between 15 and 25 mg/kg/day of ethambutol. The incidence increases with higher doses (15% of patients receiving 50 mg/kg/day) and when usual doses are used in the presence of moderate to severe renal impairment (37,127,128). Recovery is usually complete when the drug is discontinued.

The optic neuritis manifested in this patient is probably due to the combination of a higher dosage (20 mg/kg) of ethambutol and her mildly impaired renal function (estimated ClCr 50 ml/min). Since ethambutol probably adds no additional benefit to the INH-rifampin regimen (see Question 4), it could be discontinued (32–35). However, if the ethambutol is to be continued, it should be stopped until she has recovered from the optic neuritis. Ethambutol may then be re-started at a dosage of 900 mg/day (15 mg/kg). Since ethambutol is partially excreted by the kidney (50%), her serum creatinine should be monitored at least weekly and the dosage interval of ethambutol increased based on the decline in creatinine clearance (eg, ClCr 10–50 ml/min—24 to 36 hours, less than 10 ml/min—48 hours) (129). Her visual acuity should be closely monitored by periodic tests. The patient should be urged to contact her physician immediately if there are any changes in her vision (128).

This patient's elevated serum uric acid may also be attributed to her ethambutol and probably her decline in renal function. Approximately 50% of the patients receiving ethambutol experience an increase in serum uric acid due to decreased renal excretion (130). This effect would certainly be intensified in the presence of renal insufficiency. Asymptomatic hyperuricemia secondary to drugs does not usually require treatment, since a relationship between this condition and renal stone formation, renal damage, or gouty arthritis has not been demonstrated (131). This patient should be examined for causes of her increased serum creatinine. Rifampin has been shown to cause acute renal failure (see Question 15).

18. *PAS.* Would PAS (para-aminosalicylic acid) be an appropriate alternative to ethambutol for the patient in Question 17?

PAS is less expensive than ethambutol. However, the small economic savings hardly compensate for the high incidence of side effects associated with its use. Patients unwilling to tolerate troublesome side effects do not continue therapy, and higher health costs ensue because of the need for retreatment. In one study, the patient drop-out rate from treatment with INH plus PAS was 33%, as compared to an 8% to 10% drop-out rate respectively for INH 6 mg/kg and ethambutol 15 mg/kg (132). Furthermore, the combination of INH and PAS was less effective than the INH and ethambutol combination (132). In other studies of two and three drug regimens, PAS use was associated with the highest incidence of nausea, vomiting, diarrhea, and epigastric distress (133,134). For these reasons and because newer, more effective agents (ie, rifampin, ethambutol) are available, PAS is no longer used as a primary drug. However, according to an official statement of the American Thoracic Society, PAS may be preferable to ethambutol when used in combination with INH for the treatment of young children, because the changes in visual acuity which can occur with ethambutol are difficult to monitor in this age group (54,135). Children also seem to tolerate PAS better than adults.

19. *Treatment Failure.* A 27-year-old American Indian male is seen in the outpatient tuberculosis clinic for a routine follow-up visit. Four months ago, he was placed on isoniazid and rifampin for cavitary tuberculosis of the right lung. He is still producing copious sputum which on smear reveals many acid-fast bacilli. On questioning, the patient said that he only took his medication sporadically. How should tuberculosis be treated in patients such as this?

Treatment failure should be considered whenever sputum cultures remain positive four to six months after initiation of therapy, or whenever chest x-rays indicate progression of the disease (10). This patient can certainly be considered a treatment failure, because many acid-fast bacilli were present on the sputum smear which should have been negative about six to eight weeks after therapy was begun. Treatment failures can result from deficient host immune response, inappropriate therapy, drug-resistant organisms, or poor patient compliance. Lack of patient compliance in completing an antitubercular course of therapy probably represents the most important factor contributing to the unsuccessful treatment of this disease (12,136). In most cases, it is the patient who suffers the consequences of non-compliance. However, with tuberculosis, society suffers as well. Therefore, it is essential to devise special treatment programs to render unreliable patients non-infectious.

The best clinical results have been obtained with a combination of daily chemotherapy for the first two to three months followed by fully supervised intermittent therapy. Although it is very clear that twice-weekly intermittent therapy is adequate for success, some clinicians recommend a three-time-a-week regimen so that if one visit is missed, the patient would still be effectively treated (10). Dosage adjustments would have to be made in order to prevent drug toxicity.

Directly administered intermittent therapy provides one effective option for ensuring an adequate therapeutic regimen. In such programs, health personnel can visit the patient at home or at work, if necessary, to administer the needed antitubercular medications two or three times a week in doses larger than the usual daily dose (47,135,137–140).

This patient has a history of non-compliance and would be an excellent candidate for supervised intermittent therapy. Adequate sputum specimens should be collected prior to initiation of a retreatment chemotherapy program, and drug sensitivity tests should be performed. The results from susceptibility testing will be delayed for about six to eight weeks, but therapy should begin immediately with at least two drugs which he has not previously received. A single, new, potentially effective drug must never be added to a regimen that has already failed, because the further development of resistance must be avoided (2,10,15,135). Since this patient has been receiving isoniazid and rifampin, streptomycin and pyrazinamide should be added to the daily regimen until drug susceptibility tests are received. It may be necessary to hospitalize this patient initially until it is determined how well he tolerates the additional drugs.

If the bacilli are not resistant to any of these drugs, the streptomycin and pyrazinamide can be discontinued. The INH and rifampin should be given twice a week under supervision until the sputum culture has been negative for at least six months (2).

If INH-resistant organisms are found, treatment should be continued with the four-drug regimen according to the principles outlined in Question 5. If ethambutol is substituted for either streptomycin or pyrazinamide, therapy should be extended for 18 to 24 months (125).

20. *Pregnancy.* **A 25-year-old Caucasian woman who is being treated with INH 15 mg/kg and rifampin 600 mg twice a week for uncomplicated pulmonary TB thinks that she might be pregnant. Her obstetrician is concerned about the possible teratogenic effects of INH and rifampin and urges her to have a therapeutic abortion. Are these drugs teratogenic, and should she have an abortion?**

Isoniazid, rifampin, ethambutol, and streptomycin have all been reported to be teratogenic in animals, but no direct correlation with human malformation has been reported. Animal data can suggest that a drug may be teratogenic, but because of genetic and environmental differences, these data cannot always be extrapolated to humans (141). Ideally, all drugs should be discontinued during pregnancy. However, offspring of women with untreated pulmonary tuberculosis reportedly have a higher incidence of congenital defects than offspring of women receiving treatment (142). Furthermore, the untreated patient is a community health hazard and has a greater chance of dying from the tuberculosis herself.

A comprehensive review of the literature by Snider et al reveals that INH, rifampin, and ethambutol in normal dosages are all relatively safe to use during pregnancy (143). All pregnant women receiving INH should also receive pyridoxine 50 to 100 mg daily because of the possibility of CNS toxicity. Rifampin has only been used in a small number of pregnant patients. The incidence of limb malformations was slightly increased but was not statistically different from the control population. Several infants were reported to have hypoprothrombinemia or increased tendency to hemorrhage.

Streptomycin should not be used during pregnancy except as a last alternative. It has been associated with mild to severe ototoxicity in the infant. This ototoxicity can occur throughout the gestational period and is not confined to the first trimester. With the exception of streptomycin ototoxicity, the occurrence of birth defects in women being treated for TB with the above agents is no greater than that of healthy pregnant women. (See Table 5.)

Table 5.

PREGNANCY OUTCOMES AMONG WOMEN RECEIVING ANTITUBERCULOUS
THERAPY AND IN A NORMAL POPULATION*

Drug	Spontaneous Abortion (%)	Stillbirth (%)	Premature Birth (%)	Malformed Infant (%)
Isoniazid	0.34	0.61	1.83	1.09
Ethambutol	0.16	0.78	4.08	2.19
Rifampin	1.67	2.15	0.48	3.35
Streptomycin	0.97	0	0	16.91
Normal Populations	6.8†	2.2‡	7.1‡	1.4–6.0§ 2.3–13.8‖

*Rates expressed as percentages of all conceptions that were not electively aborted.
†Based on fetal deaths at 12 to 20 weeks' gestation, Werner EE, Bierman JM, French FE. The children of Kauai. Honolulu: University of Hawaii Press. 1971.
‡Based on Collaborative Perinatal Study data for whites. Niswander KR, Gordon M. The women and their pregnancies. Washington, DC: USGPO, 1972:40.
§Based on reports in 16 series of malformations noted at birth. Reviewed in: Hakasalo JK. Cumulative detection rates of congenital malformations in a 10-year study. Acta Pathol Microbiol Scand [A] 1973; Suppl 242:12.
‖Cumulative rates of malformations detected by 5 yr of age. Ibid.

Reprinted with permission from Snider DE et al: Treatment of tuberculosis during pregnancy. Am Rev Respir Dis. 1980; 122:65.

Therapeutic abortion is not necessary in the TB patient who becomes pregnant. The benefits versus the risks should be discussed with the patient, and she should decide whether to continue the pregnancy or to have a therapeutic abortion.

21. *Pediatric Patients.* **A 6-year-old child is admitted to the emergency room with nausea and vomiting. The child has been receiving INH 15 mg/kg and rifampin 20 mg/kg for about two months. Laboratory data reveal an SGOT of 80 U/L (Normal 7–40 mU/ml) and a serum bilirubin of 1.5 mg/dl (Normal 0–1.0 mg/dl). Are these dosages and drugs appropriate for this child? What is the incidence of hepatotoxicity of INH-rifampin regimens in children?**

The short-course chemotherapy regimen recently adopted by the American Thoracic Society and the Center for Disease Control may be effective in children; however, there is only limited experience in this group (53,54). It is recommended that pediatric patients receive INH 10 mg/kg (max 300 mg) and rifampin 10–20 mg/kg (max 600 mg) daily. As with adults, ethambutol (15 mg/kg/daily) should be added to the regimen if drug resistance is suspected. In children who cannot be monitored for visual acuity, PAS 200–300 mg/kg (max 12 gm) or streptomycin 20 mg/kg (max 1 gm) daily should be used as a substitute for ethambutol (54).

Since the frequency of hepatotoxic reactions to rifampin was unknown in children, a follow-up report by the CDC suggested limiting the dosage of rifampin to 15 mg/kg/daily (54). Further study of this problem found that hepatotoxic reactions were six times more frequent in children receiving isoniazid and rifampin than among those receiving INH with other drugs. Most of these reactions occurred in the first 90 days, and in the majority of patients recommended dosage guidelines were exceeded (144). The overall hepatotoxicity rate of the INH-rifampin combinations was about 3.2%.

In this patient, the dosages of both INH and rifampin were probably excessive. The drugs should be discontinued until clinical symptoms of hepatotoxicity are resolved and laboratory values return to normal. Therapy should be resumed with INH 10 mg/kg and rifampin 15 mg/kg daily. The child should be closely monitored for recurrence of hepatotoxicity.

22. *Tuberculous Meningitis.* **A 54-year-old male is brought to the emergency room fol-**

lowing a four day period in which he progressively became disoriented, febrile to 105° F, and obtunded. He also had severe headaches during this time. Physical examination revealed some nuchal rigidity and a positive Brudzinski sign (neck resistant to flexion). An initial diagnosis of possible meningitis was made and a lumbar puncture ordered. The cerebrospinal fluid (CSF) appeared turbid, and laboratory analysis revealed an elevated protein concentration of 200 mg/dl, a decreased glucose concentration of 30 mg/dl, and a white blood cell count of 500/cu mm (85% lymphocytes). A Gram's stain of the spinal fluid was negative, but a Ziehl-Neelsen stain was positive for acid-fast bacilli. Other laboratory tests were within normal limits. A diagnosis of tuberculous meningitis was made. Discuss tuberculous meningitis. How should this man be treated?

Tuberculous meningitis in older persons is usually due to hematogenous dissemination of tubercle bacilli from a primary site, usually in the lungs. In its early stages, tuberculous meningitis is often confused with aseptic meningitis, since the Gram's stain is negative (2,28).

The most common symptoms of tuberculous meningitis are headache, fever, restlessness, irritability, nausea, and vomiting. A positive Brudzinski sign and neck stiffness may be present. The cerebrospinal fluid (CSF) is usually turbid with increased protein, decreased glucose, and an increase in white blood cells with a predominance of lymphocytes (28). Acid-fast bacilli are cultured from the CSF in only about 20–37% of cases (28,145). The presence of tryptophan in the CSF is evidence of possible tuberculous meningitis (2).

Early recognition and treatment is essential to a favorable outcome. In a study by Kennedy et al, four of five patients whose treatment was delayed for seven or more days died (145). Treatment must usually be based on a suspected diagnosis of tuberculous meningitis and must be started before culture and sensitivity reports are received. At least two and probably three drugs should be used since irreversible brain damage or death may occur as soon as two weeks after the onset of infection (not clinical symptoms) (146).

Treatment should be initiated in this man with INH 10 mg/kg/day and rifampin 10 mg/kg/day (max 600 mg). Streptomycin 1 gm per day intramuscularly in combination with pyrazinamide 500 mg three times a day may be given for the first two to three months with the INH-rifampin regimen (147,148). Both INH and rifampin penetrate into the cerebrospinal fluid and have been proven to reduce the morbidity and mortality associated with tuberculous meningitis (149–151). Streptomycin penetrates poorly even in inflamed meninges, but in combination with pyrazinamide appears to be extremely effective (37,148). After meningeal irritation has subsided (two to three months), this combination should be discontinued because of toxicity and because streptomycin does not penetrate the normal meninges very well. See Table 6 for a list of the most commonly used drugs and their cerebrospinal fluid concentrations.

Treatment with INH and rifampin should be continued 18 to 24 months. In addition, pyridoxine 10 to 50 mg/day should be given to this patient to prevent the occurrence of peripheral neuropathy secondary to INH. It should also be remembered that rifampin may impart a red to orange color to the spinal fluid.

The use of corticosteroids in the initial treatment of tuberculous meningitis is questionable. They are used to reduce the intracranial pressure associated with cerebral edema (146). Prednisone 60 to 80 mg daily is recommended in patients who are in a coma or have subarachnoid block or spinal fluid pressures greater than 300 mm H_2O (152). The dosage of prednisone can be tapered slowly after symptoms subside. Corticosteroids are not indicated for this patient at this time.

Pediatric patients should be treated with INH 15 to 20 mg/kg/day and rifampin 15 to 20 mg/kg/day (max 600 mg) (153). The dosage of INH should be reduced by 50% after the first four weeks of treatment (154). Streptomycin may be used in addition to the INH-rifampin regimen for the first four to six weeks in dosages of 40 mg/kg/day (max 1 gm) given intramuscularly in two divided doses.

Table 6.

CONCENTRATION LEVELS OF THE COMMON ANTITUBERCULAR AGENTS

	Cerebrospinal Fluid Concentrations (mcg/ml)	Minimum Inhibitory Concentrations
Isoniazid	2–5	0.05–0.2
Ethambutol	1–2	1–2
Rifampin	2–4	0.5
Pyrazinamide	60	20

References

1. Bates JH: Diagnosis of tuberculosis. Chest. 1979; 76(suppl):757.
2. Stead WW et al: Tuberculosis. In *Harrison's Principles of Internal Medicine,* 9th ed, edited by K. Isselbacher et al, McGraw-Hill, New York, 1980, p 700.
3. Abeles H: The early discharge of tuberculosis patients with sputum containing acid fast bacilli. Am Rev Respir Dis. 1973; 108:975.
4. American Thoracic Society: Guidelines for work for patients with tuberculosis. Am Rev Respir Dis. 1973; 108:160.
5. Bates JH: Ambulatory treatment of TB: An idea whose time has come. Am Rev Respir Dis. 1974; 109:317.
6. Brooks SM et al: A pilot study concerning the infection risk of sputum positive tuberculosis patients on chemotherapy. Am Rev Respir Dis. 1973; 108:799.
7. Gunnells JJ et al: Infectivity of sputum positive TB patients on chemotherapy. Am Rev Respir Dis. 1974; 109:323.
8. Oatway WH: Early discharge of patients with active TB. Am Rev Respir Dis. 1974; 109:321.
9. Bates JH et al: Effect of chemotherapy on infectiousness of tuberculosis. N Engl J Med. 1974; 290:459.
10. Reichman LB et al: Practical management and control of tuberculosis. Med Clin North Am. 1977; 61:1185.
11. Stead WW: Control of tuberculosis in institutions. Chest. 1979; 76(suppl):797.
12. Sbarbaro JA: Tuberculosis: The new challenge to the practicing clinician. Chest. 1975; 68(suppl):436.
13. Farer LS: The public health aspects of tuberculosis. Semin Respir Med. 1981; 2:175.
14. American Thoracic Society: Diagnostic standards and classification of tuberculosis and other mycobacterial diseases (14th edition). Am Rev Respir Dis. 1981; 123:343.
15. Glassroth J et al: Tuberculosis in the 1980's. N Engl J Med. 1980; 302:1441.
16. Sbarbaro JA: Tuberculosis. Med Clin North Am. 1980; 64:417.
17. Comstock GW et al: The competing risks of tuberculosis and hepatitis for adult tuberculin reactors. Am Rev Respir Dis. 1975; 11:573.
18. Center for Disease Control: Tuberculosis—United States: Current trends. Morbid Mortal Weekly Rep. 1981; 30:325.
19. Center for Disease Control: Follow-up on tuberculosis among Indochinese refugees. Morbid Mortal Weekly Rep. 1980; 29:573.
20. Center for Disease Control: Guidelines for prevention of TB transmission in hospitals. (HEW publication no. (CDC) 79-8371) 1979.
21. Bates JH: The changing scene in tuberculosis. N Engl J Med. 1977; 297:610.
22. Leff A et al: Tuberculosis: A chemotherapeutic triumph but a persistent socioeconomic problem. Arch Intern Med. 1979; 139:1375.
23. Reichman LB: Tuberculin skin testing: The state of the art. Chest. 1979; 76(suppl):764.
24. Wijsmuller G et al: The tuberculin test effects of storage and methods of delivery on reaction size. Am Rev Respir Dis. 1973; 107:267.
25. Harrison BDW et al: Tuberculin reaction in adult Nigerians with sputum positive pulmonary TB. Lancet. 1975; 1:421.
26. Rooney J Jr et al: Further observation on tuberculin reactions in active tuberculosis. Am J Med. 1976; 60:517.
27. Nash DR et al: Anergy in pulmonary tuberculosis. Chest. 1980; 77:32.
28. Fernandez E: The clinical presentation and diagnosis of tuberculosis. Semin Respir Med. 1981; 2:202.
29. MacGregor RR: A year's experience with tuberculosis in a private urban teaching hospital in the post sanatorium era. Am J Med. 1975; 58:221.
30. Greenbaum M et al: The accuracy of diagnosing pulmonary tuberculosis at a teaching hospital. Am Rev Respir Dis. 1980; 121:477.
31. Newman R et al: Rifampin in initial treatment of pulmonary tuberculosis. Am Rev Respir Dis. 1974; 109:216.
32. Second East African/British Medical Research Council: Controlled clinical trial of four 6-month regimens of chemotherapy for pulmonary tuberculosis. Am Rev Respir Dis. 1976; 114:471.
33. Stead WW et al: Contribution of a third drug to various two drug regimens in the treatment of tuberculosis. Am Rev Respir Dis. 1980; 121:463. (Abstract).
34. Fox W et al: Short-course chemotherapy for pulmonary tuberculosis. Am Rev Respir Dis. 1975; 111:325.
35. Hong Kong Chest Service/British Medical Research Council: Controlled trial of 6-month and 8-month regimens in the treatment of pulmonary tuberculosis: the results up to 24 months. Tubercule. 1979; 60:201.
36. Long MW et al: U.S. Public Health Service cooperative trial of three rifampin-isoniazid regimens in treatment of pulmonary tuberculosis. Am Rev Respir Dis. 1979; 119:879.
37. Mandell GL et al: Antimicrobial agents: Drugs used in the chemotherapy of tuberculosis and leprosy. In *The Pharmacological Basis of Therapeutics,* 6th ed, edited by AG Gilman, L Goodman, and A Gilman, Macmillan, New York, 1980, p 1200.
38. Mitchison DA: Basic mechanisms of chemotherapy. Chest. 1979; 76(suppl):771.
39. Dickinson JM et al: Experimental models to explain the high sterilizing activity of rifampin in the chemotherapy of tuberculosis. Am Rev Respir Dis. 1981; 123:367.
40. Stradling P et al: Twice-weekly streptomycin plus isoniazid for tuberculosis. Tubercule. 1970; 51:44.
41. Hong Kong Chest Service/British Medical Research Council: Controlled trial of 6-month and 8-month regimens in the treatment of pulmonary tuberculosis. Am Rev Respir Dis. 1978; 118:219.
42. Jindani A et al: The bactericidal activity of drugs in patients with pulmonary tuberculosis. Am Rev Respir Dis. 1980; 121:939.
43. East African/British Medical Research Council: Cooperative investigation: Controlled clinical trial of five short-course (4 month) chemotherapy regimens in pulmonary tuberculosis. Lancet. 1978; 2:334.
44. Hong Kong Chest Service/British Medical Research Council: Controlled trial of four thrice-weekly regimens and a daily regimen all given for 6 months for pulmonary tuberculosis. Lancet. 1981; 1:171.
45. British Thoracic and Tuberculosis Association: Short-course chemotherapy in pulmonary tuberculosis. Lancet. 1976; 2:1102.

46. Singapore Tuberculosis Service/British Medical Research Council: Controlled trial of intermittent regimens of rifampin plus isoniazid for pulmonary tuberculosis in Singapore: the results up to 30 months. Am Rev Respir Dis. 1977; 116:807.

47. Dutt AK et al: Short-course chemotherapy for tuberculosis with largely twice-weekly isoniazid-rifampin. Chest. 1979; 75:441.

48. East African/British Medical Research Council: Controlled clinical trial of four short-course regimens of chemotherapy for two durations in the treatment of pulmonary tuberculosis—first report. Am Rev Respir Dis. 1978; 118:39.

49. Hong Kong Chest Service/British Medical Research Council: Controlled trial of 6-month and 9-month regimens of daily and intermittent streptomycin plus isoniazid plus pyrazinamide for pulmonary tuberculosis in Hong Kong. Am Rev Respir Dis. 1977; 115:727.

50. Zierski M et al: Short-course (6 month) cooperative tuberculosis study in Poland: results 18 months after completion of treatment. Am Rev Respir Dis. 1980; 122:879.

51. East African/British Medical Research Council Study: Results at 5 years of a controlled comparison of a 6-month and a standard 18-month regimen of chemotherapy for pulmonary tuberculosis. Am Rev Respir Dis. 1977; 116:3.

52. American Thoracic Society and The Center for Disease Control: Guidelines for short-course tuberculosis chemotherapy. Am Rev Respir Dis. 1980; 121:611.

53. Center for Disease Control: Guidelines for short-course tuberculosis chemotherapy. Morbid Mortal Weekly Rep. 1980; 29:97.

54. Center for Disease Control: Follow-up on guidelines for short-course tuberculosis chemotherapy. Morbid Mortal Weekly Rep. 1980; 29:183.

55. Stead WW et al: An advance in treatment of tuberculosis. Ann Intern Med. 1980; 93:364.

56. Moulding TS et al: The treatment of tuberculosis. Semin Respir Med. 1981; 2:215.

57. Dutt AK et al: Short-course treatment regimens for patients with tuberculosis. Arch Intern Med. 1980; 140:827.

58. Johnston RF et al: State of the art review: The impact of chemotherapy on the care of patients with tuberculosis. Am Rev Respir Dis. 1974; 109:636.

59. Leff A et al: Outpatient treatment of advanced pulmonary tuberculosis without initial hospitalization. Am Rev Respir Dis. 1974; 109:697.

60. Byrd RB et al: Toxic effects of isoniazid in tuberculosis chemoprophylaxis. JAMA. 1979; 241:1239.

61. Byrd RB et al: Isoniazid chemoprophylaxis. Arch Intern Med. 1977; 137:1130.

62. American Thoracic Society: Preventive therapy of tuberculosis infection. Am Rev Respir Dis. 1974; 110:371.

63. Falk A et al: Prophylaxis with isoniazid in inactive tuberculosis. Chest. 1978; 73:44.

64. Taylor WC et al: Should young adults with a positive tuberculin test take isoniazid? Ann Intern Med. 1981; 94:808.

65. Comstock GW: Evaluating isoniazid preventive therapy: the need for more data. Ann Intern Med. 1981; 94:817 (editorial).

66. Curry FJ: Prophylactic effect of INH in young tuberculin reactors. N Engl J Med. 1967; 277:562.

67. Mitchell JR et al: Increased incidence of isoniazid hepatitis in rapid acetylators. Possible relation to hydrazine metabolites. Clin Pharmacol Ther. 1975; 18:70.

68. Mitchell JR et al: Acetylation rates and monthly liver function tests during one year of isoniazid preventive therapy. Chest. 1975; 68:181.

69. Mitchell JR et al: Isoniazid liver injury—clinical spectrum, pathology, and probable pathogenesis. Ann Intern Med. 1976; 84:181.

70. Maddrey WC et al: Isoniazid hepatitis. Ann Intern Med. 1973; 79:1.

71. Black M: Isoniazid and the liver. Am Rev Respir Dis. 1974; 110:1.

72. Byrd RB et al: Isoniazid chemoprophylaxis. Arch Intern Med. 1977; 137:1130.

73. Ellard GA: Variations between individuals and populations in the acetylation of isoniazid and its significance for the treatment of pulmonary tuberculosis: Clin Pharmacol Ther. 1976; 19:610.

74. Dickinson DS et al: The effect of acetylation status on isoniazid hepatitis. Am Rev Respir Dis. 1977; 115 (suppl):395.

75. Ellard GA et al: The hepatic toxicity of isoniazid among rapid and slow acetylators of the drug. Am Rev Respir Dis. 1978; 118:628.

76. Kopanoff DE et al: Isoniazid-related hepatitis. Am Rev Respir Dis. 1978; 117:991.

77. Dash LA et al: Isoniazid preventive therapy. Am Rev Respir Dis. 1980; 121:1039.

78. Comstock GW et al: Tuberculin conversions; True or false. Am Rev Respir Dis. 1978; 118:215.

79. Thompson NJ et al: The booster phenomenon in serial tuberculin testing. Am Rev Respir Dis. 1979; 119:587.

80. Richards NM et al: Tuberculin test conversions during repeated skin testing, associated with sensitivity to nontuberculosis mycobacteria. Am Rev Respir Dis. 1979; 120:59.

81. Atkinson ML et al: TB testing for hospital employees: New recommendations. Hospital Medical Staff. 1979; 8:16.

82. American Thoracic Society: Screening for pulmonary tuberculosis in institutions. Am Rev Respir Dis. 1977; 115:901.

83. Farer LS et al: CDC recommends 2-step TB skin testing for hospital employees. Hospital Infection Control. 1979; 6:1.

84. Kopanoff DE et al: A continuing survey of tuberculosis primary drug resistance in the United States. March 1975 to November 1977. Am Rev Respir Dis. 1978; 118:835.

85. Center for Disease Control: Primary resistance to antituberculosis drugs—United States. Morbid Mortal Weekly Rep. 1980; 29:345.

86. Center for Disease Control: Drug resistant tuberculosis in Mississippi. Morbid Mortal Weekly Rep. 1977; 26:417.

87. Center for Disease Control: Follow-up on drug-resistant tuberculosis—Mississippi. Morbid Mortal Weekly Rep. 1980; 29:602.

88. Hong Kong TB Treatment Services/British Medical Research Council: Controlled trial of 6 and 9 month regimens of daily and intermittent streptomycin plus INH plus pyrazinamide for pulmonary TB in Hong Kong. Tubercule. 1975; 56:81.

89. Lim BT et al: Ethambutol and capreomycin in the retreatment of advanced pulmonary TB. Am Rev Respir Dis. 1969; 99:793.

90. Fairshter RD et al: Failure of INH prophylaxis after exposure to INH-resistant tuberculosis. Am Rev Respir Dis. 1975; 112:37.

91. Byrd RB: Tuberculosis chemoprophylaxis (letter). Ann Intern Med. 1977; 87:792.

92. Reichman LB et al: Tuberculosis in the foreign born. Am Rev Respir Dis. 1977; 116:561.

93. Koplan JP et al: Choice of preventive treatment for isoniazid-resistant tuberculosis infection. JAMA. 1980; 244:2736.

94. Center for Disease Control: Recommendation of the Public Health Service Advisory Committee—BCG vaccinations. Morbid Mortal Weekly Rep. 1975; 24:69.

95. Editorial: BCG vaccination. Br Med J. 1975; 4:603.

96. Center for Disease Control: Recommendations of the Public Health Service Advisory Committee on Immunization Practices: BCG vaccine. Morbid Mortal Weekly Rep. 1979; 28:241.

97. Spencer DJ et al: BCG vaccines for tuberculosis. An official statement of the American Thoracic Society and Center for Disease Control. Am Rev Respir Dis. 1975; 112:478.

98. Mackay A et al: Fatal disseminated BCG infection in an 18-year old boy. Lancet. 1980; 2:1332.

99. Goldman IL et al: Isoniazid: A review with emphasis on adverse effects. Chest. 1972; 62:71.

100. Katz GA et al: Large doses of pyridoxine in the treatment of massive ingestion of isoniazid. Am Rev Respir Dis. 1970; 101:991.

101. Cohen LK et al: Isoniazid-induced acne and pellagra. Arch Dermatol. 1974; 109:377.

101a. Girling DJ: Adverse effects of antituberculosis drugs. Drugs. 1982; 23:56.

102. Jacobs NF et al: Spiking fever from isoniazid simulating a septic process. JAMA. 1977; 238:1759.

103. Good AE et al: Rheumatic symptoms during tuberculosis therapy, a manifestation of isoniazid toxicity. Ann Intern Med. 1965; 63:800.

104. Alarcon-Segovia D: Drug-induced lupus syndromes. Mayo Clin Proc. 1969; 44:664.

105. Addington WW: The side effects and interactions of antituberculosis drugs. Chest. 1979; 76(suppl):782.

106. Dutt AK et al: Treatment of pulmonary tuberculosis with short-course, intermittent chemotherapy using rifampin-isoniazid. Am Rev Respir Dis. 1977; 115(suppl):396.

107. Sanders WE: Rifampin. Ann Intern Med. 1976; 85:82.

108. Zierski M et al: Side-effects of drug regimens used in short-course chemotherapy for pulmonary tuberculosis. A controlled clinical study. Tubercule. 1980; 61:41.

109. Girling DJ: Adverse reactions to rifampicin in antituberculosis regimens. J Antimicrob Chemother. 1977; 3:115.

110. Aquinas SM et al: Adverse reactions to daily and intermittent rifampicin regimens for pulmonary tuberculosis in Hong Kong. Br Med J. 1972; 1:765.

111. Gronhagen-Riska C et al: Predisposing factors in hepatitis induced by isoniazid-rifampin treatment of tuberculosis. Am Rev Respir Dis. 1978; 118:461.

112. Cross FS et al: Rifampin-isoniazid therapy of alcoholic and nonalcoholic tuberculosis patients in a U.S. Public Health Service cooperative therapy trial. Am Rev Respir Dis. 1980; 122:349.

113. Campese VM et al: Acute renal failure during intermittent rifampin therapy. Nephron. 1973; 10:256.

114. Nessi R et al: Acute renal failure after rifampin: A case report and survey of the literature. Nephron. 1976; 16:148.

115. Chan WC et al: Renal failure during intermittent rifampin therapy. Tubercule. 1975; 56:191.

116. Warrington RJ et al: Insidious rifampin-associated renal failure with light-chain proteinuria. Arch Intern Med. 1977; 137:927.

117. Bansal VK et al: Prolonged renal failure after rifampin. Am Rev Respir Dis. 1977; 116:137.

118. Bennett WM et al: Drug therapy in renal failure: Dosing guidelines for adults. Ann Intern Med. 1980; 93 (Part 1):62.

119. Andrew OT et al: Tuberculosis in patients with end-stage renal disease. Am J Med. 1980; 68:59.

120. Skolnick JL et al: Rifampicin, oral contraceptives, and pregnancy. JAMA. 1976; 236:1382.

121. Novi C et al: Rifampin and digoxin: Possible drug interaction in a dialysis patient. JAMA. 1980; 244:2521 (letter).

122. Zilly W et al: Pharmacokinetic interactions with rifampin. Clin Pharmacokinetics. 1977; 2:61.

122a. Ochs HR et al: Diazepam interaction with antituberculosis drugs. Clin Pharmacol Ther. 1981; 29:671.

122b. Twum-Barima Y et al: Quinidine-rifampin interaction. N Engl J Med. 1981; 304:1466.

123. Fauci AS et al: Glucocorticosteroid therapy: Mechanisms of action and clinical considerations. Ann Intern Med. 1976; 84:304.

124. Center for Disease Control: Tuberculosis in a school teacher—Pennsylvania. Morbid Mortal Weekly Rep. 1980; 29:586.

125. Stead WW et al: Chemotherapy for tuberculosis. Ann Intern Med. 1981; 94:138 (letter).

126. Farer LS: Chemotherapy for tuberculosis. Ann Intern Med. 1981; 94:137 (letter).

127. Leibold JE: The ocular toxicity of ethambutol and its relation to dose. Ann NY Acad Sci. 1966; 135:904.

128. Van Scoy RE: Antituberculosis agents—isoniazid, rifampin, streptomycin, ethambutol. Mayo Clin Proc. 1977; 52:694.

129. Bennett WM: Drug therapy in renal failure: Dosing guidelines for adults. Ann Intern Med. 1980; 93 (Part 1):62.

130. Postlethwaite AE et al: Hyperuricemia due to ethambutol. N Engl J Med. 1972; 286:761.

131. Liang MH et al: Asymptomatic hyperuricemia: The case for conservative management. Ann Intern Med. 1978; 88:666.

132. Bobrowitz ID et al: Ethambutol-isoniazid vs PAS-isoniazid in the original treatment of pulmonary tuberculosis. Am Rev Respir Dis. 1967; 96:428.

133. Bobrowitz ID et al: Ethambutol compound to streptomycin in the original treatment of advanced pulmonary tuberculosis. Chest. 1971; 60:14.

134. Doster B et al: Ethambutol in the initial treatment of pulmonary TB. Am Rev Respir Dis. 1973; 107:177.

135. Bailey WC et al: Treatment of mycobacterial disease: An official statement of the American Thoracic Society. Am Rev Respir Dis. 1977; 115:185.

136. Addington WW: Patient compliance: The most serious remaining problem in the control of tuberculosis in the United States. Chest. 1979; 76(suppl):741.

137. Curry FJ: The effect of acceptable and adequate outpatient treatment on the length of hospitalization and on readmissions for relapse or reactivation of pulmonary TB. Chest. 1973; 63:536.

138. Hudson LD et al: Twice weekly tuberculosis chemotherapy. JAMA. 1973; 223:139.

139. Sbarbaro JA et al: High dose ethambutol: An oral alternate for intermittent chemotherapy. Am Rev Respir Dis. 1974; 110:91.

140. Fox W: The chemotherapy of pulmonary tuberculosis: A review. Chest. 1979; 76(suppl):785.

141. Pagliaro LA et al: Teratogenesis. In *Problems in Pediatric Drug Therapy,* edited by L Pagliaro and R Levin, Drug Intelligence, Hamilton, 1979, p 3.

142. Warkany J: Antituberculosis drugs: Teratogen update. Teratology. 1979; 20:133.

143. Snider DE et al: Treatment of tuberculosis during pregnancy. Am Rev Respir Dis. 1980; 122:65.

144. Center for Disease Control: Adverse drug reactions among children treated for tuberculosis. Morbid Mortal Weekly Rep. 1980; 29:589.

145. Kennedy DH et al: Tuberculous meningitis. JAMA. 1979; 241:264.

146. Oill PA et al: Infectious disease emergencies: Part 1—Patients presenting with an altered state of consciousness. West J Med. 1976; 125:36.

147. Fallon RJ: The treatment of tuberculosis meningitis. J Antimicrob Chemo. 1978; 4:1.

148. Forgan-Smith R et al: Pyrazinamide and other drugs in tuberculous meningitis. Lancet. 1973; 2:374.

149. Sippel JE et al: Rifampin concentrations in CSF of patients with TB meningitis. Am Rev Respir Dis. 1974; 109:579.

150. Sumaya CV et al: Tuberculosis meningitis in children during the isoniazid era. J Pediatr. 1975; 87:43.

151. Visudhipan P et al: Evaluation of rifampicin in the treatment of tuberculosis meningitis in children. J Pediatr. 1975; 87:983.

152. Prez RD: Extrapulmonary tuberculosis. In *Cecil Textbook of Medicine,* 15th ed, edited by P Beeson, W McDermont and J Wyngaarden, WB Saunders, Philadelphia, 1979, p 491.

153. McKenzie MS et al: Drug treatment of tuberculous meningitis in childhood. Clin Pediatr (Phila). 1979; 18:75.

154. Kutt H et al: Neurological diseases. In *Drug Treatment,* 2nd ed, edited by G Avery, ADIS Press, Sydney (Australia), 1980, p 1010.

Chapter 34

Central Nervous System Infections

John C. Rotschafer

Anatomy and Physiology

Many predisposing factors contribute to the development of central nervous system (CNS) infection. The lack of specific humoral immunity, congenital or traumatic structural defects, history of previous viral infections, stress, season of the year, and age all play important roles in determining the type of infectious process that a patient will develop.

In order to appreciate the pathogenesis, morbidity, and therapeutic management problems associated with CNS infections, a basic understanding of CNS anatomy and physiology is required. In this presentation of infections of the central nervous system, only a limited review of central nervous system anatomy and physiology is possible. If the reader is unfamiliar with the CNS anatomy a more detailed review of the subject may be helpful before proceeding (13–16).

Meninges. The brain and spinal cord are encased in skeletal bone. The brain is suspended in this casing by cerebrospinal fluid (CSF) and surrounded by the meninges. The meninges are comprised of three separate membranes: dura mater, arachnoid, and pia mater. The *dura mater* or pachymeninges lies directly beneath the skeletal structure encompassing the CNS. Within the skull, the dura mater is directly adherent to the periosteum. Under the dura mater are the two membranes collectively referred to as the leptomeninges: the arachnoid and pia mater. The *pia mater* is in direct contact with the brain tissue, while the *arachnoid* lies between the dura mater and the pia mater. The subarachnoid space which is between the arachnoid and the pia mater contains the cerebrospinal fluid (see Figure 1).

Cerebral Spinal Fluid. Eighty-five percent of the CSF is produced within the lateral and fourth ventricles by the choroid plexus. The remaining 15% is formed by diffusion of fluid across the meninges. The probenecid-sensitive active transport mechanism of the choroid plexus can pump weak organic acids (eg, penicillin) from the system. Dysfunction of the choroid plexus is responsible for the elevated protein and decreased glucose concentrations which are observed with various infectious processes. The volume of the cerebrospinal fluid within the CNS is age-dependent and estimated to be approximately 40–60 ml in infants, 60–100 ml in young children, 80–100 ml in older children, and 110–160 ml in adults. The estimated rate of production of CSF fluid by the choroid plexus is approximately 0.5 ml/min. Once formed, CSF flows unidirectionally from the lateral ventricles to the 3rd and 4th ventricles and then passes into the subarachnoid space through the foramina of Magendie and Luschka. During this passage, cerebrospinal fluid can be removed by the arachnoid villi or by the vertebral venous plexus. Therefore, direct administration of a drug into the cerebrospinal fluid will result in therapeutic concentrations downstream from the site of injection but will not result in significant concentrations above the point at which the drug is instilled into the cerebrospinal fluid. Hence, lumbar injection does not result in significant ventricular concentrations. Also see Questions 19 and 20.

Definitions

Central nervous system infection is broadly categorized as septic or aseptic disease. **Septic or bacterial infection** usually is the result of a pri-

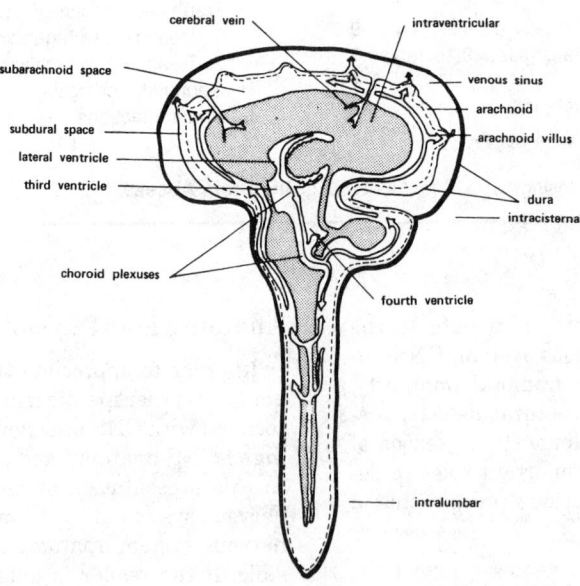

Figure 1. Diagram of the CNS.

mary focus of infection elsewhere in the body, such as pneumonia, pharyngitis, urinary tract infection, bacteremia, otitis media, sinusitis, or mastoiditis. Bacteria from these sites of infection reach the central nervous system most commonly by hematogenous spread. Bacteria also may gain entrance into the CNS from parameningeal infections such as otitis media or sinusitis, where the organisms invade from the primary point of infection because of their proximity to the meninges. Yet another method of bacterial invasion is through congenital or traumatic defects in the meninges. When treating CNS infections, it is of paramount importance that the primary source as well as infecting organism be identified. Chemotherapeutic intervention frequently begins before culture results are available. Because of the substantial morbidity and mortality associated with these infections, prompt diagnosis and treatment are mandatory to effect a favorable clinical outcome.

The term **aseptic central nervous system infection** is a misnomer implying that no infectious process exists. The term has also been misused to imply a viral infection. With regard to central nervous system infection, the term aseptic is nothing more than a broad categorical expression for any process not readily identified on routine bacterial culture. This classification encompasses viral, fungal, yeast, *M. tuberculosis* (tuberculosis), and *T. pallidum* (syphilis) infections, amebiasis, malignancy, sarcoid, and a variety of chemicals that may cause signs or symptoms of central nervous system infection.

It is important to differentiate between septic and aseptic processes because bacterial infections usually result in rapid deterioration and death of the patient. Aseptic and 75% of septic infections tend to be more subacute and allow additional time for diagnostic testing (3). Frequently, in the case of viral CNS infection, no chemotherapeutic intervention is required and the disease is allowed to run a natural and self-limited course. Some patients may have signs and symptoms consistent with meningeal irritation and may have evidence of increased intracranial pressure, but will have normal CSF upon examination. This condition is referred to as *meningism* and is frequently associated with influenza. These symptoms of meningitis will spontaneously resolve without treatment and further concern is generally not warranted.

MENINGITIS

Etiology

The types of organisms causing meningitis are clearly associated with patient age (Table 1). Enteric gram-negative organisms, most often *Escherichia coli,* are found almost exclusively during the neonatal period. Later in childhood, the most predominant organism causing meningitis is *Hemophilus influenzae,* while in adults the most common organism is *Streptococcus pneumoniae* (pneumococcus). In adults, almost all bacterial meningitis is caused by only three organisms, *S. pneumoniae* (pneumococcus), *Neisseria meningitidis* (meningococcus), and *H. influenzae.* These relationships between causative organism and patient age are very useful when antibiotics must be started without the results of CSF culture.

Certain clinical situations, however, may prompt modification of the therapeutic management plan. The incidence of nosocomial CNS infection and organisms resistant to commonly used antibiotics is increasing and therapy for the usual pathogens may not be effective. Nosocomial CNS infection heightens the clinician's suspicion of staphylococcus and gram-negative bacterial infections. Patients with CSF shunts often have shunt infections, meningitis, and ventriculitis due to *Staphylococcus epidermidis.* Evidence of open

Table 1.[12]

MENINGITIS: ORGANISMS AND PATIENT AGE

Age of the Patient	Most Likely Organism
0–1 month	E. coli
	Klebsiella sp.
	Enterobacter sp.
	Group B Streptococcus
1 month–4 years	H. influenzae
	N. meningitidis
	S. pneumoniae
5–9 years	N. meningitidis
	H. influenzae
	S. pneumoniae
10–29 years	N. meningitidis
	S. pneumoniae
	H. influenzae
30–70 years	S. pneumoniae
	N. meningitidis

head trauma dictates staphylococcal and gram-negative antibiotic coverage. Thus, integration of the physical exam, laboratory data, past medical history, and the age of the patient allows clinicians to predict with a great deal of accuracy the potential bacterial pathogen. With this knowledge, appropriate antibiotics can be selected to cover the anticipated microorganisms.

Pathogenesis and Diagnosis

Meningitis represents an infection of the sub-arachnoid space. As the infection progresses, the entire surface area of the leptomeninges may become involved. Once the process crosses the foramina of Luschka and Magendie, ventriculitis ensues. As the infection progresses, intracranial pressure may increase, resulting in papilledema. Therefore, careful examination of the eye grounds is mandatory prior to any attempt at lumbar puncture. Lumbar puncture during an episode of increased intracranial pressure may result in brain herniation due to the sudden release of pressure with needle insertion. Evidence of papilledema should prompt an investigation of other anatomical defects such as mass lesions, subdural empyema or hematoma, tumor, or drug-induced pseudotumor cerebri. A head CT scan can be useful in differentiating meningitis from a space occupying lesion.

Signs and Symptoms. The patient with meningitis will follow a course of acute or subacute illness. In acute disease, signs and symptoms of meningeal irritation may appear within 24 hours; while in subacute disease, symptoms may gradually appear over a period of one week. The most common symptoms of the central nervous system irritation include emesis, chills, backache, stiff neck, fever, headache, and changes in mental status. Many of these symptoms may overlap with an underlying infection. In this situation, examination of the cerebrospinal fluid may ultimately allow the diagnosis to be made.

CSF Findings. Perhaps one of the most rapid and useful tests available to the clinician is the Gram's stain for microorganisms (23,24). If an organism is seen on Gram's stain, immediate information is available as to whether the infecting pathogen is gram-positive or gram-negative. Combining this knowledge with the clinical situation and the age of the patient, rational antibiotic coverage can be selected.

The results of cerebrospinal fluid chemistries which are compatible with bacterial meningitis include an elevated cerebrospinal fluid white count (normal < 5 WBC/mm^3) and a differential white count which is primarily polymorphonuclear instead of mononuclear (1,3,5,7). Normally, the cerebrospinal fluid glucose level is approximately $\frac{1}{2}$ to $\frac{2}{3}$ of the simultaneous peripheral glucose (1,3,5,7). Also, the protein concentration, which should be below 50 mg/dl, is elevated (1,3,5,7). While the cerebrospinal fluid chemistry and white cell count data are helpful in separating infectious from noninfectious processes, they are not entirely reliable because other disease processes may mimic purulent disease and produce similar laboratory findings. The elevated peripheral white blood cell count with a shift to the left also is indicative of a systemic infection.

Other supplemental laboratory tests that may be ordered to confirm the presence of a systemic infection include the following: A *quellung reaction* test may prove particularly useful in identifying organisms when specific antisera are available and when organisms are encapsulated. Antiserum is added to the patient's body fluid sample (eg, sputum or CSF) which contains the suspected pathogen. Upon microscopic examination, capsular swelling will be observed if the antiserum contains antibodies against the organism which is present (24). *Counter-immunoelectrophoresis (CIE)* is another method for rapid determination of some bacterial pathogens (25–28). A sample of the clinical specimen is placed in a well on a gel plate opposite a number of different antisera while an electrical charge is generated over the plate. The clinical specimen and the antisera travel in opposite directions across the gel medium. When the microorganism comes in contact with the respective antisera, a zone of precipitation is formed and the presence of that pathogen is confirmed. The *limulus test* utilizes a chemical obtained from the horseshoe crab. This chemical reagent is added to the clinical specimen of cerebrospinal fluid to determine the presence of a gram-negative endotoxin (29–33).

Other tests that may be useful to determine if the patient has meningitis or a partial meningitis are the *cerebrospinal fluid lactate* concentration and *cerebrospinal fluid pH* (34,35). Elevated cerebrospinal fluid lactate concentration and a decreased cerebrospinal fluid pH suggest the presence of bacterial infection. However, a significant correlation between elevated CSF lactate concentrations and meningitis has been disputed (36).

When the initial lumbar puncture is equivocal or the diagnosis of meningitis is entertained, a repeat lumbar puncture may confirm the earlier suspicion or demonstrate a change in cerebrospinal fluid chemistry or cell count. A repeat lumbar puncture also can serve as an objective measurement for the success or failure of initial antibiotic therapy for meningitis (37).

When attempting to document a central nervous system infection, the clinician also must seek out the likely primary cause and mechanism by which the pathogen entered the central nervous system. Likely foci are otic, paranasal sinus, pulmonary, cardiac, or urinary tract infection. Frequently, no source can be identified. The differential diagnosis of meningitis must include attempts to rule out tumor, subdural empyema, cerebral infarction, mycotic aneurysms, extradural abscesses, and other aseptic diseases. Evaluation of these problems may necessitate skull, mastoid, paranasal sinus, and chest x-rays. Electroencephalograms, brain scans, and computerized axial tomography with and without contrast media also may be useful in the diagnosis and location of potential lesions within the central nervous system. The time interval between the patient entering the hospital, the diagnosis of central nervous system infection, and the initiation of appropriate antibiotic therapy should be minimal.

Treatment Principles

Antibiotics comprise the primary therapy of meningitis; however, when selecting antibiotics, the clinician must be aware of their ability to penetrate to the site of infection as well as their spectrum of antibacterial activity.

Two major mechanisms determine the exchange of various chemicals between the blood, brain, and cerebrospinal fluid (17–21). The *blood-brain barrier* is composed of capillary endothelial tissue that is joined with such tight intracellular junctions that the only effective way for a drug to pass from capillary blood to brain tissue is by direct passage through the capillary endothelial cell. Once having passed this barrier, the drug must then cross the glial cells which envelop the capillaries of the brain (17–19). The passage of chemical substances between the brain and cerebrospinal fluid (*blood-CSF barrier*) is controlled by the choroid plexus (17–21). The ependymal cells of the choroid plexus function in a similar capacity to renal tubular epithelial cells and possess secretory properties. This active transport mechanism within the choroid plexus can be substantially inhibited by probenecid. The selective nature of the choroid plexus to control drug passage is substantially altered by inflammation during an infection.

The penetration of antibiotics into cerebrospinal fluid and brain tissue is crucial to the successful management of central nervous system infection. However, the current medical literature concerning antibiotic passage into these tissues and fluids is limited and at times confusing. Most of this literature is based upon small study populations or anecdotal reports of patients with various diseases and co-existing complications. Many of these reports failed to document the central nervous system infection or focused exclusively upon healthy human volunteers. Study designs and methodologies differed, as did routes of antibiotic administration, use of standardized antibiotic dosages, use of co-existing antibiotics, use of various pharmacokinetic models describing antibiotic behavior, use of antimicrobial assays which measured metabolites, the degree of central nervous system inflammation, variability in antibiotic protein binding characteristics, variability in plasma and CSF pH, and the timing of blood samples drawn in relationship to the dose. Usually, CNS drug penetration is reported as a percent of the simultaneous serum levels in the CSF. Although a useful reference point, the simultaneously obtained serum sample does not truly reflect the cerebrospinal fluid concentration as this is a function of the serum concentration time profile prior to the drawing of the serum specimen.

For an antibiotic to penetrate into the central nervous system, there must be a suitable combination of properties that will allow passage from the blood into the brain tissue or cerebrospinal fluid (see Table 2). Most antibiotics enter the cerebrospinal fluid through the choroid plexus. This epithelial tissue is relatively impermeable to lipid-insoluble drugs. Antibiotics entering cerebrospinal fluid generally pass by active transport. Antibiotics poorly bound to protein, possessing a high oil-water partition coefficient (>0.03), of small molecular weight, and not significantly ionized

Table 2.

Therapeutic antibiotic concentrations obtained without inflamed meninges:
   Sulfonamides
   Trimethoprim
   Chloramphenicol
   Isoniazid
   Rifampin

Therapeutic antibiotic concentrations likely only with inflamed meninges:
   Penicillin G
   Ampicillin
   Ticarcillin
   Carbenicillin

Therapeutic antibiotic concentrations not likely regardless of state of meninges:
   Amikacin
   Streptomycin
   Gentamicin
   Kanamycin
   Tobramycin
   Polymyxin
   Lincomycin
   Clindamycin
   Cephalosporins*

* some 3rd generation cephalosporins have been used successfully to treat patients with meningitis

at body pH are likely to pass readily into the cerebrospinal fluid (21). Meningeal inflammation also improves antibiotic penetration. However, as inflammation subsides, the amount of antibiotic crossing the meninges decreases. In central nervous system infections where meningeal inflammation may not be present (abscesses), antibiotics must be selected for their ability to penetrate the CNS without the presence of inflammation. Antimicrobials not possessing these desirable central nervous system penetrating properties should not be administered intravenously and should be directly instilled into the central nervous system. The three routes of direct instillation are intralumbar, intracisternal, and intraventricular (21). In this situation, the potential morbidity and mortality associated with direct physical CNS instillation and the potential irritating properties of the drug product, vehicle, and preservatives must be considered.

Streptococcus pneumoniae Meningitis

1. L.T., 32-year-old alcoholic black male with a history of sickle cell disease, was involved in an automobile accident five years ago. A splenectomy was performed at that time because of traumatic injury to his abdomen. He had an uneventful recovery and has led a normal life for the last five years. He now presents with a history of headache, cough, pleuritic chest pain, a single shaking rigor and fever. He also complains of a stiff neck and has been "drowsy" for the past 24 hours. During neurological examination, he was placed in a supine position and asked to touch his chin to his chest but he was unable to do so. The physician then placed a hand under the patient's neck and lifted the patient's head forward toward the chest. During this maneuver, flexion was noted in the patient's knees and hips, and the patient's entire upper torso was lifted forward without substantial bending of the neck. The physician then placed the patient back in the supine position and moved to the foot of the bed where the patient's leg was bent toward the chest so that his thigh formed a right angle with the trunk of his body. The physician then attempted extension of the leg, but this was performed with some difficulty and caused the patient great pain in the hamstring region of his leg. This hamstring pain recurred when the patient attempted to perform a straight leg raising exercise. The rest of the physical examination was essentially normal except for some rales and rhonchi heard on auscultation of the chest. Examination of the eye grounds revealed no papilledema.

After finishing the physical examination, laboratory work was ordered. The results of both the sputum and CSF Gram's stains show the presence of gram-positive diplococci. The India ink stain is negative. The cerebrospinal fluid cell count and chemistries are as follows: 120 WBC/mm^3; 85% polymorphonuclear cells (PMN) and 15% mononuclear cells; protein 180 mg/dl; and glucose 20 mg/dl with a simultaneous peripheral glucose of 100 mg/dl. The patient's peripheral white count is 15,000/mm^3 with a differential of 20% bands, 63% segmented PMNs, and 17% lymphocytes.

What pertinent findings from the physical examination and laboratory results are suggestive of central nervous system infection?

The patient's history indicates that he probably has pneumonia and a possible central nervous system infection. The headache, fever, stiff neck, and changes in his mental status all suggest central nervous system infection. However, the patient's cough, pleuritic chest pain, and history of rigor may be symptoms of his pneumonia. The patient's inability to touch his chin to his chest is suggestive of nuchal rigidity (22). This is supported later in the physical examination when lifting the patient's neck elevated the upper torso from a supine position. Within this case are classic descriptions of signs of meningeal irritation: maneuvering the patient's neck forward resulted in the flexion of the patient's knees/hips (Brudzinski's sign) and extension or leg elevation resulted in a painful hamstring reflex (Kernig's sign) (22). The absence of papilledema probably rules out significant elevation of intracranial pressure and thereby allows a lumbar puncture with minimal risk of brain herniation.

The fact that this patient has gram-positive diplococci both in his sputum and cerebrospinal fluid suggests a primary infection of pneumococcal pneumonia with a secondary pneumococcal meningitis. The results of L.T.'s cerebrospinal fluid

chemistries are also compatible with bacterial meningitis. He has an elevated white cell count with a predominance of PMN's, a decreased CSF glucose level relative to the serum level (hypoglycorrhachia) and an elevated CSF protein.

2. Does this patient have any factors which predisposed him to pneumococcal meningitis? How should he be treated?

Streptococcus pneumoniae (pneumococcus) is the most common cause of meningitis in adults. Many underlying factors predispose patients to the development of this type of meningitis which is associated with about a 30% mortality. Patients such as L.T. with a history of trauma, ethanol abuse, pre-existing viral pneumonia, sickle cell disease, and splenectomy are especially susceptible to pneumococcal disease. *Streptococcus pneumoniae* also is frequently associated with "recurrent meningitis" secondary to undetected miniscule skull fractures of the cribriform plate, sinuses, or mastoid (38,39). Detection of cerebrospinal fluid leaks through these fractures usually requires surgical intervention and the use of tracer compounds such as indigo carmine or radiolabeled substances (40–42).

Penicillin G (see Tables 3 & 4) is the drug of choice for the treatment of *Streptococcus pneu-*

Table 3.

SUGGESTED PARENTERAL ANTIMICROBIAL AGENTS FOR THE TREATMENT OF MENINGITIS

Microorganism	Drug of Choice	
	First	Second
Streptococcus (Group B)	Penicillin G or Ampicillin	Chloramphenicol
Streptococcus pneumoniae	Penicillin G	Chloramphenicol
Staphylococcus aureus		
Penicillin G sensitive	Penicillin G	Vancomycin
Penicillin G resistant	Penicillinase Resistant Penicillin	Vancomycin
Methicillin resistant	Vancomycin	
Neisseria meningitidis	Penicillin G	Chloramphenicol
Hemophilus influenzae	Ampicillin & Chloramphenicol	
Escherichia coli	Ampicillin	Chloramphenicol
Pseudomonas aeruginosa	Carbenicillin or Ticarcillin & Gentamicin or Tobramycin	Moxalactam
Listeria monocytogenes	Ampicillin	Chloramphenicol

Table 4.

DOSAGE RECOMMENDATIONS° FOR THE TREATMENT OF MENINGITIS

	Total Daily Dose	Number of doses per day
Ampicillin	200–400 mg/kg/day	6
Penicillin G	200,000–250,000 units/kg/day	6
Chloramphenicol[+]	100 mg/kg/day	4
Methicillin	200 mg/kg/day	6
Gentamicin[*+]	5–7.5 mg/kg/day	3
Tobramycin[*+]	5–7.5 mg/kg/day	3
Vancomycin[+]	30–40 mg/kg/day	4
Carbenicillin	400–500 mg/kg/day	6
Ticarcillin	200–300 mg/kg/day	6

°Excludes Neonates

*Intraventricular or intrathecal administration recommended with parenteral
   use

+Serum levels should be monitored during therapy

moniae despite some isolated reports of penicillin-resistant pneumococci (43–46). These small outbreaks of resistant pneumococci could potentially have a significant impact on antibiotic selection for this disease in the future.

3. *Prophylaxis*. What prophylaxis should this splenectomized patient receive to prevent future pneumococcal infections?

A pneumococcal vaccine is now available for patients who are at high risk for the development of pneumococcal infections. These include: splenectomized patients or patients with splenic dysfunction (eg, sickle cell disease), patients with chronic cardiopulmonary disorders, and other serious underlying chronic diseases (140,141). Although this vaccine does not protect the patient from all pneumococcal subtypes, it does contain antigen for the most common and most virulent isolates. One injection should produce suitable antibody titiers against these forms of pneumococci for five years.

Two groups of patients who are at high risk for developing pneumococcal infection do not respond optimally to the vaccine. Infants and children less than two years of age have slight or absent antibody responses to the vaccine. Patients undergoing chemotherapy for Hodgkin's disease also have a poor serological response to the vaccine (141). Additionally, even though antibody response may be adequate in some normal or splenectomized older children, vaccination may not enhance serum opsonin activity against certain types of pneumococci. Little evidence exists to support the widespread use of the vaccine in groups other than sickle cell patients. Two large scale clinical trials in the 1970's demonstrated no protective benefit in high-risk, institutionalized patients nor in an elderly, non-institutionalized population (141).

The patient in this case would probably benefit from vaccination since he is young, at risk, and is likely to be able to mount an adequate serologic response.

N. meningitidis Meningitis

4. An unresponsive four-year-old white female was brought to the Emergency Room by her mother. The patient had been in her

usual state of good health prior to this admission. Past medical history reveals the patient had normal childhood diseases without any significant medical problems. On physical examination, vital signs were: pulse 98 beats/minute; respirations 32/minute; temperature 104° F rectally, and blood pressure of 80/40 mm Hg. The child was cyanotic and noted to have extensive purpuric lesions over the trunk and extremities of her body. The remainder of the physical examination was unremarkable except for pronounced nuchal rigidity. A toxicology screen, a complete blood cell count with differential, blood gasses, an electrolyte battery, two sets of blood cultures, a urine culture, and a lumbar puncture for cell count, chemistry, and culture were ordered.

The Gram's stain of the cerebrospinal fluid reveals many polymorphonuclear cells but no microorganisms. Chemistry and cell counts of the cerebrospinal fluid are consistent with bacterial meningitis. Therapy is immediately begun with ampicillin and chloramphenicol. Despite aggressive management and life support the child dies within six hours of presenting to the Emergency Room. Culture of the cerebrospinal fluid 48 hours later revealed the presence of *Neisseria meningitidis.*

How does this patient's clinical course compare with the typical presentation of *N. meningitidis* meningitis?

The features outlined in this case report are not unusual for a patient with this type of meningitis (1–8,12). This disease tends to occur primarily in children and young adults. There appears to be a seasonal preference for meningococcal disease with more cases being reported in the winter and spring. There seems to be a male predominance for this disease, with males having almost twice the incidence of females. The clinical course tends to be quite severe. Patients present with fever, malaise, abdominal pain, purpura, cyanosis, and hypotension; 14% of patients will expire within the first 24 hours of therapy (1–8).

5. *Transmission.* What is the most common source of *N. meningitidis* infection and how is the disease transmitted?

The most likely source of this infection is the patient's own nasopharyngeal flora. The disease is transmitted by direct contact or droplet transmission (48–49). Particular serogroups of *N.*

meningitidis, namely A and C, are associated with epidemic outbreaks of disease, especially in confined populations such as military bases. The most likely serotype in the nonepidemic situation is group B. Once coming in contact with *N. meningitidis* (meningococcus), incubation generally takes 2–10 days. There are three identifiable stages of infection. The organism will first localize in the nasopharynx. At some point organisms may gain access into the blood stream. Once hematogenously disseminated, the organisms can seed the meninges, resulting in this devastating disease. Most of the patients recovering from *N. meningitidis* meningitis experience residual motor or intellectual deficits. With extensive cranial nerve involvement, blindness, deafness, or strabismus may result.

6. Was the four-year-old child described in this case treated appropriately?

The initial choice of chloramphenicol and ampicillin in this patient was appropriate in view of the fact that *Hemophilus influenzae* is a common etiologic agent for meningitis in this age group, although *N. meningitidis* and pneumococcus must also be considered (also see Questions 8 and 9). If the child had survived, it would have been appropriate to change the antibiotic regimen to penicillin G as described in Tables 3 and 4.

7. *Prophylaxis.* Should prophylactic measures be taken with this patient's household contacts or school classmates?

The goal of antibiotic prophylaxis is to rid the nasopharynx of *N. meningitidis.* Carrier rates in a normal setting may range from 3 to 30%, while carrier rates in this epidemic situation may range as high as 90% (43–47). Sulfadiazine, penicillin G, and erythromycin were utilized for prophylaxis of *N. meningitidis*; however, these antibiotics are no longer routinely recommended. The current suggested drug of choice for meningococcal prophylaxis is rifampin 600 mg twice daily for two days in adults (47–49). This dosage must be modified for children (53). Minocycline had been extensively used for prophylaxis, but the high incidence of vertigo, nausea and emesis associated with its use has resulted in its replacement by rifampin (53,55). Prophylaxis is suggested only for those persons having intimate contact with the patient, such as family members; school classmates not having direct contact with the patient do not require prophylactic therapy (52–55). A vaccine also is available for those patients at high risk for *N. meningitidis* infection (56,57). For obvious reasons, the vaccine cannot be used in those situations requiring immediate protection, and it should be useful only for groups A and C, but not for Group B, *N. meningitidis* (56,57).

Hemophilus influenzae Meningitis

8. A four-year-old black female was brought back to the Pediatric Clinic by her mother with a four day history of an earache. The patient had been evaluated four days ago in clinic and received a prescription for ampicillin. According to the mother, the antibiotic was administered as directed but the child has not responded. The patient was unusually lethargic over the last day and has been febrile with temperatures up to 103–104° F orally. Meningeal irritation was noted on physical examination and the patient is now hospitalized to rule out meningitis. Based on the child's age and history, what is the most likely microorganism responsible for this patient's condition and what is the risk of morbidity?

The most likely organism, based on the child's age, would be *H. influenzae*. The primary focus of this infection would seem to be the child's otitis media, and the route of organism dissemination would appear to be extension of a parameningeal focus of infection or bacteremia. Although the source of this infection may be otitis media, other primary foci of infections must be ruled out. *H. influenzae* colonizes the upper respiratory tract and evidence of pharyngitis, immunodeficiency, trauma, or a cerebrospinal fluid leak must be ruled out. *H. influenzae* is the most common organism associated with meningitis in young children between one month and four years of age. Approximately 10–20% of these strains of *H. influenzae* are beta-lactamase-producing (59). The disease has an estimated mortality rate of 8%. Morbidity, primarily motor and intellectual deficits, exist in 30–50% of those patients surviving.

9. *Antibiotic Therapy.* The patient is initially treated with intravenous chloramphenicol (25 mg/kg every six hours) and ampicillin (50 mg/kg every four hours). Why was this antibiotic combination chosen for initial therapy?

The combination of a bacteriostatic and bactericidal antibiotic is theoretically undesirable.

Penicillins are bactericidal because they inhibit cell wall formation, which requires active protein synthesis. Chloramphenicol, however, inhibits protein synthesis and may prevent the necessary cell activity for penicillins to be effective. Whether this theoretical antagonism may be responsible for a higher incidence of sequelae following the use of this combination of antibiotics (60,61) or whether this combination results in synergism (62) needs to be resolved by controlled studies.

The current rationale for initial antibiotic coverage with these two antibiotics is based upon the increasing frequency of ampicillin-resistant *H. influenzae*. The incidence of ampicillin-resistant *H. influenzae* is estimated to be about 10–20%. Therefore, this initial therapy must provide antibiotic coverage for this possibility. When bacterial culture and sensitivity results are known, one of these antibiotics can be discontinued.

10. Assuming the organism responsible for this meningitis is susceptible to ampicillin, how successful would ampicillin alone be, as compared to chloramphenicol alone?

Patients with ampicillin-sensitive *H. influenzae* meningitis who are treated solely with ampicillin will have the same clinical outcome as patients treated with chloramphenicol (62–65). Chloramphenicol, although regarded as a bacteriostatic antibiotic, is bactericidal against many strains of *H. influenzae*. Therefore, use of either antimicrobial agent for this particular pathogen would seem to be equally effective when used alone.

11. *Monitoring of Chloramphenicol Therapy.* What objective clinical data should be monitored in this patient to detect early chloramphenicol adverse effects?

Numerous cases of chloramphenicol-induced aplastic anemia have been reported since this drug was first made available in 1949 (66–72). Since this period of time, two specific forms of chloramphenicol-related hematologic toxicity have been identified (71).

Dose-Related Hematologic Toxicity. The first and most common is a reversible bone marrow suppression. This form of chloramphenicol toxicity has been described as a maturation arrest within the marrow, resulting in a vacuolization of erythroid and myeloid precursors. This is associated with a reticulocytopenia. Clinically, this results in anemia, leukopenia, and thrombocytopenia. Monitoring increases of plasma iron content and increases in the percent saturation of iron binding globulins may allow for early detection of this process. This reversible bone marrow depression also appears to be dose-related. Doses of chloramphenicol in excess of four grams a day result in significant changes in reticulocyte count, plasma radiolabelled iron, serum iron, and platelet counts (68). This dose-related toxicity appears to be due to inhibition of an enzyme found within the mitochondrial membrane (71).

Aplastic Anemia. The second form of hematologic toxicity associated with chloramphenicol therapy is aplastic anemia. This nonreversible phenomenon which results in pancytopenia is not dose-related, and the estimated mortality rate is in excess of 50%. There appears to be a latent period of two weeks to 12 months between the time at which the chloramphenicol is discontinued and the onset of pancytopenia. The aplastic anemia might be due to a direct inhibition of DNA synthesis because inhibition of DNA synthesis does not occur in normal patients unless the chloramphenicol concentration is greater than 100 mcg/ml (71). Patients who subsequently develop aplastic anemia may be particularly sensitive to this effect of chloramphenicol because chloramphenicol concentrations of 25–50 mcg/ml could inhibit DNA. This same degree of sensitivity to chloramphenicol has been demonstrated between siblings with aplastic anemia and their parents (71). Therefore, there may be some genetic link to this effect of chloramphenicol. The nitrobenzene moiety of chloramphenicol also may be responsible for the aplastic reaction (71). Thiamphenicol, an analog of chloramphenicol which lacks the nitrobenzene moiety, inhibits mitochondrial protein synthesis but not DNA synthesis. Chloramphenicol-induced aplastic anemia also may be limited to the oral dosage form because aplastic anemia had not been reported after parenteral administration of the drug (73). Although five cases of aplastic anemia attributable to parenteral chloramphenicol have been reported (70), these patients also received oral chloramphenicol at one point or were at risk of developing aplastic anemia for other reasons. The data from yet another report suggests that blacks may be more prone to the development of chloramphenicol-induced aplastic anemia (67).

12. When and how should chloramphenicol serum levels be monitored in this patient?

How can serum levels be used to calculate a dose of chloramphenicol?

The monitoring of chloramphenicol serum concentrations to prevent dose-related toxicity has been suggested, because chloramphenicol levels greater than or equal to 25 mcg/ml are associated with a higher incidence of dose-related bone marrow suppression. Therefore, peak chloramphenicol serum concentrations should be maintained below 25 mcg/ml. While single point peak serum sampling may be useful, individualized pharmacokinetic dosage adjustments require the serum concentrations be at steady-state. However, serum concentrations obtained 5–6 hours after the first dose can be used to estimate chloramphenicol clearance (Figure 2) (74). From this estimated clearance, a dose can be calculated assuming a desired mean steady-state serum concentration (Cpss) of 15 mg/L.

The following equation can be used for dosage adjustment: Dose (mg/kg/day) = Cpss (mg/L) × chloramphenicol clearance (L/kg/hr) × 24 hrs/day. This method of calculation is not recommended if the 5–6 hour serum concentration following the first dose is greater than 13.5 mg/L or less than 2 mg/L. This method is useful because it allows

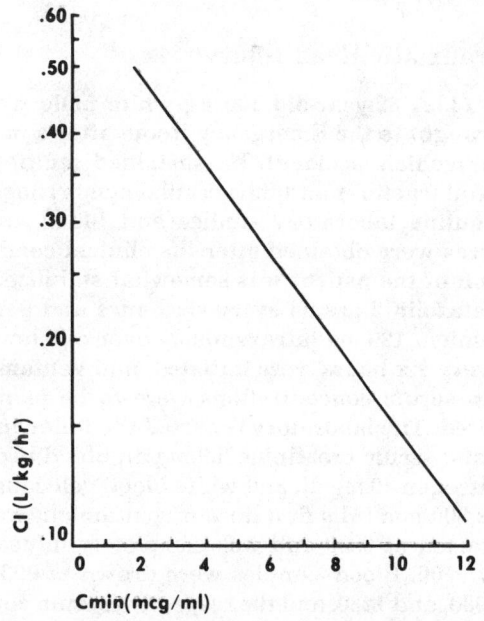

Figure 2. The relationship between the log of chloramphenicol clearance (Cl) and the chloramphenicol serum concentration (C$_{min}$) observed 6 hours after a 25 mg/kg intravenous dose.

dosage adjustment after the first dose of medication and requires only a single serum sample. Obviously, changes in the patient's cardiovascular, hepatic, or renal status will require re-evaluation of the patient's chloramphenicol therapy. Furthermore, follow-up monitoring is desirable to document the accuracy of the original observations.

Before measuring serum concentrations of chloramphenicol, the laboratory should be contacted to determine how the assay is to be performed. Because most clinical laboratories utilize a microbiological assay, it may be useful to determine whether other antibiotics which are being administered concomitantly will interfere with the assay, and whether the laboratory can successfully modify the assay procedure to accommodate for the presence of these other antibiotics.

13. *Prophylaxis.* Should close contacts of this patient receive antimicrobial prophylaxis?

Children less than four years old who are close contacts of a patient who develops this type of meningitis are at risk of developing meningitis due to colonization. Children who are at risk should receive rifampin prophylaxis (20 mg/kg once daily for four days). This treatment modality is 95% effective in eradicating the nasopharyngeal carrier state (58).

Traumatic Head Injury

14. A 32-year-old 100 kg white male was brought to the Emergency Room after a motor vehicle accident. He sustained multiple skull fractures and intracranial hemorrhage. Routine laboratory studies and blood cultures were obtained after the clinical condition of the patient was somewhat stabilized. Cefazolin 2 grams every six hours and gentamicin 120 mg intravenously over one hour every six hours were initiated, and gentamicin serum concentrations were to be monitored. The laboratory reported the following data: serum creatinine 0.9 mg/dl, blood urea nitrogen 40 mg/dl, and white blood cell count 22,300/mm³. His first dose of gentamicin was started at 0800 and was completely infused at 0900. Blood samples were drawn at 0930, 1030, and 1230, and the respective serum concentrations were 3.3, 2.2, and 1.1 mcg/ml. Based on these data, how does the volume of distribution and plasma half-life of genta-

micin in this patient compare to reported normal values?

Many different methods for adjustment of aminoglycoside dosages have been suggested (76–78). Nomograms and formulas are commonly utilized because of the ease at which dose and dosage intervals are selected. These methods do not account for interpatient and intrapatient variation in distribution volume and drug clearance, and the use of these abbreviated methods may be associated with subtherapeutic or potentially toxic serum concentrations. Although these methods are useful when initiating therapy they should not replace aminoglycoside serum concentration monitoring.

Plotting the serum concentration time data on log linear (semi-log) paper results in an estimated half-life of 1.9 hours with a corresponding Kd (0.693/1.9 hr) of 0.36 hr⁻¹. The extrapolated peak serum concentration at the end of the infusion is estimated to be 3.9 mcg/ml. Using the Sawchuk-Zaske method for one-compartment analyses, the volume of distribution is calculated to be 25.85 L or 0.26 L/kg of whole body weight (75) (See Table 5.). Both the half-life and volume of distribution are well within reported ranges for these respective parameters.

15. *Gentamicin Dosage Calculation.* What would be a suitable gentamicin dose and dosage interval for this patient with a suspected bacteremia?

Using the Sawchuk-Zaske method (Table 5) with this patient's data, a peak gentamicin serum concentration of 8 mcg/ml with a corresponding trough concentration of 1.3 mcg/ml is possible if the gentamicin is administered every six hours (allowing one of the six hours for drug infusion). The calculated dose which would produce this peak of 8 mcg/ml under these circumstances is 219 mg. Therefore, this patient should receive a 220 mg dose of gentamicin administered intravenously over one hour every six hours to produce a peak gentamicin serum concentration of 8.04 mcg/ml and a trough of 1.31 mcg/ml. If a more conservative or aggressive approach is desired, the dose and dosage interval can be modified.

16. If this patient were obese, would further dosage modification be required?

Using this particular method of dosage calculation, the patient's volume of distribution of gen-

Table 5.[75]

PHARMACOKINETIC FORMULAS FOR THE
SAWCHUK-ZASKE ONE-COMPARTMENT
AMINOGLYCOSIDE MODEL

Distribution Volume

$$Vd = \frac{Ko}{Kd} \times \frac{1 - e^{-kdt'}}{Cp_{max} - (Cp_{min}e^{-kdt'})}$$

Where:

Vd	=	distribution volume (liters/kg)
Kd	=	elimination rate (hours^{-1})
Ko	=	infusion rate (mg/kg/hr)
Cp_{max}	=	peak serum level (mcg/ml)
Cp_{min}	=	trough serum level (mcg/ml)
t'	=	infusion period (hours)
T	=	dosing interval (hours)

Infusion Rate

$$Ko = Kd\ Vd\ Cp_{max}\frac{(1 - e^{-kdT})}{(1 - e^{-kdt'})}$$

Dosage Interval

$$T = \frac{-1}{Kd} \times Ln\left(\frac{Cp_{min}}{Cp_{max}}\right) + t'$$

Dose

$$Dose = K_o \times t'$$

tamicin is calculated in liters. The value of 25.85 L would remain the same whether the patient's volume were stated in terms of L/kg of whole body weight or L/kg of lean body weight. Therefore, dosage modifications would not be required.

If the patient's volume of distribution were estimated without serum concentration time data, then allowance must be made for the contribution of lean body weight and that portion of body weight which is essentially adipose tissue. Because of the reduction in extracellular fluid per unit mass of adipose tissue, fractional estimates of body weight tend to overestimate the aminoglycoside volume of distribution. Some authors have suggested that volume of distribution be estimated as a percent of ideal body weight and adipose mass (79–81).

It should be appreciated that these studies represent relatively small numbers of patients and that when confronted with this particular situation, actual measurement of patient volume of distribution using serum concentration time data is highly recommended.

17. If this patient demonstrated a substantial degree of ascites, would a modification of dose be required?

The presence of ascites will increase the volume of distribution because ascitic fluid represents an expansion of extracellular fluid and because the peritoneal membrane will allow aminoglycoside passage (82–86). Aminoglycoside concentrations in ascitic fluid are approximately 54–60% of a simultaneous serum concentration (87).

Use of a one compartment model in measuring volume of distribution early in the patient's illness will tend to underestimate the actual value until equilibrium is established between serum and ascitic fluid. A two-compartment pharmacokinetic model, while providing more exact data as to the nature of the volume of distribution, generally is not clinically applicable due to the extended sampling time which is required. Therefore, when using a one-compartment model to characterize the volume of distribution early in an ascitic patient's clinical course, it should be appreciated that this value will probably increase and that frequent serum concentration monitoring is necessary to make modifications in the patient's course of therapy as the size of this compartment increases or decreases.

18. Is gentamicin and cefazolin a reasonable antibiotic combination for this patient?

Central nervous system trauma is associated with a high incidence of gram-positive and gram-negative infections. For this reason, antibiotic selection should be based upon antimicrobial spectrum and the ability of the selected antibiotic to successfully penetrate the central nervous system. While cefazolin and gentamicin may possess the desired antibacterial activity, antibiotic levels achieved in cerebrospinal fluid rarely exceed the minimum inhibiting concentration (88,138). Because of impaired opsonic activity, low complement levels, reduced immunoglobulin levels and the acidic milieu of purulent cerebrospinal fluid, some investigators have suggested the need to achieve aminoglycoside levels 7 to 30 times the bacterial minimum inhibiting concentration (133–139). The current literature suggests that only intraventricular administration is capable of reaching and maintaining aminoglycoside concentrations of this magnitude throughout the central nervous system (14,21,88). Because intraventricular administration represents an invasive neurosurgical procedure, most physicians avoid using aminoglycosides if possible and instead prefer parenteral antibiotics such as the third generation cephalosporins (135). While this patient may not at present have meningitis or ventriculitis, he is certainly at increased risk of developing this type of infection. Should antibiotics be prescribed, attention should be directed toward the degree of central nervous system penetration as well as the antimicrobial spectrum.

19. Assuming that the patient now has a central nervous system infection and that because of an allergic condition he cannot receive parenteral antibiotics such as the third generation cephalosporins, at what point along the central nervous system can direct administration of aminoglycosides be accomplished?

There are three points along the central nervous system at which drugs may be directly in-

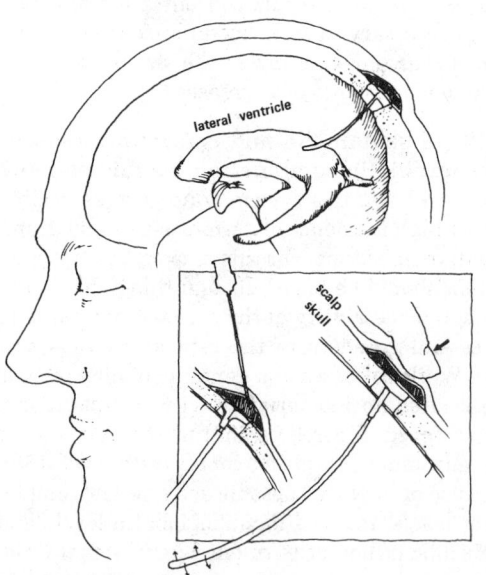

Figure 3. Subcutaneous Cerebrospinal Fluid Reservoir.

stilled into cerebrospinal fluid (88–109). These routes of administration are the intraventricular, intracisternal, and intralumbar. Intraventricular antibiotic administration requires surgical placement of a subcutaneous reservoir with an attached catheter that is placed directly into one of the lateral ventricles (89) (Figure 3). Once the reservoir is in place, the antibiotic is injected directly into this compartment, and by gentle compression of this chamber against the skull, the drug passes through the catheter directly into the ventricle. (Dosages are presented in Table 6.) On some occasions, direct needle instillation of the antibiotic into the ventricle has been performed. This practice occurs most commonly in neonates and is associated with morbidity and potential mortality (107,135). The second method of direct antibiotic instillation is to pass the needle along one side of the cervical vertebra through the dura mater into the cisterna and instill the drug directly there. The last and most common method of central nervous system antibiotic administration is intralumbar or intrathecal administration. This procedure is accomplished by passing a needle into the subarachnoid space in the lower portion of the spinal cord where the antibiotic is directly injected into the cerebrospinal fluid.

20. Place into perspective the advantages and disadvantages of intrathecal and intraventricular antibiotic administration.

Cerebrospinal fluid antibiotic levels are generally at or below the minimum inhibiting concentration for infecting pathogens when aminoglycosides are administered solely by the peripheral route (138). Kaiser demonstrated that levels of gentamicin and tobramycin varied from 0–0.9 mcg/ml in the lumbar, cisternal, and ventricular cerebrospinal fluid while concomitant serum levels ranged from 1.9 to 7.0 mcg/ml (88). Similar results have been reported by other investigators (92,94,95).

Hydrocephalus may affect the pharmacokinetics of aminoglycosides in the CSF by reduced drug clearance and increased CSF volume. When cerebrospinal fluid shunts fail to function because of obstruction, the intraventricular volume increases and prevents dissemination of aminoglycosides beyond the obstruction. Also see Question 22.

Because of the unidirectional flow of cerebrospinal fluids, adequate distribution of antibiotics

Table 6.
INTRAVENTRICULAR DOSAGES[+]

	McLaurin[117]	Wald[116]	Salmon[**121]	Sells[118]
Methicillin	25–100 mg	100 mg	50 mg	*
Chloramphenicol	25–50 mg	*	50 mg	50–100 mg
Cephalothin	25–100 mg	25–100 mg	50 mg	*
Ampicillin	10–25 mg	50 mg	25 mg	*
Gentamicin	2–4 mg	1–8 mg	4 mg	2–4 mg
Nafcillin	*	75	*	*

[+]Combined with rigorous parenteral treatment
*No recommendation made
**Recommendation if head circumference/cerebral mantle ratio ≥ 2

throughout the cerebrospinal fluids can only be assured if the drug is administered directly into the ventricle. Obviously, administration of aminoglycoside directly into the ventricle is associated with more morbidity than administration by the intralumbar route. However, because of concern for a concomitant ventriculitis associated with meningitis, it is imperative that adequate concentrations of antibiotic be obtained throughout the cerebrospinal fluid. There are few comparative studies identifying the relative merits of concomitant parenteral and direct central nervous system routes of injection of antibiotics versus parenteral therapy alone. McCracken conducted one such study in a pediatric population using parenteral plus intralumbar versus parenteral therapy alone (106). In this study, he was unable to demonstrate any difference in outcome between the two treatment groups. This study was criticized, however, for the relatively small amount of aminoglycoside administered intrathecally. In a later study, McCracken compared intraventricular therapy combined with parenteral therapy versus parenteral therapy alone (107). In this study there was substantially more mortality in the group treated with intraventricular gentamicin. However, subcutaneous reservoirs were not generally used and aminoglycoside was administered by daily needle ventricular taps, making this daily traumatic event of uncertain contribution to the overall mortality (110,111,138,139).

For obvious reasons, antibiotics which possess both suitable activity and central nervous system penetrating properties which allow parenteral administration should be used whenever possible (See Table 2). The parenteral combination of trimethoprim and sulfamethoxazole may be useful

in this capacity. In addition, preliminary reports suggest that some parenteral third generation cephalosporins are capable of producing therapeutic concentrations within the cerebrospinal fluid (112,135). However, when aminoglycoside therapy is required, the current literature suggests that the only reasonable means of assuring adequate aminoglycoside concentration throughout the cerebrospinal fluid is use of the intraventricular route. There are preservative-free intrathecal products available for gentamicin and tobramycin. Although no such specific product exists as of yet for amikacin, the parenteral products contain no harmful preservatives and can be used for direct CNS instillation. The suggested intraventricular dose for tobramycin and gentamicin is approximately 0.03 mg/ml of estimated cerebrospinal fluid (3). Somewhat higher doses have been suggested by other investigators (Table 6). For amikacin, the recommended dose is 0.10 mg/ml of estimated cerebrospinal fluid (3). In most cases, a 24-hour dosage interval is used. In all cases, assay for antibiotic concentration at the lumbar level should be performed to assure adequate distribution after intraventricular administration. Trough intraventricular concentrations have also been suggested; however, great care must be exercised to avoid residual aminoglycoside contamination. Currently, all commonly used cerebrospinal fluid ventricular shunts have a subcutaneous port for convenient ventricular antibiotic administration.

Neonatal Meningitis

21. The patient is a 2-day-old, 2,000 gram male infant, the product of a 28-week-preg-

nancy. The patient's mother is a 16-year-old diabetic female who had sporadic prenatal care. The child has been lethargic and difficult to feed over the last two days. The nurses have observed some questionable seizure activity and a fullness of the fontanelle. His rectal temperatures over the last day have been 99° F. Past medical history is significant in that the child's mother presented to the emergency room with premature rupture of membranes and onset of labor. After a 17-hour labor, the child was delivered vaginally. Meconium staining was noted at the time of delivery. One-and five-minute Apgar scores were 3 and 7, respectively. The child was immediately taken to the neonatal intensive care and placed in an isolette. Ampicillin 50 mg/kg every six hours and tobramycin 2.5 mg/kg every eight hours were started after blood, CSF, and urine cultures were obtained. What clinical data from this patient are compatible with neonatal meningitis?

Typically, neonatal meningitis presents in one of two fashions, either early or late onset. Early onset generally occurs within the first week of life (as in this case) and is a fulminant multisystem illness. High risk mothers (eg, diabetics) with premature rupture of membranes or onset of labor often predispose their infant to early onset neonatal meningitis. Mothers with a peripartum genital or urinary tract infection also predispose the child to this complication. Generally, the neonates are of low birth weight and delivered prematurely. Traumatic delivery also is commonly associated with early onset neonatal meningitis. The infecting organisms (Group B Streptococcus and enteric gram-negative rods) are acquired from the birth canal during delivery. Mortality associated with this type of presentation is estimated to be 20–50%. The second or late onset type of neonatal meningitis generally occurs after one week but can occur as early as 4 days after birth. Unlike the early onset type of meningitis, there is generally no history of obstetric complication. The bacteria causing the disease are acquired from human contact or through the hospital environment and not from the birth canal. Mortality in this type of presentation is somewhat lower and estimated to be about 10–20%.

The presentation of meningitis in the neonate is completely different from that in the adult. Few clinical symptoms are apparent on physical examination. Generally, the diagnosis is based on subjective findings such as lethargy, difficulty in feeding, and emesis. Physical examination reveals few objective findings; the presence of hypothermia or a bulging fontanelle suggests the need for further evaluation for meningitis. There is also a significant difference in both the CSF chemistry and cell count in neonates as compared to adults.

The incidence of meningitis is highest during the first month of life for the infant. Socioeconomic status, host-susceptibility, nursery and obstetric practices, and the general state of the mother's health all play important roles in the pathogenesis of neonatal meningitis.

Under normal circumstances, the infant is protected from maternal genital flora by the amniotic membrane. Premature rupture of this membrane accompanied by delayed delivery allows vaginal bacteria to ascend and cause inflammation of the fetal membranes, umbilical cord, and placenta. The aspiration of infected amniotic fluid predisposes the fetus to the onset of sepsis. The presence of meconium increases the ability of the amniotic fluid to support pathogenic bacteria such as E. coli and other organisms. After 26 weeks gestation, the concentration of immunoglobulins (IgA and IgG) begins to increase and provides protection to the amniotic fluid against invasion by these bacteria. Neonatal skin or nasopharyngeal contamination can seed organisms into the blood stream, ultimately resulting in meningitis. The most common organisms causing neonatal meningitis are E. coli, Group B Streptococcus, and L. monocytogenes. However, geographical differences in the type of organisms producing meningitis in this age group may vary. The reduced amount of immunoglobulin IgM in premature infants with low birth weight also may play an important role in the newborns' inability to defend against gram-negative bacteria invasion. As with adults, successful management depends on rapid diagnosis and implementation of appropriate antibiotic therapy. Special situations such as immunological disorders, history of neurosurgical procedures of trauma, or the presence of cerebrospinal fluid shunt may modify standard treatment plans.

Shunt Infections

22. A 7-year-old female with a previous history of hydrocephalus presents with a two day history of fever and neck stiffness one

month after ventriculoperitoneal shunt placement. Her physical examination is consistent with meningitis, and cerebrospinal fluid cultures obtained on admission revealed *Staphylococcus epidermidis*. She is immediately started on intravenous methicillin 100 mg/kg/day and given 50 mg methicillin intraventricularly. Why is the treatment of shunt infections in a patient like this so difficult?

Cerebrospinal fluid buildup associated with hydrocephalus causes intracranial hypertension which may result in brain tissue being pressed against the periosteum of the skull and subsequent brain tissue necrosis (113). Cerebrospinal fluid shunts, such as this, relieve increased pressure by diverting cerebrospinal fluid from the ventricle to a site outside the central nervous system. In this case, the ventriculoperitoneal shunt diverts cerebrospinal fluid to the peritoneal cavity. The shunt is a foreign appliance where bacteria can perpetuate, and surgical placement of these shunts is associated with a 6–39% incidence of bacterial contamination. The organisms most commonly responsible for this type of central nervous system infection are *S. epidermidis, S. aureus, H. influenzae, Klebsiella sp.,* and *Enterococcus.*

Shunt infections are usually treated with high dose systemic antibiotics. However, the lack of inflammation associated with this disease results in poor antibiotic penetration. Therefore, this approach to therapy is usually modified to include direct administration of antibiotics through a subcutaneous port in the shunt. Complete or partial surgical removal of the cerebrospinal fluid shunt is not always advisable and can cause a number of problems. Once the shunt is removed, the patient can again experience intracranial hypertension and will have to undergo surgery at a later date to replace the shunt. Usually, immediate shunt replacement is not possible due to the existence of infection. Furthermore, the ventricles are too small at this point to consider surgical replacement. Lastly, with vascular access shunts, removal sacrifices the vein and prevents future use of this route for shunting. Therefore, systemic antibiotics with concomitant intraventricular injections through the access port of the cerebrospinal fluid shunt often is preferred over surgical shunt removal. Approximately 50% of these infections can be cured with antibiotics used in this fashion (114–121).

Antibiotic toxicity from direct intraventricular administration is relatively rare, and chemical irritation has been minimal. Nevertheless, intraventricular cephalothin has been associated with seizure activity. Recommended intraventricular dosages of antibiotics are presented in Table 6. In most clinical situations, aggressive systemic antibiotic therapy should accompany the direct intraventricular injection of antibiotics. If these procedures are unsuccessful, surgical correction will be required.

BRAIN ABSCESS

23. An 8-year-old female with congenital cyanotic heart disease presents to the hospital with nausea, emesis, and fever. The patient has been progressively lethargic over the last day and at times required vigorous stimulation to arouse her. She has pronounced weakness in the left leg and has a recent history of focal seizures beginning in the left arm. She has a pronounced nuchal rigidity, and examination of her eye grounds reveals papilledema. Angiography indicates a mass lesion in the right frontal lobe. She is taken to the operating room where excision of the suspected abscess is attempted. The abscess cavity could not be evacuated as the contents have already eroded into the lateral ventricle. Twelve hours after the surgical procedure, the patient is pronounced dead. How does this patient compare to the typical presentation of a patient with a brain abscess?

The most common clinical presentation is that of headache, history of a recent onset of a seizure disorder, mild obtundation, fever, papilledema, and a focal neurological finding. While the infection itself certainly can represent a life-threatening condition, as in this patient, the most common danger of abscess formation is not from the infection itself but from the mass lesion effect (121–131). This central nervous sytem disease is almost always fatal when surgical evacuation of the abscess cavity is not possible. The overall estimated mortality for brain abscess is 30–60% (129). For those patients surviving, estimated morbidity is approximately 50%, consisting primarily of permanent neurological deficits such as hemiparesis, monoparesis, incomplete aphasia, or seizure disorder (129). Abscess formation generally results from a parameningeal focus of infection, metastatic hematogenous spread, or a late complication from penetrating traumatic injury to the central nervous system. Abscess formation frequently occurs after pulmonary infection or congenital heart disease when the organisms are seeded into the central nervous sytem from the blood stream. Localization of brain abscesses is generally possible through the use of a CT scan, electroencephalogram, brain scan, and arteriography. The usual location of an abscess is in the frontal and parietal lobes. Prior to anaerobic culture technique, abscess formation was generally felt to be associated with aerobic streptococci or staphylococci. More recently, it has been found that anaerobes account for 90% of nontraumatic abscesses. While aerobic staphylococci, streptococci, and gram-negative rods play an important role in abscess formation, anaerobic streptococci and bacteroides species are more important (124). Treatment of these infections is aimed at relieving the mass lesion effect. If at all possible, surgical removal of the entire abscess accompanied with aggressive antibiotic management is the desired procedure. Patients with an inoperable abscess or those who have multiple abscesses have a much graver prognosis than those with abscesses that can be entirely removed.

Antibiotic coverage perioperatively and postoperatively is imperative for successful management of this condition. While many antibiotics such as penicillin G, ampicillin, chloramphenicol, lincomycin, and methicillin penetrate into the abscess cavity in therapeutic concentrations, the poor antibiotic activity within the abscess makes it highly unlikely that antibiotic therapy itself will result in therapeutic cure. Antibiotics undoubtedly suppress the microbial spread, but they cannot eradicate the primary site of infection. The purulent milieu present in the cavity (pH, tissue products, and enzymes) ultimately prevent an antibiotic cure even though therapeutically effective antibiotic concentrations can be demonstrated at this site of infection (126). Antibiotics such as cloxacillin, aminoglycosides, nafcillin, and cephaloridine have poor abscess penetrating properties. Antibiotics such as rifampin, metronidazole, sulfa drugs, and trimethoprim penetrate the central nervous system and may be useful in treating these infections. Since inflammation of the meninges may not be present, antibiotics dependent on meningeal irritation for passage should be avoided. Although chloramphenicol penetrates the central nervous system relatively well, the respective concentrations produced in the abscess may be somewhat sporadic. Nafcillin penetrates very poorly and should not be used (126). Direct instillation of antibiotics into the abscess cavity is to be discouraged.

References

1. Marr JJ: Bacterial meningitis. In *Infectious Diseases,* edited by JJ Marr, Little, Brown and Company, Boston, 1973, p 53.
2. Klein JO et al: Bacterial infections. In *Infectious Diseases of the Fetus and Newborn Infant,* edited by JS Remington and JO Klein, W.B. Saunders Company, Philadelphia, 1976, p 747.
3. McGee ZA et al: Acute meningitis. In *Principles and Practice of Infectious Diseases,* edited by GL Mandell, RG Douglas, and JE Bennett, John Wiley and Sons, New York, 1979, p 738.
4. Hyslop NE et al: Bacterial meningitis. Postgrad Med. 1975; 58:120.
5. Hambleton G et al: Diagnosis and management of bacterial meningitis. Drugs. 1974; 8:15.
6. Carpenter RR et al: The clinical spectrum of bacterial meningitis. Am J Med. 1962; 33:262.
7. Smith DH et al: Diagnosis and treatment of bacterial meningitis: a symposium. Pediatrics. 1973; 52:586.
8. Nankervis GA: Bacterial meningitis. Med Clin North Am. 1974; 58:581.
9. Karandanis D et al: Recent survey of infectious meningitis in adults: Review of laboratory findings in bacterial, tuberculous, and aseptic meningitis. South Med J. 1976; 69:449.
10. Benner EJ et al: Acute bacterial meningitis. In *Infectious Diseases,* edited by PD Hoeprich, Harper and Row, Hagerstown, 1972, p 931.
11. Wehrle PF: Meningitis. In *Communicable and Infectious Diseases,* 7th ed, edited by FH Top and PF Wehrle, C.V. Mosby Company, St. Louis, 1972, p 401.
12. Geiseler PJ et al: Community acquired purulent meningitis: a review of 1,316 cases during the antibiotic era, 1954–1976. Reviews of Infect Dis. 1980; 2:725.
13. Crouch JE: The nervous system. In *Functional Human Anatomy,* 2nd ed, Lea and Febiger, Philadelphia, 1972, p 477.
14. Greenlee JE: Anatomic considerations in central nervous system infections. In *Principles and Practice of Infectious Diseases,* edited by GL Mandell, RG Douglas, and JE Bennett, John Wiley and Sons, New York, 1979, p 725.

15. Carpenter MB: Meninges and cerebrospinal fluid. In *Core Text of Neuroanatomy*, 2nd ed, edited by MB Carpenter, Williams and Wilkens, Baltimore, 1978, p 1.

16. Matzke HA et al: Gross anatomy of the central nervous system. In *Pathology of the Central Nervous System*, vol 1, edited by J Minckler, McGraw-Hill Book Company, New York, 1968, p 90.

17. Richards ML et al: Antimicrobial penetration into cerebrospinal fluid. Drug Intell Clin Pharm. 1981; 15:341.

18. Kramer PW et al: Antibiotic penetration of the brain, a comparative study. J Neurosurg. 1969; 31:295.

19. Barling RWA et al: The penetration of antibiotics into cerebrospinal fluid and brain tissue. J Antimicrob Chemother. 1978; 4:203.

20. Schanker LS: Passage of drugs into and out of the central nervous system. Antimicrob Agent Chemother. 1965; 5:1044.

21. Allinson RR et al: Intrathecal drug therapy. Drug Intell Clin Pharm. 1978; 12:347.

22. Brody IA et al: The signs of Kernig and Brudzinski. Arch Neurol. 1969; 21:215.

23. Provine H et al: The gram-stained smear and its interpretation. Hosp Pract. 1974; 9:85.

24. Gardner P et al: The specimen. In *Manual of Acute Bacterial Infections*, edited by P Gardner and HT Provine, Little, Brown and Company, Boston, 1975, p 165.

25. Coonrod JD et al: Determination of etiology of bacterial meningitis by counter-immunoelectrophoresis. Lancet. 1972; 1:1154.

26. Ingram DL et al: Countercurrent immunoelectrophoresis in the diagnosis of systemic disease caused by *Hemophilus influenzae* Type B. J Pediatr. 1972; 81:1156.

27. Greenwood BM et al: Countercurrent immunoelectrophoresis in the diagnosis of meningococcal infections. Lancet. 1971; 2:519.

28. Edwards EA et al: Diagnosis of bacterial meningitis by counterimmunoelectrophoresis. J Lab Clin Med. 1972; 80:449.

29. Ross S et al: Limulus lysate test for gram-negative bacterial meningitis bedside application. JAMA. 1975; 233:1366.

30. Nachum R et al: Rapid detection of gram-negative bacterial meningitis by the limulus lysate test. N Engl J Med. 1973; 289:931.

31. Levin J et al: The role of endotoxin in extracellular coagulations of limulus blood. Ball Hopkins Hosp. 1965; 115:265.

32. Martinez GL et al: Clinical experience on the detection of endotoxinemia with the limulus test. J Infect Dis. 1973; 127:102.

33. Stumacher R et al: Limitation of the usefulness of the limulus assay for endotoxin. N Engl J Med. 1973; 288:1261.

34. Bland RD et al: Cerebrospinal fluid lactic acid level and pH in meningitis. Am J Dis Child. 1974; 128:151.

35. Brook I et al: Measurement of lactic acid in cerebrospinal fluid of patients with infections of the central nervous system. J Infect Dis. 1978; 137:384.

36. Rutledge J et al: Is the CSF lactate measurement useful in the management of children with suspected bacterial meningitis. J Pediatr. 1981; 98:20.

37. Feigin RD et al: Value of repeat lumber puncture in the differential diagnosis of meningitis. N Engl J Med. 1973; 289:571.

38. Whitecar JP et al: Recurrent pneumococcal meningitis: a review of the literature and studies on a patient who recovered from eleven attacks caused by five serotypes of *Diplococcus pneumoniae*. N Engl J Med. 1966; 274:1285.

39. Levin S et al: Pneumococcal meningitis: the problem of the unseen cerebrospinal fluid leak. Am J Med Sci. 1972; 264:319.

40. Hull HF et al: Glucorrhea revisted. JAMA. 1975; 234:1052.

41. Hudson WR et al: Cerebrospinal rhinorrhea: diagnosis and management. South Med J. 1975; 68:1520.

42. Kosoy J et al: Glucose in nasal secretions diagnostic significance. Arch Otolaryngol. 1972; 95:225.

43. Applebaum PC et al: *Streptococcus pneumoniae* resistant to penicillin and chloramphenicol. Lancet. 1977; 2:995.

44. Anon: Follow-up on multiple-antibiotic-resistant pneumococci-South Africa. Morbidity Mortality Weekly Report. 1978; 27:1.

45. Anon: Penicillin-resistant *Streptococcus pneumoniae*—Minnesota. Morbidity Mortality Weekly Report. 1977; 26:345.

46. Anon: Multiple resistant pneumococcus—Colorado. Morbidity Mortality Weekly Report. 1981; 30:197.

47. Advisory Committee on Immunization Practices: pneumococcal polysaccharide vaccine. Morbidity Mortality Weekly Report. 1978; 27:25.

48. Greenfield S et al: Meningococcal carriage in a population of "normal" families. J Infect Dis. 1971; 123:67.

49. Kaiser AB et al: Sero-epidemiology and chemoprophylaxis of disease due to sulfonamide-resistant Neisseria meningitidis in a civilian population. J Infect Dis. 1974; 130:217.

50. Bell WE et al: Meningococcal meningitis: Past and present concepts. Mil Med. 1971; 136:601.

51. Artenstein MS et al: The risk of exposure to a patient with meningococcal meningitis. Mil Med. 1968; 133:474.

52. The Meningococcal Disease Surveillance Group: Analysis of endemic Meningococcal disease by serogroup and evaluation of chemoprophylaxis. J Infect Dis. 1976; 134:201.

53. Hendeles L et al: The prevention of meningococcal disease in the community. Drug Intell Clin Pharm. 1978; 12:278.

54. Sanders WE: Rifampin. Ann Intern Med. 1976; 85:82.

55. Allen JC: Minocycline. Ann Intern Med. 1976; 85:482.

56. Artenstein MS et al: Prevention of meningococcal disease by group C polysaccharide vaccine. N Engl J Med. 1970; 282:417.

57. Anon: Preventing spread of meningococcal disease. Med Let Drugs Ther. 1981; 23:37.

58. Cox F et al: Rifampin prophylaxis for contacts of *Haemophilus influenzae* type B disease. JAMA. 1981; 245:1043.

59. Crosson FJ et al: Acute otitis media caused by ampicillin-resistant *Haemophilus influenzae* type B. JAMA. 1976; 236:2778.

60. Lepper MH et al: Treatment of pneumococci meningitis with penicillin compared with penicillin plus aureomycin. Arch Intern Med. 1951; 88:489.

61. Lindberg J et al: Long-term outcome of *Hemophilis influenzae* meningitis related to antibiotic treatment. Pediatrics. 1977; 60:1.

62. Feldman WE: Effect of ampicillin and chloramphenicol against *Haemophilus influenzae*. Pediatrics. 1978; 61:406.

63. Girgis NI et al: Ampicillin compared with penicillin and chloramphenicol combined in the treatment of bacterial meningitis. J Trop Med Hyg. 1972; 75:154.

64. Schulkind ML et al: A comparison of ampicillin and chloramphenicol therapy in *Hemophilus influenzae* meningitis. Pediatrics. 1971; 48:411.

65. Overturf GD et al: Bacterial meningitis: which regimen? Drugs. 1979; 18:65.

66. Lewis CN et al: Chloramphenicol (Chloromycetin) in relation to blood dyscrasias with observations on other drugs. Antibiotics and Chemother. 1952; 2:601.

67. Wallerstein RO et al: Statewide study of chloramphenicol therapy and fatal aplastic anemia. JAMA. 1969; 208:2045.

68. Scott JL et al: A controlled double-blind study of hematologic toxicity of chloramphenicol. N Engl J Med. 1965; 272:1137.

69. Best WR: Chloramphenicol-associated blood dyscrasias. JAMA. 1967; 201:99.

70. Polin HB et al: Chloramphenicol. NY State J of Med. 1977; 77:378.

71. Yunis AA: Chloramphenicol-induced bone marrow suppression. Semin Hematol. 1973; 10:225.

72. Snyder MJ et al: The clinical use of chloramphenicol. Med Clin North Am. 1970; 54:1187.

73. Holt R: The bacterial degradation of chloramphenicol. Lancet. 1967; 1:1259.

74. Koup JR et al: Rapid elimination of chloramphenicol clearance in infants and children. Clin Pharmacokinetics. 1981; 6:83.

75. Sawchuk RJ et al: Kinetic model for gentamicin dosing with the use of individual patient parameters. Clin Pharmacol Ther. 1977; 21:362.

76. Sarubbi RA et al: Amikacin serum concentrations: prediction of levels and dosage guidelines. Ann Intern Med. 1978; 89:612.

77. Hull JH et al: Gentamicin serum concentrations: pharmacokinetic predictions. Ann Intern Med. 1976; 85:183.

78. Chan RA et al: Gentamicin therapy in renal failure: a nomogram for dosage. Ann Intern Med. 1972; 76:773.

79. Blouin RA et al: Tobramycin pharmacokinetics in morbidly obese patients. Clin Pharmacol Ther. 1979; 26:508.

80. Schwartz SN et al: A controlled investigation of the pharmacokinetics of gentamicin and tobramycin in obese subjects. J Infect Dis. 1978; 138:499.

81. Sketris I et al: Effect of obesity on gentamicin pharmacokinetics. J Clin Pharm. 1981; (in press).

82. Gill MA et al: Altered gentamicin distribution in ascitic patients. Am J Hosp Pharm. 1979; 36:1704.

83. Lanao JM et al: The influence of ascites on the pharmacokinetics of amikacin. Intern J Clin Pharm Ther and Tox. 1980; 18:57.

84. Pitt HA et al: Gentamicin levels in the human biliary tract. J Infect Dis. 1973; 127:299.

85. Spicehandler JR et al: Pharmacokinetics of amikacin and netilmicin in cirrhotic subjects. In *Current Chemotherapy and Infectious Disease,* edited by JD Nelson and C. Grassi, American Society for Microbiology, Washington, 1980, p 693.

86. Michelson PA: Altered gentamicin distribution in ascitic patients. Am J Hosp Pharm. 1980; 37:625.

87. Gerding DN et al: Antibiotic concentrations in ascitic fluid of patients with ascites and bacterial peritonitis. Ann Intern Med. 1977; 86:708.

88. Kaiser AD: Aminoglycoside therapy of gram-negative bacillary meningitis. N Engl J Med. 1975; 293:1215.

89. Ratcheson RA et al: Experience with the subcutaneous cerebrospinal-fluid reservoir. N Engl J Med. 1968; 279:1026.

90. Rodriquez V et al: Gentamicin sulfate distribution in body fluids. Clin Pharmacol Ther. 1970; 11:275.

91. Moellering RC et al: Relationship of intraventricular gentamicin levels to cure meningitis. J Pediatr. 1972; 81:534.

92. Vacek V et al: Penetration of antibiotics into cerebrospinal fluid in inflammatory conditions, 3. gentamicin. Int J Clin Pharm. 1969; 2:277.

93. Lee EL et al: Intraventricular chemotherapy in neonatal meningitis. J Pediatr. 1977; 91:991.

94. Goiten K et al: Penetration of parenterally administered gentamicin into the cerebrospinal fluid in experimental meningitis. Chemotherapy. 1975; 21:181.

95. Pickering LK et al: Intraventricular and parenteral gentamicin therapy for ventriculitis in children. Am J Dis Child. 1978; 132:480.

96. Kaiser AB et al: Treatment of gram-negative meningitis and ventriculitis. N Engl J Med. 1976; 294:673.

97. Wirt TC et al: Intraventricular administration of amikacin for complicated gram-negative meningitis and ventriculitis. J Neurosurg. 1979; 50:95.

98. Saad AF et al: Intracisternal and intrathecal injections of gentamicin in Enterobacter Meningitis. Arch Intern Med. 1974; 124:738.

99. Anon: Intralumbar and intraventricular therapy of bacterial meningitis. Med Let Drugs Ther. 1977; 19:93.

100. Mangi RJ et al: Treatment of gram-negative bacillary meningitis with intrathecal gentamicin. Yale J Biol Med. 1977; 50:31.

101. Yeung CY et al: Intrathecal antibiotic therapy for neonatal meningitis. Arch Dis Child. 1976; 51:686.

102. Hollifield JW et al: Gram-negative bacillary meningitis therapy: Polyradiculitis following intralumbar aminoglycoside administration. JAMA. 1976; 236:1284.

103. Wantanbe I et al: Neurotoxicity of intrathecal gentamicin: A case report and experimental study. Ann Neurol. 1978; 4:566.

104. Kourtopoulos H et al: Intraventricular treatment of *Serratia marcescens* meningitis with gentamicin. Scand J Infect Dis. 1976; 8:57.

105. Shuman RD et al: Intrathecal gentamicin for refractory gram-positive meningitis. JAMA. 1978; 240:469.

106. McCracken GH et al: A controlled study of intrathecal antibiotic therapy in gram-negative enteric meningitis of infancy. Report of the Neonatal Meningitis Cooperative Study Group. J Pediatr. 1976; 89:66.

107. McCracken GH et al: Intraventricular gentamicin therapy in gram-negative bacillary meningitis in infancy. Lancet. 1980; 1:787.

108. Sklaver AR et al: Amikacin therapy of gram-negative bacteremia and meningitis treatment in diseases due to multiple resistant bacilli. Arch Intern Med. 1978; 138:713.

109. Trujillo H et al: Amikacin concentration in the cerebrospinal fluid of children with acute bacterial meningitis.J Int Med Res. 1979; 7:45.

110. Swartz MN: Intraventricular use of aminoglycosides in the treatment of gram-negative bacillary meningitis. J Infect Dis. 1981; 143:293.

111. Wright PF et al: The pharmacokinetics and efficacy of an aminoglycoside administered into the cerebral ventricles in neonates: Implications for further evaluation of this route of therapy in meningitis. J Infect Dis. 1981; 143:141.

112. Landesman SH et al: Diffusion of a new Beta-Lactam (LY127935) into cerebrospinal fluid, implications for therapy of gram-negative bacillary meningitis. Am J Med. 1980; 69:92.

113. Shurtleff DB et al: Characteristics of the various CSF shunt systems. Clin Pediatr. 1978; 17:154.

114. Schoenbaum SC et al: Infections of cerebrospinal fluid shunts: Epidemiology, clinical manifestations, and therapy. J Infect Dis. 1975; 131:543.

115. Venes JL: Control of shunt infection report of 150 consecutive cases. J Neurosurg. 1976; 45:311.

116. Wald SL et al: Cerebrospinal fluid antibiotic levels during treatment of shunt infections. J Neurosurg. 1980; 52:41.

117. McLaurin RL: Infected cerebrospinal fluid shunts. Surg Neurol. 1973; 1:191.

118. Sells CJ et al: Gram-negative cerebrospinal fluid shunt-associated infections. Pediatrics. 1977; 59:613.

119. Shurtleff DB et al: Therapy of Staphylococcus epidermidis infections associated with cerebrospinal fluid shunts. Pediatrics. 1974; 53:55.

120. George R et al: Long-term analysis of cerebrospinal fluid shunt infections a 25-year experience. J Neurosurg. 1979; 51:804.

121. Salmon JH: Ventriculitis complicating meningitis. Am J Dis Child. 1972; 124:35.

122. Samson DS et al: A current review of brain abscess. Am J Med. 1973; 54:201.

123. Beller AJ et al: Brain abscess. J Neurol, Neurosurg, and Psychiatry. 1973; 36:757.

124. DeLouvois J et al: Bacteriology of abscesses of the central nervous system: a multicentre prospective study. Br Med J. 1977; 2:981.

125. Jefferson AA et al: Intracranial abscesses: A review of treated patients over 20 years. Quart J Med. 1977; XLVI:389.

126. Black P et al: Penetration of brain abscess by systematically administered antibiotics. J Neurosurg. 1973; 38:705.

127. Gregory DH et al: Metastatic brain abscesses. Arch Intern Med. 1967; 119:25.

128. DeLouvois J et al: Antibiotic treatment of abscesses of the central nervous system. Br Med J. 1977; 2:985.

129. Karandanis D et al: Factors associated with mortality in brain abscess. Arch Intern Med. 1975; 135:1145.

130. Morgan H et al: Experience with 88 consecutive cases of brain abscess. J Neurosurg. 1973; 38:699.

131. Brewer NS et al: Brain abscess: a review of recent experience. Ann Intern Med. 1975; 82:571.

132. Richards ML et al: Antimicrobial penetration into cerebrospinal fluid. Drug Intell Clin Pharm. 1981; 15:341.

133. Simberkoff MS et al: Absence of detectable bactericidal and opsonic activities in normal and infected human cerebrospinal fluids. J Lab Clin Med. 1980; 95:362.

134. Tofte RW et al: Opsonic activity of normal human cerebrospinal fluid for selected bacterial species. Infect Immuno. 1979; 26:1093.

135. Landesman SH et al: Past and current roles for cephalosporin antibiotics in treatment of meningitis: Emphasis on use in gram-negative bacillary meningitis. Am J Med. 1981; 71:693.

136. Strausbaugh LJ et al: Factors influencing the therapy of experimental proteus mirabilis meningitis in rabbits. J Infect Dis. 1978; 137:251.

137. McCracken GH: The rate of bacteriologic response to antimicrobial therapy in neonatal meningitis. Am J Dis Child. 1972; 123:547.

138. Swartz MN: Intraventricular use of aminoglycosides in the treatment of gram-negative bacillary meningitis: Conflicting views. J Infect Dis. 1981; 143:293.

139. Wright PF et al: The pharmacokinetics of an aminoglycoside administered into the cerebral ventricles in neonates: Implications for further evaluation of this route of therapy in meningitis. J Infect Dis. 1981; 143:141.

140. Anonymous: Pneumococcal polysaccharide vaccine. Morbidity Mortality Weekly Report. 1978; 27:25.

141. Hirschmann JV et al: Pneumococcal vaccine in the United States. JAMA. 1981; 246:1428.

Chapter 35

Endocarditis

B. Joseph Guglielmo

Pathogenesis (1)

Infective endocarditis can be defined as a microbial infection of cardiac valves or other endocardial tissue. Animal experimentation has demonstrated that several independent events are required for the development of infective endocarditis.

First, the endocardial surface must be altered to produce a suitable site for bacterial attach-ment and colonization. These alterations may include trauma, turbulence, or forms of exogenous stress. When associated with valvular insufficiency, infective endocarditis classically occurs on the atrial surface of the mitral valve and the ventricular surface of the aortic valve. Lesions associated with high degrees of turbulence, such as stenotic valves, readily create conditions which enhance bacterial attachment, whereas defects with a large surface area (eg, large ventricular septal defect), low flow states, or conditions with minimal turbulence, such as congestive heart failure with atrial fibrillation, are rarely implicated in endocarditis.

After suitable surface changes on the valve have occurred, platelets and fibrin are deposited, forming the lesion of nonbacterial thrombotic endocarditis (NBTE). Certain organisms such as enterococci, *viridans* streptococci, *Staphylococcus aureus*, *Staphylococcus epidermidis* and *Pseudomonas aeruginosa* can readily adhere to and colonize the NBTE lesion. Once colonization occurs, the vegetation enlarges by further platelet-fibrin deposition and continued bacterial proliferation. The bacterial colonies are found beneath the vegetation surface. Phagocyte infiltration is minimal, producing an environment of impaired host resistance. These conditions allow for unimpaired bacterial growth and colony counts of 10^9–10^{10} bacteria/gm of tissue. With continued unhindered growth of bacteria, severe compromise of hemodynamic function, peripheral embolization, and other complications are frequent sequelae.

Classification (1)

Until recently, endocarditis was classified as "acute" or "subacute" based on the usual progression of untreated disease. The acute form of the disease generally consists of systemic "toxicity," fever, leukocytosis, and, if left untreated, often results in death in several days to six weeks. *Staphylococcus aureus* and other virulent pathogens are most commonly associated with this infection and have the capacity to produce disease on previously undamaged valves. Conversely, subacute endocarditis is commonly associated with a history of prior valvular disease and a less fulminant course consisting of low grade fever, night sweats, weight loss, and vague systemic complaints. The subacute disease is classically caused by *viridans* streptococci. Scheld and Sande (1) state "although useful conceptually, this classification (acute vs subacute) ignores the nonbacterial forms of infective endocarditis and the frequent overlap in manifestations by individual organisms such as the enterococci. A classification based on the etiologic agent is preferable since it has implications for the course usually followed, the likelihood of preexisting heart disease, and the appropriate antimicrobial agent(s) to use."

Epidemiology (1)

Infective endocarditis is relatively uncommon, accounting for approximately 1 case/1000 hospital admissions. An average of 54% of the cases occur in patients 31–60 years of age, 26% in patients less than 30 years of age, and 21% in patients older than 60 years. The disease remains uncommon in children.

While rheumatic heart disease has been the underlying lesion in 37–76% of the infections in the last two decades, other congenital heart lesions such as Tetralogy of Fallot and ventricular septal defects are implicated in 6–24% of the cases. Additionally, "nosocomial endocarditis" secondary to newer therapeutic modalities (intravenous catheters, hyperalimentation lines, pacemakers, dialysis shunts, etc.) has emerged. As many as 28% of reported cases of endocarditis are nosocomial in origin (2). Degenerative cardiac lesions, idiopathic hypertrophic subaortic stenosis (IHSS), and mitral valve prolapse also appear to predispose an individual to infective endocarditis.

The heart valve involved seems to be dependent on predisposing disease as well as infecting organisms. In endocarditis associated with rheumatic heart disease, the mitral valve is involved in more than 85% of cases, with *viridans* streptococci the most common organism (1). However, the tricuspid valve is most commonly involved (3) in staphylococcal endocarditis associated with intravenous drug abuse with no underlying cardiac lesion.

VIRIDANS STREPTOCOCCAL ENDOCARDITIS

Clinical Manifestations and Diagnosis

1. R.T., a 31-year-old male, is admitted to the medical center with chief complaints of lethargy, fever and weight loss. He had been in excellent health until 3 months prior to admission, when symptoms of fatigue, arthralgias and low grade fever resulted in a visit to his private physician. A 10-day course of cephalexin 500 mg po qid eliminated all of the above symptoms. However, 5 days after completion of therapy, he "relapsed." A new prescription of the above resulted in transient cure, but once again, his symptoms recurred after discontinuing therapy. Of sig-

nificance in his past medical history is rheumatic fever at age 10 as well as a heart murmur first noticed at the age of 17. Two months prior to the onset of his initial symptoms, he underwent extensive dental procedures including gingivectomy.

Physical examination revealed a 70 kg black male with a blood pressure of 160/60 mm Hg, a pulse of 85/min, and a temperature of 38.5°C. Head, ears, eyes, nose, and throat examination revealed the presence of Roth spots, and there was a grade III/VI diastolic murmur with aortic regurgitation on auscultation. He had a palpable spleen, Osler's nodes on the finger pads of his left hand and Janeway lesions on the sole of his left foot. With the exception of a headache, his neurologic examination was within normal limits.

Admitting laboratory results were as follows: Hematocrit 37%; Hemoglobin 12 gm/dl; White Blood Cell Count 7000/mm³ with 65% PMN's, 2% Bands, 5% Monocytes and 3% Eosinophils; Blood Urea Nitrogen 16 mg/dl, Creatinine 1.0 mg/dl, Erythrocyte Sedimentation Rate 49 mm/hr, and positive Rheumatoid Factor. A urinalysis revealed 10–15 Red Blood Cells per high power field. The results of an echocardiogram were negative.

Six blood cultures were drawn over three days and the results are pending. Penicillin 20 million units per day IV and streptomycin 500 mg every 12 hours IM are started.

What clinical manifestations in patient R.T. are consistent with endocarditis? What are other common manifestations?

Included in R.T.'s chief complaints are malaise, fever, and weight loss. Fever is present in 90% of reported cases of infective endocarditis, with temperatures rarely in excess of 103°F except in the "acute" form. The weight loss and malaise are also consistent with endocarditis, with a reported incidence of 25%. Other common nonspecific symptoms include anorexia, chills, weakness, nausea, and night sweats (2).

The two-month time interval between R.T.'s gingivectomy, an event which is likely to produce bacteremia, and the onset of the above symptoms is consistent with previously reported data. However, this incubation period may be as short as two weeks (1).

Several peripheral manifestations of disease are evident in R.T. These include Roth spots, which are oval, pale retinal lesions surrounded by hemmorrhage usually located near the optic nerve, and Osler's nodes, which are painful nodular lesions similar to wheals that develop most commonly on the pads of the fingers and toes or on the palms and soles. The latter are erythematous and have slightly white centers; they differ from Janeway lesions in their tenderness and lack of hemorrhagic appearance. While splinter hemorrhages are widely described as being diagnostic of endocarditis, the specificity of this sign is low. In fact, of all patients admitted to hospitals, 10 to 66% have splinter hemorrhages and the highest incidence is in patients with mitral stenosis without endocarditis and in patients receiving hemodialysis. Petechiae as well as nail clubbing are also common signs of subacute forms of endocarditis, with a reported incidence of 15–50% (4,5).

Heart murmurs occur in over 85% of cases but may be absent in right-sided endocarditis or mural infection. The arthralgias and splenomegaly seen on R.T.'s physical examination are also common signs and symptoms consistent with endocarditis (1,2).

While not currently evident in R.T., congestive heart failure (CHF) is the leading cause of death in patients with endocarditis. Major embolic episodes involving the spleen, kidney, coronary arteries, and brain are second only to CHF as complications of endocarditis and occur in at least one-third of the cases (4,5). Neurologic manifestations of cerebral embolization may be minor (headache as seen in this patient) or significant (eg, hemiplegia, seizures, or toxic encephalopathy) (6).

Renal manifestations of embolization may include infarctions of portions of the kidney from large emboli, or focal glomerulonephritis which is probably due to either small emboli or immune complexes. Although not related to emboli, diffuse glomerulonephritis is also common and frequently results in renal insufficiency (4).

Laboratory findings in more prolonged disease may show anemia of chronic disease. Leukocytosis is usually only seen in acute disease. The erythrocyte sedimentation rate (ESR) is nearly always elevated, while rheumatoid factor (RF) is positive in approximately 50% of cases. The urinalysis (UA) is frequently abnormal, with proteinuria, microscopic hematuria, and RBC casts (7).

The echocardiogram is an often used test in the diagnosis of infective endocarditis. However, the test suffers from poor sensitivity. It does not distinguish between active and inactive cases, and as observed in R.T., false negative as well as false positive results occur (8). It does appear to be useful as a prognostic indicator and may identify patients who require surgical intervention. Individuals with endocarditis who have vegetations large enough to be documented by echocardiogram have a higher incidence of CHF and major embolic phenomena and most frequently require surgery. Based on the above criteria, this patient's negative echocardiogram and lack of heart failure suggest he is not a likely surgical candidate (9).

2. Comment on the number of blood cultures which were obtained from R.T.

The subacute nature of R.T.'s disease coupled with the importance of identifying the pathogen suggest that drawing several cultures over two to three days is appropriate. If the patient had been more acutely ill, it would have been more appropriate to obtain five to six the first day followed by immediate initiation of appropriate antibiotic therapy (1).

When antibiotics have been administered in the previous two weeks, the rate of positive cultures declines. Since R.T. recently completed a course of cephalexin, additional cultures may be needed (1,8).

It has been suggested that five blood cultures are necessary to diagnose the majority of cases of bacterial endocarditis; however, Belli demonstrated that most cases are diagnosed with the first culture. After five cultures are drawn, appropriate antibiotic therapy should be started in an attempt to reduce valve damage and other complications of endocarditis (10).

Treatment

3. The results of R.T.'s blood cultures return with four out of the six growing *viridans* streptococci sensitive to penicillin. How is sensitivity determined? Discuss the major methods of treating this infection with antibiotics. What would be most appropriate for this patient?

Viridans streptococci are the organisms most frequently isolated in infective endocarditis, constituting at least 45% of all cases. In addition, these organisms are responsible for the majority

of cases of subacute bacterial endocarditis (11).

At least 80% of these organisms are sensitive to penicillin (12); however, the estimate may be closer to 90%. Blount has subcategorized *S. viridans* into "sensitive," "moderately sensitive," and "relatively resistant" strains. An organism is considered sensitive to penicillin if it is inhibited by less than 0.1 unit/ml and moderately sensitive if it is inhibited by 0.1–1.0 unit/ml. Relatively resistant organisms require > 1 unit/ml for inhibition of growth (13). Nonenterococcal group D streptococci show essentially the same sensitivity to penicillin (14). (See Table 1.)

The most commonly used tests to determine whether *S. viridans* and other bacteria are sensitive to a given antibiotic are the minimum inhibitory concentration (MIC) and, to a lesser ex-

Table 1.

MINIMUM INHIBITORY CONCENTRATION FOR
ORGANISMS COMMONLY IMPLICATED
IN INFECTIVE ENDOCARDITIS

Organism-Antibiotics	Usual MIC (mcg/ml)
S. viridans	
Penicillin	0.01
Cephalothin	0.5
Cefazolin	0.5–1.0
Vancomycin	0.312–1.25
Clindamycin	0.02
S. aureus (penicillinase producer)	
Nafcillin	0.25–1.0
Oxacillin	0.4
Methicillin	2.0
Cephalothin	0.5
Cefazolin	0.5
Clindamycin	0.1
Vancomycin	0.2–2
Tobramycin/gentamicin	0.1–4.0
Enterococcus	
Penicillin	2.0
Ampicillin	1.0–5.0
Vancomycin	0.3–2.5
P. aeruginosa	
Tobramycin	0.12–2.0
Gentamicin	0.25–2.0
Amikacin	1.6–12.5
Carbenicillin	50
Ticarcillin	25

(Abstracted from Kucers A and Bennett N: *The Use of Antibiotics*. 3rd Ed. JB Lippincott Company, Philadelphia, 1979.

tent, the minimum bactericidal concentration (MBC).

The MIC is determined by culturing the infecting organisms in a broth culture for 24 hours. The least amount of antibiotic needed to prevent turbidity in the broth (growth) is defined as the MIC.

The MBC is the lowest concentration of antibiotic needed to kill 99.9% or more of the bacteria by 24 hours (11). Table 1 lists organisms known to commonly produce endocarditis and their usual MIC's. It is important to emphasize that the sensitivity of an organism to a particular antibiotic may vary widely at different institutions. Thus, it is emphasized that the practicing clinician have a knowledge of the sensitivity of bacterial isolates at his or her own institution.

In vitro synergy has been well documented with the combination of penicillin and an aminoglycoside against nonenterococcal group D species (14,15) and viridans streptococci (16–18). Sande has documented that S. viridans are eradicated more rapidly with a penicillin-aminoglycoside combination than with penicillin alone (17). Watanakunakorn et al indicate that kanamycin, gentamicin or tobramycin offer no therapeutic advantages over the older aminoglycoside, streptomycin, for synergy against viridans streptococci (15).

The combination of penicillin 10–20 million units IV daily or procaine penicillin 1.2 million units q 6 h IM for 4 weeks with streptomycin 500 mg q 12 h IM for the initial two weeks of therapy has been used successfully to treat over 200 patients with "penicillin-sensitive" streptococcal endocarditis with no relapses (12).

Although past evidence indicates that short-term therapy may be ineffective in the treatment of infective endocarditis due to these organisms (19), Wilson and colleagues successfully treated 33 cases with only two weeks of antibiotic therapy, utilizing procaine penicillin 1.2 million units q 6 h IM and streptomycin 500 mg q 12 h IM. No relapses were observed and a decrease in the cost of therapy was documented (20). More recently, the same investigators reported their results in 91 patients using the same regimen. Seventy cases were caused by viridans streptococci and 21 by the nonenterococcal group D streptococcus, S. bovis. No relapses were observed. In those patients who required surgery for congestive heart failure, all had evidence of endocarditis at oper-

ation. However, gram-stained smears and cultures of the excised valves were negative in all cases (21).

Since these bacteria are so sensitive to penicillin and the potential toxicities of streptomycin may be significant, the need for aminoglycosides has been evaluated. Two recent studies suggest that the use of aminoglycosides may be unnecessary (22,23). The reported failure of penicillin therapy alone in the past (relapse rate of 5%) may have been complicated by the fact that several of the treatment "failures" were given inadequate doses of penicillin, or were partially treated with bacteriostatic agents such as tetracyclines (24). Additionally, some of these patients may have been infected with organisms which were only moderately sensitive or relatively resistant to penicillin G. Karchmer noted only one relapse among 99 patients with nonenterococcal streptococcal endocarditis treated with single agent therapy (penicillin, cephalothin, or vancomycin) for 30 days (23). In a similar study, relapse occurred in only 2 of 49 patients after four weeks of penicillin alone compared to 0/18 receiving combination therapy. Both relapses occurred in a group of 13 patients that had symptoms for longer than three months (22).

In patients with more severe and chronic disease or in those infected by more resistant organisms, the combination of four weeks of penicillin with two weeks streptomycin should be the treatment of choice. In patients 65 years of age or older and in individuals with renal failure or previous vestibular problems, streptomycin should probably be avoided. Four weeks of penicillin therapy is most appropriate in this group of patients. In the penicillin-allergic patient, cephalothin 2.0 gm q 4 h IV or cefazolin 1.0–2.0 gm q 6 h IV for four weeks, or vancomycin 500 mg q 6 h IV alone for four weeks are all appropriate alternatives (25–27). This patient is relatively young and has no renal or vestibular disease; thus, any of the above mentioned alternatives are reasonable. If his symptoms had been present for longer than three months or if the streptococcus had been only moderately sensitive to penicillin, combination therapy for four weeks would have been indicated. (See Table 2.)

4. Serum Bactericidal Titers. It is elected to use penicillin alone in the treatment of R.T.'s endocarditis; however, after continued fever

Table 2.

SUGGESTED REGIMENS FOR THERAPY OF ENDOCARDITIS DUE TO VIRIDANS STREPTOCOCCI AND
GROUP D NON-ENTEROCOCCAL STREPTOCOCCI[27]

Antibiotic	Dosage	Route	Duration
1. Aqueous crystalline penicillin G	10–20 MU/day either continuously or in equally divided doses every 4 hours	IV	4 weeks
2. Aqueous crystalline penicillin G*	10–20 MU/day either continuously or in equally divided doses every 4 hours	IV	4 weeks
or			
Procaine penicillin G	1.2 MU every 6 hours	IM	4 weeks
plus			
Streptomycin	10 mg/kg (not to exceed 500 mg) every 12 hours	IM	2 weeks
or			
Gentamicin	1 mg/kg every 8 hours	IM/IV	2 weeks
3. Aqueous crystalline penicillin G*	10–20 MU/day either continuously or in equally divided doses every 4 hours	IV	2 weeks
or			
Procaine penicillin G	1.2 MU every 6 hours	IM	2 weeks
plus			
Streptomycin	10 mg/kg (not to exceed 500 mg) every 12 hours	IM	2 weeks
or			
Gentamicin (Tobramycin)	1 mg/kg every 8 hours	IM/IV	2 weeks
If Penicillin-Allergic:			
1. Vancomycin	10 mg/kg (not to exceed 500 mg) every 6 hours	IV	4 weeks
2. Cephalothin**	2.0 gm every 4 hours	IV	4 weeks
or			
Cefazolin**	1.0 gm every 6–8 hours	IV	4 weeks

*Age more than 65 years or renal or VIIIth nerve impairment are relative contraindications to the use of streptomycin.

**Potential cross-allergicity between penicillins and cephalosporins should be kept in mind.

and lack of clinical improvement, "serum bactericidal titers" (SBT) are ordered. An order for a "peak" SBT is written. Comment on the use and timing of the titer in R.T. How do these titers differ from MIC's and MBC's?

The clinical roles of the minimum inhibitory concentration (MIC), minimum bactericidal concentration (MBC), and serum bactericidal titer (SBT) in the treatment of serious infection are controversial.

While the MIC and MBC have been valuable in the management of infection, there are laboratory related peculiarities that may affect their determination. It is well established that the type of growth medium may cause significant differences in the observed bactericidal activity of an-

tibiotics (28,29). (Also see the discussion of MIC and MBC in the previous question.)

Serum bactericidal titers were first used by Schlicter and colleagues in 1947. These investigators theorized that adequate therapy might be better based on the action of the patient's own serum, during antibiotic administration, against the specific organism isolated (30). Serial two-fold dilutions of the patient's serum containing the administered antibiotic are prepared. A standard inoculum of the patient's infecting organism is transferred to each tube and the tubes are incubated at 37°C for 24 hours. Those tubes showing no visible growth and the last tube showing growth are subcultured onto agar plates and incubated for an additional 24 hrs. The subculture which reveals a marked (99.9%) reduction in the inoculum from the control is the bactericidal endpoint. The results of the SBT are expressed as the highest dilution of serum which is bactericidal (11).

While many clinicians elect to use the SBT in the treatment of endocarditis (23,31–33), efficacy has never been shown to correlate well with a particular titer (34). Furthermore, there is discrepancy as to the proper timing of these levels. While some investigators utilize "trough" levels immediately before antibiotic administration (23,30), others suggest "peak" levels are most appropriate (11,35,36). Other clinicians have used both peak and trough SBT in their investigations (31,37). Two investigative reports have suggested that improved outcome is best correlated with a peak SBT greater than or equal to 1:8 (38,39).

Patients with normal renal function, such as R.T., may have little or no antibiotic in the blood at the nadir of the administration schedule. Since efficacy has been best correlated with peak titers, it seems more appropriate that the sample be obtained immediately after the penicillin dose. A variety of factors may affect the outcome of this test, but the principal difficulty in interpretation is dependent on bacterial inoculum size. The larger the size of the inoculum, the less effective the antibiotic appears (40). Another factor that may radically change the test results occurs when more than one antibiotic effective against the infecting organism is present. The timing of the peak SBT may radically alter the results, depending on the selected antibiotic.

5. Synergy. Since R.T.'s infecting organism is found to be only moderately sensitive to penicillin, streptomycin is added in an attempt to achieve synergy. Define synergy and its implications in the treatment of endocarditis.

The rationale surrounding the use of any antibiotic combination is four-fold: to achieve broad-spectrum empiric antibiotic coverage in critically ill patients with undefined bacterial infection; to treat mixed bacterial infections; to prevent the emergence of resistant strains; and to achieve an additive or synergistic effect against a single organism. When one uses antibiotic combinations in an attempt to augment antimicrobial action, one of four results may be expected: indifference, an additive effect, synergy, or antagonism.

Synergy is defined as inhibition resulting from a combination of less than one-half the amount of each drug required to inhibit the organism when used alone. Because the inherent error of this method includes a single two-fold dilution of each antibiotic, a significant synergistic effect requires that inhibition result from a combination of one-fourth or less of the inhibitory concentrations of each drug. If one-half of an inhibitory concentration of each drug is required to produce inhibition, the effect is "additive," and if more than one-half of each is necessary, then the drugs are "antagonistic" (41).

Beta-lactam antibiotics or vancomycin in combination with aminoglycosides have been shown to display *in vitro* synergism against the three organisms most commonly associated with infective endocarditis (*S. aureus, S. viridans,* enterococcus). This *in vitro* effect does not guarantee increased clinical efficacy *in vivo*. However, as mentioned previously, since this organism is only moderately sensitive to penicillin, the synergistic effect of streptomycin may result in increased therapeutic efficacy.

CULTURE-NEGATIVE ENDOCARDITIS

6. If R.T.'s blood cultures had been negative, how would he have been managed diagnostically and therapeutically?

The phenomenon of active endocarditis with negative blood cultures has been observed in 10–15% of reported cases. The most common causes of "culture-negative" endocarditis include organisms with special growth characteristics (eg, fastidious bacteria such as anaerobes and other slow growing organisms). Fungi such as *Histoplasma, Aspergillus,* and *Candida,* as well as the etiologic agent of Q-fever, are also common causative agents (2,42).

Poor blood sampling technique is a frequent cause of negative blood cultures; this is particularly a problem with anaerobic cultures. Antibiotic administration prior to culture also correlates with negative blood cultures in endocarditis (42,43). This patient received a course of cephalosporins just prior to hospitalization, which increases the likelihood that his blood cultures may be negative.

Use of the following guidelines should improve the diagnosis and treatment of culture-negative endocarditis:

A. Continue routine cultures and subcultures for up to 21 days to isolate slow-growing or nutritionally fastidious organisms.

B. If the patient is not acutely compromised, hold all antibiotics until positive cultures are obtained.

C. In patients who have received antibiotics, an effort should be made to inactivate the antibiotics which may have been carried over into the culture flask from the patient's blood. The addition of a beta-lactamase (penicillinase) to the medium may be helpful in patients who have received penicillins or cephalosporins.

D. Rule out fungal infections with the use of appropriate culture media, arterial blood cultures, and appropriate serologies.

E. Rule out other infectious agents (Q-fever, *Brucella,* etc).

F. If cultures continue to be negative and endocarditis is strongly suspected, initiate therapy with a combination of penicillin and streptomycin or gentamicin. If staphylococcus is strongly suspected, add a semisynthetic penicillin such as nafcillin to the above regimen (42–45). If the patient responds clinically, treatment should be continued for four to six weeks.

ENTEROCOCCAL ENDOCARDITIS

7. N.B. is a patient who presents with signs and symptoms similar to those observed in R.T. (see Question 1). However, the organism isolated in his case is enterococcus rather than *S. viridans.* How will this change the choice of antibiotics?

Enterococci, especially *Streptococcus faecalis,* are etiologic agents in 10–15% of infective endocarditis cases and are associated with a mortality rate of 20–50% (46). Unlike *viridans* streptococci, experimental evidence suggests the need for combination therapy. Penicillins, semisynthetic penicillins, cephalosporins, vancomycin, and aminoglycosides rarely are bactericidal when used alone against enterococcus (47). However, the synergistic combination of penicillins and aminoglycosides is well established in this disease (47–50). Cephalosporins (51–53) and anti-staphylococcal penicillins (54–57) have shown synergism against enterococcus when used with aminoglycosides, but rarely is the combination bactericidal. These combinations should not be used therapeutically because the doses of cephalosporin or semisynthetic penicillin would be prohibi-

tively high. On the other hand, vancomycin has been shown to be effective when used in combination with aminoglycosides against the enterococcus (58–59).

The choice of aminoglycoside is a controversial subject in the treatment of enterococcal endocarditis. Several papers have documented a high level of streptomycin resistance, defined as an MIC of greater than 2000 mcg/ml (60–62). Watanakunakorn studied the synergy of penicillin-aminoglycoside combinations against 33 strains of enterococci and found that a combination of penicillin 20 mcg/ml and streptomycin 20 mcg/ml displayed synergism against only 20 of the strains. However, the combination of penicillin 20 mcg/ml and gentamicin 4 mcg/ml was synergistic against all strains tested (48). Other investigators have observed similar results (63–65). Using an animal model, Carrizosa observed that a combination of penicillin and gentamicin was more effective than penicillin plus streptomycin in the treatment of streptomycin-resistant enterococcal endocarditis (66). The value of sensitivity testing can be observed in a recently reported case of *S. faecalis* endocarditis which failed to respond to a combination of ampicillin and gentamicin. Laboratory testing showed *in vitro* resistance to this combination, but sensitivity to a combination of ampicillin and tobramycin. The patient was eventually cured with the latter combination (67).

Ampicillin is two to four times as active as penicillin against enterococci *in vitro,* and some clinicians prefer this agent. However, experimental studies have failed to show clinically significant differences between these penicillins (47,50).

The most widely-used regimen in the treatment of enterococcal endocarditis consists of 15–20 million units daily of intravenous penicillin G for 6 weeks, combined with streptomycin 1.0 gm q 12 h IM for the initial 2 weeks followed by 500 mg q 12 h IM for the final 4 weeks (25,26). However, the results of Tompsett and others have shown that a total of 4 weeks of antibiotic therapy may be sufficient (68).

While some clinicians routinely use a penicillin-gentamicin regimen for all cases of enterococcal endocarditis, other investigators believe this regimen should be considered only for those strains which are highly resistant to streptomycin (25). Furthermore, the relative toxicities of streptomycin and gentamicin (see Question 9) must be considered for each respective patient.

Table 3.

SUGGESTED REGIMENS FOR THERAPY OF ENDOCARDITIS DUE TO ENTEROCOCCUS
(STREPTOCOCCUS FAECALIS)[25]

Antibiotic	Dosage	Route	Duration
1. Penicillin	20 MU/day in equally divided doses every 4 hours	IV	4–6 weeks
or			
Ampicillin	1.5–2.0 gm every 4 hours	IV	4–6 weeks
plus			
Streptomycin	10 mg/kg (not to exceed 500 mg) every 12 hours	IM	4–6 weeks
or			
Gentamicin (Tobramycin)	1 mg/kg every 8 hours	IM/IV	4–6 weeks
If Penicillin-Allergic:			
1. Vancomycin	10 mg/kg (not to exceed 500 mg) every 6 hours	IV	4–6 weeks
plus			
Streptomycin	10 mg/kg (not to exceed 500 mg) every 12 hours	IM	4–6 weeks
or			
Gentamicin (Tobramycin)	1 mg/kg every 8 hours	IM/IV	4–6 weeks

In those patients allergic to penicillin, a combination of vancomycin 500 mg q 6 h IV with an aminoglycoside is the treatment of choice (25). While experience with this regimen is limited, the experimental (47) and clinical evidence (69) suggests the above choice is appropriate. (See Tables 1 and 3.)

Penicillin Toxicity

8. What is the appropriate dose of penicillin to treat N.B.'s enterococcal endocarditis if his creatinine clearance is 20 ml/min? What dose-related toxicities associated with penicillin should be anticipated?

It is well known that penicillin is excreted primarily unchanged in the urine and accumulates in those individuals with impaired renal function. A mean serum concentration of 20 mcg/ml is sufficient to treat serious streptococcal infections including enterococcus and lacks serious toxicity. Bryan et al (178) have developed the following equation to approximate the daily dose in millions of units (MU) which will achieve this concentration:

$$\text{Dose (MU/day)} = 3.2 + \frac{Cl_{Cr}}{7}$$

Therefore, the calculated dose for N.B., who has a creatinine clearance of 20 ml/min, is six million units/day, or one million units every four hours:

$$\text{Dose (MU/day)} = 3.2 + \frac{20}{7}$$
$$= 6 \text{ MU/day}$$

The major toxicities associated with penicillin are neurologic in nature and include seizures (179,180), hallucinations (with procaine penicillin) (181), and coma (180). However, prolongation of the bleeding time has been reported in a uremic patient receiving 10 million units of penicillin G per day (182). ADP-induced platelet aggregation is consistently abnormal with doses of 24 million units of penicillin G daily in normal volunteers (183). Thus, certain hemostatic defects may accompany high doses of penicillin G or "normal" doses in patients with concomitant renal failure. Renal function should be carefully monitored, therefore, in patients receiving penicillin G.

Aminoglycosides

9. *Toxicity.* Enterococcal endocarditis is diagnosed in an elderly patient with impaired hearing and an aminoglycoside must be added to his penicillin treatment. Which

aminoglycoside would be most appropriate?

The likely aminoglycoside should be chosen from streptomycin, tobramycin, or gentamicin. Amikacin should be reserved for gram-negative infections resistant to the usual aminoglycosides. The choice of aminoglycoside should be based on each agent's relative toxicity and efficacy.

Nephrotoxicity. Nephrotoxicity is a serious concern with aminoglycoside therapy. Streptomycin appears to be the least nephrotoxic aminoglycoside, and recent literature, while controversial, suggests that tobramycin may be less toxic than gentamicin. For more detailed information on aminoglycoside nephrotoxicity see the chapter entitled Kidney Diseases.

Ototoxicity. Ototoxicity is a serious complication of aminoglycoside therapy which may affect either the auditory (cochlear) or vestibular functions of the ear. Cochlear damage appears to be a result of hair cell loss in the organ of Corti beginning at the basilar turn of the cochlea and progressing toward the apex. Injury to other cochlear structures has been demonstrated, but direct toxicity to the hair cells appears to be the primary mechanism. Once hair cells are lost, no regeneration can occur; however, the fact that recovery from cochlear toxicity occurs suggests an additional reversible mechanism of ototoxicity. The mechanism of vestibular toxicity is less understood but felt to be related to aminoglycoside accumulation in melanin granules in specific cells (70). It has been postulated that ototoxicity relates to the accumulation of aminoglycoside in the inner ear. Stupp has documented that aminoglycosides are concentrated in perilymph and have an elimination half-life of 15 hours from that space (71).

It is widely claimed that streptomycin may be more toxic to vestibular function, while gentamicin and tobramycin are more cochlear-toxic (72). Until recently however, none of these drugs had been clinically compared in humans to determine their relative toxicity. Fee compared tobramycin to gentamicin in 113 patients. Drug dosage was based on kidney function and aminoglycoside serum levels. While this study suffers from the same limitations inherent in the nephrotoxicity studies (eg, definition of ototoxicity criteria, etc.), the results suggest that tobramycin is less toxic to the vestibular apparatus than gentamicin. There was no observed difference in auditory toxicity between the two drugs (70). Thus, it is not pos-

sible to differentiate between the various aminoglycosides in terms of auditory (cochlear) toxicity. The aminoglycoside of choice in the above patient with enterococcal endocarditis and impaired hearing should be based on the most efficacious drug. While it may be argued that serum gentamicin and tobramycin levels are easier to monitor, the correlation between serum levels and toxicity is controversial (see Question 10).

10. Serum Levels. "Peak" and "trough" aminoglycoside levels are ordered. What is the usefulness of aminoglycoside serum levels?

Aminoglycoside levels are widely used in the management of infectious diseases. The primary reasons for monitoring serum levels are to assure "therapeutic" levels and to avoid potential toxicity associated with excessive levels. It is most commonly suggested that one obtain "peak" and "trough" levels. A peak serum level should be drawn one hour after an intramuscular injection or immediately following intravenous infusions (one hour or less) to avoid the rapid distribution phase (see the Clinical Pharmacokinetics chapter). The trough serum level should be drawn immediately prior to the dose. Since the trough represents a time of relative distribution equilibrium between blood and tissue, this level is most useful in predicting drug accumulation (73).

Only peak serum levels have been found to correlate with therapeutic efficacy. Studying patients with pseudomonas bacteremia, Jackson and Riff observed that peak serum gentamicin levels ≤ 2 mcg/ml were ineffective in controlling infection, while concentrations ≥ 4 mcg/ml were successful in all patients but leukemics (74). Noone and colleagues observed that peak serum gentamicin levels ≥ 5 mcg/ml adequately treated septicemia, urinary tract infection and wound infection. Peak levels ≥ 8 mcg/ml correlated best with effective treatment of pneumonia (75). In one investigation, 52 gram-negative bacteremias were observed in patients receiving an appropriate antibiotic against their infecting organism as tested by disc diffusion. Subinhibitory serum levels were documented in 20 of 42 patients studied, reinforcing the need for adequate antibiotic levels (76).

The association of elevated serum trough levels with nephrotoxicity revolves around the studies of Dahlgren (77) and Goodman (78). In the former study, 8 of 21 patients with trough gentamicin levels ≥ 2 mcg/ml developed an elevated serum creatinine; this did not occur in any patients with trough levels less than 2 mcg/ml. Rising serum creatinine levels were seen in two out of six patients with trough levels of 3–4 mcg/ml and five out of five patients with trough levels greater than 4 mcg/ml. However, this correlation between trough levels and elevated serum creatinine levels was not statistically significant. In Goodman's investigation, gentamicin trough levels greater than 4 mcg/ml were significantly associated with nephrotoxicity. However, in this study as well as that of Dahlgren, the occurrence of high trough levels in association with elevated serum creatinine might be interpreted as a sign of renal damage rather than the cause of it.

Elevated trough levels have also been reported to be associated with ototoxicity (79). Nordstrum found a significant relationship between trough levels greater than 3 mcg/ml and ototoxicity. However, those patients who developed ototoxicity had significantly higher serum creatinine levels prior to and during therapy as well as a longer duration of aminoglycoside therapy (80). In a similar study, there was a significant correlation between ototoxicity and serum amikacin peak levels greater than 32 mcg/ml and trough levels greater than 10 mcg/ml. Again, ototoxic patients received larger total doses for more prolonged periods of time (81).

Thus, limited information suggests that peak serum gentamicin levels of 5–8 mcg/ml are necessary for maximal therapeutic efficacy. The treatment of pneumonia may require higher levels than UTI's and wound infections. Gentamicin levels greater than 8 mcg/ml have never been shown to be therapeutically superior to lower levels. Although excessive serum levels have not been significantly correlated with toxicity, levels greatly exceeding 8 mcg/ml should be avoided.

While there appears to be a relationship between gentamicin trough levels greater than 2–3 mcg/ml and toxicity, "breakthrough" bacteremia secondary to inadequate antibiotic levels is possible if antibiotic dosages are adjusted too low to prevent toxicity.

STAPHYLOCOCCAL ENDOCARDITIS

11. A.G., a 22-year-old, 60 kg male who abuses amphetamine and heroin intravenously, presents to the county hospital emer-gency room with recent complaints of chest pain, cough, and dyspnea. He also notes spiking fevers and severe headache.

Physical examination reveals a 60 kg white male with a blood pressure of 120/70 mm Hg, a pulse of 100/min, and a temperature of 39.7°C. Ophthalmologic examination reveals hemorrhagic retinal exudates, and the cardiovascular examination reveals a grade IV/VI holosystolic murmur. Abdominal examination reveals hepato-splenomegaly. Petechiae were observed around the clavicle and lower neck area. The patient complains of severe headache and is confused.

Admitting laboratory values include the following: Hematocrit 40%; Hemoglobin 13.5 gm/dl; White Blood Count 13,500/mm^3, with 83% PMN's, 5% Bands, and 12% Lymphocytes. The BUN was 21 mg/dl and the creatinine was 2.4 mg/dl. A urinalysis revealed 50 RBC's per high power field and 2+ protein. Six blood cultures were drawn and the results are pending. His drug history reveals an allergy to ampicillin.

How does this patient's presentation differ from the *viridans* streptococcus case of bacterial endocarditis?

The frequency of valvular involvement in drug addicts differs markedly from that disease in nonaddicts. The tricuspid valve alone or in combination with others is involved in 52.2%, the aortic valve alone in 18.5%, the mitral valve alone in 10.8%, and both aortic and mitral valves in 12.5% of cases. In those series where most cases of narcotic-associated endocarditis involve the tricuspid valve, pleuritic chest pain, cough, and dyspnea, as displayed by this individual, are seen in the majority of patients (3).

A.G. presents with signs and symptoms that are consistent with an acute infection. He is confused, has a higher temperature, and a more pronounced leukocytosis. The duration of illness in these patients is usually one week or less (3,82).

12. It has been stated that addicts with endocarditis, such as this patient, have a better prognosis than nonaddicts. Why might this discrepancy exist?

The reasons for this phenomenon relate to age, existence of prior heart disease, and type of valve infected (82–4). The average age of patients with narcotic-associated endocarditis is 29, whereas the average age of patients in the general population with endocarditis is closer to 50. Most nonaddict patients with endocarditis have an underlying cardiac abnormality that predisposes them to infection. The intravenous drug abusers, however, more commonly have normal cardiac anatomy and generally present with endocarditis caused by microorganisms capable of attacking normal valves. The increased virulence of these bacteria accounts for the frequent presentation of acute infection. Nonaddicts are generally infected with less virulent organisms capable of infecting only abnormal valves (3). As discussed earlier, the bacteria most likely to produce endocarditis in the nonaddict are streptococci (55–60%), both *viridans* and enterococci (85). However, *Staphylococcus aureus* is the most common infecting organism (60–65%) in narcotic addicts, followed by streptococci, gram-negative bacilli, and fungi (3,85).

The most important prognostic variable in endocarditis is the type of valve infected. Patients with rheumatic valvulitis most often have aortic and mitral valve infection. The tricuspid valve is most commonly involved in endocarditis associated with IV drug abuse (83,87,88). The hemodynamic consequences of aortic or mitral involvement (eg, severe heart failure) are much more devastating than those associated with a pure right-sided infection. However, it should be emphasized that addicts also can have involvement of the left side of the heart. When the aortic or mitral valve is involved in addicts with acute endocarditis, mortality approaches 50% (3).

Penicillin Allergy

13. What is the risk of using penicillin or the cephalosporin derivatives in the treatment of A.G.'s infection, considering he has a history of "ampicillin allergy?"

An accurate drug history is critical in assessing the risk of using penicillin in a "penicillin-allergic" patient. Estimates of the frequency of penicillin allergy range from 1–10% of patients treated (169). The allergic manifestations range from immediate hypersensitivity reactions, such as anaphylaxis, to delayed-onset, serum sickness-like reactions. Mild cutaneous manifestations are most frequent. A dose-related hemolytic anemia, although rare, has been associated with penicillin administration (170). As many as 75% of the

deaths due to anaphylactic reactions in the United States have been associated with penicillin (171). These reactions appear to occur most frequently when penicillin is given by the parenteral route (172). Urticarial eruptions and angioedema may present as immediate hypersensitivity reactions (Type I); however, recurrent urticarial eruptions have been associated with delayed-onset, serum sickness-like reactions as well (170). The risk versus benefit of using penicillin in the "penicillin-allergic" patient must be based on the relative severity of the reaction reported.

Skin Testing. Often, after an accurate history, the severity of the allergy may remain uncertain. In these instances, skin testing may be warranted to make the diagnosis of penicillin hypersensitivity.

The major metabolite of penicillin is the penicilloyl group. It is referred to as the "major determinant" and is felt to be the antigen responsible for accelerated reactions, but not anaphylaxis. Relatively little of the penicillin is degraded to other breakdown products (the "minor determinants"). These minor determinants are probably responsible for anaphylaxis and other immediate systemic reactions. Thus, both penicilloyl as well as a minor determinant mixture must be utilized to detect potential reactors.

A commercial skin test preparation containing penicilloyl-polylysine is available. A minor determinant mixture is not readily available; however, freshly reconstituted solutions of penicillin G may be utilized. It has been suggested that the use of penicilloyl-polylysine in combination with a penicillin solution will detect 90-95% of those potential anaphylactic reactors (170).

Desensitization. If a patient such as A.G. is found to be severely allergic to penicillin by history or by skin testing and it is necessary that he receive penicillin despite this history, desensitization may be considered.

One protocol begins desensitization with low doses of intradermal or oral penicillin. Doses are doubled at 20 minute intervals until an intradermal or oral dose of 50,000 units is achieved. At this point, low doses of subcutaneous penicillin are administered. These subcutaneous doses are increased gradually until a dose of 500,000 units is reached. A dose of one million units is then given intramuscularly, and after a 20 minute interval, full doses of intravenous penicillin may be administered (173).

Ampicillin Rash. A patient who is truly allergic to penicillin should be considered allergic to all penicillin derivatives. The same is not the case for patients such as A.G. who report allergies to ampicillin. Ampicillin therapy is associated with a higher incidence of maculopapular rash compared with other penicillins. This reaction appears to occur more commonly in patients with infectious mononucleosis or lymphatic leukemia and in those patients receiving concomitant allopurinol therapy. The rash usually occurs within four days of the initiation of ampicillin therapy and may often resolve despite continuation of therapy (174).

Cephalosporin Cross-Sensitivity. Individuals who are allergic to penicillin are approximately four times more likely to develop an allergic reaction to a cephalosporin than those individuals who have no penicillin allergy (175). In other words, 5–16% of patients allergic to penicillins develop allergic reactions to the cephalosporins (176). Anaphylaxis has occurred in penicillin-allergic patients who have been given cephalosporins (177).

In summary, an accurate history of A.G.'s "ampicillin allergy" is mandatory. The decision to use penicillin or the cephalosporins will depend on the severity of A.G.'s ampicillin allergy relative to his need for treatment with these antibiotics.

Treatment

14. Six out of six blood cultures return positive for *Staphylococcus aureus*. The medical intern asks whether nafcillin or cefazolin would be the antibiotic of choice.

Experimentally, the semisynthetic penicillins and cephalosporins have been the antibiotics most studied in the treatment of *S. aureus* endocarditis. Methicillin, nafcillin, and oxacillin are equally effective in eliminating staphylococci from cardiac vegetations (89). When cephalosporins are compared to anti-staphylococcal penicillins, the results are variable. Cefazolin (20 mg/kg q 6–8 h), cephalothin (40 mg/kg q 6 h) and methicillin (40 mg/kg q 6 h) have all been found to be effective in the treatment of experimental endocarditis; however, the semisynthetic penicillins result in more rapid sterilization of vegetations (36,90). A more recent study indicates that ceforanide and cefazolin are as effective as methicillin and nafcillin (91). Comparisons between individual cephalosporins indicate that cefazolin is the most susceptible to inactivation by beta-lactamase (92–95). Goldman observed that significantly fewer cefazolin-treated animals with *S. aureus* endocarditis survived when compared to a similar cephalothin-treated group. It was suggested that reported failures of cefazolin in the treatment of staphylococcal endocarditis might be due to beta-lactamase inactivation of the drug (96).

While there have been case reports of treatment failures with cephalosporins (97–99), the drugs have generally been effective in the treatment of staphylococcal endocarditis (98,100). It is the opinion of this author that the experience *in vivo* with semisynthetic penicillins (101–103) coupled with the above-mentioned occasional *in vitro* superiority of penicillins over cephalosporins suggest that nafcillin or oxacillin are the beta-lactam antibiotics of choice in this situation. Although methicillin is effective, it is nephrotoxic and should be avoided. Doses of 100–150 mg/kg/day for 4–6 weeks are suggested (25) for A.G., assuming his history of allergy to ampicillin is consistent with a simple maculopapular rash (or less). Otherwise, vancomycin is recommended as an alternative. (See Tables 1 and 4.)

15. Is there any therapeutic advantage in adding an aminoglycoside to this patient's therapy?

The addition of an aminoglycoside to nafcillin or methicillin enhances the effect of these penicillins against *Staphylococcus aureus, in vitro* (104). Experimentally, the combination significantly increases the rate of bacterial killing in valvular vegetations when compared to nafcillin alone (105–106).

While there have been case reports in patients documenting an increased clinical response from this combination (107), two major studies indicate the benefit of adding an aminoglycoside may be small. Abrams et al studied 25 episodes of staphylococcal endocarditis in drug abusers. There were no treatment failures or relapses in either the single agent or the combination groups. Mean days to defervescence were also similar (6–7 days) (103). Sande and colleagues also noted no difference in survival or relapse rates in addicts or nonaddicts when treated with nafcillin versus nafcillin-gentamicin. However, in the combination group it took a shorter time to defervesce and to clear bac-

Table 4.

SUGGESTED REGIMENS FOR THERAPY OF ENDOCARDITIS DUE TO STAPHYLOCOCCUS AUREUS[25]

Antibiotic	Dose	Route	Duration
1. Nafcillin methicillin or oxacillin	1.5 gm every 4 hours	IV	4–6 weeks
2. Nafcillin *plus*	1.5 gm every 4 hours	IV	4–6 weeks
Gentamicin or tobramycin	1 mg/kg every 8 hours	IM/IV	1 week
If Penicillin Allergic:			
1. Vancomycin	10 mg/kg (not to exceed 500 mg) every 6 hours	IV	4–6 weeks
2. Cephalothin* or	2.0 gm every 4 hours	IV	4–6 weeks
Cefazolin*	1.0 gm every 6 hours	IV	4–6 weeks

*Potential cross-allergicity between penicillins and cephalosporins must be kept in mind.

teremia in patients with tricuspid valve infection (102).

Thus, while the addition of an aminoglycoside for several days may result in a more rapid clearance of bacteremia and a shorter time to defervescence, there is no evidence that this alters the overall course of disease. Some authorities, however, elect to add 3–5 mg/kg/day of gentamicin or tobramycin for 7–10 days to the semisynthetic penicillin regimen, especially in an acutely ill patient (102). (See Tables 1 and 4.)

16. *Tolerance.* After 10 days of nafcillin therapy, the patient appears to be responding well to therapy. However, the MIC of the organism to nafcillin is determined to be 0.5 mcg/ml, while the MBC is 16 mcg/ml. The physician notes this might be a "tolerant organism." What is tolerance, and how should therapy be directed against such an organism?

The phenomenon of tolerance is defined as the characteristic of a microorganism to have a marked dissociation between the minimum inhibitory concentration (MIC) and the minimum bactericidal concentration (MBC). As defined earlier in this chapter, the MBC is the lowest concentration necessary to kill 99.9% or more of an inoculum of bacteria by 24 hours. Tolerant bacteria generally require 48 hours or more to achieve a 99.9% kill rate (108). Thus, bactericidal activity exists, but the rate of killing is much slower in the tolerant strain.

Tolerance has been noted almost exclusively in *Staphylococcus aureus,* with a prevalence of as much as 60% (108–110). The antibiotics most often associated with tolerance are the cephalosporins and semisynthetic penicillins (108–111). However, tolerance to aminoglycosides (111) and vancomycin (112–114) has been noted as well. Conversion of nontolerant to tolerant *S. aureus* has been observed in some reports, suggesting that tolerance may be mediated by a bacteriophage (115).

Several case reports have reported failures in the treatment of *Staphylococcus aureus* endocarditis with vancomycin. In each case, serum antibiotic levels greatly exceeded the MIC, but a great disparity between the MIC and MBC was noted. After the addition of supplementary antibiotics, there was clinical and laboratory evidence of improvement (112–114). An experimental study of tolerance in staphylococcal endocarditis showed methicillin to have the same efficacy against tolerant strains as nontolerant strains of *S. aureus.* In addition, those animals injected with a tolerant strain survived significantly longer than those injected with a nontolerant strain, suggesting a greater virulence in the nontolerant microorganism (116). Two recent investigations have documented increased morbidity and mortality in patients infected with tolerant staphylococcus when compared with non-tolerant strains (117–118). Rajashekaraiah and colleagues studied the clinical significance of tolerant strains of *Staphylococcus aureus* in 50 cases of endocarditis. Although fever was more prolonged and the complication rate higher in infection due to tolerant *S. aureus,* no significant difference in mortality was noted (110).

Thus, the clinical relevance of tolerant staphylococci is still uncertain. While some investigators suggest that the phenomenon is clinically significant, the majority of patients infected with tolerant strains have been treated successfully with beta-lactam antibiotics (110,116–118). A reasonable approach to the treatment of serious infections caused by tolerant strains would be to initially utilize antibiotics to which the specific infecting organism is known to be susceptible (by MIC). Only if there is a lack of documented improvement following this therapy should one elect to substitute or add other potentially less effective or more toxic antibiotics. Since this patient is responding clinically to the current therapy and the organism is sensitive by MIC, no changes in antibiotic therapy are indicated.

17. *Oral Therapy.* **After three weeks of nafcillin therapy, the patient is refusing continued intravenous therapy and threatens to sign out against medical advice. Can oral dicloxacillin be used for the remainder of the patient's therapy? Is oral antibiotic therapy effective in endocarditis and would it be appropriate in this patient?**

The treatment of infective endocarditis demands at least two weeks, but more often four to six weeks of parenteral antimicrobial therapy. The cost of prolonged hospitalization, frequent loss of intravenous sites for administration of antibiotic, or lack of a parenteral form of certain antibiotics (eg, rifampin) have encouraged clinicians to utilize oral antibiotic therapy in the treatment of endocarditis.

Oral penicillin V has been shown to be only marginally effective in combination with intramuscular streptomycin in the treatment of subacute bacterial endocarditis (119). However, Parker et al have observed excellent results in the treatment of staphylococcal endocarditis with a combination of intravenous and oral antibiotic therapy. Utilizing a mean duration of 16.4 days of parenteral anti-staphylococcal therapy with a mean of 26 days of appropriate oral therapy, these investigators were able to cure 35 cases of endocarditis in patients unable to tolerate intravenous therapy (120).

Rifampin has been shown to be an effective

adjunct in combination with other agents in the treatment of staphylococcal endocarditis, especially that due to *S. epidermidis* (121,123,124). A regimen of oral amoxicillin and intramuscular gentamicin has been used to treat enterococcal endocarditis (122). *Bacteroides fragilis* endocarditis has been successfully treated with oral metronidazole, the only available antimicrobial consistently bactericidal against this organism (125).

Thus, while parenteral therapy is preferable in the treatment of endocarditis, oral antibiotics may be useful in certain clinical settings. If this patient refuses the remainder of intravenous nafcillin therapy and appears clinically stable, one to three weeks of dicloxacillin 500 mg q 6 h is a reasonable alternative.

18. The cultures of the previously mentioned staphylococcus show excellent sensitivity to nafcillin, cephalosporins, clindamycin, gentamicin, tobramycin, and vancomycin. Could an aminoglycoside or clindamycin be used as single agents to treat this infection?

Aminoglycosides used alone in the treatment of staphylococcal endocarditis have been shown experimentally to be ineffective in reducing the bacterial population of vegetations. Miller observed that animals with staphylococcal endocarditis were persistently bacteremic when treated with an aminoglycoside alone (106). These observations are consistent with those of other investigators (105). Furthermore, it has been shown that within 24 hours, subpopulations of *S. aureus* can be isolated which are capable of growth in concentrations of aminoglycoside which are as much as eight times above the MIC for the parent strain (126). Thus, the relative inefficacy of the aminoglycosides and their potential toxicity make them inappropriate choices as single-agents in the therapy of staphylococcal endocarditis.

The relative lack of *in vitro* bactericidal activity suggests that erythromycin and clindamycin are also not first-line drugs in the treatment of this infection; however, clindamycin has been shown to be occasionally effective in the treatment of staphylococcal endocarditis (127).

19. *Vancomycin.* **The patient in the case above was treated successfully, but returns six months later with similar complaints. Blood cultures are obtained and nafcillin therapy is reinstituted. Forty-eight hours later, the patient has not improved and culture and**

sensitivity testing reveals *Staphylococcus aureus* which is resistant to nafcillin. Therapy is to be changed to vancomycin. Discuss the dosing and potential side effects of vancomycin in this patient. (See Question 11. Assume all admitting laboratory reports are the same.)

Vancomycin in doses of 15–20 mg/kg/day intravenously remains the drug of choice in nafcillin-resistant staphylococcal endocarditis (25). This is documented by the excellent *in vitro* and *in vivo* experience with the drug in this disease state (128–130).

Vancomycin is excreted primarily unchanged by the kidneys, with a serum half-life of approximately six hours in patients with normal renal function. However, in renal impairment, the half-life may be as long as six to nine days. Therefore the following equation has been suggested to approximate a serum concentration of 20 mcg/ml in patients with renal impairment (131):

$$\frac{\text{Maintenance Dose}}{\text{(mg/day)}} = (Cl_{Cr})(15) + 150 \quad \text{(Eq. 1)}$$

Thus, utilizing the following equation for creatinine clearance (see chapter on Clinical Pharmacokinetics):

$$Cl_{Cr} = \frac{(140-\text{Age})(\text{Wt in kg})}{(72)(Sr_{Cr})} \quad \text{(Eq. 2)}$$

we derive a clearance of 40 ml/min for A.G. Substituting this clearance into the first equation, a maintenance dose of 750 mg daily or 250 mg q 8 h IV is calculated.

Side effects and toxicities of vancomycin are both acute and chronic. Although vancomycin preparations have been purified since the 1950's, *fever, phlebitis,* and *extravasation* have been associated with its administration. The use of a dilute solution (500 mg in 100–200 ml saline) appears to reduce most of these complications (132). *Hypotension* is a commonly reported side effect which is related to the rate of intravenous injection. Thus, it is recommended that vancomycin be administered over 30 minutes, with frequent monitoring of the patient's blood pressure and heart rate (133).

Ototoxicity is the most serious complication of vancomycin therapy and appears to be related to serum levels greater than 80 mcg/ml. Cautious monitoring of vancomycin levels and adjustment

of the dose relative to renal function are, therefore, important. Most authorities attempt to keep peak levels below 30 mcg/ml (132). The incidence of *nephrotoxicity* has been low since the reformulation of the product. However, patients receiving concomitant aminoglycosides should be closely monitored for this potential toxicity (132).

GRAM-NEGATIVE ENDOCARDITIS

20. B.G., a 35-year-old intravenous amphetamine abuser recently admitted to the hospital with presumed endocarditis, has failed to improve on empiric therapy with nafcillin, penicillin, and gentamicin. His temperature has been spiking up to 39.8° over the last 48 hours.

Physical examination shows a thin, cachetic-looking individual in acute distress with chief complaints of acute pleuritic pain and symptoms of moderate heart failure.

His blood culture results return growing *Pseudomonas aeruginosa* resistant to gentamicin but sensitive to tobramycin. Renal function tests are normal with a serum creatinine of 1.0 mg/dl.

Why are gram-negative organisms not more common as infecting agents in endocarditis? How should gram-negative endocarditis be managed? Make specific recommendations for this patient.

With the recent increase in intravenous drug abuse and number of prosthetic valve replacements, the prevalence of gram-negative endocarditis has increased from 1.7% in the 1960's to 7% currently. The organism most commonly implicated is *Pseudomonas aeruginosa* (31,134,135), followed by *Serratia marcescens* (136,137), *Pseudomonas cepacia, Enterobacter sp.* and *Haemophilus influenzae* or *parainfluenzae*, in that order (138).

Reasons for the prevalence of gram-positive bacteria and to a lesser extent *P. aeruginosa* as causes of most cases of infective endocarditis are two-fold. First, gram-negative bacteria cause bacteremia far less frequently than gram-positive cocci. Secondly, these organisms have a capacity to adhere to valve leaflets, whereas organisms such as *E. coli* and *K. pneumoniae* do not (139). Further experimentation with streptococci has shown that dextran may be implicated in the pathogenesis of this disease. Parker et al found that dextran-positive streptococci were more likely to produce endocarditis than dextran-negative species (140). Scheld and investigators have observed experimentally that *S. sanguis* is less able to produce infective endocarditis after treatment with dextranase (an enzyme which removes dextran from the bacterial cell surface) (141).

Treatment recommendations are difficult to make due to the limited experience with gram-negative endocarditis as well as the multitude of organisms known to produce this disease. However, certain guidelines can be suggested. For endocarditis secondary to *Pseudomonas aeruginosa,* experimental evidence suggests a need for combination therapy with carbenicillin or ticarcillin plus an aminoglycoside (142). Reyes utilized carbenicillin 30 gm/day and gentamicin or tobramycin 2.5–5.0 mg/kg/day and observed that only 5 of 20 patients were cured. They suggested that a combination of medical therapy and surgical intervention was necessary for cure (134). More recently, the same group of investigators reported an increased cure rate and decreased overall mortality with a combination of high dose aminoglycoside therapy (8 mg/kg/day) and carbenicillin in the previously described dose. Nine of 14 patients (64%) were treated medically and the overall mortality was reduced from 50% to 14%. However, 9 of the 14 patients treated in this manner suffered diminished vestibular, auditory, or renal function (135). Thus, B.G. should be started on carbenicillin 30 gm/day or ticarcillin 18–24 gm/day in conjunction with tobramycin 5 mg/kg/day. If the patient responds poorly, surgery may be indicated.

Experience with *Serratia marsescens* in the San Francisco Bay Area reaffirms the necessity for drug combinations in the treatment of most forms of gram-negative endocarditis. Gentamicin in combination with carbenicillin or chloramphenicol has been shown to be the most appropriate therapy (137). For infections due to gram-negative organisms susceptible to ampicillin or penicillin G, high doses of single agents producing serum bactericidal titers of at least 1:8 have been suggested (138).

21. *Surgical Therapy.* The patient continues to have positive blood cultures despite maximal medical management. Additionally, worsening heart failure as well as cerebral embolic phenomena are now noted. What factors suggest the need for surgery in addition to medical management of infective endocarditis and which of these factors are present in B.G.?

Certain subgroups of patients with infective endocarditis require early surgical intervention. Appreciable or worsening congestive heart failure is the most commonly suggested indication for valve replacement (143,144). Recurrent systemic emboli, as well as infection uncontrolled by adequate antibiotic therapy are additional findings which indicate the need for surgery (145,146). Virulence of the organism is also an important consideration. Fungal endocarditis mandates valve replacement, and infections due to gram-negative bacilli (such as *P. aeruginosa*) often require surgery for cure (145). Some clinicians feel that all patients with an established diagnosis of endocarditis caused by gram-positive bacteria which are not highly sensitive to penicillin, penicillin derivatives, or cephalosporins should also be considered probable candidates for surgery (147). Acquired heart block and annular/myocardial abscesses are also high-risk conditions that require surgical intervention for valve replacement (147). Dehiscence or mechanical failure of a prosthetic valve necessitate immediate operative treatment (145). B.G.'s worsening heart failure, embolization, and lack of response to therapy strongly suggest the need for surgery.

PROSTHETIC VALVE ENDOCARDITIS

22. S.K. is a 53-year-old woman with a history of placement of a Bjork-Shiley (mechanical) prosthesis one month ago. She now presents to her cardiologist with complaints of fever, lethargy and anorexia which have persisted over the last week. On physical examination, a regurgitant murmur suggests prosthetic valve dysfunction. The impression is prosthetic valve endocarditis. What is prosthetic valve endocarditis and how should it be managed in this patient?

The incidence of prosthetic valve endocarditis (PVE) ranges from 0–9.5% among published series, with an average of 2.3%. Early prosthetic valve infection, defined as endocarditis occurring within two months of valve replacement, has an average reported prevalence of 1.1%. There are many variables which may influence the rate of early prosthetic valve infection. The presurgical condition of the patient, skill of the surgeon, choice of prosthetic valve, the length of time the patient is subjected to extra-corporeal circulation, the sterility of the heart-lung machine, and the development of a postoperative extracardiac infection are all significant factors (148). Categorization of PVE into early and late endocarditis is important because early prosthetic valve endocarditis is associated with a significantly higher mortality (72%) than late prosthetic valve endocarditis (45.4%) (148–50). The instability of patients in the immediate postoperative period as well as the increased virulence of "early" infecting organisms contribute to this discrepancy.

The aortic valve is infected at a significantly higher rate than the mitral, and while the overall rate of endocarditis appears to be no higher in mechanical valves than heterograft tissue valves, the rate of *early* PVE may be higher in tissue valves than mechanical prostheses. However, infection of mechanical valves appears to be more readily managed medically than infection of tissue valves (151).

The most common infecting organism in PVE is *Staphylococcus epidermis* which is often methicillin-resistant; it accounts for 27.4% of the early cases and 22.9% of the late cases. *Staphylococcus aureus,* gram-negative bacilli, and fungi (in order of frequency) are the next most common infecting agents in early PVE, while streptococci appear to be the most common bacteria associated with late disease (148,149,152–154).

In the patient with acute PVE, methicillin-resistant staphylococci, streptococci, and gram-negative bacteria are the primary pathogens. Thus, a combination of vancomycin and an aminoglycoside is appropriate empiric therapy pending the receipt of culture results.

Once the infecting organism is known, experimental evidence suggests that combination therapy is superior to single-agent chemotherapy. Pelletier noted that the combination of penicillin and streptomycin was significantly better than penicillin alone in eradicating *Streptococcus sanguis* in experimental PVE. Additionally, the greater the delay before initiation of antibiotics, the greater the duration of therapy that is required for clinical and bacteriologic cure (155). This reinforces the need for early recognition and immediate initiation of therapy in patients with PVE.

Based on the previously mentioned definitions, this patient's endocarditis should be classified as "early". Vancomycin and tobramycin or gentamicin should be started immediately, pending identification of the organism. The patient's subsequent clinical course will ultimately determine her need for surgery.

23. The results of one of the blood cultures grows *Staphylococcus epidermidis* resistant to methicillin and cefazolin but sensitive to vancomycin and gentamicin. Could the above organism be a "contaminant" or is it likely to be the actual pathogen?

The presence of *Staphyloccocus epidermidis* in blood cultures has generally been felt to be due to contamination during venipuncture. However, recent experience with prosthetic valve endocarditis and vascular graft infections documents the potential of *Staphyloccocus epidermidis* as a pathogen. These organisms can be highly resistant to methicillin, with estimates ranging from 10% to 63% of isolates (156,157).

Methicillin-resistant strains are also highly resistant to other antibiotics, making effective antimicrobial therapy a difficult undertaking. Cephalosporins and other semisynthetic penicillins are often ineffective. Vancomycin, gentamicin, and rifampin have been shown to have the most activity against these organisms (158). However, the emergence of strains resistant to rifampin (156,159) and gentamicin (157) precludes the use of these agents alone. Additionally, *in vivo* evidence documents the occasional lack of efficacy of vancomycin when used alone (123–4). Thus, some authorities suggest a combination of vancomycin, rifampin, and gentamicin in the treatment of *S. epidermidis* endocarditis (25). This combination has been shown to be effective and appears to prevent the emergence of rifampin and gentamicin resistant strains *in vivo* (124,157). Thus, while only one of the above blood cultures is positive for *S. epidermidis,* empiric therapy against this organism must be started.

24. Six out of six blood cultures finally return positive for *Candida albicans.* As a result, it is presumed that this patient has fungal endocarditis involving her prosthetic valve. Discuss the proper management of fungal endocarditis.

The devastating effects of fungal endocarditis are evidenced by the high mortality associated with this disease. Rubinstein has noted that despite the availability of antifungal antibiotics and surgery, over 80% of patients with documented fungal endocarditis die of this infection. It is a disease most commonly noted in narcotic addicts and patients with prosthetic valve endocarditis; *Candida* and *Aspergillus* species are the most common infecting organisms (160).

Medical management alone with amphotericin B, flucytosine, and other antifungal agents is rarely curative. Valve tissue penetration of amphotericin B is very poor (161), and viable organisms have been cultured from surgically excised valves despite prolonged preoperative amphotericin B therapy and sterile blood cultures (162). The results of all studies suggest that a combination of pre- and postoperative amphotericin B (as discussed in the chapter on Infections in the Compromised Host) in conjunction with early surgical excision is the most appropriate means of curing fungal endocarditis (160–4).

PREVENTION OF ENDOCARDITIS

25. T.N. is a 26-year-old patient with a previous history of rheumatic heart disease, with a murmur first noted at age 17. He is scheduled for sigmoidoscopy as part of a work-up for GI bleeding. Should the patient receive prophylactic antibiotics for this procedure? Briefly describe the American Heart Association recommendations for the prevention of endocarditis.

Dental procedures and instrumentation or surgery involving the upper respiratory tract, genitourinary tract, and lower gastrointestinal tract may be associated with transient bacteremia (165). Prevention of bacterial endocarditis has been reviewed by the American Heart Association (AHA), which suggests the following chemoprophylactic regimens for these procedures (166):

DENTAL PROCEDURES AND UPPER RESPIRATORY TRACT SURGICAL PROCEDURES

Since *Streptoccus viridans* is the most commonly implicated organism in bacterial endocarditis following these procedures, antibiotic prophylaxis should be directed against this organism. This prophylaxis is recommended for all dental procedures (including routine professional cleaning) that are likely to produce gingival bleeding.

Regimen A
Parenteral-Oral Combined

Adults: Aqueous crystalline penicillin G 1 MU IM mixed with procaine penicillin G 600,000 U IM 30 minutes to 1 hour prior to procedure, then penicillin V 500 mg po q 6 h × 8 doses.

Children: Aqueous crystalline penicillin G 30,000 U/kg IM mixed with procaine penicillin G 600,000 U IM 30 minutes to 1 hour prior to the procedure, then penicillin V 250 mg po q 6 h × 8 doses.

Oral

Adults: Penicillin V 2.0 gm po 30 minutes to 1 hour prior to the procedure, then 500 mg po q 6 h × 8 doses.

Children: Same as above. If < 60 lbs. give 1.0 gm po 30 minutes to 1 hour prior to the procedure, then 250 mg po q 6 h × 8 doses.

If Allergic to Penicillin
Parenteral-Oral Combined

Adults: Vancomycin 1.0 gm IV over 30 minutes to 1 hour. Start initial infusion 1/2 to 1 hour prior to procedure, then erythromycin 500 mg po q 6 h × 8 doses.

Children: Vancomycin 20 mg/kg IV over 30 minutes to 1 hour, then erythromycin 10 mg/kg q 6 h × 8 doses.

Oral

Adults: Erythromycin 1.0 gm po 1½ to 2 hours prior to the procedure, then 500 mg po q 6 h × 8 doses.

Children: Erythromycin 20 mg/kg po, then 10 mg/kg q 6 h × 8 doses.

Regimen B

Adults: Aqueous crystalline penicillin G 1 MU IM mixed with procaine penicillin G 600,000 U IM *plus* streptomycin 1.0 gm IM given 30 minutes to 1 hour prior to the procedure, then penicillin V 500 mg po q 6 h × 8 doses.

Children: Aqueous crystalline penicillin G 30,000 U/kg IM mixed with procaine penicillin G 600,000 U IM *plus* streptomycin 20 mg/kg IM, then penicillin V 500 mg po q 6 h × 8 doses. If < 60 lbs penicillin V 250 mg po q 6 h × 8 doses.

If Allergic to Penicillin

Vancomycin IV *with* subsequent erythromycin po (as outlined above).

Regimen B is suggested for prophylaxis of prosthetic heart valves while either A or B is recommended for other congenital heart defects and valvular disease. It is important to note that patients receiving continuous oral penicillin for secondary prevention of rheumatic fever may harbor alpha hemolytic streptococci *(Streptococci viridans)* in the oral cavity which are relatively resistant to penicillin (166). While it is likely that the doses of penicillin recommended in Regimen A are adequate to control these organisms, the clinician may utilize Regimen B or choose erythromycin. The recent observations of two documented cases of endocarditis due to resistant *viridans* streptococci after oral penicillin prophylaxis suggests these recommendations may be correct (167).

GENITOURINARY TRACT AND GASTROINTESTINAL TRACT SURGERY OR INSTRUMENTATION

Enterococci are the microorganisms most frequently responsible for endocarditis following genitourinary tract and gastrointestinal tract surgery or manipulation. Although bacteremia and sepsis with gram-negative bacteria may follow GU or GI procedures, these organisms rarely cause endocarditis. Thus, chemoprophylaxis should be directed primarily against enterococci.

Adults: Aqueous crystalline penicillin G 2 MU IM/IV or ampicillin 1.0 gm IM/IV *plus* gentamicin 1.5 mg/kg (not to exceed 80 mg) IM/IV or streptomycin 1.0 gm IM.

Children: Aqueous crystalline penicillin G 30,000/kg IM/IV or ampicillin 50 mg/kg IM/IV *plus* gentamicin 2.0 mg/kg IM/IV or streptomycin 20 mg/kg IM.

Give initial doses 30 minutes to 1 hour prior to procedure. If gentamicin is used then give a similar dose of gentamicin and penicillin (or ampicillin) every 8 hours for two additional doses. If streptomycin is used then give a similar dose of streptomycin and penicillin (or ampicillin) every 12 hours for two additional doses.

If Allergic to Penicillin

Adults: Vancomycin 1.0 gram IV over 30 minutes to 1 hour *plus* streptomycin 1.0 gm IM. A single dose of these antibiotics begun 30 minutes to one hour prior to the procedure is probably sufficient, but the same dose may be repeated in 12 hours.

Children: Vancomycin 20 mg/kg IV *plus* streptomycin 20 mg/kg IM. (timing same as adults).

Based upon currently available evidence, the following procedures do *not* require antibiotic prophylaxis in most patients with underlying heart disease: uncomplicated vaginal delivery, upper GI endoscopy (without biopsy), percutaneous liver biopsy, proctoscopy, sigmoidoscopy, barium enema, pelvic examination, dilation and curettage of the uterus, and uncomplicated insertion or removal of intrauterine devices. Therefore, the above-mentioned patient does not require prophylaxis based on AHA guidelines.

No controlled clinical trials exist to assess the appropriateness of above guidelines for prevention of endocarditis in man. Only through the experimental animal model has any direct information been made available to document the efficacy of the presently available regimen. Thus, it is not surprising that over 300 individual cases of apparent failure to prophylactic therapy have been recorded in the literature (168).

References

1. Scheld WM et al: Endocarditis and intravascular infections. In *Principles and Practice of Infectious Diseases*, 1st ed., edited by G. Mandell, R. Douglas and J. Bennett, John Wiley and Sons, New York, 1979, p 653–65.
2. Pelletier LL et al: Infective endocarditis. A review of 125 cases from the University of Washington Hospitals, 1963–72. Medicine. 1977; 56:287.
3. Reisberg BE: Infective endocarditis in the narcotic addict. Progr Cardiovasc Dis. 1979; 22:193.
4. Heffner JE: Extracardiac manifestations of bacterial endocarditis. West J Med. 1979; 131:85.
5. Lerner PI et al: Infective endocarditis in the antibiotic era. N Engl J Med. 1966; 274:199, 259, 323, 388.
6. Pruitt AA et al: Neurologic complications of bacterial endocarditis. Medicine. 1978; 57:329.
7. Garvey GJ et al: Infective endocarditis—an evolving disease. Medicine. 1978; 57:105.
8. Miller MH et al: Infective endocarditis: new diagnostic techniques. Am Heart J. 1978; 96:123.
9. Davis RS et al: The demonstration of vegetations by echocardiography in bacterial endocarditis. An indication for early surgical intervention. Am J Med. 1980; 69:53.
10. Belli J et al: The number of blood cultures necessary to diagnose most cases of bacterial endocarditis. Am J Med Sci. 1956; 232:284.
11. Wilson WR et al: Infective endocarditis: therapeutic considerations. Am Heart J. 1980; 100:689.
12. Wolfe JC et al: Penicillin-sensitive streptococcal endocarditis. *In vitro* and clinical observations on penicillin-streptomycin therapy. Ann Intern Med. 1974; 81:178.
13. Blount JG: Bacterial endocarditis. Am J Med. 1965; 38:909.
14. Watanakunakorn C: Streptococcus bovis endocarditis. Am J Med. 1974; 56:256.
15. Watanakunakorn C et al: Synergism with aminoglycosides of penicillin, ampicillin and vancomycin against non-enterococcal group-D streptococci and viridans streptococci. J Med Microbiol. 1977; 10:133.
16. Durack DT et al: Chemotherapy of experimental streptococcal endocarditis. J Clin Invest. 1974; 53:829.
17. Sande MA et al: Penicillin-aminoglycoside synergy in experimental streptococcus viridans endocarditis. J Infect Dis. 1974; 129:572.

18. Duperval R et al: Bactericidal activity of combinations of penicillin or clindamycin with gentamicin or streptomycin against species of viridans streptococci. Antimicrob Agents Chemother. 1975; 8:673.

19. Tompsett R et al: Short term penicillin and dihydrostreptomycin therapy of streptococcal endocarditis. Results of the treatment of thirty five patients. Am J Med. 1958; 24:57.

20. Wilson WR et al: Short-term intramuscular therapy with procaine penicillin plus streptomycin for infective endocarditis due to viridans streptococci. Circulation. 1978; 57:1158.

21. Wilson WR et al: Short-term therapy for streptococcal infective endocarditis. Combined intramuscular administration. JAMA. 1981; 245:360.

22. Malacoff RF et al: Streptococcal endocarditis (nonenterococcal, non group A). Single vs. combination therapy. JAMA. 1979; 241:1807.

23. Karchmer AW et al: Single-antibiotic therapy for streptococcal endocarditis. JAMA. 1979; 241:1801.

24. Hoppes WL: Treatment of bacterial endocarditis caused by penicillin-sensitive streptococci. Arch Intern Med. 1977; 137:1122.

25. Sande MA et al: Combination antibiotic therapy of bacterial endocarditis. Ann Intern Med. 1980; 92:390.

26. Kaye D: Antibiotic treatment of streptococcal endocarditis. Am J Med. 1980; 69:650.

27. Bisno AL et al: AHA Committee Report. Treatment of infective endocarditis due to viridans streptococci. Circulation. 1981; 63:730A.

28. Peterson LR et al: Medium-dependent variation in bactericidal activity of antibiotics against susceptible staphylococcus aureus. Antimicrob Agents Chemother. 1978; 13:665.

29. Pursiano TA et al: Effect of assay medium on the antibacterial activity of certain penicillins and cephalosporins. Antimicrob Agents Chemother. 1973; 3:33.

30. Schlicter JG et al: A method of determining the effective therapeutic level in the treatment of subacute bacterial endocarditis with penicillin. Am Heart J. 1947; 34:209.

31. Myerowitz PD et al: Earlier operation for left sided pseudomonas endocarditis in drug addicts. J Thorac Cardiovasc Surg. 1979; 77:577.

32. Reymann MT et al: Persistent bacteremia in staphylococcal endocarditis. Am J Med. 1978; 65:729.

33. Bryan CS et al: Gram-negative bacillary endocarditis. Interpretation of the serum bactericidal tests. Am J Med. 1975; 58:209.

34. Hyams DE: Antibiotic therapy of staphylococcal endocarditis. Ann Intern Med. 1979; 91:492.

35. Archer G et al: Experimental endocarditis due to pseudomonas aeruginosa. II. Therapy with carbenicillin and gentamicin. J Infect Dis. 1977; 136:327.

36. Carrizosa J et al: Treatment of experimental staphylococcus aureus endocarditis: comparison of cephalothin, cefazolin, and methicillin. Antimicrob Agents Chemother. 1978; 13:74.

37. Parker RH et al: Intravenous followed by oral antimicrobial therapy for staphylococcal endocarditis. Ann Intern Med. 1980; 93:832.

38. Klastersky J et al: Antibacterial activity in serum and urine as a therapeutic guide in bacterial infections. J Infect Dis. 1974; 129:187.

39. Carrizosa J et al: Antibiotic concentrations in serum, serum bactericidal activity, and results of therapy of streptococcal endocarditis in rabbits. Antimicrob Agents Chemother. 1977; 12:479.

40. Jawetz E: Assay of antibacterial activity in serum. Am J Dis Child. 1962; 103:81.

41. Rahal JJ: Antibiotic combinations: the clinical relevance of synergy and antagonism. Medicine. 1978; 57:179.

42. Cannady PB et al: Negative blood cultures in infective endocarditis. South Med J. 1976; 69:1420.

43. Pesanti EL et al: Infective endocarditis with negative blood cultures. An analysis of 52 cases. Am J Med. 1979; 66:43.

44. Parkey GA: The prevention and treatment of bacterial endocarditis. Am Heart J. 1979; 98:102.

45. Casey JI et al: Infective endocarditis: Part II. Current Therapy. Am Heart J. 1978; 96:263.

46. Mandell GL et al: Enterococcal endocarditis. An analysis of 38 patients observed at the New York Hospital-Cornell Medical Center. Arch Intern Med. 1970; 125:258.

47. Wilkowske CJ et al: Antibiotic synergism: enhanced susceptibility of group D streptococci to certain antibiotic combinations. Antimicrob Agents Chemother. 1970; 195.

48. Watanakunakorn C: Penicillin combined with gentamicin or streptomycin: synergy against enterococci. J Infect Dis. 1971; 124:581.

49. Hook EW et al: Antimicrobial therapy of experimental enterococcal endocarditis. Antimicrob Agents Chemother. 1975; 8:564.

50. Fekety FR et al: Antibiotic synergism: enhanced susceptibility of enterococci to combinations of streptomycin and penicillins or cephalosporins. Antimicrob Agents Chemother. 1966; 156.

51. Abrutyn E et al: Cephalothin-gentamicin synergism in experimental enterococcal endocarditis. J Antimicrob Chemother. 1978; 4:153.

52. Weinstein AJ et al: Studies of cephalothin-aminoglycoside synergism against enterococci. Antimicrob Agents Chemother. 1975; 7:522.

53. Weinstein AJ et al: Cephalosporin-aminoglycoside synergism in experimental enterococcal endocarditis. Antimicrob Agents Chemother. 1976; 9:983.

54. Glew RH et al: Effect of protein binding on the activity of penicillins in combination with gentamicin against enterococci. Antimicrob Agents Chemother. 1979; 15:87.

55. Lincoln LJ et al: Penicillinase-resistant penicillins plus gentamicin in experimental enterococcal endocarditis. Antimicrob Agents Chemother. 1977; 12:484.

56. Marier RL et al: Synergism of oxacillin and gentamicin against enterococci. Antimicrob Agents Chemother. 1975; 8:571.

57. Glew RH et al: Comparative synergistic activity of nafcillin, oxacillin and methicillin in combination with gentamicin against enterococci. Antimicrob Agents Chemother. 1975; 7:828.

58. Westenfelder GO et al: Vancomycin-streptomycin synergism in enterococcal endocarditis. JAMA. 1973; 223:37.

59. Watanakunakorn C et al: Synergism of vancomycin-gentamicin. Antimicrob Agents Chemother. 1973; 4:120.

60. Standiford HD et al: Antibiotic synergy of enterococci. Relation to inhibitory concentration. Arch Intern Med. 1970; 126:255.

61. **Moellering RC et al: Prevalence of high-level resistance to aminoglycosides in clinical isolates of enterococci. Antimicrob Agents Chemother. 1970; 335.**

62. Iannini PB et al: Effects of ampicillin-amikacin and ampicillin-rifampin on enterococci. Antimicrob Agents Chemother. 1976; 9:448.

63. Serra P et al: Synergistic treatment of enterococcal endocarditis. *In vitro* and *in vivo* studies. Arch Intern Med. 1977; 137:1562.

64. Moellering RC et al: Synergy of penicillin and gentamicin against enterococci. J Infect Dis. 1971; 124: S207.

65. Moellering RC et al: Penicillin-tobramycin synergism against enterococci: a comparison with penicillin and gentamicin. Antimicrob Agents Chemother. 1973; 3:526.

66. Carrizosa J et al: Antibiotic synergism in enterococcal endocarditis. J Lab Clin Med. 1976; 88:132.

67. Moellering RC et al: A novel mechanism of resistance to penicillin-gentamicin synergism in Streptococcus faecalis. J Infect Dis. 1980; 141:81.

68. Tompsett R et al: Enterococcal endocarditis: duration and mode of treatment. Trans Am Clin Assoc. 1977; 89:49.

69. Cook FV et al: Treatment of bacterial endocarditis with vancomycin. Am J Med Sci. 1978; 276:153.

70. Fee WE: Aminoglycoside ototoxicity in the human. Laryngoscope. 1980; 40 Suppl 24 Part 2:1.

71. Stupp H et al: Inner ear concentrations and ototoxicity of different antibiotics in local and systemic application. Audiology. 1973; 12:350.

72. Meuwissen JH et al: The ototoxic antibiotics: a survey of current knowledge. Clin Pediatr. 1967; 6:262.

73. Mangione A et al: Therapeutic monitoring of aminoglycoside antibiotics: an approach. Ther Drug Monitoring. 1980; 2:159.

74. Jackson GG et al: Pseudomonas bacteremia, pharmacologic and other bases for failure of treatment with gentamicin. J Infect Dis. 1971; 124 (Suppl) S185-91.

75. Noone P et al: Experience in monitoring gentamicin therapy during treatment of serious gram-negative sepsis. Br Med J. 1974; 1:477.

76. Anderson ET et al: Simultaneous antibiotic levels in "breakthrough" gram-negative rod bacteremia. Am J Med. 1976; 61:493.

77. Dahlgren JG et al: Gentamicin blood levels: a guide to nephrotoxicity. Antimicrob Agents Chemother. 1975; 8:58.

78. Goodman EI et al: Prospective comparative study of variable dosage and variable frequency regimens for administration of gentamicin. Antimicrob Agents Chemother. 1975; 8:434.

79. Benck G et al: Retrospective study of the ototoxicity of gentamicin. Acta Pathol Microbiol Scand. 1973; B81 (Suppl) 241:54.

80. Nordstrom L et al: Prospective study of the ototoxicity of gentamicin. Acta Pathol Microbiol Scand. 1973; B81 (Suppl) 241:58.

81. Black RS et al: Ototoxicity of amikacin. Antimicrob Agents Chemother. 1976; 9:956.

82. Menda KB et al: Favorable experience with bacterial endocarditis in heroin addicts. Ann Intern Med. 1973; 78:25.

83. Sklaver AR et al: Staphylococcal endocarditis in addicts. South Med J. 1978; 71:638.

84. Watanakunakorn C et al: Prognostic factors in staphylococcus aureus endocarditis and results of therapy with a penicillin and gentamicin. Am J Med Sci. 1977; 273:133.

85. Thell R et al: Bacterial endocarditis in subjects 60 years of age and older. Circulation. 1975; 51:174.

86. Hiratzka LF et al: Operative experience with infective endocarditis. Drug users compared to nondrug users. J Thorac Cardiovasc Surg. 1979; 77:355.

87. Banks T et al: Infective endocarditis in heroin addicts. Am J Med. 1973; 55:444.

88. Tuazon CU et al: Staphylococcal endocarditis in drug users. Clinical and microbiologic aspects. Arch Intern Med. 1975; 135:1555.

89. Egert J et al: Comparison of methicillin, nafcillin and oxacillin in therapy of Staphylococcus aureus endocarditis in rabbits. J Lab Clin Med. 1977; 89:1262.

90. Carrizosa J et al: Effectiveness of nafcillin, methicillin and cephalothin in experimental Staphylococcus aureus endocarditis. Antimicrob Agents Chemother. 1979; 15:735.

91. Carrizosa J et al: Comparison of ceforanide, cefazolin, methicillin, and nafcillin in Staphylococcus aureus endocarditis therapy in rabbits. Antimicrob Agents Chemother. 1980; 18:562.

92. Fong IW et al: Relative inactivation by Staphylococcus aureus of eight cephalosporin antibiotics. Antimicrob Agents Chemother. 1976; 9:939.

93. Farrar WE et al: Antistaphylococcal activity and β-lactamase resistance of newer cephalosporin. J Infect Dis. 1976; 133:691.

94. Regamey C et al: Inactivation of cefazolin, cephaloridine, and cephalothin by methicillin-sensitive and methicillin-resistant strains of Staphylococcus aureus. J Infect Dis. 1975; 131:291.

95. Sabath LD et al: Effect of inoculum and of beta-lactamase on the antistaphylococcal activity of thirteen penicillins and cephalosporins. Antimicrob Agents Chemother. 1975; 8:344.

96. Goldman PL et al: Importance of beta-lactamase inactivation in the treatment of experimental endocarditis caused by Staphylococcus aureus. J Infect Dis. 1980; 141:331.

97. Bryant RE et al: Unsuccessful treatment of staphylococcal endocarditis with cefazolin. JAMA. 1977; 237:569.

98. Quinn EL et al: Clinical experiences with cefazolin and other cephalosporins in bacterial endocarditis. J Infect Dis. 1973; 128:S386.

99. Burgess HA et al: Failure of cephaloridine in a case of staphylococcal endocarditis. Br Med J. 1966; 2:1244.

100. Reinarz JA et al: Evaluation of cefazolin in the treatment of bacterial endocarditis and bacteremia. J Infect Dis. 1973; 128:S392.

101. Masur H et al: Nafcillin therapy for Staphylococcus aureus endocarditis. Antimicrob Agents Chemother. 1978; 14:457.

102. Sande MA et al: Endocarditis Collaborative Group. 11th International Congress on Antimicrobial Agents and Chemotherapy, Boston, 1979.

103. Abrams B et al: Single or combination therapy of staphylococcal endocarditis in intravenous drug abusers'. Ann Intern Med. 1979; 90:789.

104. Watanakunakorn C et al: Enhancement of the effects of antistaphylococcal antibiotics by aminoglycosides. Antimicrob Agents Chemother. 1974; 6:802.

105. Sande MA et al: Nafcillin-gentamicin synergism in experimental staphylococcal endocarditis. J Lab Clin Med. 1976; 88:118.

106. Miller MH et al: Single and combination antibiotic therapy of Staphylococcus aureus experimental endocarditis: emergence of gentamicin-resistant mutants. Antimicrob Agents Chemother. 1978; 14:336.

107. Murray HW et al: Combination antibiotic therapy in staphylococcal endocarditis. The use of methicillin sodium-gentamicin sulfate therapy. Arch Intern Med. 1976; 136:480.

108. Mayhall CG et al: Variation in the susceptibilities of strains of Staphylococcus aureus to oxacillin, cephalothin, and gentamicin. Antimicrob Agents Chemother. 1976; 10:707.

109. Bradley JJ et al: Incidence and characteristics of antibiotic-tolerant strains of Staphylococcus aureus. Antimicrob Agents Chemother. 1978; 13:1052.

110. Rajashekaraiah KR et al: Clinical significance of tolerant strains of Staphylococcus aureus in patients with endocarditis. Ann Intern Med. 1980; 93:796.

111. Watanakunakorn C et al: Antibiotic tolerant Staphylococcus aureus. J Antimicrob Chemother. 1978; 4:561.

112. Massanari RM et al: The efficacy of rifampin as adjunctive therapy in selected cases of staphylococcal endocarditis. Chest. 1978; 73:371.

113. Falville RJ et al: Staphylococcus aureus endocarditis. Combined therapy with vancomycin and rifampin. JAMA. 1978; 240:1963.

114. Gopal V et al: Failure of vancomycin treatment in Staphylococcus aureus endocarditis. JAMA. 1976; 236:1604.

115. Bradley HE et al: Tolerance in Staphylococcus aureus: evidence for bacteriophage role. J Infect Dis. 180; 141:233.

116. Goldman PL et al: Significance of methicillin tolerance in experimental Staphylococcus endocarditis. Antimicrob Agents Chemother. 1979; 15:802.

117. Hilty MD et al: Oxacillin-tolerant Staphylococcal bacteremia in children. J Pediatr. 1980; 96:1035.

118. Denny AE et al: Serious Staphylococcal infections with strains tolerant to bactericidal antibiotics. Arch Intern Med. 1979; 139:1026.

119. Quinn EL et al: Subacute bacterial endocarditis. Clinical and laboratory observations in 27 consecutive cases treated with penicillin V by mouth. N Engl J Med. 1961; 264:835.

120. Parker RH et al: Intravenous followed by oral antimicrobial therapy for staphylococcal endocarditis. Ann Intern Med. 1980; 93:832.

121. Lidji M et al: Bacterial endocarditis on a prosthetic valve. Chest. 1978; 74:224.

122. Seligman SJ: Treatment of enterococcal endocarditis with oral amoxicillin and intramuscular gentamicin. J Infect Dis. 1974; 124:S213.

123. George T et al: Rifampin in the management of early prosthetic Staphylococcus epidermidis endocarditis. Ann Thorac Surg. 1980; 29:74.

124. Archer GL et al: Rifampin therapy of Staphylococcus epidermidis. JAMA. 1978; 240:751.

125. Galgiani JN et al: Bacteroides fragilis endocarditis, bacteremia and other infections treated with oral or intravenous metronidazole. Am J Med. 1978; 65:284.

126. Wilson SG et al: Selection and characterization of strains of Staphylococcus aureus displaying unusual resistance to aminoglycosides. Antimicrob Agents Chemother. 1976; 10:519.

127. Cherubin CE et al: Clindamycin in infective endocarditis. JAMA. 1978; 239:626.

128. Cook FV et al: Treatment of bacterial endocarditis with vancomycin. Am J Med Sci. 1978; 276:153.

129. Hook EW et al: Vancomycin therapy of bacterial endocarditis. Am J Med. 1978; 64:411.

130. Esposito AL et al: Vancomycin—a second look. JAMA. 1977; 238:1756.

131. Nielsen HF et al: Renal excretion of vancomycin in kidney disease. Acta Med Scand. 1975; 197:261.

132. Cook FV et al: Vancomycin revisited. Ann Intern Med. 1978; 88:813.

133. Newfield P et al: Hazards of rapid administration of vancomycin. Ann Intern Med. 1979; 91:581.

134. Reyes MP et al: Pseudomonas endocarditis in the Deroit Medical Center 1969–1972. Medicine. 1973; 52:173.

135. Reyes MP et al: Treatment of patients with pseudomonas endocarditis with high dose aminoglycoside and carbenicillin therapy. Medicine. 1978; 57:57.

136. Williams JC et al: Serratia marsescens endocarditis. Arch Intern Med. 1970; 125:1038.

137. Mills J et al: Serratia marsescens endocarditis: a regional illness associated with intravenous drug abuse. Ann Intern Med. 1976; 84:29.

138. Cohen PS et al: Infective endocarditis caused by gram-negative bacteria: a review of the literature, 1945–1977. Progr Cardiovasc Dis. 1980; 22:205.

139. Gould K et al: Adherence of bacteria to heart valves in vitro. J Clin Invest. 1975; 56:1364.

140. Parker MT et al: Streptococci and aerococci associated with systemic infection in man. J Med Microbiol. 1976; 9:275.

141. Scheld WM et al: Bacterial adherence in the pathogenesis of endocarditis. Interaction of bacterial dextran, platelets and fibrin. J Clin Invest. 1978; 61:1394.

142. Archer G et al: Experimental endocarditis due to Pseudomonas aeruginosa. II. Therapy with carbenicillin and gentamicin. J Infect Dis. 1977; 136:327.

143. Wilson WR et al: Valve replacement in patients with active infective endocarditis. Circulation. 1978; 58:585.

144. Wilson WR et al: Cardiac valve replacement in congestive heart failure due to infective endocarditis. Mayo Clin Proc. 1979; 54:223.

145. Stinson EB: Surgical treatment of infective endocarditis. Progr Cardiovasc Dis. 1979; 22:145.

146. McAnulty JH et al: Surgery for infective endocarditis. JAMA. 1979; 242:77.

147. Richardson JV et al: Treatment of infective endocarditis: a 10-year comparative analysis. Circulation. 1978; 58:589.

148. Watanakunakorn C: Prosthetic valve infective endocarditis. Progr Cardiovasc Dis. 1979; 22:181.

149. Dismukes WE et al: Prosthetic valve endocarditis. Analysis of 38 cases. Circulation. 1973; 48:365.

150. Wilson WR et al: Prosthetic valve endocarditis. Ann Intern Med. 1975; 82:751.

151. Rossiter SJ et al: Prosthetic valve endocarditis. Comparison of heterograft tissue valves and mechanical valves. J Thorac Cardiovasc Surg. 1978; 76:795.

152. Downham WH et al: Endocarditis associated with procaine valve xeno-grafts. Arch Intern Med. 1979; 139:1350.

153. Kaplan EL et al: A collaborative study of infective endocarditis in the 1970's. Emphasis on infections in patients who have undergone cardiovascular surgery. Circulation. 1979; 59:327.

154. Slaughter L et al: Prosthetic valvular endocarditis. A 12-year review. Circulation. 1973; 47:1319.

155. Pelletier LL et al: Chemotherapy of experimental streptococcal endocarditis. V. Effect of duration of infection and retained intracardiac catheter on response to treatment. J Lab Clin Med. 1976; 87:692.

156. Archer GL: Antimicrobial susceptibility and selection of resistance among Staphylococcus epidermides isolates recovered from patients with infections of indwelling foreign devices. Antimicrob Agents Chemother. 1978; 14:353.

157. Lowy FD et al: Antibiotic activity in vitro against methicillin-resistant Staphylococcus epidermidis and therapy of an experimental infection. Antimicrob Agents Chemother. 1979; 16:314.

158. Sabath LD et al: Methicillin resistance of Staphylococcus aureus and Staphylococcus epidermidis. Antimicrob Agents Chemother. 1968; 302.

159. Vasquez GJ et al: Antibiotic therapy of experimental Staphylococcus epidermidis endocarditis. Antimicrob Agents Chemother. 1980; 17:280.

160. Rubinstein E et al: Fungal endocarditis: Analysis of 24 cases and review of the literature. Medicine. 1975; 54:331.

161. Rubinstein E et al: Tissue penetration of amphotericin B in Candida endocarditis. Chest. 1974; 66:376.

162. Utley JR et al: Valve replacement for bacterial and fungal endocarditis. A comparative study. Circulation. 1973; 47,48 (Suppl 3):42.

163. Harris PD et al: Fungal endocarditis secondary to drug addiction. Recent concepts in diagnosis and therapy. J Thorac Cardiovasc Surg. 1972; 63:980.

164. Galgiani JN et al: Fungal endocarditis: need for guidelines in evaluating therapy. J Thorac Cardiovasc Surg. 1977; 73:293.

165. Everett ED et al: Transient bacteremia and endocarditis prophylaxis. A review. Medicine. 1977; 56:61.

166. Kaplan EL et al: AHA Committee Report. Prevention of bacterial endocarditis. Circulation. 1977; 56:139A.

167. Parillo JE et al: Endocarditis due to resistant viridans streptococci during oral penicillin chemoprophylaxis. N Engl J Med. 1979; 300:296.

168. Bisno AL et al: Failure of prophylaxis for bacterial endocarditis: American Heart Association Registry. Am J Cardiol. 1980; 45:186.

169. Van Arsdel PP: Allergic reactions to penicillin. JAMA. 1965; 191:238.

170. Erffmeyer JE: Adverse reactions to penicillin. Ann Allergy. 1981; 47:288.

171. Delage C et al: Anaphylactic deaths. A clinicopathologic study of 43 cases. J Forensic Sci. 1972; 17:525.

172. Parker CW: Drug allergy. N Engl J Med. 1975; 292:511,732,957.

173. Anon: Penicillin allergy. Med Lett Drugs Ther. 1978; 20:13.

174. Kagan BM: Ampicillin rash. West J Med. 1977; 126:333.

175. Petz LD: Immunologic cross-reactivity between penicillins and cephalosporins: A review. J Infect Dis. 1978; 137(Suppl):S74.

176. Moellering RC et al: Drug therapy. The newer cephalosporins. N Engl J Med. 1976; 294:24.

177. Scholand JF et al: Anaphylaxis to cephalothin in a patient allergic to penicillin. JAMA. 1968; 206:130.

178. Bryan CS et al: "Comparably massive" penicillin G therapy in renal failure. Ann Intern Med. 1975; 82:189.

179. Whelton A et al: Carbenicillin-induced acidosis and seizures. JAMA. 1971; 218:1942.

180. Smith H et al: Neurotoxicity and 'massive' intravenous therapy with penicillin. Arch Intern Med. 1967; 120:47.

181. Green RL et al: Elevated plasma procaine concentrations after administration of procaine penicillin G. N Engl J Med. 1974; 291:223.

182. Androssy K et al: Penicillin-induced coagulation disorder. Lancet. 1976; ii:1039.

183. Brown CH et al: Defective platelet function following the administration of penicillin compounds. Blood. 1976; 47:949.

Chapter 36

Urinary Tract Infections

—— Kermit J. Fendler and Julia K. Elenbaas ——

This chapter will begin with a brief review of urinary tract infections (UTIs), but it will primarily focus on the management of patients with UTIs. For a more detailed discussion of the etiology, pathophysiology, and diagnosis of UTIs, the reader is referred to some excellent texts and review articles (1–7).

Definitions. UTIs encompass a spectrum of clinical entities that includes pyelonephritis, cystitis, prostatitis, and urethritis (2).

Pyelonephritis is defined as an inflammatory process of the kidney and its adjacent structures (the renal pelvis). No specific etiologic agent is noted as responsible in this broad definition, but it is frequently used to mean a bacterial infection of the kidney. Pyelonephritis may be either acute or chronic.

Cystitis is defined as an inflammatory process confined to the urinary bladder. Bacteria are the most common etiologic agents.

Prostatitis designates various inflammatory conditions affecting the prostate, including acute and chronic infections with specific bacteria and, more commonly, instances in which signs and symptoms of prostatic inflammation are present but no specific organisms can be detected.

Urethritis is defined as an inflammation of the urethra. In males, the etiologic organisms most commonly implicated are *Neisseria gonorrhoeae, Ureaplasma urealyticum,* and *Chlamydiae.* In females, introital bacteria, principally *Escherichia coli,* and *Chlamydiae* may be causative agents.

Bacteriuria refers to the presence of bacteria in the urine. It is found in most cases of UTI, both symptomatic and asymptomatic.

Epidemiology. Infections of the urinary tract (UTIs) occur frequently in both community and hospital environments and are the most common bacterial infections in humans (1). Bacteriuria occurs in about 1–2% of school-age females, and is about 30 times more prevalent in females than in males of the same age (2). The incidence of symptomatic bacteriuria peaks between the ages of 15 and 24 in females; it then persists at a lower rate throughout life (8). Approximately 10 to 20% of women in the general population will experience a UTI during their lifetime (3). Women have more UTIs than men probably because of anatomical and physiological differences. The female urethra is relatively short, which allows bacteria easy access to the bladder. In contrast, males are partly protected because of a longer urethra and the presence of antimicrobial substances in prostatic secretions (1,9).

The incidence of UTIs in neonates is about 1%, and most neonatal cases of UTIs occur in males (10). Many of these patients prove to have congenital structural abnormalities. The mortality rate among newborns with UTIs is about 10–11% (11).

UTIs again become a problem for males after the age of 50, when prostatic obstruction, urethral instrumentation, and surgery influence the infection rate. Infection at an earlier age in a male is rare and requires careful evaluation for the presence of urinary tract pathology (2,3).

In general, 10–20% of the elderly living at home have bacteriuria. This increases to 20–25% in extended care facilities, 30% in hospitals, and 35–40% in long-stay hospitals. The frequency of infection also tends to rise with increasing age for those 65 years of age and older. Most of the UTIs in these patients are asymptomatic. The reasons for higher UTI rates in elderly people include the high prevalence of prostatitis in males, poor bladder emptying, and fecal incontinence in very old patients (12).

Etiology. Most UTIs are caused by gram-negative aerobic bacilli from the intestinal tract. *E. coli* account for 80% of non-institutionally acquired uncomplicated urinary tract infections, and other Enterobacteriaceae such as *Klebsiella, Enterobacter,* and *Proteus mirabilis* also are common pathogens. *Pseudomonas aeruginosa,* coagulase-negative staphylococci (eg, *S. epidermidis*), and group D streptococci (including enterococci) account for the remaining 5 to 10% of cases. Diphtheroids, microaerophilic streptococci, and non-group D alpha-hemolytic streptococci are usually considered contaminants.

Hospital-acquired urinary tract infections and those associated with urinary tract pathological abnormalities are so-called complicated infections. *E. coli* is still the most prevalent etiologic organism; but there is a higher incidence of infection with other organisms, especially those more refractory to the commonly used antimicrobial agents, such as *Pseudomonas, Proteus, Providencia, Morganella, Klebsiella, Enterobacter, Citrobacter, Serratia,* and *Acinetobacter.* UTIs due to *Staphylococcus aureus* are usually a result of a generalized staphylococcal infection with bacteremia (2).

Pathogenesis. The most common pathway for the spread of bacteria to the urinary tract is the ascending route. A UTI usually begins with heavy and persistent colonization of the vaginal vestibule with intestinal bacteria, especially in women with recurrent UTIs. Once introital colonization has occurred, colonization of the urethra leads to retrograde infection of the bladder (9).

Even with urethral colonization, the bladder has certain defense mechanisms which prevent further spread of the infection. Micturition washes bacteria out of the bladder and is effective if urine can flow freely and the bladder can be emptied completely. Elements in the urine, including organic acids which contribute to a low pH, and urea, which contributes to a high osmolality, also are antibacterial. The bladder mucosa also has antibacterial properties (1,9).

Focal renal involvement may result from the spread of bacteria via the ureters, and may be facilitated by the presence of vesicoureteral reflux or decreased ureteral peristalsis. Reflux can be produced by cystitis alone or by anatomic defects. Ureteral peristalsis is decreased by pregnancy, ureteral obstruction, or gram-negative bacterial endotoxins (1).

Predisposing Factors. Extremes of age, female gender, pregnancy, instrumentation, urinary tract obstruction, neurologic dysfunction, and renal disease are predisposing factors for the development of UTIs.

The incidence of bacteriuria in pregnant women is 4–10%, which is at least twice that of similarly aged nonpregnant women (1). The incidence of acute symptomatic pyelonephritis in pregnant women with untreated bacteriuria is also high. Factors that render the pregnant female more susceptible to symptomatic disease are not known, although hormones and anatomical changes are implicated (13).

Instrumentation, such as urethral and ureteral catheterization, micturating cystourethrography, and cystoscopy, predisposes to UTIs (6,14). Patients undergoing surgical procedures of the urinary tract, such as transurethral prostatectomy, are also at greater risk of developing UTIs (15).

Any obstruction to the free flow of urine (eg, ureteral stenosis, stones, tumor) or mechanical difficulty in evacuating the bladder (eg, prostatic hypertrophy, urethral stricture) predispose patients to UTIs. Furthermore, infections associated with ureteral or renal pelvic obstruction can lead to rapid destruction of the kidney and sepsis (6).

Renal disease increases the susceptibility of the kidney to infection (6). Renal transplant patients demonstrate a high incidence of asymptomatic bacteriuria (16).

Patients with spinal cord injuries, stroke, atherosclerosis, or diabetes may have neurological dysfunctions which frequently result in UTIs. The neurological dysfunction allows pooling of urine, and subsequent catheter use is required. Furthermore, prolonged immobilization facilitates hypercalciuria and stone formation in some of these patients (6).

Other factors which may increase the risk of developing a UTI are less convincing. For example, diabetes mellitus has been associated with UTIs, but recent studies in adult diabetics have yielded conflicting results (17–20). Furthermore, the prevalence of UTIs in juvenile diabetics is similar to that in the general population of school-age children (2,21,22). Another example is sexual intercourse. In recent years, some studies tended to support an association between sexual intercourse and UTIs (23–25), but these studies have not yet adequately established a causal relationship (26).

Clinical Presentation. Symptoms commonly associated with lower UTIs (eg, cystitis) include burning on urination (dysuria), frequent urination, and suprapubic pain. Patients with acute pyelonephritis may also present with loin pain, costovertebral angle tenderness, fever, chills, nausea, vomiting, and blood in the urine (1).

These signs and symptoms correlate poorly both with the actual presence of a UTI and with the extent of the infection. For example, symptoms common in lower UTIs are often the only positive findings in upper UTIs (i.e., pyelonephritis) (1).

Microscopic examination of the urine sediment in patients with documented UTIs reveals the presence of many bacteria (usually more than 20) per high-power field (HPF). A Gram's stain of the unspun urine will show at least one organism per immersion oil field and will usually correlate with a positive urine culture. Pyuria, the presence of at least 5–10 WBCs per HPF in the urine, is frequently present in UTIs but is nonspecific for infection. For example, WBCs from the vaginal area are often contaminants of urine samples. However, WBC casts in the urine strongly suggest an acute pyelonephritis (2).

Diagnosis. The major criterion used for the diagnosis of a UTI is the urine culture. However, proper interpretation of these cultures depends upon appropriate urine collection techniques. Urinating into a sterile collection cup is the most practical method of urine collection. This method of urine specimen collection is especially useful for males but is less useful in female patients because contamination is extremely difficult to avoid (2). The external urethral area first must be thoroughly cleaned and rinsed before collecting the urine specimen after initiation of the urine stream (hence "midstream").

Suprapubic bladder aspiration, although unpleasant from a patient's point of view, is generally not painful and is very reliable. It is not practical for routine office or clinic practice, but may be especially useful when voided urine samples repeatedly yield questionable results, or when patients have voiding problems. Since contamination is negligible, any number of bacteria found by this method reflects infection (2).

Urinary catheterization yields fairly reliable results if performed carefully. Infections may result from the procedure itself because organisms may be introduced into the bladder at the time of catheterization (27).

Urine cultures in the bacteriology laboratory are usually evaluated by the pour plate or streak plate method. Greater than 10^5 colonies of bacteria per ml cultured from a midstream urine specimen confirms the presence of a UTI. A single carefully collected urine specimen provides 80% reliability, and two consecutive cultures of the same organism are virtually diagnostic (2). The criterion of greater than 10^5 colonies per ml is not absolute and may be too restrictive (28).

New, simplified culture methods such as the filter-paper method (eg, Testuria-R), dip-slide method (eg, Uricult), and pad-culture method (Microstix) are as reliable as the traditional laboratory methods for bacterial identification and quantification. The filter-paper method is relatively inexpensive, but it does not differentiate between gram-positive and gram-negative organisms. The dip-slide and pad-culture methods are both accurate, differentiate between gram-positive and gram-negative organisms, and are similar in cost. The dip-slide method has the added advantages of ease in storage and a nitrite indicator pad (discussed below).

Chemical tests are also available as rapid, inexpensive methods to screen for bacteriuria. They are useful in self-screening for asymptomatic bacteriuria at home, especially in patients with recurrent UTIs. The most common test is the nitrite test (Griess Test), which detects urinary nitrite formation from reduction of normally present nitrates by bacteria. At least 10^5 bacteria per ml are necessary to form enough nitrite to react with a reagent to produce a pink color. Some false positive and false negative results occur, but accuracy is enhanced by use of the first morning specimen and by repeat testing. Since this test is a color method, phenazopyridine and methylene blue-containing medications can interfere with the test interpretation (27,29).

Overview of Treatment. Treatment of UTIs is usually successful if the proper antimicrobial agent is administered and if the patient has no underlying complicating factors. The major therapeutic problem posed by UTIs is recurrence. Because recurrent infections tend to be asymptomatic, medical treatment either may be overlooked by the practitioner or may be neglected by the patient.

Many antimicrobial agents are useful in the prevention and treatment of UTIs; however, only those medications which are used specifically in the treatment of UTIs will be presented in this chapter. The reader should consult Tables 1–3 of this chapter for specific information regarding various drugs, indications, doses, and adverse effects.

Uncomplicated Acute UTI

1. A 20-year-old female (married, no children) with no previous history of UTI, complains of burning on urination, frequent urination of small amounts, and bladder pain. She has no fever or costovertebral angle tenderness. A clean-catch midstream urine sample shows gram-negative rods on Gram's stain. A culture and sensitivity (C&S) test is ordered, and the results of a stat urinalysis are as follows:

Appearance:	Straw-colored
Specific gravity:	1.015
pH:	8.0
Protein:	negative
Glucose:	negative
Ketones:	negative
Bilirubin:	negative
Blood:	negative
WBC's:	10–15/HPF
RBC's:	0–1/HPF
Bacteria:	many/HPF
Epithelial cells:	3–5/HPF

Based on these findings, the assessment is that the patient probably has cystitis. What should be the treatment plan at this time?

Drug treatment of an uncomplicated acute cystitis is often started before C&S results are known because the most likely infecting organism and its sensitivity to antibiotics can be predicted. As noted earlier, about 90% of community-acquired infections are caused by the Enterobacteriaceae (especially *E. coli*). Approximately 80% of community-acquired *E. coli* are sensitive to ampicillin, amoxicillin, the tetracyclines, or the sulfonamides, and these agents have continued to be the drugs of choice for initial infections. Alternative medications and doses can be found in Table 1.

2. How long should therapy be continued in this patient?

About 85% of outpatients with acute, uncomplicated, initial UTIs can be treated successfully with a 7–14 day course of oral medications (1). A urine culture and sensitivity should be obtained prior to antibacterial therapy and repeated 2–3 weeks after the completion of therapy (2,6), although this practice is frequently omitted in young patients with a first UTI.

The duration of therapy for urinary tract infections is controversial. The conventional 7–14 day course of antibiotic therapy may be excessive for patients with uncomplicated infections. Bladder instillation with 100 ml of 0.2% neomycin has eradicated infections in patients with bacteria restricted to the bladder (39). In addition, a three-day course of amoxicillin was shown to be as effective as a ten-day course for treating women with lower-tract UTI symptoms and significant bacteriuria (40). Even a single dose of an antibiotic may be as effective as longer courses in a select group of patients, primarily adult females with acute uncomplicated UTI's (41,45–47). Although one study favored multiple-dose therapy, this study may be discounted because 50% of the patients were more than 40 years of age (41).

The advantages of single-dose treatment of UTIs include: improved compliance, cost savings, proven efficacy in a defined population of patients (i.e., young women with acute, uncomplicated UTIs), minimal side effects, and a potentially decreased incidence of bacterial resistance associated with antibiotic overuse. Furthermore, failure to eradicate the organism with a single dose of an antibiotic may help to identify patients who require more intensive investigations of their urinary tract. Studies using localization procedures (bladder washout or ACB test) and radiographic procedures (IVP, micturating cystourethrography) have suggested that bladder infections are usually cured by a single dose of an antibiotic, while kidney infections are not (42–45,48,49).

There are also some concerns about single-dose therapy (50). Sample sizes in comparative studies have been relatively small. The long-range effect of single-dose therapy on recurrence rates needs more extensive evaluation. The safety of single-dose therapy in patients with "silent" kidney infections needs to be evaluated as to whether patients will develop more deeply seated infection, bacteremia, or renal impairment. This latter point may not be a real problem; one study noted that most of the patients with a positive ACB test who failed on single-dose therapy failed on the conventional 7–14 days of antibiotic treatment as well (45).

Single-dose antibiotic therapy of UTIs may be considered in young women with acute uncomplicated UTIs. Patients with systemic manifestations of infection, renal disease, anatomical abnormalities of the urinary tract, diabetes mellitus, pregnancy, history of antibiotic resistance, and history of relapse on single-dose therapy should be treated with conventional antibacterial therapy for 7–14 days. Since this young female patient does not have any of these contraindications to single-dose therapy, her acute uncomplicated UTI can be treated either with amoxicillin 3.0 gm or with the combination of trimethoprim 480 mg and sulfamethoxazole 2400 mg (3 double strength tablets of Bactrim or Septra). A urine culture and sensitivity should be obtained in 1–2 weeks.

3. Conventional therapy with sulfisoxazole was prescribed for this patient in a dose of 2 gm stat, then 1 gm qid for 10 days. Is sulfisoxazole the sulfonamide of choice?

Different sulfonamides do not result in different clinical outcomes in patients with UTIs, but sulfisoxazole is often considered the agent of choice. Although one might predict that sulfisoxazole would be most efficacious because it is excreted into the urine more rapidly than long-acting compounds such as sulfamethoxazole, there is no concrete evidence to document its clinical "superiority." Cost is the major factor affecting one's choice of a sulfonamide (51).

4. What is the rationale and necessity for the "stat" 2 gm dose of sulfisoxazole? If sulfamethoxazole were used, would a loading dose be required?

The 2 gm loading dose is recommended in the manufacturer's product literature but is unnecessary and probably represents a "carry-over" from earlier days when long-acting sulfonamides were in use. A single oral dose of sulfisoxazole is well absorbed, and peak serum levels are reached in

Table 1.

COMMONLY USED ORAL ANTIMICROBIAL AGENTS FOR ACUTE URINARY TRACT INFECTIONS[31,32,32-38]

Drug	Usual Dose		Pregnancy	Breast Milk (BM)	Comments
	Adult	Pediatric			
Amoxicillin	0.25 gm q8h or 3.0 gm single dose	20–40 mg/kg/d in 3 doses	crosses placenta $\frac{(cord)}{(maternal)} = 30\%$	small amount present	Drug of choice for acute uncomplicated infections
Ampicillin	0.25–0.5 gm qid	50–100 mg/kg/d in 4 doses	crosses placenta	variable amount $\frac{(BM)}{(serum)} < 1{-}30\%$	Same as amoxicillin
Carbenicillin	0.382–0.764 gm qid	50–65 mg/kg/d in 4 doses			Drug of choice for pseudomonal infection; alternate choice for organisms resistant to other agents
Cefadroxil	0.5–1.0 gm bid	15–30 mg/kg/d in 4 doses	crosses placenta		Alternate choice for patients allergic to penicillins, although cross hypersensitivity can occur. Drug of choice for coagulase negative staphylococcus
Cephalexin	0.25–0.5 gm qid		crosses placenta	enters breast milk	
Cephradine	0.25–0.5 gm qid		crosses placenta $\frac{(cord)}{(maternal)} = 10\%$	$\frac{(BM)}{(serum)} = 20\%$	
Cinoxacin	0.5 gm bid				Alternate choice; resistance may develop rapidly
Nalidixic Acid	1.0 gm qid	50 mg/kg/d in 4 doses	manufacturer reports safety in 2nd and 3rd trimesters	variable amounts; not detectable to 4 mcg/ml; hemolytic anemia reported; use with caution	Same as cinoxacin
Nitrofurantoin	0.05–0.1 gm qid	5–7 mg/kg/d in 4 doses	no reports of transfer or adverse effect	variable amounts; not detectable to 30%; may cause hemolysis in G6PD deficient baby	Alternate choice

Drug	Dose (adult)	Dose (pediatric)	Placental transfer	Breast milk	Comments
Doxycycline	0.1 gm bid			$\dfrac{(BM)}{(serum)} = 30\text{--}40\%$	Effective for acute urethral syndrome. Avoid in children less than 8 years old. Alters bowel flora to favor resistant organisms, reducing its effectiveness in recurrence
Tetracycline	0.25 gm qid		avoid throughout pregnancy; deposition into and deformities of bone and teeth may occur	$\dfrac{(BM)}{(serum)} = 20\text{--}140\%$ risk may be decreased by binding to milk calcium, but is best to avoid	
Sulfisoxazole	0.5–1.0 gm qid	50–100 mg/kg/d in 4 doses	crosses placenta; avoid near term; displacement of bilirubin may lead to hyperbilirubinemia and kernicterus	enters breast milk; displacement of bilirubin may lead to neonate jaundice; may cause hemolysis in G6PD deficient baby	Drug of choice for acute uncomplicated infections. Alters bowel flora to favor resistant organisms, reducing its effectiveness in recurrence
Sulfamethoxazole	1.0 gm bid	60 mg/kg/d in 2 doses			
Trimethoprim	0.1 gm bid		crosses placenta $\dfrac{(cord)}{(maternal)} = 60\%$	$\dfrac{(BM)}{(serum)} >1$	Alternate choice
Trimethoprim plus Sulfamethoxazole	0.16 + 0.8 gm bid or 0.48 + 2.4 gm single dose				TMP-SMX should be reserved for recurrent infections

30–120 minutes. The elimination half-life is 3–6 hours, and 70% of the drug appears in the urine as the free, active form. Because it is rapidly absorbed and appears in high concentrations in the urine, a loading dose of sulfisoxazole is not particularly advantageous and need not be given (51,52).

Sulfamethoxazole is not as completely or rapidly absorbed as sulfisoxazole. Peak serum levels are achieved within 4–6 hours, the elimination half-life of sulfamethoxazole is approximately 9–12 hours, and about 50% of the drug appears in the urine as the free, active form. Because of its longer half-life, sulfamethoxazole is generally administered only twice daily. Despite these pharmacokinetic differences, a loading dose of sulfamethoxazole is also probably unnecessary because most patients with cystitis are not critically ill (51,52).

5. Culture and sensitivity studies in this patient show a few *Klebsiella* and greater than 10^5/ml *Proteus mirabilis* which are sensitive to ampicillin, cephalosporins, trimethoprim, trimethoprim-sulfamethoxazole, and gentamicin. The *Proteus* also are intermediately sensitive to sulfonamides, carbenicillin, and nalidixic acid; and resistant to tetracycline. Based on the clinical presentation and the recent culture and sensitivity reports, did the patient have a true urinary tract infection?

As noted earlier, more than 10^5 colonies of bacteria/ml cultured from a midstream urine specimen confirms the diagnosis of UTI. Thus, therapy was definitely indicated in this patient. However, this criterion is not absolute. In performing suprapubic aspirations in over 900 women who had greater than 10^5 colonies per ml cultured from midstream urine samples, Little et al observed that over 90% of the gram-negative infections and about 70% of the gram-positive infections could be confirmed (53). In patients with midstream urine cultures of 10^4–10^5 colonies per ml, suprapubic aspiration confirmed 74% of gram-negative infections and about 30% of gram-positive infections. Low midstream urine concentrations of a single organism may be an early infection, dilution of a true infection, or evidence of an extraluminal infection. In any case, a true infection may be present, especially if the organism is gram-negative.

The presence of mixed flora (two or more organisms) is rare except in severely debilitated individuals. The presence of mixed flora frequently suggests contamination, and a repeat specimen should be obtained.

6. Two days later, when the patient returns for her scheduled clinic appointment, she is completely free of symptoms. Another urine specimen is obtained, and microscopic examination reveals no bacteria. Considering that the organism demonstrated only intermediate sensitivity to sulfonamides, should this patient continue her sulfisoxazole therapy?

Bacterial susceptibility to different antimicrobial drugs is usually tested by placing antibacterial impregnated discs on an agar surface which has been seeded with the infecting organism. Bacterial sensitivity, or susceptibility, is indicated by a zone of inhibited growth around the disk containing the drug. Most discs are impregnated with a quantity of drug which correlates with achievable *serum* concentrations. However, drugs useful in the treatment of UTIs are primarily excreted by the kidney, and urine concentrations of these drugs may be 20–100 times greater than the serum concentration. Therefore, a particular organism which is only intermediately sensitive, or even "resistant" to the concentration of antibacterial drug in the testing disk, might be very sensitive to the high concentration of drug in the urine (54). Furthermore, *in vitro* and *in vivo* sensitivity may correlate poorly.

When antimicrobial therapy is empirically chosen without the benefit of culture and sensitivity testing results, the patient is in essence serving as her own "sensitivity study." If the infecting organism is sensitive, the urine will be sterile in 24 and certainly by 48 hours. If a urine specimen collected 48 hours after initiation of therapy is not sterile and the patient has been taking the medication properly, either the antibiotic is inappropriate or the focus of infection is deeper (eg, pyelonephritis, abscess, obstruction). Because the urine specimen in this patient now is sterile, the appropriate antimicrobial is being used (regardless of sensitivity studies), and the full course of therapy should be completed (2).

Hospital-Acquired Acute UTI

7. An alert 70-year-old female with chest pain was hospitalized to rule out acute myocardial infarction. This is her third hospi-

talization for chest pain in the last six months. Two days after admission, she complained of burning on urination and bladder pain. Ampicillin 250 mg orally every six hours was ordered after microscopic examination of the urine indicated the presence of a urinary tract infection. Was this empiric ampicillin therapy appropriate?

The sensitivity of community-acquired pathogenic bacteria to antimicrobial agents differs from hospital-acquired bacteria, and this antibacterial susceptibility frequently varies from one hospital to another. Therefore, the microbiology department of a particular hospital should be consulted to determine current trends in the susceptibility of bacteria acquired in that setting. In general, *E. coli* is still the predominant urinary tract infecting organism, but there is an increased incidence of infections caused by other gram-negative bacteria such as *Proteus* and *Pseudomonas.*

Repeated courses of antibiotic therapy, anatomic defects of the urinary tract, old age, and repetitive exposure to the hospital environment are associated with a higher incidence of antibiotic resistance. In particular, *Pseudomonas, Proteus, Providencia, Morganella, Klebsiella, Enterobacter, Acinetobacter,* and *Serratia* are difficult to eradicate because they usually are less susceptible to commonly used antimicrobial agents. This particular patient is elderly, hospitalized, and repetitively exposed to potentially resistant organisms during her multiple hospitalizations. However, if prompt treatment is deemed necessary, as in this case, ampicillin is a reasonable first choice because *E. coli* is still the most likely causative agent. When culture and sensitivity results are available, a different agent may be required (1,2).

Acute Pyelonephritis

8. A 45-year-old female diabetic comes to the emergency room complaining of frequent urination, fever, shaking chills, and flank pain. She takes 20 units of NPH insulin subcutaneously every morning. Positive physical findings include a temperature of 103°F, a pulse of 110/min, blood pressure of 90/60 mm Hg, and costovertebral angle (CVA) tenderness. A Gram's stain of the patient's urine reveals gram-negative rods, and a stat urinalysis demonstrates glucosuria, macroscopic hematuria, 20–25 WBC's/hpf, numerous bac-

teria/hpf, and the presence of WBC casts. The patient also has a blood sugar of 400 mg/dl. The patient is admitted to the hospital with a diagnosis of acute bacterial pyelonephritis, and routine laboratory tests including an SMA, a CBC with differential, and specimens of urine and blood for culture and sensitivity are ordered. The patient is started on an IV of normal saline, one gram of ampicillin IV every 6 hours, and a rainbow schedule of regular insulin based on every-6-hour blood sugars. Why is this patient predisposed to the development of pyelonephritis?

There is some evidence for a higher incidence of renal infection in diabetic patients, possibly because of altered antibacterial defense mechanisms in these patients and because of bladder catheterizations when these patients are hospitalized (55). Histologic findings of chronic pyelonephritis also are more common in diabetics, despite the uncertain relationship of this finding to bacterial infection (56). UTIs are major complicating factors in the increased incidence of perinephritis, perinephric abscess, and acute papillary necrosis observed in individuals with diabetes (57).

9. Why was this patient with a urinary tract infection hospitalized?

The management of the *acutely febrile individual* who may have evidence of an upper urinary tract infection (eg, flank pain) centers around the need for hospitalization. Although the majority of patients with clinical pyelonephritis can be managed as outpatients, the need for hospitalization is often dependent on the social situation as well as the ability of the individual to maintain an adequate fluid intake and to tolerate oral medications. Most patients with evidence of bacteremia (eg, shaking chills) or any evidence of endotoxemia (eg, hypotension) should be hospitalized. It is usually prudent to hospitalize the febrile diabetic patient who has a urinary tract infection. This patient should be hospitalized because she is *acutely ill* with a high temperature, a rapid pulse, hypotension, shaking chills, and hyperglycemia.

10. Why might parenteral ampicillin be inappropriate for this patient?

The majority of patients with a urinary tract infection who are seen by a primary care clinician will be afebrile, not seriously ill, have no mechanical complications, and will have had neither a prior infection nor a previous urine culture. For such individuals without indications for hospitalization or without suspicions of a pyelonephritis, an inexpensive oral agent such as a sulfonamide, tetracycline, or ampicillin will usually suffice. However, in the acutely ill patient with pyelonephritis and suspected bacteremia, the worst should be expected (eg, the infection may be caused by a gram-negative bacillus which may be resistant to many drugs). Thus, the use of ampicillin in this patient may be questioned. She is acutely ill, bacteremic, diabetic, and has gram-negative organisms in her urine. Patients with diabetes, as well as patients receiving corticosteroids, are prone to colonization with unusual organisms. Therefore, this patient should be treated with a parenteral aminoglycoside or cephalosporin rather than ampicillin. Since most hospital laboratories will be able to substantiate or refute this hypothesis within 48 hours, the aminoglycoside or cephalosporin can be discontinued if other rational therapy is more appropriate.

11. Would it be more appropriate to achieve bactericidal concentrations in the urine or in the serum for this patient?

When the renal parenchyma is infected (eg, pyelonephritis as opposed to uncomplicated cystitis), adequate tissue concentrations of the antimicrobial agents may be needed. Although it is not clear whether renal parenchymal concentrations of antibiotics correlate best with blood or urine concentrations, vigorous treatment with a bactericidal drug to which the organism is sensitive is advisable (see Table 2). Patients requiring hospitalization should be treated with parenteral antibiotics for 3–5 days, or until they have been afebrile for 24–48 hours. This should be followed with a course of oral antibiotics for at least 10–14 days. Specimens for culture and sensitivity should be obtained on the second day of therapy (to rule out treatment failure), 2–3 weeks after the completion of therapy, and again at 3 months (1,6).

Acute Urethral Syndrome

12. A 22-year-old female complains of increased frequency and painful urination. Urinalysis reveals 10–15 WBC's/hpf, but no bacteria are seen on a Gram's stain of the urine. Phenazopyridine 200 mg three times daily is prescribed. What would be a reason-

Table 2.

ANTIMICROBIAL AGENTS USED IN THE TREATMENT OF ACUTE BACTERIAL PYELONEPHRITIS[2,31,32]

Drug	Adult Daily Dose		Pediatric Daily Dose		Usual Dosage Interval
	Oral	Parenteral	Oral	Parenteral	
Ampicillin	2 gm	2–4 gm	100 mg/kg	50–100 mg/kg	q 6h
Amoxicillin	1.5 gm	—	40 mg/kg	—	q 8h
Trimethoprim plus Sulfamethoxazole	320 mg TMP 1600 mg SMX	—	8 mg/kg TMP 40 mg/kg SMX	—	q 12h
Gentamicin	—	3–5 mg/kg	—	6–7.5 mg/kg	q 8h
Tobramycin	—	3–5 mg/kg	—	3–5 mg/kg	q 8h
Amikacin	—	15 mg/kg	—	15 mg/kg	q 8–12h
Cephalothin	—	2–6 gm	—	40–80 mg/kg	q 4–6h
Cephradine	2–4 gm	2–4 gm	25–50 mg/kg	50–100 mg/kg	q 6h
Cefazolin	—	1.5–4 gm	—	25–50 mg/kg	q 6–8h
Cephapirin	—	2–6 gm	—	40–80 mg/kg	q 4–6h
Cefamandole	—	1.5–6 gm	—	50–100 mg/kg	q 4–8h
Cefoxitin	—	4–8 gm	—	80–160 mg/kg	q 4–8h
Cefotaxime	—	2–6 gm	—	—	q 6–8h
Cephalexin	2–4 gm	—	25–50 mg/kg	—	

able assessment of this patient's clinical presentation?

Not all patients who present with symptoms of urinary tract infections (increased frequency of urination, pain on voiding, and urgency) actually have a bacterial infection. In several studies of general practice populations (227), as many as 50% of women presenting with these problems were found to have insignificant bacteriuria. In one study, 8% of women presenting with dysuria were found to have gonorrhea and 17% vaginitis. Thus, urinary tract infections cannot be differentiated from other causes of these symptoms without a careful examination of the patient and the urine.

The absence of an organism on Gram's stain may mean that the urine specimen is sterile or that the concentration of the organism in the urine sample is small. Patients with dysuria who do not have greater than 10^5 colonies of bacteria per ml of cultured urine are generally said to have acute urethral syndrome (28,58). In one study of 59 patients with the acute urethral syndrome, 27 had true infection confirmed by pure isolates from suprapubic aspiration (28). Of the remaining 32 patients, 11 had evidence of recent chlamydial infection either by isolation of the organism or by raised antibody titer. Furthermore, pyuria (greater than 8 leukocytes/ml) in conjunction with clinical symptoms of UTI but with less than 10^5 bacteria in the urine was associated with either an *E. coli* or chlamydial infection in the majority of cases. In contrast, very few infections could be documented if pyuria was not present. Thus, patients with the acute urethral syndrome may or may not have a true infection, based on the presence or absence of pyuria. Since this patient has 10–15 WBC's/hpf in her urine and is symptomatic, an infection cannot be ruled out with absolute certainty despite the absence of bacteria on a Gram's stain of the urine.

13. Should this patient be treated with antibiotics?

A double-blind, placebo-controlled study evaluated the use of doxycycline 100 mg twice daily in patients with the acute urethral syndrome (59). Clinical cure of bacteriuria and pyuria was significantly greater in the doxycycline-treated group. The doxycycline did not alter symptoms in patients without pyuria. Since *E. coli,* other coliforms, and *Chlamydia trachomatis* are the usual causes of acute urethral syndrome, antibiotic therapy, which includes chlamydial coverage, may be a reasonable initial treatment in patients presenting with urinary tract symptoms if pyuria is also present. All tetracyclines and sulfonamides with or without trimethoprim probably will also be proven effective, but only doxycycline has been studied in the acute urethral syndrome at this time.

14. Why is phenazopyridine inappropriate for this patient?

Phenazopyridine (Pyridium), a urinary tract analgesic, is often prescribed alone or concurrently with an antibacterial agent for the symptomatic relief of dysuria. It is commonly found in fixed combination with antimicrobials such as sulfisoxazole (Azo-Gantrisin), sulfamethoxazole (Azo-Gantanol), and tetracycline (Azotrex). Although 200 mg three times daily may relieve dysuria in patients (60–62), it is ineffective in the management of true urinary tract infections. Therefore, this drug, by itself, probably would not be of value to this patient if an infection is present.

In an uncontrolled study, 50% of patients experienced relief of urinary symptoms when treated with phenazopyridine and antibacterials if infection was suspected (61). Likewise, phenazopyridine improved urinary symptoms better than methylene blue; however, the majority of patients received antibacterial agents concurrently (62). More recently, comparisons of phenazopyridine to flavoxate for symptomatic relief of urinary disorders (63) have noted similar relief of specific symptoms in most cases, but again, both antibiotics and systemic analgesics were permitted. The logical study should compare symptomatic relief with appropriate antibacterial therapy plus phenazopyridine to relief with antibacterial therapy alone, but such a study has not been published.

15. What adverse effects have been associated with phenazopyridine?

Phenazopyridine is an azo dye and may discolor the urine to an orange-red, orange-brown, or red color which can cause staining of clothes. Other adverse effects of phenazopyridine occur as a result of acute overdose or chronic ingestion by elderly patients or patients with decreased renal function. Phenazopyridine can produce methemoglobin *in vitro* (64,65), and accumulation may account for the toxicity associated with chronic dosing in elderly patients (68). *In vivo,* about 50% of phenazopyridine is metabolized to aniline, which can cause methemoglobinemia and hemolytic anemia. Therefore, acute overdose or chronic ingestion of phenazopyridine might lead to the accumulation of aniline and subsequent methemoglobinemia or hemolytic anemia. Interestingly, the aniline produced by ingestion of 200 mg phenazopyridine three times daily exceeds the 35 mg maximal allowable dose of aniline (68). The hemolytic anemia following ingestion of phenazopyridine occurs primarily in patients with G6PD deficiency.

Rare cases of acute renal failure have occurred in elderly patients, especially when large doses were used in the presence of impaired renal function (66,67). The acute renal failure occurred within days of initiating therapy and reversed one to two weeks after drug discontinuance.

Cases of allergic hepatitis have been rare following brief exposure to phenazopyridine. A fever spike with nausea and abdominal pain were common initial symptoms, and re-exposure to phenazopyridine resulted in recurrence of symptoms within 24 hours (69–71).

Asymptomatic Bacteriuria

16. An asymptomatic 6-year-old schoolgirl is found to have significant bacteriuria on routine screening. Should she be treated with an antimicrobial agent?

The management of patients with asymptomatic bacteriuria depends upon the clinical setting in which it is found. Asymptomatic bacteriuria occurs in a heterogeneous group of patients with different prognoses and risks. Some patients will have significant bacteriuria ($>10^5$ bacteria/ml of urine) without pyuria. Others may have pyuria without significant bacteriuria. The patients in this latter group probably have self-limiting infections and do not require treatment if asymptomatic. However, asymptomatic patients with significant bacteriuria and pyuria subsequently may develop overt pyelonephritis, and therapy is probably warranted if significant bacteriuria is confirmed on successive cultures (6).

Although the management of asymptomatic bacteriuria is varied, the potential for long-term complications from UTIs must be considered. UTIs in infants and preschool children (predominantly girls) are occasionally associated with renal tissue damage during the growth phase of this organ. Although the risk of significant chronic renal disease in a child is small (76), a clubbed calyx,

kidney scarring, or gross destruction may result (7,72–75). Asymptomatic bacteriuria of childhood also is important because it may be a manifestation of mechanical disease and, therefore, should be fully evaluated. Thus, screening for bacteriuria in young females and treating those with positive cultures, regardless of their clinical presentation, seems reasonable. Furthermore, treatment of this 6-year-old girl is important, because if any renal damage occurs as a result of asymptomatic bacteriuria, it frequently occurs during childhood.

17. The decision to treat the asymptomatic bacteriuria of the 6-year-old girl in the previous question was primarily based upon increased probability of renal damage during childhood. What other population groups should be treated for asymptomatic bacteriuria?

In the absence of urinary tract obstruction, UTIs in adults rarely, if ever, lead to progressive renal damage (72,78). Therefore, asymptomatic bacteriuria may be ignored in adult patients who have no evidence of mechanical obstruction or renal insufficiency. However, aggressive antimicrobial therapy is appropriate during pregnancy. As many as 40% of pregnant women with asymptomatic bacteriuria later develop symptomatic urinary tract infections, particularly pyelonephritis. In addition, a lower birth weight has been associated with asymptomatic bacteriuria (175,226). Treatment may be chosen on the basis of the *in vitro* susceptibility testing by selecting the least expensive and least toxic agent. Tetracyclines are to be avoided because they may stain and weaken the forming dentition of the unborn child. Sulfonamides are to be avoided in late pregnancy because they can contribute to kernicterus in the neonate (also see Questions 35–36).

Bacteriuria also has been associated with excess mortality in a relatively select population of elderly patients (79). Nevertheless, therapy of asymptomatic bacteriuria in the elderly is by no means mandatory in the absence of obstruction (80). The UTI can be cured in these patients, but frequent relapse and reinfection requires continual retreatment or chronic suppressive therapy. As a result, some practitioners have opted to withhold therapy in the asymptomatic older patient when the expense, side effects, and potential complications of drug therapy might outweigh the theoretical benefits (4,81).

Recurrent UTI

18. A 28-year-old female with a history of recurrent infections was recently treated for an *E. coli* UTI with ampicillin 250 mg every six hours orally for 10 days. A repeat urinalysis was scheduled, but she cancelled her appointment because she "felt fine." Six weeks later, she returned to the clinic with signs and symptoms of another UTI. The only other medication she has taken is an oral contraceptive. Why would culture and sensitivity testing of a urine sample be especially useful at this time?

Repeat culture and sensitivity data should aid in the determination of whether this infection represents a relapse or a reinfection. Relapse refers to a recurrence of bacteriuria caused by the same microorganism that was present before the initiation of therapy. Most relapses appear within one to two weeks after the completion of therapy and are assumed to be due to the persistence of the organism in the urinary tract. Reinfection implies recurrence of bacteriuria with a different microorganism. Reinfections may occur at any time during or after the completion of treatment, but most appear several weeks to several months later. Approximately 80% of recurrences are due to reinfection (78,80). These reinfections generally are due to introital colonization with Enterobacteriaceae from the intestinal tract (82).

19. Is there an association between this patient's use of oral contraceptives and her risk of contracting a UTI?

The available literature does not appear to support an association between oral contraceptive use and UTIs. The incidence of bacteriuria in 12,000 healthy women taking oral contraceptives was 2.4%, as compared to a 1.6% incidence among those who had never taken oral contraceptives (83). Although greater sexual activity among the oral contraceptive users might account at least in part for these findings, there was a positive correlation between the dose of estrogen and the frequency of bacteriuria. However, the overall incidence of bacteriuria in this study was low compared to that expected for the general population (2 to 10%). Furthermore, a small prospective study involving eighty-two women demonstrated no difference between oral contraceptive users and non-users with respect to bacteriuria (84). Finally, birth control methodologies do not

appear to affect the rate or duration of bacteria in the urine following sexual intercourse (25).

Ureteral dilatation similar to that noted in pregnancy has been observed in some women taking oral contraceptives, and the stasis of urine may facilitate the rise of bacteria from the lower tract and cause infection (85,86). However, ureteral dilatation is not consistently observed in UTI patients who are taking oral contraceptives (87).

20. Pending the C&S results, what therapy should be instituted in this patient?

This patient has a history of recurrent infections and now probably has a reinfection. Therefore, ampicillin may be a reasonable choice once again. If this patient had been initially treated with a sulfonamide or a tetracycline, it would be advisable to switch to a different agent, because bacteria frequently develop resistance to these drugs. The probability that a resistant organism will be responsible for the infection increases when the interval between infectious episodes is short, because if several months elapse between each episode of antimicrobial therapy, normal fecal bacterial flora will have been re-established.

The alteration of fecal flora caused by the sulfonamides and tetracyclines makes these drugs poor choices for repeated use in cases of frequent reinfection, especially when C&S results are not known. The development of bacterial resistance may also limit the usefulness of these agents for chronic antimicrobial therapy (88).

21. What other drugs may be useful for this patient's recurrent infections?

Nitrofurantoin is effective against 80–90% of *E. coli* strains. It does not significantly alter the fecal or introital flora, and the development of resistance from previously sensitive strains does not occur. Therefore, it is generally a useful agent for the treatment of recurrent *E. coli* infections. Culture and sensitivity testing should not be neglected, however. Reinfection can involve a new organism, and other infecting organisms such as *P. mirabilis* or *Klebsiella* tend to be somewhat resistant to nitrofurantoin (31).

Nalidixic acid is effective against a broad spectrum of gram-negative bacteria commonly infecting the urinary tract, including *E. coli, Proteus, Klebsiella,* and *Enterobacter. Pseudomonas, Staphylococci,* and *Strep. fecalis* are not sensitive to nalidixic acid at concentrations achievable in the urine. Nalidixic acid might be most effective for UTIs secondary to *Klebsiella* or indole-positive *Proteus,* and in penicillin-allergic individuals who have *Proteus mirabilis* infections (89). The usefulness of nalidixic acid can be limited by the rapid development of resistant organisms. The frequency of this occurrence is disputed. In an evaluation of fifty patients treated with nalidixic acid, thirteen (26%) developed resistant strains of the same species and serotype that were sensitive to the drug prior to treatment (90). Others have reported a lower incidence (6–14%) of resistance (91,92). The resistance generally appears within 2–3 days, is extremely stable, nontransferable, and is thought to result from a single-step mutation (90). Although the possibility of rapid emergence of resistant bacteria during therapy with nalidixic acid has been of concern, several investigations now suggest that inordinate selection of resistant bacterial strains and treatment failure do not occur when full therapeutic dosages of 4 grams/day are administered (224,225). Furthermore, the incidence of nalidixic acid-resistant strains within a community has not increased (93).

Cinoxacin is similar to nalidixic acid, but *E. coli* are more sensitive to low concentrations of cinoxacin than to nalidixic acid (94). Essentially all *E. coli* strains as well as *Klebsiella, Enterobacter, Proteus,* and *Serratia* are inhibited at 8 mcg/ml, but much higher concentrations are achieved in the urine (95). Thus, the clinical superiority of cinoxacin over nalidixic acid is questionable because high concentrations of both drugs are achieved in the urine (96). *E. coli* resistance to cinoxacin has been demonstrated *in vitro* and occurs at a rate similar to that of nalidixic acid (95,96). Although the development of resistance has not been a problem during clinical treatment, this potential risk should be considered because other agents are available for UTIs. Unlike nalidixic acid, which is dosed four times daily, cinoxacin can be given twice daily.

Trimethoprim and **trimethoprim-sulfamethoxazole** also are useful in this setting. Carbenicillin and the cephalosporins are unnecessary unless the results of *in vitro* sensitivity tests indicate that they offer a distinct advantage over less costly agents (2).

22. Greater than 10⁵/ml *Proteus mirabilis*, sensitive to ampicillin, was noted in this patient's urine. One week after completing her second course of ampicillin therapy, signs and symptoms of a UTI again appeared. What additional clinical evaluative procedures should be performed at this time?

One should first attempt to rule out causes for relapse. Inadequate therapy resulting from patient non-compliance with the prescribed treatment, inappropriate antibiotic selection, or bacterial resistance to the prescribed agent should be considered if significant bacteriuria persists in spite of treatment. Subsequently, structural abnormalities of the urinary tract should be ruled out. Infected kidney stones and unilateral atrophic kidneys are common but correctable abnormalities in females. Since *P. mirabilis* is the most common organism found in infected stones, repeated *Proteus* infections should raise the index of suspicion for an infected stone which is "seeding" the bladder (97). Finally, one must consider renal infections, which cause the great majority of relapsing UTIs (98). Chronic bacterial prostatitis, which is common in males, need not be considered because this patient is female.

Radiologic investigation, by intravenous pyelography (IVP) or micturating cystourethrography, is helpful in uncovering urinary tract abnormalities such as polycystic kidneys, stones, papillary necrosis, chronic atrophic pyelonephritis, or reflux that are amenable to surgery. Therefore, these diagnostic evaluations are normally reserved for children; males younger than 50 years of age; and patients with UTIs in association with bacteremia, ureteral colic, or passage of stones, because these populations are most likely to have surgically correctable lesions. Routine radiological assessment in adult women and elderly males with UTIs is usually not indicated (99).

23. What localization studies are needed to evaluate this patient's UTI?

There is some evidence that the treatment outcome of urinary tract infections is dictated by the anatomic site of the infection. As a result, a variety of both direct and indirect methods have been developed to assist in the localization of urinary tract infections to either the kidney or to the bladder. Ureteral catherization and bladder washout technique are direct methods for localizing UTIs; and indirect methods include serum antibodies, urine concentration test, urinary enzyme excretion, and the detection of antibody-coated bacteria in the urine. The majority of these methods are not clinically applicable because the test is either too cumbersome or not sufficiently sensitive or specific. Only the antibody-coated bacteria (ACB) assay has clinical applicability at this time (100).

The ACB assay is based on the premise that bacteria in the kidney stimulate an immune response, whereas bacteria localized to the bladder do not. Thus, with renal infections, bacteria become coated with a specific antibody which can be detected in the urine by direct immunofluorescence. Antibody-coated bacteria have been demonstrated in various types of patients with UTIs (55,101–104).

The ACB assay correlated well with the site of infection in early studies (105,106) which used the bladder washout technique as a comparative procedure; however, when the ACB test is compared to ureteral catheterization (the reference standard among localization procedures) the results are not as encouraging (107,108). The overall probability that a patient with a positive ACB assay will have a renal infection is 81.3%, and the probability that a patient with negative ACB test will have bladder bacteriuria is 78.8% (109). Thus, approximately 20% of ACB assays result in both false-positives and false-negatives. Prostatic infection in males (110), rectal and vaginal contamination of the urine in children (111), heavy proteinuria (112), urinary tract tumors or stones (107,113), chronic vesicostomy tubes (114), and ileal conduits (115) may cause false-positive ACB assays. In addition, the antibody-coated bacteria in the urine may not be specific for kidney infections, but instead may only represent a local immune response to bacterial invasion of the uroepithelium at any site along the urinary tract (107,116,117). Thus, a bladder infection with mucosal invasion might yield a false-positive ACB test. False-negatives occur when the time interval between bacterial invasion and urine sampling is not sufficient to allow for an immune response. For example, in experimental pyelonephritis in rabbits, it takes eleven days before antibodies are found in the urine (118). Finally, variations in the criteria used by different investigators for determining a positive ACB test may be contributing to the inaccuracies (117) of this assay.

Although afebrile patients with only lower urinary tract symptomatology may actually have an upper urinary tract infection, localization of this patient's UTI is impractical at this time.

24. Pending C&S results, what would be a reasonable medication for this patient at this time?

This patient should be treated with a bactericidal agent because of the possibility of renal involvement. An antimicrobial with a low order of bacterial resistance also would be desirable because of the frequency of this patient's urinary tract infections. Therefore, trimethoprim-sulfamethoxazole (TMP-SMX) would be a reasonable choice.

Gram-positive and gram-negative microorganisms, with the notable exceptions of *Pseudomonas aeruginosa* and anaerobes are generally susceptible to TMP-SMX. The efficacy of this drug combination largely depends on the sensitivity of the organism to trimethoprim, although *Neisseria gonorrheae* are relatively more susceptible to the sulfonamide. Individually, trimethoprim and sulfamethoxazole are bacteriostatic, but in combination they are bactericidal against most organisms (119). Furthermore, this combination is almost uniformly successful in the treatment of UTI, even against organisms that were originally resistant to either agent alone. In one study, 78% of patients with recurrent, persistent infections unresponsive to treatment with sulfamethoxazole and trimethoprim separately responded to the combination (120). Most urinary pathogens seem susceptible to this drug combination.

The ratio of trimethoprim to sulfamethoxazole in the available products is 1:5 (eg, 80 mg trimethoprim/400 mg sulfamethoxazole in the tablet). This has been chosen to achieve an approximate 1:20 ratio of peak serum concentrations of the two drugs, which is optimal for synergistic activity against most microorganisms. However, trimethoprim has a much larger distribution volume than sulfamethoxazole, so the concentration ratios achieved in other tissues and fluids (eg, urine) vary. Nevertheless, bactericidal activity is still potentiated with drug ratios ranging from 1:5 to 1:40 *in vitro* (121–123). The urine concentrations of trimethoprim and sulfamethoxazole far exceed the MIC values for most susceptible urinary pathogens, and probably account for the combination's effectiveness in the management of UTIs (124).

25. How long should this therapy be continued?

The duration of therapy of relapsing infections is usually about 14 days. However, a six week course of therapy has been associated with a better cure rate than a two week course of therapy for patients with renal infections who relapse (82). Some recommend even longer courses of therapy ranging from six months to one year. These prolonged courses generally should be reserved for children, adults who have continuous symptoms, or adults who are at high risk of developing progressive renal damage. Therefore, this patient should be treated for at least two weeks and perhaps as long as six weeks.

26. This patient was previously treated with TMP-SMX for a UTI and experienced nausea and vomiting after taking the medication. Would trimethoprim alone be an appropriate substitute?

Trimethoprim alone and trimethoprim in combination with sulfamethoxazole are active *in vitro* against many of the Enterobacteriaceae associated with UTIs. TMP-SMX is more active against these organisms when combined in a ratio of 1:20, which is optimal for synergistic activity (129). Due to pharmacokinetic differences, however, the ratio of trimethoprim to sulfamethoxazole in the urine following standard doses is 1:1, and this ratio is probably not synergistic (130–132). In addition, clinical studies have failed to show a difference in the bacteriological response to UTIs between two tablets of TMP-SMX bid and trimethoprim 200 mg bid (133–136). Thus, trimethoprim is an effective alternative to TMP-SMX in the management of both chronic and acute UTIs. It would be especially appropriate for this patient because gastrointestinal intolerance to TMP-SMX is most commonly attributed to the sulfamethoxazole component, and trimethoprim is probably associated with a lower incidence of adverse effects. There is some concern for the potential development of resistant organisms (139) to trimethoprim, but studies using trimethoprim alone have failed to demonstrate a significant increase in the resistance of bacteria (137,138).

Currently, trimethoprim is approved only for acute uncomplicated UTIs in a dosage of 100 mg bid for ten days. Published clinical studies, however, generally have used 200 mg bid for varying lengths of time. Although trimethoprim use is increasing, the combination of trimethoprim with sulfamethoxazole may be more advantageous in treating chronic UTIs of patients with structural abnormalities of the genitourinary tract (126).

27. The patient was successfully treated with trimethoprim. Would subsequent prophylactic antimicrobial therapy be appropriate?

Chronic urinary tract infections may be managed by treating each recurrent infection with an appropriate antibacterial for a specific period of time or by administering chronic, low-dose, prophylactic therapy.

The frequency of urinary infections is probably the main determinant of whether chronic suppressive therapy should be used. Data suggest that repeated treatment of recurrent infection will eventually result in a decreased incidence of subsequent infections (2). Furthermore, according to the U.S. Public Health Cooperative Study, the incidence of recurrent infections was significantly less (30%) in males taking chronic antimicrobials than in males taking placebo (20%) over one year (140). More recently, the use of a decision analysis model (141) determined that from a pure cost effectiveness standpoint, women having more than one episode of cystitis per year benefit from antimicrobial prophylaxis. Prophylaxis of women with three or more episodes of cystitis per year is clearly more cost effective than treatment of individual infections. Therefore, chronic antimicrobial prophylaxis should be considered in any patient with two or more episodes of UTI per year.

The duration of prophylactic therapy is also determined by the frequency of infection. Women with three or more UTIs in the 12 months prior to a six-month course of antimicrobial prophylaxis have a significantly higher recurrence rate (75%) in the six months following prophylaxis than women who had two infections in the 12 months before prophylaxis (26%) (142). Prophylaxis should be continued for six months in patients with less than three UTIs per year and at least 12 months for those with three or more UTIs per year. Prior to chronic antimicrobial suppressive therapy, active infections must be completely eradicated by an appropriate course of antibiotic therapy. The low doses of antimicrobials used for chronic prophylaxis suppress bacterial growth, but do not eliminate active infection. Furthermore, surgically correctible anatomical deformities which predispose the patient to recurrent infections (eg, obstruction, stones) and renal infections should be ruled out. Patients with urologic abnormalities respond poorly to prophylactic therapy (137, 143).

Age should also be considered when contemplating chronic antimicrobial therapy. An asymptomatic, elderly patient taking many other medications is not a candidate for chronic prophylactic treatment (81,144), but suppressive therapy is indicated in the young patient (141).

Since this 28-year-old female has a history of recurrent UTIs, has had at least three UTIs in the past few months, has been extensively evaluated, and has just been successfully treated with trimethoprim, a 12-month course of antimicrobial prophylaxis would seem reasonable. She also should be evaluated at regular intervals for recurrences of urinary tract infections and for the development of resistant organisms (3).

28. Methenamine mandelate 1.0 gram four times daily is prescribed as a course of antimicrobial prophylaxis for this patient. Why is it desirable to monitor this patient's urine pH while she is being treated with this drug?

Methenamine is hydrolyzed to formaldehyde in an acid medium, and it is the formaldehyde which is the active component of both methenamine mandelate (Mandelamine) and methenamine hippurate (Hiprex, Urex). Although both the mandelic acid and the hippuric acid components of these two products have bacteriostatic activity in large doses, they probably do not exert any antibacterial effect at commonly utilized dosages. It is doubtful that these agents contribute anything more than their effect on urine pH. A low pH alone is bacteriostatic, so both these salts might have some additive effect with the formaldehyde if the urine pH is sufficiently acidified (145).

The metabolism of methenamine to formaldehyde varies considerably and can be decreased by a urine pH greater than 6.5, an increased urine volume (high fluid intake or diuretics), or a low urine specific gravity (146,147). When methenamine hippurate 1.0 gram twice daily is administered, urine formaldehyde concentrations are greatest at a pH of 5.5 or less. Therefore, regular monitoring of urine pH would be desirable to assure that the urine pH is sufficiently acidic to allow for adequate formaldehyde formation. Such monitoring would be especially appropriate in this patient with a history of *Proteus* infections of her urinary tract. Urease-splitting microorganisms, such as *Proteus* tend to raise the pH of the urine and thus inhibit the release of formaldehyde.

29. Why is the prescription of ascorbic acid 500 mg qid unnecessary in this situation?

Ammonium chloride, methionine, and ascorbic acid are sometimes used in an attempt to acidify the urine of patients receiving methenamine because a low urine pH is essential to the conversion of methenamine to formaldehyde (2). Ammonium chloride, 2.0–3.0 grams four times daily, effectively lowers urine pH, but its effect is reversed within two days by renal compensatory mechanisms (148). Methionine is effective in doses of 8–12 gm daily, but it is unpalatable and gastrointestinal irritation limits its usefulness (2). Therefore, the most commonly used urinary acidifier is ascorbic acid. However, there is considerable variability in the extent to which ascorbic acid lowers the urine pH, and the mean decrease in urine pH is often insignificant. Nahata et al observed that 4 to 6 gm of ascorbic acid daily did not significantly alter the urine pH in ten healthy persons (149). Similar results were observed in children and in patients with neurogenic bladders, all of whom had sterile urines at the time of study (148,150). In another study, ascorbic acid increased the titratable urine acid, but urine pH values were not provided, and all patients were fasting or on a low calorie diet (151).

The goal of acidification during methenamine therapy is to achieve a urine pH of 5.5 to maximize formaldehyde formation. Only 30% of the patients achieved this pH goal in one study (150), and the overall mean pH did not fall below 5.99 in another (149). In a survey of geriatric patients on 1–2 gm of ascorbic acid with methenamine hippurate or mandelate, only 35% of patients had a urine pH below 5.5 (152). Even with ascorbic acid, the pH of the urine fluctuates considerably throughout the day (148). Although, in one trial, the combined use of methenamine mandelate with ascorbic acid tended to keep the mean urine pH lower than it was with ascorbic acid alone, methenamine mandelate alone was not studied, and whether the ascorbic acid made a significant contribution to the acidity generated by the antibacterial agents could not be determined. In another study, the urine pH was significantly lower in patients receiving ascorbic acid in combination with methenamine mandelate than in untreated patients, but again the enhancement of acidity beyond that achieved by methenamine alone was not documented (151). In summary, there appears to be no substantiation of an enhanced effect of methenamine salts by ascorbic acid. The pH of the urine should be monitored in patients receiving methenamine salts, and high doses of antacids, which can alkalinize the urine, should be avoided in patients taking methenamine (153).

30. The patient admits she has difficulty in taking her methenamine mandelate four times a day. What would be an alternative therapeutic plan?

Numerous drugs have been used for chronic antimicrobial therapy, but only a few have been examined in well-designed studies. The U.S. Public Health Cooperative Study compared sulfamethizole, nitrofurantoin, methenamine mandelate, and placebo in 249 males over a two-year period. The side effects resulting from the long-term use of these agents were negligible and the emergence of resistant organisms was not significant (140). However, a surprisingly higher mortality rate unrelated to infection occurred in the sulfamethizole group. Methenamine was superior in delaying recurrence after one year of treatment, but the differences among all drugs and placebo became negligible on longer therapy. More recently, TMP-SMX, trimethoprim, and nitrofurantoin were compared to placebo in a randomized, double-blind, six month trial of urinary prophylaxis (142). All three drugs were equally effective and significantly better than placebo in preventing infections during therapy. They were also well tolerated.

There is some evidence to suggest that trimethoprim-sulfamethoxazole (TMP-SMX) may be the drug of choice for chronic antimicrobial therapy. In a crossover study of 40 females comparing TMP-SMX, one-half tablet daily, to methenamine mandelate 500 mg qid, sulfamethoxazole 500 mg daily, and placebo, the incidence of recurrence was significantly less in those patients treated with TMP-SMX as compared to those treated with the other regimens over a one-year period (154). Kalowski et al also observed that TMP-SMX, one tablet daily, was superior to one gram of methenamine hippurate daily (143). In another study, one-half tablet of TMP-SMX daily for six months in women with histories of recurrent UTI yielded a lower incidence of positive vaginal and fecal cultures during therapy than a 100 mg/day regimen of nitrofurantoin for a similar time period. This was associated with a lower order of bacterial resistance to both anti-infectives (155). Furthermore, one-half tablet of TMP-SMX given only

three times a week also is an effective, well-tolerated prophylactic regimen (156). Successful prophylaxis, however, is significantly decreased in patients with urological abnormalities or renal dysfunction (143,157). Also, infections which are not eradicated by a short-term therapeutic trial of TMP-SMX are not likely to respond to a long-term regimen (157). Finally, enterococci may colonize introitally in patients on chronic TMP-SMX (154,142).

When selecting a drug for chronic antimicrobial therapy, one must consider efficacy, likelihood that resistant organisms will develop, long-term toxicity, and convenience to the patient. The most commonly used agents are listed in Table 3. Sulfonamides are generally not recommended for prophylaxis because they alter the normal fecal flora and frequently select out resistant organisms (88). Methenamine and nitrofurantoin were considered equally effective in the U.S. Public Health Cooperative Study; however, the results in this population of males cannot be extrapolated to the more common female population. The dosing for methenamine is less convenient than the once daily dosing used with nitrofurantoin.

Based on the available information, it appears that this patient could be switched to TMP-SMX. Although she has a history of gastrointestinal distress due to this drug, this may not be a problem with the lower doses used for prophylaxis. If it is, trimethoprim alone would also be effective (134,142,158,159).

Prostatitis

Prostatitis is a common but poorly understood entity. Many clinicians group all prostatic diseases into one category; but in fact, there are a variety of types of prostatitis as a result of different etiologies. The most prevalent forms include acute and chronic bacterial prostatitis, chronic calculous prostatitis, nonbacterial prostatitis, and prostatodynia (160).

Acute bacterial prostatitis is characterized by the sudden onset of chills and fever, perineal and low back pain, urinary urgency and frequency, nocturia, dysuria, and generalized malaise and prostration. Patients may also complain of myalgias, arthralgias, and symptoms of bladder outlet obstruction. Rectal examination usually discloses an exquisitely tender, swollen prostate that is firm and warm to the touch. The causative organisms can generally be identified by culture of the voided urine, and are usually similar in type and inci-

Table 3.

ANTIMICROBIAL AGENTS COMMONLY USED FOR CHRONIC PROPHYLAXIS
AGAINST RECURRENT UTIs[2,156]

Drug	Adult Dose	Pediatric Dose	Comments
Methenamine Mandelate	1 gm qid	5 years or less: 250 mg/30 lb qid 6–12 years: 500 mg qid	
Methenamine Hippurate	1 gm bid	6–12 years: 500 mg–1 gm bid	
Nitrofurantoin	50–100 mg hs	1.25–1.75 mg/kg hs	Contraindicated in infants less than one month of age
Trimethoprim	100 mg hs	—	Not recommended in children under 12 years of age
Trimethoprim 80 mg plus Sulfamethoxazole 400 mg	one-half to one tablet hs or 3 times a week	1–2 mg/kg trimethoprim + 5–10 mg/kg sulfamethoxazole hs	Not recommended for use in infants less than 2 months of age

dence to those that cause UTIs. In acute bacterial prostatitis, prostatic massage should be avoided because of patient discomfort and the risk of bacteremia (161).

Chronic bacterial prostatitis is one of the most common causes of recurrent UTI in men. Except in males with spinal cord injuries, infectious stones, or obstructive abnormalities of the urinary tract, recurrent infections are almost assuredly relapses due to persistence of bacteria in the prostate. Normally, males secrete a prostatic antibacterial factor; however, this substance is absent in men with chronic prostatitis (162). Simple UTIs will often eventually involve the prostate gland, where bacteria are difficult to eradicate.

The clinical manifestations of chronic bacterial prostatitis are highly variable. In fact, many patients are asymptomatic. The disease is usually suspected when a male treated for a UTI relapses. The diagnosis is confirmed by examination of expressed prostatic secretions (163). To ensure accurate localization (i.e., to distinguish prostatic from urethral bacteria), segmented urine samples are taken. The first 10 ml of voided urine represents the urethral sample, the midstream urine collected represents the bladder sample, and the first 10 ml voided immediately after prostatic massage represents the prostate sample. When the bladder sample is sterile or nearly so, bacterial prostatitis is diagnosed if the bacterial count in the prostate sample is at least

one logarithm greater than that in the urethral sample. The bacterial pathogens responsible for chronic prostatitis are often similar to those of acute prostatitis and of UTIs in general (161).

31. A 60-year-old male experienced his first UTI at age 40, with symptoms of frequency, dysuria, nocturia, perineal pain, chills and fever, but no flank pain. Acute prostatitis was diagnosed. *E. coli* were cultured from the urine, and treatment with a sulfonamide was successful. After 12 asymptomatic years, acute prostatitis due to *E. coli* recurred and again responded to sulfonamide therapy. Two more *E. coli* infections occurred over the next eight years. The fourth infection responded to sulfonamides but recurred two weeks after the medication was discontinued. Were sulfonamides appropriate treatment of this patient's acute episodes of bacterial prostatitis?

Any appropriate antibacterial drug, including sulfonamides, can be used for the treatment of acute bacterial prostatitis because the diffuse intense inflammation of the prostate gland allows many drugs to readily penetrate into the prostatic fluid (162). Antimicrobial therapy, however, should be continued for about a month to prevent the development of chronic prostatitis (161).

In retrospect, sulfonamides certainly were appropriate for this patient simply because they were effective in the treatment of his infections.

32. What would be a reasonable antimicrobial for treatment of this patient's present recurrence?

Most antibiotics are acidic and do not readily cross the prostatic epithelium into the alkaline prostatic fluid because inflammation is minimal with chronic prostatitis in contrast to acute prostatitis. Trimethoprim, clindamycin, erythromycin, oleandomycin, and rosamicin are the only antibiotics that achieve high prostatic concentrations in dog experiments (164). However, the pH of normal human prostatic fluid is higher than that in the dog, and even higher in the presence of chronic bacterial prostatitis (165). Theoretically, this increased alkalinity should impair the diffusion of trimethoprim and enhance the diffusion of the tetracyclines, certain sulfonamides, and the macrolide antibiotics such as erythromycin. Nevertheless, TMP-SMX has the best documented cure rates in the treatment of chronic bacterial prostatitis. Long-term therapy of 4–16 weeks with TMP-SMX is associated with a cure rate of 32–71%, which significantly exceeds the cure rate after short-term therapy of 2 weeks or less (164). In two other studies, cure rates of recurrent UTIs were better in the men who received prolonged TMP-SMX therapy for six or twelve weeks than in those who received 10 or 14 days of treatment (166,167). Some of the patients in these studies had underlying renal or bladder pathology without apparent prostatic involvement, so the results do not necessarily apply only to men with chronic bacterial prostatitis.

Although limited, some studies have reported success with erythromycin and minocycline in the treatment of chronic bacterial prostatitis (168,179). In addition, one investigator has experimented with direct perineal injections of antibiotics into prostatic lobes (170). More experience with these therapies is needed. Therefore, it would be reasonable to treat this man with TMP-SMX for 6–12 weeks.

In the event of treatment failure, chronic low-dose therapy with TMP-SMX, nitrofurantoin, or acidifying agents can alleviate the symptoms of episodic bladder infection associated with chronic bacterial prostatitis. Infections eventually recur with greater frequency in most of these patients, although some become asymptomatic, even in the presence of chronic bacteriuria. Chronic, low-dose antibacterial therapy sterilizes the bladder, alleviates symptoms, confines bacteria to the prostate, and inhibits infection and damage to the rest of the urinary tract. Chronic bacterial prostatitis is one of the few indications for continuous antibiotic therapy.

Sexual Intercourse; Pregnancy

33. On routine screening, asymptomatic bacteriuria is noted in a 30-year-old pregnant woman in her first trimester. Five years ago, during her first pregnancy, she developed acute bacterial pyelonephritis which required hospitalization and treatment with parenteral antibiotics. Since that time, she has had recurrent UTIs, apparently related to sexual intercourse. These subsided when she began taking a single dose of nitrofurantoin after coitus, but she discontinued the practice prior to this pregnancy because she was afraid of what it might do to the fetus. What is the association between sexual intercourse and the occurrence of UTIs?

Although recent studies tend to support an association between sexual intercourse and UTIs (23–25), a causal relationship has not been adequately established (26). Studies do indicate that introital (vaginal vestibule and urethral mucosa) bacterial colonization by fecal bacteria has a definite role in recurrent infection. There is an increase in the number of introital enterobacteria immediately prior to urinary tract infection, and they are identical serotypically to the infecting bacteria cultured from the urinary tract. It appears that there is a high risk of UTI after sexual intercourse only if the appropriate organisms, primarily Enterobacteriaceae, are present in the region beforehand (26).

Since UTIs are uncommon in males, transmission of an infection from the male to the female is unlikely. Occasionally, bacteria harbored under the foreskin of an uncircumcised male may be transmitted to his partner in intercourse (3).

34. Was it rational to manage these infections with a single dose of an antibiotic after intercourse?

Post-coital antibiotic prophylaxis is often recommended when a UTI is thought to result from sexual intercourse. Theoretically, a single dose of antimicrobial produces bactericidal activity in the urine before bacteria have a chance to multiply. The patient empties her bladder just after intercourse and before taking the medication to minimize the number of bacteria present in the bladder and to eliminate unnecessary dilution of the drug in the urine. Since most drugs effective in UTIs are rapidly excreted by the kidney and reach high urinary concentrations, this regimen appears reasonable and does lower the incidence of post-coital infections. However, it has the same drawbacks as any other type of antibiotic prophylaxis, and is not recommended in patients with an abnormal urinary tract or decreased renal function. It is also important to treat symptomatic infection with appropriate therapy before beginning prophylaxis.

A single nightly dose of 50 mg nitrofurantoin inhibited bacterial growth in a double-blind trial of 50 women with histories of recurrent urinary tract infections. Of 37 women with normal intravenous pyelograms (IVP), only one became infected over a trial period of 10–183 weeks, and only five of the patients with abnormal IVP's became infected over 14–260 weeks of therapy (171). In another study (172), nitrofurantoin, cephalexin, nalidixic acid, sulfonamide, and penicillin all decreased the frequency of bacteriuria, but nitrofurantoin and cephalexin were the most effective.

35. Since the patient has an asymptomatic UTI at this time, should treatment be withheld because of her pregnancy?

Acute symptomatic pyelonephritis may develop in pregnant women with untreated bacteriuria. In an evaluation of 265 bacteriuric pregnant patients, there was a 25% incidence of acute pyelonephritis in the untreated group and a 3% incidence in the treated group (173). Another study reported comparative rates of 19% and 0%, respectively (174). Thus, proper treatment greatly reduces this complication. In addition, there is evidence that maternal UTIs during pregnancy are associated with an increase in prenatal mortality rates and more frequent pre-term deliveries (175). Although a cause and effect relationship has not been established, this is an important consideration, and it strengthens the argument for treating maternal UTIs.

Screening for bacteriuria in pregnancy is appropriate because of the high incidence of bacteriuria (1) which is often present early in pregnancy but rarely later (176). The high frequency of bacteria early in pregnancy may be an expression of asymptomatic bacteriuria existing before conception (13). In partial support of this hypothesis, UTIs during pregnancy appear to be more common in women with a history of childhood bacteriuria than in women without such a history (72).

36. Which antimicrobial agents are contraindicated in this patient?

As indicated in Table 1, *tetracyclines* are contraindicated in pregnant women and in nursing mothers because they can cause permanent yellow, grayish-brown or brown discoloration of the teeth in the fetus or nursing infant. In addition, tetracyclines have been associated with the development of fatty liver and nephropathy in the pregnant female. Tetracyclines should be avoided in pregnancy whenever possible.

Sulfonamides and sulfonamide combinations (eg, TMP-SMX) can cause kernicterus in neonates if given to mothers during the third trimester of pregnancy or to lactating women. The sulfonamides displace unconjugated bilirubin from plasma albumin and thereby allow increased bilirubin to enter the brain and induce encephalopathy in the newborn. Sulfonamides in breast milk can cause hemolytic anemia in infants with G6PD deficiency.

Teratogenicity attributed to *TMP-SMX* has not been reported to date, although it has been used only minimally during pregnancy (133,137). The total number of females taking the preparation during the first trimester, when the fetus is most susceptible to teratogenic effects, is too small for a conclusive statement about its safety. Fetal malformations have been associated with the use of other folic acid antagonists, so it may be best to avoid the use of TMP-SMX and trimethoprim during pregnancy or during the nursing period.

Clinically, teratogenic effects of *nitrofurantoin* are not known; however, *in vitro* investigations suggest a slight mutagenic potential. Nitrofurantoin could also cause hemolytic anemia in a G6PD-deficient nursing infant; however, only very small amounts have been detected in breast milk (178).

Adverse genetic effects from *nalidixic acid* in man are unknown, but it increases the rate of mutation and gene modification in insects. It is advisable not to give nalidixic acid during the first month of pregnancy. In addition, it too can cause hemolytic anemia in a G6PD-deficient nursing infant (178).

The *penicillins,* the *cephalosporins,* and the *aminoglycosides* appear to be relatively safe to use during pregnancy. These drugs, along with the others listed in Table 1, cross the placental barrier and thus the risk of toxicity or teratogenicity to the fetus must always be considered before deciding to treat a pregnant female with a UTI.

In this case, ampicillin or sulfisoxazole could be prescribed for treatment of the patient's UTI. The patient was correct in discontinuing her nitrofurantoin before pregnancy, since the risk to the fetus, though small, tends to offset the advantage of antimicrobial prophylaxis. However, the patient must receive proper follow-up care.

Urinary Catheters

Catheter-induced UTIs are the most common type of hospital-acquired infection. Catheterization and other forms of urologic instrumentation are involved in 75% of all hospital-acquired UTIs, and catheter-associated UTI is said to account for 30% of all nosocomial infections. These UTIs are also the major cause of gram-negative bacteremia (179,180).

Infection may occur by bacterial entry from several routes related to the catheter. The urethral meatus and the distal third of the urethra are normally colonized by bacteria, and the initial catheter insertion can introduce bacteria into the bladder. Bacterial contamination at the catheter junctions or in the urine collection bag may lead to migration of bacteria through the catheter lumen to the bladder, thus initiating infection (180). The extraluminal space in the urethra has also been considered a potential route of contamination (181). The risk of infection is directly related to catheter insertion technique, care of the catheter, duration of catheterization, and the susceptibility of the patient. Diagnostic or single, short-term catheterization is associated with a much lower risk of infection than indwelling, long-term catheterization. Despite careful technique, there is always the risk of contaminating a sterile bladder with urethral bacteria. The incidence of infection following a single catheterization is 1% in healthy young women and 20% in debilitated patients (182). Each reinsertion of the catheter on an intermittent basis introduces a risk of infection.

The risk of infection from an indwelling catheter is well-recognized. In the open drainage system, where the urine is collected in an unattached receptacle, the sterility of the unit is disrupted. Consequently, the most careful and aseptic insertion techniques will not prevent infection, and 50% of patients are infected within 24 hours and nearly 100% of patients are infected after four days, with an open system (183).

Infections can be dramatically reduced by the closed sterile drainage system, which is the most common type of catheter currently in use. With this system, the drainage tube leads from the catheter directly to a closed plastic collection bag. The overall incidence of infection from the closed system with careful insertion and maintenance is about 20%; the risk increases with time to 50% after 14 days of catheterization. If the system is accidentally disconnected or contaminated, the infection rate is similar to that of an open system (184).

The condom catheter avoids the potential risk of contaminating the bladder which occurs with initial insertion of the indwelling catheter and allows urine flow through the urethra, which discourages upward migration of bacteria through the periurethral space. Hirsh et al observed that no infections occurred with condom catheters placed for 7–58 days in comatose or paraplegic patients, but occurred in 53% of alert patients in whom tampering of the catheter was evident (185). Thus, the condom catheter might be a consideration in incontinent male patients if manipulation of the catheter is minimal.

Bacterial contamination of the bladder with meatal and urethral flora when the catheter is inserted accounts for the infections following single diagnostic catheterizations and probably the early infections from indwelling catheters. Therefore, the periurethral area should be carefully cleansed with soap and water followed by some type of antiseptic solution. An iodophor solution is often recommended, but benzalkonium chloride should be avoided because it is ineffective against some gram-negative organisms (180).

With the advent of closed drainage systems, infections by the luminal route have been reduced considerably, and contamination by meatal bacteria via the extraluminal space may now play a larger role in catheter infections. Garibaldi et al demonstrated that bacteriuria occurred with significantly greater frequency in those patients having positive meatal cultures than in those with negative cultures (181). In addition, the infecting organism was of the same species as the meatal culture of 94 of 110 infections with positive meatal cultures. However, prospective placebo-controlled studies fail to demonstrate control of infection by locally applied medicated lubricants. Reduction in infection rate was not observed by lubricating the catheter with polymyxin and benzalkonium chloride prior to insertion, or by inserting antiseptic-impregnated catheters (186). Specially perforated catheters which facilitated daily urethral lubrication with polymyxin B or placebo also failed to demonstrate differences in infection rate (187). It appears, however, that the lubrication itself, with or without an anti-infective agent, had a protective effect against bacteriuria in women.

Recommendations for catheter care, published by the Center for Disease Control (180), emphasize the importance of asepsis and sterility at insertion as well as proper maintenance. A closed drainage system should never be disconnected, because contamination may be initiated from the connection site (179,188,189). Likewise, to avoid reflux the collection bag should be positioned to maintain a downward flow. Since cross-infection among catheterized patients can occur, catheterized patients should be separated. It is particularly important to separate bacteriuric catheterized patients from non-infected catheterized patients (190). The rate of infection in post-trauma spinal cord injury patients has been reduced considerably by intermittent catheterization, a sterile technique which also encourages bladder control during rehabilitation (182).

37. An 18-year-old male was hospitalized following a diving accident which resulted in a spinal cord injury with paralysis. Included among a number of initial interventions was insertion of a Foley catheter with a closed drainage system because of bladder incontinence. Two weeks after admission to the hospital, the patient was noted to have an asymptomatic UTI. How should this be treated?

Systemic antibiotic therapy selected specifically for the infecting organism will result in a sterile urine (184,191). However, reinfection, often by a resistant organism, occurs in one-third to one-half of these cases if closed drainage catheterization is continued during therapy (191). For this reason, it is generally recommended that systemic antimicrobial therapy begin after the catheter is removed, or with catheter in place if its removal is soon anticipated (2). Since bacteriuria is inevitable in long-term catheterization, Kunin suggests that the asymptomatic patient be left

untreated to avoid the complication of recolonization and potential bacteremia by highly resistant organisms (2). The strictest adherence to good catheter care is the primary concern in the chronically catheterized patient. Recatheterization with a new, sterile unit is necessary whenever contamination is suspected.

38. A 0.25% acetic acid solution for catheter irrigation is prescribed to prevent the spread of infection. How effective are constant bladder irrigations with antibacterial or antiseptic solutions in preventing infection?

Antibacterial bladder instillation with 0.25% acetic acid or a combination of neomycin and polymyxin (Neosporin GU irrigant) is quite effective in preventing infection in the open drainage system. The incidence of infection can be reduced from 100% to less than 20% (183). In a very limited prospective study of six patients catheterized for a period of less than two days, constant bladder rinse with one liter of 0.25% acetic acid daily resulted in one infection (192). A urine pH less than 5 is necessary for the antibacterial effect of acetic acid (193).

Constant irrigation with neosporin 40 mg and polymyxin 20 mg per liter prevented infections after short-term (less than 3 days), open drainage catheterization in 10 patients (192). However, infection rates are considerably lower in patients catheterized for less than 10 days (6 to 22%) than in those catheterized longer than 10 days (more than 60 to 70%) (194,195).

Regular irrigation with acetic acid has resulted in systemic absorption of acetic acid from the bladder (195). In contrast, 10 days of instillation with Neosporin GU irrigant did not result in detectable concentrations of polymyxin in the serum, and the observed neomycin concentrations of 0.1 ug/ml were well below the toxic range. Clinical toxicity was not observed in patients irrigated with neomycin and polymyxin for up to 72 days (195).

Although the combination of bladder irrigation and closed drainage catheterization should be additive in preventing bladder infection, this speculation has not been proven. The closed drainage system in itself results in an infection rate comparable to that of irrigation with an open system (about 20% after one week) (184,188). There was also a 20% infection rate in patients with closed systems receiving continuous bladder irrigation with neomycin 40 mg plus polymyxin

B 20 mg per liter (196,197). A prospective comparison of irrigation and nonirrigation further supported the lack of advantage in irrigating a closed drainage system (189). Interestingly, infection occurred more frequently on days that catheter junctions were disconnected, suggesting the importance of this site in closed systems.

39. What other modes of antimicrobial prophylaxis might be useful for this patient with the closed system indwelling catheter?

Two additional means of controlling infection with indwelling catheters are the addition of antiseptics to the drainage bag and the administration of oral systemic antibiotics.

The addition of antiseptics to the drainage bag has been examined as a means of decreasing the risk of infection from this source because the drainage bag is usually infected prior to bladder infection (188). Although infections were minimal during the first four days of catheterization, the rate increased after four days, despite continued addition of antiseptics to the drainage bag. Therefore, other etiologies of infection are probably more important with chronic catheterization (198,199).

The benefits of systemic antibiotics in preventing catheter-induced UTIs have not been clarified. Studies using closed drainage systems and diligent catheter care indicate that systemic antibiotics decrease the daily and overall incidence of infection in patients with sterile urines prior to catheterization (179,184,197,200). The preventive effect of the antimicrobial agents is greatest for short-term catheterizations or during the first four to seven days of catheterizations (179,197). Thereafter, the rate of infection increases. Although the overall infection rate remains lower than that of the patients not given systemic antibiotics, the emergence of resistant organisms is significant. Therefore, in deciding to use systemic antimicrobials, one must consider the patient's underlying diseases or risk factors, duration of catheterization, and the potential complications of drug toxicity or resistant organisms which may result from the chronic use of antimicrobial agents.

Renal Failure

40. A 55-year-old male with a history of hypertension and chronic renal failure develops a UTI. His creatinine clearance, determined from a recent 24 hour urine collection, is 20 ml/min. What antimicrobial agent and what dose should be prescribed?

The major problem encountered in selecting an antimicrobial agent for the treatment of UTI in a patient with renal failure is achievement of adequate urine concentrations of the drug without causing systemic toxicity. This problem could be readily overcome *if* (a) the drug was inherently nontoxic, even at high serum concentrations, making dosage adjustments unnecessary, (b) the drug was excreted unchanged in the urine (i.e., not metabolized), and (c) the drug was eliminated by renal tubular secretion so that high levels could be achieved in the urine. Unfortunately, no such "ideal" drug exists.

Nitrofurantoin, doxycycline, and many of the sulfonamides are substantially metabolized by the liver. Such drugs are usually not recovered in high concentrations in the urine and generally yield low levels in the urine of uremic patients. Tetracycline and the aminoglycosides are handled almost exclusively by the kidneys. The dosage reduction that is necessary to avoid toxicity in uremic patients will also result in inadequate urine concentrations. The penicillins, the cephalosporins, and trimethoprim are metabolized by the liver and also eliminated by the kidney to a significant extent. These agents most closely meet the criteria for an "ideal" drug mentioned above.

As illustrated in Table 4, a number of antimicrobial agents could be used in this patient. Some would require changes in the dosing interval; others would not. However, based on pharmacokinetic considerations, a penicillin (eg, ampicillin), a cephalosporin, or trimethoprim would be preferred. TMP-SMX would also be effective; but, in patients with renal failure, the activity of sulfamethoxazole in the urine is decreased. This alters the optimal trimethoprim/sulfamethoxazole ratio and may diminish the synergism between the two agents (2).

Adverse Drug Effects

Table 5 lists the adverse effects associated with the commonly used antimicrobial agents in the treatment of UTIs. Some of these adverse effects are illustrated and discussed in the following cases.

41. *Sulfonamide Hemolytic Anemia.* A 65-year-old black male with an eight-year history of congestive heart failure (CHF) was admitted to the hospital with increasing shortness of breath. His hematocrit was stable at 39–43%, and his total serum bilirubin

was reported to be 0.8 mg/dl. Sixteen days after admission, a UTI due to *E. coli* was discovered, and the patient was treated with sulfisoxazole 4 gm daily. Twenty days after admission, the hematocrit suddenly dropped to 25% and the hemoglobin to 8.4 gm/dl. There were no signs of bleeding, but his sclerae became icteric. Twenty-three days after admission, the hematocrit was still 25%, but the reticulocyte count had risen to 6.6%, and the bilirubin was 3.0 mg/dl. Sulfisoxazole was discontinued, and over a period of two weeks the hematocrit steadily rose to 40%. What mechanism might explain this patient's sulfonamide-induced hemolytic anemia?

Hemolytic anemia is associated with sulfonamide administration and can be mediated by a number of mechanisms including (203): abnormally high blood levels, acquired hypersensitivity as reflected by the development of a positive Coombs' test, genetically determined abnormalities of red blood cell metabolism (eg, deficiency of glucose-6-phosphate-dehydrogenase); or the presence of an "unstable" hemoglobin in the red blood cell (eg, Hemoglobin Zurich, Hemoglobin Towns, Hemoglobin H).

In this case, hemolytic anemia due to glucose-6-phosphate-dehydrogenase (G6PD) deficiency could be confirmed by measuring red blood cell levels of this enzyme. G6PD deficiency is more fully discussed in the chapter on Anemias. Although the defect appears to be most common and most severe in Mediterranean males, one variant affects as many as 11% of American Black males (204).

The acute hemolytic anemia induced by sulfonamides in G6PD-deficient individuals does not appear to be a dose-related phenomenon. It is usually abrupt in onset and occurs within the first week of therapy. Typical symptoms include nausea, fever, vertigo, jaundice, hepatosplenomegaly, and, occasionally, hypotension. Hematocrit and hemoglobin values may fall precipitously and may be reduced to 30–50% of the normal values; leukocytosis and reticulocytosis are common; and acute renal failure may result from the hypotension and hemolysis. A mild hemolytic episode is characterized by reticulocytosis without a significant fall in hemoglobin or hematocrit (204,205). Several other urinary tract antimicrobials such as nalidixic acid, nitrofurantoin, and TMP-SMX also induce G6PD-deficiency hemolysis (204).

Clinical illness as well as drug administration may precipitate hemolysis in patients with G6PD deficiency. Patients with chronic bacterial infections of the urinary or upper respiratory tract who receive chronic or repetitive courses of certain drugs are particularly predisposed to hemolysis (204).

Individuals with enzyme deficiencies, especially those associated with the pentose-phosphate shunt (as is G6PD), can develop hemolytic reactions when taking drugs commonly used to treat UTIs. Anemia in a female with a deficiency of glutathione peroxidase who received a sulfonamide and nitrofurantoin has been reported (206). Future use of sulfonamides, nitrofurantoin, or nalidixic acid should be avoided in this patient.

42. *Sulfonamide Rash and Interaction with a Sulfonylurea.* A 45-year-old obese diabetic female on tolbutamide 2 grams daily developed an acute UTI, for which sulfisoxazole 500 mg qid for 10 days was prescribed. Seven days later she appeared in the emergency room with a pruritic maculopapular rash and fever. She also complained of nausea and lightheadedness. Is the rash in this patient typical of sulfonamides?

Rash is one of the more common adverse effects noted after sulfonamide administration, and about 2% of patients treated with sulfisoxazole will develop a rash. A variety of hypersensitivity skin and mucous membrane reactions have been reported, including morbilliform, scarlatinal, urticarial, erysipeloid, pemphigoid, purpuric, and petechial rashes. Erythema nodosum, exfoliative dermatitis, photosensitivity reactions, and the Stevens-Johnson syndrome are also associated with sulfonamides. Skin eruptions usually appear after one week of treatment, although a more rapid onset may occur in a sensitized person (51).

Drug fever is also common with sulfonamide therapy, occurring in as many as 3% of patients receiving sulfisoxazole. It most often occurs between the seventh and tenth day of treatment, and may be accompanied by headache, chills, malaise, pruritus, and skin rash. Discontinuation of sulfonamide administration is generally followed by rapid defervescence (51).

43. Why might the nausea and lightheadedness in this patient be drug-related?

This patient's subjective complaints may be a result of hypoglycemia induced by the interaction of sulfisoxazole and tolbutamide. A three- to fourfold prolongation of hypoglycemic activity by sulfonylureas has been reported in patients re-

Table 4.

DOSE ADJUSTMENTS FOR UTI IN PATIENTS WITH RENAL FAILURE[201,202]

Drug	Usual Dosing Interval (hours)	Adjusted Dosing Interval for GFR:			Comments
		>50	20–50	<20	
Amoxicillin	8	8	8	8	Normal dosing required for adequate urine concentration.
Ampicillin	6	6	6	6	Normal dosing required for adequate urine concentration.
Carbenicillin	4	4	6–12	ineffective	4.7 mEq Na/gm; requires electrolyte monitoring in renal failure.
Cefadroxil	12	—	—	—	—
Cefazolin	8	8	12	ineffective at <10	—
Cephalexin	6	6	6	ineffective at <10	—
Cephalothin	6	6	6	ineffective	—
Cephradine	6	—	—	—	—
Cinoxacin	6	8	12	24	—
Doxycycline	12	12	12	avoid	Urine concentrations become inadequate, but renal tissue levels remain high.
Gentamicin	8	8–12	12–24	ineffective	Accumulation leads to nephrotoxicity and ototoxicity.
Methenamine Mandelate	6	6	ineffective	ineffective	No data in renal failure to assure adequacy of formaldehyde formation.
Methenamine Hippurate	12	12	avoid	avoid	
Nalidixic Acid	6	6	6	ineffective	—
Nitrofurantoin	6	6	avoid	avoid	Urinary levels are inadequate at $Cr_{Cl} < 50$ ml/min. Neuropathy occurs more often in patients with renal failure.
Sulfamethoxazole	12	12	12	12	Normal dosing necessary to achieve levels, but serum elevations occur; consider alternative.
Sulfisoxazole	6	6	6	6	
Tetracycline	6	avoid	avoid	avoid	Catabolic effect can cause rises in BUN and acidosis. Up to 6.5 mEq Na/gm; requires electrolyte monitoring in renal failure.

Table 4. (continued)

DOSE ADJUSTMENTS FOR UTI IN PATIENTS WITH RENAL FAILURE[201,202]

Drug	Usual Dosing Interval (hours)	Adjusted Dosing Interval for GFR:			Comments
		>50	20–50	<20	
Ticarcillin	4–6	4–6	8	12	—
Tobramycin	8	8–12	12–24	ineffective	Accumulation leads to nephrotoxicity and ototoxicity.
Trimethoprim	12	12	12	12	Serum accumulation can occur at $Cr_{Cl} < 10$ ml/min, but adverse consequences not reported.
Trimethoprim plus Sulfamethoxazole	12	12	12	24	Rare cases of nephrotoxicity reported in patients with normal and impaired renal function.

ceiving sulfisoxazole or other antibacterial sulfonamides concurrently (207). It has been suggested that the increased and prolonged hypoglycemia is due either to protein displacement or to a decrease in the rate of metabolism of the sulfonylurea (208).

The hypersensitivity reactions and possible tolbutamide interaction that occurred in this patient signify that she should avoid sulfonamides. An alternate drug should be used for future acute UTIs.

44. *TMP-SMX Folate Deficiency.* A 50-year-old epileptic female has been taking TMP-SMX nightly for three months for chronic recurrent UTI prophylaxis. She takes phenytoin 300 mg daily with effective control of her seizures. Further history reveals that she also takes diazepam 2 mg tid, smokes one pack of cigarettes per day, and drinks one pint of gin daily. Routine CBC after a clinic visit shows hemoglobin 9 gm/dl, hematocrit 30%, MCV 105 cubic microns, and MCHC 32%. How could TMP-SMX account for this patient's megaloblastic anemia?

On rare occasions, folate-deficiency megaloblastic anemia has been associated with the use of TMP-SMX (121,122). The ability of the sulfonamides to inhibit folic acid synthesis occurs only in the bacterial cell and does not affect, to a significant degree, human cell processes. Although trimethoprim has a greater affinity for the bacterial and protozoal cell, when given in high doses,

it may also affect folic acid utilization in man (31). It is especially a potential problem in patients with known or questionably deficient folic acid stores, such as pregnant women, the elderly, patients with malabsorption or malnutrition, alcoholics, patients receiving anticonvulsants, or those with chronic hemolysis (such as sickle-cell disease). Concomitant administration of folic acid will reverse these effects without interfering with antimicrobial activity (121,122). It is doubtful that significant folate deficiency would occur with short-term therapy in patients without the above risk factors.

In this patient, both phenytoin and alcohol undoubtedly contributed to folate deficiency anemia. Whether or not TMP-SMX was a significant factor may be questioned, but an alternate chronic prophylactic UTI agent may be preferable in a patient already at risk for folate deficiency.

45. *TMP-SMX Warfarin Interaction.* A 50-year-old asthmatic patient was admitted to the hospital for acute asthma which had progressively worsened over the previous two weeks. The patient was placed on IV aminophylline and metaproterenol by nebulization. Other medications included warfarin for deep vein thrombophlebitis that occurred three months ago and hydrochlorothiazide for mild hypertension. During her hospitalization, the patient developed an acute UTI, and TMP-SMX twice daily was given pending culture and sensitivity (C&S) results. Three

Table 5.

ADVERSE EFFECTS OF DRUGS USED IN THE TREATMENT OF UTIs[32,33,178]

Drug	Frequent	Occasional	Rare
Amoxicillin		diarrhea, allergic reactions[1]	pseudomembranous colitis
Ampicillin	non-allergic rash, diarrhea	allergic reactions	pseudomembranous colitis
Carbenicillin and Ticarcillin			hypokalemic alkalosis, sodium overload, bleeding disorders, hepatitis
Cephalosporins		nausea, diarrhea, allergic reactions	hemolytic anemia
Cinoxacin		nausea, rash	
Nalidixic Acid	rash	nausea, vomiting & diarrhea, CNS disturbance (visual problems, headache, dizziness, seizures, hallucinations), G6PD-deficiency hemolytic anemia	cholestatic jaundice, blood dyscrasias, arthralgias, lupus syndrome
Nitrofurantoin	nausea & vomiting	allergic pneumonitis, G6PD-deficiency hemolytic anemia, peripheral neuropathy	cholestatic jaundice, hepatitis, trigeminal neuralgia
Methenamine Mandelate and Methenamine Hippurate	nausea & vomiting	dysuria, allergic reactions	
Gentamicin and Tobramycin		renal toxicity, vestibular toxicity	auditory toxicity
Doxycycline and Tetracycline	nausea, vomiting, diarrhea, bone & teeth deformity in fetus and children up to 8 years of age, yeast superinfections	malabsorption, increased azotemia in renal failure, esophageal ulcers, photosensitivity, allergic reactions	enterocolitis, intracranial hypertension
Sulfisoxazole and Sulfamethoxazole	rash, photosensitivity, drug fever	kernicterus in newborn, G6PD-deficiency hemolytic anemia	pseudomembranous colitis, Stevens Johnson syndrome, blood dyscrasias, crystalluria
Trimethoprim	rash, nausea		blood dyscrasias

[1]allergic reactions = rash, urticaria, anaphylaxis, serum sickness

days later, the C&S reports showed *E. coli* sensitive to ampicillin, tetracycline, nitrofurantoin, TMP-SMX, carbenicillin, and gentamicin. At this time, a prolongation of the prothrombin time to 38 seconds (control: 12 seconds) was noted. Because a TMP-SMX-warfarin interaction was suspected, warfarin was withheld for two days and ampicillin 500 mg qid was given instead of the TMP-SMX. Subsequently the prothrombin time was maintained at 22 seconds during the remainder of the hospitalization. Why was this problem attributed to a drug interaction?

TMP-SMX can potentiate the anticoagulant effects of racemic warfarin (the form that is administered to humans) (209,210). There is recent evidence that TMP-SMX has a stereoselective interaction with warfarin, causing a greater increase in serum levels of the more potent levorotatory warfarin enantiomorph and a decrease in the less potent dextrorotatory enantiomorph (211). The net effect is no change in the total warfarin level, but a higher concentration of the potent enantiomorph and an increase in the prothrombin time. Although a few cases of sulfonamide-induced hypoprothrombinemia have been reported, current evidence does not rule out the possibility that trimethoprim may play a role in the reports of TMP-SMX-induced hypoprothrombinemia (212).

46. *Nitrofurantoin GI Disturbance.* A 45-year-old female who weighs 110 pounds is placed on nitrofurantoin 100 mg qid for 14 days for an acute UTI. The patient complains of nausea and gastrointestinal upset after the ingestion of each dose of nitrofurantoin. How can this effect be minimized?

Nausea is a fairly frequent complication of nitrofurantoin therapy, and the patient's compliance with the prescribed regimen may be severely affected by this common side effect. It is not fully known whether the mechanism by which nitrofurantoin produces nausea is central or local, but a central component may be present because nausea occurs after parenteral administration. Several approaches can be used to decrease nitrofurantoin-induced nausea:

Take each dose with food: All manufacturers of nitrofurantoin recommend that the drug be taken with food or milk. If the nausea is a locally-mediated effect, the food may be helpful by serving as a buffer; if the nausea is centrally-mediated, then food may be helpful by slowing the rate of absorption and lowering the peak serum concentration of the drug. Interestingly, however, food increases the bioavailability of nitrofurantoin. In a single-dose crossover study, urinary excretion of various products of nitrofurantoin were considerably lower in the fasting state than when administered after a meal (213). There was significant variation among the products. There do not appear to be any published studies to determine whether or not the net effect of slower but increased absorption with meals decreases nausea as compared to the lesser absorption while fasting.

Change to a macrocrystalline product: A study of the incidence of nitrofurantoin adverse effects demonstrated significantly fewer adverse effects with the use of the macrocrystalline preparation than with the crystalline preparation (17% vs 39%) (214). The cure rate did not differ significantly.

The larger particle size of the macrocrystalline preparation results in a slower rate of dissolution and absorption, and lower serum levels. Unfortunately, patients were not instructed when to take their medications in this study (214). The total absorption of the macrocrystalline form is less than that of the crystalline form during the fasting state (213,215,216). However, the amount absorbed is equivalent when taken after meals (213). A disadvantage of the macrocrystalline form is the cost, which may be two to ten times that of the crystalline form, depending on the product source.

Lower the dose: Nausea and vomiting appear to be dose-related; they occur more frequently in small persons (217). The minimum effective dose of nitrofurantoin is generally stated to be 5 mg/kg/day; the average dose is usually 7 mg/kg/day. At daily doses above 7 mg/kg, the incidence of nausea appears to increase markedly, so the dose in this 110 lb (50 kg) patient could be decreased.

47. *Nitrofurantoin Pneumonitis.* The patient tolerated the macrocrystalline form taken with meals and continued her regimen. However, ten days later she presented with dyspnea, tachypnea, coughing, and wheezing. Examination revealed a temperature of 38.4°C, pulse of 115 beats/min, and soft inspiratory and expiratory rhonchi with a few bibasilar rales. Nitrofurantoin administration was stopped, and intravenous aminophylline and steroids were administered. Symptoms gradually disappeared after a few days; however, rechallenge with a single 50 mg dose of nitrofurantoin caused a recurrence of the respiratory distress. What is the nature of the apparent nitrofurantoin-induced respiratory reaction which occurred in this patient?

Several hundred cases of nitrofurantoin-induced pulmonary reactions have been reported (218–220). Acute, subacute, and chronic reactions have been described. The acute form illustrated by this case often manifests within several days of initiating the drug with a sudden flu-like syndrome consisting of fever, dyspnea, and cough. The subacute form tends to occur after at least a month of exposure; symptoms include fever and dyspnea. The chronic form tends to be a more insidious process with milder dyspnea and low-grade fever. In all forms, rales are commonly heard and pulmonary infiltrates can be demonstrated on chest x-ray. Although eosinophilia frequently occurs with the acute form, it may be absent with the subacute and chronic forms (219). Antinuclear antibodies are elevated in the latter two forms. Discontinuation of nitrofurantoin results in complete recovery after several weeks; permanent fibrotic changes may persist with the chronic pulmonary reaction, however. Although steroids are frequently administered when the adverse reaction is diagnosed, their efficacy has not been demonstrated. Rechallenge with oral nitrofurantoin results in rapid reappearance of pulmonary symptoms in those who suffered an acute reaction.

48. *Nitrofurantoin Neurotoxicity.* A 55-year-old female has been taking nitrofurantoin 100 mg qid for an acute UTI. Pertinent history includes hypertension and moderate renal failure. Medications include methyldopa, hydrochlorothiazide, and allopurinol. On the tenth day of therapy, she complains that both her hands and feet feel numb and weak. Physical examination shows marked sensory loss to hands and feet, as well as absent ankle reflexes, although knee and arm reflexes are present. What are the characteristics of the neuropathy which is associated with nitrofurantoin therapy?

Peripheral neuropathy is usually characterized by symmetrical dysesthesia and paresthesia in the distal extremities which progresses in a central and ascending fashion. In a review of 137 published cases (221), the following characteristics of this adverse effect were noted. It usually occurred within the first 45 days of treatment, although neuropathy was recognized up to 42 days after discontinuation of therapy in 16%. Symptom severity was unrelated to the total nitrofurantoin dose. Reversibility was related to severity and, in some cases, occurred months after drug withdrawal. Thirteen patients had permanent neuropathy. Also, a large proportion of patients had pre-existing renal failure, but neuropathy has been reported in patients with normal renal function as well (220).

Nitrofurantoin excretion is impaired in renal failure; however, serum levels do not rise proportionately, suggesting that the drug might be sequestered in an extravascular space. It has been postulated that neurotoxicity is due to accumulation of nitrofurantoin in neural tissue (223), or that toxic metabolites are involved (221). In view of the inability to achieve adequate urinary concentrations of nitrofurantoin even in mild renal failure (See Table 4), this patient should not be given this drug.

References

1. Rubin RH: Infections of the urinary tract. In *Scientific American Medicine,* edited by E Rubenstein, DD Federman, Scientific American, New York, 1980, p XXXIII-1.

2. Kunin CM: *Detection, Prevention and Management of Urinary Tract Infections,* 3rd ed, Lea & Febiger, Philadelphia, 1979.

3. Stamey TA: *Pathogenesis and Treatment of Urinary Tract Infections,* Williams & Wilkins, Baltimore, 1980.

4. Turck M: Therapeutic guidelines in the management of urinary tract infections and pyelonephritis. Urol Clin North Am. 1975; 2:943.

5. Fass RJ et al: Urinary tract infections. Practical aspects of diagnosis and treatment. JAMA. 1973; 225:1509.

6. Riff LJM: Evaluation and treatment of urinary infection. Med Clin North Am. 1978; 62:1183.

7. Brumfitt W: Urinary infection. Med Soc Trans. 1974; 90:105.

8. Sabath LD et al: Urinary tract infections in the female. Obstet Gynecol. 1980; 55(5 Suppl):162s.

9. Mulholland SG: Lower urinary tract antibacterial defense mechanisms. Invest Urol. 1979; 17:93.

10. Abbot GD: Neonatal bacteriuria: A prospective study in 1,460 infants. Br Med J. 1972; 1:267.

11. Pascual JF: Neonatal urinary tract infection. Contr Nephrol. 1979; 15:41.

12. Kaye D: Urinary tract infections in the elderly. Bull NY Acad Med. 1980; 56:209.

13. Andriole VT: Urinary tract infections in pregnancy. Urol Clin North Am. 1975; 2:485.

14. Maskell R et al: Urinary infection after micturating cystography. Lancet. 1978; 2:1191.

15. Collste LG et al: Urinary infection and transurethral prostatectomy. Scand J Urol Nephrol. 1978; 12:7.

16. Ramsey DE et al: Urinary tract infections in kidney transplant recipients. JAMA. 1979; 114:1022.

17. Vejlsgaard R: Studies on urinary infections in diabetics. Acta Med Scand. 1966; 179:173.

18. Vejlsgaard R: Studies on urinary infections in diabetics. III. Acta Med Scand. 1973; 193:337.

19. Ooi BJ et al: Prevalence and site of bacteriuria in diabetes mellitus. Postgrad Med J. 1974; 50:497.

20. O'Sullivan DS et al: Urinary tract infections. A comparative study in diabetics and the general population. Br Med J. 1961; 1:786.

21. Etzwiler DD: Incidence of urinary tract infections among juvenile diabetics. JAMA. 1965; 191:81.

22. Pometta D et al: Asymptomatic bacteriuria in diabetes mellitus. N Engl J Med. 1967; 276:1118.

23. Kunin CM et al: An epidemiologic study of bacteriuria and blood pressure among nuns and working women. N Engl J Med. 1968; 278:635.

24. Bran JL et al: Entrance of bacteria into the female urinary bladder. N Engl J Med. 1972; 286:626.

25. Buckley RM et al: Urine bacterial counts after sexual intercourse. N Engl J Med. 1978; 298:321.

26. Kunin CM: Sexual intercourse and urinary infections. (Editorial) N Engl J Med. 1978; 298:336.

27. Schaeffer AJ: Office laboratory. Urol Clin North Am. 1980 Feb; 7:29.

28. Stamm WE et al: Causes of acute urethral syndrome in women. N Engl J Med. 1980; 303:409.

29. Kunin CM: New methods in detecting urinary tract infections. Urol Clin North Am. 1975 Oct; 2:423.

30. Keys TF: Antimicrobials commonly used for urinary tract infections. Mayo Clin Proc. 1977; 52:680.

31. Kucers A et al: *The Use of Antibiotics*, 3rd Ed, Heinemann, London, 1979, p 701.

32. Abramowicz M (Ed): *Handbook of Antimicrobial Therapy*, Medical Letter, New Rochelle, 1980.

33. Hays DP: Teratogenesis: A review of the basic principles with a discussion of selected agents, Parts I–III. Drug Intell Clin Pharm. 1981; 15:444,542,639.

34. Anderson PO: Drugs in breast feeding—A review. Drug Intell Clin Pharm. 1977; 11:200.

35. Conte JE et al: *Manual of Antibiotics and Infectious Disease,* 4th ed, Lea & Febiger, Philadelphia, 1981.

36. Craft I et al: Maternal-fetal cephradine transfer in pregnancy. Antimic Ag Chemother. 1978; 14:924.

37. Reid DNJ et al: Maternal and transplacental kinetics of trimethoprim and sulfamethoxazole, separately and in combination. Can Med Assoc J. 1975; 112:675.

38. Mischler TW et al: Cephradine and epicillin in body fluids of lactating and pregnant women. J Reprod Med. 1978; 21:130.

39. Boutros P et al: Localization of urinary infection. Am J Obstet Gynecol. 1972; 112:379.

40. Charlton CAC et al: Three-day and ten-day chemotherapy for urinary tract infections in general practice. Br Med J. 1976; 1:124.

41. Leigh DA et al: Treatment of domiciliary urinary tract infection with a single dose of amoxycillin (letter). J Antimicrob Chemother. 1980; 6:403.

42. Bailey RR et al: Treatment of urinary tract infection with a single dose of amoxycillin. Nephron. 1977; 18:316.

43. Bailey RR et al: Treatment of urinary tract infection with a single dose of trimethoprim-sulfamethoxazole. Can Med Assoc J. 1978; 118:551.

44. Fang LST et al: Efficacy of single-dose and conventional amoxicillin therapy in urinary tract infection localized by the antibody-coated bacteria technic. N Engl J Med. 1978; 298:413.

45. Rubin RH et al: Single-dose amoxicillin therapy for urinary tract infection. JAMA. 1980; 244:561.

46. Anderson JD et al: The use of a single 1-g dose of amoxycillin for the treatment of acute urinary tract infections (letter). Antimicrob Chemother. 1979; 5:481.

47. Bailey RR et al: Treatment of uncomplicated urinary tract infections with a single dose of co-trimoxazole. NZ Med J. 1980; 92:285.

48. Ronald AR et al: Bacteriuria localization and response to single-dose therapy in women. JAMA. 1976; 235:1854.

49. Fairley KF et al: Single-dose therapy in management of urinary tract infection. Med J Aust. 1978; 2:75.

50. Stamm WE: Single-dose treatment of cystitis (editorial). JAMA. 1980; 244:591.

51. Weinstein L et al: The sulfonamides. N Engl J Med. 1960; 263:793.

52. Van Petten GR et al: Studies on the physiologic availabilities and metabolism of sulfonamides. J Clin Pharmacol. 1971; 11:27.

53. Little PJ et al: Significance of bacterial and white cell counts in midstream urines. J Clin Pathol. 1980; 33:58.

54. Stamey TA et al: The localization and treatment of urinary tract infections. Medicine. 1965; 44:1.

55. Forland M et al: Urinary tract infections in patients with diabetes mellitus. JAMA. 1977; 238:1924.

56. Thornton GF: Infections and diabetes. Med Clin North Am. 1971; 55:931.

57. Plevin SN et al: Perinephrotic abscess in diabetic patients. J Urol. 1970; 103:538.

58. Sanford JP: Urinary tract symptoms and infections. Ann Rev Med. 1975; 26:485.

59. Stamm WE et al: Treatment of acute urethral syndrome. N Engl J Med. 1981; 304:956.

60. Kirwin TJ et al: The effects of Pyridium in certain urogenital infections. Am J Surg. 1943; 62:330.

61. Spinelli AN et al: A new medication for relief of urinary symptoms: A preliminary report. J Am Geriatr Soc. 1964; 12:771.

62. Trickett PC: Ancillary use of phenazopyridine (Pyridium) in urinary tract infections. Curr Ther Res. 1970; 12:441.

63. Gould S: Urinary tract disorders. Clinical comparison of flavoxate and phenazopyridine. Urology. 1975; 5:612.

64. Nathan DM et al: Acute methemoglobinemia and hemolytic anemia with phenazopyridine. Arch Intern Med. 1977; 137:1636.

65. Greenberg MS et al: Methemoglobinemia and Heinz body hemolytic anemia due to phenylazopyridine hydrochloride. N Engl J Med. 1964; 271:431.

66. Alano FA et al: Acute renal failure and pigmentation due to phenazopyridine (Pyridium). Ann Intern Med. 1970; 72:89.

67. Eybel CE et al: Skin pigmentation and acute renal failure in a patient receiving phenazopyridine therapy. JAMA. 1974; 228:1027.

68. Johnson WJ et al: The metabolism and excretion of phenazopyridine hydrochloride in animals and man. Toxicol Appl Pharmacol. 1976; 37:371.

69. Hood JW et al: Jaundice caused by phenazopyridine hydrochloride. JAMA. 1966; 198:116.

70. Goldfinger SF et al: Hypersensitivity hepatitis due to phenazopyridine hydrochloride. N Engl J Med. 1972; 286:1090.

71. Badley BWD: Phenazopyridine-induced hepatitis. Br Med J. 1976; 2:850.

72. Gillenwater JY et al: Natural history of bacteriuria in school girls. N Engl J Med. 1979; 301:396.

73. Bailey RR: The relationship of vesico-ureteric reflux to urinary tract infection and chronic pyelonephritis-reflux nephropathy. Clin Nephrol. 1973; 1:132.

74. MacGregor ME et al: Childhood urinary infection associated with vesico-ureteric reflux. Quart J Med. 1975; 175:481.

75. Smellie J et al: Vesico-ureteral reflux and renal scarring. Kidney Int. 1975; 8:565.

76. Kass EH et al: Bacteriuria and renal disease. J Infect Dis. 1969; 120:27.

77. Freedman LR: Natural history of urinary tract infections in adults. Kidney Int. 1975; 8:596.

78. Santoro J et al: Recurrent urinary tract infections. Pathogenesis and management. Med Clin North Am. 1978; 62:1005.

79. Dontas AS et al: Bacteriuria and survival in old age. N Engl J Med. 1981; 304:939.

80. Fang LST et al: Localization and antibiotic management of urinary tract infection. Ann Rev Med. 1979; 30:225.

81. Lindemeyer RI et al: Factors determining the outcome of chemotherapy in infections of the urinary tract. Ann Intern Med. 1963; 58:201.

82. Turck M et al: Relapse and reinfection in chronic bacteriuria. II. The correlation between site of infection and pattern of recurrence in chronic bacteriuria. N Engl J Med. 1968; 287:422.

83. Takahashi M et al: Bacteriuria and oral contraceptives. JAMA. 1974; 227:762.

84. Corriere JN et al: Bacteriuria in young women. Urology. 1973; 2:539.

85. Marshall S et al: Ureteral dilatation following use of oral contraceptives. JAMA. 1966; 198:782.

86. O'Grady F et al: Kinetics of urinary tract infections. Br J Urol. 1966; 38:149.

87. Corriere JN: Effect of anovulatory drugs on the human urinary tract and urinary tract infections. Obstet Gynecol. 1970; 35:211.

88. Lincoln K et al: Resistant urinary tract infections resulting from changes in resistance pattern of fecal flora induced by sulfonamide and hospital environment. Br Med J. 1970; 3:305.

89. Stamey TA et al: Clinical use of nalidixic acid: A review and some observations. Invest Urol. 1969; 6:582.

90. Ronald AR et al: A critical evaluation of nalidixic acid in urinary tract infections. N Engl J Med. 1966; 275:1081.

91. Barlow AM: Nalidixic acid in infection of the urinary tract. Br Med J. 1963; 2:1308.

92. Reese L: Nalidixic acid in the treatment of urinary infections. Can Med Assoc J. 1965; 92:394.

93. Brumfitt W et al: Observations on bacterial sensitivities to nalidixic acid and critical comments on the 6-center survey. Postgrad Med J. 1971; 47(suppl):16.

94. Barnham M et al: In vitro susceptibility of urinary isolates of Escherichia coli to cinoxacin. J Antimicrob Chemother. 1979; 5:413.

95. Lumish RM et al: Cinoxacin: In vitro antibacterial studies of a new organic acid. Antimicrob Ag Chemother. 1975; 7:159.

96. Giamarellou G et al: Antibacterial activity of cinoxacin in vitro. Antimicrob Ag Chemother. 1975; 7:688.

97. Brumfitt W: Recent developments in the treatment of urinary tract infections. J Infect Dis. 1969; 120:61.

98. Turck M et al: Relapse and reinfection in chronic bacteriuria. N Engl J Med. 1966; 275:70.

99. Aascher AW: Investigation and differential diagnosis. In The Challenge of Urinary Tract Infections, Grune & Stratton, New York, 1980, p 83.

100. Thomas V et al: Antibody-coated bacteria in the urine and the site of urinary-tract infection. N Engl J Med. 1974; 290:588.

101. Rubin RH et al: Usefulness of the antibody-coated bacteria assay in the management of urinary tract infection in the renal transplant patient. Transplantation. 1979; 27:18.

102. Keren DF et al: Antibody-coated bacteria as an indication of the site of urinary tract infection in renal transplant recipients receiving immunosuppressive agents. Am J Med. 1977; 63:855.

103. Riedasch G et al: Antibody coating of urinary bacteria in transplanted patients. Nephron. 1978; 20:267.

104. Newman E et al: Urinary tract infection in patients with spinal cord lesions: Antibody-coated bacteria tests as a diagnostic aid. Arch Phys Med Rehabil. 1980; 61:406.

105. Jones SR et al: Localization of urinary-tract infections by detection of antibody-coated bacteria in urine sediment. N Engl J Med. 1974; 290:591.

106. Harding GKM et al: Urinary tract localization in women. JAMA. 1978; 240:1147.

107. Riedasch G et al: Antibody coating of urinary bacteria: Relation to site of infection and invasion of uroepithelium. Clin Nephrol. 1978; 10:239.

108. Hawthorne NJ et al: Accuracy of antibody-coated bacteria test in recurrent urinary tract infections. Mayo Clin Proc. 1978; 53:651.

109. Mundt KA et al: Identification of site of urinary tract infections by antibody-coated bacteria assay. Lancet. 1979; 2:1172.

110. Jones SR: Prostatitis as a cause of antibody-coated bacteria in urine. N Engl J Med. 1974; 291:365.

111. Montplaisir S et al: Antibody-coated bacteria in contaminated urine specimen (letter). N Engl J Med. 1977; 296:758.

112. Brande R et al: Proteinuria and antibody-coated bacteria in the urine (letter). N Engl J Med. 1977; 297:617.

113. Forsum U et al: A clinical evaluation of a test for antibody-coated bacteria in the urine. Scand J Urol Nephrol. 1978; 12:45.

114. Bagley DH et al: Antibody-coated bacteria in urine (letter). Urology. 1980; 15:216.

115. Woodside JR et al: Antibody-coated bacteria in urine of patients with ileal conduit urinary diversion. Urology. 1978; 11:472.

116. Rumans LW et al: The relationship of antibody-coated bacteria to clinical syndromes. Arch Intern Med. 1978; 138:1077.

117. Gleckman R: A critical review of the antibody-coated bacteria test. J Urol. 1979; 122:770.

118. Smith JW et al: Significance of antibody-coated bacteria in urinary sediment in experimental pyelonephritis. J Infect Dis. 1977; 135:577.

119. Brumfitt W et al: Trimethoprim-sulfamethoxazole. The present position. J Infect Dis. 1973; 128Suppl:S778.

120. Cox CE et al: Combined trimethoprim-sulfamethoxazole therapy of urinary tract infection. Postgrad Med J. 1969; 45Suppl:65.

121. Wormser GP et al: Trimethoprim-sulfamethoxazole in the United States. Ann Intern Med. 1979; 91:420.

122. Gleckman R et al: Drug therapy reviews: Trimethoprim-sulfamethoxazole. Am J Hosp Pharm. 1979; 36:893.

123. Rubin RH et al: Trimethoprim-sulfamethoxazole. N Engl J Med. 1980; 303:426.

124. Patel RB et al: Clinical pharmacokinetics of co-trimoxazole (trimethoprim-sulfamethoxazole). Clin Pharmacokinetics. 1980; 5:405.

125. Cosgrove MD et al: Ampicillin vs trimethoprim-sulfamethoxazole in chronic uninary tract infection. J Urol. 1974; 111:670.

126. Gleckman RA: A cooperative controlled study of the use of trimethoprim-sulfamethoxazole in chronic urinary tract infections. J Infect Dis. 1973; 128Suppl:S647.

127. Gleckman RA: Trimethoprim-sulfamethoxazole vs ampicillin in chronic urinary tract infections. JAMA. 1975; 233:427.

128. Harding GKM et al: Efficacy of trimethoprim-sulfamethoxazole in bacteriuria. J Infect Dis. 1973; 128Suppl:S641.

129. Kuehler R et al: The in vitro demonstration of the efficacy of trimethoprim as an antibacterial agent in a comparative bacteriological study on the effects of trimethoprim, sulfamethoxazole, and the combination trimethoprim-sulfamethoxazole. Chemotherapy. 1973; 18:242.

130. Greenwood D et al: Activity and interaction of trimethoprim and sulfamethoxazole against Escherichia coli. J Clin Path. 1976; 29:162.

131. Anderson JD et al: Failure to demonstrate an advantage in combining sulfamethoxazole with trimethoprim in an experimental model of urinary infection. J Clin Path. 1974; 27:619.

132. Stokes A et al: Effect of thymidine on activity of trimethoprim and sulfamethoxazole. J Clin Path. 1978; 31:165.

133. Brumfitt W et al: Double-blind trial to compare ampicillin, cephalexin, co-trimoxazole and trimethoprim in treatment of urinary infection. Br Med J. 1972; 2:673.

134. Mannisto PT: Comparison of oxolinic acid, trimethoprim, and trimethoprim-sulfamethoxazole in the treatment and long-term control of urinary tract infection. Curr Ther Res. 1976; 20:645.

135. Seneca H et al: Chronic urinary tract infections. Remission rates with trimethoprim and/or sulfamethoxazole or indanyl carbenicillin. NY State J Med. 1974; 74:494.

136. Koch UJ et al: Efficacy of trimethoprim, sulfamethoxazole and the combination of both in acute urinary tract infection. Chemotherapy. 1973; 19:314.

137. Editorial: Trimethoprim. Lancet. 1980; 1:519.

138. Huovinen P et al: Trimethoprim resistance in Finland after five years' use of plain trimethoprim. Br Med J. 1980; 1:72.

139. Editorial: Bacterial resistance to trimethoprim. Br Med J. 1980; 281:571.

140. Freeman RB et al: Long-term therapy for chronic bacteriuria in men. Ann Intern Med. 1975; 83:133.

141. Stamm WE et al: Is antimicrobial prophylaxis of urinary tract infections cost-effective? Ann Intern Med. 1981; 94:251.

142. Stamm WE et al: Antimicrobial prophylaxis of recurrent urinary tract infections. A double-blind, placebo-controlled trial. Ann Intern Med. 1980; 92:770.

143. Kalowski S et al: Controlled trial comparing co-trimoxazole and methenamine hippurate in the prevention of recurrent urinary tract infections. Med J Aust. 1975; 1:585.

144. Turck M: Localizing site of recurrent urinary tract infections. Urol Clin North Am. 1975; 2:433.

145. Hamilton-Miller JMT et al: Methenamine and its salts as urinary tract antiseptics. Invest Urol. 1977; 14:287.

146. Katul MG et al: Antibacterial activity of methenamine hippurate. J Urol. 1970; 104:320.

147. Miller H et al: Antibacterial correlates of urine drug levels of hexamethylenetetramine and formaldehyde. Invest Urol. 1970; 8:21.

148. Travis LB et al: Urinary acidification with ascorbic acid. J Pediatr. 1965; 67:1176.

149. Nahata MC et al: Effect of ascorbic acid on urine pH in man. Am J Hosp Pharm. 1977; 34:1234.

150. Hetey SK et al: Effect of ascorbic acid on urine pH in patients with injured spinal cords. Am J Hosp Pharm. 1980; 37:235.

151. Murphy FJ: Ascorbic acid as a urinary acidifying agent: 1: Comparison with the ketogenic effect of fasting. J Urol. 1965; 94:297.

152. Naccarto DV: Appraisal of ascorbic acid for acidifying the urine of methenamine-treated geriatric patients. J Am Geriatr Soc. 1979; 27:34.

153. Gibaldi M et al: Effect of antacids on pH of urine. Clin Pharmacol Ther. 1974; 16:520.

154. Harding GKM et al: A controlled study of antimicrobial prophylaxis of recurrent urinary infection in women. N Engl J Med. 1974; 291:597.

155. Stamey TA et al: Prophylactic efficacy of nitrofurantoin macrocrystals and trimethoprim-sulfamethoxazole in urinary infections. Biologic effects on the vaginal and rectal flora. N Engl J Med. 1977; 296:780.

156. Harding GKM et al: Prophylaxis of recurrent urinary tract infection in female patients. Efficacy of low-dose, thrice-weekly therapy with trimethoprim-sulfamethoxazole. JAMA. 1979; 242:1975.

157. O'Grady F et al: Long-term treatment of persistent or recurrent urinary tract infection with trimethoprim-sulfamethoxazole. J Infect Dis. 1973; 128Suppl:S652.

158. Kunin CM et al: Trimethoprim therapy for urinary tract infection. Long-term prophylaxis in a uremic patient. JAMA. 1978; 239:2588.

159. Iwarson S et al: Long-term low-dose trimethoprim prophylaxis in patients with recurrent urinary tract infections (letter). J Antimicrob Chemother. 1979; 5:316.

160. Meares EM: Prostatitis and related diseases. DM. 1980; 26:1.

161. Meares EM: Prostatitis. Ann Rev Med. 1979; 30:279.

162. Drach GW: Prostatitis. Man's hidden infection. Urol Clin North Am. 1975; 2:499.

163. Meares EM et al: Bacteriologic localization patterns in bacterial prostatitis and urethritis. Invest Urol. 1968; 5:492.

164. Meares EM: Prostatitis syndromes: New perspectives about old woes. J Urol. 1980; 123:141.

165. Fair WR et al: A re-appraisal of treatment in chronic bacterial prostatitis. J Urol. 1979; 121:437.

166. Smith JW et al: Recurrent urinary tract infections in men: Characteristics and response to therapy. Ann Intern Med. 1979; 91:544.

167. Gleckman R et al: Therapy of recurrent invasive urinary-tract infections of men. N Engl J Med. 1979; 301:878.

168. Mobley DF: Erythromycin plus sodium bicarbonate in chronic bacterial prostatitis. Urology. 1974; 3:60.

169. Paulson DF et al: Trimethoprim-sulfamethoxazole and minocycline hydrochloride in the treatment of culture-proved bacterial prostatitis. J Urol. 1978; 120:184.

170. Baert L: Re: A re-appraisal of treatment in chronic bacterial prostatitis (letter). J Urol. 1980; 123:606.

171. Bailey RR et al: Prevention of urinary tract infection with low-dose nitrofurantoin. Lancet. 1971; 2:1112.

172. Vosti KL: Recurrent urinary tract infections. JAMA. 1975; 231:934.

173. Little PJ: Incidence of urinary infection in 5000 pregnant women. Lancet. 1966; 2:925.

174. Bailey RR: Urinary infections in pregnancy. NZ Med J. 1970; 71:216.

175. Naeye RL: Causes of the excessive rates of prenatal mortality and prematurity in pregnancies complicated by maternal urinary tract infections. N Engl J Med. 1979; 300:819.

176. Norden DW et al: Bacteriuria of pregnancy—A critical appraisal. Ann Rev Med. 1978; 19:431.

177. Williams JD et al: Treatment of bacteriuria in pregnant women with sulfamethoxazole and trimethoprim. Postgrad Med J. 1969; 45Suppl:71.

178. Dukes MNG (Ed): *Meyler's Side Effects of Drugs*, vol 8 & 9, Excerpta Medica, New York, 1975, 1980.

179. Garibaldi RA et al: Factors predisposing to bacteriuria during indwelling urethral catheterization. N Engl J Med. 1974; 291:215.

180. Stamm WE: Guidelines for prevention of catheter-associated urinary tract infections. Ann Intern Med. 1975; 82:386.

181. Garibaldi RA et al: Meatal colonization and catheter-associated bacteriuria. N Engl J Med. 1980; 303:316.

182. Kunin CM: Urinary tract infections. Surg Clin North Am. 1980; 60:223.

183. Andriole VT: Hospital-acquired urinary infections and the indwelling catheter. Urol Clin North Am. 1975; 2:451.

184. Kunin CM et al: Prevention of catheter-induced urinary tract infections by sterile closed drainage. N Engl J Med. 1966; 274:1155.

185. Hirsh DD et al: Do condom catheter collecting systems cause urinary tract infection? JAMA. 1979; 242:340.

186. Butler HK et al: Evaluation of polymixin catheter lubricant and impregnated catheters. J Urol. 1968; 100:560.

187. Kunin CM et al: Evaluation of an intraurethral lubricating catheter in prevention of catheter-induced urinary tract infections. J Urol. 1971; 106:928.

188. Thornton GF et al: Bacteriuria during indwelling catheter drainage. JAMA. 1970; 214:339.

189. Warren JW et al: Antibiotic irrigation and catheter-associated urinary tract infections. N Engl J Med. 1978; 299:570.

190. Maki DG et al: Prevention of catheter-associated urinary tract infection. JAMA. 1972; 221:1270.

191. Butler HK et al: Evaluation of specific systemic antimicrobial therapy in patients while on closed catheter drainage. J Urol. 1968; 100:567.

192. Martin CM et al: Bacteriuria prevention after indwelling urinary catheterization. Arch Intern Med. 1962; 110:703.

193. Kass EH et al: Prevention of infection of urinary tract in presence of indwelling catheter. JAMA. 1959; 169:1181.

194. Meyers MS et al: Controlled trial of nitrofurazone and neomycin-polymixin as constant bladder rinses for prevention of postindwelling catheterization bacteriuria. Antimicrob Ag Chemother. 1964; 571.

195. Thornton GF et al: Bacteriuria during indwelling catheter drainage. JAMA. 1966; 195:179.

196. Gladstone JL et al: Prevention of bacteriuria resulting from indwelling catheters. J Urol. 1968; 99:458.

197. Keresteci AG et al: Indwelling catheter infection. Can Med Assoc J. 1973; 109:711.

198. Eaizels M et al: Decreased incidence of bacteriuria associated with periodic instillation of hydrogen peroxide into the urethral catheter drainage bag. J Urol. 1980; 123:841.

199. Webb JK et al: Closed urinary drainage into plastic bags containing antiseptic. Br J Urol. 1968; 40:585.

200. Shapiro SR et al: Catheter-associated urinary tract infections: Incidence and a new approach to prevention. J Urol. 1974; 112:659.

201. Bennett WM et al: *Drugs and Renal Disease,* Vol 2, Churchill-Livingstone, New York, 1978.

202. Anderson RJ et al: *Clinical Use of Drugs in Renal Failure,* CC Thomas, Springfield, Ill, 1976.

203. Zinkham WH: Unstable hemoglobins and the selective hemolytic action of sulfonamides. Arch Intern Med. 1977; 137:1365.

204. Burka ET et al: Clinical spectrum of hemolytic anemia associated with glucose-6-phosphate dehydrogenase deficiency. Ann Intern Med. 1966; 64:817.

205. Heinrich RA et al: A pharmacological study of a new sulfonamide in G6PD-deficient subjects. J Clin Pharmacol. 1971; 11:428.

206. Steinberg M et al: Acute hemolytic anemia associated with erythrocyte glutathrone-peroxidase deficiency. Arch Intern Med. 1970; 125:302.

207. Holbrooke SS: Drug-induced hypoglycemia. A review based on 473 cases. Diabetes. 1972; 21:955.

208. Pond SM et al: Mechanisms of inhibition of tolbutamide metabolism: Phenylbutazone, oxyphenbutazone, sulfaphenazole. Clin Pharmacol Ther. 1977; 22:573.

209. O'Reilly RA et al: Racemic warfarin and trimethoprim-sulfamethoxazole interaction in humans. Ann Intern Med. 1979; 91:34.

210. Kaufman JM et al: Potentiation of warfarin by trimethoprim-sulfamethoxazole. Urol. 1980; 16:601.

211. O'Reilly RA: Stereoselective interaction of trimethoprim-sulfamethoxazole with the separated enantiomorphs of racemic warfarin in man. N Engl J Med. 1980; 302:33.

212. Hansten PD: *Drug Interactions,* 4th Ed, Lea & Febiger, Philadelphia, 1979, p 57.

213. Rosenberg HA et al: The influence of food on nitrofurantoin bioavailability. Clin Pharmacol Ther. 1976; 20:227.

214. Kalowski S et al: Crystalline and macrocrystalline nitrofurantoin in the treatment of urinary tract infections. N Engl J Med. 1974; 290:385.

215. Conklin JD et al: Urinary drug excretion in man during oral dosage of different nitrofurantoin formulations. Clin Pharmacol Ther. 1969; 10:534.

216. Hailey FJ et al: Gastrointestinal tolerance to a new macrocrystalline form of nitrofurantoin: A collaborative study. Curr Ther Res. 1967; 9:600.

217. Koch-Weser J et al: Adverse reactions to sulfisoxazole, sulfamethoxazole, and nitrofurantoin. Arch Intern Med. 1971; 128:399.

218. Hailey FJ et al: Pleuropneumonic reactions to nitrofurantoin. N Engl J Med. 1969; 281:1087.

219. Sovijarvi ARA et al: Nitrofurantoin-induced acute, subacute, and chronic pulmonary reactions. Scand J Resp Dis. 1977; 58:41.

220. Gleckman R et al: Drug therapy reviews: Nitrofurantoin. Am J Hosp Pharm. 1979; 36:342.

221. Toole JF et al: Nitrofurantoin polyneuropathy. Neurology. 1973; 23:554.

222. Jacknowitz AI et al: Nitrofurantoin polyneuropathy: Report of two cases. Am J Hosp Pharm. 1979; 34:759.

223. Felts JH et al: Neural, hematologic, and bacteriologic effects of nitrofurantoin in renal insufficiency. Am JMed. 1971; 51:331.

224. Cederberg A et al: Nalidixic acid in urinary tract infections with particular reference to the emergence of resistance. Scand J Infect Dis. 1974; 6:259.

225. Stamey TA et al: Resistance to nalidixic acid: a misconception due to under-dosage. JAMA. 1976; 236:1857.

226. Zinner SH: Bacteriuria and babies revisited. N Engl J Med. 1979; 300:853.

227. Dans PE et al: Dysuria in women. Johns Hopkins Med J. 1976; 138:13.

Chapter 37

Sexually Transmitted Diseases

Michael L. Ryan and Richard F. de Leon

The importance of sexually transmitted diseases to the health care practitioner stems from both their high frequency of occurrence and their associated morbidity. The spectrum of sexually transmitted diseases has expanded greatly since the onset of the "sexual revolution." Nongonococcal urethritis (NGU) and herpes genitalis, which are not even reportable diseases in the United

States, are now as prevalent as gonorrhea and syphilis. Sexually transmitted diseases can be seen in every population, from adults to pediatric patients and from heterosexuals to homosexuals. The morbidity associated with sexually transmitted diseases can be severe, as seen with gonorrhea (PID, infertility) and neonatal herpes (blindness, spastic paralysis).

NONGONOCOCCAL URETHRITIS

Nongonococcal urethritis (NGU) is probably the most common sexually transmitted disease in the United States today (1,2,5). In several European countries, NGU is reported to occur with a frequency twice that of gonorrhea (1–4). Unlike gonococcal urethritis, NGU occurs more frequently in the educated, heterosexual white male population (1,6).

NGU, which formerly was referred to as non-specific urethritis, has been demonstrated to have a microbiological etiology. However, out of the multitude of organisms that have been associated, only *Chlamydia trachomatis* has been shown to have a causal relationship.

Chlamydia trachomatis is responsible for about 40–50% of all cases of NGU (1,7–10). Specific serotypes of *C. trachomatis* are responsible for hyperendemic blinding trachoma, lymphogranuloma venereum, NGU, proctitis, and epididymitis in men (6,9). The complications of *C. trachomatis* infection in the female include cervicitis, which usually is asymptomatic, salpingitis with subsequent nongonococcal pelvic inflammatory disease, and hypertrophic erosion of the cervix (6,9). Transmission to a neonate during passage through a chlamydia-infected birth canal results in both inclusion conjunctivitis and chlamydial pneumonia in the newborn (3,6).

C. trachomatis, an intracellular obligate parasite, is a difficult organism to demonstrate in clinical specimens, requiring cell culture techniques which are not routinely available to the practitioner. It is sensitive to tetracyclines and to erythromycin, but is unresponsive to penicillin, cephalosporins, aminoglycosides, and metronidazole therapy (3,10–12). Trimethoprim-sulfamethoxazole may be useful for the treatment of chlamydial NGU, although it is rarely used for this purpose (11,13).

Ureaplasma urealyticum, a coccobacillary organism, may be the cause of 25–40% of all cases

of NGU (10,12,15). In one study of 289 men with NGU, *U. urealyticum* was cultured in 58% of patients, 29% of whom had concurrent *C. trachomatis* infections (14). However, since only 35% of patients who are culture positive for *U. urealyticum* have symptomatic NGU, the exact pathogenic role of *U. urealyticum* in the disease state is still unclear (1,6,7). Most strains of *U. urealyticum* are sensitive to tetracyclines and erythromycin (10,14,17). However, tetracycline-resistant *U. urealyticum* have been reported with increasing frequency over the past few years (14,18–20).

Together, *C. trachomatis* and *U. urealyticum* account for no more than 70–80% of all reported cases of NGU. The other 20–30% of reported cases are thought to be due to either *Corynebacterium genitalium* type 1, which is also sensitive to tetracyclines and erythromycin, *Trichomonas vaginalis,* herpes simplex virus, *Candida albicans,* or secondary infections following an underlying urological problem such as urethral stricture (3, 7,10,21).

1. T.K. is a 26-year-old sexually active white male with complaints of mild dysuria, urgency, and a mucoid-like urethral discharge 15 days after intercourse. The patient did not present with fever, lymphadenopathy, penile lesions nor hematuria. A gram-stained smear of an anterior urethral specimen showed the presence of 20 PMN's per high power field and no intracellular gram-negative diplococci. What subjective and objective clinical data in this patient are compatible with NGU?

A patient may present with either gonococcal or nongonococcal urethritis. In fact, many patients will have both infections simultaneously, thereby accounting for the reported 30–40% incidence of post-gonococcal urethritis (urethritis acquired after penicillin therapy of gonococcal urethritis) (22). NGU is usually milder in nature than gonococcal urethritis and typically presents with a moderate mucopurulent urethral discharge and mild dysuria 8–20 days after intercourse with a new sexual partner. The discharge, which can be seen after urethral milking or after long periods without urination, is either clear or white in color and is usually mucoid (65% of patients) in consistency (1,3,6). Urgency, frequency, hematuria and genital irritation may also be present. Gonococcal urethritis is more abrupt in onset, having an incubation period of 2–9 days, and is usually associated with a higher degree of dysuria and a more profuse and purulent (80% of patients) urethral discharge (1,3,6,8).

It is impossible to accurately distinguish between NGU and gonococcal urethritis on the basis of clinical history and symptomatology alone. Since laboratory facilities for isolating the two major causes of NGU (*C. trachomatis* and *U. urealyticum)* are not routinely available at this time, the diagnosis of NGU is currently made by exclusion. A Gram's stain of the urethral discharge is examined for the presence of four or more polymorphonuclear leukocytes per oil-immersion field, confirming the suspicion of urethritis and the absence of typical intracellular gram-negative diplococci, thus excluding the diagnosis of gonococcal urethritis. In approximately 15% of the cases, the Gram's stain will reveal extracellular gram-negative cocci; in these cases the Gram's stain is considered not to be diagnostic and cultures are required (6,8). Since the small amount of discharge usually associated with NGU is easily washed away with urination, it is advisable to obtain all specimens via urethral stripping at least two hours after micturation (10).

2. How should T.K. be treated?

Since *C. trachomatis* and *U. urealyticum* account for approximately 75% of all NGU and 70% of all post-gonococcal urethritis (PGU), it is not surprising that tetracycline is the drug of choice for the treatment of NGU (1,3,10). Tetracycline is usually administered at a dose of 250 mg four times a day for 7–14 days (3,6,10,12). However, if there is any uncertainty as to whether the urethritis is nongonococcal or gonococcal in origin, then tetracycline in doses adequate to treat both conditions (0.5 grams four times a day for 7–14 days) is indicated (3,6).

Up to 70% of all female contacts of males with NGU are culture positive for *Chlamydia trachomatis* even though they may be asymptomatic. Therefore, concurrent therapy of all sexual partners is required. If the patient is unable to comply with the tetracycline dosage schedule, treatment with either minocycline (200 mg loading dose followed by 100 mg twice a day for 14 days) or doxycycline (200 mg loading dose followed by 100 mg daily for 14 days) is indicated. Erythromycin, 250 mg four times a day for two weeks, is the therapy of choice for patients who are either pregnant or unable to tolerate tetracyclines (1,10). Patient counseling on the disease state should emphasize the need to avoid further sexual activity until the prescribed course of therapy has been completed in order to prevent re-infection. If this is impossible, a condom may provide sufficient protection, although this has not yet been thoroughly evaluated.

3. T.K. was treated with tetracycline 250 mg four times a day for 14 days. T.K. remained asymptomatic for eight days following completion of his therapy, when he again complained of dysuria and a mucoid-like urethral discharge. How should T.K.'s recurrent infection be treated?

The major problem with the treatment of NGU is the high rate of recurrent infections. Up to 40% of patients will experience a recurrent infection within six weeks (29). This is especially true if the original infection was nonchlamydial in etiology (14). The majority of this high failure rate is due to a lack of patient compliance with medication regimens, failure to treat the sexual partner(s) adequately, or re-infection from a new sexual partner. Other causes of treatment failure include tetracycline-resistant *Ureaplasma urealyticum*, infection with either *Trichomonas vaginalis* or herpes simplex virus, urethral stricture or chronic prostatitis (1,10,14).

If lack of compliance or failure to treat the sexual partner is the cause of the patient's recurrent infection, retreatment of both the patient and his or her sexual partner with the same antibiotic dosage regimen is indicated (1,6). If therapy has been completed appropriately, trichomonas and herpes simplex infections should be ruled out; and if necessary, a urologist should be consulted to exclude stricture and prostatitis as possible causes of the patient's recurrent urethritis. If all the above mentioned causes of recurrent NGU have been ruled out, retreatment with either high-dose tetracycline (500 mg four times a day for three weeks) or erythromycin, at the same dosage schedule, is indicated (22).

GONORRHEA

Gonorrhea is one of the most common sexually transmitted diseases in the United States today. The incidence of gonorrhea tripled between 1965 and 1975 (30). However, due to the more frequent use of approved therapeutic regimens, improved contact tracing, asymptomatic screening programs, and increased public awareness, there has been no further increase in the incidence of gonorrhea since 1975. Presently there are one million cases of reported gonorrhea and two million unreported cases occurring in the United States annually (30–32). In addition, the VD Branch of the Center for Disease Control (CDC) estimates that there are presently 800,000 cases of asymptomatic, undetected gonorrhea in the U.S. female population.

4. J.C. is a 23-year-old male naval officer, recently stationed in the Philippines, with complaints of urgency and frequency of urination, meatal pain, and a milky urethral discharge. He reports to our clinic with his pregnant wife, B.C., who is asymptomatic. What subjective clinical data in J.C. and B.C. are consistent with the diagnosis of gonorrhea? What are the consequences of untreated gonorrhea?

Gonorrhea is caused by *Neisseria gonorrhoeae*, a gram-negative diplococcus. In males, gonorrhea becomes clinically apparent four to ten days after contact with an infected source. A milky discharge associated with meatal pain (especially when voiding) and urinary frequency are the first signs of infection. The discharge, which is caused by an irritating endotoxin released by the dying gonococcus, may become more profuse and blood-tinged as the infection progresses. Extension of the infection to the seminal vesicles, epididymis, and prostate may occur if the condition is untreated. Urethral stricture after repeated attacks, and sterility after epididymitis, are now rare complications of gonococcal infection due to the effectiveness of antibiotics.

Patients with asymptomatic disease serve as reservoirs for the infection. At one time, only females were thought to have asymptomatic gonorrhea, but asymptomatic male carriers (10%) are becoming significant (33–36). Approximately 75% of all females with gonorrhea are asymptomatic, although a purulent discharge is often seen (33). Urgency, frequency, and dysuria also may occur.

Although lower genital tract symptoms in women may disappear within a month, the patient remains infected and becomes an asymptomatic carrier of gonorrhea if untreated. Eventually, salpingitis with fibrosis and scarring of fallopian tubes may result in sterility. Pelvic inflammatory disease (PID) is a further complication of untreated gonorrhea (see Question 11). Other complications include gonococcal arthritis

(Question 12) and gonococcal ophthalmia neonatorum (Questions 13 & 14).

5. No intracellular gram-negative diplococci were seen on the Gram's stain of J.C.'s urethral exudate. Upon questioning, it was revealed that J.C. was taking tetracycline 250 mg three times a day for acne. Could J.C.'s tetracycline therapy have affected the results of his Gram's stain and should his wife receive a urethral smear? How can the diagnosis be established?

In a male, a purulent urethral discharge occurring 4 to 10 days after sexual contact is sufficient evidence to make a presumptive diagnosis of gonorrhea (37). The subsequent demonstration of intracellular gram-negative diplococci in the Gram's stained exudate confirms the diagnosis. If the Gram's stain is negative, the exudate should be cultured on Thayer-Martin (TM) medium, an enriched chocolate agar to which vancomycin, colistimethate, and nystatin have been added (38). If the patient has taken penicillin, tetracycline or other antibiotics 3 to 4 hours before the urethral smear, charcteristic gonococci will not be apparent and a culture will be required for the diagnosis of the infection (33). Cultures from both the oral and anal orifice should also be obtained if warranted by history.

A urethral smear should not be used to diagnose gonorrhea in a female (33). Due to the presence of other gram-negative diplococci and the relative scarcity of gonococci on the cervix during an infection, urethral smears are highly inaccurate in diagnosing gonorrhea in a female. The most useful test for the screening of women with asymptomatic gonorrhea is an endocervical culture, which is positive in 80% of cases (39). This test should be a part of every pelvic examination of sexually active women. After treatment, the anal canal should be cultured as a test-of-cure, since the organism persists here in approximately 25% of treatment failures. Nevertheless, diagnosing gonorrhea in women from cultures is a major problem because vaginal and rectal organisms commonly overgrow and obscure the gonococcus. Swarming overgrowths of *Proteus* and other organisms with colonial morphology resembling *N. gonorrhoeae* that are not inhibited by the TM medium make the diagnosis of gonorrhea sometimes difficult. Additonally, the vancomycin and colistin in the TM medium can inhibit as many as 8% of the cultures with a definite population of gonococci. Therefore, a completely satisfactory laboratory method for the diagnosis of gonococci is probably dependent upon the development of a specific diagnostic antiserum or a specific serological technique (40).

6. B.C. is totally asymptomatic and the results of her endocervical culture are pending. Should B.C. be treated, and how does one determine if the drug therapy of gonorrhea has been effective?

Since approximately 75% of all females and 10% of all males who have gonorrhea are asymptomatic, it is important to trace all sexual contacts of patients with gonorrhea and to treat them appropriately.

The absence of discharge and other symptoms following therapy is inadequate proof of cure. For males, smears of genital and anal secretions should be made 3 to 7 days after treatment. If the smear is positive, then retreatment is indicated. If it is negative, then a repeat culture on Thayer-Martin medium should be obtained; a positive culture is indication for retreatment.

For women, repeat cultures should be taken from the endocervical canal, anus, and pharynx if warranted by history. Two successive negative cultures are required for proof of cure following antigonorrheal therapy.

7. Taking into consideration that B.C. is both pregnant and allergic to penicillin, how should B.C.'s and J.C.'s uncomplicated gonorrhea be treated? Compare the various treatment regimens for gonorrhea.

In 1979 the CDC revised their recommended treatment schedules for gonorrhea (Table 1). The most important change is the expansion of the drug regimens of choice to include not only aqueous procaine penicillin G (4.8 million units IM) with probenecid (1 gram orally) but both tetracycline (0.5 gm orally four times a day for 5 days) and either ampicillin 3.5 gm or amoxicillin 3.0 gm, with probenecid 1 gm. The lack of significant differences in failure rates between these three therapies (3% for APPG-probenecid, 4% for tetracycline, and 7% for ampicillin-probenecid or amoxicillin-probenecid) (22) and the problems associated with APPG regimen prompted the change in recommended therapy. However, these three therapies do not have the same restrictions and advantages; thus the final decision as to the most appropriate therapy is patient specific.

Aqueous procaine penicillin G with probenecid (APPG-probenecid) therapy offers the advantages of single-dose one-time therapy, safety in pregnancy, spirocheticidal activity, and effectiveness against genital, pharyngeal, and anorectal gonorrhea. Long-acting penicillins such as benzathine penicillin should not be used for the treatment of gonorrhea, because they do not achieve adequate tissue levels, and low serum levels of penicillin serve only to select out resistant gonococci (41). Oral penicillin preparations

Table 1.

CENTER FOR DISEASE CONTROL RECOMMENDATIONS FOR
TREATMENT OF UNCOMPLICATED GONORRHEA (22,52)

Drug	Regimen	Success Rate
Aqueous procaine Penicillin G (APPG)	4.8 million units IM in two injections at one visit plus 1.0 gm probenecid by mouth	96.8%
Tetracycline	0.5 gm four times a day for five days	96.8%
Ampicillin Amoxicillin	3.5 gm ampicillin, or 3.0 gm amoxicillin each with 1.0 gm probenecid given simultaneously at one visit	92.8%

Patients who are allergic to the penicillins or probenecid should be treated with oral tetracycline as above. Patients who cannot tolerate tetracycline may be treated with spectinomycin 2.0 gm in one intramuscular injection.

Patients who fail therapy with penicillin, ampicillin, amoxicillin, or tetracycline should be treated with 2.0 gm of spectinomycin intramuscularly.

such as penicillin V are also not recommended for the treatment of gonorrhea. The problems associated with APPG-probenecid therapy include anaphylactoid reactions, especially in those patients who are allergic to penicillin (B.C. is allergic), acute psychotic procaine reactions (0.1% of patients) (42), and pain with IM administration. APPG-probenecid therapy is also not effective against *C. trachomatis* and the use of APPG-probenecid therapy may result in post-gonococcal urethritis. Therefore, APPG-probenecid therapy is best used in patients who are unreliable and cannot be expected to comply with a prescribed outpatient therapeutic regimen or to return for test-of-cure cultures. APPG-probenecid is also indicated in homosexual or heterosexual patients who have multiple foci (anorectal, pharyngeal) of gonococcal infection.

Tetracycline (0.5 gm orally four times a day for five days) is effective therapy for uncomplicated genital and pharyngeal gonorrhea, incubating syphilis and *Chlamydia trachomatis* as well (43). The major problem with tetracycline therapy is compliance with the complete five day regimen. Therefore, tetracycline is recommended for reliable patients and is the treatment of choice for patients who are allergic to penicillin or who have concomitant NGU. Tetracycline, which has a failure rate of 15%, is not as effective as APPG-probenecid or spectinomycin for the treatment of anorectal gonorrhea (44). Tetracycline is contraindicated in pregnant women (B.C. is pregnant). The 1.5 gm loading dose of tetracycline previously recommended by the CDC is not of any therapeutic value and has been deleted from the current CDC dosing guidelines (45).

Congeners of tetracycline (demeclocycline, doxycycline, and minocycline) have been used to treat uncomplicated gonorrhea. The primary advantage of these long-acting tetracyclines over the hydrochloride salt is that they may be given less frequently (twice daily), which may improve patient compliance. The long-acting tetracyclines are, however, no more effective than generic tetracycline hydrochloride in eradicating uncomplicated gonorrheal infections of the urethra and are frequently more expensive. The following dosage regimens have been employed for the long-acting tetracyclines:

   a. doxycycline 300 mg po daily for four days.
   b. minocycline 100 mg every 12 hours for 3 days.

Ampicillin 3.5 gm or *amoxicillin* 3.0 gm, each with 1 gm of probenecid is only slightly less effective than APPG-probenecid or tetracycline for the treatment of uncomplicated genital gonorrhea. Therefore, ampicillin-probenecid or amoxicillin-probenecid provide effective oral therapy for the non-compliant patient. Since neither of these one-time oral penicillin therapies is effective for the treatment of pharyngeal or anorectal gonorrhea, they should be used with caution in homosexual or heterosexual patients who engage in oral-genital or rectal intercourse. Both ampicillin-probenecid and amoxicillin-probenecid therapy are contraindicated in patients who are allergic to penicillin.

Spectinomycin is not a first-line drug for the treatment of gonorrhea. It should be reserved for the treatment of patients who either fail treatment with penicillin, ampicillin, amoxicillin or tetracycline or in penicillin allergic patients who are unable to tolerate or comply with the prescribed tetracycline dosage schedule. Spectinomycin is given as a 2 gm IM injection and is not effective in the treatment of pharyngeal gonorrhea, incubating syphilis, or *Chlamydia trachomatis* (43).

Erythromycin (0.5 gm four times a day for four days) has been shown to have a failure rate of up to 24% and has been deleted from the present CDC recommendations (46). *Spectinomycin, 2 gm IM, is currently recommended for pregnant penicillin-allergic patients.*

8. *Penicillinase-producing Neisseria gonorrhea.* J.C. was treated with 4.8 million units of aqueous procaine penicillin G IM plus 1 gm of probenecid by mouth; B.C. was treated with 2 gm of spectinomycin IM. Three weeks later, J.C. still complained of urgency, dysuria, and a milky urethral discharge. Multiple intracellular gram-negative diplococci were present on the Gram's stain of J.C.'s urethral discharge. A check of J.C.'s test-of-cure culture revealed numerous penicillinase-producing *Neisseria gonorrhoeae* (PPNG). How should J.C. and B.C. be treated?

The first cases of penicillinase-producing *Neisseria gonorrhoeae* (PPNG) infection were reported in the United States in 1976 (30,47). The code for this beta-lactamase enzyme is contained within a 4.4 milidalton plasmid (30). Those gonococci whose genomes contain this intermediate sized plasmid are totally resistant to penicillin and often are resistant to tetracycline as well (48–

50). PPNG are especially prevalent in South East Asia, the Far East, and West Africa. In the United States, PPNG strains account for a very small percentage (0.6%) of all gonococcal infections. However, the rate of occurrence of PPNG within the United States continues to rise, having increased 167% from 1980 to 1981 (221).

Due to the relative infrequency of penicillinase-producing strains of *Neisseria gonorrhoeae* within the United States today, one need not consider these organisms in the initial management of uncomplicated genital gonorrhea. However, all patients, especially those who have or whose sexual contacts have recently traveled to areas where PPNG is endemic, should receive test-of-cure cultures for β-lactamase production. Patients whose test-of-cure culture yields strains of PPNG should be treated with spectinomycin, 2 gm IM in a single injection. Although cases of spectinomycin-resistant gonococci have been reported (51,222), resistance to spectinomycin is rare. Those patients with documented spectinomycin-resistant PPNG should be treated with either cefoxitin (2 gm IM) with probenecid (1 gm po), or trimethoprim-sulfamethoxazole (nine tablets of 400 mg SMX and 80 mg TMP taken orally in single daily doses for 3 days) (222,240).

9. Anorectal and Pharyngeal Gonorrhea. M.B. is a 24-year-old sexually active homosexual male with a two-month history of perianal itching, painful defecation, constipation, a bloody mucoid rectal discharge and a sore throat. On physical examination, sigmoidoscopy revealed severe mucosal inflammation but no apparent ulcers or fissures. Stool examination for parasites was negative and a VDRL was nonreactive. Delayed fluorescent antibody test of rectal cultures and a pharyngeal culture both revealed *Neisseria gonorrhoeae*. How should M.B. be managed?

Gonorrhea, syphilis, anal warts, and various sexually transmitted enteric diseases occur much more frequently in homosexual than heterosexual men (165–169). In VD clinics in the United States gonorrhea is reported to occur in 19% of male heterosexual patients as compared to 30% of all homosexual male patients (165). Syphilis and anal warts occur in homosexual men with a frequency approximately two and ten times higher, respectively, than that in heterosexual men (165). However, not all sexually transmitted diseases occur more frequently in homosexual men. In fact,

NGU, genital herpes, and genital warts all occur with a significantly lower frequency in the homosexual population (165). The exact reasons for the higher prevalence of various sexually transmitted disease states among the homosexual population are not known for certain. However, the increased promiscuity and anonymity of male homosexual partners, the more frequent use of rectal and oral orifices for the attainment of sexual pleasure, and the high incidence of asymptomatic carrier states associated with these diseases are all thought to be contributory (166, 168,170).

The most prevalent sexually transmitted disease among the gay male population is gonorrhea. Unlike the heterosexual male population, where 99.9% of all gonococcal infections are penile, anorectal (46.8%) and pharyngeal (15%) gonococcal infections frequently occur in male homosexuals (169). Since 80–90% of all pharyngeal and 70–90% of all anorectal gonococcal infections, as opposed to only 7% of all penile gonococcal infections, are asymptomatic, there is a large reservoir of asymptomatic carriers in the homosexual male population (92,170–173). Anorectal gonorrhea, which is usually asymptomatic, may present with signs of perianal pruritus, pain or irritation upon defecation, a brownish yellow or bloody mucoid discharge, and constipation (170,171). Severe symptoms and complications of anorectal gonorrhea, such as tenesmus, ischiorectal abscess, rectal stricture, fistulas, and/or fissures are rare, occurring in less than 2% of patients with anorectal gonorrhea (170,174). Symptomatic anorectal gonorrhea, which is diagnosed by a delayed fluorescent antibody test of rectal cultures, is often confused with other intestinal disorders such as radiation- or drug-induced proctitis, colitis, intestinal cancer or amebiasis. As with anorectal gonorrhea, the majority of pharyngeal gonococcal infections are asymptomatic. However, patients may complain of symptoms ranging from a mild sore throat to an acute febrile tonsilitis (172–174).

The treatment of choice for both anorectal and pharyngeal gonorrhea is 4.8 million units of aqueous procaine penicillin G IM plus 1 gram of probenecid orally (52). This therapy is 97% effective (166,44). Alternative oral therapy for anorectal gonorrhea includes 3.5 grams of ampicillin plus 1 gram of probenecid both given orally once, then repeated in 12 hours. This two-dose ampicillin and probenecid therapy has been shown to have a failure rate of only 1.6%, as opposed to 10–15% with single dose therapy (44,175). Patients with anorectal gonorrhea who are allergic to penicillin should be treated with 2 grams of spectinomycin hydrochloride IM, which is nearly 100% effective for anorectal gonorrhea but lacks spirocheticidal activity (44,171,175,176).

Both spectinomycin and single-dose ampicillin plus probenecid therapy are ineffective for the treatment of pharyngeal gonorrhea (178–181). Patients with pharyngeal gonorrhea who are allergic to penicillin should be treated with either trimethoprim (80 mg) and sulfamethoxazole (400 mg) two tablets twice a day for seven days, or tetracycline 500 mg four times a day for five days (174,182). All patients with either anorectal or pharyngeal gonorrhea should be advised to avoid sexual activity until repeat cultures in 2–4 weeks are negative. Cultures should be obtained from sexual partners of patients with documented anorectal or pharyngeal gonorrhea even if they are presently asymptomatic.

10. What other sexually transmitted diseases are prevalent in the homosexual male population?

Nearly half of all reported cases of male **syphilis** are due to homosexual contact, approximately half of which are anorectal infections (168, 169,183). Primary anorectal syphilis usually results in chancres which are painless and not routinely visible, thereby resulting in a high frequency of asymptomatic infections. However, anorectal chancres may be extremely painful. Homosexual men have also been shown to have a higher prevalence of **hepatitis B** surface antigen and antibody than heterosexual males (184–186). Transmission of the virus, which has been found in both saliva and semen, is thought to occur by means of oral-anal sexual contact (184). The **"gay bowel syndrome"** is made up of more than simply anorectal gonorrhea and syphilis. Amebiasis, shigellosis, perianal warts, *Giardia lamblia, Campylobacter fetus,* as well as various traumatic injuries are all found with a much higher frequency in the homosexual male population.

11. *Pelvic Inflammatory Disease.* B.O. is a 19-year-old sexually active female with complaints of mild dysuria, a purulent vaginal discharge, fever (38°C), and moderately se-

vere bilateral lower abdominal pain of three days duration. Laboratory examinations showed a normal VDRL and urinalysis. A pregnancy test performed at this time was negative. The peripheral white blood cell count was mildly elevated (11,000) with 70% polymorphonuclear leukocytes. A cervical Gram's stain revealed numerous intracellular gram-negative diplococci with *Neisseria gonorrhoeae* found on culture. How should B.O. be treated?

Pelvic inflammatory disease (PID), which is a complication of gonorrhea, occurs in up to 10% of females with gonococcal infections (54,55). In fact, *N. gonorrhoeae* is the causative organism in over half of the reported cases of PID within the United States (231). PID results when gonococci migrate from the cervix into the uterus and through the fallopian tubes into either the peritoneal cavity (peritonitis) or bowel surfaces. Abscess formation may occur in the pelvic or abdominal cavity and in one or both of the fallopian tubes. Tubal occlusion and fibrosis secondary to fallopian tube inflammation (salpingitis) has been shown to result in infertility in up to 13% of women with their initial episode of PID and in 35–75% of women with recurrent PID (232).

Acute PID is manifested by severe cramp-like, non-radiating lower abdominal pain of short duration accompanied by chills, fever, leukocytosis, and a purulent endocervical exudate (56,57,233). Typical gram-negative diplococci are seen in 67% of patients with gonococcal PID (121). Treatment of these patients varies with the severity of the infection.

Mild cases of either salpingitis or epididymitis can be treated similarly on an outpatient basis. Due to its broader nongonococcal spectrum and the inherent difficulties in distinguishing among gonococcal, chlamydial, and other nongonococcal causes of PID, many clinicians prefer to use tetracycline (500 mg four times a day for 10 days) for the treatment of all cases of mild salpingitis and epididymitis. However, if a gram-stained smear of endocervical material reveals numerous intracellular gram-negative diplococci, then therapy with either APPG 4.8 million units intramuscularly, followed by ampicillin 0.5 gm (or amoxicillin 0.5 gm) orally four times a day for 10 days; or ampicillin 3.5 gm (or amoxicillin 3.0 gm) with probenecid 1 gm, followed by ampicillin 0.5 gm (or amoxicillin 0.5 gm) orally four times a day for 10 days would be appropriate.

Patients with moderate to severe PID should be hospitalized and treated with parenteral antibiotics. Patients may be treated with either aqueous crystalline penicillin G, 20 million units given intravenously each day until the fever, pain and leukocytosis improve, followed by ampicillin 0.5 gm orally four times a day for 10 days; or 0.25 gm of IV tetracycline four times a day until improvement occurs, followed by 0.5 gm orally four times a day for 10 days. The IV tetracycline dosage may need to be adjusted for patients with renal insufficiency.

12. *Gonococcal Bacteremia*. S.P. is a 28-year-old sexually active female who was seen for stiffness and pain of the wrists and fever (38°C). Physical examination revealed no abnormalities with the exception of a diffuse pinpoint erythematous macular rash over the legs and forearms. A latex fixation test for rheumatoid factor was negative. Cultures of the blood, urethra and rectum were negative for *Neisseria gonorrhoeae*, and the patient was discharged on aspirin 650 mg every four hours as needed. The rash was noted to disappear over the next week and the joint pain subsided substantially. However, three weeks later the patient complained of severe bilateral wrist and knee pain, fever, and malaise. On physical examination both knee and wrist joints were found to be hot, red, and obviously swollen; a diffuse vesiculopustular rash appeared on the patient's legs and forearms, and the patient had a fever of 38.5° C. A tap of the right knee effusion revealed a WBC count of 14,000/cu mm, with 80% PMN leukocytes and a negative Gram's stain. Cultures of the skin lesions, blood, urethra and rectum were again negative. However, *N. gonorrhoeae* were found on both throat and synovial fluid cultures. Chest radiograph, echocardiogram and EKG were all normal, and no murmur could be appreciated. How should S.P. be managed?

Gonococcal bacteremia occurs in 1–3% of women and 1% of men with gonorrhea. The most common manifestation of gonococcemia is the gonococcal arthritis-dermatitis syndrome. Gonococcal arthritis, which is the most common cause of infectious arthritis (58), is five times more common in women than men (59). Initial symptoms include fever, occasional chills, a mild tenosynovitis of the small joints, and skin lesions that are petechial, papular, pustular, and hemorrhagic in appearance, and involving primarily the distal extremities (60,235). Untreated, these initial symptoms of disseminated gonococcal infection will usually clear spontaneously within a week. However, within 2–3 weeks characteristic skin lesions reappear with increased polyarticular pain and swelling of the large joints (knee, wrists). If untreated, erosion of the cartilage and adjacent bony structures may occur (60). Cultures of skin lesions and synovial fluid are positive in approximately two-thirds of patients, with the probability of positive blood cultures decreasing dramatically as the disease progresses (30,235).

Mild cases of gonococcal arthritis may be treated on an outpatient basis with either:

—Ampicillin 3.5 gm or amoxicillin 3.0 gm orally, each with probenecid 1 gm, followed by ampicillin 0.5 gm or amoxicillin 0.5 gm four times a day for seven days.

—Tetracycline 500 mg orally four times a day for seven days.

—Spectinomycin 2 gm IM twice a day for three days.

—Erythromycin 0.5 gm orally four times a day for seven days.

Severe cases of gonococcal arthritis and bacteremia require treatment with IV aqueous crystalline penicillin G 10 million units daily for three days, followed by ampicillin or amoxicillin, 500 mg orally four times a day for four days (52).

A small number of patients with disseminated gonococcal infections will go on to develop gonococcal endocarditis or meningitis (30). The incidence of gonococcal endocarditis has declined with the introduction of antibiotics. Gonococcal endocarditis primarily involves the pulmonary valve, resulting in septic emboli, valve damage, congestive heart failure and uremia. Gonococcal meningitis mimics meningococcal meningitis and may occur in adults with genitourinary gonorrhea or in infected newborns (34).

Gonococcal endocarditis and meningitis require high-dose IV penicillin therapy. Aqueous crystalline penicillin G 10 million units IV daily until improvement occurs, followed by ampicillin 0.5 gm four times a day for seven days is indicated for both disease states. In penicillin-allergic patients with gonococcal endocarditis, desensitization and administration of penicillin is indicated. Chloramphenicol (4–6 gm/day for 10 days) may be used in penicillin-allergic patients with gonococcal meningitis (52).

**13. *Gonococcal Ophthalmia Neonatorum.*
T.P. is a 2,060 gm newborn whose mother had
a documented gonococcal infection at term.
What prophylactic therapy should T.P. receive for gonococcal ophthalmia?**

Whether a maternal gonococcal infection has
been documented or not, all newborns should be
treated prophylactically for gonococcal ophthalmia neonatorum. The need for this prophylactic
therapy is based upon the high frequency of
asymptomatic female gonococcal infections and
the potentially severe consequences of gonococcal
ophthalmia neonatorum. The infection is usually
acquired as the fetus passes through an infected
birth canal. However, ascending infections are
known to occur, and infants delivered by cesarean
section should also receive prophylactic therapy
(223).

The instillation of 1% silver nitrate drops at
birth has been the standard of therapy for the
past 100 years, and has been shown to decrease
the incidence of gonococcal ophthalmia neonatorum from 13 to 0.5% (223–226). However, therapy with silver nitrate frequently results in the
development of chemical conjunctivitis. As many
as 90% of infants treated with 1% silver nitrate
will develop a mild form of conjunctivitis (227).
The conjunctivitis usually appears within 6 hours
of therapy and clears spontaneously within 24
hours after a single irrigation with warm isotonic
saline (227). However, the symptoms of chemical
conjunctivitis (eye discharge, swelling and redness) can persist and may potentially mask an
underlying bacterial infection.

Due to the frequent development of chemical
conjunctivitis associated with silver nitrate therapy and the increasing frequency of chlamydial
conjunctivitis, the Center for Disease Control
(CDC) and the American Academy of Pediatrics
(AAP) have recently expanded their list of approved agents for the prophylactic therapy of gonococcal ophthalmia neonatorum. The new guidelines state that "1% silver nitrate solution in a
single-dose ampule or single-use tubes of an
ophthalmic ointment containing 1% tetracycline
or 0.5% erythromycin are effective and acceptable regimens for prophylaxis of gonococcal
ophthalmia neonatorum" (52,223). Flushing of the
eyes with sodium chloride or sterile water after
the instillation of these agents has been shown
not to decrease the incidence of chemical conjunctivitis and may in fact decrease the efficacy
of prophylactic therapy (227). Therefore, it is rec-

ommended that the newborn's eyes not be flushed
following the instillation of any of the prophylactic medications (52,223).

Erythromycin and tetracycline ophthalmic
ointments have been shown to be as effective, but
no more effective than silver nitrate for the prophylaxis of gonococcal conjunctivitis (227). However, erythromycin and tetracycline ophthalmic
ointments are more effective than silver nitrate
in preventing chlamydial conjunctivitis, which has
been shown to account for twice as many neonatal conjunctival infections as gonococcal conjunctivitis (228,229). Antibiotic ointments are also
associated with a lower frequency of chemical
conjunctivitis than silver nitrate therapy (227).
However, antibiotic ointments do result in approximately a 10% incidence of late onset conjunctivitis and may needlessly sensitize the infant to these antibiotics (65,227,230). In addition,
the widespread use of tetracycline and erythromycin antibiotics may result in an increased frequency of neonatal eye infections which are resistant to tetracycline and/or erythromycin
antibiotic prophylaxis.

Treatment failures are known to occur with tetracycline and erythromycin as well as silver nitrate prophylaxis (2% of reported cases) (229).
Treatment failures have resulted from inappropriately applied drugs or ointment, well-established infections at the time of delivery, the flushing of eyes following instillation of the prophylactic
agent, and resistant organisms. Prophylaxis alone
is therefore insufficient for infants born to mothers with documented gonococcal infections. These
infants should, in addition to prophylaxis, receive
aqueous crystalline Penicillin G intravenously or
intramuscularly in a single dose of 50,000 units
for full-term infants or 20,000 units for low birth
weight infants (52,223).

**14. T.P. was treated with 1% silver nitrate
drops at birth. Three days later T.P. developed increasing inflammation and discharge
from the left eye. A Gram's stain of the discharge revealed gram-negative intra- and extracellular diplococci and a presumptive diagnosis of gonococcal ophthalmia was made.
How should T.P. be treated?**

Gonococcal ophthalmia neonatorum characteristically develops 1–3 days after birth. Initially
a profuse purulent conjunctival discharge is seen,
followed by the development of moderate to severe edema and hyperemia of the eyelids (234).

The diagnosis of gonococcal ophthalmia neonatorum is based upon the clinical history of the patient, and Gram's stains and cultures of the discharge (234). However, one should not await culture results before initiating therapy in a patient whose clinical history and Gram's stain are suggestive of gonococcal infection, since the infection can rapidly progress to irreversible corneal scarring and eventual blindness.

Gonococcal ophthalmia is highly contagious and all patients should be hospitalized and isolated for 24 hours after initiating therapy. Neonates with gonococcal ophthalmia should receive aqueous crystalline penicillin G 50,000 units/kg per day in two divided doses intravenously for seven days. Saline irrigation of the eyes should be performed as needed. Topical antibiotic preparations are insufficient when used alone and not required when appropriate systemic antibiotic therapy is given (52,223). Neonatal disseminated gonococcal infection should be treated with aqueous crystalline penicillin G 75,000–100,000 units/kg per day intravenously in 2–3 divided doses for seven days. Meningitis should be treated with aqueous crystalline penicillin G 100,000 units/kg per day, divided into 3 or 4 intravenous doses, and continued for at least 10 days (52,223).

HERPES GENITALIS

Herpes genitalis is a disease that has been known since the beginning of mankind but was rarely diagnosed prior to 1965 (67). However, today well over 40% of all genital ulcers are the result of herpes simplex virus infection (68,69). In fact, herpes genitalis is the third most common sexually transmitted disease, behind only gonorrhea and nongonococcal urethritis (67,70–73).

Herpes simplex virus (HSV) is a DNA-containing virus which belongs to the family Herpesviridae. Epstein-Barr virus, cytomegalovirus, and varicella zoster virus are three other members of this family which also infect human cells. HSV is divided into two immunologically distinct serotypes, HSV-1 and HSV-2. HSV-1, which is associated predominantly with infections above the waist, is the primary cause of herpes labilis (fever blisters), herpes keratitis, and herpetic encephalitis. Genital herpes and neonatal herpes are primarily the result of HSV-2 infections. However, these anatomical boundaries are not exclusive in that genital HSV-1 as well as oral HSV-2 infections have been reported. In fact, 10–15% of all reported cases of genital herpes are due to HSV-1 infections acquired through oral sex (75–77).

15. B.J. is a 28-year-old sexually active male with complaints of painful penile lesions and lymphadenopathy. The lesions were vesicular and limited to the scrotum, glans and shaft of the penis. The onset of the lesions was preceded by a period of fever, malaise, and itching. Tzank smear of the lesions yielded multinucleated giant cells characteristic of herpes simplex virus infection. What subjective and objective clinical data in this patient are compatible with herpes genitalis? Will the infection recur?

Most initial episodes of genital herpes, especially in the male, are symptomatic. The symptoms usually start about a week after the initial exposure with prodromal signs of tingling, itching, paresthesia, and/or genital burning (67, 76,78,80,81). The prodromal stage, which can last from a few hours to several days, is followed by the appearance of numerous vesicles. The vesicles eventually erupt, resulting in painful genital ulcers. The lesions are usually limited to the glans, corona prepuce and shaft of the penis in the male, and to the vulva and vagina in the female. However, lesions can occur on the buttocks, thighs and urethra (76,83).

The most common complaint of individuals suffering from genital herpes is genital pain. The pain and edema associated with genital herpetic lesions, especially if they are secondarily infected, can be severe enough to result in dysuria and urinary retention. Systemic symptoms of fever, headache, lymphadenopathy, and malaise often accompany the primary infection (76,77,80). In primary infections, the local symptoms of pain, itching, and urethral or vaginal discharge last from 11–14 days, with a complete disappearance of lesions in 3–6 weeks (76,81,84).

The most disturbing problem associated with mucocutaneous genital herpes is the tendency for the infection to recur. During the initial exposure, the herpes simplex virus establishes itself intracellularly within the host's sensory ganglion cells (9,10,19,20). Since the latent infection is intracellular, it is protected from the host's humoral and cellular immune responses and will most likely persist for the lifetime of the patient. Although this latent virus may remain dormant indefinitely, it usually will undergo intermittent periods of viral replication and migration, resulting in recurrent infections. Various stimuli, such as emotional stress, menstruation, sunlight, trauma and viral infections, are known to elicit such recurrences (72,75,88).

Most patients (50–80%) will experience a recurrence within three months of their initial infection (75,76,81). The rate of repeat infections varies among individual patients; however, less than 10% of patients will have more than four such episodes per year for the first two years and some patients may never experience a recurrence (88).

Recurrent infections usually appear at or near the site of the initial infection and involve fewer lesions than primary infections (76,78). Systemic symptoms such as lymphadenopathy, fever, and malaise are milder in nature and are less frequently associated with recurrent than with primary infections (76,81,83,89). The duration of local symptoms such as pain and itching (4–5 days) and the lesions themselves (7–10 days) is less than with primary infections (76,78,82,89). Generally, recurrent infections are less severe than primary infections and will reappear less frequently with time.

16. B.J. states that this is the first time he has had such lesions and that he has had only one sexual partner for the last 14 months. His sexually active female partner has no prior history of herpes genitalis or any other venereal disease. The couple is very curious as to how B.J. acquired his infection. How is HSV transmitted?

Transmission of HSV occurs by direct contact with active lesions (75,90,91). Genital HSV-2 infections are usually acquired through sexual intercourse, whereas genital HSV-1 infections are acquired via oral-genital sexual practices. The popularity of rectal intercourse among male homosexuals can result in severe problems with defecation due to anorectal herpes (88,92,93). Condoms are presently thought to act as an effective barrier to viral transmission, although no definitive research has yet been conducted to establish this (68,75,88).

A patient with genital herpes is contagious only when he or she is shedding the virus. The patient will begin to shed virus during the prodromal phase, which may be several hours to days before the actual lesions first appear (91). Lesions are most contagious during the ulcerative phase and will continue to shed virus until the lesions are entirely healed and have disappeared (88,91).

It is possible to acquire a herpes genitalis infection from an individual who has never had symptomatic genital lesions. States of asymptomatic viral shedding are reported to occur in up to 14% of women with recurrent genital herpes and are probably due to limited infections involving the cervix and/or vagina (88,89). Males are thought to have a lower incidence of asymptomatic infections, about 1%, although recent studies testing the secretions of the male genitourinary tract indicate that the rate may be as high as 15% (93–95).

17. A herpes simplex virus complement fixation antibody test of B.J.'s serum taken on day 1 of the illness was negative. However, twenty days later the herpes simplex virus antibody titer was 615. Viral cultures of B.J.'s genital lesions grew HSV-2. A genital pap smear and serological antibody detection tests were negative in B.J.'s asymptomatic sexual partner. How are these laboratory tests to be interpreted?

The accuracy with which herpes genitalis can be diagnosed without the aid of laboratory tests is generally quite good, especially if the infection is recurrent in nature. However, due to the potentially severe psychological and physiological ramifications of such a diagnosis, either virological and/or serological confirmation of the diagnosis should be obtained (88,91).

There is presently no definitive laboratory test available for the diagnosis of herpes genitalis, since false positives and/or negatives are associated with all the present diagnostic tests. Viral culture of the vesicular lesions, requiring 1–4 days, is the most accurate laboratory test available (75, 76,80,88). Routine Pap smears, which have a sensitivity approximately 2/3 that of viral cultures, are quite useful in diagnosing asymptomatic carriers (76,88). Other tests used to diagnose herpes genitalis include serological antibody detection, giemsa-stained and Tzank smears of lesional extracts, which are approximately half as sensitive as Pap smears. False negative serological tests are frequently encountered in patients whose infections are quiescent, and false positive results are often encountered due to the prevalence of herpes labialis infections in the general population and the antigenic similarity between HSV-1 and HSV-2 (76–80). Primary HSV infections are characterized by a fourfold or greater rise in the herpes simplex virus antibody titer.

18. *Neonatal Herpes.* A.P., a 26-year-old female in her 32nd week of gestation, was hospitalized with complaints of painful genital lesions, headache, fever, increased vaginal discharge, and dysuria of one week's duration. On physical examination, multiple ulcerative lesions were present on the cervix, vulva, labia minora and thighs. How should this pregnant patient with genital herpes be managed?

Neonatal herpes is a devastating systemic infection of the newborn. Sixty-five percent of infants who acquire neonatal herpes will die, and severe neurological toxicities and/or blindness occur in up to 50% of those infants who survive (68,76,88,96,98). The diagnosis of neonatal herpes is often missed since characteristic herpetic lesions, which are not limited to the genitals and may involve any external site including the eyes and oral cavity, appear in only 54% of infants with neonatal herpes (97). Therefore, neonatal herpes should be ruled out in any severely ill newborn whose mother or her sexual contacts are known to have genital herpes.

HSV-2 is the cause of approximately 75% of all neonatal herpes, with HSV-1 accounting for the remaining 25% (88). The herpes simplex 2 virus is usually transmitted to the newborn during passage through an infected birth canal, although ascending infections in newborns delivered by cesarean section six hours after the membranes have ruptured have been known to occur (75,88,96–98).

There is a 40–60% chance of acquired neonatal herpes infection in infants born to mothers with an active herpes genitalis infection at term unless the infant is delivered by cesarean section within 4–6 hours after the membranes have ruptured (96,98). Herpes genitalis infections in pregnant females occur three times more frequently than in non-pregnant females, with 0.1% of all pregnant females experiencing an active genital herpes infection at or near term (96,98,100,101). Unfortunately, a large percentage (36%) of those infections occurring during pregnancy are limited to the cervix and are totally asymptomatic (98).

Although the drug therapy for neonatal herpes has progressed rapidly over the last few years, the best therapy for neonatal herpes remains pre-vention. Pregnant patients who have a history of herpes genitalis themselves or whose sexual partners(s) have such history should receive weekly pelvic examinations after the thirty-second week of gestation to determine the presence of asymptomatic genital infections (88,96). If the mother has an active herpes genitalis infection at the time of delivery, cesarean section should be performed within four hours after the membranes have ruptured in order to prevent exposure of the neonate to the virus (96,98,99,104).

Other complications associated with herpes genitalis in pregnancy include a threefold increase in the chance of spontaneous abortion for maternal HSV infections occurring during the first 20 weeks of gestation (98). This figure increases significantly with the severity of the infection, being as high as a fivefold increase for maternal infections which are primary (98). The rate of premature deliveries is also increased twofold by the presence of a primary genital herpes infection in the mother after the 20th week of gestation (98). An early concern about the mutagenic potential of HSV infections acquired during the first trimester of pregnancy has not been sufficiently established to currently recommend abortion as a therapeutic alternative to these patients (88).

19. While in the emergency room, A.P.'s membranes ruptured and the child was delivered by cesarean section 36 hours later. Cultures of the uterine fluid, cord blood and placenta at the time of delivery were negative. However, cultures of the mother's lesions were positive for HSV-2.

The baby presented as a normal 1600 gm infant whose hospital course was routine until the onset of fever and diarrhea on day 4. A lumbar puncture performed at this time was positive for HSV-2 and vesicles first appeared on the trunk and face on day 8. The baby continued to suffer from progressive liver enlargement and secondary convulsions and died at 12 weeks secondary to adrenal insufficiency. Autopsy revealed focal necrosis of the liver and adrenal glands as well as CNS involvement. How should this infant have been treated?

Neonatal herpes first appears in the infant as a mild fever and diarrhea 2-10 days after birth (96,102). Herpetic lesions, if they are to appear, will do so 1–3 weeks after birth. This is rapidly followed by necrotic involvement of the liver, adrenal glands, lungs and central nervous system resulting in jaundice, convulsions, and respiratory and adrenal failure.

Infants born to mothers with documented herpes genitalis at term should be isolated and monitored closely for any signs of HSV infection. Vidarabine (Ara-A), 15 mg/kg/day by IV infusion over 12 hours for 10 days, is the therapy of choice in those infants with documented HSV infection (106). Vidarabine reduces the mortality of disseminated neonatal herpes from 74% to 38% and localized infections from 50% to 10%. It also significantly reduces the morbidity in those infants who do survive (106). The vidarabine infusion should be started within three days of the onset of the infection in order to provide maximum efficacy (106,109).

Vidarabine therapy is of little therapeutic benefit in patients whose infections have progressed to the comatose stage (236). Therefore, empiric therapy with vidarabine is indicated in infants born to women with a history of herpes genitalis, especially if the maternal infection was active at term, who develop symptomatology consistent with neonatal herpes infection (236–238). Whether vidarabine therapy should be stopped if brain biopsies and other viral cultures are still negative after five days of therapy is still controversial (236–238,245).

Vidarabine is associated with a variety of toxicities including nausea, vomiting, diarrhea, fluid overload, thrombocytopenia, leukopenia, liver dysfunction, and CNS toxicities. Unlike other antiviral agents, such as IDU and Ara-C, these adverse effects are minimal with neonatal dosages of vidarabine (106,108,109). However, one should closely monitor the WBC and platelet counts, hemoglobin, bilirubin and SGOT levels in patients receiving vidarabine. Further studies are presently underway to determine the efficacy of high dose vidarabine (20–25 mg/kg/day) and acyclovir in the treatment of neonatal herpes.

20. Complications of Herpes Genitalis. M.F. is a 23-year-old sexually active female student with a history of frequent and severe recurrences of genital herpes since her initial infection three year ago. The patient has tried numerous therapies including topical ether, small pox vaccinations, photoinactivation, and BCG vaccines. None of these therapies has provided M.F. with any relief of her symptoms, nor have they decreased the frequency of her recurrences. M.F. has read much in the lay press concerning herpes and is concerned about the possible complications of the disease, especially cervical cancer. What are the potential complications of herpes genitalis?

Present research indicates that HSV-2 may be an oncogenic agent responsible for carcinoma of the cervix. The theoretical association between HSV-2 and carcinoma of the cervix is based primarily upon the following facts: females with carcinoma of the cervix show a higher frequency of antibodies to HSV-2 present than do cancer free controls (37% and 7.1% respectively) (110,111); females with a history of HSV-2 infection have a greater incidence of premalignant cervical changes than women without a history of HSV-2 infection (112,113); and some herpes viruses are known to be oncogenic in laboratory animals (111,114). However, data from other excellent studies have cast doubts upon these correlations (115,116). At present, it is recommended that women with a history of genital HSV-2 infection receive a routine Pap smear every six months to a year, to detect the presence of malignant cervical changes as early as possible (67,88,110,111).

Ulcerative herpetic lesions may become secondarily infected, usually with either monilia, *Staphylococcus aureus* or streptococcus, resulting in a more severe and prolonged illness (67,76). Other rare but possible complications of herpes genitalis include visceral herpes (usually seen in the neonate), aseptic meningitis, herpetic laryngitis, and herpetic keratitis (68,111).

21. Treatment of Genital Herpes. M.F. returns to clinic with complaints of recurrent herpetic lesions of the genitals for the second time in the past month. How should M.F. be managed?

The great anxiety commonly associated with the diagnosis of genital herpes is due to the fact that there is presently no effective treatment available for the condition (67,68,75,76,86,88). Therapies ranging from antiviral agents to photoinactivation to vaccines have been tried but none has yet been shown to be efficacious in either decreasing the severity of symptoms or decreasing the frequency of recurrent infections.

Antiviral agents such as adenine arabinoside (Ara-A) and idoxuridine (IDU), which act by inhibiting DNA synthesis and are effective in the treatment of neonatal herpes and herpetic keratitis, are ineffective in the treatment of herpes genitalis (82,119–121). High-dose IDU (5–20%) in dimethylsulfoxide (DMSO) may be effective in decreasing the duration of active lesions and viral shedding; however, this therapy is considered to have a very high carcinogenic potential and probably will not become available in the U.S. (12,123).

Photoinactivation, once the therapy of choice for the treatment of severe genital herpes, has fallen into disfavor over the past few years. Early studies demonstrated that herpes viruses were capable of absorbing and forming complexes with various vital dyes, and that the virus itself could be inactivated by exposing such complexes to either incandescent or fluorescent light (137). However, in recent controlled double-blind studies photoinactivation was found to be no more effective than a placebo in reducing the duration or frequency of recurrent infections (124,126). These studies, coupled with the possible oncogenic potential of the therapy itself, have discouraged the use of photoinactivation for the treatment of herpes genitalis (75,76,88,124).

Ether, chloroform, nonoxynol 9, and other lipid solvents have been used in the treatment of herpes genitalis. These agents act by disrupting the lipid-containing viral envelope required for the virus to invade the host cell. The application of ether to herpetic lesions is associated with severe pain and has not yet been shown to be of any therapeutic value (76,127). Likewise, nonoxynol 9, a nonionic surface active agent known to be virucidal *in vitro,* does not affect either the frequency or duration of recurrent infections (128,129).

Both humoral and cellular immune systems are known to play an important role in ameliorating genital herpes infections. Thus, researchers have attempted to decrease the frequency and duration of recurrent herpes infections by increasing the host's resistance to HSV. None of these immunostimulator therapies, including vaccines (130), BCG (138), and levamisole (131), has yet to be shown to be efficacious in the treatment of mucocutaneous genital herpes. Zupidon, a heat inactivated HSV-2 vaccine indicated for the treatment of recurrent herpes genitalis due to HSV-2, has recently become available in Europe. However, the efficacy of this vaccine has not yet been established (111).

A series of uncontrolled observations published by Griffith in 1977 indicated that lysine, in doses of 312–1,200 mg per day, was highly effective in the treatment of mucocutaneous herpes simplex infections (241). These observations, coupled with tissue culture studies which showed that lysine suppresses both the replication and cytopathogenicity of HSV, raised new hopes for lysine as a therapeutic agent for the treatment of herpes (242). However, two excellent double-blind, placebo-controlled, randomized studies performed by Milman have clearly demonstrated that lysine is no more effective than a placebo in decreasing either the duration of active HSV lesions or the frequency of their recurrences (243,244).

There are several medications that are currently undergoing investigation which have potential for the treatment of herpes genitalis. Acyclovir (acyloguanosine) is a new antiviral agent with a much larger therapeutic index than that of previous antiviral agents (132,133). Acyclovir is essentially a prodrug that is converted to its active form, acyclovir triphosphate, within the viral infected cell by a viral DNA-coded thymidine kinase (139). Acyclovir triphosphate, which has a 30-fold greater affinity for viral than mammalian DNA polymerase, selectively blocks viral DNA replication (132,133,139). Acyclovir, given by IV infusion, is effective in the treatment of corneal herpetic keratitis, herpes encephalitis, and cutaneous and disseminated HSV infections in cancer patients (133–135). Further studies are currently underway to assess the efficacy of topical acyclovir in the treatment of mucocutaneous herpes genitalis.

Another experimental approach to the treatment of genital herpes is Herpigon with ultrasound (70). Herpigon is a combination of zinc, tannic acid and urea in a cream base (HEB). A study by Fahim in 1980 showed that Herpigon, when administered by ultrasound, was effective in both promoting the healing of active lesions and significantly reducing the rate of recurrent infections (70).

Most genital herpes infections, unless the patient is immunocompromised or the lesions have become secondarily infected, are benign and will heal spontaneously. The patient should be instructed to keep the involved areas clean and dry. In order to prevent autoinoculation, the patient should be told not to touch the lesions and to wash his or her hands immediately afterwards if they should do so. Local anesthetics provide relief from the pain of genital lesions; however, they should be avoided if possible since they counteract efforts to keep the lesions dry. Local corticosteroid therapy is contraindicated due to its potential to cause secondary bacterial infections of the lesions (76,88).

Patient counseling is an important facet in the therapy of genital herpes. Faced with the social realities of the disease, patients have been known to suffer severe psychological disturbances leading to attempted suicide (88,91). Health care practitioners should attempt to recognize these patients and to relieve their feelings of guilt and anxiety. In individuals with frequent recurrences, efforts should be made to identify and avoid stimulatory factors such as sunlight, trauma, or emotional stress. The limitations of therapy and the decreased severity and frequency of recurrences with time should be explained to the patient. The periods of infectivity and the need to avoid sexual activity during these times should also be emphasized. Women with herpes genitalis should be scheduled for a routine Pap smear every six months to a year and should be instructed to discuss the problem with their physician should they become pregnant.

SYPHILIS

The prevalence of primary and secondary syphilis in the United States has increased dramatically (26.3%) since 1977 (140). However, the number of reported cases of syphilis in women fell 19.1% from 1969 to 1980, with a corresponding decrease in congenital syphilis (140). The astonishing increase in the rate of male syphilis, 50.8% from 1969 to 1980, is primarily the result of a tremendous increase in homosexually acquired syphilitic infections in males, 187.2% from 1969 to 1980 (140).

Clinical Course

Primary Stage. The incubation period of syphilis varies from 10 to 90 days. During this incubation period the patient is not infectious, although fetal infections have resulted from an incubating maternal infection. The first clinical expression of primary syphilis is the development of a primary chancre at the invasion site about three weeks after the initial exposure. The chancre, which begins as a painless papule, is characteristically ulcerated, raised, nontender, and filled with numerous spirochetes. Since they are painless (unless secondarily infected), occur in obscure sites (the cervix is most commonly in-

volved in the female), and are masked by subtherapeutic doses of commonly used antibiotics, primary chancres are frequently missed by the patient. Unnoticed and untreated, the primary chancre will resolve spontaneously in two to six weeks. Primary syphilis is the most infectious stage and lasts six to eight weeks.

Secondary Stage. A widespread maculopapular skin rash, frequently involving the palms of the hands and the soles of the feet in addition to the trunk and extremities, marks the beginning of the secondary stage. Mucous membranes may also be involved; and the patient may complain of fatigue, malaise, headache, and fever during this time. Patients with secondary syphilis are infectious to others. If untreated, the lesions of secondary syphilis heal spontaneously in four to 12 weeks. This is the beginning of the latent stage of the disease.

Latent Stage. During the latent stage there are no clinical lesions, the darkfield examination is negative, and the cerebrospinal fluid examination is normal. Positive nontreponemal and treponemal serologic tests are the only manifestations of the disease during this stage. The latent stage is divided into the early latent (less than four years duration) and late latent (more than four years duration) phases. The early latent phase is infectious if there is relapse to the secondary stage, while the late latent stage is considered to be noninfectious.

Late Consequences. The lesions of late syphilis involve virtually every organ system and tissue. The skeletal system is affected in about 5% of patients with late syphilis. Involvement of the cardiovascular and central nervous systems (the most serious of complications) is responsible for 90% of deaths due to syphilis. The cardiovascular system may be affected as late as 20 to 30 years after acquisition of the infection. *Treponema pallidum* may invade the media of the ascending aorta, causing tissue destruction and loss of elasticity which ultimately may lead to aneurysm formation. Rupture of the aneurysm will cause death.

Neurosyphilis has a broad range of symptoms. Headache, vomiting, and malaise are symptoms of a meningitis that usually respond to appropriate therapy. Invasion of nervous system tissues by *T. pallidum* produces general paresis, tabes dorsalis, or optic atrophy. General paresis (dementia paralytica) usually occurs 10 to 25 years after the primary lesion. The disease begins with loss of memory, confusion and impaired judgment, and progresses rapidly to the point where the patient is physically, socially and mentally disabled. General paresis is usually fatal within three years of its onset.

Tabes dorsalis (locomotor ataxia) may become evident 10 to 20 years after the primary lesion. Destruction of portions of the nervous system affects the patient's sense of joint position and results in a characteristic gait. "Lightning pains," sharp jabs of pain, are experienced by most patients with tabes dorsalis.

Congenital Syphilis. Syphilis may be transmitted from the infected mother to the fetus. Congenital syphilis may be manifested by severe dehydration and malnutrition. Roentgenographs of the long bones may demonstrate bone destruction and osteochondritis. Late congenital syphilis involving the CNS may appear as late as 20 years after birth. Eighth nerve deafness, optic atrophy, and juvenile paresis may also occur.

Laboratory Evaluation

Darkfield Examination. Darkfield microscopy provides the earliest means of diagnosing syphilis during the primary stage. The patient's immune response to the infection may not be sufficiently developed early in the disease process; consequently, serologic tests would be of no use.

Serous material obtained from the suspected syphilitic lesion is viewed through a microscope fitted with a darkfield condenser. Objects viewed through such equipment appear to be brightly illuminated when placed against a black background. A positive diagnosis is made if organisms of the characteristic morphology and motility of *T. pallidum* are observed. Darkfield examination of oral lesions may be unreliable, since *T. microdentium,* a non-pathogen that is part of the normal flora of the mouth, is morphologically indistinguishable from *T. pallidum.*

Serologic Tests. Serologic tests, unlike darkfield examination, are associated with varying rates of false positive and negative results during the different stages of syphilis. Therefore, in order to interpret the results of serologic tests for syphilis, one must understand their limitations. Darkfield examination is the test of choice for early-lesion syphilis. Serological tests for syphilis first become reactive during the primary stage, approximately four to eight weeks after the initial infection.

However, the patient's immune response is not yet reliable enough to exclude syphilis in patients with negative serological tests (see Table 2). Patients with positive histories and physical examinations but negative darkfield examination and serology should receive repeat serologic tests in two to four weeks. Serologic tests are most reliable during secondary syphilis, when reagin levels are highest. The reagin levels fall slowly during latent syphilis, resulting in a decreasing reliability of serologic testing. There are two types of tests used for the serodiagnosis of syphilis: nontreponemal tests, which measure serum concentrations of a reagin (a lipoidal antigen that is generated as part of a nonspecific immune response to an infectious or noninfectious disease), and treponemal tests, which detect the presence of antibodies specific for *T. pallidum* (141).

Nontreponemal Tests. Nontreponemal tests, unlike treponemal tests, are not specific for *T. pallidum* but can be quantified. Nontreponemal tests are inexpensive and useful for screening large numbers of people. There are presently three different types of nontreponemal tests: the Venereal Disease Research Laboratory (VDRL) test, the Rapid Plasma Reagin (RPR) Card test, and the Automated Reagin Test (ART). The VDRL test is the most widely used of these nontreponemal tests.

The quantitative VDRL is much more useful than the qualitative test. Serum is geometrically diluted and the test is repeated on each dilution. The value reported is the most dilute serum concentration having a positive reaction. Subsequent testing may be used to follow the progress of the disease or the effectiveness of therapy. If the titer of a patient receiving therapy increases by two dilutions or more, eg, from a dilution of 1:4 to 1:16, the therapy is ineffective and another

Table 2.

FALSE NEGATIVE RESULTS
WITH VDRL AND FTA-ABS TESTS

Stage of Syphilis	Percentage of False Negative Results	
	VDRL	FTA-Abs
Primary	24%	14%
Secondary	<0.1%	<0.1%
Early Latent	5%	1%
Late Latent	28%	5%

treatment regimen must be instituted. Usually, effective therapy will decrease the titer and eventually return the patient to a seronegative state. Patients usually become seronegative six to 12 months after treatment for primary syphilis and 12 to 24 months after therapy for secondary syphilis. Patients treated with oral tetracycline or erythromycin are less likely to become seronegative (141). Therapy is considered adequate in patients who never become seronegative if the titer decreases fourfold (142). Quantitative VDRL tests are also required for those patients who remain serofast (ie, have a consistent reactivity at the same titer for an indefinite period, perhaps for life); two dilution deviations in either direction from the "steady state" titer are indicative of disease relapse or return to seronegativity. False positives can result from technical error, a variety of disease states (see Table 3), vaccinations, immunizations, IV narcotic abuse, and pregnancy (141–143).

Treponemal Tests. Specific treponemal tests are used to help distinguish between a biological false positive and a true positive test for syphilis, to assist in establishing a diagnosis of syphilis in those patients without clinical manifestations of syphilis, and to establish the diagnosis of syphilis in patients with evidence of the disease. The Fluorescent Treponemal Antibody Absorption (FTA-Abs) test is the most commonly used treponemal

test. Since the results of the FTA-Abs test, like all treponemal tests, cannot be quantified, the test is of no value in determining the effectiveness of therapy. Although the FTA-Abs test may lead to false negative results in primary syphilis, it is considerably more reliable than the VDRL test in detecting latent syphilis.

The Treponema Pallidum Immobilization (TPI) test and the Microhemagglutination (MHA-TP) test are two other treponemal tests. The TPI test is not routinely used because of its cost and complexity. The MHA-TP test, which is not as sensitive as the FTA-Abs test in primary syphilis, is commonly used.

Treatment

The drug of choice for the treatment of all stages of syphilis is penicillin (144,145). Every effort should be made to rule out penicillin allergy before choosing other antibiotics which have been studied much less extensively than penicillin in the treatment of syphilis. If penicillin is contraindicated, the alternatives are tetracycline or erythromycin, each at 500 mg orally four times a day for 15 days. Since *T. pallidum* has not developed resistance to antibiotic treatment, drug regimens have not changed substantially over the years.

Primary, secondary, and latent syphilis (with a negative CSF) of less than one year's duration is best treated with a single intramuscular dose of 2.4 MU of benzathine penicillin G. Alternately, aqueous procaine penicillin G can be administered intramuscularly 600,000 units daily for eight days (144). Latent syphilis, neurosyphilis, and cardiovascular syphilis are treated with 2.4 MU of intramuscular benzathine penicillin G on the first visit. This dose is repeated twice at seven-day intervals. Aqueous procaine penicillin G 600,000 units intramuscularly daily for 15 days can be used as an alternative (144). Patients who are allergic to penicillin and who have syphilis of more than one year's duration (latent syphilis, neurosyphilis, or cardiovascular syphilis) should be treated with either tetracycline or erythromycin, 500 mg four times a day for 30 days (144).

Once treatment is initiated, *T. pallidum* disappears from the infected lesions within 24 hours (146). Repeat physical examinations and quantitative VDRL tests should be performed at 1, 3, 6, 9, 12, 18, and 24 months (145). Return of le-

Table 3.

CAUSES OF FALSE POSITIVE
VDRL AND FTA-ABS TESTS

VDRL	FTA-Abs
Technical error	Technical error
Other spirochetal (yaws, bejel, pinta)	Genital herpes
	Heroin addiction
Lupus erythematosus	Leprosy
Hasimoto's thyroiditis	Mononucleosis
Malaria	Collagen vascular diseases
Mononucleosis	Pregnancy
Pregnancy	
Vaccinations	
Immunizations	
IV narcotic abuse	

sions or a two-dilution increase in titer indicates the need for retreatment due to relapse or reinfection. In two years, all but a small percentage of patients with early syphilis become seronegative. If the disease is treated during the late stages, complete seroreversal may not occur; and while the disease process may have been halted, the damage that may have been done to the cardiovascular system or nervous system cannot be reversed.

22. *Syphilis During Pregnancy.* N.W. is a 27-year-old pregnant woman in the 19th week of gestation who has a positive VDRL and a positive FTA-Abs. How should N.W. be managed? How would management be altered in the face of penicillin allergy?

Because transmission of syphilis to the fetus does not take place until the fifth month of gestation (149), treatment before the 18th week of gestation almost always prevents fetal infection. Therapy initiated after 18 weeks of gestation will cure the fetal spirochetemia, but may not prevent the development of congenital syphilis. If the mother is left untreated, the fetus may be aborted, stillborn, or may be born with congenital syphilis.

Pregnancy may cause false-positive reactions to both the nontreponemal (150,151) and the treponemal tests (152). A patient who is seropositive does not necessarily require therapy if, for example, she has been treated adequately, has no significant increase in titer (two dilutions or more), and has no signs of relapse. The patient who has recently become seropositive, developed a two-dilution increase in titer, or shows signs of relapse or reinfection must be treated. During pregnancy, the patient should be followed with monthly quantitative VDRL titers to evaluate the effectiveness of therapy; therafter, she should be followed as any other syphilitic patient.

The treatment of the pregnant patient with syphilis is the same as for other patients with the disease. Penicillin is the drug of choice (153). Primary, secondary, and latent syphilis of less than one year's duration may be treated with 2.4 million units of benzathine penicillin G given intramuscularly at a single session, or 4.8 million units total of aqueous procaine penicillin G given intramuscularly in divided doses of 600,000 units daily for eight days (144). Latent syphilis of more than one year's duration, cardiovascular, late-benign, and neurosyphilis should be treated with

three successive weekly intramuscular injections of 2.4 million units of benzathine penicillin G for a total of 7.2 million units. Aqueous procaine penicillin G may also be used if 600,000 units are given intramuscularly each day for 15 days (144).

Tetracycline should be avoided during pregnancy because of its effects on the fetus (tooth staining and damage to the long bones) and its association with maternal liver and kidney damage (154–157). Erythromycin has been used with success in the treatment of pregnant patients with syphilis. Doses range from 250 to 500 mg orally four times daily for 15 days (149,153). Erythromycin, however, achieves only 6 to 20% of the maternal blood levels in the fetus (158,159). This may explain why some patients treated with erythromycin aborted or gave birth to stillborn infants. Therefore, documentation of penicillin allergy is especially important before resorting to erythromycin. The estolate salt of erythromycin, like the tetracyclines, is not recommended because of potential adverse effects on the mother and fetus (144). Clindamycin may be a more satisfactory alternative to penicillin than erythromycin, because it crosses the placental barrier more readily and predictably (160).

Cephaloridine may also be used for the pregnant syphilitic patient with penicillin allergy. It has been used in early syphilis in doses of 0.5 to 2 gm given intramuscularly daily for three to 32 days (161,162). A regimen of 0.5 gm given intramuscularly daily for 10 days was found to be effective in patients with early syphilis (163). Cephalexin provides an effective oral cephalosporin alternative for the treatment of pregnant syphilitic patients. Cephalexin, at dosages of 500 mg four times a day for 15 days, is as effective as erythromycin or tetracycline in the treatment of primary and secondary syphilis (136).

If the VDRL performed on cord blood of the fetus is positive, both the FTA-Abs and FTA-Abs IgM should be performed. Because both the VDRL and FTA-Abs tests may become positive as a result of the passive transfer of antibodies in maternal blood to the fetus, the FTA-Abs IgM is the most reliable test for the detection of congenital syphilis (164). The test relies on the detection of antitreponemal antibodies produced in utero by the fetus in response to *T. pallidum* infections. Since IgM does not cross the placenta, the presence of this antibody indicates that the fetus is infected by spirochetes. The newborn with congenital syphilis and a normal CSF can be treated with benzathine penicillin G 50,000 units/kg in a single dose (144). Infants with congenital syphilis should have a CSF examination before treatment and should return for repeat quantitative nontreponemal tests three, six, and 12 months after treatment. Additional guidelines for the treatment of congenital syphilis can be found with the Center for Disease Control (144).

23. *Jarisch-Herxheimer Reaction.* N.W. was treated with an IM injection of 2.4 million units of benzathine penicillin G. Six hours later N.W. complained of diffuse myalgias, chills, sore throat, headache and an exacerbation of her rash. N.W.'s respiratory rate was 20/minute and her blood pressure was 130/80 mm Hg. How should N.W. be managed?

The Jarisch-Herxheimer reaction is a benign, self-limiting complication of treponemal antibiotic therapy due to the sudden release of antigenic substances from rapidly killed treponemes. The reaction is not an allergic reaction to penicillin and patients should not be labeled as such (239). The reaction characteristically occurs six to eight hours after the first penicillin dose and subsides spontaneously in 18 to 24 hours (142,239). The Jarisch-Herxheimer reaction occurs in up to 50% of patients with primary syphilis and 75% of patients with secondary syphilis (140). The resulting fever, malaise, shaking chills, headache, myalgias, and a worsening of the syphilitic lesions may be controlled with the use of antipyretics or corticosteroids. Penicillin allergy may also be a treatment complication. Incidence of penicillin allergy in venereal disease clinics is 6.61 cases per 1,000 patients (147), which is slightly below the 1% incidence in the general population (148).

TRICHOMONIASIS

Trichomoniasis is a sexually transmitted disease caused by the protozoan *Trichomonas vaginalis.* Although the organism has been known to survive on moist surfaces for several hours, transmission is almost exclusively by sexual intercourse (190). About 24.6% of all women over the age of twenty have smears which are positive for *Trichomonas vaginalis* (191,192).

24. N.J. is a 32-year-old female with a two month history of vaginal itching and burning and a recent onset of a profuse yellow leukorrhea. A wet mount examination of vaginal secretions revealed numerous trichomonads and the diagnosis of trichomoniasis was made. What subjective and objective clinical data support this diagnosis?

Trichomoniasis in the female is usually symptomatic, although asymptomatic carrier states are known to occur. The female patient usually presents with persistent or recurrent vaginal itching and/or burning. Vaginal discharge, which is usually increased profusely, is creamy yellow to green in color and has a fetid odor. Examination of the vaginal epithelium commonly reveals inflammatory changes and possible petechial bleeding. Trichomonas infections in the male commonly involve the prostate and urethra and are usually asymptomatic, although symptomatic NGU secondary to *Trichomonas vaginalis* has been reported.

Laboratory confirmation of trichomoniasis is easily obtained by the presence of motile trichomonads on a fresh mounted or giemsa-stained preparation of vaginal secretions. The organism is also found in samples of freshly voided urine, prostatic and/or urethral secretions (193).

25. How should N.J.'s trichomoniasis be treated?

The drug of choice for the treatment of *Trichomonas vaginalis* is oral metronidazole. It is essential that the patient and all his or her sexual partners are treated simultaneously with the same dosage regimen. Metronidazole, 250 mg three times a day for seven days, is the most commonly prescribed dosage regimen, curing 90–95% of documented cases (194–196). However, five days of this program or a single 2 gm dose are equally effective, curing 85–90% of documented cases (194,196–201).

Treatment failures have been reported in 10–20% of patients treated with metronidazole. Most cases of persistent or recurrent trichomoniasis are due to either poor compliance, which can be alleviated by treatment with a single 2 gm dose, or reinfection, usually due to the failure to treat the sexual partner(s) simultaneously. Other possible, but certainly rare, causes of recurrent trichomoniasis include inadequate absorption of the drug and the presence of aerobic organisms such as *K. aerogenes, E. coli,* or *S. fecalis* which have the potential to absorb and inactivate metronidazole (202,203).

Since the development of a more accurate *in vitro* assay several years ago, the reports of metronidazole-resistant strains of *Trichomonas vaginalis* have increased significantly (204–207). Such strains of *T. vaginalis* are responsible for an as yet unknown percentage of cases of persistent trichomoniasis. Since such resistant strains of *T. vaginalis* are sensitive to higher serum levels of metronidazole, a trial of metronidazole at a higher dosage schedule would seem prudent in those cases of recurrent trichomoniasis where compliance and failure to treat the sexual partner(s) have been ruled out as possible causative factors (202).

26. N.J. was treated with metronidazole 250 mg three times a day for seven days. On the fourth day of therapy, while attending a party for a friend, N.J. developed a severe headache, followed by nausea, sweating and dizziness. Could N.J.'s symptoms be caused by her drug therapy?

Minor side effects associated with metronidazole therapy include nausea, vomiting (especially with single dose therapy), headache, skin rashes, and alcohol intolerance (194,197,208). The alcohol intolerance is due to a metronidazole-induced inhibition of aldehyde dehydrogenase, resulting in the buildup of high serum acetaldehyde levels. Severe "antabuse reactions" secondary to concomitant use of metronidazole and ethyl alcohol are not common. However, patients should still be warned about the possibility of nausea, vomiting, flushing, and respiratory distress following ethanol ingestion (209,210). More serious side effects associated with metronidazole therapy include transient leukopenia with prolonged therapy and peripheral neuropathy, both of which are rare and generally reversible if therapy is stopped immediately (197,211,212).

27. S.G., a 31-year-old female, is in her first trimester of pregnancy and has a history of recurrent trichomoniasis. She now complains of mild vaginal itching and burning, and a small amount of frothy yellow-green leukorrhea. The preliminary diagnosis of trichomoniasis is confirmed by a wet mount examination of vaginal secretions which revealed numerous trichomonads. S.G. has read much of the lay press on metronidazole and is concerned about her safety as well as that of her fetus. How should S.G. be treated?

Recent studies indicating that metronidazole is carcinogenic in rodents and mutagenic in bacteria have cast doubts upon its use in the treatment of trichomoniasis. Several studies have documented that long-term high-dose metronidazole in laboratory mice may cause an increase in the frequency of pulmonary and hepatic tumors (197,213). However, these data are difficult to extrapolate to humans and, in fact, no increase in the incidence of cancer in human patients treated with metronidazole has yet been documented (197,214,215).

Although studies in laboratory animals and bacteria have indicated that metronidazole has a mutagenic potential, human studies have not documented any significant increase in congenital defects in infants due to the maternal use of metronidazole during pregnancy (216,217). However, studies to date have not involved a sufficient number of patients to completely rule out any congenital risk to the fetus. In fact, a study by Peterson in 1966 suggested that the use of metronidazole during the first trimester of pregnancy may lead to an increased risk of fetal abnormalities (216). All that can be said at present is that the use of metronidazole is contraindicated during the first trimester of pregnancy and should be avoided if possible during the second and third trimesters. If the pregnant patient is symptomatic and local therapy is required, then vaginal creams or douches are indicated.

Alternative therapy for the treatment of *Trichomonas vaginalis* in the U.S. presently involves the use of vaginal creams, furazolidone-niferoxime combination (Tricofuran) and clotrimazole (Gyne-Lotrimin) being the most commonly prescribed. However, these agents are not as effective as oral metronidazole, since they are unable to reach all sites of infection (218,219). Therefore, a trial of vinegar or other acidifying douches, which act by restoring the pH of the vagina to 4.5–5 and avoidance of restrictive clothing are usually advocated first before local therapy in those cases where metronidazole is contraindicated (217,220).

References

1. Melo JC: Nongonococcal urethritis. J Key Med Assoc. 1979; 77:520.
2. Venereal Disease Control Div: Non reported sexually transmitted diseases. United States. Morb Mort Weekly Rep. 1979; 28:61.
3. Felman YM et al: Nongonococcal urethritis: a clinical review. JAMA. 1981; 245:381.
4. Willcox RR: How suitable are available pharmaceuticals for the treatment of sexually transmitted diseases? 1. Conditions presenting as genital discharges. Br J Vener Dis. 1977; 55:314.
5. Melton LS: Comparative incidence of gonorrhea and nongonococcal urethritis. Am J Epidermiol. 1976; 104:535.
6. McCormack WM: Nongonococcal urethritis. Infect Dis Pract. 1978; 1:1.
7. Holmes KK et al: Etiology of nongonococcal urethritis. N Engl J Med. 1975; 292:1199.
8. Jacobs NF et al: Gonococcal and nongonococcal urethritis in men. Clinical and laboratory differentials. Ann Intern Med. 1975; 82:7.
9. Schachter J: Chlamydial infections. N Engl J Med. 1978; 298:428; 490; 540.
10. Oriel JD: Management of nongonococcal urethritis. Drugs. 1979; 18:398.
11. Paavonen J et al: Treatment of nongonococcal urethritis with trimethoprim-sulphadiazine and with placebo. A double-blind partner controlled study. Br J Vener Dis. 1980; 56:101.
12. Bowie WR et al: Tetracycline in nongonococcal urethritis. Br J Vener Dis. 1980; 56:332.
13. Kuo C-C et al: Antimicrobial activity of several antibiotics and a sulfonamide against Chlamydia trachomatis organisms in cell culture. Antimicrob Agents Chemother. 1977; 12:80.
14. Stimson JB et al: Tetracycline-resistant Ureaplasma urealyticum: a cause of persistent nongonococcal urethritis. Ann Intern Med. 1981; 94:192.
15. Loufalik ED et al: Treatment of nongonococcal urethritis with rifampicin as a means of clearing the role of Ureaplasma urealyticum. Br J Vener Dis. 1979; 55:36.
16. Bowie WR et al: Etiology of nongonococcal urethritis: evidence for Chlamydia trachomatis and Ureaplasma urealyticum. J Clin Invest. 1977; 59:735.
17. McCormack WM et al: The genital mycoplasmas. N Engl J Med. 1973; 288:78.
18. Ford DK et al: Nonspecific urethritis associated with a tetracycline-resistant T-mycoplasma. Br J Vener Dis. 1974; 50:373.
19. Evans RT et al: The incidence of tetracycline-resistant strains of Ureaplasma urealyticum. J Antimicrob Chemother. 1978; 4:57.
20. Spasepen MS et al: Tetracycline-resistant T-mycoplasmas (Ureaplasma urealyticum) from patients with a history of reproductive failure. Antimicrob Agents Chemother. 1976; 9:1012.
21. Furness G et al: Corynebacterium genitalium (non-specific Corynebacterium): biologic reactions differentiating commensals of the urogenital tract from the pathogens responsible for urethritis. Invest Urol. 1977; 15:23.

22. Handsfield HH: The latest protocols for sexually transmitted infections. Drug Therapy. 1979; June:43.
23. Berger RE et al: Chlamydia trachomatis as a cause of acute 'idiopathic' epididymitis. N Engl J Med. 1978; 298:301.
24. Goldmeier D et al: Isolation of Chlamydia trachomatis from throat and rectum of homosexual men. Br J Vener Dis. 1977; 53:184.
25. Beem MO et al: Respiratory-tract colonization and a distinctive pneumonia syndrome in infants infected with Chlamydia trachomatis. N Engl J Med. 1977; 296:306.
26. Treharne JD et al: Antibodies to Chlamydia trachomatis in acute salpingitis. Br J Vener Dis. 1979; 55:26.
27. Harrison HR et al: Chlamydia trachomatis infant pneumonia: comparison with matched controls and other infant pneumonitis. N Engl J Med. 1978; 298:702.
28. Stramm WE: Annual update on managing sexually transmitted diseases. Modern Medicine. 1979; October:95.
29. Handsfield HH et al: Differences in the therapeutic response of chlamydia-positive and chlamydia-negative forms of nongonococcal urethritis. J Amer Vener Dis Assoc. 1976; 2:5.
30. Wiesner PJ: Gonorrhea. Cutis. 1981; 27:249.
31. Fiumara NJ: Treating gonorrhea. Am Fam Physician. 1979; 23:123.
32. Fleming WL et al: National survey of venereal disease treated by physicians in 1968. JAMA. 1970; 211:1827.
33. Fiumara NJ: The sexually transmissible diseases. DM. 1978; 25:1.
34. Pariser H et al: Asymptomatic gonorrhea in the male. South Med J. 1964; 56:688.
35. Pariser H et al: Gonorrhea—frequently unrecognized reservoirs. South Med J. 1964; 5b:688.
36. Pariser H: Asymptomatic gonorrhea. Med Clin North Am. 1972; 56:1127.
37. Ashamalia G et al: Recent clinicolaboratory observations in the treatment of acute gonococcal urethritis in men. JAMA. 1966; 195:1115.
38. Thayer JD et al: Improved medium selective for cultivation of N. gonorrhoeae and N. meningitides. Pub Health Rep. 1966; 81:559.
39. LaLuna F et al: Gonococcal pharyngitis and arthritis. Ann Intern Med. 1971; 75:649.
40. Anthony BF et al: Gonococcal infections—laboratory, clinical, and epidemiological aspects. West J Med. 1974; 120:456.
41. Willcox R: A survey of problems in the antibiotic treatment of gonorrhea with special references to Southeast Asia. Br J Vener Dis. 1970; 46:217.
42. Downham TF: Systemic toxic reactions to procaine penicillin G. Sex Trans Dis. 1978; 5:4.
43. McCormack WM: Treatment of gonorrhea. Ann Intern Med. 1979; 90:845.
44. Sands M: Treatment of anorectal gonorrhea infections in men. JAMA. 1980; 243:1143.
45. Judson FN et al: Tetracycline in the treatment of uncomplicated male gonorrhea. Sex Trans Dis. 1976; 3:56.
46. Brown JT et al: Comparison of erythromycin base and estolate in gonococcal urethritis. JAMA. 1977; 238:1371.

47. Siegal MS et al: Penicillinase-producing Neisseria gonorrhoeae: Results of surveillance in the United States. J Infect Dis. 1978; 137:170.

48. The Medical Letter: Treatment of gonorrhea. 1979; 21:66.

49. Phillips I et al: In vitro activity of twelve antibacterial agents against Neisseria gonorrhoeae. Lancet. 1970; 1:263.

50. Reyn A et al: Relationships between the sensitivities in vitro of Neisseria gonorrhoeae to spiramycin, penicillin, streptomycin, tetracycline, and erythromycin. Br J Vener Dis. 1969; 45:223.

51. Reyn A et al: Spectinomycin hydrochloride in the treatment of gonorrhea. Observations of resistant strains of Neisseria gonorrhoeae. Br J Vener Dis. 1973; 49:54.

52. Center for Disease Control: Gonorrhea: CDC-recommended treatment schedules, 1979. J Infect Dis. 1979; 139:496.

53. Sattler FR et al: Therapy of gonorrhea. Comparison of trimetho-trimethoprim-sulfamethoxazole and ampicillin. JAMA. 1978; 240:2267.

54. Johnson DW et al: Antibiotic treatment of asymptomatic gonorrhea in hospitalized women. N Eng J Med. 1970; 283:1.

55. Rees R et al: Gonococcal salpingitis. Br J Vener Dis. 1969; 45:205.

56. Benson RC: Gynecology and obstetrics. In Current Diagnosis and Treatment, Ed by H Brainert et al, Lange Medical Publications, Palo Alto, California, 1969; p 433.

57. Jacobsen L et al: Objectivized diagnosis of acute pelvic inflammatory disease. Am J Obstet Gynecol. 1969; 105:1088.

58. Cooke CL et al: Gonococcal arthritis. JAMA. 1971; 217:204.

59. Goobar JE et al: Rheumatological manifestations of gonorrhea. AIR. 1964; 7:11.

60. Kraus SJ: Complications of gonococcal infection. Med Clin North Am. 1972; 56:115.

61. Holmes KK et al: The gonococcal arthritis-dermatitis syndrome. Ann Intern Med. 1971; 75:470.

62. Branham SE et al: Gonococcic meningitis. JAMA. 1938; 110:1804.

63. Harbin T et al: Gonococcal conjunctivitis. Ann Ophth. 1974; 6:221.

64. Anon: Prophylaxis of gonococca, ophthalmia. Med Let Drugs Ther. 1970; 12:38.

65. Holmes KK: Gonococcal infection—clinical, epidemiologic, and laboratory perspectives. Adv Intern Med. 1974; 19:259.

66. Kaufman RE et al: National gonorrhea therapy monitoring study: treatment results. N Engl J Med. 1976; 294:1.

67. Amstey MS: Genital herpes virus infection. Clin Obstet Gynecol. 1975; 18:89.

68. Ramirez CH et al: Sexually transmitted disease part II syphilis, chlamydias, herpes and scabies. Bol Assoc Med PR. 1980; 72:530.

69. Nahmias A et al: Antigentic and biological differences in herpesvirus hominis. Progr Med Virol. 1968; 10:110.

70. Fahim MS et al: Treatment of genital herpes simplex virus in male patients. Arch Androl. 1980; 4:79.

71. Guinan ME et al: The course of untreated recurrent genital herpes simplex infection in 27 women. N Engl J Med. 1981; 304:759.

72. Brown ZA et al: Clinical and virologic course of herpes simplex genitalis. West J Med. 1979; 130:414.

73. Gardner HL et al: Herpes genitalis: clinical features. Clin Obstet Gynecol. 1972; 15:896.

74. Rawls WE et al: Genital herpes in two social groups. Am J Obstet Gynecol. 1971; 110:682.

75. Rosenthal MS: Genital herpes simplex virus infections. Primary Care. 1979; 6:517.

76. Davis LG et al: Genital herpes simplex virus infections: clinical course and attempted therapy. Am J Hosp Pharm. 1981; 38:825.

77. Chang T et al: Genital herpes. JAMA. 1974; 229:544.

78. Kaufman RH et al: Clinical features of herpes genitalis. Cancer Res. 1973; 33:1446.

79. Dolin R et al: Genital herpes simplex virus type 1 infection—variability in modes of spread. J Am Vener Dis Assoc. 1975; 2:13.

80. Nahmias AJ et al: Infection with herpes-simplex viruses 1 & 2. N Engl J Med. 1973; 269:667; 1973; 289:719; 1973; 289:781.

81. Fleury FJ: Clinical management of genital herpes. Contemp Obstet Gynecol. 1976; 7:36.

82. Adams HG et al: Genital herpetic infection in men and women: clinical course and effect of topical application of adenine arabinoside. J Infect Dis. 1976; 133 (suppl):A151.

83. Nahmias AJ et al: Genital herpetic infection—the old and the new. In Sexually Transmitted Diseases. Catherall RD, Nichol CS, eds, London, Acapeuic Press, 1976, p 135.

84. Corey L et al: Cellular immune response in genital herpes simplex virus infection. N Engl J Med. 1978; 299:986.

85. Baringer JR: Recovery of herpes simplex virus from human sacral ganglions. N Engl J Med. 1974; 828:291.

86. Adams HG: Treatment of genital infections with herpes virus hominis. Sex Trans Dis. 1977; 4:160.

87. Notkins AL: Immune mechanisms by which the spread of viral infections is stopped. Cell Immunol. 1974; 11:478.

88. Nahmias AJ et al: Herpes simplex viruses 1 & 2—basic and clinical aspects. DM. 1979; 15:1.

89. Rahray MC et al: Recurrent genital herpes among women: symptomatic vs asymptomatic viral shedding. Br J Vener Dis. 1978; 54:262.

90. Aurealian L: The "virus of love" and cancer. Am J Med Technol. 1974; 40:496.

91. Hamilton R: The Herpes Book, J.P. Tarchar, Inc. 1980.

92. Merino HI et al: An innovative program of venereal disease case-finding, treatment and education for a population of gay men. Sex Trans Dis. 1977; Apr-June:50.

93. Carr G et al: Anal warts in a population of gay men in New York City. Sex Trans Dis. 1977; Apr-June:56.

94. Centifanto YM et al: Herpesvirus type 2 in the male genitourinary tract. Science. 1972; 178:318.

95. Jeansson S et al: Genital herpes hominis infection: a venereal disease? Lancet. 1970; 1:1064.

96. Kibrick S: Herpes simplex infection at term. What to do with mother, newborn, and nursery personnel. JAMA. 1980; 243:157.

97. Nahmias AJ et al: Infection of the newborn with herpesvirus hominis. Adv Pediatr. 1970; 17:185.

98. Nahmias AJ et al: Perinatal risk associated with maternal genital herpes simplex virus infections. Am J Obstet Gynecol. 1971; 110:825.

99. Josey WE et al: Viral and virus-like infections of the female genital tract. Clin Obstet Gynecol. 1969; 12:161.

100. Hanshaw JB: Herpesvirus hominis infection in the fetus and the newborn. Am J Dis Child. 1971; 110:825.

101. Nahmias AJ et al: Significance of herpes simplex virus infection during pregnancy. Clin Obstet Gynecol. 1972; 15:929.

102. Lerner AM: Infections with herpes simplex virus. In *Harrison's Principles of Internal Medicine,* McGraw-Hill Book Co., New York, 8th edition, 1977, p 1023.

103. Amstey MS: Management of pregnancy complicated by genital herpes virus infection. Obstet Gynecol. 1971; 37:515.

104. Light IJ et al: Neonatal herpes simplex infection following delivery by cesarean section. Obstet Gynecol. 1974; 44:496.

105. Visintine AM et al: Genital herpes. Perinatal Care. 1978; 2:32.

106. Whitley RJ et al: Vidarabine therapy of neonatal herpes simplex virus infection. Pediatrics. 1980; 66:495.

107. Boston Interhospital Virus Study Group—A NIAID-sponsored cooperative antiviral clinical study: failure of high dose 5-iddo-2'-Deoxyuridine in the therapy of herpes simplex virus encephalitis: evidence of unacceptable toxicity. N Engl J Med. 1975; 292:559.

108. Stevens DA et al: Adverse effect of cytosine arabinoside on disseminated zoster in a controlled trial. N Engl J Med. 1973; 289:873.

109. Chien LT: Antiviral chemotherapy and neonatal herpes simplex virus infection: a pilot study—experience with adenine arabinoside (ARA-A). Pediatrics. 1975; 55:678.

110. Centifanto YM et al: Relationship of herpes simplex genital infection and carcinoma of the cervix: population studies. Am J Obstet Gynecol. 1971; 110:690.

111. Wise TG et al: Editorial: herpes simplex vaccines. J Infect Dis. 1977; 136:706.

112. Naib ZM et al: Cytology and histopathology of cervical herpes simplex infection. Cancer. 1973; 19:1026.

113. Rawls WE: The association of herpes virus type 2 and carcinoma of the uterine cervix. Am J Epideuriol. 1969; 89:547.

114. Purchase HG: Role of herpes virus in Marek's disease, a malignant lymphoma of chickens. Ped Proc. 1972; 31:1634.

115. Adams E et al: Sero-epidemiological studies of herpesvirus type 2 and carcinoma of the cervix. 1. case-control matching. J Natl Cancer Inst. 1971; 47:941.

116. Amstay MS et al: Herpes virus cervicitis and neoplasia. Cancer. 1973; 32:1321.

117. Murray DP: Genital herpes. Br Med J. 1980; August:455.

118. Beilby JW et al: Herpes virus hominis infection of the cervix associated with gonorrhea. Lancet. 1968; 1:1065.

119. Goodman EL et al: Prospective double-blind evaluation of topical adenine arabinoside in male herpes progenitalis. Antimicro Agents Chemother. 1975; 8:6937.

120. Taylor PK et al: Comparison of the treatment of herpes genitalis in men with proflanine photoinactivation, idoxuridine ointment, and normal saline. Br J Vener Dis. 1975; 51:125.

121. Kibrick S et al: Topical idoxuridine in recurrent herpes simplex. Ann NY Acad. 1970; 173:83.

122. Parker JD: A double-blind trial of idoxuridine in recurrent genital herpes. J Antimicrob Chemother. 1977; Suppl:A131.

123. MacCullum FO et al: Herpes simplex virus skin infection in man treated with idoxuridine in dimethy/sulfoxide. Results of a double-blind controlled trial. Br Med J. 1966; 2:805.

124. Roone AP et al: Neutralized photoinactivation in the treatment of herpes genitalis. Br J Vener Dis. 1975; 51:13.

125. Meyers MG et al: Failure of neutral red photodynamic inactivation in recurrent herpes simplex virus infections. N Engl J Med. 1975; 293:945.

126. Kaufman RH et al: Treatment of genital herpes simplex virus infection with photodynamic inactivation. Am J Obstet Gynecol. 1978; 132:861.

127. Corey L et al: Ineffectiveness of topical ether for the treatment of genital herpes simplex virus infection. N Engl J Med. 1978; 299:237.

128. Vontuer LA et al: Clinical course and diagnosis of genital herpes simplex virus infection and evaluation of topical surfactant therapy. Am J Obstet Gynecol. 1979; 133:548.

129. Friedrich EG et al: Effect of providine-iodine on herpes genitalis. Obstet Gynecol. 1975; 45:337.

130. Blank H et al: Experimental human reinfection with herpes simplex virus. J Invest Dermatol. 1973; 61:223.

131. Chang TW et al: Treatment with levamisole of recurrent herpes genitalis. Antimicrob Agents Chemother. 1978; 13:809.

132. Gunby P: New anti-herpes virus drug being tested. JAMA. 1980; 243:1315.

133. Selby PJ et al: Parenteral acyclovir therapy for herpes virus infections in man. Lancet. 1979; December:1267.

134. Sara R et al: Acyclovir prophylaxis of herpes-simplex virus infections. A randomized, double-blind, controlled trial in bone marrow-transplant recipients. N Engl J Med. 1981; 305:63.

135. Jones BR et al: Efficacy of acycloguanosine against herpes simplex corneal ulcers. Lancet. 1979; i:243.

136. Duncan WC et al: Cephalexin therapy for infectious syphilis. Arch Dermatol. 1974; 110:77.

137. Wallis C et al: Herpes genitalis: venereal aspects. Clin Obstet Gynecol. 1972; 15:912.

138. Corey L et al: Trial of BCG vaccine for the prevention of genital herpes. Paper presented to 16th annual ICAAC, Chicago IL, 1976; Oct. 29.

139. Elion GB et al: Selectivity of an antiherpetic agent, 9-(2-hydroxyethoxymethyl) quanine. Proc Nat Acad Sci USA. 1977; 74:5716.

140. Center for Disease Control: Syphilis trends in the United States. MMWR. 1981; 30:441.

141. Felman YM et al: Syphilis serology today. Arch Dermatol. 1980; 116:84.

142. Templeton WC et al: A clinical approach to the choice of antimicrobial agents, case number 12: fever and a cutaneous eruption. J Kentucky Med Assoc. 1979; December:649.

143. Felman YM et al: Questions physicians ask concerning syphilis serologies. NY State J Med. 1979; December:2063.

144. Anon: Syphilis—CDC recommended treatment schedules, 1976. USPHS MMWR. 1976; 25:101.

145. Drusin LM: The diagnosis and treatment of infections and latent syphilis. Med Clin North Am. 1972; 56:1161.

146. Guthe T: Treponemal disease. In Cecil-Loeb *Textbook of Medicine,* Ed. by PB Beeson and W McDermott, W.B. Saunders, Philadelphia. 1971, p 655.

147. Rudolph AH et al: Penicillin reactions among patients in venereal disease clinics: a national survey. JAMA. 1973; 223:499.

148. Minkin W et al: Incidence of immediate systemic penicillin reactions. Military Med. 1968; 133:557.

149. Holdern WR et al: Syphilis in pregnancy. Med Clin North Am. 1972; 56:1151.

150. Boak RA et al: Biologic false-positive reactions for syphilis in pregnancy as determined by the Treponema pallidum immobilization test. Surg Gynecol Obstet. 1955; 101:751.

151. Tuffaneli DL et al: Fluorescent treponemal antibody absorption tests. Studies of false positive reactions to tests for syphilis. N Engl J Med 1967; 276:258.

152. Salo OP et al: False-positive serological tests for syphilis in pregnancy. Acta Derm Venerol. 1969; 49:332.

153. Anon: Treatment and prevention of syphilis and gonorrhea. Drugs Ther. 1971; 13:85.

154. Kline AH et al: Transplacental effect of tetracycline on teeth. JAMA. 1964; 188:178.

155. Pflug GR: Toxicities associated with tetracycline therapy. Am J Pharm. 1963; 135:438.

156. Clendenning WE: Complications of tetracycline therapy. Arch Derm. 1965; 91:628.

157. Dowling HF et al: Hepatic reactions to tetracycline. JAMA. 1964; 188:307.

158. South MA et al: Failure of erythromycin estolate therapy in utero syphilis. JAMA. 1964; 190:70.

159. Weinstein L: Antibiotics: Miscellaneous antibiotic agents. In *The Pharmacological Basis of Therapeutics*, 4th ed, Ed by LS Goodman and A Gilman, The Macmillan Co, New York, 1970.

160. Philipson A et al: Transplacental passage of erythromycin and clindamycin. N Engl J Med. 1973; 288:1219.

161. Flarer F: On the antitreponemic action of cephaloridine. Postgrad Med J. 1967; 43(Suppl):133.

162. Gonzallez-Ochoa A et al: The treatment of early syphilis with cephaloridine. Postgrad Med J. 1967; 43(Suppl):134.

163. Glicksman JM et al: Parenteral cephaloridine treatment of patients with early syphilis. Arch Intern Med. 1968; 121:342.

164. Mamunes P et al: Early diagnosis of neonatal syphilis. Am J Dis Child. 1970; 120:17.

165. Judson FN et al: Comparative prevalence rates of sexually transmitted diseases in heterosexual and homosexual men. Am J Epidemiol. 1980; 112:836.

166. Babb RR: Sexually transmitted infections in homosexual men. Post Grad Med. 1979; 65:215.

167. Owen WF: Sexually transmitted diseases and traumatic problems in homosexual men. Ann Intern Med. 1980; 92:805.

168. Judson FN: Sexually transmitted disease in gay men. Sex Trans Dis. 1977; April-June:76.

169. British Co-Operative Clinical Group: Homosexuality and venereal disease in the United Kingdom. A second survey. Br J Vener Dis. 1980; 56:6.

170. Klein ES et al: Anorectal gonorrhea. Ann Intern Med. 1977; 86:340.

171. Fluker JL et al: Rectal gonorrhea in male homosexuals. Presentation and therapy. Br J Vener Dis. 1980; 56:397.

172. Wiesner PJ: Gonococcal pharyngeal infections. Clin Obstet Gynecol. 1975; 18:121.

173. Bro-Jorgensen A et al: Gonococcal pharyngeal infections: Report of 110 cases. Br J Vener Dis. 1973; 49:491.

174. Owen RL et al: Rectal and pharyngeal gonorrhea in homosexual men. JAMA. 1972; 220:1315.

175. Sands M et al: Therapy of anorectal gonorrhea in men. West J Med. 1980; 133:469.

176. Fiumara NJ: The treatment of gonococcal proctitis: An evaluation of 173 patients treated with 4 grams of spectinomycin. JAMA. 1978; 239:735.

177. Lebedeff DA et al: Rectal gonorrhea in men: Diagnosis and treatment. Ann Intern Med. 1980; 92:463.

178. Karney WW et al: Comparative therapeutic and pharmacological evaluation of amoxicillin and ampicillin plus probenecid for the treatment of gonorrhea. Antimicrob Agents Chemother. 1974; 5:114.

179. Karney WW et al: Single-dose oral therapy for uncomplicated gonorrhea: Comparison of amoxicillin and ampicillin given with and without probenecid. J Infect Dis. 1974; 129(Suppl):250.

180. Wiesner PJ et al: Clinical spectrum of pharyngeal gonococcal infection. N Engl J Med. 1973; 288:181.

181. Karney WW et al: Spectinomycin versus tetracycline for the treatment of gonorrhea. N Engl J Med. 1977; 296:889.

182. Di Caprio JM et al: Ampicillin therapy for pharyngeal gonorrhea. JAMA. 1978; 239:1631.

183. Henderson RH: Improving sexually transmitted disease health services for gays; a national prospective. Sex Trans Dis. 1977; 4:58.

184. Corey L et al: Sexual transmission of hepatitis A in homosexual men. N Engl J Med. 1980; 302:435.

185. Szmuness W et al: On the role of sexual behavior in the spread of hepatitis B infection. Ann Intern Med. 1975; 83:489.

186. Dietzman DE et al: Hepatitis B surface antigen (H Bs Ag) and antibody to H Bs Ag. Prevalence in homosexual and heterosexual men. JAMA. 1977; 238:2625.

187. Willcox RR: The rectum as viewed by the venerologist. Br J Vener Dis. 1981; 57:1.

188. Schmerin MJ et al: Giardiasis: Association with homosexuality. Ann Intern Med. 1978; 88:801.

189. Quinn TC et al: Campylobacter proctitis in a homosexual man. Ann Intern Med. 1980; 93:458.

190. Burrow GN et al: *Medical Complications During Pregnancy*. WB Saunders Co, Philadelphia. 1975; p 471.

191. Manorama HT et al: Single-dose oral treatment of vaginal trichomoniasis with tinidazole and metronidazole. J Intern Med Res. 1978; 6:46.

192. Novak ER: Novak's *Textbook of Gynecology*, 9th ed, Williams & Williams Co, Baltimore, 1975, p 214.

193. Plorde JJ: Minor protozoan diseases. In *Harrison's Principles of Internal Medicine*, 9th ed, McGraw-Hill Books Co, New York, 1980, p 887.

194. Hager WD et al: Metronidazole for vaginal trichomoniasis. Seven-day vs single-dose regimens. JAMA. 1980; 244:1219.

195. Keighly EE: Trichomoniasis in a closed community: efficacy of metronidazole. Br Med J. 1971; 1:207.

196. Pereyra AJ et al: Urogenital trichomoniasis: treatment with metronidazole in 2,002 incarcerated women. Obstet Gynecol. 1964; 24:499.

197. Goldman P: Metronidazole. N Engl J Med. 1980; 303:1212.

198. Nicol ES et al: Flagyl (8823RP) in the treatment of trichomoniasis. Br J Vener Dis. 1960; 36:152.

199. Dykers JR: Single-dose metronidazole for trichomonal vaginitis: patient and consort. N Engl J Med. 1975; 293:23.

200. Czonka GW: Trichomonal vaginitis treated with one dose of metronidazole. Br J Vener Dis. 1971; 47:456.

201. Ross SM: Single and triple dose treatment of trichomonas infection of the vagina. Br J Vener Dis. 1973; 49:475.

202. Muller M et al: Three metronidazole-resistant strains of Trichomonas vaginalis from the United States. Am J Obstet Gynecol. 1980; 138:808.

203. Kane PO et al: Absorption and excretion of metronidazole. II studies on primary failures. Br J Vener Dis. 1961; 37:276.

204. Edwards DI et al: Inactivation of metronidazole by aerobic organisms. J Antimicrob Chemother. 1979; 5:315.

205. Meingassner JG et al: Studies on strain sensitivity of Trichomonas vaginalis to metronidazole. Br J Vener Dis. 1978; 54:72.

206. de Carneri I et al: In vitro resistance to metronidazole induced on four recently isolated strains of Trichomonas vaginalis. Drug Res. 1971; 3:377.

207. Meingassner JG et al: Assay conditions and the demonstration of nitromidazole resistance in trichomonads foetus. Antimicrob Agents Chemother. 1978; 13:1.

208. Katz M: Parasitic infections. J Pediatr. 1976; 87:165.

209. Penick SB: Metronidazole in the treatment of alcoholism. Am J Psychiatry. 1969; 125:1063.

210. Gupta NK: Effect of metronidazole on liver alcohol dehydrogenase. Biochem Pharmacol. 1970; 19:2805.

211. Coxin A et al: Metronidazole-induced sensory neuropathy. J Neurol, Neurosurg and Psychiatr. 1976; 39:403.

212. Karlsson IJ et al: Metronidazole neuropathy. Br Med J. 1977; 2:832.

213. Rustia M et al: Experimental induction of hepatomas, mammary tumors, and other tumors with methronidazole in non inbred sas. mrc(wi)Br rats. J Natl Cancer Inst. 1979; 63:863.

214. Beard CM et al: Lack of evidence for cancer due to the use of metronidazole. N Engl J Med. 1979; 301:519.

215. Friedman GD: Cancer after metronidazole. N Engl J Med. 1980; 302:519.

216. Peterson WF et al: Metronidazole in pregnancy. Am J Obstet Gynecol. 1966; 94:343.

217. Rodin P et al: Metronidazole and pregnancy. Br J Vener Dis. 1966; 42:210.

218. Rein MF et al: Trichomoniasis, candidiasis, and the minor venereal diseases. Clin Obstet Gynecol. 1975; 18:73.

219. Dunlop EMC: Sexually transmitted diseases. Clin Obstet Gynecol. 1977; 4:451.

220. Anon: Is flagyl dangerous? Med Let Drugs Ther. 1975; 17:53.

221. Venereal Disease Control Div: Infections due to penicillinase-producing Neiserria gonorrhoeae—Florida. MMWR. 1981; 30:245.

222. Venereal Disease Control Div: Spectinomycin-resistant penicillinase producing Neisseria gonorrhoeae—California. MMWR. 1981; 30:221.

223. American Academy of Pediatrics: Prophylaxis and treatment of neonatal gonococcal infections. Pediatrics. 1980; 65:1047.

224. Shaw EB: Comment on silver nitrate prophylaxis. Pediatrics. 1977; 60:773.

225. Crede KSF: Die Verhutung der Augentzundung der Neugeborenen. Arch Gynaek. 1881; 17:50.

226. Hornblass A: Severe silver nitrate ocular damage. NY State J Med. 1976; 76:1875.

227. Nishida H et al: Silver nitrate ophthalmic solution and chemical conjunctivitis. Pediatrics. 1975; 56:368.

228. Hammerschiag MR et al: Erythromycin ointment for ocular prophylaxis of neonatal chlamydial infection. JAMA. 1980; 244:2291.

229. Armstrong JH et al: Ophthalmia neonatorum: A chart review. Pediatrics. 1976; 57:884.

230. Lyle DJ: Allergic reaction of previously sensitized eye to parenteral penicillin. Am J Ophthalmol. 1948; 31:1490.

231. Eschenbach DA et al: Polymicrobial etiology of acute pelvic inflammatory disease. N Engl J Med. 1975; 293:166.

232. Westrom L et al: Effect of acute pelvic inflammatory disease on infertility. Am J Obstet Gynecol. 1975; 121:707.

233. Smith MS et al: Pelvic inflammatory disease. A review. Clin Pediatr. 1980; 19:791.

234. Thatcher RW: Treatment of acute gonococcal conjunctivitis. Ann Ophthalmol. 1978; 10:445.

235. Bayer AS: Gonococcal arthritis syndromes. An update on diagnosis and management. Postgrad Med. 1980; 67:200.

236. Whitley RJ et al: Adenine arabinoside therapy of biopsy-proved herpes simplex encephalitis. National Institute of Allergy & Infectious Diseases Collaborative Antiviral Study. N Engl J Med. 1977; 297:289.

237. Barza M et al: The decision to biopsy, treat, or wait in suspected herpes encephalitis. Ann Intern Med. 1980; 92:641.

238. Lauter CB: Herpes simplex encephalitis: A great clinical challenge. Ann Intern Med. 1980; 93:696.

239. Meislin HW et al: Jarisch-Herxheimer reaction case report. JACEP. 1976; 5:779.

240. Berg SW et al: Cefoxitin as a single-dose treatment for urethritis caused by penicillinase-producing Neisseria gonorrhoeae. N Engl J Med. 1979; 301:509.

241. Griffith RS et al: A multicentered study of lysine therapy in herpes simplex infections. Dermatologica. 1978; 156:257.

242. Tankersley RW et al: Amino acid requirements of herpes simplex virus in human cells. J Bact. 1964; 87:609.

243. Milman N et al: Failure of lysine treatment in recurrent herpes simplex labialis. Lancet. 1978; 2:942.

244. Milman N et al: Lysine prophylaxis in recurrent herpes simplex labialis: A double-blind, controlled crossover study. Acta Derm Venereol (Stockh). 1980; 60:85.

245. Landry ML et al: Duration of vidarabine therapy in biopsy-negative herpes simplex encephalitis. JAMA. 1982; 247:332.

Chapter 38

Infection in the Compromised Host

——— Mary E. Russo ———

Patients with congenital or acquired defects in immunocompetence are considered abnormal or compromised hosts, and they are at high risk of becoming infected. The critical role of infection in the compromised host is demonstrated by the fact that it is the leading cause of morbidity and mortality in patients with underlying neoplastic disease. In 450 patients with hematologic malignancies who were autopsied at the National Cancer Institute between 1965 and 1971 (1), approximately 79% were infected at the time of death. This high incidence has been corroborated by other large studies (2–4). Between 50 and 70% of patients with acute and chronic leukemias, lymphomas, and solid tumors die of infection. In fact, during initial remission induction therapy for acute leukemia, patients may spend more than 20 consecutive days neutropenic; about 60% of them become infected, and the resultant mortality rate is 25%. Moreover, about 50% of the patients with multiple myeloma have infectious complications during chemotherapy, and 60% of these are fatal. Infection is, therefore, one of the most significant problems we face in managing the compromised host.

The following case studies illustrate the predisposing factors to infection in the compromised host, special considerations for antibiotic therapy and infection prevention measures, and guidelines for appropriate management of fever in the neutropenic patient. The two major areas discussed in this chapter are bacterial infection and *Pneumocystis carinii* pneumonitis.

BACTERIAL INFECTION IN A COMPROMISED HOST

1. L.B. is a 45-year-old male who was referred to the University Hospital because of an abnormal chest x-ray which was taken one week ago. He is an adult-onset diabetic controlled with diet. He was well until six months prior to admission when he began to notice extreme fatigue at the end of a day's work and gradually increasing anorexia. He sought medical help two weeks ago with a chief complaint of weakness and cough. He lost 20 pounds in the last three months and was experiencing frequent night sweats and fever. His cough became more severe and was productive of a moderate amount of white mucoid sputum. He has smoked 2–3 packs of cigarettes a day for the last 25 years. His private physician obtained a chest x-ray which revealed mediastinal widening, and he was referred for further evaluation.

Upon admission to the hospital, this thin, chronically ill-appearing man was complaining of fatigue, cough, and lower back pain. Vital signs were temperature 37° C, respiration 20/minute, pulse 90 beats/minute, and blood pressure 112/60 mm Hg. Several anterior cervical nodes up to 1.5 cm in diameter were present bilaterally. A left, hard, nontender 2 cm supraclavicular node was present. Chest was hyperresonant with terminal expiratory wheezes in the right mid-lung field. The heart was normal. The liver and spleen were slightly palpable but non-tender. The extremities showed obvious wasting.

Laboratory data revealed: hematocrit 35 vol%, hemoglobin 10.8 gm/dl, white blood cells 6,000/mm^3 with 62% polymorphonuclear leukocytes, 14% bands, 10% lymphocytes, 10% monocytes, 2% eosinophils, and 2% basophils. Sedimentation rate was elevated at 87 mm/hr, and alkaline phosphatase was increased. His blood glucose was 180 mg/dl, and albumin was 2.5 gm/dl. Other laboratory parameters were within normal limits. Chest x-ray revealed a large right superior mediastinal mass. An intravenous pyelogram showed the right kidney to be displaced inferiorly. An electrocardiogram was normal. The bone marrow was hypercellular with increased megakaryocytes and a marked shift in the myeloid element. Right scaline lymph node biopsy revealed mixed cellularity Hodgkin's lymphoma. Pulmonary function tests showed mild obstructive lung disease. Air broncho-gram demonstrated the left main stem bronchus to be narrower than the right, and there was mild obstruction in this area. X-rays of the lumbar vertebrae and pelvis showed definite areas of osteoblastic activity.

Assessment at this time was Stage IVB Hodgkin's disease. Because of respiratory difficulties secondary to the mediastinal mass, it was decided to radiate the mass and also start him on a MOPP-Bleo regimen (nitrogen mustard, vincristine, procarbazine, and prednisone, with bleomycin added on days 1 and 8). On the tenth day of therapy his white blood cell count was 800/mm^3 with 20% polymorphonuclear leukocytes, and his platelet count was 40,000/mm^3. He was nauseated and vomiting guaiac-positive coffee-ground material. His blood glucose was elevated at 280 mg/dl, and he was started on NPH insulin 10 units in the morning.

What is the single most important factor predisposing L.B. to infection? List the etiologies for this.

Neutropenia is the major factor associated with infection. The most likely causes in L.B. are chemotherapy and radiation-induced bone marrow suppression (4–6). Other patients may become neutropenic because of tumor invasion of the bone marrow. The frequency of infection is inversely related to the absolute number of circulating neutrophils (7). The absolute neutrophil count (ANC) is calculated by multiplying the percent polymorphonuclear leukocytes and the percent bands by the total WBC count. The ANC in L.B. is 20 percent of 800, or 160/mm^3. The frequency of infection increases dramatically with ANC $\leq$ 500/mm^3. Patients with profound neutropenia (ANC $\leq$ 100/mm^3) for $\geq$ 3 weeks may all become infected. The degree, duration, rate of change, and nadir of neutropenia are important prognostic indicators of infection and subsequent response to antibiotic therapy. Table 1 shows the frequency of infection and mortality rate at various levels of neutropenia.

2. What other factors in this patient make him a compromised host and susceptible to infection?

L.B. exhibits abnormalities in three major host defense systems. First, his integument-mucosal barrier is altered (4). The skin and mucous membranes are the first line of defense against bacterial and fungal invasion. Disruption of these mechanical barriers in L.B. is demonstrated by his guaiac-positive emesis and indicates a break in the mucosal lining of the gastrointestinal (GI) tract. This can result from stress ulceration and chemotherapy-induced mucositis. L.B.'s pulmonary defense mechanisms are affected by cigarette smoke which can depress mucociliary transport, increase mucous production, and decrease function of alveolar macrophages. Obstruction to bronchopulmonary drainage by the tumor mass also predisposes L.B. to infection distal to the site of obstruction. In one series of 816 autopsies, 67% of the fatal infections were due to ulcerated or necrotic tumors which compressed or obstructed the urinary, alimentary, or respiratory tracts (4). These infections seldom respond to antibiotics unless the obstruction is alleviated. Radiation therapy in L.B. should decrease the size of his tumor. However, radiation pneumonitis may occur and further alter the mucosal barrier in the tracheobronchial tree (4). Breaks in the integumentary barrier by intravenous catheters, which are used to administer chemotherapy, are potential sites for infection. This is especially important when infusing very irritating solutions such as nitrogen mustard.

Secondly, antibody-mediated immunity in L.B. is altered by his chemotherapy and his underlying disorders; altered antibody-mediated immunity can result in abnormal production and function of phagocytes and complement (8–10). Abnormal chemotaxis occurs in diabetes mellitus and Hodgkin's disease, and abnormal granulocyte adherence is associated with the administration of corticosteroids. His weight loss and wasted appearance are suggestive of protein-calorie malnutrition which can cause hypocomplementemia and add to his deficient host defenses.

Finally, T-lymphocyte and macrophage function, the major processes in cellular immunity, are affected by Hodgkin's disease and steroid therapy (8–10).

3. Besides these factors, what other defects in the host defense system can occur? Why is it important to know these?

The list of factors resulting in abnormal immunocompetence is extensive. An outline of the major areas with representative examples is presented in Table 2. If the compromised patient, like

Table 1.

INFECTION AND MORTALITY RATES ASSOCIATED WITH
NEUTROPENIA IN CANCER PATIENTS

Absolute Neutrophil Count (ANC/mm³) During First Week of Infection	Infection Rate	Mortality Rate
> 1000	3% 10% patient days 49–68% of febrile episodes	32%
500–1000	8% 20% patient days 63% of febrile episodes	30%
100–500	13% 37% patient days 63% of febrile episodes	46%
< 100	19% 53% patient days 67% of febrile episodes	80–90%
> 1000 and declines but stays > 1000	4%	
> 1000 and declines to		
1000	10%	
< 1000	14%	
500	19%	
< 100	28%	72%
< 1000 and declines to any level	28%	59%
< 1000 and increases but stays < 1000		40%
< 1000 and increases to > 1000		27–32%

Adapted from references: 7,13,14,21,26

L.B., can be categorized according to his deficiencies in host defenses, it will help to determine the type of organisms to which he is most susceptible. This will then allow the clinician to select a rational empiric antibiotic regimen when infection is suspected.

4. Over the last few days, L.B. has complained of increasing shortness of breath. Chest x-ray shows a decrease in the mediastinal mass and a few patchy interstitial infiltrates in the right lower lung field. On the evening of the tenth day of therapy he spikes a temperature to 39° C. How would you evaluate his fever?

Fever is the predominant sign of infection in patients with underlying malignancies (11–15). Approximately 50–80% of the patients with a leukemia, lymphoma, or solid tumor develop fever as the initial sign of infection. This is noted especially in those patients with advanced malignancies.

It is important, however, to exclude other causes of fever such as transfusion reactions, the underlying neoplasm, and chemotherapy-induced febrile episodes (13,16). Extravascular hemolysis associated with incompatibilities in the Rh system can cause mild febrile reactions and malaise during the transfusion and for a few hours thereafter. Antipyretics can be administered at this time; however, the temperature should be rechecked 6–8 hours after discontinuing antipyretics to determine whether the febrile episode was a transient effect. Malignancies can cause fever, although such fevers are usually low grade in nature. Many of the drugs used in chemotherapy regimens also induce febrile reactions for a few hours after administration. Bleomycin is the most

Table 2.

CLASSIFICATION OF IMMUNODEFICIENCY STATES

I.   Antibody-mediated immunity (phagocytes, complement, B lymphocytes, T-helper cells, T-suppressor cells)
  A.   Congenital
  B.   Acquired
    1. Malignancies (acute and chronic leukemias, non-Hodgkin's lymphoma, multiple myeloma)
    2. Alcoholism
    3. Collagen vascular diseases
    4. Burns
    5. Acute infections
    6. Neonatal infections
    7. Sickle-cell disease
    8. Protein-calorie malnutrition
    9. Renal diseases
    10. Hepatic diseases
    11. Granulomatous diseases
    12. Diabetes mellitus
    13. Macroglobulinemia
    14. Splenectomy
  C.   Drug-induced
    1. Neutropenia (multiple drugs, in particular, antineoplastic agents)
    2. Abnormal function
      a. Colchicine
      b. Tetracycline
      c. Cyclophosphamide
      d. Corticosteroids
      e. Aspirin
      f. Chloramphenicol
      g. Phenylbutazone
      h. Azathioprine
II. Cellular-mediated immunity
  A.   Congenital
  B.   Acquired
    1. Hodgkin's lymphoma
    2. Sezary syndrome (erythrodermia)
    3. Protein-calorie malnutrition
  C.   Drug-induced
    1. Corticosteroids
    2. Azathioprine
    3. Cyclophosphamide

Adapted from, Grieco MH: Introduction to the abnormal host and complicating infections. In *Infections in the Abnormal Host*, 1st edition, edited by MH Grieco, Yorke Medical Books, New York, p 1.

commonly implicated agent and causes fever in up to one-third of treated patients (17). Temperatures as high as 40° C have been recorded. The onset is usually 3–5 hours after administration, and duration is up to an hour. Since L.B. received bleomycin two days earlier, it would not be a consideration in him.

5. Besides fever, what are the other clinical manifestations of infection in L.B.?

This patient exhibits increasing shortness of breath and patchy infiltrates on the chest x-ray, suggesting a possible pneumonia. Other signs associated with pneumonia, such as cough, sputum production, purulence on Gram's stain, rales, and consolidation on physical exam and chest x-ray, are not apparent in L.B.

Clinical manifestations of infection are dramatically altered in the neutropenic patient. Physical findings of exudates, ulceration, fissure, local heat, and swelling are significantly less common in anorectal and local skin infections (11,18); cough, sputum production, and purulence occur significantly less often with pneumonias (11,14,15); and dysuria, frequency, and pyuria are significantly decreased in the setting of urinary tract infections (11). The neutropenic patient, however, exhibits fever and bacteremia more commonly during these infectious episodes.

6. How common is pneumonia in a compromised host? What are the major sites of infection?

Pneumonias and septicemias account for over 80% of the infections in cancer patients, and these infections are especially common in those with hematologic malignancies (1–4). In these cases, pneumonias are usually secondary to hematogenous spread. The frequency of septicemias in a general hospital population is 1/100 for non-cancer patients, 2/100 for solid tumors, and 45/100 for hematologic malignancies. Over one-half of the fatal infections in patients with gastrointestinal or genitourinary cancers are due to septicemias, whereas over 75% of the fatal infections in patients with cancer of the head, neck, and lungs are due to pneumonias (4).

Other sites of infection, though less frequent, present special problems for the cancer patient. They include cellulitis, urinary tract infection, meningitis, enterocolitis, and perirectal infections. The latter is an important source of septicemia (18).

7. L.B. was initially categorized as having alterations in his host defenses that included impaired integument-mucosal barrier, altered antibody-mediated immunity, impaired cellular defenses, and, most importantly, neutropenia. To which bacterial organisms is he most susceptible?

The majority of bacterial infections in the neutropenic patient are due to gram-negative bacilli (3,4,13–15,17,19–21). The most common pathogens in this group are *Escherichia coli, Klebsiella-Enterobacter* species and *Pseudomonas aeruginosa.* While all of these organisms can colonize the hospitalized patient, *P. aeruginosa* most frequently progresses to bacteremia (22,23). Moreover, *in vitro* studies demonstrate that some antineoplastic agents may suppress non-*Pseudomonas* organisms in the GI tract and permit overgrowth of the pathogen (24,25). The mortality rate following the onset of bacteremia with *Pseudomonas* species is close to 50% in the first 48 hours. The incidence of fatal infections with *Klebsiella* species and *E. coli* varies between 18 and 25% during this time (12). *Staphylococcus aureus* is the most common gram-positive organism, occurring in up to 23% of the cases (19–21). Anaerobic infections are relatively uncommon with less than 5% incidence (13).

The underlying malignant disorder can influence the type of organism found. For example, infections with intracellular bacteria, such as *Salmonella* and *Listeria*, are common in Hodgkin's and non-Hodgkin's lymphoma than in other types of cancer (9,10). Table 3 shows the association between various malignancies and bacterial pathogens.

8. Since mortality from infection is high in a neutropenic patient, empiric antibiotic therapy is indicated. What general principles of antibiotic therapy should be considered in L.B.?

Once cultures are obtained, the selection of an antibiotic regimen should be based upon two general principles: the use of *bactericidal* drugs and the use of a *synergistic combination* of antibiotics (5,12,26–28).

Bactericidal Antibiotics. Because of abnormal host defense mechanisms in the compromised patient, the antibiotics used should be able to kill the organism and not merely inhibit its growth. The latter effect relies upon the body's intact immunologic defenses to eradicate the organism. This

Table 3.

ASSOCIATION BETWEEN VARIOUS MALIGNANCIES AND BACTERIAL PATHOGENS

Malignancy	Gram-negative	Gram-positive	Anaerobes	Intracellular organisms*
Acute leukemias	+ +	+ esp. *Staphylococci*	−	+ esp. *Salmonella* and tuberculosis
Chronic lymphocytic leukemia	+	+ esp. pneumococci	−	−
Lymphomas (including Hodgkin's)	+ +	+ esp. *Staphylococci*	+	+ +
Multiple myeloma	+ +	+ + esp. pneumococci	−	−
Solid tumors	+ +	+ + esp. *Staphylococci*	+ +	+ + esp. *Salmonella*

*Intracellular organisms = *Listeria, Salmonella,* tuberculosis

is abnormal in the neutropenic patient with an underlying malignancy.

Synergistic Combinations of Antibiotics. The use of synergistic combinations of antibiotics is associated with a better clinical response than single drugs or combination regimens which are only additive or antagonistic. In one study, the combination of gentamicin and carbenicillin resulted in an 83% success rate, whereas each antibiotic used alone was successful 57 and 50% of the time, respectively (29). Klastersky et al (30) demonstrated a failure rate of only 18% in cancer patients treated with combination antibiotics which showed *in vitro* synergy. The failure rate was significantly higher (47%) when non-synergistic antibiotics were used. Lau et al (31) also found an 18% mortality rate with synergistic regimens. Additive combinations resulted in 44% mortality, and when the organism was not responsive to one or both antibiotics, the mortality rates were 71 and 100%, respectively. Table 4 demonstrates various antibiotic combinations which are synergistic against the most common infecting organisms. In general, various two-drug regimens of an aminoglycoside, a penicillin, or a cephalosporin are synergistic against *E. coli, Klebsiella* species, *P. aeruginosa*, and *S. aureus*.

9. Which combination of antibiotics would you recommend to initiate therapy in L.B.? Is there a difference between two-drug versus three-drug regimens?

In the setting of a presumed infection that is not yet microbiologically documented, there are no significant differences among two-drug combinations that include two of the following antibiotic classes: penicillins (carbenicillin or ticarcillin), aminoglycosides (gentamicin, tobramycin, or amikacin), and cephalosporins (cephalothin, cefazolin). Response rates between 60 and 95% are achieved in most studies with no single combination achieving significantly better outcomes (19,21,31–34). In bacteriologically documented infections, approximately 45–80% of the patients responded to these two-drug regimens (19,20,29, 31–34). The trend, however, favors the use of an aminoglycoside and a penicillin which is effective against *Pseudomonas aeruginosa* (19,32). Only one series had a lower response rate (36–55%) with two-drug therapy in both documented and undocumented infections in neutropenic patients (32).

Three-drug regimens utilizing one drug from each of the above antibiotic classes results in a similar response rate to two-drug regimens and ranges from 50 to 80% (35–37). Therefore, no advantage is gained by using three antibiotics as initial therapy. Tattersall et al (38) tried various five-drug combinations as initial therapy, but only 53% of the patients with documented infections responded.

Based on these studies, a combination of gentamicin, tobramycin, or amikacin, and carbenicillin or ticarcillin are rational choices for initial empiric therapy. The sensitivity patterns in the

Table 4.

SYNERGISTIC BACTERICIDAL ANTIBIOTIC COMBINATIONS FOR COMMON
BACTERIAL PATHOGENS IN THE COMPROMISED HOST

Bacterial pathogens	Synergistic combinations*
Escherichia coli	Gent, tobra, or amik and carb, ticar, amp, or ceph
Klebsiella pneumoniae	Gent, tobra, or amik and ceph
Pseudomonas aeruginosa	Gent, tobra, or amik and carb or ticar
Staphylococcus aureus	Penase pen and gent, tobra, amik, or rif; vanc and rif, gent, tobra, or amik; ceph and gent, tobra, or amik

*Gent = gentamicin; tobra = tobramycin; amik = amikacin; carb = carbenicillin; ticar = ticarcillin; amp = ampicillin; ceph = cephalosporins; penase pen = penicillinase-resistant penicillins; vanc = vancomycin; rif = rifampin

hospital where the patient is being treated should be considered when choosing the aminoglycoside. A rational antibiotic combination for L.B. would be gentamicin and ticarcillin.

10. After two days cultures are negative, and L.B. is still spiking a temperature. He remains neutropenic at this time. How long should antibiotic therapy be continued? Should the regimen be changed?

Only two studies have tried to establish the appropriate duration of antibiotic therapy in the compromised host. An early study in cancer patients by Rodriquez et al (16) determined that patients with presumed infection who became afebrile after four days of therapy with a combination of carbenicillin and cephalothin should be continued on antibiotics for an additional three to five days. None of the patients in this group died. However, two of the 30 patients who were afebrile after four days and randomized to discontinue antibiotic therapy died of *Klebsiella* sepsis. The majority of patients who remained febrile after four days of antibiotic therapy responded to the addition of gentamicin. In a more recent series by Pizzo et al (39), 33 patients who were still neutropenic but became afebrile after seven days of triple drug therapy (cephalothin, gentamicin, and carbenicillin) were randomized to either continue antibiotics until their ANC was >500/mm³ or stop therapy. Patients maintained on antibiotic therapy had no further infectious sequelae. The median duration of granulocytopenia in these patients was 12 days (range 9–25

days). Forty-one percent of the patients (7 of 17) who had antibiotics discontinued became febrile within two to five days of stopping therapy. Five of these patients had a documented infection, and two of them died. Based upon these limited data, a flow diagram outlining a rational approach to managing fever in L.B. is presented in Fig. 1.

Problems with Antibiotic Therapy

11. *Aminoglycoside-Cephalosporin Nephrotoxicity.* M.P. is a 65-year-old male with chronic myelogenous leukemia in blastic transformation. He underwent intensive chemotherapy and is currently profoundly neutropenic (ANC <100/mm³) and febrile (39° C). Because he "broke out in hives" the last time he received penicillin, M.P. was started on cephalothin and gentamicin for his fever. *Klebsiella pneumoniae* was eventually cultured from his blood. One week later his serum creatinine rose to 1.9 mg/dl (0.9 mg/dl on admission) and his blood urea nitrogen increased to 28 mg/dl (12 mg/dl on admission). What is the most likely cause of his decreasing renal function?

This situation appears to be the result of enhanced nephrotoxicity from the combination of cephalothin and gentamicin. While most of the early data on cephalosporin nephrotoxicity dealt with cephaloridine, there are some reports of acute renal failure in patients treated with cephalothin and gentamicin (40–43). Other studies have also observed azotemia and increased serum creati-

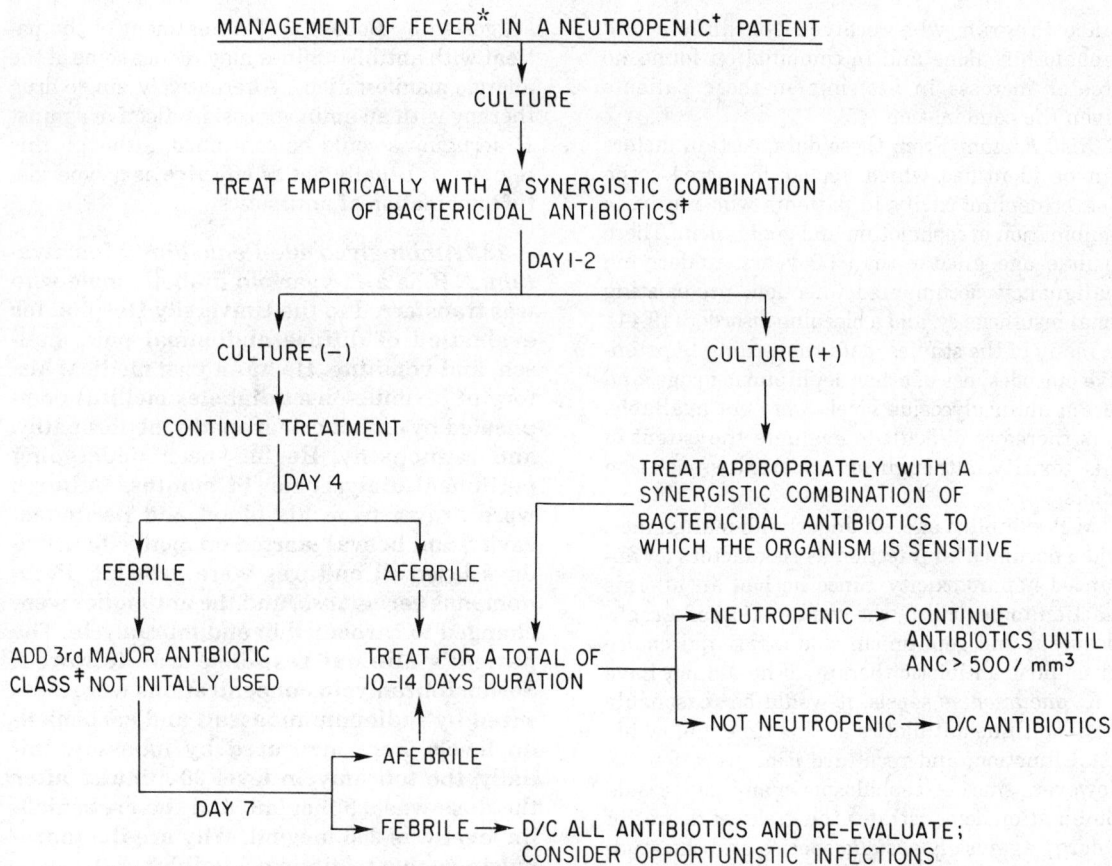

Figure 1. Algorithm for the management of fever in a neutropenic patient.

* Fever = temperature > 38.3°C and not temporally related to transfusions or chemotherapeutic drugs known to cause febrile reactions.

⁺ Neutropenic = absolute neutrophil count (ANC) ≤ 500/mm³

‡ Major antibiotic classes include penicillins (carbenicillin or ticarcillin), aminoglycosides (gentamicin, tobramycin or amikacin), and cephalosporins (cephalothin, cefazolin).

See text for discussion of synergistic combinations.

nine with cephalothin aminoglycoside combinations. The EORTC trial found that 16% of the patients treated with gentamicin and cephalothin exhibited azotemia as compared to a 6% incidence with cephalothin and carbenicillin and a 3% incidence with carbenicillin and gentamicin (19). Klastersky et al (32) found a 21% incidence of azotemia in patients given cephalothin and tobramycin as compared to a 2% and 6% incidence with ticarcillin/cephalothin and ticarcillin/tobramycin, respectively. In a series reported by Plager (44), 33 of 69 patients who died within two weeks of receiving cephalothin and gentamicin in com-

bination were found to have histologic evidence of renal tubule injury. Of the 208 postmortem examinations evaluated, 13 patients received either drug alone without evidence of primary tubular damage. Seventeen patients, however, demonstrated histopathologic features similar to those seen with the cephalothin/gentamicin combination. These were attributed to sustained hypotension, cisplatinum therapy, and hypercalcemia. One patient received cephalothin and kanamycin, and no cause was identified in five patients. In contrast, a retrospective analysis of over 1,000 patients in the Boston Collaborative Drug Surveillance Program who received gentamicin and cephalothin alone and in combination found no greater increase in azotemia in those patients given the combination (45).

Risk Factors. From these data, certain factors can be identified which appear to increase the risk of nephrotoxicity in patients who receive a combination of cephalothin and gentamicin. These include age greater than 60 years, underlying malignancy, documented infection, pre-existing renal insufficiency, and a bleeding disorder (19,44). In many of the studies, data concerning hypotensive episodes, use of other nephrotoxic drugs, and serum aminoglycoside levels were not available. It is therefore difficult to evaluate the extent of this toxicity, although an apparent association exists.

M.P. exhibited age, an underlying malignancy, and a documented infection as risk factors for enhanced nephrotoxicity. Since he had an allergic reaction to penicillin, the combination of a cephalosporin and gentamicin was a rational choice for empiric antibiotic therapy. If he did not have a *K. pneumoniae* sepsis, it would be reasonable to discontinue antibiotics at this time, follow his renal function, and reculture if he were febrile. However, since a cephalosporin/aminoglycoside combination demonstrates the greatest degree of synergy against *Klebsiella* species and the studies evaluated for nephrotoxicity implicate either cephaloridine or cephalothin, an alternative cephalosporin, such as cefazolin, could be used. It is unknown whether cefazolin, cephapirin, and other newer cephalosporins used in combination with the aminoglycosides increase the incidence of nephrotoxicity. Currently, reports of these are rare.

12. *Penicillin Allergy.* R.D. is a 20-year-old female with AML who is in blast crisis. She spiked a temperature to 40° C two days ago and was started on cephalothin and tobramycin. She had an urticarial reaction to penicillin one year ago. Blood and sputum cultures are growing *Pseudomonas aeruginosa.* What would you recommend?

The best combination of antibiotics against *P. aeruginosa* is carbenicillin or ticarcillin in combination with gentamicin, tobramycin, or amikacin. Since there is a high mortality rate associated with *Pseudomonas* sepsis and pneumonia, desensitization to carbenicillin or ticarcillin is

suggested by Bodey (2). Pretreatment of the patient with antihistamines may reduce some of the allergic manifestations. Alternatively, single drug therapy with an aminoglycoside effective against *P. aeruginosa* could be continued, although this regimen is usually not as effective as a synergistic combination of antibiotics.

13. *Aminoglycoside-Penicillin Inactivation.* A.R. is a 41-year-old diabetic male who was transferred to the University Hospital for evaluation of diffuse abdominal pain, nausea, and vomiting. He has a past medical history of juvenile-onset diabetes mellitus complicated by diabetic neuropathy, nephropathy, and retinopathy. He has been undergoing peritoneal dialysis for 14 months. Cultures were drawn from his blood and peritoneal cavity, and he was started on methicillin. Two days later all cultures were growing *Pseudomonas aeruginosa,* and the antibiotics were changed to carbenicillin and tobramycin. The patient's clinical response was followed. Serum tobramycin concentrations were measured by radioimmunoassay, and carbenicillin levels were measured by bioassay. Initially, the tobramycin level 30 minutes after the dose was 0.8 mcg/ml, and the carbenicillin level was 256 mcg/ml. Why are the tobramycin concentrations negligible?

A number of reports demonstrate that a high penicillin-to-aminoglycoside dosage or serum ratio for a prolonged period of time results in chemical inactivation of both compounds (46–51). This occurs *in vitro* when both drugs are physically mixed together and *in vivo* in patients with poor renal function where excretion of the drugs is delayed. An irreversible and inactive complex is formed. The beta-lactam ring of the penicillin is opened by the methylamino group on the aminoglycoside (52). Two biologically inactive compounds are subsequently formed. The aminoglycoside-penicillin combination most affected by this reaction is tobramycin-carbenicillin, while the combination least affected is amikacin-ticarcillin (53,54). *In vitro* studies have shown this reaction to be time, temperature, and medium dependent, but pH independent. With a longer contact time, a higher temperature, and a lower solute concentration in the medium, there will be a greater degree of inactivation. *In vivo*, the inactivation of both antibiotics has been shown in patients with end-stage renal disease in whom excretion of the drugs is delayed. Higher concentrations and prolonged contact times in these patients simulate the *in vitro* model, and subsequent inactivation occurs. Therefore, the most likely reason for the low tobramycin level in A.R. is *in vivo* inactivation. It seems reasonable to adjust the dose so that adequate levels of active antibiotic are achieved. However, it is not known whether the inactive complex that is formed has any toxic potential. Weibert et al (51) reported one patient who became deaf after prolonged gentamicin therapy even though the serum levels were consistently less than 2 mcg/ml. Further studies are necessary to determine the potential toxicity of the microbiologically inactive complex.

14. What other factors affect the laboratory determination of antibiotic serum concentrations?

Other factors that should be considered to explain abnormally low serum concentrations include decreased recovery rate of the antibiotic from uremic sera, heparin-aminoglycoside complexation, and *in vitro* inactivation during the assay procedure (55–57). These have been discussed in detail elsewhere (57). Particular attention should also be given to the handling of the sample once it is drawn from the patient. Inactivation of tobramycin in the presence of high concentrations of carbenicillin can occur if the sample is left at room temperature prior to assay (58). When abnormally high antibiotic concentrations are reported, the possibility that concurrent chemotherapy is affecting the assay methods should be considered. Wright et al (59) demonstrated that certain antineoplastic drugs such as 5-fluorouracil can interfere with routine microbiological assay methods for cephalothin and result in almost a 100% error.

Prognostic Indicators for Antibiotic Response

15. A.D. is a 14-year-old male who was referred for evaluation and treatment of probable acute lymphoblastic leukemia (ALL). About one month prior to admission, the patient and his parents noticed increasing bruisability. Two days ago he developed a fever of 39.5° C which did not return to normal. Upon admission to the hospital his white blood cell count was 20,900/mm³ with 2% polymorphonuclear leukocytes, 38% lymphocytes, and 60% blasts. Bone marrow revealed 90% lymphoblasts, and a diagnosis of ALL was confirmed. Cultures were obtained, and he was started on a chemotherapy regimen. Gentamicin and methicillin were also begun. On day 4 the blood and urine cultures grew out *Pseudomonas aeruginosa* and *Escherichia coli*. His antibiotics were changed to gentamicin and carbenicillin. The white blood cell count at this time was 2970/mm³ with 1% polymorphonuclear leukocytes. What are the major prognostic indicators in A.D. that will determine his response to therapy?

The most important factor that will determine A.D.'s response to therapy is the change in ANC (6). No change or a decrease in the ANC during the first week of infection is a poor prognostic sign (14,19,20,35,60). A.D. had an ANC of 418/mm³ on admission which decreased to 30/mm³ on his fourth day of hospitalization. In one series, 88% of the patients with gram-negative bacteremia improved if the ANC increased, whereas only 22% improved if there was no change or a decrease (61). Other prognostic indicators include the type of organism and the source of infection. In the EORTC trial (19), 55% of the patients recovered from infections due to a single gram-negative organism, whereas only 18% recovered from polymicrobic infections with gram-negative bacilli. Patients with gram-positive infections have the greatest chance of recovery (13,19,20). Higher mortality rates are also associated with intra-abdominal and pulmonary foci (21). Finally, patients in shock, elderly patients, and those with underlying problems such as renal insufficiency, diabetes mellitus, malignancies, and other chronic debilitating diseases have a poorer prognosis (19,20,61).

16. Would granulocyte transfusions be useful in the treatment of A.D.?

Granulocyte transfusions have been shown to improve short-term survival in neutropenic patients with documented infections (62–65). Because of the high cost and the potential side effects to the donor and the recipient (discussed in Question 20), the decision to initiate granulocyte transfusion should be based upon some predetermined guidelines (66,67). The overall clinical status of the patient and the likelihood of bone marrow recovery are important considerations. If aggressive therapy is planned and the patient has a documented gram-negative septicemia that is not responding to appropriate antibiotic therapy, then granulocyte transfusions should be considered if the bone marrow is not likley to recover within the first week of infection. Limited data suggest that at least four transfusions should be given, but data on the dose, timing, and frequency of transfusions are lacking (65,68). The most important factor in successful treatment is bone marrow recovery and an increase in the ANC.

Since A.D. has a documented gram-negative infection and his antibiotics have just been changed to an appropriate two-drug regimen, his clinical status should be re-evaluated over the next 24–48 hours. If a documented improvement in clinical signs and symptoms is not found, then granulocyte transfusions would be reasonable in A.D., because his ANC is not likely to increase during the first week of infection, and aggressive therapy is planned to induce a remission.

17. *Effects on Platelet Function.* Four days after his antibiotics were changed, A.D. developed epistaxis and multiple petechiae on his lower extremities. His coagulation times were normal, and his platelet count was 25,000/mm³. What are some of the potential causes for his bleeding?

The two most likely reasons for his bleeding episode are thrombocytopenia and carbenicillin-induced alterations in platelet function. The hemostatic defect produced by carbenicillin, namely defective platelet function, has been found in patients and healthy volunteers given the usual daily dose of 300–600 mg/kg. Brown et al (69) found abnormal adenosine-diphosphate (ADP)-induced platelet aggregation in all of 11 healthy volunteers. Six subjects had abnormal epinephrine-induced aggregation, and five had abnormal collagen-induced aggregation. Bleeding times (BT) were prolonged in the majority of cases. Three of the volunteers who received 600 mg/kg/day and two of the patients who received 340 and 375 mg/kg/day developed clinical bleeding episodes. This was demonstrated by fresh blood in gastric secretions and occult fecal blood loss in the volunteers. Bleeding from the nose and gastrointestinal and urinary tracts was seen in one patient, and the other had bleeding from a surgical wound.

18. Is there an advantage to using ticarcillin in this circumstance?

Ticarcillin is two- to fourfold more active against *P. aeruginosa* strains than carbenicillin, and the recommended dosage of ticarcillin is approximately 150–300 mg/kg/day (70). Since the effects of ticarcillin and carbenicillin on platelet function appear to be dose-related, ticarcillin should cause less problems with platelet aggregation. Brown et al (71) evaluated platelet function in 17 volunteers receiving 100–300 mg/kg ticarcillin daily. While all of the subjects exhibited abnormal bleeding times and ADP-induced aggregation, only the 200 and 300 mg/kg dose had a significant effect on bleeding time and the 300 mg/kg dose had a significant effect on ADP-induced aggregation. The hemostatic defect produced by the highest dose of ticarcillin was similar to that produced by 300–600 mg/kg/day carbenicillin in their previous work. These lower doses of ticarcillin are within the therapeutic range and exhibit only mild defects in platelet function. Therefore, ticarcillin may have less side effects than carbenicillin in patients who are at risk for bleeding.

19. What are some of the other adverse reactions associated with carbenicillin and ticarcillin? Should their dosages be adjusted in renal or hepatic failure?

Both of these antibiotics have a high sodium content. Approximately 5 mEq of sodium is contained in each gram of carbenicillin or ticarcillin. The usual daily dose of carbenicillin in patients with normal renal function is 30 grams given in six divided doses. This results in 150 mEq of sodium administered daily or the equivalent of one liter of normal saline. Since the usual dose of ticarcillin is one-half the dose of carbenicillin, half the amount of sodium is given. The high sodium content is a potential problem for patients with salt and water retention such as those with congestive heart failure, renal failure, and hypertension. Because of the large amount of sodium delivered to the renal tubules, the kidneys reabsorb sodium and excrete potassium. The antibiotics themselves are non-absorbable anions which also cause potassium excretion. Both of these factors result in hypokalemia. Patients who become hypokalemic and patients who are receiving digitalis glycosides should be given potassium supplementation. Although not yet supported by controlled studies, ticarcillin should exhibit less sodium and water retention and less hypokalemia than carbenicillin because of its lower dose. Both of these antibiotics also exhibit toxicities and side effects similar to the other penicillins.

Carbenicillin and ticarcillin are both excreted by the kidneys. They undergo some elimination via the hepatobiliary tract. Their half-lives (t½) are prolonged in renal failure (normal carbenicillin t½ = 1.5 hr, renal failure = 10–20 hr; normal ticarcillin t½ = 1–1.5 hr, renal failure = 16 hr). Hoffman et al (72) suggest adjusting carbenicillin dosages in the following manner: creatinine clearance (Cl_{Cr}) 10–30 ml/min, 2–4 gm q 6–12 hrs; Cl_{Cr} ≤ 10 ml/min, 2 gm q 12 hr; Cl_{Cr} ≤ 10 ml/min plus hepatic dysfunction, 2 gm q 24 hr. An additional maintenance dose is required after hemodialysis. Since the half-life of ticarcillin is prolonged similarly, comparable dosage adjustments can be made using one-half the recommended dose of carbenicillin (73).

20. Do the newer semisynthetic penicillins, piperacillin and mezlocillin, offer any advantages over current antibiotic regimens when treating presumed infection in the neutropenic patient?

When considering the bacterial organisms commonly found in neutropenic patients, piperacillin and mezlocillin show greater *in vitro* activity against *Pseudomonas aeruginosa* and *Klebsiella pneumoniae* than currently available penicillins and greater activity than the cephalosporins against *P. aeruginosa*. Moreover, piperacillin is more active than mezlocillin against *P. aeruginosa*. Both drugs demonstrate little activity against penicillinase-producing *Staphylococcus aureus* (114).

Mezlocillin was evaluated in two studies as a single agent in empiric therapy for febrile, granulocytopenic cancer patients (115,116). It was found to be inadequate when used alone. Response rates ranged from 46–50%. However, a combination of mezlocillin and gentamicin treatment in this population was efficacious in one report (117).

Piperacillin and mezlocillin have broader activity than currently available penicillins and cephalosporins and they are less toxic than aminoglycosides. However, they are not recommended as single agents in neutropenic patients. Comparative studies of these drugs in combination with aminoglycosides or other antibiotics in this population of patients are not yet available.

INFECTION PREVENTION

21. W.M. is a 60-year-old man who was admitted to the hospital because of dyspnea on exertion and recurrence of easy bruisability and epistaxis. Ten years prior to admission he was diagnosed as having polycythemia vera (P. vera) and was treated with phlebotomies and radioactive phosphorus (P^{32}). He did well until two years ago when he again became symptomatic. Treatment with chlorambucil was begun with resolution of symptoms over the next few months. He was continued on a regimen of chlorambucil 10 mg daily for 30 days followed by a one month rest period.

Physical examination is pertinent for a pale individual with petechiae over his extremities and conjunctivae. His spleen is enlarged to three finger-breadths below the left costal margin. Laboratory parameters demonstate: hemoglobin 8 gm/dl, hematocrit 26 vol%, white blood cells 34,500/mm³ with 10% polymorphonuclear leukocytes, 26% lymphocytes, 2% monocytes, 2% eosinophils, and 60% blasts. Bone marrow biopsy shows a marrow cavity packed with blasts. His uric acid is 17 mg/dl.

Assessment at this time is acute myeloblastic leukemia probably secondary to treatment of P. vera. Therapy will be initiated with allopurinol and a chemotherapy regimen of adriamycin, vincristine, cytosine arabinoside, and prednisone.

W.M. is at high risk of becoming infected. What measures can be used for prophylaxis against infection? Define their rationale and list their disadvantages.

Five modalities have been used with varying success as infection prevention techniques in granulocytopenic patients. These include protected environments, microbial suppression, colonization resistance, attenuation of chemotherapy-inducd neutropenia, and granulocyte transfusions.

Protected Environments. The rationale for using protected environments (PE), such as laminar air flow rooms (LAFR) or "Life Islands" in conjunction with sterile food, water, and supplies is to decrease the number of ambient organisms and protect the patient from acquiring new potential pathogens (74). The majority of infections arise from the patient's endogenous flora, of which over half of the organisms are acquired during hospitalization (22). Since almost 70% of the cultures taken in LAFR are sterile, PE would serve to decrease the number of organisms to which the patient is exposed (75). This is especially important for *Pseudomonas aeruginosa*, since colonization with this organism increases the chance of developing infection twofold (22). LAFR and "Life Islands" are equipped with high-efficiency particulate air filters which remove organisms greater than 0.3μ from the air. The main difference between these two types of PE is that LAFR have a unidirectional, or laminar, air flow which reduces air turbulence and directs the flow away from the patient, visitors, and staff. "Life Islands" are plastic tent-enclosed beds which do not have adequate air circulation. These isolation units allow endogenous microbial flora to accumulate and recontaminate the environment. This can be minimized by concomitant use of microbial suppression techniques (76,77). The disadvantages of PE are expense and psychological impact on the patient (74,76). Almost a decade ago, the cost of PE was estimated at $300 to $500 a day. This did not include the specially trained personnel to staff the environment. Psychologically, the feeling of entrapment and loss of privacy in the "Life Island" units can be detrimental to the patient and is poorly tolerated. Acceptance of LAFR is much better.

Microbial Suppression. Microbial suppression decreases the patient's endogenous flora with the administration of prophylactic oral nonabsorbable antibiotics (PA) alone or in combination with topical and orificial antisepsis (74,76). Between 40 and 87% of aerobic and anaerobic stool cultures become negative in patients treated with PA, compared to less than 3% of untreated controls (75,77). Fungi are more difficult to eradicate, with only 30–60% of the cultures becoming negative (75,78). PA are usually effective in suppressing microbial flora and occasionally in eliminating them. The most popular regimen is gentamicin, vancomycin, and nystatin (GVN), although a variety of combinations have been used (74). The oral nonabsorbable antibiotics are not tolerated by some patients because of poor taste, anorexia, and varying degrees of nausea, vomit-

ing, and diarrhea. In one study, the GVN regimen was discontinued because of these side effects (79). The cost of these regimens is expensive, exceeding $100 per day. However, the most significant problems are development of resistant organisms and an increased infection rate upon discontinuation of the antibiotics during periods of granulocytopenia (80,81). Since microbial suppression creates a microbial vacuum, the patient is likely to acquire and become colonized with organisms, such as gram-negative bacilli, that are resistant to aminoglycosides. In one series, 30% of the acquired gram-negative bacilli were resistant to gentamicin. In another study, no resistant organisms were detected (81). Discontinuation of PA while the patient is granulocytopenic can result in rapid colonization of the alimentary tract with potential pathogens before recovery of the normal flora. An increased incidence of severe and fatal infections has been reported in many of these cases.

Colonization Resistance. Colonization resistance is another approach towards infection prevention and involves the selective suppression of aerobic microbial flora in the alimentary tract. The capacity of the remaining anaerobic flora to prevent colonization of the gastrointestinal tract by potential pathogens is termed "colonization resistance" (74). Drugs such as trimethoprim-sulfamethoxazole (TMP-SMX), nalidixic acid, oxolinic acid, and pipemidic acid are capable of doing this. Sulfa drugs have the potential for causing allergic reactions, and nalidixic acid may cause mild nausea. These agents, however, are better tolerated than PA regimens such as GVN, and there is little or no overgrowth of naturally-resistant organisms. While TMP-SMX, a folic acid antagonist, can potentially prolong bone marrow recovery time in granulocytopenic patients, limited data have not demonstrated this (79).

Attenuation of Chemotherapy-induced Neutropenia. The attenuation of chemotherapy-induced granulocytopenia would be expected to decrease the infection rate, since neutropenia is the single most important factor associated with infection in compromised hosts. Lithium carbonate was found serendipitously to cause a reversible neutrophilic leukocytosis in schizophrenic patients (82). The maximum response occurs 7–10 days after initiation of treatment and returns to pre-treatment levels a week after discontinuation of therapy. Although plasma lithium concentrations of 0.5–1.0 mEq/L appear to be effective, plasma lithium concentrations do not appear to correlate with the magnitude of the neutrophil increase. The proposed mechanism is stimulation of monocyte colony-stimulating factor (CSF) with subsequent proliferation of marrow myeloid elements (83). This results in an increased total body neutrophil pool, including bone marrow, circulating, and marginal pools, and a decreased daily turnover rate with resultant increased half-life of neutrophils (84). These cells maintain the properties of migration, chemotaxis, and phagocytosis, although one study suggests a decrease in bactericidal activity (85). The side effects associated with lithium therapy include gastrointestinal distress, tremor, lethargy, confusion, and mild diabetes insipidus. Other abnormalities, such as chromosome aberrations, selective lymphocytopenia, erythroid hypoplasia, carcinogenesis, and severe myelotoxicity, are potential problems for which there are negative or conflicting reports in the small number of patients studied (83).

Granulocyte Transfusions. The rationale for the use of prophylactic granulocyte transfusions is also based on the quantitative inverse relationship between levels of circulating neutrophils and the incidence of infection. The quality and quantity of granulocyte transfusions may affect the patients's response (66,68). For example, ABO matching and leukocyte alloantibody determinations are important to minimize transfusion reactions, sensitization to whole blood or platelets, and pulmonary reactions. These latter effects can be manifested as respiratory insufficiency from volume overload, sequestration of granulocytes in a pulmonary lesion, interaction between circulating endotoxins and granulocytes resulting in "shock lung," or leukoagglutination reactions causing intravascular aggregation and subsequent embolization of granulocytes into the lungs. Recovery rates of transfused granulocytes also appear to be dependent upon these factors and HL-A typing. However, it is unclear as to whether a demonstrable increment in circulating neutrophils after transfusion is necessary for a beneficial effect, since this does not take into account the unmeasured marginal neutrophil pool and the sequestered cells. The quality of granulocytes procured by differential sedimentation is generally good and without functional alterations. The use of reversible adhesion techniques (filtration leukapheresis) results in a variable product morphologically, with some alteration in chemotactic and bactericidal activity. The significance of this in terms of clinical efficacy is unknown (66). This method also causes a higher incidence of transfusion reactions which can be minimized by slowing the infusion rate and pretreating the recipient with antipyretics, antihistamines, or corticosteroids. Other problems include the transmission of mononucleosis, cytomegalovirus, malaria, toxoplasmosis, hepatitis, and immunocompetent lymphocytes. In the latter case, a graft-versus-host disease can occur; however, irradiation of the granulocytes before transfusion should decrease the severity of this reaction. Data from UCLA show that cytomegalovirus infections were significantly increased in their bone marrow transplant patients who were receiving prophylactic granulocyte transfusions (86). Some patients receive transfusions from donors with chronic myelogenous leukemia (CML) because of the large numbers of granulocytes in these individuals. There is the potential for engraftment of CML stem cells in the recipient, and Philadelphia chromosome abnormalities have been seen occasionally.

In addition to the adverse reactions in the recipient, the donor may also be affected (66). Citrate toxicity manifesting as hypocalcemia can occur from the acid citrate dextrose or citrate phosphate dextrose which are used as anticoagulants during the collection process. Methods employed to increase granulocyte yield, such as systemic corticosteroids or etiocholanolone, can potentially cause problems. In particular, fever, chills, and pain on intramuscular injection of etiocholanolone have been described. A single dose of a corticosteroid, however, should not cause any major problems. Mild symptoms of volume overload may occur when hydroxyethyl starch is used as a rouleauxing agent to increase the efficiency of RBC separation from WBC. Other side effects include traumatic intravascular hemolysis secondary to roller pumps used in moving blood during the procedure and increased pulmonary artery pressure and decreased oxygen tension secondary to leukoagglutination in the lungs. It is postulated that this latter effect is caused by complement activation by the nylon fiber filters used in filtration leukapheresis. Finally, the cost of collection and transfusion of granulocytes is prohibitive.

In summary, the utility of these prophylactic measures is to decrease infection rate and allow additional treatment to be given which might otherwise be withheld because of infection.

22. What is the effect of each of these modalities on the incidence of infection?

The majority of the randomized, controlled studies demonstrate that the "total protected environment," utilizing LAFR or "Life Islands" in conjunction with PA, results in a significant decrease in infection rate (76,77,80,87). Only one randomized, controlled study has evaluated PE alone, and it demonstrated a significant decrease in the incidence of infection (77). Randomized comparisons of PA alone with control and PE-PA groups demonstrate a significant effect in only half of the studies (75–77,80,88,89).

The use of selective microbial suppression, or colonization resistance, has been studied in two small randomized, controlled series (79,90). A significant reduction in infection rate and febrile episodes was noted. The antibiotic combination used most often is TMP-SMX. The dose of TMP-SMX is 320 mg TMP and 1600 mg SMX (two tablets twice daily or one double-strength tablet twice daily).

The use of lithium carbonate in daily doses of 300–1000 mg can attenuate neutropenia secondary to chemotherapy. However, only one of five studies demonstrated a significant decrease in infection rate compared to a control group (82,91).

The incidence of infection with prophylactic granulocyte transfusions was significantly decreased in only one randomized, controlled study (92). Survival, however, was not improved. Little is known about the quantity of neutrophils required to prevent infection. Some authors suggest that at least 1×10^{10} neutrophils are needed to achieve a measurable quantity in the blood (66). They could be given daily for the duration of the neutropenia; however, these are only empiric guidelines.

23. Which regimen should be used for infection prevention in W.M.?

Based upon the available literature, TMP-SMX has the best risk-to-benefit and cost-to-benefit ratios of the five modalities discussed. However, only small numbers of patients have been studied, and long term adverse effects are unknown. Additional well-designed trials are necessary to establish whether TMP-SMX is the best mode of treatment for infection prevention. It is important to realize that none of these measures appreciably affects remission rates, duration of remission, and long-term survival in patients with acute leukemias. As chemotherapy for these malignancies improves, infection prevention measures may allow more intensive regimens to be administered.

24. Besides these specific modalities, what general principles of infection prevention should be considered in W.M.?

Some general principles of infection prevention that can be used in W.M. have been outlined by Levine et al (1). These include avoidance of hospitalization for procedures that can be performed in outpatients to reduce colonization by gram-negative bacilli, avoidance of invasive procedures such as urinary catheterization and intravenous lines to minimize iatrogenic infection, and maintenance of good nutrition. Additional measures include respiratory toilet and good humidification for patients with pulmonary disease, control of diabetes mellitus, and treatment of underlying diseases that contribute to immunodeficiency states, if possible. Immunizations should also be considered.

PNEUMOCYSTIS CARINII PNEUMONIA

25. S.T. is a 46-year-old, 60 kg male with renal failure secondary to chronic glomerulonephritis who underwent renal transplantation about two months ago. The kidney was of cadaveric origin, and tissue typing showed incompatibility with two major transplantation antigens. The first seven postoperative weeks were characterized by severe rejection episodes, and an average of 150 mg of prednisone per day was required. Azathioprine was given in varying dosage schedules according to the peripheral leukocyte count. The patient was discharged on the fiftieth post-transplantation day with prednisone 30 mg daily and azathioprine. The creatinine clearance was 45–60 ml/minute.

On the sixtieth post-transplantation day, the patient was readmitted because of fever of one day's duration and a minimal nonproductive cough. Physical examination revealed a temperature 102.6° F, cyanosis, and tachypnea of 40–45 respirations/minute. Examination of the chest revealed no abnor-

malities. **Laboratory studies showed a white blood cell count of 1400/mm³. The creatinine clearance was 50 ml/min. A chest x-ray was within normal limits. Routine cultures of blood, sputum, and urine were unrevealing. The daily immunosuppressive therapy was continued at 30 mg of prednisone and intermittent azathioprine. Fever to 102–104° F continued with chills each afternoon. The arterial PO₂ was 44 mm Hg and the PCO₂ was 32 mm Hg. The diffusing capacity was 8% (normal greater than 70%). Bronchoscopy performed on the sixty-fifth day revealed no abnormality. Brush biopsy specimens were taken, and methenamine silver stain showed *Pneumocystis carinii*. The chest x-ray at this time showed progression to bilateral diffuse patchy alveolar infiltrates.**

On the sixty-eighth day the patient was started on trimethoprim (TMP) 20 mg/kg and sulfamethoxazole (SMX) 100 mg/kg per day. By the seventy-first day clearing of chest x-ray was marked, and the patient became afebrile. There was a gradual improvement in the PO₂ over the first week of treatment. The PCO₂ remained normal. TMP/SMX was continued for 14 days. Serum levels of TMP and SMX were obtained and showed concentrations of 10 mcg/ml TMP and 140 mcg/ml SMX at two hours after a dose. The dosages of TMP/SMX were not adjusted, and the prednisone dosage was not changed throughout the course of the pneumonia. The patient was discharged on the ninetieth post-transplantation day, at which time chest x-ray showed only minimal residual bilateral pulmonary infiltrates.

What is *Pneumocystis carinii* pneumonitis, and why was S.T. at risk for developing this infection?

Pneumocystis carinii is a ubiquitous organism that does not yet have a definitive taxonomic classification. It is currently listed in the phylum Protozoa under the class Sporozoa (93). The pneumonitis appears to result from reactivation of a latent infection in children and adults and not as a primary infection. This is suggestd by the fact that almost two-thirds of children have humoral antibodies to *P. carinii* by age four (94). The natural habitat, mode of transmission, and portal of entry are unknown. It rarely occurs in healthy individuals. The incidence in immunocompro-

mised patients ranges from 2–15%, and it is the major cause of death in patients with ALL in remission (90,95,96). The lung is the major organ affected, and rarely does disseminated infection occur.

Microbiologically, *P. carinii* exists as three forms: a cyst (thick-walled which stains with methenamine silver nitrate or toluidine blue 0 stain), a trophozoite (thin-walled which stains with polychrome methylene blue), and a sporozoite (intra-cystic structure which stains with polychrome methylene blue) (94). The trophozoite attaches to the host cell, enlarges into a pre-cyst form, and then detaches and becomes a mature, thick-walled cyst. The sporozoites exit through the wall of the cyst. The host cell then degenerates. The affinity of the trophozoites for the alveolar septae results in a pneumonitis with marked impairment of gas exchange.

S.T. was at risk for developing pneumocystis because of intense immunosuppression with corticosteroids and azathioprine which were being used to treat his renal transplant rejection. Since pneumocystis was first diagnosed in humans in 1956, certain high risk groups have been identified (94,97). They include premature infants, children at their nadir of immunocompetence (2–3 months of age), individuals with protein-calorie malnutrition, congenital immunodeficiency states (primarily cellular, but also humoral), and acquired immunodeficient states. The latter group are those with underlying malignancies (especially those with ALL in remission) who are being treated with chemotherapy and irradiation, and organ transplant patients undergoing intense immunosuppressive therapy. Hughes et al (98) demonstrated that the incidence of pneumocystis was related to the number of chemotherapeutic agents used for maintenance therapy. Of 149 children with ALL in remission receiving one, two, three, or four drugs, 5.0, 2.3, 2.2, and 22.4%, respectively, developed *P. carinii* pneumonitis. It has also been found that approximately 60% of the patients with steroid-associated pneumocystis infections had their dose decreased or discontinued shortly before the onset of symptoms (93). S.T. would fall into this category since he had his prednisone dose tapered from 150 mg to 30 mg over the first seven post-transplantation weeks.

26. What characteristic signs and symptoms of pneumocystis did S.T. exhibit?

S.T. complained of fever and non-productive cough. He was tachypneic and had signs of cyanosis. There were no rales on chest examination. He was hypoxic with a PO_2 of 44 mm Hg and a normal PCO_2. Diffusing capacity was low, indicating poor gas exchange. Chest x-ray eventually showed bilateral, diffuse, patchy alveolar infiltrates. These findings are typical of pneumocystis as well as other types of opportunistic pneumonias in the compromised host (93,94,99,100). In addition to the clinical features seen in S.T., some patients rapidly progress to respiratory decompensation with respiratory rates up to 80–100/min, intercostal retractions, and nasal flaring. They may require assisted or controlled ventilatory support.

The signs and symptoms demonstrated by S.T. are typical of the mild child-adult sporadic type of pneumocystosis. This is different from the infantile epidemic infections seen primarily in Europe. A comparison of these two types of infections is shown in Table 5 (94,97).

27. How is pneumocystis diagnosed?

When the clinical presentation of the patient suggests pneumocystis, the diagnosis can be made by staining a specimen from the lung for the presence of cysts (93,100–102). The best results have been obtained when tissue from open lung biopsy is stained with methenamine silver nitrate or toluidine blue O for identification of thick-walled cysts. Giemsa, Wright, Gram-Weigert, or polychrome methylene blue stains can be used to see thin-walled cysts. Fluorescein-labelled antibody techniques have no advantage over staining methods. Transbronchial biopsy and endobronchial brush biopsy can also be used to obtain lung specimens although they are ≤ 80–90% as dependable as open lung biopsy. Transthoracic needle aspiration gives an 87% yield if one specimen is

Table 5.

CLINICAL FEATURES OF THE TWO FORMS OF
PNEUMOCYSTIS CARINII PNEUMONITIS

Clinical features	Child-adult type	Infantile type
Type	Sporadic	Epidemic
Onset	Acute, fulminating	Insidious

High risk groups	Immunosuppressed
	    Cancer
	    Organ transplant
	    Congenital
	    Corticosteroids
	    Antineoplastics
		Premature infants
		Marasmic infants 2–6 months old
		Protein-calorie malnutrition
		Immunocompetence nadir at 2–3
		    months old

Signs and symptoms	Fever Tachypnea Cough Intercostal retractions Nasal flaring Cyanosis Rales absent	Diarrhea Failure to thrive Poor feeding Tachypnea Intercostal retractions Cyanosis Fever absent Rales absent

Chest x-ray findings	Hyperexpanded lung
	Diffuse bilateral pulmonary
	    infiltrates starting in hilum
	    and progressing peripherally
		Hyperexpanded lung
		Diffuse bilateral pulmonary
		    infiltrates starting in hilum
		    and progressing peripherally

Mortality untreated	90–100%	50%
Mortality treated	~ 25%	~ 3%

Adapted from references: 93,94,97

obtained and a 95% yield with two specimens. Other methods which are used include staining of transtrachial aspirates, gastric contents, sputum, pharyngeal secretions, and bronchopulmonary lavage samples. These results are quite variable, and they usually are low yield procedures. Other antibody techniques, such as complement-fixation and indirect immunofluorescence, are also variable.

28. What antibiotics can be used to treat pneumocystis?

Pentamidine isethionate is an aromatic diamidine compound that was one of the first drugs used to treat pneumocystis (93,94). It is an experimental antibiotic for parenteral use only and can be obtained from the Center for Disease Control (CDC) in Atlanta, Georgia. Studies have demonstrated a 68–75% recovery rate from pneumocystis with pentamidine (103). It has decreased the mortality rate from nearly 100% to 25% at best in the child-adult form and from 50% to about 3% in the infantile-epidemic form (94). The mechanism of action is not known, although animal studies suggest an inhibition of dihydrofolate reductase. Pentamidine is usually given as a 4 mg/kg intramuscular dose once a day for 14 days.

A combination of pyrimethamine and a sulfonamide appears to be effective against *P. carinii;* however, sufficient clinical trials are lacking to recommend this combination (93,94).

The combination of trimethoprim-sulfamethoxazole (TMP-SMX) in a dosage regimen of 20 mg/kg TMP and 100 mg/kg SMX given in four divided doses per day for 14 days results in a 75% recovery rate from pneumocystis (103). This is comparable to results achiveable with pentamidine. TMP-SMX can be given orally by mouth or via a nasogastric tube. However, in patients who are unable to take the drug orally or in cases where absorption may be affected, such as an adynamic ileus, the intravenous preparation can be obtained from Hoffman La-Roche, Inc. in Nutley, New Jersey (104–106). This is still an investigational form of the drug. The mechanism of action of SMX, a structural analogue of para-aminobenzoic acid, is interference with the synthesis of dihydropteroic acid. TMP acts on a later step in folate metabolism. It is a structural analogue of the pteridine portion of dihydrofolic acid

and interferes with the formation of tetrahydrofolic acid.

Para-amino benzoic acid

Sulfonamides | dihydropteroate synthetase

Dihydropteroic acid

dihydrofolate synthetase

Dihydrofolic acid

Trimethoprim | dihydrofolate reductase

Tetrahydrofolic acid

The two antibiotics are synergistic when used in combination (107).

29. What are the differences in side effects between pentamidine and TMP-SMX?

In over 1,000 patients given TMP-SMX for the treatment of pneumocystis or for chemoprophylaxis, only 5–10% exhibited adverse reactions (96,103,108). These patients experienced skin rashes, hives, erythema multiforme, Stevens-Johnson syndrome, mild gastrointestinal complaints, and some hematologic abnormalities. The latter side effect was manifested as neutropenia or thrombocytopenia. In approximately 400 patients treated with pentamidine, 47% had adverse reactions (109). These included impaired renal function (24%), injection site reactions (18%), liver dysfunction (10%), hypotension (10%), hypoglycemia (6%), hematologic disturbances (4%) such as thrombocytopenia and coagulation abnormalities, skin rashes (2%), and hypocalcemia (1%). In one study of 50 children in whom pentamidine and TMP-SMX were compared, TMP-SMX had minimal adverse effects in comparison to pentamidine (103).

30. Why were plasma levels of TMP-SMX monitored in ST? How should they be interpreted?

Limited data suggest that response to TMP-SMX therapy within the first 24–72 hours is greater with TMP levels of 3–5 mcg/ml and SMX levels of 100–150 mcg/ml at 1.5–2 hours after the dose (103,106,110). In one study, Hughes et al (103) found that children who did not respond to

TMP-SMX within the first three days of therapy had lower plasma concentrations. It is therefore recommended that TMP-SMX plasma concentrations be monitored. In two groups of patients, this may be of particular benefit. Miser el al (104) noted that some critically ill patients with pneumocystis who had undergone lung biopsy developed ileus. This resulted in low levels of TMP because of altered absorption of the antibiotic. In this case, the intravenous form TMP-SMX or use of pentamidine would be indicated. Another group who would benefit from plasma drug level determinations are renal failure patients (111). About half the dose of TMP is excreted unchanged in the urine, whereas only a small portion of SMX is eliminated as active drug. Eighty percent of the SMX which is excreted is in the form of inactive metabolites (107). Appropriate dosage adjustments should be made to minimize toxicity of these agents in patients with renal insufficiency, and blood levels can be used to determine the extent of dosage reduction. Because of the difference in metabolic fate of each compound, it may be necessary to utilize the individual components and not the combination product. Trimethoprim and sulfamethoxazole are both commercially available as individual drugs if needed.

31. Would pentamidine be a better choice in patients with renal insufficiency?

Pentamidine offers no advantage to TMP-SMX in this circumstance. It is primarily excreted unchanged by the kidneys, and recommendations for dosage adjustments in renal failure are not available (112).

32. What prognostic indications did S.T. exhibit which suggested a good chance for recovery from his *P. carinii* pneumonitis?

A good response to therapy is indicated by defervescence within two to four days of initiating treatment, resolution of the pulmonary infiltrate beginning the second to fifth day of treatment with nearly complete clearing of the chest x-ray by three weeks, and improved oxygenation by the eighth day (105). All of these indicators were seen in S.T. Most of the studies evaluating the effects of treatment considered crossover to the alternate therapy if improvement in these signs and symptoms was not seen in the first 72 hours of treatment (103).

33. F.J. is a 16-year-old female with ALL in remission who is scheduled for maintenance chemotherapy. Since she is at high risk for developing pneumocystis, chemoprophylactic measures are being considered. What forms of chemoprophylaxis are available? What is the risk-to-benefit ratio of treatment?

A variety of measures have been tried as chemoprophylaxis for pneumocystis. These include immunization, pentamidine, rifampin, pyrimethamine-sulfadiazine combination, clindamycin, and TMP-SMX (90). Only TMP-SMX in a dosage schedule of 4–5 mg/kg (or 150 mg/m^2) TMP and 20–25 mg/kg (or 750 mg/m^2) SMX given daily in two divided doses has been shown to be effective in preventing pneumocystis. This continuous low dose regimen was evaluated in a double-blind, randomized, placebo-controlled study in 160 high risk cancer patients (90). None of the 80 patients receiving TMP-SMX developed pneumocystis, whereas 21% of the placebo group became infected. TMP-SMX also significantly reduced the incidence of bacterial sepsis in the treated group. Oral candidiasis was the only side effect noted. In another series of 229 patients treated for about two years with continuous low-dose TMP-SMX, none developed pneumocystis; complications included neutropenia (4.8%), rash (3.5%), and gastrointestinal distress (1.3%) (96). For selected high risk groups of patients, chemoprophylaxis with TMP-SMX is effective and well-tolerated.

34. Which patients appear to be at greater risk of developing the hematologic side effects of TMP-SMX?

Thrombocytopenia and neutropenia are significantly more common in patients receiving prophylactic regimens of TMP-SMX who are also receiving azathioprine (113). In this study, renal allograft recipients undergoing immunosuppressive therapy with azathioprine were compared to similar groups of patients receiving TMP-SMX for either treatment of a urinary tract infection (6–16 days of therapy) or prophylaxis for pneumocystis (≥ 22 days of therapy). There was a significant increase in the incidence of thrombocytopenia and neutropenia in the prophylaxis group. The proposed mechanism for this effect is enhanced bone marrow suppression from the combined antimetabolite properties of 6-mercaptopurine, the active moiety of azathioprine, and the antifolate effects of TMP-SMX. Since organ transplant patients are at high risk of developing pneumocystis because of the intense immunosup-pressive regimens employed, further studies are necessary in this group to determine the risk-to-benefit ratio of chemoprophylaxis with TMP-SMX.

References

1. Levine AS et al: Hematologic malignancies and other marrow failure states: progress in the management of complicating infections. Semin Hematol. 1974; 11:141.
2. Bodey GP: Infections in cancer patients. Can Treat Rep. 1975; 2:89.
3. Chang H et al: Causes of death in adults with acute leukemia. Medicine. 1976; 55:259.
4. Inagaki J et al: Causes of death in cancer patients. Cancer. 1974; 33:568.
5. Dilworth JA et al: Infections in patients with cancer. Semin Oncol. 1975; 2:349.
6. Yancey RS: Complications of cancer chemotherapy. Can Bull. 1980; 5:168.
7. Bodey GP et al: Quantitative relationships between circulating leukocytes and infection in patients with acute leukemia. Ann Intern Med. 1966; 64:328.
8. Grieco MH: Introduction to the abnormal host and complicating infections. In *Infections in the Abnormal Host*, 1st ed, edited by MH Grieco, Yorke Medical Books, New York, 1980, p 1.
9. Neu HC: The role of cellular and humoral factors in infections. Clin Hematol. 1976; 5:449.
10. Harris J et al: Impaired immunoresponsiveness in tumor patients. Ann NY Acad Sci. 1974; 230:56.
11. Sickles EA et al: Clinical presentation of infection in granulocytopenic patients. Arch Intern Med. 1975; 135:715.
12. Ketchel SJ et al: Acute infections in cancer patients. Semin Oncol. 1978; 5:167.
13. Bodey GP et al: Fever and infection in leukemia patients. A study of 494 consecutive patients. Cancer. 1978; 41:1610.
14. Valdivieso M et al: Gram-negative bacillary pneumonia in the compromised host. Medicine. 1977; 56:241.
15. Sickles EA et al: Pneumonia in acute leukemia. Ann Intern Med. 1973; 79:528.
16. Rodriguez V et al: Management of fever of unknown origin in patients with neoplasms and neutropenia. Cancer. 1973; 32:1007.
17. Shastri S et al: Clinical study with bleomycin. Cancer. 1971; 28:1142.
18. Schimpff SC et al: Rectal abscesses in cancer patients. Lancet. 1972; 2:844.
19. The EORTC International Antimicrobial Therapy Project Group: Three antibiotic regimens in the treatment of infection in febrile, granulocytopenic patients with cancer. J Infect Dis. 1978; 137:14.
20. Schimpff SC et al: Ticarcillin in combination with cephalothin or gentamicin as empiric antibiotic therapy in granulocytopenic cancer patients. Antimicrob Agents Chemother. 1976; 10:837.
21. Singer C et al: Bacteremia and fungemia complicating neoplastic disease. Am J Med. 1977; 62:731.
22. Schimpff SC et al: Origin of infection in acute nonlymphocytic leukemia. Significance of hospital acquisition of potential pathogens. Ann Intern Med. 1972; 77:707.
23. Schimpff SC et al: Significance of *Pseudomonas aeruginosa* in the patient with leukemia or lymphoma. J Infect Dis. 1974; 130(suppl):S24.
24. Goldschmidt MC et al: Effect of chemotherapeutic agents upon microorganisms isolated from cancer patients. Antimicrob Agents Chemother. 1972; 1:348.
25. Metcalfe D et al: Effects of methotrexate on Group A beta hemolytic streptococci and streptococcal infection. Cancer. 1972; 30:588.
26. Rodriguez V et al: Antibacterial therapy—special considerations in neutropenic patients. Clin Hematol. 1976; 5:347.
27. Klastersky J: The use of synergistic combinations of antibiotics in patients with hematological diseases. Clin Hematol. 1976; 5:361.
28. Rahal JJ: Antibiotic combinations: the clinical relevance of synergy and antagonism. Medicine. 1978; 57:179.
29. Klastersky J et al: Therapy with carbenicillin and gentamicin for patients with cancer and severe infections caused by gram-negative rods. Cancer. 1973; 31:331.
30. Klastersky J et al: Clinical significance of in vitro synergism between antibiotics in gram-negative infections. Antimicrob Agents Chemother. 1972; 2:470.
31. Lau WK et al: Comparative efficacy and toxicity of amikacin/carbenicillin versus gentamicin/carbenicillin in leukopenic patients. A randomized prospective trial. Am J Med. 1977; 62:959.
32. Klastersky J et al: Empiric therapy for cancer patients: comparative study of ticarcillin-tobramycin, ticarcillin-cephalothin, and cephalothin-tobramycin. Antimicrob Agents Chemother. 1975; 7:640.
33. Keating MJ et al: A randomized comparative trial of three aminoglycosides—comparison of continuous infusions of gentamicin, amikacin and sisomicin combined with carbenicillin in the treatment of infections in neutropenic patients with malignancies. Medicine. 1979; 59:159.
34. Middleman EL et al: Antibiotic combinations for infections in neutropenic patients. Evaluation of carbenicillin plus either cephalothin or kanamycin. Cancer. 1972; 30:573.
35. Klastersky J et al: Carbenicillin, cefazolin, and amikacin as an empiric therapy for febrile granulocytopenic cancer patients. Can Treat Rep. 1977; 61:1433.
36. Klastersky J et al: Gram-negative infections in cancer. Study of empiric therapy comparing carbenicillin-cephalothin with and without gentamicin. JAMA. 1974; 227:45.
37. Bloomfield CD et al: Cephalothin, carbenicillin, and gentamicin combination therapy for febrile patients with acute non-lymphocytic leukemia. Cancer. 1974; 34:431.
38. Tattersall MNH et al: Initial therapy with combination of five antibiotics in febrile patients with leukemia and neutropenia. Lancet. 1972; 1:162.

39. Pizzo PA et al: Duration of empiric antibiotic therapy in granulocytopenic patients with cancer. Am J Med. 1979; 67:194.

40. Fillastre JP et al: Acute renal failure associated with combined gentamicin and cephalothin therapy. Br Med J. 1973; 2:396.

41. Bobrow SN et al: Anuria and acute tubular necrosis associated with gentamicin and cephalothin. JAMA. 1972; 222:1546.

42. Kleinknecht D et al: Acute renal failure after high doses of gentamicin and cephalothin (letter). Lancet. 1973; 1:1129.

43. Cabanillas F et al: Nephrotoxicity of combined cephalothin-gentamicin regimen. Arch Intern Med. 1975; 135:850.

44. Plager JE: Association of renal injury with combined cephalothin-gentamicin therapy among patients severly ill with malignant disease. Cancer. 1976; 37:1937.

45. Fanning WL et al: Gentamicin- and cephalothin-associated rises in blood urea nitrogen. Antimicrob Agents Chemother. 1976; 10:80.

46. McLaughlin JE et al: Clinical and laboratory evidence for inactivation of gentamicin by carbenicillin. Lancet. 1971; 1:261.

47. Noone P et al: Therapeutic implications of interaction of gentamicin and penicillins. Lancet. 1971; 2:575.

48. Davies M et al: Interactions of carbenicillin and ticarcillin with gentamicin. Antimicrob Agents Chemother. 1975; 7:431.

49. Ervin FR et al: Inactivation of gentamicin by penicillins in patients with renal failure. Antimicrob Agents Chemother. 1976; 9:1004.

50. Riff LJ et al: Laboratory and clinical conditions for gentamicin inactivation by carbenicillin. Arch Intern Med. 1972; 130:887.

51. Weibert R et al: Carbenicillin inactivation of aminoglycosides in patients with severe renal failure. Trans Am Soc Artif Int Org. 1976; 22:439.

52. Waitz JA et al: Biological aspects of the interaction between gentamicin and carbenicillin. J Antibiot. 1972; 25:219.

53. Pickering LK et al: Effects of time and concentration upon interaction between gentamicin, tobramycin, netilmicin or amikacin and carbenicillin or ticarcillin. Antimicrob Agents Chemother. 1979; 15:592.

54. Holt HA et al: Interactions between aminoglycoside antibiotics and carbenicillin or ticarcillin. Infection. 1976; 4:107.

55. Stessman J et al: Error in recovery rate of aminoglycosides from uremic sera. Chemother. 1977; 23:142.

56. Yourassowsky E et al: Effect of heparin on gentamicin concentration in the blood. Clin Chim Acta. 1972; 42:189.

57. Russo ME: Penicillin-aminoglycoside inactivation: another possible mechanism of interaction. Am J Hosp Pharm. 1980; 37:702.

58. Polk RE et al: Mail order tobramycin serum levels: low values caused by ticarcillin (letter). Am J Hosp Pharm. 1980; 37:920.

59. Wright DN et al: Bioassay of antibiotics in body fluids from patients receiving cancer chemotherapeutic agents. Antimicrob Agents Chemo. 1980; 17:417.

60. Valdivieso M et al: Amikacin therapy of severe infections produced by gram-negative bacilli resistant to gentamicin. Am J Med Sci. 1977; 273:177.

61. Schimpff SC et al: Empiric antibiotic therapy. Can Treat Rep. 1978; 62:673.

62. Herzig RH et al: Successful granulocyte transfusion therapy for gram-negative septicemia. A prospectively randomized controlled study. N Engl J Med. 1977; 296:701.

63. Alavi JB et al: A randomized clinical trial of granulocyte transfusions for infection in acute leukemia. N Engl J Med. 1977; 296:706.

64. Vogler WR et al: A controlled study of the efficacy of granulocyte transfusions in patients with neutropenia. Am J Med. 1977; 63:548.

65. Graw RG et al: Normal granulocyte transfusion therapy: treatment of septicemia due to gram-negative bacteremia. N Engl J Med. 1972; 287:367.

66. Higby DJ et al: Granulocyte transfusions: current status. Blood. 1980; 55:2.

67. Boggs DR: Neutrophils in the blood bank (editorial). N Engl J Med. 1977; 296:748.

68. Boggs DR: Transfusion of neutrophils as prevention or treatment of infection in patients with neutropenia. N Engl J Med. 1974; 290:1055.

69. Brown III CH et al: The hemostatic defect produced by carbenicillin. N Engl J Med. 1974; 291:265.

70. Neu HC et al: Comparative in vitro activity and clinical pharmacology of ticarcillin and carbenicillin. Antimicrob Agents Chemother. 1975; 8:457.

71. Brown III CH et al: Study of the effects of ticarcillin on blood coagulation and platelet function. Antimicrob Agents Chemother. 1975; 7:652.

72. Hoffman TA et al: Pharmacodynamics of carbenicillin in hepatic and renal failure. Ann Intern Med. 1970; 73:173.

73. Parry MF et al: Pharmacokinetics of ticarcillin in patients with abnormal renal function. J Infect Dis. 1976; 133:46.

74. Schimpff SC: Infection prevention during profound granulocytopenia. New approaches to alimentary canal microbial suppression. Ann Intern Med. 1980; 93:358.

75. Levine AS et al: Protected environments and prophylactic antibiotics. A prospective controlled study of their utility in the therapy of acute leukemia. N Engl J Med. 1973; 288:477.

76. Pizzo PA et al: The utility of protected-environment regimens for the compromised host: a critical assessment. Prog Hematol. 1977; 10:311.

77. Yates JW et al: A controlled study of isolation and endogenous microbial suppression in acute myelocytic leukemia patients. Cancer. 1973; 32:1490.

78. Bodey GP et al: Effect of prophylactic measures on the microbial flora of patients in protected environment units. Medicine. 1974; 53:209.

79. Gurwith MJ et al: A prospective controlled investigation of prophylactic trimethoprim/sulfamethoxazole in hospitalized granulocytopenic patients. Am J Med. 1979; 66:248.

80. Schimpff SC et al: Infection prevention in acute nonlymphocytic leukemia. Laminar air flow room reverse isolation with oral, nonabsorbable antibiotic prophylaxis. Ann Intern Med. 1975; 82:351.

81. Hahn DM et al: Infection in acute leukemia patients receiving oral nonabsorbable antibiotics. Antimicrob Agents Chemother. 1978; 13:958.

82. Shopsin B et al: Lithium and leukocytosis. Clin Pharmacol Ther. 1971; 12:923.

83. Lee M et al: Attenuation of chemotherapy-induced neutropenia with lithium carbonate. Am J Hosp Pharm. 1980; 37:1066.

84. Rothstein G et al: Effect of lithium on neutrophil mass and production. N Engl J Med. 1978; 298:178.

85. Friedenberg WR et al: The effect of lithium carbonate on lymphocyte, granulocyte, and platelet function. Cancer. 1980; 45:91.

86. Winston DJ et al: Prophylactic granulocyte transfusions during human bone marrow transplantation. Am J Med. 1980; 68:893.

87. Bodey GP et al: Protected environment-prophylactic antibiotic program for malignant lymphoma. Randomized trial during chemotherapy to induce remissions. Am J Med. 1979; 66:74.

88. Storring RA et al: Oral non-absorbed antibiotics prevent infection in acute non-lymphoblastic leukemia. Lancet. 1977; 2:837.

89. Reiter B et al: Use of oral antimicrobials during remission induction in adult patients with acute non-lymphoblastic leukemias (Abstract). Clin Res. 1973; 21:652.

90. Hughes WT et al: Successful chemoprophylaxis for *Pneumocystis carinii* pneumonitis. N Engl J Med. 1977; 297:1419.

91. Lyman G et al: The use of lithium carbonate to reduce infection and leukopenia during systemic chemotherapy. N Engl J Med. 1980; 302:257.

92. Clift RA et al: Granulocyte transfusions for the prevention of infection in patients receiving bone-marrow transplants. N Engl J Med. 1978; 298:1052.

93. Ryning FW et al: *Pneumocystis carinii, Toxoplasma gondii,* cytomegalovirus and the compromised host. West J Med. 1979; 130:18.

94. Hughes WT: Pneumocystis pneumonia: a plague of the immunocompromised. Johns Hop Med J. 1978; 143:184.

95. Hughes WT: Prophylaxis for pneumocystis pneumonia (letter). N Engl J Med. 1978; 298:853.

96. Harris RE et al: Prevention of pneumocystis pneumonia. Am J Dis Child. 1980; 134:35.

97. Hughes WT: *Pneumocystis carinii* pneumonia. N Engl J Med. 1977; 297:1381.

98. Hughes WT et al: Intensity of immunosuppressive therapy and the incidence of *Pneumocystis carinii* pneumonitis. Cancer. 1975; 36:2004.

99. Stagno S et al: *Pneumocystis carinii* pneumonitis in young immunocompetent infants. Pediatrics. 1980; 66:56.

100. Michaelis LL et al: Pneumocystis pneumonia: the importance of early open lung biopsy. Ann Surg. 1976; 183:301.

101. Lau WK et al: *Pneumocystis carinii* pneumonia. Diagnosis by examination of pulmonary secretions. JAMA. 1976; 236:2399.

102. Hughes WT: Current status of laboratory diagnosis of *Pneumocystis carinii* pneumonitis. CRC Crit Rev Clin Lab Sci. 1975; 6:145.

103. Hughes WT et al: Comparison of pentamidine isethionate and trimethoprim-sulfamethoxazole in the treatment of *Pneumocystis carinii* pneumonia. J Pediatr. 1978; 92:285.

104. Miser JS et al: Management of *P. carinii* pneumonitis (letter). N Engl J Med. 1977; 296:47.

105. Lau WK et al: Trimethoprim-sulfamethoxazole treatment of *Pneumocystis carinii* pneumonia in adults. N Engl J Med. 1976; 295:716.

106. Winston DJ et al: Trimethoprim-sulfamethoxazole for the treatment of *Pneumocystis carinii* pneumonia. Ann Intern Med. 1980; 92:762.

107. Wormser GP et al: Trimethoprim-sulfamethoxazole in the United States. Ann Intern Med. 1979; 91:420.

108. Wilber RB et al: Chemoprophylaxis for *Pneumocystis carinii* pneumonitis. Am J Dis Child. 1980; 134:643.

109. Walzer PD et al: *Pneumocystis carinii* pneumonia in the United States. Ann Intern Med. 1974; 80:83.

110. Hughes WT et al: Treatment of *Pneumocystis carinii* pneumonitis with trimethoprim-sulfamethoxazole. Can Med Assoc J. 1975; 112(suppl):47S.

111. Bourgault A et al: Trimethoprim with sulfamethoxazole for treatment of infection with *Pneumocystis carinii* in renal insufficiency. Chest. 1978; 74:91.

112. Waalkes TP et al: Pharmacology of pentamidine. NCI Monograph. 1976; 43:171.

113. Bradley PP et al: Neutropenia and thrombocytopenia in renal allograft recipients treated with trimethoprim-sulfamethoxazole. Ann Intern Med. 1980; 93:560.

114. Russo Jr J et al: A comparative review of two new wide spectrum penicillins: mezlocillin and piperacillin. Clinical Pharmacy (in press).

115. Issell BF et al: Mezlocillin for treatment of infections in cancer patients. Antimicrob Agents Chemother. 1980; 17:1008.

116. Wade JC et al: Potential of mezlocillin as empiric single agent therapy in febrile granulocytopenic cancer patients. Antimicrob Agents Chemother. 1980; 18:299.

117. Melikan V et al: Mezlocillin and gentamicin in the treatment of infections in seriously ill and immunosuppressed patients. J Antimicrob Chemother. 1981; 7:657.

Chapter 39

Opportunistic Fungal and Viral Infections

Catherine Angell Sohn

OPPORTUNISTIC FUNGAL INFECTIONS

Fungal infections are becoming more prevalent because the development of effective antibacterial and chemotherapeutic drugs has increased the survival of immunocompromised hosts (see Table 1) (1). Fungi pathogenic to man are classified into three groups according to the kinds of disease they cause. Primary pathogens cause potentially serious systemic (deep) mycotic infections in otherwise healthy persons; secondary pathogens are more likely to produce opportunistic mycoses in the immunocompromised host; and superficial mycoses are contagious and generally occur in the skin, hair, or nails (2). This chapter will discuss the first two types of fungal infections. The latter are discussed in the chapter on Skin Diseases.

Systemic fungal infections such as histoplasmosis and coccidioidomycosis may begin as primary pulmonary infection in an otherwise healthy person. Infection is acquired by inhalation of dust particles containing organisms from the soil in an endemic area. Although this usually results in asymptomatic pulmonary infection, rarely it will disseminate to the skin and cause granuloma and hypersensitivity reactions.

Patient Populations at Risk. Opportunistic fungal infections such as candidiasis, cryptococcosis, *Mucor* infections, and aspergillosis can be serious, life-threatening infections in the compromised host. Patients at high risk for these opportunistic mycoses include those with a defective or impaired cell-mediated immune system, such as patients with leukemia and lymphoma or those receiving radiation therapy. The use of long-term suppressive doses of corticosteroids (for asthma, rheumatoid arthritis, collagen vascular disease, or to renal transplant patients) also impedes the body's normal defense mechanisms against invasion of fungal pathogens. Broad spectrum antibiotics destroy or reduce the normal bacterial flora of the oral pharynx, gastrointestinal tract, and the skin, allowing fungi to multiply unchecked and invade the host. Diabetic ketoacidosis inhibits the mobilization or phagocytic function of neutrophilis, facilitating progressive invasion by mycotic organisms such as *Mucor* species. Intravenous catheters, transtracheal tubes, and hyperalimentation lines facilitate the entry of fungi into the body (3–6).

Diagnosis. The diagnosis of fungal infections requires a high index of suspicion toward patients with medical and social histories which place them at risk. Skin tests are not diagnostic and only indicate that the patient has had prior contact with the organism. Many of the serologic tests for antibody are available on a restricted basis and have limited usefulness. Therefore, diagnosis relies heavily on isolation of the organism from body fluids or tissues. Positive cultures of the sputum, wounds, and urine may indicate only colonization, and positive blood cultures may only reflect transient fungemia. However, isolation of fungi from otherwise sterile fluids or tissues such as the bone marrow, cerebral spinal fluid (CSF), or lung tissue indicates the presence of an infection requiring treatment with antifungal agents. When biopsy demonstrates deep tissue invasion by fungi,

Table 1.

SUMMARY OF RECORDED CASES AND PROJECTED HOSPITALIZATION RATES FOR SYSTEMIC MYCOSES, 1976

	Primary Diagnosis		Secondary Diagnosis	
	# Cases	Projected Rate (per 10^6)	# Cases	Projected Rate (per 10^6)
Histoplasmosis	639	8.35	1,244	5.51
Coccidioidomycosis	897	12.56	453	2.57
Aspergillosis	164	1.92	259	2.42
Cryptococcosis	87	1.40	60	1.09
Disseminated Candidiasis	15	0.20	136	1.24
Sporotrichosis	30	0.34	18	0.08
Blastomycosis	15	0.18	6	0.02
Actinomycosis	136	1.93	115	0.66

From: Fraser: Aspergillosis and systemic mycosis. JAMA. 1979; 12:1631.

serious fungal infection is confirmed by clinical symptoms of disease (2,7–10).

Early diagnosis of fungal infections and prompt antifungal therapy are important factors in determining patient prognosis. Aisner et al demonstrated that diagnosis of invasive aspergillosis within 72 hours of the appearance of pulmonary or sinus infiltrates and initiation of amphotericin B therapy within 96 hours was associated with a better response rate than when the diagnosis was delayed (two weeks or more) (7).

To aid in early diagnosis and treatment, some cancer centers have evaluated and now utilize surveillance culture data in high risk, immunocompromised, neutropenic patients. Attempts are made to isolate fungi from urine, stool, and respiratory specimens twice weekly. Organisms isolated in these renal transplant and cancer patients included *Candida* species and *Aspergillus*. Sanford found that positive surveillance cultures for *Candida tropicalis* correlated with the presence of systemic disease, but *Candida albicans* was such a common colonizing organism (67% of patients) that positive cultures did not correlate with systemic infection. No patient was colonized with *Aspergillus*. Negative surveillance cultures were associated with the absence of systemic disease for both *C. albicans* and *C. tropicalis*. They concluded that surveillance culture data in high risk, immunocompromised patients can aid in early diagnosis of systemic fungal infection and allow prompt initiation of antifungal therapy (8).

Candidiasis

Candida albicans, a yeast, is part of the normal body flora in many patients. It can cause superficial infections in otherwise normal patients (eg, vulvovaginal candidiasis), especially when there is local tissue damage. In immunocompromised patients, the toxic effects of chemotherapy to the skin and gastrointestinal tract, local irritation and fibrosis from radiation therapy, or skin maceration from wound dressings, allow the yeast to invade the surrounding tissue and the bloodstream (3,9).

Candida species can often be found in expectorated sputum or in the urine of a patient with a foley catheter in place. It is postulated that candidal species from the skin or environment colonize these sites and that their presence alone does not indicate systemic infection. Hospitalized patients may experience transient episodes of fungemia. In both of these situations, colonization and transient fungemia, the question is not which drug to use, but whether or not treatment is indicated (6).

Diagnosis. Current criteria for the diagnosis of serious candidal infection which warrants aggressive antifungal therapy include (3,7–10):

a. a single positive blood culture with evidence of peripheral dissemination of candidemia, such as endophthalmitis, osteomyelitis, arthritis, myocarditis, meningitis, or macronodular skin lesions with surrounding erythematous halos;

b. multiple positive blood cultures in a symptomatic high risk patient;

c. a single positive culture from a normally sterile body fluid such as the CSF or intraocular fluid;

d. serologic demonstration of rising precipitans titers or conversion of a negative value to a positive one in the appropriate clinical setting.

Titers are suggestive of disease because they indicate the body is reacting to a "foreign" substance. There are, however, patients with "positive" titers who do not have systemic disease. In these cases, a positive titer is only indicative of prior exposure to the fungal organism, not the presence of current infection. In contrast, patients with active disease often have "false negative" titers. This makes the use of these tests unreliable for the accurate diagnosis of systemic disease.

Agglutinating antibody studies lack specificity in that a severely immunocompromised patient may not be able to mount an antibody response even in the face of disseminated candidiasis. It has been estimated that a premortem diagnosis is established early enough for timely institution of appropriate therapy in only 15–40% of cases (3).

The most promising diagnostic tool may be the new investigational antigen assay that is reportedly able to differentiate between transient and serious fungemia (11).

Candida Septicemia. Candida septicemia develops most frequently in patients who have had:

a. foley or indwelling intravenous catheters inserted for prolonged periods of time,

b. have recently received a course of broad spectrum antibiotics, and

c. have leukemia or lymphoma.

Clinical manifestations of candidal septicemia may include fever and chills unresponsive to antibiotics, pulmonary infiltrates, endophthalmitis with decreased vision, and skin lesions (3). Because of the high risk of candidal infections, most long-term hyperalimentation patients should have routine biweekly ophthalmologic exams to look for early evidence of candidemia and endophthalmitis (6).

Candida Endocarditis. Candida endocarditis is occurring with increasing frequency in the following clinical situations: heroin addiction, postprosthetic heart valve replacement; following major surgery; broad-spectrum antibiotic use; in patients with prolonged indwelling intravenous catheters for nutritional, therapeutic, or diagnostic purposes; and in patients with concurrent or pre-existent bacterial endocarditis, following intratracheal intubation or urethral instrumentation in patients with valvular or cardiac structural abnormalities (12,13). Diagnosis should be suspected if the patient exhibits any of the clinical manifestations of candidemia and has any of the usual symptoms of endocarditis (see the chapter on Endocarditis). The diagnosis of fungal endocarditis should also be considered if an echocardiogram demonstrates large valvular vegetations or large emboli to major vessels or if endophthalmitis is present in a high risk patient with fever, chills, and cardiac murmur who has multiple positive blood cultures for Candida. However, fungal endocarditis may occur without concurrent fungemia and must be considered in these settings using clinical signs and symptoms, precipitans titers, and *Candida* antigen data.

1. *Disseminated Candidiasis.* L.G. is a 55-year-old woman who had abdominal surgery eight weeks ago following massive trauma suffered in an automobile accident and is currently receiving intravenous hyperalimentation. Two weeks ago, pyelonephritis and sepsis due to *E. coli* were treated with ampicillin and gentamicin for ten days. She now complains of recurrent fevers, chills, increasing shortness of breath, weakness, and blurred vision. Her past medical history was significant for hypertension controlled with hydrochlorothiazide 100 mg daily and asthma managed with theophylline 600 mg daily, terbutaline 7.5 mg daily, and prednisone 10 mg every other day.

The patient's temperature was 101°F, her blood pressure was 155/95 mm Hg with a pulse of 100/min, and she had a respiratory rate of 28/min. She is 5′7″ and weighs 41 kg.

Physical examination revealed a dyspneic, malnourished woman in respiratory distress. A small, white perimacular lesion was seen in the left eye. Cardiac examination confirmed the presence of a mitral valve flow murmur that had increased in intensity since her initial admission. She was noted to have 3+ pitting edema in the extremities, and her cervical veins were distended. Pulses were absent in the lower extremities. Multiple abdominal sutures were healing without drainage or signs of inflammation. The patient had a subclavian line in place and a foley catheter was draining normally.

Laboratory data obtained included a hemoglobin concentration of 8 gm/dl and a white blood count of 9,600/mm^3 with 30% neutrophils, 63% lymphocytes, 5% monocytes, and 2% eosinophils. The urea nitrogen was 20 mg/dl, the serum creatinine was 1.4 mg/dl, and electrolytes were within normal limits (Na: 140 mEq/L, K: 4.0 mEq/L, Cl: 99 mEq/L, HCO$_3$: 24 mEq/L). Chest x-ray revealed an enlarged left ventricle; no infiltrates were seen, and a subclavian line was in place. EKG also suggested left ventricular failure. The urinalysis was noncontributory; no bacterial or fungal growth were reported. Two blood cultures drawn on successive days grew *Candida albicans* as did cultures of the subclavian catheter tip. *Candida* precipitans were positive at a titer of 1:8 (normal: negative).

Visual acuity was measured to be 20/70 in the left eye and 20/30 in the right eye.

What signs, symptoms, and laboratory tests in this patient are consistent with the diagnosis of disseminated candidiasis and *Candida* endocarditis?

L.G. has symptoms of recurrent fevers, chills, increasing weakness and shortness of breath, and blurred vision. Candidemia manifests clinically with signs and symptoms like those seen in bacterial sepsis. In this case, her temperature of 101°F, an elevated white blood cell count with increased lymphocytes, positive blood cultures for yeast, and positive serology demonstrate candidemia. The presence of blurred vision and the left eye infiltrate indicate *Candida* endophthalmitis as a site of dissemination. Her chest x-ray, EKG, symptoms of dyspnea, weakness, peripheral edema, and a cardiac murmur, in the presence of blood cultures growing yeast, suggest *Candida* endocarditis.

2. What factors present in this patient predisposed her to disseminated candidiasis and *Candida* endocarditis?

Prolonged intravenous hyperalimentation following severe trauma and surgery is a major risk factor for disseminated candidiasis in this patient, because the subclavian catheter can provide an access site to her bloodstream. Malnutrition, massive trauma, and corticosteroid therapy compromised her ability to inactivate and eliminate *Candida* that invaded the bloodstream. Bacterial sepsis and the prior course of broad spectrum antibiotics which suppressed enteric bacteria and allowed yeast to proliferate are also factors associated with the development of disseminated candidiasis. Hematogenous *Candida* endophthalmitis following candidemia is now recognized as a risk of intravenous hyperalimentation; if untreated, it may lead to loss of vision (18).

Other risk factors, not seen in this patient, include prior cancer chemotherapy, radiation therapy, high doses of corticosteroids, and uncontrolled diabetes mellitus. When symptoms of sepsis occur in these patients, both bacterial and fungal cultures should be obtained.

In patients with prior valvular heart disease, structural abnormalities, or prosthesis, the risk of endocarditis is increased following candidemia (13). Because of her many risk factors and symptoms of cardiac failure, an echocardiogram was obtained which demonstrated mycotic vegetations on the mitral valve leaflets. She did not have other clinical evidence of endocarditis such as Roth spots, Janeway lesions, or splinter hemorrhages.

Positive precipitans titers in this patient are compatible with infection but cannot be relied upon solely because of the high incidence of false positive titers. Agglutinating antibodies and tests for antigenemia, which are more specific for infection, were not obtained.

3. *Treatment.* What agents are available for the treatment of disseminated candidiasis and candidal endocarditis?

Intravenous amphotericin B is the drug of choice for disseminated candidiasis (including endophthalmitis) and for candidal endocarditis (14–19).

In severely ill, immunocompromised hosts with disseminated candidiasis and for *Candida* meningitis and endocarditis, flucytosine may be added to amphotericin B if *in vitro* synergy can be demonstrated (21,22). It is not used as a single agent because almost 50% of *Candida* species are resistant (21). Rifampin has also been shown to provide *in vitro* synergy against *Candida albicans, Aspergillus,* and histoplasmosis (23,24).

The imidazole derivatives, intravenous miconazole and oral ketoconazole are the available alternatives to amphotericin B in a patient who fails to respond to amphotericin, refuses further amphotericin B because of severe side effects (anemia, hypokalemia, etc.), or has developed severe amphotericin B renal failure or dose-related renal tubular acidosis. Miconazole has been used successfully in many cases of candidemia, although relapses are a major limitation to wider use. Large scale, comparative clinical studies using ketoconazole in disseminated candidiasis have not yet been reported. (15,25,26) (See Table 2) (Also see Questions 15–16)

In addition to intravenous amphotericin B, nearly all patients with endocarditis require cardiac surgery to remove the mycotic vegetations from the affected valve or to have the valve replaced. The presence of heart failure and the suggestion of emboli as indicated by the absence of pulses in her legs are indications for surgical valve replacement. Antifungal chemotherapy alone is insufficient for the treatment of fungal endocarditis. Patients should be treated with amphotericin B prior to, during, and following surgery for a prolonged period to avoid relapses (26a). The vegetations formed on the heart valve are large and friable so that embolic episodes, as illustrated in this case, often occur. In addition, it has been demonstrated that there is very little penetration of amphotericin B into avascular fibrin clots (14).

Amphotericin B (AmB). Amphotericin B is a polyene antibiotic that is stabilized with desoxycholate and forms a colloidal suspension when added to water. It is the most effective and widely used antifungal agent and acts by binding to the sterol content of the fungal cell membrane (primarily ergosterol). This allows leakage of intracellular contents including potassium and magnesium. It also binds to the cholesterol in human cells to a lesser degree. This affinity for tissues may be the mechanism for some of the toxicities

Table 2.

DRUGS FOR SYSTEMIC FUNGAL INFECTIONS

Drugs	Available Dosage Form	Mechanism of Action	Indications	Doses	Major Side Effects	Comments
Amphotericin B (AmB) (15,27–46)	50 mg per vial for reconstitution for intravenous use or irrigation (Fungizone)	Binds sterol in fungal cell wall, disrupts membrane and causes leakage of cellular contents	Drug of choice for all systemic mycoses including Cryptococcosis Disseminated Candidiasis Histoplasmosis Aspergillosis Coccidioidomycosis	Intravenous:* For systemic infections, 0.3–1.0 mg/kg/day to total dose of 1 to 4 gm <u>Dosage Schedule for Amphotericin B</u> Intravenous: (34) Critically Ill Patients (Regimen A) Test dose (1 mg) — Day 1 0.25 mg/kg — Day 1 0.5 mg/kg — Day 2 0.75 mg/kg — Day 3 Increase dose or maintain, as tolerated by patient. Alternate Procedure (Regimen B) Test dose (1 mg) — Day 1 5 mg — Day 1 10 mg — Day 2 15 mg — Day 3 20 mg — Day 4 25 mg — Day 5 30 mg — Day 6 Increase dose by 5 mg increments or maintain, as tolerated by patient. Intrathecal: 1. Reconstitute 50 mg vial in 150 ml D_5W to give a concentration of 0.3 mg/ml. Intrathecal dose: 0.5 mg (16.6 ml) is combined with CSF disadvantage: arachnoiditis 2. 0.5 mg dose is prepared in hyperbaric $D_{10}W$ and administered intrathecally with the patient's head lowered (Trendelenburg's position) to facilitate penetration to cistern and ventricles. Bladder Irrigation: 1. 50 mg is diluted in 1000 ml and infused daily as a continuous bladder irrigation over 24 hours using a triple lumen catheter. 2. 15 mg is diluted in 100 ml and instilled daily into patient's bladder and allowed to remain until voiding. Intraperitoneal: 1–5 mg is diluted in the dialysate daily to treat post-operative or peritoneal dialysis associated Candida infection.	<u>Acute:</u> Fever Chills Nausea/vomiting Headache Thrombophlebitis <u>Chronic:</u> Anemia—suppression of erythropoietin (44) Hypokalemia/ hypomagnesemia Renal Tubular Acidosis—disruption of renal tubular cell membrane (45,46) Renal Failure—renal artery spasm leading to ischemia	Toxicities and patient tolerance may limit duration of therapy. *Daily dose and rate of infusion are governed by patient's tolerance to drug side effects, renal function and clinical status.
Miconazole (25,48–50)	10 ml ampules containing 10 mg/ml (100 mg/ 10 ml) for intravenous use (Monistat)	Dose dependent. At low concentrations purine transport is inhibited; at higher concentrations damages fungal cell wall and permeability is increased; at higher concentrations, damages endoplasmic reticulum	Coccidioidomycosis Cryptococcosis Candidiasis	Intravenous: 1800–3600 mg/day for 3 to >20 weeks 1200–2400 mg/day for 3 to >12 weeks 600–1800 mg/day for 1 to >20 weeks 200 mg every 8 hr. increased to 25–30 mg/kg/ day as tolerated by patient. Doses up to 4 gm/ day have been used. Dosages are usually divided into three infusions per day and infused over 30 to 60 minutes Intrathecal: 20 mg daily of undiluted solution in addition to full intravenous doses (47,49) Bladder Irrigation: 200 mg diluted and instilled daily in appropriate volume (25)	Thrombophlebitis— due to vehicle Anemia Thrombocytosis— (mechanism unknown)—platelet count may reach 1,000,000/mm³ Hyponatremia—may be due to SIADH secretion Hyperlipidemia—due to polyethoxylated castor oil vehicle	Relapses and persistence of positive cultures following therapy limit usefulness. Higher doses may improve "cure" rate.

Table 2. (continued)
DRUGS FOR SYSTEMIC FUNGAL INFECTIONS

Drugs	Available Dosage Form	Mechanism of Action	Indications	Doses	Major Side Effects	Comments
Flucytosine (5-Fluorocytosine) (22,51–53)	250 mg and 500 mg oral capsules (Ancobon)	After penetrating fungal cell wall converted to 5-fluorouracil which interferes with nucleic acid synthesis	In combination with AmB for cryptococcal meningitis, cutaneous and mucocutaneous candidiasis and candida UTI's	100–150 mg/kg/day in four divided doses. UTI can be treated with doses of 50–75 mg/kg/day.	GI: nausea, vomiting *Agranulocytosis/ Aplastic Anemia *Hepatotoxicity (*dose related)	Resistance precludes use as sole agent. Dosage must be reduced if CrCl less than 40 ml/min.
Ketoconazole (26,54,54a, 54b,54c)	200 mg oral tablets (Nizoral)	impairs synthesis of ergosterol (major component of fungal cell wall)	Candidiasis Chronic mucocutaneous candidiasis Oral thrush Candiduria Coccidioidomycosis Histoplasmosis Paracoccidioidomycosis	200 mg daily up to 400 mg daily if insufficient response	nausea, vomiting (decreased if taken with meals) abdominal pain less frequently: pruritus, headache, dizziness, constipation, diarrhea, transient rises in liver enzymes	Inadequate duration of treatment may lead to poor response and early recurrence of clinical symptoms. Minimum treatment for systemic mycoses is six months, chronic mucocutaneous candidiasis usually requires maintenance therapy. No adjustment necessary in renal failure Gastric acidity is required to solubilize the oral tablets; therefore, the manufacturer recommends antacids, anticholinergics and H_2 antagonists be administered 2 hours following ketoconazole administration.

associated with AmB and also accounts for its long half-life of 15 days (15,28–33).

4. *Administration of Amphotericin B.* A diagnosis of disseminated candidiasis with candidal endocarditis is made. The following orders are written: Amphotericin B 1 mg IV to be followed by 10 mg IV on day 1. Day 2: 20 mg. Day 3: 30 mg. What precautions must be observed in preparing and administering this drug?

The pharmacist should reconstitute a vial of AmB with 10 ml of sterile water for injection to give a final concentration of 5 mg/ml of colloidal suspension. To avoid precipitation, the water should contain no preservative or bacteriostatic agent. The reconsistituted suspension should be kept under refrigeration and used within one week. The test dose of 1 mg should be diluted in 150 ml of 5% dextrose in water (D5W) and infused slowly over 2 to 6 hours. AmB should never be added to saline-containing solutions, because the colloidal suspension would precipitate (33,34). Subsequent daily doses of AmB should be diluted in 500 ml of D5W and administered over 4 to 6 hours. It is not necessary to cover the solution or intravenous tubing to protect them from deterioration caused by light if the drug is used within 24 hours (34a). An in-line filter would disrupt the colloidal suspension and should not be used. AmB cannot be administered via the same line as the hyperalimentation because of electrolyte incompatibility.

Initially, AmB should be administered into alternating veins, as distal as possible, using scalp vein needles, to minimize the occurrence of phlebitis. Heparin, 100 to 1000 units, may be added to the AmB infusion to reduce the frequency of this reaction (15).

5. The patient became nauseated and developed chills during the administration of the 10 mg dose of AmB which was given over 2 hours. How should these symptoms be evaluated? What recommendations can be made to help prevent or decrease these symptoms?

Immediate reactions to AmB include nausea, fever, chills, and headache and occur in 20 to 90% of adult recipients (33). The fever and chills associated with the AmB infusion can be prevented by the prophylactic administration of 900 mg of aspirin or acetaminophen. This dose may be repeated in 3 hours and 25 or 50 mg of hydrocortisone can also be added to the AmB to decrease these symptoms. It was recently demonstrated that intravenous meperidine given during the administration of AmB may minimize the severity and duration of severe fever and chills unresponsive to premedication with analgesics, antihistamines, and hydrocortisone. The dose should be titrated for each patient; an average dose of 45 mg has been shown effective after 30 minutes in cancer patients receiving therapeutic doses of AmB (41).

Nausea and vomiting should be treated with standard doses of prochlorperazine (5–10 mg IM) or diphenhydramine (25–50 mg) when symptoms develop and prior to future infusions.

Slow infusion over 4 to 6 hours is often recommended to help decrease these acute symptoms. This may be especially appropriate when doses of 0.25 mg/kg/day are used to initiate therapy in critically ill patients (such as this patient). Gradual increase in the daily dose as in Regimen B of Table 2 is an attempt to make the patient less likely to develop severe hypersensitivity or adverse reactions. These may be dose-related reactions to the desoxycholate used to form a colloidal solution or to the colloidal suspension itself.

6. *Monitoring of Therapy.* The patient was taken to surgery and her mitral valve was replaced with a porcine prosthesis. Amphotericin B 24 mg daily (0.6 mg/kg/day) was continued. Flucytosine 1.0 gm four times daily was added when synergy was demonstrated. Hyperalimentation was discontinued. What parameters should be monitored to assess the efficacy of drug therapy?

The patient's fever, white blood cell count, and differential should return to normal. Clinical symptoms of fever, weakness, shortness of breath, and blurred vision should gradually resolve. Blood cultures should remain sterile. Symptoms of heart failure should disappear following cardiac surgery.

7. What is a therapeutic dose of amphotericin B for disseminated candidiasis? How long should treatment be continued? What are the endpoints of therapy?

There is no universal agreement on the daily or total dose of AmB. Recommendations have been arrived at empirically, and in the past a total dose of AmB has been used. Unfortunately, there are no good objective data on the appropriate length of therapy for *Candida* and most other fungal infection (with the exception of cryptococcal meningitis). Toxicities and patient tolerance often limit the duration of therapy. Generally accepted recommendations include daily doses of up to 1 mg/kg to a total dose of 1.5 to 2 grams given over 6 to 12 weeks (3,9,15).

8. The patient is responding clinically to valve replacement, and AmB therapy has been continued for four weeks at 24 mg per day. She now is reported to have the following laboratory abnormalities: hemoglobin 9.0 gm/dl; hematocrit: 28%; reticulocyte count: 0.3%; potassium: 2.5 mEq/L; bicarbonate: 23 mEq/L; blood urea nitrogen: 31 mg/dl; serum creatinine: 2.3 mg/dl; urine specific gravity: 1.007. Evaluate each of her problems and make recommendations for management.

This patient has developed anemia, hypokalemia, and renal damage, problems that are commonly seen with prolonged amphotericin B administration. The patient has a reduced hemoglobin, hematocrit, and reticulocyte count.

Anemia. (hemoglobin: 9.0 gm/dl, hematocrit: 28%, retic count: 0.3%). Normochromic, normocytic anemia occurs in more than 95% of patients treated with long-term, therapeutic doses of amphotericin B and may be due to inhibition of erythropoietin production. Amphotericin-induced renal damage may contribute to this condition, but the degree of anemia does not always correlate with the level of azotemia. The reticulocyte count remains inappropriately low in relation to the hematocrit. This is characteristic of amphotericin-induced anemia and may help to differentiate it from other causes of anemia (44).

The hematocrit has been observed to fall to a mean value of 26% by the fourth to sixth week of therapy and returns toward baseline following the completion of a course of AmB therapy. The anemia does not usually warrant discontinuation of amphotericin, but if the hematocrit drops much below 26% or if the patient develops severe symptoms of hypoxemia, blood transfusions may become necessary to allow the patient to complete a course of therapy (15).

Renal Damage. Renal damage is the most serious toxic effect of AmB. The nephrotoxicity may be secondary to a drug-induced renal vasoconstriction resulting in ischemia and a secondary decrease in glomerular filtration rate (GFR). The GFR initially falls to about 40% of baseline in nearly all patients, but then it stabilizes at 20 to 60% of baseline and remains at this level

throughout the course of therapy (15). Serum levels of AmB do not rise with impaired renal function because the drug is not renally excreted. However, if the serum creatinine rises to greater than 3 mg/dl and if the renal failure is felt to be due to the drug, amphotericin should be discontinued for 24 to 48 hours, if the patient's clinical condition allows, to prevent further damage. When the serum creatinine returns to ≤2 mg/dl, therapy can be reinstituted at 50 to 100% of the previous daily dosage and increased gradually according to the patient's tolerance. It should be noted that these guidelines have been developed empirically, based on past anecdotal experience that has been successful. A serum creatinine value of 3 mg/dl was chosen to indicate a significant decrease in renal function for a patient with an initial value in the normal range. The drug can be given to patients with renal impairment (serum creatinine greater than 3 mg/dl). Corresponding values to indicate a decline in renal function should be chosen at the onset of AmB treatment (15,29,30).

Attempts at reducing the nephrotoxicity from amphotericin B by using mannitol (25 mg) to increase renal blood flow and glomerular filtration rate have proved unsuccessful (42). Furthermore, mannitol itself has been shown to induce renal lesions. Alternate day administration has been recommended by some authorities, but reports on the benefits of this approach are conflicting. Adequate hydration and adjustment of the daily dose remain the most reliable means for avoiding or minimizing azotemia (14,46).

Hypokalemia. Excessive potassium loss occurs frequently and requires monitoring in all patients. Twenty-five percent of patients will require potassium supplementation to prevent cardiac and neurologic sequelae. Daily doses of up to 100 mEq may be required to maintain a normal potassium level (15,45). If vomiting or diarrhea are present, higher doses may be required.

Renal Tubular Acidosis. Hypokalemia may precede azotemia and a more serious, but less frequent, type of amphotericin-induced nephrotoxicity, renal tubular acidosis (RTA). This has been shown to be due to selective damage to the distal nephrons and may be associated with AmB binding to the cholesterol content of the cells. RTA is characterized by cylindruria, impaired acid secretion, and inability to concentrate the urine (45,46).

Hypocalcemia (due to calcium phosphate deposits in the renal parenchyma), *hypomagnesemia,* and rarely, *systemic acidosis* may develop as a result of amphotericin inhibition of bicarbonate reabsorption in the renal tubules. Patients given less than a two gram total dose may exhibit a partial or reversible RTA, while a total dose of greater than four grams has been associated with a more permanent and total RTA which may necessitate discontinuance of therapy. Prevention of dehydration and hypokalemia help reduce the nephrotoxic effects of this drug (45,46).

Since this patient's creatinine is 2.3 mg/dl, no change in dosage is necessary at this time. Potassium supplements, starting at 80 mEq per day should be administered. The clinician should continue to monitor the following laboratory values for evidence of further deterioration in renal function: serum creatinine, blood urea nitrogen, urine specific gravity, urinary casts and protein, serum potassium, magnesium, and calcium.

9. Sequential Use of Leukocyte Transfusions and Amphotericin B. A.M., a 19-year-old male who was severely neutropenic following his last course of chemotherapy for acute myelogenous leukemia, developed fevers, chills, hypotension, and gram-negative sepsis (*E. coli* isolated from urine and blood cultures). He remained febrile (102.5°F) and neutropenic (WBC: 400/mm³) for five days while receiving carbenicillin and tobramycin at which time daily leukocyte transfusions were begun. On day seven when *Candida* was reported growing in two out of two blood cultures, amphotericin B therapy was initiated. Following the third dose, the patient complained of shortness of breath, rapid breathing, and coughed up small amounts of blood. He required intubation and assisted ventilation because of progressive hypoxia. Chest x-ray revealed diffuse infiltrates.

Could this reaction be related to his antiinfective therapy? How could it have been prevented?

Investigators at the National Institutes of Health recently reported an increased risk for acute pulmonary deterioration when amphotericin B was administered following leukocyte transfusion (WBC therapy). To determine a cause and effect relationship, they retrospectively reviewed the occurrence of acute pulmonary symptoms (dyspnea, hypoxemia, and diffuse interstitial pulmonary infiltrates) in patients with bone marrow aplasia, prolonged neutropenia, and life-threatening sepsis and found the following incidence of pulmonary deterioration:

Amphotericin B following WBC therapy	64%
Amphotericin B alone	0%
WBC therapy alone	6%

The authors concluded that the sequential use of leukocyte transfusions and amphotericin B therapy is associated with an increased risk of acute pulmonary distress symptoms in profoundly neutropenic patients with fever of unknown cause. They recommended:

a. caution in the use of amphotericin in leukocyte recipients;

b. separating the infusion of amphotericin as far as possible from the time of a leukocyte transfusion; and

c. slow administration of amphotericin while the patient is closely monitored for respiratory depression (55).

10. Candida Esophagitis. J.B. is a 60-year-old white male who was admitted to the hospital with a chief complaint of dysphagia (he can't swallow any food) and a 14-pound weight loss over the past two weeks. He denies hematemesis, hemoptysis, melena, chills, or syncope.

His past medical history is significant for the fact that he was diagnosed as having squamous cell carcinoma of the lung 11 months prior to admission and underwent a right upper lobectomy followed by radiation therapy to the head and neck region for metastases to the temporal lobe. Three weeks prior to admission, the patient received a seven day course of ampicillin (500 mg qid) for an *E. coli* urinary tract infection.

On physical examination, the patient was noted to have a temperature of 99°F, a blood pressure of 120/90 mm Hg, a pulse of 88/min, and a respiratory rate of 18/min. Endoscopic examination revealed inflammation along the esophagus, two linear swallow ulcers near the gastro-esophageal junction, and whitish collections in the esophagus with friable tissue underneath. A KOH smear of this material revealed hyphae consistent with *Candida*.

A laboratory report indicated that the patient had a hematocrit of 40%, a hemoglobin concentration of 13.7 gm/dl, and white blood cell count of 10,900/mm³ with 64% neutrophils, 11% basophils, and 25% lymphocytes. The blood urea nitrogen was 11 mg/dl and the creatinine was 0.4 mg/dl.

A diagnosis of *Candida* esophagitis was made.

What factors predisposed this patient to the development of *Candida* esophagitis?

Malignancy and radiation therapy may have eroded the oral and esophageal mucosa, thereby facilitating invasion by *Candida*. Also, oral antibiotic therapy suppressed normal oral bacterial flora allowing for overgrowth of *Candida* species (56,57).

11. What therapies, if any, should be recommended for this patient?

Since this patient has severe disabling symptoms of dysphasia, odynophasia, and secondary weight loss, antifungal therapy should be instituted to alleviate symptoms and prevent fungal dissemination into the blood stream and systemic infection. J.B. does not yet have signs of fungemia (fever, chills, or hypotension), but blood cultures may still be obtained to rule out candidemia. (See Table 3.)

Oral nystatin is usually tried first because of its greatest safety and because it is designed to apply the drug locally to the affected mucosa (56). Low doses of intravenous amphotericin have been shown effective in the management of *Candida* esophagitis without the significant side effects associated with the full dose regimens used for systemic fungal infection (56,57). Ketoconazole, 200 mg daily, is now approved for oral thrush and has the advantage of being orally effective and well tolerated. Miconazole has also been reported to be of benefit in treating a patient with a two year history of esophageal candidiasis (58). However, because miconazole penetrates into sputum poorly and because this use is not widespread, this treatment cannot be recommended at this time.

If this patient does not respond to oral nystatin suspension in 24 to 48 hours or to oral ketoconazole 200 mg daily, low dose amphotericin should be initiated at a daily dose of 10 mg. Therapy should be continued 48 hours after the patient's symptoms resolve or cultures become negative. The goals of therapy are to alleviate symptoms so that the patient can eat and swallow and to prevent dissemination of fungi into the blood stream.

Cryptococcal Meningitis

12. R.M., a 49-year-old male, was admitted to the hospital with a one month history of headache (which has been unresponsive to aspirin), fevers, and increasing confusion and weakness over the past two months.

His past medical history is significant for a diagnosis of polyarteritis nodosa with rapidly progressive glomerular nephritis. This has been controlled with daily cyclophosphamide and prednisone for the last 18 months. He has adult onset diabetes mellitus which has been controlled on diet and a 19-year history of hypertension which has been

Table 3.

TREATMENT ALTERNATIVES FOR CANDIDA ESOPHAGITIS

Drug	Dosage Regimen
Nystatin Oral Suspension (56)	200,000 units (2.0 ml of 100,000 units/ml) every two hours
Nystatin Vaginal Tablets	Hold one tablet in mouth until dissolved. Repeat every 2–4 hours.
Amphotericin B (57)	1–15 mg IV daily until symptoms resolve (usually less than 14 days required)
Ketoconazole (54c)	200 mg orally per day for 1–2 weeks
Clotrimazole Troches* (59) (*Investigational use only)	10 mg or 50 mg dissolved orally five times daily

controlled on furosemide and clonidine. He also has congestive heart failure which is being treated with digoxin 0.125 mg daily. His weight is 80 kg.

He has an 80-pack-year history of smoking. Physical examination revealed a temperature of 100°F, a blood pressure of 135/90 mm Hg, a pulse of 80/min, and his respiratory rate was 17/min. His neck was supple, and he was well oriented to person, time, and place.

Laboratory data included sodium: 136 mEq/L, potassium: 5.4 mEq/L, chloride: 106 mEq/L, bicarbonate: 28 mEq/L. BUN was 65 mg/dl and serum creatinine was 3.7 mg/dl (creatinine clearance = 25 ml/min). His hemoglobin was normal; white blood cell count was 5000/mm³ with 85% neutrophils, 4% bands, and 9% lymphocytes.

Lumbar puncture revealed a CSF glucose of 36 mg/dl (normal: 50–85 mg/dl), protein: 60 mg/dl (normal: 10–45 mg/dl, and white blood cell count: 300/mm³ with 20% neutrophils and 80% lymphocytes (normal: 0–5 lymphocytes/mm³). India ink stain (looking for fungi and yeast forms) and Gram's stain of the CSF were negative. Cryptococcal antigen was positive at a titer of > 1:512 (normal: negative titers) and *Cryptococcus neoformans* was grown on culture.

No masses were detected on CAT scan and no bacteria or fungi were grown on blood cultures.

What clinical manifestations and laboratory evidence of cryptococcal meningitis does this patient demonstrate? What criteria establish the diagnosis of cryptococcal meningitis?

R.M. has complaints of weakness, increasing confusion, headache, and a history of fevers. Fungal meningitis characteristically develops gradually over several weeks to months, but may present with an acute course similar to bacterial meningitis. Other symptoms typical of cryptococcal meningitis not seen in this patient include motor weakness and focal neurologic findings. Even with widespread cryptococcosis, the usual routine laboratory tests (hematocrit, white blood count, erythrocyte sedimentation rate) may not reveal any abnormality as in this patient. Analysis of cerebral spinal fluid (CSF) will almost always reveal CNS involvement. Opening pressure is often elevated, the protein concentration is usually increased, glucose may be lowered, and there is generally a lymphocytosis of 40–400 WBC/mm³ with lymphocytes outnumbering neutrophils. India ink staining of the CSF may reveal the *Cryptococcus* in 50% of cases. Because of the few number of organisms, it is useful to analyze the CSF for cryptococcal antigen titers.

The diagnosis of cryptococcal meningitis can be made if the organism is detected by culture from the CSF or if CSF cryptococcal antigen titers are elevated in association with the above clinical symptoms. This patient has clinical symptoms of meningitis and the time course is compatible with a chronic infection. In addition, R.M. has a low grade fever (100°F) and an abnormal lumbar puncture. A cryptococcal antigen of < 1:512 and a positive CSF culture for the organism established the diagnosis in this symptomatic patient (20,60,61).

13. What treatment regimens should be recommended for this patient with cryptococcal meningitis? How will the patient's renal function influence the selection and dosing of antifungal agents?

This patient should receive a combination regimen of amphotericin B and flucytosine for six weeks. Bennett recently demonstrated that the combination regimen of low doses of amphotericin B (0.3 mg/kg/day) and 5-flucytosine (5FC) was at least as effective in curing or improving symptoms when compared to a higher dose of amphotericin B (0.6 mg/kg/day) alone for a longer duration of therapy (10 weeks) (See Table 4.) Overall, 68% (23/34 patients) were cured or improved with the combination and 47% (15/32 patients) with amphotericin B alone. In this small study, it appeared that low doses (0.3 mg/kg/day) of amphotericin B were relatively free of toxic effects to the kidney and bone marrow (20).

Because this patient has an elevated baseline serum creatinine, a new endpoint for a deterioration in renal function will have to be established, for example, a serum creatinine of 5 or 6 mg/dl. Poor renal function is not a contraindication to the use of amphotericin. Because it is not eliminated renally, serum levels of the drug do not accumulate. However, administration may have to be temporarily discontinued to prevent any further decline in renal function due to amphotericin damage. Flucytosine, however, is primarily excreted by glomerular filtration, and the

Table 4.

SUMMARY OF CRYPTOCOCCAL MENINGITIS STUDY [20]

	Amphotericin B	Amphotericin B plus Flucytosine
Regimen	0.4 mg/kg/day × 70 days	0.3 mg/kg/day × 6 wk
		150 mg/kg/day × 6 wk
Total Dose		
Amphotericin B	21–35 mg/kg	9.4–15.7 mg/kg
Flucytosine	0	3150–7820 mg/kg
*Cured (no. of patients)	7	13
†Improved	4	3
††Relapsed	5	1
Failed Full Course	6	2
Died during therapy	5	5
	27	24

*Cures: No evidence of active cryptococcosis, including lumbar puncture at 1 year

†Improved: Negative cultures for *Cryptococcus neoformans* at discharge—less than 1 year follow-up

††Relapsed: Discharged as improved, but readmitted with positive urine or CSF cultures.

dosage must be appropriately reduced to prevent accumulation and subsequent toxicity. Therefore, this patient should be treated with amphotericin B 24 mg IV per day and flucytosine 1 to 2 gm po twice daily. (See Table 5 for reduced dosage of 5FC.) (53)

14. How does flucytosine act as an antimycotic agent? What are the major side effects of flucytosine therapy?

Flucytosine (5FC), a purine analogue, is proposed to act via activation to the antimetabolite, 5-fluorouracil (5FU) (52). Within the yeast cell, an enzyme, cytosine deaminase, facilitates this conversion which stops further cellular replication. Since the enzyme is not present within human cells, the toxicity to human cells is low.

The major side effects, which are relatively minor as compared to amphotericin B, include: gastrointestinal (rare nausea, diarrhea), hematologic (bone marrow suppression), and hepatotoxicity (transient rises in SGOT with rare hepatocellular necrosis) (15,51,52). The latter two appear to be related to higher doses and serum levels. The presumed mechanism of toxicity is due to the accumulation of the antimetabolite 5FU. It is desirable to achieve peak concentrations greater than 30 mcg/ml and less than 100 mcg/ml two hours following an oral dose to insure efficacy and minimize toxicity (53). In the cryptococcal meningitis study, all seven cases of drug toxicity were ascribed to flucytosine and included

Table 5.

DOSING OF 5-FLUCYTOSINE IN RENAL FAILURE [53]

Creatinine Clearance (ml/min)	Dose (mg/kg)	Dosing Interval (hours)
greater than 40	25–50	6
20–40	25–50	12
10–20	25–50	24
less than 10	50	24–48
	Interval according to the serum concentration of the drug	
Hemodialysis	25–50	48–72

leukopenia, thrombocytopenia, diarrhea, and rash (20).

15. What alternate therapy to amphotericin B and flucytosine is available?

Miconazole. Eight weeks of intravenous miconazole, 400 mg every 8 hours, has also been reported to cure and resolve neurologic sequelae in a patient with cryptococcal meningitis and cerebral cryptococcoma who had relapsed after a previous course of amphotericin B (920 mg total dose) and 5FC. Neurosurgical drainage could not be performed in the patient because of the location of the cerebral mass (62). Miconazole therapy may prove to be effective in future large scale studies.

Ketoconazole. Ketoconazole, a new oral imidazole derivative, is a potent inhibitor of erogosterol synthesis in *Candida albicans* and a wide range of fungal pathogens (26,54). MIC's for most organisms are less than 1 mcg/ml and are easily achievable with the usual daily oral doses of 200–400 mg. Peak blood levels of 3–6 mcg/ml are reached 2 hours after an oral dose, and a serum half-life of 2 hours has been noted. Limited clinical studies in man have documented efficacy in resolving chronic mucocutaneous candidiasis, histoplasmosis, and coccidioidomycosis when 200 mg/day was administered for up to 180 days. Minor side effects observed to date include nausea and vomiting, which may be decreased when ketoconazole is taken with meals, abdominal pain and, less frequently, headache, dizziness and transient mild elevations in liver enzymes.

A more moderate and slower response to ketoconazole has been observed in coccidioidomycosis than in paracoccidioidomycosis and histoplasmosis (50% of patients cured or markedly improved in 42 weeks).

Because ketoconazole requires gastric acidity to solubilize the oral tablets, the manufacturer recommends that antacids, anticholinergics, or H_2 antagonists not be given until two hours after ketoconazole administration. In cases of achlorhydria, patients should be instructed to dissolve each tablet in 4 ml aqueous solution of 0.2N HCl; this mixture should be ingested through a plastic straw to avoid contact with the teeth and be followed by a glass of water.

Thus, ketoconazole appears to offer a broad spectrum of antimycotic activity, oral administration, and little toxicity that may allow prolonged therapy to prevent the relapses seen following intravenous antifungal therapy.

16. Why is miconazole not more widely used to treat systemic fungal infections?

Clinical studies with miconazole have been limited, and as yet, no large scale, comparative trials to amphotericin B have been published. Individual case reports and reports from small series of patients have claimed up to 60 to 80% efficacy in clearing candidal infections, although reports of zero to 100% response have also been published. The difficulty in evaluating these data is the diverse nature of the patients' underlying diseases and the extent of clinical infection at the time therapy with miconazole was instituted. Dif-

ferent criteria for diagnosis and "cure" were used by various investigators. In addition, many of the "failures" received relatively low doses (200–1600 mg/day) of the drug. It is possible that larger doses of 3 to 4 grams per day may be more effective in the treatment of serious fungal infections. However, it should be noted that the majority of these patients were severely ill and often amphotericin B failures when miconazole was begun. Therefore, the drug has been most widely evaluated in patients with a high chance for failure. Large numbers of lower risk patients with a good prognosis for cure, currently given other antifungal therapy, have not been included in miconazole evaluations to date.

The major limitations to the widespread or initial therapeutic use of miconazole are relapses following therapy or the persistence of positive fungal cultures despite weeks of therapy. This could be due to inadequate daily dosage or treatment duration, because miconazole requires intravenous administration, usually three times daily, to maintain adequate blood levels. Thus a patient must remain hospitalized for prolonged therapy. Often the patient begins to feel well and is anxious to go home, especially if weeks of amphotericin therapy preceded the use of miconazole (25).

17. If miconazole therapy must be used as an alternative to amphotericin B, what toxic and adverse effects should be monitored?

The manufacturer (Janssen Pharmaceutica) has collated overall figures on the incidence of side effects during treatment with systemic miconazole from various published and unpublished reports (25):

	USA Studies	non-USA Studies
Phlebitis	28%	6%
Pruritus	21%	2%
Nausea	18%	2%
Fever/Chills	11%	0.5%

Phlebitis, pruritus, nausea, and fevers and chills are the most common adverse reactions reported in U.S. studies. The higher incidence in this country may be due to the use of higher doses and the commercially available buffered product. Hyponatremia (average decrease: 11 mEq/L), anemia, and nausea/vomiting are more frequently reported in some series than in others. Occasionally, hyperlipidemia is reported and is presumed to be due to the vehicle, a polyethoxylated castor oil derivative which itself has been shown to produce this effect in animal studies. Thrombocytosis has been reported in a small number of patients, and therefore, the platelet count should be monitored during therapy. Kidney, liver, and bone marrow toxicity have not been reported with up to four months of therapy, which makes miconazole appear to be a safe alternative when patients become toxic from amphotericin B and/or flucytosine.

To prospectively evaluate the occurrence of adverse effects, the following parameters should be monitored in patients receiving intravenous miconazole for serious fungal infections: temperature, hematocrit, electrolytes, serum triglycerides and platelet count.

18. *Drug Interactions*. What potential drug interactions should be monitored in this patient receiving antifungal therapy? What recommendations can be made for monitoring other patients for drug interactions?

Amphotericin B and prednisone may induce *hypokalemia* which may enhance digitalis toxicity. Therefore, this patient should receive supplemental potassium to maintain his serum potassium greater than 3.5 mEq/L if the potassium level falls. This is less likely to occur due to his impaired renal function than in other patients with normal renal function. The patient should also be monitored for hypokalemia due to the additive effects of carbenicillin or ticarcillin should such therapy become necessary for future concurrent bacterial infections. The *nephrotoxicity* of amphotericin B may further reduce renal function in this patient with prior damage and could lead to the accumulation of 5FC and subsequent toxicity (15,45).

If miconazole must be used, additive *bone marrow suppression* with cyclophosphamide may occur. The red and white blood cell count with differential and platelet counts should be monitored and adjustments in therapy made should the patient become severely anemic, leukopenic, or thrombocytopenic (25).

Miconazole has been shown to increase the *anticoagulant effect* of warfarin. Therefore, if a patient is receiving both drugs, the prothrombin time must be monitored, and warfarin dosage must be adjusted both at the start and the end of micon-

azole therapy to avoid potential bleeding or clotting episodes.

Aspergillosis

19. *Invasive Aspergillus Pneumonia*. T.C., a 22-year-old female with acute lymphocytic leukemia (ALL) diagnosed 11 months prior to admission (PTA), presents with fever, cough, increasing weakness, and right-sided pleuritic chest pain after receiving multiple cycles of chemotherapeutic agents including Ara-C, vincristine, prednisone, daunomycin and l-asparaginase. The last course of l-asparaginase and prednisone was administered 12 days prior to admission.

Her temperature was 103°F, blood pressure was 110/70 mm Hg, pulse was 120/min, and respiratory rate was 20/min. Her weight was 50 kg.

Physical examination revealed substernal, post-cervical, and supraclavicular nodules on the right side. Crackles and decreased breath sounds were noted at the base of the right lung. A new, right midline infiltrate in the right, lower lobe was detected on chest x-ray.

Laboratory data included a hemoglobin of 8.6 gm/dl, a hematocrit of 24%, and a white blood cell count of 700/mm^3 with 46% neutrophils, 33% bands, 7% blasts, and 14% lymphocytes. Her platelet count was 79,000/mm^3. Electrolytes were within normal limits, and her serum creatinine was 0.7 mg/dl.

Gram's stain of her sputum revealed 3 to 4 WBC per high powered field, but no predominant organism was seen. Urinalysis was normal. Sputum stains for acid fast bacilli were negative. Blood and urine cultures were sent and treatment initiated with carbenicillin and gentamicin. The patient remained symptomatic for three days while receiving these antibiotics, hydration, and pulmonary toilet.

Bronchoscopy then revealed local tissue and blood vessel invasion with branching gram-negative filamentous elements. Cultures of this material grew *Aspergillus flavis*. Blood and urine cultures were negative.

What signs and symptoms in this patient are consistent with aspergillosis? What are the predisposing factors to this type of infection?

This patient presented with fever, increasing

weakness, and pulmonary symptoms of cough and right-sided pleuritic chest which were consistent with lobar pneumonia. Hemoptysis and other signs of necrotizing bronchitis or lobar pneumonia may also be present in other patients with this type of aspergillosis.

Aspergillosis may present in one of three forms. a) Bronchopulmonary aspergillosis is a hypersensitivity syndrome resembling asthma and is treated with steroids. b) Benign secondary infection may occur as *Aspergillus* colonization of a persistent chronic cavitary lesion (also called "fungus ball"); no treatment is warranted. c) The most serious form is invasive necrotizing bronchopneumonia in which *Aspergillus* invades blood vessels and local lung tissue, resulting in necrosis and, potentially, thromboemboli. This patient illustrates the latter type of aspergillosis which must be managed with antifungal therapy and surgery (1,10,63).

Invasive necrotizing pneumonia with *Aspergillus fumigans* or *flavis* occurs in patients with malignancy, especially those with leukemia who are receiving concurrent cytotoxic chemotherapy or corticosteroids (illustrated by this patient). Pulmonary edema and pulmonary fibrosis due to radiation therapy are also risk factors though not present in this case (4,5,10,63).

20. What treatment would be appropriate for this patient with invasive aspergillosis?

Amphotericin B should be administered in a dose of 0.5–0.8 mg/kg/day. Daily doses should be rapidly advanced to the full therapeutic range. This patient was initially given a 5 mg test dose over 4 hours. Subsequent daily doses were 10 mg, 20 mg, 40 mg. The early institution of therapy resulted in clinical resolution of her symptoms and negative follow-up sputum cultures. She received six weeks of amphotericin B and her next cycle of chemotherapy was given on schedule.

Predissemination Coccidioidomycosis

This infection is caused by the fungus *Coccidioides immitans* which is endemic to the soil of the arid southwestern United States and the central San Joaquin Valley of California. Infection results from inhalation of dust particles containing arthrospores which cause an inflammatory response in the bronchi and lungs. Mild primary infection, also known as "Valley Fever" may present with acute pulmonary symptoms resembling

pneumonia; cough, fever, and chest pain associated with arthralgias and skin rash resolve in 3 to 8 weeks. Fifty percent of the population in these endemic areas may have had a subclinical infection to which the body responded with a cell-mediated, localized granulomatous reaction that is responsible for life-long immunity under normal circumstances.

From the initial pulmonary lesion, the disease may disseminate to the skin, bone, meninges, lymph nodes, and visceral organs in certain high risk groups in whom the primary disease is more severe and dissemination is more frequent. These include infants, pregnant women in their third trimester, debilitated adults, patients receiving corticosteroids or immunosuppressive drugs, and certain dark-skinned groups including Filipinos, blacks, and Mexicans (64–66).

21. T.M., a 62-year-old Filipino male who has recently moved to central California, presents with chief complaints of dry cough, aching joints, fever with night sweats, and pleuritic chest pain which have increased over the last four weeks. His past medical history is significant for severe rheumatoid arthritis managed with ibuprofen 3200 mg/day, cyclophosphamide 70 mg/day, and prednisone 10 mg/day, and hypertension controlled with furosemide 120 mg/day and clonidine 0.6 mg/day.

His temperature was 101°F, blood pressure was 145/90 mm Hg with a pulse of 80/min, and respiratory rate was 26/min. Physical exam revealed paratracheal adenopathy, decreased breath sounds bilaterally, and severely deformed joints.

Pertinent laboratory data included a white blood cell count of 8,700/mm³ with 2% eosinophils, 65% neutrophils, 30% lymphocytes, and 3% monocytes; an erythrocyte sedimentation rate (ESR) of 70 mm/hours; and a serum creatinine of 1.9 mg/dl. Complement-fixing antibody (CFA) titer for *Coccidioides* was 1:64. There was no reaction to PPD skin testing for tuberculosis. Chest x-ray revealed a right middle lobe infiltrate with mediastinal and paratracheal adenopathy. Sputum culture grew *Coccidioides immitis*.

What signs and symptoms consistent with coccidioidomycosis are present in this patient?

This patient has symptoms of cough, pleuritic chest pain, fevers, night sweats, and arthralgias which are typical of severe primary coccidioidomycosis. His chest x-ray findings of infiltration with adenopathy are also consistent with the diagnosis. High positive CFA titers (1:32 or greater) and positive sputum cultures indicate severe primary disease.

22. What therapy, if any, should be recommended for this patient?

This patient's immunosuppressive drug therapy (cyclophosphamide and prednisone) in addition to his ethnic background place him at high risk for dissemination which has a high incidence of morbidity and mortality. He should receive amphotericin B therapy because of the development of respiratory symptoms, chest x-ray evidence of disease, and positive CFA titers and cultures for *Coccidioides immitans*. The total dose and duration of treatment remain largely empiric. Most clinicians recommend a total intravenous dose of one to four grams. Local instillation may improve tissue penetration and has been used for patients with a pulmonary cavity, osteomyelitis, or meningitis. After a total of one gram of amphotericin B has been administered, this patient should be reevaluated. If his symptoms and pulmonary infiltrate have resolved and the CFA has dropped, therapy may be discontinued.

Nocardiosis

Nocardia asteroides is classified as a bacteria-like fungi. Structurally it is a complex fungal-like organism, but it is susceptible to antibiotic therapy. It is an uncommon cause of infections that usually originate in the lungs and have a marked potential to spread to the brain. Infection may occur in adults who may have an underlying neoplasm or have been receiving immunosuppressive therapy and also in otherwise normal hosts (67).

23. *Pulmonary Nocardiosis*. J.P., a 42-year-old male, was admitted to the hospital with a five week history of fevers, cough, and shortness of breath. His symptoms did not resolve after a ten day course of oral ampicillin.

His past medical history is significant for alcoholic liver disease and chronic active hepatitis for which he is taking azathioprine

and prednisone. His temperature on admission was 101°F, blood pressure was 115/75 mm Hg, pulse was 100/min, and respiratory rate was 24/min. Physical findings included dullness to percussion in the right middle and lower lobe lung fields, hepatosplenomegaly, and a normal neurologic examination.

Arterial blood gases were reported as pH: 7.5, P_aO_2: 72 mm Hg, and P_aCO_2: 33 mm Hg on room air. Other laboratory findings included a normal white blood cell count and a serum creatinine of 1.3 mg/dl. Gram stain of the sputum revealed normal flora.

Chest x-ray revealed a necrotizing lesion with possible abscess and cavitation in the right middle and lower lobes with effusions. Gram's stain of this fluid revealed gram-positive filaments. *Nocardia asteroides* grew on culture.

What signs and symptoms in this case are consistent with pulmonary nocardial infection?

This patient has non-specific pulmonary symptoms of cough and shortness of breath with fevers. Physical examination and chest x-ray detected involvement of the right lung.

Nocardial infections may present as bronchopneumonia with empyema or abscess as was illustrated in this patient. Poorly encapsulated brain abscesses may also be found with metastatic infection.

The diagnosis is confirmed by culture and when gram-positive filaments and hyphae are seen in sputum, bronchial washings, pulmonary fluid, in tissue, or from material drained from a brain abscess.

24. What therapy should be recommended for nocardial infection?

Standard therapy of nocardial infections has been 6–9 grams per day of sulfadiazine to achieve serum sulfonamide levels of 10–15 mg/dl. Sulfadiazine penetrates well into the CSF, but it has the disadvantage of low urine solubility. The incidence of crystalluria can be reduced by high fluid intake and sodium bicarbonate alkalinization of the urine. Overall survival for patients given this therapy has been 55–75% for pulmonary infection and 13% survival for those with CNS involvement. Relapse is a major problem following initial resolution of symptoms.

25. What alternatives in therapy are available for the treatment of nocardiosis?

Trimethoprim-sulfamethoxazole has been used with success in a limited number of patients. A recent review of the literature revealed 18 cases who were treated with this drug. An overall mortality rate of 11% in this small number of patients compared favorably to sulfadiazine results (68–71). The dosages used ranged from 6 to 16 tablets (regular strength) per day. Because of the importance of adequate levels and the low level of toxicity, most authors recommend 2–4 regular strength tablets four times daily.

Other therapies that have been tried based solely on *in vitro* susceptibility data in isolated case reports include high doses of ampicillin, cycloserine, chloramphenicol, and minocycline (72).

26. How long should treatment be continued? What are endpoints of therapy?

The major limitation to the interpretation of data on the therapy for nocardial infection is that patients often relapse after discontinuing therapy. Because oral trimethoprim-sulfamethoxazole achieves therapeutic levels, the treatment regimen can be continued for several months. A minimum of 6 weeks is recommended, but most authors suggest that 6–12 months or more may be necessary to achieve cure without relapse or appearance of metastatic foci. Any abnormalities initially present on chest x-ray or brain scan must be resolved before discontinuing treatment.

VIRAL INFECTIONS

Viruses are unique in that they are intracellular parasites. Because peak replication and dissemination occur prior to the development of symptoms and because recovery usually occurs without treatment, development of antiviral therapy and design of clinical studies to evaluate therapeutic response have been limited (77–79).

The Herpes family of viruses is responsible for significant infection. *Herpes simplex* can cause cold sores in and around the mouth, genital ulcers, and, in rare cases, encephalitis. *Cytomegalovirus* (CMV) is pathogenic to neonates and to transplant patients and others receiving immunosuppressive therapy. When pathogenic, CMV can cause an illness similar to mononucleosis, as well as severe pneumonia or organ rejection reactions (73–76).

27. *Herpes Encephalitis.* C.B., a 12-year-old white female with acute lymphocytic leukemia, was admitted to the hospital with a chief complaint of fever, sore throat, malaise, nausea, vomiting, and increasing confusion over the last four days. She developed left-sided motor weakness and had two episodes of loss of consciousness.

Physical examination revealed a temperature of 39.8°C, a blood pressure of 120/70 mm Hg, a pulse of 115/min, and a respiratory rate of 24/min. Small vesicles were detected on her trunk and around her mouth.

Laboratory data on admission included a white blood cell count of $400/mm^3$ with only lymphocytes and monocytes seen, a sodium of 135 mEq/L, a potassium of 2.8 mEq/L, and a serum creatinine of 1.1 mg/dl.

Brain scan revealed a mass in the right temporal lobe. *Herpes simplex* was isolated from the biopsy material from this lesion.

What clinical features and criteria confirmed a diagnosis of herpes simplex encephalitis in this child? What treatment is available?

This child has fever, nausea, vomiting, confusion and increasing lethargy with left-sided focal neurologic findings. In general, patients may present acutely with febrile encephalopathy, disordered mentation, focal neurologic symptoms, paresis, seizures, and coma. Lesions are most frequent in the temporal lobe and are localized by EEG, arteriogram, or brain scan. Definitive diagnosis requires isolation of the herpes virus from a brain biopsy specimen.

The need for a brain biopsy for diagnosis of *Herpes simplex* encephalitis has been challenged since the availability of effective treatment with vidarabine. It has been argued that the drug should be instituted when clinical evidence suggests the diagnosis. In a follow-up study, the Collaborative Antiviral Study Group found that only 57% of patients who underwent brain biopsy for clinically suspected disease were found to have *Herpes simplex* encephalitis on biopsy (75). The procedure is necessary to rule out other causes of acute encephalopathy such as vasculitis, brain abscess, or tumor which respond to *alternative* therapies. Because the brain biopsy missed only 5.4% of the cases who did have herpes encephalitis, a negative biopsy will avoid the use of vidarabine and the high volume of fluid necessary for administration in patients who have cerebral edema.

28. How has vidarabine compared to placebo in the treatment of *Herpes simplex* encephalitis? What factors correlate with best prognosis?

Vidarabine, 15 mg/kg/day IV for 10 days was compared to placebo in a national collaborative study of patients who had the clinical symptoms listed above and who had undergone brain biopsy (74). Overall, the mortality rate in biopsy-proven cases was 28% in the drug-treated group versus 70% in the placebo group. However, it is most important to consider neurologic sequelae in patients who survived. These included personality changes, dysphagia, incontinence, hemiparesis, and seizures. Prognosis for least morbidity and mortality was clearly related to age and to the level of consciousness when treatment was begun, not to duration of symptoms or the presence of paresis and seizures. In patients presenting initially with only lethargy, less than 20% suffered severe neurologic sequelae or death. In contrast, 100% of patients who were comatose at the time therapy was initiated either died or suffered severe sequelae which required institutionalization for care.

29. What are the side effects and limitations of vidarabine therapy?

Vidarabine is a poorly soluble inhibitor of viral DNA synthesis. Because of this, the drug must be diluted to 0.7 mg/ml or less and administered by intravenous infusion over 12 hours. This fluid load (3–5 liters/day) may be undesirable in patients with edema, congestive heart failure, and hypertension.

Adverse reactions to vidarabine include nausea/vomiting, diarrhea, skin rashes, and hallucinations. The major limiting toxic reaction is bone marrow suppression which appears to be dose related. It is rarely reported at 10–15 mg/kg/day and is much more frequent at higher doses and in patients who are already immunocompromised (74–81,83).

30. For what other diseases is vidarabine therapy effective?

A national collaborative study investigated the use of vidarabine for *Herpes zoster,* or shingles, in the immunocompromised host. In these patients with lymphomas, leukemia, and solid tumors, five days of vidarabine 10 mg/kg/day was compared in a crossover design study to placebo. Because of this, each patient was given active drug at some time. However, given this limitation which excluded the potential to evaluate postherpetic neuralgias, vidarabine given in the first five days was associated with faster resolution of acute pain, faster viral clearance of vesicles, more rapid cessation of new vesicle formation, and quicker time to total healing. Factors that did not correlate with vidarabine therapy were resolution of erythema and temperature (80).

Vidarabine was found to be of greatest benefit in the leukemia and lymphoma cancer patients who were at higher risk for dissemination and had a slower natural healing rate (as compared to patients with solid tumor). Younger (less than 35 years), immunosuppressed patients have a more prolonged natural course of herpes zoster infection but responded better to treatment. Vidarabine therapy was not useful in accelerating healing if started more than six days after onset of disease because pustulation had usually begun. At the doses used, 10 mg/kg/day, vidarabine had minimal adverse effects on the bone marrow, kidney, or liver. Antiviral therapy is not recommended for the non-immunocompromised host with *Herpes zoster.*

31. What alternative antiviral agents are available?

Acyclovir, a DNA analog which inhibits replication of the herpes viruses, has greater selectivity for viral replication than vidarabine (79). This is because the drug, also known as acycloguanosine, is activated within the viral cell by viral thymidine kinase. It has the advantage of greater solubility (can be administered intravenously over one hour every eight hours), and minimal toxicity has been reported to date. Limited reports have attested to efficacy in encephalitis, pneumonia, and cutaneous infections (84–89).

References

1. Fraser DW et al: Aspergillosis and other systemic mycoses: The growing problem. JAMA. 1979; 242:1631.
2. Johnson JE: Mycotic infections: Guidelines for differential diagnosis. Drug Therapy. 1978; 8:33.
3. Edwards JE et al: Severe candidal infections: Clinical perspective, immune defense mechanisms, and current concepts of therapy. Ann Intern Med. 1978; 89:91.
4. Williams DM et al: Pulmonary infection in the compromised host. State of the art. AM Rev Respir Dis. 1976; 114:359 and 1976; 114:593.
5. Krick JA et al: Opportunistic invasive fungal infections in patients with leukemia and lymphoma. Clin Haematol. 1976; 5:549.
6. Klein JJ et al: Hospital-acquired fungemia. Am J Med. 1979; 67:51.
7. Aisner J et al: Treatment of invasive aspergillosis: Relation of early diagnosis and treatment to response. Ann Intern Med. 1977; 86:539.
8. Sanford GR et al: The value of fungal surveillance cultures as predictors of systemic fungal infections. J Infect Dis. 1980; 142:503.
9. Edwards JE: Candida species. In *Principles and Practice of Infectious Diseases*, 1st ed, edited by GL Mandell, RG Douglas, JE Bennett, John Wiley and Sons, Inc., New York, 1979, p 1981.
10. Edwards JE: Asperigillus species. Ibid. p 2002.
11. Weiner MN et al: Mannan antigenemia in the diagnosis of invasive Candida infections. J Clin Invest. 1976; 58:1045.
12. Rubinstein E et al: Fungal endocarditis. Medicine. 1975; 54:331.
13. Seelig MS et al: Fungal endocarditis: Patients at risk and their treatment. Postgrad Med J. 1979; 55:632.
14. Rubinstein E et al: Tissue penetration of amphotericin B in candida endocarditis. Chest. 1974; 66:376.
15. Medoff G et al: Strategies in the treatment of systemic fungal infections. N Engl J Med. 1980; 302:145.
16. Bennett JE: Chemotherapy of systemic mycosis. N Engl J Med. 1974; 290:30, and 1974; 290:320.
17. Medoff G et al: Selecting the appropriate antifungal agent. Drug Therapy. 1978; 8:55.
18. Fishman LS et al: Hematogenous candida endophthalmitis—a complication of candidemia. N Engl J Med. 1972; 286:675.
19. Montgomerie JZ et al: Association of infection due to candida albicans with intravenous hyperalimentation. J Infect Dis. 1978; 137:197.
20. Bennett JE et al: A comparison of amphotericin B alone with flucytosine in the treatment of cryptococcal meningitis. N Engl J Med. 1979; 301:126.
21. Montgomerie JZ et al: Synergism of amphotericin B and 5-fluorocytosine for candida species. J Infect Dis. 1979; 123:82.
22. Fass RJ et al: Flucytosine in the treatment of cryptococcal and candida mycoses. Ann Intern Med. 1971; 74:535.
23. Beggs WH et al: Synergistic action of amphotericin B and rifampin against candida species. J Infect Dis. 1976; 133:206.

24. Kwan CN et al: Potentiation of the antifungal effects of antibiotics by amphotericin B. Antimicrobial Ag Chemother. 1972; 2:61.
25. Hell RC et al: Miconazole: a preliminary review of its therapeutic efficacy in systemic fungal infections. Drugs. 1980; 19:7.
26. Borelli D et al: Ketoconazole, an oral antifungal: Laboratory and clinical assessment of imidazole drugs. Postgrad Med J. 1979; 55:657.
26a. Galgiani JN et al: Fungal endocarditis: Need for guidelines in evaluating therapy. J Thor Cardiovasc Surg. 1977; 73:293.
27. Sande MA et al: Miscellaneous antibacterial agents; antifungal and antiviral agents. In *The Pharmacological Basis of Therapeutics*, 6th ed, edited by AG Gilman, LS Goodman, MacMillan, New York, 1980, p 1233.
28. Sarosi GA et al: Treatment of fungal diseases. Am Rev Respir Dis. 1979; 120:1393.
29. Craven PC et al: Excretion pathways of amphotericin B. J Infect Dis. 1979; 140:329.
30. Atkinson AJ et al: Amphotericin B pharmacokinetics in humans. Antimicrob Ag Chemother. 1978; 13:271.
31. Polak A: Pharmacokinetics of amphotericin B and flucytosine. Postgrad Med J. 1979; 55:667.
32. Goodman JS et al: Amphotericin B—specifics of administration. Modern Treatment. 1970; 7:581.
33. Meade KH: Clinical pharmacology and therapeutic use of antimycotic drugs. Am J Hosp Pharm. 1979; 36:1326.
34. Conte JE et al: Antibiotics. In *Manual of Antibiotics and Infectious Diseases*, 4th edition, edited by JE Conti and SL Barriere, Lea and Febiger, Philadelphia, 1981, p 1.
34a. Shadomy S et al: Light sensitivity of prepared solutions of amphotericin B. Am Rev Resp Dis. 1973; 107:33.
35. Alazraki NP et al: Use of hyperbaric solution for administration of intrathecal amphotericin B. N Engl J Med. 1974; 290:641.
36. Wise GJ et al: Candidal cystitis. Management by continuous bladder irrigation with amphotericin B. JAMA. 1973; 224:1636.
37. Goldman HJ et al: Monilial cystitis—effective treatment with instillations of amphotericin B. JAMA. 1969; 174:97.
38. Janosko EO et al: Evaluation and treatment of urinary candidiasis. Southern Med J. 1979; 72:1578.
39. Bortolussi RA et al: Treatment of candida peritonitis by peritoneal lavage with amphotericin B. J Pediatr. 1975; 87:987.
40. Anon: Amphotericin B toxicity. Clinical Staff Conference. Am J Med. 1964; 61:334.
41. Burks LC et al: Meperidine for the treatment of shaking chills and fever. Arch Intern Med. 1980; 140:483.
42. Bullock WE et al: Can mannitol reduce amphotericin B nephrotoxicity? Antimicrob Ag Chemother. 1976; 10:555.
43. Brandiss MW et al: Anemia induced by amphotericin B. JAMA. 1964; 189:663.
44. MacGregor RR et al: Erythropoietin concentration in amphotericin B-induced anemia. Antimicrob Ag Chemother. 1978; 14:270.

45. Douglas JB et al: Nephrotoxic effects of amphotericin B, including renal tubular acidosis. Am J Med. 1969; 46:154.

46. McCurdy DI et al: Renal tubular acidosis due to amphotericin B. N Engl J Med. 1968; 278:124.

47. Sung JP et al: Intravenous and intrathecal miconazole therapy for systemic mycoses. West J Med. 1977; 126:5.

48. Stevens DA: Miconazole in the treatment of systemic fungal disease. Am Rev Respir Dis. 1977; 116:801.

49. Deresinski SC et al: Treatment of fungal meningitis with miconazole. Arch Intern Med. 1977; 137:1180.

50. Brincker H: Prophylactic treatment with miconazole in patients highly predisposed to fungal infections. Acta Med Scan. 1978; 204:123.

51. Bennett JE: Flucytosine. Ann Intern Med. 1977; 86:379.

52. Block ER: Pharmacologic studies of 5-fluorocytosine. Antimicrob Ag Chemother. 1972; 1:476.

53. Schonebeck J et al: Pharmacokinetic studies of oral antimycotic agent 5-fluorocytosine in individuals with normal and impaired kidney function. Chemother. 1973; 18:321.

54. Van Den Bossche H et al: In vitro and in vivo effects of the antimycotic drug ketoconazole on sterol syntheses. Antimicrob Ag Chemother. 1980; 17:922.

54a. Package insert: Nizoral. Janssen Pharmaceutica—June 1981.

54b. Graybill JR et al: Ketoconazole: A major innovation for treatment of fungal diseases. (editorial) Ann Intern Med. 1980; 93:921.

54c. Symoens J et al: An evaluation of two years' clinical experience with ketoconazole. Reviews Infect Dis. 1980; 2:674.

55. Wright DG et al: Lethal pulmonary reactions associated with the combined use of amphotericin B and leukocyte transfusions. N Engl J Med. 1981; 304:1185.

56. Kodsi BE et al: Candida esophagitis. Gastroenterology. 1976; 71:715.

57. Medoff G et al: A new therapeutic approach to candida infections. Arch Intern Med. 1972; 120:241.

58. Rutgeerts L et al: Intravenous miconazole in the treatment of chronic esophageal candidiasis. Gastroenterology. 1977; 72:316.

59. Yap BS et al: Oropharyngeal candidiasis treated with a troche form of clotrimazole. Arch Intern Med. 1979; 139:656.

60. Diamond RD: Cryptococcus neoformans. In Principles and Practice of Infectious Diseases. 1st ed, edited by GL Mandell, RG Douglas, JE Bennett, John Wiley & Sons, Inc., New York, 1979, p 2023.

61. Bennett JE: Cryptococcosis. In Textbook of Medicine, 15th ed, edited by PB Beeson, W McDermott, JB Wyngaarden, Saunders, Philadelphia, 1979, p 543.

62. Weinstein L et al: Successful treatment of cerebral cryptococcoma and meningitis with miconazole. Ann Intern Med. 1980; 93:569.

63. Pennington JE: Aspergillus pneumonia in hematologic malignancy. Arch Intern Med. 1977; 137:769.

64. Drutz D et al: State of the art: coccidioidomycosis. Am Rev Resp Dis. 1978; 117:559 and 117:727.

65. Goldstein E: Miliary and disseminated coccidioidomycosis. Ann Intern Med. 1978; 89:365.

66. Einstein HE: Coccidioidomycosis. Basics of RD. Am Thoracic Society. 1980; 9:1.

67. Frazier AR: Nocardiosis. Mayo Clin Proc. 1975; 50:657.

68. Rosett W et al: Recent experience with nocardial infections. Am J Med Sci. 1979; 276:279.

69. Cook FV et al: Treatment of nocardia asteroides infection with trimethoprim sulfamethoxazole. Southern Med J. 1978; 71:512.

70. Maderazo EG et al: Treatment of nocardial infection with trimethoprim and sulfamethoxazole. Am J Med. 1974; 57:671.

71. Bennett JE: Factors influencing susceptibility of nocardia species to trimethoprim-sulfamethoxazole. Antimicrob Ag Chemother. 1978; 13:624.

72. Wren MV: Apparent cure of intracranial nocardia with minocycline. Arch Intern Med. 1979; 139:241.

73. Hirsch MS: Herpes simplex virus. In Principles and Practice of Infectious Diseases, 1st ed, edited by GL Mandell, RG Douglas, JE Bennett, John Wiley Sons, Inc., New York, 1979, p 1283.

74. Whitley RJ et al: Adenine arabinoside therapy of biopsy-proved herpes simplex encephalitis. N Engl J Med. 1977; 297:289.

75. Whitley RJ et al: Vidarabine therapy and diagnostic problems. N Engl J Med. 1981; 304:313.

76. Alford CA et al: Treatment of infection due to herpes virus in humans: a critical review of the state of the art. J Infect Dis. 1976; 133:A101.

77. Whitley RJ et al: Developmental aspects of selected antiviral chemotherapeutic agents. Ann Rev Microbiol. 1978; 32:285.

78. Hermans PE: Antiviral agents. Mayo Clin Proc. 1977; 5:683.

79. Koch-Weser J: Antiviral agents. N Engl J Med. 1980; 302:903.

80. Whitley RJ et al: Adenine arabinoside therapy of herpes zoster in the immunosuppressed; NIAID Collaborative Antiviral Study. N Engl J Med. 1976; 294:1193.

81. Lauter CB et al: Microbiologic assays and neurological toxicity during the use of adenine arabinoside in humans. J Infect Dis. 1976; 134:75.

82. Chang TW: A caution on treatment of encephalitis and vidarabine. N Engl J Med. 1979; 300:796.

83. Vidarabine for herpes simplex encephalitis. Medical Letter, 1979; 21:17.

84. Collins P et al: The activity in vitro against herpes virus of 9-(2-hydroxyethoxymethyl) guanine (acycloguanosine), a new antiviral agent. J Antimicrob Chemother. 1979; 5:431.

85. Kaufman HE et al: Effect of 9-(2-hydroxyethoxymethyl) guanine on herpes virus-induced keratitis and iritis in rabbits. Antimicrob Ag Chemother. 1978; 14:842.

86. O'Meara A et al: Acyclovir for treatment of mucocutaneous herpes infection in a child with leukemia (letter). Lancet. 1979; 2:1196.

87. deMiranda P et al: Acyclovir kinetics after intravenous infusion. Clin Pharmacol Ther. 1979; 26:718.

88. Jones BR et al: Efficacy of acycloguanosine (Wellcome 248U) against herpes simplex corneal ulcers. Lancet. 1979; 1:243.

89. Goldman JM et al: Acycloguanosine for viral pneumonia (letter). Lancet. 1979; 1:820.

Chapter 40

Parasitic Infections

Kent E. Lieginger

MALARIA

Most cases of malaria reported in the United States are found in travelers recently exposed to mosquitos in endemic areas. Additionally, transmission may occur in drug addicts sharing needles and syringes or by blood transfusions. Rarely, infection is caused congenitally or by mosquito transmission from imported cases. Delays often occur in the recognition and treatment of malaria because American physicians fail to consider this in their differential diagnosis. The delay in initiation of therapy is responsible for the difference in mortality rates recorded in American civilian hospitals versus military hospitals. The mortality in civilian hospitals is 8.5% versus 0.7% in military hospitals (1). Physicians also neglect to advise travelers of the need to receive chemoprophylaxis for malaria when traveling to endemic areas (1,2).

Life Cycle. The plasmodia which cause malaria *(P. vivax, P. ovale, P. malariae, P. falciparum)* go through a number of morphological changes with multiplication of the organisms in man and in insect vectors. Man is infected by the saliva of a female anopheline mosquito that contains the infective sporozoite forms. The sporozoites enter the liver cells where they multiply. After approximately seven to ten days, multiple small forms break out of the liver cells into the blood and subsequently enter red blood cells. The dormancy of the infection in the liver cells explains relapses in malaria caused by *Plasmodium vivax* and *Plasmodium ovale.* While in the red blood cells the organisms produce multiple infective merozoites. Upon bursting of the erythrocyte, this form can enter new red blood cells. The duration of this cycle is approximately two days for *P. vivax, P. ovale,* and *P. falciparum* and three days for *P. malariae.* This phase of the cycle presents clinically as episodic febrile attacks. Some of these merozoites become sexual forms or gametocytes which when consumed by mosquitos complete the life cycle (3,4,6).

In malaria caused by transfusion, or the sharing of needles and syringes by drug addicts, red blood cells containing the parasites directly enter the blood stream. Since there is no hepatic stage, relapses do not occur (3–5).

Epidemiology. Infections caused by malaria species normally occur between 45 degrees north and 40 degrees south latitude. Infections caused by *P. vivax* are more widely distributed than other types. *P. malariae* is found in temperate areas and also in the sub-tropics; it is comparatively rare. *P. falciparum* is found in all tropical areas. *P. ovale* is uncommon; most cases are found in Africa.

Malaria remains endemic in many countries including Africa, Central America, the Caribbean Islands (only Haiti and the Dominican Republic), South America (except Chile and Uruguay), Europe (including Turkey and the Soviet Union), Asia (west of the Indian sub-continent, except Cyprus, Israel, and Lebanon), Indian sub-continent, Eastern Asia and Oceania (except Australia, Hong Kong, Japan, Macao, New Zealand). Within these countries, large cities and high altitude areas are often malaria free. Also, at cer-

tain times of the year malaria is not transmitted (3,4).

Drug Resistance. Malaria produced by chloroquine-resistant *P. falciparum* was reported in Columbia in 1961. Since then, many countries have reported chloroquine resistance. These areas include the western hemisphere (Brazil, Columbia, Panama, Surinam, and Venezuela), and Asia (Burma, Cambodia, India, Indonesia, Laos, Malaysia, Nepal, Philippines, Singapore, Thailand and Vietnam) (3,4). There have been a small number of cases of resistance to chloroquine reported in Africa (Kenya and Tanzania); however, the prevalence of these strains in these two areas is not known (11,12).

1. *Acute Malaria.* B.L. is a 28-year-old woman with a chief complaint of sporadic chills and fever of four days duration. Two months prior to admission she returned from a trip to Haiti where she spent a great deal of time in the countryside observing the lives of the inhabitants. Four days prior to admission, she experienced an episode of fever and shaking chills. Three days prior to admission, she had a normal temperature in the morning but developed a fever of 102°F and shaking chills in the afternoon which subsided again by that evening. This pattern repeated itself the day before admission. Two days prior to admission, she was diagnosed as having influenza and was told to drink plenty of fluids and to get some rest. On the day of admission, the patient's temperature rose to 105°F and she experienced a shaking chill. Physical examination revealed a well-developed woman who was acutely ill; heart and lung examination were normal. Abdominal examination was within normal limits except for a slightly enlarged spleen. The blood pressure was 136/85 mm Hg, the pulse 120/min, respiratory rate 20/min, and the temperature 103.4°F. Pertinent laboratory findings included: hemoglobin 14 gm/dl; erythrocyte sedimentation rate 15 mm/hr; white blood cell count 6,650 with 80% neutrophils, 19% lymphocytes, and 1% monocytes; platelets 60,000; and bilirubin 1.2 mg/dl. Urinalysis revealed a specific gravity of 1.015 and 1–2 white blood cells per high power field. There was no glucose or albumin present in

the urine. **Thick and thin blood smear show** *Plasmodium vivax* **trophozoites. What subjective and objective information in the above case are consistent with malaria?**

The patient has explained to her physician the pattern of recurrent fever and chills. She also has a history of travel to a malarious area. Even though she returned from her trip two months ago, this would not exclude malaria as a possible diagnosis; however, it would aid in the diagnosis of the species of the infecting plasmodium. In one study, the time after return to the United States that travelers became ill was shortest for *P. falciparum* (6). Eighty-two percent of those infected with *P. falciparum* were diagnosed within one month after arrival; only 35% of *P. vivax* infections occurred in the first month. One percent of the patients infected with *P. falciparum* developed illness after six months from the time of their return to this country. In contrast, patients who were infected with the other three species of plasmodia (17 to 28% of those studied) became ill six months or more after their return (6).

The patient's elevated temperature, low hemoglobin, slightly elevated bilirubin, and the thick and thin smear showing *P. vivax* trophozoites lead to the diagnosis of *Plasmodium vivax* malaria. Sometimes this is referred to as benign tertian malaria.

2. *Treatment*. What drug treatment should this patient receive? Discuss the regimens for other infective species of plasmodia.

Selection of the proper drug for the treatment of malaria is dependent upon the infecting species, mode of transmission, and where the infection was acquired. If the infection is caused by *P. vivax, P. ovale, P. malariae,* or sensitive strains of *P. falciparum,* chloroquine phosphate 1 gm (600 mg base) orally, followed by 500 mg (300 mg base) after six hours and 500 mg daily for two days is the appropriate regimen (4,8–10). Patients infected with *P. vivax* or *P. ovale* (except patients infected by transfusion or shared needles, only having the erythrocytic form of the disease) require additional treatment with primaquine phosphate 26.3 mg (15 mg base) daily for 14 days given after completion of the chloroquine regimen. The pediatric dose for chloroquine is 10 mg per kg (base) not to exceed 600 mg (base) initially, followed by half this amount on subsequent doses

(8). The pediatric dose of primaquine is 0.3 mg/kg (base) daily for 14 days (8).

Infection with *P. falciparum* should be considered a medical emergency and prompt therapy is required to prevent complications and death. Extremely ill patients who cannot take oral medication should receive chloroquine hydrochloride IM or IV in a dose of 250 mg (200 mg base) every six hours until oral therapy is possible. The parenteral form can be obtained from the Center for Disease Control. If the patient does not show a prompt response to chloroquine, then parasite resistance must be considered. Chloroquine resistance must be presumed in patients infected with *P. falciparum* contracted in areas with known resistant strains (see Drug Resistance, above). Resistant strains should be treated with quinine 650 mg orally three times daily for 14 days combined with 25 mg of pyrimethamine orally twice daily for three days plus sulfadiazine 500 mg orally four times daily for five days (4,8). In patients too ill to receive oral medication, quinine can be given intravenously, 600 mg in 300 ml of normal saline over thirty minutes every eight hours until oral therapy is possible. Pediatric doses are as follows: for quinine, 25 mg/kg/day divided into three doses; pyrimethamine, 6.25 mg/day for less than 10 kg, 12.5 mg/day for 10 to 20 kg, 25 mg/day for 20 to 40 kg; and for sulfadiazine, 100 to 200 mg/kg/day divided into four doses. The parenteral pediatric dose of quinine dihydrochloride is 25 mg/kg/day divided into two doses given six to eight hours apart. The maximum daily dose is 1800 mg/day (8).

3. *Prophylaxis.* B.T. is an airline pilot who has been assigned to several international routes. He is given free travel for his family and would like to know which medications he and his family should take for chemoprophylaxis against malaria and in what doses they should be taken. He is especially concerned about the dosage for his sons who are two and four years old.

All persons traveling to endemic areas run the risk of aquiring malaria. If the pilot and his family will be visiting such an area, they should follow general protective measures. These measures include remaining in well-screened areas between dusk and dawn and sleeping under mosquito netting. When outside, the risk can be reduced by wearing clothing which covers the arms and legs and also by using mosquito repellent on exposed areas of the skin. Chloroquine phosphate is the drug of choice for suppression of the disease caused by *P. vivax, P. malariae, P. ovale* and sensitive strains of *P. falciparum*. The recommended adult dosage is 500 mg (300 mg base) orally once weekly (11a). The dosage for children is 5 mg/kg (base) once weekly (12). This should be initiated one to two weeks prior to entering a malarious area and continued for six weeks after leaving. Brohult (13) recommends taking 600 mg (base) for the first four weeks of prophylaxis and then reducing the weekly dose to 300 mg (base) thereafter. However, the CDC does not recommend this higher dosage. This dose is believed to provide more reliably protective blood levels during the first month of therapy (14). The CDC's recommendations are probably adequate when chloroquine is dosed two weeks before entering the malarious area. This allows steady state blood levels of chloroquine to be reached prior to exposure. Therapy should begin prior to entering the malarious area for several reasons. Chloroquine's half-life is approximately 3 days when dosed weekly (14a), and therefore it should be dosed early to allow steady state blood levels to be reached. Secondly, early dosing would allow any early adverse reaction to occur prior to the traveler's departure so their family physician can manage the problem. Lastly, this helps establish a regular pattern of drug administration.

Chloroquine is active only against erythrocytic stages of malaria. It suppresses the clinical symptoms of a malarial infection without preventing the infection. In other words, it prevents the clinical symptoms of a malarial infection by eliminating parasites from the blood stream without eliminating the exoerythrocytic stages. For *P. falciparum* and *P. malariae,* which have no persistant exoerythrocytic phase, chloroquine will usually produce a suppressive cure after leaving the malarious area. Said another way, it eliminates all parasites from the body by suppressive treatment which is continued longer than the natural duration of the exoerythrocytic stages. Infrequently, delayed attacks caused by these two species can occur after six weeks. Travelers should be aware of this; if a fever develops after completion of the prophylactic regimen, they should report their possible malaria exposure to their physician immediately.

Because of the prolonged exoerythrocytic stages of *P. vivax* and *P. ovale,* delayed malarial attacks can occur as long as four years after discontinuance of chloroquine suppressive therapy. These can be prevented by the addition of primaquine to the regimen. This drug is active against the exoerythrocytic stages of the parasites. Primaquine prophylaxis is somewhat controversial and the decision to add primaquine should consider both the intensity of the exposure to *P. vivax* and *P. ovale* and the potential risk of primaquine toxicity (11a). If travelers remain in urban areas and stay in the tourist routes, the intensity of malaria exposure is usually low. Adverse reactions to primaquine may pose problems in some ethnic groups. For these reasons primaquine prophylaxis is recommended only in travelers who are heavily exposed to mosquitos and in those in whom G6PD deficiency has been excluded (11a). There is doubt as to whether G6PD deficiency protects against the more severe forms of malaria (15). The dosage of primaquine is 26.3 mg (15 mg base) daily for 14 days or 79 mg (45 mg base) once weekly for eight weeks, starting the last two weeks of or following a course of suppression with chloroquine (11a). The pediatric dosage is 0.3 mg/kg/day (base) for 14 days or 0.9 mg/kg/weekly (base) for eight weeks.

When traveling to areas where chloroquine-resistant strains of *P. falciparum* have been reported (see Drug Resistance), the most effective drug for suppression is a fixed combination of pyrimethamine and sulfadoxine (Fansidar) (11a). This drug is not available in this country, but it can be obtained in most countries with known chloroquine-resistant malaria (12). Travelers should begin taking chloroquine one to two weeks before entering a malarious area and prior to obtaining pyrimethamine-sulfadoxine (11a,12). The dosage is pyrimethamine 50 mg and sulfadoxine 1000 mg orally once every two weeks. The drug is active against the erythrocytic stages and will produce a suppressive cure when continued for six weeks after returning from a malarious area. Strains of *P. vivax* which are resistant to pyrimethamine have been reported and some authorities recommend adding chloroquine to a course of pyrimethamine-sulfadoxine (16).

Like chloroquine, pyrimethamine-sulfadoxine will not prevent delayed attacks due to persistent exoerythrocytic stages of *P. vivax* or *P. ovale* when suppression is discontinued. In such cases, primaquine prophylaxis may be needed (11a). For pregnant travelers, chemoprophylaxis is not contraindicated. Neither chloroquine nor any of the other four aminoquinolines have been associated with teratogenic effects when given in prophylactic doses. Pyrimethamine has been associated with congenital defects in animals (11a).

When chemoprophylaxis is necessary in children, it should be noted that chloroquine has an extremely bitter taste and is not available in liquid form in this country. Therefore, tablets must be crushed, scored, or broken and then dissolved. Chocolate syrup is one of the better vehicles. Chloroquine syrup (Nivaquine) can be purchased outside this country and can be used in children visiting malarious areas for long periods of time (11a).

4. Is there a vaccine available for the airline pilot and his family?

Several problems exist in developing a malaria vaccine. Studies of malaria vaccines that involve human subjects who may be partially immune to malaria can provide useful information. However, the results may not be pertinent to nonimmune subjects (17). Of the vaccines researched, the only one successful in humans is the sporozoite vaccine (18,19). There are problems in extending these limited successes to the development of a practical vaccine. First, immunity to sporozoites confers no protection against erythrocytic infection. Secondly, this immunity lasts for approximately three months. The most serious difficulty in the development of the vaccine is the relative unavailability of antigen except for the limited number of sporozoites that can be obtained from infected mosquitos (20). Also, vaccines may show varying degrees of effectiveness in relation to different strains, species, intensities of parasite inocula, and hosts (17). At this time no vaccines are commercially available.

5. *Side Effects.* What kind of side effects and toxicities can the airline pilot expect while taking chloroquine or pyrimethamine for malaria chemoprophylaxis?

The side effects of chloroquine resemble mild cinchonism, and may be reduced by taking the medication with a meal. They include vertigo, malaise, anorexia, diarrhea, headache, blurring of vision, pruritus and urticaria (24).

When chloroquine is used in high doses for long periods of time, such as in rheumatoid arthritis, it may cause a severe and non-reversible retinopathy. This has never been reported in association with prophylactic doses of chloroquine (300 mg base weekly) (11a). Although a few patients with the early stages of retinopathy may show regression, occasionally a patient with a more advanced stage of the disease may show progression upon discontinuance of therapy (27). It is this author's opinion that individuals receiving prophylaxis for many years should receive periodic ophthalmological examinations.

Pyrimethamine is well tolerated and no serious adverse reactions have been reported in studies of four to six months duration (33–36). The combination product does contain a sulfonamide and should not be given to patients with a known contraindication to one of the sulfa drugs. Large doses of pyrimethamine given for long periods of time may lead to folic acid deficiency, but folate can be supplemented to rectify the hematologic abnormality without disrupting the drug's therapeutic effect (37). However, long-term use of this drug is discouraged until more information becomes available on its yet unknown deleterious effects (11a).

6. *G6PD.* A 30-year-old Black male with a documented Glucose-6-Phosphate-Dehydrogenase (G6PD) deficiency is infected with *P. vivax.* Characterize the reaction that patients with G6PD deficiency may experience while taking primaquine.

Hemolysis occurring at the initiation of therapy can cause a low grade fever, malaise, weakness and chills lasting approximately two to three days. It is estimated that over one hundred million people are affected with G6PD deficiency (28); these include Blacks, Indians, Chinese, Sardinians, Jews, Greeks, and Iranians (28–30). This phenomenon, which is commonly referred to as primaquine sensitivity, is an inborn error of metabolism transmitted by a gene of partial dominance located on the X chromosome. The reduced amounts of Glucose-6-Phosphate-Dehydrogenase results in hemolysis of the red blood cells, which may lead to the above clinical signs. If enough hemolysis occurs, it could lead to clinical jaundice or yellowing of the sclera and epidermis.

The amount of hemolysis occurring with primaquine therapy is dependent upon three factors: the degree of G6PD deficiency, the age of the erythrocyte population, and the size of the dose. Because the gene is carried on the X chromosome, heterozygous males and homozygous females have the full expression of the disease. Also Caucasians affected by the deficiency, especially those from the Mediterranean, have a more severe hemolysis (28). The first cells to hemolyze are the older red blood cells because they contain less G6PD. Therefore, with small daily doses of primaquine (15 mg base) the hemolysis will be self-limiting, because the older cells will have already hemolyzed. The hemolytic reaction associated with the ingestion of 30 mg base daily would be more severe than that associated with 15 mg daily. Cahn (30) has shown that the reaction to weekly doses of 45 mg of base in primaquine-sensitive patients is mild.

In endemic areas of falciparum malaria, approximately 20% of the population carry this gene trait. It has been said that this may confer a small degree of protection (31) against malaria caused by falciparum. However, others suggest that the deficiency provides no protection (31). The data suggest that it may even increase the risk of severe disease in females (32).

AMEBIASIS

Amebiasis has long been known as a disease acquired by travelers while visiting foreign countries whose sanitation standards are not equal to those of the United States (1a). The disease has also been acquired in rural areas of the United States, in the southern states, in lower social economic groups, and in institutions for the mentally retarded (2a). Today, amebiasis is described in male homosexuals in San Francisco and New York with increasing frequency (3a,4a,5a). The infection is usually asymptomatic, but it may become symptomatic, producing dysentery, an intestinal mass, or lesions outside the intestines, generally liver abscesses.

Life cycle. The amebic cyst is the infective stage of *Entamoeba histolytica* and is usually ingested in food and drink contaminated by feces from an infected individual. Cysts passing through the intestines are subjected to digestive secretions and the wall of the cyst is broken down. It then provides the multiplying stage or trophozoite. These trophozoites are not infective to other individuals. However, they may invade the tissue of the large intestine where they multiply and

produce ulcerative lesions. Trophozoites can be carried to the liver via the portal system, causing abscess, and can spread either contiguously or hematogenously to other areas such as the lungs or brain. Cysts are formed again when the trophozoites are carried towards the rectum where the fecal material is dehydrated. Once excreted, they are in the infective form (6a).

7. *Amebic Liver Abscess.* A 27-year-old homosexual male seeks attention at the medical center. He describes a two-week history of bloody diarrhea and several days of fever. Physical examination reveals a temperature of 101.6°F with no chest abnormalities; the liver is slightly tender. The laboratory values are as follows: hematocrit 50%, leukocyte count 12,000 with a normal differential, bilirubin 1.1 mg/dl, alkaline phosphatase 138 IU per liter (nl<90), SGOT 240 units/dl (nl<280), SGPT 530 units/dl (nl<300). Cultures for *Neisseria gonorrhaeae* and other bacterial pathogens were negative. A liver scan showed a single 5 cm defect in the dome of the right lobe. Trophozoites of *Entamoeba histolytica* were found on examination of the stool, and rectal biopsies showed numerous organisms. The indirect hemagglutination titer for amebae drawn during the acute illness was positive at 1:4096.

What would be the most appropriate drug therapy for this patient? Explain the rationale behind the various drug regimens.

Drugs available for the treatment of amebiasis can be grouped according to their sites of action. Drugs effective against organisms located in the lumen (in the fecal material) include iodoquinol, diloxanide furoate, and paromomycin. These agents are not active against parasites in tissues such as the bowel wall or liver cells. Dehydroemetine and emetine are effective against parasites located in tissues. When administered parenterally, but they lack effectiveness against luminal organisms (38). Although metronidazole is active against organisms located in the bowel lumen, bowel wall, and in tissue (41,44–46), metronidazole is not as effective as other luminal amebicides (38–41). Chloroquine is active only against organisms in the liver (38). (See Tables 1 and 2.)

The patient in the above case should be treated with metronidazole 750 mg orally three times daily

Table 1.
TREATMENT OF AMEBIC INFECTIONS (38,47)

Infection	Drug of Choice	Alternate
Asymptomatic Intestinal	diloxanide	iodoquinol
Mild to Moderate Intestinal	diloxanide or iodoquinol, plus tetracycline, plus chloroquine	metronidazole, plus diloxanide furoate or iodoquinol
Severe Intestinal	metronidazole plus diloxanide furoate or iodoquinol	tetracycline, plus diloxanide furoate or iodoquinol or dehydroemetine; followed by tetracycline plus diloxanide furoate or iodoquinol; followed by chloroquine

Dphpable: Center for Disease Control
Dosages: (404) 329-3670 – daytime

diloxanide:	500 mg orally three times daily for ten days
iodoquinol:	650 mg orally three times daily for twenty-one days
tetracycline:	250 mg orally four times daily for ten days
chloroquine:	250 mg (salt) twice daily for fourteen days
metronidazole:	750 mg orally three times daily for ten days

Table 2.
PEDIATRIC DOSAGES FOR AMEBIASIS (47)

Drugs	Doses
diloxanide furoate	20 mg/kg/day in three doses (Not to children under two years of age)
iodoquinol	40 mg/kg/day in three doses
metronidazole	50 mg/kg/day in three doses
chloroquine	10 mg/kg/day (base)
dehydroemetine	1–1.5 mg/kg/day in two doses (maximum 90 mg/day)

for 5–10 days. Because of metronidazole's poor luminal amebicide activity, the course of metronidazole should be followed by diloxanide furoate 500 mg orally three times daily for 10 days, or iodoquinol 650 mg orally three times daily for 21 days (38,42). Diloxanide must be obtained from the Center for Disease Control (CDC) in Atlanta, Georgia. The patient should begin to respond to the metronidazole in the first 72 hours of therapy (38,43). If response does not occur, therapy should be changed to dehydroemetine 1 mg per kg intramuscularly or subcutaneously daily for 10 days (maximum daily dose is 100 mg; this drug is also available from the CDC), plus chloroquine 500

mg (salt) twice daily for two days and then 250 mg (salt) twice daily for 26 days, plus diloxanide or diiodohydroxyquine in the dosages already mentioned (38).

Dehydroemetine (available from the CDC) and emetine are equally effective, but dehydroemetine may be less cardiotoxic (62,63). Electrocardiographic changes are common, but severe toxicity is rare. Cardiac toxicity will usually appear seven days after initiation of therapy (65). Toxicity has also been reported after cessation of therapy (66).

8. *Stool Examination.* A homosexual male has been experiencing abdominal discomfort for nearly two months. His symptoms include anorexia, bloating, and periods of diarrhea followed by constipation. He has seen two community physicians prior to his visit to the medical center today. Several specimens sent for ova and parasites have been negative. What problems exist in the identification of ova and parasites in the stool?

The demonstration of *E. histolytica* in the stool is the only positive proof of intestinal amebiasis. Examination takes a great deal of time and is more difficult than searching fecal material for other pathogens. Unfortunately, many laboratories lack personnel trained in parasitology. Specimens may be misinterpreted for several reasons:

Trophozoites will lyse and be unrecognizable when left standing at room temperature. Ideally, specimens should be viewed within one hour of passage; if this is unrealistic, the specimen should be stored in the refrigerator at 4°C or preserved in formalin or a polyvinyl alcohol fixative (48).

Other problems include the examination of stools containing interfering substances. These include tetracycline, sulfonamides, antiprotozoal agents, castor oil, magnesium hydroxide, barium sulfate, hypertonic salt, soap or tap water enemas, and bismuth or kaolin compounds (49).

Another common error is the misidentification of white blood cells in the stool as trophozoites or cysts of *E. histolytica* (50,51). Occasionally, cysts or trophozoites of *E. hartmanni*, a nonpathogenic ameba, are mistaken for those of the pathogen *E. histolytica.*

The trophozoites and cysts can be most easily found during the acute phase of diarrhea when examining a fresh stool specimen (42). The clinician should obtain three stool specimens, taken every other day, from a patient. Ideally, the third specimen should be obtained following a purge induced by 10 ounces of magnesium citrate.

9. *Metronidazole Safety.* **T.R. was recently diagnosed as having amebiasis and was treated with metronidazole. Since then she has heard that it can cause cancer. Is metronidazole carcinogenic?**

Metronidazole has been reported to significantly increase the number of pulmonary tumors in rats and mice given high doses for long periods of time (52). Other studies have shown that metronidazole may cause hepatocarcinomas and mammary tumors in rats (52,53). It has also been shown to be mutagenic in the Ames Salmonella bacterial test system (54,55). This finding was significant because of the correlation between the compound's mutagenicity for these bacteria and its carcinogenicity in animals (55). Other tests in rats and hamsters and also tests for chromosomal abnormalities have been negative (52,56,57). Two retrospective studies of women treated with metronidazole for trichomoniasis, one for 10 years of follow-up (58) and the other for a shorter follow-up period (59), have failed to show an increased incidence of cancer. These negative findings do not establish the safety of metronidazole because the latent period for carcinogenesis in humans may be 20 years or more (60). In conclusion, metronidazole should be viewed as a poten-

tially hazardous drug and should be reserved as an alternate drug for mild to moderate intestinal amebiasis. However, metronidazole is considered the drug of choice for the treatment of severe colitis, hepatic abscess, and extraintestinal amebiasis, since the use of alternative drugs may be less efficacious and more toxic (60).

10. *SMON.* **A 40-year-old importer who recently visited the Sudan, received a course of clioquinol (iodochlorhydroxyquin) therapy for amebiasis. The regimen was 500 mg three times daily for 21 days. Two days prior to his visit to the clinic he began noticing numbness in his fingers and today he notices decreased visual acuity. What do these symptoms suggest?**

The patient could be experiencing a neurotoxic syndrome secondary to clioquinol therapy. The syndrome termed SMON (subacute myelo-optic neuropathy) may present as peripheral neuropathy or myelopathy (68); infrequently, cerebral manifestations have occurred (69). Symptoms range from minimal dysesthesia to death and include optic atrophy (68). Patients generally improve upon discontinuation of the drug, although they may experience some residual effects (70). The optic atrophy may progess to blindness even after the drug has been discontinued (71). Symptoms develop in 1% of those patients taking 750–1500 mg per day for less than two weeks (72,73). Thirty-five percent of patients taking doses 750–1500 mg per day for longer than two weeks will develop symptoms (72,74).

No cases of this syndrome have been reported with iodoquinol (diiodohydroxyquin) when used at the dosage now recommended. When iodoquinol was given in high doses for longer periods of time to children being treated for acrodermatitis enteropathica, the syndrome did develop (75).

In this patient who has received potentially toxic doses of clioquinol, the drug should be discontinued and possibly the symptoms will resolve.

GIARDIASIS

Until approximately 40 years ago *Giardia lamblia* was considered an intestinal commensal organism. Since that time, outbreaks of giardiasis have been reported in Colorado (1b), Utah and other Rocky Mountain states (2b,3b). Reports of infections in travelers to Russia (4b), Europe, the

Middle East (5b), and Viet Nam have been noted (6b). Several reports suggest giardiasis is sexually transmitted and is not uncommon in homosexuals (7,8a,9a). Giardia is the most common pathogenic intestinal parasite reported to the Center for Disease Control in Atlanta, Georgia (10a). The rate of positive stool cultures of giardia ranges from 0 to 10% for individual states, and averages 4.1% for the United States (10a). Fortunately, if recognized, this pathogen can be treated effectively with relatively nontoxic medication.

Life Cycle. *Giardia lamblia* lives in the upper part of the small intestine of man. This parasite has two forms, the trophozoite and the cyst. The trophozoites are seen in duodenal aspirates and diarrheal stool when transit times are rapid. They are never seen in formed stool. Trophozoite resistance to local conditions and the stimulus for cyst-formation are unknown (5b).

The stools of infected individuals usually contain the cyst forms, the infectious stage of the parasite. Cysts are viable in water for longer than three months (5b).

Infection is spread by direct fecal-oral contamination or by transmission of cysts in food or water. After ingestion, the organisms divide in the upper gastrointestinal tract (5b).

11. *Giardiasis.* **R.T. returned from a trip around the world last month. While crossing the Middle East he experienced a bout of "gastroenteritis." This consisted of one to two weeks of diarrhea which produced approximately 5 to 7 stools per day. The stools were foul smelling, watery, and tended to float in the toilet. However, at no time did he see blood or mucous in the stools. Since that time he describes alternating periods of constipation and diarrhea and an uneasy feeling in his stomach. He currently weighs 10–15 pounds less than he did prior to his departure and his current bowel habits are much different than before his trip. Because of his travel history and symptoms, a CBC, three stool samples for ova and parasites, and stool cultures were ordered. The CBC was normal, stool for ova and parasites showed** *Giardia lamblia* **cysts, and stool cultures were negative. Discuss the normal presentation of giardiasis. Which of R.T.'s symptoms correlate with the usual picture of giardiasis?**

R.T.'s symptoms are classic for giardial infections. Unlike the diarrhea of bacterial origin, the onset of giardial diarrhea is usually late, beginning one to three weeks after the onset of infection. The stools are loose, greasy, and occasionally watery in nature. The diarrhea may be persistent, or intermittent, and may be associated with marked weight loss. Patients often complain of upper abdominal discomfort, bloating and nausea. Eosinophilia and an elevated white blood cell count are seldom seen (5b,76,77). These acute symptoms are followed by a chronic form of the disease which is characterized by a relentless or intermittent course of mushy stools, with periodic constipation, abdominal distention and flatulence, and a slightly increased or normal number of stools. If not treated correctly, giardiasis may persist for months or years with exacerbations and remissions (78).

12. If R.T.'s stools for ova and parasites had been negative, what other tests could have been performed to obtain a positive diagnosis of giardiasis?

Negative stools would require sampling of the duodenal contents either by intubation and aspiration or by the use of the string test (Enterotest) (79). The string test consists of a gelatin capsule packed with 140 cm of nylon line. The capsule is swallowed by the patient and the free end of the line is secured to the face and left in position for four hours. In 95% of the cases the line fully extends and reaches the duodenum by peristaltic action. On removal of the line by traction, the distal section of the line is saturated with bile-stained mucous. This mucous is then examined for the presence of *Giardia lamblia* trophozoites. This technique has been shown to be as effective as duodenal aspiration for detection of *Giardia lamblia* (80).

13. *Treatment.* **What drug therapy should R.T. receive?**

The drug of choice for this patient is *quinacrine* (Atabrine). Quinacrine has been used to treat giardiasis for forty years and is still considered by many to be the drug of choice (5b,76,81–83). This drug provides cure rates of 90% or more in patients with giardiasis (76,81). The adult dosage is 100 mg orally three times daily for five to seven days; the dosage for children is 2 mg/kg three times daily for five days (76,81,83). With this dosage, side effects are few. They consist of gastrointestinal disturbances, headaches, and rarely, a slight yellow discoloration of the skin and sclerae (76,81,82). With the doses formerly used for malaria, a toxic psychoses developed in 1.5% of the patients receiving this drug (76,81).

The only other drug approved by the Food and Drug Administration for the treatment of giardiasis is *furazolidone.* It is available in suspension form, and although effective, it is not as well tolerated as other drugs. The dosage is 5 mg/kg/day given four times daily for 10 days. Side effects commonly seen are gastrointestinal disturbances, morbilliform rashes, and darkening of the urine (81,82). The drug can cause hemolysis in G6PD deficient patients (81,82).

Metronidazole, although not approved by the FDA for giardiasis, produces cure rates of 70 to 100% depending upon the dosage schedule. When 250 mg is given three times daily for seven to ten days, it is slightly less effective than quinacrine but better tolerated (76,84,85).

Three weeks after completion of the regimen, stools should be checked for ova and parasites. Treatment failure would necessitate a second course of quinacrine or metronidazole, which is highly effective if used in larger doses than those usually recommended (750 mg orally three times daily for ten days) (5b).

ENTEROBIASIS

Enterobius vermicularis, known as pinworm, threadworm, seatworm, oxyuriasis, or enterobiasis, is the most common parasite worldwide. It is the fourth most prevalent parasite in the United States (10a). In comparison to most other helminth infections, enterobiasis is more bothersome than an actual health hazard (1c). The infection is most common in children and occurs most frequently in crowded institutional settings (2c). Fortunately, the host can be treated and cured with nontoxic agents. Frequently patients must be retreated for recurrence of this intestinal parasite.

Life Cycle. *Enterobius vermicularis* is threadlike in appearance and is approximately 1 cm in length. After ingestion, eggs hatch in the upper intestines. The larvae then migrate to the ileum. Mating of the worm occurs in the lower portion of the small intestine, and the female then migrates into the lower bowel. The female moves out the anus and deposits her eggs in the perianal

area. The eggs cause an anal pruritus, and scratching leads to rectal-oral transmission; thus, the life-cycle is completed (3c).

14. *Enterobiasis.* **P.C. is a 7-year-old girl whose mother is an elementary school teacher. P.C. has been extremely irritable and unattentive for the past two months and has been experiencing insomnia and episodes of enuresis. Upon questioning, it is learned that she is also experiencing perianal itching. Because of the child's symptoms and age and the mother's occupation, an adhesive tape test was performed. This revealed *Enterobius vermicularis* eggs.**

Is this patient's age typical of those with enterobiasis? What is the most likely source of this infection? Explain the adhesive tape test used to make this diagnosis.

Enterobiasis is commonly seen in children five to nine years of age (4c). However, the infection can be seen in all age groups; estimates of prevalence suggest rates of 30% in children compared with 16% in adults (2c). The source of P.C.'s infection may have been her mother, who may have been infected at her work place. The close contact and the use of common towels and crowded, though not necessarily unsanitary conditions, can increase the spread of this infection.

The adhesive tape test used in the diagnosis is preferably performed in the morning. A two inch strip of adhesive tape is repeatedly pressed against the perianal and perineal skin. With the adhesive side down, the tape is placed onto a drop of toluene on a microscope slide. This is then examined for the presence of eggs. When performed once, it yields 50%, three times 90%, five times 99% of the positive cases. Since P.C. was positively diagnosed, other members of her family should also be examined (4c).

15. *Treatment.* **What drug therapy would be most appropriate for P.C.'s enterobiasis? What other measures should be discussed with P.C.'s mother?**

The most appropriate drug for P.C. would be *mebendazole (Vermox).* This drug is extremely effective for enterobiasis infections with cure rates of 90–100% (93). Studies in children and adults demonstrated it to have fewer side effects than other anthelmintics (94,95). Although mebendazole is remarkably free of side effects, mild nausea, vomiting, diarrhea, and abdominal pain have been reported. Less than 10% of drug is absorbed (1c,93) after an oral dose. Because of the low bioavailability, the dosage is the same for patients of all ages. The dose is 100 mg as a single dose and should be repeated in two weeks. Because of inadequate data, it is not recommended for children less than two years of age.

There is a social stigma associated with parasitic infections. Hence, after the diagnosis is made, the patient should be counseled regarding the prevalence and the harmlessness of the infection. Enterobiasis is unaffected by the most stringent of sanitary measures (96), and infection frequently recurs despite effective anthelmintic therapy (97).

16. What alternative drugs could be used in this enterobiasis infection?

Pyrvinium pamoate (Povan) given as a single dose of 5 mg/kg (maximum 250 mg) is highly effective in the treatment of enterobiasis (1c,89). Cure rates range from 90 to 100% (89). Pyrvinium occasionally causes nausea, vomiting (emesis occurs more frequently with the suspension than with the tablets) (89), diarrhea, and dizziness. This drug is a red dye and it will color the stool red for several days; spilled suspension or vomitus following ingestion of pyrvinium will result in permanent staining of clothing. Tablets should be swallowed whole to prevent tooth staining.

Pyrantel pamoate (Antiminth), when given as a single dose of 10 mg/kg (base) (maximum 1 gm) and then repeated in two weeks, is equally as efficacious as pyrvinium pamoate (89). However, pyrantel produces fewer side effects than pyrvinium (90,91). Pyrantel offers the additional advantage of not staining clothing red. Side effects include nausea, vomiting, diarrhea, abdominal cramping, and transient elevation of SGOT levels in approximately 2 to 4% of the patients treated (92). The FDA has tentatively accepted its advisory review panel's recommendation to move pyrantel pamoate to non-prescription status (103).

Piperazine (Antepar) is no longer recommended for the treatment of enterobiasis (1c,4c,86) because it must be dosed daily for seven days and because of frequent adverse reactions such as vomiting, diarrhea, urticaria, tremor, dizziness, visual disturbances and weakness (87). When given orally at a dose of 65 mg/kg/day (maximum daily dose of 2.5 gm) for seven days it produces cures in 95% of the cases treated (88).

Gentian violet is the only nonprescription product available for the treatment of enterobiasis. The drug produces side effects in 14 to 28% of the patients. Furthermore, this drug may act as a carcinogen by interacting with DNA in cultured cells (98–101). In light of these problems and the availability of other products, gentian violet is not recommended for the treatment of enterobiasis (1c,102).

References

1. Heineman HS: The clinical syndrome of malaria in the United States. A current review of diagnosis and treatment by American physicians. Arch Intern Med. 1972; 129:607.

1a. Curtis KJ et al: Infection and parasitic diseases, In *Gastrointestinal Diseases* by M Sleisenger, J Fordtran, WB Saunders, Philadelphia, 1978.

1b. Moore GT et al: Epidemic giardiasis at a ski resort. N Engl J Med. 1969; 281:402.

1c. Committee on Drugs: Commentary on anthelmintics. Pediatrics. 1978; 62:251.

2. Barrett-Connor E: Chemoprophylaxis in malaria. Ann Intern Med. 1978; 89:417.

2a. Brooke MN: Epidemiology of amebiasis in the United States. JAMA. 1964; 188:519.

2b. Center for Disease Control: MMWR. 1974; 23:78.

2c. Warren KS: Helmintic diseases endemic in United States. Am J Trop Med Hyg. 1974; 23:723.

3. Young MD: Malaria. In *Tropical Medicine,* 5th ed, edited by G Hunter, JC Swartzwelder, DF Clyde, WB Saunders, Philadelphia, 1976, p 353.

3a. Schermin MJ et al: Amebiasis—an increasing problem among homosexuals in New York City. JAMA. 1977; 238:1386.

3b. Center for Disease Control: MMWR. 1974; 23:397.

3c. Hunter G: Intestinal nematodes, In *Tropical Medicine,* 5th ed, edited by G Hunter, JC Swartzwelder, DF Clyde, WB Saunders, Philadelphia, 1976, p 461.

4. Butler T: Algorithms in the diagnosis and management of exotic diseases. XIII. Malaria. J Infect Dis. 1976; 133:721.

4a. Dritz SK et al: Patterns of sexually transmitted enteric disease in a city. Lancet. 1977; 2:3.

4b. Brodsky RE et al: Giardiasis in American travelers to the Soviet Union. J Infect Dis. 1974; 130:319.

4c. Warren KS et al: Algorithms in the diagnosis and management of exotic disease. V. Enterobiasis. J Infect Dis. 1975; 132:229.

5. Miller LH: Current prospects and problems for a malaria vaccine. J Infect Dis. 1977; 135:855.

5a. Unger KW: Amebiasis (letter). N Engl J Med. 1978; 298:148.

5b. Mahmoud AAF et al: Algorithms in the diagnosis and management of exotic diseases. II. Giardiasis. J Infect Dis. 1975; 131:621.

6. Shaw PK et al: Malaria surveillance in the United States 1974. J Infect Dis. 1976; 133:19.

6a. Hunter G: Amebiasis, In *Tropical Medicine,* 5th ed, edited by G. Hunter, JC Swartzwelder, DF Clyde, WB Saunders, Philadelphia, 1976, p 329.

6b. Butler T et al: Chronic and recurrent diarrhea in American servicemen in Viet Nam. Arch Intern Med. 1973; 32:373.

7. Schnerin MJ et al: Giardiasis associated with homosexuals. Ann Intern Med. 1978; 88:801.

8. Drugs for parasitic infections. In *Handbook of Antibicrobial Therapy.* The Medical Letter, New Rochelle, 1974, p 60.

8a. Mildavan D et al: Venereal transmission of enteric pathogens in male homosexuals. JAMA. 1977; 238:1387.

9. Young MD: Malaria. In *Tropical Medicine,* 5th ed, edited by G Hunter, JC Swartzwelder, DF Clyde, WB Saunders, Philadelphia, 1976, p 353.

9a. Hurwitzal et al: Venereal transmission of intestinal parasites. West J Med. 1978; 128:89.

10. Clyde DF: Malaria. In *Current Therapy 1980,* edited by HF Conn, WB Saunders, Philadelphia, 1980, p 38.

10a. Intestinal Parasites Surveillance, Annual Summary. US Department of Health, Education, Welfare, Center for Disease Control (Atlanta, GA): Publication # (CDC) 1978, 1979–8352.

11. Center for Disease Control: MMWR. 1979; 27:463.

11a. Center for Disease Control: MMWR. 1979; 27: supplement.

12. Medical Letter. Malaria chemoprophylaxis. 1979; 21:72.

13. Brohult J et al: Weekly malaria prophylaxis: 300 mg or 600 mg chloroquine base. Lancet. 1979; 2:522.

14. Berliner RW et al: The physiological disposition, antimalarial activity, and toxicity of some derivatives of 4-aminoquinolines. J Clin Invest. 1948; 27:98.

14a. Rocco IM: Drugs used in the chemotherapy of malaria. In *The Pharmacological Basis of Therapeutics,* 6th Ed ed by A. Gilman, L Goodman. MacMillan, New York, 1980; p 1044.

15. Martin SK et al: Severe malaria and G6PD deficiency: a reappraisal of the malaria-G6PD hypothesis. Lancet. 1979; Vol 1:524.

16. Pearlman EJ et al: The suppression of plasmodium falciparum and plasmodium vivax parasitemias by sulfadoxine-pyrimethamine combination. Am J Trop Med Hyg. 1977; 26:1108.

17. Powell RD: Malaria vaccine development. Bull WHO. 1979; 57(supple 1):273.

18. Clyde DF et al: Immunization of man against sporozoite-induced falciparum malaria. Am J Med Sci. 1973; 266:169.

19. Clyde DF et al: Specificity of protection of man immunized against sporozoite-induced falciparum malaria. Am J Med Sci. 1973; 266:398.

20. Miller LH: Current prospects and problems for a malaria vaccine. J Infect Dis. 1977; 135:855.

21. Young MD: Malaria. In *Tropical Medicine,* 5th ed, edited by G Hunter, JC Swartzwelder, DF Clyde, WB Saunders, Philadelphia, 1976, p 394.

22. Catchpool JF: Antiprotozoal drugs. In *Review of Medical Pharmacology,* 7th ed, edited by FH Meyer, E Jawetz, A Goldfein, Lange, Los Altos, 1980, p 623.

23. Young MD: Malaria. In *Tropical Medicine,* 5th ed, edited by G Hunter, JC Swartzwelder, DF Clyde, WB Saunders, Philadelphia, 1976, p 395.

24. Catchpool JF: Antiprotozoal drugs. In *Review of Medical Pharmacology,* 7th ed, edited by FH Meyer, E Jawetz, A Goldfein, Lange, Los Altos, 1980, p 625.

25. Ogawas et al: Progression of retinopathy long after cessation of chloroquine therapy. Lancet. 1979; 2:1408.

26. Catchpool JF: Antiprotozoal drugs. In *Review of Medical Pharmacology,* 7th ed, edited by FH Meyer, E Jawetz, A Goldfein, Lange, Los Altos, 1980, p 624.

27. Rinkle JR et al: Long term course of chloroquine retinopathy after cessation of medication. Am J Ophthalmol. 1979; 88:1.

28. Catchpool JF: Antiprotozoal drugs. In *Review of Medical Pharmacology,* 7th ed, edited by FH Meyer, E Jawetz, A Goldfein, Lange, Los Altos, 1980, p 628.

29. Beutler E: Hemolytic effect of primaquine and related compounds: a review. J Hem. 1959; 14:103.

30. Cahn NM: The tolerance to large weekly doses of primaquine and amodiaquine in primaquine-sensitive and non-sensitive subjects. Am J Trop Med Hyg. 1962; 11:605.

31. Catchpool JF: Antiprotozoal drugs. In *Review of Medical Pharmacology,* 7th ed, edited by FH Meyer, E Jawetz, A Goldfein, Lange, Los Altos, 1980, p 629.

32. Bienzie U: G6PD and malaria: greater resistance of females heterozygous for enzyme deficiency and of males with non deficient variant. Lancet. 1972; 7742:107.

33. Pearlman EJ et al: Chemosuppressive field trials in Thailand. III. Suppression of plasmodium falciparum and plasmodium vivax parasitemias by a sulfadoxine-pyrimethamine combination. Am J Trop Med Hyg. 1977; 26:1108.

34. O'Holohand DR et al: Malaria suppression and prophylaxis on a Malayan rubber estate: sulfomethoxine-pyrimethamine single monthly dose vs. chloroquine single weekly dose. South Asian J Trop Med Pub Health. 1971; 2:164.

35. Ebisawai I et al: Malaria at Nam Ngum Dam construction site in Laos: suppression with combinations of sulfonamides and pyrimethamine. Jpn J Exp Med. 1971; 41:209.

36. Pearlman EJ et al: Prevention of chloroquine-resistant falciparum malaria. Ann Intern Med. 1975; 82:590.

37. Catchpool JF: Antiprotozoal drugs. In *Review of Medical Pharmacology,* 7th ed, edited by FH Meyer, E Jawetz, A Goldfein, Lange, Los Altos, 1980, p 631.

38. Catchpool JF: Antiprotozoal drugs. In *Review of Medical Pharmacology,* 7th ed, edited by FH Meyer, E Jawetz, A Goldfein, Lange, Los Altos, 1980, p 632.

39. Hunter G: Malaria. In *Tropical Medicine.* 5th ed, edited by G Hunter, JC Swartzwelder, DF Clyde, WB Saunders, Philadelphia, 1976, p 336.

40. Weber DM: Amebic abscess of liver following metronidazole therapy. JAMA. 1971; 216:1339.

41. Everett ED: Metronidazole and amebiasis. Am J Dig Dis. 1974; 19:626.

42. Johnston TS: Diagnosis and treatment of five parasites. Drug Intell Clin Pharm. 1981; 15:103.

43. Ylvisaker JT et al: Sexually acquired amebic colitis and liver abscess. West J Med. 1980; 132:153.

44. Adam EB et al: Invasive amebiasis-II. Amebic liver abscess and its complications. Medicine. 1977; 56:325.

45. Cohen JG et al: Comparison of metronidazole and chloroquine in the treatment of amebic liver abscess—a controlled trial period. Gastroenterology. 1965; 69:35.

46. Adam EB et al: Invasive amebiasis-I. Amebic dysentery and its complications. Medicine. 1977; 56:315.

47. Drugs for parasitic infections. *Handbook of Antimicrobial Therapy.* The Medical Letter, New Rochelle, 1974, p 53.

48. Krogstad DJ et al: Current concepts in parasitology: amebiasis. N Engl J Med. 1978; 298:262.

49. Juniper K Jr: Parasitic diseases of the intestinal tract. In *Gastroenterologic Medicine,* edited M Paulson, Lea, Febiger, Philadelphia, 1969, p 472.

50. Krogstad DJ et al: Amebiasis: Epidemiologic studies in the United States. Ann Intern Med. 1978; 88:89.

51. Tucker PC et al: Amebic colitis mistaken for inflammatory bowel disease. Arch Intern Med. 1975; 135:681.

52. Roe JFC: A critical appraisal of the toxicology of metronidazole. In *Metronidazole,* first edition, edited by I Phillips, J Collier, Academic Press, London, 1979, p 215.

53. Rustia M et al: Experimental induction of hepatomas, mammary tumors, and other tumors with metronidazole in noninbred SAS: NRC (Wl) BR rats. J Natl Cancer Inst. 1979; 63:863.

54. Rosenkranzs et al: Mutagenicity of metronidazole: activation by mammalian liver microsomes. Biochem Biophys Res Commun. 1975; 66:520.

55. McCan J et al: Detection of carcinogens at mutagens in the salmonella/microsome test: assay of 300 chemicals. Proc Natl Acad Sci USA. 1976; 73:950.

56. Bost RG: Metronidazole: Mammalian mutagenicity. In *Metronidazole: Proceedings of the International Medtronidazole Conference,* edited by SM Finegold, Excerpta Medica, Amsterdam, 1977, p 126.

57. Lambert B et al: Absence of genotoxic effects of metronidazole and two of its urinary metabolites on human lymphocytes in vitro. Mutation Res. 1979; 67:281.

58. Beard CM et al: Lack of evidence for cancer due to the use of metronidazole. N Engl J Med. 1979; 301:519.

59. Friedman GD: Cancer after metronidazole. N Engl J Med. 1980; 302:519.

60. Catchpool JF: Antiprotozoal drugs. In *Review of Medical Pharmacology,* 7th ed, edited by FH Meyer, E Jawetz, A Goldfein, Lange, Los Altos, 1980, p 639.

61. Finegold SM: Metronidazole. Ann Intern Med. 1980; 93:585.

62. Powell SJ et al: A comparative trial of dehydroemetine and emetine hydrochloride in identical dosage in amebic liver abscess. Ann Trop Med Parasitol. 1967; 61:26.

63. Catchpool JF: Antiprotozoal drugs. In *Review of Medical Pharmacology,* 7th ed, edited by FH Meyer, E Jawetz, A Goldfein, Lange, Los Altos, 1980, p 634.

64. Sharad CS et al: Cardiovascular toxicity of emetine and dehydroemetine. Indian Pract. 1971; 24:237.

65. Paine A et al: Electrocardiographic changes due to emetine therapy. Trans R Soc Trop Med Hyg. 1968; 62:221.

66. Lister GD: Delayed myocardial intoxication following the administration of dehydroemetine hydrochloride. J Trop Med Hyg. 1968; 71:219.

67. Catchpool JF: Antiprotozoal drugs. In *Review of Medical Pharmacology,* 7th ed, edited by FH Meyer, E Jawetz, A Goldfein, Lange, Los Altos, 1980, p 636.

68. Oakley GP: The neurotoxicity of the halogenated hydroxyquinolines. JAMA. 1973; 225:395.

69. Sobue I et al: Myeloneuropathy with abdominal disorders in Japan. Neurology. 1971; 21:168.

70. Selby G: Subacute myelo-optico-neuropathy in Australia. Lancet. 1972; 1:123.

71. Strandvik B et al: Amaurosis after broxyquinoline. Lancet. 1968; 1:922.

72. Tsubaki T et al: Neurological syndrome associated with clinoquinol. Lancet. 1971; 1:696.

73. Nakae K et al: Subacute myelo-optico-neuropathy (SMON) in Japan. Lancet. 1971; 2:510.

74. Yoshitake Y et al: Subacute myelo-optico-neuropathy, a new neurological disease prevailing in Japan. Jap J Med Sci Bio. 1971; 24:195.

75. Committee on Drugs: Blindness and neuropathy from diiodohydroxyquin-like drugs. Pediatrics. 1974; 54:378.

76. Wolfe MS: Giardiasis. N Engl J Med. 1978; 298:319.

77. Jacobowski W: *Proceedings of the National Symposium on Waterborne Transmission of Giardiasis,* Cincinnati, Ohio, September 18–20, 1978. EPA (Wash DC) publication # EPA-600-9-79-001 Govt Printing Office 1979, p 39.

78. Peterson H: Giardiasis. Scand J Gastroenterol. 1972; 7(suppl):14.

79. Beal CB et al: A new technique for sampling duodenal contents. Demonstration of upper small bowel pathogens. Am J Trop Med Hyg. 1970; 19:349.

80. Bezjak B: Evaluation of a new technique for sampling duodenal contents in parasitologic diagnosis. Am J Digest Dis. 1972; 17:848.

81. Sealy DP et al: Giardiasis: a common and underdiagnosed enteric pathogen. J Fam Pract. 1981; 12:47.

82. Blumenthal DS: Intestinal parasites. In *Current Therapy 1980,* edited by HF Gann, WB Saunders, Philadelphia, 1980, p 405.

83. Drugs for parasitic infections. *Handbook of Antimicrobial Therapy,* The Medical Letter, New Rochelle, 1974, p 56.

84. Wolfe MS: Giardiasis. JAMA. 1975; 233:1362.

85. Wolfe MS: Giardiasis. Pediatr Clin North Am. 1979; 26:295.

86. Goldsmith RS: Anthelmintic drugs. In *Review of Medical Pharmacology,* 7th ed, edited by FH Meyer, E Jawetz, A Goldfein, Lange, Los Altos, 1980, p 666.

87. Most H: Treatment of common parasitic infections of man encountered in the United States Pt. I. N Engl J Med. 1972; 287:495.

88. Goldsmith RS: Anthelmintic drugs. In *Review of Medical Pharmacology,* 7th ed, edited by FH Meyer, E Jawetz, A Goldfein, Lange, Los Altos, 1980, p 667.

89. Goldsmith RS: Anthelmintic drugs. In *Review of Medical Pharmacology,* 7th ed, edited by FH Meyer, E Jawetz, A Goldfein, Lange, Los Altos, 1980, p 669.

90. Bell WJ et al: Comparison of pyrantel pamoate, piperazine phosphate in the treatment of ascariasis. Am J Trop Med Hyg. 1971; 20:584.

91. Farahnanidian I et al: Comparative studies in the evaluation of the effects of new anthelmintics on various intestinal helminthiasis in Iran. Chemotherapy. 1977; 23:98.

92. Pitts NE et al: Antiminth (pyrantal pamoate): the clinical evaluation of a new broad-spectrum anthelmintic. Clin Pediatr. 1974; 13:87.

93. Goldsmith RS: Anthelmintic drugs. In *Review of Medical Pharmacology,* 7th ed, edited by FH Meyer, E Jawetz, A Goldfein, Lange, Los Altos, 1980, p 660.

94. Maqbool S et al: Treatment of trichuriasis with a new drug, mebendazole. J Pedriatr. 1975; 86:463.

95. Wolfe MS et al: Mebendazole: treatment of trichuriasis and ascariasis in Bahamian children. JAMA. 1974; 230:408.

96. Sawitz W et al: Studies on the epidemiology of oxyuriasis. South Med J. 1940; 33:913.

97. Matsen JM et al: Reinfection in enterobiasis (pinworm infection) Am J Dis Child. 1969; 118:576.

98. Rozenbranz HR et al: Possible hazards in the use of gentian violet. Br Med J. 1971; 3:702.

99. Au W: Cytogenic toxicity of gentian violet and crystal violet on mammalian cells in vitro. Mutation Res. 1978; 58:269.

100. Hsu TC: Cytogenic assays of chemical clastogens using mammalian cells in culture. Mutation Res. 1971; 45:233.

101. Au W: Further study of the genetic toxicity of gentian violet. Mutation Res. 1979; 66:103.

102. Pettinato FA: Anthelmintic products. *Handbook of Non Prescription Drugs,* American Pharmaceutical Association, Washington DC, 7th ed (in press).

103. Federal Register. 1980; 45:59445.

Chapter 41

Anemias

Nancy E. Korman

Anemia is defined as a reduction in red cell mass. However, because it is difficult to measure the red cell mass accurately, anemia is more practically defined as a decrease in the red blood cell concentration per unit volume of blood, which is represented by a decrease in hemoglobin concentration.

Anemia is not a disease in the strict sense of the word, but a symptom which has many causes. Its occurrence is associated with several nutritional deficiencies, acute and chronic diseases, and exogenous factors such as drugs. Consequently, anemia is one of the most common problems encountered in clinical medicine.

Since anemia can be caused by many pathologic conditions, it can be classified on a pathophysiological basis as seen in Table 1. This table categorizes anemia into (a) anemia due to decreased red cell production, (b) anemia due to increased red cell destruction, and (c) anemia due to acute blood loss. Anemia due to decreased red cell production can be further subdivided into (i) anemias due to disturbances in stem-cell proliferation or differentiation and (ii) anemia due to disturbances in mature or differentiated cells.

Anemias can also be classified according to the morphological appearance of the red blood cell. This latter approach is practical as well as simple and subdivides anemias into: (a) microcytic, hypochromic, (b) normocytic, and (c) macrocytic. On the basis of this type of classification, a simple microscopic evaluation of the peripheral blood smear can provide valuable information leading to the diagnosis of macrocytic anemias due to vitamin B-12 or folic acid deficiencies, or to a microcytic anemia such as that of iron deficiency.

Pathophysiology. Anemic patients suffer from tissue hypoxia because of the low oxygen-carrying capacity of the reduced red cell mass. The body compensates to offset the effects of this decreased oxygen-carrying capacity by increasing tissue perfusion to vital organs such as the brain, heart, and kidneys by shunting blood from non-vital organs such as cutaneous tissues. Pallor of the skin results and is the most obvious sign of anemia. The most reliable sites to examine for pallor are mucous membranes, the conjunctivae, and nail beds. Additionally, the skin may lose its elasticity and develop a dry, wrinkled appearance.

If the anemia is severe (ie, hemoglobin less than 7 gm/dl), cardiac output rises with an increase in both heart rate and stroke volume. In addition, the kidneys secrete erythropoietin which stimulates red cell production. The respiratory rate also increases. Of all of the compensatory mechanisms, increased vital organ tissue perfusion and increased erythropoietin secretion are the most efficient. The increased respiratory rate is relatively ineffective in increasing oxygen delivery to the tissues.

Secondary complications can arise from these compensatory effects. For example, excessive car-

Table 1.

PHYSIOLOGIC CLASSIFICATION OF ANEMIA
(Modified from Wintrobe)

I. Deficient red cell production
  A. Deficiency of essential substances
    1. Iron, copper*, cobalt*
    2. Vitamin B_{12}; folic acid; pyridoxine*, riboflavin*; Vitamin E*; pantothenic acid*; protein deficiencies*
    3. Inadequate supply of plasma iron
      a. Block in discharge of iron from red cell (unknown cause) as in anemia of chronic disorders
      b. Absence of circulating transferrin
  B. Bone marrow failure—aplastic anemia; irradiation; tumor; cancer chemotherapeutic agents; sideroblastic anemias
  C. Endocrine deficiency—pituitary; thyroid; adrenal; testicular
II. Excessive red cell destruction
  A. Hemolytic anemias
    1. Intrinsic—hereditary spherocytosis; glucose 6 phosphate dehydrogenase (G6PD) deficiency; paroxysmal nocturnal hemoglobinuria (PNH); complement dependent abnormalities
    2. Extrinsic—Coombs' positive; autoimmune reactions
III. Anemias with both increased destruction and decreased production
  A. Anemias of chronic disease (renal, liver, connective tissue disorders; infection; malignancy)
  B. Hemoglobinopathies (eg, sickle cell)
  C. Thalassemias

*experimentally induced

diac hyperactivity in severely anemic patients can result in systolic murmurs, angina pectoris, high-output congestive heart failure, pulmonary congestion, ascites, and edema. Thus, anemia is generally not well tolerated in patients with cardiac disease. Uncorrected tissue hypoxia per se can lead to a number of complications related to the cardiovascular, central nervous, respiratory, and gastrointestinal systems. These specific problems include angina, intermittent claudication, muscular cramps, headache, tinnitus, faintness, orthopnea, dyspnea, and diffuse abdominal pain. Orthopnea and dyspnea are characteristic complications of anemia.

Laboratory Diagnosis. The usual diagnostic workup of anemia includes: hematocrit, hemoglobin, total iron binding capacity, as well as serum iron, folate, and B-12 levels. Urinalysis is useful to determine the presence of hemoglobinuria or red blood cells. Stool guaiac tests should be performed to determine if gastrointestinal bleeding may be the cause of anemia. In most cases, these test results will provide enough information to manage the common "treatable" anemias, which are associated with iron, folate, and B-12 deficiency. Normal values for common hematologic tests are given in Table 2.

If all of the above tests do not reveal an obvious cause for anemia, diseases such as collagen vascular disease, malignancy, chronic infection, endocrine disorders, drug-induced red cell destruction, and several other etiologies must be considered.

When uncertainty exists as to the cause of anemia, bone marrow examination is performed. The specimen is examined for iron stores and nucleated erythroid precursors. A myeloid-to-erythroid (M/E) ratio can also be obtained. The M/E ratio relates the percentage of neutrophil precursors to the percentage of nucleated erythroid precursors. The normal M/E ratio in men is 1.5:1 to 3.3:1. An increase in the M/E ratio indicates a decreased percentage of nucleated red cells and decreased red cell production. Various malignancies, as well as each type of anemia, have a characteristic M/E ratio. Table 3 provides a relatively complex flow diagram for the work-up of anemia.

Numerous types of anemias are encountered in clinical medicine. This chapter will be limited to the most common treatable anemias and drug-induced anemias. Anemias secondary to congenital disorders will not be discussed. Before proceeding, the reader should review the basic hematologic laboratory tests in the chapter entitled Interpretation of Clinical Laboratory Tests.

IRON DEFICIENCY ANEMIA

Before iron deficiency is manifested as anemia, a large amount of iron must be lost. The body contains a total of approximately 3.5 gm of iron. Of this, 2.5 gm is present in hemoglobin, and the remainder exists as stores in the reticuloendothelial system (bone marrow, spleen, liver). Only a small fraction is present in the plasma (100–150 mcg/dl), bound to the transport protein, transferrin. Free iron is extremely toxic.

Despite the continuing rapid turnover of red blood cells, iron stores are well preserved. The loss of iron from urine, sweat, and sloughing of intestinal mucosal cells containing ferritin is 0.5 to 1.0 mg per day. In women, menstruation adds another 0.5 to 1.0 mg to the daily iron loss. Pregnancy and lactation are other common sources of iron loss.

Approximately 10% of dietary iron is absorbed in individuals with adequate iron stores. Thus, if 1.0 mg of elemental iron is lost daily, the amount of ingested iron which will replace that loss will be approximately 10 mg. For menstruating and lactating women, the daily iron requirement may be as high as 20 mg.

Since the average American diet contains approximately 6 mg of elemental iron per 1000 kcal, a minimum of 1500 kcal will supply the daily iron requirement. Among the foodstuffs highest in iron are liver, heart, Brewer's yeast, egg yolks, and dried beans. Non-green vegetables and milk products contain the lowest quantities of iron.

Iron is primarily absorbed from the duodenum and upper jejunum by an active transport mech-

Table 2.
NORMAL HEMATOLOGIC VALUES

Ferritin	12–250 mcg/L
Folate	7–18 mcg/ml
Haptoglobin	40–180 mg/dl
Hematocrit	
males	42–48%
females	38–44%
Hemoglobin	
males	13–18 gm/dl
females	12–16 gm/dl
Hemoglobin (serum)	< 5 mg/dl
Hemopexin	50–100 mg/dl
Iron (Fe)	50–150 mcg/dl
Iron Binding Capacity (TIBC)	250–400 mcg/dl
Mean Corpuscular Hemoglobin Concentration (MCHC)	32–36%
Mean Corpuscular Volume (MCV)	82–92 microns^3
Reticulocyte Count	0.5–1.5%
Vitamin B-12	> 200 pg/ml

Table 3.

LABORATORY DIAGNOSIS OF ANEMIA

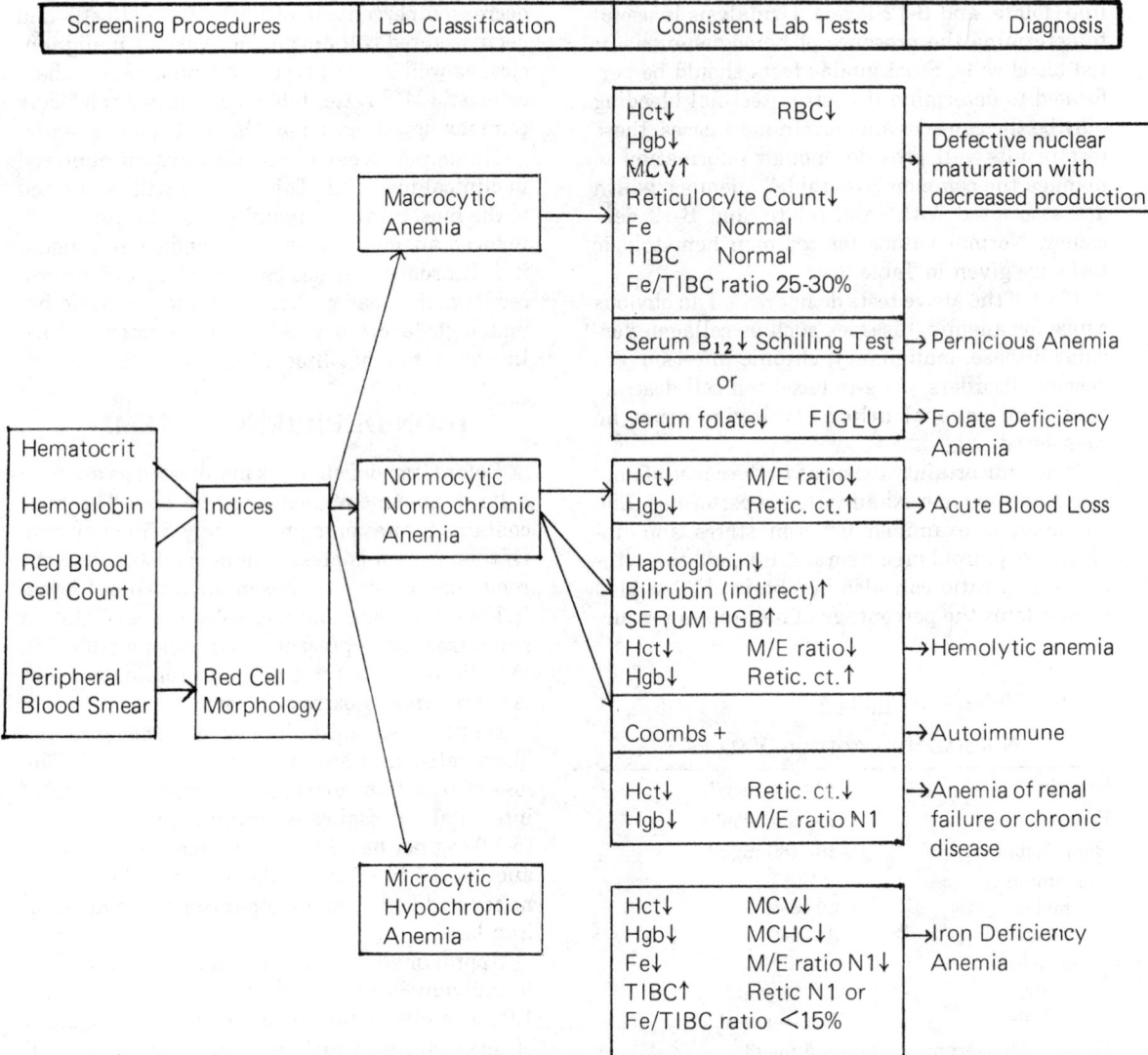

Screening Procedures	Lab Classification	Consistent Lab Tests	Diagnosis

Hematocrit
Hemoglobin
Red Blood Cell Count
Peripheral Blood Smear → Indices / Red Cell Morphology

Macrocytic Anemia:
Hct↓   RBC↓
Hgb↓
MCV↑
Reticulocyte Count↓
Fe   Normal
TIBC   Normal
Fe/TIBC ratio 25-30%
→ Defective nuclear maturation with decreased production

Serum B_{12}↓ Schilling Test → Pernicious Anemia
or
Serum folate↓   FIGLU → Folate Deficiency Anemia

Normocytic Normochromic Anemia:
Hct↓   M/E ratio↓
Hgb↓   Retic. ct.↑
→ Acute Blood Loss

Haptoglobin↓
Bilirubin (indirect)↑
SERUM HGB↑
Hct↓   M/E ratio↓
Hgb↓   Retic. ct.↑
→ Hemolytic anemia

Coombs + → Autoimmune

Hct↓   Retic. ct.↓
Hgb↓   M/E ratio N1
→ Anemia of renal failure or chronic disease

Microcytic Hypochromic Anemia:
Hct↓   MCV↓
Hgb↓   MCHC↓
Fe↓   M/E ratio N1↓
TIBC↑   Retic N1 or
Fe/TIBC ratio <15%
→ Iron Deficiency Anemia

anism. Dietary iron (which is primarily in the ferric state) is converted to the more readily absorbed ferrous form in the acid milieu of the stomach. The ferrous form is bound to the transport protein, transferrin which takes the iron to the bone marrow where it is incorporated into the hemoglobin of mature red blood cells. A portion of the iron is bound in the intestinal lumen to another protein, ferritin.

Several factors may alter the absorption of iron. Absorption is enhanced (20–30%) when storage iron is depleted or when erythropoiesis occurs at a more rapid rate. Gastrectomy, vagotomy, or antacids effectively block the conversion of the ferric form of iron to the ferrous state, thereby diminishing iron absorption. Certain foods and drugs can complex with iron and decrease its absorption. Finally, animal sources of iron are better absorbed than plant sources.

There are several causes of iron deficiency. *Blood loss,* whether it be from menstruation or another source, constitutes the most important cause of iron deficiency and subsequent anemia. One milliliter of packed red cells contains approximately 1 mg of iron and 1 ml of whole blood contains about 0.5 mg of iron. Common causes of chronic blood loss include peptic ulcer disease, hemorrhoids, ingestion of gastrointestinal irritants, menstruation, multiple pregnancies, and multiple blood donations.

Increased requirements for iron which are not met by usual dietary intakes occur in pregnant and lactating women and in children. In pregnancy, maternal iron is diverted to the fetus for production of its red blood cell mass. Maternal iron provides infants born at full term with sufficient iron stores until six months of age (1). Between six months and three years of age, children are prone to develop iron deficiency due to their threefold increase in blood volume, rapid growth, and poor dietary iron intake. Milk and certain vegetables contain relatively little iron and may also complex any ingested iron and make it unavailable for absorption. Infant cereals are fortified with iron and are excellent dietary sources for iron (see Table 4). Generally, full-term infants require about 1 mg of iron per day (2); however, premature infants do not receive their complete complement of maternal iron and require greater amounts of iron during their first year of life. If an iron deficiency develops, 10 to 20 mg of elemental iron should be administered in divided daily doses (3). Table 5 provides a listing of some pediatric iron dosage forms and the appropriate daily pediatric dose.

Inadequate dietary intake is another common

Table 4.
IRON CONTENT OF VARIOUS TYPES OF INFANT FOODS

Type of Food	Fe Content (mg/oz)
Breast milk	0.03
Whole milk	0.02
Pablum	9.0
Gerber	14.0
Vegetable purees	0.2
Meat	0.8

modified from Fairbanks (3)

contributory cause of iron deficiency. This is commonly observed in females whose caloric intakes are inadequate to meet daily iron requirements. Consequently, most women of childbearing age have depleted iron stores (300 mg) as compared to men (1000 mg). Elderly patients also have a decreased caloric intake which decreases their ingestion of iron. Additionally, their diets frequently contain large portions of cereal which contain phytates that bind iron and prevent its absorption. Alcoholics who ingest most of their calories in the form of alcohol also have inadequate intakes of iron.

Because males have larger iron stores, a greater caloric intake than women and children, and no exogenous sources of blood loss, iron deficiency is relatively uncommon. A finding of iron deficiency in this population warrants a search for an underlying disease.

Table 5.
DOSE AND IRON CONTENT OF PEDIATRIC IRON PREPARATIONS

	Trade Name	Amount (mg/ml)	Iron Content (mg/ml)	Dose to Provide 20 mg of Elemental Iron	Monthly Cost**
Ferrous Sulfate					
elixir	Feosol	44	8.8	2.3 ml qd	$3.45
drops	Fer-in-Sol	125	25	0.8 ml qd	$4.76
syrup	Fer-in Sol	18	3.6	5.6 ml qd	$4.95
Ferrous Gluconate					
elixir	Fergon	60	7	2.85 ml qd	$3.79

There are other iron preparations which may be equally efficacious. The above preparations are not being endorsed.

*Modified from Levin (1).

**Cost plus a prescription fee of $3.00. The fee will vary among pharmacies.

The cost for each drug was based on Blue Book, 1982.

1. *Iron Deficiency Anemia.* A 35-year-old woman is seen in the clinic with a chief complaint of weakness, dizziness, and epigastric pain. She has a five year history of peptic ulcer disease and uses antacids frequently. She also has a ten year history of heavy menses and chronic headaches. She has four children aged 1, 3, 5, and 7.

Current medications include tetracycline 250 mg bid for acne, allopurinol 300 mg daily for urate nephrolithiasis, daily use of aspirin for headaches, and antacids.

The review of systems is positive for decreased exercise tolerance and dysphagia with solid foods. Dysphagia has been present for the past six months.

Physical examination reveals a pale, lethargic white female appearing older than her stated age with a regular heart rate of 100 beats per minute. Her examination is notable for pale nail beds, koilonychia, and splenomegaly.

Significant laboratory results include: hemoglobin 8 gm/dl; hematocrit 27%; mean corpuscular hemoglobin concentration (MCHC) 25%; mean corpuscular volume (MCV) 24 microns^3; serum iron 35 mcg/dl; iron binding capacity (TIBC) 450 mcg/dl; serum ferritin 5 mcg/L; 4+ guaiac stools; platelet count 800,000 mm^3; reticulocyte count 0.2%.

The diagnosis of an iron deficiency anemia is made. The plan is to perform an upper GI series with a small bowel follow through (SBFT) to work-up the persistent epigastric pain.

What factors predispose this patient to iron deficiency anemia?

There are several factors present in this patient which predispose her to iron deficiency. First and foremost is blood loss. Her history of heavy menses and the 4+ stool guaiac indicate menstrual and gastrointestinal sources of blood loss. The gastrointestinal blood loss may be secondary to the patient's heavy use of salicylates and/or recurrent peptic ulcer disease.

The patient has had four children, and most women of childbearing age have a borderline iron deficiency which becomes more evident during pregnancy when 85 to 90% develop clinically significant iron deficiency (4). Iron requirements during pregnancy are approximately doubled (5,6). Thus her iron stores have been repeatedly taxed

in recent years. Lastly, her absorption of dietary iron may be inadequate. Antacids and tetracycline may complex with iron and impair absorption. (For a discussion of these potential interactions, see Question 6.)

2. Identify the signs, symptoms, and laboratory tests which are typical of iron deficiency in this patient.

This patient's constitutional symptoms of weakness and dizziness could be a result of her severe anemia. Generally, until the anemia is severe, such constitutional symptoms occur with equal frequency in the non-anemic population. The most important signs and symptoms of iron deficiency anemia are related to the cardiovascular system and are a reflection of the imbalance between the ongoing demands for oxygen against an ever diminishing oxygen supply. The patient's increased heart rate and decreased exercise tolerance are evidence of tissue anoxia and the subsequent cardiovascular response. The patient's pale nail beds and koilonychia, or spoon-shaped nails, are signs of iron deficiency anemia. Dysphagia to solid foods, as this patient described, was first noted in the early 1900's in middle-aged women with hypochromic anemia and represents a web or stricture at the junction between the hypopharynx and esophagus. The dysphagia will not be corrected by iron replacement and dilatation of the involved esophagus segment is necessary. The splenomegaly noted in this patient is a less common sign of iron deficiency and is found in approximately 10% of all patients with iron deficiency anemia.

Iron deficiency which has not yet progressed to anemia is usually diagnosed on the basis of laboratory tests, while iron deficiency with anemia may manifest itself clinically as well as chemically. The first evidence of iron deficiency is the depletion of storage iron, which is distributed primarily in the reticuloendothelial system. Ferritin, an iron storage compound, is found primarily intracellularly, but serum levels can be detected by radioimmunoassay. In the absence of liver disease and some malignancies, serum ferritin is a very sensitive indicator of iron stores (7,8). Thus, the serum ferritin and total iron-binding capacity are modified before clinical manifestations of anemia are apparent. This is illustrated by this patient. Similarly, the bone marrow is depleted of hemosiderin granules which contain approximately 25 to 30% iron.

After the depletion of iron in the storage compartment, iron is not as readily available for heme and hemoglobin synthesis, and thus the effect on erythrocyte production is manifested in the peripheral blood smear. In severe deficiency, the red blood cells become hypochromic (low mean corpuscular hemoglobin concentration—MCHC) and microcytic (low mean corpuscular volume—MCV). The indices usually do not become abnormal until the hemoglobin concentration falls below 12 gm/dl in males or 10 gm/dl in females. This patient's corpuscular indices indicate that her anemia is hypochromic and microcytic.

Other changes in the peripheral blood include neutropenia (10%), thrombocytopenia, or thrombocytosis. The latter has been reported in 50 to 75% of patients with hypochromic anemia secondary to chronic blood loss. Thrombocytosis is present in this patient; the platelet count will return to normal after treatment. The reticulocyte count is usually normal or low in iron deficiency anemia, and this patient's reticulocyte count is only 0.2% (normal: 0.5–1.5%).

Iron deficiency anemia is most commonly associated with a low serum iron and an elevated total iron-binding capacity (TIBC). If both the TIBC and serum iron are low, then these laboratory findings are more consistent with the abnormalities found in various infections, inflammatory disorders, and neoplastic states. Except when due to acute blood loss, a low serum iron in the absence of an elevated TIBC should be supplemented with a bone marrow aspiration and specific iron stain before an anemia is attributed solely to iron deficiency (9–11). This patient's low serum iron and elevated TIBC are, therefore, typical of the laboratory findings associated with iron deficiency anemia. Besides examining the absolute values reported for serum iron and TIBC, the ratio of the serum iron concentration to the TIBC should be determined [(SeFe/TIBC) × 100]. This ratio is termed the transferrin saturation ratio, and with iron deficiency this ratio falls below 15%. The patient's calculated transferrin saturation ratio is 7.8% and is consistent with iron deficiency anemia. Most clinicians begin iron therapy when the ratio is less than 10%, even if the peripheral indices (MCHC, MCV) are not abnormal.

In the workup of a microcytic, hypochromic anemia the stool should be examined for occult blood loss with a stool guaiac test. The patient's 4+ stool guaiac suggests blood loss via the gastrointestinal tract and therefore the patient is scheduled for an upper GI series.

In conclusion, the patient's signs, symptoms, and laboratory findings all support the diagnosis of an iron deficiency anemia.

3. How should this patient's iron-deficiency anemia be treated? What dosage of iron should be given?

The primary treatment of this patient should be directed toward control of the cause of anemia, which in this case is probably due to gastrointestinal blood loss. After the underlying cause has been managed, the patient should be given supplemental iron to correct the anemia and replenish her stores (12).

The usual dose of ferrous sulfate is one tablet (325 mg) three times daily between meals. Actually, one can calculate the approximate daily dose of elemental iron which is required if no iron is being lost by bleeding (13). The calculations are based upon the fact that the maximal rate of hemoglobin regeneration is about 0.256 gm/100 ml per day.

Elemental Iron (mg/day)

$$= \frac{0.25 \text{ gm Hgb}}{100 \text{ ml blood/day}} \times \frac{5000 \text{ ml}}{\text{blood}} \times \frac{3.4 \text{ mg Fe}}{1 \text{ gm Hgb}}$$

$$= \frac{40 \text{ mg Fe/day}}{20\% \text{ absorption}}$$

$$= 200 \text{ mg Fe/day}$$

$= 1000 \text{ mg } FeSO_4/\text{day since } FeSO_4 \text{ contains } 20\%$ elemental iron

$= 325 \text{ mg } FeSO_4 \text{ tid}$

This patient should receive iron therapy for approximately six months to insure adequate repletion of iron stores. During the first month of therapy, as much as 35 mg of elemental iron is absorbed daily; however, with time, a smaller percentage of iron is absorbed. By the third month, only about 5 to 10 mg of elemental iron is absorbed daily.

4. *Iron Product Selection.* Are there any major differences between iron products? Which is the product of choice?

Salt Form. A number of factors must be considered when selecting an iron product. First, the form of the iron is important, because the ferrous form is absorbed three times more readily than the ferric form. Therefore, only a ferrous salt should be selected. Several ferrous iron salts are available. Brise and Hallberg examined the absorption of ferrous sulfate, ferrous gluconate, and ferrous fumarate; on a mg for mg basis all three salts are absorbed almost equally (14). A significant difference between these three salt forms is the quantity of elemental iron each contains. Table 6 compares the number of tablets of ferrous sulfate, gluconate, and fumarate required to provide the necessary daily adult dose of 180 to 200 mg of elemental iron. If compliance is enhanced when the patient takes the smallest number of tablets, then ferrous sulfate or ferrous fumarate are the better choices.

Product formulation is of considerable importance in product selection. There is a common misbelief that the more expensive sustained-release iron preparations are inherently better. Sustained release preparations fall into three groups: (a) those claimed to increase gastrointestinal tolerance or decrease side effects, (b) those formulated to increase bioavailability, and (c) those with adjuvants claimed to enhance absorption. These preparations supposedly need only be given once daily and thus have the theoretical advantage of improving compliance.

Anecdotal claims that sustained release iron preparations cause fewer gastrointestinal side effects have not been substantiated by controlled studies (15). Furthermore, sustained release iron products tend to transport iron past the duodenum and proximal jejunum and thereby reduce

the absorption of iron (16). Thus, it is not surprising that clinical trials demonstrate poor absorption and poor hematological responses to ferrous sulfate sustained release capsules (17,18). Likewise, Ferro-Sequel, Vitron-C, Feosol Spansule, and enteric-coated ferrous sulfate release iron into gastric and duodenal fluids poorly (4,19). Fero-Gradumet is the only long-acting iron preparation which has been documented to induce an adequate hematologic response.

Many iron supplements contain adjuvants which are included in the formulation to either enhance absorption or decrease side effects. Ascorbic acid is added to some products to enhance iron absorption (20,21). Ascorbic acid maintains iron in the ferrous state and forms a soluble chelate with trivalent iron to enhance ferric iron absorption (22,23). Ascorbic acid, in doses of 500 to 1000 mg, only increases iron absorption by 10%. Doses of 100 mg of ascorbic acid do not significantly increase the absorption of iron. Table 7 lists a number of iron/vitamin C combinations. The small amount of ascorbic acid contained in these products would not be expected to significantly enhance iron's absorption, and therefore, these exceedingly expensive combinations cannot be recommended.

Other iron products contain stool softeners or other adjuvants to diminish side effects such as constipation. Generally, these products contain inadequate doses of adjuvants and/or iron and are

Table 6.

IRON CONTENT OF VARIOUS IRON SALTS

Drug	Dose (mg)	Iron Content (mg)	% Fe	Daily Dose (tablets)
Ferrous Gluconate	325 mg	37	11	6
Ferrous Fumarate	200 mg	66	33	3
Ferrous Sulfate	325 mg	65	20	3
Fero-Gradumet (slow release FeSO₄)	525 mg	105	20	2

Table 7.

HEMATINICS CONTAINING VITAMIN C

Drug	Amt. Vit. C (mg)	Amount of Elemental Iron (mg)	Cost* ($)
Fero-Grad 500	500	105	7.21
Fergon Plus	75	58	12.92
Vitron C	125	66	6.11
Mol-Iron W/C Chronospules	150	78	5.56
Theragran Hematinic	100	67	11.44
Iberet 500	500	105	12.22
Stuartinic	500	100	9.93
Ferrous Sulfate (plain)	—	65	3.49

*Based on 180–200 mg daily iron. Cost based on 1980 Redbook, including a prescription fee of $3.00.

unwarranted. Stool softeners should be pre-scribed only if needed and in the appropriate dose.

Cost is an important factor in determining the oral iron preparation of choice. Table 8 compares the relative monthly cost of various oral iron preparations. The sustained release preparations are much more expensive than ferrous sulfate, ferrous gluconate, and ferrous fumarate tablets. Thus, it is clear that the most efficacious, least expensive agents are ferrous sulfate, gluconate, or fumarate.

5. What are the goals of iron therapy? How should the patient be monitored?

The goal of therapy in the treatment of iron deficiency anemia is to correct the hemoglobin and hematocrit and replete iron stores (24). This process requires approximately six months of oral iron therapy.

If doses of elemental iron are adequate, the re-ticulocyte response may begin within four days and peak between the seventh and tenth day of therapy. Thereafter, the reticulocyte count falls off rapidly to normal after 15 days of therapy (24). Therefore, the most convenient index to monitor in outpatients is the hemoglobin response. The hemoglobin should be increased by 2 gm/dl and the hematocrit by 6% in three weeks.

Table 8.

COMPARATIVE COST OF VARIOUS
IRON PREPARATIONS

Drug	Amt. (mg)	Iron Content (mg)	Monthly Cost ($)
Ferrous Sulfate	325	65	3.49
Ferrous Gluconate	325	37	4.65
Ferrous Fumarate	200	66	3.13
Ferrous Sulfate (enteric coat)	325	65	3.99
Feosol tablets	200	60	3.56
Feosol Spansules	167	50	10.72
Ferronord	250	40	14.70
Fero-Gradumet	525	105	6.51
Mol-Iron Chronosule	390	78	9.79

Determined on the basis of 180–200 mg daily of ele-mental iron plus a prescription fee of $3.00. The fee will vary among pharmacies. The cost for each drug was based on American Druggist Redbook, 1980.

6. *Patient Information.* What kind of information should be transmitted to the patient upon dispensing oral iron?

This patient has four children. It is important that she understand that iron is a very poisonous drug (see Poisonings chapter). Iron should be dis-pensed in a childproof container and should be stored in a locked cabinet away from her children.

The patient should be told that oral iron ther-apy will produce black stools. In fact, compliance can be determined by the presence of black stools and/or constipation. If these changes are not pres-ent, then the patient is probably not taking her medication (25).

Iron tablets should be taken on an empty stom-ach, because meals can decrease absorption by 40 to 50% (26). On the other hand, if gastric intol-erance to iron does occur and strategies to de-crease intolerance fail (Question 7), the patient can be instructed to take the iron with meals. Since a smaller percentage of iron is absorbed with increasing doses (21,27,28), iron should be given in divided doses rather than one large daily dose. The doses should be spaced at least four hours apart, because the absorption of oral iron returns to normal four hours after the last dose (29). Consumption of fad diets may impair ab-sorption of iron. Certain foods containing oxa-lates, phytates (spinach), and phosphate complex with iron and inhibit its absorption (27).

Several potential drug interactions exist for this patient, and she should be counselled as to the proper way of taking her various medications. She is taking *antacids* which may decrease iron ab-sorption; therefore, she should be advised to take her iron one hour before the antacid dose. The mechanism of this interaction is unknown, but it may be that the antacid forms an insoluble com-plex with iron. This interaction has been reported with antacids containing calcium, magnesium, and aluminum cations (30). Antacids theoretically will also prevent conversion of ferric ion to the re-duced, absorbable ferrous state. Further docu-mentation of the clinical significance of this iron-antacid interaction is needed, but based on the available literature, it is advisable to space the iron and antacid doses apart. The patient has been prescribed *tetracycline* for the treatment of acne. The absorption of both iron and tetracycline is decreased when they are administered concomi-tantly. When the two drugs must be taken to-gether, the iron should be taken three hours before or two hours after the tetracycline dose (31). Lastly, the patient has been prescribed *allopurinol*. The manufacturer states that iron and allopurinol should not be used together, because the latter has been shown to increase hepatic storage of iron in animals. Short-term and long-term allopurinol therapy has not produced an increase in iron absorption, serum iron levels, liver storage, or an alteration of ferro-kinetics. Therefore, the clinical significance of this drug-drug interaction is minimal and should not deter the clinician from treating iron deficiency with ferrous sulfate (32–35).

7. *Gastric Intolerance.* The patient described above was given ferrous sulfate 325 mg to be taken four times a day. Based on a friend's recommendation, she took 3 grams of vitamin C with each dose of iron. Two weeks later she returns to clinic complaining of severe nausea and epigastric pain. What factors are involved in gastrointestinal side effects from iron, and how can these side effects be decreased?

Gastrointestinal side effects of oral iron include nausea, epigastric pain, constipation, abdominal cramps, and diarrhea. Constipation does not appear to be related to dose, but side effects such as nausea and epigastric pain occur more frequently as the quantity of soluble elemental iron in contact with the stomach and duodenum increases. Many studies comparing the incidence of gastrointestinal effects caused by various iron salts have not been well controlled. However, a double-blind controlled study (36) compared an equal quantity (222 mg of elemental iron per day) administered as one of three salts, gluconate, fumarate, or sulfate to placebo. The incidence of gastrointestinal side effects with placebo was 13%. Each of the three iron salts caused a 25% incidence of gastrointestinal side effects. Therefore, no difference in gastrointestinal side effects among these three salts was seen when equivalent elemental doses of iron were administered. In another study (37), about 15% of patients taking 200 mg daily of elemental iron reported gastrointestinal intolerance; none of these patients experienced this problem with daily doses of 100 mg of elemental iron.

Many patients tolerate the equivalent of 180 mg of elemental iron daily. If gastric intolerance to oral iron does occur, it would be advisable to utilize the technique first popularized by Pierre

Blaud in 1832. Oral iron therapy is begun with a single tablet of ferrous sulfate 325 mg daily and the dose is gradually increased in increments of one tablet per day every two to three days until a full therapeutic dose of ferrous sulfate 325 mg three times daily is reached.

The patient in question was prescribed a high dose of elemental iron, approximately 240 mg per day, and this high dose could certainly be responsible for the epigastric pain the patient was experiencing. The patient's concomitant use of vitamin C with the iron further increased the quantity of iron absorbed and contributed to the severe gastrointestinal discomfort she described. The vitamin C therapy should be discontinued and the dosing of ferrous sulfate decreased to three times a day. If necessary, Blaud's technique of incremental increases in dose should be employed.

8. *Parenteral Iron Therapy.* B.T., a 60-year-old male, is seen in the emergency room with a chief complaint of black stools and progressive weakness over the last two months. He has a 30-year history of regional enteritis and a one-year history of osteoarthritis which is being treated with ibuprofen (Motrin).

Significant laboratory results are hemoglobin 8 gm/dl; hematocrit 24.2%; serum iron 34 mcg/dl; iron binding capacity (TIBC) 418 mcg/dl; 3+ guaiac stools; peripheral smear— hypochromic, microcytic red cells, and an increase in nucleated red cells.

The diagnosis of an iron deficiency is made. The physician prescribes ferrous sulfate 325 mg three times a day. Two weeks later the patient returns to his physician's office. The patient complains of severe epigastric pain which he attributes to the iron. Laboratory studies reveal a reticulocyte count of 1% and a hemoglobin of 8 gm/dl, unchanged from two weeks ago.

What factors are present in this patient which would contribute to a treatment failure with oral iron therapy?

The patient may be experiencing continued blood loss secondary to his use of ibuprofen. The patient's non-steroidal antiinflammatory agent should be stopped and the patient switched temporarily to enteric coated aspirin or another non-steroidal agent. The patient's guaiac positive stools require further diagnostic work-up.

The patient's inflammatory bowel disease could have resulted in a malabsorption of the iron. Additionally, the patient is probably noncompliant, since the oral iron caused severe epigastric pain.

9. Can parenteral iron be used to treat this patient's iron deficiency? Which preparation and route would be preferable?

Although oral iron therapy is generally preferred, parenteral iron is indicated in specific situations as illustrated by this case. Patients with malabsorption syndromes (eg, sprue), duodenal or upper small intestine resection, ulcerative colitis, regional enteritis, patients with continued blood loss with inadequate maintenance of hemoglobin values by oral iron, and non-compliant patients are candidates for parenteral therapy.

Available intramuscular preparations include iron-dextran (Imferon) and iron sorbitex (Jectofer). Iron sorbitex is only given intramuscularly, because iron from this complex is readily mobilized and may be toxic if given intravenously. To prevent iron overload, no more than 100 mg of iron sorbitex should be given at one time. Iron-dextran (Imferon) is a much more tightly bound complex and is more slowly released; it is the preferred product (38).

One concern does exist regarding the use of parenteral iron in this particular patient. The patient carries the diagnosis of osteoarthritis. Rheumatoid arthritis should be ruled out, because the administration of iron-dextran to patients with rheumatoid arthritis may exacerbate their symptoms (39). The explanation for this adverse effect is unclear, but it appears to be related to a delayed hypersensitivity reaction to the dextran in Imferon. During exacerbations of symptoms, the erythrocyte sedimentation rate increases. Although well-controlled studies are lacking, caution should be exercised when using iron dextran in this group of patients. Block (40) claims that 80 to 90% of patients with active inflammatory disease will develop severe reactions.

Iron-dextran can be given by the intravenous or intramuscular route, but the intramuscular route possesses certain disadvantages. Intramuscular iron-dextran must be given by deep injection into the gluteal mass using a Z-track technique. Staining and pain at the site of injection are commonly encountered. Other problems of IM injection of iron include slow absorption of the drug from the muscle, sterile abscesses, and hematomas. Additionally, intramuscular iron-dextran may cause localized sarcomas (41). The maximum volume of iron-dextran which can be

administered into one intramuscular site is 2 ml (100 mg iron). Thus, many injections are needed to complete a single course of therapy.

In contrast, intravenous administration of iron-dextran avoids many of the above problems of intramuscular injection. Systemic reactions are not more common but include fever, chills, backache, myalgia, dizziness, syncope, rash, urticaria, and anaphylaxis. Despite published opinions to the contrary, intravenous iron-dextran is not clinically more allergenic than the intramuscular preparation. In fact, if a patient is allergic to iron-dextran, the intravenous infusion can be stopped immediately, whereas the absorption of iron-dextran from IM sites continues over a prolonged period. Reactions resulting from IM injections will therefore be more difficult to control (42–44).

10. What is the total dose of parenteral iron-dextran needed for B.T. to restore hemoglobin to normal and replenish iron stores? (B.T. weighs 60 kg, his hemoglobin is 8 gm/dl, and his hematocrit is 24.2%.)

Several formulas can be used to calculate iron deficits (38,43,45). One formula used to calculate the iron dose is:

$$\text{Iron deficit (mg)} = (\text{wt in kg})(70 \text{ ml/kg})(0.45 - \frac{\text{Hct}}{100}) \quad \text{(Eq. 1)}$$

where Hct is the observed hematocrit. This equation calculates the packed RBC deficit in milliliters and is based upon the assumption that for each ml of blood which is lost, 1 mg of iron must be replaced. This is derived from the following information:

a. Blood volume is equal to 70 ml/kg.
b. Each gram of hemoglobin contains 0.35% iron. If the mean corpuscular hemoglobin concentration (Hgb/Hct $\times$ 100) is assumed to be 33 gm/dl of packed RBC's, then each milliliter or gram of packed RBC's contains approximately 1 mg of iron.

An additional amount of iron equalling 10 mg/kg (minimum 600 mg) must be added to this calculated amount to replete iron stores.

A second method of calculating total doses of iron is as follows:

$$\text{Total iron (mg)} = (0.3)(\text{wt in lbs})(100 - \frac{100\text{Hgb}}{14.8}) \quad \text{(Eq. 2)}$$

where Hgb is the patient's observed hemoglobin in gm/dl. Eq. 2 provides the total dose of iron necessary to replete stores and correct the hemo-globin in one calculation and is the more com-monly utilized formula.

The last method of calculating total iron dose is:

$$\text{Total iron (gm)} = (0.255)(14.8 - \text{observed Hgb}) \qquad \text{(Eq. 3)}$$

Eq. 3 is based on an average 70 kg individual and assumes that 0.255 gm iron must be replaced for each gram of hemoglobin deficit. It does not take into account variations in weight and attendant alterations in blood volume.

The following chart compares total dose cal-culations for iron obtained at various body weights.

Weight (kg)	Eq. 1 (mg)	Eq. 2* (mg)	Eq. 3 (mg)
50	1083	1516	1734
60	1180	1819	1734
70	1376	2130	1734
80	1573	2425	1734

*Calculations include stores.

Eq. 2 possesses certain advantages compared with Eq. 1 and 3. It allows one to calculate the total dose of iron, including stores, in one simple step and it includes body weight as a variable in the calculation of the required iron dose. Utiliz-ing Eq. 2, B.T. will require 1,819 mg of parenteral iron-dextran.

11. It is decided to administer the entire dose of Imferon at once. What parenteral form of Imferon should be employed to prepare an intravenous total dose infusion? What pre-cautions should be taken?

Two dosage forms of Imferon are available and both contain 50 mg of elemental iron per milli-liter. One is supplied in multiple dose vials and contains phenol 0.5% as a preservative. The pack-age insert warns that this multidose vial should only be used for intramuscular injection. If a total dose of iron-dextran (2.0 gm or 40 ml) from this dosage form were given to a patient, the amount of phenol given would be 200 mg. Phenol is well absorbed from any route of administration, and systemic reactions consist of respiratory insuffi-ciency, central nervous system depression and circulatory failure (46). The toxic dose of phenol for adults is estimated to be 8 to 15 gm (47). Thus, a 200 mg dose of phenol is unlikely to produce

systemic toxicity, but it would be prudent to avoid the phenol. Imferon is also available in ampules without preservatives and should be used for all IV Imferon dosing.

There are two methods of administering the total dose of parenteral iron: by infusion and by bolus injection of the undiluted drug. Unfortu-nately, neither of the parenteral iron products commercially available in the United States is FDA approved for total dose intravenous infu-sion. The package insert for iron-dextran (Im-feron) only provides instructions for the intrave-nous administration of a maximum dose of 2 ml per day (45). A 70 kg individual would require ten to fifteen days of such therapy to receive his total dose. The insert guidelines are in dramatic opposition to the actual clinical practice of total dose intravenous infusion or bolus administra-tion. Though no data are available which indicate increased hazards with total dose administration, the clinician must recognize that this mode of administration is not approved by the Food and Drug Administration.

There does exist a very small risk that par-enteral iron-dextran may cause systemic side ef-fects such as thrombophlebitis, flushing, head-ache, nausea, vomiting, bronchospasm, urticaria and arthralgia, and intravenous infusions of iron-dextran should be given in a manner that avoids or minimizes systemic reactions. Moderate to se-vere local phlebitis occurs in 5% of patients (48). This incidence can be reduced to 2% if normal saline is used as the diluent. Mild phlebitis occurs in 15 to 25% of patients. The incidence of phebitis is also minimized if the infusion time is confined to 4 to 5 hours (43,49). Phlebitis has not occurred after direct IV injection of undiluted iron dextran. Concomitant administration of heparin and hy-drocortisone do not decrease the incidence of gen-eralized reactions (43,49). Anaphylactoid reac-tions have been reported but are extremely rare. These reactions include bronchospasm, urticaria, and severe dyspnea. These symptoms respond readily to the intravenous administration of 0.3 to 0.4 ml of 1:1000 epinephrine plus 1000 mg hy-drocortisone phosphate for shock, if present.

Intravenous infusion of iron-dextran has re-cently become very popular, but it appears that direct intravenous injection of undiluted iron dex-tran is equally efficacious and safe. Direct IV in-jection should not be given any faster than 50 mg/minute. The following protocol applies to both infusion and direct intravenous injection and will minimize systemic reactions (42,49):

a. Exclude allergic patients (ie, asthmatics).

b. Precede infusion or injection by an antihistamine one-half hour before administration.

c. For infusion, dilute iron-dextran in normal saline (if possible) or 5% dextrose to make a concentration not exceeding 5 gm/dl (50 mg/ml). Use an infusion set which delivers 60 drops per milliliter.

d. Give a test dose: Infusion—10 drops/minute for 20 minutes under supervision.

e. Increase the infusion rate to 45 drops/minute provided no reaction occurs.

f. The direct injection should be given slowly and should not exceed 50 mg/minute.

12. Describe the predicted hematological response from intravenous iron-dextran. Does it produce a response which differs from oral or intramuscular iron replacement?

The rate of hemoglobin regeneration is essentially equivalent whether iron is given orally, intramuscularly, or intravenously. The anticipated response to oral or intramuscular iron replenishment is a two- to three-fold increase in marrow production (50). At steady state, intravenous iron also increases marrow production two to three times normal; however, a transient increase in marrow production of as much as four to eight times normal may occur during the first 7 to 10 days after an intravenous infusion. Thus, the response rate following intravenous administration may be slightly faster (43,50).

The reticulocyte count increases by about the fourth day, usually peaks at 5 to 15% in about a week, and returns to normal about one week later. The rate of rise in hemoglobin is approximately 1 gm/dl per week; the hemoglobin usually peaks about eight weeks after either parenteral or oral iron therapy. (Also see Question 5.)

MEGALOBLASTIC ANEMIAS

Megaloblastic anemias are characterized by impaired DNA synthesis which results in *ineffective erythropoiesis*. Megaloblastic red blood cells tend to be destroyed in the bone marrow in excessive numbers. The red blood cells that emerge from the bone marrow are large and oval in appearance. The most common causes of megalo-

blastic anemias are deficiencies in vitamin B-12 and/or folic acid.

Vitamin B-12 Deficiency Anemia

The normal body stores of vitamin B-12 are approximately 4000 mcg. Since the minimum daily requirement is only about 2 mcg per day, several years must elapse before deficiency occurs. Vitamin B-12 is fairly ubiquitous in our diets. It is found in all animal products (meat and dairy products). Except in strict vegetarians, dietary insufficiency is rarely a cause of vitamin B-12 deficiency. Impaired absorption is the usual cause.

The absorption of vitamin B-12 occurs by two processes: passive diffusion and complexing with intrinsic factor. Passive diffusion operates independently of intrinsic factor and is important only when vitamin B-12 is present in greater than normal concentrations. Intrinsic factor binds vitamin B-12 and prevents degradation by gastrointestinal microorganisms.

After vitamin B-12 is absorbed, it is bound to a specific beta-globulin and transported to the liver and other organs. Fifty to ninety percent of the total body stores of B-12 are found in the liver. Vitamin B-12 is then converted in the liver to co-enzyme B-12; co-enzyme B-12 has a variety of metabolic functions which include hematopoiesis, maintenance of myelin throughout the entire nervous system, and production of all epithelial cells.

Although 3–8 mcg of vitamin B-12 are excreted into the gastrointestinal tract daily by biliary excretion, only 1 mcg per day is lost in the feces. At an intraluminal pH greater than 6.0, intrinsic factor binds with the majority of the excreted vitamin B-12, and this bound B-12 is then reabsorbed in the terminal ileum. Daily urinary losses of vitamin B-12 are exceedingly small (at the most, approximately 0.2 mcg per day).

Classical vitamin B-12 deficiency, or pernicious anemia, represents an inherited or acquired lack of intrinsic factor. Without intrinsic factor, vitamin B-12 absorption and reabsorption cannot occur. Autoantibodies directed against the gastric mucosa have been noted in some patients with pernicious anemia. Another situation in which a vitamin B-12 deficiency anemia will develop is after total gastrectomy. This surgical procedure removes the source of intrinsic factor, and subsequently the same hematological and neurological abnormalities as seen in pernicious anemia will ensue. Other factors which may lead to vitamin B-12 deficiency include fish tapeworm infestation and small bowel bacterial overgrowth in patients with blind loops, strictures, or diverticuli. In both instances, the worm or bacteria compete with the human host for vitamin B-12. Rarely, drugs may lead to vitamin B-12 malabsorption (Table 9). Once intrinsic factor and/or vitamin B-12 are no longer available, a gradual decline occurs in vitamin B-12 stores. The onset of the pernicious anemia is insidious. In most instances two of the following diagnostic triad of symptoms are encountered: weakness, sore tongue, and numbness or tingling in the extremities. Anorexia, pallor, or pale yellow complexion, and shortness of breath on exertion are also bothersome and may overshadow the diagnostic triad. In addition, the patient usually has not felt well for the past six months to a year.

Schilling Test. The diagnosis of pernicious anemia is substantiated by evaluation of the absorption of vitamin B-12 (Schilling Test). A radioactive tracer dose of vitamin B-12 is given orally, and the measurement of urinary excretion of radioactivity reveals the degree of absorption. In patients with pernicious anemia, 0 to 7% of the administered dose is excreted. The normal range is 15 to 40%. The patient should be fasted overnight and urine collected for 24 hours. Since very little radioactivity will be excreted, 100 mcg of unlabeled vitamin B-12 is given parenterally two hours after the oral dose to serve as a "flushing dose." This allows the excretion of radioactive B-12. This test cannot be performed in patients with severe renal dysfunction since the excretion of labeled vitamin B-12 depends on an adequate urinary output and an accurate urine collection (51–53).

13. *Pernicious Anemia.* D.L. is a 60-year-old, blue-eyed male of Norwegian descent who is seen by his private physician because of a one-year history of weakness and emotional instability. The patient also complains of a painful tongue, alternating constipation and diarrhea, and feet feeling like "pins and needles."

The pertinent findings on physical examination are: pallor, pronounced yellow coloration of the patient's skin; scleral icterus; beefy, red tongue; loss of vibratory sense in his lower extremities; disturbed position sense; muscle weakness; and ataxia.

Significant laboratory findings include: hemoglobin 7 gm/dl; hematocrit 22%; MCV 105 microns[3]; MCHC 32%; poikilocytosis and anisocytosis on smear; WBC 4200/mm[3]; platelets 105,000/mm[3]; serum iron 80 mcg/dl; TIBC 300 mcg/dl; serum vitamin B-12 100 pg/ml; serum folate 10 mcg/ml; Schilling test less than 4% excretion.

What signs, symptoms, and laboratory findings are typical of pernicious anemia in this patient?

Signs and Symptoms. D.L.'s signs and symptoms are classical for pernicious anemia. Pernicious anemia remains the most common cause of megaloblastic anemia in temperate climates. Among individuals of Scandinavian, English, and Irish ancestry, the incidence is 0.13%. The disease occurs equally in both sexes, and the average age of onset is 60 years. Pernicious anemia develops as a result of inability of the stomach to secrete intrinsic factor, and characteristic findings include megaloblastic anemia, neurological damage, and diminished or abolished secretion of gastric juice. D.L.'s yellow skin and scleral icterus, his painful and red tongue, his loss of vibratory sense in his lower extremities, vertigo, his emotional symptoms, and his GI symptoms are all typical.

Laboratory Findings. The significantly elevated MCV (macrocytosis) suggests the presence of a megaloblastic anemia. The serum folate and vitamin B-12 should always be evaluated when the MCV is elevated. In this case, the serum folate is normal, but the B-12 level is low (see Table 2).

Table 9.

DRUGS WHICH DECREASE ABSORPTION OF VITAMIN B$_{12}$

Drug	% of Patients with Decreased B$_{12}$ absorption	Ref.
Colchicine	92	(68)
KCl tablets (slow release)	36	(69)
Anticonvulsants	—	(70)
Phenformin	46	(71)
Neomycin	—	(72)
p-aminosalicylic acid	—	(73)

Megaloblastic anemias are characterized by ineffective erythropoiesis. The poikilocytosis and anisocytosis observed in the blood smear indicate that the erythrocytes are of abnormal shape and size, respectively. In a megaloblastic anemia such as seen in this patient, the bone marrow suffers from a maturation arrest and is subsequently filled with precursors of platelets and of the myeloid (white blood) series. Peripherally, a leukopenia and thrombocytopenia may be noted as in this patient's case. The patient's low serum B-12 level (100 pg/ml) is indicative of pernicious anemia, and the diagnosis is confirmed by the results of the Schilling Test (less than 4% excretion in this case).

14. How should this patient's pernicious anemia be treated?

This patient should receive parenteral vitamin B-12 in sufficient doses to provide not only the daily requirement of approximately 2 mcg, but also about 2000 to 5000 mcg (average 4000 mcg) to replenish liver stores.

Since 30% of vitamin B-12 is bound to plasma transcobalamin I and cellular binding sites, single intravenous and intramuscular doses in excess of 100 mcg exceed the binding capacity, resulting in rapid renal excretion of the unbound fraction (56). Intramuscular administration of vitamin B-12 leads to slower systemic absorption and greater retention of this vitamin such that 11% of cyanocobalamin and 33% of hydroxycobalamin remain 28 days after administration of a 100 mcg dose (57).

Even though hydroxycobalamin provides higher and more sustained blood levels than cyanocobalamin, there is no clinical evidence that it is any more effective in normalizing the hematocrit (58). In fact, hydroxycobalamin administration has been associated with the development of transcobalamin II—vitamin B-12 complex antibodies; therefore hydroxycobalamin therapy is not recommended (59). Despite the common belief that cyanocobalamin therapy must be initiated with a loading dose of 1000 mcg of cyanocobalamin daily for several days, this practice is unnecessary. As previously indicated, ninety percent of this loading dose is excreted due to the saturation of transcobalamin and tissue binding sites. Rather, in the treatment of this patient's pernicious anemia, 100 mcg of IM cyanocobalamin should be given daily for two to three weeks in order to replete stores (60). The patient's reticulocyte count

should be monitored to assure that appropriate hematological response occurs. After repletion of stores, life-long cyanocobalamin therapy is needed to maintain these stores. Cyanocobalamin 100 mcg IM is then administered every two to four weeks for life. To assess the adequacy of therapy, serum vitamin B-12 and peripheral blood counts should be obtained every three to six months.

15. What factors affect the oral absorption of vitamin B-12? Compare oral products available. Is oral vitamin B-12 therapy an effective alternative to parenteral therapy?

The maximal amount of vitamin B-12 which can be absorbed from a single oral dose or meal is 2 to 3 mcg, although 5 to 15 mcg of this vitamin is absorbed daily from the average American diet. The percent of vitamin B-12 absorbed decreases with increasing doses. Absorption of a 1–2 mcg dose is 50%; absorption of a 20 mcg dose is 5% (61). Doses of 100 mcg or more must be ingested to absorb 5 mcg of vitamin B-12. Refractoriness to oral vitamin B-12 occurs and is due to antibody production against vitamin B-12-intrinsic factor substances derived from hog mucosa (62). Therefore, preparations containing hog mucosal intrinsic factor are ineffective (see Table 10).

Some of the preparations listed in Table 10 do not contain intrinsic factor derived from hog mucosa, and successful treatment of pernicious anemia with high dose oral cyanocobalamin therapy has been reported (63). However, because of the risk of non-compliance and subsequent serious adverse consequences, oral vitamin B-12 therapy cannot be routinely recommended. Oral vitamin B-12 should be reserved for those patients in whom hemorrhagic complications from parenteral B-12 therapy are a significant risk. Patients receiving

Table 10.

ORAL VITAMIN B_{12} PREPARATIONS

Preparation	Amount B-12 (mcg)	Intrinsic Factor (hog mucosa)
Vitamin B-12 (various)	10–1000	No
Redisol	50	No
Trophite	12	No
Trinsicon	15	Yes
Lextron	2	Yes
Ferro-Zem	15	Yes

oral vitamin B-12 therapy should be monitored more frequently to ensure compliance with therapy.

16. What is the expected response to therapy with vitamin B-12? How should D.L. be monitored?

If therapy is administered in optimal doses described above and no complicating disease is present, the patient will become more alert within 48 hours. The soreness of tongue also usually improves within 48 hours, and the tongue returns to normal after two to three weeks (64). Reticulocytosis is related to the degree of anemia, but usually values peak after five to eight days of therapy. At this time the hematocrit begins to increase and returns to normal values after four to eight weeks of treatment (65). Since vitamin B-12 deficiency can result in irreversible neurological damage, neurological symptoms may not be fully corrected even by optimal therapy.

17. *Anemias after Gastrectomy.* A patient has just undergone a total gastrectomy for recurrent non-healing ulcers. What form(s) of anemia would be expected to develop in a post-gastrectomy patient? Should he receive prophylactic vitamin B-12?

Partial or total gastrectomy often results in anemia (66,67). Most commonly a microcytic, hypochromic anemia due to *iron deficiency* develops. Iron deficiency in gastrectomy patients occurs due to lack of gastric acid which normally enhances iron's absorption by increasing conversion of iron to the ferrous state.

Vitamin B-12 deficiency anemia will most certainly occur in this patient. After a total gastrectomy, the source of intrinsic factor secretion is lost, and oral vitamin B-12 absorption will be impaired. The hematological and neurological abnormalities associated with B-12 deficiency will not develop for 760 to 900 days, the time required to deplete the existing vitamin B-12 stores. Parenteral prophylactic vitamin B-12 should be administered to this post-total gastrectomy patient following the guidelines discussed in Question 14.

The patient may also develop a *folate deficiency* in association with the vitamin B-12 deficiency, because vitamin B-12-dependent synthesis of methionine is blocked. Folate, which is normally converted to active tetrahydrofolate during methionine synthesis, becomes "trapped" as inactive N-5 methyl tetrahydrofolate. Thus, a modest, functional deficiency of folate coenzymes develops. The patient's folate level should be checked annually to screen for folate deficiency.

Folic Acid Deficiency Anemia

Folate is abundant in virtually all food sources, especially fresh green vegetables, yeast, and liver. However, prolonged cooking destroys folate. The average American diet provides 50 to 2000 mcg of folate per day. The minimum daily adult requirement is 50 mcg, but because absorption is less than complete, 200 mcg of folate is the recommended daily intake. Folate requirements are increased in conditions in which the metabolic rate and rate of cellular division are increased (eg, pregnancy, infection, hemolytic anemia). The daily requirement during pregnancy is 400 mcg; the requirement during lactation is 300 mcg.

Dietary folic acid (FA) is in the polyglutamate form and must be enzymatically deconjugated in the gastrointestinal tract to the monoglutamate form before it is absorbed. Once absorbed, the inactive dihydrofolate (FH_2) must be converted to active tetrahydrofolate (FH_4, folinic acid) by dihydrofolate reductase (DHRF). Folate coenzymes are concerned with nearly all mammalian metabolic systems in which there is a transfer of a one-carbon unit.

In contrast to the body's large stores of vitamin B-12, the body's folate stores are relatively small, approximately 5 to 10 mg. Therefore, deficiency and subsequent megaloblastic anemia may occur within three to four months of abolishment of folate intake.

There are three situations in which folate deficiency is most commonly observed. In *alcoholics,* the daily intake of the folate contained in food may be restricted or absent, and the recirculation of folate through the enterohepatic cycle may be impaired due to alcohol's untoward effect on hepatic cells. Folate deficiency may develop during *the third trimester of pregnancy* as a result of a marginal diet and the rapid metabolism of the fetus. In any condition of *rapid cellular turnover* (eg, hemolytic anemias, hemoglobinopathies, sideroblastic anemia, leukemias, multiple myeloma) and a marginal diet, folate deficiency will develop because folate coenzymes are involved in so many metabolic pathways. Folate deficiency may also occur with chronic hemodialysis, diseases which impair absorption from the small intestine (eg, regional enteritis), extensive jejunal resections, or drugs that inhibit dihydrofolate reductase (eg, methotrexate).

Diagnosis of folate deficiency is important before therapy is initiated, because large doses of folate can reverse the hematological abnormalities caused by vitamin B-12 deficiency without correcting the neurological damage. Thus, the indiscriminate use of "shotgun hematinic" preparations is dangerous.

18. Folate Deficiency Anemia. R.P. is a 42-year-old male with a 15-year history of alcohol abuse and a five-year history of seizure disorder. The patient complains of weakness, indigestion, and diarrhea. Pertinent laboratory data include: hematocrit 26%, MCV 103 microns³, MCHC 31%, serum folate 2 mcg/ml, serum vitamin B-12 250 pg/ml, reticulocyte count 1%, platelet count 95,000/mm³, WBC 4200/mm³. Current medications include phenytoin 400 mg daily and phenobarbital 90 mg daily. Alcohol consumption is approximately one quart of whiskey per day. The diagnosis is folate deficiency anemia. What laboratory findings typical of folate deficiency are illustrated by this patient? What other laboratory findings would be expected?

This case illustrates many of the laboratory findings typical of folic acid deficiency anemia, including a severely depressed serum folate level, macrocytosis, a low reticulocyte count, and low white blood cell and platelet counts. Other laboratory findings not described in this patient, but characteristic of folic acid deficiency are: hypersegmentation of mature granulocytes, a hypercellular bone marrow with M/E ratio 1:1 or less, anisocytosis, and poikilocytosis (93). A more definitive diagnostic test to evaluate folate body stores is the red blood cell folate. Red cell folate levels generally better reflect tissue stores of folate than do serum levels. The red cell folate generally correlates better with the degree of anemia and is less prone to interference than the serum assay (94). Unfortunately, red cell folate assays are not as readily available as serum assays.

19. What factors predisposed R.P. to this folate deficiency anemia?

Alcoholism may lead to a poor diet with a resultant nutritional folate deficiency (75). Alcoholism, and more specifically cirrhosis, may result in a decreased ability of the liver to store folate and in an increased urinary excretion of folate. In addition, R.P.'s anticonvulsant therapy may have contributed to his folate deficiency. Phenytoin can produce a malabsorption of folate (76).

20. Drug-Induced Folate Deficiency. What other drugs may cause folate deficiency?

Like phenytoin, many other "group A" drugs (see Fig. 1 and Table 11) lower serum folate by inhibiting deconjugase enzymes in the gastrointestinal tract (76–78,100). Usually drugs which lead to malabsorption of folate do not produce megaloblastic changes in red blood cells except when high doses are given for prolonged periods of time or when pretreatment folate stores are already decreased (79). Decreased serum folate occurs in 75% of patients taking anticonvulsants (77,80). Folate deficiency induced by "group A" drugs may be treated or prevented with the administration of 1 mg folic acid daily since all pharmaceutical folate products are in the readily absorbable monoglutamate form.

Other drugs ("group B" drugs; see Fig. 1 and Table 11) may produce altered folate metabolism

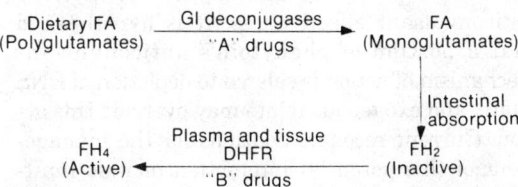

Figure 1. Sites of action for drugs which induce a folate deficiency.

Table 11.

DRUGS WHICH ALTER SERUM FOLATE LEVELS

Group A Drugs	Ref.	Group B Drugs	Ref.
Malabsorption		*Folate Antagonism*	
Phenytoin	76	Methotrexate	89
Primidone	77	Pyrimethamine	90
Barbiturates	77	Pentamidine	83
Oral contraceptives		Trimethoprim	81,91
(with mestranol)	78	Triamterene	92
Ethanol	83		
Isoniazid	87		
Cycloserine	87		
Glutethimide	88		

by binding to intracellular dihydrofolate reductase (DHFR), thus blocking the formation of active tetrahydrofolate. In mammalian cells, this effect is significant only with high doses (81) or when the patient is already deficient in folate. Methotrexate is the most potent inhibitor of DHFR, but megaloblastic anemia does not occur when leucovorin rescue (folinic acid) is employed with methotrexate.

21. How should R.P.'s folate deficiency anemia be treated?

The estimated total body folate store is 5 to 10 mg. Therefore, 1 mg of folic acid given daily for two to three weeks should be more than adequate to replace this patient's storage pool of folate. The patient should then be reassessed after the course of therapy to determine response to therapy and to determine if the cause of the folate deficiency has been corrected. Since the patient is maintained on chronic phenytoin therapy, supplementation with folic acid 1 mg daily will probably be required as long as the patient remains on the anticonvulsant. Some hypothetical and clinical data suggest that folic acid may increase the metabolism of phenytoin and decrease phenytoin's anticonvulsant effectiveness. It is hypothesized that a portion of phenytoin's anticonvulsant mechanism of action is related to depletion of CNS folate, and exogenous folate may override this action. Current recommendations for the management of this potential interaction include limiting the daily dose of folate to 1 mg orally and observing the patient for increased frequency of seizures (95–97).

22. What are the goals of therapy, and what response to therapy should be anticipated?

The goals of therapy are the correction of anemia, improvement in constitutional symptoms, and abolishment of diarrhea. With the institution of folate therapy, diarrhea should reverse within several days. A reticulocyte response will begin in three to five days with a peak response in five to ten days. The hematocrit will begin to rise about two weeks after institution of therapy (93).

ANEMIA OF CHRONIC DISEASE

23. A 46-year-old woman with a 10-year history of seropositive rheumatoid arthritis is being seen for her routine examination. A complete blood count includes the following data: hemoglobin 10.3 gm/dl, hematocrit 33%, MCV 80 microns³, and MCHC 30%. The peripheral smear shows normochromic and normocytic cells. The patient's only complaints are waxing and waning arthralgias and morning stiffness. Her only medication is enteric coated aspirin 975 mg four times a day. What is the most likely cause of this patient's anemia? What is the appropriate treatment?

From the data provided, this appears to be an anemia of chronic disease. This anemia is generally normocytic, normochromic and develops when a disease has persisted for longer than one or two months. Diseases associated with anemia of chronic disease include chronic infections (eg, subacute bacterial endocarditis or tuberculosis), malignancy (eg, multiple myeloma), and chronic inflammatory conditions (eg, rheumatoid arthritis). Generally, the anemia is mild. Hypochromia may or may not be present, and red cell size is generally normal. The reticulocyte count will usually be low or normal. Both serum iron and total iron binding capacity are decreased, and transferrin saturation is usually below normal. If a bone marrow aspirate is performed, hemosiderin content is elevated. Three factors are hypothesized to be responsible for the anemia of chronic disease: (A) impaired release of iron from reticuloendothelial stores; (B) decreased erythrocyte life span; and (C) impaired bone marrow response in the face of a decreased erythrocyte life span.

The anemia of chronic disease does not respond to treatment with iron, vitamin B-12, or folic acid. Therapy is directed at treatment of the underlying disease. As in this patient, the anemia is usually asymptomatic.

MIXED ANEMIAS

24. A 33-year-old woman in her eighth month of pregnancy complains of extreme lethargy at a routine obstetric visit. Her complete blood count is reported as: hematocrit 28%, hemoglobin 7 gm/dl, MCV 90 microns³, reticulocytes 0.5%. Other laboratory results include: serum folate 4 mcg/ml, serum vitamin B-12 400 pg/ml, serum iron 30 mcg/dl, and TIBC 440 mcg/dl. A peripheral smear dem-

onstrates macrocytosis, hypersegmented granulocytes, hypochromia, and microcytosis. The patient has not been taking the prescribed iron and folate supplements. Can the red cell indices be correlated with the peripheral smear? What other factors should be considered in the etiology of this mixed anemia?

This patient's macrocytic RBCs and microcytic RBCs offset each other, and the resultant MCV is read as being normal. The red cell indices only reflect average values and should be considered as one of several diagnostic tools. Accordingly, a peripheral blood smear should be examined to ascertain morphology and pathology. In this case, the patient appears to have a combined iron and folate deficiency anemia.

Many patients do not present with a single cause of anemia, and there are many examples of situations in which a mixed anemia will occur, including pregnancy. As previously discussed in this chapter, pregnancy imposes increased iron and folate requirements. Folate deficiency anemia may occur by the third trimester (93). This patient will require iron and folate therapy: folate 1 mg daily and ferrous sulfate 325 mg three times daily.

Another factor to consider in the etiology of a mixed anemia is heavy alcohol consumption. Alcoholics may develop iron deficiency secondary to alcohol's effects on the gastrointestinal tract and subsequent acute and chronic blood loss. Nutritional folic acid deficiency is also common among alcoholics and may lead to a megaloblastic anemia. Further, alcohol ingestion may lead to a suppression of erythropoiesis (99). Other situations in which a mixed anemia will occur include patients with chronic renal failure or gastrointestinal disorders.

HEMOLYTIC ANEMIAS

A hemolytic anemia is characterized by an increased rate of red cell destruction and normally responsive bone marrow. If the hemolysis is mild, the bone marrow, which is able to increase RBC production six to eight fold, may be able to compensate for the increased RBC destruction. Eventually destruction will overwhelm the bone marrow's compensatory ability and symptomatic anemia will ensue.

Intracorpuscular (intrinsic) disorders resulting in hemolysis are related to a hereditary defect in the red cell membrane, enzymes, or the hemoglobin molecule. An example of a red cell membrane disorder is hereditary spherocytosis. The most significant disorder of the hemoglobin molecule is hemoglobin S which results in sickle cell trait and disease.

Extracorpuscular disorders are acquired and are the result of an environmental factor which leads to hemolysis. These factors can be either immunological or traumatic in origin. Immunological mechanisms are responsible for the development of idiopathic autoimmune hemolytic anemia and drug-induced hemolytic anemias. Mechanical destruction of red blood cells by prosthetic heart valves will produce a traumatic hemolytic anemia.

Altered red cells may be destroyed by (a) colloid osmotic lysis, (b) primary perforation of the red cell membrane, (c) fragmentation, or (d) red cell phagocytosis (51).

If destruction occurs in the plasma, the process is termed intravascular hemolysis. If the red cells are sequestered or trapped in certain regions of the circulation (spleen, liver, bone marrow), the process is termed extravascular hemolysis (51).

Extravascular hemolysis is the more common type of hemolytic anemia and examples include autoimmune idiopathic and drug-induced hemolytic anemias. Extravascular hemolysis represents an exaggeration of the normal mechanism for the removal of red cells, and with this sort of hemolysis the red cells are recognized as abnormal by the reticuloendothelial system and are prematurely phagocytosed. With the destruction of red cells in the reticuloendothelial system, hemoglobin dissociates to form heme and globin. Heme is metabolized to biliverdin, and carbon monoxide and iron are released into the plasma. Since the sole source of carbon monoxide is from the destruction of red cells, carbon monoxide production is employed as a means of measuring red cell survival. Biliverdin is reduced to bilirubin and then undergoes glucuronide conjugation in the liver to bilirubin diglucuronide. Following biliary excretion, bilirubin diglucuronide is reduced to urobilinogen, and approximately 10% of the urobilinogen then undergoes enterohepatic recirculation. With extravascular hemolysis, the liver's ability to conjugate bilirubin is exceeded and unconjugated, or indirect, bilirubin accumulates. The clinical presentation of extravascular hemolysis includes jaundice not associated with pruritus. The jaundice is usually mild to moderate in intensity and is most readily appreciated in the sclerae. Because the bilirubin is unconjugated and does not appear in the urine, the jaundice is termed acholuric.

In contrast to extravascular hemolysis, intravascular hemolysis is relatively rare, is generally an acute process, and occurs with gross injuries to red cells (eg, trauma-induced or complement fixed). Examples of intravascular hemolysis include the hemolysis associated with the administration of an incompatible blood transfusion, hemolytic-uremic syndrome, and paroxysmal nocturnal hemoglobinuria.

When intravascular hemolysis is the major site of destruction, hemoglobin is delivered directly to the plasma, and hemoglobin elimination follows a different metabolic pathway from extravascular hemolysis. Haptoglobin is a collective term for the alphaglobulins which bind hemoglobin in the plasma. The molecular relationship of haptoglobin to hemoglobin is 1:1 but depends on the concentration of each component. When haptoglobin is absent or completely saturated, hemoglobin circulates briefly then is either dissociated into heme and globin, removed in the liver, or excreted by the kidney. Unbound hemoglobin is filtered by the glomerulus and may exceed the reabsorption maximum in the proximal renal tubules, resulting in hemoglobinuria (51,102). Some of the unbound hemoglobin is metabolized to methemoglobin which subsequently dissociates to ferriheme and globin. A plasma beta-glucoprotein, hemopexin, binds ferriheme in a one-to-one molar ratio and thus prevents the glomerular filtration of the small ferriheme molecule. The ferriheme-hemopexin complex is then taken up by the hepatic parenchymal cells and removed. With intravascular hemolysis, the plasma hemopexin falls. The hemopexin level is not as sensitive an indicator of hemolysis as haptoglobin, but is a good index to the severity of hemolysis since minor episodes of hemolysis will not alter the hemopexin level. Other laboratory findings associated with intravascular hemolysis include methemalbuminemia, hemosiderinuria, and hemoglobinemia and are more commonly encountered with episodes of severe intravascular hemolysis.

With hemolysis, the bone marrow is stimulated to increase red cell production and the marrow becomes hyperplastic and undergoes erythroid hyperplasia. As a result of the compensatory efforts of the bone marrow, increased numbers of young red cells or reticulocytes appear in the peripheral circulation. Reticulocytes, which normally comprise 0.5 to 1.5% of the red cells, increase to 10 or 20% in hemolysis. However, the reticulocyte count must always be related to the hematocrit. Thus, a reticulocyte count of 24% at a hematocrit of 15 gm/dl is equivalent to a reticulocyte count of 8% at a hematocrit of 45 gm/dl (51,12). Various morphologic changes of the erythrocyte may be seen on peripheral smear and vary with the cause of hemolysis.

Other findings consistent with a hemolytic anemia may include an elevated serum lactate dehydrogenase, and with hereditary hemolytic anemias, the marrow hyperplasia may result in certain bony changes evident upon x-ray examination.

Once it has been ascertained that the anemia is indeed hemolytic, then the etiology must be determined. The patient is evaluated for the presence of hemoglobin SS, G6PD deficiency, and antibodies. One such antibody test is the Coombs' test.

The Coombs' or antiglobulin test is an *in vitro* test used to detect the presence of coating antibodies against human erythrocytes. The two major types of erythrocyte coatings detected by this test are IgG, and C3b and C3d of the complement system. When these antibodies are present on the red blood cell surface, the antiglobulin reagents react to these proteins and the erythrocytes agglutinate (103).

Coombs' serum is prepared by the injection of human globulins into rabbits or goats. Subsequently, serum from these animals is collected. The direct Coombs' test is a one step procedure. A sample of the patient's red blood cells is collected and washed to remove any non-immunologically bound antibody. The washed erythrocytes are then combined with Coombs' serum. If agglutination occurs, the direct Coombs' test is positive. The direct Coombs' test is used in the diagnosis of hemolytic disorders of newborns such as erythroblastosis fetalis, hemolytic disorders of adults including acquired autoimmune hemolytic anemia, and hemolytic transfusion reactions (103).

The indirect Coombs' test is a two-stage procedure. The first step can be performed by two different methods. If one wishes to detect auto-antibodies in the serum of a patient, red blood cells of known antigenic composition are exposed to the patient's serum containing unknown antibodies. After a sufficient contact time has passed, the exposed erythrocytes are washed and combined with Coombs' serum. If agglutination occurs, the indirect Coombs' test is positive and confirms that a now identified circulating antibody was present in the patient's serum. On the other hand, if one wishes to detect certain red blood cell antigens, serum containing specific known antibodies is combined with erythrocytes of unknown antigenic composition. After exposure, these red cells are added to Coombs' serum. If agglutination occurs, the indirect Coombs' is positive and antigens coating the patient's erythrocytes will have been identified. The indirect Coombs' test is used in the detection of autoantibodies in serum or certain weak antigens on red blood cells, such as D^u, or incomplete antigens, such as Duffy, Kidd, or Kell (103). Drugs associated with a positive direct Coombs' test and hemolytic anemia include: cephalosporins, isoniazid, levodopa, methyldopa, penicillins, phenacetin, quinidine, quinine, rifampin, sulfonamides, and sulfonylureas.

Therapy is aimed at treating the underlying cause of the hemolytic anemia. Shock should be treated with fluid therapy to maintain fluid balance and reverse any renal damage. Transfusion of blood may be difficult, because matching of blood is tedious if antibodies are present.

The following series of questions will deal with the treatment of autoimmune idiopathic hemolytic anemia and a much rarer form of hemolytic anemia, drug-induced, and its several etiologies.

25. Idiopathic Autoimmune Hemolytic Anemia. A 42-year-old male was hospitalized with a ten day history of weakness, malaise, dark colored urine, and jaundice. Laboratory data included: hemoglobin 7.2 gm/dl, hematocrit 19%, WBC 9,600/mm³, and reticulocyte count 1.1%; the indirect bilirubin was 2.5 mg/dl; the direct Coombs' test was 2+ and the indirect Coombs' test was negative. A Cr⁵¹ red cell survival test resulted in a half life of 15 to 16 days (nl: 27 to 33 days). The diagnosis was idiopathic autoimmune hemolytic anemia. What are the causes of autoimmune hemolytic anemia and how is it treated?

Autoimmune hemolytic anemia is due to immunological factors in the red cell's environment and frequently is secondary to lymphomas, chronic lymphocytic leukemia, infections, rheumatoid arthritis, or other disorders. It also may be induced by drugs, or if no cause is readily discernible, it simply is categorized as idiopathic (104).

Prednisone 60 to 80 mg per day for 10 days is commonly used to treat autoimmune hemolytic anemia. Larger corticosteroid doses do not produce additional therapeutic benefits. Once a remission with steroids has been attained, the steroid should be tapered slowly over several months to a dose which will produce minimal side effects (10 mg prednisone daily) and prevent a recurrence of the anemia. As many as 84% of patients achieved partial or complete remission with a single course of corticosteroid therapy in one study. However, when the dose of prednisone was tapered to 10 to 15 mg per day, only 16% remained in remission. If the patient fails to respond to a ten day course of corticosteroid therapy, splenectomy is then a viable therapeutic alternative. Splenectomy can induce a remission in 44% of patients and is therefore sometimes utilized as an adjunct to steroid therapy in patients with relapsing autoimmune hemolytic anemia (104). Although splenectomized patients have twice the mortality of steroid-treated patients, this may simply reflect the fact that patients who failed to respond to the corticosteroids tend to be more severely affected (105). When splenectomy is contraindicated and when steroids result in therapeutic failure, cyclophosphamide 50 mg bid on alternative days is effective (104).

Drug-Induced Hemolytic Anemias

26. G6PD Deficiency. A 28-year-old journalist has returned from Southeast Asia to the United States. He has the diagnosis of malaria falciparum and is begun on primaquine and chloroquine therapy. One week later he feels extremely weak, his urine is dark brown, and the sclera of his eyes appear yellow. What may be the cause of these signs and symptoms?

The primary consideration in this case is the probable occurrence of drug-induced hemolysis with concurrent hyperbilirubinemia and jaundice. Primaquine is the classic drug which elicits hemolysis in hereditary G6PD deficiency. Hemolysis and anemia may be caused by a variety of oxidant drugs in patients with glucose-6-phosphate dehydrogenase (G6PD) deficiency (106–108), but the severity and incidence of the reaction varies substantially depending upon (a) the genotype of G6PD and (b) the racial characteristics of the subject exposed to the drug.

There are two types of G6PD enzymes, types A and B. The "normal" G6PD is type B and makes up the most common enzyme in all population groups. However, there are substantial differences in the occurrence of variant enzymes in various population groups. Approximately one-third of Black Americans have the type A G6PD variant and only have 5 to 15% of the needed enzyme activity within their red blood cells. Other groups, such as Mediterranean Jews or Chinese also have a high prevalence of G6PD deficient activity, and their cells often contain less than 1% of normal G6PD activity. The lower the enzyme activity, the more severe the hemolytic reaction.

Hemolysis occurs in G6PD deficiency because G6PD is necessary to reduce nicotinamide adenine diphosphate (NADP) to NADPH at a normal rate. NADPH protects red blood cells from oxidation by keeping glutathione in a reduced state and thus prevents glutathione from complexing with hemoglobin and denaturing it. Denatured hemoglobin precipitates within the red cell as Heinz bodies, and the red cells are lysed. Exposure to certain drugs (Table 12) with oxidant properties significantly increases the amount of glutathione free radicals that can bind to sulfhydryl groups on the hemoglobin molecule. Therefore, the severity of the hemolysis after drug exposure is greater in those subjects who have very low levels of G6PD enzyme activity, and thus NADPH, than in those who have moderate to normal enzyme activity.

The bone marrow responds to hemolysis by producing young red cells. In the type A G6PD deficiency seen in Black Americans, these young red cells have normal enzyme activity and are resistant to hemolysis. The deficiency occurs in only the old or mature red cells. As a result, hemolysis is self-limiting in Black people, despite continued therapy with the offending agent. In the Mediterranean Jews with type B G6PD deficiency, the deficiency exists in all red cells and chronic, severe hemolysis occurs and drug therapy must be discontinued (106,108).

Table 12 lists the drug and average doses that

reportedly elicit hemolysis due to G6PD deficiency. Several oxidant drugs have not been reported to produce significant hemolysis in G6PD deficiency and these include: aspirin, ascorbic acid, chloroquine, dimercaprol, diphenhydramine, menadione, methylene blue, para-aminobenzoic acid, procainamide, probenecid, sulfadiazine, sulfamerazine, sulfisoxazole, sulfathiazole, sodium sulfoxone, tripelennamine, pyrimethamine, quinine, and quinacrine.

If primaquine were continued at the same dose, the clinical course of hemolysis would typically occur in three phases: the acute, recovery, and equilibrium phases. The acute phase generally begins one to three days after the start of drug administration. Heinz bodies are present at this time, and urine may be positive for hemoglobin. During the acute phase, systemic symptoms include weakness, mild abdominal or back pain, and slight jaundice. At four to six days after the initiation of drug administration, the reticulocyte count is increased, indicating bone marrow compensation. The recovery phase begins seven to ten days after drug administration with rising hemo-

Table 12.

DRUGS PRODUCING CLINICALLY SIGNIFICANT HEMOLYSIS IN PATIENTS WITH G6PD DEFICIENCY

Drug	Trade Name	Dose
Acetanilid		3.6 gm
Diaminodiphenylsulfone	Dapsone	25–200 mg
Furazolidone	Tricofuron	400 mg
Furmethonol	Altafur	1.0 gm
Nalidixic acid	NegGram	
Neoarsphenamine	Neosalvarsan	600 mg
Nitrofurantion	Furadantin, Macrodantin	400 mg
Nitrofurazone	Furacin	1.5 gm
Pamaquine		
Aminoquine	Plasmoquine	30 mg
Pentaquine		30 mg
Primaquine		30 mg
Sulfacetamide	Sulamyd	
Sulfamethoxypyrimidine		
Sulfanilamide		3.6–5.0 gm
Sulfapyridine		4.0 gm
Sulfasalazine	Azulfidine	6.9 gm

globin and hematocrit (after a nadir of 25 to 35% decrease of pre-drug levels). The patient should begin to feel better clinically. The equilibrium phase begins about 40 days after primaquine therapy and consists of full hematologic and clinical recovery. However, if the dose of primaquine is increased, a new episode of hemolysis will occur.

27. **Hypophosphatemic Hemolytic Anemia.** E.O., a 47-year-old man, was hospitalized with abdominal pain, vomiting, and diarrhea of one week duration. The patient had recently become depressed after a laryngectomy for squamous cell carcinoma of the larynx. Since that surgery, he had not eaten routinely, but did ingest a fifth of whiskey per day. On admission, physical examination was significant for profound muscle weakness and tremulousness. Laboratory studies confirmed the diagnosis of acute pancreatitis. Approximately twenty-four hours after admission, serum phosphorous was noted to be less than 0.1 mg/dl. The initial hematocrit was 44% and over the next five days it dropped to 25%. Serum bilirubin rose to 8.0 mg/dl, and the reticulocyte count rose up to 9%. Workup of the hemolytic anemia was negative, and included: direct and indirect Coombs', serum B-12, serum folate, cold agglutinins, G6PD, and pyruvic kinase. What was the cause of the hemolytic anemia?

Severe hypophosphatemia, secondary to starvation and alcoholism, was initially manifested in this patient as muscular weakness. The hypophosphatemia was not treated for several days and a significant hemolysis ensued.

Hemolytic anemia secondary to hypophosphatemia is believed to be due to decreased levels of erythrocyte adenosine triphosphate (ATP) which maintains red cell membrane integrity and plasticity. ADP (adenosine diphosphate) is phosphorylated to ATP by inorganic phosphorous. The reservoir of phosphorous for phosphorylation is extracellular and is transmitted intracellularly by passive diffusion.

In vitro studies indicate that when ATP levels fall below 15% of normal, the erythrocyte membrane becomes rigid (109); however, it is unusual for ATP levels to fall below 40% of normal even in the presence of significant hypophosphatemia. Serum phosphorous levels must be extremely depressed (below 0.2 mg/dl) before ATP production

is affected enough to induce hemolysis. An ATP level of 11% of normal was detected in a patient with a serum phosphorous of 0.1 mg/dl, and hemolytic anemia developed secondary to the hypophosphatemia (109).

Hypophosphatemia not only depresses ATP concentrations, but also levels of 2,3 diphosphoglycerate (2,3 DPG). Low levels of 2,3 DPG shift the oxy-hemoglobin saturation curve to the left, resulting in tissue anoxia (109).

28. How should the above hypophosphatemic hemolytic anemia be treated?

The severe hemolytic anemia secondary to hypophosphatemia is readily reversible with the parenteral or oral administration of phosphates. Parenteral therapy may be preferred, especially if other signs of severe hypophosphatemia such as coma or convulsions are present. If oral therapy is utilized, Fleet's Phopho-Soda 15 to 30 ml (80 to 160 mEq of phosphate) is given three times a day. If parenteral medication is necessary, monobasic potassium phosphate 60 mEq is administered by continuous infusion over eight hours for a total of twenty-four hours or longer (110) with careful monitoring of potassium values as well as clinical response. Oral or parenteral phosphate replenishment should not be overzealous, as hyperphosphatemia and the resultant hypocalcemia and metastatic calcification must be avoided (111). Red cell survival improves within two to three days after correction of the serum phosphorous level (109).

29. What drugs can induce hypophosphatemic hemolytic anemia?

Drug-induced causes of hypophosphatemia include aluminum-containing antacids, phosphate-poor total parenteral nutrition solutions, thiazide diuretics, estrogens, and androgens (112). As little as 90 ml of an aluminum-containing antacid, four times daily for thirty to ninety days, can produce symptomatic hypophosphatemia (113) by binding phosphate in the gastrointestinal tract. When phosphate-poor total parenteral nutrition solutions are administered, severe hypophosphatemia can develop within five to fourteen days (114). Phosphate is required for anabolism, and serum phosphorous will remain within normal limits when 20 mEq of phosphate is administered for each 1000 kilocalories (115,116).

30. *Haptene Type Hemolysis.* A 40-year-old woman was hospitalized with a systolic murmur, low grade fever, fatigue, night sweats, and joint pain. The diagnosis was subacute bacterial endocarditis, and penicillin G five million units IV every 4 hours was instituted. After five days of therapy the hematocrit dropped from 39% to 27% and the hemoglobin dropped from 13 gm/dl to 9 gm/dl. The serum bilirubin rose from 0.8 mg/dl to 1.8 mg/dl (1.5 mg/dl indirect), the reticulocyte count rose from 2% to 9%, and the serum haptoglobin was 5 mg/dl. Additionally, the direct Coombs' test was positive and the indirect test was negative. What is the problem and what should be done?

This patient is experiencing the haptene type of hemolytic anemia which occurs in patients receiving more than 20 million units per day of intravenous penicillin. Not all patients receiving this dose develop IgG antibody (positive direct Coombs' test), nor do those who develop antibody necessarily have evidence of hemolysis (117–119).

A number of drugs which act as haptenes become antigenic when they combine with the red cell membrane. IgG antibody reacts with the drug—red cell complex producing hemolysis (117,120). The direct Coombs' test is usually positive while the indirect is negative (121). The penicillins and cephalosporins bind to red cells strongly and are good examples of this type of immune-induced hemolytic anemia (122). The patient produces antibodies against the drug—red cell complex and thus coats them with immunoglobulins, with or without complement. The complement system may also be stimulated (123).

The symptoms of this patient are of mild to moderate severity; in many cases of haptene type hemolytic anemia, symptoms are not evident. In cases of severe hemolytic anemia, shaking, chills, high fever, shock, jaundice, palpitations, dyspnea, cyanosis, cardiomegaly, anuria, as well as pain in the abdomen, back, or extremities may develop. Clinical signs of hemolytic anemia include hemoglobinuria, red urine, dark stools, hyperbilirubinemia (indirect), reticulocytosis, and splenomegaly (55).

The treatment of a haptene-type hemolytic anemia is discontinuation of the drug. Transfusion may be required depending on the degree of anemia. In this case, the patient does not need transfusions because she is asymptomatic from the hemolytic process. Corticosteroids are not effective in immune-induced hemolytic anemias (51).

31. *Innocent Bystander Type of Hemolysis.* A 71-year-old woman is started on quinine sulfate 300 mg three times daily for leg cramps due to arteriosclerotic vascular disease. Four days after the initiation of therapy she returns with what she believes to be the flu (chills, abdominal pain, and diarrhea). She also asks if her new medicine (quinine) can cause red discoloration of the urine. Could any of her complaints be associated with quinine therapy?

Quinine has been reported to produce hemolytic anemia in many instances (124). The clinical findings of this drug-induced hemolysis may occur from 1 to 5 days after initiation of therapy and include fever, chills, and hemoglobinuria. Quinine therapy should be stopped.

32. Describe the mechanism by which quinine produces red cell hemolysis.

Unlike haptene-induced hemolytic anemia from penicillin, quinine produces the innocent bystander type of hemolysis where the drug binds to an antibody (Ab), usually of the IgM type, to form an immune complex which then attaches to the erythrocyte membrane. Neither the drug nor the antibody alone have a high affinity for the red cell. After attachment of the immune complex to the red cell membrane, complement (C′) interacts with the drug-Ab-membrane and stimulates anti-C′ antibodies which lyse the red blood cell with dissociation of the drug-Ab complex. The dissociated drug-Ab complex which was released into the plasma then goes on to initiate the reaction on other red cells. The small number of drug-Ab complexes accounts for a negative Coombs' test (antigamma globulin). However, the immune reaction becomes positive with anti-C′ serum (125).

The dose of quinine need not be large to produce acute hemolysis, hemoglobinuria, and hemoglobinemia. However, prior drug exposure is required to elicit the reaction.

Several drugs produce hemolysis by the innocent bystander mechanism and include: chlorpromazine, insulin, melphalan, isoniazid, quinidine, quinine, rifampin, and sulfonamide. Most of these drug reactions are mediated by IgM (121), although some are of the IgG type (126). Most of these drugs also produce immune-induced thrombocytopenia. It has been proposed that IgM antibodies are responsible for hemolysis, while IgG antibodies are responsible for thrombocytopenic reactions (127).

As in haptene-induced hemolysis, discontinuing the drug results in rapid reversal of clinical symptoms. If the anemia is severe (hematocrit less than 20%) transfusions should be given.

33. *Autoimmune Hemolysis.* **A 67-year-old man with Parkinson's disease was started on two grams of levodopa daily in March because of poor control with anticholinergics. By November, his hematocrit had dropped from 45% to 37%. By February of the following year, he noticed jaundice, weakness, and anorexia. His hematocrit was 19%, a reticulocyte count was 36%, total bilirubin was 5.6 mg/dl (4.1 mg/dl indirect), and Coombs' tests (direct and indirect) were 4+ positive. What type of anemia has developed? Explain the mechanism involved.**

An autoimmune type of hemolytic anemia is evident in this case. It differs from the "haptene" and "innocent bystander" type in that the direct and indirect Coombs' with antiglobulin G are positive (125). In addition, the IgG antibody can be obtained by eluting the Coombs' positive red cells which will then react with normal red blood cells without the addition of drug. These antibodies have an Rh-type specificity (51).

In a large study, the positive direct Coombs' test developed in 9% of patients receiving an average dose of five grams of levodopa (128). Most of these patients became positive between 90 and 360 days after therapy was initiated. Hemolytic anemia to both levodopa and alphamethyldopa is rare, but the clinical presentation and duration of antiglobulin response make it an interesting problem. The symptoms and hematologic values (hematocrit and reticulocytes) usually return to normal within two months after discontinuing therapy; however, the Coombs' test can remain positive for many years (119,129).

References

1. Levin R: Iron deficiency anemia in the pediatric patient. Am Pharm Assoc J. 1971; NS11:670.
2. Lowe C et al: Iron balance and requirements in infancy. Pediatrics. 1969; 43:134.
3. Fairbank V: Iron deficiency. In *Hematology*, edited by W Williams, McGraw-Hill, New York, 1972, p 311.
4. Beutler E: Iron deficiency. In *Hematology*, edited by W Williams, McGraw-Hill, New York, 1972, p 316.
5. Beal R: Hematinics: pathophysiological and clinical aspects. Drugs. 1971; 2:190.
6. Brown E: Clinical pharmacology of drugs used in the treatment of iron deficiency anemia. Pharmacol Physicians. 1968; 2:11.
7. Lipschitz DA et al: A clinical evaluation of serum ferritin as an index of iron stores. N Engl J Med. 1974; 290:1213.
8. Jacobs A et al: Ferritin in serum: clinical and biochemical implications. N Engl J Med. 1975; 292:951.
9. Stojceski T et al: Studies on the serum iron-binding capacity. J Clin Pathol. 1965; 18:446.
10. Bainton DF et al: The diagnosis of iron deficiency anemia. Am J Med. 1974; 37:62.
11. Fairbanks VF: Iron deficiency: still a diagnostic challenge. Med Clin North Am. 1970; 54:903.
12. Hillman R et al: Erythropoiesis: normal and abnormal. Semin Hematol. 1967; 4:327.
13. Bothwell T: Iron deficiency. Med J Aust. 1972; 2:433.
14. Brise H et al: Absorbability of different iron compounds. Acta Med Scan. 1962; 171(suppl 376):23.
15. O'Sullivan D et al: Oral iron compounds, a therapeutic comparison. Lancet. 1955; 2:482.
16. Middleton E et al: Studies on the absorption of orally administered iron from sustained-release preparations. N Engl J Med. 1966; 274:136.
17. Beutler E et al: Doses and dosing. N Engl J Med. 1966; 274:136.
18. Bothwell T et al: Factors affecting iron absorption. J Lab Clin Med. 1958; 51:24.
19. Beutler E: Iron deficiency. In *Hematology*, edited by W Williams, McGraw-Hill, New York, 1972, p 308.
20. Beal R: Hematinics: clinical pharmacological and therapeutic agents. Drugs. 1971; 2:207.
21. Bothwell T et al: The intestine in iron absorption. Am J Digest Dis. 1957; 1:145.
22. Conrad M et al: Ascorbic acid chelates in iron absorption, a role for hydrochloric acid and bile. Gastroenterology. 1968; 55:35.
23. Pollack S et al: Iron absorption: effects of sugars and reducing agents. Blood. 1964; 24:577.
24. Giorgio A: Current concepts of iron metabolism and iron deficiency anemia. Med Clin North Am. 1970; 54:1399.
25. American Medical Association: Council on foods and nutrition. JAMA. 1968; 203:61.
26. Brise H et al: Iron absorption studies. Acta Med Scan. 1962; 171(suppl 376):1.
27. Beutler E: Iron metabolism. In *Hematology*, edited by W Williams, McGraw-Hill, New York, 1972, p 129.

28. Smith M et al: Absorption of inorganic iron from graded doses. Br J Hemat. 1958; 4:428.

29. Brown EB Jr et al: Studies in iron transportation and metabolism. XI. Critical analysis of mucosal block by large doses of inorganic iron in human subjects. J Lab Clin Med. 1958; 52:335.

30. Hall G et al: Inhibition of iron absorption by magnesium trisilicate. Med J Aust. 1969; 2:95.

31. Neuvonen P et al: Interference of iron with the absorption of tetracyclines in man. Br Med J. 1970; 4:532.

32. Boyett J et al: Allopurinol and iron metabolism in man. Blood. 1968; 32:460.

33. Davis P et al: Effect of allopurinol on radioiron absorption in man. Lancet. 1966; 2:470.

34. Emmerson B: Effects of allopurinol on iron metabolism in man. Ann Rheum Dis. 1966; 25:700.

35. Powell L: Effects of allopurinol on iron storage in the rat. Ann Rheum Dis. 1966; 25:697.

36. Hallberg L et al: Studies on oral iron therapy. Acta Med Scan. 1966; (suppl):459.

37. Beutler E: Clinical Disorders of Iron Metabolism (Monograph). Grune & Stratton, New York, 1963.

38. Savin M: A practical approach to the treatment of iron deficiency. Rational Drug Therapy. 1977; 11:1.

39. Lloyd K: Reactions to total dose infusion of iron dextran in rheumatoid arthritis. Br Med J. 1970; 2:323.

40. Block M: Using IV iron. In Iron: A Total Clinical Learning Experience, edited by W Crosby, Medcom series, New York, 1972.

41. Robertson AG et al: Intramuscular iron and local oncogenesis. Br Med J. 1977; 1:946.

42. Cade J et al: The use of iron dextran by total dose infusion. Med J Aust. 1968; 1:716.

43. Wallerstein R: Intravenous iron dextran complex. Blood. 1968; 32:690.

44. Will G et al: The treatment of iron deficiency anemia by iron-dextran infusion: a radio-isotope study. Br J Haematol. 1968; 14:61.

45. Package insert—Imferon (Lakeside Co.)

46. Gleason M et al: Section 3. therapeutics index: phenol. In Clinical Toxicology of Commercial Products, edited by M Gleason et al, Williams and Wilkins Co., 1969, p 189.

47. Esplin D: Antiseptics and disinfectants: fungicides, ectoparasiticides. In Pharmacologic Basis of Therapeutics, edited by L Goodman and A Gilman, MacMillan Co., New York, 1970, p 1035.

48. Bonnar J: Anemia in Obstetrics: an evaluation of treatment by iron dextran infusion. Br Med J. 1965; 3:1030.

49. Newcombe R: Precautions in the intravenous use of iron dextran. Postgrad Med. 1967; 43:372.

50. Hillman R et al: Control of marrow production by the level of iron supply. J Clin Invest. 1969; 48:454.

51. Harris J: The Red Cell, Harvard Press, Cambridge, Mass., 1972, p 559.

52. Rath C et al: Effect of renal disease on the Schilling test. N Engl J Med. 1957; 256:111.

53. Schilling R et al: Intrinsic factor studies, III: further observations utilizing the urinary radioactivity test in subjects with achlorhydria, pernicious anemia, or a total gastrectomy. J Lab Clin Med. 1955; 45:926.

54. Harris J: The Red Cell, Harvard Press, Cambridge, Mass., 1972, p 559.

55. Wintrobe M: Principles of Internal Medicine, 6th ed, McGraw-Hill, New York, 1970, p 1614.

56. Beck W: Vitamin B12 deficiency. In Hematology, edited by W Williams, McGraw-Hill, New York, 1972, p 256.

57. Boddy K et al: Retention of cyanocobalamin, hydroxycobalamin after parenteral administration. Lancet. 1968; 2:710.

58. Chalmers J et al: Comparison of hydroxycobalamin and cyanocobalamin in pernicious anemia. Lancet. 1965; 2:1305.

59. Skouby et al: Antibody to transcobalamin II and B-12 binding capacity in patients treated with hydroxycobalamin. Blood. 1971; 38:769–774.

60. Hillman RS: Vitamin B-12, folic acid, and the treatment of megaloblastic anemias. In The Pharmacological Basis of Therapeutics, edited by A Gilman, Macmillan, New York, 1980, p 1337.

61. Chanarin I: Absorption of cobalamins. J Clin Pathol. 1971; 5(suppl 24):60.

62. Lowenstein L et al: An immunologic basis for acquired resistance to oral administration of hog intrinsic factor and vitamin B12 in pernicious anemia. J Clin Invest. 1961; 40:1656.

63. Berlin R et al: Vitamin B12: body stores during oral and parenteral treatment of pernicious anemia. Acta Med Scand. 1978; 204:81.

64. Schieve JR et al: Response of lingual manifestations of pernicious anemia to pteroylglutamic and vitamin B12. J Lab Clin Med. 1949; 34:439.

65. Issacs R et al: Standards for red blood cell increases after liver and stomach therapy in pernicious anemia. JAMA. 1938; 111:2291.

66. Lous P et al: The absorption of vitamin B12 following partial gastrectomy. Acta Med Scand. 1959; 164:407.

67. Chanarin I: The Megaloblastic Anemias, Blackwell Scientific Pub., Oxford, England, 1969, p 282.

68. Webb D et al: Mechanism of vitamin B12 malabsorption in patients receiving colchicine. N Engl J Med. 1968; 279:845.

69. Salokannel S et al: Malabsorption of vitamin B12 during treatment with slow release KCL. Acta Med Scand. 1970; 187:431.

70. Lees F: Radioactive vitamin B12 absorption in the megaloblastic anemia caused by anticonvulsant drugs. Quart J Med. 1961; 30:231.

71. Tomkin G et al: Malabsorption of vitamin B12 in diabetic patients treated with phenformin. Br Med J. 1973; 3:673.

72. Jacobson E et al: An experimental malabsorption syndrome induced by neomycin. Am J Med. 1960; 28:524.

73. Hess D et al: Para-aminosalicylic acid-induced intestinal malabsorption. Clin Res. 1970; 18:77.

74. Herbert V et al: Correlation of folate deficiency with alcoholism and associated macrocytosis, anemia, and liver disease. Ann Intern Med. 1963; 58:977.

75. Eichner ER et al: Folate balance in dietary-induced megaloblastic anemia. N Engl J Med. 1971; 284:933.

76. Hoffbrand A et al: Mechanism of folate deficiency in patients receiving phenytoin. Lancet. 1968; 2:528.

77. Klipstein F: Subnormal serum folate and macrocytosis associated with anticonvulsant drug therapy. Blood. 1964; 23:68.

78. Streiff R: Malabsorption of polyglutamic folic acid secondary to oral contraceptives. Clin Res. 1969; 17:71.

79. Waxman S: Metabolic approach to the diagnosis of megaloblastic anemias. Med Clin North Am. 1973; 57:315.

80. Reynolds E et al: Anticonvulsant therapy, megaloblastic hemopoiesis and folic acid metabolism. Quart J Med. 1966; 35:521.

81. Whitman A: Effect of prolonged administration of trimethoprim-sulfamethoxazole. Postgrad Med. 1969; 45:46(suppl).

82. Jenkins GC et al: A hematological study of patients receiving long-term treatment with trimethoprim and sulphonamide. J Clin Pathol. 1970; 23:392.

83. Waxman S et al: Drugs, toxins, and dietary amino acids affecting vitamin B_{12} or folic acid absorption and utilization. Am J Med. 1970; 48:599.

84. Herbert V: Drugs effective in megaloblastic anemia. In *Pharmacological Basis of Therapeutics*, edited by L Goodman and A Gilman, MacMillan Co., New York, 1970, p 1414.

85. Herbert V: Drugs effective in megaloblastic anemia. In *Pharmacological Basis of Therapeutics*, edited by L Goodman and A Gilman, MacMillan Co., New York, 1970, p 1397.

86. Frei E et al: A new approach to cancer chemotherapy with methotrexate. N Engl J Med. 1975; 292:846.

87. Klipstein F et al: Folate deficiency associated with drug therapy for tuberculosis. Blood. 1967; 29:697.

88. Pearson D: Megaloblastic anemia due to glutethimide. Lancet. 1965; 1:110.

89. Bertino J et al: Studies on the inhibition of dihydrofolate reductase by the folate antagonists. J Biol Chem. 1964; 239:497.

90. Waxman S et al: Mechanism of pyrimethamine-induced megaloblastosis in human bone marrow. N Engl J Med. 1969; 280:1316.

91. Sive J et al: Effect of trimethoprim on folate-dependent DNA synthesis in human bone marrow. J Clin Pathol. 1972; 25:194.

92. Corcino J et al: Mechanism of triamterene-induced megaloblastosis. Ann Intern Med. 1970; 73:419.

93. Strieff R: Folic acid deficiency anemia. Semin Hematol. 1970; 7:23.

94. Carmel R: The laboratory diagnosis of megaloblastic anemias. West J Med. 1978; 128:294.

95. Reynolds EH: Anticonvulsants, folic acid, and epilepsy. Lancet. 1973; 1:1376.

96. Baylis EM et al: Influence of folic acid on blood-phenytoin levels. Lancet. 1971; 1:62.

97. Glazko AJ: Antiepileptic drugs: biotransformation, metabolism, and serum half-life. Epilepsia. 1975; 16:367.

98. Wintrobe M: The anemia of chronic disorders and the sideroblastic anemias. In *Clinical Hematology*, 7th ed, edited by M Wintrobe, Philadelphia, 1974, p 677.

99. Halsted CA: The effect of alcoholism on the absorption of folic acid. J Lab Clin Med. 1967; 69:116.

100. Rosenberg I et al: Impairment of intestinal deconjugation of dietary folate: a possible explanation of megaloblastic anemia associated with phenytoin therapy. Lancet. 1968; 2:530.

101. Weed R et al: Membrane alteration leading to red cell destruction. Am J Med. 1966; 41:681.

102. Wintrobe M: The hemolytic disorders: general consideration. In *Clinical Hematology*, 7th ed, edited by M Wintrobe, Philadelphia, 1974, p 893.

103. Wintrobe M: Immunohemolytic anemias. In *Clinical Hematology*, 7th ed, edited by M Wintrobe, Philadelphia, 1974, p 893.

104. Chaplin H et al: Autoimmune hemolytic anemia. Arch Intern Med. 1977; 137:346.

105. Allgood JW et al: Idiopathic acquired autoimmune hemolytic anemia: a review of 47 cases treated from 1955 through 1965. Am J Med. 1967; 43:254.

106. Beutler E: Glucose 6-phosphate deficiency. In *Hematology*, edited by W Williams, McGraw-Hill, New York, 1972, p 395.

107. Beutler E: Drug-induced hemolytic anemia. Pharmacol Rev. 1969; 21:73.

108. Pannacciulli I et al: The course of experimentally-induced hemolytic anemia in a primaquine-sensitive caucasian. A case study. Blood. 1965; 25:92.

109. Jacob HS et al: Acute hemolytic anemia with rigid cells in hypophosphatemia. N Engl J Med. 1971; 285:1446.

110. Klock JC et al: Hemolytic anemia and somatic cell dysfunction in severe hypophosphatemia. Arch Intern Med. 1974; 134:360.

111. Goldsmith R et al: Inorganic phosphate treatment of hypercalcemia of diverse etiologies. N Engl J Med. 1966; 274:1.

112. Fitzgerald F: Hypophosphatemia. West J Med. 1975; 122:482.

113. Lotz M et al: Evidence for a phosphorous-depletion syndrome in man. N Engl J Med. 1968; 278:409.

114. Silvis SE et al: Paresthesia, weakness, seizures, and hypophosphatemia in patients receiving hyperalimentation. Gastroenterology. 1972; 62:513.

115. Rudman D et al: Elemental balances during intravenous hyperalimentation of underweight adult subjects. J Clin Invest. 1976; 55:94.

116. Sheldon GF et al: Phosphate depletion and repletion: Relation to parenteral nutrition and oxygen transport. Ann Surg. 1975; 182:683.

117. Petz L et al: Coombs' positive hemolytic anemia caused by penicillin administration. N Engl J Med. 1966; 274:171.

118. White J et al: Penicillin-induced hemolytic anemia. Br J Hematol. 1968; 3:26.

119. Worlledge S: Immunologic drug-induced hemolytic anemias. Semin Hematol. 1973; 10:327.

120. Kerr R et al: Two mechanisms of erythrocyte destruction in penicillin-induced hemolytic anemia. N Engl J Med. 1972; 287:1322.

121. Croft J et al: Coombs' test positivity induced by drugs. Ann Intern Med. 1968; 68:176.

122. Spath P: Studies on the immune response to penicillin and cephalothin in humans. Part I and II. J Immunol. 1971; 107:1209.

123. Kerr R et al: Erythrocyte-bound C_5 and C_6 in autoimmune hemolytic anemia. J Immunol. 1971; 107:1209.

124. Muirhead E et al: Drug-dependent Coombs' (antiglobulin) test and anemia. Observations on quinine and phenacetin. Arch Intern Med. 1958; 101:82.

125. Garratty G: Drug-related problems. In *A Seminar on Problems Encountered in Pretransfusion Tests*. American Assoc of Blood Banks, Washington, D.C., 1972, p 33.

126. Eisner E et al: Quinine-induced thrombocytopenic purpura due to an IgM and IgG antibody. Transfusion. 1972; 12:317.

127. Shulman N: Mechanism of blood destruction in individuals sensitized to foreign antigens. Trans Assoc Am Physicians. 1963; 76:72.

128. Joseph C: Occurrence of positive Coombs' test in patients with levodopa. N Engl J Med. 1972; 286:1401.

129. Territo M et al: Autoimmune hemolytic anemia due to levodopa therapy. JAMA. 1973; 226:1347.

ACKNOWLEDGMENT: The contributions of Dr. Robert J. Ignoffo are sincerely appreciated. Portions of his work which appeared in an earlier edition of this textbook have been included into this present chapter.

Chapter 42

Oncology

Robert J. Ignoffo

The pioneering research of Gilman in 1946 and Farber in 1948 established that cures could be achieved in the treatment of advanced cancers with the use of systemic chemotherapy (1,2). More recent advances have demonstrated that patients with widely metastatic disease may have long-lasting remissions with dramatic lengthening of their survival time (3). These achievements have led researchers to continue to devise new agents, new regimens, and modalities to further increase the chances for cancer patients to assume a normal lifespan. After a brief review of basic concepts that led to these achievements, this chapter will illustrate some of the problems that are commonly encountered in the application of chemotherapy. For detailed information on individual disease entities, the reader is referred to the cancer texts by Carter (4) and Haskell (5).

Cancer is a set of neoplastic disorders consisting of over 300 distinct disease entities. Approximately one in four Americans will contract cancer in their lifetime. It ranks second to cardiovascular diseases in mortality. Fortunately, approximately one-third of diagnosed patients can be cured with surgery or irradiation. Those who are less fortunate will develop a constellation of signs and symptoms consistent with advanced disease.

Most patients seek medical attention when symptoms such as pain, weight loss, bleeding, malaise, or an abnormal tissue growth stimulate such action. The ability of the clinician to detect cancer has improved dramatically in recent years with the advent of new radiologic techniques, tumor markers, and diagnostic techniques.

The patient with an abnormal mass will usually undergo a basic examination that includes a physical examination, a chest x-ray, a blood chemistry panel, and an evaluation of the pathology of the tumor from a biopsy specimen. Other tests will be included depending on the normal pattern of metastatic spread. For example, patients with Hodgkin's disease (a lymphatic cancer) will also undergo a lymphangiogram to detect non-clinical sites of involvement (eg, inguinal or abdominal lymph nodes) and a bone marrow aspirate plus biopsy. The results of these tests assist in the staging of the disease, and the pathologic or histologic grading of the tumor. Table 1 lists several common cancers and their usual sites of metastases.

The objectives of staging are to determine: the aggressiveness of the tumor cell type, whether it

Table 1.

COMMON CANCERS AND SITES OF METASTASES

Cancer	Primary	Secondary
Breast		
Premenopause	Liver, Lung	Brain
Postmenopause	Bone, Soft tissue	Lung
Colon	Liver	Lung
		Brain
Pancreas	Liver	Adrenal
		Lung
Hodgkin's	Lymph nodes	Bone marrow
	Stomach	Lung
	Liver	
Lung	Liver	Brain
	Bone	

has spread (metastasized), where it has metastasized, and prognosis. For example, the 5-year survival for a patient with breast cancer closely relates to the stage of disease (Figure 1). As illustrated, a cancer which is more advanced at the time of diagnosis (eg, stage IV) carries a poorer prognosis than one which is diagnosed at an early stage.

Several staging classifications currently exist, but the most useful one is the TNM system. Table 2 describes this classification system which grades the status of the tumor, lymph nodes, and metastasis. This classification provides a uniform method of staging for all involved in the care of the patient.

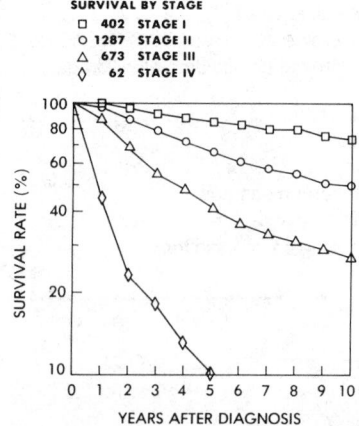

Figure 1. Staging and Survival in Breast Cancer.

Table 2.

TNM STAGING CLASSIFICATION

Tumor
  T_1 - Mass less than 2 cm
  T_2 - Mass between 2 and 4 cm
  T_3 - Mass greater than 4 cm

Node
  N_0 - negative regional lymph node
  N_1 - positive regional lymph node
  N_2 - positive distant lymph node

Metastases
  M_0 - no metastases
  M_1 - evident metastases

Example: A breast cancer patient with 4 cm primary
         lesion, 4 of 20 axillary lymph nodes
         positive, and bone metastases is classified
         as $T_3N_1M_1$.

The treatment of cancer has advanced considerably in recent years. More than 40 cytotoxic drugs and hormonal agents are commercially available, some of which have substantially changed the natural history of some cancers. For example, cisplatin and doxorubicin are cytotoxic agents with a broad spectrum of activity which have increased the survival of advanced cancer of the testes and breast, respectively. Other modalities, such as immunotherapy, are less well established and await further study.

Tumor Growth (7,8)

To understand why chemotherapy works, one must understand normal as well as tumor cell growth. Both normal and tumor cells increase in size by proceeding through several phases of growth which are depicted by the cell cycle (Figure 2). The "business" portion of cell cycle occurs during the **S-phase** (nucleic acid synthesis) when DNA doubles in content in preparation for cell division. During the pre-mitotic (GAP 2) or **G_2-phase,** additional protein and RNA synthesis occur; this phase is necessary for the formation of the mitotic spindle. Then, in **M-phase** (mitosis) the cell divides its nuclear material to form two new cells which can do one of three things: 1) go back in cycle into the **G_1-phase** (GAP 1) where enzymes are formed prior to S-phase; 2) mature and then die, or 3) go into a resting state called

G_0-phase (GAP OUT). It is important to consider these phases because they are critical to the action of some chemotherapeutic agents. Agents that kill cells only during a particular phase, such as S-phase or DNA synthesis, are called phase-specific or cell-cycle specific (CCS). Those drugs with cytotoxic effects that are independent of any cellular phase are called phase-nonspecific or cell-cycle nonspecific (CCNS). The importance of these distinctions is apparent when one considers that agents which are most effective during S-phase are usually ineffective inhibitors of slowly-dividing cells, such as those in large bulky tumors.

The relative duration of time spent by the cell in each phase is another important factor and has been approximately determined for each phase: S-phase (10–20 hours), G_2 (2–10 hours), G_1 (variable—18 hrs average). These times affect the doubling of a tumor cell population. The doubling time is that time for a mass to double in size and is related to the number of cells actually dividing, termed the growth fraction. Other cell compartments also influence tumor growth and thus the doubling time (Figure 3). The cell populations in compartments B and C decrease the growth fraction of cells and include hypoxic, nutritionally deficient, or resting G_0 cells. These cells are generally less sensitive to antineoplastic drugs or irradiation. Unfortunately, some tumors, usually large tumors, may have a large fraction of cells in the resting state.

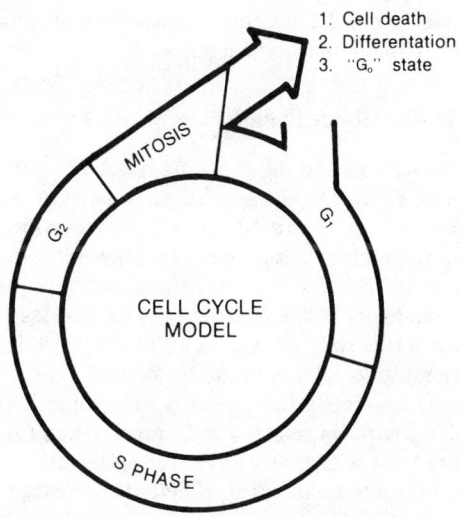

Figure 2. Phases of The Cell Cycle.

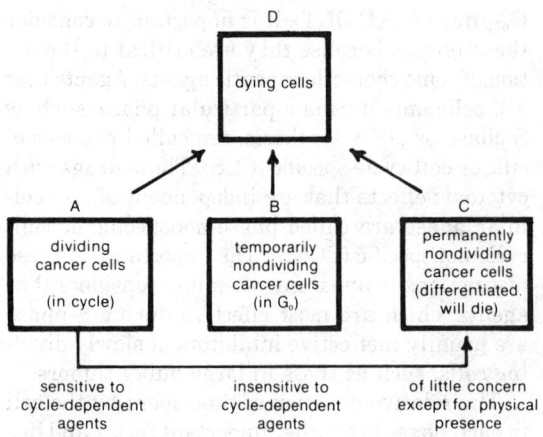

Figure 3. Relationship of Cell Compartments and Cell Loss.

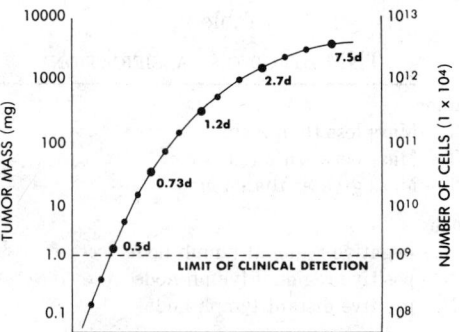

Figure 4. Gompertzian Cell Growth.

Tumor growth often follows *Gompertzian growth* kinetics (Figure 4) in which early tumor cell growth is rapid and has a high growth fraction and rapid doubling time. As the tumor enlarges, it begins to outgrow its blood and nutrient supply and its growth rate decreases and reaches a plateau phase of growth. Some tumors, such as multiple myeloma, closely follow this pattern of growth (8).

Therefore, the selection of an agent(s) may depend on whether the disease is at an early or advanced stage. It should be apparent that an advanced tumor with a low growth fraction should respond better to a phase-nonspecific than to a phase-specific agent, and vice-versa for a small tumor. Table 3 lists the commonly used phase-specific and nonspecific agents.

Cell Kill Hypothesis

Tumor size and mass can be related to clinical events. When the disease is diagnosed at an early stage such as carcinoma *in situ*, the earliest lesion producing symptoms probably consists of about 10^9 cells, which is equivalent to 1 cubic centimeter or 1 gram of tumor; late disease contains $\sim 10^{12}$ cells, which is 1000 cm^3 or 1 kg of tumor and usually is lethal to the host. The number of tumor cells and its mass is shown in Figure 4 along with its relation to Gompertzian growth. If a patient is at a very advanced stage (10^{12} cells) and is treated with very effective chemotherapy (cell kill 99.9%, or three-log), the patient will probably have a complete response. However, 10^9

Table 3.

CLASSIFICATION BY CELL-CYCLE ACTION

Phase-Specific Agents (CCS)	Phase-Nonspecific Agents (CCNS)
Asparaginase	Actinomycin D
Azathioprine	Bleomycin*
Bleomycin*	Busulfan
Cytarabine	Carmustine (BCNU)
Hydroxyurea	Chlorambucil
Mercaptopurine	Cisplatin
Methotrexate	Cyclophosphamide
Thioguanine	Dacarbazine (DTIC)
Vinblastine	Daunorubicin
Vincristine	Doxorubicin
Vindesine	Fluorouracil
	Hexamethylmelamine
	Lomustine (CCNU)
	Melphalan (L-PAM)
	Nitrogen mustard
	Procarbazine
	Thiotepa

*Bleomycin has properties of both CCS and CCNS.

tumor cells still remain and will undoubtedly regrow without further therapy. Thus, one should not confuse a complete response with cure.

An important principle in chemotherapy is that drugs kill a *fraction* of cells, which can vary from a few up to 99.999% of tumor cells, with the fraction killed being related to the dose of the drug administered. This fraction is described by first-order kinetics or exponential (logarithmic) cell kill. Therefore, a one-log to a three-log kill is equivalent to a 90 and 99.9% cell kill, respectively.

Principles of Cancer Chemotherapy (10)

In order to maximize the effectiveness of chemotherapy, the following principles should be considered:

A. Chemotherapy should be started when the tumor burden is low and growth fraction is high.

B. Debulking procedures, such as surgery and radiation, should be performed before chemotherapy, whenever possible.

C. Combinations of antineoplastic drugs generally will kill a larger percentage of tumor cells than single agent treatment.

D. Drug scheduling is very important. For the same dose of drug, intermittent dosing with rest periods for bone marrow recovery are less toxic to host tissue than continuous daily dosing. An intermittent schedule can often be repeated over several months as long as the maximum tolerable dose already has been determined.

E. Patients should be dosed to either response or toxicity, whichever comes first, before a change in therapy is considered.

F. The benefits from chemotherapy must be greater than the toxicity induced.

G. CCS and CCNS drugs should be administered in the appropriate schedule. A phase- (or cell-cycle)-non-specific drug (CCNS) is usually schedule-independent, because it is most effective when given in large, intermittent dosage schedule. In contrast, a phase- (or cell-cycle)-specific agent (CCS) is most effective when given in a continuous prolonged schedule and is usually schedule-dependent.

CLINICAL USE OF ANTICANCER DRUGS

The above principles form the basis for the use of antineoplastic agents in the clinical setting. The oncologist or hematologist will generally select a therapy which is considered a "first-line" treatment, or he may design a therapy specifically for the patient. In the latter situation, a deviation from first-line therapy may occur be-

cause of the presence of some form of organ dysfunction which may preclude treatment with a particular drug. For example, methotrexate may be contraindicated in a patient with severe renal dysfunction or a pleural effusion. Some commonly used chemotherapy regimens are listed in Table 4, and potentially curable cancers are listed in Table 5.

The selection of a chemotherapy program may depend upon factors that could affect the response to a drug or combination of drugs. For example, when a first-time chemotherapy regimen for a "curable" cancer has failed and the disease has become advanced, it is often difficult to salvage a cure. Previous chemotherapy may affect subsequent drug selection, because drugs from similar pharmacologic classes will not usually be chosen. Furthermore, an inadequate bone marrow reserve may not allow adequate dosing of the more potent myelosuppressive agents, or myelosuppressive therapy may increase the risk of further bacteremia and sepsis in a patient with a preexisting infection. Finally, tumors which have failed to respond to several chemotherapy programs are unlikely to respond to further therapy. A list of factors which affect drug selection appears in Table 6.

Classification of Anticancer Drugs

Cytotoxic, hormonal, and immune response modifying drugs comprise the three major categories of anticancer drugs.

Cytotoxic Agents. These drugs can be classified in various ways, but the most common are by biochemical mechanisms of action, by cell-cycle kinetic action(s), and by in vivo cell-culture, animal-model systems.

According to one classification based upon mechanisms of action, cytotoxic drugs can:

A. Interfere with the biosynthesis of DNA, RNA, and proteins:
  1. Folic acid antagonists (methotrexate, aminopterin)
  2. Purine antagonists (6-mercaptopurine, 6-thioguanine)
  3. Pyrimidine antagonists (5-fluorouracil, FUdR, ftorafur, cytarabine, 5-azacytidine, 6-azauridine, hydroxyurea, guanazole)
  4. Miscellaneous [nitrosoureas (carmustine, lomustine, semustine, streptozotocin), procarbazine]

Table 4.

Commonly Used Combination Regimens

Cancer	Acronym	Drugs*	Doses	Frequency Response Rate
Bladder	Cisca	Pt	100 mg/m^2 d 2 IV	Q 3 wks
		CTX	650 mg/m^2 d 1 IV	
		Adria	50 mg/m^2 d 1 IV	
Breast	CMF	CTX	100 mg/m^2/d × 14 po	Q 4 wks
		MTX	40 mg/m^2/d 1, 8 IV	
		FU	400 mg/m^2 d 1, 8 IV	
	CAF	CTX	100 mg/m^2/d × 14 po	Q 4 wks
		Adria	30 mg/m^2 d 1, 8 IV	
		FU	400 mg/m^2 d 1, 8 IV	
Colorectal	—	FU	400 mg/m^2 weekly IV	Weekly
		MeCCNU	175 mg/m^2 d 1 IV	Q 6 wks
Hodgkin's	MOPP	NM	6 mg/m^2 d 1, 8 IV	Q 4 wks
		Onc	1.4 mg/m^2 d 1, 8 IV	
		PROC	100 mg/m^2 d 1–14 po	
		Pred	40 mg/m^2 d 1–14 po	
Leukemia				
ALL	VP	VCR	2 mg/m^2 q wk IV × 4	As needed
		Pred	2.2 mg/kg po d 1–28.	
	OAP	Onc	1 mg d 1, 8, 15, 22 IV	As needed
		Ara C	100 mg/m^2 d 1–10 IV infusion	
		Pred	100 mg/d dl–5 po	
AML	DA	Dauno	45 mg/m^2 d 1–3	As needed
		Ara C	100 mg/m^2 d 1–10 IV infusion	
Lymphoma				
Favorable	CHL	CHLOR	0.4 mg/kg (pulse)	Q 4 wks daily
		CHLOR	8–12 mg/d × 6 wks	
Unfavorable	C-MOPP	CTX	400 mg/m^2 d 1, 8 IV	Q 4 wks
		ONC	1.5 mg/m^2 d 1, 8 IV (2 mg max)	
		PROC	100 mg/m^2 d 1–14 po	
		Pred	40 mg/m^2 d 1–14 po	
	CHOP	CTX	750 mg/m^2 d 1 IV	Q 3 wks
		H (Adria)	50 mg/m^2 d 1 IV	
		Onc	1.4 mg/m^2 d 1 (max 2 mg)	
		Pred	100 mg/d d 1–5	
	CVP	CTX	400 mg/m^2 d 2–6 po	Q 3 wks
		VCR	1.4 mg/m^2 dl	
		Pred	100 mg/m^2 d 2–6 po	
Ovary	HexaCAF	Hexa	150 mg/m^2 d 1–14 po	Q 4 wks
		CTX	150 mg/m^2 d 1–14 po	
		MTX	40 mg/m^2 d 1, 8 IV	
		FU	600 mg/m^2 d 1, 8 IV	
	FAM	FU	600 mg/m^2 d 1, 8, 28, 35	Q 8 wks
		Adria	30 mg/m^2 d 1, 28 IV	
		Mito-C	10 mg/m^2 d 1 only IV	

Table 4. (continued)

COMMONLY USED COMBINATION REGIMENS

Cancer	Acronym	Drugs*	Doses	Frequency Response Rate
Sarcoma	—	Adria	60 mg/m^2 d 1 IV	Q 3 wks
		DTIC	250 mg/m^2 d 1–5 IV	

*Drug Abbreviations: Adria (Adriamycin); Ara C (Cytarabine); CHLOR (Chlorambucil); CTX (cyclophosphamide); Dauno (Daunorubicin); DTIC (dacarbazine); FU (5-Fluorouracil); Hexa (Hexamethylmelamine); MeCCNU (Semustine); MTX (methotrexate); Mito-C (mitomycin-C); NM (Nitrogen Mustard); Onc (Vincristine); Pred (Prednisone); PROC (Procarbazine); Pt (Cisplatin); VCR (Vincristine)

B. Inhibit protein synthesis:
   1. Enzyme (L-asparaginase)

C. Interfere with the replication, transcription and translation of DNA:
   1. Alkylators (nitrogen mustard, cyclophosphamide)
   2. Other alkylators (pipobroman, dibromodulcitol, galaclitol, diamminodichloroplatinum, mitomycin-C, nitrosoureas, imidazole carboxamide, ICRF-159)
   3. Interfere with transcription (actinomycin-D, daunomycin, doxorubicin, carminomycin)
   4. Translation inhibitors (puromycin)

D. Enhance radiomimetic effects (bleomycin, streptonigran)

E. Interfere with the mitotic spindle (vincristine, vinblastine, etoposide, teniposide)

Hormones. Although hormones do not possess cytotoxic action, they can cause tumor regression by altering the hormonal milieu. These agents are primarily effective against tumors that arise from hormone-responsive tissue (11). Drugs used therapeutically against such tumors are listed in Table 7.

Immune Modifying Agents. The immune system is essential for the total eradication of tumor cells; investigational immune modifying agents are listed in Table 8. These agents may be useful only if the tumor burden is less than 10^6 cells. Therefore, the rationale for immunotherapy is based upon its use as an adjuvant to surgery, radiotherapy, or chemotherapy. The potentially useful immunoadjuvants are nonspecific because they indirectly augment immune responses to all

Table 5.

DISEASES WHERE CURES ARE ACHIEVABLE OR SURVIVAL SUBSTANTIALLY PROLONGED

Disease	Therapy*
Lymphoma	CHOP + XRT
Choriocarcinoma (Women)	Methotrexate, Act-D
ALL (childhood)	VCR + Pred
Hodgkin's disease	MOPP
Testicular carcinoma	PVB (platinum, vinblastine, bleomycin)
Ewing's sarcoma	VCR + Act-D + XRT

*Abbreviations: Act-D (Actinomycin D); XRT (Radiotherapy); others in Table 4.

Table 6.

FACTORS AFFECTING DRUG SELECTION

1. Curability of the cancer
2. Previous chemotherapy
3. Previous radiotherapy
4. Bone marrow reserve
5. Nutritional status
6. Performance status
7. Organ dysfunction
8. Concurrent problems
   a. Infections
   b. Malignant effusions
   c. Metabolic abnormalities (hypercalcemia)
9. Tumor resistance
10. Psychosocial aspects
11. Expected tolerance

Table 7.

HORMONES IN THE TREATMENT OF CANCER

Disease	Therapy/Drug
Breast Cancer	Estrogens
	Diethylstilbestrol (DES)
	Ethinylestradiol (EE)
	Antiestrogens
	Tamoxifen
	Androgens
	Calusterone
	Fluoxymesterone
	Testosterone esters
	Testolactone
	Progestins
	Medroxyprogesterone
	Megestrol
	Norethisterone
	Glucocorticoids
	Prednisone
	Medical adrenalectomy
	Aminoglutethimide
Renal cell cancer	Progestins (see drugs above)
Endometrial cancer	Progestins
	Antiestrogens
Prostatic carcinoma	Estrogens

Table 8.

IMMUNE MODIFYING AGENTS

BCG
C. Parvum
Interferon
Levamisole
MER (Methanol Extraction Residue of BCG)
Thymosin

cancers and not to a particular cancer cell. The results with immunotherapy have been generally disappointing, and its use has diminished dramatically in recent years.

Tumor Markers

1. **A 28-year-old male has the diagnosis of testicular embryonal cell carcinoma. Clinical evidence of metastatic disease is lacking and his blood chemistries are within normal limits except for elevated serum concentrations of alpha-fetoprotein (α-FP) and human chorionic gonadotropin (β-HCG). What is the clinical importance of these elevations in α-FP and β-HCG?**

Some types of tumors can increase the secretion of endogenous tissue substances which may or may not have pharmacologic activity. These substances, usually hormones or polypeptide proteins, can act as tumor markers for diagnosis or for monitoring the disease process (11).

In this case, α-FP and β-HCG are not usually found in the normal male. The α-FP and β-HCG

are tumor-specific proteins which are *not* hormonally active. Their presence in the blood suggests metastatic dissemination of this patient's testicular cancer despite the absence of other clinical evidence which might implicate metastasis. Thus, the stage of this patient's disease and his prognosis are worse than would be the case if no tumor markers were found. Other tumor markers are listed in Table 9.

Bone Marrow Suppression

2. **A 55-year-old, 70-kg female with breast carcinoma and lung metastases was treated with 5-FU, mitomycin-C, adriamycin, and vincristine. Her complete blood count (CBC) is shown below. Her platelets fell to their lowest value (nadir) on day 21, and epistaxis was noted on that same day.**

	Day 1	21	28	42
WBC	4300	3500	4100	4500
Hematocrit	38.6%	35.7%	38%	38%
Platelets	154,000	44,000	60,000	220,000
Mitomycin-C	25 mg	0	0	18 mg
5-FU	700 mg	0	0	700 mg
Vincristine	2 mg	0	2 mg	2 mg
Adriamycin	40 mg	0	0	40 mg

Which agent was probably responsible for the decrease in platelet count?

Several antineoplastic drugs exert selective effects on one hematologic element more than another. In this case, mitomycin-C was probably the agent that caused the platelet count to fall to its lowest value (nadir) 21 days after initiation of therapy (12). The nitrosoureas, thiotepa, and methotrexate also depress platelets more selectively than leukocytes. Other agents, such as busulfan and cyclophosphamide, spare the platelets at the expense of leukocyctes.

Table 9.

TUMOR MARKERS IN MALIGNANCY

Marker Substance	Acronym	Tumor(s) Associated
Carcinoembryonic antigen	CEA	Carcinomas of breast, lung, pancreas, stomach, colon, rectum
Alphafetoprotein	α-FP	Hepatoma, embryonal carcinoma of testis
Human chorionic gonadotropin (beta subunit)	β-HCG	Choriocarcinoma, carcinoma of testis
Acid Phosphatase	—	Prostatic carcinoma
Estrogen Receptor	ER	Carcinoma of breast, liver, prostate, ovary
Progesterone Receptor	PR	Carcinomas of breast, uterus, ovary
Ectopic hormones	—	Various neoplasms (see paraneoplastic syndromes, Table 21)
Immunoglobulins	IgG IgM IgA IgE	Multiple Myeloma

In a single dose of 12 mg/kg or less, 5-fluorouracil (5-FU) is relatively nontoxic to the bone marrow. Also, the typical nadir from 5-FU appears by day 7–10. In contrast, mitomycin in doses of 15 mg/m² can produce substantial leukocyte or platelet count depression with mean time to nadir of about 25 to 30 days and recovery usually by about the forty-second day (12). It appears that this patient's pattern of bone marrow suppression was primarily due to mitomycin-C.

Other drugs with different patterns of bone marrow suppression and recovery are shown in Table 10 and Figure 5. As can be seen, two patterns exist (13). Following the administration of cyclophosphamide, cytarabine, methotrexate, nitrogen mustard, vinblastine, cisplatin, and doxorubicin, the leukocyte count falls to its nadir in 8 to 10 days and recovers by day 17 to 21. With the nitrosoureas, melphalan, chlorambucil, and thiotepa, the leukocytes decrease in a biphasic wave pattern on day 8 to 10 and again on day 28 with recovery by 6 weeks.

3. Why was vincristine administered on day 28 when the patient's platelet count was only 60,000?

Bone marrow suppression is the most common dose-limiting toxicity of chemotherapy. Therefore, the pattern of leukocyte or platelet depression for each drug is an important consideration in determining the most effective, yet maximally

tolerable, dosage schedule. When bone marrow is especially sensitive to certain agents, drugs such as vincristine which have little or no effect on the marrow elements should be utilized. Although the platelet count was 60,000 in this patient, the administration of vincristine would not be expected to suppress the platelet count any further.

Other cytotoxic drugs with relatively little effect on the bone marrow (14) are listed in Table 11. With these drugs, dosages need not be modified because of myelosuppression. Of the agents

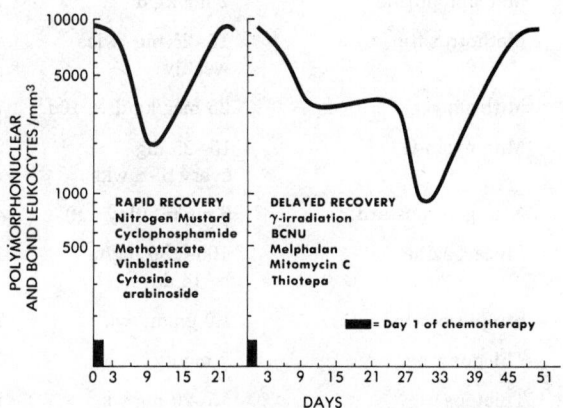

Figure 5. Leukopenia from Chemotherapy: Patterns of Toxicity and Recovery. (Modified from Bergsagel, ref 13.)

listed in Table 11, both vincristine and methotrexate are active against this patient's breast
cancer, but vincristine is considerably less bone
marrow suppressive than methotrexate.

**4. Were the doses of 5-FU and mitomycin-
C on day 42 adequately reduced to reflect the
degree of myelosuppression in this patient?**
The dosage of mitomycin-C was decreased about

Table 10.

MYELOSUPPRESSIVE EFFECTS FROM CHEMOTHERAPY

Drug	Dose	Onset (days)	Nadir (days)	Recovery (days)	Severity (Qualitative)
Actinomycin D	0.1 mg/kg/d	7	14	21–28	moderate
Adriamycin	60 mg/m^2	10	14	21–24	moderate
Ara-C (cytarabine)	100–150 mg/m^2	4–7	14–18	21	severe
BCNU (carmustine)	100–150 mg/m^2	7	14	42–50	severe
Bleomycin	10 mg/m^2	4–7	10	18	none
Busulfan	4–6 mg/d	7	14–21	28	moderate
CCNU (lomustine)	100–150 mg/m^2	14	21	42	severe on platelets
Chlorambucil	0.2 mg/kg/d	7	10–14	21	moderate
Cisplatin	100 mg/m^2	10	14	21	moderate
Cyclophosphamide	1–1.5 gm/m^2 every 3 weeks	7	10–14	21	moderate
DTIC (dacarbazine)	200–400 mg/m^2 × 5d every 4 wks	7	10–14	24	mild
Etoposide (VP-16)	80–100 mg/m^2	10	16	21	moderate
Fluorouracil	15–20 mg/kg/wk	7–10	14	16–24	mild
Hexamethylmelamine	6 mg/kg/d	14	21	28	mild
Melphalan	12–18 mg/d every 6–7 weeks	7	10–18	42–50	moderate
Mercaptopurine	2 mg/kg/d	7–10	14	21	moderate
Methotrexate	15–25 mg twice weekly	4–7	14	21	mild
Mithramycin	25 mcg/kg/d × 10d	7	14	21–28	moderate
Mitomycin-C	15–25 mg every 6–8 wks	21	36	42–56	severe on platelets
Nitrogen mustard	6 mg/m^2 (day 1,8)	4–7	10	21–28	severe
Procarbazine	100–150 mg/m^2 × 14 days	14	21	28	moderate
Streptozotocin	1.0 gm/m^2/wk	7	14	21	mild
Thioguanine	2 mg/kg	7–10	14	21	moderate
Thiotepa	15–20 mg/wk	10	14	28	platelets severe
Vinblastine	5 mg/m^2/wk	7	10	17	moderate
	0.2 mg/kg	7	10	17	severe
Vincristine	1–2 mg/wk	NA	NA	NA	

Table 11.

CHEMOTHERAPEUTIC AGENTS OR
DOSAGE REGIMENS
WHICH ARE RELATIVELY BONE MARROW SPARING
WHEN USED ALONE

Bleomycin
Corticosteroids
Cyclophosphamide (platelet-sparing only)
Ftorafur
Hexamethylmelamine
ICRF-159
Methotrexate with citrovorum factor rescue
Streptozotocin
Vincristine
VM-26

25% because of the risk of hemorrhage. On day 21, the patient's platelet count decreased to 44,000/mm³, her hematocrit decreased by about 3%, and an episode of epistaxis was noted. The nadir of the WBC count also occurred on the twenty-first day after initiation of chemotherapy, but a nadir of 3500/mm³ is acceptable. In most clinical settings, it is desirable to maintain the granulocyte and platelet counts at more than 2,000 and 50,000/mm³, respectively.

Doses of medications can be adjusted either on the basis of the present WBC and platelet counts or on the nadir of these two blood elements. According to the following guidelines which are commonly utilized at the University of California, San Francisco, this patient would not have received such a large second dose of mitomycin-C if the nadir of the platelet count is the major determinant:

Leukocytes	Platelets	% dose
4,000/mm³	120,000/mm³	100
3,000–3,999	100,000–119,000	75
2,500–2,999	75,000–99,000	25–50
2,500	75,000	0

However, in this case, the platelet and WBC counts recovered fully to baseline levels, and delay of further therapy could have led to relapse of the disease between treatment courses (15). Thus, an argument can be made for treating this patient despite the above guidelines. The potential for toxicity, however, may be greater (15,16), and for that reason the dose of mitomicin-C was decreased.

ADVERSE EFFECTS OF CHEMOTHERAPY

Anthracycline Cardiac Toxicity

5. D.A., a 63-year-old female, has bronchogenic carcinoma with regional recurrence and metastatic disease. After receiving 4500 rads of cobalt[60] to her chest over 45 days, systemic chemotherapy is planned with doxorubicin (45 mg/m² every 3 weeks) and cyclophosphamide (750 mg every 3 weeks). Upon interview, it was ascertained that the patient is taking digoxin 0.25 mg daily, hydrochlorothiazide 50 mg daily, and supplemental potassium for heart failure. Pertinent past medical history includes a myocardial infarction six years ago. Why is this patient especially susceptible to the toxicity of doxorubicin?

The major dose-limiting toxicity for the anthracycline, doxorubicin (adriamycin), results from its direct effect on myocardial tissue (17). In adults, the incidence (and probably the severity) of doxorubicin-induced congestive heart failure (CHF) is directly related to the cumulative dose of this anthracycline. The incidence is approximately 3% at 400 mg/m², 7% at 550 mg/m², and 18% at 700 mg/m² (18). Patients have also developed CHF after a single dose of doxorubicin or daunorubicin (50 mg/m²). In children, a similar dose-related incidence of CHF is evident and enhanced by irradiation to the chest. Children under 10 years of age appear to be at greater risk for toxicity at doses less than 550 mg/m² (19).

Several risk factors may enhance the cardiotoxic potential of anthracyclines (18,20). Patients who receive mediastinal or left chest wall irradiation have a higher incidence of cardiomyopathy at lower cumulative doses. Also, concurrent cyclophosphamide, prior cardiac disease, hypertension, and aortic stenosis increase the risk of anthracycline cardiomyopathy (21,22). This patient has several of these risk factors. (The cardiotoxic effects of the anthracyclines are also discussed in the chapter entitled Pediatric Oncology.)

6. If CHF develops, how should it be managed?

The early reports of doxorubicin-induced heart failure suggested that it was often refractory to treatment and frequently fatal (23). However, with cardiomyopathy being a recognized complication of anthracycline usage, the drug is now discontinued at the earliest sign of CHF and the patient is treated with digitalis glycosides and diuretic therapy. Thus, mortality from cardiac failure is now uncommon.

7. What objective data might be of value in predicting doxorubicin-induced CHF?

Even though most patients will not develop CHF, typical myocardial lesions probably occur in all patients given 240 mg/m^2 or more of doxorubicin (24). However, it is uncertain which of these patients will go on to develop symptoms. Predicting those patients at risk is best demonstrated by endomyocardial biopsies which often show early myocardial damage, but this technique has limited practical usefulness. Noninvasive techniques, such as radionuclide scanning with exercise testing, might be more readily accepted if studies can confirm accurate predictions of early or late toxicity. This monitoring test may be useful for diagnosis and follow-up evaluation of ventricular function (25).

8. The usual dose of doxorubicin ranges from 45–60 mg/m^2 every three weeks or 15–20 mg/m^2 weekly. Which dosage regimen would be best for this patient?

When doxorubicin is administered in a weekly schedule, the incidence of CHF decreases threefold compared to a single dose given every three weeks (26). This substantial reduction in myocardial toxicity may be due to the lower peak concentrations which result from more frequent administration of smaller doses. As such, continuous infusion doxorubicin, which results in very low plasma levels of the drug compared to rapid intravenous injections, may also produce a much lower incidence of CHF (27,28). Doxorubicin by infusion, however, requires indwelling intravenous catheterization, and other practical considerations generally make this approach difficult. Therefore, the weekly dosage regimen may be preferable for this patient who is more susceptible to doxorubicin cardiotoxicity. However, even though weekly dosing is safer, its therapeutic efficacy remains to be established.

9. About 24 hours after receiving her first dose of 45 mg/m^2 of doxorubicin, patient D.A. experienced an episode of tachycardia which persisted for 12 hours. Can her next dose of doxorubicin be safely given in three weeks?

A second form of anthracycline (doxorubicin or daunorubicin) cardiotoxicity consists of acute ar-

rhythmias which occur in approximately one-third of patients (21). These arrhythmias are usually transient, asymptomatic, and do not require modification of the doxorubicin treatment. In some patients with a prior history of severe arrhythmias, anthracyclines may have to be discontinued. In patients with abnormal electrocardiograms *prior* to doxorubicin therapy, the incidence of new electrocardiogram abnormalities increases from 15% to 43%; however, electrocardiogram abnormalities per se are not predictive of doxorubicin-induced CHF or cardiomyopathy (21). This patient should be followed closely for signs of severe arrhythmia lasting longer than 24 hours and if present, therapy should be discontinued.

Pulmonary Toxicity

Several cytotoxic drugs (Table 12) are associated with respiratory dysfunction (29–31). The onset of clinical symptoms is usually insidious and is generally characterized by nonproductive cough, fever, dyspnea, tachypnea, and interstitial infiltrates on the chest x-ray. The pulmonary toxicity usually develops after these drugs have been administered for several years and appears to be related to direct cell damage. In contrast, some drugs, such as asparaginase, mercaptopurine, and methotrexate, are associated with rapid onset of pulmonary symptoms which probably are representative of an allergic pulmonary reaction.

Bleomycin classically produces fine bibasilar rales as its earliest sign of pulmonary toxicity. The chest x-ray usually shows a diffuse interstitial infiltrate consistent with pneumonitis. Approximately 10% of patients will develop this toxicity and, of these patients, 10% will die from progressive respiratory failure (32). In most cases, respiratory dysfunction improves if bleomycin is discontinued at the first sign of toxicity. Even though the chest x-ray and pulmonary function are usually abnormal at the time of diagnosis, these tests are not predictive of impending toxicity. The best predictor may be lung diffusing capacity (DCO) which measures the ability of the alveoli to transport oxygen (33).

The risk of bleomycin pulmonary toxicity is increased in patients more than 60 years of age, and in patients with concurrent or recent lung irradiation, concurrent chemotherapy, or preexisting pulmonary disease (30,32,34,35). Bleomycin lung toxicity is more common with doses greater than 200 mg/m², but it also has occurred at doses as low as 50 mg. Corticosteroids may be clinically helpful in early cases of pneumonitis.

Hypersensitivity Reactions

10. **A 32-year-old female with acute lymphoblastic leukemia is hospitalized for induction chemotherapy with vincristine, prednisone, and L-asparaginase. Approximately four hours after drug administration, a fever of 39°C is noted. A chest x-ray is normal, and the CBC reveals 50,000 white cells with 5% granulocytes, 20% lymphocytes. Cultures are obtained from blood, sputum, and urine. Ticarcillin and tobramycin are started, but cultures are negative and antibiotics are discontinued three days later. A second dose of L-asparaginase is given and the patient again spikes a fever to 39°C. What may be the cause of this patient's fever and how should it be treated?**

In granulocytopenic patients, fever most often indicates life-threatening bacterial infection, and broad-spectrum antibiotics are usually initiated immediately. However, cytotoxic agents such as vincristine, bleomycin, and L-asparaginase are also frequently associated with febrile reactions (36).

Table 12.

PULMONARY TOXICITY FROM CHEMOTHERAPY (data from refs. 52,53,54)

Drug	Incidence or No. Case Reports	Pathology	Drug Schedule	Onset	Reversibility/ Treatment
Asparaginase	22%	Uncertain	Daily × 7	Rapid (days)	(+) antihistamines
Azathioprine	Rare	Alveolitis	Daily	Moderate (wks)	(+) steroids
Bleomycin	10%	Pneumonitis, interstitial fibrosis	Weekly	Delayed (months)	(+)(−) avoid total doses > 200 mg/m²
Busulfan	24 cases up to 1978	Interstitial fibrosis	Daily	Insidious (yrs)	(−) steroids ineffective
Carmustine	11 cases up to 1980	Interstitial fibrosis	Intermittent (q 4 wks)	Insidious (yrs)	(−)
Chlorambucil	4 cases	Interstitial fibrosis	Daily	Delayed (months)	(−)
Cyclophosphamide	2 cases	Interstitial fibrosis	Daily	Insidious (yrs)	(−)
Melphalan	2 cases	Interstitial fibrosis	Daily	Insidious (yrs)	(−)
Mercaptopurine	Rare	Interstitial pneumonitis	Daily	Rapid (days)	(+) discontinuation
Methotrexate	Uncommon	Alveolitis	Daily/ Biweekly	Rapid (days)	(+) prednisone 30 mg/d
Mitomycin C	12 cases	Alveolar cell hypertrophy	Intermittent (q 4–6 wks)	Moderate (8–30 wks)	(+)(−) steroids
Procarbazine	2 cases	Alveolitis	Daily	Delayed (months)	(+) discontinuation
Semustine	1 case	Interstitial fibrosis	Intermittent (q 4–6 wks)	Delayed	(?)

The fever usually occurs two to six hours after drug administration and probably reflects an allergic response. Because chemotherapy often involves a combination of drugs, it is difficult to attribute these febrile reactions to any one specific agent. In this particular case, the febrile episode probably is a drug reaction caused by L-asparaginase since infection appears to have been ruled out and the fever reappeared immediately after a second dose of this drug. Other cytotoxic agents that produce febrile reactions are listed in Table 13.

Antipyretics may mask a clinical sign of infection and should probably be avoided in leukopenic patients, who are at high risk for infection. However, fever may enhance platelet destruction and increase the risk of hemorrhage as well. If an infection has been ruled out, antipyretics may be used to treat an allergic febrile reaction. Antihistamines (eg, diphenhydramine) 30–60 minutes prior to L-asparaginase therapy also may be useful in this patient.

11. A 32-year-old male with diffuse histiocytic lymphoma (Stage IV) was treated with cyclophosphamide, doxorubicin, vincristine, prednisone, and bleomycin (CHOP-BLEO).

Table 13.

CHEMOTHERAPEUTIC AGENTS
WHICH PRODUCE FEVER

Agent	Route of Administration
Adriamycin	Intravenous
L-Asparaginase	Intravenous
Azathioprine	Oral
Bleomycin	Intramuscular; intravenous
Chlorambucil	Oral
Cyclophosphamide	Intravenous
Cytosine Arabinoside	Intravenous
Dacarbazine	Intravenous
Dactinomycin	Intravenous
Daunomycin	Intravenous
6-Mercaptopurine	Intravenous; oral
Methotrexate	Intramuscular; intrathecal; intravenous
Mithramycin	Intravenous
Procarbazine	Intravenous; oral
Quinacrine	Intracavitary
Vinblastine	Intra-arterial; intravenous
Vincristine	Intravenous

One hour after administration of these drugs the patient complained of urticaria, dizziness and was markedly hypotensive. What drug was the most likely cause of this symptom complex?

Occasionally, chemotherapy with agents such as bleomycin, L-asparaginase, cisplatin, intravenous melphalan, zinostatin, and teniposide (VM-26) can cause hypersensitivity reactions. In this case, bleomycin appears to be implicated because of the "pseudoanaphylactic" pattern (37). These reactions may be mild or life-threatening. The most severe reactions occur in patients with lymphoma, and the prevalence is 1 to 8% (32,38,39). These reactions usually occur after intravenous injections (38), although a fatal reaction after an intramuscular injection has been reported (41).

Severe hypersensitivity reactions have occurred after test doses of bleomycin as well as after several doses of the drug (41). One of our patients experienced an anaphylactic reaction after the twentieth dose of bleomycin. This reaction was successfully treated with epinephrine and diphenhydramine.

Renal/Bladder Toxicity

12. M.P. is a 62-year-old female with carcinoma of the ovary metastatic to the pelvis. She is being treated with her third course of chemotherapy with doxorubicin 50 mg IV, cisplatin 150 mg IV infusion over six hours, and cyclophosphamide 700 mg IV. In addition, she is given prophylactic prochlorperazine as an antiemetic. Serum electrolyte concentrations are as follows: sodium 138 mEq/L, potassium 4.2 mEq/L, chloride 100 mEq/L, bicarbonate 28 mEq/L, and magnesium 2.7 mEq/L. Her serum creatinine is 1.1 mg/dl; one week later her serum creatinine increases to 2.5 mg/dl, and urinalysis reveals tubular casts. During her previous course of chemotherapy, she developed a gram-negative urinary tract infection and was treated with cefazolin and tobramycin. How does cisplatin-induced nephrotoxicity usually appear, and what clinical data implicate this drug as the cause of nephrotoxicity in this patient?

Cisplatin induces proximal renal tubular damage (42) in as many as 40% of patients. In these patients, the blood urea nitrogen (BUN) and serum creatinine concentrations usually increase within

4 to 30 days after initiation of therapy and usually peak between the tenth and twentieth day (43). The renal function usually deteriorates progressively after each course of cisplatin. In patients treated with 100 mg/m^2 of cisplatin every four weeks, the creatinine clearance may decrease by approximately 50% by the end of the fourth course of therapy (45). Although the renal function usually begins to improve two to four weeks after therapy, it does not completely recover to its pretreatment level. Thus, cisplatin nephrotoxicity is probably permanent and simulates renal damage from other heavy metals such as mercury (46). Pathologic analysis demonstrates a heavy metal type of renal lesion consisting of tubular necrosis, interstitial edema, and tubular degeneration.

Patients who have recently received other nephrotoxic agents, such as furosemide, aminoglycosides, or cephalothin, are at greater risk for developing cisplatin-induced acute renal failure (44). This patient received both a cephalosporin and an aminoglycoside during her previous course of chemotherapy. Furthermore, the tubular casts which were noted in the urine of this patient suggest renal tubular necrosis, and such casts are consistent with cisplatin nephrotoxicity.

13. What therapeutic interventions might have been utilized in an attempt to minimize or prevent the cisplatin nephrotoxicity in this patient?

Hydration and forced diuresis seem to decrease the incidence of cisplatin renal dysfunction by about four-fold (47,48). Apparently, these endeavors dilute the concentration of cisplatin in the renal tubular filtrate and also may decrease the accumulation of the drug within the proximal renal tissue. Although such therapy should increase the renal excretion of cisplatin, studies have not been conclusive (49,50). Nevertheless, forced diuresis with 25 gm of mannitol or 20 mg of furosemide in addition to parenteral fluid hydration to maintain a urine output of at least 125 ml/hour might have been reasonable for this patient.

14. Patient M.P. complains of burning during urination and red urine on the day after chemotherapy. Moderate hematuria (25 RBC's per HPF) is confirmed by urinalysis. What would be a reasonable assessment of this problem?

Although doxorubicin (and daunorubicin) is excreted into the urine in sufficient amounts to impart a red or orange-red color to the urine (51–53), this patient's hematuria would more likely be due to cyclophosphamide-induced hemorrhagic cystitis. Approximately 5% of cyclophosphamide-treated patients will develop signs of bladder toxicity, and it occurs most commonly in those with concurrent dehydration or renal dysfunction (54). The onset of hematuria may start as early as the first day or as late as four months after treatment. Early onset of cyclophosphamide-induced hemorrhagic cystitis usually is associated with high-dose intermittent treatment, while a late onset usually is associated with chronic low doses (55). Bladder damage is usually dose-related and is most common when doses are greater than 40 mg/kg. Bladder toxicity is manifested by dysuria, urinary frequency, or minor hematuria (55), or it may be severe enough to cause gross blood loss and even mortality. Such severe blood loss requires surgical urinary diversion (54). (Cyclophosphamide-induced bladder toxicity is also discussed in the chapter entitled Pediatric Oncology.)

15. What therapeutic interventions might be appropriate for the management of this patient's bladder toxicity?

Cyclophosphamide-induced bladder damage is caused by active drug metabolites. When present in high concentrations for a prolonged period of time, these metabolites alkylate bladder mucosal tissue (55,56). Therefore, this cystitis may be prevented by decreasing the urine concentration of these metabolites through hydration, diuresis, and frequent voiding (58). Furthermore, frequent urinary voiding diminishes the contact time between alkylating metabolites and the bladder mucosa. Thus, administration of cyclophosphamide in the early morning hours, as opposed to bedtime hours, would facilitate frequent urine voiding. Another method to decrease urinary concentrations of cyclophosphamide metabolites is to divide the daily dose into two or three fractions.

Patient M.P.'s hematuria does not require surgical intervention at this time because the hematuria does not seem to be severe. In situations of moderate cyclophosphamide-induced hematuria which does not respond to the above therapeutic modalities, bladder instillation of a 1 to 4% solution of formalin is effective in about 80%

of patients (56). Higher concentrations of formalin are best avoided because of major complications such as papillary necrosis, hydronephrosis, or fatal peritoneal extravasation. The formalin bladder instillation is thought to coagulate bladder protein, debride the bladder mucosa, and stimulate bladder tissue regeneration (56). Experimentally, N-acetylcysteine also has been used in animals because studies suggest it might neutralize alkylating metabolites (57).

16. Patient M.P. had received four courses of CTX + Adria + cisplatin, but her carcinoma was not responding. Methotrexate is now being considered. Her serum creatinine is 3.2 mg/dl, creatinine clearance 20 ml/min, and urine pH 6.0. Why does this renal impairment make the use of methotrexate hazardous?

Although 50–80% of methotrexate is excreted renally in the first 12 hours after administration (59,60), small methotrexate doses (250 mg/m^2 or less) generally are *not* associated with increased nephrotoxicity. Large doses, however, can precipitate acute renal failure because of drug crystallization in the renal tubule (61). The crystallization has been attributed to the low aqueous solubility of methotrexate and its 7-hydroxy metabolite (62). Methotrexate and its metabolite are approximately 20-fold and 10-fold more soluble, respectively, at a pH of 7 than at pH 5 (62). Therefore, alkalinization of the urine and efforts to ensure adequate hydration of the patient have been included into protocols in order to decrease the risk of crystal nephropathy from high-dose therapy (63,64).

In patients with creatinine clearances of less than 50 ml/min, methotrexate renal clearance may be decreased and enhanced systemic cytotoxicity may result. Thus, methotrexate is relatively contraindicated in this patient. Other nephrotoxic anticancer drugs such as those listed in Table 14 should be avoided in this patient.

Table 14.

RENAL AND URINARY TOXICITY FROM ANTINEOPLASTIC DRUGS*

Drug	Site	Pathology	Incidence	Onset	Recovery	Management
Cisplatin	Kidney	Tubular necrosis	10%–40%	1–4 weeks	2–4 weeks	Prehydration with saline with or without mannitol and furosemide
Cyclophosphamide	Bladder, ureter	Cystitis	5%	2–3 days	3–5 days	Hydration with 1–2 liters of fluid
Methotrexate (1–10 gm/m^2)	Renal pelvis	Tubular obstruction from drug precipitation	5%	6–12 hours	1–7 days	Prevention: prehydration with saline; alkalinization of urine with sodium bicarbonate or acetazolamide
Mithramycin (daily doses)	Kidney	Tubular necrosis	20%	7–14 days	1–4 weeks	Alternate-day therapy produces much lower incidence of nephrotoxicity
Semustine (> 1500 mg total dose)	Kidney	Tubular necrosis	50%	14–18 months	Months	General supportive care; dose related
Streptozotocin	Kidney	Tubular necrosis	30%–40%	7–14 days	1–4 weeks	Dosing every 3–4 weeks may allow greater recovery

*Modified from See-Lasley and Ignoffo, ref. 203 p. 270.

Vesicant Reactions

Many cytoxic agents cause local tissue necrosis when extravasated at the site of injection (Table 15). This iatrogenic complication develops in about 2 to 5% of patients when vesicant anticancer drugs are administered (65); however, it probably occurs in less than 1% of patients when experienced personnel administer these agents by standard protocol (Table 16).

Of these, doxorubicin is the most notorious of all the cytotoxic drugs in producing severe tissue necrosis upon extravasation because healing occurs very slowly, if at all. Surgical debridement and skin grafting (66,67) may be required if doxorubicin, mitomycin-C, or actinomycin-D (68) are extravasated. Vincristine, vinblastine, and nitrogen mustard produce severe local pain and erythema of rapid onset, usually within 24 hours of extravasation (65), but these drugs usually do not cause as extensive tissue destruction as doxorubicin.

Treatment of extravasation reactions must be undertaken immediately, regardless of the agent. Some anticancer drugs have specific antidotes, while others only have theoretical antidotes which are unproven clinically but may be of psychological benefit to both the patient and clinician. Mechlorethamine, vincristine, and doxorubicin have recommended antidotes (65). Other clinicians elect to observe the patient and not use local antidotes.

17. What course of action should be taken if patient M.P. complained of pain and erythema at the site of chemotherapy injection?

In patient M.P., doxorubicin is probably the cause of this problem because of three prescribed chemotherapy drugs, doxorubicin is the only one

with vesicant properties. Sodium bicarbonate and a glucocorticoid may be administered to the extravasation site to counteract the local cytotoxic properties of doxorubicin (69,70). Although the effectiveness of sodium bicarbonate is debated (71,72), most oncology teams currently instill $NaHCO_3$ locally. Additionally, the manufacturer claims that this technique has inhibited severe skin necrosis in 13 of 15 cases (73). A small dose of hydrocortisone phosphate has been effective in managing doxorubicin-induced lesions in the mouse model (71) and may be worthy of a trial in patients because it is of relatively low risk.

M.P. may be treated as described in Table 17. Instillation of 2–4 ml of $NaHCO_3$, a small dose of hydrocortisone phosphate (25 mg), and weekly followup visits are all appropriate interventions. If the lesion proceeds to local pain, induration,

Table 15.

VESICANT ANTICANCER DRUGS

Carmustine (phlebitis)
Dactinomycin
Daunorubicin
Doxorubicin (Adriamycin)
Etoposide (VP-16)
Mechlorethamine
Mithramycin
Mitomycin C
Vinblastine
Vincristine
Vindesine

Table 16.

GUIDELINES FOR ADMINISTERING CHEMOTHERAPY*

1. Dilute the drug in the appropriate amount of diluent to avoid high concentrations.
2. Select an infusion site in the following order of preference: forearm > dorsum of hand > wrist > antecubital fossa.
3. Insert a 20 or 21 gauge "butterfly" needle (one venipuncture only) into the vein.
4. Lightly tape the tubing of the "butterfly" distal to the needle. Do not obscure the injection site by covering it with tape.
5. Administer 5 ml of normal saline solution (NS) and withdraw a small amount of blood to test vein integrity and flow. Observe for extravasation.
6. If extravasation of NS is obvious, select another site (the other arm, or lateral or proximal to the initial site in that arm). Avoid a distal point on the same vein because of the potential for extravasation "upstream."
7. Administer the drug over at least 3 minutes or approximately 5 ml per minute. Withdraw blood once for each 1 to 2 ml of solution administered to assure proper needle placement. Repeatedly ask the patient if he feels any pain or burning.
8. Follow the drug injection with 5 to 10 ml or more of a saline infusion to flush tubing and needle of all drug.
9. If multiple drugs are prescribed, inject the nonvesicant agents first. If all drugs are vesicants, inject the one with the least amount of diluent first. Separate each administered drug with 3 to 5 ml of saline.

*From Ignoffo, ref. 195 p. 365.

and initial necrosis (usually by day 10), surgical excision and skin grafting should be considered.

Nausea and Vomiting

18. Why was it appropriate for patient M.P. to receive an antiemetic prophylactically?

Nausea and vomiting from chemotherapy is one of the side effects most dreaded by patients; however, not all cytotoxic drugs induce this adverse effect. It appears that the cytotoxic drugs can be classified into three groups of high, moderate, and low emetogenic potential (Table 18) (74). The highly emetogenic drugs, cisplatin, doxorubicin, and dacarbazine, often cause severe fluid and electrolyte imbalances, and patients probably should be hospitalized as a precaution. Thus, antiemetic prophylaxis clearly was indicated for patient M.P.

19. What antiemetics are effective in the management of chemotherapy-induced nausea and vomiting?

The *phenothiazines* have been the most widely used antiemetics for either chemotherapy- or ra-

Table 17.

MANAGEMENT OF CHEMOTHERAPY EXTRAVASATION*

1. Stop injection immediately, leaving needle in place.
2. Withdraw 3 to 5 ml of blood and solution (if possible).
3. Administer 25 mg hydrocortisone into the needle (optional) and remove needle.
4. With a 27-gauge TB syringe, aspirate any extravasated solution not removed by procedure (2).
5. Purposely administer the antidote subcutaneously in a "pin-cushion" manner in the extravasated area (use 4 to 5 injections).
6. Apply cold compresses for 1 hour to allow time for the antidote to interact with the vesicant.
7. Apply warm compresses at the extravasated site for 1 hour.**
8. Follow-up should be obtained weekly (or earlier if mechlorethamine), observing for signs of inflammation and necrosis.
9. Surgical excision should be considered at the first sign of tissue breakdown or ulceration.

*From Ignoffo, ref. 195, p. 365.
**It is well known that drug absorption from subcutaneous or intramuscular injections is enhanced in the presence of heat and decreased by cold. Some clinicians prefer cold over heat in the setting of extravasation. In our opinion, a combination of initial cold compresses followed by heat may be more rational than either method alone.

diation-induced nausea and vomiting (75,76), and their clinical use is presented in the chapter entitled Nausea and Vomiting. When phenothiazines are ineffective, other classes of agents are necessary.

The *butyrophenones,* haloperidol and droperidol, are probably as effective as phenothiazines in relieving nausea and vomiting, but clinicians have had less experience with these agents (77). Although extrapyramidal adverse effects may be more readily associated with these drugs (77) than with some classes of phenothiazines, these adverse effects are by no means predictable (78). Furthermore, these drugs have benefited 65% and 74% of cisplatin- and doxorubicin-treated patients, respectively; and haloperidol was effective in 54% of patients who previously did not respond optimally to prochlorperazine (78).

The anesthetic agent, droperidol, inhibits emesis in postsurgical patients, and reportedly is effective in cisplatin-treated patients refractory to standard antiemetics when given in IV doses of 0.5 mg one hour prior to cisplatin infusion and every four hours for the next one to five days (79). In this particular trial, the only noted side effect was mild somnolence which was tolerable. The antiemetic action of droperidol probably results from blocking the transmission of dopamine in the CTZ (80).

Several *antihistaminic drugs* have been used in chemotherapy-induced emesis, but these agents are no more effective than placebo. Trimethobenzamide (Tigan) and benzquinamide (Emete-Con) are used frequently in prochlorperazine failures, but only the latter agent appears to have sufficient activity against the more emetogenic cytotoxic drugs (81).

Metoclopramide (Reglan), a procainamide derivative, has both central (on the vomiting center) and peripheral (increasing gastric emptying time) antiemetic actions. Although metoclopramide in low doses was less effective than phenothiazines against chemotherapy-induced vomiting (75), 20 mg every four hours was 70% effective in cisplatin-induced vomiting refractory to standard antiemetics (82). Studies at Sloan-Kettering and New York University have demonstrated the efficacy and safety of metoclopramide in adults even when given in large doses of 1 to 2 mg/kg every 2–3 hours (83,214).

Glucocorticosteroids also may be of benefit in chemotherapy-induced emesis. The glucocorticoids are thought to inhibit the release of pros-

Table 18.
EMETIC POTENTIAL OF ANTINEOPLASTIC DRUGS*

Severe**	Moderate**	Mild-to-none**
Azacytidine (rapid injection)	Azacytidine (slow infusion)	Bleomycin
Carmustine	Cytarabine	Busulfan
Cisplatin	Etoposide	Chlorambucil
Cyclophosphamide (high-dose parenteral)	Hexamethylmelamine	Fluorouracil
Dacarbazine	Mitotane	Hydroxyurea
Dactinomycin	Procarbazine	L-Asparaginase
Daunorubicin	Razoxane	Melphlan
Doxorubicin	Teniposide	Mercaptopurine
Lomustine	Thiotepa	Methotrexate
Mechlorethamine	Vinblastine	Mitomycin C
Mithramycin		Thioguanine
Semustine		Vincristine
Streptozotocin		

*From Ignoffo, ref. 195, p. 265.
**The listing of agents is based on the frequency and severity of nausea and vomiting. That is, severe includes a frequency of >75% incidence of vomiting, usually with retching; moderate is between 25% and 75% vomiting; and mild is either nausea or less than 25% vomiting.

taglandins which are stimulated by the direct gastrointestinal toxicity of chemotherapy drugs. Dexamethasone and methylprednisolone relieved emesis in about 70% of patients (84,85); however, these studies were uncontrolled and were not stratified with regard to emetogenic drugs.

The *cannabinoids*, delta-9-tetrahydrocannabinol (Δ^9-THC) and a derivative, nabilone, have very good antiemetic activity against chemotherapy-induced nausea and vomiting. The cannabinoids decrease or eliminate vomiting episodes in about 70% of patients (86); and patients who respond either experience a euphoric "high" or achieve blood concentrations greater than 5 mcg/ml (87). THC is at least as effective as phenothiazines in preventing vomiting from chemotherapy of high emetic potential and more effective against agents of low or moderate emetic potential (88,89). More adverse effects occurred in the THC-treated versus the prochlorperazine-treated group and were most common in patients over 50 years of age (90). Several studies are ongoing (in 13 different states) to define the role of THC in the prevention of chemotherapy-induced emesis (91). In our experience, THC has been useful for chemotherapy of mild to moderate emetogenic potential and in younger, marijuana-experienced patients.

Neurotoxicity

Several cytotoxic drugs may cause neurologic disorders (92) and are listed in Table 19. The most common neuropathy occurs in the peripheral nervous system and usually consists of bilateral, symmetrical paresthesias, numbness, or motor weakness. Central nervous system neuropathies usually consist of confusion, somnolence, or facial nerve palsies; and autonomic neuropathies generally manifest as constipation, ileus, or urinary retention. These neuropathies usually are reversible upon discontinuation of therapy.

20. A.L., a 59-year-old white female with acute lymphoblastic leukemia, is hospitalized for induction chemotherapy. Vincristine 2 mg IV push every week, prednisone 100 mg daily, L-asparaginase 15,000 units daily for 14 days, and allopurinol 300 mg tid for three days to be followed by 300 mg/day are ordered. Laboratory data obtained at the time of hospital admission include: a white blood cell count of 120,000/mm^3 with 9% granulocytes, 11% lymphocytes, and 80% "blast" cells; and a uric acid of 7.5 mg/dl. After three weeks of therapy the patient complains of paresthesia

(numbness) in the fingers and the soles of her feet. She finds it difficult to "sense" her feet when walking, and trying to stand from a sitting position requires great effort. The patient also complains of severe constipation. The patient has been disoriented to time and place on several occasions. On physical examination, the deep tendon reflexes are abnormal, and the proximal thigh muscles and ankles are weak. Cranial nerves are intact. What is the probable cause of this patient's paresthesias, and must therapy be discontinued?

Neurologic dysfunction is commonly associated with vinca alkaloids, especially after 6–8 mg of vincristine have been administered (92). Symptoms initially consist of distal paresthesias, loss of ankle jerks, or depression of deep tendon reflexes. Areflexia occurs in about 50 to 70% of patients treated with the drug for 3 to 4 weeks (92), and about 60% of patients treated with weekly vincristine will develop paresthesias within the first two weeks of treatment (93). Sensory loss is uncommon (4%) with usual doses. Paresthesias are not dose-limiting and may not require discontinuation of therapy. Motor weakness, however, can be disabling and is a dose-limiting toxicity of vincristine. It is characterized by weakness in dorsiflexors of the toes and ankles, and extensors of the wrists and fingers (94). About 20–36% of patients develop weakness, and some may go on to develop muscle wasting. This condition is partially or completely reversible, but recovery may take several months (92). (The reader should also consult the chapter entitled Pediatric Oncology.)

21. What is the significance of the examination of the cranial nerves in this patient?

Cranial nerve toxicity occurs in 1 to 10% of patients receiving vinca alkaloids and consists of ptosis or ophthalmoplegia. This toxicity probably is a result of damage to the third cranial nerve (95,96). Toxicity to other cranial nerves may result in trigeminal neuralgia (VII), facial palsy (V), and depressed corneal reflexes (96). Furthermore, vocal cord paralysis may develop in about 1% of patients receiving vinca alkaloids. Another uncommon neurologic side effect is jaw pain, which may occur after the first or second injection (97). None of these findings are evident in this patient, and the cranial nerves in this patient are intact.

22. Why should this patient's constipation have been expected?

Vincristine also can be toxic to the autonomic nerves. Constipation occurs in 46% of patients; ileus is rare but may be particularly severe. Moreover, bladder atony develops in 4% of patients and may be common in patients older than 60 years of age (98).

23. Which drug is the most likely cause of this patient's disorientation?

L-asparaginase is frequently associated with central nervous system (CNS) toxicity, which usually manifests as lethargy and confusion (92). However, severe cerebral dysfunction may occasionally occur, resulting in stupor or coma, excessive somnolence, disorientation, hallucinations, or severe depression. Both early (within 2 days) or delayed (about 1 week) signs of enceph-

Table 19.

NEUROLOGIC TOXICITY FROM CHEMOTHERAPY

Drug	Type	Incidence
Asparaginase	CNS	13–40%
Cisplatin	PNS	uncommon
Hexamethylmelamine	PNS	33%
Methotrexate (intrathecal)	CNS	20%
Procarbazine	CNS	5%
Vinblastine	ANS, CNS, PNS	10%
Vincristine	ANS, CNS, PNS	50%

ANS: autonomic nervous system
CNS: central nervous system
PNS: peripheral nervous system

alopathy may occur secondary to L-asparaginase (99,100). The acute syndrome usually clears rapidly (1–2 days), but the delayed form may last several weeks.

The frequency and severity of CNS symptoms appear to be greater for high-dose regimens of L-asparaginase (92). At doses of 200 IU/kg the incidence is about 13%, compared to about 40% for doses of 1000–5000 IU/kg. Most current protocols utilize lower doses of the drug.

Hepatotoxicity

24. A blood chemistry from patient A.L. on day 21 reveals: SGOT 120 U/ml, LDH 350 U/ml, alkaline phosphatase 140 IU/L, serum albumin 2.6 gm/dl, serum bilirubin 1.8 mg/dl, and prothrombin time 16 seconds. What course of action is necessitated by these findings?

These chemical abnormalities are indicative of hepatic dysfunction and probably are due to L-asparaginase therapy. Hepatotoxicity from L-asparaginase occurs in more than 75% of patients and appears to be related to the drug's effect on hepatic metabolism and protein synthesis (101, 102). Several liver function tests are affected, including albumin (decreased in 70 to 80% of patients), alkaline phosphatase (increased up to 5-fold in 30–45%), SGOT or SGPT (increased in about 40%), bilirubin (increased in 60%), and bromsulfophthalein (increased in 60 to 80%) (103). Clotting abnormalities are frequent and manifested by decreased fibrinogen in over 90%, prolonged prothrombin time in 20–30%, and prolonged partial thromboplastin time in about 80% of patients (102,104). Despite these clotting abnormalities, bleeding seldom occurs (6% of cases) and the hepatic damage is reversible.

The hepatic lesion appears morphologically as diffuse fatty metamorphosis and is evident in up to 80% of autopsied patients (103). The liver toxicity most likely involves both L-asparagine depletion and inhibition of protein synthesis. The latter effect is reflected by the high incidence of hypoalbuminemia, hypocholesterolemia, and decreased synthesis of clotting proteins.

Fortunately, the hepatotoxic effects of L-asparaginase regress rapidly, usually within 2 weeks after stopping therapy (105). In the event of severe symptoms such as bleeding or hypovolemia,

Table 20.

HEPATIC TOXICITY FROM ANTINEOPLASTIC DRUGS

Drug	Dosing	Incidence*
Asparaginase	Daily × 3–7	80%
Azathioprine	Daily	Uncommon
Azacytidine	Daily × 5	Common
Bleomycin	Intermittent	Rare
Carmustine	Intermittent	Common
Cyclophosphamide	Intermittent	Rare
Cytarabine	Daily × 5–10	Uncommon
Dacarbazine	Intermittent	Uncommon
Daunorubicin	Daily × 3	Uncommon
Doxorubicin	Intermittent	Rare
Etoposide	Daily × 3	Rare
Mercaptopurine	Daily	Common
Methotrexate	Daily	Common
	Weekly	Rare
	High-Dose	Rare
Mithramycin	Daily × 10	Very common
	Intermittent	Uncommon
Mitomycin C	Intermittent	Rare
Streptozotocin	Intermittent	Common

*Very common ≦ 75%; Common 20–75%; Uncommon 1–20%; Rare = <1%.

fresh frozen plasma with active clotting factors and albumin should be administered.

Other cancer chemotherapeutic agents also are associated with hepatotoxicity; however, their effects on the liver are generally more mild (Table 20). The increased serum transaminase concentrations usually reverse within 14 days after discontinuation of therapy (103).

CHRONIC CANCER PAIN

Pain is a common problem in cancer patients. It occurs in about one-third of those with metastatic disease, and it is especially prominent when the malignancy spreads to the bones and nerves (106). In contrast to acute pain from trauma, pain in the cancer patient is usually chronic and persistent. Ultimately, the pain elicits a syndrome consisting of anxiety and depression in addition to the pain itself. Unless pain is controlled, a cycle of ache and agony, which perpetuates itself, often develops. Thus, the strategy should be to treat not only the pain, but also the psychological variables which can increase pain.

Although some factors which influence the perception of pain may be psychological, these variables are nevertheless real. Thus, psychosocial therapy and adjunctive drug therapy also may be directed at the anxiety, fear, and depression which sometimes accompany chronic cancer pain (107,108). There may even be a pharmacologic basis for inclusion of tricyclic antidepressants and phenothiazines in treating patients with chronic pain. In chronic pain, 5-hydroxytryptamine (5-HT) and dopamine, which are known to be neuromodulators of pain, are increased and decreased, respectively, leading to decrease in the pain threshold (109). 5-HT is blocked by phenothiazines, and dopamine is increased by tricyclic antidepressants (109). Clinical trials with these agents are limited but appear to support the use of these drugs in some patients (109,110).

Principles of chronic pain management are reviewed in the literature, and generally include the following recommendations: a) determine the underlying pathology; b) treat the underlying pain with specific therapy (eg, chemotherapy or radiation); and c) initiate analgesic therapy only when palliative treatment is required or when specific treatment no longer controls pain (108,111,112).

Selection of the appropriate analgesic is critical for successful pain control (113). Most patients with chronic pain can be controlled with oral analgesics. The severity of pain, described as mild, moderate, or severe, usually determines the initial selection of the analgesic(s). Nonnarcotic analgesics such as salicylates, acetaminophen, or nonsteroidal anti-inflammatory agents are often effective in mild pain. Moderate pain is best treated with codeine or its derivatives in combination with aspirin or acetaminophen. Potent narcotics such as morphine, hydromorphone, or methadone are usually reserved for severe pain. In patients with excruciating pain, parenteral morphine or hydromorphone may be necessary. (The chapter entitled Pain also should be consulted.)

The following general principles of analgesic therapy should be considered when dosing analgesics, particularly narcotics.

1. Avoid "as needed" or "prn" orders, which tend to increase anxiety by delaying the onset of pain relief.
2. Give appropriate doses and avoid underdosing patients (a common problem among house staff) (114).
3. Administer analgesics regularly because addiction is uncommon in chronic pain states.
4. In patients with severe renal or hepatic dysfunction, avoid analgesics with a long biologic half-lives, such as methadone or levorphanol, or those which are metabolized to toxic metabolites, such as meperidine.
5. After pain control has been stabilized for 3–5 days, begin a tapering program until pain reappears. Then, increase the dose slightly.
6. Dose the drugs according to their duration of action, usually every 4 to 6 hours.
7. Know how to interchange analgesics by use of approximate equivalent doses.
8. Patients receiving narcotics should be given concurrent laxatives or stool softeners to prevent constipation.

25. P.B., a 65-year-old female, has breast cancer which is metastatic to the pelvic bones. Her cancer has stabilized with combination therapy consisting of cyclophosphamide, methotrexate, and fluorouracil; however, her major complaint at this time is severe hip bone pain. She has been treated with two Percodan (oxycodone 5 mg and 225 mg aspirin)

tablets every six hours, but this medication provides only slight pain relief for about two hours. The Percodan has been discontinued and replaced with hydromorphone 2.0 mg po four times daily prn. This latter medication also fails to relieve her pain. What would be a reasonable plan to improve her pain control?

The above principles concerning "prn" orders and underdosing seem to have been violated. Furthermore, two tablets of Percodan contain 10 mg of oxycodone and provide analgesia which is comparable to about 2.0 mg of hydromorphone. So it is not surprising that the 2.0 mg dose of hydromorphone was as ineffective as the two Percodan tablets.

The treatment of worsening pain usually is more successful when equivalent doses of analgesics can be increased by 25–50%. There is little risk of inducing either hemodynamic or respiratory adverse effects in patients who have been treated chronically (usually more than two weeks) with narcotics. This method usually controls pain within 48 hours and interrupts the ache/agony cycle as well. In addition, the patients' new confidence in the drug therapy will allow them to concentrate on the more positive aspects of living, rather than on the negative aspects of pain. Thus, a more appropriate plan would be to increase the hydromorphone dose to 4.0 mg every four hours instead of four times daily as needed. The patient may also be considered for oral morphine therapy. For a detailed discussion of the use of oral morphine in cancer pain, refer to the chapter entitled Pain.

26. Patient P.B. did benefit from the increased hydromorphone dose. However, she later developed a pathologic fracture of her left hip and now requires 20 mg of IV morphine every three hours. These large doses seem to depress her respirations for several minutes after the dose. Would a slow intravenous infusion of morphine be useful in this situation?

Morphine infusions are being used with increasing frequency in the management of refractory chronic pain (115–118). This method of administration has the advantage of controlling pain without inducing excessive sedation or respiratory depression. Most clinicians begin with 10 mg of morphine per hour and gradually increase the dose up to 80 mg per hour if necessary. The disadvantages of this approach are constant monitoring of flow rate, vascular access, and dependence on the intravenous route.

27. Which narcotic analgesics would not be appropriate in this patient?

Some narcotic agents have pharmacologic properties that are undesirable in the treatment of chronic cancer pain. Meperidine, which has a short duration of action (less than 4 hours), should not be used. In addition, the major meperidine metabolite, normeperidine, lowers the seizure threshold and may induce seizures in patients with brain metastases (119). Pentazocine, which is equivalent to aspirin in potency, also should not be used in cancer patients because of the high incidence of dysphoria and hallucinations associated with its use.

28. Would nonsteroidal anti-inflammatory drugs be useful in this patient?

Some tumors, especially those that invade bone, have been associated with prostaglandin E_2 production. Therefore, drugs such as ibuprofen or naproxen may be effective (120). In one study, 100 mg of zomepirac was equivalent to Percodan in providing relief to patients with chronic cancer pain (121). Therefore, a nonsteroidal agent should be added to this patient's pain management plan.

HYPERCALCEMIA

29. A 55-year-old male with a history multiple myeloma is brought to the clinic by a family member because of severe disorientation and confusion. Prior to admission, the patient reportedly was very thirsty and urinating frequently; he now appears to be severely dehydrated. What is the likely cause of this patient's symptoms?

The symptoms of nausea, vomiting, polyuria, and polydipsia are consistent with hypercalcemia. A serum calcium should be obtained immediately to confirm this assessment. If the serum calcium is greater than 14 mg/dl, therapy must be initiated immediately and the patient should be hospitalized because of the possibility of cardiovascular complications.

Hypercalcemia is generally caused by the presence of osteolytic bone metastases and is most commonly associated with multiple myeloma, breast cancer, and leukemia (122,123). The hypercalcemia which occasionally occurs with bronchogenic carcinomas may be due to the release of a parathyroid hormone-like substance. Tumors associated with paraneoplastic syndromes of hypercalcemia are listed in Table 21. Other humoral substances such as prostaglandins which stimulate bone resorption may be released by some tumors (124,125).

30. The patient's serum calcium is 14.0 mg/dl. What therapeutic interventions are available and which are indicated in this patient?

Prompt treatment according to the guidelines in Table 22 is required to prevent subsequent stupor, confusion, coma, renal failure, or cardiac arrythmias. General measures should include mobilization, adequate hydration with normal saline, low dietary calcium intake (eg, milk, cheese), and treatment of the underlying malignancy. Intravenous saline with furosemide diuresis is indicated and should be rapidly effective (126,127).

This patient's hypercalcemia probably results from an osteoclast activating factor which is associated with his multiple myeloma. His hypercalcemia, therefore, theoretically might not respond to mithramycin as readily as hypercalcemia which is presumably due to a parathyroid-like hormone secreting tumor. Nevertheless mithramycin is effective in most cases of hypercalcemia; it inhibits bone resorption (128) within two days

after an intravenous dose of 25 mcg/kg. If a favorable response (60%) is not seen in three days, the dose may be repeated. The usual toxic effects of mithramycin on the bone marrow, liver and kidney are seldom encountered after only one or two doses (128).

Hypercalcemia caused by increased prostaglandin release (renal cell carcinoma, squamous-cell lung cancer, and ovarian carcinoma) can be effectively treated with prostaglandin inhibitors such as aspirin and indomethacin (129,130). Indomethacin in a dose of 25 mg twice daily significantly reduces the serum calcium within three days in such cases.

Calcitonin can be used in refractory cases of hypercalcemia. It is administered as a continuous infusion in plastic IV bags (glass binds the drug) in doses of 2–8 MRC units/kg over 24 hours (123). Its hypocalcemic effect is transient but may be prolonged by the concurrent use of glucocorticoids. Calcitonin appears to be the fourth-line agent after fluids, loop diuretics, and mithramycin.

Dichloromethylene diphosphonate is an analog of pyrophosphate, which is a naturally occurring inhibitor of bone resorption. It appears to slow both the dissolution and mineralization of bone. When administered in IV doses of 2.5 mg/kg initially followed by 5.0 mg/kg thereafter, the serum calcium begins to decrease within two days

Table 21.

PARANEOPLASTIC SYNDROMES

Syndrome	Substance	Tumors Frequently Associated
Hypercalcemia	Prostaglandin	Lung cancer
	Parathormone	Lung cancer Lymphoma Renal adenocarcinoma
	Osteoclast activating factor	Multiple myeloma
Inappropriate ADH	ADH	Oat Cell Lung cancer
Cushing's	ACTH	Oat Cell Lung cancer Thymoma Islet cell pancreatic Bronchial carcinoid

Table 22.
MANAGEMENT OF HYPERCALCEMIA IN MALIGNANT DISEASE

A. Mild cases:
1. Normal saline infusion for rehydration and increased urinary calcium (Na^+ competitively inhibits tubular reabsorption of Ca^{++})
2. Loop Diuretics
   a. Furosemide, or
   b. Ethacrynic acid
3. Corticosteroids: if high Ca^{++} due to osteolytic lesions
   a. Hydrocortisone 300–500 mg/liter every 8 hours, or
   b. Prednisone 40–100 mg in divided doses, taper after lowering of calcium
B. Severe cases (arrhythmias, CNS disorientation):
1. Normal saline, furosemide as in A.1 and A.2
2. Mithramycin 25 micrograms per kg IV. Repeat in 48 hours if no response, or
3. Calcitonin (Calcimar) 2–8 units per kg by IV infusion over 24 hours (use plastic IV bag, avoid glass because of adsorption)
C. In cases of renal failure:
1. Hemodialysis
2. Peritoneal dialysis

of the start of treatment and reaches normal levels within a week (132). This investigational drug is undergoing extensive study because of its apparent effectiveness and lack of serious toxicity. Other miscellaneous agents such as parenteral sodium sulfate and phosphate generally are used only after other therapy has failed (123).

31. What treatment may be helpful in maintaining this patient's serum calcium within normal limits when he is discharged from the hospital?

When the patient's serum calcium has decreased to normal levels, oral phosphates, such as Fleet's Phosphosoda or neutral phosphate (Neutro-Phos), in divided doses of four grams per day usually are effective in binding excess calcium from the gut (122).

Glucocorticoids also are effective in about 80% of patients with osteolytic bone lesions, but long-term therapy is associated with numerous adverse effects including the predisposition of patients to infections (131). Thus, glucocorticoids should be used only after oral phosphates have become ineffective (123).

MALIGNANT EFFUSIONS

32. A 35-year-old female with poorly differentiated diffuse lymphoma is hospitalized with shortness of breath (SOB) and weakness. The cardiac examination is normal, and a chest x-ray reveals pleural fluid which is not loculated on a supine film. Thoracentesis and drainage produce 1500 ml of hazy, pink fluid. The analysis of the pleural fluid shows: protein 4.5 gm/dl, lactic dehydrogenase 370 U/ml, white blood cells 2,600/m³, red blood cells 110,000/mm³, and specific gravity of 2.025. A complete blood count analysis shows a white blood cell count of 3,200/mm³, platelets 180,000/mm³, and hematocrit of 36%. This is the second hospitalization for the management of this patient's effusion. Over the last 24 hours she has improved with less SOB, but by the second day the fluid has reaccumulated and her condition has worsened. Chemotherapy (cyclophosphamide, doxorubicin, and vincristine) was administered seven days prior to admission. What is the cause of this patient's pleural effusion? Does she have a transudative or an exudative effusion?

Malignancy is responsible for nearly one-half of all cases of pleural effusion (133). Of the pleural effusions which are associated with malignancies, 30% are caused by breast cancer, 29% by lung cancer, 12% by lymphoma, 4% by ovarian cancer, and 25% by other neoplasms (134). In most cases, the pleural fluid takes on the character of an exudate rather than a transudate; differentiation is based on the following criteria (134,135):

Pleural Fluid	Exudate	Transudate
Appearance	Cloudy	Clear
WBC/mm³	> 1,000	< 1,000
RBC/mm³	> 100,000	< 100,000
Spec. Gravity	> 1.016	< 1.016
Protein (total)	> 3.6 gm/dl	< 3.6 gm/dl
LDH (fluid: serum)	> 0.6	< 0.6

It appears from the results of pleural fluid analysis that the patient has an exudative effusion. This differentiation between an exudate or a transudate is important in the diagnostic evaluation of a patient.

33. What is the goal in the management of this patient's effusion?

The primary goal of treatment is palliation of symptoms (decreased dyspnea, cough, and pain). Systemic chemotherapy should be tried initially in patients with highly responsive tumors, such as lymphomas or breast cancer. Since this patient already is receiving combination chemotherapy, adjunctive local treatment would be reasonable. The local treatment of malignant effusions primarily involves repeated thoracentesis and closed-tube thoracostomy drainage with or without a sclerosing agent (133). The sclerosing agents are administered through a thoracostomy tube and the patient is rotated every 10 to 15 minutes for one to two hours. The sclerosing agent then is removed by suction drainage. The success of sclerosing therapy is dependent upon good local coverage of the pleural surfaces.

34. What sclerosing agent would be a reasonable choice for use in this patient?

The effectiveness of a sclerosing agent depends primarily upon its ability to cause an adhesive pleuritis and obliteration of small pleural blood vessels, rather than upon its specific antineoplastic activity (133).

Tetracycline is the least toxic sclerosing agent and is associated with the lowest rate of relapse (136). Some cytotoxic drugs such as nitrogen mustard, thiotepa, and bleomycin also are effective, but these are associated with about a 40 to 60% relapse rate within four months of therapy. The antimalarial, quinacrine (Atabrine) is as effective as nitrogen mustard, but the parenteral form is no longer commercially available in the United States (137).

In this case, tetracycline is the sclerosing agent of choice because of its relative lack of systemic toxicity. Nitrogen mustard and thiotepa would not be good choices because about 30% is absorbed into the systemic circulation (138) and either drug might enhance the myelosuppression in this patient who already is receiving chemotherapy.

MALIGNANT MENINGITIS

35. R.C. is a 40-year-old female with a nine-month history of acute myelogenous leukemia. She has been in complete remission and is currently on maintenance chemotherapy with IV cytarabine and oral thioguanine. She is seen in the clinic and now complains of frontal headache and a stiff neck which has lasted for about one week. Decreased plantar reflexes and neck stiffness are noted during her physical examination. All blood chemistries are within normal limits. Bone marrow aspirate and biopsy are normal.

A lumbar fluid aspiration reveals slightly xanthochromic fluid and an opening pressure of 190 mm H_2O. The cell count is 90 white blood cells/mm^3 with several blast cells and 10 blood cells/mm^3. Chemical analysis of this fluid reveals 70 mg/dl protein and 45 mg/dl glucose. Microbiological cultures of the spinal fluid are negative not only for bacteria, but also for acid-fast bacteria and fungi. The assessment is leukemic meningitis. Why has this patient developed leukemic meningitis in the face of bone marrow remission?

Even though cancer chemotherapy frequently produces complete remission, malignant cells can reside in "sanctuary" sites, such as the central nervous system (CNS). The reappearance of disease arising from "sanctuaries" appears to be related to the inability of certain cytotoxic agents to cross the blood-brain barrier to sterilize nests of cells in the brain. Meningeal cancer occurs in about 4% of all cancers, but is most common in leukemia (139). Untreated, it develops in about 20% of adult leukemia and 80% of childhood leukemia (140). The solid tumors that most often metastasize to the meninges include breast, testicular, lung, gastric, and pancreatic cancers as well as non-Hodgkin's lymphoma of unfavorable histology.

36. What clinical data would be suggestive of malignant meningitis?

The clinical signs of meningeal involvement usually include headache, cranial nerve palsies, mental changes, or seizures. Ocular signs of increased intracranial pressure also may be evident. Analysis of the cerebrospinal fluid establishes the diagnosis when malignant cells are present along with elevated protein and decreased glucose concentrations. The analysis of the cerebrospinal fluid in patient R.C. is consistent with meningeal leukemia.

37. What would be a reasonable plan for the management of this patient's leukemic meningitis?

Cranial irradiation and intrathecal chemotherapy are the two primary treatment modalities for meningeal cancer (141), and both are appropriate for this patient. Although methotrexate, cytarabine, and thiotepa are all commonly utilized intrathecally, methotrexate is particularly effective in leukemic patients (141). Methotrexate, however, is less effective when tumor cells metastasize into tissues beyond the meninges because this drug does not penetrate tissues well. Since methotrexate penetrates into only about three millimeters of tissue, sterilization of deep-seated malignant cells is less likely (142). Nevertheless, intrathecal methotrexate is still probably an excellent choice for leukemic meningitis. This patient should receive 12 mg of methotrexate twice weekly until leukemic cells are cleared from the cerebrospinal fluid, and then once a month for an additional three to six months.

38. What pharmacokinetic properties of methotrexate need to be considered when using this drug in the treatment of central nervous system leukemia?

Methotrexate elimination from the cerebrospinal fluid (CSF) is biphasic, with an initial half-life of four hours and a slower phase half-life of 14 hours. In adults, methotrexate distributes into an apparent volume of distribution in the CSF of about 400 ml (144,145).

The disappearance of methotrexate from CSF may be influenced by several factors: 1) total CSF outflow; 2) CSF flow between subarachnoid and ventricular spaces; 3) diffusion of extracellular fluid (ECF) to and from the parenchyma; and 4) choroidal transport of ECF (146). It appears the total CSF flow is the most important of these factors. In patients with active meningeal disease, bulk flow is often impaired and may result in delayed CSF clearance (143,144).

The unidirectional flow characteristics of cerebrospinal fluid also affect the ventricular concentration of drugs such as methotrexate; in fact, intraventricular concentrations of methotrexate frequently are substantially less than corresponding lumbar concentrations. As a result, some clinicians recommend direct intraventricular administration of methotrexate through an Ommaya reservoir to circumvent the problem of uneven methotrexate distribution between ventricular and lumbar spaces (143).

The intrathecal dosing of methotrexate probably should be based upon the apparent fluid volume in the brain rather than upon total body surface area, because the CNS fluid volume plateaus by age three as contrasted to the sixteen to twenty years of age before body surface area plateaus (147). (Also see the chapter entitled Pediatric Oncology.)

39. What toxicities might be expected from the intrathecal administration of methotrexate?

The primary adverse effects of intrathecal methotrexate are meningeal irritation, nerve palsies or paralysis, and encephalopathy. These neurotoxic syndromes appear to be associated with high concentrations of the drug in the CSF (147,148). Patients who develop neurotoxicity tend to be older and have overt meningeal disease and decreased clearance of methotrexate (147).

40. This patient received 18 mg of intrathecal methotrexate, and on the fourth day after administration, the CSF methotrexate concentration was 5×10^{-7} moles/liter. Should another dose of methotrexate be given to the patient?

In patients receiving multiple doses of intrathecal methotrexate (ie, once or twice weekly), CSF methotrexate concentrations should be assayed before each intrathecal dose is administered. The guidelines by Bleyer should be used to adjust the interval between doses of methotrexate (Figure 6). If CSF levels are greater than 1×10^{-7} moles/liter on day 4 (point A) or 1×10^{-8} moles/liter on day 8 (point B), the patient is not clearing methotrexate appropriately and another

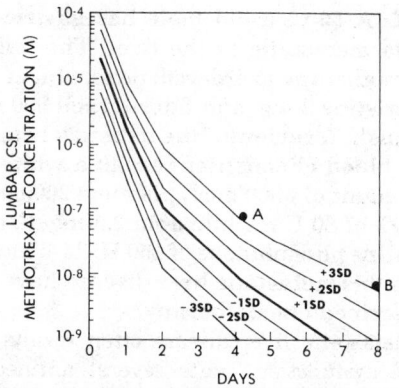

Figure 6. CSF Methotrexate Levels after 12 mg/m². (Modified from Bleyer, ref 149 with permission.)

dose of methotrexate should not be administered until the level has fallen to less than 1×10^{-8} moles/liter (149). Subsequent doses of methotrexate should be decreased such that the methotrexate level falls below 1×10^{-7} moles/liter by day 4.

The patient should probably receive systemic calcium leucovorin in a dose of 10 mg/m^2 every six hours for four doses to prevent systemic bone marrow toxicity (149). See Questions 44–50 concerning leucovorin rescue.

41. After several doses of intrathecal methotrexate, leukemic cells are still present in the CSF. What other cytotoxic agents can be used for leukemic meningitis?

Cytarabine, an alternative to methotrexate, is used in doses of 5 to 70 mg/m^2 up to three times weekly. CNS toxicity (headache and nausea) is uncommon with intrathecal cytarabine, but is more common when daily doses are greater than 30 mg/m^2 (151). The CSF half-life of cytarabine ranges from 2–11 hours (152), and CSF concentrations between 0.01 and 0.15 mg/ml are cytotoxic (153). Assuming a CNS volume of about 400 ml and a half-life of two hours, a 100 mg dose would remain therapeutic for about 21 hours and a 50 mg dose for about 19 hours. Thus, a dose of 30 mg/m^2 is probably more than adequate and may avoid potential neurotoxicity. Although thiotepa has also been used intrathecally in doses of 1 to 10 mg/m^2 once or twice weekly for carcinomatous meningitis (154,155), experience with this agent is much less than with methotrexate or cytarabine.

CHEMOTHERAPY IN HEPATIC DYSFUNCTION

42. A 60-year-old male has gastric carcinoma metastatic to the liver. The following chemotherapy is ordered: doxorubicin 80 mg, vincristine 2 mg, and fluorouracil 600 mg, all IV push. A review of the patient's hemogram and blood chemistries reveal: a white blood cell count of 6000/mm^3, platelets 200,000/mm^3, SGOT of 80 U/ml, bilirubin 2.5 mg/dl, and an alkaline phosphatase of 250 IU/L. What effect does this metastatic liver disease have on the prescribed chemotherapy?

Metastatic liver disease often results in hepatic dysfunction. Since several antineoplastic drugs are inactivated by the liver, a decrease in total body clearance may be evident in patients with hepatic dysfunction (159). Drugs which may be affected include doxorubicin and vincristine since both are excreted primarily via the biliary route.

The use of normal doses of doxorubicin, in the face of hyperbilirubinemia, has been reported to produce severe bone marrow suppression and subsequent infectious complications (160). The guidelines for dose reduction are depicted in Table 24 at the end of the chapter. Thus, an appropriate dose reduction would be 50% to 40 mg.

In contrast, an established guideline for vincristine is less well defined. However, since 40% of an administered dose is excreted in the bile within two hours, patients with biliary obstruction or a bilirubin greater than 3 mg/dl should probably not receive full doses of the drug, if at all (161). It is uncertain if dose modification is necessary in patients with hepatic metastases, but doses probably should be reduced if concurrent jaundice is present.

The last agent for consideration is fluorouracil, which is primarily metabolized by the liver and intracellular enzymes to CO_2, urea, and ammonia. About 80% of a dose is degraded by the liver and excreted in the lungs as CO_2 (162). Only 15% of unchanged drug is excreted by the kidneys. Thus, neither hepatic nor renal dysfunction require dose modification of 5-FU.

CHEMOTHERAPY IN RENAL DYSFUNCTION

43. A 45-year-old, 65 kg female has adenocarcinoma of the ovary with an abdominal mass that is producing bladder obstruction. Her BUN and serum creatinine are 70 and 5 mg/dl, respectively. The following antineoplastic drugs are being considered for therapy: doxorubicin, cyclophosphamide, cisplatin, and methotrexate (MTX). Which of these drugs are contraindicated and which require dosage adjustments because of her renal status?

Several chemotherapeutic agents are excreted by the kidney; however, there are few guidelines for use in patients with renal dysfunction (156). A list of the commonly-used agents and their pharmacokinetic parameters is shown in Table 24 at the end of this chapter.

Since this patient has an estimated creatinine clearance of less than 50 ml/min, and cisplatin and methotrexate are primarily excreted by the kidney, their use in this patient presents a risk of enhanced cytotoxicity. Cyclophosphamide is primarily metabolized in the liver, but its metabolites, which are excreted by the kidneys, have cytotoxic activity (157).

Since cyclophosphamide and its metabolites are eliminated solely by the kidney and the drug is truly indicated, the usual dosage may be decreased by use of the following equation from Tozer (158):

$$Q = 1 - [(f_e)(1 - k_f)] \qquad \text{(Eq. 1)}$$

where Q = dosage reduction factor; f_e = fraction or renal excretion of active drug or metabolite; and k_f = fraction of normal creatinine clearance (Cl_{cr}). The f_e for cyclophosphamide and metabolites in a 48-hour period is estimated at 0.75. K_f can be estimated by use of the equations for Cl_{cr} below:

$$Cl_{cr} \text{ (males)} = \frac{140 - age}{serum\ cr} \times \frac{Pt.Wt.(kg)}{70\ kg} \qquad \text{(Eq. 2)}$$

$$Cl_{cr} \text{ (females)} = Cl_{cr} \text{ (males)} \times 0.85 \qquad \text{(Eq. 3)}$$

Thus, this patient has an estimated creatinine clearance of 15 ml/min and a K_f of 0.15. The dose reduction factor is calculated as:

$$Q = 1 - [(.75)(1 - .15)] = 0.36$$

Therefore, 36% of a usual dose of cyclophosphamide may be given. Further adjustment may be needed after follow-up evaluation.

Although this patient has moderate to severe renal dysfunction, the risk of cyclophosphamide cystitis is not greater than in the normal patient if fluid intake and urine output are sufficient (1.5 to 2 liters per day). The cisplatin, however, is not recommended for this patient or any patient with a Cl_{cr} less than 50 ml/min because of its nephrotoxic potential. Methotrexate also is excreted renally, but the above equation may not be appropriate because intracellular toxicity usually correlates best with the slow terminal phase half-life of this drug. Thus, methotrexate should be avoided in patients with moderate or severe renal

dysfunction until studies indicate that it can be safely administered to these patients.

Other agents which should be used with caution in patients with renal dysfunction include carmustine, dacarbazine, hydroxyurea, mercaptopurine, mithramycin, streptozotocin, and thioguanine.

The doxorubicin may be administered in full dosage to this patient, since most of the drug is metabolized (85%) to inactive metabolites and excreted in the bile.

HIGH-DOSE METHOTREXATE WITH LEUCOVORIN RESCUE

44. R.A. is a 24-year-old male with osteogenic sarcoma of the femur. The patient undergoes surgical removal of the tumor and regional lymphadenectomy. The plan is for postoperative high-dose methotrexate (HD-MTX) in a dose of 10 grams over six hours followed by leucovorin rescue. All serum chemistries, including liver and renal function are within the normal range. However, a chest x-ray reveals pleural effusion. The serum creatinine is 1.0 mg/dl. The patient weighs 70 kg and is somewhat dehydrated. Why is leucovorin included in the planned HDMTX therapy?

Methotrexate (MTX) is cytotoxic as a result of its intracellular inhibition of the enzyme dihydrofolate reductase (DHFR) (148). With conventional doses, the drug is actively transported across the cell membrane (163); however, with *high doses,* when serum concentrations are 100 to 1000 times greater, the drug can enter the cell by passive diffusion (164). Some tumors that lack an active transport system and are suspected to be resistant to conventional doses may respond to HDMTX, but the resultant high concentrations are also toxic to normal cells. Thus, leucovorin must be used in this patient.

45. How does leucovorin rescue normal cells, and when should it be administered to this patient?

Leucovorin (folinic acid, citrovorum factor) "rescues" cells from the cytotoxic effect of MTX by bypassing the block to DHFR. Its ability to reverse the toxicity of MTX, however, is dependent on the same active transport mechanism as MTX (165). Extracellularly, leucovorin must compete with MTX for transport into the cell (166). Therefore, it will be most effective when serum concentrations of leucovorin are greater than MTX, which occurs 2 to 18 hours after MTX is completed. Once within the cell, it enhances MTX efflux and dissociation from DHFR. This effect may be greater in normal cells than in tumor cells (166).

46. Describe the methodology of HDMTX plus leucovorin to be given in this patient. How does this compare with other high dose regimens?

HDMTX regimens vary extensively and range from 500 mg/m² to 10 gm/m² given as an infusion from 1 up to 42 hours (167). Calcium leucovorin is administered usually in doses of 10 mg/m² starting 2 to 40 hours after completion of the MTX infusion. Leucovorin should not be given concurrently with MTX because concentrations of leucovorin are not high enough to effectively compete with MTX (168). Leucovorin is usually continued for at least 72 hours or until serum MTX concentrations fall below 5×10^{-8}M. This patient will have very high serum levels at the end of the infusion and these high serum concentrations should fall to 1×10^{-7}M by 24 hours after the end of the infusion.

47. What clinical parameters should be monitored to evaluate toxicity from HDMTX in this patient?

The major adverse effects of HDMTX may be decreased granulocytes or platelets, mucosities, diarrhea, decreased urine output (elevated creatinine), and increased liver function tests.

Even though high-dose regimens of MTX may use 1000 times the amount of drug compared to conventional-dose regimens, the incidence of myelosuppression is only about 6% and gastrointestinal toxicity is only about 30% (169,170). However, nephropathy due to urinary drug crystallization may occasionally occur in dehydrated patients. Occasional hepatic necrosis has also been reported, usually in patients with delayed plasma clearance of MTX. Mortality has been reported in about 6% of patients treated with HDMTX (171).

48. What effect may this patient's pleural effusion and hydration status have on MTX toxicity?

This patient may have delayed plasma clearance or elevated MTX concentrations and be at high risk for toxicity (172). His pleural effusion will decrease body clearance of MTX by decreasing drug transport back into the central circulation for excretion by the kidneys (173). Since the kidneys eliminate 50–90% of MTX over 48 hours, renal dysfunction results in elevated concentrations by decreasing renal tubular secretion and, thus, clearance of MTX (174). This patient's renal function is normal; however, dehydration and aciduria increase the risk of MTX crystal formation in the renal tubule after high-dose therapy (172). In order to minimize the risk of toxicity in these clinical situations, measures must be taken to either maximize drug clearance or prevent lethal damage to cells with adequate rescue therapy (168). Therefore, serum methotrexate levels should be closely monitored and urinary alkalinization to pH 6.5 or higher with sodium bicarbonate (100 mEq over 2–4 hours) should be instituted prior to MTX administration.

49. If MTX serum concentrations are to be monitored, what concentrations would be expected after the completion of therapy?

MTX distributes into two compartments: the mean initial Vd = 0.18 L/kg; mean steady-state Vd = 0.6–0.8 L/kg (175,176). The initial phase half-life and terminal phase are 1.8 and 10 hours, respectively (167,177). The approximate peak concentrations from various HDMTX regimens are listed in Table 23 (178).

The serum levels during the first 18–24 hours after MTX administration decrease to a concentration of about 5×10^{-6} M because of renal clearance. After 24 hours, clearance of MTX is primarily from intracellular loss and at 48 hours plasma concentrations range from 5×10^{-7}M to 1×10^{-8}M (179,180).

Table 23.
PLASMA LEVELS AFTER
HIGH DOSE METHOTREXATE

Regimen (gm/m²)	Infusion Period (hrs)	Peak Concentrations ($\times 10^{-6}$M)
0.5	1	75
0.5	24	3
1–5	6	25–125
1–5	24	6–30
5–10	6	125–250
5–10	24	30–60

Using a k_α of 0.385 hrs^{-1} (t½ α of 1.8 hrs), a k_β of 0.069 hrs^{-1} (t½ β of 10 hrs), and a peak concentration of 125×10^{-6}, one can estimate a 24 and 48 hour concentration as follows:

$$
\begin{aligned}
C_{p24^\circ} &= C_{pk} \times e^{-k\alpha t} & \text{(Eq. 4)} \\
&= 125 \times e^{(-.385 \times 24)} \\
&= 0.121 \times 10^{-6} \text{ M } (1.2 \times 10^{-7} \text{ M})
\end{aligned}
$$

$$
\begin{aligned}
C_{p48^\circ} &= C_{p24^\circ} \times e^{-k\beta t} & \text{(Eq. 5)} \\
&= 0.121 \times e^{-.069\,(24)} \\
&= 0.023 \times 10^{-6} \text{ M } (2.3 \times 10^{-8} \text{ M})
\end{aligned}
$$

Thus, at 24 hours, calcium leucovorin (10 mg/m^2 per dose) will effectively rescue MTX toxicity. The guidelines by Bleyer and Nirenberg illustrate the dose of leucovorin which should be used if MTX concentrations are higher than predicted (181,182). If the 24-hour MTX level is greater than 5×10^{-6} M, leucovorin dosage should be increased to 50 mg/m^2. If greater than 1×10^{-6} M at 48 hours, leucovorin dosage should be increased to 100 mg/m^2.

BREAST CANCER

50. A 56-year-old female has carcinoma of her left breast. This malignancy has metastasized to several ribs. An assay for estrogen-receptors is strongly positive and therapy with tamoxifen 10 mg bid is initiated. Why is estrogen receptor status important to the treatment of this patient?

Hormone dependence of breast cancer has been known for several years (196); however, the relatively recent finding of protein receptors in breast cancer tissue has enhanced the predictability of breast cancer responsiveness to hormone therapy (197).

Prior to the development of the estrogen receptor (ER) assay, the overall beneficial response to hormone therapy of breast cancers ranged between 20 and 40% (199,200). With the ER assay, the response rates for ER$^+$ tumors and ER$^-$ tumors are 60% and 8%, respectively (201). Therefore, positive ER status increases a clinician's ability to correctly select patients likely to respond to hormone therapy.

Estrogen receptor status is based upon the concept that hormones bind to protein receptors in the cytoplasm of the targeted cell with high affinity and specificity (198). The hormone-receptor complex then binds to nuclear chromatin and alters transcription as well as the synthesis of messenger RNA (see Figure 7). Therefore, hormone-receptor binding is essential to the cytotoxicity of these hormones, because the absence of hormone receptors results in the inability of the tumor cell to respond to exogenous hormone.

51. Would the estrogen, diethylstilbestrol (DES) be as effective as the antiestrogen, tamoxifen in this patient?

Yes. Estrogens are as effective as antiestrogens, but better patient tolerance with tamoxifen has made it the preferred agent (202). The mechanism of antiestrogens in postmenopausal patients is not completely understood, but these drugs bind to hormone receptors in the cytosol of tumor specimens and inhibit DNA transcription (203). Tamoxifen is the antiestrogen of choice in the treatment of breast cancer. In doses of 10–20 mg twice daily, it produces 50 to 60% objective regression in ER-positive metastatic disease (204).

52. Diethylstilbesterol and tamoxifen were initially beneficial to the patient. Will halotestin (an androgen) or megestrol (a progestin) be effective in this patient?

Yes, other additive hormones are usually beneficial after an initial hormone response. If estrogens or antiestrogens had initially failed, the

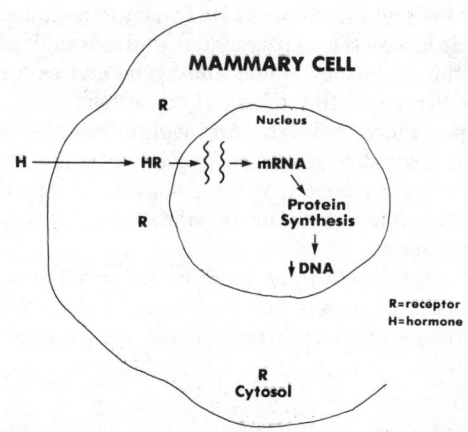

Figure 7. Mechanism of Hormone Binding to Receptor Protein on DNA in Mammary Receptor Protein on DNA in Mammary Tissue. R = receptor; H = hormone.

patient would probably not respond to other hormones.

Before the advent of antiestrogens, androgens were commonly used in the postmenopausal patient with breast cancer (205). Because of their poorly tolerated side effects and lower response rates (33% in ER$^+$) compared to estrogens or antiestrogens, androgens are being used less frequently than before in the hormonal treatment of breast cancer. Like other hormones, responses to androgens are usually observed within six weeks of initiating therapy (206).

The progestins are effective in 20 to 40% of unselected postmenopausal patients (200,207). It is likely that the response rate for progestins is greater in the ER$^+$ or PR$^+$ (progesterone receptor) patient. Studies are in progress to define the role of progesterone receptor status in response to therapy.

53. The patient is also being considered for either surgical or medical adrenalectomy after initially responding to tamoxifen. What role does adrenalectomy play in this patient's care?

Surgical adrenalectomy is effective in more than 50% of ER$^+$ positive patients (208); however, it also is associated with a 5 to 10% risk of mortality. Many oncologists prefer medical adrenalectomy which is predictive for surgical adrenalectomy and effective in almost 50% of ER$^+$ patients and avoids complications from surgery (209). Medical adrenalectomy can be accomplished with the use of aminoglutethimide, which inhibits steroidogenesis by blocking the adrenal conversion of cholesterol to pregnenolone and ultimately to estrone and estradiol (210). Thus, aminoglutethimide decreases extragonadal and adrenal production of estrogens and androgens and as a result decreases the effects of those hormones on breast cancer growth. Aminoglutethimide produces 26 to 55% responses in ER$^+$ patients (211). Objective remissions range from 3 to 20 months in duration and occur primarily in soft-tissue metastases.

Aminoglutethimide inhibits not only the synthesis of estrogens and androgens, but also the synthesis of glucocorticoids and mineralocorti-

coids. Because cortisol production is particularly suppressed, the pituitary responds by increasing its secretion of ACTH, which can override the therapeutic effect of the drug. Thus, patients must be given concurrent corticosteroids. Occasionally, patients may also require concurrent mineralocorticoids (fludrocortisone). The current agent of choice is hydrocortisone given in physiologic doses. Dexamethasone may also be used but must be given in supraphysiologic doses (3 mg daily) because aminoglutethimide increases its hepatic metabolism three-fold (212).

Adrenal suppression from aminoglutethimide is rapidly reversible after discontinuation of therapy, but patients should be monitored for adequate recovery by measurements of serum cortisol or dihydroepiandrostenedione (DHEA) (213).

54. A 37-year-old pre-menopausal patient has breast cancer metastatic to the bones. Her estrogen receptor status is positive. What is the preferred treatment for this patient? What therapy should be considered for subsequent relapse?

If the patient is a good surgical candidate, she should have a bilateral oophorectomy to remove the estrogen-rich hormonal milieu. About 40% of such patients respond, and the mean duration of response is about 12 months. Following relapse from previous response, either medical or surgical adrenalectomy or hypophysectomy is of benefit to another 40%. After another relapse, progestins are used for a 20% response rate. Androgens should be avoided because peripheral metabolism converts them to estrogens which can exacerbate premenopausal disease.

55. A breast cancer patient relapses after oophorectomy with metastases to the liver. She is ER negative. What is the next alternative for treatment?

This patient should be treated with antineoplastic drugs such as cyclophosphamide, methotrexate, and fluorouracil. The doses of these drugs are listed in Table 4. About 50 to 60% of patients will respond to this treatment, and the duration of remission is about 8 to 12 months.

Table 24.

PHARMACOKINETIC PARAMETERS FOR ANTINEOPLASTIC DRUGS

Drug	Distribution	Site of Metabolism	Excretion	Conditions Requiring Dose Reduction or Avoidance
Asparaginase	Vd = 4–5 liters; primarily plasma, Lymph 25%, CSF 1%; t½ = 8–30 hrs	Uncertain, plasma elimination by reticulo-endothelial system	Uncertain	No correlation of clearance with renal or hepatic dysfunction
Azacytidine	Vd = 0.6–1.1 L/kg; Ascites = plasma after 6 hours; CSF/plasma < 10%; t½ = 3.4–6.2 hrs	Liver; metabolites unknown	Renal, 20% parent compound plus metabolites	Hepatic dysfunction
Bleomycin	Vd = 20 liters; Liver, kidney, tissue uptake; Low CSF/plasma ratio; t½ (α) = 10–20 min, t½ (β) = 2–4 hrs	Liver, kidney, tissue biotransformation	Renal, 20–60% active drug	Renal Dysfunction: Cr 1.5–2.0: 50% dose Cr 2.5–4.0: 25% dose Cr 4–10: 10–20% dose
Busulfan	Vd unknown; tissue uptake uncertain; tumor, lung, hematologic elements; t½ = rapid, 90% degradation in 3 minutes	Plasma and liver biotransformation; metabolites unknown	Renal, 25–35% as methanesulfonic acid; no parent drug	Uncertain
Carmustine	Vd = probably large (> body water); lipid, liver, gut, bone marrow; CSF/plasma > 50%; t½ = 5 min for parent compound; t½ = 27–72 hrs for metabolites	Liver, to active metabolites	Renal, 60–80% of metabolites in 96 hrs	Renal dysfunction; uncertain guidelines
Chlorambucil	Oral absorption: rapid; Vd = 0.2 L/kg; protein bound; extensive in liver and tissues; CSF/plasma = low; t½ (α) = 30–80 min t½ (β) = 7–21 hrs	Liver; metabolite is aminophenyl acetic acid	Renal, 50% unchanged drug	Renal dysfunction; uncertain guidelines
Cisplatin	Highly protein bound in plasma, kidneys, and liver; Low CSF/plasma ratio; t½ (α) = 30–77 min t½ (β) = 14–73 hrs	Intracellular, to mono- and diaquo-complex	Renal, 20% at 24 hrs, 30% at 48 hrs	Renal dysfunction

Table 24. (continued)

PHARMACOKINETIC PARAMETERS FOR ANTINEOPLASTIC DRUGS

Drug	Distribution	Site of Metabolism	Excretion	Conditions Requiring Dose Reduction or Avoidance
Cyclophosphamide	Oral absorption: 31–66% Protein binding = 50% as alkylating metabolites. Distributes into plasma, bone marrow, liver, and kidney. Low CSF/plasma ratio; $t\frac{1}{2}$ = 4 to 6.5 hrs	Hepatic activation by microsomal enzymes to active metabolites (88%); possible interactions with phenobarbital, phenytoin, allopurinol, and corticosteroids	Renal: 10% and 12% of parent compound at 24 and 48 hrs, respectively; 50–70% of metabolites at 24 and 48 hrs, respectively; f_r = 0.15; renal clearance: 11 ml/min or 15% of Cl_{Cr}	Renal dysfunction: avoid with Cl_{Cr} of less than 30 ml/min; decrease dose proportionate to decrease in Cl_{Cr}
Cytarabine	Oral absorption: 20%, but not usually used by this route. Protein binding: low Distribution: liver, lymphatic, bone marrow; CSF/plasma ratio = 0.4 after 5 day continuous infusion; $t\frac{1}{2}$ (α) = 10 min $t\frac{1}{2}$ (β) = 140 min CSF $t\frac{1}{2}$ = 2–11 hrs	Hepatic and plasma deamination to inactive uracil arabinoside	Renal: unchanged ARA-C = 4–10%, metabolites = 90%	None established for either renal or hepatic dysfunction
Dacarbazine	Oral absorption: poor and erratic; distributes into liver, kidney, lymphatics, and bone marrow; protein binding = 5%; CSF/plasma ratio is low; $t\frac{1}{2}$ (α) = 35 min $t\frac{1}{2}$ (β) = 5 hrs	Hepatic demethylation to *active* aminoimidazole carboximide (50% conversion in 6 hrs); potential interaction with enzyme inducers, such as phenobarbital and phenytoin	50% unchanged and 50% metabolites at 6 hours; tubular secretion of metabolites	Hepatic and renal dysfunction increases $t\frac{1}{2}$ (β) to 7.2 hours; decrease dose proportionate to decrease in Cl_{Cr} or serum bilirubin
Daunorubicin	Protein binding extensive to liver, heart and hematopoietic tissues; large Vd; CSF/plasma ratio is low; $t\frac{1}{2}$ (α) = 40 min $t\frac{1}{2}$ (β) = 46–55 hrs	Hepatic and cellular metabolism to daunomycinol (active) by reductase enzyme	Renal: 25% unchanged in 5 days; biliary 75% in 5 days	Hepatic dysfunction: *Serum bilirubin* *Dose reduction* <1.2 mg/dl 0 1.2–3.0 mg/dl 25% >3.0 mg/dl 50%

Table 24. (continued)

PHARMACOKINETIC PARAMETERS FOR ANTINEOPLASTIC DRUGS

Drug	Distribution	Site of Metabolism	Excretion	Conditions Requiring Dose Reduction or Avoidance
Doxorubicin	Distribution into liver, heart, bone marrow, and poietic cells; large Vd; Protein binding unknown; CSF/plasma ratio is low; $t\frac{1}{2}$ (α) = 30 min $t\frac{1}{2}$ (β) = 3 hrs $t\frac{1}{2}$ (δ) = 15 hrs $t\frac{1}{2}$ (δ) (metabolites) = 30 hrs	Hepatic and cellular metabolism to adriamycinol	Renal: 6% unchanged; biliary: 80% unchanged	Hepatic dysfunction: *Serum bilirubin* / *Dose reduction* <1.2 mg/dl — 0; 1.2–3.0 mg/dl — 50%; >3.0 mg/dl — 75%
Etoposide (VP-16)	Oral absorption: 40%; protein binding: >90% to albumin; Vd = 0.33 L/kg; distributes into intestine, liver, kidney, thyroid, lung, skin, bone marrow; low CSF/plasma ratio (0.04); $t\frac{1}{2}$ (α) = 2.8 hrs $t\frac{1}{2}$ (β) = 11.5–15 hrs	Site of catabolism unknown; major metabolite is 4'-demethyl derivative (probably inactive)	Renal: 45–70% as unchanged drug; fecal: 53% as metabolite and 1–16% unchanged	Uncertain, but hepatic dysfunction might increase systemic toxicity (eg, myelosuppression)
Fluorouracil	Oral absorption: 50–80%, erratic, especially in acidic solutions; protein binding: low; Vd = 0.25–0.33 L/kg; distributes into GI tract, body water; CSF/plasma ratio low; $t\frac{1}{2}$ = 10–20 min	Intracellular activation to active monophosphate nucleoside; enzyme catabolism by liver to dihydro-5-FU with further breakdown to CO_2, urea, ammonia	Renal: Up to 15% unchanged drug; pulmonary: 60–80% as CO_2	None; even though the liver is a major metabolic site, other tissues are capable of detoxification
Hexamethylmelamine	Oral absorption variable; protein binding unknown; Vd unknown; distributes into liver, brain, intestine; CSF/plasma high; $t\frac{1}{2}$ = 4.6–10.2 hr (Ave. 6.9)	Liver, probably microsomal enzymes; demethylated to pentamethylmelamine and other metabolites	Renal: 60% of metabolites in 24 hrs, >90% in 72 hrs; fecal: trace; pulmonary: trace	Probably severe hepatic dysfunction

Table 24. (continued)

PHARMACOKINETIC PARAMETERS FOR ANTINEOPLASTIC DRUGS

Drug	Distribution	Site of Metabolism	Excretion	Conditions Requiring Dose Reduction or Avoidance
Hydroxyurea	Oral absorption is complete; Vd is unknown; distributes into gut, brain, kidney, lung; $t\frac{1}{2} = 3$ hr	Liver, to urea or CO_2	Renal: 80% as unchanged drug or urea	Renal failure
Lomustine (CCNU)	Oral absorption is rapid; Vd is probably large; distributes into fat; CSF/plasma ratio = 0.25; $t\frac{1}{2} = 5$ min $t\frac{1}{2}$ metabolites = 1–3 days	Biotransformed nonenzymatically to cyclohexyl and chloroethyl metabolites (active) in the liver, microsomal hydroxylation	Renal: 50% cyclohexyl or chloroethyl metabolites in 12–24 hrs; 75% degradation products in 96 hrs	Unknown
Mechlorethamine	IV only Vd is unknown; distributes into plasma, water; $t\frac{1}{2} = 15$ min	Plasma, chemical hydrolysis to reactive electrophilic alkylating moieties	Renal: 50% inactive metabolites in 24 hrs	Unknown
Melphalan	Oral absorption: erratic and incomplete. Vd = 44 liters (body water) Protein binding = 50–60% $t\frac{1}{2}(\alpha) = 8$ min $t\frac{1}{2}(\beta) = \sim 2$ hrs	Plasma and cellular degradation to monohydroxy- and dihydroxy-metabolites	Renal: 13% unchanged in 24 hrs; Fecal: 20–50% of oral dose excreted over 6 days as unchanged or metabolized drug	Unknown
Mercaptopurine	Oral absorption is rapid and complete; $t\frac{1}{2} = 1.5$ hrs; half-lives of metabolites unknown	Hepatic methylation and oxidation (xanthine oxidase)	Renal: 50% of oral dose as unchanged drug and metabolites	Concurrent allopurinol is metabolized by xanthine oxidase; thus, 6-MP dosage should be decreased by 67–75%
Methotrexate	Oral absorption: Up to 30 mg complete absorption; doses > 30 mg, absorption decreases to 20–30% of a parenteral dose; Vd = 0.6–1 L/kg; Vd (IT) = 400 ml $t\frac{1}{2}(\alpha) = 45$ min $t\frac{1}{2}(\beta) = 2$–4 hrs IV $t\frac{1}{2}(\delta) = 10$–27 hrs $t\frac{1}{2}(IT) = 4.5$–14 hrs	In high doses (>1 gm), 10% metabolized to 7-hydroxy-methotrexate	Primarily unchanged; Renal: Low doses ~ 90% High doses ~ 50–70% Tubular secretion: $Cl_{MTX} \approx 120$–180 ml/min	Renal dysfunction: $Cl_{Cr} < 70$ ml/min-avoid MTX; drug interactions: probenicid, sulfonamides, salicylates decrease Cl_{MTX} by 25, 39, and 63%, respectively

Table 24. (continued)

PHARMACOKINETIC PARAMETERS FOR ANTINEOPLASTIC DRUGS

Drug	Distribution	Site of Metabolism	Excretion	Conditions Requiring Dose Reduction or Avoidance
Misonidazole	Oral absorption is rapid and complete; $Vd = 0.6$ L/kg; $t\frac{1}{2} = 10–12$ hrs; tumor levels ~ 80% of plasma levels	Liver: microsomal enzymes to desmethylmisonidazole (active)	Renal: 12–65% of drug and metabolites over 24 hours	Renal or hepatic dysfunction; Dehydration—patients must be able to take oral fluids
Mithramycin	Rapid, over 80% of drug removed from plasma in 3 hours into tissues; Vd is probably large	Unknown	Renal: ~ 25% of parent compound in 2 hours	Renal dysfunction
Mitomycin C	$Vd = ~ 0.6$ L/kg; $t\frac{1}{2} = 10–20$ min	Liver, active metabolites	Renal: 6% unchanged drug	Unknown
Procarbazine	Oral absorption is rapid and complete; Vd is probably large; readily enters CSF; $t\frac{1}{2}$ (parent compound) = 7 min	Liver, microsomal metabolism and erythrocyte metabolism to active metabolites	Renal: ~ 25% of dose in urine in 24 hours—most as a metabolite	Avoid alcohol because of "Antabuse-like" reaction; avoid tyramine-containing foods
Semustine (MeCCNU)	Oral absorption is rapid and complete; $Vd = 3.25$ L/kg; $Cl = 56$ ml/min (Ave.); CSF/plasma ratio: high; $t\frac{1}{2}$ (parent compound) = rapid	Liver: hydroxylation to active intermediates	Renal: Up to 60% of an oral dose excreted in the urine as metabolites	Cumulative myelosuppression: repeated dosing should be no more frequent than once every 6 weeks; liver dysfunction may lead to prolonged clearance of active metabolites and enhanced myelosuppression
Streptozotocin	Vd is probably large because of rapid clearance of intact drug; tumor penetration high; drug metabolites concentrate in kidney, liver and tumor; CSF/plasma ratio: high; $t\frac{1}{2}$ (parent compound) = 15–35 min $t\frac{1}{2}$ (metabolite) = 6 min (distrib phase), 3.5 hr (plasma phase), 40 hr (terminal phase)	Liver, active and inactive metabolites	Renal: 15% of dose excreted in urine; Lung: expired to a significant but not quantitated amount	Renal dysfunction: nephrotoxic agent

Table 24. (continued)

PHARMACOKINETIC PARAMETERS FOR ANTINEOPLASTIC DRUGS

Drug	Distribution	Site of Metabolism	Excretion	Conditions Requiring Dose Reduction or Avoidance
Tamoxifen	Oral absorption is rapid and complete; Vd is unknown; $t_{\frac{1}{2}} (\alpha) = 16$ hrs $t_{\frac{1}{2}} (\beta) = 35$ hrs $t_{\frac{1}{2}} (\delta) = 100$ hrs	Liver, conjugated and hydroxylated; metabolites are active; metabolite plasma concentrations are similar to concurrent tamoxifen levels	Renal: small amount of parent compound in urine; about 30% of oral dose as hydroxylated metabolite	None
Tegafur (FTORAFUR)	Oral absorption is rapid and complete; Vd = 0.4–0.8 L/kg; CSF/plasma ratio: high; $t_{\frac{1}{2}} = 6$–16 hrs; plasma clearance = 50 ml/kg/hr	Liver: hepatic activation to significant amount of the total dose; less than 5% as FU; several hydroxylated metabolites	Renal: 10–30% in the urine as metabolites; Lung: 60–80% respired as CO_2	Liver dysfunction prolongs half-life and may lead to increased toxicity
Thioguanine	Oral absorption is slow; peak plasma levels occur 10–12 hours after dose	Liver: metabolites include thioxanthine, thiouric acid, and methylthioguanine	Renal: 20–60% of parent compound and metabolites in the urine in 24 hours	Liver and renal dysfunction may delay clearance of active compound and enhance toxicity
Thiotepa	Unknown; plasma clearance of parent compound is rapid but pharmacologic half-life is long (7 days or longer)	Liver: some hepatic inactivation	Renal: almost 100% of unchanged drug in the urine in 48 hours	Renal dysfunction may delay urinary excretion of active compound
Vinblastine	Vd = 18–25 liters; distributes into platelets, leukocytes and other tissues rapidly; CSF/plasma ratio: low $t_{\frac{1}{2}} (\alpha) = 35$ min $t_{\frac{1}{2}} (\beta) = 53$ min $t_{\frac{1}{2}} (\delta) = 19$ hr	Liver: partial metabolism to deacetyl vinblastine (active)	Renal: about 33% excreted in urine in 3 days; fecal: 21% in stool via biliary excretion in 3 days	Biliary obstruction (hyperbilirubinemia): toxicity greatly increased; reduce dosage by at least 50% of usual dose
Vincristine	Vd = body water; distributes into red cells and and other tissues rapidly; $t_{\frac{1}{2}} (\alpha) = 1$ min $t_{\frac{1}{2}} (\beta) = 7.4$ min $t_{\frac{1}{2}} (\delta) = 2.6$ hrs	Liver: about 50% of drug metabolized to inactive metabolite	Renal: about 12% excreted in the urine as active and inactive compounds; Fecal: 60–70% excreted in stool via biliary clearance	Biliary obstruction (hyperbilirubinemia): toxicity greatly increased; reduce dosage by at least 50–75% of usual dose

References

1. Gilman A et al: The biologic actions and therapeutic applications of -chloroethyl amines and sulfides. Science. 1946; 103:409.

2. Farber S: Temporary remissions in acute leukemia in children produced by folic acid antagonist, 4-aminopteroylglutamic acid. N Engl J Med. 1948; 238:787.

3. DeVita VT et al: Combination chemotherapy in the treatment of advanced Hodgkin's Disease. Ann Intern Med. 1970; 73:881.

4. Carter SK: In *Chemotherapy of Cancer 2nd Ed.,* edited by SK Carter, Wiley & Sons, 1981.

5. Haskell CM: In *Cancer Treatment,* edited by M Cline and CM Haskell, Saunders, Philadelphia, 1980, p 3.

6. Cancer Facts and Figures 1980. American Cancer Society, New York, 1980.

7. Haskell CM: Principles of Cancer Chemotherapy. In *Cancer Treatment,* edited by M Cline and CM Haskell, Saunders, Philadelphia, 1980, p 38.

8. Valeriote FA: The role of cell kinetics in cancer chemotherapy. Semin Oncol. 1977; 4:217.

9. Salmon SE: Expansion of the growth fraction in multiple myeloma with alkylating agents. Blood. 1975; 45:119.

10. Haskell CM: Principles of cancer chemotherapy. In *Cancer Treatment,* edited by C Haskell and M Cline, Saunders, Philadelphia, 1980, p 27.

11. Lippman M: Steroid hormone receptors in human malignancy. Life Sci. 1976; 18:143.

12. Crooke ST el al: Mitomycin-C: A review. Cancer Treatment Reviews. 1976; 3:121.

13. Bergsagel DE: An assessment of massive-dose chemotherapy of malignant disease. Can Med Assoc J. 1971; 104:31.

14. Cadman E: Toxicity of chemotherapeutic agents. In *Cancer: A Comprehensive Treatise,* Vol 5, edited by FF Becker, Plenum Press, New York, 1977, p 59.

15. Rosenoff SH: Recovery of normal hematopoietic tissue and tumor following injury from cyclophosphamide. Blood. 1975; 45:465.

16. Vogler WR: The effect of methotrexate on granulocyte stem cells and granulopoiesis. Cancer Res. 1973; 33:1628.

17. Lenaz L: Cardiotoxicity of adriamycin and related anthracyclines. Cancer Treat Rev. 1976; 3:111.

18. Von Hoff DD et al: Risk factors for doxorubicin-induced congestive heart failure. Ann Intern Med. 1979; 91:710.

19. Pratt CB et al: Age-related adriamycin cardiotoxicity in children. Cancer Treat Rep. 1978; 62:1381.

20. Bristow MR et al: Early anthracycline cardiotoxicity. Amer J Med. 1978; 65:823.

21. Minow RA et al: Adriamycin cardiomyopathy—risk factors. Cancer. 1977; 39:1397.

22. Bristow MR et al: Clinical spectrum of anthracycline antibiotic cardiotoxicity. Cancer Treat Rep. 1978; 62:873.

23. Blum RH et al: Adriamycin: A new anticancer drug with significant clinical activity. Ann Intern Med. 1974; 80:249.

24. Bristow MR et al; Doxorubicin cardiomyopathy evaluated by phonocardiography, endomyocardial biopsy, and cardiac catheterization. Ann Intern Med. 1978; 88:168.

25. Gottdiener JS et al: Doxorubicin cardiotoxicity: assessment of late left ventricular dysfunction by radionuclide cineangiography. Ann Intern Med. 1981; 94:430.

26. Chlebowski RT: Adriamycin (Doxorubicin) cardiotoxicity: A review. West J Med. 1979; 131:364.

27. Legha SS: Adriamycin by continuous IV infusion. Northern California Oncology Group, Scientific Meeting. San Francisco, California. April 17, 1981.

28. Legha SS et al: Augmentation of adriamycin's therapeutic index by prolonged continuous IV infusion for advanced breast cancer. Proc Am Assoc Cancer Res. 1979; 20:261 (abst. 1059).

29. Weiss RB et al: Cytotoxic drug-induced pulmonary disease. Update 1980. Am J Med. 1980; 68:259.

30. Collis CH: Lung damage from cytotoxic drugs. Cancer Chemother Pharmacol. 1980; 4:17.

31. Sostman HD et al: Cytotoxic drug-induced lung disease. Am J Med. 1977; 62:608.

32. Blum RH et al: A clinical review of bleomycin—A new antineoplastic agent. Cancer. 1973; 31:903.

33. Comis RL et al: Single breath CO diffusion capacity as an indicator of subclinical bleomycin pulmonary toxicity in testicular cancer patients. Proc Am Assoc Cancer Res. 1978; 19:236.

34. Samuels ML et al: Large-dose bleomycin therapy and pulmonary toxicity: a possible role of prior radiotherapy. JAMA. 1976; 235:1117.

35. Nygard K et al: Pulmonary complication from bleomycin, irradiation, surgery for oesophageal cancer. Cancer. 1978; 41:17.

36. Prince RA et al: Antineoplastic agents as a cause of fever. Drug Intell Clin Pharm. 1975; 9:124.

37. Weiss RB et al: Hypersensitivity reactions to cancer chemotherapeutic agents. Ann Intern Med. 1981; 94:66.

38. Hass CD et al: Phase II evaluation of bleomycin: a Southwest Oncology Group Study. Cancer. 1976; 38:8.

39. Durkin WJ et al: Treatment of advanced lymphomas with bleomycin (NSC-125066). Oncology. 1976; 33:140.

40. Ma DD et al: Cytotoxic-induced fulminant hyperpyrexia. Cancer. 1980; 45:2249.

41. Blenoxane Product Brochure, 1981.

42. Talby RW et al: Clinical evaluation of toxic effects of cis-diamminedichloroplatinum (NSC-119875) phase I clinical study. Cancer Chemother Rep. 1973; 57:465.

43. Hardaker WT et al: Platinum nephrotoxicity. Cancer. 1974; 34:1030.

44. Gonzales-Vitale JC et al: Acute renal failure after cis-dichloroammineplatinum (II) and gentamicin-cephalothin therapies. Cancer Treat Rep. 1978; 62:693.

45. Dentino M et al: Long term effect of cis-diamminedichloride platinum (CDDP) on renal function and structure in man. Cancer. 1978; 41:1274.

46. Madias NE et al: Platinum nephrotoxicity. Am J Med. 1978; 65:307.

47. Hayes D et al: Amelioration of renal toxicity of high-dose cis-platinum by mannitol-induced diuresis. Proc Am Assoc Cancer Res. 1976; 17:171.

48. Einhorn LH et al: Cis-diamminedichloroplatinum, vinblastine, and bleomycin. Combination chemotherapy in disseminated testicular cancer. Ann Intern Med. 1977; 87:293.

49. Frick GA et al: Renal excretion kinetics of high-dose cis-dichloroammine platinum (II) administered with hydration and mannitol diuresis. Cancer Treat Rep. 1979; 63:13.

50. Rainey JM et al: Safe, rapid administration schedule for cis-platinum-mannitol. Med Pediatr Oncol. 1978; 4:371.

51. Bachur NR et al: Adriamycin (NSC-123127) pharmacology. Cancer Chemother Rep. Part 3, 1975; 6:153.

52. Alberts DS et al: The pharmacokinetics of daunomycin in man. Clin Pharmacol Ther. 1971; 12:96.

53. Huffman DH et al: Daunorubicin metabolism in acute non-lymphatic leukemia. Clin Pharmacol Ther. 1972; 13:895.

54. Berkson GM et al: Severe cystitis induced by cyclophosphamide. JAMA. 1973; 225:605.

55. Rubin JS et al: Cyclophosphamide hemorrhagic cystitis. J Urol. 1966; 96:313.

56. Shrom SH et al: Formalin treatment for intractable hemorrhagic cystitis. Cancer. 1976; 38:1785.

57. Tolley DA: The effect of N-acetyl cysteine on cyclophosphamide cystitis. Br J Urol. 1977; 49:659.

58. Buckner CD et al: High-dose cyclophosphamide therapy for malignant disease: Toxicity, tumor response, and the effects of stored autologous marrow. Cancer. 1972; 29:357.

59. Huffman DH: Pharmacokinetics of methotrexate. Clin Pharmacol Ther. 1973; 14:572.

60. Bleyer WA: The clinical pharmacology of methotrexate. Cancer. 1978; 41:36.

61. Stoller RG et al: Pharmacokinetics of high-dose methotrexate (NSC-740). Cancer Chemother Rep. 1975; 6:19.

62. Jacobs SA et al: 7-Hydroxymethotrexate as a urinary metabolite in human subjects and rhesus monkeys receiving high-dose methotrexate. J Clin Invest. 1976; 57:534.

63. Nirenberg A et al: High dose methotrexate with citrovorum factor rescue: Predictive value of serum MTX concentrations and corrective measures to avert toxicity. Cancer Treat Rep. 1977; 61:779.

64. Pitman SW et al: Weekly methotrexate—calcium leucovorin rescue: Effect of alkalinization; pharmacokinetics in the CNS; and use in CNS non-Hodgkin's lymphoma. Cancer Treat Rep. 1977; 61:695.

65. Ignoffo RJ et al: Treatment of local toxicities from cancer chemotherapeutic agents. Cancer Treat Rev. 1980; 7:17.

66. Rudolph R et al: Skin ulcers due to adriamycin. Cancer. 1976; 38:1087.

67. Reilly JJ et al: Clinical course and management of accidental adriamycin extravasation. Cancer. 1977; 40:2053.

68. DeGregorio M et al: Mitomycin extravasation reactions in the rabbit model. Publication in preparation.

69. Zveig JI et al: An apparently effective counter-measure for doxorubicin extravasation (Letter). JAMA. 1978; 239:2116.

70. Bartkowski-Dodds L et al: Use of sodium bicarbonate as a means of ameliorating doxorubicin-induced dermal necrosis in rats. Cancer Chemother Pharmacol. 1980; 4:179.

71. Dorr RT et al: The limited role of corticosteroids in ameliorating experimental doxorubicin skin toxicity in the mouse. Cancer Chemother Pharmacol. 1980; 5:17.

72. Ignoffo RJ et al: A model for skin toxicity of antineoplastic drug: doxorubicin, mitomycin-C, and vincristine (abst.). Clinical Res. April 1981.

73. Luce JK: Adria Laboratories. Personal communication 1980.

74. Sallan SE et al: Antiemetics in patients receiving chemotherapy for cancer. N Engl J Med. 1980; 302:135.

75. Moertel CG et al: A controlled clinical evaluation of antiemetic drugs. JAMA. 1963; 186:116.

76. Moertel CG et al: Controlled clinical studies of orally administered antiemetic drugs. Gastroenterology. 1969; 57:262.

77. Plotkin DA et al: Haloperidol in the treatment of nausea and vomiting due to cytotoxic drug administration. Curr Ther Res. 1973; 15:599.

78. Neidhart JA et al: Specific antiemetics for specific cancer chemotherapeutic agents. Cancer. 1981; 47:1439.

79. Grossman B et al: Droperidol prevents nausea and vomiting from cis-platinum. N Engl J Med. 1979; 301:47.

80. Edmonds-Seal J et al: Pharmacology of drugs used in neuroleptic analgesia. Br J Anaesth. 1970; 42:207.

81. Harris JG et al: Nausea and vomiting and cancer treatment. CA–A Cancer Journal for Clinicians. 1978; 28:194.

82. Kahn T et al: A single dose of metoclopramide in the control of vomiting from cis-dichloroammine-platinum (II) in man. Cancer Treat Rep. 1978; 62:1106.

83. Gralla RJ et al: High dose metoclopramide: effective antiemetic against cisplatin (DDP) in randomized trials vs. placebo and prochlorperazine (PCP). Proc Am Soc Clin Onc. 1981; 22:420 (abst. C-344).

84. Baker JJ et al: Comparison of dexamethasone plus prochlorperazine to placebo plus prochlorperazine as antiemetics for cancer chemotherapy. Proc Am Soc Clin Oncol. 1980; 21:339 (abst. C-81).

85. Rich WM et al: Methylprednisolone as an antiemetic drug during cancer chemotherapy. Gynecol Oncol. 1980; 9:193.

86. Davignon JP: Delta-9-tetrahydrocannabinol: comments on antiemetic trials. Front Radiat Ther Onc. 1981; 15:148.

87. Chang AE et al: Delta-9-tetrahydrocannabinol as an antiemetic in cancer patients receiving high-dose methotrexate. A prospective randomized evaluation. Ann Intern Med. 1979; 91:819.

88. Frytak S et al: Delta-9-tetrahydrocannabinol as an antiemetic for patients receiving cancer chemotherapy. A comparison with prochlorperazine and a placebo. Ann Intern Med. 1979; 91:825.

89. Lucas VS et al: Δ^9-Tetrahydrocannabinol for refractory vomiting induced by cancer chemotherapy. JAMA. 1980; 243:1241.

90. Chang AE et al: A prospective evaluation of Delta-9-tetrahydrocannabinol as an antiemetic in patients receiving adriamycin and cytoxan chemotherapy. Cancer. 1981; 47:1746.

91. National Cancer Institute: Dr. Daniel Hoth—personal communication.

92. Weiss HD et al: Neurotoxicity of commonly used antineoplastic agents. N Engl J Med. 1974; 297:127.

93. Holland JF et al: Vincristine treatment of advanced cancer: a cooperative study of 392 cases. Cancer Res. 1973; 33:1258.

94. Casey EB et al: Vincristine neuropathy: clinical and electrophysiological observations. Brain. 1973; 96:69.

95. Albert DM et al: Ocular complications of vincristine therapy. Arch Ophthalmol. 1967; 78:709.

96. Rosenthal S et al: Vincristine neurotoxicity. Ann Intern Med. 1974; 80:733.

97. Haggard ME et al: Vincristine in acute leukemia of childhood. Cancer. 1968; 22:438.

98. Sandler SG et al: Vincristine-induced neuropathy: a clinical study of fifty leukemic patients. Neurology (Minreap.). 1969; 19:367.

99. Pratt CB et al: Low-dosage asparaginase treatment of childhood acute lymphocytic leukemia. Am J Dis Child. 1971; 121:406.

100. Ohnuma T et al: Biochemical and pharmacological studies with asparaginase in man. Cancer Res. 1970; 30:2297.

101. Zubrod CG: The clinical toxicities of L-asparaginase in treatment of leukemia and lymphoma. Pediatrics. 1970; 45:555.

102. Haskell CM et al: L-asparaginase. Therapeutic and toxic effects in patients with antineoplastic disease. N Engl J Med. 1969; 281:1028.

103. Menard DB et al: Antineoplastic agents and the liver. Gastroenterology. 1980; 78:142.

104. Oettgen HF et al: Toxicity of *E. Coli* L-asparaginase in man. Cancer. 1970; 25:253.

105. Pratt CB et al: Duration and severity of fatty metamorphosis of the liver following L-asparaginase therapy. Cancer. 1971; 28:361.

106. Foley KM: Pain syndromes in patients with cancer. In *Advances in Pain Research,* Vol. 3, edited by J Bonica, Raven Press, New York, 1979, p 59.

107. Twycross RG: Overview of analgesia. In *Advances in Pain Research,* Volume 3, edited by J Bonica, Raven Press, New York, 1979, p 617.

108. Lipman AG: Drug therapy in chronic pain. J Contin Educ Hosp Clin Pharm. 1979, Sept/Oct issue: p 11.

109. Budd K: Psychotropic drugs in the treatment of chronic pain. Anaesthesia. 1978; 33:531.

110. Halpern LM: Psychotropics, ataractics, and related drugs (in pain). In *Advances in Pain Research,* Volume 2, edited by J Bonica, Raven Press, New York, 1977, p 276.

111. Catalano RB: The medical approach to management of pain caused by cancer. Semin Oncol. 1975; 2:379.

112. Reuler JB et al: The chronic pain syndrome: Misconceptions and management. Ann Intern Med. 1980; 93:588.

113. Moertel CG: Treatment of cancer pain with orally administered medications. JAMA. 1980; 244:2448.

114. Marks RM et al: Undertreatment of medical inpatients with narcotic analgesics. Ann Intern Med. 1973; 78:173.

115. See-Lasley K et al: Pain management. In *Manual of Oncology Therapeutics,* edited by K See-Lasley and R Ignoffo, Mosby, St. Louis, 1981, p 319.

116. Frazer D: Intravenous morphine infusion for chronic pain. (Letter) Ann Intern Med. 1980; 93:781.

117. Ensworth S: Morphine IV infusion for chronic pain. (Letter) Drug Intell Clin Pharm. 1979; 13:297.

118. Miser AW et al: Continuous intravenous infusion of morphine sulfate for control of severe pain in children with terminal malignancy. J Pediatr. 1980; 96:930.

119. Szeto HH et al: Accumulation of normeperidine, an active metabolite of neperidine, in patients with renal failure or cancer. Ann Intern Med. 1977; 86:738.

120. Twycross RG: Bone pain in advanced cancer. Topics in Therapeutics. 1978; 4:94.

121. Stambough JE et al: Double-blind comparisons of zomepirac and oxycodone with APC in cancer pain. J Clin Pharmacol. 1980; 20:261.

122. Chopra D et al: Hypercalcemia and malignant disease. Med Clin N Am. 1975; 59:441.

123. Mazzaferri EL et al: Treatment of hypercalcemia associated with malignancy. Semin Oncol. 1978; 5:141.

124. Powell D et al: Nonparathyroid humoral hypercalcemia in patients with neoplastic diseases. N Engl J Med. 1973; 289:176.

125. Seyberth HW et al: Prostaglandins as mediators of hypercalcemia associated with cancer. N Engl J Med. 1975; 293:1278.

126. Muggia FM et al: Hypercalcemia associated with neoplastic disease. Ann Intern Med. 1970; 73:281.

127. Suki WN et al: Acute treatment of hypercalcemia with furosemide. N Engl J Med. 1970; 283:836.

128. Slayton RE: New approach to the treatment of hypercalcemia: The effect of short-term treatment with mithramycin. Clin Pharmcol Ther. 1971; 12:833.

129. Brereton HD et al: Indomethacin-responsive hypercalcemia in a patient with renal-cell adenocarcinoma. N Engl J Med. 1974; 291:83.

130. Tashjian AH: Tumor humors and the hypercalcemia of cancer. N Engl J Med. 1974; 290:905.

131. Jessiman AG: Hypercalcemia in carcinoma of the breast. Ann Surg. 1963; 157:377.

132. Jacobs TP et al: Hypercalcemia of malignancy: Treatment with intravenous dichloromethylene diphosphonate. Ann Intern Med. 1981; 94:312.

133. Friedman MA et al: Malignant pleural effusions. Cancer Treat Rev. 1978; 5:49.

134. Leff A et al: Pleural effusion from malignancy. Ann Intern Med. 1978; 88:532.

135. Light LW et al: Cells in pleural fluid. Arch Intern Med. 1973; 132:854.

136. Wallach HW et al: Intrapleural tetracycline for malignant pleural effusion. Chest. 1975; 68:510.

137. Borja ER et al: Single-dose quinacrine (Atabrine) and thoracostomy in control of pleural effusion in patients with metastatic disease. Cancer. 1973; 31:899.

138. Dollinger MR: Management of recurrent malignant effusions. Cancer. 1972; 22:138.

139. Posner JB: Management of central nervous system metastases. Semin Oncol. 1977; 4:81.

140. Dawson DM et al: Neurologic complications of acute leukemia in adults: changing rate. Ann Intern Med. 1973; 79:541.

141. Pochedly C: Treatment of meningeal leukemia. Hospital Practice. 1976; November, p 123.

142. Blasberg RG et al: Intrathecal chemotherapy-brain-tissue profiles after ventriculo cisternal perfusion. J Pharmacol Exp Ther. 1975; 195:73.

143. Shapiro WR et al: Methotrexate: Distribution in cerebrospinal fluid after intravenous, ventricular and lumbar injections. N Engl J Med. 1975; 293:161.

144. Bleyer WA et al: Pharmacokinetics and neurotoxicity of intrathecal methotrexate therapy. N Engl J Med. 1973; 289:770.

145. Bleyer WA et al: Clinical pharmacology of intrathecal methotrexate: I. Pharmacokinetics in non-toxic patients after lumbar injection. Cancer Treat Rep. 1977; 61:703.

146. Evans WE: Methotrexate. In *Applied Pharmacokinetics: Principles of Therapeutic Drug Monitoring,* edited by WE Evans, JJ Schentag, and WJ Jusko, Applied Therapeutics Inc., San Francisco, 1980, p 526.

147. Bleyer WA: Clinical pharmacology of intrathecal methotrexate: II. An improved dosage regimen derived from age-related pharmacokinetics. Cancer Treat Rep. 1977; 61:1419.

148. Pochedly C: Neurotoxicity due to CNS therapy for leukemia. Med Pediatr Oncol. 1977; 3:101.

149. Bleyer WA: Methotrexate clinical pharmacology, current status and therapeutic guidelines. Cancer Treat Rev. 1977; 4:87.

150. Evans WE: Methotrexate. In *Applied Pharmacokinetics: Principles of Therapeutic Drug Monitoring,* edited by WE Evans, JJ Schentag, and WJ Jusko, Applied Therapeutics Inc., San Francisco, 1980, p 533.

151. Band PR et al: Treatment of central nervous system leukemia with intrathecal cytosine arabinoside. Cancer. 1973; 32:744.

152. Ho DH et al: Clinical pharmacology of 1-α-D arabinofuranosylcytosine. Clin Pharmacol Ther. 1971; 12:944.

153. Wan SH et al: Pharmacokinetics of 1-α-D arabinofuranosylcytosine in humans. Cancer Res. 1974; 34:392.

154. Gutin PH: Intrathecal thio-tepa in the treatment of malignant meningeal disease. Cancer. 1976; 38:1471.

155. Gutin PH et al: Treatment of malignant meningeal disease with intrathecal thio-tepa. Cancer Treat Rep. 1977; 61:885.

156. Anderson RJ et al: Immunosuppressive and antineoplastic agents. In *Clinical Use of Drugs in Renal Failure,* edited by RJ Anderson, JG Gambertoglio, and RW Schrier, Charles Thomas Publishing Co., Springfield, IL 1976, p 173.

157. Cohen JL: Pharmacokinetics of cyclophosphamide in man. Br J Pharmacol. 1971; 43:677.

158. Tozer TN: Nomogram for modification of dosage regimens with chronic renal function impairment. J Pharmacokinetics Biopharm. 1974; 2:13.

159. Spreafico F et al: Drug disposition during development. In *Antineoplastic Agents,* edited by PL Morselli, Spectrum Publications, New York, 1977, p 101.

160. Benjamin RS: Adriamycin chemotherapy—efficacy, safety and pharmacologic basis of an intermittent single high-dose schedule. Cancer. 1974; 33:19.

161. Jackson DV et al: Biliary excretion of vincristine. Clin Pharmacol Ther. 1978; 24:101.

162. Macmillan WE et al: Pharmacokinetics of fluorouracil in humans. Cancer Res. 1978; 38:3479.

163. Goldman ID: Analysis of the cytotoxic determinants for methotrexate: A role for free: intracellular drug. Cancer Chemother Rep. Part 3, 1975; 6:51.

164. Djerassi I: High dose methotrexate and citrovorum rescue: Background and rationale. Cancer Chemother Rep. Part 3, 1975; 6:3.

165. Pinedo HM et al: Role of drug concentration, duration of exposure and endogenous metabolites in determining methotrexate cytotoxicity. Cancer Treat Rep. 1977; 61:709.

166. Goldman ID: The membrane transport of methotrexate (NSC-740) and other folate compounds: relevance to rescue protocols. Cancer Chemother Rep. Part 3, 1975; 6:63.

167. Isacoff WH: High dose methotrexate therapy of solid tumors. Med Pediatr Oncol. 1976; 2:319.

168. Bertino JR: Techniques in cancer chemotherapy. Use of leucovorin and other rescue agents after methotrexate treatment. Semin Oncol. 1977; 4:203.

169. Stoller RG et al: A clinical and pharmacologic study of high dose methotrexate with minimal leucovorin rescue. Cancer Res. 1979; 39:908.

170. Hande KR et al: Pharmacology and pharmacokinetics of high dose methotrexate. In *Clinical Pharmacology of Antineoplastic Drugs,* edited by HM Pinedo, Elsevier/North Holland, Amsterdam, 1978, p 97.

171. Von Hoff DD et al: Incidence of drug-related deaths secondary to high-dose methotrexate and citrovorum factor administration. Cancer Treat Rep. 1977; 61:745.

172. Evans WE et al: Pharmacokinetic monitoring of high dose methotrexate: Early recognition of high-risk patients. Cancer Chemother Pharmacol. 1979; 3:161.

173. Evans WE et al: Effect of pleural effusion on high dose methotrexate kinetics. Clin Pharmacol Ther. 1978; 24:68.

174. Shen DD et al: Clinical pharmacokinetics of methotrexate. Clin Pharmacokinetics. 1978; 3:1.

175. Lerne PR et al: Kinetic model for the disposition and metabolism of moderate and high-dose methotrexate (NSC-740) in man. Cancer Chemother Rep. 1975: 59:811.

176. Pratt CB et al: High-dose methotrexate used alone and in combination for measurable and primary metastatic osteosarcoma. Cancer Treat Rep. 1980; 64:11.

177. Stoller RG et al: Pharmacokinetics of high dose methotrexate. Cancer Chemother Rep. Part 3, 1975; 6:19.

178. Tattersall MH et al: Clinical pharmacology of high dose methotrexate (NSC-740). Cancer Chemother Rep. 1975; 6:25.

179. Stoller RG et al: Use of plasma pharmacokinetics to predict and prevent methotrexate toxicity. N Engl J Med. 1977; 297:630.

180. Isacoff WH et al: Pharmacokinetics of high-dose methotrexate with citrovorum factor rescue. Cancer Treat Rep. 1977; 61:1665.

181. Bleyer WA: The clinical pharmacology of methotrexate: new applications of an old drug. Cancer. 1978; 41:36.

182. Nirenberg A et al: High dose methotrexate with CF rescue: Predictive value of serum methotrexate concentrations and corrective measures to avert toxicity. Cancer Treat Rep. 1977; 61:779.

183. Liegler DG et al: The effect of organic acids on renal clearance of methotrexate in man. Clin Pharmacol Ther. 1969; 10:849.

184. Rodrigues V et al: Management of fever of unknown origin in patients with neoplasms and neutropenia. Cancer. 1973; 32:1007.

185. Bodey GP: Infections in cancer patients. Cancer Treat Rev. 1975; 2:89.

186. Whitecar JP et al: Replacement of platelets and granulocytes in patients with myelosuppression. In *Cancer Chemotherapy II,* edited by I Brodsky, Grune and Stratton, New York, 1972, p 287.

187. Gaydos LA et al: The quantitative relation between platelet count and hemorrhage in patients with acute leukemia. N Engl J Med. 1962; 266:905.

188. Aisner J: Platelet transfusion therapy. Med Clin N Am. 1977; 61:1133.

189. DeConti RC: Use of allopurinol for prevention and control of hyperuricemia in patients with neoplastic disease. N Engl J Med. 1966; 274:481.

190. Maher JF et al: Hyperuricemia complicating leukemia: treatment with allopurinol and dialysis. Arch Intern Med. 1969; 123:198.

191. Krakoff IH: Use of allopurinol in preventing hyperuricemia in leukemia and lymphoma. Cancer. 1966; 19:1489.

192. Hande K et al: Allopurinol kinetics. Clin Pharmacol Ther. 1978; 23:598.

193. Boston Collaborative Drug Surveillance Program: Interaction in relation to bone marrow depression. JAMA. 1974; 227:1036.

194. Herrington RT et al: Uric acid nephropathy in leukemia. N Engl J Med. 1966; 266:934.

195. Ignoffo RJ: Adverse reactions to anticancer drugs. In *Manual of Oncology Therapeutics*, edited by K See-Lasley and R Ignoffo, Mosby & Co., 1981, p 249.

196. McGuire WL: Hormone dependence in breast cancer. Metabolism. 1974; 23:175.

197. McGuire WL et al: Current status of estrogen and progesterone receptors in breast cancer. Cancer. 1977; 39:2934.

198. Legha SS et al: Hormonal therapy of breast cancer: new approaches and concepts. Ann Intern Med. 1978; 88:69.

199. McGuire WL et al: Estrogen receptors. In *Estrogen Receptors in Human Breast Cancer*, edited by WL McGuire, Raven Press, 1975, p 1.

200. Kennedy BJ: Hormonal therapies in breast cancer. Semin Oncol. 1974; 1:119.

201. McGuire WL: Current status of estrogen receptors in human breast cancer. Cancer. 1975; 36:638.

202. Ingle JN et al: Randomized clinical trial of diethylstilbestrol versus tamoxifen in postmenopausal women with advanced heart cancer. N Engl J Med. 1981; 304:16.

203. Lippman M et al: The effects of estrogens and antiestrogens on hormone-responsive human breast cancer in long-term tissue culture. Cancer Res. 1976; 36:4595.

204. Kiang DT et al: Tamoxifen (antiestrogen) therapy in advanced breast cancer. Ann Intern Med. 1978; 88:69.

205. Henderson IC et al: Cancer of the breast. N Engl J Med. 1980; 302:78.

206. Talley RW et al: A dose-response evaluation of androgens in the treatment of metastatic breast cancer. Cancer. 1973; 32:315.

207. Edelstyn GA: Norethisterone acetate in advanced breast cancer. Cancer. 1973; 32:1317.

208. Lipton A et al: Medical adrenalectomy using aminoglutethimide and dexamethasone in advanced breast cancer. Cancer. 1974; 33:503.

209. Newsome HH et al: Medical and surgical adrenalectomy in patients with advanced breast carcinoma. Cancer. 1977; 39:542.

210. Fishman LM et al: Effects of aminoglutethimide on adrenal function in man. J Clin Endocrinol Metab. 1967; 27:481.

211. Smith IE et al: Aminoglutethimide in treatment of metastatic breast cancer. Lancet. 1978; 2:646.

212. Santen RJ et al: Kinetic, hormonal and clinical studies with aminoglutethimide in breast cancer. Cancer. 1977; 39:2948.

213. Griffiths CT et al: Preliminary trial of aminoglutethimide in breast cancer. Cancer. 1973; 32:31.

214. Gralla RM et al: Antiemetic efficacy of high-dose metoclopramide: Randomized trials with placebo and prochlorperazine in patients with chemotherapy-induced nausea and vomiting. N Engl J Med. 1981; 305:906.

Chapter 43

Pediatric Oncology

William E. Evans and Gary C. Yee

In the United States, cancer kills more children between 1 and 14 years of age than any other disease. For every million children under 15 years of age, approximately 111 new cases of cancer will be diagnosed (1). The most common childhood cancer is leukemia, comprising about 30% of all childhood malignancies. Approximately 77% of childhood leukemia cases at St. Jude Children's Research Hospital are diagnosed as acute lymphocytic leukemia (ALL) and 20% as acute nonlymphocytic (ANLL; also called acute myelocytic leukemia, or AML). In American children less than 15 years of age, the incidence of Wilms' tumor, soft tissue sarcoma, sarcoma of bone, Hodgkin's disease, non-Hodgkin's lymphoma, and neuroblastoma is reported to be similar to that of acute nonlymphocytic leukemia (2).

Prior to the introduction of aminopterin as treatment for acute leukemia in 1948, a child with acute leukemia had a median survival of about two to four months. The use of aminopterin to induce temporary remissions marked the beginning of the current era of therapy for acute leukemia, during which time numerous antineoplastic agents have been developed and become available for clinical use. Concurrent with the development of better treatment modalities for leukemia and other malignancies has been the improvement of therapy for the complications of treatment, such as infections. These developments, coupled with an increased understanding of the biology of malignant diseases, have led to improvement in the prognosis of many childhood malignancies. The most striking example of this is childhood ALL, where the therapeutic approach has changed from one of palliation of an almost universally fatal disease to current approaches aimed at long-term, disease-free survival and cure. Several reviews have summarized the current status of the treatment of childhood cancers, particularly ALL (3–8).

This chapter emphasizes the chemotherapy of

childhood neoplastic diseases. Other components of treatment are also briefly described to provide a perspective of the total therapeutic approach to these diseases and the importance of chemotherapy in each. Results of clinical trials currently in progress will undoubtedly alter the current therapy of many childhood cancers and hopefully lead to further improvement in responses to treatment.

ACUTE LYMPHOCYTIC LEUKEMIA

Before discussing specific patient cases, a brief introduction of acute lymphocytic leukemia (ALL) is warranted. Acute lymphocytic leukemia can be defined as a hematologic neoplasm characterized by accumulation of immature lymphoid cells in the bone marrow and resulting in impairment of normal stem cell function. As will be discussed in subsequent questions, the term ALL encompasses a heterogeneous group of diseases with distinct clinical, biochemical, and immunological characteristics, some of which have prognostic significance.

The clinical manifestations of ALL are usually related to replacement of normal hematopoietic cells in the bone marrow by leukemia cells. The initial symptoms are usually non-specific and are sometimes indistinguishable from symptoms of a viral infection. Common manifestations early in the disease are anorexia, irritability, and lethargy. Pallor, bleeding, bruising, and fever are usually the findings that cause patients to seek medical attention. On physical examination, hepatosplenomegaly and lymphadenopathy may be present. Bone pain and arthralgias, due to infiltration with leukemic blasts, occur in about one-fourth of the patients. Peripheral blood counts usually show a leukocyte count of less than 10,000/mm^3, a platelet count of less than 25,000/mm^3, and mild anemia. Lymphoblasts are usually easily detected in blood smears from patients with leukocyte counts greater than 5000/mm^3. The anemia is almost always normocytic and normochromic, with evidence of inadequate marrow cell production.

Although these clinical and laboratory features are helpful in the diagnosis, definitive diagnosis is made from examination of an adequate bone marrow specimen. This specimen almost always shows virtually complete replacement of normal cell elements by leukemic blast cells. Subclassification of patients with ALL is now possible based on a combination of clinical and/or laboratory findings at diagnosis. These subgroups have prognostic significance, as discussed in Question 17.

The therapeutic approach for ALL has been developed only recently, with the crucial phases of treatment being remission induction, preventive central nervous system (CNS) therapy, and systemic continuation therapy. Although specific cases for each individual phase will be discussed in detail, the effectiveness and toxicity of one phase can affect the efficacy of other phases. Some treatment programs include intensification or consolidation phases after remission induction; however, the benefit of these additional phases has not been proven.

Remission Induction

1. **A.B.C. is a 10-year-old white boy with pallor, lethargy, normochromic normocytic anemia, and thrombocytopenia who was referred with a probable diagnosis of acute leukemia after his physician noted a preponderance of immature, poorly differentiated lymphocytes in his peripheral blood. A diagnosis of acute lymphoblastic leukemia was established following examination of a bone marrow aspirate. At diagnosis, the patient's white blood cell count was 80,000/mm^3, there was no mediastinal mass on chest x-ray, no leukemia cells found in the cerebrospinal fluid, and his lymphoblasts did not produce spontaneous rosette formations when incubated with sheep erythrocytes. He was started on remission induction chemotherapy with prednisone, vincristine, and L-asparaginase. What is the goal of remission induction chemotherapy and what drugs are currently used for remission induction? How effective are these agents in inducing remission and how long will it take?**

The immediate goal of remission induction therapy for children with acute lymphocytic leukemia is to rapidly reduce the number of leukemic cells and allow for normal marrow regeneration while producing the least drug-related toxicity. Attainment of this goal is based on examination of an adequate bone marrow specimen. There are approximately one trillion (10^{12}) cells at the time of diagnosis and a reduction of 99.99% occurs with disease remission (8).

Drugs that have been used for remission induction therapy in children with acute lymphocytic leukemia (ALL) include prednisone (PRED), vincristine (VCR), L-asparaginase (L-ASP), daunomycin (DAUNO), etoposide (VM26), cytosine arabinoside (ARA-C), methotrexate (MTX), cyclophosphamide (CYCLO), and 6-mercaptopurine (6MP) (9–12). The ideal drug would be cytotoxic only to leukemic cells, have no effect on the proliferative activity of normal cells, and be cell-cycle nonspecific. Although no drug presently possesses all of these ideal characteristics, prednisone, vincristine, and L-asparaginase most closely meet these criteria.

As a single agent, prednisone will induce complete remission in approximately 50% of previously untreated children with ALL, while vincristine alone will induce remission in approximately 80% of patients (8). When administered in a multiple-drug induction regimen, these two agents induce remission in about 90% of children with previously untreated ALL (13–16). The addition of a third agent, usually L-ASP or DAUNO, or a fourth agent results in induction rates as high as 95–98% (17–22). The addition of these agents has been associated with more severe toxicity and even early death. A complete remission is usually achieved within four weeks when a combination of three agents is used.

2. Since the addition of a third cancer chemotherapeutic agent for remission induction has been associated with more severe toxicity, should A.B.C. have been treated with only two agents?

Although a slight increase in the remission induction rate is achieved with these three- and four-drug regimens, the primary reason for including a third remission induction drug (or an intensive phase with two additional drugs) is that it increases leukemia-free survival. The importance of the intensity of remission induction therapy on the length of continuous complete remission (CCR) is based on an analysis of studies in which the major variable was the type of remission induction therapy (23). Only 38% of patients who received two drugs for remission induction were in CCR after 30 months, compared to 50–60% of those receiving either three-drug induction or an intensive phase early in remission. There is no advantage to adding a fourth agent for remission induction or to using an intensification

phase if a three-drug regimen has been used. It is currently recommended that remission induction therapy should consist of three of the first-line drugs or include an intensive phase (with additional drugs) early in remission. Since 6MP and MTX are useful in maintenance therapy regimens, three-drug induction regimens with PRED, VCR, and L-ASP or DAUNO are preferable for standard-risk ALL patients such as A.B.C. As will be discussed later, remission induction for high-risk patients is less effective (80%) when these same drugs are used. Thus, response to remission induction therapy, as well as the length of leukemia-free survival, is worse in some subpopulations of patients with ALL. Children who fail to attain complete remission with standard remission induction therapy have a poor prognosis; however, the combination of VM-26 and ARA-C may be effective in these cases (25). Identification of these "high-risk" patients and possible modifications of therapy are discussed in Question 17.

3. *Allopurinol.* Prior to starting remission induction chemotherapy in A.B.C., oral allopurinol 200 mg/m²/day in two divided doses was given. What is the rationale for giving allopurinol?

The accelerated degradation on nucleoprotein following leukemia cell lysis by chemotherapy often results in increased uric acid production (26–27). Uric acid nephropathy, which may occur in association with acute increases in uric acid production, has been reported to be the most common cause of acute renal failure in patients with leukemia (28). Allopurinol, when given 12–48 hours before oncolytic therapy is started and continued for the duration of remission induction chemotherapy, is clearly effective in reducing serum and urinary uric acid levels (29–31). The administration of allopurinol suppresses uric acid formation by inhibiting xanthine oxidase, the enzyme that catalyzes the oxidative conversion of hypoxanthine to xanthine and xanthine to uric acid (32–33). Oral sodium bicarbonate in doses of 4–6 gm/m²/day or greater is commonly used to alkalinize the urine, thereby increasing the solubility of uric acid and reducing the likelihood of uric acid precipitation in the renal tubules and collecting ducts (26). Vigorous fluid intake sufficient to maintain good urine flow is also essential in preventing urate nephropathy.

4. Will allopurinol interact with any of the cancer chemotherapeutic agents currently prescribed for A.B.C.? Can any interaction be anticipated with any of the other agents commonly used for remission induction chemotherapy of ALL?

The inhibition of xanthine oxidase by allopurinol suppresses the metabolic pathway responsible for the oxidative conversion of *6-Mercaptopurine* (6MP) to 6-thiouric acid, a noncarcinostatic metabolite (34). The mechanism of this interaction and its significance remains to be determined, since studies have been unable to show a change in the half-life or area under the plasma concentration-time curve of 6MP as a result of allopurinol administration (35). Current recommendations are that doses of 6MP be reduced by 50–75% when administered concomitantly with allopurinol (35–37). *Azathioprine*, an immunosuppressive agent used primarily as an adjunct for prevention of rejection of kidney homografts, is converted *in vivo* to 6MP. Similar cautions and dosage adjustments should be observed when azathioprine is administered concomitantly with allopurinol.

Retrospective data from the Boston Collaborative Drug Surveillance Program indicate that cancer patients treated with allopurinol and cyclophosphamide have a greater incidence of bone marrow suppression than those treated with cyclophosphamide alone (38). Human studies by Bagley et al demonstrated a significantly longer cyclophosphamide half-life in four patients who received allopurinol when compared to those receiving only cyclophosphamide (39). They were unable to demonstrate any difference in urinary excretion of intact cyclophosphamide, peak plasma levels of alkylating metabolites or the fraction of injected cyclophosphamide appearing as alkylating metabolites in the urine within 24 hours.

5. *Vincristine Neurotoxicity.* D.E.F. is a 21-year-old male with ALL diagnosed in November 1976. He obtained a complete remission with VCR, PRED, DAUNO, and L-ASP therapy. Cranial irradiation was successfully completed and maintenance therapy with 6-MP and MTX was begun in January 1977. Leukemic relapse in the bone marrow was documented in February 1978 and he achieved another complete remission with PRED, DAUNO, and VCR. Maintenance therapy with weekly VCR and CYCLO was begun in March 1978. A second marrow relapse was documented in October 1979 and he received PRED, VCR, and VM-26.

In February 1980, the patient began to complain of his "knee giving way." This became progressively worse and eventually disabled him from walking except for short distances. The weakness was noted to be primarily from the knees down. Neurological exam revealed severe bilateral foot drop, depressed deep tendon reflexes (DTR), "stocking-like" depression of the pin-prick test, and decreased vibratory sensation. Nerve conduction studies documented a generalized, sensorimotor peripheral neuropathy, predominating in the lower extremities. What is the most likely cause of these neurological abnormalities?

The most probable cause of this patient's neurological abnormalities is vincristine. Vincristine is almost always incorporated in remission induction regimens for ALL because it is highly efficacious and produces minimal myelosuppression. However, the drug is unusual among antineoplastic agents because neurotoxicity is frequently the dose-limiting toxic effect (40–42).

The earliest and most consistent objective manifestation of vincristine neurotoxicity is suppression of the Achilles-tendon reflex (43–45). Quantitative measurement of the Achilles reflex reveals that maximal reflex depression occurs about 17 days after a single dose, with the reflex returning to normal in one to three months (43). Paresthesia involving the feet or hands (or both) is an early subjective manifestation of vincristine neurotoxicity, often occurring within the first few weeks of therapy (46). These symptoms disappear if the drug is stopped at the onset of paresthesia, although this may require several months in some patients (44). Patients usually retain intact perception of vibration, pin-prick, position sense, and two-point discrimination, although, as indicated by this patient, deficits in sensation can occur (44–55).

Motor involvement is one of the most disabling manifestations of vincristine neurotoxicity. Characteristically, the weakness impairs the dorsiflexors of the toes and ankles, and the extensors of the fingers and wrists (43,46). The loss of deep tendon reflexes almost invariably precedes the onset of objective weakness. The weakness may be more pronounced in the lower than in the upper extremities as illustrated by D.E.F., and is often manifested by a characteristic broad-based, slapping gait, or foot drop, due to weakness of the ankle and toe dorsiflexors (45). Muscle wasting may accompany the weakness, but is usually absent (45,46). The weakness is generally partially or even completely reversible, but recovery after discontinuation of therapy is often slow, requiring months.

Cranial nerves may also be affected. Bilateral ptosis without pupillary or other oculomotor dysfunction, diplopia, and apparent abducens nerve palsies have been observed (45). Ocular findings have occasionally been the first evidence of serious vincristine neurotoxicity (47). Bilateral vocal cord paresis or paralysis may also be caused by vincristine therapy (48).

The earliest symptoms of vincristine toxicity are often colicky abdominal pain and constipation. These complaints are common, being reported in one-third to one-half of cases (44–45). The acute gastrointestinal symptoms occur within a few days of vincristine administration and precede the earliest signs of peripheral neuropathy, such as reflex depression, by several days. The constipation is sometimes troublesome and may cause fecal impaction high in the colon. At St. Jude Children's Research Hospital, patients are routinely given dioctyl sodium sulfosuccinate (Colace) during remission induction therapy with vincristine. In some cases, an adynamic ileus may develop (44–45). Other less frequent manifestations of autonomic dysfunction include bladder atony with urinary retention, impotence, and orthostatic hypotension (49–50).

Peripheral nerve dysfunction appears to be the predominant clinical manifestation of vincristine neurotoxicity. There is no known therapy for the neuropathy other than reducing the dose or discontinuing the medication; empiric thiamine and vitamin B-12 therapy have not been of benefit (51).

The electrophysiology and pathology of vincristine neurotoxicity have not been well-described. Only slight decreases, within the normal limits, have been detected in motor or sensory nerve conduction velocities (43,46,52–53). The preservation of normal nerve conduction in the presence of clinically severe neuropathy suggests that axonal degeneration rather than segmental demyelinization is the primary lesion.

In summary, several important generalizations can be made about the clinical manifestations of vincristine neurotoxicity. First, the signs and symptoms of neuropathy are usually symmetrical, as illustrated by D.E.F. Strictly unilateral weakness, areflexia, or sensory changes are not consistent with a diagnosis of vincristine neurotoxicity. Second, there is a direct relation between dose and toxicity; as the total dose increases, the frequency of neurotoxic symptoms increases (10,44,54). A single inadvertent massive overdose can produce a serious degree of neurologic impairment (55). Consequently, in patients with liver dysfunction, unusually severe neurotoxic reactions may develop after routine doses of vincristine, probably due to impaired hepatic inactivation of the drug (45,48). Thirdly, although the majority of patients whose tumors regress on vincristine therapy will experience at least mild to moderate neurotoxicity (43), this toxicity is not related to tumor responsiveness (56). Finally, the manifestations of vincristine neuropathy are partially or completely reversible when the dosage is lowered or the drug discontinued. Thus, loss of deep tendon reflexes and paresthesia alone are not sufficient indications for discontinuing therapy before completion of an adequate therapeutic trial of vincristine.

6. G.H.I., a 4-year-old white boy with the diagnosis of acute lymphocytic leukemia, was placed on induction therapy consisting of prednisone 40 mg/m²/day for 28 days, vincristine 1.5 mg/m²/wk for 4 doses, and daunomycin 25 mg/m²/wk IV for 4 doses. During the third week of therapy the patient's appetite and fluid intake decreased and his abdomen became distended. Approximately 12 hours after the onset of symptoms the patient became increasingly lethargic with a loss of deep tendon reflexes. Shortly thereafter he experienced a generalized seizure. Laboratory data revealed the patient to be hyponatremic (serum sodium 120 mEq/L), with a serum osmolality of 235 mOsm/L. His urinary loss of sodium was excessive (urine sodium 112 mEq/L). Urine osmolality was 525 mOsm/L and the specific gravity was 1.030. Renal function tests were within normal limits (serum creatinine 0.5mg/100 ml; blood urea nitrogen 9.1 mg/100 ml). Other laboratory data included serum potassium 3.9 mEq/L, chloride 82 mEq/L, HCO₃ 25 mEq/L, and glucose 110 mg/100 ml. The patient was subsequently diagnosed as having inappropriate antidiuretic hormone (ADH) syndrome and was successfully treated

by fluid restriction. Discuss the component of this patient's induction chemotherapy which may be related to the inappropriate ADH syndrome.

The association between hyponatremia and vincristine therapy was first described by Fine et al (57); subsequently, cases of vincristine-induced inappropriate antidiuretic hormone secretion (IADHS) have been reported in both children (58–60) and adults (61–63). Suskind et al demonstrated increased levels of plasma antidiuretic hormone in a patient receiving vincristine who developed the syndrome of inappropriate ADH, and confirmed the diagnosis of IADHS by using both bioassay and radioimmunoassay (59). The precise mechanism by which vincristine produces an inappropriate secretion of ADH remains unclear. Some speculate that vincristine has a direct toxic effect on the supraoptic or paraventricular nuclei of the hypothalamus, the neurohypophyseal tract, or perhaps even on the posterior pituitary gland (58). There may be a close relationship between the dose-related neurotoxicity of vincristine and vincristine-induced inappropriate antidiuretic hormone secretion (43).

For the patient presented above, the seizures were most likely related to the severe hyponatremia, although seizures may occur secondary to the direct neurotoxicity of vincristine (10,64).

In summary, inappropriate ADH secretion induced by vincristine is probably a dose-related, reversible toxicity which occurs infrequently. The mechanism may be a direct neurotoxic effect on the central nervous system at the sites of antidiuretic hormone storage and/or formation.

7. *L-Asparaginase Reactions.* J.K.L. is a 4-year-old white boy who was diagnosed as having acute lymphocytic leukemia. Remission induction therapy was begun with prednisone 40 mg/m²/day in three divided doses for 28 days, VCR 1.5 mg/m²/wk for four doses, and L-asparaginase (L-ASP) 10,000 U/m² for four doses. Immediately following the administration of the second dose of L-ASP, the patient became dyspneic and cyanotic. Shortly thereafter he lost consciousness and his blood pressure dropped to 100/60 mm Hg. The patient was treated with oxygen by mask and intravenous diphenhydramine and epinephrine. Following a second dose of epinephrine, the patient improved rapidly and

his blood pressure returned to normal. Was this a drug-related reaction, and if so, what alternative drug would you recommend for future administration in this patient?

L-asparaginase is an enzyme with a molecular weight of approximately 130,000. The majority of L-asparaginase in clinical use today is obtained from *Escherischia coli*. Since this drug is a large molecular weight foreign protein, one of the most serious adverse effects is the occurrence of anaphylactoid reactions. Peterson and associates demonstrated passive hemagglutinating antibodies to L-ASP in all patients who had an allergic reaction, at least one day before the reaction occurred; such antibodies were absent in all patients who did not manifest a reaction (65).

Asparaginase prepared from *Erwinia carotovora* also possesses antileukemic properties, and it is presently the only asparaginase available for clinical use that has been reported to be antigenically different from *E. coli* asparaginase (66–68). Although not entirely without risk, *Erwinia carotovora* asparaginase has been administered to patients who are allergic to the *E. coli* asparaginase without a significant degree of immunologic cross-reaction (69).

The incidence of acute hypersensitivity reactions to *E. coli* asparaginase varies widely in published studies, ranging from 5 to 33% of treated patients (70–85). When all patients reported in these published studies are combined, there have been 284 "allergic reactions" in 1442 patients, or an incidence of 19.7% of treated patients. However, it is apparent from these studies that several variables may influence the incidence of anaphylactoid reactions to asparaginase.

It has been suggested that the risk of "hypersensitivity reactions" increases with continuing administration of asparaginase or with re-administration following a period of no asparaginase therapy (70,75). Oettgen et al (78) report that the risk of reactions is dose-related, while Jaffe et al (73) suggest that the risk is unrelated to dose or schedule. Nesbit et al have reported that the concomitant administration of 6-mercaptopurine significantly reduces the incidence of allergic reactions when compared to patients given asparaginase alone (5.1% versus 27%) (76). Land et al reported a trend toward fewer reactions in patients receiving concurrent prednisone-vincristine, although the difference was not statistically significant (7% versus 14%, p > 0.05) (74). A similar observation described by Jacqiullatt et al was also not statistically confirmed (72). Conversely, Jaffe et al (73) and Dellinger et al (70) have reported that concurrent prednisone therapy or pretreatment with corticosteroids does not avert asparaginase reactions.

The Children's Cancer Study Group (CCSG) compared the efficacy and toxicity of intravenous (IV) versus intramuscular (IM) asparaginase as a single agent for treatment of acute leukemia relapse in 153 children (77). Using a three-times-weekly schedule, response rates were comparable with the two routes of administration, and overall toxicity was lower with IM asparaginase. The incidence of "sensitivity reactions" was 37.5% with IV asparaginase and 31.5% with IM administration. However, when patients experiencing only abdominal pain and/or fever are excluded, reactions occurred in 28.8% with IV asparaginase and 12.3% with IM. The fact that the most severe category of sensitivity reactions ("anaphylaxis") was not observed with IM asparaginase in the CCSG study is provocative, but awaits confirmation (77).

All investigators assessing the value of pretreatment skin tests agree that this is not a reliable means of predicting hypersensitivity reactions (71,73,78–80,83). A study at our institution (85) demonstrated that a 50 IU intravenous test dose of asparaginase rarely results in a reaction ($< 1\%$) and yields false negative results in more than 80% of patients who have an anaphylactoid reaction. Thus, the use of a 50 IU IV test dose is no better than previously reported results using interdermal skin tests.

There is general agreement that fatal reactions are rare, being reported in only two of 1737 patients described in the published literature reviewed above (84). The low incidence of fatal reactions is probably related to careful observation of all patients and rapid treatment of those patients manifesting anaphylactoid reactions. Published data on hypersensitivity reactions to *Erwinia* asparaginase are much less extensive, precluding determination of the incidence and risk factors.

Data derived from a study at St. Jude Children's Research Hospital provide clarification of several of the above controversies regarding the incidence and risk factors of anaphylactoid reactions to *E. coli* and *Erwinia* asparaginase (85). First, the incidence of anaphylactoid reactions to *E. coli* asparaginase is about 15% of treated patients, although subgroups of these patients were at significantly greater risk. It was evident that the risk of an anaphylactoid reaction to *E. coli* asparaginase was significantly greater in patients who were not receiving concomitant prednisone-vincristine therapy (6.3% versus 23%, $P<0.01$) and in patients who had a hiatus of at least one month between courses of *E. coli* asparaginase (13% versus 37%, $P<0.01$). Second, it was observed that the risk of anaphylactoid reactions to *Erwinia* asparaginase was significantly greater in patients who had previously reacted to *E. coli* asparaginase (4% versus 26%, $P<0.01$), and that the risk of a reaction was related to the total number of asparaginase doses given. The greater risk of *Erwinia* anaphylactoid reactions in patients previously reacting to *E. coli* asparaginase is in contrast to previous reports of no cross-reactivity (70). However, the increased reaction rate to *Erwinia* asparaginase in those patients with prior reactions to *E. coli* asparaginase must be interpreted cautiously, since these patients may have been more sensitive to all foreign antigens. A lower risk of anaphylactoid reactions to either asparaginase in ALL patients was apparently due to fewer variables associated with increased risk of a reaction in this group; specifically, the smaller number of asparaginase doses given ALL patients, the greater proportion of ALL patients receiving concomitant prednisone-vincristine, and the smaller proportion of ALL patients with prior reactions to *E. coli* asparaginase. Therefore, J.K.L. could possibly be treated with *Erwinia* asparaginase without a reaction, although the 26% incidence of a reaction to *Erwinia* asparaginase in this situation is significantly greater than his original chance of developing a reaction to *E. coli* asparaginase. Intramuscular administration and the coadministration of prednisone and vincristine would also be rational recommendations.

8. M.N.O. is a 17-year-old male with standard-risk ALL diagnosed in December 1980. He was begun on VCR, PRED, and L-ASP remission induction therapy. He received his four doses of L-ASP 10,000 U/m² on days 4, 8, 12, and 15 without unusual toxicity. After his last L-ASP dose, the patient complained of vomiting and diarrhea. Except for a mildly elevated total bilirubin and SGPT, laboratory tests were within normal limits. Serum amylase was 35 MIU (normal range 20–191

MIU). No fever or abdominal pain were noted initially, and he was treated symptomatically for probable gastroenteritis. The next day abdominal pain developed, and he was given acetaminophen with codeine with apparent relief. Then his hands became cold, he became hypothermic, and one hour later he suddenly stopped breathing. Autopsy showed severe fulminant generalized acute hemorrhagic pancreatitis affecting all areas of the pancreas. Is pancreatitis associated with the use of any of the drugs that the patient received?

Corticosteroids and L-asparaginase, two drugs commonly included in remission induction combination regimens, have been associated with the occurrence of acute hemorrhagic pancreatitis (86–87). The incidence of this serious toxic effect ranges from 0–18% (71–74,78–80,88–89). The wide range in incidence may be due to differences in the source of L-asparaginase, dosage, dosage schedule, and diagnostic criteria. Five to ten percent of patients treated have evidence of mild pancreatitis on postmortem examination (74,78). However, some patients with clinical or laboratory evidence of pancreatitis have no evidence of pancreatic damage at autopsy (89).

Although serum amylase levels are usually elevated in patients with clinically evident pancreatitis, they are usually normal prior to the onset of symptoms and, as shown by this patient, are not predictive of the occurrence of acute fatal hemorrhagic pancreatitis (74). Patients can also exhibit transient hyperglycemia and, in rare instances, diabetic ketoacidosis has been reported (74,89). These abnormalities in glucose tolerance may be exacerbated by concomitant high-dose corticosteroid therapy.

Unfortunately, clinical signs and symptoms suggestive of pancreatitis are usually not present until fulminant disease is evident. Patients generally complain of severe abdominal pain, nausea and vomiting. In severe cases such as M.N.O.'s, clinical signs and symptoms characteristic of shock occur. Death ensues quickly unless adequate circulation is restored with volume-expanding fluids. No specific treatment is indicated except for temporary or permanent discontinuation of L-asparaginase therapy. The decision to continue L-asparaginase therapy depends on the severity of pancreatic toxicity, the availability of other chemotherapeutic agents, and the status of the patient's leukemia. Obviously, permanent discontinuation is necessary in patients with severe cases. No data are available concerning the use of alternate sources of L-asparaginase, such as *Erwinia carotovora* asparaginase.

The role of steroids in the pathogenesis of pancreatitis is not clear; however, one study suggests that L-asparaginase is the primary etiologic agent (90). These investigators found that 14 out of 104 patients treated with L-asparaginase developed clinical or autopsy evidence of pancreatitis. In contrast, in a comparison group of 32 patients with leukemia receiving steroids but not L-asparaginase, 6% had evidence of pancreatic fat necrosis, but none had pathologic evidence of acute pancreatitis.

9. *Relapse.* P.Q.R. is a 6-year-old black girl who was diagnosed with acute lymphocytic leukemia at the age of four. After successful remission induction therapy and CNS preventive therapy with cranial irradiation and intrathecal methotrexate, maintenance chemotherapy was begun with methotrexate and mercaptopurine. After 1½ years of continuous complete remission, the patient was diagnosed as having a relapse of her leukemia following a routine marrow examination. What is the incidence and prognosis of leukemic relapse?

In a recent reappraisal of 639 consecutive, newly diagnosed children with ALL treated from 1962 to 1975 at St. Jude Children's Research Hospital, it was found that nearly 60% of patients relapsed (91). However, some of the patients treated in the early sixties obviously received inadequate therapy based on present-day standards. These differences in treatment modalities (e.g., CNS irradiation) and combination regimens probably account for the wide range of reported relapse rates (91–93). For example, only 16% of patients treated as part of Total Therapy Studies I-IV (1962–1967) were in continuous complete remission for 2½ years, whereas 50–60% of children treated in Total Therapy Studies V, VI, and VIII were in continuous complete remission over a comparable period (91). Furthermore, patients now classified as "high-risk" patients were treated in the same way as "standard-risk" patients, and, as will be discussed in Question 17, these patients are not comparable to "standard-risk" patients with regard to the initial remission induction rate and relapse rate. Most of the treatment protocols today attempt to divide patients into several categories according to their estimated risk of relapse.

Relapse of leukemia at any site worsens the prognosis for survival, but bone marrow relapses are the most ominous and are usually fatal (94–95). Unfortunately, marrow relapses represent the major source of treatment failure in patients who have received adequate preventive CNS therapy (22–23,93,96–97). Although 20% of the patients with bone marrow relapses complain of generalized bone pain, the vast majority (80%) are asymptomatic as illustrated by P.Q.R. (94). Physical and roentgenographic findings, as well as complete blood counts, were unremarkable in about one-half of the children with marrow relapse (94). This emphasizes the importance of regular (about every 3–6 months) marrow examinations in children with ALL during the first 3–6 years of therapy.

10. What is the expected response to reinduction therapy? What factors influence response to reinduction therapy?

Although the overall prognosis is poor, treatment of marrow relapses has improved. The incorporation of promising investigational agents, such as VM-26, into combination regimens has also improved the prognosis for children with recurrent ALL (98).

In general, the likelihood of response to reinduction therapy decreases with each relapse and with repeated attempts to induce remission (99). Aur and associates reported a 12-month median duration of complete remission following reinduction therapy (100). Six of the 16 children studied were surviving after 46 to 50 months and four of these patients were no longer receiving chemotherapy. These patients were initially treated prior to 1969 and therefore had received less intensive therapy for initial remission induction and maintenance. The likelihood of response to reinduction therapy for hematologic relapse is probably greater in patients who have received less intensive initial therapy (101). Similarly, there is a greater likelihood of achieving a second remission if the patient is a "standard-risk" patient at diagnosis and if they have had a prolonged first remission (102).

More recent studies conducted in patients who received more intensive remission induction therapy indicate that the response to reinduction

therapy and the duration of second remissions is significantly better in patients who relapse following cessation of therapy versus those who relapse while receiving maintenance therapy, like PQR. Results of reinduction therapy for patients who initially received preventive central nervous system (CNS) therapy and 30 months of combination chemotherapy indicate that of the 17 patients who developed hematologic relapse *following cessation* of therapy, complete bone marrow remissions were achieved in 16 using vincristine, prednisone and adriamycin (103). The median duration of the second hematologic remissions was 216 days. The fact that the second hematologic remission was terminated by an equal number of CNS and hematologic relapses indicated that a second course of preventive CNS therapy was needed.

These responses were significantly better than those achieved in seven patients who relapsed *while receiving* maintenance chemotherapy. These seven children received the same treatment as those patients who relapsed after therapy was stopped. Reinduction of remission was achieved in only four of these patients (57%) and the median duration of second remission was only 50 days (103). All seven of the patients who relapsed while receiving maintenance therapy eventually died with active leukemia. In contrast, four of the 17 patients who developed recurrent ALL following cessation of therapy had their therapy electively stopped for a second time after 30–44 months of continuous second bone marrow remission (104). All four of these patients experienced an isolated extramedullary relapse. Relapse in the bone marrow was associated with a poor prognosis, eight of nine patients relapsing in the bone marrow for the second time have died. Certain patient variables were of value in predicting the length of second hematologic remission. Specifically, an initial complete remission duration of less than 3 years, relapse occurring within 6 months of cessation of therapy, and the presence of hematologic plus extramedullary sites of relapse all proved to be unfavorable prognostic indicators.

In conclusion, reinduction of remission can usually be achieved following relapse and is more easily achieved in patients who relapse following cessation of therapy. Likewise, the duration of the second remission is significantly longer in patients who relapse after elective cessation of therapy versus those who relapse while receiving maintenance therapy as did P.Q.R. These results also indicate that a second course of CNS preventive therapy with intrathecal methotrexate and cytosine arabinoside significantly reduces the incidence of CNS relapse in second remissions. Although almost all patients who have an initial marrow relapse have an extremely poor prognosis with current therapy, the results of these studies are encouraging, and the use of new treatment approaches may allow selected patients to achieve long-term leukemia-free survival. Remission induction therapy should be successful in P.Q.R. (~ 80%) and it would not be unusual for her to have a prolonged second remission, although her relapse while receiving maintenance chemotherapy is an unfavorable prognostic feature.

Preventive CNS Therapy

11. As described above, P.Q.R. received intrathecal methotrexate with cranial irradiation as initial preventive CNS therapy. Why is CNS preventive therapy used? What are the complications and pharmacokinetics of intrathecally administered methotrexate, and how can patients receiving this form of therapy be monitored?

Central nervous system prophylaxis with tumoricidal doses of cranial irradiation and intrathecal methotrexate (IT MTX) reduces the frequency of CNS leukemia from greater than 50% to less than 10% and results in a significant prolongation of complete remission (Table 1) (13,96). When this form of CNS preventive therapy is used, as illustrated by P.Q.R., all patients who attain remission after induction therapy are promptly entered on a program of cranial irradiation (2400 rads) over two and a half weeks and intrathecal methotrexate 12 mg/m^2 twice weekly for five doses. Thus, the fact that P.Q.R. did not have her disease relapse in the CNS is related to the CNS preventive therapy she received at diagnosis. As discussed in Question 12, other programs of CNS preventive therapy may use intrathecal MTX with high-dose intravenous MTX or intrathecal MTX plus intensive multi-drug systemic therapy.

Neurological complications attributable to intrathecal MTX include chemical arachnoiditis, motor dysfunction, and necrotizing leukoencephalopathy (Table 2) (40,105–107). These toxicities can be divided into acute, subacute, and

Table 1.

PREVENTIVE CNS TREATMENT IN ACUTE LYMPHOCYTIC LEUKEMIA

Studies and Years[a]	Preventive CNS Therapy[b]	Frequency of Initial CNS Relapse	Median Duration of Hematological Remission (months)
I-II (1962–63)	500 rads CrSp	3/13 (23%)	14
III (1964–65)	1200 rads CrSp	12/24 (50%)	22
IV (1965–67)	None	25/42 (60%)	19
V (1967–68)	2400 rads Cr + ITMTX	3/31 (10%)	107+
VI (1968–1970)	a) 2400 rads CrSp b) None	2/45 (4%) 33/49 (67%)	86+ 53
VII (1970–71)	a) 2400 rads Cr + ITMTX b) 2400 rads CrSp	8/45 (18%) 3/49 (6%)	24 23
VIII (1972–75)	2400 rads Cr + ITMTX	27/268 (10%)	–[c]

[a] Refers to St. Jude Total Therapy Studies
[b] Cr = Cranial, CrSp = Craniospinal, ITMTX = Intrathecal Methotrexate
[c] Too early to evaluate

Table 2.

METHOTREXATE NEUROTOXICITY

Type	Onset	Intrathecal Methotrexate	Systemic Methotrexate
Acute	Hours	Arachnoiditis (chemical meningitis, acute toxic syndrome)	Encephalopathy (only with very high intravenous doses)
Subacute	Days to weeks	Motor Dysfunction Syndrome: Spinal Cord weakness paralysis Brain seizures cerebellar dysfunction cranial nerve palsies	Seizures
Delayed	Months to years	Necrotizing leukoencephalopathy	Necrotizing leukoencephalopathy

chronic, depending on their clinical pattern. The most common form of toxicity is chemical arachnoiditis, an acute syndrome characterized by fever, back pain, dizziness, neck stiffness, vomiting, and headache (108–113). Cerebrospinal fluid examination shows elevated pressure, increased protein, and pleocytosis. Signs and symptoms of meningeal irritation begin within hours after a dose and generally subside within several days.

The subacute neurotoxicity of intrathecal MTX occurs a few weeks after therapy and characteristically presents as motor dysfunction of the spinal cord (paresis, paraplegia, or quadriplegia) or brain (cerebellar dysfunction, seizures, or cranial nerve palsies) (114–121). All the reported cases have occurred after multiple doses (> 5), and neurotoxicity occurs most frequently in patients receiving intensive intrathecal MTX two to three times per week. Although it has been proposed that MTX neurotoxicity is related to the presence of preservatives in the commercial perparation, most investigators feel that the more serious neurotoxicities are not attributable to these agents (108). However, methotrexate is currently available without preservatives, and a freshly prepared preservative-free intrathecal preparation should be used. It has also been suggested that the use of an "unphysiological" ionic content MTX solution may contribute to these toxicities (113).

The neurotoxicity of intrathecal MTX can be correlated with prolonged exposure of the CNS to excessive concentrations of MTX (130). Older children (> 10 years of age) may be predisposed to MTX neurotoxicity because the ratio of the dose to cerebrospinal fluid volume is high. Similarly,

children with active meningeal leukemia may also be predisposed because the elimination of the drug from the cerebrospinal fluid may be impaired. The half-life of intrathecal methotrexate in the cerebrospinal fluid is 12–18 hours in patients without neurotoxicity. Methotrexate levels in the cerebrospinal fluid of toxic patients range from 1.5 to 100 times higher than the corresponding mean value for non-toxic patients (130). P.Q.R., because of her age and the absence of active meningeal leukemia, would be at low risk of developing methotrexate-related neurotoxicity. It is conceivable that monitoring methotrexate levels in the cerebrospinal fluid (CSF) at the time of an intrathecal administration (ie, CSF obtained during the spinal tap for the next scheduled dose) may assist in calculating subsequent doses and reducing toxicity. Although this is usually not necessary when intrathecal MTX is given as routine preventive therapy, it may prove valuable when treating active meningeal leukemia.

The human disposition of intrathecal (IT) MTX in the cerebrospinal fluid is difficult to assess because of the need for repeated lumbar punctures to obtain serial CSF samples from individual patients. For this reason, very few studies report pharmacokinetic parameters derived from serial CSF concentrations. Assessment of CSF MTX disposition is further complicated by the uneven distribution of IT MTX between lumbar and ventricular CSF, and the intrinsic difficulties in obtaining ventricular CSF samples. Despite these limitations, some potentially useful information about the CSF disposition of IT MTX is available. Bleyer and coworkers measured lumbar CSF MTX concentrations in 76 patients given intrathecal MTX, with serial samples assessed in five of these patients (131). All patients were given the same dosage of 12 mg/m^2, in an injection volume of 12 ml/m^2 up to a maximum of 18 ml. None of these patients had evidence of active CNS disease. When the lumbar CSF MTX concentrations measured at various times (12 to 96 hours) after an intrathecal dose (for 76 patients) were collectively used to simulate CSF disposition, a biphasic disappearance curve was produced. Half-lives of 4.5 hours and 14 hours were estimated during the intervals of 4 to 36 and 48 to 96 hours after the injection, respectively. These two half-life values were similar to values estimated from serial concentrations measured in one patient. Concurrent MTX concentrations in plasma (resulting from the intrathecal dose) reached a peak of about 10^{-7} M between 3 and 12 hours after the intrathecal injection, and declined in parallel with the CSF concentrations. The terminal CSF half-life of MTX appears to be longer in patients with active meningeal leukemia (132), which is consistent with previous observations that CSF MTX concentrations and the likelihood of neurotoxicity are greater in patients with active meningeal leukemia or meningeal carcinomatosis (130,133). The disappearance of MTX from lumbar CSF is apparently dependent upon a number of physiologic processes including: (a) bulk flow removal via normal pathways of CSF absorption, (b) bulk flow distribution within the subarachnoid and ventricular CSF, (c) diffusion throughout the extracellular fluid of the brain parenchyma and spinal cord, (d) diffusion from the extracellular fluid into the capillaries of the brain and spinal cord, and (e) absorption from ventricular fluid by the energy-dependent transport process of the choroid plexus (105). It has been hypothesized that delayed clearance of MTX from the CSF of patients with active meningeal disease is due to impairment of bulk flow removal of MTX. The rate of decline in CSF MTX concentrations can also be prolonged by either probenecid (134) or vincristine (135).

The dose of intrathecal MTX is usually based on the patient's body surface area (12 mg/m^2) and is usually the same whether the drug is used for preventive CNS therapy or for the treatment of active meningeal leukemia (the dosing interval may be altered when MTX CSF elimination is delayed by active meningeal disease). However, the CSF volume of children older than 3 years approaches that of adults, while body surface area does not plateau at adult levels until 16 to 20 years of age. Thus, CSF concentrations of MTX after intrathecal administration of 12 mg/m^2 are generally higher as age increases from 3 to 20 years (132). This may partially explain the increased risk of neurotoxicity in older patients given intrathecal MTX (130). It has been proposed that all patients greater than 3 years of age be given the same dose of MTX (12 mg) and not a dosage based on body surface area.

Methotrexate may also be given intraventricularly, and at least one study has indicated that the distribution of methotrexate in CSF is more reliable when the drug is administered intraventricularly via an indwelling intraventricular subcutaneous reservoir, compared to intrathecal administration (133). However, the distribution of intrathecal MTX in this study was sufficient to achieve therapeutic levels in the ventricular CSF and may have been significantly better had the volume of the intrathecal preparation been larger. Rieselbach et al reported that the volume of the injected solution is an important factor in attaining widespread distribution following intrathecal administration (136). Body position may also influence MTX distribution in the CSF; following intralumbar MTX administration, animals placed in either Trendelenburg or flat position had ventricular CSF MTX concentrations which were 1000-fold higher than those achieved when the animals were placed in the upright position (137). Although subarachnoid and ventricular distribution of methotrexate may not be critical when cranial irradiation is given concomitantly for CNS prophylaxis, uniform cerebrospinal fluid distribution is essential if methotrexate is used alone for the prophylaxis of CNS leukemia.

In summary, the clinical benefits and precise criteria for using measured CSF methotrexate concentrations as therapeutic guidelines for intrathecal MTX have not been clearly established. Although sometimes administered with IT MTX, leucovorin is usually not necessary and may even be detrimental, since 5-methyltetrahydrofolate (a leucovorin metabolite) readily enters the CSF (138). This reduced folate metabolite is active as a rescue agent, and may thereby diminish the CNS activity of intrathecal MTX. Therefore, when leucovorin is given to negate any systemic effect of intrathecal MTX, it should probably be delayed for 24 to 36 hours after the intrathecal dose to minimize any effect the leucovorin may have on the CNS efficacy.

12. S.T.U. is a 12-year-old with ALL diagnosed in 1973. After receiving remission induction therapy, 2400 rads cranial irradiation with intrathecal MTX and two-drug maintenance therapy, all therapy was stopped after 2½ years of continuous complete remission. In 1980, his teacher at school noted that he had difficulty paying attention. She also noted that he frequently became frustrated because of difficulty in mathematical skills. Neuropsychologic testing showed no abnormalities in gross intellectual function. Computerized tomography brain scans were normal. What are the long-term toxic effects of CNS irradiation in survivors of ALL? What alternate methods of CNS preventive therapy are being studied to possibly minimize these adverse neurologic effects?

As discussed in Question 11, the importance of CNS prophylaxis has been clearly shown by investigators at St. Jude Children's Research Hospital (Table 1) (13,96,139–140) and other institutions. Although the risk of relapse in the CNS is reduced from about 50% (if preventive CNS therapy is not given) to less than 10%, this multimodality treatment regimen does carry some risk of CNS damage. As previously discussed, the most acute and serious form of toxicity is necrotizing leukoencephalopathy, which is extremely rare with current therapy. However, since children with ALL treated with current treatment programs are now surviving for long periods following cessation of therapy, more subtle neurologic abnormalities have become evident in some patients (141).

The initial study evaluating neuropsychologic function reported no significant differences between children receiving 2400 rads cranial irradiation and controls (142). However, the follow-up was less than two years in that study. More recent studies have shown that one-third to one-half of these children have a shortened attention span, poor short-term memory, and specific deficits in learning, particularly mathematical skills (143–144). Children who were diagnosed at age six or younger appeared to be particularly susceptible to the adverse effects of irradiation. McIntosh et al also found that children receiving 2400 rads cranial irradiation were at risk for de-

veloping seizures followed by abnormalities in motor, perceptual, behavioral, or language development (145).

The recent use of computed tomography (CT) now enables clinicians to monitor more closely for early neurologic abnormalities. Numerous studies indicate the presence of abnormal CT brain scans in a significant proportion of patients receiving cranial irradiation (146). At present there are no clinical or laboratory tests which can accurately predict which children are likely to experience neuropsychologic problems. Patients who develop "somnolence syndrome" shortly after CNS prophylaxis (148) or those who have increased cerebrospinal levels of myelin base protein (149) may be at greater risk for developing neurotoxicity. However, prospective studies involving large numbers of patients are needed to assess these predictors of neuropsychological toxicity.

In view of these adverse CNS effects, alternative methods of preventing CNS leukemia are being explored. It is important that these methods be not only less toxic, but also of comparable efficacy when compared to the present standard of 2400 rads cranial irradiation and intrathecal MTX. The use of intrathecal MTX alone without aggressive multidrug therapy during maintenance is ineffective in preventing CNS relapse, even in patients who have low WBC counts ($< 20,000/mm^3$) (128). Treatment programs which include a consolidation phase, an intensive continuation regimen, and periodic intrathecal MTX without cranial irradiation have resulted in CNS relapse rates comparable to cranial irradiation and intrathecal MTX 18,93). However, this treatment is complicated and involves many drugs; the treatment plan uses three drugs for remission induction, four drugs for consolidation, and eight drugs for maintenance therapy. The use of 1800 rads instead of 2400 rads cranial irradiation with intrathecal MTX is also being investigated (150). Preliminary results indicate that, in the majority of patients, 1800 rads are equivalent to 2400 rads in preventing CNS relapse. However, in patients with an initial WBC of $> 50,000/mm^3$, 1800 rads may not provide adequate CNS preventive therapy. Studies to determine whether the neurotoxic effects of 1800 rads are less than that observed with 2400 rads have not been reported.

One of the most promising new approaches is the use of "intermediate" or "moderate-dose" MTX as prolonged intravenous infusions with intrathecal MTX (128,151–153). CNS irradiation is omitted in an attempt to decrease treatment-related neurotoxicity. Methotrexate doses of 500–1000 mg/m^2 are infused over at least 24 hours, in an attempt to achieve and maintain cytotoxic levels of MTX throughout the cerebrospinal fluid (154). Low dose leucovorin rescue is also included with each MTX course. These prolonged MTX infusions may also help to control leukemic disease in other sites such as the bone marrow and testes. Preliminary results indicate that this approach may be superior to conventional therapy for standard-risk patients; however, longer follow-up is necessary before definite conclusions can be reached (155). Although serious abnormalities were not detected with CT brain scans in one series (156), additional investigations are necessary before CT brain scan abnormalities can be totally ruled out as a consequence of this therapy. The pharmacokinetics of moderate-dose MTX are also being evaluated as a component of this investigation. Preliminary results in over 50 children indicate marked interpatient variability in steady-state serum MTX concentration, systemic MTX clearance, and area under the MTX concentration-time curve. Studies attempting to correlate these pharmacokinetic parameters with continuous complete remission and toxicity are in progress.

13. *Remission Maintenance*. S.T.U. received two-drug maintenance therapy consisting of oral 6-mercaptopurine 50 mg/m^2/day and oral methotrexate 25 mg/m^2/weekly. The dosages were adjusted according to the white blood cell count; the white blood cell count usually remained between 2000 and 3500/mm^3. Regardless of the type or number of drugs used for remission induction therapy of acute lymphocytic leukemia, relapse occurs in the great majority of patients if therapy is stopped immediately after remission induction. What drugs most effectively prolong remissions? What have been the results of combination chemotherapy regimens for maintaining remission?

The efficacy of individual drugs in maintaining remissions has been reviewed by Goldin (157). Methotrexate is the single most effective agent for prolonging the duration of remission of ALL. Intermittent, IV administration of methotrexate is superior to daily, oral administration of metho-

trexate (158–159). Mercaptopurine is the next most effective single agent, followed by cyclophosphamide. Other, less effective single agents include vincristine, cytosine arabinoside, daunomycin, and L-asparaginase. Many of the newer drugs with documented antileukemic activity have never been tested as single agents for initial remission maintenance, since it is now clearly evident that single drug therapy is inferior to combination chemotherapy.

The development of resistance and subsequent relapse following remission maintenance therapy with single agents led to the evaluation of multiple-drug maintenance therapy. Combination chemotherapy for remission maintenance was designed to take advantage of the different mechanisms of action and toxicities of the effective maintenance-therapy drugs. In any given schedule, the efficacy of a single- or multiple-drug regimen is related to dosage (15,157,160–162). The first controlled study of single versus combination maintenance chemotherapy reported that the median duration of remission in childhood ALL was the same whether methotrexate and mercaptopurine were given alone or in combination (163). Subsequently, however, prolongation of the remission period was reported in studies using multiple-drug maintenance therapy (157,164).

Another effort to improve remission maintenance therapy was the administration of "pulse doses" of drugs which had different mechanisms of action, to further reduce the residual leukemia cell population. Both positive and negative results have been reported in studies evaluating the additive effects of pulse therapy (161,165–166); however, comparative studies have indicated that with an adequate induction and continuation regimen, pulses do not significantly improve the duration of remission (23,96).

14. Is there any advantage of adding a third or fourth drug to maintenance therapy?

The St. Jude Children's Research Hospital Total Therapy Study VIII was designed to answer the question: "does the advantage of multiple agent chemotherapy outweigh the disadvantage of administering (in combination) each of these agents at a less than maximally tolerated dosage (22)?" In other words, if two or more effective drugs are administered in combination, then the dosage of each drug must usually be reduced to limit host toxicity. Therefore, each drug is being given at a dosage lower than its maximum tolerated dosage as a single agent, which might offset the advantages of combination therapy. After attaining a complete remission and receiving preventive CNS therapy, patients were randomized to receive either (a) methotrexate, (b) methotrexate + mercaptopurine, (c) methotrexate + mercaptopurine + cyclophosphamide or (d) methotrexate + mercaptopurine + cyclophosphamide + cytosine arabinoside (22). Dosage adjustments were made to keep the leukocyte count between 2000 and 3500/mm³. The group receiving only methotrexate was closed shortly after the initiation of the study because of an unusually high incidence of subacute leukoencephalopathy (Table 3). This toxicity was subsequently attributed to the systemic administration of higher dosages (50–60 mg/m²) of MTX after cranial irradiation in this group of patients. Results indicated that remission duration and the proportion of patients who were in continuous complete remission for 30 months and were able to electively stop therapy were similar for patients receiving two-, three-, and four-drug maintenance therapy (22). As expected, patients receiving four-drug maintenance therapy had the greatest degree of immunosuppression, resulting in a higher incidence of infections, particularly *Pneumocystis carinii* pneumonia and disseminated varicella-zoster (Table 3) (22,167). This randomized study demonstrates that the addition of a third or fourth drug to the daily mercaptopurine and weekly methotrexate regimen does not prolong remission duration but only adds to the risk of complications. Similar studies indicate that more aggressive regimens are not necessarily more efficacious but add to chemotherapy-related complications (168). Therefore, it is not recommended that a third or fourth drug be added to S.T.U.'s regimen.

Although three or four drugs given *together* did not prove to be better than the two-drug combination of MTX and 6-MP, this does not completely rule out the need for additional drugs for maintenance chemotherapy. Even with the best current therapy, more than one-third of "standard-risk" ALL patients (see Question 17) will experience a leukemic relapse while receiving maintenance therapy. These relapses are likely due to the emergence of drug-resistant leukemic blasts. New regimens are needed to prevent the emergence of these resistant cells while not jeopardizing the remaining patients for whom current treatment is adequate for long-term disease control and cure. One approach is the use of rotating two-drug combinations which have different mechanisms of cytotoxicity. Such an approach would be consistent with the cytokinetic rationale proposed by Skipper et al (169). Other approaches which have been tried include the use of intensive intermittent combination therapy every three weeks (97). Although follow-up has been short, results using this approach are com-

Table 3.

RESULTS OF ST. JUDE TOTAL THERAPY STUDY VIII

	MTX	MTX + 6MP	Maintenance Regimen[a] MTX + 6MP + CTX	MTX + 6MP + CTX + Ara-C
No. of patients	20	68	70	70
No. patients with 30 months of CCR[a]	4	45	38	41
No. patients with Pneumocystis carinii pneumonia	0	1	7	19
No. patients with disseminated Varicella-Zoster	0	8	16	20
No. patients with leukoencephalopathy	9	0	0	0
Total no. of hospitalizations	13	25	49	72

[a] Abbreviations used: MTX = methotrexate, 6MP = 6-mercaptopurine, CTX = cyclophosphamide, Ara-C = cytosine arabinoside, CCR = continuous complete remission

parable to other effective continuation regimens. The ideal approach would be to identify those patients who are likely to relapse and treat them more aggressively. As will be discussed in Question 17, certain clinical and laboratory features at initial diagnosis correlate with the likelihood of long-term disease-free survival with current therapy.

Another important issue concerning maintenance chemotherapy, aside from the optimal number of drugs, is how aggressively one needs to use these drug combinations during remission. This was addressed, from the standpoint of drug dosage, in an early study (St. Jude Total Therapy IV) which randomized patients after remission induction to receive either maximum tolerated dosages (WBC count between 2000 and 3500/mm^3) or only half-dosages of methotrexate, mercaptopurine, cyclophosphamide, and vincristine. Although only 42 patients were studied, the results were clear; almost half of the full-dosage group was still in hematologic remission after three years, compared to only 20% in the half-dosage group (15). This is consistent with other studies establishing the steep dose-response relationship for antineoplastic agents and the need to use a maximally tolerated drug dosage of cancer chemotherapy (157,160–162). This concept may also provide another rationale for using high-dose methotrexate with leucovorin rescue in children who have not had cranial irradiation. (Note: High doses of MTX cannot be given to patients who have received cranial irradiation because of the risk of leukoencephalopathy.)

15. Cessation of Maintenance Therapy. S.T.U. had his chemotherapy stopped in October 1975 after 30 months of continous complete remission. What are the criteria and rationale for cessation of maintenance therapy? Should S.T.U.'s maintenance chemotherapy have been continued?

It is clear that if therapy is stopped immediately after remission is induced, there is a high frequency of relapse regardless of the induction regimen used (92,160,170–173). With continued therapy, the proportion of patients in complete remission declines in an exponential fashion for the first 2 to 3 years of remission but levels off thereafter (164). There is also evidence that after a period of time, continued administration of maintenance chemotherapy may not eradicate, but

only suppress, the remaining leukemia cells and a more resistant clone could eventually emerge and proliferate (174). Moreover, these drugs are immunosuppressive and place the patient at increased risk for fatal opportunistic infections despite leukemic control (17–176). With approximately 50% of children with ALL achieving continued remissions for many years after cessation of therapy, potential delayed consequences of chemotherapy are an additional concern. Delayed toxicities may include secondary malignancies; hepatic, pulmonary, skeletal and cardiovascular toxicities; prolonged immunosuppression; sterility; and adverse effects on the central nervous system (177). The actual significance of these potential delayed consequences of therapy cannot be determined until a larger number of patients with childhood ALL reach adulthood.

When single- or multiple-drug maintenance therapy is stopped after 6 weeks to 14 months of remission, 50% of patients relapse within 2 to 10 months (178). Patients who receive adequate remission induction, prophylactic CNS therapy, and maintenance chemotherapy, and who remain in continuous complete remission for 2½ years, have about a 16% risk of relapse within the first year after therapy is stopped, and about 2–3% during the second to fourth year (91). Similar results have been reported from other institutions (179–180). These data make possible an operational definition of cure, a point that may be useful in comparing the effectiveness of alternative modes of therapy. Another study assessed the value of continuing therapy for a total of 5 years, and the most recent report suggests a lower relapse rate when compared to patients whose treatment is stopped at 3 years (181). Since many of these children were treated prior to the development of currently accepted chemotherapy, longer follow-up is needed to determine if these early results are due to the elimination of late relapse or merely the delay of relapse.

The ultimate goal of continuation therapy is the total eradication of all leukemia cells. Unfortunately, there is presently no way to determine when this goal has been achieved in an individual patient, since as many as one billion leukemia cells may be present but completely undetectable following remission induction. It is clear that new therapeutic strategies are required to accomplish this goal in a greater majority of children with acute lymphocytic leukemia.

In conclusion, current data indicate that patients should be continued on remission maintenance chemotherapy for at least 2 to 3 years, after which time the benefits of chemotherapy may not exceed the risks. It is important to note that some patients have had recurrence of their disease as late as 11 years after diagnosis (187).

A rebound lymphocytosis, which may be confused with relapse, may also occur after discontinuation of remission maintenance chemotherapy for acute lymphocytic leukemia (182). This rebound lymphocytosis varies in degree and duration and is accompanied by a recovery of immunocompetence (183).

16. With current therapy for ALL, can one identify clinical features which are related to the length of remission *following* cessation of therapy?

Certain clinical features may aid in predicting the length of complete remission after cessation of therapy. George et al found that race, initial leukocyte count, age at diagnosis, capability of lymphoblasts to form rosettes with sheep erythrocytes, and the presence or absence of a mediastinal mass were *not* helpful in identifying those patients who are at increased risk for relapse after therapy is electively stopped (91). However, sex proved to be an important prognostic variable; 33% of boys relapsed within 4 years after cessation of therapy as compared to 15% of girls. Other studies have reported similar results (181,184). Some of this increased relapse rate in boys is related to testicular relapse, but not all of the increased risk can be accounted for by this site. Prolonging maintenance therapy beyond 2½–3 years has been suggested as one method of decreasing the frequency of testicular relapse, however, longer follow-up is needed to determine if testicular relapse is merely being delayed and also whether the potential benefit outweighs the added risk of continuing therapy beyond 2½–3 years (185–186). Although major advances have been made in the treatment of relapses occurring after cessation of therapy (see Questions 9–10), the long-term prognosis remains poor (91,104).

Prognostic Criteria at Diagnosis

17. J.K.L. is a 12-year-old black male who presents with a two-week history of "feeling tired." Initial evaluation revealed anemia and thrombocytopenia, with a white cell count of 140,000/mm³. Most of these cells were immature lymphoblasts. After arrival at St. Jude Children's Research Hospital, chest roentgenogram revealed a mediastinal mass, and *in vitro* studies showed that the lymphoblasts spontaneously formed rosettes with sheep erythrocytes. J.K.L. was classified as having "high-risk" ALL, and remission induction treatment was initiated with VM-26 and cytosine arabinoside, followed by prednisone, vincristine, and L-asparaginase. Why did this patient receive more intensive remission induction therapy, and what is the significance of J.K.L.'s clinical and laboratory features?

Early attempts to identify prognostic criteria at the time of diagnosis suggested that a high initial white blood cell count, massive hepatosplenomegaly, central nervous system involvement, and an age of less than one year or greater than ten years were poor prognostic factors (172,188–189). Also, the likelihood of inducing remission and the median duration of remission are less in Negro children as compared to Caucasian children (190). (Note: The prognostic features discussed in Question 16 relate to the outcome after elective cessation of therapy, whereas this question addresses prognostic features relative to the probability of long-term continuous complete remission.)

Simone analyzed the relationship of a variety of initial features and the outcome of therapy in 363 children with acute lymphocytic leukemia (191). The criteria for evaluating the prognostic significance of a given feature was whether the patient attained or exceeded the median duration of complete remission, hematologic remission, or survival for all patients studied. In general, patients with more massive or extensive disease at diagnosis had a poorer response to therapy. Specific factors at the time of diagnosis associated with poor prognosis included: CNS involvement, spleen enlargement greater than 5 cm below the costal margin, initial leukocyte count above 100,000/mm³, and mediastinal involvement. Children who were over ten years of age at the time of diagnosis and Negro children had a poorer prognosis. Also, children who were under two years of age at the time of diagnosis or who had hepatomegaly greater than 5 cm below the costal margin were less likely to attain at least three years of continuous complete remission. It is important to realize, however, that with the exception of early CNS involvement, there were patients with each of the poor prognostic factors who had excellent responses to therapy.

A major advance in the understanding of leukemia cell biology came in 1974 with the demonstration of E-rosette-forming lymphoblasts in patients with ALL (192). It had previously been shown that the major subpopulation of normal circulating lymphocytes bears surface receptors that generate rosettes when incubated with sheep erythrocytes (E+). These cells are now known as T (thymus-derived)-lymphocytes because processing in the thymus is necessary for maturation. The demonstration of a corresponding T-lymphoblast was the first evidence for variation in the cell lineage in acute lymphocytic leukemia.

Since the initial report of Sen and Borella of the clinical importance of lymphoblasts with T-cell markers in childhood leukemia, numerous studies have attempted to assess the prognostic value of cell surface markers (193–195). Specific surface markers on lymphoblasts have been related to the prognosis of acute lymphocytic leukemia in children (196). Patients were categorized in one study as having T-marker lymphoblasts, B-marker lymphoblasts, or null lymphoblasts. T-cells were identified by spontaneous rosette formation with sheep erythrocytes (E+) and B-cells by the presence of surface immunoglobulin. Of 37 patients evaluated, eight had T-marker lymphoblasts, 28 had no markers, and one had B-marker lymphoblasts. Poor prognostic factors were found in 7 of 17 patients with null lymphoblasts and all of the patients with T-marker lymphoblasts. A mediastinal mass was not found in any patients with null lymphoblasts, but was found in the one child with B-marker lymphoblasts and in 5 of 7 patients with T-marker lymphoblasts. There was no statistically significant difference in the proliferative activity of the lymphoblasts among the three groups of patients as measured by the mitotic index and labeling index. In general, patients with T-marker lymphoblasts had a poorer prognosis than those with null lymphoblasts. Subsequent studies have clearly established that patients with T-cell leukemia, as defined by E+ lymphoblasts, are at greater risk for treatment failure (197).

Analysis of clinical trials at St. Jude Children's Research Hospital has made it possible to define a group of "high-risk" patients (median duration of complete remission less than one year) by a combination of clinical and laboratory findings at diagnosis: (a) leukocyte count greater than $100,000/mm^3$, (b) mediastinal mass, (c) CNS involvement, or (d) E-rosette-forming lymphoblasts. Although the presence of only one of these findings places patients in this "high-risk" group, most "high-risk" patients have two or more of these features (198). Fortunately, these "high-risk" patients constitute only about 20% of newly diagnosed cases of ALL at our institution.

It is important to recognize that the definition of "high-risk" ALL has not been standardized; therefore the percentage of newly diagnosed patients placed in this category may vary from institution to institution. For example, some institutions consider patients with initial leukocyte counts greater than $20,000/mm^3$ to be "high-risk" patients, whereas patients with WBC counts between 20,000 and $100,000/mm^3$ are considered "standard-risk" at our institution (128). When evaluating published studies assessing new treatment regimens for ALL, one must carefully assess the definition of "standard" and "high-risk" patients for each study. Moreover, these definitions of "standard-" and "high-risk" ALL are based on outcome of treatment with currently available therapy, and will likely undergo revision as new and better treatment is developed.

Presently, "high-risk" patients, as defined at our institution, have a less than 20% chance that their disease will remain in complete remission for $2^1/_2$ years, with a median duration of complete remission of only 7 months (199). The efficacy of initial remission induction therapy is also lower in this group of patients (~80%) when compared to "standard-risk" patients. Other investigators have reported similar results in a group of 141 "high-risk" (WBC > $100,000/mm^3$) ALL patients (200). Because of these clear differences in treatment outcome in these two categories of patients, current studies at our institution are evaluating more aggressive therapy for the "high-risk" patients. The response of "high-risk" patients to contemporary therapy for "standard-risk" ALL is unacceptable.

In addition to the categorization of ALL patients using the clinical and laboratory findings described above, morphologic, cytoplasmic, cytogenetic, nuclear, and cell surface characteristics of lymphoblasts have been investigated as possible prognostic indicators and as a tool to better define the biologic correlates of prognosis (193–195).

There is some morphologic heterogeneity within the diagnostic category of acute lymphoblastic leukemia. These subtypes of ALL are recognized in the French-American-British (FAB) classification: L-1 (the most common), with small-cell predominance, scanty cytoplasm and dense, homogeneous chromatin; L-2, with a heterogeneous cell population, most being larger and having greater amounts of cytoplasm; and L-3 (very rare), with large, uniform, basophilic and vacuolated cells with round nuclei and dense granular chromatin having one or more prominent nucleoli (201). A retrospective analysis has indicated that patients in the L-1 category have a superior outcome, even when other clinical prognostic features are taken into account (202).

Studies which probably have the greatest potential value in refining the classification of acute lymphoblastic leukemia are those evaluating the heterogeneity in expression of cell surface markers (Table 4). This is a logical outgrowth of the initial recognition of E-rosette-forming lymphoblasts in some cases of ALL. Surface markers indicating various phases of lymphoid differentiation are now being used systematically to characterize blast cells from all new patients as a means to develop more detailed classifications for patients with ALL. Approximately 20% of childhood acute lymphocytic leukemias are clas-

sified as T-cell leukemia. However, not all the lymphoblasts are E-rosette-forming; some express only T-cell antigens, evidence of definite but more primitive T-cell origin (203). More recent investigations using monoclonal antibodies have demonstrated the presence of multiple T-cell antigen expression reflecting orderly phases of T-cell differentiation (204). Use of these new methods of identifying cell surface antigens have led to subgroups of acute T-cell leukemia which may prove clinically important (205).

Differentiation of B-cell lymphoblast to the level of surface immunoglobulin expression is extremely rare, occurring in no more than 2% of children with acute lymphocytic leukemia (206). However, this variant of the disease is important to recognize because of its remarkably aggressive clinical course and the extremely small likelihood of a good response to therapy. Because of its apparent similarity with Burkitt's lymphoma in a leukemic phase, these patients are treated aggressively as part of lymphoma treatment protocols.

The remaining 75–80% of cases, formerly labelled as cases of "null-cell" (or non-T-non-B) acute lymphocytic leukemia, can now be further subdivided based on the expression of a common lymphoid stem cell antigen. This antigen was first described by Greaves and is known as the "common" ALL antigen or "Greaves antigen" (207–210). These leukemias represent earlier stages of lymphoid differentiation than the T- or B-lym-

Table 4.

BIOLOGIC CLASSIFICATION OF ACUTE LYMPHOCYTIC LEUKEMIA

Leukemia Blast Cell Type	Approximate Percent of Patients	Usual Cell Characteristics	Risk Assessment
Common ALL	65	Common ALL antigen, Ia-like antigen, cytoplasmic corticosteroid binding, nuclear TdT activity	Standard
Pre-B-cell ALL[a]		Above characteristics with cytoplasmic IgM	
T-cell ALL	20	T-cell antigen, 50% have E^+ blasts, reduced cytoplasmic corticosteroid binding, nuclear TdT activity, acid phosphatase positive	High
B-cell ALL	<5	Surface Ig positive, Ia-like antigen	High
Undifferentiated[b]	10	May have Ia-like antigen	Variable

[a]Approximately 20% of ALL patients have blast cells with cytoplasmic IgM demonstrable by immunofluorescence. Studies to date indicate no clinical differences from patients with common ALL not having this feature.
[b]This group currently cannot be identified by defined cell marker systems. It is probably heterogenous and the clinical outcome is variable.

phocyte counterparts described above. Approximately 65–70% of new cases of ALL are non-T, non-B and react with the "common" ALL antigen. The remaining 10–15% of cases are non-T, non-B and lack the markers of "common" ALL. These latter cases are currently referred to as undifferentiated or "true-null" disease. It is important to note that the pattern of surface antigen expression may be different at the time of diagnosis and the time of relapse (211–212). Such changes should not necessarily be interpreted as evidence that more than one leukemic clone is involved, since it could also be explained by modulation in the predominant cell type by emergence of a drug resistant cell line following periods of maintenance therapy.

It is also clear that the presence of the previously described clinical high-risk features is related to cell surface markers. For example, a leukocyte count greater than 50,000, a mediastinal mass, or early CNS leukemia are all much more common in patients with T-cell disease when compared to patients with "common" ALL (196–198). Given the same therapy, failure of remission induction therapy and early disease relapse are more frequent in patients with T-cell disease. Likewise, B-cell leukemia is a much more aggressive and refractory form of the disease. Based on preliminary results, most patients with "common" ALL remain in continuous complete remission, while patients with undifferentiated disease may be at greater risk for treatment failure (207,213,4).

Sufficient information is currently lacking to establish the clinical relevance of the sub-subgroups of T-cell and common forms of ALL. It is not yet established that the newer antigenic markers of T-cell differentiation carry the same independent prognostic significance as the E-rosette-positive disease. Another recently described subgroup of patients are those with demonstrable cytoplasmic immunoglobin M and evidence of commitment to B-cell differentiation (eg, "pre-B" ALL) (214). This subgroup (about 20% of ALL patients) is comprised largely of patients previously categorized as "common-ALL" or undifferentiated ALL. Although initial studies (215) indicated no clinical differences from patients with "common" ALL not having this feature, more extensive studies are needed to determine whether these patients have a poorer prognosis than true

"common-ALL" patients, as has been suggested by preliminary results of more recent studies.

It is apparent that a wealth of new information has been generated which more clearly demonstrates that childhood acute lymphocytic leukemia is a heterogeneous disease. These studies and the ongoing development and application of more sophisticated clinical and laboratory methods of classifying acute lymphocytic leukemia have provided new insights into the biological basis of therapeutic failures. Knowledge of the prognostic significance of these clinical and biological variables is of obvious importance when attempting to evaluate results of new treatment approaches for acute lymphocytic leukemia. Likewise, this information may prove useful in determining which patients require more aggressive therapy, as well as identifying a group of patients who will do well with less treatment.

Adriamycin Cardiotoxicity

18. X.Y.Z. is a 10-year-old boy with high-risk acute lymphocytic leukemia who achieved initial remission following prednisone, vincristine, and L-asparaginase therapy. Maintenance therapy consisted of methotrexate and mercaptopurine. After 10 months of continuous complete remission, he had a hematologic relapse, but was successfully treated with prednisone, vincristine, and adriamycin for remission reinduction. Since this patient failed remission maintenance with methotrexate and mercaptopurine but has responded to prednisone, vincristine, adriamycin, should adriamycin be used (in combination with another agent) for long-term remission maintenance therapy of this patient? If so, what is the major complication of long-term administration of adriamycin, and what factors have been associated with an increased risk of developing this toxicity?

Adriamycin is an anthracycline antibiotic which may produce several transient toxic effects including nausea, vomiting, stomatitis, alopecia, and myelosuppression (216–221). However, the use of adriamycin has been limited primarily by the severe dose-dependent cardiomyopathy that may occur with repeated administration (222–224). The cardiotoxicity is manifested both by acute, transient, and usually benign electrocardiographic changes and by a chronic, cumulative dose-dependent, and potentially fatal cardiomyopathy. The most frequently observed electrocardiographic abnormalities are supraventricular tachycardia, atrial and ventricular extrasystoles, ST-T wave changes, and decrease in QRS voltage (216–218,225–227). With the exception of decreased QRS voltage, these abnormalities are usually reversible within 1–2 months. Electrocardiographic changes occur in approximately 10–30% of patients receiving adriamycin and are more common in patients with pre-existing heart disease (216,218,225,227).

In contrast to the transient electrocardiographic changes, the chronic toxicity of cardiomyopathy carries significant morbidity and mortality. Patients with adriamycin-induced cardiomyopathy usually present suddenly with signs and symptoms characteristic of congestive heart failure. Before the cardiotoxicity was widely recognized, the course was characterized by rapid progression, generally leading to death in a few weeks (216–217,225). However, anthracycline therapy is now discontinued at the first appearance of signs or symptoms of possible congestive heart failure, if not sooner. Treatment with digitalis glycosides and diuretics is often effective, although some patients can still experience rapidly progressive cardiac failure. The cardiomyopathy can occur at any time during the course of therapy and has been reported to occur as long as 23 months after discontinuation of adriamycin therapy (228). Since X.Y.Z. is a "high-risk" ALL patient and the prognosis becomes worse with each relapse, the most effective agents should be administered as early in the stage of the disease as possible. Therefore, X.Y.Z. was continued on adriamycin as part of maintenance therapy.

19. Now that X.Y.Z. is receiving adriamycin as part of maintenance therapy, how should he be followed for the development of cardiotoxicity? Are there any clinical features which place him at higher risk for developing cardiotoxicity? What measures have been tried to prevent this toxic effect?

There is a clear relationship between the cumulative dosage of adriamycin and the incidence of cardiomyopathy (Table 5) (229, 230). Although the overall incidence is less than 1%, the frequency of cardiomyopathy is markedly increased at total cumulative dosages above 550 mg/m^2, so that a clinician who chooses to exceed this dosage level must carefully weigh the risk against the anticipated benefit. In addition, other syndromes of cardiac dysfunction such as pericarditis-myocarditis and possible precipitation of myocardial infarction have been reported following one or two courses of anthracycline therapy (231).

The risk of developing cardiomyopathy has been reported to increase in patients with uncontrolled hypertension or in patients who have received prior or concurrent mediastinal radiotherapy, and possibly in patients receiving concurrent cyclophosphamide. In these patients, it has been recommended that the total cumulative dose be limited to 400–450 mg/m^2 (226,228–230,232–237). The incidence of cardiotoxicity in adults is greater with increasing age and may be attributed to a higher frequency of pre-existing heart disease in elderly patients (228,230,238). Children may be more susceptible to the cardiotoxic effect of anthracyclines than adults (Table 5) (230,238–239); the reasons for this higher risk are not known, although several hypotheses have been proposed (240). Concomitant or prior use of other chemotherapeutic agents has also been implicated as risk factors; however, these reports involve small numbers of patients or retrospective analysis and require further documentation (229,240–242).

The exact mechanism of adriamycin cardiotoxicity is unknown, but several mechanisms have been proposed (243). These include: (a) interference with DNA-directed DNA or RNA synthesis, especially in the myocardial mitochondria and capillary epithelium; (b) inhibition of mitochondrial phosphorylation; (c) calcium accumulation in the myocardium secondary to alteration in membrane permeability or inhibition of membrane Na$^+$K$^+$ATPase; (d) an autoimmune process; (e) accumulation of toxic metabolites; or (f) free radical formation in the heart.

Numerous procedures have been evaluated for predicting which patients will develop cardiotoxicity. These include changes in electrocardiogram voltage (225,232), systolic time intervals measured from phonocardiograms (244–246), and ejection fractions determined from echocardiograms (236,247–248). Unfortunately, none of these tests have been shown to accurately predict which patients will develop cardiomyopathy. Recent studies have indicated that other procedures may be of value in determining when clinically significant cardiotoxicity has developed, and these procedures provide information early enough to modify or discontinue anthracycline therapy (228,235–237,249). Alexander et al evaluated left ventricular function using serial ejection fractions derived from radionuclide angiography (235). Patients with mild, moderate, and severe cardiotoxicity were classified according to clinical criteria and declines in ejection fractions. In five patients who developed severe cardiotoxicity, radionuclide evidence of declines in ejection fractions was present before clinical signs and symptoms appeared. These trends were then applied prospectively to discontinue adriamycin in six patients with moderate cardiotoxicity. The cumulative adriamycin dosage in these patients ranged from 460 to 900 mg/m^2 and was comparable to the cumulative dosage in the patients experiencing severe cardiotoxicity. With a mean follow-up interval of over two months, no clinical evidence of congestive heart failure has appeared and ejec-

tion fractions have subsequently increased. However, even if the ejection fraction returned to normal and clinical signs improved, further adriamycin therapy should be administered with extreme caution since additional drug can precipitate fatal congestive heart failure (249).

Serial endomyocardial biopsies with quantitative assessment of morphologic changes may provide the most specific evaluation of cardiotoxicity (228,233,236–237). The incidence of cardiotoxicity, as defined by abnormalities with cardiac catheterization or the presence of clinical signs and symptoms, increased as morphologic changes became more severe (236). Serial biopsies usually showed pathologic changes during continued adriamycin therapy. The predictive value of this technique has not been prospectively evaluated. Patients with a +3 pathology score (scale 0 to +3) should not receive additional adriamycin since nine of 10 of these patients had evidence of cardiotoxicity. On the other hand, no patients with scores of 0 and only one of 25 patients with scores

Table 5.

CUMULATIVE RISK OF DEVELOPING DOXORUBICIN (ADRIAMYCIN)-INDUCED CONGESTIVE HEART FAILURE[a]

Cumulative Dose	Weekly Schedule[b]				Every 3-Week Schedule[b]			
	0–14	15–39	40–59	60+	0–14	15–39	40–59	60+
mg/m^2								
50	0.0	0.0	0.1	0.1	0.2	0.1	0.3	0.4
100	0.1	0.1	0.2	0.3	0.4	0.2	0.7	1.0
150	0.2	0.1	0.2	0.4	0.6	0.3	1.0	1.5
200	0.2	0.1	0.3	0.5	0.9	0.4	1.3	2.1
250	0.3	0.1	0.4	0.6	1.0	0.5	1.5	2.4
300	0.4	0.2	0.6	0.9	1.5	0.7	2.2	3.4
350	0.4	0.2	0.6	0.9	1.5	0.8	2.3	3.6
400	0.5	0.3	0.7	1.2	1.9	1.0	2.3	4.6
450	0.7	0.3	1.0	1.6	2.6	1.3	3.4	6.1
500	1.0	0.5	1.5	2.3	3.8	2.0	5.8	8.9
550	1.5	0.8	2.4	3.7	6.1	3.1	9.1	13.9
600	2.6	1.3	3.9	6.1	10.0	5.2	14.9	22.4
650	3.3	1.7	5.0	7.7	12.6	6.6	18.6	27.5
700	5.7	3.0	8.7	13.2	21.2	11.3	30.5	43.5
750	8.4	4.3	12.6	19.0	29.8	16.4	41.8	57.2
800	10.1	5.2	15.0	22.5	34.7	19.4	47.9	64.0
850	13.2	6.9	19.6	28.9	43.5	25.1	58.3	74.6
900	15.1	8.0	22.2	32.5	48.2	28.4	63.3	79.0
950	16.9	9.0	24.7	35.9	52.5	31.4	68.0	83.1

[a]This table can be used to estimate risk of developing doxorubicin-induced congestive heart failure if total dose of doxorubicin received, dose schedule, and patient's age are known. For example, for a 30-year-old patient on an every 3-week schedule of doxorubicin administration who has received a total dose of 300 mg/m^2, the probability of developing drug-induced congestive heart failure is 0.7. (Reproduced with permission from reference 230.)

[b]Age groups, in years.

of +1 have developed cardiotoxicity without subsequent treatment, suggesting that these patients can safely tolerate more anthracycline therapy. Decisions concerning patients with pathology scores of +2 are difficult, although treatment is usually discontinued (236). These impressive data, if confirmed in larger prospective studies with longer follow-up, may provide an accurate method of assessing cardiac muscle damage and aid in therapeutic decisions concerning additional therapy.

Various drugs used to counteract adriamycin or daunomycin cardiotoxicity appear promising; however, these drugs have been evaluated only in experimental animal models and confirmation in prospective clinical trials is needed. The most promising agents tested are two free radical scavengers, alpha-tocopherol (Vitamin E) (250–252) and N-acetyl-L-cysteine (Mucomyst) (250,253). Anthracyclines are believed to form a superoxide radical ion when exposed to microsomal enzymes and NADPH, which then goes on to initiate a free radical chain reaction resulting in myocardial damage (254). Since both alpha-tocopherol and N-acetyl-L-cysteine are free radical scavengers, this chain of events is disrupted. Other compounds being studied to ameliorate cardiotoxicity include co-enzyme Q10 (ubiquinone) (255) and carnitine (256). There is also increasing evidence that cardiotoxicity is schedule-dependent and that lower, more frequent doses may be less harmful (230,244,257–258). This suggests that pharmacokinetic parameters (peak levels, area under curve, metabolite production) may correlate better with cardiotoxicity than total cumulative dose, which has been supported by clinical studies demonstrating less cardiotoxicity when adriamycin was given by continuous infusion versus bolus injections.

Cyclophosphamide Bladder Toxicity

20. G.H.I. is a 4-year-old girl with ALL diagnosed in 1977. Following remission induction therapy and CNS preventive therapy, she received maintenance therapy with cyclophosphamide, 6-mercaptopurine, and methotrexate. After several months of maintenance therapy, she began to complain of pain when urinating and noted her urine was a reddish color. Could this be a toxic manifestation of her drug therapy? If so, how should she be treated?

Cyclophosphamide has many side effects which are commonly encountered with other antineoplastic drugs including nausea, vomiting, anorexia, leukopenia, and alopecia (259). However, it is the only alkylating agent exhibiting bladder toxicity. Although it is not clear whether nornitrogen mustard (260) or acrolein (261–262) or both are the etiologic agents, most agree that this troublesome side effect is caused by contact of irritating metabolites with the bladder mucosa. The bladder toxicity most commonly manifests itself as bacteriologically sterile hemorrhagic cystitis, but cases of transitional cell carcinoma (263–264), squamous cell carcinoma (265), fibrosis (266), and severe epithelial atypia (267) have been reported.

The incidence of cyclophosphamide-induced hemorrhagic cystitis varies depending on the patient population and diagnostic criteria, but most large series show an incidence of less than 10% when strict diagnostic criteria are used (268–270). The onset of the cystitis is variable and usually exceeds several months, although cases have occurred following only one dose (271) and as long as four years after initiation of therapy (272). There is no exact relationship with the total dose administered. However, studies utilizing large intravenous doses of cyclophosphamide report an incidence of 20–63% (273–274).

In one study, 25 of 314 (8%) children with acute lymphocytic leukemia developed well documented hemorrhagic cystitis, which was usually mild and transient, although one death occurred secondary to bladder hemorrhage (269). There was no correlation between the total dose administered and the severity of the cystitis, nor was there a correlation between the frequency of cyclophosphamide-induced cystitis and age, sex, or route of administration. Nineteen of the 25 cases occurred in the spring and summer months. It was suggested that this may have been related to a poorer state of hydration during these months, resulting in a higher concentration of active metabolites in the urine. However, this could not be documented by urine specific gravity determinations. Also, cyclophosphamide-induced cystitis was found to be twice as frequent in black children as in white.

Other investigators reported a significantly increased frequency and severity of urinary-bladder toxicity in children receiving pelvic irradiation with simultaneous cyclophosphamide (270). The incidence of bladder toxicity was 34% in patients who received both pelvic irradiation and cyclophosphamide, compared to 8% in patients who received cyclophosphamide with radiotherapy outside the pelvic region. Since the reported frequency of urinary-bladder toxicity from pelvic irradiation ranges from 2.5–12%, cyclophosphamide and pelvic irradiation may act synergistically to produce bladder toxicity. It is therefore recommended that an alkylating agent other than cyclophosphamide be considered when patients are receiving or will receive radiotherapy to the pelvic region.

The course of cyclophosphamide-induced hemorrhagic cystitis is usually benign, although death from massive refractory hemorrhage has occurred (269,275–280). Occasionally, 50 to 60 units of blood have been required over a period of weeks to maintain an adequate hematocrit. Patients with hemorrhagic cystitis initially go through an asymptomatic stage characterized by microscopic hematuria seen only on urinalysis. Some of these patients then progress to a symptomatic stage characterized by complaints of brief, episodic periods of painful urination, frequency and hematuria which usually subsides over a period of several days or weeks upon discontinuation of the drug. The decision to re-institute cyclophosphamide therapy depends on the severity of the cystitis, the availability of equally efficacious drugs, the therapeutic response of the tumor being treated, and the pathology of the bladder. If irreversible bladder wall fibrosis is seen, the risk of bleeding is high if cyclophosphamide is restarted; however, if no morphologic alterations are seen on the bladder wall, cyclophosphamide can often be safely given later (266).

Specific treatment is usually unnecessary except for bed rest, transfusions if needed, analgesics, and discontinuation of the drug. Some clinicians have tried other modes of treatment such as antispasmodics (281), steroids (282–284), mannitol diuresis (285), and aminocaproic acid (272,278,280). Local instillation of formalin has been effective in some refractory cases and acts by causing coagulation of proliferating telangiectactic capillaries (286–289). This initial tissue destruction produces sloughing of the bladder mucosa followed by replacement by normal tissue. Others have also tried local instillation of silver nitrate, electro-cauterization of bladder blood vessels, and intravesical hydrostatic pressure (270,284,290–293). If the above measures fail, surgical urinary diversion is required to prevent continued urine contact with the bladder mucosa (280).

Two animal studies have shown that use of N-acetylcysteine protects against the development of cystitis, but human studies are needed to confirm its efficacy (294–296). Current efforts to prevent the occurrence of cyclophosphamide-induced cystitis include the administration of intravenous fluids immediately following administration of intravenous cyclophosphamide and education of parents to have their children drink large amounts of liquids the day of drug administration and void just before going to bed. These represent efforts to reduce the concentration of alkylating metabolites in the urine and reduce the duration of bladder exposure to these active metabolites.

ACUTE MYELOCYTIC LEUKEMIA

Acute myelocytic leukemia (AML, acute granulocytic leukemia, acute nonlymphocytic leukemia) is a neoplastic disease of the blood-forming organs characterized by proliferation of precursors and other immature cells of the myeloid series. Often the term acute nonlymphocytic leukemia (ANLL) is used to collectively refer to acute myelocytic, myelomonocytic, monocytic, progranulocytic, and erythroleukemia, since the therapy for all of these is currently the same. At our institution, AML represents approximately 20% of all cases of leukemia (297). The treatment of AML has been the subject of excellent reviews, to which the reader is referred for further details of other components of its therapy (298–299).

The disease, like ALL, is characterized by infiltration of bone marrow and other organs by immature precursors of the involved white cell line. This eventually produces dysfunction of the infiltrated organs, with resultant anemia, granulocytopenia, and thrombocytopenia. If untreated, the disease is rapidly fatal with a median survival of less than two months.

The first therapeutic goal in the treatment of AML is to induce a complete remission. Successful remission induction therapy produces a reduction of leukemic cells to undetectable levels, with restoration of normal bone marrow function, normalization of hemoglobin, platelet and granulocyte counts, resolution of hepatosplenomegaly and normalization of the patient's performance status.

21. B.C.D. is a 12-year-old white boy who presented with a normochromic-normocytic anemia, splenomegaly and occasional bone pain. At presentation, his total white blood cell count was 94,000/mm³ with a predominance of myeloblasts. A bone marrow aspirate revealed a hypercellular marrow with predominant myeloblasts, leading to a diagnosis of acute myelocytic leukemia. What is the current chemotherapy for this disease, and what is the expected outcome of therapy?

Currently, the two best drugs for remission induction therapy are daunomycin (daunorubicin) and cytosine arabinoside (Ara-C). Daunomycin is considered the most effective single agent for AML, with complete remission rates of 35 to 50% when given in a dosage of 45 to 60 mg/m² daily for three consecutive days (300–303). Adriamycin has not been as extensively evaluated because of early reports indicating that it was not as active for AML as daunomycin (304). However, more recent clinical trials indicate that comparable response rates can be obtained with adriamycin, using two-thirds the dosage of daunomycin (305–307). Whether this lower total anthracycline dosage (mg/m²) actually constitutes an advantage to using adriamycin for remission induction of AML remains to be confirmed in a larger number of patients. In our institution, as well as other institutions, adriamycin has produced more acute toxicities (eg, stomatitis) than daunomycin when given with Ara-C for remission induction (307).

Cytosine arabinoside, a pyrimidine analogue that inhibits DNA synthesis, has a short biological half-life and is active primarily against proliferating cells during S phase of the cell cycle. Its antileukemic effect is apparently dose- and schedule-dependent. When administered for five to seven days in a dosage of 100 to 200 mg/m² per day by continuous infusion or by intermittent intravenous injections every 12 hours, the complete response rate for AML is approximately 25–38% (308–312). Since cytosine arabinoside was available prior to the anthracyclines, early multiple-drug induction regimens included Ara-C with 6-thioguanine or vincristine and prednisone. These combinations resulted in complete response rates of 35–50% (312–316).

Currently, the most widely used and effective remission induction therapy includes an intensive course of an anthracycline and Ara-C, which produces complete response rates of 60–84% (300,317–321). Either daunomycin (45–60 mg/m²) or adriamycin (30 mg/m²) is given daily for three days followed by (or overlapping with) Ara-C given either as a continuous infusion (100 mg/m²/day) or by intravenous bolus (100 mg/m² every 12 hours) for five to seven days.

Other drugs which have activity for AML and have been used in some induction regimens and for patients who fail first-line drugs include: 6-thioguanine, vincristine, methotrexate, prednisone, and 6-mercaptopurine. Particularly promising is the introduction of several investigational drugs which have been found to be active in refractory AML. These include VP-16 (324), 5-azacytidine (325), and m-AMSA (326). Use of these drugs in remission induction or during maintenance therapy may prolong the duration of continuous complete remission and, in some patients, may even achieve cure of their leukemia (327).

22. What are the major complications which can be anticipated from B.C.D.'s induction chemotherapy?

Although this intensive induction therapy yields improved response rates, it also produces a long period of marrow aplasia with the attendant risk of infectious diseases. Bleeding and bacterial infections are major complications of this induction therapy. The development of aggressive antibiotic therapy and granulocyte transfusions has decreased the mortality of treatment-related complications (323); however, despite these improvements in supportive care, 10–15% of patients receiving remission induction die from infection (321). Remission induction therapy of AML is generally more successful in younger patients than in older patients (> 50 years) (322).

23. B.C.D. received remission therapy as described above with success. Is maintenance therapy indicated for patients with AML?

In contrast to ALL, the value of maintenance therapy after achieving a complete remission has not been established. Randomized trials evaluating the role of maintenance therapy have produced conflicting results. One trial of 26 patients reported a median remission duration of 6.7 months without maintenance chemotherapy versus 10.3 months for patients administered maintenance chemotherapy (Ara-C, 6-TG), but all patients relapsed by three years (328). A larger study by the Southeast Cancer Study Group reported no difference in the remission duration of the control group and those administered BCNU 50 mg/m^2 every 4 weeks and Ara-C 100 mg/m^2 weekly as maintenance chemotherapy (329). However, this study did not use aggressive maintenance chemotherapy by current standards, which may partially explain its apparent lack of effectiveness. These results are supported by data from Lewis et al, who also found no significant differences in survival in maintained versus unmaintained patients less than 50 years of age (330). Several uncontrolled studies have shown similar durations of continuous complete remission despite wide variation in the intensity of maintenance therapy used (331–335). Therefore, the value of maintenance therapy is still under investigation, and patients such as B.C.D. should receive therapy according to a clinical protocol designed to answer this or other unresolved questions about the management of AML.

24. Is CNS prophylactic therapy indicated for B.C.D.?

Central nervous system involvement is not uncommon in patients with AML; the incidence of clinically evident CNS disease is about 10% (300,336–339). The increasing incidence of CNS involvement in patients with AML is probably related to longer survival with current systemic therapy. Unlike ALL, for which CNS preventive therapy is critical for long-term survival, the role of CNS prophylactic therapy for AML is uncertain. The primary obstacle to long-term survival is presently not CNS relapse, but bone marrow relapse. However, as more effective remission maintenance regimens are developed, CNS prophylactic therapy may become increasingly important.

25. Since response to standard chemotherapeutic regimens is so dismal, what other approaches to the management of AML have been tried? What is the rationale for their use?

Despite attainment of a complete remission with intensive anthracycline/cytosine arabinoside remission induction, approximately one-half of these patients will relapse in 12–18 months. This is in contrast to the encouraging results in childhood ALL, where over one-half of all standard-risk patients will be "cured" of their disease. Because of these dismal results, several clinical or laboratory approaches are being investigated. Recently, studies have identified several features at diagnosis which predict the length of continuous complete remission (339). Similarly, *in vitro* sensitivity of bone marrow specimens to selected drugs (340) and measurement of pharmacokinetic parameters (341–342) may also aid in predicting response. If these factors prove to be useful, more intensive chemotherapeutic regimens may be administered to patients who are likely to experience early relapse.

The role of late intensification chemotherapy represents another attempt to prolong remission duration. With this approach, patients in remission for several months (generally about 12 months) receive late intensive courses of chemotherapy. The rationale of this approach is based on the hypothesis that, in most patients, leukemic relapse is caused by myeloblasts which have become resistant to maintenance therapy. Therefore, administration of effective drugs that the patient has not received previously may eradicate these residual leukemic cells. Several studies using this approach have reported encouraging results; however, these studies are uncontrolled and follow-up is short (343–345). In a recent update of results, the median duration of remission was about three years, and 40% remain in complete remission for over five years (345).

Another chemotherapeutic approach involves the use of non-crossresistant, sequential drug combinations during maintenance therapy (321). This approach is based on experimental data indicating that at a given point ("nadir"), further killing of chemotherapeutically sensitive cells is counterbalanced by the overgrowth of resistant cells, resulting in clinically detectable relapse. If chemotherapy is empirically alternated at this "nadir," resistant cells may be killed and the remission prolonged. This approach is currently being tested in our institution. Obviously, this approach requires the availability of several effective drugs with different mechanisms of action. Investigational agents, such as VP-16, 5-azacytidine, and m-AMSA may prove especially useful in this regard (324–326).

Immunotherapy has been tried in several trials based on the selective cytotoxic effect of an immune response on leukemia-specific antigens, which was not observed on normal cells. Because immunotherapy is most effective against small numbers of tumor cells, this form of therapy has been incorporated into remission maintenance regimens. Preliminary results in some trials evaluating immunotherapy suggest some benefit in prolonging remission in patients with AML (346–347). However, most of the trials have shown no beneficial effect of immunotherapy. Controlled, randomized trials of large numbers of patients are needed before immunotherapy can be recommended.

Finally, bone-marrow transplantation may be an effective form of therapy in selected patients with AML. This form of therapy is based on the premise that the leukemia-infiltrated bone marrow can be destroyed and replaced by normal bone marrow. Several reviews have been recently published, and the reader is referred there for greater detail (347–349). Allogeneic bone-marrow transplantation from an HLA-matched sibling yields a disease-free survival comparable to that achieved with chemotherapy (350). Patients with AML who receive transplantation during their first remission or from an identical twin are even more likely to experience long-term disease-free control (351–352). However, several problems limit the success of bone-marrow transplantation, including graft-versus-host disease, recurrent leukemia, interstitial pneumonitis, and immunodeficiency. Autologous bone-marrow transplantation may be useful in patients lacking a suitable donor, and this approach is attractive because of the lack of immunological complications (353). Conversely, mild graft-versus-host reactions may be related to a favorable outcome of this therapy. In summary, the precise role of bone-marrow transplantation is unclear (354–355); however, this technique may offer an opportunity for some patients with AML to achieve prolonged leukemia-free survival and possibly cure.

NON-HODGKIN'S LYMPHOMA

26. R.S.T. is a 13-year-old boy who is admitted because of a several week history of cramping epigastric and left upper quadrant pain and also for evaluation of "coffee-ground" emesis. Further work-up revealed diffuse undifferentiated lymphoma, Burkitt's type, involving the stomach and retroperitoneal area. Following additional studies, he was found to have Stage III disease. Unfortunately, his tumor was unresectable. How

should R.S.T. be managed? What is the response to chemotherapy?

Non-Hodgkin's lymphoma (NHL) is a neoplastic disease of lymphoreticular cells which exhibits a spectrum of clinical syndromes dependent upon the site of primary tumor involvement, extent of disease at diagnosis and, to a lesser extent, histologic type. Lymphomas are the third most common malignancy affecting white children in the United States (2). In the previous two decades, the overall two-year survival in childhood NHL was 20–30% (356–358); however, with current intensive combined-modality regimens, over one-half of children survive for two years (359–363). Children with localized disease (Stages I and II) do significantly better than patients with generalized disease (Stages III and IV). In our institution, the two-year disease-free survival is 90% for Stages I–II versus 39% for Stages III–IV (363). Unfortunately, about 70% of all cases of childhood NHL are Stage III–IV (364). The therapy of childhood NHL has been the subject of several excellent reviews, to which the reader is referred for additional details (364–366).

While the extent of the disease is an important determinant of outcome, there is no such consensus regarding the importance of histologic classification. In contrast to adult NHL, where nodular lymphomas comprise about 45% of all NHL, nodular lymphomas are rare in children but have a good prognosis (367–368). Greater than 95% of all cases of childhood NHL have a diffuse histologic pattern. It has been concluded by several investigators that either (a) the prognostic value of histology has not been established, (b) the histology exerts no independent prognostic influence, or (c) at the very least, histology should not be used to determine management. Most institutions presently use a modification of the Rappaport classification (diffuse or nodular), and the cytological classification (lymphocytic or histiocytic), although the functional classification of the non-Hodgkin's lymphomas is currently under revision (369).

The ability to detect cell-surface markers has aided in characterizing childhood NHL (193–194). As with childhood ALL, childhood NHL can be divided into at least three subgroups: T cell, B cell, and "null" or non-T, non-B cell (370–371). Whereas the majority of ALL is non-T, non-B cell (eg, common ALL), most cases of childhood NHL are T- or B-cell in character. In adults with diffuse histiocytic lymphoma, approximately 76% were B-cell in origin, 8% T-cell, and the remainder either histiocytic by surface marker or undefined (371). It is not known if a similar distribution is also seen in children with diffuse histiocytic lymphoma. Children with either B-cell or T-cell NHL have a poorer prognosis than those with "null-cell" NHL.

Combined-modality therapy is usually given to all children with NHL. Only 30–50% of children with localized (Stage I–II) NHL treated with radiation alone experience long-term disease-free survival, as compared to 80% or greater when combination chemotherapy is added (372). The role of combined-modality therapy in Stage III–IV disease is less clear, since the major cause of treatment failure in these patients is relapse in unirradiated areas. Randomized studies indicate that in these patients with advanced disease, the addition of radiotherapy does not improve remission duration, but only adds to toxicity (363). Conventional therapy over the past two decades has cured roughly one-third of all children with NHL (356–358,379). Survival of children with localized disease is consistently better than children with generalized disease. Recent studies show that approximately 90% of children with Stage I disease are curable if an intensive multiple drug chemotherapy regimen is combined with radiation (359–363,378–380). This is in contrast to the less than 40% two-year survival of patients with Stage III and IV disease (359–363,378–379). It has been recommended that treatment of children with NHL should be determined by the primary anatomic location and extent of disease (365). This is based on the extremely poor prognosis of patients with unresectable abdominal or mediastinal NHL (364). Because there are differences in histology, clinical behavior, and chemotherapeutic sensitivity between NHL in adults and children, improvement in the response of children with generalized disease is unlikely to result from the application of therapeutic innovations introduced in the treatment of adults with NHL.

Since childhood NHL is often a generalized disease at diagnosis, as in R.S.T., chemotherapy plays an important role in remission induction. Combination chemotherapy is superior to single-agent chemotherapy in malignant lymphomas, with the most active agents against NHL being alkylating agents, vinca alkaloids, adriamycin, bleomycin, and corticosteroids (373). Several combinations of active agents have been used in remission induction; these regimens have been patterned from successful results in adults with NHL (373–376). Examples of such combinations are cyclophosphamide, vincristine, and prednisone (CVP), CVP plus hydroxydaunomycin (adriamycin) (CHOP), CVP plus procarbazine (C-MOPP), and CHOP plus bleomycin (BACOP). At St. Jude Children's Research Hospital, use of radiotherapy with CVP or CHOP, depending on stage, produces a 88% complete response rate (363).

Following remission induction with chemotherapy or chemotherapy and radiotherapy, maintenance therapy is used for 18–24 months. Because of the excellent results in patients with Stage I–II disease, there are studies underway to determine if shorter periods of maintenance therapy can produce similar results with less toxicity. Furthermore, in these patients with localized disease, the role of lower-dose radiotherapy during remission induction is also being examined.

Since 1971, children with NHL at Memorial Sloan-Kettering Cancer Center have been treated with the LSA-L$_2$ protocol (362,377–378). The initial results of the LSA-L$_2$ protocol were excellent, with 80% of children with all stages of disease alive and free of disease at 40 months. A recent update continues to show excellent results, with over 70% of the children off therapy and free of disease at 70 months (378). This complex treatment protocol is divided into an induction phase, consolidation phase, and maintenance phase, and includes ten different drugs. The authors concluded that the main factor in the survival of children with NHL is therapy and that it must be early, aggressive, prolonged, and include surgery, irradiation, and chemotherapy. However, comparison of the results of this series to others is difficult because of the large number of patients with Stage IV disease (40%) and the high percentage of patients with nodular lymphoma (14%). Many of the patients with Stage IV disease (on the basis of initial bone marrow involvement) would be considered leukemic by conventional criteria and would therefore be expected to have a very good response to therapy.

NEUROBLASTOMA

Neuroblastoma is the most common extracranial solid tumor in infancy and childhood, comprising 7–14% of childhood malignancies and 15–

50% of neonatal malignancies (2,381–382). Neuroblastoma arises in the sympathetic nervous system, and usually presents as an abdominal mass (383–385). An additional 15–20% of patients present with a mediastinal mass. Despite the progress that has been made during the past two decades for other childhood cancers, the prognosis in patients with neuroblastoma remains poor due to the frequency of disseminated disease at diagnosis; 70% of children over one year of age and 40–50% of those under one year of age have disseminated disease at diagnosis (385).

The prognosis of children with neuroblastoma is influenced primarily by age, stage, and, possibly, primary site of disease (383,385). Younger children (less than one year of age) tend to respond more favorably than older children. The prognostic effect of primary site of disease is difficult to evaluate, since patients with abdominal neuroblastomas almost always have metastatic disease at diagnosis. In contrast, children with neuroblastoma involving the head, neck, or pelvis can often be treated with complete surgical resection. It is also important to realize that neuroblastoma has the highest rate of spontaneous remission of any human malignancy (387). The basis for this phenomenon is unknown, although investigators have proposed various hypotheses to explain its occurrence (388).

The treatment of neuroblastoma includes surgery, radiation therapy, and chemotherapy. The roles of each of these components on therapy have been recently reviewed in detail (384). Another modality of therapy that is currently under investigation is immunotherapy with BCG (bacillus Calmette Guérin) plus irradiated tumor cells.

27. L.M.N. is a 2-year-old child who was admitted for evaluation of vague abdominal pain that had persisted for several weeks. IVP showed a laterally displaced right kidney with a large mass displacing both kidneys and extending up to the liver. A biopsy of the abdominal mass revealed neuroblastoma and he was transferred to St. Jude Hospital for further evaluation. Numerous scans and a bone marrow aspirate were normal. How should L.M.N. be treated? What are the current results of treatment regimens for neuroblastoma?

Vincristine, adriamycin, and cyclophosphamide are currently the most effective agents used to treat patients with disseminated disease (218,389–390). The response rate to combination chemotherapy with vincristine and cyclophosphamide is reported in three series to be 32, 28, and 38% (391–393). Sawitsky reported a 55% response rate with these two drugs and noted similar results whether the drugs were given sequentially, concurrently, or in an alternate week schedule (394). Other drugs which have been reported to have antitumor activity for neuroblastoma include DTIC, VM-26, and cisplatin (395–398).

The most effective combination for neuroblastoma at this time is cyclophosphamide and adriamycin. Green et al have reported a 52% complete response rate in 68 children with disseminated neuroblastoma treated with this combination (399). Although comparable complete response rates have been reported from other studies, the criteria for complete response differed significantly (400). Green and co-workers (399) defined a complete remission as total regression of all apparent tumor for four months, whereas the Children's Cancer Study Group (400) required only a one month duration of complete remission. Furthermore, approximately 70% of children in the latter series received radiotherapy, while in the series by Green et al, radiotherapy was withheld until response to chemotherapy could be evaluated. The regimen used by Green et al is recommended for L.M.N.: cyclophosphamide (150 mg/m^2/day for seven days) followed by adriamycin (35 mg/m^2/day on day eight). This regimen is well-tolerated and is based on cell-kinetic principles; preliminary data indicate a high correlation between cell-kinetic perturbations and clinical response (401). The median survival for complete responders is 22 months, with some children surviving for more than five years (399). The combination of cisplatin and VM-26 has proved to be useful in patients failing to attain a complete response to cyclophosphamide and adriamycin (402), and this combination is currently being evaluated as an addition to first-line therapy.

WILMS' TUMOR

Wilms' tumor is the most common intra-abdominal childhood tumor and has an incidence in white children similar to neuroblastoma (2). This tumor, also called nephroblastoma, originates in the kidney and represents one of the success stories in pediatric oncology (403). Disease-free survival of children with Wilms' tumor has improved from 32% with surgery alone, to 47% with the addition of radiotherapy, to 80–90% with combined-modality therapy (404–407).

Although the overall survival is excellent, some subgroups of Wilms' tumor are associated with a poor prognosis. Sarcomatous or anaplastic patterns, which account for about 11% of all Wilms' tumors, are associated with a poor prognosis (407–410). Approximately 10–15% of children with Wilms' tumor have distant metastatic disease at diagnosis and have a two-year disease-free survival of 54% with modern treatment, as compared to 84–95% for tumor confined to the kidney or abdomen (407).

28. K.L.M. is a 20-month-old male referred to St. Jude Hospital for evaluation of an abdominal mass. He did not complain of abdominal pain and his appetite was normal. An exploratory laparotomy was performed, followed by right radical nephrectomy for probable Wilms' tumor. Pathologic examination confirmed the diagnosis: Wilms' tumor, non-sarcomatous type. Because the tumor had probably penetrated the peritoneum and tumor was noted in the right renal vein, a diagnosis of Stage III Wilms' tumor was made. How will this child be managed? What is the expected prognosis for this child with present chemotherapy?

Chemotherapy plays an important role in the management of Wilms' tumor. The most active single agents are vincristine (411–412), actinomycin D (404,413), and adriamycin (218). When actinomycin D was given as a single agent on the day of surgery, the two-year survival was 89%, whereas only about 50% of patients not given the drug survived (414). Wolff et al then conducted a randomized study comparing the efficacy of single versus multiple courses of actinomycin D (413,415). Patients receiving actinomycin D over a 15 month period experienced a longer disease-free survival as compared to those given the drug only on the day of surgery. However, because of the good response to alternate chemotherapy and radiotherapy among patients who relapsed, the overall survival was not affected by multiple-dose treatment (413). About this same time, vincristine was shown to be effective in patients with

Wilms' tumor refractory to actinomycin D (412). Pediatric oncologists were divided concerning the efficacy of actinomycin D versus vincristine, as well as the role of radiotherapy. Because patient numbers were limited, the National Wilms' Tumor Study Group was formed to study this and other unresolved questions.

The first National Wilms' Tumor study dealt with the need for postoperative radiation therapy and the choice of postoperative chemotherapy regimens (405). In children with tumor confined to the kidney (Group I), the need for postoperative radiotherapy appeared to vary according to age. In children less than 2-years-old, irradiation is unnecessary; however, for children ≥ 2-years-old, the four-year disease-free survival was 76% for the group receiving radiotherapy versus 57% for the group receiving actinomycin D alone. In patients with more advanced disease but still confined to the abdomen (Group II–III), the combination of actinomycin D, vincristine, and postoperative radiation was clearly shown to improve disease-free and overall survival compared to radiation therapy with either agent alone. For patients with distant metastases (Group IV), no advantage was seen with administering vincristine preoperatively.

The second National Wilms' Tumor Study sought to establish whether the addition of vincristine to actinomycin D in Group I children would produce results comparable to only actinomycin D with radiotherapy (407). Because of the increasing awareness of long-term toxicity associated with cancer treatment, the efficacy of six months of treatment was compared to 15 months in this low-risk group. For Groups II–IV, the study evaluated the added benefit of adriamycin to the established regimen of actinomycin D and vincristine. Postoperative radiation was used in all but Group I patients. In Group I patients, six months of actinomycin D and vincristine was as effective as 15 months of therapy with the same drugs. In patients with more advanced disease (Groups II–IV), the addition of adriamycin prolonged disease-free survival, as well as toxicity, when compared to actinomycin D and vincristine. The disease-free and overall survival at two years for the adriamycin-containing regimen was 77% and 84%, respectively. These studies clearly demonstrate that many children with Wilms' tumor will, with modern therapy, experience long-term disease-free survival, and possibly cure. Therapy for the 11% of patients with unfavorable histology was clearly inadequate; only about 35% of these patients were free of disease at two years. In contrast, because of the risk of long-term complications, the goal for patients with favorable histology is to use the least intensive treatment necessary to produce long-term disease-free survival (416–417).

The third National Wilms' Tumor Study is now underway. Some of the major questions this study will try to answer are: (a) In patients with favorable histology Group I Wilms' tumor, can even shorter courses of actinomycin D and vincristine be used without sacrificing therapeutic effectiveness? (b) In patients with favorable histology Group II–III disease, is postoperative radiotherapy necessary, and if so, at what dosage? Also, what is the role of adriamycin? (c) In patients with Group IV disease (any histology) or unfavorable histology (any stage), does the addition of cyclophosphamide to adriamycin, actinomycin D, and vincristine improve the results?

OSTEOSARCOMA

Osteosarcoma is the most common malignant bone tumor of childhood. The tumor can arise in any bone, but most commonly affects the long bones of the arm or leg. Osteosarcoma represents one of the greatest challenges to chemotherapists because it most commonly affects young people during their second decade of life and also because of the limited number of drugs effective against this cancer.

Various approaches to the medical treatment of osteosarcoma have been attempted in the past 50 years. In the largest series of pediatric patients with this tumor, there was a 17% five-year disease-free survival rate, with a median post-amputation survival time of 8½ months for patients who died (418). Radiation therapy followed by delayed amputation did not extend the lives nor improve the results of treatment of patients with this tumor (419). Metastases were usually noted in the lungs during the first year following surgical removal of the primary tumor. Development of pulmonary metastases and ultimate outcome were found to be unrelated to sex, race, preoperative duration of symptoms, or preoperative radiation therapy. Based on the dismal results despite complete surgical removal and the lack of clinically detectable metastatic disease at diagnosis, a new approach was needed.

It became apparent that the great majority of patients with osteosarcoma had clinically undetectable metastases ("micrometastases") at the time of diagnosis. It was reasoned that these micrometastases should be treated aggressively with combination chemotherapy. Cell-kinetic studies also supported this concept, indicating that the proportion of rapidly proliferating cells in the tumor would be highest when the tumor burden was low. Therefore, chemotherapy administered immediately after surgery ("adjuvant chemotherapy") when the neoplastic cells were most sensitive would provide the best chance for long-term survival and cure. This combined-modality approach is now used in most institutions (420–423), although its value over surgery alone has recently been questioned (424–427).

29. B.D.D. is a 14-year-old male who bruised his right knee while playing basketball. The pain and swelling persisted over several weeks, and he sought the advice of a physician. Radiographic studies revealed increased uptake in the distal femur, and a biopsy was obtained. Pathologic examination revealed osteosarcoma. Careful CAT scans of both lungs revealed no evidence of metastatic disease. The patient's right leg was amputated and, after allowing for post-surgical healing, chemotherapy consisting of high-dose methotrexate with leucovorin rescue (HDMTX), adriamycin, and cyclophosphamide was initiated. What is the rationale for aggressive chemotherapy in patients with osteosarcoma without evidence of distant metastatic disease?

In 1972, Jaffe adapted the use of high-dose methotrexate-leucovorin rescue to adjuvant chemotherapy for osteosarcoma after noting two complete and two partial responses in ten patients with pulmonary metastases (428). These investigators used high-dose methotrexate and oral leucovorin in a method first advocated by Djerassi for the treatment of acute lymphocytic leukemia and lung cancer (429). Jaffe et al also advocated the administration of vincristine 30 minutes prior to methotrexate infusions in an attempt to increase the intracellular concentrations of high-dose methotrexate (430), a combination that now appears to be without good rationale and potentially harmful (431–432). Using this regimen, approximately 60% of treated patients were free of pulmonary metastases, as compared to only 20% of patients ("historical controls") treated by amputation alone (433–434).

During this same period of time, several investigators observed the response of the pulmonary metastases of osteosarcoma following treatment with the antitumor antibiotic, adriamycin (435–437). They adapted the use of adjuvant adriamycin to their patients who were free of obvious pulmonary metastases at the time of the diagnosis, and early results were most encouraging, indicating that about 50% of patients treated with adjuvant chemotherapy were disease-free two years after diagnosis (438). Recent reports using either high-dose methotrexate or adriamycin as single agents indicate that 30–40% of patients receiving adjuvant therapy are free of disease at five years (439–440). Although a variety of drugs have since been tried, alone and in combination (441–442), adriamycin and high-dose methotrexate are currently considered the most active and are now included in most combination regimens (443–448).

However, investigators at the Mayo Clinic raised serious questions about the efficacy of adjuvant chemotherapy for osteosarcoma when they reported a 50% two-year disease-free survival rate for their patients treated with surgery alone between 1972 and 1974 (449). This 50% figure is comparable to the results reported with adjuvant chemotherapy (442–448) and substantially better than the 25% two-year disease-free survival with surgery alone achieved at the Mayo Clinic from 1963–1972 (449). The exact reason for this improvement without adjuvant chemotherapy at the Mayo Clinic is not clear, but likely relates to better techniques (CAT scans) for detecting metastatic disease at diagnosis, and possibly to changing patient referral patterns. Interpretation of this observation is confounded by disparate results at other institutions whose two-year relapse-free survival rates following surgery alone were 16%, 19%, and 20% at M.D. Anderson (447), Sidney Farber (433) and Memorial Sloan-Kettering (418, 450), respectively. Moreover, these institutions now enter essentially all newly diagnosed patients onto adjuvant chemotherapy protocols, precluding any analysis of surgery alone during the same time period as the Mayo experience.

Since none of the initial clinical trials evaluating adjuvant chemotherapy were randomized controlled studies, all results must be interpreted based on the historical controls. At the time these initial studies were conducted (1971–1975), the use of historical controls seemed warranted since results with surgery alone had been consistently poor, and the number of available patients per year very small (about 1000/year in the U.S.). Now, a decade later, the value of adjuvant chemotherapy for osteosarcoma is still unclear, and will remain so until the historical control issue is resolved or until an adequate prospective randomized clinical trial is performed.

Such a controlled clinical trial was initiated at the Mayo Clinic in 1976, and preliminary results have been presented (451). Unfortunately, only a small number of patients referred to the Mayo Clinic consented to be enrolled in the study (about 50% of eligible patients). The preliminary results in these 37 patients were that 50% of all patients were disease-free two years after surgery alone (no adjuvant therapy), and 75% are estimated to survive for two years. There was no difference in the estimated disease-free survival between this group and those who received adjuvant therapy. The seriousness of this dilemma and the provocative preliminary results of the Mayo Clinic study have led the National Cancer Institute to initiate a multi-institutional clinical trial to address this problem, although it will be some time before it is resolved.

Meanwhile, Rosen and coworkers at Memorial Sloan-Kettering have reported a 68% disease-free 2½-year survival rate among 31 patients treated with preoperative chemotherapy (3 months of high-dose methotrexate with leucovorin rescue, and adriamycin), followed by surgical ablation (not amputation) and five additional months of postoperative chemotherapy (high-dose methotrexate, adriamycin, cyclophosphamide) (452). Histologic examination of the primary tumor at surgery indicated a more complete response to chemotherapy by the 21 disease-free survivors and has been suggested as a guideline for dosage escalation of methotrexate in the "non-responders." These investigators stress the efficacy of chemotherapy (especially methotrexate) when used in appropriately high dosages and offer a provocative alternative to amputation. If these data are supported by additional independent clinical trials and the en bloc resection of tumor with prosthetic bone replacement results in reduced morbidity when compared to amputation, this approach to the treatment of osteosarcoma will be an attractive alternative to radical surgery regardless of the outcome of the historical control dilemma.

ACKNOWLEDGMENTS: The authors wish to thank the many investigators at St. Jude Children's Research Hospital for helpful comments and Ms. Fabrienne Holloway for the typing of the manuscript.

References

1. Silverberg E: Cancer statistics, 1981. CA-A Journal for Clinicians. 1981; 31:13.
2. Young JL et al: Incidence of malignant tumors in U.S. children. J Pediatr. 1975; 86:254.
3. Mauer AM: Therapy of acute lymphoblastic leukemia in childhood. Blood. 1980; 56:1.
4. Bowman WP: Childhood acute lymphocytic leukemia: progress and problems in treatment. Can Med Assoc J. 1981; 124:129.
5. Frei E et al: Acute lymphoblastic leukemia: treatment. Cancer. 1978; 42:828.
6. Miller DR: Acute lymphoblastic leukemia. Pediatr Clin North Am. 1980; 27:525.
7. Mauer AM et al: Current progress in the treatment of the child with cancer. J Pediatr. 1977; 91:525.
8. Mauer AM et al: The current status of the treatment of childhood acute lymphoblastic leukemia. Can Treat Rev. 1976; 3:17.
9. Fernbach DJ et al: Chemotherapy of acute leukemia in childhood: Comparison of cyclophosphamide and mercaptopurine. N Engl J Med. 1966; 275:451.
10. Hardisty RM et al: Vincristine and prednisone for the induction of remissions in acute childhood leukemia. Br Med J. 1969; 2:662.
11. Krivit W et al: Induction of remission in acute leukemia of childhood by combination of prednisone and either 6-mercaptopurine or methotrexate. J Pediatr. 1966; 68:965.
12. Matthews RN et al: Daunorubicin results in childhood leukemia. Arch Dis Child. 1972; 47:272.
13. Aur RJA et al: Central nervous system therapy and combination chemotherapy of childhood lymphocytic leukemia. Blood. 1971; 37:272.
14. George P et al: A study of "total therapy" of acute lymphocytic leukemia in children. J Pediatr. 1968; 72:399.
15. Pinkel D et al: Drug dosage and remission duration in childhood lymphocytic leukemia. Cancer. 1971; 27:247.
16. Pinkel D: Five-year follow-up of "total therapy" of childhood lymphocytic leukemia. JAMA. 1971; 216:648.
17. Aur RJA et al: A comparative study of central nervous system irradiation and early remission of childhood acute lymphocytic leukemia. Cancer. 1972; 29:381.
18. Hagbin M et al: Intensive chemotherapy in children with acute lymphoblastic leukemia (L-2 Protocol). Cancer. 1974; 33:1491.
19. Komp DM et al: Cyclophosphamide-asparaginase-vincristine-prednisone induction therapy in childhood acute lymphocytic and nonlymphocytic leukemia. Cancer. 1976; 37:1243.
20. Ortega JA et al: L-asparaginase, vincristine, and prednisone for induction of first remission in acute lymphocytic leukemia. Cancer Res. 1977; 37:535.
21. Sallan SE et al: Clinical and cytokinetic aspects of remission induction of childhood acute lymphoblastic leukemia (ALL): Addition of an anthracycline to vincristine and prednisone. Med Pediatr Oncol. 1977; 3:281.
22. Aur RJA et al: Childhood acute lymphocytic leukemia—study VIII. Cancer. 1978; 42:2133.
23. Simone JV: Factors that influence haematological remission duration in acute lymphocytic leukemia. Br J Haematol. 1976; 32:465.
24. Aur RJA et al: Multiple combination therapy for childhood acute lymphocytic leukemia (ALL). Blood. 1978; 52:238.
25. Rivera G et al: VM-26 and cytosine arabinoside combination chemotherapy for initial induction failures in childhood lymphocytic leukemia. Cancer. 1980; 46:1727.
26. Rieselbach RE et al: Uric acid excretion and renal function in the acute hyperuricemia of leukemia. Am J Med. 1964; 37:872.
27. Lynch EC: Uric acid metabolism in proliferative diseases of the marrow. Arch Intern Med. 1962; 109:43.
28. Frei E et al: Renal complications of neoplastic disease. J Chronic Dis. 1963; 16:757.
29. Deconti RC et al: Use of allopurinol for prevention and control of hyperuricemia in patients with neoplastic disease. N Engl J Med. 1966; 274:481.
30. Krakoff IH: Use of allopurinol in preventing hyperuricemia in leukemia and lymphoma. Cancer. 1966; 19:1489.
31. Muggia FM et al: Allopurinol in the treatment of neoplastic disease complicated by hyperuricemia. Arch Intern Med. 1967; 120:12.
32. Rundles RW et al: Allopurinol in the treatment of gout. Ann Intern Med. 1966; 64:229.
33. Yu TF et al: Effect of allopurinol on serum and urinary uric acid in primary and secondary gout. Am J Med. 1964; 37:885.
34. Elion GB et al: Relationship between metabolic fates and antitumor activities of thiopurines. Cancer Res. 1963; 23:1207.
35. Coffey JJ et al: Effect of allopurinol on the pharmacokinetics of 6-mercaptopurine (NSC 755) in cancer patients. Cancer Res. 1972; 32:1283.
36. Levine AS et al: Combination therapy with 6-mercaptopurine and allopurinol during induction and maintenance of remission of acute leukemia in children. Cancer Chemother Rep. 1969; 53:53.
37. Rundles RW et al: Effects of xanthine oxidase inhibitor on thiopurine metabolism, hyperuricemia, and gout. Trans Assoc Am Physicians. 1963; 76:126.
38. Boston Collaborative Drug Surveillance Program: Allopurinol and cytotoxic drugs. Interaction and relation to bone marrow suppression. JAMA. 1974; 227:1036.

39. Bagley CM et al: Clinical pharmacology of cyclophosphamide. Cancer Res. 1973; 33:226.

40. Weiss HD et al: Neurotoxicity of commonly used antineoplastic agents. N Engl J Med. 1974; 291:75 and 127.

41. Allen JC: The effects of cancer therapy on the nervous system. J Pediatr. 1978; 93:903.

42. Rosenthal S et al: Vincristine neurotoxicity. Ann Intern Med. 1974; 80:733.

43. Casey EB et al: Vincristine neuropathy: Clinical and electrophysiological observations. Brain. 1973; 96:69.

44. Holland JF et al: Vincristine treatment of advanced cancer: A cooperative study of 392 cases. Cancer Res. 1973; 33:1258.

45. Sandler SG et al: Vincristine-induced neuropathy: A clinical study of fifty leukemia patients. Neurology. 1969; 19:367.

46. Bradley WG et al: The neuromyopathy of vincristine in man: clinical, electrophysiological and pathological studies. J Neurol Sci. 1970; 10:107.

47. Albert DM et al: Ocular complications of vincristine therapy. Arch Ophthalmol. 1967; 78:709.

48. Bohannon RA et al: Vincristine in the treatment of lymphomas and leukemias. Cancer Res. 1963; 23:613.

49. Carmichael SM et al: Orthostatic hypotension during vincristine therapy. Arch Intern Med. 1973; 126:290.

50. Gottlieb RJ et al: Vincristine-induced bladder atony. Cancer. 1971; 28:674.

51. Gubisch NJ et al: Experience with vincristine in solid tumors. Cancer Chemother Rep. 1963; 32:19.

52. McLeod JG et al: Vincristine neuropathy: an electrophysiological and histological study. J Neurol Neurosurg Psychiatry. 1969; 32:297.

53. Tobin W et al: Neurophysiological alterations induced by vincristine (NSC-67574). Cancer Chemother Rep. 1968; 52:519.

54. Carbone PP et al: Clinical studies with vincristine. Blood. 1963; 21:640.

55. Berenson MP: Recovery after inadvertent massive overdosage of vincristine (NSC-67574). Cancer Chemother Rep. 1971; 55:525.

56. Sutow WW et al: Combination of vincristine and prednisone in therapy of acute leukemia in children. J Pediatr. 1968; 73:426.

57. Fine RN et al: Hyponatremia and vincristine therapy. Am J Dis Child. 1966; 112:256.

58. Slater LM et al: Vincristine neurotoxicity and hyponatremia. Cancer. 1969; 23:122.

59. Suskind RM et al: Syndrome of inappropriate secretion of antidiuretic hormone produced by vincristine toxicity (with bioassay of ADH level). J Pediatr. 1972; 81:90.

60. Nicholson RG et al: Hyponatremia in association with vincristine therapy. Can Med Assoc J. 1972; 106:356.

61. Robertson GL et al: Vincristine neurotoxicity and abnormal secretion of antidiuretic hormone. Arch Intern Med. 1973; 132:717.

62. Oldham RK et al: Vincristine-induced syndrome of inappropriate secretion of antidiuretic hormone. South Med J. 1972; 65:1010.

63. Cutting HO: Inappropriate secretion of antidiuretic hormone secondary to vincristine therapy. Am J Med. 1971; 51:269.

64. Johnson FL et al: Seizures associated with vincristine sulfate therapy. J Pediatr. 1973; 82:699.

65. Peterson RG et al: Immunological responses to L-asparaginase. J Clin Invest. 1971; 50:1080.

66. Capizzi RL et al: L-asparaginase. Ann Rev Med. 1970; 21:433.

67. Beard MEJ et al: L-asparaginase in treatment of acute leukemia and lymphosarcoma. Br Med J. 1970; 1:191.

68. Wade HE et al: A new L-asparaginase with antitumor activity. Lancet. 1968; 11:766.

69. Ohnuma T et al: *Erwinia carotovora* asparaginase in patients with prior anaphylaxis to asparaginase from *E. coli*. Cancer. 1972; 30:376.

70. Dellinger CT et al: Comparison of anaphylactic reactions to asparaginase derived from *Escherichia coli* and from *Erwinia* cultures. Cancer. 1976; 38:1843.

71. Haskell CM et al: L-asparaginase therapeutic and toxic effects in patients with neoplastic disease. N Engl J Med. 1969; 281:1028.

72. Jacquillat C et al: Treatment of acute leukemia with L-asparaginase preliminary results on 84 cases. Recent Results Cancer Res. 1970; 33:263.

73. Jaffe N et al: L-asparaginase in the treatment of neoplastic diseases in children. Cancer Res. 1971; 31:942.

74. Land VJ et al: Toxicity of L-asparaginase in children with advanced leukemia. Cancer. 1972; 30:339.

75. Mathe G et al: The place of the L-asparaginase in the treatment of acute leukemia. Recent Results Cancer Res. 1970; 33:279.

76. Nesbit M et al: Reduction of sensitivity reactions produced by L-asparaginase by combinations with 6-mercaptopurine. Proc AACR and ASCO. 1971; 11:39.

77. Nesbit M et al: Evaluation of intramuscular versus intravenous administration of L-asparaginase in childhood leukemia. Am J Pediatr Hematol Oncol. 1979; 1:9.

78. Oettgen HF et al: Toxicity of *E. coli* L-asparaginase in man. Cancer. 1970; 25:253.

79. Pratt CB et al: Low-dosage asparaginase treatment of childhood acute lymphocytic leukemia. Am J Dis Child. 1971; 121:406.

80. Pratt CB et al: Comparisons of daily versus weekly L-asparaginase for the treatment of childhood acute leukemia. J Pediatr. 1970; 77:474.

81. Rutler DA et al: Toxicity of asparaginase. Lancet. 1975; 1:1293.

82. Steuber CP et al: Use of L-asparaginase and cytosine arabinoside for refractory acute lymphocytic leukemia with particular reference to T-cell leukemia. Med Pediatr Oncol. 1978; 5:33.

83. Whitecar JP et al: L-asparaginase. N Engl J Med. 1970; 282:732.

84. Zubrod CG: The clinical toxicities of L-asparaginase in the treatment of leukemia and lymphoma. Pediatrics. 1970; 45:555.

85. Evans WE et al: Anaphylactoid reactions to *E. coli* and *Erwinia* asparaginase in children with leukemia and lymphoma. Cancer. 1982; 49:1378.

86. Mallory A: Drug-induced pancreatitis: A critical review. Gastroenterology. 1980; 78:813.

87. Nakashima Y et al: Drug-induced acute pancreatitis. Surg Gynecol Obstet. 1977; 145:105.

88. Ohnuma T et al: Biochemical and pharmacological studies with asparaginase in man. Cancer Res. 1970; 30:2297.

89. Weetman RM et al: Latent onset of clinical pancreatitis in children receiving L-asparaginase therapy. Cancer. 1974; 34:780.

90. Loeb E et al: Treatment of acute leukemia with L-asparaginase. Recent Results Cancer Res. 1970; 33:204.

91. George SL et al: A reappraisal of the results of stopping therapy in childhood leukemia. N Engl J Med. 1979; 300:269.

92. Lonsdale D et al: Interrupted vs. contained maintenance therapy in childhood acute leukemia. Cancer. 1975; 36:341.

93. Haghbin M et al: A long-term clinical follow-up of children with acute lymphoblastic leukemia treated with intensive chemotherapy regimens. Cancer. 1980; 46:241.

94. Rivera G et al: Recurrent childhood lymphocytic leukemia: clinical and cytokinetic studies of cytosine arabinoside and methotrexate for maintenance of second hematological remission. Cancer. 1978; 42:2521.

95. Reaman G et al: Improved treatment results in the management of single and multiple relapses of acute lymphoblastic leukemia. Cancer. 1980; 45:3090.

96. Aur RJA et al: Comparison of two methods of preventing central nervous system leukemia. Blood. 1973; 42:349.

97. Sallan SE et al: Intermittent combination chemotherapy with adriamycin for childhood acute lymphoblastic leukemia: clinical results. Blood. 1978; 51:425.

98. Rivera G et al: Combined VM-26 and cytosine arabinoside in treatment of refractory childhood lymphocytic leukemia. Cancer. 1980; 45:1284.

99. Lane DM et al: Remission induction in childhood leukemia with a second course vincristine and prednisone therapy. Cancer Chemother Rep. 1970; 54:113.

100. Aur RJA et al: Response to combination therapy after relapse in childhood acute lymphocytic leukemia. Cancer. 1972; 30:334.

101. Jacquillat MW et al: Evaluation of 216 four-year survivors of acute leukemia. Cancer. 1973; 32:286.

102. Herson J et al: Vincristine and prednisone vs vincristine, L-asparaginase, and prednisone for second remission induction of acute lymphocytic leukemia in children. Med Pediatr Oncol. 1979; 6:317.

103. Rivera G et al: Recurrent childhood lymphocytic leukemia following cessation of therapy. Cancer. 1976; 37:1679.

104. Rivera G et al: Second cessation of therapy in childhood lymphocytic leukemia. Blood. 1979; 53:1114.

105. Bleyer WA: Current status of intrathecal chemotherapy for human meningeal neoplasms. National Cancer Institute Monograph No. 1977; 46:171.

106. Pochedly C: Neurotoxicity due to CNS therapy for leukemia. Med Pediatr Oncol. 1977; 3:101.

107. Pizzo PA et al: Neurotoxicities of current leukemia therapy. Am J Pediatr Hematol Oncol. 1979; 1:127.

108. Duttera MJ et al: Irradiation, methotrexate toxicity, and the treatment of meningeal leukemia. Lancet. 1973; 2:703.

109. Mott MG et al: Methotrexate meningitis. Lancet. 1972; 2:656.

110. Sullivan MP et al: Clinical investigations in the treatment of meningeal leukemia: radiation therapy regimen vs. conventional intrathecal methotrexate. Blood. 1969; 34:301.

111. Rosner F et al: Intrathecal methotrexate. Lancet. 1970; 1:249.

112. Naiman JL et al: Intrathecal methotrexate. Lancet. 1970; 1:571.

113. Geiser CF et al: Adverse effects of intrathecal methotrexate in children with acute leukemia in remission. Blood. 1975; 45:189.

114. Back EH: Death after intrathecal methotrexate. Lancet. 1969; 2:1005.

115. Bagshawe KD et al: Intrathecal methotrexate. Lancet. 1969; 2:1258.

116. Baum ES et al: Intrathecal methotrexate. Lancet. 1971; 1:649.

117. Pasquinucci G et al: Intrathecal methotrexate. Lancet. 1970; 1:309.

118. Saiki JH et al: Paraplegia following intrathecal chemotherapy. Cancer. 1972; 29:370.

119. Gagliano R et al: Paraplegia following intrathecal methotrexate: report of a case and review of the literature. Cancer. 1976; 37:1663.

120. Luddy RD et al: Paraplegia following intrathecal methotrexate. J Pediatr. 1973; 83:988.

121. Thompson SW et al: Paraplegia following intrathecal antileukemia therapy. Neurology. 1971; 21:454.

122. Kay HE et al: Encephalopathy in acute leukemia associated with methotrexate therapy. Arch Dis Child. 1972; 47:344.

123. Price RA et al: The central nervous system in childhood leukemia. II. Subacute leukoencephalopathy. Cancer. 1975; 35:306.

124. Rubinstein LJ et al: Disseminated necrotizing leukoencephalopathy: a complication of treated central nervous system leukemia and lymphoma. Cancer. 1975; 35:291.

125. Novell H et al: Leukoencephalopathy following the administration of methotrexate into the cerebrospinal fluid in the treatment of primary brain tumors. Cancer. 1974; 33:923.

126. Shapiro WR et al: Necrotizing encephalopathy following intraventricular instillation of methotrexate. Arch Neurol. 1973; 28:96.

127. Smith B: Brain damage after intrathecal methotrexate. J Neurol Neurosurg Psychiatry. 1975; 38:810.

128. Green DM et al: Comparison of three methods of central-nervous-system prophylaxis in childhood acute lymphoblastic leukemia. Lancet. 1980; 1:1398.

129. Abelson HT: Methotrexate and central nervous system toxicity. Cancer Treat Rep. 1978; 62:1999.

130. Bleyer WA et al: Neurotoxicity and elevated cerebrospinal-fluid methotrexate concentration in meningeal leukemia. N Engl J Med. 1973; 289:770.

131. Bleyer WA et al: Clinical pharmacology of intrathecal methotrexate. I. Pharmacokinetics in non-toxic patients after lumbar injection. Cancer Treat Rep. 1977; 61:703.

132. Bleyer WA: Clinical pharmacology of intrathecal methotrexate. II. An improved dosage schedule derived from age-related pharmacokinetics. Cancer Treat Rep. 1977; 61:1419.

133. Shapiro WR et al: Methotrexate distribution in cerebrospinal fluid after intravenous, ventricular and lumbar injections. N Engl J Med. 1975; 293:161.

134. Spector R: Inhibition of methotrexate transport from cerebrospinal fluid by probenecid. Cancer Treat Rep. 1976; 60:913.

135. Tejada F et al: Vincristine effect on methotrexate cerebrospinal fluid concentration. Cancer Treat Rep. 1979; 63:143.

136. Rieselbach RE et al: Subarachnoid distribution of drugs after lumbar injection. N Engl J Med. 1967; 267:1273.

137. Echelberger CK et al: Influence of body position on ventricular cerebrospinal fluid methotrexate concentration following intralumbar administration. Proc AACR and ASCO. 1981; 22:365.

138. Levitt M et al: Transport characteristics of folates in cerebrospinal fluid; a study utilizing doubly labeled 5-methyltetrahydrofolate and 5-formyltetrahydrofolate. J Clin Invest. 1971; 50:1301.

139. Simone JV: Preventive central-nervous-system therapy in acute leukemia. N Engl J Med. 1973; 289:1248.

140. Kun LE et al: Meningeal leukemia—control versus cure. Int J Radiat Oncol Biol Phys. 1977; 2:371.

141. Kirs PJ et al: Neuromotor and neuropsychological manifestations of "total therapy" in children with acute lymphoblastic leukemia. Cancer Treat Rev. 1980; 7:85.

142. Soni SS et al: Effects of central-nervous-system irradiation on neuropsychologic functioning of children with acute lymphocytic leukemia. N Engl J Med. 1975; 293:113.

143. Eiser C et al: Retrospective study of intellectual development in children treated for acute lymphoblastic leukaemia. Arch Dis Child. 1977; 52:525.

144. Eiser C: Intellectual abilities among survivors of childhood leukaemia as a function of CNS irradiation. Arch Dis Child. 1978; 53:391.

145. McIntosh S et al: Chronic neurologic disturbance in childhood leukemia. Cancer. 1976; 37:853.

146. Peylan-Ramu N et al: Abnormal CT scans of the brain in asymptomatic children with acute lymphocytic leukemia after prophylactic treatment of the central nervous system with radiation and intrathecal chemotherapy. N Engl J Med. 1978; 298:815.

147. Enzmann DR et al: Enlargement of subarachnoid spaces and lateral ventricles in pediatric patients undergoing chemotherapy. J Pediatr. 1978; 92:535.

148. Ch'ien LT et al: Long-term neurological implications of somnolence syndrome in children with acute lymphocytic leukemia. Ann Neurol. 1980; 8:273.

149. Gangji D et al: Leukoencephalopathy and elevated levels of myelin basic protein in the cerebrospinal fluid of patients with acute lymphoblastic leukemia. N Engl J Med. 1980; 303:19.

150. Nesbit ME et al: Presymptomatic central nervous system therapy in previously untreated childhood acute lymphoblastic leukaemia: comparison of 1800 rad and 2400 rad. Lancet. 1981; 1:461.

151. Freeman AI et al: High-dose methotrexate in acute lymphocytic leukemia. Cancer Treat Rep. 1977; 61:727.

152. Moe PJ et al: High dose methotrexate in acute lymphocytic leukemia in children. Acta Paediatr Scand. 1978; 67:265.

153. Moe PJ et al: Intermediate dose methotrexate in childhood acute lymphocytic leukemia in Norway. Acta Paediatr Scand. 1981; 70:73.

154. Shapiro WR et al: Methotrexate distribution in cerebrospinal fluid after intravenous, ventricular and lumbar injections. N Engl J Med. 1975; 293:161.

155. Bowman WP: Personal communication, 1981.

156. Ochs JJ et al: Computed tomography brain scans in children with acute lymphocytic leukemia receiving methotrexate alone as central nervous system prophylaxis. Cancer. 1980; 45:2274.

157. Goldin A et al: The chemotherapy of human and animal acute leukemia. Cancer Chemother Rep. 1971; 55:309.

158. Acute Leukemia Group B: New treatment schedule with improved survival in childhood leukemia. JAMA. 1965; 194:75.

159. Perrin JCS et al: Intravenous methotrexate (amethopterin) therapy in the treatment of acute leukemia. Pediatrics. 1963; 31:833.

160. Holland JF et al: Chemotherapy of acute lymphocytic leukemia of childhood. Cancer. 1972; 30:1480.

161. Leikin SL et al: The use of combination therapy in leukemia remission. Cancer. 1969; 24:427.

162. Frei E et al: Dose: a critical factor in cancer chemotherapy. Am J Med. 1980; 69:585.

163. Frei E III et al: Studies of sequential and combination anti-metabolite therapy in acute leukemia: 6-mercaptopurine and methotrexate, from the acute leukemia group B. Blood. 1961; 18:431.

164. Simone JV et al: "Total Therapy" studies of acute lymphocytic leukemia in children: current results and prospects for cure. Cancer. 1972; 30:1488.

165. Miller DR et al: Additive therapy in the maintenance of remission in acute lymphoblastic leukemia in childhood: The effect of initial leucocyte count. Cancer. 1974; 34:508.

166. Fernbach DJ et al: Long-term results of reinforcement therapy in children with acute leukemia. Cancer. 1975; 36:1552.

167. Hughes WT et al: Intensity of immunosuppressive therapy and the incidence of Pneumocystis carinii pneumonitis. Cancer. 1975; 36:2004.

168. Berry DH et al: Comparison of prednisolone, vincristine, methotrexate and 6-mercaptopurine vs. 6-mercaptopurine and prednisone maintenance therapy in childhood acute leukemia. Cancer. 1980; 46:1098.

169. Skipper H: On further testing of a strategy aimed at reducing treatment failures due to overgrowth of drug-resistant neoplastic cells. South Res Inst Booklet. 1978; 8.

170. Henderson ES: Combination chemotherapy of acute lymphocytic leukemia of childhood. Cancer Res. 1967; 27:2570.

171. Henderson ES et al: Evidence that drugs in multiple combinations have materially advanced the treatment of human malignancies. Cancer Res. 1969; 29:2272.

172. Wolff JA et al: Prednisone therapy of acute childhood leukemia: Prognosis and duration of response in 330 treated patients. J Pediatr. 1967; 70:626.

173. MRC Working Party on Leukemia in Childhood: Treatment of acute lymphoblastic leukaemia: effect of variation in length of treatment on duration of remission. Br Med J. 1977; 2:495.

174. Krivit W et al: The need for chemotherapy after prolonged complete remission in acute leukemia of childhood. J Pediatr. 1970; 76:138.

175. Hughes WT et al: Infectious disease in children with cancer. Pediatr Clin North Am. 1974; 21:3.

176. Simone JV: Fatalities during remission of childhood leukemia. Blood. 1972; 39:759.

177. Proceedings of the National Cancer Institute Conference on the delayed consequences of cancer therapy: Proven and Potential. Cancer. 1976; 37:999.

178. Simone JV: Treatment of children with acute lymphocytic leukemia. Adv Pediatr. 1972; 19:13.

179. Moe PJ: Cessation of therapy in childhood leukemia: a survey of 160 cases from the Nordic countries. Acta Paediatr Scand. 1978; 67:145.

180. Mandelli F et al: Discontinuing therapy in childhood acute lymphocytic leukemia. Cancer. 1980; 46:1319.

181. Baum E et al: Relapse rates following cessation of chemotherapy during complete remission of acute lymphocytic leukemia. Med Pediatr Oncol. 1979; 7:25.

182. Borella L et al: Immunologic rebound after cessation of long-term chemotherapy in acute leukemia. Blood. 1972; 40:42.

183. Green AA et al: Immunological rebound after cessation of long-term chemotherapy in acute leukemia II. In vitro response to phytohemagglutin and antigens by peripheral blood and bone marrow. Blood. 1973; 42:99.

184. Report to the Medical Research Council by the Working Party on Leukaemia in Childhood: Effects of varying radiation schedule, cyclophosphamide treatment, and duration of treatment in acute lymphoblastic leukaemia. Br Med J. 1978; 2:787.

185. Nesbit ME et al: Testicular relapse in childhood acute lymphoblastic leukemia: association wth pretreatment patient characteristics and treatment. Cancer. 1980; 45:2009.

186. Land VJ et al: Long-term survival in childhood acute leukemia: "late" relapses. Med Pediatr Oncol. 1979; 7:19.

187. Feldman F et al: Acute leukemia relapse after prolonged remission. J Pediatr. 1970; 76:926.

188. Freireich EJ: Factors influencing patient selection for chemotherapy studies of acute leukemia. J Chron Dis. 1962; 15:251.

189. Miller DR: Prognostic factors in childhood leukemia. J Pediatr. 1975; 87:672.

190. Walters T et al: Poor prognosis in Negro children with acute lymphocytic leukemia. Cancer. 1972; 29:210.

191. Simone JV et al: Initial features and prognosis in 363 children with acute lymphocytic leukemia. Cancer. 1972; 30:2099.

192. Sen L and Borella L: Clinical importance of lymphoblasts with T-markers in childhood acute leukemia. N Engl J Med. 1975; 293:828.

193. Bowman WP et al: Cell markers in lymphomas and leukemias. Adv Intern Med. 1980; 25:391.

194. Aisenberg AC: Cell-surface markers in lymphoproliferative disease. N Engl J Med. 1981; 304:331.

195. Humphrey GB et al: Cell surface markers in acute lymphoblastic leukemia. Ann Clin Lab Sci. 1980; 10:169.

196. Tsukimoto I et al: Surface markers and prognostic factors in acute lymphoblastic leukemia. N Engl J Med. 1976; 294:245.

197. Dow LW et al: Initial prognostic factors and lymphoblast-erythrocyte rosette formation in 109 children with acute lymphoblastic leukemia. Blood. 1977; 50:671.

198. Bowman WP et al: Cell markers in acute lymphocytic leukemia: a clinical perspective. Cancer Res. 1981; 41:4794.

199. Dahl GV et al: High-risk acute lymphocytic leukemia (ALL): problem of early relapse. (Abst. 510) Blood. 1978; 52:244.

200. Harousseau JL et al: High-risk acute lymphocytic leukemia: a study of 141 cases with initial white blood cell counts over 100,000/cu mm. Cancer. 1980; 46:1996.

201. Bennett JM et al: Proposals for the classification of acute leukaemias. Br J Haematol. 1976; 33:451.

202. Wagner VM et al: Correlation of the FAB morphologic criteria and prognosis in acute lymphocytic leukemia of childhood. Am J Pediatr Hematol Oncol. 1979; 1:103.

203. Thiel E et al: T-cell-antigen positive, E-rosette negative acute lymphoblastic leukemia. Blut. 1978; 36:363.

204. Reinherz EL et al: Regulation of the immune response—inducer and suppressor T-lymphocyte subsets in human beings. N Engl J Med. 1980; 303:370.

205. Reinherz EL et al: Subset derivation of T-cell acute lymphoblastic leukemia in man. J Clin Invest. 1979; 64:392.

206. Flandrin G et al: Acute leukemia with Burkitt's tumor cells: a study of six cases with special reference to lymphocyte surface markers. Blood. 1975; 45:183.

207. Chessells JM et al: Acute lymphoblastic leukaemia in children: classification and prognosis. Lancet. 1977; 2:1307.

208. Greaves MF et al: Antisera to acute lymphoblastic leukemia cells. Clin Immunol Immunopathol. 1975; 4:67.

209. Roberts M et al: Acute lymphoblastic leukaemia (ALL) associated antigen-I. Expression in different haematopoietic malignancies. Leuk Res. 1978; 2:105.

210. Pesando JM et al: Leukemia-associated antigens in ALL. Blood. 1979; 54:1240.

211. Greaves MF et al: Acute lymphoblastic leukemia associated antigen. III. Alterations in expression during treatment and in relapse. Leuk Res. 1980; 4:1.

212. Goldstone AH et al: Clonal identification in acute lymphoblastic leukemia. Blood. 1979; 53:892.

213. Sallan SE et al: Cell surface antigens: prognostic implications in childhood acute lymphoblastic leukemia. Blood. 1980; 55;395.

214. Vogler LB et al: Pre-B-cell leukemia: a new phenotype of childhood lymphoblastic leukemia. N Engl J Med. 1978; 298:872.

215. Crist W et al: Clinical and laboratory characterization of pre-B cell leukemia in children. Blood. 1979; (Abst.482) 54:183a.

216. O'Bryan RM et al: Phase II evaluation of adriamycin in human neoplastic disease. Cancer. 1973; 32:1.

217. Middleman E et al: Clinical trials with adriamycin. Cancer. 1971; 28:844.

218. Tan C et al: Adriamycin—an antitumor antibiotic in the treatment of neoplastic diseases. Cancer. 1973; 32:9.

219. Wang JJ et al: Therapeutic effect and toxicity of adriamycin in patients with neoplastic diseases. Cancer. 1971; 28:837.

220. Carter SK: Adriamycin—a review. J Natl Cancer Inst. 1975; 55:1265.

221. Rinehart JJ et al: Adriamycin in 87 patients with osteosarcoma. Cancer Chemother Rep. (Part 3) 1975; 6:305.

222. Henderson IC et al: Adriamycin cardiotoxicity. Am Heart J. 1980; 99:671.

223. Ghione M et al: Cardiotoxic effects of antitumor agents. Cancer Chemother Pharmacol. 1978; 1:25.

224. Lenaz L et al: Cardiotoxicity of adriamycin and related anthracyclines. Cancer Treat Rev. 1976; 3:111.

225. Lefrak EA et al: A clinopathologic analysis of adriamycin cardiotoxicity. Cancer. 1973; 32:302.

226. Dindogiu A et al: Electrocardiographic changes following adriamycin treatment. Med Pediatr Oncol. 1978; 5:65.

227. Gilladoga AC et al: The cardiotoxicity of adriamycin and daunomycin in children. Cancer. 1976; 37:1070.

228. Bristow MR et al: Doxorubicin cardiomyopathy: Evaluation by phonocardiography, endomyocardial biopsy, and cardiac catheterization. Ann Intern Med. 1978; 88:168.

229. Praga C et al: Adriamycin cardiotoxicity: A survey of 1273 patients. Cancer Treat Rep. 1979; 63:827.

230. Von Hoff DD et al: Analysis of risk factors for development of doxorubicin-induced congestive heart failure. Ann Intern Med. 1979; 91:710.

231. Bristow MR et al: Early anthracycline cardiotoxicity. Am J Med. 1978; 65:823.

232. Minow RA et al: Adriamycin cardiomyopathy—risk factors. Cancer. 1977; 39:1397.

233. Billingham ME et al: Adriamycin cardiotoxicity: endomyocardial biopsy evidence of enhancement by irradiation. Am J Surg Pathol. 1977; 1:17.

234. Kinsella TJ et al: Adriamycin cardiotoxicity in stage IV breast cancer: possible enhancement with prior left chest radiation therapy. Int J Radiatr Oncol Biol Phys. 1979; 5:1997.

235. Alexander J et al: Serial assessment of doxorubicin cardiotoxicity with quantitative radionuclide angiocardiography. N Engl J Med. 1979; 300:278.

236. Mason JW et al: Invasive and noninvasive methods of assessing adriamycin cardiotoxic effects in man: superiority of histopathologic assessment using endomyocardial biopsy. Cancer Treat Rep. 1978; 62:857.

237. Billingham ME et al: Anthracycline cardiomyopathy monitored by morphologic changes. Cancer Treat Rep. 1978; 62:865.

238. Von Hoff DD et al: Daunomycin-induced cardiotoxicity in children and adults. Am J Med. 1977; 62:200.

239. Pratt CB et al: Age-related adriamycin cardiotoxicity in children. Cancer Treat Rep. 1978; 62:1381.

240. Mosijczuk AD et al: Anthracycline cardiomyopathy in children. Cancer. 1979; 44:1582.

241. Buzdar AU et al: Adriamycin and mitomycin C: Possible synergistic cardiotoxicity. Cancer Treat Rep. 1978; 62:1005.

242. Kushner JP et al: Cardiomyopathy after widely separated courses of adriamycin exacerbated by actinomycin D and mitomycin. Cancer. 1975; 36:1577.

243. Reich SD et al: Clinical correlations of adriamycin pharmacology. Pharmacol Ther. 1978; 2(C):239.

244. Rinehart JJ et al: Adriamycin cardiotoxicity in man. Ann Intern Med. 1974; 81:475.

245. Al-Ismail SAD et al: Systolic time interval as index of schedule-dependent doxorubicin cardiotoxicity in patients with acute myelogenous leukemia. Br Med J. 1979; 1:1392.

246. Balcerzak SP et al: Systolic time intervals in monitoring adriamycin-induced cardiotoxicity. Cancer Treat Rep. 1978; 62:893.

247. Ramos A et al: Echocardiographic evaluation of adriamycin cardiotoxicity in children. Cancer Treat Rep. 1976; 60:1281.

248. Bloom KR et al: Echocardiography in adriamycin cardiotoxicity. Cancer. 1978; 41:1265.

249. Ritchie JL et al: Anthracycline cardiotoxicity: clinical and pathologic outcomes assessed by radionuclide ejection fraction. Cancer. 1980; 46:1109.

250. Kimball JC et al: Vitamin E and N-acetyl-L-cysteine modification of adriamycin toxicities. Proc AACR and ASCO. 1979; 20:188.

251. Sonneveld P et al: Effect of alpha-tocopherol on the cardiotoxicity of adriamycin in the rat. Cancer Treat Rep. 1976; 60:691.

252. Myers CE et al: Adriamycin: amelioration of toxicity by alpha-tocopherol. Cancer Treat Rep. 1976; 60:961.

253. Doroshow JH et al: The prevention of doxorubicin cardiac toxicity by N-acetyl-L-cysteine. Proc AACR and ASCO. 1979; 20:253.

254. Myers CE et al: Adriamycin: the role of lipid peroxidation in cardiac toxicity and tumor response. Science. 1977; 197:1965.

255. Cortes EP et al: Adriamycin cardiotoxicity: early detection by systolic time interval and possible prevention by coenzyme Q10. Cancer Treat Rep. 1978; 62:887.

256. Vick J et al: Potentiation of the cytotoxicity of adriamycin by the cardio-protective drug carnitine. Proc AACR and ASCO. 1978; 19:148.

257. Weiss AJ et al: Studies on adriamycin using a weekly regimen demonstrating its clinical effectiveness and lack of cardiac toxicity. Cancer Treat Rep. 1976; 60:813.

258. Legha SS et al: Augmentation of adriamycin's therapeutic index by prolonged continuous intravenous infusion for advanced breast cancer. Proc AACR and ASCO. 1979; 20:261.

259. Friedman OM et al: Cyclophosphamide and related phosphoramide mustards: current status and future prospects. Adv Cancer Chemother. 1979; 1:145.

260. Colvin M et al: Alkylating properties of phosphoramide mustard. Cancer Res. 1976; 36:1121.

261. Cox PJ: Cyclophosphamide cystitis—identification of acrolein as the causative agent. Biochem Pharmacol. 1979; 28:2045.

262. Brock N et al: Acrolein, the causative factor of nontoxic side-effects of cyclophosphamide, ifosfamide, trofosfamide and sufosfamide. Arzneim Forsch. 1979; 29:659.

263. Richtsmeier AJ: Urinary bladder tumors after cyclophosphamide. N Engl J Med. 1975; 293:1045.

264. Worth PHL: Cyclophosphamide and the bladder. Br Med J. 1971; 3:182.

265. Wall RL et al: Carcinoma of the urinary bladder in patients receiving cyclophosphamide. N Engl J Med. 1975; 293:271.

266. Johnson WW et al: Urinary bladder fibrosis and telangiectasia associated with long-term cyclophosphamide therapy. N Engl J Med. 1971; 284:290.

267. Aptekar RG et al: Cyclophosphamide-induced, nonhemorrhagic cystitis with abnormal bladder cells. Arthritis Rheum. 1972; 15:530.

268. Goldman RL et al: Hemorrhagic cystitis and cytomegalic inclusions in the bladder associated with cyclophosphamide therapy. Cancer. 1970; 25:7.

269. Lawrence HJ et al: Cyclophosphamide-induced hemorrhagic cystitis in children with leukemia. Cancer. 1975; 36:1572.

270. Jayalakshmamma B and Pinkel D: Urinary bladder toxicity following pelvic irradiation and simultaneous cyclophosphamide therapy. Cancer. 1976; 38:701.

271. Marsh FP et al: Cyclophosphamide necrosis of bladder causing calcification, contracture and reflux, treated by colocystoplasty. Br J Urol. 1971; 43:324.

272. Foad BSI et al: Urinary bladder complications with cyclophosphamide therapy. Arch Intern Med. 1976; 136:616.

273. Mullins GM et al: High-dose cyclophosphamide therapy in solid tumors. Cancer. 1975; 36:1950.

274. Buckner CD et al: High-dose cyclophosphamide therapy for malignant disease. Cancer. 1972; 29:357.

275. Pearlman CK: Cystitis due to Cytoxan: Case report. J Urol. 1966; 95:713.

276. Reynolds RD et al: Hemorrhagic cystitis due to cyclophosphamide. J Urol. 1969; 101:45.

277. Wiseman JC et al: Cyclophosphamide and haemorrhagic cystitis. Med J Aust. 1971; 2:576.

278. Liedberg CF et al: Cyclophosphamide hemorrhagic cystitis. Scand J Urol Nephrol. 1970; 4:183.

279. Hutter AM et al: Cyclophosphamide and severe hemorrhagic cystitis. NY State J Med. 1969; 69:305.

280. Berkson BM et al: Severe cystitis induced by cyclophosphamide, role of surgical management. JAMA. 1973; 225:605.

281. Reeve TS: Treatment of malignant disease with an alkylating agent: Review of 100 patients treated with "Endoxan." Med J Aust. 1961; 1:686.

282. Golin AL et al: Cyclophosphamide hemorrhagic cystitis requiring urinary diversion. J Urol. 1977; 118:110.

283. Bennett AH: Cyclophosphamide and hemorrhagic cystitis. J Urol. 1974; 111:603.

284. Pauwels RPE et al: Therapy in Cytoxan hemorrhagic cystitis. Urol Int. 1970; 25:187.

285. Anderson EE et al: Cyclophosphamide and hemorrhagic cystitis. J Urol. 1967; 97:857.

286. Mahboubi S et al: Ureteritis cystica after treatment of cyclophosphamide induced hemorrhagic cystitis. Urology. 1976; 7:521.

287. Firlit CF: Intractable hemorrhagic cystitis secondary to extensive carcinomatosis: management with formalin solution. J Urol. 1973; 110:57.

288. Shah BC et al: Intravesical instillation of formalin for the management of intractable hematuria. J Urol. 1973; 110:519.

289. Stein M et al: Uncontrollable hemorrhage secondary to bladder carcinoma and cyclophosphamide cystitis: Mt. Sinai hospital experience with intravesical formalin instillation. NY State J Med. 1978; 78:1056.

290. Ansell ID et al: Carcinoma of the bladder complicating cyclophosphamide therapy. Br J Urol. 1975; 47:413.

291. Lapides J: Treatment of delayed intractable hemorrhagic cystitis following radiation or chemotherapy. J Urol. 1970; 104:707.

292. Holstein P et al: Intravesical hydrostatic pressure treatment: new method for control of bleeding from the bladder mucosa. J Urol. 1973; 109:234.

293. Kumar APM et al: Silver nitrate irrigation to control bladder hemorrhage in children receiving cancer therapy. J Urol. 1976; 116:85.

294. Primack A: Amelioration of cyclophosphamide-induced cystitis. J Natl Cancer Inst. 1971; 47:224.

295. Levy L et al: Effect of N-acetylcysteine on some aspects of cyclophosphamide-induced toxicity and immunosuppression. Biochem Pharmacol. 1977; 26:1015.

296. Tolley DA: The effect of N-acetylcysteine on cyclophosphamide cystitis. Br J Urol. 1977; 49:659.

297. Choi S and Simone JV: Acute non-lymphocytic leukemia in 171 children. Med Pediatr Oncol. 1976; 2:119.

298. Gale RP et al: Advances in the treatment of acute myelogenous leukemia. N Engl J Med. 1979; 300:1189.

299. Kobrinsky NL et al: Acute nonlymphocytic leukemia. Pediatr Clin North Am. 1980; 27:345.

300. Weil M et al: Acute granulocytic leukemia: treatment of the disease. Arch Intern Med. 1976; 136:1389.

301. Weil M et al: Daunorubicin in the therapy of acute granulocytic leukemia. Cancer Res. 1973; 33:921.

302. Wiernik PH et al: Randomized clinical comparison of daunorubicin, cytosine arabinoside (NSC-82151) alone with a combination of daunorubicin, cytosine arabinoside (NSC-63878), 6-thioguanine (NSC-752), and pyrimethamine (NSC-3061) for the treatment of acute nonlymphocytic leukemia. Cancer Treat Rep. 1976; 60:41.

303. Wiernik PH et al: A randomized clinical trial of daunorubicin and the combination of prednisone, vincristine, 6-mercaptopurine, and methotrexate in adult acute nonlymphocytic leukemia. Cancer Res. 1972; 32:2023.

304. Cortes E et al: Adriamycin in the treatment of acute myelocytic leukemia. Cancer Chemother Rep. 1972; 56:237.

305. McCredie KB et al: Chemoimmunotherapy of adult acute leukemia. Cancer. 1981; 47:1256.

306. Preisler HD et al: Adriamycin-cytosine arabinoside therapy for adult acute myelocytic leukemia. Cancer Treat Rep. 1977; 61:89.

307. Yates JW et al: A study of daunorubicin vs adriamycin induction and monthly vs bimonthly maintenance in acute myelocytic leukemia from CALGB. Proc AACR and ASCO. 1981; 22:487.

308. Ellison RR et al: Arabinosyl cytosine: a useful agent in the treatment of acute leukemia in adults. Blood. 1968; 32:507.

309. Wang JJ et al: Prolonged infusion of arabinosyl cytosine in childhood leukemia. Cancer. 1970; 25:1.

310. Southwest Oncology Group: Cytarabine for acute leukemia in adults: effects of schedule on therapeutic response. Arch Intern Med. 1974; 133:251.

311. Bodey GP et al: Chemotherapy of acute leukemia: comparison of cytarabine alone and in combination with vincristine, prednisone and cyclophosphamide. Arch Intern Med. 1974; 133:260.

312. Carey RW et al: Comparative study of cytosine arabinoside therapy alone and combined with thioguanine, mercaptopurine or daunorubicin in acute myelocytic leukemia. Cancer. 1975; 36:1560.

313. Clarkson BD et al: Treatment of acute leukemia in adults. Cancer. 1975; 36:775.

314. Gee TS et al: Treatment of adult acute leukemia with arabinosyl cytosine and thioguanine. Cancer. 1969; 23:1019.

315. Lewis JP et al: Randomized clinical trial of cytosine arabinoside and 6-thioguanine in remission induction and consolidation of adult nonlymphocytic adult leukemia. Cancer. 1977; 39:1387.

316. Medical Research Council: Treatment of acute myeloid leukemia with daunorubicin, cytosine arabinoside, mercaptopurine, L-asparaginase, prednisone and thioguanine: results of treatment with five multiple-drug schedules. Br J Haematol. 1974; 27:373.

317. Holland JF et al: Acute myelocytic leukemia. Arch Intern Med. 1976; 136:1377.

318. Glucksberg H et al: Combination chemotherapy for acute nonlymphoblastic leukemia in adults. Cancer Chemother Rep. 1975; 59:1131.

319. Gale RP et al: High remission-induction rate in acute myeloid leukemia. Lancet. 1977; 1:497.

320. Cassileth PA et al: Chemotherapy for adult acute non-lymphocytic leukemia with daunorubicin and cytosine arabinoside. Cancer Treat Rep. 1977; 61:1441.

321. Weinstein HJ et al: Treatment of acute myelogenous leukemia in children and adults. N Engl J Med. 1980; 303:473.

322. Gehan EA et al: Prognostic factors in acute leukemia. Semin Oncol. 1976; 3:271.

323. Levine AS et al: Recent developments in the supportive therapy of acute myelogenous leukemia. Cancer. 1978; 42:883.

324. Mathe G et al: Two epipodophyllotoxin derivatives, VM-26 and VP16213, in the treatment of leukemias, hematosarcomas, and lymphomas. Cancer. 1974; 34:985.

325. Saiki J et al: 5-azacytidine in acute leukemia. Cancer. 1978; 42:2111.

326. Legha SS et al: 4'-(9-Acridinylamino)methanesulfon-m-anisidide (AMSA): a new drug effective in the treatment of adult acute leukemia. Ann Intern Med. 1980; 93(Part 1):17.

327. Bloomfield CD: Treatment of adult nonlymphocytic leukemia—1980. Ann Intern Med. 1980; 93(Part 1):133.

328. Emburg SH et al: Remission maintenance therapy in acute myelogenous leukemia. West J Med. 1977; 126:267.

329. Omura GA et al: A combined clinical trial of chemotherapy vs BCG immunotherapy vs no further therapy in remission maintenance of acute myelogenous leukemia (AML). Proc AACR and ASCO. 1977; 18:272.

330. Lewis JP et al: Maintenance management of acute nonlymphocytic leukemia (ANLL). Cancer Clin Trials. 1981; 4:115.

331. Vaughan WP et al: Long chemotherapy-free remissions after single-cycle timed-sequential chemotherapy for acute myelocytic leukemia. Cancer. 1980; 45:859.

332. Peterson BA et al: Intensive five-drug combination chemotherapy for adult acute non-lymphocytic leukemia. Cancer. 1980; 46:663.

333. Coltman CA et al: Chemotherapy of acute leukemia: a comparison of vincristine, cytarabine, and prednisone alone and in combination with cyclophosphamide or daunorubicin. Arch Intern Med. 1978; 138:1342.

334. Skeel RT et al: Cyclophosphamide, cytosine arabinoside and methotrexate versus cytosine arabinoside and thioguanine for acute non-lymphocytic leukemia in adults. Cancer. 1980; 45:224.

335. Wiernik PH et al: A comparative trial of daunorubicin, cytosine arabinoside, and thioguanine, and a combination of the three agents for the treatment of acute myelocytic leukemia. Med Pediatr Oncol. 1979; 6:261.

336. Wolk RW et al: The incidence of central nervous system leukemia in adults with acute leukemia. Cancer. 1974; 33:863.

337. Dawson DM et al: Neurological complications of acute leukemia in adults: changing rate. Ann Intern Med. 1973; 79:541.

338. Law IP et al: Adult acute leukemia: frequency of central nervous system involvement in long term survivors. Cancer. 1977; 40:1304.

339. Keating MJ et al: Factors related to length of complete remission in adult acute leukemia. Cancer. 1980; 45:2017.

340. Preisler HD: Prediction of response to chemotherapy in acute myelocytic leukemia. Blood. 1980; 56:361.

341. Rustum Y et al: Correlation between leukemic cell retention of 1-beta-D-arabinosyl-cytosine-5'-triphosphate and response to therapy. Cancer Res. 1979; 39:42.

342. Greene W et al: High-dose daunorubicin therapy for acute nonlymphocytic leukemia: correlation of response and toxicity with pharmacokinetics and intracellular daunorubicin reductase activity. Cancer. 1972; 30:1419.

343. Bodey GP et al: Late intensification therapy for acute leukemia in remission: chemotherapy and immunotherapy. JAMA. 1976; 234:1021.

344. Glucksberg H et al: Intensification therapy for acute non-lymphocytic leukemia (AML) in adults. Proc AACR and ASCO. 1981; 22:232.

345. Bodey GP et al: Prolonged remission in adults with acute leukemia following late intensification chemotherapy and immunotherapy. Cancer. 1981; 47:1937.

346. Oettgen HF et al: Immunotherapy of cancer. N Engl J Med. 1977; 297:484.

347. Thomas ED et al: Marrow transplantation in the treatment of acute leukemia. Adv Cancer Res. 1978; 27:269.

348. Thomas ED et al: Current status of bone marrow transplantation for aplastic anemia and acute leukemia. Blood. 1977; 49:671.

349. Thomas ED: Current status of marrow transplantation for aplastic anemia and acute leukemia. Am J Clin Pathol. 1979; 72:887.

350. Thomas ED et al: One hundred patients with acute leukemia treated by chemotherapy, total body irradiation, and allogeneic marrow transplantation. Blood. 1977; 49:511.

351. Fefer A et al: Bone marrow transplantation for refractory acute leukemia in 34 patients with identical twins. Blood. 1981; 57:421.

352. Thomas ED et al: Marrow transplantation for acute B nonlymphoblastic leukemia in first remission. N Engl J Med. 1979; 301:597.

353. Graze PR et al: Autotransplantation for leukemia and solid tumors. Transplant Proc. 1978; 10:177.

354. Various authors: Marrow transplantation for acute nonlymphoblastic leukemia. N Engl J Med. 1980; 302:408.

355. Various authors: Marrow transplantation and acute nonlymphocytic leukemia. Ann Intern Med. 1980; 93:778.

356. Glatstein E et al: Non-Hodgkin's lymphomas. VI. Results of treatment in children. Cancer. 1974; 34:204.

357. Lemerle M et al: Lymphosarcoma and reticulum cell sarcoma in children. Retrospective study of 172 cases. Cancer. 1973; 32: 1499.

358. Murphy SB et al: A study of childhood non-Hodgkin's lymphoma. Cancer. 1975; 36:2121.

359. Brecher ML et al: Non-Hodgkin's lymphoma in children. Cancer. 1978; 41:1997.

360. Carabell SC et al: The role of radiation therapy in the treatment of pediatric non-Hodgkin's lymphomas. Cancer. 1978; 42:2193.

361. Lau BM et al: Childhood malignant lymphoma. Favourable outlook with aggressive combination chemotherapy and radiotherapy. Eur J Cancer. 1977; 13:1237.

362. Wollner N et al: Non-Hodgkin's lymphoma in children. A comparative study of two modalities of therapy. Cancer. 1976; 37:123.

363. Murphy SB et al: A randomized trial of combined modality therapy of childhood non-Hodgkin's lymphoma. Cancer. 1980; 45:630.

364. Murphy SB: The management of childhood non-Hodgkin's lymphoma. Cancer Treat Rep. 1977; 61:1161.

365. Murphy SB: Childhood non-Hodgkin's lymphoma. N Engl J Med. 1978; 299:1446.

366. Murphy SB: Classification, staging and end-results of treatment of childhood non-Hodgkin's lymphomas: dissimilarities from lymphomas in adults. Semin Oncol. 1980; 7:332.

367. Jones SE et al: Non-Hodgkin's lymphomas. IV. Clinicopathologic correlation in 405 cases. Cancer. 1973; 31:806.

368. Frizzera G et al: Follicular (nodular) lymphoma in childhood: a rare clinical-pathological entity. Cancer. 1979; 44:2218.

369. Nathwani BN: A critical analysis of the classifications of non-Hodgkin's lymphomas. Cancer. 1979; 44:347.

370. Coccia PF et al: Prognostic significance of surface marker analysis in childhood non-Hodgkin's lymphoproliferative malignancies. Am J Hematol. 1976; 1:405.

371. Stein RS et al: Correlations between immunologic markers and histopathologic classifications: clinical implications. Semin Oncol. 1980; 7:244.

372. Jenkin RDT: Radiation in the treatment of non-Hodgkin's lymphoma in children. Semin Oncol. 1977; 4:311.

373. Bonadonna G et al: Recent trends in the treatment of non-Hodgkin's lymphomas. Eur J Cancer. 1976; 12:661.

374. Canellos GP et al: Chemotherapy of the non-Hodgkin's lymphomas. Cancer. 1978; 42:932.

375. Sweet DL et al: The treatment of histiocytic lymphoma. Semin Oncol. 1980; 7:302.

376. Lewis BJ et al: Combination therapy of the lymphomas. Semin Hematol. 1978; 15:431.

377. Wollner N et al: Non-Hodgkin's lymphoma in children: Results of treatment with LAS-L2 Protocol. Br J Cancer. 1975; 31:337.

378. Wollner N et al: Non-Hodgkin's lymphoma in children. Cancer. 1979; 44:1990.

379. Pinkel D et al: Non-Hodgkin's lymphoma in children. Br J Cancer. 1975; 31:298.

380. Aur RJA: Therapy of localized and regional lymphosarcoma of childhood. Cancer. 1971; 27:1328.

381. Dargeon HW: Neuroblastoma. J Pediatr. 1962; 61:456.

382. Evans AR: Congenital neuroblastoma. J Clin Pathol. 1965; 18:54.

383. Holland T et al: The current mechanism of neuroblastoma. J Urol. 1980; 124:579.

384. Jaffe N: Neuroblastoma: Review of the literature and an examination of factors contributing to its enigmatic character. Cancer Treat Rev. 1976; 3:61.

385. Hayes FA et al: Neuroblastoma. In Practice of Pediatrics III (Chapter 77), Harper and Row, pp 1–6.

386. Breslow N et al: Statistical estimation of prognosis for children with neuroblastoma. Cancer Res. 1971; 31:2098.

387. Everson TC and Cole WH: In *Spontaneous Regression of Cancer*. WB Saunders Co., Philadelphia, pp 11–87, 1966.

388. Knudson AG et al: Regression of neuroblastoma IV-S: a genetic hypothesis. N Engl J Med. 1980; 302:1254.

389. Thurman WG et al: Cyclophosphamide therapy in childhood neuroblastoma. N Engl J Med. 1964; 270:1336.

390. Windmiller J et al: Vincristine sulfate in the treatment of neuroblastoma in children. Am J Dis Child. 1966; 11:75.

391. Evans AE et al: Vincristine sulfate and cyclophosphamide for children with metastatic neuroblastoma. JAMA. 1969; 207:1325.

392. Pinkel D et al: Survival of children with neuroblastoma treated with combination chemotherapy. J Pediatr. 1968; 73:928.

393. Sullivan MP et al: Evaluation of vincristine sulfate and cyclophosphamide chemotherapy for metastatic neuroblastoma. Pediatrics. 1969; 44:685.

394. Sawitsky A: Vincristine and cyclophosphamide therapy in generalized neuroblastoma. Am J Dis Child. 1970; 119:308.

395. Finklestein JZ et al: 5-(3,3-Dimethyl-1-1-triazeno) imidazole-4-carboxamide (NSC-45388) in the treatment of solid tumors in children. Cancer Chemother Rep. 1975; 59:351.

396. Nitsche R et al: Cis-diamminedichloroplatinum (NSC-119875) in childhood malignancies. A Southwest Oncology Group Study. Med Pediatr Oncol. 1978; 4:127.

397. Bleyer WA et al: Phase II study of VM-26 in acute leukemia, neuroblastoma, and other refractory childhood malignancies: a report from the Children's Cancer Study Group. Cancer Treat Rep. 1979; 63:977.

398. Rivera G et al: Epipodophyllotoxin VM-26 in the treatment of childhood neuroblastoma. Cancer Treat Rep. 1977; 61:1243.

399. Green AA et al: Sequential cyclophosphamide and adriamycin for induction of complete remissions in children with disseminated neuroblastoma. Cancer. 1982; 48:2310.

400. Finklestein JZ et al: Multiagent chemotherapy for children with metastatic neuroblastoma: a report from Children's Cancer Study Group. Med Pediatr Oncol. 1979; 6:179.

401. Hayes FA et al: Correlation of cell kinetic and clinical response to chemotherapy in disseminated neuroblastoma. Cancer Res. 1977; 37:3766.

402. Hayes FA et al: Clinical evaluation of sequentially scheduled cisplatin and VM-26 in neuroblastoma; response and toxicity. Cancer. 1982; 48:1715.

403. Green DM et al: Wilms' tumor—a model of a curable pediatric malignant solid tumor. Cancer Treat Rev. 1977; 5:143.

404. Farber S: Chemotherapy in the treatment of leukemia and Wilms' tumor. JAMA. 1966; 198:826.

405. D'Angio GJ et al: The treatment of Wilms' tumor. Cancer. 1976; 38:633.

406. D'Angio GJ et al: Wilms' tumor: an update. Cancer. 1980; 45:1791.

407. D'Angio GJ et al: The treatment of Wilms' tumor: results of the second national Wilms' tumor study. Cancer. 1981; 47:2302.

408. Beckwith JB et al: Histopathology and prognosis of Wilms' tumor. Results from the First National Wilms' Tumor Study. Cancer. 1978; 41:1937.

409. Morgan E et al: Undifferentiated sarcoma of the kidney. A tumor of childhood with histopathologic and clinical characteristics distinct from Wilms' tumor. Cancer. 1978; 42:1916.

410. Breslow NE et al: Wilms' tumor: prognostic factors for patients without metastases at diagnosis—Results of the National Wilms' Tumor Study. Cancer. 1978; 41:1577.

411. Sullivan MP et al: Vincristine sulfate in management of Wilms' tumor. JAMA. 1967; 202:38.

412. Vietti TJ et al: Vincristine sulfate and radiation therapy in metastatic Wilms' tumor. Cancer. 1970; 25:12.

413. Wolff JA et al: Long-term evaluation of single versus multiple courses of actinomycin D therapy of Wilms' tumor. N Engl J Med. 1974; 290:84.

414. Burgert EO et al: Dactinomycin in Wilms' tumor. JAMA. 1967; 199:464.

415. Wolff JA et al: Single versus multiple dose dactinomycin therapy of Wilms' tumor. N Engl J Med. 1968; 279:290.

416. Miller RW: Leukemia in survivors of Wilms' tumor. J Pediatr. 1975; 87:505.

417. Jaffe N et al: Childhood urologic cancer therapy related sequelae and their impact on management. Cancer. 1980; 45:1815.

418. Marcove RC et al: Osteogenic sarcoma under the age of twenty-one. J Bone Joint Surg. 1962; 52:42.

419. Friedman MA et al: The theory of osteogenic sarcoma: current status and thoughts for the future. J Surg Oncol. 1972; 4:482.

420. Jaffe N: The potential of combined modality approaches for the treatment of malignant bone tumors in children. Cancer Treat Rev. 1975; 2:33.

421. Weiss RB et al: Multimodal primary cancer treatment (adjuvant chemotherapy): Current results and future prospects. Ann Intern Med. 1979; 91:251.

422. Frei E et al: Adjuvant chemotherapy of osteogenic sarcoma: progress and perspectives. J Natl Cancer Inst. 1978; 60:3.

423. Sutuw WW: Multidrug chemotherapy in osteosarcoma. Clin Orthop. 1980; 153:67.

424. Carter SK: The dilemma of adjuvant chemotherapy for osteogenic sarcoma. Cancer Clin Trials. 1980; 3:29.

425. Muggia FM et al: Five years of adjuvant treatment of osteosarcoma: more questions than answers. Cancer Treat Rep. 1978; 62:301.

426. Kolata GB: Dilemma in cancer treatment. Science. 1980; 209:792.

427. Edmonson JH et al: Methotrexate as adjuvant treatment for primary osteosarcoma. N Engl J Med. 1980; 303:642.

428. Jaffe N: Recent advances in the chemotherapy of metastatic osteogenic sarcoma. Cancer. 1972; 30:1627.

429. Djreassi I: High-dose methotrexate (NSC 740) and citrovorum factor (NSC 3590) rescue: background and rationale. Cancer Chemother Rep. 1975; (Part 3)6:3.

430. Zager RF et al: The effects of antibiotics and cancer chemotherapeutic agents on the cellular transport and antitumor activity of methotrexate in L1210 murine leukemia. Cancer Res. 1973; 33:1670.

431. Evans WE et al: Unproven efficacy of vincristine-methotrexate combination therapy. Am J Hosp Pharm. 1978; 35:779.

432. Ridgway D et al: Vincristine in the etiology of toxicity of high-dose methotrexate therapy. Cancer. 1980; 46:2571.

433. Jaffe N et al: Adjuvant methotrexate and citrovorum-factor treatment of osteogenic sarcoma. N Engl J Med. 1974; 291:994.

434. Jaffe N et al: High-dose methotrexate with citrovorum factor in osteogenic sarcoma—progress report II. Cancer Treat Rep. 1977; 61:675.

435. Cortes EP et al: Doxorubicin in disseminated osteosarcoma. J Am Med Assoc. 1972; 221:1132.

436. Pratt CB et al: Doxorubicin in treatment of malignant solid tumors in children. Am J Dis Child. 1974; 127:534.

437. Wang J et al: Therapeutic effect and toxicity of adriamycin in patients with neoplastic disease. Cancer. 1971; 28:837.

438. Cortes EP et al: Amputation and adriamycin in primary osteosarcoma. N Engl J Med. 1974; 291:998.

439. Cortes EP et al: Amputation and adriamycin in primary osteosarcoma: a 5-year report. Cancer Treat Rep. 1978; 62:271.

440. Jaffe N et al: High-dose methotrexate in osteogenic sarcoma: a 5-year experience. Cancer Treat Rep. 1978; 62:259.

441. Ochs JJ et al: Cis-dichlorodiammineplatinum (II) in advanced osteogenic sarcoma. Cancer Treat Rep. 1978; 62:239.

442. Ettinger LJ et al: Adjuvant adriamycin and cis-diaminedichloroplatinum (cis-platinum) in primary osteosarcoma. Cancer. 1981; 47:248.

443. Eilber FR et al: Adjuvant therapy for osteosarcoma: preoperative and postoperative treatment. Cancer Treat Rep. 1978; 62:213.

444. Etcubanas E et al: Adjuvant chemotherapy for osteogenic sarcoma. Cancer Treat Rep. 1978; 62:283.

445. Pratt CB et al: Combination chemotherapy for osteosarcoma. Cancer Treat Rep. 1978; 62:251.

446. Rosenberg SA et al: The treatment of osteogenic sarcoma. I. Effect of adjuvant high-dose methotrexate following amputation. Cancer Treat Rep. 1979; 63:739.

447. Sutow WW et al: Multidrug adjuvant chemotherapy for osteosarcoma: interim report of the Southwest Oncology Group studies. Cancer Treat Rep. 1978; 62:265.

448. Pratt CB et al: Osteosarcoma—outcome of therapy for 100 patients at St. Jude Children's Research Hospital 1973–1980. Proc AACR and ASCO. 1981; 22:428.

449. Taylor WF et al: Trends and variability in survival from osteosarcoma. Mayo Clin Proc. 1978; 53:695.

450. Marcove RC: En bloc resection of osteogenic sarcoma. Cancer Treat Rep. 1978; 62:225.

451. Edmonson JH et al: Post-surgical treatment of primary osteosarcoma of bone—comparison of high dose methotrexate vs observation: preliminary report. Proc AACR and ASCO. 1980; 21:476.

452. Rosen G et al: Primary osteogenic sarcoma—the rationale for preoperative chemotherapy and delayed surgery. Cancer. 1979; 43:2163.

Chapter 44

Psychoses

Larry Ereshefsky and Glen L. Stimmel

Systematic drug therapy monitoring of the psychiatric patient requires specialized skills and knowledge. The assessment of therapeutic efficacy and adverse drug effects is most efficiently accomplished by blending traditional medical record or patient profile reviews with direct patient contact and observation (1). The technique of mental status examination is a structured, reproducible evaluation of the patient. This chapter will use terminology based on mental status assessment observations, defining nomenclature but not elaborating on the mechanics of the process itself. The reader is referred elsewhere for reviews on interviewing techniques (2–4).

Psychotic disorders are one of the major psychiatric classifications where drug therapy is the mainstay of contemporary treatment. Psychosis is a descriptor useful in categorizing the severity of a behavioral disturbance. It can best be defined as the inability of the person to function in our society (provide food, clothing, and shelter) due to a loss of reality testing, affective function (mood disorders), or orientation. Schizophrenia and schizophreniform disorders have a combined prevalence of 1–2% and comprise the majority of psychotic behavioral manifestations treated with antipsychotic (neuroleptic, major tranquilizer) agents (5).

Antipsychotic agents are useful in non-schizophrenic psychoses (eg, mania, psychotic depression, psychotic organic brain syndrome), but a discussion of their use in these disorders is beyond the scope of this chapter. The symptoms of psychosis amenable to neuroleptic treatment "cut across" psychiatric diagnostic labels. Therefore a target symptom approach to drug therapy for psychosis, using schizophrenia as a common example, is advocated throughout the chapter. Comments regarding the efficacy, limitations, adverse effects, and precautions of neuroleptic drug use in the treatment of schizophrenia apply to these other indications as well.

SCHIZOPHRENIA

Schizophrenia is a cluster of related difficulties in behavior, thoughts, and feelings. It has a chronic, fluctuating course. Clinical manifestations in a patient may be similar to or very different from those in other schizophrenics. Schizophrenic patients may be floridly psychotic, yet at other times they may be in total control of their behavior,

thoughts, and feelings. Commonly encountered symptoms of schizophrenia (6) include Bleuler's 4 A's: autism (preoccupation with internal stimuli), inappropriate affect (emotional responsiveness), associational disturbances (illogical or idiosyncratic thought processes), and ambivalence (opposing, contradictory thinking). Schneider identified symptoms which are among the most commonly observed in the acutely psychotic patient. These symptoms include: ego boundary disruptions such as depersonalization, out-of-body experiences, made impulses ("people control me"), thought broadcast or insertion (described as resembling ESP), and hallucinations. Delusions (fixed false beliefs) are constructed to explain the psychotic experience. Mendel, in seeking to establish precision in the diagnosis of schizophrenia, has identified the following three basic disabilities of function which are the trademark of schizophrenia (7). Whether in psychotic exacerbation or remission, schizophrenics show difficulties in: (a.) anxiety management, (b.) interpersonal relationships, and (c.) learning from experience (failure of historicity). The symptoms of psychosis are secondary to these three disabilities and essentially represent attempts at restitution, or are the physiological or psychological consequence of these disabilities. No single schizophrenic will demonstrate all of these symptoms. The schizophrenic's presentation is extremely variable from day to day and from exacerbation to exacerbation.

Schizophrenia is best described as being one type of psychosis. Schizophrenia is the most common of the functional psychoses. Other functional psychoses include the major affective disorders, paranoid states, and reactive psychosis. There is also a wide variety of organic psychoses: dementias, alcoholic psychosis, and psychoses associated with cerebral, intracranial and cerebral vascular disturbances, endocrine and metabolic disorders, systemic infection, drug or poison intoxication, and childbirth (8).

Diagnosis. The patient's presentation during a psychotic episode does *not* clearly dictate the diagnosis. Psychosis can be thought of as a common final pathway for severe mental illness, and most of the psychotic behaviors are nonspecific (9). Current psychiatric diagnostic criteria as outlined in the Diagnostic and Statistical Manual for Psychiatric Disorders, Third Edition (DSM-III) reflect this controversy (10). Differentiation of manic episodes and drug-induced psychosis from schizophrenia is among the most commonly encountered diagnostic and treatment dilemmas (11).

Crucial to the diagnosis of schizophrenia is the concept of chronicity. The *course* of the illness is more important in the differential diagnosis than the number and severity of presenting symptoms. DSM-III outlines the schizophrenic's course as deteriorating over time in such areas as work, social relations, and self-care. The signs of illness should be present for at least six months, and a residual impairment should be observed in the spheres of social behavior, perceptual experiences, affective responses, and thought processes. In contrast, schizophreniform illness meets all the criteria for schizophrenia, except the duration of illness is greater than two weeks but less than 6 months. Brief reactive psychosis is behaviorally similar to schizophrenia; it lasts more than a few hours but less than two weeks.

Many classification systems have been proposed for schizophrenia, based upon symptomatology, perceived etiology, and premorbid condition. DSM-III redefines schizophrenia, incorporating many of the criteria from the research diagnostic criteria of Feighner and colleagues. These new categories are described below (10).

Disorganized schizophrenia is characterized by marked incoherence with a nonresponsive (flat), inappropriate or silly affective presentation. There are no well developed (systematized) delusions, although diffuse or poorly thought-out (fragmentary) delusions and hallucinations are common. Associated features include grimaces and other repetitive unconscious behaviors (stereotypical mannerisms), hypochondriacal complaints, and extreme social withdrawal. In other classification systems this type is termed hebephrenic.

Catatonic schizophrenia is characterized by marked psychomotor disturbances which can present as stupor, rigidity, strange body language (posturing), or excitement. Sometimes there is rapid alternation between the extremes of excitement and stupor. Noncommunicativeness (mutism) is particularly common. Associated features include stereotypy and a unique form of posturing with rigidity in which the patient's extremities when placed in a given position slowly fall to their sides like molten wax (waxy flexibility).

Paranoid schizophrenia is manifested by prominent persecutory or grandiose delusions, or hallucinations with a persecutory or grandiose content. Associated features include anxiety, anger, argumentativeness, and violence. Many individuals will express doubts or fears concerning their gender identity. Preoccupation with homosexual ideation is quite common.

Undifferentiated schizophrenia, the largest category, is used for the diagnosis whenever prominent psychotic symptoms cannot be classified in any category previously listed. Therefore, this is a category of schizophrenia in which an individual's clinical behavior matches portions of more than one of the descriptions listed above.

Residual schizophrenia is a category which is used when there has been at least one previous episode. The clinical picture should be one of emotional blunting, social withdrawal, eccentric behavior, illogical thinking, and loosening of associations. Prominent psychotic symptoms should be absent, though impairment in daily living skills is commonly observed.

Progression of Symptoms. Prior to the onset of psychotic symptomatology, schizophrenic patients commonly undergo subtle changes in their behavior (12,13). During early stages, patients commonly feel worried, unhappy, and anxious. They perceive a "nervousness about their thoughts and interactions with others." They can be suspicious of close associates and frequently do not make friends easily, if at all. They gradually become withdrawn and can have difficulty in finishing their education or in maintaining employment. This pattern of behavior is classified as schizoid. As time passes, patients will spend increasing amounts of time ruminating about seemingly trivial associations and significances. The initial denial of mental illness will not prevent a gradual increase in levels of anxiety. Intensification of the psychotic process, often precipitated by environmental stress, causes a panic state. At this point the first signs of mental illness will become readily apparent. Psychic disorganization ensues, causing a retreat into fantasy (primary process thinking) which leads to impaired reality testing. Personal appearance is ignored; sex and religion usually become frequent topics of rumination. Finally, they find relief in false beliefs, simple defenses, symbolic interpretations, grandiose and paranoid ideation, and further interpersonal retreat. Patients often describe "special" experiences; for example, colors seem brighter, sounds seem louder, and thoughts come more clearly. This *schizophreniform cognitive mode* is a descriptive model characterizing the initial thought and information processing disturbances believed to be fundamental to the psychotic process (14). A defective limbic system "filter" is postulated to be the cause of this schizophreniform cognitive mode (15).

One can view drug therapy as an attempt to improve limbic function, allowing an individual to handle increased stress levels. The schizophrenic will learn behaviors that minimize stress. Social withdrawal, seeming amotivation, and blunted affect can all be viewed as a schizophrenic's attempt to "hold himself together." These behaviors are secondary to the overload of affects, thoughts, and sensory perceptions considered part of the schizophreniform cognitive mode. Delusions and paranoid ideation can be classified as acute or chronic. The chronic schizophrenic accepts his delusions as the "reason or explanation" for his illness. These delusions form a framework around which the person can build as unstressed a life as possible (14).

Mechanism of Antipsychotic Drug Action. The biochemical, neuroanatomic cause of the "core symptoms" discussed is postulated to be limbic system dysfunction. An understanding of the progression of the schizophrenic process is necessary for evaluation of drug effects (14).

Although the exact mechanism of antipsychotic activity of neuroleptic drugs has not been identified, much data have accumulated to suggest central dopaminergic receptor blockade of the limbic system as an essential feature for drug effect (16–18). It has been shown that the antipsychotic, extrapyramidal, and antiemetic effects of neuroleptic drugs are related to their interactions with central dopaminergic receptors. There appears to be more than one type of dopamine receptor in the CNS. Receptor binding studies suggest that differential affinities of antipsychotic agents for limbic (therapeutic effects) and nigrostriatal (extrapyramidal side effects) dopamine receptors may lead to a breakthrough in the treatment of psychosis with less extrapyramidal symptoms and tardive dyskinesia (19). Understanding of the antipsychotic agents' effects on neurotransmitters is useful in explaining and predicting many of their clinical and toxic effects (20).

The descriptions of patients which follow are based on the authors' clinical experiences. The overall treatment philosophy is conservative. The literature contains contradictions, periodic reversals in treatment philosophies, and redefini-

tions of diagnostic criteria. The clinician must carefully evaluate the psychiatric literature and integrate and conceptualize the information into a working model that is continuously modified by clinical experience and new information.

The following case history reflects many of the typical features of the schizophrenic patient and will serve as the basis for the questions that follow.

1. *Description of Schizophrenia.* **P.L., a 29-year-old single unemployed male, was committed by the court to an acute psychiatric ward after standing on a window sill and threatening to jump. The patient complained of being frightened and of hearing voices which told him to kill himself. (Admission date July 1979.)**

History of Present Illness: The patient cannot relate the exact events leading up to hospitalization. He wants protection from the people trying to "mess up his mind." He stopped taking his medication one month after his discharge from a California state hospital. He felt an urge to make it on his own and moved to San Antonio. He rented a motel room, found a job distributing leaflets, and "kept to myself, minded my own business." Two weeks prior to admission, the patient began to hear voices telling him to prepare for his mission to save the United States from the Communists. The patient reports a progressive increase in anxiety, suspiciousness of people, and inability to sleep at night. He reports strange experiences such as "the radio's music contains coded messages, people are reading my mind, colors seem brighter, and sounds are clearer than usual." The policeman who removed him from the windowsill noted strange stereotypical movements where the patient would "freeze up," stare towards the sky and raise and lower his hands over his head repeatedly.

Past Medical History: In 1970 he was hospitalized for four months in Dallas because of a "nervous breakdown." He states he received electroconvulsive therapy (ECT) and chlorpromazine (Thorazine). "Thorazine made me a zombie." In 1972, he underwent surgery on his arm after jumping from a car in a suicide attempt. In 1973, he was hospitalized for three months after a suicide attempt with diet pills. From February to May 1974, he was hos-

pitalized in Texas for "nervous problems and hearing voices." During his last admission, he received thiothixene (Navane) 10 mg three times a day, which he describes as "good stuff."

Family History: A brother was treated for "nerves" with thiothixene and "did well."

Personal History: The patient denies any childhood problems such as bedwetting, fire-setting, or phobias. At age 16 he was seen by a child psychiatrist because of destructive behavior and was treated with medication. In 1970 he was engaged to a girl who worked as a stripper; he terminated his relationship with her and then started homosexual involvements. He denies any recent homosexual experiences. He has worked odd jobs, never holding a single job for more than six months.

Physical Examination on Admission: Unremarkable.

Mental Status Examination on Admission: *Appearance and Behavior:* He presents as a somewhat thin, disheveled individual, talking in a monotone voice and displaying marked motor restlessness. Despite the warm temperature in the interviewer's office, he refuses to take off his long coat and hat. His pants and shirt are on inside out. *Mood:* Very anxious and fretful, concerned that he has failed his mission and that the CIA is after him to kill him. While talking about the CIA, he laughs and smiles. *Sensorium:* Oriented to time, place, and person. *Thoughts:* The patient is suspicious. He demands to see the examiner's medical license, asking if the room is "bugged." His associations are loosened (his train of thought jumps around: "Why am I here? The time of day is wrong for supper. They aren't here yet, and I should be watching out for them. Why are you writing notes—are you a spy?"). He complains that the CIA

has let him down and now he must complete his mission on his own. Voices (auditory hallucinations) tell him what to do and he "cannot disobey these commands." Insight and judgment are poor. Motivation for treatment is absent and the patient denies mental illness. He appears to have suicidal ideation.

Provisional Diagnosis: Schizophrenia, paranoid type, chronic course with acute exacerbation (from Diagnostic and Statistical Manual of Mental Disorders, 3rd Edition).

What is P.L.'s prognosis? What factors in P.L.'s past psychiatric history are consistent with schizophrenia?

The age of onset of psychotic symptoms (20-years-old), the course of P.L.'s illness, and the symptoms are all consistent with schizophrenia. Typical ages of onset for schizophrenia range from late adolescence to the early 30's (21). The chronic course of the disorder, with acute exacerbations as manifested by repeated hospitalizations, further supports the diagnosis (7). His family history of a brother with psychiatric problems responsive to thiothixene is also consistent with the diagnosis.

Childhood adjustment problems (poor premorbid history) followed by socially inappropriate relationships indicate that a poor prognosis is likely in this individual (22,23). A structured environment may be required when he has regained his highest level of functioning. P.L.'s self-care skills and coping abilities are probably not adequate to allow him to lead a "normal life" (eg, marriage, children, steady employment). Nonetheless, with antipsychotic medications, the need for long-term custodial care in a psychiatric facility will be greatly reduced. Predictors for good and poor prognosis in schizophrenics, sometimes designated as reactive and process schizophrenia, are listed in Table 1.

Table 1.

PROGNOSTICATORS OF OUTCOME FOR SCHIZOPHRENICS

Feature	Good Prognosis	Poor Prognosis
Premorbid adjustment	Good	Poor
Precipitating factors	Present	Absent
Onset of symptoms	Sudden	Insidious
Family history	Positive for Affective Illness	Positive for Schizophrenia
Sensorium	Clear	Dream-like
Affective symptoms	Present	Blunted affect

2. What target symptoms of schizophrenia are present in P.L.? How are target symptoms utilized in therapy?

P.L. demonstrates the following target symptoms: agitation, anxiety, paranoid delusions ("The CIA is after me"), loose associations ("Why am I here? The time of day is wrong for supper."), auditory hallucinations (voices tell him what to do), illusions (radio music contains messages), paranoid ideation with suspiciousness ("Are you a spy? Is the room bugged?"), made impulses (voices tell him to jump off buildings), grandiosity (mission to save the United States), poor self-care skills (clothes inside out, dirty and disheveled appearance), and limited insight and judgment (denies being sick).

Target symptoms are utilized as monitoring parameters for drug therapy. They are not meant to be diagnostic for a single category of mental disease. Assessment of abnormal functioning in all spheres of the mental status examination is useful in the management of drug therapy (14). Changes in target symptoms are among the most important criteria for assessment of drug therapy. Typical target symptoms observed in schizophrenia are listed in Table 2.

NEUROLEPTIC THERAPY

3. Which of P.L.'s target symptoms are likely to respond to drug therapy?

Table 3 lists common target symptoms in order of probability of drug responsiveness. Symptoms of anxiety, sensory, thought, and affective overload respond best to antipsychotic agents (eg, agitation, hostility, hallucinations, paranoia); long-term learned responses to illness are much less amenable to drug therapy (amotivation, blunted affect, or social withdrawal) (24). Clearly, the younger schizophrenic less set in his ways will respond better in all spheres of function to drug therapy.

4. How long will it usually take for a patient like P.L. to respond to drug therapy?

Initial response to neuroleptics in P.L. would be expected to occur within two to seven days. Lehman (25) postulates that there are four stages to the schizophrenic's response to drug therapy. During the initial stage, termed *medicated cooperation,* the patient responds to the calming properties of the major tranquilizers. This stage usu-

Table 2.

TARGET SYMPTOMS OF SCHIZOPHRENIA BY MENTAL STATUS EXAM

Appearance
  Bizarre or disheveled
  Poor hygiene
Behavior
  Distractability
  Bizarre actions
  Restlessness
  Suicidal or Assaultive
  Insomnia
Mood and Affect
  Inappropriate emotional responsiveness (blunted or flat)
  Agitation
  Anxiety
Sensorium
  Usually unimpaired (time, place, person)
Intellectual Function
  Average intelligence
  Poor insight
  Poor judgment
Thought Processes
  Loosened associations (disconnected thoughts and illogical thinking)
  Delusional ideation (fixed false beliefs)
  Hallucinations (perception of sensory stimulus not there)
  Concrete interpretations (cannot do abstract thinking)
  Suspiciousness
  Ideas of reference (incorrect interpretation of events as having reference to one's self)
  Illusions (misperception of a real stimulus)

ally occurs within the first week of therapy. The second stage, *improved socialization,* usually occurs within the first two to six weeks of drug therapy. During the socialization stage, the patient begins to obey ward or society rules and begins to act in a socially appropriate fashion. Many severely ill schizophrenics never achieve totally normal socialization. The third stage is the *elimination of thought disorder* and this can occur within any time frame. During this phase the individual will begin to think and behave more normally. This is due to a decrease in delusions, associational disturbances, paranoid ideation, and sensory overload. Many individuals can function in our society even though their thought disorder is not entirely eliminated. It is more important

Table 3.

RELATIVE RESPONSIVENESS OF TARGET SYMPTOMS TO DRUG THERAPY

Most Responsive

Combativeness and Hostility
Tension and Hyperactivity
Hallucinations
Sleep
Appetite
Dress
Delusions
Social Skills
Affect
Realistic Planning
Judgment
Insight

Least Responsive

for an individual to be able to handle his handicap than to completely eradicate the persistent hallucination or delusion that is refractory to drug therapy. The final stage is the *maintenance therapy* stage, and this is the period of time where an individual can most benefit from non-drug therapies. Behavior modification, vocational training, and resocialization training are important additional steps to allow the patient to function at a higher level than drug therapy alone would allow. Initially, response to behavioral control can be hastened by a more aggressive, high-dose therapy and/or parenteral administration of the more potent neuroleptic drugs (26).

5. *Drug Selection.* Why would thiothixene be a reasonable choice of neuroleptics for P.L.?

Previous response is the best prognosticator for therapeutic success in subsequent exacerbations of a schizophrenic process (25). Additionally, the metabolic and pharmacodynamic variables affecting an antipsychotic drug's effects appear to be genetically transmitted. Therefore, therapeutic and side effects in P.L. should be similar to those seen in his brother (27).

The preponderance of clinical evidence demonstrates therapeutic equivalence for all the commonly marketed neuroleptic agents when adequate dosages are utilized (25). Potency equivalents and daily dosages for the antipsychotic agents, although established and validated in clinical epidemiologic studies, are imprecise (28–30) (see Table 4). When a flexible dosage regimen is used to

titrate the chosen agent to maximum effect, all neuroleptics will demonstrate *statistical* equivalence in a study population. In a specific individual, one agent may work while another will not. Reasons for this *individual* inequivalence include pharmacokinetic and pharmacodynamic differences as well as possible multiple etiologies of the patient's schizophrenia. Obtaining the patient's past medication history is an extremely important step in the selection of an antipsychotic drug.

This patient's subjective response to neuroleptics should also be utilized in deciding on a specific agent. P.L. states: "Thorazine made me a zombie; Navane was good stuff." Patients' subjective responses to single doses of neuroleptics have been evaluated for their relationship with positive treatment outcomes (31). Patients who experience a pleasurable response or a reduction in their symptoms, consistent with a psychological desire to get well (ego syntonic), improve more quickly and refuse their medications less often than those who experience an unpleasant response or a change in symptoms which is contrary to their desires (ego dystonic) after a single test dose of neuroleptic (31).

In the absence of a treatment history (family or patient), the side effect spectra of the various antipsychotic agents constitute an important selection criterion. Although most neuroleptic drugs are qualitatively similar in their adverse effects, clinically significant differences do exist among the various agents. The relative incidences of the most commonly encountered adverse effects are summarized in Table 5. The goal of product selection is to match the individual patient's medical history, psychiatric target symptoms, and social situation to the drug side effect profile (15,25,28,31).

6. P.L. is agitated and anxious; why would the choice of a sedating neuroleptic be inappropriate for him?

The anxiety, agitation, and insomnia experienced by this patient are secondary to his psychosis and should therefore respond to neuroleptic therapy. By successfully treating the psychotic process with a neuroleptic agent, the secondary psychological symptoms will abate. All antipsychotics *calm* the distraught schizophrenic patient. Therefore, sedation is not needed in the majority of anxious, psychotic patients.

Neuroleptics are categorized as high and low potency agents (Table 5). The lower potency drugs

Table 4.

ANTIPSYCHOTIC DRUG DOSAGE AND RELATIVE POTENCY* BY CHEMICAL CLASS

Chemical Class Drug Name (Trade Name)	Acute	Chronic	Range	Traditional Equivalence	Acute Dose (mg/day)	Maintenance Dose (mg/day)
Phenothiazines						
Aliphatic type:						
chlorpromazine (Thorazine)	100	100	100	100	400–1500[+]	200–100
Piperidine type:						
Thioridazine (Mellaril)	107	96	72–116	100	400–800	200–800
Piperazine type:						
perphenazine (Trilafon)	8.5	9.0	7.7–10	10	32–96[+]	16–48
trifluoperazine (Stelazine)	2.8	3.4	2.1–6.2	5	20–100	10–40
fluphenazine (Prolixin)	1.2	1.4	1.0–1.5	2	20–80	5–40
Non-Phenothiazines						
Thioxanthene:						
thiothixene (Navane)	3.4	3.1	1.3–5.4	4	20–100[+]	5–40
Butyrophenone:						
haloperidol (Haldol)	2.8	2.3	0.3–3.5	2	20–100	5–40
Dibenzoxazepine:						
loxapine (Loxitane)	10	8.8	7.5–10	10	50–250[+]	25–100
Dihydroindolone:						
molindone (Moban)	7.6	4.4	3.1–10	10	50–400	25–100

[+]Dosage can be exceeded with caution.
*Acute, chronic and range of antipsychotic potencies derived from Ref. 30.

Table 5.

RELATIVE INCIDENCE OF ANTIPSYCHOTIC DRUG ADVERSE EFFECTS

	Sedation	Extrapyramidal Symptoms	Anticholinergic	Cardiovascular
Low Potency Agents				
chlorpromazine	high	moderate	moderate	high*
thioridazine	high	low	high	high*
High Potency Agents				
trifluoperazine	low	high	low	low
fluphenazine	low	very high	low	low
thiothixene	low	high	low	low
haloperidol	very low	very high	very low	very low
loxapine	moderate	high	low	moderate[+]
molindone	very low	high	low	low

+ orthostatic hypotension; not arrhythmogenic in overdose
* orthostatic hypotension; arrhythmias can occur in overdose

(eg, chlorpromazine and thioridazine) are less "clean" pharmacologically. Increased dermatologic, cardiac, autonomic, and central nervous system side effects and toxicities are observed with these less specific agents. Sedation, anticholinergic effects, and orthostatic hypotension are adverse reactions commonly seen upon the initiation of low potency neuroleptic treatment. These side effects can obscure or interfere with the patient's psychiatric assessment because of drug-induced alterations in consciousness. Additionally, patients suspected of drug abuse, intoxication, or withdrawal are at greater risk for adverse drug reactions if low potency agents are utilized. High potency agents (eg, haloperidol and thiothixene) have less side effects, though extrapyramidal symptoms, a direct extension of the dopamine blockade, are more frequent. Patients without a drug history documenting a response to low potency agents should receive a high potency agent as the treatment of choice (32).

A common exception to this rule is the patient with severe insomnia and anxiety who is refractory to non-sedating neuroleptics. Sedating agents (eg, chlorpromazine) would decrease the need for adjunctive medications.

P.L. was started on thiothixene 10 mg every morning and 20 mg at bedtime. Adjunctive sedative-hypnotic agents were not required. After the first week of therapy, the thiothixene was changed to 30 mg at bedtime. A decrease in paranoia and hallucinations with a corresponding increase in reality testing was slowly achieved over the course of hospitalization.

7. *Monitoring of Drug Therapy.* What subjective and objective clinical data should be monitored or reviewed to detect the occurrence of the four most common major side effects (sedation, extrapyramidal symptoms, anticholinergic effects, and cardiovascular toxicity) of antipsychotic medications?

The relative incidence of the four most commonly encountered adverse effects for the neuroleptic agents are summarized in Table 5 (15,25,28). Thus, clinicians should first of all determine which of these four adverse effects would be the most likely to occur with the neuroleptic agent about to be prescribed. For example, haloperidol would most likely cause extrapyramidal symptoms (EPS); chlorpromazine and thioridazine would most likely cause cardiovascular toxicity or sedation; and thioridazine would be most likely to cause anti-cholinergic effects. Secondly, the individual's past medical history should be reviewed. For the individual with a history of severe EPS, an agent such as haloperidol or trifluoperazine would probably be undesirable, and in this situation the medication should be changed to thioridazine which has a lower incidence of EPS. For the patient with prostatic hypertrophy, chronic constipation, or narrow angle glaucoma, thioridazine would probably be undesirable, and the medication should be switched to an agent less likely to precipitate anticholinergic effects (such as haloperidol or thiothixene). Unfortunately, none of the antipsychotic agents is without at least one of these adverse effects. The decision to choose one agent over another always entails trading one side effect for another (15).

If the patient's past medical history is not helpful in predicting adverse effects, then clinicians must still be alert for the appearance of these four most common side effects. *Extrapyramidal symptoms* are best detected by observing the patient's movements. Tremor, festinating gait, drooling, muscle spasms, jitteriness or motor restlessness, and repetitive involuntary movements are all indicators of extrapyramidal system dysfunction. *Cardiovascular toxicity* can best be checked by vital sign measurements, including pulse and blood pressure readings in both the standing and supine or sitting positions. Patients at risk for cardiac toxicity (the elderly or those with preexisting cardiovascular diseases) should receive serial electrocardiograms. Patient complaints of dizziness or palpitations should be taken seriously and followed up with vital signs and an electrocardiogram. *Anticholinergic effects* are best determined by asking the patient about perceived autonomic nervous system function. Complaints of dry mouth, constipation, or urinary hesitancy should alert the clinician to the possibility of anticholinergic side effects. *Sedation* is also best assessed by asking the patient to describe his level of alertness. Special attention should be paid to those individuals who "lay around all day and do not cause any trouble." These individuals may be lethargic secondary to oversedation.

8. *Possible Drug-Induced Psychosis.* T.C. is a 28-year-old, single, unemployed male who lives with his parents. Because of violent outbursts and bizarre behavior, he was committed to an acute psychiatric ward at the State Hospital at his parents' request. His mother

claimed that he is a "drug addict." She reported finding empty prescription vials for trihexyphenidyl and Dexedrine. Admission date was January 1981.

History of Present Illness: The patient was brought in by the local police in handcuffs; he had physically assaulted the policeman who transported him to the hospital. He explained that the policemen are part of the Air Force's plot to keep him from his house where he was monitoring secret experiments going on beneath his home. He claimed to have had a receiver and tape recorder implanted into his head so that he could receive orders from the President without anyone else hearing them. "The Air Force recently found out that I was keeping tabs on them, so they started beaming X-rays at me to make me sick. I can feel the rays come out of the light bulbs. They also are jamming my receiver, sending laughter and loud noise to drown out the President. Now they have enlisted my family to stop me by slipping me LSD and poisoning my food." He denied suicidal or homicidal ideation.

Previous Illness: In 1973 he was hospitalized for three weeks because he "freaked out" after being discharged from the Air Force for psychiatric reasons. In 1975, he was hospitalized for aggressive behavior following the use of marijuana and LSD; he was discharged on haloperidol 20 mg every evening at bedtime.

Family History: His sister was hospitalized three times for schizophrenia, chronic undifferentiated type.

Personal History: His developmental history is unremarkable. He is one of two children with a normal childhood and adolescence. While at college, he began to smoke marijuana regularly and occasionally used amphetamines, phencyclidine, and LSD.

Physical Examination on Admission: Within normal limits except for vital signs: pulse 110 and regular, blood pressure 160/100 mm Hg.

Mental Status Examination on Admission: *Appearance and Behavior:* He was a well-groomed male who looked his stated age and was in apparent discomfort. His speech was rapid and nervous. At times he stopped talking quite abruptly (blocking) and looked around the room. He could not sit still and asked permission to pace while being interviewed. Supportive communication and an environment of low sensory stimulation only made T.C. more agitated. *Mood:* He was nervous and frightened; he asked "Will I be put to death now that the Air Force has caught me?" *Affect:* Flat and expressionless. *Sensorium:* Oriented to time and person. *Intelligence:* Normal, though difficult to evaluate due to the patient's distractibility and preoccupation with internal stimuli. *Thought:* His associations were tight (coherent), and he denied hallucinations and delusions. His thought content focused around his mission and it was apparent that he was experiencing auditory hallucinations and blocking. He had persecutory and grandiose delusions.

Provisional Diagnosis: Paranoid schizophrenia, acute exacerbation. Rule out drug-induced or exacerbated psychosis.

Treatment: The patient received diazepam 15 mg po. Two hours later he remained acutely psychotic and anxious.

How can one differentiate between a drug-induced psychosis and schizophrenia in this patient?

Although the patient described being "slipped LSD," it was unclear whether this was a delusion or a misinterpretation of his own drug abuse pattern. Many drugs cause psychotic symptoms in both normal and schizophrenic individuals. Psychotomimetic drugs do not usually induce schizophrenia in individuals without endogenous psychiatric disorders. Drug-induced psychotic symptoms (eg, hallucinations and paranoid delusions) are common in "normals," but they usually lack the chronic behavioral aspects of schizophrenia. Schizophrenic patients on psychotomimetic agents can experience an exacerbation of their psychotic process and their mental status will deteriorate. On discontinuation of the offending drug, mental functioning usually returns to its previous level. In individuals predisposed to psychiatric illness (latent thought disorder), the psychotogenic effects of the drugs may unmask the underlying process (15).

Central Nervous System Stimulants (33–35). Amphetamines are considered the prototypical central nervous system stimulant agents. An acute, toxic amphetamine psychosis following one or two extremely large doses is not generally confused with schizophrenia because of the organic component which is present: delirium, disorientation, confusion, visual hallucinations, and autonomic nervous system findings (increased pulse and blood pressure). It is the non-toxic amphetamine psychosis, occurring with prolonged stimulant use, that can resemble schizophrenia. Initially in this chronic abuse pattern, the drug's effects include anorexia, euphoria, and increased psychomotor activity. Tolerance to these effects occurs, and the abuser gradually increases his dose. Individuals develop stereotyped, ritualized movements such as picking at the skin and pulling of the hair. With continued abuse and increasing dosage, patients can become suspicious and eventually develop paranoid delusions as well as auditory and visual hallucinations. The subtle difference between nontoxic amphetamine psychosis and paranoid schizophrenia is that the former often lacks the thought disorders and affective components typically found in schizophrenia, and that evaluation of the longitudinal history of the patient's premorbid and post-hospitalization function can distinguish the two etiologies. Acute drug-induced behavioral disturbances remit quickly once the offending agent is withdrawn. If an individual continues to be psychotic one to two weeks after the suspected ingestion, then a functional cause for the behavior should be considered.

This patient's vital signs and drug abuse history indicate that a possibility of a drug ingestion exists. However, based on the patient's psychiatric history, a drug-exacerbated schizophrenic process is most likely the correct diagnosis. The hospitalization in 1973 (pre-drug use), chronic delusions, hallucinations, and a flat affect, coupled with the family history for schizophrenia in a sister, further substantiate this conclusion.

Phencyclidine (36–38). Phencyclidine (PCP or angel dust) has demonstrated an increasing popularity among drug abusers. Reports of PCP-induced psychosis are frequent. PCP intoxication (as well as intoxication with other substances) must be excluded, especially in young adults or adolescents experiencing an acute psychotic episode, before the diagnosis of schizophrenia is assigned. PCP-induced psychosis frequently presents with dose-related abnormalities including ataxia, nystagmus, hyperreflexia, hypertension, and, rarely, seizures. Behaviorally, the patient can demonstrate any of the symptoms of schizophrenia from mute catatonic withdrawal to agitated, paranoid or violent outbursts. Environmental hypersensitivity can manifest itself as spontaneous disrobing or increased agitation when stimulated. Sensory deprivation is often the only treatment necessary. The psychosis usually persists for less

than three days, and the autonomic and central nervous system findings can help in establishing a differential diagnosis. This patient's chronic clinical course, lack of neurologic findings, and the elaborate delusions argue against PCP intoxication. A urine or blood test for PCP would be the only definitive means of disproving intoxication.

LSD (39). LSD (lysergic acid diethlyamide) can cause many adverse effects including panic states, "flash-backs," and psychosis. LSD-induced psychosis is most commonly seen in patients with a schizophrenic or borderline diagnosis (37).

In T.C., exacerbation or unmasking of the underlying psychiatric state by LSD was reported in 1975. Visual hallucinations usually dominate the intoxication. This patient did not report visual hallucinations. Benzodiazepines or "talking the patient down" can calm the individual experiencing a "bad trip." These two interventions were not successful in T.C.

Anticholinergic Agents (atropine, benztropine, antihistamines, tricyclic antidepressants) (40). When ingested in large quantity (toxic doses) anticholinergic agents can produce a delirium with psychosis. The "organic" psychosis (see Question 31) and physiological findings (hyperpyrexia, flushed appearance, mydriasis, tachycardia) aid in the differential diagnosis between functional and toxic psychoses (see Question 31). T.C. did not have the classic physiological evidence for anticholinergic excess. Physical findings usually precede severe psychological reactions to anticholinergic agents. (Also see the chapter on Drug Abuse.)

9. What are T.C.'s target symptoms? What are the initial goals of therapy for this patient?

T.C.'s major target symptoms include thought insertion, auditory hallucinations, persecutory and grandiose delusions, paranoid ideation, anxiety, agitation, blocking, and poor insight and judgment. The violent outbursts and bizarre behavior at home can be viewed as an attempt to deal with the voices.

Antipsychotic medication should be the mainstay of treatment to initially control this patient's acute psychotic symptomatology. The acute, agitated, psychotic patient can be calmed within 24 to 72 hours after initiation of antipsychotic drug therapy (25). The potentially combative or hostile patient should be aggressively dosed with antipsychotic medications. Restoration of normal sleep patterns and the rapid reduction of panic or anxiety states is a high priority. After one to two weeks of therapy, the patient should begin to socialize with the staff and other patients. T.C. demonstrates rapid speech with an agitated motor level. He is distractible and preoccupied with internal stimuli (hallucinations and paranoid ideation). He is obviously in distress and at one point asked "Will I be put to death now that the Air Force has caught me?" These symptoms are among the most responsive to antipsychotic medications and are a clear indication for aggressive therapy.

10. *High Dose Haloperidol.* What drug, dose, schedule, and route should be employed in treating T.C.'s psychosis?

T.C. does not appear to have antisocial behavior, but he manifests dangerous, destructive behavior because of his severe thought disorder. Therefore, a high potency, non-sedating antipsychotic agent would be preferable. Based on his previous history, haloperidol would be a reasonable choice.

Intramuscular therapy may be necessary for the agitated, floridly psychotic patient. The "high potency" antipsychotics are preferred to the "low potency" agents because they have fewer dose-limiting adverse effects (27,32). Additionally, the injectable high potency agents obtain more antipsychotic effect per dose than the lower potency agents. If this patient refuses oral medication ("it's poisoned"), then haloperidol, 5 mg per ml, may be given intramuscularly (5–10 mg) every one-half to one hour as needed to calm him. The onset of activity is rapid, and the hourly injections can rapidly calm the patient as well as assist in determining the acute oral starting dose. Initially, the medication is titrated to alleviate the agitation and insomnia or hostility and *not* to control the psychotic thought process (41). The technique of administering hourly injections until control of agitation is achieved is commonly called *rapid neuroleptization.*

If T.C. accepts oral medications but demonstrates marked agitation, then the *high dose induction oral therapy* technique should be considered. Using haloperidol as an example, the patient is started on 10–20 mg orally the first day and the haloperidol is increased by 10–20 mg increments *daily* or *every other day.* Typical effective doses range from 40 to 100 mg/day. Utilizing either of these aggressive techniques, the goal is rapid control of the acute symptoms which render the patient dangerous. Once calming is achieved,

careful monitoring for oversedation should be initiated. Overshooting the optimum dose in the early phase of treatment is preferable to violent or dangerous behavior. However, in the later phases of treatment, downward titration to the lowest effective dose should be attempted.

Based on T.C.'s previous response to haloperidol 20 mg/day, one would expect that moderate doses of antipsychotic agents would be needed to calm him. During the first one to three days of antipsychotic therapy, a flexible dosage titration regimen is best.

11. Is high dose therapy routinely recommended for patients such as T.C.?

The issue of high versus low dosage regimens is still unresolved in the literature. Possible benefits of using high dose, aggressive treatment regimens include: reduced duration of hospitalization, increased use of hospital beds and more rapid patient turnover, treatment of acute psychotic episodes in specialized units with patient admissions lasting only 1–3 days, early participation of patient in psychotherapeutic and rehabilitative programs, early establishment of staff/patient rapport, decreased risk for institutionalization of the patient, and decreased risk of staff or patient morbidity due to violence (42,43).

Recent studies indicate that low to moderate dosages of antipsychotic medication are sufficient for the majority of acutely ill individuals (44,45). High dose, rapid neuroleptization should therefore be reserved for those individuals who do not respond to one or two injections of medication and where the environment is not sufficiently structured to maintain these patients. Prior to the use of aggressive antipsychotic therapy, careful physical and laboratory assessment should be completed to rule out medical causes of psychosis.

12. Eight hours after admission, T.C. struck out at the staff, threatening to kill them all. Rapid neuroleptization was ordered, and he received haloperidol 10 mg intramuscularly every hour for six doses. He was then placed on haloperidol concentrate, 40 mg po twice daily. Was this initial dosage conversion to oral haloperidol appropriate? Why was the concentrate used?

Haloperidol has an oral bioavailability of approximately 60–70%. Therefore the dosage conversion was appropriate (46). The use of concentrate is recommended in the initial treatment phase to decrease the chance of patient noncompliance or "cheeking" of medications. The technique of rapid neuroleptization utilized in this patient usually requires that the individual receive adequate follow-up with oral medications within the first 24 hours of intramuscular therapy. If he had been given a lower dosage of oral haloperidol (eg, 20 mg per day), then the chances of his becoming reagitated or violent would have been greatly increased.

13. *Dosage Evaluation.* After receiving haloperidol concentrate 40 mg po twice daily for two weeks, T.C. continued to be delusional and nervous but was no longer violent. He denied ever having a receiver in his head. He was sleeping through the night and socializing with staff. He could concentrate on performing tasks during occupational and recreational therapy classes. Should the dose of neuroleptic be increased?

T.C.'s remaining target symptoms (chronic delusions about the Air Force) are ones which are generally slow to show response and may not be drug-treatable. While the haloperidol could be further increased towards 100 mg/day, little additional response would be expected. Antipsychotic drug therapy for acute psychosis usually results in a rapid initial phase of symptom amelioration followed by a much slower period of gradual behavioral restitution. This patient's denial of past symptoms following remission is not uncommon in poorly insightful patients and is not a sign of worsening.

14. Under what circumstances would a dosage increase be appropriate? When would another drug be considered?

If acute symptoms (agitation, distractibility, insomnia) were still present after several weeks of therapy at 80 mg/day, a further dosage increase to 100 mg or more per day could be considered. Although the FDA has set the maximum dose of haloperidol at 100 mg, there are no absolute daily maximum dosages for any neuroleptic agent (except thioridazine) (47). If T.C. had demonstrated assaultive or agitated behavior after four weeks of therapy on haloperidol 80–100 mg/day, then a change to another high potency antipsychotic agent would be indicated. The conversion from one antipsychotic agent to another is not well defined in the literature. Table 4 lists common dos-

age ranges for acute and maintenance doses of neuroleptic drugs and the relative potencies of these drugs (48–50). However, because individuals may vary in their response to these drugs, dosage conversions based on Table 4 at this high a dosage level are not recommended. Instead, a moderate dosage of the new drug (eg, loxapine 100–150 mg/day) would be preferable.

15. *Once-Daily Dosing.* Prior to discharge, T.C.'s medication was changed to haloperidol 60 mg at bedtime. What are the advantages of once-daily administration of antipsychotic drugs?

The benefits of once-daily dosing include increased patient compliance, lower cost (fewer tablets), decreased nursing error among inpatients, decreased experience of side effects (peak blood levels occur while the patient is asleep), and decreased need for adjunctive hypnotics. For most patients, these advantages outweigh any disadvantages (49); disadvantages include patient reluctance to ingest many tablets at once and the possibility of drug-induced disturbances in sleep patterns. The prolonged action of these drugs makes once-daily dosing reasonable. Most important is the fact that the primary reason for rehospitalization of schizophrenic patients is poor compliance with medication. Once-daily dosing is associated with a higher compliance rate than multiple-daily dosing. However, during the initial dosage titration phase, divided dosing is recommended (50a).

16. *Polypharmacy.* P.P., a 58-year-old woman with the diagnosis of schizophrenia, residual type, was discharged from the hospital after her ninth admission; her total accrued length of stay in that institution was 25 years. Her mental status presentation was basically nonpsychotic, with poor social skills, blunted affect, and limited insight and judgment. Her discharge medications included chlorpromazine 50 mg bid, trifluoperazine 2 mg tid, flurazepam 30 mg qhs, docusate sodium 100 mg qhs, benztropine 2 mg qhs, and doxepin 25 mg bid. Doxepin had been administered at this dosage for five years and the doxepin plus desmethyldoxepin plasma level was 25 ng/ml (subtherapeutic). How could this patient's drug therapy be improved?

This drug regimen is a classic example of "polypharmacy." In patients who are institutionalized for long periods of time, such polypharmacy is often the result of adding another drug for each new problem encountered without reviewing and optimizing the previous therapy. This psychotropic dosing regimen is confusing for the patient, pharmacologically irrational, and guarantees noncompliance. The use of two or more antipsychotics is usually not justifiable. There is little evidence in the literature which suggests that several neuroleptics are better than one when equivalent dosages are used (51–53). Polypharmacy has evolved as a result of clinical practice rather than research. It illustrates the partial effectiveness of these agents in treating schizophrenia.

An advantage of using a single neuroleptic drug is that side effects can be anticipated (Table 5). Multiple neuroleptic administration can increase the number of side effects experienced by the patient as well as make the recognition and management of side effects and dose titration more difficult (54). The use of lower doses does not guarantee a reduced incidence of side effects. Dose versus response relationships for these agents are unpredictable and reflect the wide variability of pharmacokinetic and pharmacodynamic responses among individuals. The antidepressant medication is not indicated and can worsen the patient's mental status. Antidepressants have been reported to increase hostility, paranoia and agitation in schizophrenic patients (55). However, the dose of antidepressant based on the plasma levels is subtherapeutic (56). Combinations of antipsychotics and antidepressant drugs can lead to an increased incidence of side effects because of additive sedative, anticholinergic, and orthostatic hypotensive effects.

The hypnotic flurazepam should not be administered on a chronic basis. Accumulation of the long-acting active metabolite could lead to significant excess sedation or affective dulling in this individual (57). Although some patients may require routine use of a stool softener, simplification of the drug regimen to one with less anticholinergic effects might be possible. Before drugs are used to treat constipation, high fiber diet, exercise, and increased water consumption should be tried.

In addition to discontinuation of all but the antipsychotic drugs, two rational simplifications of this patient's treatment regimen are possible: If extrapyramidal symptoms are the major pre-senting side effect, or if sedation is required, then her antipsychotic medication could be given as thioridazine 200 mg every night at bedtime. If anticholinergic effects are the major problem, then her drug therapy could be changed to trifluoperazine 10 mg every night at bedtime. In either case, she would be maintained on an equivalent dose of antipsychotic medication.

17. Duration of Therapy. Is long-term therapy indicated in this individual? Should P.P. continue to receive neuroleptic therapy?

The need for long-term maintenance neuroleptic therapy for chronic schizophrenic patients is well established (25,58,59). A significantly higher incidence of psychotic exacerbations occurs in patients whose neuroleptic therapy is terminated than in patients maintained on therapy (45). However, these findings are primarily based on studies of short to intermediate duration, and few guidelines have been elaborated for long-term maintenance therapy of several years or even decades. One study of eight years duration did show a significant benefit from chlorpromazine after four years, but noted that the effect of maintenance therapy seemed to decrease with the passage of time (60). Although maintenance neuroleptic therapy consistently shows significant prolongation of symptom remission, there remains up to one half of the patients studied who show no exacerbation of psychotic symptoms after being without medications for four to eight months. Unfortunately, no reliable predictors have been elucidated which can distinguish between patients who will maintain remission and those who will relapse (61,62).

The value of maintenance neuroleptic therapy can also be assessed in terms of schizophrenic subtypes and prognosis groups (45,63). Extremely poor prognosis and extremely good prognosis schizophrenic patients will not benefit greatly from long-term maintenance neuroleptic therapy. Long-term therapy is of greatest benefit to the chronic schizophrenic patient with fair to good prognosis who manifests intermittent psychotic episodes (64,65). P.P. probably fits into the category of residual schizophrenia with a poor prognosis. Based on DSM-III, this is a chronic non-psychotic classification where functional impairment remains in the areas of social and self-care skills while the overt psychosis is abated. The value of maintenance therapy in this individual can be determined by evaluating her past history. If previous hospitalizations were the result of noncompliance with antipsychotic drugs, then the patient should be maintained on the minimum effective dose. At present, the only way to ascertain this minimum effective dose is by downward titration of medications, watching for relapse. At the first signs or symptoms of psychosis, the dosage should be increased. Typical maintenance doses for stable schizophrenic outpatients range from 2 to 40 mg/day of trifluoperazine or its equivalent.

18. *Depot Fluphenazine.* N.L., a 27-year-old woman, was admitted to the psychiatric ward for her fourth acute schizophrenic episode in four years. Her compliance with medications as an outpatient has been poor, and she has poor insight into her illness. She attends outpatient follow-up only when individual therapy sessions are planned. During this hospitalization, she responded well to two weeks of haloperidol 20 mg twice daily. The treatment team then decided to try long-acting fluphenazine for outpatient follow-up. What factors make this patient a good candidate for depot fluphenazine therapy? When should depot fluphenazine be used?

Several factors make N.L. a potentially good candidate for a long-acting fluphenazine preparation. Her high frequency of psychotic episodes clearly suggests the need for maintenance neuroleptic therapy, and her past history of noncompliance to medication as an outpatient makes oral medication a poor choice (28). A positive response to continued individual contacts can be coordinated with scheduled injection appointments which will favorably influence compliance. Lastly, poor insight into her illness contributes to her noncompliance with oral medications. Patients who cannot understand the need for their medication are aware only of adverse effects and often comply poorly.

Another indication for long-acting fluphenazine, which is not present in this patient, is poor response to oral medication. Up to 40% of chronic drug-refractory schizophrenics treated with oral chlorpromazine have low serum levels, and many respond when given parenteral neuroleptics (66,67). This variability may be due to induction of hepatic enzymes, altered metabolic transformation, or significant metabolism within the gastrointestinal tract (68,69). On a practical basis,

these patients cannot be given short-acting parenteral hydrochloride preparations of neuroleptics for long-term therapy. Therefore long-acting depot fluphenazine is clearly indicated on a trial basis for refractory schizophrenics.

19. Which of the two currently available depot preparations, fluphenazine enanthate and fluphenazine decanoate, would be the better choice for N.L.?

The decanoate ester of fluphenazine offers several advantages over the enanthate and is therefore the preferred preparation. The two preparations are identical in terms of efficacy, just as are all other antipsychotics. When fluphenazine-induced EEG changes were compared, peak effects from the enanthate occurred after one week, while peak effects for the decanoate ester occurred after two weeks (70). The duration of clinical effect from the decanoate ester is as much as two weeks longer than that of the enanthate ester (71). A 25 mg intramuscular injection of fluphenazine decanoate provides sustained serum levels of 0.1 to 0.5 ng/ml for a period of one to four weeks (72,73). Typical plasma levels in responding schizophrenics range from 0.5 to 2.8 ng/ml. Fluphenazine plasma levels from the enanthate preparation are more variable and not as long-lasting. The decanoate ester also causes a slightly lower incidence of extrapyramidal effects when compared with the enanthate ester (74).

20. How should N.L.'s 20 mg twice daily oral haloperidol be converted to a comparable dose of fluphenazine decanoate?

N.L. is taking 40 mg of haloperidol per day, which is essentially equal to 40 mg of fluphenazine per day (Table 4). However, there is no exact conversion factor between oral fluphenazine and the long-acting injections. The dosage of fluphenazine decanoate is best estimated as if it were a separate drug. There are formulae for conversion in the literature, but they suffer from many questionable assumptions. One such method follows (75):

Multiply the daily oral dose of fluphenazine or its equivalent by the intended dosing interval (in days). Divide by 4 (assume that the parenteral form is 4 times more bioavailable than the oral form). Reduce by one-third as a "safety margin" to avoid extrapyramidal effects from too high a blood level, and round off to the nearest one-half milliliter increment (12.5 mg). For example, the equivalent of oral fluphenazine 40 mg daily given as fluphenazine decanoate injection every 7 days would be:

$$\frac{2}{3}\left(\frac{40 \text{ mg/day} \times 7 \text{ days}}{4}\right) \cong 50 \text{ mg (2 ml)}$$

A practical, useful conversion developed from extensive clinical use of fluphenazine decanoate is to take the daily dose of oral fluphenazine or its equivalent, round the daily dose up to the next 0.5 ml amount of fluphenazine decanoate (12.5 mg), and give that amount weekly (or every other week). This approach is based on the observation that 20–80 mg of oral fluphenazine is needed for treatment of an acute psychotic episode, and that the typical dosage range for fluphenazine decanoate is 25–100 mg. The clinical validity of this empirical method is substantiated by the close agreement obtained by the equation above and this simpler method.

Thus, N.L. should receive 50 mg of fluphenazine decanoate each week. Rather than abruptly stopping the haloperidol, it should be tapered off rapidly over one to three days after the injection is given. Despite contradictory reports in the earlier literature, peak levels of fluphenazine may occur within hours after a depot injection (69,70). Nonetheless, overlap of the oral medication and the depot injection appears safe and clinically appropriate until further pharmacokinetic studies are undertaken to elucidate a more appropriate transition plan.

When patients are taking a low potency neuroleptic (eg, chlorpromazine), it is desirable to switch them to oral fluphenazine at an equivalent dosage before the depot injection is given. After several days on oral fluphenazine therapy, most severe idiosyncratic reactions would be expected to have occurred. Once a depot form of the drug is administered to the patient, severe side effects can persist for weeks. For reasons which are not clear, individuals sometimes respond differently to "equivalent" agents. In N.L., the pharmacologic similarity of haloperidol and fluphenazine allows a direct conversion to the decanoate. The initial injections should be given on a weekly basis. Based on the patient's clinical condition, the injection interval can subsequently be lengthened to two weeks. This is the usual dosage interval used in clinical practice. Acutely ill schizo-

phrenics require more frequent injections than do chronic schizophrenic patients (76).

21. Could fluphenazine decanoate or enanthate have been used for treatment of N.L.'s acute psychotic episode?

While the efficacy of long-acting fluphenazine for chronic maintenance therapy of psychosis is widely accepted, its usefulness in the treatment of acute psychotic episodes is less well established (77). One study suggests that fluphenazine enanthate, alone or combined with an oral neuroleptic during the acute psychotic episode, is more effective than chlorpromazine alone (78). Although differences in efficacy can be attributed to inequivalent doses, fluphenazine enanthate probably is effective in the treatment of acute psychosis. Despite these reports, the use of long-acting fluphenazine for treatment of acute psychotic episodes cannot be recommended. It makes little sense to use a long-acting preparation when initial neuroleptic therapy requires the flexible dosage titration which is obtainable only with oral and intramuscular hydrochloride preparations. When severe toxicity occurs after depot administration, the effects remain for days and often weeks. Severe extrapyramidal reactions caused by fluphenazine decanoate may persist for up to one month and occasionally do not respond to conventional antiparkinsonian therapy (79). A malignant neuroleptic syndrome has been reported, and its occurrence after depot injection makes management more difficult (80). Therefore the acute use of depot fluphenazine does not seem appropriate. In individuals in whom aggressive fluphenazine decanoate is to be initiated (eg, the acutely psychotic patient who has already been shown to be refractory to conventional oral therapy), it is advised that a one or two day trial of intramuscular fluphenazine hydrochloride be utilized before the decanoate is given.

NEUROLEPTIC SIDE EFFECTS

Extrapyramidal Symptoms

22. *Dystonia.* B.F., a 19-year-old male, was admitted to the county hospital complaining of insomnia and auditory hallucinations of three weeks duration. His behavior was observed to be appropriate, and he was not dangerous to himself or to others. He was ad-

mitted as a voluntary patient and placed on haloperidol 5 mg IM every hour as needed for agitation, up to a maximum of five doses in 24 hours. On the second day of hospitalization, he was more agitated and confused than during the initial mental status examination. At one point, he picked up a chair and threatened to throw it at the staff. He was then given haloperidol 5 mg IM which was repeated in one hour. This appeared to calm him and no routine medications were ordered at that time. On the following day (16 hours later), the patient complained of his neck being bent to the left side and so stiff that he could not straighten it. He stated that his tongue felt so thick that he could not speak clearly, and that his muscles throughout his back and neck were sore and tight. What is this neuroleptic adverse effect? What pathophysiologic and neurochemical mechanisms are involved?

This adverse effect should be identified as torticollis, a dystonic reaction which involves the muscles of the neck unilaterally. Acute dystonic reactions are of sudden onset and usually take place within 24–48 hours after the start of medication. The incidence is greater in younger people and in males (82,83). A study of 1152 psychiatric inpatients who received a phenothiazine, thioxanthine, or a butyrophenone reported a 10.1% incidence of dystonia (84). Torticollis was the most frequently observed extrapyramidal side effect, followed in order by swollen tongue, trismus, oculogyric crisis, and opisthotonus. Haloperidol was most frequently associated with dystonia, followed by piperazine phenothiazines, chlorpromazine, and thioridazine. The time course in this patient is consistent with dystonia.

Extrapyramidal effects are a result of postsynaptic dopaminergic blockade by neuroleptics in the corpus striatum (85). Increased dopamine turnover also appears to correlate with dystonic reactions. A simplified model of the corpus striatum and substantia nigra which relates the influences of cholinergic, dopaminergic, and gamma-aminobutyric acid systems (GABA) is presented in Figure 1 (86). Normal motor activity depends upon a balance between the striatal cholinergic and dopaminergic systems. Neuroleptic drugs upset this balance by diminishing dopaminergic activity in the striatum, causing a net cholinergic excess which manifests clinically as extrapyram-

idal effects. The role of the GABA pathways is not as clearly understood as those of the dopaminergic and cholinergic pathways. It appears that GABA plays an important auto-feedback role in maintaining normal basal ganglia function. The feedback system represented in Figure 1 accounts for the observed lack of extrapyramidal reactions in the majority of patients receiving neuroleptic drugs. The effects of the drugs in the nigro-striatal region are related to their movement disorder side effects and not to their therapeutic efficacy. Many individuals respond quite well to antipsychotic agents (demonstrating dopaminergic effect in the limbic system) without clinically apparent extrapyramidal symptoms. Therefore these GABA pathways may play an important role in mitigating the adverse effects of dopamine blockade in the basal ganglia.

23. How should B.F.'s neuroleptic-induced dystonia be treated?

Parenteral anticholinergic agents are the most efficacious and rational treatment for neuroleptic-induced dystonias (49). Of all the extrapyramidal symptoms, dystonias are most responsive to treatment. Improvement is usually observed within ten minutes and peak effects occur in 30 minutes (87,88).

The choice of intravenous versus intramuscular anticholinergic therapy is difficult to make due to the paucity of clinical comparisons. Response to the treatment of post-encephalitic oculogyric crisis with benztropine mesylate occurred within 15 minutes after IV therapy and 30 after following IM therapy (89). Diphenhydramine is equally effective in the treatment of acute dystonic reactions. Alternately, benzodiazepines are effective for acute EPS (eg, lorazepam 0.025–0.05 mg/kg IM).

An important consideration in the treatment of neuroleptic-induced dystonias is the patient's reaction to this acute stress. The paranoid, psychotic individual will respond with a marked increase in agitation, anxiety, and assaultiveness. Other patients may be so traumatized by this negative experience that they will refuse all medications. It is therefore important that the most rapid treatment be utilized to relieve the dystonia. If a single injection of 2 mg of benztropine mesylate is not sufficient, then a repeat dose of 2 mg given IM or IV in 30 minutes is appropriate. The usual dose of diphenhydramine is 50 mg IM

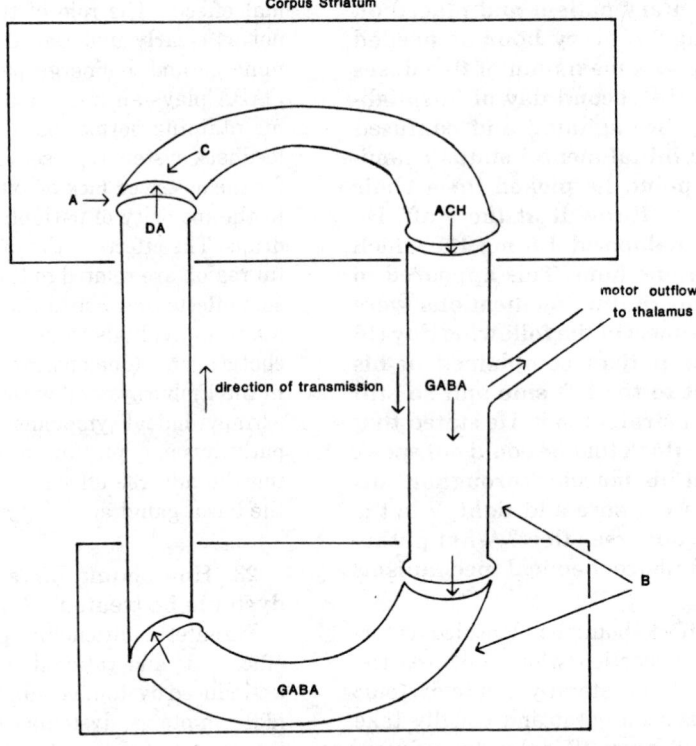

Figure 1. Simplified model of neurotransmitter "wiring diagram" for the corpus striatum and substantia nigra. Modified from ref. 83.

I.   Normal movements occur when dopamine (DA) and acetylcholine (ACH) are in balance and GABA outflow to thalamus is normal.

II. Antipsychotic drug therapy (A) blocks the post-synaptic DA receptor, causing the imbalance of less DA effect than ACH effect. GABA outflow is increased; pseudoparkinsonism occurs.

III. Two GABA neurons (B) in series mitigate DA blockade by the antipsychotic agent (eg, feedback loop).

IV. Denervation hypersensitivity of post-synaptic DA receptor (C) causes the imbalance of more DA effect than ACH. GABA outflow is reduced and tardive dyskinesia occurs.

or IV. In this patient, without severe behavioral reaction to the dystonia, benztropine 2 mg IM or diphenhydramine 50 mg IM would be the best treatment. Oral anticholinergic agents should be given to this patient for at least three days. This is based on the assumption that no further neuroleptic therapy is administered and that the biological effect of the neuroleptic lasts one to three days. If the dystonic reaction occurs during the initiation phase of antipsychotic therapy, then anticholinergic agents should be maintained for one to three months. After that time the anticholinergic agent should be tapered and discontinued (90).

24. During the remaining two months of B.F.'s hospitalization, he was treated with haloperidol oral concentrate 5 mg twice daily and benztropine tablets 2 mg twice daily. He discontinued these medications after he left the hospital. Six months after discharge, he was begun on haloperidol 10 mg oral concentrate twice daily at an outpatient clinic because of bizarre, disorganized behavior. Why should B.F. receive prophylactic antiparkinsonian agents? How long should prophylaxis continue?

Since B.F. experienced extrapyramidal effects upon initiation of the same medication eight months previously (the dystonic reaction described in Question 22), he is currently at risk for similar problems. Patients who discontinue routine administration of antipsychotic medication will reexperience initial adverse effects upon reinitiation of therapy. Furthermore, prevention of adverse effects is important in facilitating subsequent compliance with drug therapy. A study of why schizophrenics are reluctant to take their medications revealed that 89% of the noncompliant patients had experienced extrapyramidal effects as compared to only 20% of the compliant patients. The overall conclusion was that reluctance to take neuroleptic medication was significantly associated with extrapyramidal effects, most notably akathisia (93). Thus B.F. will be more likely to discontinue therapy if he experiences another significant adverse effect from the haloperidol. Haloperidol has a high incidence of extrapyramidal effects, particularly dystonias and akathisia.

Although the issue of prophylactic anticholinergic agents has received much attention in the literature, clinicians still vary greatly in their clinical use of these agents. It has been clearly established that after three months of neuroleptic therapy, the vast majority of patients do not need anticholinergic agents. One study of 403 patients withdrawn from antiparkinson agents after more than three months of therapy found that 82% did not require them (90). Similar studies show that the majority of patients do not need antiparkinson drugs. The remaining area of controversy is the initial three months of therapy (91,92).

Since B.F. has not been taking any medication for the past six months, his susceptibility to adverse extrapyramidal effects has returned to baseline, and he should again receive prophylactic benztropine for as long as three months after haloperidol is reinstituted.

25. What differences exist among the available anticholinergic antiparkinsonian drugs?

Table 6 lists the more commonly used antiparkinson drugs and their relative potencies. No differences in efficacy have been established among the anticholinergic drugs (94). The primary difference of clinical significance is duration of effect, with benztropine having the longest duration. Benztropine can be dosed once daily, while the other drugs must be dosed three or four times

Table 6.

ESTIMATED EQUIVALENT
DOSES OF ANTIPARKINSON AGENTS

Anticholinergic	
benztropine (Cogentin)	2 mg
trihexyphenidyl (Artane)	5 mg
biperiden (Akineton)	4 mg
procyclidine (Kemadrin)	5 mg
diphenhydramine (Benadryl)	50 mg
Dopaminergic	
amantadine (Symmetrel)	100 mg
Gabaminergic	
lorazepam (Ativan)	2 mg
diazepam (Valium)	10 mg

daily (100). Euphoria and hallucinations have been attributed more frequently to trihexyphenidyl than benztropine (87). Benztropine, diphenhydramine, and biperiden are available in parenteral dosage forms, while trihexyphenidyl is not. Trihexyphenidyl is less sedating than the other agents.

26. If B.F. were intolerant to the anticholinergic effects of benztropine, what treatment alternative could be utilized?

As depicted in Figure 1, extrapyramidal effects are the result of postsynaptic dopaminergic blockade by neuroleptics in the corpus striatum. Normal motor activity depends on the balance between striatal cholinergic and dopaminergic systems. Therefore the balance can be restored by the administration of an anticholinergic agent which results in the restoration of relative equality of dopaminergic and cholinergic effects. Although levodopa might seem to be suitable as a treatment alternative for extrapyramidal adverse effects, it does not restore the relative deficit of dopamine because of the neuroleptic blockade of striatal dopaminergic receptors.

In patients who are intolerant to anticholinergic agents, or who are refractory to their effects, amantadine (Symmetrel) is a suitable alternative (94). Amantadine is a putative dopaminergic agonist which is apparently more specific for nigro-striatal dopamine receptors than limbic receptors. In recommended doses it very rarely causes exacerbation of the psychotic state, but it is as effective as standard doses of anticholinergic antiparkinson agents (95). Its exact mechanism of action in the treatment of neuroleptic-induced extrapyramidal symptoms has not been completely elucidated.

The onset of amantadine's beneficial effects usually occurs within 24 hours. The usual starting dose is 100 mg twice daily. Although the dose can be titrated up to 300–400 mg/day, a higher incidence of side effects is observed at these higher dosages. The most common side effects include tremor, slurred speech, ataxia, depression, hallucinations, insomnia, and hyperexcitability. These effects are rarely seen in neuroleptic-treated patients who are given amantadine 100 mg twice daily. Other side effects which occur infrequently include skin rash, exzematoid dermatitis, photosensitization, visual disturbances, dryness of the mouth, dyspnea, nausea, vomiting, constipation, urinary retention, and orthostatic hypotension. Amantadine does possess weak anticholinergic activity, and any anticholinergic agents being given in addition to amantadine will have additive effects. Amantadine therapy should be considered for patients with benign prostatic hypertrophy, patients who are experiencing anticholinergic effects which have led to functional impairment (eg, blurred vision, urinary retention), and patients with extrapyramidal symptoms which are refractory to anticholinergic agents given without amantadine (eg, not responsive to benztropine 6–8 mg/day).

A potential advantage of amantadine is that by lessening dopaminergic blockade at the nigrostriatal receptors, the extent of dopamine receptor supersensitivity due to denervation hypersensitivity may be mitigated (96). If this observation is confirmed, then amantadine might be useful in preventing tardive dyskinesia. A disadvantage of amantadine is that it costs 10–15 times more than equivalent anticholinergic treatment. Therefore amantadine is not recommended as the drug of choice for neuroleptic-induced extrapyramidal symptoms except in the instances outlined above.

27. Why do neuroleptic drugs differ in their ability to cause extrapyramidal effects, and why is the incidence of extrapyramidal effects not directly dose-related?

The individual neuroleptic drugs differ in their propensity for causing extrapyramidal side effects (see Table 5). It has been suggested that all neuroleptic drugs have the same tendency to elicit extrapyramidal effects by virtue of their striatal-dopaminergic receptor blockade, but that they differ in incidence of extrapyramidal effects only because they differ in inherent anticholinergic activity (97). When the anticholinergic and extrapyramidal effects in Table 5 are compared, an inverse relationship is noted. Haloperidol causes a high incidence of extrapyramidal effects because it has low inherent anticholinergic activity. Thioridazine is associated with a low incidence of extrapyramidal effects because it is also a potent anticholinergic agent.

However, receptor binding studies in laboratory animals have challenged this relatively useful but simplistic view of neuroleptic drug effects (17). Dopamine receptor blockade by various neuroleptics apparently varies both in extent and specificity. Therefore differences in extrapyramidal effects may be due to differences in preferential blockade of striatal dopamine receptors as well as specific anticholinergic properties.

Over the past twenty years, high-dose therapy with neuroleptics has become acceptable treatment for some patients. Practitioners employing high-dose treatment have noted that extrapyramidal effects are not strictly dose related, and in some cases extrapyramidal effects from high-dose therapy may be less than with moderate-dose therapy. As the dosage is increased, dopaminergic blockade increases nonlinearly (approaching an asymptote) but anticholinergic activity increases significantly (linearly). Anticholinergic effects appear to be purely dose related. With increasing anticholinergic activity, and minimal change in striatal dopamine activity, extrapyramidal effects are stabilized or even decreased (80).

28. Akathisia. After six weeks of haloperidol 20 mg daily (without benztropine), B.F. complained of persistent anxiety and difficulty in falling asleep. He was visibly agitated and unable to sit still during the interview. He asked for more medication. How can a differential diagnosis be made between reemerging psychosis and akathisia? How should he be treated?

Akathisia is described as the subjective desire to be in constant motion, typically manifest by the patient's constant pacing or inability to sit still. Mild akathisia may be virtually impossible to distinguish from anxiety, while the patient with severe akathisia may be restless to the point of agitation and panic. The differential diagnosis between reemerging psychosis and akathisia is extremely difficult to make in some patients; akathisia is sometimes mistaken for psychotic agitation. Based on the information presented, it is likely that B.F. is experiencing akathisia. The time course of six weeks is consistent with akathisia as the presenting symptomatology, and he was not given prophylactic anticholinergic medication. Haloperidol is more likely to cause akathisia as compared to other extrapyramidal manifestations, and B.F. did not present with other symptoms suggestive of psychosis. For these reasons, akathisia should be the provisional diagnosis, and anticholinergic therapy should be instituted. If treatment with an anticholinergic agent in standard antiparkinson doses (eg, benztropine 4–6 mg/day) is successful, then the diagnosis of akathisia is confirmed. Conversely, if an antipsychotic agent administered on a prn basis for the nervousness reduces the level of agitation and anxiety, then psychiatric causes for the restlessness are more likely.

Akathisia is the most common extrapyramidal effect induced by neuroleptics; its incidence has been cited at 21.2% (87). The incidence is probably higher today because of the more widespread use of high potency agents such as haloperidol and fluphenazine. Akathisia is among the most commonly cited causes for poor compliance with drug therapy (83,85).

29. Assuming that B.F. is experiencing akathisia and response to treatment is poor, what can be done?

On occasion, akathisias show little response to treatment with anticholinergic agents. It appears that akathisias are among the most difficult extrapyramidal symptoms to treat successfully (82). If anticholinergic agents have been pushed to maximal dosage levels without adequate response, oral amantadine, diphenhydramine, or diazepam can be added as an adjunct. As a last resort, the dosage of the neuroleptic must be lowered or the neuroleptic drug changed to one that will not cause this effect in the patient being treated (83,99).

30. Despite treatment with larger than usual doses of benztropine (6 mg/day), B.F.'s akathisia was still present. Since he did not exhibit any anticholinergic side effects, would it be reasonable to continue increasing the dose of benztropine?

Receptor binding assay studies for anticholinergic drugs have identified the inadequacy of standard dosage regimens in some individuals. Although the alleviation of neuroleptic-induced extrapyramidal symptoms correlates positively with anticholinergic drug plasma levels, patients administered standard doses of benztropine may exhibit a greater than 10-fold variation in their plasma levels. Benztropine may not follow first-order kinetics. Small increases in dosage can cause large increases in plasma levels. Individual titration of the dosage regimen based on clinical monitoring is necessary. Patients demonstrating extrapyramidal symptoms without anticholinergic side effects should have their dosage of benztropine increased to as high as 8–12 mg/day. Further kinetic studies are required to refine dosing recommendations.

31. Anticholinergic Toxicity. Because of his persistent akathisia, B.F.'s benztropine was increased to 4 mg po twice daily. Two days later his condition deteriorated. He was confused, agitated, and combative. He was picking at his clothes, claiming that there were bugs crawling under his skin. What is the most likely cause of this change in his mental status? How should he be treated?

B.F. appears to be experiencing acute CNS toxicity from the combined effects of the increased dose of benztropine and the anticholinergic effects of the haloperidol (101). The acuteness of the syndrome coupled with the organic picture of disorientation, confusion, and tactile hallucinations differentiates it from a worsening of the schizophrenic process. Mental status changes which are typical of anticholinergic intoxication include a high incidence of disorientation, confusion, agitation, and picking or plucking movements; classic physiologic manifestations include mydriasis, dry mucous membranes, and tachycardia (102). Complete neuropsychiatric recovery occurs within one or two days of anticholinergic drug discontinuation in more than one-half of cases. Drug treatment is rarely indicated, but if agitation must be controlled, benzodiazepines can be used. Neuroleptic drugs are relatively contraindicated because of their anticholinergic activity.

32. Pseudoparkinsonism. B.F. recovered from his anticholinergic delirium and was placed on benztropine 3 mg twice daily and amantadine 100 mg twice daily in addition to his haloperidol. One week later he complained of a rhythmical tremor of both hands

and difficulty in walking. What is this extra-pyramidal side effect? How can it be treated?

B.F. is exhibiting pseudoparkinsonism, the neuroleptic-induced equivalent to the idiopathic illness. The symptom complex is similar to the natural illness. Table 7 lists the more commonly observed symptoms (83,103). The occurrence of persistent extrapyramidal symptoms in B.F. despite maximum doses of antiparkinsonian medications necessitates a switch to a neuroleptic with less extrapyramidal side effects (eg, thioridazine) (86,97).

Tardive Dyskinesia

Tardive dyskinesia is a late-appearing, potentially irreversible neurological syndrome which is associated with antipsychotic drug use. It is characterized by involuntary, abnormal movements of the face (especially the mouth) and of the extremities (see Question 33).

Pathogenesis. The most popular theory describes the pathogenesis of tardive dyskinesia as a disuse hypersensitivity (denervation) of the postsynaptic dopamine receptors in the nigrostriatal region of the brain caused by neuroleptic receptor blockade. This dopaminergic hyperfunction results in a relative cholinergic hypofunc-

Table 7.

FEATURES OF PSEUDOPARKINSONISM

Tremor
> Worse at rest
> Pill-rolling movements of hands

Akinesia or Bradykinesia
> Slowing of body movements
> Mask-like facies

Rigidity
> Cogwheeling of extremities
> Stiffness

Postural Abnormalities
> Stooped shuffling gait
> Festinating gait
> Postural instability

Autonomic Manifestations
> Salivary drooling
> Perspiration
> Seborrhea

Abnormal Reflexes
> Palmomental
> Glabellar

tion. It is theorized that dopamine receptor blockade causes an increase in the number of binding sites and perhaps a slight alteration in the sensitivity of the receptors to dopamine (19,104). Figure 1 demonstrates the relationship between dopaminergic, cholinergic, and gamma-aminobutyric acid mediated neurons. Utilizing this postulated pathophysiology, it is apparent that tardive dyskinesia and pseudoparkinsonism (acute extrapyramidal symptoms) are opposites in terms of neurotransmitter function in the extrapyramidal system (97). This theory, although attractive in its ability to explain the etiology of tardive dyskinesia, extrapyramidal symptoms and the treatment modalities for extrapyramidal symptoms, does not adequately explain all aspects of tardive dyskinesia. This theory best explains the transient withdrawal dyskinesias but does not explain the irreversible symptoms found after drug discontinuation. Further, this theory cannot explain the presence of tardive dyskinesia and pseudoparkinsonism in the same patient at the same time. This simplification does not take into consideration the presence of presynaptic dopaminergic auto-receptors or the presence of two types of dopamine receptors (105). Nonetheless, this model does allow the clinician to predict and assess the potential impact of various chemotherapies on the movement disorder being treated (104). In this model, the major defect is not an excess of dopamine in the synaptic cleft. Rather, it is an exaggerated response to the existing dopamine released into the synapse which accounts for the movements.

Numerous epidemiologic studies have attempted to identify risk factors in the development of tardive dyskinesia (85). The incidence of tardive dyskinesia seems to increase with increasing age. This may be due to increased sensitivity of older patients to neuroleptic drugs. There appears to be a greater incidence of tardive dyskinesia in females than in males. Studies have indicated that tardive dyskinesia is more common in patients who have a history of acute extrapyramidal symptoms or prolonged anticholinergic therapy. Preexisting organic brain syndrome may also predispose individuals to tardive dyskinesia. These variables, though potentially important, are overshadowed by the strong correlation of duration of therapy, daily dosage, and total cumulative dosage received by the patients (106). Prolonged treatment with high dosages of neuroleptics is generally thought to increase the incidence of tardive dyskinesia. However, case reports indicate that tardive dyskinesia can occur in as short a time interval as after three to six months of neuroleptic therapy.

Treatment. Specific treatment approaches to tardive dyskinesia should relate to the striatal dopaminergic, cholinergic, and gabaminergic systems (Fig. 1) (104). Since the dopaminergic influence predominates, balance can be achieved by either decreasing the dopaminergic activity or increasing the cholinergic activity (19,107,108). Both treatment approaches have been evaluated clinically. More recently, use of agents that facilitate or increase GABA have been advocated (86).

Drugs which are capable of decreasing dopaminergic activity include *dopamine depletors* such as reserpine and *dopamine blockers* such as neuroleptics. Neuroleptic agents effectively mask tardive dyskinesia but carry the risk of further exacerbating the dysfunction. Of the dopamine depleting drugs, the most useful seem to be tetrabenazine and reserpine (109). Reserpine's effects, however, are only temporary, and dosage increases are required to maintain the patient at a movement-free state. Research is now focusing on the role of *presynaptic auto-receptors* in the control of dopamine levels in the nigro-striatal system (19). Apomorphine, a dopaminergic agonist, at low doses (subemetic) appears to preferentially stimulate presynaptic dopamine receptors. This auto-receptor stimulation leads to a decrease in dopamine production and release via a feedback mechanism (110). Analogues of apomorphine are currently being investigated for use in animal models of tardive dyskinesia.

Facilitation of cholinergic influence in the basal ganglia is another promising treatment for tardive dyskinesia. A useful agent for the prediction of success with cholinergic treatment of tardive dyskinesia is physostigmine (108). Physostigmine given in a dose of 1.0 mg IV (with repeat doses up to 4 mg) will reduce the movements. It is recommended that methylscopolamine be co-administered to block the peripheral cholinergic effects. If physostigmine causes a decrease in movements, then a trial with an orally active cholinergic agent is worthwhile (109). Deanol, at one time thought to be a precursor to acetylcholine, has produced mixed results in the treatment of tardive dyskinesia (107,108). Choline, a precursor to acetylcholine, has been demonstrated to increase levels of acetylcholine in animal brains. The typical dosage of choline is 150–200 mg/kg/day. Side effects include lacrimation, blurred vision, anorexia, diarrhea, depression, and a distinctive fishy odor. This odor is caused by the breakdown of choline to trimethylamine by gastrointestinal bacteria. The results with choline, though promising, are by no means consistent. A third cholinergic intervention is the use of lecithin (phosphatidyl choline). Lecithin is the primary dietary source of choline. It is not degraded by gut bacteria and therefore has the advantage of not producing a fishy odor. A disadvantage is that commercial lecithin products contain a variable amount of phosphatidyl choline. Therefore trials reporting dosages of lecithin are not necessarily comparable, depending on the source of the drug. Doses of lecithin equivalent to 24 grams of choline are usually necessary to control movements. Various degrees of response have been reported (111). Lecithin is currently the cholinergic agent of choice for the treatment of tardive dyskinesia (108).

Based on the current theories for tardive dyskinesia, GABA should play an important role in the negative feedback inhibition of dopamine release (24,108,109). Therefore the use of *agents which facilitate GABA* should decrease dopamine release and cause a decrease in movements. Baclofen (4-chlorophenyl-GABA) has been used in a limited number of double-blind studies (108). These studies suffer from small sample size, and it is also unclear as to baclofen's true mechanism of action. Side effects from baclofen in the usually administered doses of 60–90 mg/day are relatively severe. Typical incidences of side effects in patients receiving 60 mg/day of baclofen are muscular hypotonia 25%, sedation 20%, and muscular rigidity 15% (108). Another possible GABA facilitator is sodium valproate (valproic acid). This anticonvulsant drug appears to facilitate GABA, and placebo-controlled studies have demonstrated improvement in movement disorders (108). Dosages have ranged from 600 mg to 1600 mg per day. In most studies less than 50% of the patients responded to this therapy. The most commonly used facilitators of GABA are the benzodiazepines. Efficacy is difficult to assess because of these drugs' sedative actions. Sedation itself will often cause nonspecific improvement in movement disorder symptoms. Clonazepam has been demonstrated to improve movements when used in a dosage of 4 mg/day. Side effects include sedation, ataxia, confusion, and increased parkinsonian symptoms. Diazepam and chlordiazepoxide have been used to treat both tardive dyskinesia and Huntington's chorea. Agents that are effective in Huntington's chorea should also yield a beneficial effect in patients with iatrogenic dyskinesias.

There is currently no single efficacious treatment for tardive dyskinesia. It appears that there are subgroups of patients that are responsive to cholinergic or dopaminergic interventions and not necessarily to both (112). At the present time a trial and error approach is utilized. If one treatment approach fails, a suitable alternate treatment should be chosen from one of the other neurotransmitter categories. Polypharmacy in the treatment of tardive dyskinesia has not been evaluated. The long-term efficacy and safety of these treatments have not been established; thus, they should only be used when severe social impairment results (113). Treatments are usually only partially effective (108).

Prevention. Tardive dyskinesia is not easily treated once it becomes manifest. Therefore, prevention becomes the single most important intervention. The following guidelines should be observed when treating patients with antipsychotic drugs (114): (a) Neuroleptics should be used only for symptoms which are known to be responsive (eg, psychosis); (b) the minimum effective dose should be used; (c) patients treated with neuroleptics for more than three months should be examined to determine their need to remain on the medication and should receive a neurologic examination to detect the presence of tardive dyskinesia; (d) for those patients who develop abnormal tongue or finger movements while on neuroleptics, an assessment of the risks versus benefits should be made; (e) if tardive dyskinesia appears, the dose should be decreased or the drug discontinued; (f) anticholinergic agents should be used judiciously and discontinued if tardive dyskinesia is diagnosed; and (g) neuroleptic drugs should be completely withdrawn at least temporarily to unmask latent symptoms, particularly in patients with insipient manifestations.

Antipsychotic medications should be gradually withdrawn so that acute withdrawal dyskinesias are not exacerbated (113). Drug-free intervals ("drug holidays") should be a minimum of four weeks. Yearly drug holidays are no longer rec-

ommended (115). However, trial withdrawal should be attempted to determine if the antipsychotic is truly needed. Thirty per cent of chronic schizophrenics can be maintained without antipsychotic medications for up to one year or longer without relapsing. Many times a drug holiday simply consists of discontinuing medications while the patient is in the community. If the patient relapses and is returned to the hospital, then drug holidays are not indicated.

33. *Tardive Dyskinesia.* M.H., a 43-year-old woman, was admitted to the state hospital for the third time since age 25. She had no idea why she had been brought there from her boarding home. She had stopped her medications approximately three months prior to this admission and had become confused and threatening. She had also tried to set a car on fire, stating "I could not control myself." There was no significant medical history, and physical examination and laboratory data were within normal limits. Prior to discontinuing her medication, she had been taking thiothixene 60 mg at bedtime and trihexyphenidyl 2 mg four times daily. She had taken medication irregularly since her first admission. Of particular note was the presence of involuntary, abnormal movements. Orofacial, truncal, and extremity involvement was manifested by tongue protrusion, masticatory movements, blepharospasms (frequent blinking) and choreoathetosis (irregular, spasmodic movements mixed with constant, slow, writhing involuntary movements of the arms and legs accompanied by pelvic thrusting). What clinical data presented here are consistent with the syndrome of tardive dyskinesia? What symptoms are typical of tardive dyskinesia?

This patient's history and abnormal movements are consistent with tardive dyskinesia. Tardive dyskinesia is a syndrome characterized by involuntary movement following chronic treatment with antipsychotic drugs. Usually insidious in onset, it starts as mild tongue movements and may involve the buccal, facial, and lingual musculature. Blinking, grimacing, and arching of the eye brows are commonly seen. In severe cases, axial and appendicular muscles can be involved, causing dyskinesias which resemble chorea, athetosis, myoclonic jerks, and rotary pelvic movements. This iatrogenic disorder can be irreversible (109,114,116). M.H. presents with many of these symptoms.

34. How can tardive dyskinesia be differentiated from other dyskinesias?

Withdrawal dyskinesias are similar to tardive dyskinesia in both pathophysiology and in the movements observed, but are frequently reversible. Withdrawal dyskinesias occur upon the discontinuation or decrease in the dosage of antipsychotic medication (117). Withdrawal dyskinesias can identify patients that might be at risk for developing irreversible dyskinesias. If the movement persists for longer than three to six months, then tardive dyskinesia is a more appropriate descriptor. A differential diagnosis between tardive dyskinesia and other choreoathetoid syndromes is usually quite difficult to make in psychiatric patients (109). Oftentimes the diagnosis of tardive dyskinesia is made by the exclusion of all other possible etiologies. Drug histories are critical in determining whether the observed movements are suggestive of tardive dyskinesia. Long-term, chronic neuroleptic therapy would increase the likelihood of the observed movements being classified as tardive dyskinesia (118).

M.H. is probably not experiencing a withdrawal dyskinesia. The long-term neuroleptic treatment (three admissions) and the length of time since discontinuation of medication (three months) suggest that these movements are more correctly identified as tardive dyskinesia.

35. How can M.H.'s dyskinesia be treated?

M.H. was not begun on antipsychotic medications upon admission to the state hospital. It was decided that a drug-free period was essential to determine if the tardive dyskinesia was reversible. She received no neuroleptic drugs and was placed on diazepam 5 mg qid (GABA facilitator). The dyskinesia was still severe after four weeks of hospitalization and interfered significantly with her eating, talking, and socializing. The patient expressed great concern that she would be unable to care for herself because of the movements. She continued to hear voices that told her what to do. Because her anxiety and agitation level increased over the course of hospitalization, it was decided to reinstitute antipsychotic therapy. Thioridazine 100 mg bid was begun. Within three

weeks, the orofacial movements had decreased and the athetoid movements of the extremities had disappeared. After four months of neuroleptic therapy, the dyskinesias had recurred and the patient was again complaining of frequent, bothersome tongue, mouth, hand, and arm movements.

36. Is M.H.'s tardive dyskinesia irreversible?

Case reports and studies suggest that tardive dyskinesia remains reversible if the duration of neuroleptic drug therapy is less than two years (115). Tardive dyskinesias which develop or are discovered after two years are most likely irreversible. Irreversible dyskinesias have been reported within shorter periods of time (eg, less than 1 year).

M.H. had been maintained on neuroleptics for more than 10 years; therefore her dyskinesia is likely to be irreversible. Nonetheless, the neuroleptic was discontinued to determine if the dyskinesia was reversible. In this case, the neuroleptic medication had to be reinstituted because of the patient's worsening mental status. If antipsychotic medications are required, the minimum effective dose should be utilized to minimize further potential worsening of the dyskinesia. Thioridazine was chosen because of animal studies which indicate that it may have a more specific effect for limbic than striatal dopaminergic receptors (19). Sedating antipsychotic agents may be preferable to high potency antipsychotic agents for nonspecific behavioral control.

37. How could M.H.'s tardive dyskinesia be quantitatively assessed so that treatment interventions could be evaluated?

Many rating scales are available to objectify the assessment of a patient's tardive dyskinesia. The AIMS (Abnormal Involuntary Movement Scale) is the simplest rating scale to use (see Fig. 2). The Simpson Rating Scale is more detailed and more specific concerning assignment of severity scores (118a). An assessment of all patients on neuroleptics is recommended every 6–12 months. Early detection of dyskinesias with these scales can lead to interventions aimed at reducing the incidence of irreversibility.

Cardiovascular Side Effects

38. *Orthostatic Hypotension.* R.M., a 29-year-old woman, was being treated as an out-

**A simple method to determine
Tardive Dyskinesia Symptoms   AIMS* Examination Procedure**

Patient Identification _____   Date _____

Rated by _____

Either before or after completing the examination procedure, observe the patient unobtrusively at rest (eg, in waiting room).

The chair to be used in this examination should be a hard, firm one without arms.

After observing the patient, he may be rated on a scale of 0 (none), 1 (minimal), 2 (mild), 3 (moderate) and 4 (severe) according to the severity of symptoms.

Ask the patient whether there is anything in his/her mouth (ie, gum, candy, etc) and if there is to remove it.

Ask patient about the *current* condition of his/her teeth. Ask patient if he/she wears dentures. Do teeth or dentures bother patient *now*?

Ask patient whether he/she notices any movement in mouth, face, hands or feet. If yes, ask to describe and to what extent they *currently* bother patient or interfere with his/her activities.

| 0 | 1 | 2 | 3 | 4 | Have patient sit in chair with hands on knees, legs slightly apart and feet flat on floor. (Look at entire body for movements while in this position.) |

| 0 | 1 | 2 | 3 | 4 | Ask patient to sit with hands hanging unsupported. If male, between legs, if female and wearing a dress, hanging over knees. (Observe hands and other body areas.) |

| 0 | 1 | 2 | 3 | 4 | Ask patient to open mouth. (Observe tongue at rest within mouth.) Do this twice. |

| 0 | 1 | 2 | 3 | 4 | Ask patient to protrude tongue. (Observe abnormalities of tongue movement.) Do this twice. |

| 0 | 1 | 2 | 3 | 4 | Ask the patient to tap thumb, with each finger, as rapidly as possible for 10–15 seconds; separately with right hand, then with left hand. (Observe facial and leg movements.) |

| 0 | 1 | 2 | 3 | 4 | Flex and extend patient's left and right arms. (One at a time) |

| 0 | 1 | 2 | 3 | 4 | Ask patient to stand up. (Observe in profile. Observe all body areas again, hips included.) |

| 0 | 1 | 2 | 3 | 4 | †Ask patient to extend both arms outstretched in front with palms down. (Observe trunk, legs and mouth.) |

| 0 | 1 | 2 | 3 | 4 | †Have patient walk a few paces, turn and walk back to chair. (Observe hands and gait.) Do this twice. |

*Abnormal Involuntary Movement Scale   † Activated movements

Figure 2. Abnormal Involuntary Movement Scale.

patient with chlorpromazine 200 mg hs for paranoid schizophrenia. In addition, she was taking hydrochlorothiazide 50 mg every morning for hypertension. During one of her clinic visits, she became markedly agitated and delusional while talking about her family. At one point she smashed a chair against the wall and threatened the therapist. She was given 50 mg of chlorpromazine intramuscularly, and within 30 minutes she said she felt calmer and expressed a desire to leave the clinic. Upon getting up, she fell to the floor. The therapist elevated her legs and told her not to move. When her blood pressure was measured, it was 100/50 mm Hg standing and 100/70 mm Hg supine; her pulse was 105/min.

Why did the patient become hypotensive? What patients are at greater risk for developing this adverse effect?

Orthostatic hypotension is the most frequent neuroleptic-induced cardiovascular effect. It occurs more frequently and is most severe following the administration of an aliphatic phenothiazine (eg, chlorpromazine). It is infrequently associated with piperazine phenothiazines and is rarely associated with haloperidol or thiothixene (119–121). The mechanism by which neuroleptic drugs cause hypotension is not entirely understood. Neuroleptic drugs have alpha-adrenergic blocking effects which may contribute to orthostatic hypotension by increasing venous pooling. The loss of reflex vasoconstriction on assuming an upright position is the cause of dizziness and syncope in this patient. Some evidence suggests that neuroleptics also possess a central effect and a direct arterial effect which contributes to vasodilation (28). Patients who have a decreased vascular volume from acute hemorrhage, dehydration, or treatment with diuretic drugs are more prone to the hypotensive effects of neuroleptic drugs (120). The exact incidence and severity of neuroleptic-induced hypotension is difficult to determine, because most studies report only daily blood pressures without description of technique or patient position. Preexisting cardiovascular illness increases the risks of neuroleptic-induced hypotension (122).

39. How should this patient's hypotension be treated?

Patients who develop hypotension from neuroleptic drugs generally do not proceed to develop a shock syndrome. The hypotension can usually be treated by postural intervention (80). Placing the patient in a reverse Trendelenburg's position, thereby facilitating the return of blood from the legs, is usually all that is necessary. Volume expansion and drug treatment are only indicated when the patient develops shock.

Epinephrine should *not* be used because the neuroleptic's alpha-adrenergic blockade permits unopposed beta (vasodilation) activity and increased heart rate to predominate (25). This can progress to a worsening of the shock and myocardial ischemia. Plasma expansion with saline is usually the second intervention to be tried. When indicated, drug therapy should be a pure alpha-agonist such as phenylephrine. Norepinephrine, which possesses alpha and beta$_1$ (cardiac) effects, is an acceptable alternative (123,124).

40. How could this patient's hypotension have been prevented?

First, the use of intramuscular chlorpromazine is associated with a high incidence of alpha-blocking effects. If chlorpromazine was felt to be the only drug indicated, then the patient should have remained in a sitting or recumbent position for at least one hour. All patients, especially those being started on aliphatic and piperidine phenothiazines, should be warned about the possibility of orthostatic hypotension. This patient should have been instructed to stand up slowly to allow time for maximum circulatory compensation to occur. She should have been warned to sit up prior to standing when arising from a supine position.

At the first sign of dizziness upon arising, patients should be instructed to sit down and place their head between their legs (121). Tolerance appears to develop to a constant dosage level of antipsychotic medication; continued orthostatic hypotension is rare. Patients who experience a severe hypotensive episode should be changed to an agent with less alpha-blocking effects. Other risk factors that should be considered in the choice of a neuroleptic agent are age and concomitant medical illness and drug therapy. Drugs that cause plasma volume depletion or possess adrenergic blocking effects will predispose individuals to hypotension.

41. *Adverse Cardiac Effects.* L.G. is a 65-year-old schizophrenic who has been treated with thioridazine 200 mg at bedtime. She was hospitalized with a myocardial infarction which her cardiologist attributed to her medication. Upon questioning, she admitted that she had increased her dosage of thioridazine prior to her MI because of increasing suspiciousness and agitation; on the evening prior to her MI she had taken 700 mg of thioridazine. What phenothiazine cardiovascular toxicities could have contributed to this woman's myocardial infarction? What alternative treatment would be appropriate?

The most common cardiovascular effect of these drugs is *orthostatic hypotension* caused by alpha-adrenergic blockade. Orthostatic hypotension occurs most frequently with the low potency antipsychotic agents (eg, thioridazine, chlorpromazine). A patient who takes a large dose of thioridazine will have an acute drop in blood pressure and reflex tachycardia with poor return blood flow to the heart. These effects on the cardiovascular system can precipitate life-threatening cardiac ischemia in the predisposed individual.

Electrocardiographic changes have been observed with the phenothiazine drugs (122,123). High doses of thioridazine, and to a lesser extent, other antipsychotic drugs, can cause T wave changes and slowing of conduction (quinidine-like effect). Sinus tachycardia can occur from large doses of low potency, highly anticholinergic drugs like thioridazine. Overdoses of these drugs, particularly thioridazine, can lead to life-threatening arrhythmias.

Caution should be exercised when administering these drugs, particularly thioridazine, to elderly patients with preexisting cardiac disease. It is suggested that baseline electrocardiograms be obtained in older patients. If cardiac abnormalities are present, then a high potency drug (eg, haloperidol or thiothixene) would be the treatment of choice (130).

In this patient, the additive effects of possible preexisting cardiac pathology, increased catecholamine release associated with agitation, and the pharmacologic effects of the drug contributed to her MI. In the future she should be treated with haloperidol or thiothixene.

Temperature Regulation Dysfunction

42. M.T., a 38-year-old obese woman, has been hospitalized for the past two years for schizophrenia, chronic undifferentiated type, partially responsive to drug therapy. She has been treated with loxapine, and the dosage has been slowly increased over the past six months. For the past two months, she has received 100 mg twice daily with slow improvement in her target symptoms (agitation and hallucinations). She resists vocational and social retraining programs. She now has outside privileges. Two hours after leaving the ward to exercise, she was found lying unconscious outside. The ambient temperature was 95° F with a relative humidity of 82%. In the emergency room, her rectal temperature was 106° F, pulse was 115/min, blood pressure was 70/40 mm Hg, and respiratory rate was 28/min. The diagnosis was heat stroke. What led to the development of heat stroke in this patient?

The mechanisms of temperature control are quite complex and involve both the central and peripheral nervous system and circulatory mechanisms. Adrenergic, dopaminergic, serotonergic, and cholinergic systems are all involved in temperature regulation. Antipsychotic agents affect most of these neurotransmitter systems (126). Additionally, peripheral circulation and control of perspiration is affected by the autonomic nervous system effects of antipsychotics. The net result is poikilothermia (the ambient temperature influences body temperature) (25,125). Patients should be warned of this potential effect and especially during summer months should wear a hat, stay in the shade, and should seek a cooler environment at the first sign of weakness or overheating. Reports of hyperthermic episodes due to impaired temperature regulation in schizophrenic patients (mainly catatonia) antedates the use of antipsychotic agents (125). However, this patient probably experienced drug-induced heat stroke due to the environmental conditions (hot and humid) and due to the relatively high dose of neuroleptic.

Dermatologic Side Effects

43. What other environmental hazards are present for patients taking neuroleptics?

Excessive exposure to the sun should be avoided because of the danger of *photosensitivity*. Neuroleptic photosensitivity is thought to occur because the tricyclic structure of these agents absorbs ultraviolet energy from sunlight (25). Free radicals are formed which can damage biologic tissues. Clinically, areas of the body exposed to sunlight become erythematous and sunburned. Second degree burns are quite common with sustained exposure to sunlight. Chlorpromazine has been implicated most frequently (3%) based upon reported cases. Thiothixene has also been implicated (127). Thioridazine, however, while definitely causing skin pigmentation, has not been found to cause photosensitivity (128).

Patients should be warned of this potential effect and, especially during summer months, should wear protective clothing or use a sunscreen preparation with a high protection factor (129). (See the chapter on Skin Diseases.)

Sunlight is also involved in the *abnormal pigmentation* of skin which may occur after long-term administration of high doses of low potency phenothiazines (eg, chlorpromazine). This blue-gray pigmentation is reversible after substitution with a high potency phenothiazine or, optimally, after substitution with haloperidol, which is devoid of pigmentary effects. Pigmentation is now rare with current clinical practices. When it occurs, there is high probability of concomitant corneal and lens pigmentation.

Sex and Pregnancy

44. D.R., a 41-year-old single male, came into the community mental health center for a refill of his medication. He had been taking thioridazine 200 mg hs for eight years and was doing well. Upon further questioning, his

only complaint was a medical one. For about the last eight years, he could maintain an erection and sometimes experience orgasm while masturbating but did not ejaculate. He described a very active sex life during his 20's and 30's but now no longer feels virile or adequate. The patient last dated a woman six years ago. He blames the problem on his age but hopes he can be helped. Explain thioridazine's possible role in this patient's complaint.

Disorders of male sexual function, including impotence, decreased libido, and ejaculation disorders, have been reported with many of the neuroleptic drugs (137,138). Thioridazine has been particularly implicated in inhibition of ejaculation while not altering erection or orgasm. The proposed mechanism of ejaculation inhibition is hypothalamic sympathetic depression and peripheral alpha-adrenergic blockade. The central effect is common to all neuroleptics, but the significantly greater peripheral effects of thioridazine explain its high association with this disorder (125).

45. P.W., a 20-year-old female with schizophrenia, paranoid type, has decided that she no longer desires to take oral contraceptives. She claims "God made me to have children and I want a baby." She is concerned about the possible fetal effects of her antipsychotic medications. What are the risks of taking neuroleptic drugs during pregnancy?

Any decision concerning the use of drugs in pregnancy is a benefit-to-risk assessment. Psychotic, agitated, and disorganized individuals are not usually able to perform good pre- and postnatal care. Therefore, if the drugs are not dangerous, then a clear indication for their use is present.

In a prospective study involving 12,764 pregnant women (315 took phenothiazines), the use of an antipsychotic agent of the phenothiazine type was associated with a statistically increased risk of syndactyly, microcephaly, clubbed extremities, cleft lip, and cardiac malformations. The majority of the patients were medicated with phenothiazines uncommonly used in the United States (eg, methoxypromazine, oxomemazine). There has been one report of limb deformity with haloperidol. Subsequent retrospective studies did not find an association of haloperidol and birth defects (139). The evidence for the safety of the neuroleptic drugs in pregnancy based on large scale clinical experience indicates that the incidence of teratogenesis and mutagenesis is extremely low and approximates that in the untreated individual. Neonatal adverse reactions due to neuroleptics administered to mothers have been reported. Dystonias, withdrawal dyskinesias, and irritability occasionally occur. The lowest possible effective dose should be used, especially during the first trimester of pregnancy. Past clinical history should be evaluated to assist in the benefit-to-risk (relapse) determination. Use of non-phenothiazine antipsychotics (eg, haloperidol) is recommended due to the apparent absence of reported defects (139).

It should also be noted that neuroleptics, especially those of low potency, may produce amenorrhea, galactorrhea, and false positives with the HCG-method pregnancy test.

References

1. Dorsey R: Psychopharmacological screening criteria development project. JAMA. 1979; 241:1021.

2. Freedman AM et al: Mental status exam. In *Modern Synopsis of Psychiatry II*, edited by AM Freedman et al, Williams and Wilkins, Baltimore, 1976, pp 347–365.

3. Solomon P et al: The psychiatric examination, common psychiatric symptoms and differential diagnostic symptoms and signs. In *Handbook of Psychiatry*, edited by P Solomon et al, Lange Medical Publications, Los Altos, 1974, pp 26–100.

4. Detre TP et al: The assessment of the patient and examination, disposition and management. In *Modern Psychiatric Treatment*, edited by TP Detre et al, Lippincott, New York, 1971, pp 15–75.

5. Baldessarini RJ: Schizophrenia. N Engl J Med. 1977; 297:988.

6. Himmelhoch JM: What is schizophrenia? In Birth Defects: Original Article Series, 1978; 14:19.

7. Mendel WM: Precision in the diagnosis of schizophrenia. Psychiatria Fennica. 1975; 1:107.

8. American Psychiatric Association: *Diagnostic and Statistical Manual of Mental Disorders*, 2nd ed, Washington DC, 1968.

9. Burch EA et al: The congestive heart failure model of schizophrenia. JAMA. 1979; 241:1923.

10. American Psychiatric Association: Schizophrenic Disorders. In *Diagnostic and Statistical Manual of Mental Disorders 3rd Edition*, Washington DC, 1980, p 181.

11. Pope HG et al: Diagnosis in schizophrenia and manic depressive illness. Arch Gen Psychiatry. 1978; 35:811.

12. Donlon PT et al: Stages of schizophrenic decompensation and reintegration. J Nerv Ment Dis. 1972; 157:200.

13. Docherty JP: Stages of onset of schizophrenic psychosis. Am J Psychiatry. 1978; 135:420.

14. Detre TP et al: Schizophrenic disorders. In *Psychiatric Treatment,* edited by TP Detre et al, Lippincott Co., Philadelphia, 1971, p 109.

15. Ereshefsky L et al: Schizophrenia and psychosis. In *Manual of Drug Therapy: Essentials of Systematic Drug Monitoring,* edited by A Watanabe et al, Lea and Febiger, Philadelphia, 1981, in press.

16. Snyder SH et al: Drugs, neurotransmitters and schizophrenia. Science. 1974; 184:1243.

17. Carlsson A: Antipsychotic drugs, neurotransmitters and schizophrenia. Am J Psychiatry. 1978; 135:164.

18. Berger PA: Biochemistry and the schizophrenias: old concepts and new hypotheses. J Nerv Ment Dis. 1981; 169:90.

19. Klawans HL et al: Tardive dyskinesia: review and update. Am J Psychiatry. 1980; 137:900.

20. Stimmel GL: Neuroleptics and the corpus striatum. Dis Nerv Syst. 1976; 37:219.

21. Kolb LC: *Modern Clinical Psychiatry,* WB Saunders Co., Philadephia, 1973, p 308.

22. Shader RI et al: Approaches to schizophrenia. In *Manual of Psychiatric Therapeutics,* edited by RI Shader, Little, Brown and Company, Boston, 1976, p 63.

23. Rosebaum CP: *The Meaning of Madness,* Sciencehouse, New York, 1970, p 16.

24. NIMH Psychopharmacology Service Center Collaborative Study Group: Phenothiazine treatment in acute schizophrenia: Effectiveness. Arch Gen Psychiatry. 1964; 10:246.

25. Appleton WS et al: Before drug therapy begins, choosing an antipsychotic and principles of prescribing antipsychotics. In *Practical Clinical Psychopharmacology,* 2nd ed, edited by WS Appleton et al, Williams and Wilkins, Baltimore, 1980, p 1.

26. Meltzer HY et al: The dopamine hypothesis of schizophrenia: a review. Schizophrenia Bull. 1976; 2:19.

27. Mason AS: Basic principles in the use of antipsychotic agents. Hosp and Commun Psychiatry. 1973; 24:825.

28. Kessler KA et al: Clinical use of the antipsychotics. Am J Psychiatry. 1981; 138:202.

29. Davis JM: Recent developments in the treatment of schizophrenia. Psychiatric Ann. 1976; 6:71.

30. Wyatt RJ: Biochemistry and Schizophrenia (Part IV) The Neuroleptics. Psychopharmacology Bull. 1976; 12:5.

31. May PRA et al: Prediction of schizophrenic patients' response to pharmacotherapy. In *Psychopharmacology: A Generation of Progress,* edited by MA Lipton et al, Raven Press, New York, 1978, p 1139.

32. Zavodnick S: A pharmacological and theoretical comparison of high and low potency neuroleptics. J of Clin Psychiatry. 1978; 39(4):332.

33. Kalant OJ: *The Amphetamines: Toxicity and Addiction.* Charles C. Thomas Co., Toronto, 1963.

34. Ellenwood EH: Amphetamine psychosis: individuals, settings, and sequences. *Current Concepts of Amphetamine's Abuse,* 1972; 143, (DHEW Publication No. HSM72-9085).

35. Snyder S: A model schizophrenia mediated by catecholamines. Am J Psychiatry. 1973; 130:61.

36. Hollister LE: Phencyclidine use: Current problems. Int Drug Ther Newsl. 1979; 14:17.

37. Richards ML et al: Phencyclidine psychosis. Drug Intell Clin Pharm. 1979; 13:336.

38. Barron MB et al: Hallucinogenic drugs. Sci Am. 1964; 210:29.

39. Fink M et al: Prolonged adverse reactions to LSD in psychotic subjects. Arch Gen Psychiatry. 1966; 15:450.

40. Janowsky DS et al: Combined anticholinergic agents and atropine-like delirium. Am J Psychiatry. 1971; 129:360.

41. Donlon PT et al: Overview: efficacy and safety of the rapid neuroleptization method with injectable haloperidol. Am J Psychiatry. 1979; 136:273.

42. Donlon PT: High dose neuroleptic therapy. Int Pharmacopsychiatry. 1976; 11:235.

43. Donlon PT et al: Rapid "digitalization" of decompensated schizophrenic patients with antipsychotic agents. Am J Psychiatry. 1974; 131:310.

44. Aubree JC et al: High and very high dosage antipsychotics: a critical review. J Clin Psychiatry. 1980; 41:341.

45. Davis JM et al: Important issues in the drug treatment of schizophrenia. Schizophrenia Bull. 1980; 6:70.

46. Rubin RT et al: Serum haloperidol determinations in psychiatric patients. 1980; 37:1069.

47. McNeil Laboratories: Haldol package insert, 1975.

48. Based on clinical use of authors; modified from references 28, 29, 43.

49. Appleton WS: Third psychoactive drug usage guide. Dis Nerv Syst. 1976; 37:39.

50. Bassuk EL: Clinical application of the antipsychotic agents. In *Guide to Psychoactive Drug Use,* edited by EL Bassuk et al, Plenum Publishers, New York, 1977, p 95.

50a. Ayd FJ: Once-a-day neuroleptic and tricyclic antidepressant therapy. Int Drug Ther Newsl. 1971; 7:33.

51. Casey JF et al: Combined drug therapy of chronic schizophrenics. Am J Psychiatry. 1961; 117:997.

52. Freeman H: The therapeutic value of combinations of psychotropic drugs, a review. Psychopharmacol Bull. 1967; 4:1.

53. Merlis S et al: Polypharmacy in psychiatry: patterns of differential treatment. Am J Psychiatry. 1970; 126:1647.

54. Veterans Administration Mental Health and Behavioral Sciences Service: Antischizophrenic Drug Use, G-14, M-2, Past X, Washington DC, 1978.

55. Rampling D: Aggression: A paradoxical response to tricyclic antidepressants. Am J Psychiatry. 1978; 135:117.

56. Risch SC et al: Plasma levels of tricyclic antidepressants in clinical efficacy: review of the literature Part II. J Clin Psychiatry. 1979; 40:58.

57. Greenblatt DJ et al: Benzodiazepines Part I. N Engl J Med. 1974; 291:1011.

58. Prien RF et al: Relapse in chronic schizophrenics following abrupt withdrawal of tranquilizing medication. Br J Psychiatry. 1969; 115:679.

59. Hogarty GE et al: Drugs and social therapy in the aftercare of schizophrenic patients. Arch Gen Psychiatry. 1973; 28:54.

60. Engelhardt DM et al: Phenothiazines in prevention of psychiatric hospitalization, IV delay or prevention—a re-evaluation. Arch Gen Psychiatry. 1967; 16:98.

61. Rifkin A et al: Long term use of antipsychotic drugs. In *Progress in Psychiatric Drug Treatment,* edited by DF Klein et al, Brunner-Mazel, New York, 1975, p 387.

62. Marder SR et al: Predicting drug-free improvement in schizophrenic psychosis. Arch Gen Psychiatry. 1979; 36:1080.

63. Stephens JH: Long-term prognosis and follow-up in schizophrenia. Schizophrenia Bull. 1978; 4:25.

64. Judd LL et al: Phenothiazine effects in good premorbid schizophrenics divided into paranoid-nonparanoid status. Arch Gen Psychiatry. 1973; 29:207.

65. Leff JP et al: Trial of maintenance therapy in schizophrenia. Br Med J. 1971; 3:599.

66. Adamson L et al: Fluphenazine decanoate trial in chronic inpatient schizophrenics failing to absorb chlorpromazine. Dis Nerv Syst. 1973; 34:181.

67. Curry SH et al: Double-blind trial of fluphenazine decanoate. Lancet. 1972; 2:543.

68. Cole JO: Introduction to symposium on long-acting phenothiazines in psychiatry. Dis Nerv Syst. 1970; 31 (suppl 9):5.

69. Curry SH: Chlorpromazine: concentration in plasma, excretion in urine and duration of effect. Proc R Soc Med. 1971; 64:285.

70. Itil TM et al: EEG changes after fluphenazine enanthate and decanoate based on analogue power spectra and digital computer analysis. Psychopharmacologia. 1971; 20:230.

71. Van Praag HMM et al: Fluphenazine enanthate and fluphenazine decanoate: a comparison of their duration of action and motor side effects. Am J Psychiatry. 1970; 130:801.

72. Curry SH et al: Kinetics of fluphenazine after fluphenazine hydrochloride, enanthate and decanoate administration to man. Br J Clin Pharm. 1979; 7:325.

73. Wiles D: Tardive dyskinesia and depot fluphenazine. Br J Psychiatry. 1979; 135:382.

74. Groves JE et al: The long-acting phenothiazines. Arch Gen Psychiatry. 1975; 32:893.

75. Hollister LE: Psychiatric disorders. In *Drug Treatment: Principles and Practice of Clinical Pharmacology and Therapeutics,* 2nd ed, edited by GS Avery, Adis Press, New York, 1980, p 1081.

76. Grosser HH: Experience of psychiatric management of schizophrenia with fluphenazine decanoate. Dis Nerv Syst. 1970; 31 (suppl 9):32.

77. Ayd FJ: The depot fluphenazines: a reappraisal after ten years' clinical experience. Am J Psychiatry. 1975; 132:491.

78. Chien CP et al: Depot phenothiazine treatment in acute psychosis: a sequential comparative clinical study. Am J Psychiatry. 1973; 130:13.

79. Warner AM et al: Delayed severe extrapyramidal disturbance following frequent depot phenothiazine administration. Am J Psychiatry. 1975; 132:743.

80. Hollister LE: Adverse reactions to psychotherapeutic drugs. In *Drug Treatment of Mental Disorders,* edited by LL Simpson, Raven Press, New York, 1976, p 267.

81. Ayd FJ: Guidelines for effective and safe use of depot fluphenazines for maintenance therapy. Int Drug Ther Newsl. 1975; 10:9.

82. Coleman JH et al: Drug induced extrapyramidal effects—a review. Dis Nerv Syst. 1975; 36:591.

83. FDA Task Force Report: Neurological syndromes associated with antipsychotic drug use. Arch Gen Psychiatry. 1973; 28:463.

84. Swett C: Drug induced dystonia. Am J Psychiatry. 1975; 32:532.

85. Sovmer R et al: Extrapyramidal syndromes and other neurological side effects of psychotropic drugs. In *Psychopharmacology: A Generation of Progress,* edited by MA Lipton et al, Raven Press, New York, 1978, p 1021.

86. Ehrensing RH: Tardive dyskinesia. Arch Intern Med. 1978; 138:1261.

87. Ayd FJ: A survey of drug-induced extrapyramidal reactions. JAMA. 1961; 175:1054.

88. Sheppard C et al: Drug-induced extrapyramidal symptoms: incidence and treatment. Am J Psychiatry. 1967; 123:886.

89. Paulson G et al: Some remarks on the treatment of postencephalitic oculogyric crisis with benztropine. Int J Neuropsychiatry. 1965; 1:214.

90. Kleet CJ et al: Evaluating the long-term need for antiparkinson drugs by chronic schizophrenics. Arch Gen Psychiatry. 1972; 26:374.

91. Rifkin A et al: Akinesia. Arch Gen Psychiatry. 1975; 32:672.

92. Manos N et al: The need for continuous use of antiparkinsonian medication with chronic schizophrenic patients receiving long-term neuroleptic therapy. Am J Psychiatry. 1981; 138:184.

93. Van Putten T: Why do schizophrenic patients refuse to take their drugs? Arch Gen Psychiatry. 1974; 31:67.

94. Hoffman BF: The diagnosis and treatment of neuroleptic-induced parkinsonism. Hosp and Comm Psychiatry. 1981; 32:110.

95. Fann WE et al: Amantadine versus trihexyphenidyl in the treatment of neuroleptic-induced parkinsonism. Am J Psychiatry. 1976; 133:940.

96. Allen M et al: Amantadine reduces haloperidol-induced dopamine receptor hypersensitivity in the striatum. Eur J Pharmacology. 1980; 65:313.

97. Stimmel GL: Neuroleptics and the corpus striatum: clinical implications. Dis Nerv Syst. 1976; 37:219.

98. Gerlach J et al: Tardive dyskinesia during and following treatment with haloperidol, haloperidol plus biperiden, thioridazine, and clozapine. Psychopharmacology. 1978; 59:105.

99. Stimmel GL: Schizophrenia. J Am Pharm Assoc. 1974; 14:257.

100. Neu C et al: Antiparkinson medication in the treatment of extrapyramidal side effects. Curr Ther Res. 1972; 14:246.

101. Warnes H: Toxic psychosis due to antiparkinson drugs. Can Psychiatric Assoc J. 1967; 12:323.

102. van der Kolk B et al: Autonomic effects of psychotropic drugs. In *Psychopharmacology: A Generation of Progress,* edited by MA Lipton et al, Raven Press, New York, 1978, p 1009.

103. Duvoisin R: Parkinsonism. Ciba Clinical Symposia. 1976; 28(1):1.

104. Marsden CD et al: The pathophysiology of extrapyramidal side-effects of neuroleptic drugs. Psychol Med. 1980; 10:55.

105. Roth RH: Dopamine autoreceptors: pharmacology, function and comparison with post-synaptic dopamine receptors. Commun Psychopharmacology. 1979; 3:429.

106. Stimmel GL: Tardive dyskinesia with low dose short-term neuroleptic therapy. Am J Hosp Pharm. 1976; 33:961.

107. Kobayashi RM: Drug therapy of tardive dyskinesia. N Engl J Med. 1977; 296:257.

108. Jeste V et al: In search of treatment for tardive dyskinesia: review of the literature. Schizophrenia Bull. 1979; 5:251.

109. Baldessarini RJ et al: Tardive dyskinesia. In *Psychopharmacology: A Generation of Progress*, edited by MA Lipton et al, Raven Press, New York, 1978, p 993.

110. Christensen AV et al: Dopaminergic supersensitivity: influence of dopamine agonists, cholinergics, anticholinergics, and drugs used for the treatment of tardive dyskinesia. Psychopharmacology. 1979; 62:111.

111. Gelenberg AJ et al: Choline and lecithin in the treatment of tardive dyskinesia: preliminary results from a pilot study. Am J Psychiatry. 1979; 136:772.

112. Casey DE: Managing tardive dyskinesia. J Clin Psychiatry. 1978; 39:748.

113. Jus A: Long term treatment of tardive dyskinesia. J Clin Psychiatry. 1979; 40:72.

114. Ayd FJ: Ethical and legal dilemmas posed by tardive dyskinesia. Int Drug Ther Newsl. 1977; 12:29.

115. Jeste DV: Tardive dyskinesia—reversible and persistent. Arch Gen Psychiatry. 1979; 36:505.

116. Crane GE: Tardive dyskinesia and related neurological disorders. In *Handbook of Psychopharmacology* Vol 10, edited by LL Iversen et al, Plenum Press, New York, 1978, p 165.

117. Gardos G: Withdrawal symptoms associated with antipsychotic drugs. Am J Psychiatry. 1978; 135:1321.

118. Klawans HL: The pharmacology of tardive dyskinesias. Am J Psychiatry. 1973; 130:82.

118a. Simpson GM et al: A rating scale for tardive dyskinesia. Psychopharmacology. 1979; 64:171–9.

119. Ayd FJ: Haloperidol: fifteen years of clinical experience. Dis Nerv Syst. 1972; 33:459.

120. Ebert MH et al: Cardiovascular effects. In *Psychotropic Drug Side Effects*, edited by RI Shader et al, Williams and Wilkins Co., Baltimore, 1970, p 149.

121. Jefferson JW: Hypotension from drugs: incidence, peril, prevention. Dis Nerv Syst. 1974; 35:66.

122. Paul SM et al: Cardiotoxicity of commonly prescribed psychotherapeutic drugs: clinical implications. In: *Psychotherapeutic Drugs Part I*, edited by E Usdin et al, Marcel Dekker, New York, 1977, p 484.

123. Stimmel B: The major tranquilizers. In *Cardiovascular Effects of Mood-Altering Drugs*, edited by B Stimmel, Raven Press, New York, 1979, p 117.

124. Warens II et al: Complications of psychotropic medications in high dosage. Psychiatric Quarterly. 1971; 45:87.

125. van der Kolk B et al: Autonomic effects of psychotropic drugs. In *Psychopharmacology: A Generation of Progress*, edited by MA Lipton et al, Raven Press, New York, 1978, p 1009.

126. Jacknowitz AI: Thioridazine-induced hyperpyrexia. Am J Hosp Pharm. 1979; 36:674.

127. Appleton WS et al: Dermatological effects. In *Psychotropic Drug Side Effects*, edited by RI Shader et al, Williams and Wilkins Co., Baltimore, 1970, p 77.

128. Berger H: Pigmentation after thioridazine. Arch Derm. 1969; 100:487.

129. Koreny IC: The effect of benzophenone sunscreen lotion on chlorpromazine treated patients. Am J Psychiatry. 1969; 125:143.

130. Lipscomb PA: Cardiovascular side effects of phenothiazines and tricyclic antidepressants. Postgrad Med. 1980; 67:189.

131. Leestma JE et al: Sudden death and phenothiazines. Arch Gen Psychiatry. 1968; 18:137.

132. Peele R et al: Phenothiazine deaths: a critical review. Am J Psychiatry. 1973; 130:306.

133. Risch SC et al: Interfaces of psychopharmacology and cardiology—Part II. J Clin Psychiatry. 1981; 42:47.

134. Hansten PD: *Drug Interactions,* third edition, Lea and Febiger, Philadelphia, 1976, p 159.

135. Remick RA et al: Antipsychotic drugs and seizures. J Clin Psychiatry. 1979; 40:78.

136. Evans L: Psychological effects caused by drugs in overdose. Drugs. 1980; 19:220.

137. Blair SH et al: Effect of antipsychotic drugs on reproductive functions. Dis Nerv Syst. 1966; 27:645.

138. Ayd FJ: Neuroleptics and male sexual dysfunction. Int Drug Ther Newsl. 1979; 14:21.

139. Hays DP: Teratogenesis: a review of the basic principles with a discussion of selected agents: Part II. Drug Intell Clin Pharm. 1981; 15:542.

Chapter 45

Affective Disorders

James H. Coleman and Joseph A. Johnston

History

Hippocrates is generally credited with the first descriptions of an affective disorder, though the Old Testament describes the dysphoric mood of Job. Hippocrates is thought to have coined the term "melancholia," literally translated as "black bile." He thought that the influence of black bile and phlegm on the brain produced the depressive state which he labeled as melancholia (1).

In the second century A.D., Aretaeus made reference to melancholia and mania, noting that the conditions are often episodic but also occurred in a chronic, unremitting form. He, like Hippocrates, attributed the cause to humoral imbalance.

In 1896, Kraepelin separated the functional psychoses into two groups, the manic-depressive psychoses and dementia praecox. Undoubtedly, his work was influenced by earlier endeavors of Falret and Baillarger who both gave very accurate clinical descriptions of recurrent attacks of depression and mania. Kraepelin felt that manic-depressive psychosis was independent of social and psychological forces and that the cause of the illness was "innate" (2).

Estimates of the prevalence of primary affective disorder vary from population to population. Average estimates of those who can expect to have a primary affective disorder sometime during their lives range from 5% of men to 9% of women. One estimate for the American population puts the figure at 18%. This suggests that these disorders are possibly the most common psychiatric conditions to be encountered (3–5).

Classification

Affective disorders are disturbances of mood. These disturbances involve either depression of the mood state (depression) or elevation of the mood state (mania). Table 1 lists the current classification of affective disorders according to the *Diagnostic and Statistical Manual of Mental Disorders* (DSM III) (6). This classification should be used in order to provide more universally consistent diagnostic terminology. Inconsistent diagnostic semantics has hindered medical progress in affective disorders, and psychiatry in general, for years. Various classifications of depression have included exogenous, endogenous, reactive, nonreactive, primary, secondary, neurotic, unipolar, bipolar, and melancholic depression (7–10). These terms are no longer valid diagnoses; rather, the clinician should strive to use the DSM III classification since this will undoubtedly aid future research and will also assist in increasing the validity of retrospective studies. The *major affective disorders* include bipolar disorder and major depression (6).

Bipolar disorder refers to those patients who have had at least one manic episode. (Mania will be discussed fully later in this chapter.) They may or may not have had a major depressive episode. Bipolar affective disorder is synonymous with the old terminology—manic depressive illness. There are three types of bipolar disorder: The *mixed type* includes those patients whose clinical symptoms meet the criteria for mania and major depressive illness either intermixed or alternating every few days. The *manic type* includes those patients who are currently experiencing a manic episode. The *depressed type* includes those patients who have had one or more manic episodes and who currently are experiencing a major depressive episode (6).

Major depression includes those patients who meet the DSM III criteria for major depression. (This will be discussed in Question 1). The major depression category is further divided into single episode or recurrent episodes (6).

Other specific affective disorders include cyclothymic disorder and dysthymic disorder. *Cyclothymia* includes those individuals who have numerous periods of mood disturbances similar to both the depressive and manic syndromes but do not meet the criteria for either a manic or depressive episode due to lack of symptom severity and duration. *Dysthymic disorder* (or depressive

neurosis) includes those patients who are chronically troubled by symptoms characteristic of the depressive syndrome; however, they do not meet the criteria for the depressive syndrome due to lack of severity and duration of symptoms (6).

Atypical bipolar disorder and *atypical depression* include those individuals with manic and depressive features respectively, but whose symptoms are not sufficient for the diagnosis of bipolar disorder or major depressive illness. In the case of atypical bipolar disorder, the patient may meet the criteria for major depressive illness, but only demonstrate partial symptomatology of mania. For the diagnosis of atypical depression the patient may not meet the criteria for any other affective illness (6).

The reader is referred to the DSM III for a complete discussion of the diagnostic criteria of affective disorders (6).

Pathophysiology

No single cause or theory can successfully explain the pathogenesis of affective disorders. Mental health scholars have debated for years on the cause of affective disorders. Psychiatrists who subscribe to the psychosocial doctrine search for stressful life events or intrapsychic conflicts preceding the onset of the affective episode. Strict biological psychiatrists explain depression and mania in terms of neuronal levels of catechola-

Table 1.

AFFECTIVE DISORDERS
DIAGNOSTIC AND STATISTICAL MANUAL
OF MENTAL DISORDERS
(THIRD EDITION)

A. Major Affective Disorders
  1. Bipolar Disorder
    Mixed
    Manic
    Depressed
  2. Major Depression
    Single Episode
    Recurrent

B. Other Specific Affective Disorders
  Cyclothymic Disorder
  Dysthymic Disorder (or Depressive Neurosis)

C. Atypical Affective Disorder
  Atypical Dipolar Disorder
  Atypical Depression

mines (eg, dopamine, norepinephrine, epinephrine) and the indolamines (eg, serotonin). Acceptance of either a psychosocial doctrine or a biological doctrine alone assumes a simplistic point of view. It is more realistic to think of depression as the result of a *psychobiological final common pathway*. Using this model, affective illness is the endpoint of several processes that conceivably converge in those areas of the brain that modulate arousal, mood, motivation, and psychomotor function. The presenting clinical picture will depend on the interaction of several factors:

a. Genetic Vulnerability: A genetic role is clearly involved in major affective disorders.
b. Developmental Events: Early object loss (ie, loss of a parent) may make an individual more sensitive to certain kinds of stressful events in adult life.
c. Psychosocial Events: Certain events in adult life may overwhelm the coping mechanisms of the individual (ie, divorce or retirement).
d. Physiological Stresses: Infections, childbirth, disease states, and drugs (ie, reserpine) may directly induce physiochemical changes.
e. Personality Traits: Preexisting personality traits can influence an individual's reaction to stress including the stress of being depressed (ie, a very dependent individual will have much greater turmoil from the loss of a support system than an independent individual).

Various combinations of these factors lead to biochemical alterations of the central nervous system and account for the frequently observed features shared by individuals suffering from affective disorders (7,11). This psychobiological final common pathway model integrates all the major psychiatric models for affective illness and demonstrates that there is no singular cause for affective illness. However, from the standpoint of understanding drug action, it is useful to consider various biochemical explanations of affective disorders.

Catecholamine Hypothesis. The catecholamine hypothesis is an explanation of depression and mania based on neuronal concentrations of the catecholamines. Schildkraut formulated this hypothesis in 1965 when he stated that, "Some, if not all depressions are associated with an absolute or relative deficiency of catecholamines, particularly norepinephrine, at functionally important adrenergic receptor sites in the brain. Elation conversely may be associated with an excess of such amines" (12). Similar evidence has accumulated for the role of serotonin (13–16). As previously stated, this is a somewhat simplistic view. There are many theories involving the biogenic amines, most of which focus on the premise that alterations in the levels or metabolic fates of the biogenic amines provoke some behavior. However, there is evidence to suggest that the converse may be true; that is, alterations in social and/or psychological events (stress, etc.) can induce major changes in brain amine levels (17–19).

Permissive Hypothesis. The permissive hypothesis developed by Prange and others offers an explanation of affective disorders based more on the role of serotonin than on the catecholamines (20). This hypothesis places depression and mania on a continuum rather than on polar opposites. Depressive illness is noted to be a less severe deviation from the normal than mania. Indeed, there are clinical and biological dysfunctions shared by both manic and depressed patients. For example, depressed patients suffer from CNS arousal such as insomnia, anorexia, agitation, and increased residual intraneuronal sodium concentrations. These same conditions exist in the manic state but are more pronounced. Additionally, manic episodes are usually preceded and followed by mild depressive episodes; and occasionally, manic and depressive symptoms occur simultaneously, which can only be explained by a continuum model. By placing the permissive influence on the CNS levels of serotonin, the role of the catecholamines becomes secondary and thus determines the type of affective disorder which will be observed. These data are presented in Table 2.

Table 2.

PERMISSIVE HYPOTHESIS FOR
AFFECTIVE DISORDERS

(IA = Indoleaminergic Transmission)
(CA = Catecholaminergic Transmission)

Normal IA	+ Normal CA	=	Normal
Reduced IA	+ Normal CA	=	Predisposition to Affective Disorder
Reduced IA	+ Reduced CA	=	Depression
Reduced IA	+ Increased CA	=	Mania

Intraneuronal hypernatremia. As noted above, it may be demonstrated that depression and mania are a continuum representing a state of CNS hyperarousal, mania representing a more severe arousal than depression. Whybrow and Mendels reported that this CNS hyperarousal was commonly manifested by a lowered arousal threshold, disruption of rapid eye movement (REM) sleep patterns, and disappearance of delta or deep sleep (21). They subsequently postulated that this state of CNS hyperarousal could result from an intraneuronal hypernatremic condition. There are studies to indicate that intracellular sodium levels are increased during alcoholic inebriation, thus possibly producing some of the depressive symptomatology commonly seen in those who consume large amounts of alcohol during drinking binges (22–26). Increases in intraneuronal sodium cause the resting membrane potential to be lowered, thus producing a state of hyperarousal. This phenomenon may in part explain the seizure diathesis commonly associated with chronic alcohol abuse. It becomes easy, utilizing this model, to understand why depressed individuals seeking to "drown their sorrows" find themselves in a worsened state after using alcohol. A disordered electrolyte state may precipitate a disorder in biogenic amine function, since several of the enzyme systems involved in normal biogenic amine function are sodium dependent. Aberrant biogenic amine function may in turn produce a disturbance of the diencephalic reinforcement mechanisms with subsequent impairment in mood, psychomotor activity, appetite, sleep, and libido. Much of the research in this area is new, emerging, contradictory, and controversial (27–36).

Mechanisms of Drug Action

Lithium and the antidepressants (predominately the tricyclics) are the major psychotherapeutic agents used in the treatment of affective disorders. Antipsychotics are also used, as will be illustrated in some of the questions which follow.

Antidepressants. There are six pharmacologic categories of antidepressants: stimulants, monoamine oxidase inhibitors (MAOIs), tricyclics, tetracyclics, triazolopyridines, and tetrahydroisoquinolines. The agents which enjoy the greatest use are the tricyclic compounds, although the MAOIs are still of considerable value for some patients (37–39). As experience is gained

with the newer agents, they may become as extensively used as the tricyclic antidepressants.

The tricyclic agents, of which imipramine is the prototype, presently encompass eight agents, and more are expected in the near future. Six of these drugs have been on the market for several years. These include the tertiary amines imipramine, amitriptyline, and doxepin, and the secondary amines desipramine, nortriptyline, and protriptyline. The new tricyclic compounds, trimipramine and amoxapine, are discussed in Question 9.

According to the catecholamine hypothesis, depression involves a real or at least functional deficiency in one or more of the neurotransmitters. In normal states, neurotransmitter activity is terminated by enzymatic degradation, by catechol-o-methyltransferase (COMT) in the synaptic cleft and postsynaptic neuron, and by monoamine oxidase (MAO) in the presynaptic neuron. Neurotransmitters are also inactivated by reabsorption into the presynaptic neuron via a reuptake mechanism. This mechanism is of considerable importance, accounting for 60% of the inactivation of norepinephrine (40,41). The tricyclics apparently impede this reuptake process, thereby producing a greater quantity of the transmitter within the synaptic cleft (42). This process theoretically increases synaptic transmission. There is a latency period ranging from several days to two or three weeks before the antidepressant action becomes evident (43). Neither the formation of active metabolites nor distribution of parent drug and metabolites can account for this latency period (44,45).

There appears to be some specificity of reuptake blocking among the various tricyclics (46–48). The tertiary amine tricyclics (imipramine, amitriptyline, and doxepin) principally block the reuptake inactivation of the neurotransmitter serotonin, while the secondary amine tricyclics (desipramine, nortriptyline, and protriptyline) principally block the reuptake inactivation of the neurotransmitter norepinephrine. Theoretically, this could be of clinical importance. However, in practice these differences begin to blur, because the tertiary tricyclics are eventually demethylated to secondary tricyclics, and in this form they exert an effect on norepinephrine as well. Although attempts have been made to identify subtypes of depression which correlate with various neurotransmitter deficiencies, practical application of this research remains unclear (46–51). In clinical situations, it is common for patients to not respond to one tricyclic but to subsequently respond to another tricyclic from the same chemical class. Individual patient differences in steady-state parent compound/metabolite plasma ratios may account for these differences in response.

Lithium. The mechanism of action of lithium is unknown, although several explanations which relate to the still poorly understood pathophysiology of mania have been offered. According to the catecholamine hypothesis, norepinephrine levels are increased in mania. Lithium may facilitate the transport of norepinephrine across neuronal membranes which would decrease norepinephrine-mediated synaptic transmission. Furthermore, this effect on norepinephrine transport would tend to stabilize the synaptic concentration of norepinephrine, thus explaining the prophylactic effect of lithium for both mania and depression (52,53). It is also theorized that mania may result from increased neuronal sodium concentrations, and lithium may work by replacing some of the sodium within the neuron, lowering the sodium concentration to normal (52). Other explanations have been advanced as well, but the precise mode of action of lithium in affective disorders remains unclear (52,54–58).

MAJOR DEPRESSION

1. **C.R., a 37-year-old male, came to outpatient clinic with the chief complaint of "feeling tired." Other problems elicited during the interview included weight loss (10 pounds over the past six weeks), nausea, and occasional headaches. Physical examination was unremarkable. An upper GI series, complete blood count, SMA-12 laboratory panel, thyroid function studies, and urinalysis were ordered. The results of all these evaluations were reported as being within normal limits. When C.R. returned to the clinic the following week, a more thorough interview was performed and the following information was obtained. C.R. was experiencing insomnia characterized by early morning awakening with an inability to return to sleep. He no longer enjoyed eating, although formerly he thoroughly enjoyed food. His job had become boring; he no longer felt motivated.**

He was experiencing difficulty with his memory and recently began making notes for himself. He felt much of his problem was due to laziness and his inability to concentrate on his work. He expressed guilt over the neglect of his wife and children. When asked about his sexual relationship, he answered "I have no interest in sex and can't seem to perform anyway." He said that he no longer desired to live but would never attempt suicide. He said "I wish I could go to sleep and never wake up." At no point in the interview did C.R. use the word "depression." These symptoms began about six weeks prior to his seeking medical help and seemed to be increasing in severity. He had come to the clinic at the insistence of his wife. C.R. was given a diagnosis of major depression, single episode. What signs and symptoms of depression are illustrated by this patient?

Depression affects all aspects of bodily function. It is more common for patients to present with complaints such as weakness, headaches, or gastrointestinal disturbances than the specific complaint of "depression." The general population has little concept of the far reaching effects of depression; most individuals with major depression feel they have an organic illness (59,60). Clinicians should not overlook the importance of a psychiatric assessment in all patients, especially those without objective findings. In the above case, a more detailed initial interview could have prevented the delay that occurred in the institution of proper treatment.

The symptoms of depression can generally be divided into four categories: emotional disturbances, physiological disturbances, intellectual disturbances, and somatic complaints. (See Table 3)

The *emotional problems* presented in this case include loss of interest, feelings of worthlessness, guilt, and passive suicide wishes. Other emotional disturbances might include fear, depressed mood, agitation, irritability, social withdrawal, anhedonia (absence of pleasure from acts that would ordinarily be pleasurable), hopelessness, and self-pity. Hallucinations with depressive connotations (visions of a deceased loved one) may be present. Paranoid delusions are often present and generally involve a fear of being harmed (6).

The *physiological problems* noted in the above case included sleep disturbance, appetite disturbance, loss of energy, gastrointestinal problems, and impotence. Other physiologic disturbances frequently present include menstrual irregularities, psychomotor retardation, tachycardia, shortness of breath and others (6).

Intellectual disturbances frequently include loss of memory and concentration. Generally the memory loss is for more recent events, and sufferers complain of forgetting where they have recently placed an item or as in this case, of having

Table 3.

DEPRESSIVE SYMPTOMATOLOGY*

EMOTIONAL DISTURBANCES
  depressed mood
  loss of interest
  guilt
  fear
  worthlessness
  hopelessness
  helplessness
  anhedonia
  irritability
  social withdrawal
  self pity
  psychosis
  suicidal thoughts
  diminished libido

SOMATIC COMPLAINTS
  headaches
  backaches
  gastrointestinal complaints
  various other complaints without objective findings

PHYSIOLOGICAL DISTURBANCES
  insomnia
  hypersomnia
  anorexia
  fatigue
  anergy
  gastrointestinal dysfunction
  psychomotor agitation
  psychomotor retardation
  menstrual irregularities
  impotence

INTELLECTUAL DISTURBANCES
  decreased memory
  decreased concentration
  diminished ability to calculate and carry out intellectual tasks

*There may be some discrepancy as to which category each symptom is assigned (i.e., irritability might be due to depressed mood or psychomotor agitation)

to make notes when their memory was always reliable in the past (6).

Somatic complaints in this case included headaches, but other bodily complaints such as backaches or tingling sensations are frequently noted (6). The possibility of depression should always be considered in individuals expressing somatic complaints with an absence of objective findings.

2. Are there any laboratory procedures which are clinically useful in diagnosing depression?

Several types of testing are now possible which help in the diagnosis of affective disorders. The most clinically practical test is the 24-hour dexamethasone suppression test. A low oral dose (1–2 mg) of dexamethasone is given at midnight immediately after the drawing of a baseline serum cortisol level. A second serum cortisol level is obtained 24 hours later. In at least 40% of depressed patients the second cortisol level will not show suppression of the pituitary-adrenal axis. This is indicated by a normal or moderately elevated baseline cortisol level and no decrease in the level 24 hours after dexamethasone administration. Depressed patients who are dexamethasone nonsuppressors generally are more severely depressed and generally respond better to antidepressant therapy. This information is obviously advantageous especially since it can be obtained in most hospitals with minimal risk and discomfort to the patient. Research on this subject is still in the early stages; therefore, the clinician should use this test only as one aspect of his diagnostic process (62–64).

Less clinically practical are sleep laboratory evaluations and determinations of urinary MHPG. Although sleep laboratory research indicates that electroencephalogram patterns during sleep are altered in depressed patients as compared with normal subjects (65–68), this mode of evaluation is limited to research facilities. Since 3-methoxy-4-hydroxyphenyl glycol (MHPG) is the principal metabolic product of norepinephrine, its urinary excretion may parallel norepinephrine levels in the brain. Although urinary MHPG levels appear to be decreased before the onset and during depression, urinary MHPG assays are not clinically applicable. Exercise and/or stress may increase urinary MHPG. Furthermore, collection and assay difficulties limit the accuracy of this technique (13,40,69–72).

3. Tricyclic Antidepressants. C.R. was given a prescription for amitriptyline 50 mg tablets, #50, one at bedtime for the first three nights, then two at bedtime thereafter. He was scheduled for a return visit in two weeks. Comment on the drug selection and its dosing for this patient.

As pointed out in the introduction, it is not clinically feasible to identify biochemical subtypes of depression and select the tricyclic antidepressant which might be expected to be most specific for the presumed biochemical abnormality. Instead, drug selection must be empirical, although relative differences in side effects (eg, the considerable sedation produced by amitriptyline) might be considered.

Amitriptyline, a tertiary amine, is metabolized to the secondary amine nortriptyline, and both compounds are pharmacologically active with specificity for serotonin (reuptake blocked by amitriptyline) and norepinephrine (reuptake blocked by nortriptyline). Like other tricyclics (Table 4), amitriptyline and nortriptyline have long half-lives, and accumulation to steady-state levels requires a period of one to three weeks. The metabolism of tricyclics varies considerably among individuals (45,75,76).

Because of their long half-lives, tricyclics can be dosed once daily as was done for this patient. This approach is convenient and allows maximum sedation (and other side effects) to occur at night. If daytime anxiety had been a problem, then multiple daily dosing could have been used to take advantage of the sedative effects of this drug. Sedation from amitriptyline occurs immediately, unlike the beneficial antidepressant effects which may not be seen for days or weeks.

Institution of outpatient therapy is generally begun with 50 mg of amitriptyline or imipramine (or the equivalent dosage of another tricyclic) and increased at three- to seven-day intervals until a clinical response is obtained. Inpatient therapy can be more aggressive, beginning with 150 mg (or its equivalent) and rapidly titrating upwards until clinical response is obtained. The starting dose of 50 mg per day was appropriate for C.R., and 100 mg per day is within the usual therapeutic range (Table 4). However, a daily dosage of 150 mg per day most often results in therapeutic blood levels and antidepressant effect. Clinicians should be aware of the long half-lives of these drugs when evaluating dose response or changing from one drug to another. A limited supply of drug was dispensed (1.25 gm) because of the potentially lethal effects of overdosage of tricyclics in suicide attempts; the treatment of overdosage is discussed in the chapter on Poisonings.

4. Tricyclic Side Effects. C.R. phoned the following week to report that the medication had made his mouth dry and caused him to be slightly constipated. What suggestions can be made? Briefly outline other side effects that might be encountered during treatment with tricyclic antidepressants.

Both of C.R.'s complaints are due to the anticholinergic effects of amitriptyline. *Dry mouth* usually diminishes in intensity with continuous treatment but may never completely disappear. Sugarless hard candy or gum, lemon and glycerine swabs, or ice chips may be useful in relieving this minor side effect. Artificial saliva (eg, V.A. Oralube) may also be helpful. Fluids may also be used to relieve dry mouth, but excessive fluid intake should be avoided in patients with cardiovascular disease. In addition, pathological water intoxication has resulted from self-prescribed endeavors to relieve oral dryness by dramatically increasing fluid intake (84,85). *Constipation*, which occurs as a result of decreased gastrointestinal motility, is a common occurrence and can be treated with dioctyl sodium sulfosuccinate or milk of magnesia. Adequate fluid intake, exercise, and a high bulk diet should be tried before medication for constipation (see the chapter on Constipation and Diarrhea). Paralytic ileus requiring surgical intervention is rare but has been reported (86–89).

Anticholinergic side effects are frequent during treatment with tricyclic antidepressants. All tricyclics possess anticholinergic activity to some extent, and amitriptyline and doxepin are the most potent in this regard (83). The agents which are weakest in anticholinergic activity are desipramine, trazodone, and nomifensine; the others fall between these extremes.

Other Anticholinergic Side Effects. Difficulty in initiating urination may occur and may be aggravated in males with benign prostatic hypertrophy (90,91). Blurred vision may result from pupillary dilation and from decreased accommodation (92). These drugs can precipitate angle closure glaucoma in those with narrow angle glaucoma (92–94). An organic psychosis like that described in Questions 8 and 31 of the chapter on Psychoses can be produced by the additive anticholinergic effects of the tricyclics and other drugs that the patient may be taking (101–103). Dizziness and tachycardia are other anticholinergic effects.

Cardiovascular. Orthostatic hypotension may be a problem, especially in older patients. In addition to their anticholinergic vagolytic effects, the tricyclics have a quinidine-like effect on myocardial conduction. Furthermore, an increase in circulating catecholamines may give rise to additional cardiac problems (95–100). The pressor effects of exogenously administered sympathomimetic amines are markedly exaggerated in patients taking tricyclic antidepressants (100a).

Neurologic. A tremor which is more coarse in character than that produced by lithium may occur (109). Neither tricyclic- nor lithium-induced tremors respond to anticholinergic medication.

Psychiatric. In addition to the "anticholinergic psychosis" mentioned above, the tricyclics can aggravate a preexisting psychotic disorder and precipitate a manic attack (switch process) in bipolar patients who do not have adequate lithium levels (105,106).

Miscellaneous. Despite the pronounced anticholinergic effects of these drugs, the paradoxical complaint of excessive sweating is not uncommon. The cause is unknown.

5. *Tricyclic Plasma Levels.* The physician would like to evaluate C.R.'s tricyclic antidepressant plasma concentrations when he returns in two weeks. What practical points should be considered in the use of plasma level evaluation of tricyclic antidepressant therapy?

First, it should be remembered that although plasma level evaluation is becoming more widely employed, clinical evaluation of the patient should remain the primary point of focus. Attainment of "therapeutic levels" does not assure a positive response. Furthermore, side effects cannot be avoided by maintaining levels within the therapeutic range. However, plasma levels are valuable in determining when changes in drug dosing and drug selection are indicated.

Steady-State. These drugs have long half-lives, and plasma level evaluations undertaken too soon after a dosage change will not reflect steady-state (see Table 4).

Table 4.

TRICYCLIC AND RELATED ANTIDEPRESSANTS

	Half-Life (Hours)	Therapeutic Plasma Level (ng/ml)	Time to Reach Steady State	Recommended Dosage Range (mg/day)
AMITRIPTYLINE	17–40	*125–250	4–10 days	75–300
IMIPRAMINE	6–24	*150–300	2–5 days	75–300
DOXEPIN	8–36	*150–250	2–8 days	75–300
PROTRIPTYLINE	54–198	115–210	10 days	15–60
NORTRIPTYLINE	15–93	50–150	4–19 days	50–200
DESIPRAMINE	12–76	150–300	2–11 days	75–300
AMOXAPINE	8–30	*180	2–7 days	100–600
TRIMIPRAMINE	7–30	*180	2–6 days	75–300
TRAZODONE	4–5	N/A	3–7 days	50–600
MAPROTILINE	27–58	*200–300	6–10 days	150–300
NOMIFENSINE	2–4	N/A	2–5 days	50–200

*Parent compound plus active metabolite
N/A - not available at this writing

Active Metabolites. Many of these drugs have active metabolites, and patients will aquire plasma concentrations of both the parent compound and its active metabolite. In some patients the rate of conversion may be so great that the predominant pharmacologically active compound will be the secondary metabolite (45,75,76). The ratio of amitriptyline to its secondary metabolite (nortriptyline) varies from less than 0.25 to more than 3, while the imipramine/desipramine ratio ranges from 0.1 to 3. Although some clinicians have postulated that the relative ratios of the drugs are of key importance (76–78), the combined levels of parent drug and active metabolite are used for monitoring therapy (see Question 6).

Plasma Sampling. Sampling should be performed during the elimination phase of the drug, a minimum of 8 hours after the last dose. Vacutainer tubes should not be used, because a plasticizer in the rubber stoppers of these tubes causes spuriously low determinations. This problem can be avoided by the use of Venoject syringes and collection tubes (79,80).

Factors which Alter Plasma Concentrations. Tobacco smoking, barbiturates, chloral hydrate, trihexyphenidyl, and acidic urine pH may decrease tricyclic antidepressant plasma concentrations. On the other hand, methylphenidate, chloramphenicol, haloperidol, phenothiazines, and basic urine pH may increase tricyclic antidepressant plasma concentrations (45).

6. **When C.R. was seen again two weeks later, little clinical improvement had occurred. He was sleeping better, but his affect remained the same as two weeks previously, his memory and appetite remained poor, and he had lost another two pounds. A plasma level was drawn and subsequently reported as 100 ng/ml of amitriptyline and nortriptyline combined. How should his clinical response and plasma level be interpreted? Should the dosage be increased?**

Assuming good compliance, most patients would be expected to begin to improve at this point. Furthermore, his plasma levels suggest that another dosage increment of 50 mg would be advisable. A review of 11 studies which correlated blood levels with clinical response in a total of 321 patients determined that a steady-state range of 120 to 250 ng/ml of amitriptyline and nortriptyline combined correlates most clearly with antidepressant efficacy (45). Therapeutic plasma levels for other

tricyclics are listed in Table 4. The pharmacokinetics of the tricyclics vary considerably among individuals. For example, the bioavailability of amitriptyline may vary as much as two-fold among individuals, its clearance may vary as much as two-fold, and the clearance of nortriptyline may show as much as a four-fold difference among individuals (45). However, we now know that 100 mg per day of amitriptyline in this patient resulted in approximate steady-state levels of 100 ng/ml of amitriptyline/nortriptyline combined, and his absorption and clearance would not be expected to change. These drugs follow first-order pharmacokinetics, and as demonstrated in the pharmacokinetics chapter of this text, alterations in the maintenance dose can be expected to produce a proportional change in the steady-state plasma levels. Thus, assuming his past compliance has been good, an additional 50 mg per day of amitriptyline would be expected to bring his steady-state plasma levels within the therapeutic range. In addition to continuing to monitor clinical response, his plasma levels should be re-evaluated in another two weeks.

7. *Maintenance Therapy.* **When C.R. returned after another two weeks, after a total of four weeks of treatment with amitriptyline, he appeared much more alert and rested. His memory and ability to concentrate had almost returned to normal, and his sleep and appetite had also improved. The results of a plasma level drawn on the previous morning were reported as 155 ng/ml amitriptyline/ nortriptyline combined (desired range: 125–250 ng/ml). How long should he continue taking amitriptyline?**

There are little firm data for a conclusive answer to this question. Continued treatment with 100 to 150 mg per day of imipramine or amitriptyline for three to six months after remission is a widely applied practice because of the high rate of relapse with earlier discontinuation of drug therapy. Although dosage reduction may be possible during this maintenance phase, there is some evidence which suggests that it is desirable to maintain plasma levels within the therapeutic range during maintenance (45).

8. *MAO Inhibitors.* **C.G., a 32-year-old woman, presented with generalized fear and a feeling of impending doom. She was experiencing both initial and terminal insomnia.**

Her daily activities were greatly curtailed because she was afraid to leave her house. She had lost 15 pounds in the past two months. Her memory was not significantly impaired, but her concentration was diminished by her preoccupation with her fear. She failed to respond to treatment with doxepin 200 mg for three weeks, despite adequate plasma levels. Because she had previously failed to respond to desipramine, imipramine, perphenazine, and thiothixene, the clinician decided upon a therapeutic trial of phenelzine 15 mg tid. When should monoamine oxidase inhibitors be employed? What is their mechanism of action, and what dangers are inherent in their use?

Because of the toxicity of the monoamine oxidase (MAO) inhibitors, the tricyclic antidepressants are preferred. If there is good genetic inference that the patient will respond to MAO inhibitors better than to tricyclics (eg, response of blood relatives), or if a patient is found to be refractory to tricyclic antidepressants (as illustrated by this patient), then a MAO inhibitor may be judiciously tried. There is some evidence that when hysteria, obsessive-compulsive behavior, phobias, and anxiety neuroses accompany depression, the MAO inhibitors may be more effective than tricyclics (115–117).

Like the tricyclics, these agents increase the amount of biogenic amines available within the synaptic cleft. The mechanism of action of the MAO inhibitors differs from the tricyclics in that they block the metabolic destruction of biogenic amines by the enzyme monoamine oxidase within the presynaptic neuron. However, these agents not only inhibit MAO in the brain, but elsewhere in the body as well. Consequently, the MAO-inhibited individual is in toxic jeopardy if he consumes certain dietary amines or amine-active drugs. Although MAO inhibition occurs within a few days, the antidepressant effects of the MAO inhibitors may be delayed for two or three weeks. Orthostatic hypotension occurs with all the MAO inhibitors, and excessive central stimulation may also occur as a direct extension of the pharmacological effects of these drugs (42).

In acute MAO inhibitor toxicity it is tempting to control hypotension with sympathomimetic amines and CNS hyperexcitability with barbiturates. This action can lead to disastrous consequences. Because MAO inhibitors prevent the destruction of sympathomimetic amines, severe hypertensive crisis may ensue. Similarly, these agents may also prolong the CNS depressant effects of barbiturates, as well as narcotics, alcohol, and anticholinergic agents. Conservative, supportive treatment aimed at maintaining normal temperature, respiration, blood pressure, and proper fluid and electrolyte balance has proven most successful (42).

9. *Other Drugs.* What other drugs are employed in the treatment of depression?

Stimulants. Stimulants are used infrequently in psychiatry. Their use is attended by addiction liability, rapid development of tolerance, and a perception of unpleasantness by the depressed patient. Furthermore, the withdrawal reaction which results upon discontinuation after the development of dependence is characterized by depression. However, amphetamine has been utilized during the latency period of tricyclics (118,119). Methylphenidate appears to interfere with the enzymatic destruction of imipramine (and presumably other tricyclics), thus producing increased plasma and tissue levels (118–131). This action probably has no advantage over an increased dosage of imipramine alone. Needless to say, stimulants should not be used in combination with MAO inhibitors because of the potentially fatal hypertensive crisis which could be produced by such a combination.

Thyroid Hormone. Triiodothyronine (T_3) has been used experimentally as an adjunct to tricyclic therapy (121,139). Although triiodothyronine may shorten the lag time associated with tricyclic response and may convert non-responders to responders, cardiovascular risks are increased, and such use remains experimental.

Antipsychotic Drugs. See Question 10.

Newer Antidepressants. Five new antidepressants are available or will soon be available in the United States: trimipramine (a tricyclic), amoxapine (a tricyclic), maprotiline (a tetracyclic), nomifensine (a tetrahydroisoquinoline), and trazodone (a triazolopyridine).

Trimipramine and *amoxapine* resemble the presently available tricyclics (122–127). Their side effect profiles differ somewhat but not significantly. However, amoxapine might offer some interesting differences from the other antidepressants since it is a metabolite of loxapine (an antipsychotic); like loxapine, it blocks dopamine receptors. Therefore it is possible that amoxapine may possess neuroleptic effects as well as antidepressant effects (128,129). Like other tricyclics, it also blocks the reuptake of serotonin and norepinephrine. Several studies have shown amoxapine to possess a quicker onset of action than the other tricyclics (130,132). Clinical response may be observed as early as four days after the initiation of therapy. It also may possess less cardiotoxicity than other tricyclics (131,132).

Maprotiline is the first of the tetracyclic antidepressants to be marketed. The indications for its use and its pharmacological profile are quite similar to the existing tricyclics. It selectively inhibits the reuptake of norepinephrine with no effect on serotonin and thus would be expected to parallel desipramine in action and clinical application (133,134).

Nomifensine is a tetrahydroisoquinoline chemically unrelated to either the tricyclics or tetracyclics. It is a rather potent blocker of norepinephrine reuptake and an equally potent blocker of dopamine reuptake, while it has a weak blocking effect on the reuptake of serotonin (135). This mechanism of action would be expected to parallel that of amoxapine.

Trazodone is the first of a class of triazolopyridines to be marketed. It has little or no effect on blocking the reuptake of dopamine or norepinephrine but does exert a rather potent action on the reuptake of serotonin (136).

Both trazodone and nomifensine have less anticholinergic activity than the tricyclics and this can be a definite advantage in treatment (135–138).

The newer agents offer several potential advantages over the older products: activity on different transmitter systems; possible antipsychotic activity; decreased cardiovascular and anticholinergic effects; and a new modality for previously resistant cases. Precisely how advantageous these "new effects" are has yet to be ascertained.

10. *Psychotic Depression.* M.A., a 30-year-old female, was seen in the emergency room of city hospital in a very depressed, dysphoric state. She was withdrawn, displayed psychomotor retardation, bland affect and episodic crying. Questioning revealed that her thought content was coherent and appropriate. She related that she felt worthless, hopeless and totally devoid of any pleasurable feelings or emotional responsiveness. She expressed ideas of reference, and indicated that she had heard her name being called on several occasions only to find no one was calling to her. She admitted suicidal intent. History revealed that this was the third episode of this nature for the patient and that she was presently taking 250 mg of amitriptyline daily. There was a negative history for alcohol or other drugs. All routine laboratory tests were within normal limits. The patient was started on thiothixene 2 mg qid along with the tricyclic and began to respond after four days of therapy. Why was thiothixene added to the treatment regimen?

Depressions, per se, do not constitute an indication for antipsychotic therapy. Usually, depressions can be adequately managed with antidepressant therapy alone. However, when a depressive reaction becomes so severe as to produce poor reality testing in the afflicted individual (manifested by delusions, hallucinations, feelings of unreality, depersonalization, paranoid ideation) a major tranquilizer has a definite place in the therapeutic regimen. It is not intended that these agents be administered solely to produce rest, relaxation and sedation. These effects, though helpful, can be achieved with the proper selection of an antidepressant. Some reports have indicated that certain of the antipsychotic agents possess significant antidepressant properties (140). Those agents that have proven most efficacious in this respect are the more potent, less sedating agents. Generally, because of the attendant adverse effects associated with major tranquilizers, they should only be used if antidepressants alone fail to achieve the desired clinical response.

MANIA

11. N.M., a 28-year-old woman, was committed to the affective disorder unit because of uncontrollable and sometimes assaultive behavior. Her history revealed that she had done extremely well in life; she was voted most popular member of her high school graduating class, she achieved a high scholastic record in college, and she had been very successful in her work for a large sales corpo-

ration, becoming regional sales manager after a series of rapid promotions. There was no history of previous emotional disturbances. Her fiancé noted that she had become overly enthusiastic and amiable approximately one month prior to admission. She appeared to have unending energy and was unusually active. Her sleep decreased to 3–4 hours per night, yet she would wake up refreshed and was almost immediately involved in some activity. Her fiancé also noted that her sexual interests had increased, and she was even flirtatious with friends and strangers. He felt that this was not the patient's normal behavior and admitted to having jealous feelings. She appeared unusually happy and he suspected she might be on drugs, even though he had no evidence of this. The symptoms seemed to worsen until seven days prior to admission. At that point the patient began to go without sleep. She flew to her company's board of directors meeting with an elaborate illogical plan to triple the company's sales. When her plan was turned down, the patient became enraged and accused the board of lack of insight and ignorance. She then quit her job. She returned home and immediately withdrew her savings and spent it foolishly on a car, furniture, clothes, and even gave out five dollar bills to people on the street. At this point the patient would listen to no one. She was grossly hyperactive and stated, "I have never been better in my life and my mind is quicker than it has ever been before." Despite her elation, she was easily irritated and assaulted an individual who stopped to help when she was walking and singing on a busy intersection. She was brought to the hospital by police in a combative yet elated state. She refused to be admitted and was therefore committed. At the time of admission she was talking constantly in a loud voice, jumping quickly from one subject to another without finishing sentences. She would make sexual remarks to the male staff and generally entertained all with her witty remarks. She had evidently lost a good deal of weight as evidenced by her loose fitting clothes. Significant family history included a brother who has been treated with lithium for an unknown mental condition and maternal grandfather who committed suicide. Admis-

sion laboratory data, including a drug screen, were unremarkable. The diagnosis was bipolar affective disorder, manic. Describe the signs and symptoms of mania as they apply in this case.

The most prominent symptoms in mania are elated and/or irritable mood. At least one of these symptoms must be present for the diagnosis of mania (6). In the above case, the patient exhibited both symptoms, as is frequently the case. Experienced clinicians, upon finding themselves amused by a patient, immediately consider the possibility of mania (60). However, focusing on elated mood alone as a required criterion for mania frequently causes one to miss the diagnosis of mania in an irritable patient. Manic patients are often frustrated with the bureaucracy of medical care and as a result often present with an irritable mood even though their mood may have been elated on arrival to the treatment facility.

Increased activity is a frequent symptom. N.M. exhibited increased sexual and vocational activity. Increased activity is also frequently observed in religious, political, social, and domestic areas.

Manic patients are generally very talkative, often boisterous, presenting the clinician with some difficulty in completion of the interview. The content of the speech is generally dependent on whether the mood is elated or irritable. The elated patient is usually enjoyable to be near while the irritable individual can be very caustic and hostile. The approach to this type of patient should be delicate since violence could result from confrontation. Often the speech seems to be pressured as if the patient cannot produce his words fast enough, a condition which may be accompanied by flight of ideas or racing thoughts. These patients often jump from thought to thought and rarely finish a complete sentence. This condition differs from loose associations, because the patient is aware of which thoughts are associated and which are not.

Manics may also exhibit inflated self-esteem or grandiosity. This was illustrated in N.M. when she presented her plan to triple her company's sales. Generally manic patients feel they can accomplish any task and do it better than anyone else. Grandiosity can take on psychotic proportions when patients develop delusion systems (eg, believing they are the Virgin Mary or a well known actor).

Manic patients frequently have a decreased

need for sleep. The amount varies from patient to patient, but some go for days without sleep and continue to have excessive energy. The amount of sleep required can often serve as a guide to the severity of the manic episode.

Distractibility is common; any interruption in an interview with a manic can shift the patient's train of thought. Interviews should be conducted in a quiet area with a minimum of distractions. Likewise, the inpatient setting and staff should minimize sensory input by environmental manipulation until the patient is medicated and responding to treatment.

Manic patients frequently begin numerous tasks without finishing them. One of the most serious symptoms in manic patients is their involvement in activities which have painful, unanticipated consequences. In the above case, the patient quit her job without regard to her future. She spent her savings even though she had just lost all means of income. It was not until the patient was treated that she recognized the consequences of her actions. The most serious consequence could involve physical harm or even death resulting from promiscuous behavior or from grandiose delusions (such as the belief of immortality causing foolish risks to be taken). There are obviously numerous other possibilities. In the above case the patient was committed before physical harm occurred.

A combination of the above symptoms must persist for a minimum of one full week before the diagnosis of a manic episode can be made. Hypomania is a frequently used term which refers to patients with manic symptoms of less severity. The symptoms of mania are summarized in Table 5 (6).

Other factors which help to substantiate a diagnosis of bipolar affective disorder include:

A positive family history for affective disorders. The clinician should look for histories of depression, mania, alcoholism, and suicide in blood relatives (74). Families frequently try to hide a history of mental illness; therefore, questioning should be thoughtful and delicate.

Periods of normal behavior preceding and following affective episodes. Patients with bipolar affective illness generally function as "normal individuals" outside their periods of illness (60).

Bipolar affective disorder is often misdiagnosed due to the presence of delusions, hallucinations, flight of ideas and other symptoms which

Table 5.

SYMPTOMS OF MANIA

1. Elevated or Irritable Mood*

2. Increased Activity

3. Talkative, Sometimes with "Pressured Speech"

4. Flight of Ideas and/or Thought Racing

5. Inflated Self-esteem (Grandiosity)

6. Decreased Need for Sleep

7. Distractibility

8. Excessive Involvement in Activities that Have a High Potential for Painful Consequences

*The patient must have either or both of these symptoms to meet the criteria for mania.

are felt to be "schizophrenic symptoms." These symptoms are reported in 20% to 50% of substantiated cases of bipolar affective disorders, and they should not prejudice the clinician towards a diagnosis of schizophrenia. Cross-national and historical data suggest that over-diagnosis of schizophrenia and under-diagnosis of bipolar affective illness is a problem of considerable magnitude (141).

12. *Drug Management.* N.M. was given a 10 mg intramuscular dose of haloperidol during her initial interview. After the interview she was placed in a quiet seclusion room and monitored by the staff. Because there was no behavioral change within one hour and the staff remained concerned over the patient's safety, she was given a second 10 mg intramuscular dose of haloperidol. After approximately 30 minutes she became quiet and recumbent. Treatment was then continued with haloperidol and lithium. Why was haloperidol rather than lithium used for initial control of her symptoms? What other drugs could have been used?

Although lithium is the drug of choice for the treatment of mania, its onset of action is delayed. The clinical effects of lithium can usually be observed within 3–5 days, but its full effects in some patients may be delayed for as long as two weeks. It is often unsafe to wait several days or a week for control of manic symptoms. Antipsychotics are effective in mania and more rapidly acting than lithium. In hypomania, an antipsychotic is not generally indicated; rather, the clinician can safely wait for the clinical effects of lithium (142). Because minor tranquilizers (eg, benzodiazepines) are generally ineffective in tranquilizing manic patients, their use should not be considered.

The full spectrum of mania generally requires initial high dose antipsychotic administration. In the uncooperative patient, parenteral administration is required. Average daily doses would include 20–40 mg of haloperidol or 400–600 mg of chlorpromazine. Higher dose requirements are not infrequent, and higher doses are most often required during the initial days of treatment. The antipsychotic and lithium should be started concurrently. As symptoms abate, the antipsychotic may be tapered. The increasing neuronal concentration of lithium will gradually replace the clinical effects of the antipsychotic. Most bipolar patients can be managed on lithium alone after neuronal concentrations are adequate (142).

Minimal doses of antipsychotics should be used since they have unpleasant and sometimes permanent side effects. Conversely, properly dosed lithium patients frequently report, "I can't tell I'm taking anything." Antipsychotics and lithium are equally efficacious in mania, but the incidence of adverse effects from antipsychotics is greater (143). Long-term antipsychotic therapy for mania should be reserved for patients who cannot take lithium or for those in whom lithium is not fully effective (142). The rule of thumb for using antipsychotics is to give them only when indicated, at the lowest possible dose, and for the shortest possible interval.

Any antipsychotic can be efficacious for the treatment of mania. The most commonly used agents are chlorpromazine, haloperidol, and thiothixene. Each of these has the advantage of parenteral administration. The sedation of chlorpromazine is advantageous in manic patients. Haloperidol and thiothixene cause little sedation but have the advantage of causing far fewer cardiovascular side effects. We prefer haloperidol or thiothixene in acute mania, because the cardiovascular system is already stressed due to the hypermetabolic state of mania. Parenteral administration of the antipsychotic is likely and side effects are generally more severe with parenteral administration.

Irreversible brain damage from the combination of lithium and haloperidol has been reported (144,188) and somewhat discounted (145). Most of the cases were relatively isolated events which occurred within a much larger group of lithium-haloperidol treated patients who did not manifest such effects. Furthermore, several epidemiologic studies have failed to detect evidence supporting a lithium-haloperidol interaction. However, negative epidemiological evidence does not disprove the occurrence of this interaction in specific predisposed individuals, and one must assume that under certain conditions the combination of these drugs may be detrimental. Although a definite cause and effect relationship between the drug combination and severe CNS toxicity has not been established, sufficient evidence of an interaction exists so that one should not ignore the possibility. Therefore, some recommend that neuroleptics be used alone for initial control of acute mania symptoms and that lithium be added as the neuroleptic dosage is reduced (188).

13. After N.M. had been calmed by the second 10 mg intramuscular dose of haloperidol (Question 12), she was started on haloperidol liquid concentrate 10 mg three times daily, and an order was also written for haloperidol 10 mg IM every six hours as needed. Lithium carbonate 300 mg after meals and at bedtime was begun when laboratory values (ordered on admission) were reported as being within normal limits. How should haloperidol and lithium be dosed and monitored during the initial days and weeks of therapy?

Haloperidol. The 30 mg daily oral dose of haloperidol was chosen for N.M. because she required 20 mg of intramuscular haloperidol initially and oral dosing is somewhat less effective than intramuscular dosing. Multiple dosing was used in order to evaluate possible dosing increments. Liquid concentrate was used to decrease the chance of the patient "cheeking" the medication. An "as needed" intramuscular order was written to cover the possible need for rapid control of an exacerbation. N.M. responded well to haloperidol oral concentrate, and after two days the order was changed to haloperidol tablets 30 mg at bedtime. She remained on this regimen for one week. It was then felt that adequate intraneuronal lithium levels had been obtained and the haloperidol could be tapered. The dosage was subsequently decreased to 20 mg at bedtime for five days, then 10 mg at bedtime for five days, and then discontinued. N.M. had no problems with these dosage reductions, and she remained euthymic (normal mood) with the discontinuation of haloperidol.

Lithium. Before starting lithium, baseline complete blood count, serum sodium, potassium, fasting glucose, blood urea nitrogen, serum creatinine, T3, T4, and urinalysis should be obtained. A baseline electrocardiogram is also advisable. Because of lithium's low therapeutic index, serum levels must be used to monitor therapy. Initially, serum lithium levels should be obtained twice weekly until the dosage and serum level are stabilized. During an acute manic episode, serum levels between 1.2 and 1.5 mEq/L are desirable. Divided daily doses of 1200 to 2400 mg/day are usually required to produce these levels in patients with good renal function. Single doses larger than 600 mg should be avoided, if possible, because of the risks of nephrotoxicity (see Question 23). Once response occurs, the dosage should be decreased and the desired serum level lowered to 0.8 to 1.2 mEq/L in order to prevent toxicity. Manic patients require higher dosages of lithium (perhaps because of their higher metabolic rate) and can tolerate higher serum levels than euthymic individuals (152,153). In order to minimize dosage titration, Cooper and Simpson (154,155) recommend the use of a 24 hour lithium level after a single 600 mg oral dose for determining dosage requirements.

Lithium absorption from the gastrointestinal tract is virtually complete and is not significantly impaired by food and medications. Since lithium often causes gastric distress, it should be taken immediately after meals or with food and milk. Peak levels occur in 2 to 4 hours, and absorption is complete within 8 hours. Lithium excretion is by renal elimination. About 80% of filtered lithium is reabsorbed by the renal tubules; thus, lithium clearance is about 20% of that for creatinine. Since the half-life of lithium is about 24 hours, steady state can be expected to occur in about five days; however, excretion varies among individuals and the half-life in some patients may be shorter or considerably longer. Elderly individuals frequently have diminished renal function; therefore, lithium clearance is likely to be reduced and its half-life prolonged in these patients (152, 153,153a,158,159).

Plasma samples should be drawn in the morning 12 hours after the evening dose, to avoid elevations due to the distribution phase of the previous dose. Because peak serum levels after each dose can be two or three times higher than the steady-state concentration 8 to 12 hours after the dose, and because lithium is irritating to the gastrointestinal tract, the daily dose should be divided. Clinical monitoring (for nausea, diarrhea, sedation, and fine tremor) is as important as serum levels.

Serum levels do not necessarily correlate with intraneuronal levels. This is evidenced by the lag time of the action of lithium despite therapeutic serum levels. Erythrocyte lithium levels and saliva lithium levels have been evaluated as means of making monitoring more accurate or more convenient (160–162). However, the benefits and reliability of these techniques remain to be established.

14. N.M. subsequently required a daily lithium dosage of 1800 mg, and although a serum level of 1.3 mEq/L was attained without side effects and with only slight euphoria, she eventually developed nausea and tremor not related to dose administration by the time she had become euthymic. The dose was then reduced to 300 mg four times daily. Twenty-two days after admission she was discharged with this dose and a serum lithium level of 1.0 mEq/L. Her mood had been euthymic since the fifteenth hospital day. How often should N.M.'s lithium therapy be monitored? What discharge instructions should she receive?

Patients should receive weekly lithium determinations until manic symptoms have subsided and steady-state levels have been attained. N.M.'s lithium level of 1.0 mEq/L at a dosage of 300 mg qid probably represents steady state. However, a lithium determination one week after discharge would be helpful in verifying this and would also serve as a check on medication compliance. Thereafter, serum level determinations every two weeks, then every month and eventually every other month should be adequate.

N.M. should be instructed on the importance of continuing to take her lithium regularly. She should understand the importance of precise dosing; extra dosing could result in toxic effects because of the closeness of the therapeutic range (0.8 to 1.2 mEq/L) to the toxic range (mild to moderate reactions at 1.5 to 2.5 mEq/L and moderate to severe reactions at 2.0 to 2.5 mEq/L). Moreover, she should consume an adequate amount of fluid each day (2 or 3 quarts of water or other fluid) and avoid possible causes of dehydration such as sauna bathing. She should contact her physician if she develops diarrhea or fever, as this may result in dehydration and require a temporary decrease in dosage. Likewise, she should contact her physician should signs of moderate lithium toxicity arise: diarrhea, vomiting, tremor, mild ataxia, drowsiness, or muscular weakness.

15. *Mild Toxicity from Low Sodium Diet.* A year and a half after her discharge, N.M. came to a regularly scheduled outpatient appointment complaining of frequent loose stools, persistent nausea, and mild lethargy. Her serum lithium level was 1.4 mEq/L. Further questioning revealed that she had started a self-prescribed low salt diet two weeks previously in an effort to lose weight. The early symptoms of toxicity began four days prior to her visit. How does sodium intake affect serum lithium levels?

Approximately 80% of the glomerular filtrate of lithium is reabsorbed in the proximal tubule, competing with sodium. Although there is further absorption of sodium distally (15–20%), there is almost no absorption of lithium in the distal renal tubules. During periods of sodium depletion, the body will conserve univalent cations (sodium and lithium) and reabsorb more than 80% from the proximal tubule. This increased lithium reabsorption will cause serum levels to rise and toxicity may follow. Excessive sodium intake will cause serum lithium levels to decrease. Patients on lithium should be instructed not to change their dietary intake of sodium without medical supervision. Patients on low sodium diets can be treated with lithium if properly monitored (158,163,164).

A few old reports dealing with the treatment of lithium toxicity recommend treatment with hypertonic saline. This does little to increase lithium excretion in an acute situation. Saline should only be used in hyponatremic patients and only then with the goal of restoring normal sodium levels. Though rather large changes in sodium and fluid intake are necessary to produce significant serum lithium alterations, patients suffering from severe diarrhea, vomiting and dehydration should be carefully monitored for toxic signs (165).

16. How should this case of mild lithium toxicity be managed?

N.M.'s symptoms should disappear with cessation of the lithium. She should be told to discontinue the lithium and return to her regular dietary habits. Daily evaluation by telephone should be all that is necessary. The symptoms should disappear in 24 to 48 hours and the lithium therapy should be reinstituted at the same dose. If the symptoms do not abate in that time interval, this may be indicative of a deterioration in renal function and a prolonged half-life. Further serum levels and evaluation of renal function should then be performed.

17. What other side effects and toxic effects are seen with lithium therapy?

Lithium adverse effects can be divided into three categories: benign effects, acute toxic effects, and chronic toxic effects (See Table 6). Benign effects include a fine tremor that may persist and is unresponsive to anticholinergic therapy; however, propranolol has been successful in reducing tremor intensity in some patients (166). Nausea, anorexia, stomach irritation, and diarrhea are common complaints of lithium therapy which may be controlled by administering the drug with meals. Polyuria and excessive thirst are prominent within the first week of therapy due to sodium diuresis. Ataxia may appear, but is uncommon and usually transient.

Acute toxic effects include persistent vomiting and uncontrollable diarrhea, hypertonic muscles with hyperactive deep tendon reflexes (DTR), and prominent muscular weakness. Chorea and choreoathetoid movements (writhing movements of the limbs) are serious toxic signs. Lethargy, drowsiness, and impaired consciousness that could progress to coma are signs that must be closely monitored and corrected at the onset. Opisthotonus (spastic hyperflexion of the neck), seizures and cardiac arrhythmias portend potentially fatal problems. The benign effects are often seen with therapeutic levels, while the serious toxicities generally appear with serum levels exceeding 2.0 mEq/L (167,168).

Influenza and early lithium toxicity present similar clinical pictures. Lithium patients with suspected influenza should have a serum lithium determination and the lithium withheld until toxicity is ruled out.

Chronic toxicities are rare and include such

Table 6.

ADVERSE AND TOXIC EFFECTS OF LITHIUM

Benign Effects	Acute Toxicity	Chronic Toxicity
*Nausea	Persistent Vomiting	Goitrogenic Hypothyroidism
*Vomiting	Uncontrollable Diarrhea	Renal Tubular Necrosis
*Diarrhea	Muscular Weakness	Diabetes Insipidus Syndrome
*Anorexia	Coarse Tremor	
Polyuria	Hyperactive DTR's	
Polydipsia	Dysarthria	
Fine Tremor	Lethargy	
Weight Gain	Somnolence	
Edema	Seizures	
	Coma	
	Death	

*These symptoms are due to direct irritation of the GI tract and are generally seen following dose administration.

conditions as non-toxic goiter (see chapter on Thyroid Diseases), kidney tubular damage and a pitressin-resistant diabetes insipidus-like syndrome (see Question 21 and the chapter on Kidney Diseases) (156,169,170). Other adverse effects of lithium include a persistent leukocytosis, rash, and glucosuria (167).

One major advantage of lithium therapy not enjoyed by most psychoactive agents is the absence of interference with sexual functioning. Most patients placed on lithium therapy report no adverse effects when serum levels are within proper limits.

18. Teratogenicity. N.M. remained euthymic for 28 months. During a follow-up visit, she mentions that she and her husband would like to start a family. Should lithium be discontinued because of the risk of teratogenicity?

Lithium should not be used during pregnancy if it can be avoided, and it certainly should not be used during the first trimester and before term. An increased incidence of fetal abnormalities has been attributed to lithium in both animals and humans. The types of abnormality vary, but cleft palate is common and cardiovascular anomalies have also been reported. Lithium taken at term may also cause deleterious effects in the newborn. Lithium is excreted in breast milk, thus mothers who are taking lithium should be discouraged from breast feeding (171,172).

As in all clinical situations, risk versus benefit must be considered. A manic episode in a pregnant patient could be potentially disastrous to the fetus. In N.M.'s case, the lithium should definitely be discontinued. Her history reveals only one affective episode and it is unknown whether she will ever have another. Her positive family history makes her chances greater. Even so, the lithium should be stopped and N.M. should be monitored at monthly intervals for symptoms of depression or mania. If symptoms emerge during the pregnancy, all forms of non-drug intervention should be used including hospitalization if necessary. Lithium should be reinstated only if her condition poses possible harm to the fetus or herself.

19. Severe Lithium Toxicity. B.W., a 65-year-old male farmer, was admitted to the intensive care unit in a state of severely impaired consciousness. He was oriented as to name and place. He was minimally responsive to stimulation. His speech was sluggish and difficult to understand. Within three hours after admission, the patient became comatose. Only minimal history was obtained from the patient, but his wife revealed that B.W. had been successfully managed with lithium for eleven

years for treatment of bipolar affective disorder. In fact, his appointments at the mental health center had been at six month intervals. He missed his last appointment due to a virus infection which began about one month prior to admission. Symptoms included nausea, generalized weakness, and a tremor. After one week of increasing discomfort, the patient went to a local clinic. He neglected to tell the physician of his psychiatric history. Routine laboratory tests and a brief physical examination were performed. The patient was told he probably had a virus and that he should return to the clinic if he did not improve over the next week. Over the next week the nausea and vomiting subsided, but the patient became increasingly lethargic. He became dizzy and noted a ringing in his ears. A short time later, the patient began to have difficulty pronouncing his words and walking.

When B.W. became too weak to walk, his wife insisted on bringing him to the hospital. "Stat" laboratory data (normal ranges in parentheses) revealed a serum sodium of 153 mEq/L (135–145 mEq/L), serum potassium of 4.9 mEq/L (3.5–5.0 mEq/L), blood urea nitrogen of 64 mg/dl (8–25 mg/dl), hematocrit of 53% (45–52%), urine specific gravity of 1.035 (1.002–1.028), and serum creatinine of 2.1 mg/dl (0.6–1.5 mg/dl). The serum lithium level was 3.7 mEq/L.

What potential lithium management problems led to this patient's intoxication?

The use of lithium in the geriatric population has been associated with a high incidence of toxic effects. The half-life of lithium in geriatric patients may be as long as 36 hours because of decreased renal function in this age group. This may result in high serum levels. Furthermore, older persons appear to be somewhat more sensitive to the effects of lithium. Consequently, more frequent monitoring of serum levels is advisable for the geriatric patient (185). B.W.'s clinic appointments were six months apart despite his age of 65 years. Moreover, because he had been taking lithium for 11 years, he was at greater risk of lithium nephrotoxicity. Furthermore, there was an apparent lack of patient education. The patient and, if possible, family members should be aware of the symptoms of lithium toxicity. It is recommended that the patient keep a list of these symptoms and the clinician's phone number on his person. Patients should be informed to let all doctors know of their current medications. In this case, more careful monitoring of lithium levels and renal function and improved patient education may have prevented the serious medical sequelae.

20. Describe the management of lithium toxicity and apply it to the above case.

This case of lithium toxicity developed over a three to four week period. There is no history of a change in dose, and his laboratory data indicate both decrease in renal function and dehydration as likely causes. A small decrease in renal function without a decrease in lithium dosage would cause a gradual development of lithium toxicity. In this case the "flu-like syndrome" was the early manifestation of lithium toxicity. Lithium levels at that time were probably in the range of 1.6 mEq/L to 2.5 mEq/L. Treatment at that point would have been discontinuation of lithium with daily evaluation of the patient's symptoms. This would most likely be done on an outpatient basis. If the symptoms did not diminish by the second day, a more intensive approach would be needed.

The severity of lithium intoxication seems to depend on at least three factors: the peak of serum lithium concentration, the duration of lithium intoxication, and individual tolerance. B.W. had a prolonged period of intoxication which means that neuronal lithium had reached maximum concentration. He also had an extremely high serum lithium level. These two factors suggest a poor prognosis. Individual tolerance is only accurately evaluated by the outcome.

The general treatment for lithium toxicity includes:

(A) If it is an acute overdose and the patient is conscious, emesis should be induced. If the patient is comatose, gastric lavage is indicated. If it is a chronic development of toxicity, any attempt at removal of the drug from the gastrointestinal tract is impractical.

(B) Urinary lithium excretion can be increased by osmotic diuresis (100–200%), acetazolamide (31%), urea (36%), or aminophylline (58%).

(C) Hemodialysis is the most effective way to remove lithium from intoxicated patients. If available, it should be used in any serious intoxication. Peritoneal dialysis is not as effective, but its use should be considered if hemodialysis is not available. Hemodialysis should be used for 10–

12 hour periods and repeated as necessary. Serum lithium levels should be followed to make sure redistribution does not cause dangerously high lithium levels. Hansen et al (165), suggest a serum lithium level of 1 mEq/L 6–8 hours after cessation of dialysis is evidence of adequate treatment.

(D) Electrolyte and fluid balance must be maintained. This patient appears to be dehydrated, which could be contributing to his symptomatology.

General treatment guidelines A and B are not considered in the case of B.W. Prevention of gastric absorption is not beneficial due to the prolonged development of toxicity. Increasing urinary excretion in a case of severe lithium toxicity with diminished renal function would probably be futile. B.W. will require repeated hemodialysis and correction of his fluid and electrolyte imbalance. Any supportive treatment necessary should also be used.

As mentioned previously, sodium chloride should not be used to enhance lithium excretion. It may be used to restore normal fluid and electrolyte balance. Without proper treatment in the early stages of lithium intoxication many patients will have chronic complications. Toxic effects have been found in the brain, heart, and kidneys. Permanent neurological manifestations include ataxia and dementia. Death is possible and underscores the need for immediate treatment (171,173,174).

21. Lithium-induced Nephrogenic Diabetes Insipidus. W.T. is a 35-year-old male with a 6-year history of bipolar affective disorder. He has been treated predominately with antidepressants, but for the last two years he has been maintained successfully on lithium carbonate 900 mg bid. Lithium levels have ranged from 0.7 mEq/L to 1.05 mEq/L. For the first year of lithium therapy, W.T. had no complaints of adverse drug effects. During the second year, he began to complain of increased thirst and frequent urination which was described as only an inconvenience. The frequency gradually increased until the patient began to experience difficulty with employment and other activities due to voiding intervals of less than one hour. A 24-hour urine was obtained, and it showed a total volume of 8700 ml and a specific gravity of 1.003. Repeat 24-hour urines revealed similar results. A water-deprivation test was performed, but the patient was still unable to concentrate urine. The lithium was discontinued, and the patient's symptoms gradually improved; however, he had a manic episode and was recently hospitalized. How does lithium cause a nephrogenic diabetes insipidus, and how should this case be managed?

Lithium can cause a diabetes insipidus-like syndrome which does not respond to vasopressin, indicating the origin of the problem is within the kidney. One possible mechanism of this syndrome involves a decreased responsiveness of the tubular epithelium and the collecting duct to antidiuretic hormone. There is some evidence to suggest that it is the absolute concentration of lithium in the urine which is responsible for lithium-induced nephrogenic diabetes insipidus. Other explanations have been made, but at this point the exact mechanism of this syndrome is not known.

Management of this syndrome involves either decreasing the dose of lithium or discontinuing its use. A dose reduction can reduce or alleviate the symptoms. With cessation of therapy, reversal of the diabetes insipidus-like syndrome usually occurs. With both these alternatives the risk of an affective episode is greatly increased, as illustrated in the above case.

Lithium therapy should be reinstituted; however, W.T.'s renal symptoms will most likely reappear. If they do, W.T. should be started on hydrochlorothiazide 50 mg daily. Any sodium depletion (in this case via diuretics) can cause increased tubular absorption of lithium, and toxicity may occur. When the thiazide diuretic is started, the lithium dose must be reduced and restabilization of the lithium regimen must be accomplished. Thiazides will decrease urine volume in nephrogenic diabetes insipidus even if lithium-induced. Explanations of the thiazide diuretic's actions in this syndrome are postulated as follows: Extracellular volume is decreased due to sodium depletion, causing the renal tubule to reabsorb more water and sodium in the proximal tubule. Thiazides also decrease the glomerular filtration rate, which would decrease the fluid volume presented in the tubule. Because of potential side effects, thiazide diuretics should be used with caution. Hyponatremia and lithium toxicity are two of the most severe consequences (170,178,179).

22. How should W.T.'s lithium be adjusted with the addition of hydrochlorothiazide?

The most critical drug interactions involving lithium are associated with diuretic agents. The effect of sodium depletion on lithium excretion has already been discussed. Because of this sodium depletion, the lithium dosage must be reduced. An initial reduction of the lithium dose by 50% is suggested. Dosage can then be adjusted upwards or downwards by careful and frequent monitoring of serum lithium levels. Any diuretic dose change should be coordinated with the psychiatry clinician in consultation (180).

23. Is there any evidence of irreversible renal damage with lithium therapy, and would W.T. be more likely to have permanent damage?

Chronic functional and morphologic kidney damage is seen in a minority of patients after years of lithium therapy. Concentrating ability is the most common abnormality and may be due to a structural nephropathy. Cellular changes have been identified in the distal tubule and the collecting ducts. It is possible that higher concentration in the distal area is responsible for the cellular damage. Only minor cellular changes have been identified in the proximal area. For this reason, it is recommended that single doses greater than 600 mg not be given if at all possible. It has not been shown that these lithium-induced changes lead to chronic renal failure; however, the clinician should always monitor renal function and be aware of this potential problem. Rafaelson suggests that high 24-hour urine volumes may be the earliest warning signal (156,157,

165,181,182). This would suggest that W.T. has a potentially greater risk of having renal damage. (Also see the chapter on Kidney Diseases.)

24. *Drug Interactions.* G.H. is a 38-year-old male with essential hypertension which is currently well controlled with methyldopa 1500 mg/day. He is being started on lithium for control of a second manic episode. How should this case be managed? What other drugs may interact with lithium?

There have been several reports of enhanced lithium toxicity in patients taking *methyldopa* (183,186). Because toxicity may occur despite lithium levels which are within the therapeutic range, patients should be given this combination only with careful monitoring. If toxicity should occur, the methyldopa should be replaced with another antihypertensive rather than attempting to adjust the dose of lithium (186).

Indomethacin reduces lithium clearance by about one-third, and concomitant administration may result in lithium intoxication in patients previously stabilized on lithium alone. Therefore, patients receiving this combination should be monitored carefully (187). Because prostaglandin inhibition may be the mechanism which accounts for indomethacin's reduction in lithium excretion, patients receiving *nonsteroidal antiinflammatory drugs* should also be carefully monitored (187).

The effect of *thiazide diuretics* during lithium therapy was discussed in Questions 21–22. Hansten (184) has reviewed the effects of a number of drugs on lithium therapy; the clinical significance of these other drug interactions remains to be established.

References

1. Lewis A: Melancholia: a historical review. In *The State of Psychiatry: Essays and Addresses,* Science House, New York, 1967.

2. Kraepelin E: *Manic Depressive Insanity and Paranoia,* E.S. Livingstone, Edinburgh, 1921.

3. Helgason T: Epidemiology of mental disorders in Iceland. A psychiatric and demographic investigation of 5395 Islanders. Acta Psychiat Scand, Supp 1964; 40:173.

4. Fremming K: The expectation of mental infirmity in the sample of the Danish population. In *Occasional Papers and Eugenics,* Number 7, Cassell, London, 1951.

5. Silverman C: *The Epidemiology of Depression.* Johns Hopkins Press, Baltimore, 1968.

6. Andreason N et al: Affective disorders. In *Diagnostic and Statistical Manual of Mental Disorders,* 3rd ed, edited by JBW Williams, American Psychiatric Association, Washington, 1980, p 205.

7. Akiskal HS et al: Overview of recent research in depression. Arch Gen Psychiatry. 1975; 32:285.

8. Gruenberg EM et al: Major affective disorders. In *Diagnostic and Statistical Manual of Mental Disorders,* 2nd ed, American Psychiatric Association, Washington, 1968, p 35.

9. Akiskal HS et al: The nosological status of neurotic depression. Arch Gen Psychiatry. 1978; 35:756.

10. Klein D: A new classification of depressive disorders. Depression Notes No. 16. Sept. 1975.

11. Neborsky RJ et al: Psychopharmacologic and psycho-therapeutic interventions: An integrated treatment approach to depression. Psych Ann Supplement. 1980; 10:369.

12. Schildkraut J: The catecholamine hypothesis of affective disorders: A review of supporting evidence. Am J Psychiatry. 1965; 122:509.

13. Fawcett J: Depression at the biochemical level. Psych Ann Supplement. 1980; 10:362.

14. Lapin IP et al: Intensification of the central serotoninergic processes as a possible determinant of the thymoleptic effect. Lancet. 1969; 1:132.

15. Glassman A: Indolamines and affective disorders. Psychosom Med. 1969; 31:107.

16. Coppen A: A biochemistry of affective disorders. Br J Psych. 1967; 113:1237.

17. Barchas J et al: Brain amines: Response to psychological stress. Biochem Pharmacol. 1963; 12:1232.

18. Bliss E et al: Brain amines and emotional stress. J Psych Res. 1966; 4:189.

19. Maynert E et al: Stress-induced release of brain norepinephrine and its inhibition by drugs. J Pharmacol Exper Ther. 1964; 143:90.

20. Prange A et al: L-Tryptophan in mania: Contribution to a permissive hypothesis of affective disorders. Arch Gen Psychiatry. 1974; 30:56.

21. Whybrow P et al: Toward a biology of depression: Some suggestions from neurophysiology. Am J Psychiatry. 1969; 125:45.

22. Akiskal H et al: Diuretic-antidepressant combination in alcoholic depressives: Preliminary findings. Dis Nerv Syst. 1974; 35:207.

23. Bear DJ et al: Fluid and electrolyte balance during acute withdrawal in chronic alcoholic patients. JAMA. 1968; 204:135.

24. Butterworth A: Depression associated with alcohol withdrawal. Q J Stud Alcohol. 1971; 32:343.

25. Mayfield D et al: Alcoholism, alcohol intoxication and suicide attempts. Arch Gen Psychiatry. 1972; 27:349.

26. Shaw D et al: Brain electrolytes in depressive and alcoholic suicides. Br J Psych. 1969; 115:69.

27. Singh M: A unifying hypothesis on the biochemical basis of affective disorders. Psych Q. 1970; 44:706.

28. Whybrow P et al: Melancholia, a model in madness: A discussion of recent psychobiologic research into depressive illness. Psych Med. 1973; 4:351.

29. Klein D: Endogenomorphic depression: A conceptual and terminological revision. Arch Gen Psychiatry. 1974; 31:447.

30. Maas J: Adrenocortical steroid hormones, electrolytes and the disposition of catecholamines with particular reference to depressive states. J Psych Res. 1972; 9:227.

31. Mendels J et al: Intracellular lithium concentration and clinical response: Toward a membrane theory of depression. J Psych Res. 1973; 10:9.

32. Naylor G et al: Erythrocyte membrane cation carrier in depressive illness. Psych Med. 1973; 3:502.

33. Shaw D: Mineral metabolism, mania, and melancholia. Br Med J. 1966; 2:262.

34. Sachar E et al: Psychoendocrinology of ego disintegration. Am J Psychiatry. 1970; 126:1067.

35. Prange AJ Jr et al: Some endocrine aspects of affective disorders. J Clin Psychiatry. 1980; 41:29.

36. Frazer A et al: Metabolism of tryptophan in depressive disease. Arch Gen Psychiatry. 1973; 29:528.

37. Quitkin F et al: Monoamine oxidase inhibitors: A review of antidepressant effectiveness. Arch Gen Psychiatry. 1979; 36:749.

38. Sheehan D et al: Treatment of endogenous anxiety with phobic, hysterical and hypochondrical symptoms. Arch Gen Psychiatry. 1980; 37:51.

39. Robinson D et al: Clinical pharmacology of phenelzine. Arch Gen Psychiatry. 1978; 35:629.

40. Hollister LE et al: Subtypes of depression based on excretion of MHPG and response to nortriptyline. Arch Gen Psychiatry. 1980; 37:1107.

41. Avelrod J et al: Catecholamines. N Engl J Med. 1972; 287:237.

42. Gilman AG, Goodman LS, and Gilman A: The Pharmacological Basis of Therapeutics. 6th Edition. MacMillan Publishing Company, Inc., New York, 1980.

43. Hollister LE: Treatment of depression with drugs. Ann Intern Med. 1978; 89:78.

44. Lidbrink P et al: The effect of imipramine-like drugs on the uptake mechanisms in the central noradrenaline and 5-hydroxytryptamine neurons. Neuropharmacol. 1971; 10:521.

45. DeVane L: Tricyclic antidepressants. In Applied Pharmacokinetics: Principles of Therapeutic Drug Monitoring, edited by W Evans et al, Applied Therapeutics, Inc., San Francisco, 1980.

46. Beckman H et al: Antidepressant response to tricyclics and urinary MHPG in unipolar patients: clinical response to imipramine or amitriptyline. Arch Gen Psychiatry. 1975; 32:17.

47. Asberg M et al: "Serotonin depression"—a biochemical subgroup within the affective disorders? Science. 1976; 191:478.

48. Rosenbaum AH et al: Clinical pharmacology: 1. Drugs that alter mood. Mayo Clin Proc. 1979; 54:335.

49. Maas JW: Clinical implications of pharmacological differences among antidepressants. In Psychopharmacology: A Generation of Progress, edited by MA Lipton, A DiMascio and K Killam, Raven Press, New York, 1978, p 955.

50. Maas JW: Biogenic amines and depression: Biochemical and pharmacological separation of two types of depression. Arch Gen Psychiatry. 1975; 32:1357.

51. Maas JW: Clinical and biological heterogeneity of depressive disorders. Ann Intern Med. 1978; 88:556.

52. Bunney WE et al: Mode of action of lithium: Some biological considerations. Arch Gen Psychiatry. 1979; 36:898.

53. Schildkraut J et al: Effects of lithium on H_3-norepinephrine. Lit Sci. 1966; 5:1479.

54. Pert A et al: Long-term treatment with lithium prevents the development of dopamine receptor supersensitivity. Science. 1978; 201:171.

55. Mandell AJ et al: Asymmetry and mood, emergent properties of serotonin regulation: A proposed mechanism of action of lithium. Arch Gen Psychiatry. 1979; 36:909.

56. Cronson AJ et al: Antagonism of cocaine highs by lithium. Am J Psychiatry. 1978; 135:856.

57. Baldessarini RJ: Lithium salts. In Chemotherapy in Psychiatry, 1st ed. Harvard University Press, Cambridge, 1977, p 57.

58. Singer I et al: Mechanisms of lithium action. N Engl J Med. 1973; 289:254.

59. Cassidy WL et al: Clinical observations in manic depressive disease. JAMA. 1953; 164:1535.

60. Goodwin DW et al: Affective disorders. In *Psychiatric Diagnosis,* 2nd ed, Oxford University Press, New York, 1979, p 3.

61. Nelson JC et al: The symptoms of major depressive illness. Am J Psychiatry. 1981; 138:1.

62. Brown WA et al: The 24-hour dexamethasone suppression test in a clinical setting: Relationship to diagnosis, symptoms, and response to treatment. Am J Psychiatry. 1979; 136:543.

63. Schlesser MA et al: Genetic subtypes of unipolar primary depressive illness distinguished by hypothalmic pituitary-adrenal axis activity. Lancet. 1979; 1:739.

64. Carroll BJ et al: Neuroendocrine regulation in depression, II: Discrimination of depressed from non-depressed patients. Arch Gen Psychiatry. 1976; 33:1051.

65. Kupfer DJ et al: The application of EEG sleep for the differential diagnosis of affective disorders. Am J Psychiatry. 1978; 135:69.

66. Coble P et al: EEG sleep diagnosis of primary depression. Arch Gen Psychiatry. 1976; 33:1124.

67. Akiskal HS et al: Characterological depressions: Clinical and sleep electroencephalographic findings separating "subaffective dysthymias" from "character-spectrum disorders." Arch Gen Psychiatry. 1980; 37:777.

68. Akiskal HS: External validating criteria for psychiatric diagnosis: Their application in affective disorders. J Clin Psych. 1980; 41:6.

69. Schatzberg AF et al: Catecholamine measures for diagnosis and treatment of patients with depressive disorders. J Clin Psych. 1980; 41:35.

70. Blombery PA et al: Conversion of MHPG to vanillylmandelic acid. Arch Gen Psychiatry. 1980; 37:1000.

72. Maas JW et al: In vivo studies of the metabolism of norepinephrine in the CNS. J Pharmacol Exper Ther. 1968; 163:147.

73. Bunney WE: Psychopharmacology of the switch process in affective illness. In *Psychopharmacology: A Generation of Progress,* Raven Press, New York, 1978, p 1249.

74. Akiskal HS et al: Differentiation of primary affective illness from situational, symptomatic, and secondary depressions. Arch Gen Psychiatry. 1979; 36:635.

75. Orsulak PJ et al: Guidelines for therapeutic monitoring of tricyclic antidepressant plasma levels. Ther Drug Monitoring. 1979; 1:199.

76. Amsterdam J et al: The clinical application of tricyclic antidepressant pharmacokinetics and plasma levels. Am J Psychiatry. 1980; 137:653.

77. Braithwaite RA et al: Plasma concentration of amitriptyline and clinical response. Lancet. 1972; 1:1297.

78. Magy A et al: Quantitative determination of imipramine and desipramine in human blood plasma and direct densitometry of thin layer chromatograms. J Pharm Pharmacol. 1973; 25:599.

79. Veith RC et al: The clinical impact of blood collection methods on tricyclic antidepressants as measured by Gc/MS-SIM. Commun Psychopharmacol. 1979; 2:491.

80. Brunswick DJ et al: Reduced levels of tricyclic antidepressant in plasma from vacutainers. Commun Psychopharmacol. 1977; 1:131.

81. Silverman J et al: Clinical significance of tricyclic antidepressant plasma levels. Psychosomatics. 1979; 20:1.

82. Avery GS et al: Guide to the clinically more important drug interactions. Appendix C. In *Drug Treatment: Principles and Practice of Clinical Pharmacology and Therapeutics,* 2nd ed., edited by G Avery, Adis Press, Sydney, 1980, p 1252.

83. Snyder SH et al: Antidepressants and the muscarinic acetylcholine receptor. Arch Gen Psychiatry. 1977; 34:236.

84. Bursfield BL et al: Studies of salivation in depression. Arch Gen Psychiatry. (Chicago). 1961; 5:76.

85. Sigg EB: Autonomic side-effects induced by psychotherapeutic agents. In *Psychopharmacology, A Review of Progress, 1957–1967,* edited by D Efron, U.S. Government Printing Office, Washington, 1968, p 581.

86. Waldrup FN et al: A comparison of the therapeutic and toxic effects of thioridazine and chlorpromazine in chronic schizophrenic patients. Compr Psychiatry. 1961; 2:96.

87. Bursfield BL et al: Depressive symptom or side effect? A comparative study of symptoms during pre-treatment and treatment periods of patients on three antidepressant medications. J Nerv Ment Dis. 1962; 134:339.

88. Burkitt E et al: Paralytic ileus after amitriptyline. Br Med J. 1961; 2:1648.

89. Gander DR et al: Ileus after amitriptyline. Br Med J. 1963; 1:1160.

90. Margolis LH: Control of enuresis with imipramine. Am J Psychiatry. 1962; 119:269.

91. Belfer ML et al: Autonomic effects. In *Psychotropic Drug Side Effects,* edited by R Shader and A DiMascio, The Williams and Wilkins Company, Baltimore, 1970, p 116.

92. Belfer ML et al: Autonomic effects. In *Psychotropic Drug Side Effects,* edited by R Shader and A DiMascio, The Williams and Wilkins Company, Baltimore, 1970, p 117.

93. Rosselet E: Misuse of psychotropics blamed for increase in eye disorders. Psychiatric News. 1968; 3:3.

94. Grant WM: Ocular complications of drugs. JAMA. 1969; 207:2089.

95. Davies B et al: Effects on the heart of different tricyclic antidepressants. Exerpta Medica. 1975.

96. Williams RB et al: Cardiac complications of tricyclic antidepressant therapy. Ann Intern Med. 1971; 74:395.

97. Boston Collaborative Drug Surveillance Program Report: Adverse reactions to the tricyclic antidepressant drugs. Lancet. 1972; 1:529.

98. Moir DC et al: Cardiotoxicity of amitriptyline. Lancet. 1972; 2:561.

99. Sigg EB et al: Cardiovascular effects of imipramine. J Pharmacol Exper Ther. 1963; 141:237.

100. Cairneross KD et al: A pharmacological basis for the cardiovascular complications of imipramine medication. Med J Aust. 1962; 49:372.

100a. Hansten PD: Drug interactions affecting cardiovascular response to sympathomimetics. Drug Interactions Newsletter. 1981; 1:21.

101. Berthiaume M: Alteration of the clinical picture during tofranil therapy. Canad Psychiatric Assoc J. 1959; 4:S-187.

102. Hohn R et al: A double-blind comparison of placebo and imipramine in the treatment of depressed patients in a state hospital. J Psychiatric Res. 1961; 1:76.

103. Hudgens RW et al: Visual hallucinations with imino-dibenzyl antidepressants. JAMA. 1966; 198:81.

104. *Psychotropic Drug Side Effects,* edited by R Shader and A DiMascio, The Williams and Wilkins Company, Baltimore, 1970.

105. Bunney WE et al: The switch process from depression to mania: Relationship to drugs which alter brain amines. Lancet. 1970; 1:1022.

106. Bunney WE et al: The "switch process" in manic-depressive illness. Arch Gen Psychiatry. 1972; 27:312.

107. Keller MH et al: Effects of imipramine and thioridazine on set and attention. Dis Nerv Syst. 1966; 27:798.

108. DiMascio A et al: Behavioral toxicity. Part 1: Definition and Part II: Psychomotor functions. In *Psychotropic Drug Side Effects,* edited by R Shader and A DiMascio, The Williams and Wilkins Company, Baltimore, 1970, p 124.

109. Klerman GL et al: The tricyclic antidepressants. In *Principles of Psychopharmacology,* edited by W Clark and J delBuidice, Academic Press, New York, 1968.

110. Wood CA et al: Management of tricyclic antidepressant toxicities. Dis Nerv Syst. 1976; 37:459.

111. Prange A: The use of drugs in depression: Its theoretical and practical basis. Psych Ann. 1973; 3:56.

112. Klein D and Davis J: *Diagnosis and Drug Treatment of Psychiatric Disorders,* Williams & Wilkins, Baltimore, 1969.

113. Stockley I: Interactions of monoamine oxidase inhibitors with foods and drugs. Pharm J. 1969; 203:174.

114. Robison D et al: Aging, monoamines, and monoamine oxidase levels. Lancet. 1972; 1:290.

115. Roth M: The phobic anxiety-depersonalization syndrome and some general aetiological problems in psychiatry. J Neuropsychiatry. 1959; 1:293.

116. Raskin A et al: Depression subtypes and response to phenelzine, diazepam, and a placebo. Arch Gen Psychiatry. 1974; 30:66.

117. Davidson J et al: A pilot study of continuation therapy with phenelzine. Personal Communications, 1979.

118. Warton R et al: A potential clinical use for methylphenidate with tricyclic antidepressants. Am J Psychiatry. 1971; 127:1619.

119. Sulzer F et al: Biochemical and metabolic considerations concerning the mechanism of action of amphetamine and related compounds. In *Psychotomimetic Drugs,* edited by D Efron, Raven Press, New York, 1970, p 83.

120. Perel J et al: In vitro metabolism studies with methylphenidate. Fed Proc. 1970; 29:345.

121. Prange AJ et al: Enhancement of imipramine by thyroid stimulating hormone: clinical and theoretical implications. Am J Psychiatry. 1970; 127:191.

122. Salzmann MM: A controlled trial with a new antidepressant drug trimipramine. Br J Psychiatry. 1965; 3:1105.

123. Rifkin A et al: Comparisons of trimipramine and imipramine: A controlled study. J Clin Psychiatry. 1980; 41:124.

124. Settle EC et al: Trimipramine: Twenty years of worldwide clinical experience. J Clin Psychiatry. 1980; 41:266.

125. Steinbook RM et al: Amoxapine, imipramine and placebo: A double-blind study with pretherapy urinary 3-methoxy-4-hydroxyphenylglycol levels. Curr Ther Res. 1979; 26:490.

126. Gallant DM et al: Amoxapine: A double-blind evaluation of antidepressant activity. Curr Ther Res. 1973; 15:56.

127. Sathananthan GL et al: Amoxapine and imipramine: A double-blind study in depressed patients. Curr Ther Res. 1973; 15:919.

128. Jaffe K et al: Galactorrhea in a patient treated with amoxapine. J Clin Psychiatry. 1978; 39:821.

129. Saito S et al: General pharmacology of amoxapine. Clin Report. 1971; 5:39.

130. Fabre LF: Double-blind placebo-controlled comparison of amoxapine and imipramine in depressed outpatients. Curr Ther Res. 1977; 22:611.

131. Wilson IC et al: A double-blind clinical comparison of amoxapine, imipramine and placebo in the treatment of depression. Curr Ther Res. 1977; 22:620.

132. Holden JM et al: Amoxapine in depressive illness. Curr Med Res Opin. 1979; 6:338.

133. Pinder RM et al: Maprotiline: A review of its pharmacological properties and therapeutic efficacy in mental depressive states. Drugs. 1977; 13:321.

134. Stimmel GL: Maprotiline (Ludiomil, Ciba-Geigy Corp.). Drug Intell Clin Pharm. 1980; 14:585.

135. Warren JA: Nomifensine: A new antidepressant. Presentation to American Society of Hospital Pharmacists. San Francisco, December 9, 1980. (unpublished).

136. Feighner JP: Trazodone, a triazopyridine derivative, in primary depressive disorder. J Clin Psychiatry. 1980; 41:250.

137. Kellams JJ et al: Trazodone, a new antidepressant: Efficacy and safety in endogenous depression. J Clin Psychiatry. 1979; 40:390.

138. Gershon S et al: Lack of anticholinergic side effects with a new antidepressant—trazodone. J Clin Psychiatry. 1980; 41:100.

139. Wheatley D: Potentiation of amitriptyline by thyroid hormone. Arch Gen Psychiatry. 1972; 26:229.

140. Overall J et al: Broad spectrum screening of psychotherapeutic drugs: Thiothixene as an antipsychotic and antidepressant. Clin Pharmacol Ther. 1969; 10:36.

141. Pope HG et al: Diagnosis in schizophrenia and manic-depressive illness: A reassessment of the specificity of "schizophrenic" symptoms in the light of current research. Arch Gen Psychiatry. 1978; 35:811.

142. Goodwin FK et al: Lithium in the treatment of mania: comparisons with neuroleptics. Arch Gen Psychiatry. 1979; 36:841.

143. Prien R et al: Comparison of lithium carbonate and chlorpromazine in the treatment of mania. Arch Gen Psychiatry. 1972; 26:146.

144. Cohen W et al: Lithium carbonate, haloperidol, and irreversible brain damage. JAMA. 1974; 230:1283.

145. Ayd F: Lithium-haloperidol for mania: Is it safe or hazardous? Internat Drug Ther Newsletter. 1975; 10:8.

146. Prien RJ: Lithium in the prophylactic treatment of affective disorders. Arch Gen Psychiatry. 1979; 36:847.

147. Schou M: Lithium as a prophylactic agent in unipolar affective illness. Arch Gen Psychiatry. 1979; 36:849.

148. Mendels J: Lithium as an antidepressant. Arch Gen Psychiatry. 1979; 36:845.

149. Dunner D et al: Clinical factors in lithium carbonate prophylaxis failure. Arch Gen Psychiatry. 1974; 30:229.

150. Prien RJ: Lithium in the treatment of schizophrenia and schizoaffective disorders. Arch Gen Psychiatry. 1979; 36:852.

151. Shopsin B et al: Pharmacology—toxicology of the lithium ion. In *Lithium: Its Role in Psychiatric Research and Treatment,* edited by S Gershon and B Shopsin, Plenum Press, New York, 1973, p 107.

152. Grof P: Some practical aspects of lithium treatment. Arch Gen Psychiatry. 1979; 36:891.

153. Amdisen A: Serum level monitoring and clinical pharmacokinetics of lithium. Clin Pharmacokinetics. 1977; 2:73.

153a. Amdisen A: Lithium. In *Applied Pharmacokinetics: Principles of Therapeutic Drug Monitoring,* edited by W Evans et al, Applied Therapeutics, Inc, San Francisco, 1980.

154. Cooper TB et al: The 24-hour serum lithium level as a prognosticator of dosage requirements. Am J Psychiatry. 1973; 130:601.

155. Cooper TB et al: The 24-hour lithium level as a prognosticator of dosage requirements: a 2-year follow-up study. Am J Psychiatry. 1976; 133:440.

156. Ayd FJ: Chronic renal lesions: A hazard of long-term lithium treatment. Internat Drug Ther Newsletter. 1977; 12:#10.

157. Ayd FJ: Lithium-induced nephrotoxicity: A further report. Internat Drug Ther Newsletter. 1978; 13:#7.

158. Thomson K: Renal lithium elimination in man and active treatment of lithium poisoning. Acta Scand Psych Suppl. 1969; 207:83.

159. Ereshefsky L et al: Lithium therapy of manic depressive illness: Part I: Target symptoms, pharmacology and kinetics. Drug Intell Clin Pharm. 1979; 13:403.

160. Pandy GN et al: Lithium transport in human red blood cells. Arch Gen Psychiatry. 1979; 36:902.

161. Lee C et al: The relationship of plasma to erythrocyte lithium levels in patients taking lithium carbonate. Br J Psychiatry. 1975; 127:596.

162. Ravenscroft P et al: Saliva lithium concentrations in the management of lithium therapy. Arch Gen Psychiatry. 1978; 35:1123.

163. Fryo B et al: Pharmacokinetics of lithium in manic depressive patients. Acta Psych Scand. 1973; 49:237.

164. Himmellock JM et al: Thiazide-lithium synergy in refractory mood swings. Am J Psychiatry. 1977; 134:149.

165. Hansen HE et al: Lithium intoxication. Quar J Med. 1978; 47:123.

166. Lapierr YO: Control of lithium tremor with propranolol. Can Med Assoc J. 1976; 114:619.

167. Reisberg B et al: Side effects associated with lithium therapy. Arch Gen Psychiatry. 1979; 36:879.

168. Vacaflor L et al: Side effects and teratogenicity of lithium carbonate treatment. J Clin Pharmacol. 1970; 10:387.

169. Halmi KA et al: Effects of lithium on thyroid function. Biol Psychiatry. 1972; 5:211.

170. Juhl RP et al: Lithium-induced nephrogenic diabetes insipidus. Am J Hosp Pharm. 1976; 33:843.

171. Goldfield M et al: Lithium in pregnancy: A review with recommendations. Am J Psychiatry. 1971; 127:888.

172. Goldfield M et al: Lithium carbonate in obstetrics: Guidelines for clinical use. Am J Obstet Gynecol. 1973:116:15.

173. Wilson JHP et al: Peritoneal dialysis for lithium poisoning. Br Med J. 1971; 2:749.

174. Rumack E et al: Management I, lithium. In *Poisindex,* Micromedex, Englewood, 1980.

175. Zoffuton A et al: Lithium-induced hypothyroidism. Southern Med J. 1977; 70:#12.

176. Rogers MP et al: Clinical hypothyroidism occurring during lithium treatment. Am J Psychiatry. 1971; 128:158.

177. Forrest JN: Lithium inhibition of cAMP-mediated hormones: A caution. N Engl J Med. 1975; 292:423.

178. Levy ST et al: Lithium-induced diabetes insipidus: Manic symptoms, brain and electrolyte correlates, and chlorothiazide treatment. Am J Psychiatry. 1973; 130:1014.

179. MacNeil S et al: Lithium and the antidiuretic hormone. Br J Clin Pharmacol. 1936; 3:305.

180. Ascione FJ: Lithium with diuretics. Drug Ther. 1977; 2:53.

181. Jenner FA et al: Lithium and the question of kidney damage. Arch Gen Psychiatry. 1979; 36:888.

182. Gerner RH et al: Results of clinical renal function tests in lithium patients. Am J Psychiatry. 1980; 137:834.

183. Byrd GJ et al: Methyldopa and lithium carbonate: Suspected interaction. JAMA. 1975; 233:320.

184. Hansten PD: *Drug Interactions,* 4th ed., 1979, Lea Febiger, Philadelphia.

185. Van der Velde C: Toxicity of lithium carbonate in elderly patients. Am J Psychiatry. 1971; 127:1075.

186. Hansten PD: Lithium and methyldopa. Drug Interactions Newsletter. 1981; 1:11.

187. Hansten PD: Lithium and indomethacin. Drug Interactions Newsletter. 1981; 1:47.

188. Hansten PD: Lithium and neuroleptic agents. Drug Interactions Newsletter. 1982; 2:17.

Chapter 46

Drug Abuse

Darryl S. Inaba and Thomas W. Dunphy

Our society has only recently acknowledged a "drug problem" resulting from the use of psychoactive drugs. In reality, drugs have been used to produce altered states of consciousness in almost every society since the beginning of recorded history (1–3). "Drug abuse" and "drug addiction" are more socio-political terms than medical-pharmacological ones. As a result, the public ambiguously classifies drugs as "licit-illicit," "addicting-nonaddicting," "narcotic-nonnarcotic," or in short, "good" and "bad" (4). What is considered "drug abuse" varies greatly from culture to culture, from time to time, and from one situation to another within the same culture. For example, if barbiturates are taken to induce sleep under medical supervision, it is considered "drug use," whereas the same amount of barbiturate administered to produce euphoria is considered "drug abuse."

To avoid further confusion, we will adhere to the definition of *drug addiction* proposed by Jaffe (2): "a behavioral pattern of compulsive drug use, characterized by an overwhelming involvement with the use of a drug, the securing of its supply, and a high tendency to relapse after withdrawal."

Physical dependence will be separately defined from addiction, for within some individuals, addiction as defined here has developed without physical dependence and, conversely, physical dependence has developed without addiction (2,5). *Physical dependence,* then, will be defined as "an altered physiological state produced by the repeated administration of a drug to prevent the appearance of a stereotype withdrawal or abstinence syndrome characteristic of a particular drug" (2).

Little is known about the mechanism of compulsive drug abuse, and although many theories have been offered, none are conclusive (6–12). Moreover, the epidemiology of any drug abuse pattern is really a complex interaction between physical, psychological, and social variables. An appreciation of all these interactions is required

by any health professional involved with the management of a "drug abuser."

Recent research has produced evidence of an endogenous opioid peptide in both man and animals. Referred to in literature as POP (Pituitary Opioid Polypeptide), endorphin, enkephalin and betaendorphin, the confirmation of endogenous peptides in man with opioid-like activity will constitute a major breakthrough in the medical overview of opioid dependence and drug addiction (13–17). This would probably not, however, immediately change the current social interaction and medical treatment of the drug dependent individual.

It is the intent of this chapter to acquaint practitioners with the clinical picture, treatment modalities, and medical complications of the most common forms of drug abuse. An attempt will also be made to form a practical classification of these commonly abused drugs. The drugs of abuse can be classed into four basic groups based upon their intrinsic pharmacological actions:

  I. Depressants:
    A. Opioid analgesics
    B. Sedative-hypnotics and alcohol
  II. Stimulants (primarily derivatives and analogues of the amphetamines, and cocaine)
  III. Psychotogens and marijuana
  IV. A miscellaneous group of inhalants, glue, and solvents.

Cases and questions will be presented to give a clinical picture of the pattern of addiction and physiologic dependence seen with each class and agents.

DEPRESSANTS

Opioid Analgesics

The use of opiates (alkaloids of opium) and opioids (opiates and other chemicals which have a pharmacology analogous to opiates) by man date back some 6,000 years (18). To date, there is no better treatment for acute and chronic pain (19,20). The clinical use of the opioids is thoroughly reviewed elsewhere in this text.

1. Heroin Addiction and Withdrawal. "Harvey the Hype" has been "fixing" (intravenous injection) two "quarter bags" ($25 quantity of heroin) of street "junk" (heroin) daily. This "run" (daily use) started two weeks ago, and he occasionally treats himself to a "quarter" of either "China White" or "Persian Brown". Harvey tried to keep this "Jones" (heroin habit) down to just "chipping" (occasional use) as he must go to jail soon and must be "clean" (abstinence from drugs). He fears "kicking" (withdrawing from heroin tissue dependence) "cold turkey" (detoxifying with no medical treatment), as he has done this many times and finds the "super flu" (heroin withdrawal symptoms) very unpleasant. Is Harvey "hooked" (addicted) again to heroin such that abstinence will demonstrate opioid tissue dependence? What objective withdrawal signs might result from abstinence?

Using a standard of 10 mg of morphine (equivalent to approximately 4–6 mg of heroin), objective withdrawal signs have been demonstrated upon naloxone challenge after only two to three days of morphine administered in a dosage of 10 mg subcutaneously every four hours. Abstinence alone, however, would not be sufficient to precipitate a withdrawal syndrome from this short duration of opiate administration (22,23). Tissue dependence, as demonstrable by an objective withdrawal syndrome upon abstinence, is highly variable but usually takes two to four weeks of daily morphine administered in the above mentioned doses. Objective withdrawal signs, also known as "nonpurposive" symptoms, are almost always accompanied by a cluster of subjective or "purposive" symptomatology (Question 9). The latter symptoms demonstrate the high degree of psychic parameters involved with any form of drug addiction.

The national average of illicit street heroin purity increased in 1980 for the first time in decades. Even at the current "purer" level, the national average of street heroin is 3.7% with diluents and adulterants (both active and inactive pharmacologically) making up the other 96% (23,24).

Street heroin is most often sold in ballons containing 200 to 400 mg of powder. This quantity of heroin is often called a "dime" ($10) or "quarter" ($25) "bag" (23). Recently, a very pure form of Southwest Asia heroin known as "Persian Brown" (up to 92% heroin) and a synthetic opioid, alpha-methyl-fentanyl, misrepresented as "China White" (pure Southeast Asian heroin), have been sold in much smaller quantities called "quarters." These "quarters" consist of 25 mg of powder usually sold for $25 and packaged in wax paper or aluminum foil folded to form small envelopes called "bindles" or "cribbies." Both new forms of illicit opioids therefore represent more active drug but smaller units of distribution for sale (23–25).

"Harvey the Hype's" current "Jones," therefore, represents a mild tissue dependence with the possibility of mild objective withdrawal signs upon abstinence.

Opiate Withdrawal Symptoms. Both objective and subjective opiate withdrawal symptoms have been described in depth by various authors (2,21,26–28), but it is important to review opioid withdrawal phenomena because many therapeutic issues revolve around the treatment of this syndrome.

The severity of opiate withdrawal symptoms that appear when the drug is discontinued depend upon many factors including the particular opiate, total daily dose, interval between doses, duration of use, and the health and personality of the addict. Unlike withdrawal from barbiturate addiction, opiate withdrawal is seldom life-threatening, and most opiate withdrawal symptoms will follow a general pattern.

Six to 12 hours after the last dose of morphine or heroin (diacetylmorphine) the addict will develop symptoms of anxiety with yawning, sialorrhea, rhinorrhea, and lacrimation. There may also be profuse diaphoresis with concurrent "shaking" chills and pilomotor activity resulting in waves of "gooseflesh" of the skin (thus the term "cold turkey"). The gastrointestinal symptoms are those of anorexia, nausea, vomiting, and diarrhea with abdominal cramps.

These symptoms peak in severity 48 to 72 hours after the last dose. The most prominent symptoms are CNS hyperactivity, restlessness, and insomnia. Muscle spasms with kicking movements and pains in the bones, muscles of the back, and extremities are also characteristic.

During withdrawal the heart rate and blood

pressure may be elevated. The levels of urinary 17-ketosteroids increase (29); leukocytosis is common; and the failure to take in food and fluids, combined with vomiting, sweating, and diarrhea, can result in marked weight loss, dehydration, ketosis and acid-base imbalance. Occasionally, cardiovascular collapse will occur during the peak phase of opiate withdrawal.

The more dramatic symptoms subside after 5–10 days of abstinence even without treatment. However, there is some evidence that a return to complete physiological equilibrium may be complex and protracted (9). More data are needed to explain the especially high recidivism after acute detoxification from opiates (2,26–28,30).

2. Are the withdrawal symptoms the same for all the opioid drugs?

Physiological withdrawal symptoms from all opioid drugs are qualitatively similar. However, there seem to be quantitative differences in the onset, duration, and overall severity of the abstinence syndromes produced by various opiate drugs.

Abstinence symptoms from meperidine appear within three hours after the last dose, peak within 8 to 12 hours and persist for 3 to 5 days. Although there seem to be fewer gastrointestinal symptoms than those produced by morphine and heroin withdrawal, there is reportedly a greater degree of restlessness, nervousness, and muscular twitching when the abstinence syndrome from meperidine is at its peak intensity (31).

Codeine, semisynthetic, and synthetic opioids also produce qualitatively similar abstinence syndromes to those of heroin and morphine. Opiates with a shorter duration of action tend to produce brief, more intense abstinence syndromes, while drugs eliminated from the body at a much slower rate produce prolonged, but milder withdrawal syndromes. The abstinence syndrome of methadone is consistent for a long-acting synthetic opioid. The symptoms are not apparent for 48–72 hours after the last dose. They are qualitatively similar to those of morphine and heroin but less severe, becoming most intense around the sixth day of abstinence. All observable symptoms except for persistent anorexia and lethargy subside and are minimal after 10 to 14 days of abstinence (32).

3. J.B., a 21-year-old male who underwent bowel surgery, required morphine 10 mg

subcutaneously q 4 h prn for two weeks. Is J.B. physiologically addicted to morphine?

As previously mentioned, only mild symptoms of withdrawal, which may not even be recognized as such, will occur in patients who have received therapeutic doses of morphine several times daily for one to two weeks (2). However, withdrawal symptoms have been demonstrated in subjects receiving therapeutic doses of morphine, methadone, or heroin four times daily after only two or three days if the narcotic antagonist nalorphine is administered (33). The number of medically addicted opioid addicts who continue to seek opiates once treatment is terminated is very few. The role of physical dependence in the development of compulsive heroin or morphine abuse is apparently minor when one considers the number of patients who are made clinically dependent on opiates during hospitalizations.

4. *Medical Complications of Heroin Abuse.* A 30-year-old female was admitted into the emergency room with violent shaking and chills. She admitted that she was a heroin addict and was forced into "doing some cottons" because of an acute financial crisis. She now fears that she has contracted "cotton fever." What is "cotton fever" and what are other medical complications of heroin addiction?

When heroin is prepared for self-administration, cotton is used as a filter to trap adulterants; thus, some of the drug remains trapped within the cotton as well. These crude filters are saved, and when money or drug availability is poor, water is added to the "old cottons" to extract any remaining drug for intravenous use. "Cotton fever" is caused by an acute septicemia or an allergic reaction. The latter, caused by broken down cotton fibers or unknown foreign material, may rarely result in anaphylactoid shock and death. The reaction is usually transient and will subside within 24 hours without treatment, although systemic shock requiring acute medical intervention may also occur.

Bacterial endocarditis, embolism, septic and aseptic abscesses, thrombophlebitis, and cellulitis have also resulted from improper sterilization of injection apparatus and poor needle techniques.

The common practice of sharing "outfits" (needle and syringe) between friends has resulted in the transmission of viral hepatitis, syphilis, tetanus, and even malaria. Other complications of heroin addiction include the following: pulmonary emboli (caused by materials used to "cut" or dilute heroin); pulmonary edema; frequent upper respiratory tract infections (especially pneumonia); malnutrition and degenerative nerve changes (seen rarely and probably allergic in origin (34–42).

5. *Heroin Overdose.* **T.F., a 21-year-old male, was brought to the emergency room in a comatose condition by friends. It was alleged that T.F. had "OD'd" (overdosed) on "junk" (heroin). A quick physical examination revealed a depressed respiratory rate (6 per minute), cyanosis, and low body temperature. He had an increased heart rate (110 per minute), symmetrically miotic pupils, and a decreased blood pressure. Several "tracks" (needle scars) and some abscesses were noted on both arms. History, physical exam, the presence of Jaffe's (2) triad (coma, pinpoint pupils, and depressed respiration) were all consistent with an acute opiate overdose. What is the immediate treatment of choice in this situation?**

Unlike the acute toxicity of other depressant drugs (eg, barbiturates), there is a fairly safe and specific antidote for opiate drug overdose. However, the use of these specific narcotic antagonists should not be viewed as the sole and primary management of this situation. The general principles of cardiopulmonary resuscitation should be considered the first step in the management of these cases (26,30,91).

Although nalorphine (Nalline) and levallorphan (Lorfan) effectively antagonize opioid depressant effects, frequent undesirable side effects and their intrinsic depressant properties in large doses limit their clinical usefulness. Their most common side effect is central nervous system excitation that can progress to acute psychosis. Other toxicities include increased narcosis, writhing, diaphoresis, and loss of urinary sphincter control. Because overdose from a mixture of depressant drugs is not an uncommon occurrence, the agonist properties of these two drugs may potentiate the CNS depressant actions of non-narcotic agents (eg, barbiturates). Therefore, naloxone (Narcan) should be used instead in the treatment of opioid overdose.

Naloxone (Narcan) has little or no agonist properties of its own and is said to lack hallucin-

ogenic, miotic, and subjective effects as well. It does not produce tolerance or signs of physical dependence (92,93). Naloxone also has a very high therapeutic index. A single 3000 mg oral dose has been tolerated with no reported side effects. The normal therapeutic dosage range for naloxone is 5 to 25 mcg/kg.

Other analgesics that have been abused and have caused respiratory depression upon acute overdose are pentazocine and propoxyphene. Reportedly, naloxone is capable of antagonizing the depressant effects of pentazocine and propoxyphene as well (95). The respiratory depressant effect of cyclazocine has also been effectively antagonized by naloxone (96). The limitations of naloxone include the following:

Short Duration. Its duration of action (3–5 hours) is short relative to that of narcotics, so there is always possibility of relapse, especially in the case of methadone overdosage (92,96,97). (See the chapter on Poisonings.)

Induction of Abstinence. Naloxone is five to eight times as potent as nalorphine in its ability to precipitate an abstinence syndrome in morphine-dependent subjects. Thus, large doses of naloxone may potentially precipitate severe withdrawal symptoms in an overdosed opiate addict. These precipitated symptoms are much more severe and difficult to manage than those induced by abstinence alone (93).

Both of these limitations apply to nalorphine and levallorphan as well. Naloxone is therefore the drug of choice in the treatment of the acute opioid toxicity.

6. T.F. was brought to the emergency room by a friend who says he administered intravenous salt and milk solutions to T.F. in an attempt to revive him. What is the rationale of this maneuver and other types of "street therapy" in the treatment of the opiate overdose?

Of the many various "street" methods of resuscitation, two of the most commonly used and misunderstood are external stimulation and the intravenous administration of salt, milk, or vinegar solutions.

External stimulation techniques such as sharp slapping of the body, squeezing of sensitive areas (eg, testicles or nipples), walking the victim around, placing him in a cold shower and applying ice to the testicles may all have some benefit in borderline cases. Since opiates depress only the autonomic regulation of respiration but not its voluntary control, external stimulation of the conscious or semiconscious opioid overdosed patient may prevent apnea (2). However, such procedures may result in an airway occluded with blood, mucous, or broken teeth, as well as broken bones and lacerations from over-vigorous application. Further, methods which produce hypothermia may exacerbate pre-existing hypotension and complicate the management of the opioid overdosed patient (38,98).

Intravenous salt and vinegar solutions are thought to bind heroin and nullify its depressant effects. A volume of salt equal to the amount of heroin used is diluted with tap water and injected intravenously. These powerful sclerosing agents are painful and are frequently deposited outside the vein, causing extreme pain. Thus, painful stimulation may again be of some benefit in arousing the borderline overdosed patient. Formation of painful abscesses, sclerosing of the veins, infections, and the potentiation of pulmonary edema from a strongly hypertonic salt solution limit the usefulness of these methods (38).

Intravenous milk is also thought to reverse a heroin overdose. However, such therapy may result in microscopic pulmonary emboli, which may account in part for the lipoid pneumonia and foreign body granulomas found in the lungs of addicts (38,99).

The force-feeding of milk and vinegar to induce vomiting is thought to stimulate the overdosed heroin addict and hasten his recovery time. Emesis may stimulate the autonomic nervous system and reverse, to some extent, the hypotension induced by a depressed vasomotor center. Such therapy in unconscious and semiconscious patients probably accounts for autopsy findings of milk aspirations in the lungs of opiate overdosed patients (98,99).

The "speed reversal" or the use of intravenous amphetamines and cocaine in the treatment of heroin overdose is thought to pharmacologically antagonize the depressant drug. The use of such drugs may precipitate life-threatening convulsions which must be treated with depressant drugs, which may once again induce severe depression in the patient. Furthermore, cocaine has a narrow margin between stimulant and depressant effects, making it a very precarious antidote for the "street" treatment of opioid toxicity (38).

Each of these "street methods" for treating the acute opioid toxicity were described to point out the medical complications induced by such therapy. Medical professionals involved with management of an acute heroin overdose must be cognizant of the fact that any one or a combination of "street methods" may have already been employed to complicate the overall medical status of the patient.

Treatment of Opioid Dependence

In a book published in 1868, H.B. Day (43) wrote that there was no agreement in the medical profession as to the proper treatment of opium disease. This statement is applicable today; the treatment of heroin addiction is still beset by legal, political, and medical controversy.

The ultimate goal of most detoxification programs is to transform the narcotic addict into a responsible, drug-free, emotionally stable, and productive member of society. Although many claims have been made, no program to date fulfills all of these goals. Furthermore, all programs either have a high recidivism rate or do not produce a drug-free state within the patient. Heroin addiction, or any chronic compulsive form of drug abuse, is a symptom of a wide variety of problems within different individuals. Therefore, no single treatment modality is universally effective.

Medical management of the opioid addicts ranges from a very "liberal" opioid maintenance approach to a very conservative "cold turkey," or no medical support, approach. Between these two polarized approaches, approved and nonapproved therapies continue to develop in this field. The current available modalities are outlined below in a very general way. The two factors dealt with for each modality are those of opiate withdrawal and social rehabilitation.

7. *Methadone.* Ms. X's son has been addicted to heroin for three years. She read in a magazine article that methadone is a "cure" for heroin addiction. Not knowing what methadone is, she seeks professional information. What is the methadone approach to the treatment of opioid addiction?

This modality, pioneered by Dole and Nyswander in 1965, has been useful primarily in the rehabilitation of chronic heroin addicts (46–49). By 1970, methadone substitution was considered the treatment of choice for opiate addiction by many researchers (2,50). Although skepticism ran high, the clamor of "drug experts" and politicians for increased methadone maintenance programs (MMTP) resulted in the hasty fabrication of many such projects throughout the country. As might be expected, the effectiveness of these programs was not as good as the original ones. Also, methadone emerged as a drug of abuse and many deaths resulted from its excessive use (51–56). Thus, the methadone approach is now more conservatively viewed as an important therapeutic modality rather than as a panacea for opiate abuse (57,58). The basic pharmacology and addiction liability of methadone should be reviewed before considerations are made to incorporate this drug in the treatment of an opiate addict. Methadone is a synthetic, fully addictive, orally-acting opiate with a prolonged duration of action (12–24 hours). Pharmacologically, it is qualitatively identical with morphine and other opioid analgesics (2). Methadone plays a dual therapeutic role in the treatment of opiate addiction: that of acute detoxification and that of maintenance or long-term replacement therapy.

8. *Methadone Legal Restrictions.* Dr. Jones, a local physician, has just seen a heroin addict who has come to him for methadone treatment. Can Dr. Jones legally prescribe methadone to treat this patient's addiction? Can the pharmacist legally dispense it?

Methadone cannot be used without a special NDA (New Drug Application) permit for the treatment of addiction. The drug is also under the more restrictive IND (Investigational New Drug) status if it is to be used in pregnant women or adolescents (59).

The Food Drug and Cosmetic Law (24CFR 130.40) allows for methadone detoxification treatment for no more than 21 days and methadone maintenance treatment in excess of 21 days if the ultimate goal is to produce a drug-free patient (section 130.44). This law defines treatment programs and makes specifications for the inclusion of comprehensive patient services in addition to methadone therapy. It also allows private practitioners to develop detoxification and maintenance programs upon approval of the Federal Food and Drug Administration and the State Authority. A special permit is granted upon approval and after Federal forms FD 2632-2634 are filed.

The limitation on the dispensing of methadone only in specially licensed pharmacies was a matter of much controversy (59). A test case (August, 1976) before the Federal Courts acknowledged the legality of methadone dispensing by community pharmacies when a valid prescription is written for the treatment of pain (60). The use of methadone in the treatment of opioid addiction, however, is still limited to specific approved treatment facilities.

9. *Methadone Detoxification.* Dr. Dope has established a Methadone Treatment Medication Unit with Cure All Pharmacy. He is treating a heroin addict who claims to have a $75–100 per day "habit" of Haight-Ashbury "junk". The patient is to be started on methadone detoxification. What is the recommended methadone dose for treatment of this patient?

The quality of illicit heroin is highly variable and depends upon the geographical area from which it was obtained, its availability, and, finally, the scruples of the local "connection" or "pusher" (also see Question 1). In the Haight-Ashbury at the time of this writing, a $10 to $25 "bag" or balloon filled with heroin contains 200–400 mg of powder which is actually only 2–15% heroin. Thus, with generous reckoning, a $75 a day habit would equal about 120 mg of pure heroin. Since the quality of heroin varies greatly, it would probably be best to start methadone therapy empirically and regulate the dose on the basis of the patient's symptomatology. Usually 1 mg of methadone can substitute for 4 mg of morphine, 2 mg of heroin, or 20 mg of meperidine (2). Reduction of the dose can be started immediately. A 20% daily reduction in dose is well tolerated and causes little discomfort. The majority of patients can be completely withdrawn from opioids in less than ten days. Applying this formula to the above case, one would start with a methadone dose of 60 mg on the first day and progressively decrease it (48 mg, 38 mg, 30 mg, 24 mg, 19 mg, 15 mg, 12 mg, 10 mg) to 8 mg by the tenth day. At that time the methadone can be discontinued. The patient should be observed for a period of two or three days without medication, since the abstinence syndrome from methadone is not apparent for 48 to 72 hours after the last dose. This approach is highly controversial. Some recent research in methadone maintenance has shown that the dose of methadone is largely irrelevant to the size of the opioid habit, since 40 to 50 mg is sufficient to prevent the development of abstinence symptoms in the majority of addicts. The use of higher doses only affords the patient a high or euphoria from his daily dose of methadone (59,62). Therefore, large initial doses of methadone for allegedly large opiate "habits" are not only superfluous but also present the danger of methadone overdosage.

For habits which allegedly exceed 80 mg of pure heroin a day, a divided daily dose of 40 mg of methadone (10 mg qid) can be used initially to minimize its euphoriant properties. After two days of stabilization, the dose of methadone can be gradually reduced by 5 mg/day until the patient is drug-free by the tenth day.

For habits of less than 40 mg of heroin per day, 1 mg of methadone is administered for each 2 mg of heroin initially. Thereafter, the usual stepwise dose reduction can be instituted over the next few days of therapy. For such habits the initial dose of methadone rarely needs to exceed 15 to 20 mg (27).

Some methadone detoxification programs use adjuvant medication along with methadone therapy. Sedative-hypnotics, gastrointestinal medications, and even analgesics are used regularly in conjunction with methadone. These are usually unnecessary and an attempt should be made to differentiate between what Jaffe (2) terms "purposive" and "nonpurposive" symptoms of opioid abstinence syndromes. *Purposive symptoms* are subjective symptomatology that an addict will express in order to manipulate for some specific goal (eg, narcotic prescriptions). *Nonpurposive symptoms* are more objective symptoms or pure physiologic signs of an abstinence syndrome (eg, tremors). Other depressant drugs potentiate the euphoric properties of methadone.

10. *Methadone Maintenance.* **Dr. Dope is also interested in establishing a methadone maintenance component to his program. He has heard that doses of methadone greater than 100 mg per day are routinely needed to maintain heroin addicts. Additionally, he is unsure if he has the staffing to be able to administer daily doses of methadone. How is methadone used in maintenance therapy?**

What are Dr. Dope's alternatives for his methadone maintenance component?

Currently, the only federally approved medical treatments for heroin addiction are either methadone detoxification or methadone maintenance therapy. The ultimate goal of methadone maintenance is to produce a drug-free individual. The object of methadone maintenance is to enable an addict to escape from the illicit drug scene, thereby affording him the time to review his present life style, reorient his goals, and rehabilitate himself into a more responsible, drug-free individual. Early enthusiasm for methadone maintenance has now been tarnished by its consequent misuse as yet another drug of abuse.

During methadone maintenance, the addict is stabilized on a dose that will be sufficient to suppress heroin withdrawal symptoms for 12 to 24 hours but will not produce the euphoria or the nodding high of opiate drugs. Although a methadone maintained addict often receives a dose in excess of 100 mg, the daily dose generally needed to prevent the onset of opioid withdrawal symptoms generally need not exceed 50 mg (62). The drug is administered in single daily oral doses so that there is daily contact with the addicted patient. With the aid of daily counseling and rehabilitation it is hoped that the patient will eventually detoxify from methadone as well.

Medical staffing problems and disruption of client employment schedules brought about by the necessity of daily methadone dosing have stimulated the search for an alternative drug to methadone. "Take home" dosing, allowing addicts to obtain more than a single day's dose of methadone for self-administration, has frequently led to drug diversion and heroin recidivism. Recently, longer-acting methadone homologs such as d-acetylmethadol or 1-methadyl acetate have been developed. It is hoped that these homologs which have a duration of action from 72 to 96 hours will help to minimize the extensive medical and paramedical resources needed to carry out the present treatment programs (50,63,64). The use of these longer-acting methadone analogues is still under federal IND classification.

11. *Treatment of Pain in Methadone Maintained Patients.* **T.A., a 44-year-old male maintained on 120 mg of methadone per day, is in severe pain from an accident involving multiple fractures in his right leg. The at-**

tending emergency room physician would like to know what type and how much analgesic can be used with safety in this patient.

Although tolerance does develop to the analgesic effects of methadone in chronically maintained patients (2), clinical experience shows that conventional doses of meperidine or morphine are effective analgesics for such cases. However, one must be wary of certain potent analgesics that are also narcotic antagonists, such as pentazocine (Talwin), which may produce opioid withdrawal symptoms when used in the methadone maintained patient (2,65). Stadol and Nubain should therefore also be avoided.

Cushman (66) outlines two methods of handling methadone maintained patients who must undergo surgery. If the procedure is minor and pain is not expected to be severe or prolonged, full methadone maintenance dosages can be administered throughout the hospital stay including the day of surgery. If the procedure is major or if protracted pain is anticipated, methadone can be tapered preoperatively if possible and discontinued during the first few postoperative days. During this interval, analgesia and maintenance of the dependent state can be accomplished with frequent conventional doses of opioid analgesics. Methadone therapy can later be resumed by gradually increasing the dose to full maintenance levels.

Tolerance to the anesthetic effects of other CNS depressants is a different situation. Cross-tolerance can occur in the methadone maintained individual so that higher doses of anesthetics may be indicated; however, these should be instituted with caution (34).

12. Pregnancy Tests.
M.S., a 25-year-old female maintained on 100 mg of methadone a day, has had amenorrhea for a month and a recent positive test for pregnancy. She has not had intercourse for the last three months. Can these symptoms be due to her methadone therapy?

Although amenorrhea, anovulation, and infertility among heroin and methadone addicted women have been somewhat over-emphasized in the past, these problems may occur and the gynecologist should be aware of them (67–70).

Horowitz and associates (71) studied the effect of differing doses of methadone on various pregnancy tests. A significant number of false positive

and inconclusive tests were related to daily methadone doses when the Gravindex Slide test or the Pregnosticon Slide test were employed. High methadone doses (eg, 200–240 mg/day) resulted in the highest percentage of false positive and inconclusive tests. However, there was minimal interference with the combination UCG-Pregnosticon tube test for pregnancy at all daily dosages of methadone studied.

In this case, the type of pregnancy test used should be established. Recommendations for a second test using the combined UCG-Pregnosticon tube test should be made. If the patient is not pregnant, methadone induced amenorrhea should be offered as a possible cause of her irregular menses. Other etiologies must also be ruled out.

13. Methadone in Pregnancy.
J.R., a 28-year-old female, has been maintained on 100 mg daily doses of methadone for the past year. She is now 8 months pregnant and her obstetrician has made the following inquiries: is methadone teratogenic? Will methadone cross the placental barrier and addict the child? Should J.R. be withdrawn from methadone? Will methadone be excreted into J.R.'s breast milk? What is the treatment of an opiate addicted newborn?

Teratogenicity. Although the evidence is inconclusive, it appears that methadone is not teratogenic and that women on methadone maintenance frequently have regular menstrual periods, ovulate, conceive, and have normal pregnancies. Thirty-three percent of babies delivered to methadone maintained mothers have been premature by weight, but no congenital anomalies have been reported. Also, four-year follow-ups have demonstrated that these infants have normal physical and intellectual development (68,72).

However, there have been several reports concerning the hazards of pregnancy in the heroin addicted mother. The most commonly encountered problems included pre-eclampsia (10–15%), low birth weight (34–50%), and addiction (50–75%) of the newborn. These problems were potentiated by inadequate medical management of the addicted mother and her newborn (73).

Neonatal Addiction. Methadone crosses the placental barrier and can cause CNS and respiratory depression as well as an opiate abstinence syndrome in the neonate. In one study, 50% of the infants born to methadone maintained mothers exhibited withdrawal signs of twitching and irritability. Half of these required treatment with phenobarbital or tincture of opium. Withdrawal signs in the newborn of a heroin addicted mother will become apparent a few hours after birth; however, in the infant of a methadone maintained mother, symptoms may be delayed for up to 3 days (68,72,74).

Withdrawal During Pregnancy. At 8 months into pregnancy, J.R. should probably not be withdrawn from methadone because of the possibility of inducing methadone withdrawal symptoms. It is probably best to maintain her on methadone and take proper precautions to treat the neonate upon delivery for either narcotic depression or methadone addiction.

Breast Feeding. Methadone is excreted into the breast milk of methadone maintained mothers. The quantities, though small, may be sufficient to cause some physical dependency in infants. Therefore, breast feeding is not advised for mothers on methadone maintenance (68).

Treatment of Neonatal Addiction. Opioid withdrawal in the neonate manifests itself in a wide variety of nonspecific signs which can readily be confused with meningitis, gastroenteritis, hypocalcemia, and intracranial hemorrhage. An accurate differential diagnosis is essential for all of these life-threatening disorders in the newborn.

In general, the most common withdrawal symptoms include restlessness, tremors, a high pitched cry, hypertonicity, increased reflexes, regurgitation, and sneezing.

Management of the neonate's narcotic withdrawal syndrome entails careful attention to hydration with demand feeding, in addition to the management of the more obvious symptoms. Mild withdrawal symptoms need no treatment; however, moderate to severe symptoms may require 14 or more days of therapy.

Symptoms of physiological addiction are usually apparent within 48 hours after birth. At this time treatment can be initiated with tincture of opium (10% opium) which is preferred over paregoric since the latter contains camphor. The initial dose is 1 to 2 drops per pound of body weight; this is increased until symptoms disappear. The tincture of opium is then gradually and totally withdrawn over a one to two week period (2,25,28). Methadone has also been used in a dose of 0.5 mg every 4 to 12 hours for 3 days. Doses of these drugs should be individualized so that neither

withdrawal symptoms nor narcosis occur. Phenobarbital can be used to control major motor convulsions if they occur (28).

Prophylactic drug therapy should not be given to infants of addicts. Rather, therapy should begin when observable central nervous symptoms occur or when the infant is unable to sleep between feedings (73).

14. *Antagonist Approach.* **What is the "antagonist" or "heroin blockade" approach to the treatment of opioid addiction?**

It has been proposed that methadone (80–150 mg or more) blocks the euphoriant effects of other opioids without producing euphoria itself. This dose allegedly produces a high degree of cross-tolerance to other opiates so that it is extremely difficult to achieve euphoric effects with intravenous injection of other opioids (47). However, this role of methadone has been questioned, since addicts have been able to obtain euphoric properties from doses of 60–100 mg of methadone. Furthermore, at lower maintenance doses of methadone which do not produce euphoria, addicts have been able to reach euphoric states through the intravenous administration of other opiates. Indeed, methadone in high blocking dosages has become a secondary drug of abuse (53, 55).

The development of the true narcotic antagonists, cyclazocine and naloxone, has offered a more rational approach to heroin blockade therapy. If opiate addiction results from a process of classical and instrumental conditioning and is positively reinforced by self administration and drug seeking behavior, then narcotic antagonists may break this addiction cycle. The advantages of the narcotic antagonists are that they block the effects of heroin and other opiates, prevent the development of physiologic dependence, and afford protection from opioid overdose deaths.

Of the two antagonists available for such therapy, cyclazocine has been the most extensively studied. The disadvantages of cyclazocine are that (a) some individuals experience unpleasant subjective effects ("like LSD"), (b) it is effective only on a short-term basis because patients usually refuse to stay on the drug, (c) physiological dependence to cyclazocine may itself develop with daily doses of 4–8 mg, and (d) it is necessary to withdraw patients from all opiates before building up the dose of cyclazocine, since it can produce very severe withdrawal symptoms if it is given to an addict who is still physiologically addicted to opioids.

Naloxone (Narcan) has the advantage of being free from unpleasant subjective effects. Unfortunately, it has a short duration of action and a variable potency when taken orally. No physiologic dependence is induced by naloxone, but its expense and the need for close supervision for frequent administration of this drug make it somewhat impractical to use.

The use of narcotic antagonists in the treatment of opiate addiction is analogous to the use of disulfiram (Antabuse) in the alcoholic. It, therefore, seems reasonable that the narcotic antagonists will have limited value in the treatment of opiate addiction. As mentioned previously, it is important to treat the opiate addict and not just his use of opioid drugs. Cyclorphan and n-allyl opiate derivatives are other narcotic antagonists currently being studied (2,50,76,77), as are naltrexone (EN-1639A-Endo Labs) and BC-2605 (Bristol Labs) (78–80).

15. *Heroin Maintenance.* What is the "heroin maintenance" approach to narcotic addiction?

The British sought to humanize addict treatment and decrease crime by allowing private physicians to prescribe heroin to legally registered addicts. Unfortunately, addicts were not provided with adequate follow-up treatment and rehabilitative programs. Furthermore, they were not eligible for welfare, and daily intravenous doses of up to 250 mg of heroin were allowed.

It has been said that to support themselves, many of these licensed British addicts simply sold part of their heroin to novices, who soon became heroin-dependent. The latter eventually registered as addicts, perpetuated the cycle and thereby increased the population of heroin addicts. Although the number of reported British addicts did in fact increase, the number of narcotic-related crimes did not. It has been suggested that this approach did not actually increase the number of new addicts, but merely exposed those who had not entered into any available treatment program (39,81).

16. *Therapeutic Communities.* What is the "therapeutic community" approach to the treatment of narcotic addiction?

A modality that has been successful in the total rehabilitation of a heroin addict is the therapeutic community or what Smith and Gay (77) have termed the "third community" (the first community being the "straight world" in which an addict feels both different and alienated, and the second being the "hip drug scene" which advocates the use of psychoactive drugs as a means of problem solving and escape).

The first of such programs, Synanon, was founded in the early 1960's by Charles Dederick in Santa Monica, California. Dederick advanced the theory that the addict can change his deviant behavior patterns only by voluntarily joining a strongly disciplined but loving pseudo-family which helps him to re-experience the process of growing up (also termed as a total commitment to a new life style). The self-help regime utilizes all members of the "family" and includes physical labor. Synanon accomplishes its goals through techniques of group encounter and confrontation which they call "The Game." Synanon is an economically self-sustaining organization with many branches throughout northern California. It offers its alternative life style to all members of society and not just drug addicts.

There have been many offshoots and variations on the Synanon theme. These include Daytop Village in Staten Island, New York; the Phoenix Complex in New York City; the Gateway House in Chicago; and the Family Awareness Houses in Arizona and California.

These are long-term programs, and although they can be successful, they appeal to relatively few addicts because of the live-in and total commitment aspects. Charles Dederick felt that Synanon would be effective for only one out of every ten addicts and that Synanon members would never be able to return to the straight or hip worlds without going back to drugs. Thus, the biggest disadvantage of this approach is that it is suitable for only a few addicts. Of those addicts who are accepted and remain in such programs for more than a few weeks, 80 to 90% remain heroin-free and crime-free for at least one year. However, this number represents only a small percent of the total number of addicts who need help. The programs lose their effectiveness if addicts do not join voluntarily (50,77,82).

Other, short-term therapeutic communities have been organized like Synanon, but have placed more emphasis upon returning the addict to society. Odyssey House in New York, Walden House, Reality House, and Delancy Street in California and various other half-way houses throughout the country are oriented in this manner. Unfortunately, the same limitations and high recidivism rates that apply to Synanon also apply to these short-term therapeutic communities (83).

17. *Drug Treatment Approach.* What is the "symptomatic" or "drug treatment" approach to the management of the opioid withdrawal syndrome?

Programs like the Haight-Ashbury Drug Detoxification, Rehabilitation and Aftercare Project in San Francisco provide outpatient non-narcotic drug treatment of heroin withdrawal symptoms and place primary emphasis upon psycho-social counseling and social-vocational rehabilitation.

Outpatient treatment of heroin addicts was first instituted in the early 1900's, and 44 centers were in operation between 1919 and 1923 (84). Though some clinics were reasonably successful, the New York Clinics were a disaster with respect to organization and supervision. These created such adverse publicity that all clinics were forced to close by 1923. Some authors now believe that these outpatient clinics did not receive a fair and adequate trial (61,81,85).

A small but significant re-emergence of the outpatient treatment clinics began in the late 1960's as the heroin problem reached epidemic proportions in certain communities. Now, with better organization and increased integration of "street professionals" (ex-addicts) with "paper professionals" (physicians, psychologists, pharmacists) these outpatient clinics are reasonably successful. They service a large number of the addict population in spite of the accessibility of numerous outpatient methadone maintenance programs.

The Haight-Ashbury Drug Detoxification Project, currently under the direction of Dr. John Newmeyer, is representative of these outpatient drug treatment programs. The medical regimen is set up to treat the symptomatology of each individual heroin addict. The symptomatology is broken down into four basic categories: (a) insomnia; (b) anxiety; (c) gastrointestinal complaints; and (d) musculoskeletal aches and pains.

A formulary of medications to treat these symptoms was established by first determining which of the non-narcotic drugs were acceptable to the patient population. Of these, only those drugs which afforded the highest therapeutic index and lowest addiction liability were included. Medications are dispensed on a daily basis; the single ingestion of a whole day's and night's dose of medication is not an uncommon experience. Thus, the medications used vary with the particular group of patients who are serviced by the program. Those in current use by the Haight-Ashbury Drug Detoxification Project include the following:

(a) Chloral hydrate 1–1.5 gm, flurazepam (Dalmane) 30–60 mg, or diphenhydramine (Benadryl) 50-100 mg are used for insomnia. Both Chloral hydrate and flurazepam have been shown to have less effect on normal REM sleep patterns as compared to other commonly used sleep medications (86). Diphenhydramine, normally used as an antihistamine, has significant sedative effects which have been useful in clients who are non-responsive to other hypnotic agents. Chloral hydrate, flurazepam and diphenhydramine all have abuse potential of their own, but each has shown less tendency for misuse and abuse in this population as compared to the short-acting barbiturates, glutethimide, methaqualone, ethchlorvynol, and methyprylon.

(b) Chlordiazepoxide (Librium) 20–60 mg or phenobarbital 60–180 mg are used for anxiety. Treatment of the anxiety states associated with opioid withdrawal phenomena has offered a true challenge to the clinician. Heroin addicts often abuse heroin for its anxiolytic effects and therefore slip into a sequela of either alcohol or sedative abuse after heroin detoxification. The benzodiazepines, with their wide therapeutic index, are the safest drugs to use for anxiety in this population. Diazepam, however, seems to precipitate more patterns of chronic abuse than either chlordiazepoxide or phenobarbital in the heroin addict population of the Haight-Ashbury Free Medical Clinic. These are the only two anxiolytic agents employed in the Project's 21-day outpatient medical detoxification protocol at the current time.

(c) Belladonna alkaloids with phenobarbital (Donnatal) 4–8 tablets per day, dicyclomine (Bentyl) 40–80 mg, or prochlorperazine (Compazine) 15–30 mg are utilized for gastrointestinal complaints. The antispasmodic effects of both Donnatal and Bentyl are effective in suppressing the hyperactivity of the GI tract during opioid withdrawal. The anticholinergic properties of these medications are also effective for the treatment of rhinorrhea, sialorrhea, diaphoresis, and lacrimation of the opioid withdrawal syndrome. Compazine is more specifically used for clients exhibiting a severe emetic reaction to opioid withdrawal.

These doses represent the daily dosage dispensed for acute heroin detoxification. The time spent in this phase should not exceed one to two weeks. The doses are then reduced daily such that addicts are on no drug by the end of their third or fourth week of medical therapy. At this time the clients are encouraged to participate in social-vocational programs while psycho-social counseling is actively continued.

This approach has been effective for the population of heroin addicts seen at the Haight-Ashbury Clinic. Modifications and adaptations of this type of program are necessary if one is to extend this therapy to differing populations of heroin addicts. The effectiveness of these programs may be attributed to their accessibility to the "street population." They further serve as a primary treatment "screen" for the heroin population (60).

18. *New Drug Approaches*. What other drugs are being tried experimentally in the treatment of opiate addiction?

Propoxyphene Napsylate. As an alternative to both the methadone and the "symptomatic" approach, a propoxyphene napsylate (Darvon-N) modality has developed over the past few years. This therapy employs propoxyphene napsylate alone as either a detoxification or a maintenence agent in doses of 0.8 to 2 gm per day for the treatment of opioid addiction. All propoxyphene salts were reclassified as narcotics as of July 24, 1980 (87–90).

Clonidine. Recent research has shown withdrawal symptoms to emanate from the locus cereleus. Clonidine, an antihypertensive drug with paradoxical alpha agonistic activity, exerts its antihypertensive effect through central activity at the locus cereleus. Experiments in animals and recently on morphine addicts have demonstrated clonidine's ability to suppress opioid withdrawal symptoms in dosages of 0.1 to 0.2 mg tid and 0.2 mg hs. Though effective, one must pay careful attention to the overdose potential of clonidine in this "high risk" population. Additionally, long-term treatment with clonidine results in a tissue

dependence characterized by a morbid hypertensive withdrawal phenomenon (44,45).

The use of clonidine or propoxyphene to treat opioid addiction is currently restricted to an FDA New Drug Application.

Sedative-Hypnotics and Alcohol

Alcohol continues to be this nation's number one drug of abuse. From a sociologic, economic, and health perspective, no other drug or substance is responsible for more damage than that incurred by our socially acceptable and legal drug, alcohol. Though it is most often used appropriately and recreationally, alcohol must be recognized as a very potent drug of full scale abuse and addiction. Because the toxicology and medical complications of alcohol abuse warrant a detailed, in-depth presentation, a separate, detailed chapter on alcoholism follows this chapter.

The short-acting barbiturates have been and continue to be a prototype of sedative-hypnotic use and abuse. Increased awareness of both the toxicity and the addiction liability of barbiturates has greatly reduced the incidence of barbiturate abuse in recent years. This has resulted in a deluge of non-barbiturate sedative-hypnotics which nevertheless have qualitatively the same addiction liability and withdrawal syndrome as the barbiturates. Of special concern is the increasing use of benzodiazepines which have a greater therapeutic index than the barbiturates but may possess an even greater risk of tissue dependence upon chronic administration.

Onset of Sedative-Hypnotic Dependence. As pointed out in the discussion of hypnotics in the chapter on Anxiety and Insomnia, minor nocturnal EEG changes in the form of REM-rebound may occur after the cessation of only a few nights treatment with normal hypnotic doses of pentobarbital. However, dependence which gives rise to more obvious and more harmful signs of withdrawal requires larger doses for longer periods. After ingesting 600 mg of pentobarbital per day for one or two months, about 10% of subjects will have a single seizure on withdrawal. When subjects have ingested 900 mg to 2.2 gm per day for several months, seizures, orthostatic hypotension, and delirium occur with high frequency on withdrawal. All of the sedative-hypnotic drugs are capable of producing this abstinence syndrome (2,100). Meprobamate will induce dependence after

3.2 to 6.4 gm have been ingested for 40 days (2). Withdrawal symptoms have been seen after daily ingestion of 80 to 120 mg of oral diazepam for 42 days (101). Table 1 lists the average dosage and time interval required for dependence on the most commonly abused sedatives.

Research currently in progress by Dr. Donald Wesson in Berkeley, California, will evaluate the tissue dependence potential of long-acting benzodiazepines administered in standard daily therapeutic doses for periods of two to five years. The increased prosecution of unethical prescription practices has resulted in a number of clients entering drug programs to detoxify from chronic use of diazepam, lorazepam, oxazepam, and chlordiazepoxide. Clients who allegedly ingested only therapeutic and non-escalating doses of diazepam have been observed to experience withdrawal seizures at the Haight-Ashbury Drug Detoxification Project. The possibility of drug accumulation and resultant tissue dependence is the focus of Dr. Wesson's investigations.

During the mid 1970's there was a marked increase in methaqualone abuse in this country. Methaqualone (Sopor, Quaalude) was originally thought to be a non-addictive, non-barbiturate and mildly toxic hypnotic drug. This is reminiscent of the early history of many sedative-hypnotics (eg, meprobamate and glutethimide). Methaqualone is now known to cause full physical addiction and toxicity as seen in barbiturate abuse (102,103). It is estimated that 2 gm ingested daily for one month will produce withdrawal seizures (103).

Withdrawal from sedative-hypnotics is characterized by hyperexcitability of those physiological systems which have been depressed by the drug, and these effects may be present subclinically. It has been suggested that rebound tension and anxiety following only a few doses of short-acting sedatives may be a motivating factor for the continued use of these agents. A single large dose of alcohol in mice first raises the seizure threshold above normal and then lowers it to subnormal levels after the effect wears off (2). Since any given drug abuser will often use a variety of CNS depressants in varying use patterns, these patients must always be treated with full awareness of possible sedative-hypnotic dependence (see also Question 20).

19. Sedative-Hypnotic Dependence. An 18-year-old woman comes to a free medical clinic in a state of extreme anxiety. She has a 12-month history of intravenous "speed" (methamphetamine) use which has markedly decreased during the past three months when she began shooting "reds" (secobarbital) to treat the panic and paranoid reactions from the speed. Although they produced no "rush," they did provide some relief from her symptoms. After she developed several painful abcesses from missing the vein and heard stories of deaths from withdrawal, she began ingesting about 20 capsules per day. She has been taking these for the past two months. She would like help in kicking her "reds" habit. What sequelae might occur if she discontinues her drugs abruptly at this point? How is sedative-hypnotic addiction treated?

Abstinence Symptoms. Abstinence symptoms may be classified as minor and major. The minor symptoms, which appear within 24 hours and last three to fourteen days for a drug like secobarbital or pentobarbital, include insomnia, anxiety, tremors of the upper extremities, twitching movements, muscular weakness, anorexia, nausea, and postural hypotension. Postural hypotension may be of value in differentiating the abstinence syndrome from ordinary anxiety states.

Major symptoms appear on the second or third day and last three to fourteen days. Clonic-tonic seizures of the grand mal type may occur as isolated seizures or as status epilepticus. The psychoses that develop usually resemble the delirium tremens produced by alcohol withdrawal, with disorientation, agitation, delusions, and hallucinations. During the delirium, hyperthermia and agitation may lead to exhaustion and cardiovascular collapse. A number of deaths have been reported. With shorter acting barbiturates and meprobamate, symptoms reach their peak within two or three days. With long-acting barbiturates and benzodiazepines, symptoms take about a week to appear and are milder (2,100,104).

Treatment. Treatment is substitution therapy which is directed at preventing major symptoms and minimizing minor symptoms. The patient is stabilized on any sedative-hypnotic and tapered slowly. Wikler (100) recommends first stabilizing the patient on pentobarbital, 200 to 400 mg (orally if possible) every 4–6 hours. The doses are adjusted to prevent abstinence phenomena and to minimize barbiturate intoxication. After two or three days of such stabilization the dose is tapered slowly at a rate not exceeding 100 mg per day.

Smith and Wesson (101) recommend phenobarbital rather than shorter acting barbiturates for substitution withdrawal, because there is a wider safety margin between easily observable toxic signs and serious overdose. Also, phenobarbital has the advantage of greater urinary excretion, a factor which may be of value in a population likely to have extensive liver damage. Furthermore, it is less likely to produce euphoria than the shorter acting barbiturates. Phenobarbital 30 mg is substituted for each 100 mg of secobarbital or pentobarbital, 10 mg of diazepam, 25 mg of chlordiazepoxide, 400 mg of meprobamate, 75 mg of methaqualone, 250 mg of chloral hydrate, 200 mg of ethchlorvynol, 100 mg of methyprylon, or 125 mg of glutethimide (103). A two day stabilization period is used for the short-acting drugs, while more time is given for stabilization after switching from diazepam or chlordiazepoxide, since withdrawal symptoms from these drugs are delayed three to five days and seizures may appear as late as the eighth day. The daily dose of phenobarbital is given in four divided doses and the patient is monitored for slurred speech, nystagmus, or ataxia before each dose. The dose is omitted should any of these signs appear. Minor symptoms of withdrawal are treated with 200 mg of phenobarbital intramuscularly and the daily dose is increased. Once the patient is stabilized, the dose is tapered at a rate of 30 mg per day as long as withdrawal proceeds smoothly. Phenytoin is not incorporated into this withdrawal scheme since it will not prevent barbiturate-induced seizures in animals.

Gay and co-workers (26,30) have modified this phenobarbital substitution regimen for outpatient use, since much of the population at the Haight-Ashbury Clinic refuses to be hospitalized. This approach makes extensive use of volunteer outreach personnel who are part of the community. The volunteers have had extensive history of personal use with drugs but have proven themselves to be current non-users. These outreach personnel provide a day to day patient monitoring that would be otherwise impossible without hospitalization.

Substitution dosing of phenobarbital must be done on a symptomatic basis rather than relying on history alone, because drug abusers give notoriously inaccurate histories; some may exaggerate their histories, while others may withhold information. Also, illicitly manufactured "reds" and "yellows" vary greatly in both purity and strength. General guidelines for phenobarbital substitution are given in Table 1.

Polydrug Abuse

An increasing problem in the drug abuse field is the management of polydrug abuse. The simultaneous tissue dependence to sedative-hypnotic drugs and other depressant or stimulant drugs is an acute medical problem. The potentially lethal consequences of sedative-hypnotic drug withdrawal mandate careful medical management on an inpatient basis whenever possible. Pragmatic and economical considerations, however, unfortunately force treatment of polydrug addiction more and more to an outpatient setting.

20. *Heroin and Secobarbital.* **Dr. Smith is treating a heroin addict in his inpatient detoxification ward at County General Hospital. The addict claims he has a $75 per day heroin habit and states that he has been taking 15 "reds" (secobarbital 100 mg) a day for the last five months. How should Dr. Smith manage this patient?**

The problem of multiple drug abuse in heroin users is becoming fairly common. In an attempt to supplement their heroin or treat their withdrawal symptoms, heroin addicts may knowingly or unknowingly addict themselves to barbiturates, alcohol, or other sedative-hypnotics. Ultimately, simultaneous physical dependence to both types of depressant drugs may occur. Since withdrawal symptoms from heroin and barbiturates are clinically similar, the treatment of such cases is difficult and may be fraught with danger if both drugs are withdrawn at the same time.

On an inpatient ward, Gay and associates (30) first withdrew the patient from the barbiturate using the phenobarbital method (see Question 19 and Table 1) while preventing the development of opiate withdrawal symptoms by maintaining the patient on 30–40 mg/day of methadone. Upon completion of the barbiturate withdrawal, they then withdrew the methadone with a stepwise reduction of 5 mg per day (27).

Patients who refuse to go to hospitals for fear of police intervention are treated on a different basis. They are withdrawn off heroin first using the non-narcotic drug treatment approach (Ques-

Table 1.

SEDATIVE-HYPNOTIC DEPENDENCE

Generic Name	Common Trade Names	Common Street Names	Oral Sedating Dose	Physical Dependence Producing Dose and Time Needed To Produce Dependence	Time Before Onset of Physical Withdrawal	Peak Withdrawal Symptoms (Convulsions)	Phenobarbital Substitution Per Each Sedating Dose
A. BARBITURATES							
secobarbital	Seconal Seco-8	Reds, Red Devils, Seccies, F-40's Mexican Reds	100 mg	800–2200 mg × 35–37 days	6–12 hrs.	2–3 days	30 mg
pentobarbital	Nembutal	Yellows, Yellow Jackets, Yellow Bullets, Nebbies	100 mg	SAME	SAME	SAME	SAME
equal parts of seco- & pentobarbital	Tuinal	Rainbows, Tuies, Double Trouble	100 mg (Lilly F65)	SAME	SAME	SAME	SAME[1]
amobarbital	Amytal	Blue Heavens, Blue Dolls, Blues	65–100 mg	SAME	8–12 hrs.	2–5 days	SAME[2]
B. NON-BARBITURATE SEDATIVE-HYPNOTICS							
glutethimide	Doriden	Goof balls, Goofers	125 mg	1.5–3 gm × 30 days	6–12 hrs.	2–3 days	30 mg
methaqualone	Quaalude, Sopor, Parest, Optimil, Somnafac	Ludes, Sopes, Soapers	75 mg	2 gm × 30 days	6–12 hrs.	2–3 days	30 mg
ethchlorvynol	Placidyl	—	200 mg	1–1.5 gm × 30 days	6–12 hrs.	2–3 days	30 mg
chloral hydrate	Noctec, Somnos, Kessodrate	Jelly Beans, Miki's, Knockout Drops	250 mg	Exact dose unknown, 12 gm/day chronically has led to delirium upon sudden withdrawal	—	—	30 mg

methyprylon	Noludar		100 mg	30 gm × 30 days (Estimated)	6–12 hrs.	2–3 days	30 mg
meprobamate	Equanil, Miltown, Meprotabs	—	400 mg	1.6–3.2 gm × 270 days	8–12 hrs.	3–8 days	30 mg
diazepam	Valium	Vals	5–10 mg	80–120 mg × 42 days	12–24 hrs.	5–8 days	30 mg[3]
chlordiazepoxide	Librium, Libritabs	Libs	10–25 mg	300–600 mg × 60–80 days	12–24 hrs.	5–8 days	SAME[3]
flurazepam	Dalmane	—	15–30 mg	100–150 mg × 30 days (Estimated)	8–24 hrs.	3–8 days	SAME[3]
clorazepate	Tranxene	—	7.5–15 mg	150–180 mg × 30 days (Estimated)	12–24 hrs.	5–8 days	SAME[3]
oxazepam	Serax	—	15–30 mg	Unknown	Unknown	Unknown	SAME[3]

[1]Note for 3 grain Tuinal (Lilly F66)—60 mg of Phenobarbital would be equivalent to one (1) capsule.

[2]For 3 grain Amytal (Lilly F33)—60 mg of Phenobarbital would be equivalent to one (1) capsule.

[3]Though 30 mg will substitute for the benzodiazepines, this offers no pharmacological advantage over slow withdrawal of the addicting agent.

tion 17) (61). Meanwhile, barbiturate addiction is maintained with subintoxicating amounts of phenobarbital (30 mg for each oral hypnotic dose of the short-acting barbiturate allegedly ingested daily). After heroin withdrawal is complete, the phenobarbital is withdrawn in decrements of 30 mg/day (28).

STIMULANTS

Many drugs produce stimulation of the central nervous system. However, this section will be limited to the abuse of amphetamines and cocaine.

Amphetamines

21. *Paranoid Psychosis from Intravenous Amphetamines.* A 28-year-old, undernourished male is admitted with a diagnosis of paranoid psychosis secondary to drug abuse. He has been using methamphetamine intravenously for the past six months. He uses heroin, alcohol, and barbiturates occasionally. He was hospitalized because of a superficial knife wound received as the result of his acting upon a very complex paranoid delusional system which appears to have developed during the past few weeks and seems related to his "speed" use. Describe the typical pattern of intravenous methamphetamine use and the development of paranoid psychosis.

The user generally begins with a 10–20 mg dose of methamphetamine that is repeated at one to two hour intervals. Tolerance develops rapidly and the continuous use necessitates the injection of 100–200 mg to perpetuate the effects. The initial "flash" is likened to an intense sexual orgasm, and there is a sensation of extreme mental and physical power. During long "runs" the subject may become disorganized, paranoid, and experience unpleasant hallucinations. He may become "hung up" carrying out some nonsensical task for hours.

At later stages, abusers may be using as much as 1 gm of the dissolved crystals at one or two hour intervals. "Speed runs" may last for several days with little or no sleep. The development of tremors, pain in the muscle joints, and utter exhaustion necessitates termination of the injections. On discontinuance, the subject falls into a prolonged semicomatose state.

Paranoid psychosis may result after a single large dose of amphetamines but inevitably follows the chronic use of high doses. Visual hallucinations often originate in the peripheral visual field; these may be accompanied by auditory and tactile hallucinations. Initially, the user may be able to attribute his paranoia to amphetamines. He may even self-medicate his psychosis with heroin or barbiturates. (This patient's use of heroin, alcohol, and barbiturates may reflect such a pattern.) It is quite common for drug abusers to treat unpleasant drug effects with other drugs. Later, as amphetamine abuse becomes more intense, the abuser loses his "intellectual awareness" of his paranoia.

These paranoid thoughts, coupled with the physical hyperactivity brought about by the drug, may predispose the subject to violence. Ellinwood (106) has reviewed the role of amphetamine-induced paranoid psychosis in 13 homicide cases. Violence related to amphetamine abuse was well documented in the Haight-Ashbury district in San Francisco in 1968 and 1969.

These reactions can be produced by amphetamine, amphetamine-type drugs and cocaine (106–111).

22. How should this patient's psychotic condition be treated initially?

Treatment should begin with "talk down" therapy. Such counseling, along with benzodiazepines, has been effective in the vast majority of cases treated at the Haight-Ashbury Free Medical Clinic. Acute psychotic manifestations have also been treated with chlorpromazine (Thorazine). In cases of actual toxicity, phenothiazines raise the LD-50 and reverse many of the physical symptoms (112). If untreated, this psychosis would probably resolve over a period of several days to several weeks.

23. What sort of withdrawal course can be anticipated for this patient, and how may it be treated?

Within a week the most acute symptoms will be gone. There may be some residual confusion, memory loss and delusional ideas, but virtually all these effects will gradually resolve over a period of six to 12 months (110).

After withdrawal, abusers tend to become irritable and often experience depression. In spite of these symptoms it was long thought that there was no true withdrawal stage. However, Watson and co-workers (113) have demonstrated changes in brain chemistry and alterations in REM (rapid eye movement) sleep that correlate with the clinical depression seen on withdrawal. They found a significant decrease in urinary 3-methoxy-4-hydroxyphenylglycol (MHPG) which correlated with amphetamine withdrawal and the onset of depression. Interestingly, similar decreases in MHPG are seen in some nondrug-induced depression, and urinary MHPG is increased in mania. Although the most intense phase of the depression ends in four to five days, residual effects may last for months. Patients are better able to cope with their depression if they are told it is related to transient chemical and electrophysiological changes. Some patients respond to tricyclic antidepressants (113).

The approach to chronic amphetamine abuse detoxification used at the Haight Ashbury Free Medical Clinic is tri-phasic (114):

A. *Initial detoxification*—utilizing the traditional talk-down techniques along with sedative-hypnotic medication.

B. *Initial abstinence*—psychosocial counseling and rehabilitation, often with the employment of tricyclic antidepressants.

C. *Long-term aftercare*—prolonged follow-up with positive support therapy.

A similar approach may be used for chronic cocaine abuse.

Cocaine

24. *Acute Cocaine Toxicity.* During a rock music concert, medical help was sought for a performer who had been up all night "snorting" (administration by nasal inhalation) cocaine. The last dose had been snorted just prior to examination.

He exhibited the symptoms of chronic adrenergic overstimulation. He spoke in rapid staccato bursts and was initially quite suspicious and difficult to examine. He was pale, nervous, and his extremities were visibly shaking. His pupils were dilated (5 to 6 mm) but reactive to light. His mucous membranes were pale and dry. He was intermittently retching and had previously vomited some bile-stained mucoid material. His apical pulse was 140/minute but thready, weak, and difficult to palpate. No rhythm irregularities were noted. His hands were pale, cold, and dry.

His blood pressure, also hard to determine, was 220/160 mm Hg bilaterally. Respirations were 40/minute and somewhat shallow. Are these symptoms consistent with an intensive, prolonged binge of cocaine inhalation? What are the symptoms of cocaine toxicity?

Mild stimulation and euphoria are the usual response to cocaine inhalation. However, profound stimulation of the sympathetic nervous system, as illustrated by this individual, would be expected with larger doses.

Response to cocaine in the CNS is biphasic, beginning with stimulation in the cortex, moving downward to stimulate lower portions of the cerebrospinal axis, eventually causing cortical depression, and finally medullary depression and respiratory failure. The stimulant effects may actually be the result of depression of inhibitory neurons (115). In addition, cocaine causes peripheral sympathetic stimulation by preventing the reuptake of catecholamines (115,116). Thus, depending on the degree of toxicity, patients may present with a mixture of stimulation and depression (117,118). A rapid shallow breathing pattern may ensue, Cheyne-Stokes respirations may appear, and death may occur due to central respiratory collapse. Further, intense vasoconstriction combined with hypermetabolism may lead to hyperpyrexia. Hyperreflexia, CNS anoxia, and tonic-clonic convulsions may supervene. A CNS hemorrhage may occur.

25. How should this patient's acute cocaine toxicity be treated?

Treatment should be symptomatic with constant monitoring (127,128). This patient was first observed for 15 minutes while at rest, during which time his vital signs remained unchanged. He was given propranolol (Inderal) 1 mg intravenously. Within 60 seconds his pulse was 120/min, blood pressure was 220/120 mm Hg, and respirations were 32/min. He was given five more 1 mg doses of propranolol at one-minute intervals. Within ten minutes after the initial dose, his pulse rate was 88/min, blood pressure was 140/86 mm Hg, and respirations were 18/min. His peripheral tremors abated, and his color improved, although his extremities remained somewhat cold and dry. His pupils remained dilated (4 mm).

He was given prochlorperazine (Compazine) 10 mg IM, whereupon his retching was immediately relieved and his anxiety markedly decreased. All signs remained normal thereafter. After another 15 minutes, speaking rationally and at a normal rate, he said he felt he could "go on now." He was given a prescription for a week's supply of diazepam, and within another 15 minutes he was on stage and playing with his group.

Propranolol has been used in 1 mg intravenous increments at one-minute intervals up to a total of 8 mg (in most cases the total dose should be limited to 5 mg) with good results in a series of more than fifty cases of cocaine-induced sympathetic overstimulation (119,120). However, use should be limited to the early stimulation phase for the purpose of reversing cardiovascular effects, because use in later stages may increase the risk of seizures (121). Risks such as bronchospasm and A-V block must also be fully appreciated if a beta-blocker is to be used.

Other symptomatic treatments include: intravenous diazepam for convulsions seen in the advanced stimulation phase (care must be taken here since CNS anoxia may already exist); establishment of an airway and administration of oxygen with assisted respiration; positioning of the patient to insure cerebral blood return; and use of external cooling to treat hyperpyrexia. In all cases treatment should remain flexible and dynamic, corresponding with the symptomatic needs of the patient.

26. The patient described above was an experienced cocaine user. What factors might account for his successful dosing prior to the concert and his subsequent excess?

Although street cocaine is usually "cut" or "stepped on" with sugars, local anesthetics, talc or, occasionally, other drugs of abuse such as amphetamines, PCP, heroin, or caffeine (119,122–124), the initial dosing for this individual was probably well titrated. Street cocaine averages roughly 50–55% (123) with the average "line" running about 1/8 inch wide by 1 inch long, or approximately 25 mg of cocaine if pure or 14.5 mg if it is street cocaine (125); regular users become adept at estimating potency. However, as the night went on and some tolerance to the euphoric effects developed, he more than likely increased the amount of cocaine he was "snorting" at each dosing interval. A "line" of cocaine has been reported to contain as much as 200 mg of the drug, and at this level of use serious signs of toxicity could arise with repeated dosing (124).

A second factor which possibly contributed to the problem was accumulation from repeated doses at a dosing interval more frequent than the rate of elimination of the drug from the body. Vasoconstriction generally limits the rate of absorption after "snorting" onto the nasal mucosa. Cocaine blood levels were studied after 1.5 mg/kg was applied as a 10% solution to the nasal mucosa of surgical patients receiving the drug prior to nasal intubation (126). Plasma levels increased rapidly for 15 to 20 minutes, peaked at 15 to 60 minutes, and gradually declined over the next 3 to 5 hours. Cocaine was obtained from the nasal mucosa as long as three hours after the initial dose. The plasma half-life of cocaine in this combined elimination and absorption situation was 2.5 hours. In spite of limited absorption due to vasoconstriction, it is possible for the rate of absorption to surpass the rate of elimination (115), and this situation might be expected with repeated doses. Fortunately, excessive use is limited because cocaine is extremely expensive (roughly $100/gm). However, this case illustrates the popularity of cocaine among subjects wealthy enough to afford frequently repeated substantial doses. When possible, doses are repeated every forty minutes to maintain the most desired effect (which is probably related to increasing blood levels). Thus, doses may have accumulated to some extent and added to the stimulation experienced after being up all night. Moreover, sensitization to catecholamines by preventing their re-uptake (115,116), in the charged atmosphere of a rock concert and in a performer about to go on stage, no doubt resulted in the acute toxic effects described.

27. _Chronic Cocaine Toxicity from Continued "Free-Basing."_ A 30-year-old male executive seeks help for symptoms from chronic cocaine use. He has had a long history of recreational drug use which includes alcohol, marijuana, and cocaine. All were used at levels which did not interfere with his work or social interactions. A few months ago he was introduced to a phenomenon known as "freebasing" in which cocaine is smoked in combination with tobacco or marijuana. He described the effects of this form of cocaine intake as an incredible "orgasmic rush" which lasts for a few minutes and is then followed by the usual cocaine high for another 30–40

minutes. Over the past few months he had escalated his use of cocaine by this route to three to five cigarettes a night, usually shared with one or two friends. After a few weeks of this higher dose intake he began waking up with a feeling of depression and lethargy. To overcome this feeling he began snorting one or two lines of cocaine before work each morning and another couple during the afternoon to "keep him going." During the past week or so he has begun to experience tactile, auditory, and visual hallucinations and extreme paranoia. He wants to stop his use of cocaine, at least temporarily, but he feels he needs help. What is free-basing, and why did he develop a preference for this mode of cocaine administration?

Both hospital and illicit cocaine are the hydrochloride salt. This form, however, is easily converted to the free base, which has a lower combustion point and is hence suitable for smoking. Cocaine base has a combustion point of 98° C, as opposed to 197° C for the hydrochloride salt (127), and can be smoked when mixed with tobacco or marijuana.

When cocaine hydrochloride is dissolved in ether or acetone and combined with an aqueous solution of an alkaline substance such as sodium bicarbonate, the hydrochloride salt is cleaved off, leaving the cocaine base dissolved in the organic layer. The organic solvent is then evaporated and the remaining sludge is scraped off. Users mix about 300 mg of cocaine base with tobacco or marijuana and consume the mixture as a cigarette. This form of cocaine intake allows much higher doses of cocaine to be absorbed through the lungs than could be absorbed through the nasal mucosa (see the discussion of limited intranasal cocaine absorption due to vasoconstriction in Question 26). Thus, the smoking of cocaine base provides much more intense effects and has become increasingly popular in recent years.

28. Does cocaine cause physical dependence?

Despite early psychic rewards, true physical dependence is not seen with cocaine. The drug does, however, produce the highest degree of psychic dependence seen among recreational drugs (127,129). Although it is generally accepted that this dependence does not manifest a physical withdrawal syndrome, chronic abusers have been observed to enter into a depressive and apathetic state of consciousness sometimes accompanied by muscular cramps, headaches, and continued sleep disturbances (118,123).

29. What are the toxic signs associated with chronic, high-dose abuse of cocaine, and how did they manifest in this patient?

The toxic signs which appeared in this patient all involved the CNS and included lethargy, depression, paranoia, and hallucinations. The hallucinations seen with chronic abuse are generally described as pseudohallucinations, lacking the concomitant delusion that such events really existed. This differs from psychotic or true hallucinations which are accompanied by delusions or beliefs that the perceptions are real. Although not evident in this case, CNS toxicity can also include a true toxic psychosis similar in all clinical characteristics to that which results from chronic amphetamine abuse (130–134). The incidence of toxicity among high-dose users has been reported to be approximately 5% (123).

Although rare and not evident in this case, another manifestation of chronic cocaine abuse is perforation of the nasal septum from necrosis secondary to the vasoconstricting effects of cocaine. A more common manifestation is the drippy nose seen in chronic users. Attempts to treat this problem with long-acting nasal sprays often complicate the irritation to the nasal mucosa and lead to a severe rebound congestion which in turn encourages continued use of the nasal spray.

30. How should this patient be treated?

Treatment of this patient should be symptomatic and supportive, recognizing that like chronic amphetamine abuse three distinct phases are involved in the detoxification process (see Question 23). In general, the cocaine psychosis is of much shorter duration than that seen with amphetamines (137). If medication is needed, small doses of a benzodiazepine are sufficient for agitation and anxiety. They are also useful in affording the patient some sleep (118,124). Though somewhat controversial, tricyclic antidepressants in mild therapeutic doses given once a day at bedtime have been effective in cases of severe depression following chronic cocaine abuse. Tricyclic antidepressants should not, however, be administered during the initial detoxification phase since they may potentiate the anticholinergic crisis sometimes seen with chronic abuse (118,135).

PSYCHOTOGENS AND MARIJUANA

Drugs from widely varying pharmacological classes are capable of inducing the "psychedelic experience" (a mental state characterized by a profound sense of intensified sensory perception) if administered in adequate dosages in the proper setting. Thus, the inclusion of many differing drugs in this classification will be based upon the intended use of such drugs by the abuse population. Some of the drugs and natural products used to induce this "psychedelic experience" are listed in Table 2. Although PCP and marijuana have been included here because of the intent with which they are used, these drugs have distinct properties which make them different from the other drugs listed in this class. Thus, while LSD, mescaline, and psilocybin might be used interchangeably to produce similar effects, PCP is likely to be used for its distinct effects. Marijuana is probably the most ubiquitous of these drugs and is used both by itself and in combination with all of the other psychotogens.

The distinguishing feature of the psychotogens is their capacity to reliably induce states of altered perception, thought, and feelings that can be further described as hallucinations, illusions, perceptual distortions, or insight (2,136,137). These drugs can also be used to explore the unconscious mind and have been used in conjunction with religious, mystical, and healing rituals and experiments throughout history (138–140). Because of space limitations and the intended scope of this chapter, discussion will be limited to problems seen with the abuse of these drugs. It should, however, be kept in mind that this is only one aspect of their use.

In discussing the subjective effects of these agents, it must be remembered that there is tremendous variation both between different individuals and within the same individual on different occasions. The "set" (the individual's frame of mind and expectations) and the "setting" (outside environment including the physical surroundings and the other people present) have enormous influence on the nature of the "trip." Experienced users of psychedelics can often predetermine the nature of a trip through manipulation of these factors, although total control is virtually impossible. (A detailed discussion of the variables affecting response to these drugs can be found in Questions 31 & 32.) While this refers specifically to marijuana it is equally valid for the other psychotogens.

Marijuana

31. *Acute Anxiety Reaction from Marijuana.* The mother of a 13-year-old boy calls for information and advice regarding the following problem. She recently discovered that her son has been smoking marijuana. She initially suspected that there was something unusual going on when she began to smell a "strange odor, as if something had been burning," in his bedroom. She also began to smell it on him some evenings when he came home from school. About a week ago she found a plastic sandwich bag in his closet which contained a green leafy material that smelled "like dried hay, but different." A friend later identified this as home-grown marijuana. This evening she came home and found her son and some friends in his room. When she entered, she smelled an odor similar to the one she had noticed previously, but sweeter. The room was also full of smoke. On the floor she found a bag full of a tannish brown leafy substance tied, in small bundles about three inches long and ¼" to ½" wide, around little sticks. These were later identified as Tai Sticks, a potent form of marijuana. When she began to question her son he seemed to be confused and disoriented and became quite upset. He was crying so much and seemed so disoriented that she decided to phone for professional help. He is resting in his room now but she is still concerned and wants to know if she should bring him to the emergency room. The other boys seemed to be all right and had gone home. They did not seem to be as affected by the drug as her son. Why did the boy have an acute anxiety reaction on this occasion when it had not occurred before? Why were the other boys apparently all right?

The effects of identical doses of marijuana on human subjects are quite variable (142,143). It is not unusual for the same individual to react differently to the same dose on different occasions, nor is it uncommon for the same dose of marijuana to produce a "high" in one individual and little effect in another. Factors which affect the subjective experience obtained from marijuana

Table 2.

ABUSED PSYCHOTOGENS OF SYNTHETIC AND NATURAL ORIGIN

Common Name	Slang Names	Chemical Constituent or Composition
LSD	Acid, Big D, Sugar, Trips, Cubes, Brown Dot, Sunshine, and a multitude of names depending on the dealer	lysergic acid diethylamide
mescaline (active constituent in Peyote cactus buttons)	Mesc, Big Chief, Cactus, Peyote	3,4,5-trimethoxyphenethylamine
psilocybin (active constituent in Psilocybe mushrooms)	Silly Putty, The Mushrooms, Magic Mexican Mushroom	3 (2-dimethylamine) ethylindol-4-ol-dihydrogen phosphate
THC (one of the active cannabinoids in marijuana, hashish and kif from the Cannabis plant)	THC, Grass, Pot, Weed, Tea, Maryjane, Bhang, Boo, Bush, Dope, Hay, Joint, Dubie, J., Reefer, Roach, Panama Red, Acapulco Gold, Hash, Kif, Hash Oil, Red Oil	tetrahydrocannabinol
PCP (sernylan, sernyl)	Angel's Dust, Hog, Peace Pill, Elephant, Crystal, Crystal Joint, KJ's	phencyclidine or phenylcyclohexylpiperidine
STP, DOM	Serenity-Tranquility-Peace Pill	2,5-dimethoxy-4-methyl-phenethylamine
MDA	Love Drug	methylene dioxy amphetamine
DMA		3,4-dimethoxyphenyl-isopropylamine
TMA		trimethoxyamphetamine
MMDA		methoxymethylene + dioxyamphetamine
STP-LSD combination	Wedge Series: Orange, Purple, etc; Wedges: Harvey Wallbanger	a single-dose form combination of these two psychotogens
DMT	Businessman's Special	N,N-dimethyltryptamine
DET		diethyltryptamine
DOET		2,5-dimethoxy-4-ethylamphetamine
morning glory seeds (Rivea corymbosa)		ololiugui and lysergic acid amide
Hawaiian woodrose seeds		lysergic acid amide
nutmeg (Myristica fragrans)		myristicin
kat (Catha edulis)		cathine
ibogaine (Tabernantha iboga)		ibogine (an indole alkaloid)
belladonna		various Belladonna alkaloids

include: long-term characteristics of the user (his/her personal and physiological idiosyncracies); the immediate expectations and desires about what will happen during intoxication; past experiences with marijuana and other psychoactive drugs, as well as learned skills for modifying the drug experience; the immediate emotional state of the individual; the social and physical setting; the amount of marijuana used; and the chemical variations of the marijuana used (143).

In the above case, the boy who had the anxiety reaction was most likely a relatively naive user who had experimented with low potency, home-grown marijuana. The delta-9-THC (delta-9-tetrahydrocannabinol, the major active ingredient in marijuana) content of these leaves was probably about 0.5 to 1%, or 5-10 mg THC per "joint" (marijuana cigarette). The Tai Sticks which were smoked on the night of the reaction are made from the seedless flowering tops of the female plant, the most potent part of the plant; these have been found to contain as much as 5% delta-9-THC, or about 50 mg/joint (144). The actual potency of any sample is impossible to determine without analysis, since factors such as growing and processing conditions and genetic differences among plants can cause wide variations in potency (141). Also, since marijuana decomposes in the presence of light and heat, storage conditions can cause significant changes in potency (145). Finally, the efficiency of the delivery of a dose of marijuana by smoking can range from 20–80%, depending on how it is smoked. Most experienced users obtain approximately 50% of the available THC from a joint (42).

Despite these variables, it still can be seen that the boy in the above case more than likely received a dose of the drug which was much higher than that to which he had previously been exposed. This in itself could have caused a problem. The second factor which probably contributed to the reaction was the situation in which he found himself when his mother walked into the room. Any normal anxiety arising from this situation could well be compounded by the overwhelming effects of using a potent form of marijuana for the first time.

There are two potential reasons why the other boys did not react in the same manner. One is that the others were experienced users of high potency marijuana and were much more comfortable with the effects of the drug and better able to control their reactions. The second possibility is that as a result of the heavy use of high potency materials on a regular basis they had developed a tolerance to the effects of the drug (147–150) and thus did not experience the same intensity of effect as the naive user.

32. Is this a common reaction to marijuana? Is any treatment necessary?

Severe adverse reactions to marijuana are rare (151), but panic reactions and toxic psychosis can occur when the drug is used by persons with previously diagnosed or latent schizophrenia (152,153), by inexperienced users when using extremely high potency materials under stressful conditions, or when used in combination with other mind-altering drugs (154–156). Disorientation, depersonalization, paranoia, and confusion are the predominant features of this reaction. Most reports of such incidents have come from countries where large amounts of highly potent cannabis preparations are readily available, and this phenomenon has not been a major problem with the use of marijuana in the U.S. to date.

Less severe reactions involving anxiety, paranoia, and a general sense of dysphoria have also been reported and tend to occur more frequently in persons with chronic pain or depression, in naive users, or in older individuals who find the mind-altering effects of the drug disturbing (157,158). These reactions are generally an exaggeration of the common effects associated with a marijuana high: paresthesias, a floating sensation, depersonalization, weakness, relaxation, perceptual changes (visual, olfactory, auditory, and/or tactile), subjective slowing of time, flight of ideas, difficulty in thinking and loss of attention, loss of immediate memory, euphoria, silliness, and sleepiness (143,159,160). The anxiety which can occur is usually focused on fears of "going crazy" or "losing control." In effect, some individuals lose the perspective that they are undergoing a transient drug-induced distortion of consciousness and become acutely anxious. Any pre-existing paranoia will tend to be exaggerated. The onset of the dysphoric symptoms and their intensity seem very much related to the particular environment in which the individuals find themselves (161).

Treatment for both severe and mild anxiety reactions involves primarily non-drug interventions. It is important to place the individuals in a quiet, comfortable environment and allow them to describe their feelings. They should be provided with warm and reassuring but firm reenforcement of the transient nature of the drug effect. At all times, the individuals should be handled in a nonthreatening manner. Only in the case of extreme agitation, panic or disorientation seen with the use of very large doses by naive individuals is sedation necessary. The drug of choice would be a benzodiazepine at a dose equivalent to diazepam 5–10 mg in adults (158,162).

The boy in the above case is probably experiencing a mild anxiety reaction and would merely require reassurance and a quiet, comfortable environment in which to rest until the drug effects wear off.

33. *Duration of Effects.* How long will the effects of the drug last?

When smoked, marijuana has a rapid onset (one to ten minutes) and, generally, a duration (as measured by subjective high) of three to four hours (141,163–165). Although the kinetics of delta-9-THC and a few of the other cannabinoids have been studied (166–169), much discrepancy exists among the reported results. The difficulty in identifying delta-9-THC in body fluids and the fact that marijuana contains 419 individual compounds including 61 specific to cannabis (cannabinoids) make the clinical relevance of such data difficult to interpret (170,171).

34. *Effects on Motivation, Cognition, Perception, and Motor Performance.* A 16-year-old male admits to the regular use of marijuana and occasional use of alcohol. Over the past year his attitude toward school has become negative and his grades have deteriorated. He now wants to obtain a driver's license, and his father would like to use this opportunity to convince him to stop using marijuana. He calls for factual information to use in discussing the situation with his son. What are the effects of marijuana on motivation? What effect does marijuana have on mental abilities and motor performance? What are the effects of marijuana alone and marijuana in combination with alcohol on driving performance?

Motivation. Marijuana has been reported to cause an "amotivational syndrome" (172–174), defined as changes in personality and behavior consisting of apathy, reduced drive and ambition,

low frustration tolerance, and an unwillingness to carry out long-term goals (156). While this has been a fear long associated with the use of the drug, most studies have failed to substantiate this contention under research conditions (175–178). The psychological and motivational changes sometimes observed in marijuana users are probably best viewed as acute, transient effects evident only after particularly heavy use (179). Given the emotional lability of teenagers, it would be very difficult to entertain a cause-effect relationship in the above case.

Intellectual and Motor Performance. A much more relevant concern is the growing use of marijuana by teenagers during school hours. In many communities, it is not unusual to see kids "toke up" (smoke marijuana) before class. Acute intoxication with marijuana has been reported to cause impairment of performance on many psychomotor and cognitive tests (180–185). Even here, however, impairment of perception, cognition, and memory has been found to be related to several kinds of variables, including the dose of the drug, the level of motivation, the individual's tolerance to marijuana, and the complexity and familiarity of the task being performed. More familiar, less demanding tasks are less interfered with than are those involving new material and more difficult task requirements (186–188). A common denominator to impairment of functioning is the effect of marijuana in decreasing short-term memory (183,186,189–191). It does not, however, seem to interfere with the retrieval of information already stored in the memory (183). No permanent impairment of intellectual functioning or psychomotor performance has been found either after short-term moderate to heavy use (177,180) or after heavy long-term chronic use (175,192–194).

Driving Skills. Marijuana's effect on driving performance again seems to depend on the individual's experience with the drug (173,195,196), but definite impairment of driving skills has been observed (187,197–199). This reduction in performance is greater with marijuana and alcohol together than it is with either drug alone (200–202). Negative effects of marijuana have also been noted on simulated flying tests (203,204).

35. *Marijuana Effects on Sex and Reproduction.* A 25-year-old man presents with the following situation for your advice. He and

his wife have decided to have children, and she plans to stop using her diaphragm next month. They consider themselves to be heavy marijuana users, smoking an average of two joints per day of what he describes as sinsemilla (a high potency form of marijuana consisting of seedless flowers from the female plant and containing 3 to 5% delta-9-THC). What effects, if any, does marijuana have on reproduction and fetal development?

Effects on Male. While some researchers have reported decreased testosterone levels from marijuana use (205,206), others have been unable to substantiate this effect (207–209). There have also been several reports of abnormalities in sperm count, motility, and in the structural characteristics of sperm in heavy users of the drug (205,210–213). However, no cause and effect relationship has been established between the use of the drug and the appearance of any clinically significant sexual dysfunction, and all abnormalities in male physiology have been shown to be reversible following cessation of cannabinoid intake.

Further, major surveys of populations engaged in heavy marijuana use have indicated no evidence of sexual dysfunction in adult males who chronically use high doses of cannabis (175,192, 193,214). It would seem a significant number of clinical case reports of impotence or sterility would have been seen in populations of users if this were a clinically significant problem. On the other hand, marijuana should be considered a potential cause of sterility in a male patient who presents with this problem. To date there have been no reports of abnormal offspring attributed to marijuana use by the father (215).

Effects on Female. In women, the use of marijuana has been reported to cause an increased frequency of abnormal menstrual cycles in which they either failed to ovulate or showed possible evidence of a shortened period of potential fertility (166,215). This should be considered in women presenting with menstrual problems or in women having difficulty becoming pregnant.

Fetal and Neonatal Effects. By far the most serious concern in this situation is the potential teratogenicity of any drug intake during pregnancy. Delta-9-THC has been demonstrated to cross the placenta (211,216–218), and teratogenic effects have been reported in rats and mice receiving high doses of the substance (211,219–221). However, conclusive teratogenicity information

is limited to this animal family. No human birth defects have been associated with the use of marijuana alone (222), although still anomalies have been reported in several cases of patients who engaged in multiple drug abuse (223–225). It remains to be determined whether or not marijuana is a low level teratogen in humans, but *abstinence from unnecessary drug use during gestation is always the best policy.*

Other potential problems can exist with the use of marijuana by lactating mothers. Agalactia has been reported (211,215,226) in some cases, and cannabinoids can appear in mothers' milk, thus affecting the nursing infant.

36. *Withdrawal.* If this couple suddenly discontinues using marijuana, will there be any symptoms of drug withdrawal?

Although no withdrawal symptoms were reported after 28 days of moderate intake of marijuana containing 1 to 2% THC (227), others report a definite set of symptoms after cessation of two to 10 joints per day of marijuana containing 2% THC over periods ranging from 7 to 64 days (150,228–230). The symptoms consist of restlessness, insomnia, general irritability, anorexia, and nausea. Some subjects compared their symptoms to an influenza-like state. The specific intensity and constancy of withdrawal symptoms depend on the dose and frequency of marijuana use. Symptom intensity generally peaks 24 to 36 hours after the last dose and is markedly diminished within 96 hours; treatment is not necessary. Interestingly, in a study of Jamaicans who had smoked high potency marijuana for many years, no withdrawal was seen on discontinuation of drug use (175).

This couple might expect some signs of withdrawal during the first two to three days after cessation of drug use, but the symptoms should be mild and should cause no serious problems.

37. *Long-Term Effects.* What kinds of problems could be expected to develop in this couple if they continue to use marijuana at the same dosage over a period of years?

The three most carefully controlled studies of heavy, chronic users of cannabis were carried out in Jamaica (175), Greece (192) and in Costa Rica (193). All involved the use of much higher doses of cannabis than are currently seen in the U.S., and the subjects had used cannabis for from 17 to 25 years. Surprisingly, there were no differences between controls and users which could be attributed to marijuana. These included comparisons of blood pressure, EKG, chromosome breakage, EEG, signs of depression and neuroticism, liver function, respiratory function, hematology, motor co-ordination, memory, and general intellectual function. These results must, however, be viewed as preliminary since the number of subjects studied was small and the testing procedures may have been insensitive to some drug-induced decrements. In addition, there have been conflicting reports in shorter-term heavy users of symptoms of chronic bronchitis (231), chronic cough (232), and rhinopharyngitis ("hash throat") (154). It has also been found that marijuana smoke has a higher tar content and contains higher amounts of carcinogenic hydrocarbons such as benzopyrene than does cigarette smoke (233–236). It would, therefore, be surprising not to see some form of lung pathology in at least some of the long-term users of this substance. It has been suggested that the lack of lung pathology seen in the above mentioned chronic studies may be attributable to the fact that users in those countries do not inhale cannabis smoke as deeply and retain it in their lungs as long as do American users (237).

38. *Gynecomastia.* A 26-year-old man is admitted to the hospital for elective surgery involving the removal of excess breast tissue. He admits to the heavy use (three joints/day) of high potency marijuana. His physician would like to know if there could be any connection between the man's marijuana use and his gynecomastia.

While there have been reports of gynecomastia in heavy users of cannabis (238), studies comparing users with matched controls (205,239) indicate no causal relationship between the two. Until further evidence is gathered, however, the possibility of a link should be considered and cessation of cannabis use should be reviewed as an option in this case, especially if the gynecomastia reappears after surgery.

39. *Drug Interactions.* Are there any interactions between marijuana and drugs that may be used in conjunction with this patient's surgery?

The only clinically significant problem reported to date involving marijuana use and drugs used in surgery is the interaction of cannabis and atropine (240). A prolonged postoperative tachycardia was seen in marijuana smokers given atropine prior to anesthesia and this should be watched for in this patient. Other potential interactions involve reports that delta-9-THC has an additive effect on subjective responses and psychomotor performance when used with sedative hypnotics and that drugs metabolized by the hepatic microsomal enzyme system may have prolonged half-lives during delta-9-THC use. The clinical significance of these interactions is difficult to determine in this case.

40. Are there any other clinically significant drug interactions with marijuana?

The only other clinically significant drug interaction reported with marijuana is that seen in patients being treated with theophylline (241). Here chronic marijuana smokers were shown to have a higher rate of clearance of theophylline than nonsmokers. This effect is similar in magnitude to that found in cigarette smokers and should be taken into account when dealing with these patients.

41. Are there any other medical contraindications to the use of marijuana?

Other than the problem with the use of marijuana by schizophrenics mentioned in Question 32, the only documented contraindication to the use of marijuana is in patients with already impaired heart function (242,243). It was found that smoking marijuana decreased exercise performance until the occurrence of angina. In comparing the effects of one marijuana cigarette to those of one high nicotine cigarette, it was found that marijuana had a greater effect on decreasing exercise time until angina. The clinical significance of this problem is probably similar to that seen for susceptible individuals now smoking tobacco or drinking caffeine-containing beverages (244).

Although no studies have been performed measuring the effects of chronic marijuana smoking on persons with already existing lung pathology, this would seem to be an obvious contraindication.

Phencyclidine (PCP)

42. *Acute Phencyclidine Intoxication.* A 17-year-old female was admitted to the emer-

gency room in a comatose state. Her posture was in board-stiff extensor rigidity and her extremities showed tonic-clonic spasticity which was exacerbated by external stimuli (movement, noise). Her eyes were open and staring, nonblinking. She responded to deep pain stimuli. Blood pressure was 150/95 mm Hg, pulse was 115/min, respirations were 26/min, and oropharyngeal and bronchial secretions were markedly increased, resulting in a very moist and noisy airway.

A history obtained from friends who brought her to the ER indicated that the group had been smoking some "killer weed" (PCP/marijuana mixture) and all had become acutely intoxicated. The patient had smoked much more than the rest and had initially become very agitated and combative and later became comatose. At this point they called another friend who hadn't been smoking with them and he drove them to the hospital. What is PCP and is this response typical of acute PCP toxicity?

PCP, or phencyclidine (phenylcyclohexylpiperidine, an arylcycloalkylamine), is a potent sympathomimetic and hallucinogenic dissociative anesthetic agent. It was originally tested by Parke Davis as a non-narcotic, non-barbiturate anesthetic agent under the trade name of Sernyl. Subsequent reports of psychologically distressing emergence and postanesthetic dysphoric reactions caused the drug to be withdrawn in 1965. It was reintroduced in 1967 as Sernylan and marketed as a veterinary anesthetic until 1978 when all manufacture and sale of the drug was made illegal. Parke Davis presently markets the structurally similar anesthetic ketamine (Ketalar) which has caused adverse reactions similar to those of PCP in some patients. Ketamine has now also appeared in the streets and is being used with increased frequency as a recreational drug (245,246). The arylcyclohexylamines defy convenient classification; they appear to have mixed excitatory, sedative, cataleptoid-anesthetic, and hallucinatory properties (245,246).

PCP first appeared on the street in the Haight-Ashbury District of San Francisco during the summer of 1967. It was introduced as the "Peace Pill" and was primarily taken by the oral route. It rapidly received a bad name because of "bad trips" which occurred frequently with its use. The "bad trips" were similar to those seen with LSD but were characterized by greater physical toxicity and paranoid thinking (247,248). In recent years, however, it has reappeared as a primary drug of abuse for an increasing number of people and is primarily self-administered by smoking, usually sprinkled on marijuana, parsley, tobacco, or mint. It is also taken orally, intranasally and by intramuscular or intravenous injection. The latter routes account for the most serious toxicity. It is known under a variety of names (see Table 2).

This patient's signs and symptoms are typical of moderately severe PCP intoxication. The onset of the drug effect is rapid when smoked and profoundly incapacitating symptoms occur at relatively light levels of anesthesia (247,249,250). Because of its rapid and profound effects, intake of the drug by "snorting" (nasal inhalation) tends to be somewhat self-limiting. Oral ingestion results in more severe symptoms but is now rarely seen among sophisticated drug users, although this method may be employed in suicide attempts (249).

At lighter levels of intoxication than seen in this case patients are often "zombie-like" but combative and hostile. They can be disoriented and extremely agitated, with hallucinations, loss of motor control, nystagmus, drooling, vomiting, and diaphoresis.

43. How should this patient be treated?

One of the first things that should be done for this patient is to place her in a quiet room to reduce external stimuli as much as possible. If she were conscious, a quiet reassuring talk-down would be initiated. Ascorbic acid should be given at a dose of 0.5–1.5 gm over a 5–10 minute period approximately every six hours for the purpose of enhancing urinary excretion (250–252). Ammonium chloride (2.75 mEq/kg every 6 hours IV as a 1–2% solution) has also been used (250) but Rappolt et al (249) recommend avoiding this drug because of a concern that the ammonia breakdown products place a demanding burden on the oftentimes impaired hepatic function of the chronic drug user.

Propranolol in doses of 1 mg IV at 1–5 minute intervals (up to 10 mg) should be given to regulate hypertension and tachycardia (249). Propranolol has also been demonstrated to cross the blood brain barrier and to cause central calmative effect (253,254). Since sympathomimetic intoxication can be accompanied by acute urinary retention, urinary bladder catheterization and administration of furosemide 40 mg IV every 6 hours should be considered but weighed against the problems which may arise through stimulation of the patient (249).

Although hyperthermia was not mentioned as a problem in this case, it can occur and should be treated, with sponge bathing.

Diazepam may be administered to relieve muscle spasms. The dosage is 2.5 mg IV at 10 minute intervals up to a total of 25 mg. If this patient were conscious and cooperative, it could be administered orally in doses of 10–30 mg. Doses should be kept as low as possible to avoid respiratory depression (250). A more detailed discussion of the various stages of PCP intoxication and their treatment has been presented by Rappolt et al (249).

44. *Chronic PCP Use.* **When the friends of this patient were questioned, it was discovered that they were all chronic users of PCP. Given the severity of the effects of PCP overdosage why do some individuals become chronic users?**

Despite reports indicating that chronic users almost universally experience negative effects with the use of PCP, many seem to be willing to tolerate these effects in order to achieve the perceived positive effects of the drug. The positive effects which are sought are a heightened sensitivity to stimuli, dissociation, mood elevation, inebriation, relaxation or tranquilization, hallucinations, and euphoria (245,246). Most chronic users seem to be able to titrate their consumption to minimize the occurrence of "bad trips" (248). Among all individuals exposed to the drug, it is estimated that approximately 23% become chronic users (246).

45. What is the usual pattern of use among chronic users?

While this is far from clear, the average amount smoked per episode by the chronic user is estimated to be about 35–80 mg, usually delivered in one or two cigarettes. This amount is smoked two or three times per day with an average daily intake of approximately 220 mg (245,246). When snorted, the intake appears to be approximately 10 mg per administration with multiple administrations per episode (246). Tolerance has been

reported (245,246,248), and chronic users tend to require increasing doses of PCP to achieve a high. Doses as high as 100 mg have been seen (245). There is evidence that PCP may accumulate in the brain and fatty tissue of the body (246,247,252) and that chronic users can have overdose episodes even if an unusually high dose has not been taken (247). Frequency of use varies from weekly to daily (245,246).

46. What chronic effects could be expected in these regular users of PCP?

Chronic users almost always complain of being "spaced" and worry about turning into vegetables. They are noticeably depressed when not high. Impairment of motor and sensory functions makes many normal physical activities dangerous (246). Many users report a gradual change in their mood while using PCP. This is characterized by increased anger, irritability or violent behavior. Others report becoming more anti-social, depressed, lonely, and isolated from people. A large percentage indicate substantial memory loss while taking the drug but most report improvement within six to twelve weeks after cessation of PCP use. Many users complain of stuttering, inability to speak, and difficulty with articulation (246,248). A clearer view of the possibility of residual brain damage awaits more definitive studies.

Finally, although PCP has been reported not to cause physical dependence (245), it does have a high psychological addiction potential (245,248), and a small percentage of patients exhibit nervousness, upset stomach, shakes, and cold sweats upon cessation of PCP use (248). Furthermore, Smith et al (247) report a high incidence of prolonged depression after PCP use is stopped. PCP use is frequently resumed for the purpose of relieving the depression (247).

47. *Phencyclidine Psychosis.* **A 32-year-old male with no previous history of psychiatric illness or severe drug abuse problems presented with a three-week history of smoking some new marijuana which was described to him as "superweed." After a few days of smoking this new substance he had become paranoid, delusional, and uncharacteristically hostile. On the day of admission, he had become quite assaultive; he had beaten up his brother and attacked a stranger on the street with a knife. He was picked up by the**

police and brought to the emergency room. He presented with primary and secondary signs of a florid schizophrenic psychosis. Analysis of the "superweed" later revealed the presence of PCP. He was diagnosed as exhibiting "PCP psychosis." What is PCP psychosis, and how common is this problem?

Phencyclidine (PCP) psychosis is defined as a schizophreniform psychosis which occurs in some individuals after phencyclidine use and which persists for more than one day. The psychosis may last for days or weeks despite abstinence and it is characteristically more severe during the first few days of its course. The cardinal signs of schizophrenia are present, and unpredictable, aggressive or withdrawn behavior is evident. There is often autistic and delusional thinking, commonly including global paranoia, delusions of superhuman strength and invulnerability, as well as delusions of persecution and grandiosity. Behavior is extremely unpredictable and the patient may be cooperative one minute and violently assaultive the next (257). This syndrome seems to fall between the schizophrenic syndrome which lasts several hours in acute toxicity (247) and that seen as an exacerbation of previously existing disease in chronic schizophrenics who are exposed to PCP (246–248,257).

Like the individual in this case, these patients have no previous history of schizophrenia and most have been living lives which demonstrated a fairly high level of social integration. It appears that these individuals have a peculiar sensitivity to the psychic effects of the drug and will develop another psychosis upon re-exposure to the drug (257).

There are no reliable data as to the incidence of this phenomenon. However, in view of the increasing use of PCP, it is probably infrequent. It may be that PCP psychosis is the most dramatic of the drug's effects and therefore the one most likely to receive medical attention (245,248).

48. How should this patient with PCP psychosis be treated?

Treatment should consist of psychiatric hospitalization with isolation in a bare, locked seclusion room with frequent observation and psychologic support when appropriate. Stimuli should be reduced to a minimum. Some clinicians utilize non-phenothiazine tranquilizers such as haloperidol (247) while others use chlorpromazine in full

psychiatric dosages (257). A slow response to the most aggressive treatment is characteristic of the PCP psychosis and sets it apart from paranoid schizophrenia which responds more rapidly. Gradual changes should begin to occur after about five days of treatment, and by the tenth day of hospitalization rapid reintegration of premorbid personality and the development of insight into the events which led to hospitalization should occur. Even at this point, however, there is often some amnesia for the early events of the psychosis (257). Outpatient follow-up should continue as he is tapered off his neuroleptic medications (247,257).

LSD and Other Psychotogens.

49. *LSD Bad Trip with Flashbacks.* A 24-year-old female was seen at the Emergency Hospital in an acutely agitated state. Approximately four hours ago she ingested a pill described as a "pink wedge" with her boyfriend.

Approximately one hour after ingestion she began having illusions with objects changing shape and color. She interpreted this perceptual alteration to be very pleasurable and decided to take five other "pink wedges" to friends. While walking across the city park, she noticed moving shadows and became quite frightened, feeling that the police were after her. To avoid detection, she "dropped her stash" (ingested the five "pink wedges") and then ran back to her Haight Street apartment. She gradually became more agitated and confused as her perceptual alterations intensified, but her boyfriend was able to maintain some control by talking to her and insisting that it was "all in her head" and would pass as the drug effect wore off. This technique worked for a few hours, but the patient finally insisted on going to the emergency hospital for a "downer" as she thought she might "go crazy."

Upon registration at the Emergency Hospital, the attending physician ordered her boyfriend to leave. At this, she became more agitated and had to be restrained by a uniformed ambulance attendant. Chlorpromazine 100 mg IM was given, and when the patient became delirious, an ambulance was called and the patient was taken under restraint to General Hospital where she was admitted to the Psychiatric Ward. Her week-long hospital course was complicated by recurrent episodes of agitation and paranoia. In addition, she was found to have two fractured ribs, which were treated without complications by a consulting orthopedist.

After her discharge from General Hospital, the patient had periodic recurrences of her bad LSD experience. She sought help at the Haight-Ashbury Clinic Psychiatric Annex because she thought she was "brain-damaged." Neurological examination was negative, and the patient was seen on a weekly basis and treated with supportive psychotherapy with emphasis placed upon reassurance and abstinence from drugs. The "flashbacks" gradually faded in frequency and intensity over the next year. What is the proper management and recommended drug therapy of this "bad trip" experience?

The above case history is typical of an acute toxic reaction to a psychotogenic substance, also referred to as the "bad trip," "bum trip," "bummer," or "freak out." The term "toxic reaction" may be somewhat of a misnomer since many factors contribute to the reaction described above. These include the setting, mental status, and personality of the drug user. The "toxic" reaction is not, therefore, directly related to the dosage of the drug ingested but to a multitude of environmental and subjective factors. Furthermore, the "bad trip" cannot be reliably predicted or prevented in any given user as they have been experienced by users who have had previous "good trips." Thus, this acute anxiety reaction can be more accurately described as an adverse reaction to a psychotogenic drug rather than as a true toxic reaction (2).

A "bad trip" due to a psychotogenic drug is characterized by an acute anxiety reaction that may progress to a full scale toxic psychosis. A full description of this phenomenon has been presented by many authors (258–261). Smith (262) has further classified the "bad trip" into three distinctive types:

Body Trips. These involve distorted perceptions of the subject's physical appearance. A feeling of ugliness or dirtiness may be the precipitant factors in this type of experience.

Environmental Trips. These include distortions of the visual field surrounding the individual. Often, frightening illusions and hallucinations develop to the point that subjects lose touch of reality and believe themselves to be going insane.

Mind Trips. These involve subconscious material which surface forth into the consciousness of the individual. Identity crisis and guilt feelings cause the subject to enter into feelings of depression, failure, disgust, and suicidal states.

Under this system of classification, the experience of the above case can best be described as a bad environmental trip. The employment of many contraindicated methods of management in this particular case warrants discussion.

The initial management of the "bad trip" should consist of "talk down" therapy. The therapist attempts to convince the patient that his perceptual distortions and feelings of panic are temporary effects of the drug which should dissipate after it is metabolized. The subjective effects of LSD, which has a half life of 175 minutes, normally begin to clear 12 hours after ingestion (2). Unlike the case treated above, verbal contact should be made with the patient in a calm, reassuring, confident manner before any medication is given. This should be done in a more peaceful setting with less noise, fewer people, and less confusion than normally occur in the emergency room of a hospital. It is more important to be supportive and friendly than it is to be a clinician in the management of a "bad trip." Time should be spent asking gentle questions in an attempt to redirect the patient's thoughts towards pleasant experiences. Reassurance and reality defining is oftentimes all that is needed in the management of the "bad trip" (261,263,264).

Drug therapy of this initial anxiety reaction should only be considered after the patient is found to be refractory to the above procedures or if the patient insists that he needs something to bring him back to reality. Although chlorpromazine 50 mg IM initially, followed by 100 mg po has been the recommended therapy of choice in the past, exacerbation of the anxiety state, orthostatic hypotensive episodes, precipitation of post-psychotic depression, an increased incidence of the "flashback" phenomenon, and potentiation of the anticholinergic effects of psychotogenic drugs now limit the usefulness of phenothiazine in the initial management of the psychotogenic "bad trip" experience.

Furthermore, some clinical experience has

suggested that the therapeutic effectiveness of the phenothiazines in the management of the "bad trip" may be more dependent upon the sedative qualities of these drugs than upon their antipsychotic properties (263–267).

This conclusion suggests that the minor tranquilizers or the sedative-hypnotic drugs such as the benzodiazepines may be effectively used in the initial management of the "bad trip" (261,266,268,269).

50. Can the above case be treated for a psychotogenic drug reaction purely from the history that the patient had ingested a drug known as a "pink wedge"?

Trade names, dosage forms, dosages, purity and strength of illicit drugs vary greatly from time to time, community to community, and from dealer to dealer. Also, drugs with low marketing potential are frequently misrepresented for drugs with higher marketing potential. It has been found by chemical analysis that many samples of LSD and phencyclidine have been sold as THC or tetrahydrocannabinol (the active constituent of marijuana). It would be best to initiate therapy in the overdosed drug abuser by the symptomatology of the patient, matching these with the history of the suspected drug ingested. The "pink wedge" in this case history was analyzed to be a combination of the two psychotogenic drugs LSD and STS (2,5-dimethoxy-4-methylamphetamine, also known as DOM (264).

51. What is the incidence rate for the bad trip phenomenon and how often does it progress to the more prolonged and severe type of toxic psychosis?

As mentioned previously, "bum trips" do not seem to be totally dose-dependent in occurrence, intensity, or duration. Thus, the overall incidence rate for this experience is somewhat of a controversy. An extensive study reported psychotic reactions lasting longer than 48 hours at an incidence of 0.08% in normal subjects and 0.18% in subjects undergoing psychotherapy. The total study population consisted of 5,000 patients who had taken LSD or mescaline an aggregate of almost 25,000 times (270). This low incidence rate was subsequently challenged (260,271,272). In addition, the frequent adulteration of illicit drugs with a combination of other powerful psychotogens may be a significant factor in the precipitation of a

"bad trip," accounting for observed higher incidence rates (262).

These "bad trip" panic reactions are the most common acute adverse reaction to LSD and other psychotogenic drugs. These reactions are generally temporary and last for approximately 24 hours with LSD. However, they can also become more prolonged, lasting for more than 48 hours, and sometimes progressing even further into a long-lasting toxic psychosis (260).

Smart and Bateman (260) have estimated that approximately 50% of prolonged "bad trip" reactions resolve within 48 hours, while roughly 25% last from two to seven days, and the remaining 25% for longer periods of time, occasionally for more than one year.

These estimates are also a matter of much controversy, since some researchers believe that the prolonged psychotic reactions to psychotogenic drugs are not due to direct toxic effects but are secondary to the unmasking of pre-existing psychotic behavioral traits (273,274).

52. The patient in the above case experienced "flashbacks" which gradually faded out in a year. What is the flashback phenomenon?

The "flashback" or "free trip" is a poorly understood phenomenon described as a transient, spontaneous recurrence of certain aspects of the psychotogenic drug experience following an earlier intoxication after a period of relative normalcy (216). Flashbacks occur most frequently in the individual who has had a multitude of LSD experiences, has taken other psychoactive drugs (often major tranquilizers such as chlorpromazine), or is in the period of psychological stress (265,266,275). This phenomenon can occur sporadically or several times a day and can last from minutes to hours, or persist for as long as a year (276).

Theories attributing "flashbacks" to cumulative LSD toxicity in the CNS, persistence of a psychoactive LSD metabolite, a long-lasting retinal or optic pathway changes in the eye have been postulated. However, the more widely held view is that "flashbacks" are a mechanism learned while in the LSD state, whereby an individual reacts to stress in a novel way. It might be compared to "war neuroses" experienced by soldiers (258,266). "Flashbacks" are transient and gradually fade in frequency and intensity over time, provided the patient refrains from psychotogenic drugs.

Treatment should follow the same guidelines as the "talk down" therapy with major emphasis placed upon reassuring the patient that he is not "brain-damaged" or that he is not "going crazy." In view of the fact that various neuroleptic medications may precipitate or exacerbate the "flashback" phenomenon, medication should be conservative and offered only when the patient exhibits extreme anxiety. Shick and Smith (266) recommend the use of the minor tranquilizers or sedative-hypnotic drugs rather than major antipsychotic tranquilizers.

53. Teratogenicity. A 19-year-old female admits to the use of LSD sometime during her second trimester of pregnancy. Her obstetrician has heard that LSD is teratogenic, causing deformities of extremities to infants born to mothers who have ingested LSD. What is the role of LSD in teratogenicity?

In an extensive review of the literature, Greenblatt and Shader (258) conclude that, "at the present time the volume and quality of evidence is not adequate to either confirm or rule out the possible adverse cytogenetic effects of LSD." Like almost all drugs, the question of LSD and pregnancy unfortunately remains unresolved.

Numerous studies on pregnant laboratory animals have been reviewed. In all of these studies huge dosages of LSD were administered, results were inconsistent, and the teratogenicity of LSD seemed to be related more to the particular strain of animal and the time of administration than upon the dose of the drug (258). Two studies involving a total of 273 pregnancies in mothers who ingested LSD during their pregnancy demonstrated a low, yet significant, increased incidence of severe congenital anomalies and spontaneous abortions. However, both studies involved "high risk" populations for these anomalies and also involved mothers who probably ingested other illicit drugs as well. These studies did indicate that LSD had no effect on the incidence of fetal anomalies when it was taken by the male partner or by the female partner prior to conception (258,277).

Five case histories have reported deformities resulting from maternal ingestion of LSD during the first trimester of pregnancy. These were in mothers who ingested drugs other than LSD during this time (278–282). Conflicting with these case studies are reports by Sato and Pergament (283) documenting a normal healthy infant born to a mother who ingested LSD on the 43rd and

57th day of pregnancy—and by Warren and coworkers (284), involving a normal child whose mother ingested large doses of LSD numerous times during pregnancy.

Most authors do not recommend the use of LSD during pregnancy especially during the first trimester period, though they feel that the literature and research do not substantiate LSD as being teratogenic (258,285).

54. Other Psychotogens. What are other commonly abused psychotogens?

Mescaline (3,4,5-trimethoxyphenylethylamine) is the active component of the Peyote Cactus (*Laphophora williamsii*) which was ingested for religious practices by the Southwestern Plains Indians (288,289). The drug is generally taken orally as dried cactus buttons, tea, or gelatin capsules. Subjective effects are very similar to LSD and treatment of an acute anxiety reaction resulting from mescaline should be treated similarly. Oral doses of 5 mg/kg (generally 6–12 buttons) cause effects lasting for about 12 hours. Nausea, diaphoresis and static tremors are frequently seen with therapeutic doses (2). Available "street" or illicit mescaline is very rare although it is a highly preferred agent. Of 41 samples of "street" mescaline analyzed in the San Francisco area only two contained mescaline; the remaining samples contained LSD, PCP or no drug at all (290).

Psilocybin, the "magic Mexican mushroom" was first reported in the medical literature by Heim in 1957. In 1958 Heim, with Hoffman and co-workers, isolated o-phosphoryl-4-hydroxy-N-dimethyltryptamine from Mexican mushrooms. This compound, which they named psilocybin, has been isolated in *Psilocybe cubensis, P. mexicana, Stropharia cubensis,* and one species of the *Conocybe* genera. Other hallucinogenic fungi have been studied, some of which contain another psychotogenic compound, bufotenine (291,292). The subjective effects of psilocybin are similar to those of LSD and mescaline with a dose of 20 to 60 mg lasting from 5–6 hours (293).

MDA (3,4-methylenedioxyamphetamine) is a psychotogenic drug structurally similar to mescaline and STP which was first synthesized in the 1930's. Doses up to 150 mg are said to intensify feelings, facilitate insight, increase empathy, and heighten aesthetic enjoyment. However, it does not induce hallucinations, perceptual alterations, or cause depersonalization at this dosage (292,294).

Effects begin about 40 to 60 minutes after ingestion and generally persist for 6 to 10 hours. Marked physical exhaustion with free floating anxiety has been reported to last up to two days in some cases (295). Toxicity from MDA is somewhat more of an acute problem than it is for other psychotogens. One near fatal and two severe cases of adverse physical reactions consisting of dilated pupils, tachycardia, diaphoresis, rapid labored breathing, fever, generalized piloerection and muscular spasms have been reported in six persons who each ingested 500 mg of MDA (296).

STP derives its initials from serenity, tranquility and peace which is inappropriate to the expected pharmacologic properties of DOM or 2,5-dimethoxy-4-methyl amphetamine. Its effects are similar to LSD and include dilated pupils, increased systolic blood pressure, and a slight increase in body temperature. Five mg of STP will produce hallucinogenic effects for five to six hours. Ten mg of the drug may last for 16 to 24 hours. More prolonged reactions (up to 72 hours), a higher incidence of acute panic reactions, and an increase in the occurrence of flashback phenomena have been reported with STP; thus, the drug has low preference in the drug abuse population (262,297,298). However, the appearance of a newer 4-bromo STP derivative has been noted on the illicit drug market (299).

DMT (dimethyltryptamine) and DET (diethyltryptamine) are psychotogenic drugs with much shorter durations of action than those of other agents. Ineffective when taken orally, DMT must be smoked or inhaled into the lungs for psychotogenic effects. DMT has a 30 to 60 minute duration of action, and it also has a rapid onset; one minute when smoked and two to five minutes when snorted. The subjective effects of DMT approximate those of an LSD experience but are much shorter in duration. The popularity and availability of DMT as well as other tryptamine derivatives continues to remain below that of other psychotogenic drugs (292,300).

References

1. Efron DH et al: *Ethno-Pharmacologic Search for Psychoactive Drugs.* Public Health Service Publications No. 1645, U.S. Government Printing Office, Washington D.C., 1967.

2. Jaffe JH: Drug addiction and drug abuse. In *The Pharmacological Basis of Therapeutics,* ed 6, Edited by AG Gilman, LS Goodman and A Gilman, Macmillan, New York, 1980.

3. Lewin L: *Phantastica, Narcotic and Stimulating Drugs, Their Use and Abuse.* E.P. Dutton and Co., New York, 1964.

4. Gay GR et al: *A Free Clinic Approach to Drug Abuse.* Proceedings of 2nd National Free Clinic Council, U.S. Government Printing Office, 1973.

5. Wikler A et al: Effects of frontal lobotomy on the morphine abstinence syndrome in man: An experimental study. Arch Neurol Psych. 1952; 67:518.

6. Collier HOJ: Tolerance, physical dependence and receptors. A theory of the genesis of tolerance and physical dependence through drug changes in the number of receptors. Adv Drug Res. 1966; 3:171.

7. Goldstein A et al: Enzyme expansion theory of drug tolerance and physical dependence. Proc Assoc Resp Nerv Mental Dis. 1968; 46:265.

8. Jaffe JH et al: Pharmacological denervation supersensitivity in the central nervous system; A theory of physical dependence. Proc Assoc Resp Nerv and Mental Dis. 1968; 46:226.

9. Martin WR: A homeostatic and redundancy theory of tolerance to dependence on narcotic analgesic. Proc Assoc Resp Nerv Mental Dis. 1968; 46:206.

10. Seevers MH et al: Physiological aspects of tolerance and physical dependence. In *Physiological Pharmacology* Vol 1, The Nervous System, Part A: Central Nervous System Drugs, edited by WS Root and FG Hogman. Academic Press, Inc, New York 1963, p 565.

11. Way EL et al: Morphine tolerance, physical dependence, and synthesis of brain 5-hydroxytryptamine. Science. 1968; 162:1290.

12. Way EL et al: Simultaneous quantitative assessment of morphine tolerance and physical dependence. J Pharmacol Exp Ther. 1969; 167:1.

13. Goldstein A et al: A synthetic peptide with morphine-like pharmacologic action. Life Sciences. 1975; 17:1643.

14. Goldstein A et al: On the role of endogenous opioid peptides failure of naloxone to influence shock escape threshold in the rat. Life Sci. 1976; 18:599.

15. Hughes J et al: Identification of two related pentapeptides from the brain with potent opiate agonist activity. Nature. 1975; 258:577.

16. Pasternak GW et al: An endogenous morphine-like factor in mammalian brain. Life Sci. 1965; 16:1785.

17. Simantov R et al: A morphine-like factor 'Enkephalin' in rat brain: subcellular localization. Brain Research. 1976; 107:650.

18. Gay GR et al: Some pharmacological perspectives on the opiate narcotics with special consideration of heroin. J Psychedelic Drugs. 1971; 4:31.

19. Beaver WT: The pharmacologic basis for the choice of an analgetic. Pharmacology for Physicians. 1970; 4:1.

20. Sandoval RG et al: Narcotics and narcotic anatagonists in clinical practice. Drug Therapy. 1971; 41.

21. Jaffe JH and Martin WR in: *The Pharmacological Basis of Therapeutics,* Ed 5; Edited by L. Goodman and A. Gilman, Macmillian: New York, p 245, 1975.

22. AMA Committee on Alcoholism Addiction: Dependence on LSD and other hallucinogenic drugs. JAMA. 1967; 202:47.

23. Inaba DS et al: *Pharmacological and Toxicological Perspectives of Commonly Abused Drugs.* Medical Monograph Series, NIDA: Rockville, Md., 1978.

24. Inaba DS et al: Persian heroin in the San Francisco Bay Area: 1977-1980. Am J Drug and Alcohol Abuse. 1981; 8:123.

24a. U.S. Dept of Justice, Drug Enforcement Admin: Southwest Asian heroin: a historical and current assessment. DEA: Washington D.C., April 1980.

25. Ayers WA et al: The bogus drug: three methyl and alpha methyl fentanyl sold as "china white": J Psychoactive Drugs. 1981; 13:91.

26. Gay GR et al: Treating acute heroin toxicity. Hosp Physician. 1971; 7:50.

27. Wesson DR et al: Managing narcotic and sedative withdrawal. Hosp Physician. 1972; 8:52.

28. Wesson DR et al: Treatment techniques for narcotic withdrawal with special reference to mixed narcotic-sedative addiction. J Psychedelic Drugs. 1971; 4:118.

29. Eisenman AJ et al: Urinary 17-ketosteroid excretion during a cycle of addiction to morphine. J Pharmacol Exp Ther. 1958; 124:305.

30. Gay GR et al: A new method of outpatient treatment of barbiturate withdrawal. J Psychedelic Drugs. 1971; 3:81.

31. Isbell H et al: Clinical characteristics of addiction. Am J Med. 1953; 14:558.

32. Isbell H et al: Liability of addiction to 6-dimethylamino 4-4-diphenyl-3-heptanone (methadone, amidone or 10820) in man. Arch Intern Med. 1948; 82:262.

33. Wikler A et al: N-allyinormorphine effects in single doses and precipitation of abstinance syndromes during addiction to morphine, methadone or heroin in man (post-addicts). J Pharmacol Exp Ther. 1953; 109:8.

34. Anon: Surgical complications in the drug addict. Mod Med. 1971; 39:23.

35. Becker CE: Medical complications of heroin addiction. Calif Med. 1971; 115:42.

36. Bick RL et al: Malaria transmission among narcotic addicts. Calif Med. 1971; 115:56.

37. Dismukes W et al: Viral hepatitis associated with illicit parenteral use of drugs. JAMA. 1968; 206:1048.

38. Gay GR et al: Recognizing the battered flower child. Hosp Physician. 1972; 8:43.

39. Louria D et al: Major medical complications of heroin addiction. Ann Intern Med. 1967; 67:1.

40. Morrison W et al: The acute pulmonary edema of heroin intoxication. Radiol. 1970; 97:347.

41. Richter R et al: Transverse myelitis associated with heroin addiction. JAMA. 1968; 206:1255.

42. Sapira JD: The narcotic addict as a medical patient. Am J Med. 1968; 45:555.

43. Day HB: *The Opium Habit, With Suggestions As to Remedy.* Harper & Brothers, New York, 1868.

44. Gold MS et al: Opiate withdrawal using clonidine. JAMA. 1980; 243:343.

45. Washton AM et al: Clonidine for outpatient opiate intoxication. Lancet. 1980; 1:1078.

46. Dole VP et al: A medical treatment for diacetylmorphine addiction. JAMA. 1965; 193:646.

47. Dole VP et al: Narcotic blockade. Arch Int Med. 1966; 118:304.

48. Dole VP et al: Successful treatment of 750 criminal addicts. JAMA. 1968; 206:2708.

49. Dole VP et al: Methadone treatment of randomly selected criminal addicts. N Engl J Med. 1969; 280:1372.

50. Senay EC et al: Treatment methods for heroin addicts: A review. J Psychedelic Drugs. 1971; 3:47.

51. Aronow R et al: Childhood poisoning - an unfortunate consequence of methadone availability. JAMA. 1971; 219:321.

52. Carroll T: Diversion, urinalysis and program abuse: Introductory comments. *Fourth National Conference on Methadone Treatment. San Francisco, 1972.* National Assoc for Prevention of Addiction to Narcotics, New York, 1972, p 147.

53. Chambers C et al: An empirical assessment of the availability if illicit methadone. *Fourth National Conference on Methadone Treatment. San Francisco, 1972.* National Assoc for Prevention of Addiction to Narcotics, New York, 1972, p 149.

54. Dobbs WH et al: Problems of controlling methadone diversion in an outpatient clinic: The case of Mary Jane. *Fourth National Conference on Methadone Treatment, San Francisco, 1972.* National Assoc for Prevention of Addiction to Narcotics, New York, 1972, p 153.

55. Newmeyer JA et al: Methadone for kicking and for kicks. *Fourth National Conference on Methadone Treatment, San Francisco, 1972.* National Assoc for Prevention of Addiction to Narcotics, New York, 1972, p 461.

56. Ramer BS: Have we oversold methadone? *Fourth National Conference on Methadone Treatment. San Francisco, 1972.* National Assoc for Prevention of Addiction to Narcotics, New York, 1972, p 97.

57. Einstein S: Critical issues concerning methadone: Treatment, therapy, or what? *Fourth National Conference on Methadone Therapy, San Francisco, 1972.* National Assoc for Prevention of Addiction to Narcotics, New York, 1972, p 515.

58. Senay ED: Methadone: Some myths and hypotheses, in *It's So Good Don't Even Try It Once—Heroin in perspective,* edited by DE Smith and GR Gay, Prentice-Hall, Inc., Englewood Cliffs, NJ, 1972, p 180.

59. Sampson P: Methadone—yes or no? JAMA. 1972; 219:1275.

60. Food and Drug Administration: Personal inquiry. Nov 15, 1976.

61. Gay GR et al: Short-term heroin detoxification on an outpatient basis. Internat J Addictions. 1971; 6:241.

62. Goldstein A: The pharmacologic basis of methadone treatment. *Fourth National Conference on Methadone Treatment, San Francisco, 1972.* National Assoc for Prevention of Addiction to Narcotics, New York, 1972, p 153.

63. Jaffe JH et al: Methadone and L-methadryl acetate. Use in management of narcotics addicts. JAMA. 1971; 216:1303.

64. Jaffe JH et al: Methadryl acetate vs methadone. A double-blind study in heroin users. JAMA. 1972; 222:437.

65. Anon: Methadone in the management of heroin addiction. Medical Letter. 1972; 14:13.

66. Cushman P: Methadone maintenance therapy for heroin addiction—Some surgical considerations. Am J Surg. 1972; 123:267.

67. Blinick G et al: Menstrual function and pregnancy in narcotic addicts treated with methadone. Nature. 1968; 219:180.

68. Blinick G et al: Methadone and pregnancy. *Fourth National Conference on Methadone Therapy, San Francisco, 1972.* National Assoc for Prevention of Addiction to Narcotics, New York, 1972, p 129.

69. Blinick G et al: Pregnancy in narcotic addicts treated by medical withdrawal: The methadone detoxification program. Am J Obst Gyn. 1969; 105:997.

70. Stone ML et al: Narcotic addiction in pregnancy. Am J Obst Gyn. 1970; 109:716.

71. Horwitz CA et al: The effect of methadone on pregnancy tests. *Fourth National Conference on Methadone Treatment, San Francisco, 1972.* National Assoc for Prevention of Addiction to Narcotics, New York, 1972, p 111.

72. Blatman S et al: Obstetrical aspects through the delivery room. Presented at the Third National Conference on Methadone Treatment, November 1970.

73. Finnegan LP et al: Comprehensive care of the pregnant addict and its effect on maternal and infant outcome. Contemp Drug Prob. 1972; 1:795.

74. Wallach RC et al: Pregnancy and menstrual function in narcotics addicts treated with methadone. The methadone maintenance treatment program. Am J Obst Gyn. 1969; 105:1226.

75. Blinick G et al: Methadone maintenance, pregnancy and progeny. JAMA. 1973; 115:477.

76. Martin WR: Opioid antagonist. Pharmacol Rev. 1967; 19:463.

77. Smith DE & Gay GR, ed: *It's So Good Don't Even Try It Once—Heroin in perspective.* Prentice-Hall, Englewood Cliffs, NJ, 1972.

78. Anon: Answers to the most frequently asked question about naltrexone (EN-1639A). Connection (Institute for Social Concern - Oakland, CA) 1973; 1:1.

79. Blumberg H et al: Analgesic and narcotic antagonist properties of noroxymorphine derivatives. Toxicol Appl Pharm. 1967; 10:406.

80. Martin WR et al: Naltrexone, An Antagonist for the treatment of heroin dependence. Arch Gen Psych. 1973; 28:784.

81. Edwards G: The British approach to the treatment of heroin addiction. Lancet. 1969; 1:768.

82. Zellweger H et al: Is lysergic acid diethylamide a teratogen? Lancet. 1967; 2:1066.

83. Shure E: *Crimes Without Victims: Deviant Behavior and Public Policy.* Prentice-Hall, Englewood Cliffs, NJ, 1965.

84. Terry CE et al: *The Opium Problem.* Bureau of Social Hygiene Inc., New York, 1928.

85. Merry J: USA and British attitudes to heroin addiction and treatment centers. Brit J Addict. 1968; 63:247.

86. Kales A et al: Hypnotics and altered sleep patterns. II. All-night EEG studies of chloral hydrate, flurazepam, and methaqualone. Arch Gen Psychiatry. 1970; 23:219.

87. Inaba DS et al: The yen for N; the use of propoxyphene napsylate in the treatment of heroin addiction. West J Med. 1974; 121:106.

88. Inaba DS et al: I got a yen for that Darvon-N: A pilot study on the use of propoxyphene napsylate in the treatment of heroin addiction. Am J Drug and Alcohol Abuse. 1974; 1:67.

89. Tennant FS et al: Heroin detoxification - A comparison of propoxyphene and methadone. JAMA. 1975; 232:1019.

90. Tennant FS et al: Treatment of heroin addicts with propoxyphene napsylate. Presented before Committee on Drug Dependence—National Academy of Sciences, Chappel Hill, North Carolina, May 23, 1973.

91. Sheppard CW et al: Emergency treatment of acute depressant drug overdose. Missouri Med. 1972; 109.

92. Hasbrouch JD: The antagonism of morphine anesthesia by naloxone. Anesth Anal Curr Res. 1971; 50:954.

93. Jasinski DR et al: The human pharmacology and abuse potential of N-allylnoroxymorphine (Naloxone). J Pharmacol Exp Ther. 1967; 157:420.

94. Foldes FF et al: Studies on the specificity of narcotic antagonists. Anesth. 1965; 26:320.

95. Fuit RE et al: Antagonism of convulsive and lethal effects induced by propoxyphene. J Pharm Sci. 1966; 55:1085.

96. Jasinski DR et al: Antagonism of the subjective, behavioral, pupillary, and respiratory depressant effects of cyclazocine by naloxone. Clin Pharmacol Ther. 1968; 9:215.

97. Fink M et al: Naloxone in heroin dependence. Clin Pharmacol Ther. 1968; 9:568.

98. Baden M: Narcotic abuse: A medical examiner's view. NY State J Med. 1972; 72:834.

99. Siegal H et al: Continuing studies in the diagnosis and pathology of death from intravenous narcotism. J Forensic Sci. 1970; 15:179.

100. Wikler A: Diagnosis and treatment of drug dependence of the barbiturate type. Am J Psych. 1968; 125:758.

101. Smith DE et al: A new method for treatment of barbiturate dependence. JAMA. 1970; 213:294.

102. Inaba DS et al: Methaqualone abuse—"Luding out." JAMA. 1973; 224:1505.

103. Smith DE et al: *Diagnosis and Treatment of Adverse Reactions to Sedative-hypnotics.* US Government Printing Office. 1974.

104. Fraser HF et al: Death due to withdrawal of barbiturates. Ann Intern Med. 1953; 38:1319.

105. Berry RE: Estimating the economic costs of alcohol abuse. N Engl J Med. 1976; 295:620.

106. Ellinwood EH: Assault and homicide associated with amphetamine abuse. Am J Psych. 1971; 127:1170.

107. AMA Committee on Alcoholism and Addiction: Dependence on amphetamines and other stimulant drugs. JAMA. 1966; 197:1024.

108. Carey JT et al: A San Francisco bay area speed scene. J Health Social Behav. 1968; 9:164.

109. Ellinwood EH: Amphetamine psychosis: 1. Description of the individuals and process. J Psychedelic Drugs. 1969; 2:42.

110. Kramer JC: Introduction to amphetamine abuse. J Psychedelic Drugs. 1969; 2:8.

111. Post RM: Cocaine psychosis: a continuum model. Am J Psych. 1975; 132:225.

112. Epstein DE et al: Amphetamine poisoning. Effectiveness of chlorpromazine. N Engl J Med. 1968; 278:1361.

113. Watson R et al: Amphetamine withdrawal: Affective state, sleep patterns, and MHPG excretion. Am J Psych. 1972; 129:263.

114. Chambers CD: Some considerations for the treatment of non-narcotic drug abusers. In *Major Modalities in the Treatment of Drug Abuse*, edited by Brill and Lieberman, Little, Brown & Co., Boston, 1970.

115. Ritchie JM et al: Local anesthetics. In *The Pharmacological Basis of Therapeutics*, 6th ed, edited by AG Gilman, L Goodman, and A Gilman, Macmillan, New York, 1980, p 300.

116. Smith RB: Cocaine and catecholamine interaction. Arch Otolaryngol. 1973; 98:139.

117. Gay GR et al: Cocaine: history, epidemiology, human pharmacology, and treatment. A perspective on a new debut for an old girl. Clin Toxicol. 1975; 8:149.

118. Gay GR et al: Acute and chronic toxicology of cocaine abuse: Current sociological, treatment and rehabilitation. In *Cocaine: Chemical, Biological, Clinical, Social and Treatment Aspects*, edited by SJ Mule, CRC Press, Cleveland, 1976, p 245.

119. Gay GR et al: "An ho, ho, baby, take a whiff on me:" La dama blanca. Cocaine in current perspective. Anesth Analg. 1976; 55:582.

120. Rappolt GT et al: Propranolol in the treatment of cardiopressor effects or cocaine. N Engl J Med. 1976; 295:448.

121. Guinn C et al: Antagonism of intravenous cocaine, lethality in nonhuman primates. Clin Toxicol. 1980; 16:499.

122. Brown JK et al: Status of drug quality in the street—drug market—an update. Clin Toxicol. 1976; 9:145.

123. Siegel RK: Cocaine: recreational use and intoxication. In *NIDA Research Monograph Series 13: Cocaine*, edited by RC Petersen and RC Stillman, US Government Printing Office, Washington, D.C., 1977, p 119.

124. Wesson DR et al: Cocaine: Its use for central nervous system stimulation including recreational and medical use. In *NIDA Research Monograph Series 13: Cocaine*, edited by RC Petersen and RC Stillman, US Government Printing Office, Washington, D.C., 1977, p 138.

125. Gottlieb A: *The Pleasures of Cocaine*, Golden State Publishing Co., San Francisco, 1976, p 45.

126. Watson R et al: Amphetamine withdrawal: Affective state, sleep patterns, and MHPG excretion. Am J Psych. 1972; 129:263.

127. Archer S et al: The chemistry of cocaine and its derivatives. In *Cocaine: Chemical, Biological, Clinical, Social and Treatment Aspects*, edited by SJ Mule, CRC Press, Cleveland, Ohio, 1976, p 15.

128. Einstein S: *The Use and Misuse of Drugs*, Wadsworth, Belmonth, California, 1970.

129. Perry C: The star-spangled powder, or through history with coke spoon and nasal spray. Rolling Stone. 1972; 81.

130. Eddy N et al: Drug dependence: its significance and characteristics. Psychopharmacol Bull, 1966; 3:1.

131. Hekiman LJ et al: Characteristics of drug abuser admitted to a psychiatric hospital. JAMA. 1968; 205:125.

132. Kane FJ et al: Mania associated with the use of INH and cocaine. Am J Psychiatry. 1963; 119:1098.

133. Kramer JC et al: Amphetamine abuse: Pattern and effects of high doses taken intravenously. JAMA. 1967; 201:89.

134. Post RM: Cocaine psychosis: A continuum mode. Am J Psychiatry. 1975; 132:225.

135. Barash PG: Cocaine in clinical medicine. In *NIDA Research Monograph Series 13: Cocaine*, edited by RC Petersen and RC Stillman, US Government Printing Office, Washington, D.C., 1977, p 193.

136. Freedman DX: On the use and abuse of LSD. Arch Gen Psychiatry. 1968; 18:330.

137. Freedman DX: The psychopharmacology of hallucinogenic agents. Ann Rev Med. 1969; 20:409.

138. Lilly JC: *Center of the Cyclone*, Bantam, New York, 1972.

139. Grof S: *Realms of the Human Unconscious*, EP Dutton, New York, 1976.

140. Oakley R: *Drugs, Society, and Human Behavior*, Mosby, Saint Louis, 1978, p 344.

141. Abel EL: The pharmacology of cannabis sativa. In *The Scientific Study of Marijuana*, edited by EL Abel, Nelson-Hall, Chicago, 1976.

142. Legator MS et al: Failure to detect mutagenic effects of delta-9-THC in dominant lethal test, host mediated assay, blood-urine studies, and cytogenic evaluation with mice. In *The Pharmacology of Marijuana*, edited by MC Braude and S Szara, Raven Press, New York, 1976, p 699.

143. Tart CT: Marijuana intoxication: common experiences. Nature. 1970; 226:701.

144. Jones RT: Cannabis. In *Chemical and Biological Aspects of Drug Dependence*, edited by ST Mule and H Brill, CRC Press, Cleveland, 1972, p 66.

145. *The Extra Pharmacopoeia*, 27th ed, edited by NW Blacow, Martindale, London, 1977, p 296.

146. Manno JE et al: Comparative effects of smoking marijuana or placebo on human motor or mental performance. Clin Pharmacol Ther. 1970; 11:808.

147. Fink M et al: Quantitative EEG studies of marijuana, Delta-9-THC, and hashish in man. In *The Pharmacology of Marijuana*, edited by MC Braude and S Szara, Raven Press, New York, 1976, p 383.

148. Tashkin DP et al: Short-term effects of smoked marijuana on left ventricular function in man. Chest. 1977; 72:20.

149. Benowitz NL et al: Cardiovascular effects of prolonged delta-9-THC ingestion. Clin Pharmacol Ther. 1975; 18:287.

150. Jones RT et al: The 30 day trip—clinical studies of cannabis tolerance and dependence. In *The Pharmacology of Marijuana*, edited by MC Braude and S Szara, Raven Press, New York, 1976, p 627.

151. Abruzzi W: Drug-induced psychosis. Int J Addict. 1977; 121:183.

152. Feinberg I et al: Effects of high dosage delta-9-THC on sleep patterns in man. Clin Pharmacol Ther. 1975; 17:458.

153. Treffert DA: Marijuana use in schizophrenia, a clear hazard. Am J Psychiatry. 1978; 135:10.

154. Tennant FS et al: Psychiatric effects of hashish. Arch Gen Psychiatry. 1972; 27:133.

155. Talbott JA et al: Marijuana psychosis: acute toxic psychosis associated with the use of cannabis derivatives. In *The Scientific Study of Marijuana*, edited by EL Abel, Nelson-Hall, Chicago, 1976, p 177.

156. Abel EL: Adverse psychological effects. In *The Scientific Study of Marijuana*, edited by EL Abel, Nelson-Hall, Chicago, 1976, p 177.

157. Andrysiak T et al: Marijuana for the oncology patient. Am J Nurs. 1979; 79:1396.

158. Anderson PO et al: THC as an antiemetic; summary of prescribing information and review of the literature. California Research Advisory Panel, San Francisco, unpublished.

159. Hollister LE: Marijuana in man; three years later. Science. 1971; 172:21.

160. Halikas JA et al: Marijuana effects; a survey of regular users. JAMA. 1971; 217:692.

161. Tassinari CA et al: Neuropsychiatric syndrome of delta-9-THC and cannabis intoxication in naive subjects. In *The Pharmacology of Marijuana*, edited by MC Braude and S Szara, Raven Press, New York, 1976, p 357.

162. Rumack BH: Management of marijuana toxicity. *Poisindex*, Micromedex Inc., Englewood, Colorado, 1980.

163. Isbell H et al: Potency of marijuana. Psychopharmacologia. 1970; 11:184.

164. Weil AT et al: Clinical and psychological effects of marijuana in man. Science. 1968; 162:1234.

165. Wall ME: The chemistry and metabolism of the cannabinoids. In *National Institutes of Health: The Interagency Committee on New Therapies for Pain and Discomfort; Report to the White House*, May 1979.

166. Nahas GG: Current status of marijuana research. JAMA. 1979; 242:2775.

167. Agurell S: *Botany & Chemistry of Cannabis*, Churchill, London, 1970, p 175.

168. Wall ME et al: Metabolism of cannabinoids in man. In *The Pharmacology of Marijuana*, edited by MC Braude and S Szara, Raven Press, New York, 1976, p 93.

169. Lemberger L et al: Metabolism and disposition of delta-9-THC in man. Pharmacol Reviews. 1971; 23:371.

170. Turner CE: Chemistry and metabolism of marijuana. In *Marijuana Research Findings*, edited by RC Petersen, US Government Printing Office, Washington, DC, 1980, p 83.

171. Lee ML et al: Gas chromatography, mass spectrometric and nuclear magnetic resonance spectrometric studies on carcinogenic polynuclear aromatic hydrocarbons in tobacco and marijuana smoke condensate. Anal Chem. 1976; 48:405.

172. Kolansky H et al: Effects of marijuana on adolescents and young adults. JAMA. 1971; 216:486.

173. Mayor's Committee on Marijuana: *The Marijuana Problem in the City of New York*, Jacques Cattell Press, Lancaster, PA, 1944.

174. McGlothlin WH et al: The marijuana problem: an overview. Am J Psychiatry. 1968; 125:370.

175. Rubin V et al: *Ganja in Jamaica: the Effects of Marijuana*, Anchor/Doubleday, New York, 1976.

176. Mendelson JH et al: Operant acquisition of marijuana in man. J Pharmacol Exper Ther. 1976; 198:42.

177. Lessin PJ et al: Assessment of the chronic effects of marijuana on motivation and achievement. In *The Pharmacology of Marijuana*, edited by MC Braude and S Szara, Raven Press, New York, 1976, p 681.

178. Brill NQ et al: Marijuana use and psychosocial adaptation. Followup study of collegiate population. Arch Gen Psychiatry. 1974; 31:713.

179. Mendelson JH et al: The effects of marijuana use on human operant behavior: Individual data. In *The Pharmacology of Marijuana*, edited by MC Braude and S Szara, Raven Press, New York, 1976, p 97.

180. Vachon L et al: Marijuana effects on learning, attention and time estimation. Psychopharmacologia. 1974; 39:1.

181. Domino EF et al: Short-term neuropsychopharmacological effects of marijuana smoking in experienced male users. In *The Pharmacology of Marijuana*, edited by MC Braude and S Szara, Raven Press, New York, 1976, p 393.

182. Tinkleberg JR et al: A model of marijuana's cognitive effects. In *The Pharmacology of Marijuana*, edited by MC Braude and S Szara, Raven Press, New York, 1976, p 429.

183. Abel E: Marijuana and memory: acquisition and retrieval. Science. 1971; 173:1038.

184. Clark LD et al: Behavioral effects of marijuana: Experimental studies. Arch Gen Psychiatry. 1970; 23:193.

185. Tinkleberg J et al: Marijuana and alcohol: time production and memory function. Arch Gen Psychiatry. 1972; 27:812.

186. Abel EL et al: Marijuana and memory. Nature. 1970; 227:1151.

187. Dornbush RL et al: Marijuana, memory and perception. Am J Psychiatry. 1971; 128:194.

188. Petersen RC: *Marijuana and Health*, US Government Printing Office, Washington, DC, 1980, p 10.

189. Abel EL et al: Effects of marijuana on the solution of anagrams, memory & appetite. Nature. 1971; 23:260.

190. Miller L et al: Effects of marijuana on recall of narrative material and stroop colour-word performance. Nature. 1972; 237:172.

191. Abel E: Retrieval of information after use of marijuana. Nature. 1971; 231:58.

192. Stefanis P et al: Clinical and psychophysiological effects of cannabis in long term users. In *The Pharmacology of Marijuana*, edited by MC Braude and S Szara, Raven Press, New York, 1976, p 659.

193. Coggins WJ: The Costa Rica Cannabis Project: An interim report on the medical aspects. In *The Pharmacology of Marijuana*, edited by MC Braude and S Szara, Raven Press, New York, 1976, p 667.

194. Petersen RC: *Marijuana and Health*, US Government Printing Office, Washington, DC, 1980, p 20.

195. Weil AT et al: Clinical and psychological effects of marijuana in man. Science. 1968; 162:1234.

196. Clark LD et al: Behavioral effects of marijuana. Arch Gen Psychiatry. 1970; 23:193.

197. Crancer A et al: Comparison of the effects of marijuana and alcohol on simulated driving performance. Science. 1969; 164:851.

198. Moskowitz H: Marijuana and driving. Accident analysis and prevention. 1976; 8:21.

199. Klonoff H: Effects of marijuana on driving in a restricted area and on city streets. In *Marijuana: Effects on Human Behavior*, edited by LL Miller, Academic Press, New York, 1974, p 359.

200. Chesher GB et al: The interaction of ethanol and delta-9-THC in man. Effects on perceptual, cognitive and motor functions. Med J Aust. 1976; 2:159.

201. Chesher GB et al: Ethanol and delta-9-THC. Interactive effects on human perceptual, cognitive and motor functions. Med J Aust. 1977; 1:478.

202. Belgrave BE et al: The effect of delta-9-THC, alone and in combination with ethanol, on human performance. Psychopharmacology. 1979; 62:53.

203. Janowsky DS et al: Marijuana effects on simulated flying ability. Am J Psychiatry. 1976; 133:383.

204. Blaine JD et al: Marijuana smoking and simulated flying performance. In *The Pharmacology of Marijuana,* edited by MC Braude and S Szara, Raven Press, 1976, p 421.

205. Kolody RC et al: Depression of plasma testosterone levels after chronic intensive marijuana use. N Engl J Med. 1974; 290:872.

206. Kolodny RC et al: Depression of plasma testosterone with acute marijuana administration. In *The Pharmacology of Marijuana,* edited by MC Braude and S Szara, Raven Press, New York, 1976, p 217.

207. Mendelson JH et al: Effects of chronic marijuana use on integrated plasma testosterone and luteinizing hormone levels. J Pharmacol Exper Ther. 1978; 207:611.

208. Cushman P: Plasma testosterone levels in healthy male marijuana smokers. Amer J Drug Alc Abuse. 1975; 2:269.

209. Schaeffer DF et al: Normal plasma testosterone concentrations after smoking marijuana. N Engl J Med. 1975; 292:867.

210. Hembree WC et al: Marijuana effects upon the human testes. Clin Res. 1976; 24:272A.

211. Bloch E et al: Effects of cannabinoids on reproduction and development. Vitamin Horm. 1978; 36:203.

212. Hembree WC et al: Changes in human spermatozoa associated with high dose marijuana smoking. In *Marijuana: Biological Effects,* edited by GG Nahas and WDM Paton, Pergamon Press, New York, 1979, p 429.

213. Issidorides MR: Observations in chronic hashish users. In *Marijuana: Biological Effects,* edited by GG Nahas and WDM Paton, Pergamon Press, New York, 1979, p 377.

214. Coggins WJ et al: Health status of chronic heavy cannabis users. Ann NY Acad Sci. 1976; 282:148.

215. Petersen RC: *Marijuana and Health,* US Government Printing Office, Washington, D.C., 1980, p 15.

216. Vardaris RM et al: Chronic administration of delta-9-THC to pregnant rats. Pharmacol Biochem Behav. 1976; 4:249.

217. Harbison RD et al: Prenatal toxicity, maternal distribution and placental transfer of THC. J Pharmacol Exper Ther. 1972; 180:446.

218. Idanpaan-Heikkila J et al: Placental transfer of tritiated delta-9-THC. N Engl J Med. 1969; 281:330.

219. Borgen LA et al: Effects of synthetic delta-9-THC on pregnancy and offspring in the rat. Toxicol Appl Pharmacol. 1971; 20:480.

220. Harbison RD et al: Prenatal toxicity, maternal distribution and placental transfer of THC. J Pharmacol Exper Ther. 1972; 180:446.

221. Mantilla-Plata B et al: Teratogenic and mutagenic studies of delta-9-THC in mice. Fed Proc. 1973; 32:746.

222. Vachon L: The smoke marijuana smoking. N Engl J Med. 1976; 294:160.

223. Hecht F et al: LSD and cannabis as possible teratogens in man. Lancet. 1968; 2:1087.

224. Carakushansky G et al: LSD and cannabis as possible teratogens in man. Lancet. 1969; 1:150.

225. Bogdanoff B et al: Brain and eye abnormalities, possible sequelae to prenatal use of multiple drugs including LSD. Am J Dis Child. 1972; 123:145.

226. Pace HB et al: Teratogenesis and marijuana. Ann NY Acad Sci. 1971; 191:123.

227. Frank IM et al: Acute and cumulative effects of marijuana smoking in hospitalized subjects: A 36-day study. In *The Pharmacology of Marijuana,* edited by MC Braude and S Szara, Raven Press, New York, 1976, p 673.

228. Jones RT: THC and the marijuana-induced social "high," or the effects of the mind on marijuana. Ann NY Acad Sci. 1971; 191:155.

229. Nowlan MA et al: Tolerance to marijuana: Heart rate and subjective high. Clin Pharmacol Ther. 1977; 22:550.

230. Williams E et al: Studies in marijuana and parahexyl compound. Pub Health Rep. 1946; 61:1059.

231. Chopra IC et al: The use of cannabis drugs in India. Bull Narc. 1957; 9:4.

232. Abramson HA et al: Respiratory disorders and marijuana use. J Asthma Res. 1974; 11:97.

233. Novotny M et al: A possible chemical basis for the higher mutagenicity of marijuana smoke as compared with tobacco smoke. Experientia. 1976; 32:280.

234. Fehr KO et al: Analysis of cannabis smoke obtained under different combustion conditions. Can J Physiol Pharmacol. 1971; 50:761.

235. Fehr KO et al: Cannabis: Adverse effects on health. The Journal. 1980:11.

236. Tashkin DP et al: Respiratory status of 75 chronic marijuana smokers: Comparison with matched controls. Am Rev Respir Dis. 1978; 117:261.

237. Petersen RC: *Marijuana and Health,* US Government Printing Office, Washington, DC, p 14.

238. Harmon J et al: Gynecomastia in marijuana users: N Engl J Med. 1972; 287:936.

239. Cates W et al: Gynecomastia and cannabis smoking. A nonassociation among US army soldiers. Am J Surg. 1977; 134:613.

240. Gregg JM et al: Cardiovascular effects of cannabinol during oral surgery. Anesthesia Analg. 1976; 55:203.

241. Jusko WJ et al: Enhanced biotransformation of theophylline in marijuana and tobacco smokers. Clin Pharmacol Ther. 1978; 24:406.

242. Prakash R et al: Effects of marijuana in coronary disease. Clin Pharmacol Ther. 1976; 19:94.

243. Aronow WS et al: Effect of smoking marijuana and of smoking a high nicotine cigarette on angina pectoris. Clin Pharmacol Ther. 1975; 17:549.

244. Johnson S et al: Some cardiovascular effects of marijuana smoking in normal volunteers. Clin Pharmacol Ther. 1971; 12:762.

245. Siegel RK: Phencyclidine and ketamine intoxication: a study of four populations of recreational users. In *Phencyclidine (PCP) Abuse: An Appraisal,* edited by RC Petersen and RC Stillman, US Government Printing Office, Washington, DC, 1978, p 119.

246. Lerner SE et al: Phencyclidine use among youth: History, epidemiology, and acute and chronic intoxication. In *Phencyclidine (PCP) Abuse: An Appraisal,* edited by RC Petersen and RC Stillman, US Government Printing Office, Washington, DC, 1978, p 66.

247. Smith DE et al: The diagnosis and treatment of the PCP abuse syndrome. In *Phencyclidine (PCP) Abuse: An Appraisal,* edited by RC Petersen and RC Stillman, US Government Printing Office, Washington, DC, 1978, p 229.

248. Fauman MA et al: The psychiatric aspects of chronic phencyclidine use: a study of chronic PCP users. In *Phencyclidine (PCP) Abuse: An Appraisal,* edited by RC Petersen and RC Stillman, US Government Printing Office, Washington, DC, 1978, p 183.

249. Rappolt RT et al: Phencyclidine (PCP) intoxication: Diagnosis in stages and algorithms of treatment. Clin Toxicol. 1980; 16:509.

250. Done AK: A phencyclidine pinup. Emergency Medicine. 1978, p 179.

251. Done AK et al: The pharmacokinetics of phencyclidine in overdosage and its treatment. In *Phencyclidine (PCP) Abuse: An Appraisal,* edited by RC Petersen and RC Stillman, US Government Printing Office, Washington, DC, 1978, p 210.

252. Aronow R et al: Clinical observations during phencyclidine intoxication and treatment based on ion trapping. In *Phencyclidine (PCP) Abuse: An Appraisal,* edited by RC Petersen and RC Stillman, US Government Printing Office, Washington, DC, 1978, p 218.

253. Rappolt RT et al: A treatment plan for acute and chronic adrenergic poisoning crisis utilizing the sympatholytic effects of the beta-1 and beta-2 receptor site blocker propranolol. Clin Toxicol. 1980; 18:725.

254. Estep DL et al: Preliminary report of the effects of propranolol HC on the discomfort caused by niacin. Clin Toxicol. 1977; 11:325.

255. Luisada PV et al: Clinical management of phencyclidine. Clin Toxicol. 1976; 9:539.

256. Showalter CV et al: Clinical pharmacology of phencyclidine toxicity. Am J Psychiatry. 1977; 134:1234.

257. Luisada PV: The phencyclidine (PCP) psychosis: Phenomenology and treatment. In *Phencyclidine (PCP) Abuse: An Appraisal,* edited by RC Braude and RC Stillman, US Government Printing Office, Washington, DC, 1978, p 241.

258. Greenblatt DJ et al: Adverse effects of LSD: A current perspective. Conn Med. 1970; 34:895.

259. Langs RJ et al: Lysergic acid diethylamide (LSD-25) and schizophrenic reactions. J Nerv Ment Disorders. 1968; 147:163.

260. Smart R et al: Unfavorable reactions to LSD: A review and analysis of available case reports. Canad Med Assoc J. 1967; 97:1214.

261. Taylor RL et al: Management of "bad trips" in an evolving drug scene. JAMA. 1970; 213:422.

262. Smith DE: Editor's note. J Psychedelic Drugs. 1970; 3:5.

263. Garson OM et al: Studies in a patient with acute leukemia after lysergide treatment. Brit Med J. 1969; 2:800.

264. Martin CM: Caring for the "bad trip"- A review of current status of LSD. Hawaii Med J. 1970; 29:555.

265. Schwarz CJ: Phenothiazine-induced psychosis after LSD. Canad Med Assoc. 1971; 105:241.

266. Schick J et al: Analysis of the LSD flashback. J Psychedelic Drugs. 1970; 3:13.

267. Tec L: Phenothiazine and biperiden in LSD reactions. JAMA. 1971; 215:980.

268. Barnett BE: Diazepam treatment for LSD intoxication. Lancet. 1971; 2:270.

269. Levy RM: Diazepam for LSD intoxication. Lancet. 1971; 1:1297.

270. Cohen S: A classification of LSD complications. Psychosom. 1966; 7:182.

271. McGlothlin WH et al: LSD revisited. 10 year follow-up of medical LSD users. Arch Gen Psych. 1971; 24:35.

272. Ungerleider JT et al: The dangers of LSD. An analysis of seven month's experience in a university hospital's psychiatric service. JAMA. 1966; 197:389.

273. Hoffer A: LSD: A review of its present status. Clin Pharmacol Ther. 1964; 6:183.

274. Ungerleider JT et al: The "bad trip"- The etiology of the adverse LSD reaction. Am J Psych. 1968; 124:1483.

275. Schwarz CJ: Paradoxical responses to chlorpromazine after LSD. Psychosom. 1967; 8:210.

276. Louria D: Lysergic acid diethylamide. N Engl J Med. 1968; 278:435.

277. McGlothlin WH et al: Effect of LSD on human pregnancy. JAMA. 1970; 212:1483.

278. Assemany SR et al: Deformities in a child whose mother took LSD. Lancet. 1970; 1:1290.

279. Carakushanski G et al: Lysergide and cannabis as possible teratogens in man. Lancet. 1969; 1:150.

280. Eller JL et al: Bizarre deformities in offspring of user of lysergic acid diethylamide. N Engl J Med. 1970; 283:395.

281. Hecht F et al: Lysergic acid diethylamide and cannabis as possible teratogens in man. Lancet. 1968; 2:1087.

282. Zellweger H et al: Is lysergic acid diethylamide a teratogen? Lancet. 1967; 2:1066.

283. Sato H et al: Lysergide a teratogen? Lancet. 1968; 1:639.

284. Warren RJ et al: LSD exposure in utero. Pediat. 1970; 45:466.

285. Tjio JH et al: LSD and chromosomes: A controlled experiment. JAMA. 1969; 210:849.

286. Grossbard L et al: Acute leukemia with "Ph"-like chromosomes in a LSD user. JAMA. 1968; 205:791.

287. AMA Committee on Alcoholism Addiction: Dependence on LSD and other hallucinogenic drugs. JAMA. 1967; 202:47.

288. Der Marderosin A: Current status of hallucinogens. Am J Pharm. 1966; 138:204.

289. Frykman JH: *A New Connection,* Scrimshaw Press, San Francisco, 1971.

290. Anon: Pharmacy Chemistry Newsletter, published by Pharmacy Chemistry Laboratories, Palo Alto. 1973; 2:2.

291. Buck RW: Mushroom toxins: A brief review of the literature. N Engl J Med. 1961; 265:681.

292. Shulgin AT: Psychotomimetic agents related to the catecholamines. J Psychedelic Drugs. 1969; 2:17.

293. Lingeman R: *Drugs From A to Z: A Dictionary.* McGraw-Hill, New York, 1969.

294. Narango C et al: Evaluations of 3,4-methylenedioxyamphetamine (MDA) as a adjunct to psychotherapy. Med Pharmacol Exper. 1967; 7:359.

295. Jackson B et al: Another abusable amphetamine. JAMA. 1970; 211:830 (letter).

296. Becker CE: Medical complications of heroin addiction. Calif Med. 1971; 115:42.

297. Smith DE: Psychotomimetic amphetamines with spe-
     cial reference to STP (DOM) toxicity. J Psychedelic
     Drugs. 1969; 2:73.
298. Snyder SH et al: DOM (STP), a new hallucinogenic drug,
     and DOET: Effects in normal subjects. Am J Psych. 1968;
     125:357.
299. Shulgin AT et al: 4-bromo-2,5-dimethoxypheylisopro-
     pylamine. Analog Pharmacol. 1971; 5:103.
300. Szara S: Hallucinogenic effects and metabolism of tryp-
     tamine derivatives in man. Fed Proc. 1961; 20:885.

Chapter 47

Alcohol Abuse

Lana Gee Witt and Lawrence D. Witt

Alcohol abuse is a major health problem in the United States today. Excessive consumption of alcohol, whether in the form of beer, wine, or distilled spirits, is responsible for numerous medical complications. Every clinician, whether working in an institutional or community setting, will encounter alcoholic patients. With an understanding of the illness, its many medical complications, and their treatment, a clinician can actively participate in the prevention, detection, and management of alcoholism. He or she will be able to educate family members and the public about this disease and will be able to recognize and implement solutions for potential drug-related problems common in alcoholic patients. Such problems include non-compliance to prescribed medications, ethanol-drug interactions, and altered drug pharmacodynamics and pharmacokinetics.

The terms *alcohol abuse, alcoholism,* and *problem drinking* need to be defined. *Alcohol abuse* is a general term which encompasses the otl. ar two terms. It means misuse of alcohol which is manifested in one or more alcohol-related problems. *Alcoholism* is addiction to alcohol (the alcohol dependence syndrome). Characteristics of an alcoholic patient include psychologic dependency, development of an abstinence or withdrawal syndrome upon discontinuation of alcohol, and tolerance to the pharmacologic effects of alcohol. A *problem drinker* is one who drinks to the extent that a problem or disability occurs. These problems may be psychological, medical (acute or chronic illnesses), or social in nature. In the current literature these three terms are often used interchangeably. Patients are given the diagnosis of alcoholism whether they are being treated for alcohol withdrawal or for alcohol-related complications such as anemia, liver disease, or cardiac arrhythmias.

Alcohol is the most widely misused drug today. National statistics are available from the Department of Health and Human Services (1). The highest prevalence of alcoholism is in the 35 to 55 age range, and approximately one-tenth of American adults are problem drinkers or alcoholics. Trends indicate an alarming increase in alcohol abuse among women and youth. Several large scale studies of American high school students indicate an increase in drinking, drunkenness, alcohol-related accidents, and alcohol-related social and dependency problems (2). Only recently recognized is the significant incidence (2–10%) of alcoholism in the elderly population (60 years and older) (3).

The economic costs of alcohol-related medical problems are enormous. In 1975, $13 billion was spent on health and medical costs. A more recent estimate is that one of every five dollars spent on hospital care is for alcohol-related complications. A substantial number of deaths each year are alcohol-related. These include accidents, homicides, suicides, and various life-threatening complications. Liver cirrhosis, of which 95% of cases are alcohol-induced, was the sixth leading cause of mortality in 1975. Stated briefly, alcoholism is extremely prevalent, is a steadily rising problem, and is responsible for numerous medical complications.

Diagnosis. Alcoholism is a complex behavior disorder and a specific disease entity recognized by the medical profession (4,5). How is alcoholism diagnosed? Commonly accepted standards include the diagnostic criteria of the American Psychiatric Association (5) and the National Council on Alcoholism (NCA) (6). This latter group has attempted to identify signs and symptoms which occur early and late in the illness. These signs and symptoms were then weighted for their diagnostic significance. Table 1 summarizes the NCA's major (definite, obligatory) criteria. A person who fits any one of these criteria must be diagnosed as being an alcoholic. Minor criteria such as odor of alcohol on the breath at the time of a medical appointment, peripheral neuropathy, various laboratory abnormalities, and many others make the diagnosis probable or possible. The presently available criteria are in a continuing state of evolution, and the reader is referred to two in-depth critiques of the NCA criteria (7,8).

Alcoholism is often unrecognized and difficult to diagnose with certainty in its early stages (5). The onset of problem drinking is insidious and the progression to alcohol dependence usually requires several years. Patients do not give a reliable history of their alcohol intake or associated problems. Their drinking patterns are variable; intake may be steady or episodic with periods of sobriety. Yet, an early diagnosis holds the most promise for therapeutic interventions. One solution is to have a high index of suspicion. There is no typical alcoholic; alcoholics are heterogeneous with regard to age, sex, race, social-economic status, and personality traits. Screening tests such

Table 1.

NCA MAJOR CRITERIA FOR THE DIAGNOSIS OF ALCOHOLISM

A. **Physiological Criteria**
   Evidence of dependence:
   1. Manifestation of a withdrawal syndrome (gross tremor, hallucinosis, withdrawal seizures, delirium tremens).
   2. Evidence of tolerance to the effects of alcohol.
      a. A blood alcohol level of more than 150 mg% without gross evidence of intoxication.
      b. A history of daily consumption of one-fifth of a gallon of whiskey or an equivalent amount of wine or beer by a 180-lb person.
B. **Clinical Criteria**
   Evidence of major alcohol-associated illnesses such as alcoholic hepatitis and alcoholic cerebellar degeneration.
C. **Behavioral, Psychological, and Attitudinal Criteria**
   Evidence of psychological dependence as shown by drinking despite strong medical contraindication or social contraindication (loss of job, marriage disruption, arrest for intoxication) known to the patient.

as interviews, self-administered questionnaires, and laboratory tests (blood alcohol level, liver enzymes, macrocytosis) are being studied for early detection (9). The search for biologic markers of alcoholism continues (4,10). Investigations into the early stages of alcoholism indicate that a generally predictable order of alcoholic behaviors and experiences occurs in many patients (11). These include blackouts, loss of control of drinking, frequent morning drinking, hospitalizations, and others. Detection of these occurrences may aid in the early diagnosis of alcoholism.

Etiology. The etiology of alcoholism is the subject of considerable investigation. Certainly authorities agree that both psychological factors and socio-cultural influences interplay in some complex manner to cause alcoholism (4). However, compelling evidence suggests that a genetic component or hereditary factors may also contribute to the development of alcoholism in an individual (4,12,13). Family studies have emphasized the high prevalence of alcoholism among relatives, and four twin studies have pointed toward a genetic control of drinking behavior. In addition, several adoption studies demonstrated a higher risk of alcoholism in adoptees born to alcoholic parents compared to adoptees raised by alcoholic parents (14–17). Also, children of alcoholics had a higher risk whether raised by their alcoholic parents or by non-alcoholic foster parents. These preliminary findings seem to indicate that a person's biologic makeup, rather than the environment in which he is raised, contributes more to the development of alcoholism. How this genetic predisposition is translated physiologically or biochemically and ultimately expressed as alcohol abuse is being studied. Current research in this area is attempting to identify differences in ethanol metabolism, in ethanol's effects on brain biogenic amines, and in objective and subjective central nervous system (CNS) responses to ethanol in an alcoholic versus a non-alcoholic population. Identifying individuals with a genetic predisposition may allow for early intervention. However, not everyone with a genetic predisposition becomes an alcoholic since many factors influence its development.

Medical Complications. This chapter will focus on the common medical complications of alcohol abuse and their management. Ethanol is a multisystem toxin. Nearly all tissues and organ systems in the body are adversely affected depending upon the volume and duration of ethanol consumption as well as individual predisposing factors. Tissue damage results from several factors: ethanol's direct toxicity, concomitant malnutrition, and metabolic derangements resulting from the metabolism of ethanol (18,19). Examples of these three processes include anemia, leukopenia, and thrombocytopenia due to direct bone marrow suppression by ethanol; Wernicke's syndrome from thiamine deficiency; and hypertriglyceridemia and fatty liver resulting from excess hydrogen ion production from the oxidation of ethanol. Acetaldehyde, a reactive intermediary of ethanol metabolism, also contributes to tissue and organ damage (18,19).

The metabolism of ethanol, which occurs primarily in the liver, is depicted in Fig. 1. The alcohol dehydrogenase pathway is the main route for ethanol elimination. Chronic consumption induces the activity of the microsomal ethanol oxidizing system (MEOS) and increases its capacity. This route becomes significant when ethanol levels are high (19). Oxidation of ethanol generates an excess of hydrogen ions which are transferred to the cofactor nicotinamide adenine dinucleotide

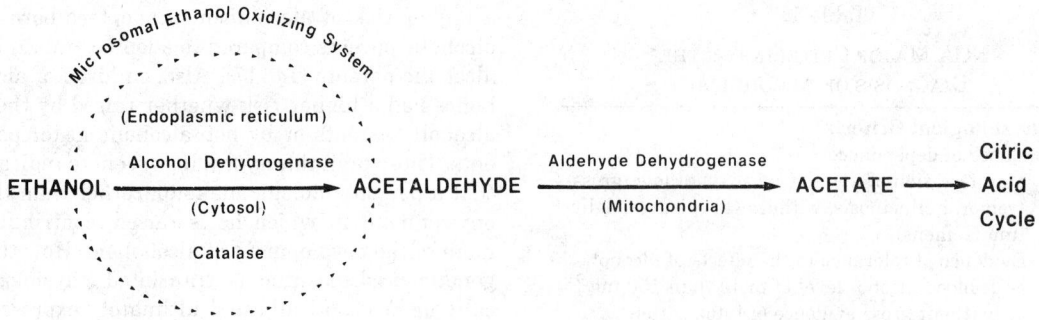

Figure 1. Hepatic Metabolism of Ethanol. Dashes indicate minor pathways.

(NAD), reducing it to NADH. This altered redox state, characterized by an elevated NADH/NAD ratio, is responsible for some of the metabolic abnormalities seen in alcoholics. These include hyperlactacidemia and secondary hyperuricemia, ketoacidosis, hypoglycemia, and hypertriglyceridemia (18,19).

ALCOHOL WITHDRAWAL SYNDROME

1. D.B., a 51-year-old male, is admitted with a chief complaint of marked tremulousness. The patient gives a history of recent heavy drinking. He states that his last drink was 12 hours ago. This patient has no other medical illnesses nor any alcohol-related medical complications. Vital signs on admission include a temperature of 100°F, a pulse of 100/min, a blood pressure of 140/100 mm Hg, and a respiratory rate of 12/min. Admitting laboratory data include the following (normal values are in parentheses): hemoglobin 12.5 gm/dl (14–18); hematocrit 42% (41–53); white cell count 3500/mm³ (5000–11,000); sodium 138 mEq/L (135–145); potassium 3.0 mEq/L (3.5–5.0); chloride 102 mEq/L (95–105); bicarbonate 28 mEq/L (24–32); calcium 10 mg/dl (8.5–10.5); phosphorus 1.8 mg/dl (2.2–4.2); and serum glucose 86 mg/dl (75–110).

Close monitoring of this patient is indicated. What signs and symptoms would indicate progression of the withdrawal syndrome?

The alcohol withdrawal syndrome, characterized by progressive hyperactivity, occurs after abrupt cessation of heavy ethanol intake. How-

ever, withdrawal symptoms may occur during drinking episodes such as in a blackout period or during a period of decreased intake. Not all drinkers experience withdrawal; its frequency and severity are dependent on the amount and length of drinking with wide individual variation (20). The withdrawal syndrome (outlined in Table 2) may be divided into four general and progressive stages which overlap in their time of onset (20,21). The majority of patients experience only mild symptoms which resolve within 48 hours.

The patient, D.B., should be monitored closely for changes in vital signs, increased tremulousness, and hyperactivity. He should be questioned about hallucinations and evaluated for orientation to person, place and time. Generalized seizures may occur.

2. What are the immediate treatment goals for this patient?

The immediate goals of treatment include suppression of the signs and symptoms of withdrawal, prevention of the progression of the alcohol withdrawal syndrome, correction of fluid and electrolyte imbalances, and provision of adequate nutrition.

3. *Drug Treatment.* What sedative-hypnotic drugs should be used to manage the alcohol withdrawal syndrome? How should they be administered and dosed?

Benzodiazepines are effective, easily administered, and the safest drugs to use in this setting. Diazepam (Valium) is most commonly used and can be given orally and intravenously (IV). Intramuscular (IM) administration is not recommended for several reasons. Because of diazepam's poor water solubility, slow or incomplete absorption may occur from the IM injection site. Also, some alcoholics have bleeding tendencies due to thrombocytopenia or hypoprothrombinemia secondary to liver disease, and in these situations IM injections should be avoided.

Diazepam should be administered frequently in small doses. D.B. should be given 10–20 mg orally every 2–4 hours until his withdrawal signs and symptoms are suppressed and he feels calm.

Table 2.

ALCOHOL WITHDRAWAL SYNDROME

Stage	Usual Onset (after last drink)	Signs and Symptoms
1	6–8 hours	Mild tremulousness, anxiety, irritability, insomnia, anorexia, nausea, vomiting, mild changes in vital signs (tachycardia, increased blood pressure and respiratory rate, fever), diaphoresis.
2	1–3 days	Marked tremors, hyperactivity, insomnia, auditory or visual hallucinations. The patient is oriented; memory and sensorium remain clear.
3	12–48 hours	Increased severity of Stage 2 symptoms. Seizure activity may occur; usually a single or multiple grand mal seizures over a short period (less than 6 hours). Status epilepticus is rare.
4	3–5 days	Delirium tremens (DTs). Marked tremor, extreme agitation requiring restraints, confusion, disorientation, hallucinations, paranoia, extreme autonomic hyperactivity (tachycardia, high fever, sweating, tachypnea). Mortality due to shock, hyperpyrexia, arrhythmias, infection or injury.

He should be sedated but awake or arousable. Diazepam should then be tapered over several days to prevent delayed withdrawal symptoms and to decrease the accumulation of the parent compound and its active metabolites.

Dosing must be individualized for each patient. Many factors in the alcoholic population make the dose requirement quite variable and unpredictable. Alcoholics will exhibit central nervous system (CNS) cross tolerance to all sedative-hypnotic drugs and may require high doses of diazepam. However, pharmacokinetic factors such as decreased protein binding due to hypoalbuminemia, increased liver metabolism due to induction of microsomal enzymes by chronic alcoholism, or reduced liver clearance due to acute ethanol intoxication or liver disease will also affect the dose required (see Questions 34 and 35).

4. Seizure Prevention. Should D.B. be given phenytoin (Dilantin) prophylactically to prevent alcohol withdrawal seizures?

No. Only 5–15% of patients undergoing withdrawal develop seizures. When seizures do occur, the seizure period is brief with a single seizure or a short burst of generalized seizures (22). Status epilepticus rarely occurs. Morbidity and mortality from these seizures can be minimized with staff preparedness and proper positioning of the patient to prevent head trauma, musculo-skeletal injury, and aspiration of gastric contents (22).

There is no indication for prophylactic anticonvulsants in this patient since he has no history of withdrawal seizures (22,23). The sole use of diazepam, which also has anticonvulsant activity, to treat the withdrawal syndrome is adequate. In one study comparing chlordiazepoxide (Librium) alone or with phenytoin, no seizures were observed in either group of 100 patients undergoing withdrawal (24). One animal study clearly demonstrated the efficacy of carbamazepine (Tegretol) in preventing withdrawal seizures (25). However, this benefit was achieved by chronic administration of the anticonvulsant and by maintaining a therapeutic serum concentration at the onset of withdrawal. It seems that effective prophylaxis necessitates either chronic administration or a rapid loading dose of an anticonvulsant at the onset of withdrawal. In light of the low incidence as well as the low morbidity and mortality of withdrawal seizures, prophylaxis with anticonvulsant drugs (except for diazepam) is not recommended.

In patients *with* a history of seizures, the issue of prophylaxis is controversial. One study involved 157 such patients with a history of adult-onset convulsions due to alcohol withdrawal and other causes. Significantly less seizure activity occurred in patients given chlordiazepoxide and phenytoin (100 mg po tid) compared to a control group that was given only chlordiazepoxide for withdrawal (26). However, it is difficult to ascribe this benefit to phenytoin since these patients achieved a mean serum phenytoin concentration of only 3–4 mg/L, which is usually considered subtherapeutic. Another study that included some patients with a history of alcohol withdrawal seizures showed no benefit in adding phenytoin to chlordiazepoxide therapy (24). More prospective studies are required before prophylactic phenytoin can be recommended for the subset of patients with a history of withdrawal seizures.

If seizure activity does develop, the patient should be given IV diazepam. Electrolyte abnormalities such as hyponatremia, hypocalcemia, hypomagnesemia, and acid-base imbalances should be corrected. For status epilepticus, an IV loading dose of phenytoin followed by maintenance doses should be given (see the Epilepsy chapter). Chronic therapy with anticonvulsants is not indicated unless the patient has another underlying seizure disorder (22). This situation is not uncommon in that a substantial number of alcoholics have idiopathic or post-traumatic epilepsy.

5. *Electrolyte Abnormalities.* What are the causes of D.B.'s electrolyte abnormalities, and how should they be treated? What other electrolyte abnormalities are commonly observed in alcoholic patients?

The hypokalemia and hypophosphatemia observed in D.B. are electrolyte abnormalities which are common in alcoholic patients (27,28). These abnormalities are due to inadequate dietary intake, enhanced urinary losses due to ethanol's diuretic effect, and losses due to vomiting and diarrhea. Chronic use of aluminum-containing antacids may also contribute to phosphate depletion. This patient may also be deficient in magnesium (27). Although the serum magnesium level is not a good indicator of total body stores, a serum magnesium level should be obtained. Of note is the fact that this patient is not hypocalcemic. Many alcoholics are low in this mineral due to hypoalbuminemia, magnesium deficiency, or vitamin D

deficiency (27,29). The patient's electrolyte deficiencies may be repleted parenterally or orally. Potassium chloride (10–20 mEq), potassium or sodium phosphate (10–20 mmoles phosphate), and magnesium sulfate (8 mEq) may be added to each liter of IV fluid to be infused over 8 hours (3 L/day). If D.B. can take oral supplementation, he should be given potassium chloride and phosphate in approximately the same doses by this route. Milk, an excellent source of phosphate, or oral phosphate preparations (Fleet's Phospho-Soda, Neutra-phos) may be used. Magnesium sulfate, available as a 50% solution, may be administered IM. The reader is referred to several clinical reviews for a more thorough discussion of these electrolyte abnormalities (30–33).

6. *Malnutrition.* What factors contribute to malnutrition in alcoholic patients?

Factors which contribute to malnutrition in the alcoholic include the following:

a. *Inadequate dietary intake* (34,35). Alcoholics commonly do not eat adequate amounts of food or ingest a diet which is disproportionately high in carbohydrates and lacking in protein, vitamins, and minerals. Except for providing calories (7 kilocalories per gram of ethanol), alcoholic beverages contribute little to normal daily nutrient requirements and often displace other foods from the diet.

b. *Impaired gastrointestinal (GI) absorption of nutrients.* Ethanol directly alters the structure and function of the intestinal membrane so that active transport and absorption of many substances are decreased. Among these are amino acids, D-xylose, glucose, thiamine, folate, and minerals (36,37).

c. Alcoholics who have had repeated bouts of pancreatitis develop *pancreatic insufficiency* and malabsorb protein and fat.

d. *Defective metabolism of nutrients.* One example is the decreased conversion of pyridoxine to its active form due to ethanol's interference with hepatic and red cell pyridoxine kinase activity (34).

e. *Decreased storage of nutrients in patients with liver disease* (34). The observed decrease in hepatic concentrations of vitamins may be secondary to decreased storage space due to fatty infiltration or fibrosis of the liver, decreased hepatic affinity, or an increased rate of release of vitamins from the liver.

7. What nutritional measures should be prescribed for D.B.?

He should be given a diet high in calories, protein, and vitamins, particularly the B vitamins. Intravenous solutions containing dextrose may be necessary in the acute phase if he is too "shaky" to eat. D.B. must be given thiamine (Vitamin B_1) before or at the same time glucose is given to avoid acutely precipitating Wernicke's syndrome. This vitamin may be given parenterally or orally. The dose is usually 50–100 mg per day (see Question 11).

DELIRIUM TREMENS AND WERNICKE'S SYNDROME

8. T.S., a 55-year-old male, was admitted to the surgical ward for diagnostic workup of a gastric carcinoma and possible surgery. The patient's long history of heavy alcohol intake was not known at the time of admission. On the second hospital day, the patient was placed on npo (nothing by mouth) restrictions and an IV was started with D-10-½NS (10% dextrose with 0.45% sodium chloride in water) at 100 ml/hr. On the third hospital day, the patient was noted to have horizontal nystagmus, ocular palsies, ataxia, and mild confusion. The next day he became incoherent, agitated, disoriented and combative, and physical restraints were required to control him. He manifested paranoid ideation and had auditory and visual hallucinations. Physical examination at this time revealed a tremulous and diaphoretic white male with a temperature of 38.5°C, a blood pressure of 140/90 mm Hg, and a pulse of 120/min. Abnormal laboratory data included mildly elevated liver enzymes: serum glutamic oxaloacetic transaminase (SGOT) 60 U/L (5–35) and total bilirubin 2 mg/dl (0.2–1.2).

A diagnosis of delirium tremens was made and orders were written for paraldehyde 10 ml po or pr q4h with chlorpromazine (Thorazine) 25 mg IM prn extreme agitation. How should delirium tremens be treated? Should paraldehyde and chlorpromazine be used?

For severe delirium tremens (DTs), the drug of choice is diazepam given IV. A suggested regimen is 10 mg followed by 5 mg every 5–15 minutes until the patient is calm (38). The patient should be checked for hypotension and respiratory depression after each dose. In one group of patients treated for DTs, the dose of IV diazepam required for initial calming ranged from 15 to 280 mg (38). A maintenance dose of 10–20 mg IV or po should be given as needed.

Paraldehyde is not recommended for several reasons. The drug is difficult to administer in that IM injections cause pain and local tissue necrosis, and IV administration may produce hypotension, respiratory depression, and pulmonary edema. Absorption is slow and erratic after oral and rectal administration (39), and local irritation may occur when the drug is administered by these routes. Also, the drug decomposes after exposure to light and air.

One study compared IV diazepam and paraldehyde administered rectally in patients with severe DTs (38). Several patients were underdosed with paraldehyde which resulted in a significantly delayed onset of effect and prolonged and extreme agitation. These patients suffered more self-injuries and caused more injuries to medical personnel than patients treated with diazepam. Overdosage resulting in apnea also occurred in several paraldehyde-treated patients. In contrast, no adverse reactions occurred in the diazepam-treated group. Large doses of paraldehyde may also cause hepatotoxicity. T.S.'s laboratory data indicate a mild hepatitis which may be worsened with paraldehyde administration.

Other drugs that should not be used for the withdrawal syndrome include ethanol, phenothiazines, antihistamines, and hydroxyzine (Atarax, Vistaril) (20,40,41). Phenothiazines such as chlorpromazine are not recommended since these drugs lower the convulsive threshold and may increase the number of seizures during alcohol withdrawal. Hypotension may also occur with chlorpromazine. Antihistamines and hydroxyzine do not reliably suppress withdrawal symptoms nor prevent the progression to DTs.

9. In view of this patient's mild liver disease, would it be preferable to treat him with oxazepam (Serax) or lorazepam (Ativan) rather than diazepam?

Oxazepam and lorazepam are benzodiazepine derivatives that are closely related to diazepam. Unlike diazepam, these compounds are shorter-acting and their metabolism is not impaired in patients with liver disease, which is a theoretical advantage in this patient whose diazepam metabolism may be slowed (42–44). However, oxazepam and lorazepam are less lipid soluble than diazepam and have a significantly slower onset of CNS effect (44). This characteristic may make them less effective in the management of delirium tremens. Furthermore, oxazepam is not available in a parenteral dosage form, and clinical trials evaluating the efficacy of these drugs in alcohol withdrawal and DTs are lacking. Therefore, this patient should be treated with diazepam as outlined in the previous question.

10. What other treatment measures are recommended for patients with DTs?

Delirium tremens is associated with a mortality rate of 5 to 25%. The causes of death include hyperpyrexia, hypotension and shock, infections, arrhythmias associated with electrolyte abnormalities, and other alcohol-associated illnesses such as acute pancreatitis or hepatitis (38). T.S. should be hydrated with IV fluids and any electrolyte deficiencies should be corrected. Antipyretics such as aspirin or acetaminophen (Tylenol) should be used to lower his fever. He must be evaluated for other illnesses mentioned above and treated appropriately.

11. Explain the patient's symptoms of nystagmus, ocular palsies, and ataxia which developed on the third hospital day. How should these be treated?

These symptoms are consistent with Wernicke's syndrome, which is due to thiamine deficiency and is characterized by ocular symptoms (paralysis of eye muscles and nystagmus), ataxia, and encephalopathy (45,46). Thiamine deficiency occurs commonly in chronic alcoholics due to inadequate intake, malabsorption, impaired hepatic storage, and decreased activation to the coenzyme, thiamine pyrophosphate (34,47–49). This vitamin is an essential cofactor in the first step of the Krebs cycle, the decarboxylation of pyruvate. Administration of glucose increases the demand for thiamine and may acutely precipitate Wernicke's syndrome in patients with marginal stores. The treatment is IV administration of thiamine at a dose of 100 mg/day. Recovery is usually very rapid with ocular symptoms completely disappearing in several hours and the ataxia resolving within several days.

After the acute symptoms have subsided, this patient may progress to a chronic phase known as Korsakoff's psychosis despite adequate thiamine replacement. Memory is severely impaired in these patients and they tend to confabulate. This latter symptom is a result of a malfunctioning brain correlating old remembered data with current situations. Subcortical lesions due to thiamine deficiency and possibly due to direct ethanol toxicity are responsible for the Wernicke-Korsakoff syndrome (50,51).

TREATMENT OF ALCOHOLISM

12. D.B., the patient described in Question 1, seeks treatment for his alcoholism. His social history reveals that he has worked steadily as a computer programmer and has a stable family environment. He attributes much of his drinking to job and financial stresses. What modalities are available to treat this patient's alcoholism?

D.B. is an excellent candidate for rehabilitation. He has acknowledged his illness and his need for help, and he has a stable social environment. Therapeutic interventions can be made at this time before any irreversible medical or psychosocial complications have occurred.

The primary goal of treatment programs is to change drinking behavior. Treatment options include:

a. Self-help groups such as Alcoholics Anonymous (AA) (52). The tenets of this group are that alcoholism is an incurable illness and recovery is achieved by alcohol abstention. Although many individuals have been helped by this widely respected organization, no statistics are kept as to its membership, effectiveness, or recovery rate, and the group's claims of success are difficult to substantiate. AA appears to be a limited resource appealing to alcoholics who desire group affiliation and who tend to develop dependent relationships (53,54).

Other self-help rehabilitation programs are sponsored by government agencies, church groups, business corporations, and other private organizations. The National Council on Alcoholism provides information and referrals through its many local offices.

b. Individual and group psychotherapy (53).

c. Family therapy.

d. Behavior modification therapy.

e. Disulfiram (Antabuse) therapy.

Though many modalities are available, there is insufficient knowledge of their relative efficacy.

Also not known is which particular treatment strategy is most likely to benefit a particular patient (53). In fact, a formal alcoholism treatment program may not be necessary in some patients. One survey of 45 cases with severe alcoholic liver disease demonstrated that primary medical care alone was sufficient for their recovery from alcoholism (55). Apparently, the impact of their severe illness along with education about alcoholism motivated these patients to abstain or significantly decrease their drinking. Regardless of the treatment chosen, follow-up care is mandatory. Alcoholism is a lifelong disease whose course is marked by periods of abstinence, moderate intake, as well as heavy drinking.

13. D.B. asks for your comments on a newspaper report stating that "controlled drinking" is a possible goal in some patients.

This highly controversial Rand Report was based on a study conducted by the Rand Corporation for the U.S. National Institute on Alcohol Abuse and Alcoholism (NIAAA) (56). The report concluded that certain patients can return to moderate ethanol consumption and control their drinking within socially accepted limits that do not cause dysfunction. Many criticisms of this study have been put forth. Some argue that the patients were not representative of the general alcoholic population but were a subset of highly motivated problem drinkers. The study's method of follow-up based on patients' self-reports is considered unreliable by many authorities. In addition, controlled drinking is contraindicated in some patients as discussed by Miller and Caddy (57). These contraindications include the following:

a. evidence of progressive liver disease;

b. evidence of other health problems that may be exacerbated by moderate alcohol use;

c. strong external demands upon the patient to abstain (eg, as a condition of probation or for reinstatement of a driver's license);

d. episodes of pathological intoxication (patient exhibits uncontrolled or bizarre behavior following even moderate alcohol use);

e. prior failure of therapy oriented toward controlled drinking;

f. use of medications which contraindicate the use of alcohol.

Total and permanent abstinence is the goal of alcoholism treatment accepted by most authorities. Only in a few patients who refuse to accept abstinence or who have repeatedly failed treatments with this goal should the therapeutic endpoint be controlled drinking (57). Although less optimal, this goal may be more feasible.

14. *Disulfiram*. The patient elects to join an AA group at work and also to take disulfiram. Discuss disulfiram's mechanism of action and its efficacy in treating alcoholism.

Disulfiram deters alcohol intake by inhibition of the enzyme aldehyde dehydrogenase. If the patient drinks while on this drug, he may suffer a disulfiram-ethanol reaction (DER) within minutes. This reaction consists of nausea, vomiting, headache, cutaneous flushing of the face and upper trunk, vasodilation, respiratory difficulties, and tachycardia. Confusion, drowsiness, and sleep usually follow with recovery within 2–4 hours. However, hypotension, shock and even death have been reported with the DER (58–61). This reaction may occur up to one week after stopping disulfiram (62). Accumulation of acetaldehyde and perhaps depletion of norepinephrine (due to inhibition of the enzyme dopamine-beta-hydroxylase by disulfiram) are responsible for this reaction (58,59). Treatment for the reaction is supportive (63).

Disulfiram is widely used and is recommended for patients with a relatively long drinking history who are older (over 40 years), socially stable, highly motivated, and not depressed (60,64). Its success in deterring alcohol consumption depends on patient compliance and a positive patient-therapist relationship (59). However, little evidence other than uncontrolled trials and anecdotes documents this drug's usefulness (60). A recent controlled, blind, prospective trial supports the idea that disulfiram may be of limited value in the treatment of alcoholism (65). The abstinence rate was equal in patients given a therapeutic dose and in a second group of patients given an identically appearing but pharmacologically inactive 1 mg dose of disulfiram. Apparently, the patients' belief that they were taking the drug and the implied threat of the disulfiram-ethanol reaction were the important deterrents to drinking. In this same study, a third control group was only given riboflavin tablets and was so informed. This group had a higher rate of drinking but this rate was not statistically different from the two disulfiram groups. The question is raised whether patients need to be subjected to the risks of disulfiram. Perhaps an inert dose or a placebo would be as effective in the treatment of alcoholism.

15. What dose of disulfiram should be prescribed for D.B.? What instructions and warnings should he be given?

This drug is administered orally and dosed at 500 mg daily for one week and then 125–250 mg daily. The following information should be given to the patient:

Prevention of DER. He should be warned of the serious nature of the DER. He must avoid all forms of alcohol while taking this drug and for at least a week after discontinuation. Included are foods (wine sauces, desserts containing alcohol) and prescription and over-the-counter (OTC) medications containing ethanol such as elixirs, tinctures, cough and cold preparations. Since alcohol absorption may occur through the skin and cause the reaction, he should also avoid mouthwashes and topical preparations such as shampoos, lotions, and colognes that contain alcohol (59,66). The patient should wear or carry identification that he is taking disulfiram.

Disulfiram Side Effects. Side effects occurring with disulfiram are mild. He may experience lethargy, fatigue, drowsiness, skin rashes, and a metallic taste in the mouth (59). Rare side effects include acute organic brain syndrome, toxic psychosis, peripheral neuropathy, optic neuritis, and hepatitis (61,67). The few reports of disulfiram hepatotoxicity indicate that the reaction is due to hypersensitivity and not related to the dose administered (68–70). These patients present with symptoms similar to viral or alcoholic hepatitis. Liver biopsy findings include hepatocellular necrosis with eosinophilic infiltration. Rechallenge with disulfiram is contraindicated since the response may be severe with extensive hepatic necrosis precipitating hepatic coma and death. Elevations of liver enzymes without clinical symptoms of hepatotoxicity have also been reported (71).

Drug Interactions. D.B. should inform his pharmacist that he is on disulfiram since it interacts with other drugs. The elimination of phenytoin is decreased and the dosage of this medication may need to be lowered (72,73). Disulfiram also augments the hypoprothrombinemic effect of warfarin and patients may require a reduction in their anticoagulant dose. This interaction cannot be explained on a pharmacokinetic basis since the metabolism of warfarin is not altered. One hypothesis is that disulfiram and its metabolites impair the formation of active prothrombin by chelating metal cations required for synthesis (74).

16. *Psychotherapeutic Drugs.* Are psychotherapeutic drugs such as major tranquilizers, antidepressants, and anti-anxiety agents indicated in this patient for control of drinking?

Based upon observations that some alcoholics suffer from psychosis, depression, or anxiety, psychotherapeutic drugs have been used to control drinking. Successes claimed in uncontrolled studies have been disproven after these drugs were subjected to rigorous trials. There is no evidence to support the use of these agents for alcoholism (75,76).

However, there are primary, often preexisting, psychiatric disorders closely associated with alcoholism as well as psychiatric sequelae of chronic alcohol abuse (77). Each individual patient needs to be evaluated for any psychopathology (which may or may not be related to his alcoholism) and appropriate psychotherapeutic agents should be used to treat any primary disorders (77).

17. *Lithium.* Does lithium have a role in the treatment of alcoholism?

Several preliminary studies have demonstrated lithium's effectiveness in decreasing alcohol consumption in chronic alcoholics, especially those with a concomitant affective disorder such as depression (78–80). Lithium's action in this setting appears to be attenuation of the patient's craving for alcohol and his subjective "high" to alcohol. Improvement in the patient's depression was not noted. The routine use of lithium for alcoholism is not recommended until more patients are evaluated for longer follow-up periods.

HEMATOLOGIC ABNORMALITIES

18. A 48-year-old female with a long history of ethanol abuse, cirrhosis and ascites is being evaluated for anemia. Her laboratory data include: hemoglobin 9.5 gm/dl (14–18), hematocrit 31% (41–53), white cell count 3000/mm³ (5000–11,000), and platelet count 80,000/mm³ (140,000–400,000). What are the common red cell abnormalities seen in alcoholics? How should this patient's anemia be evaluated?

In most alcoholic patients with anemia, the cause is multifactorial, and the anemia presents as a mixed picture. The following are commonly seen:

a. A round macrocytosis with an absent or only a slight anemia (81,82). The mean corpuscular volume (MCV) is mildly elevated in the 100–110 range (80–100). This entity is newly recognized and poorly understood and is seen in the majority of chronic alcoholics. It is not due to folate deficiency or liver disease and clears slowly after months of abstinence.

b. Megaloblastic anemia due to folate deficiency (81–83). Folate deficiency is due to inadequate dietary intake, malabsorption, and ethanol's deleterious effects on folate storage, metabolism, and transport (84–86).

c. A normocytic, normochromic anemia due to direct suppression of bone marrow production by ethanol. A reactive reticulocytosis is often seen within several days of discontinuation of drinking.

d. Iron deficiency anemia due to acute or chronic blood loss from gastritis or bleeding varices.

e. Sequestration of red blood cells and chronic mild hemolysis due to splenomegaly (87).

f. Sideroblastic anemia due to impaired iron utilization and heme synthesis. This anemia may be due to ethanol's inhibition of delta-aminolevulinic acid synthetase, a rate-limiting enzyme in heme synthesis or to a deficiency of the active form of pyridoxine (88).

There are several easy ways to evaluate this patient's anemia initially. She should abstain from alcohol, and a reactive reticulocytosis should be looked for. Her red cell indices and peripheral blood smear would indicate whether she has a macrocytic or microcytic anemia or both. In addition, hypersegmented neutrophils on the smear would indicate folate deficiency. Her stool should be guaiac tested to detect any occult GI bleeding.

19. Folate deficiency is documented in this patient by a mean corpuscular volume (MCV) of 120 (80–100), hypersegmented neutrophils on smear, and a low serum folate level. How should she be treated?

She should be encouraged to stop drinking and be given folic acid 1 mg orally per day. This dose, which far exceeds minimum daily requirements, is rational since the patient is not likely to stop drinking. Alcohol can suppress the hematopoietic response normally seen with replacement of folic acid in physiologic amounts. This block can be reversed with large doses of folic acid (89). It is unlikely that a normal hemoglobin or hematocrit can be attained in this patient. Nevertheless, all measures should be taken to replace any nutritional deficiencies (folate, iron, pyridoxine, vitamin B_{12}) and to correct any other causes of the anemia.

20. Comment on this patient's leukopenia and thrombocytopenia.

Both decreased counts and functional abnormalities in white blood cells and platelets are seen in a small percentage of alcoholics (83,90–93). These hematologic disorders contribute to an increased incidence and severity of infections and bleeding in alcoholics. The leukopenia and thrombocytopenia often reverse rapidly with the discontinuation of alcohol.

ALCOHOLIC LIVER DISEASE

21. M.W., a 51-year-old heavy drinker, is admitted with fever, anorexia, nausea, vomiting, right upper quadrant (RUQ) abdominal pain, and jaundice. The patient admits to drinking over 1 quart of whiskey daily for the past few weeks. Four months ago, the patient was noted to be a positive tuberculin reactor with fibrotic lesions on chest x-ray consistent with previous tuberculosis (TB) infection. She was started on isoniazid (INH) 300 mg per day at that time. Abnormal admitting laboratory data include: white cell count 15,000/mm³, serum glutamic oxaloacetic transaminase (SGOT) 180 U/L (5–35), serum glutamic pyruvic transaminase (SGPT) 65 U/L (5–35), total bilirubin 6 mg/dl (0.2–1.2), serum albumin 3.0 gm/dl (3.3–5.2), and prothrombin time (PT) 15 seconds (12). The differential diagnosis is alcoholic hepatitis versus INH-induced hepatitis. What are the types of alcoholic liver disease?

The three entities of alcoholic liver disease are summarized in Table 3 (94–97). Their clinical severity varies widely among patients and there is considerable overlap of the three types of liver disease in any one patient. Often alcoholic hepatitis is accompanied by fat accumulation and these two lesions may be present in an established cirrhotic liver.

22. Describe INH hepatitis. How should the diagnosis (alcoholic hepatitis versus INH hepatitis) be made in this patient?

INH hepatitis may present a clinical picture which is similar to viral hepatitis or alcoholic hepatitis. The incidence of this side effect increases with age (1.2% for ages 36–49 and 1.7% for ages over 50). It most often occurs in the first three months of treatment (50% of cases) but may occur as late as after nine months of therapy (98). Two studies indicate that alcoholism or daily alcohol consumption increases the likelihood of INH hepatotoxicity (99,100), but this contention has been challenged by a recent U.S. Public Health Service cooperative trial. In this report, the incidence was not increased in a select population of alcoholics with no pretreatment abnormalities in liver function tests as compared to a control group of nonalcoholics (101).

A liver biopsy would be the most help in distinguishing between the two diagnoses. Both alcohol and INH cause hepatocellular injury with an inflammatory response. However, in alcoholic hepatitis one would expect to find pericellular fi-

Table 3.

ALCOHOLIC LIVER DISEASE

Entity	Incidence and Onset	Signs and Symptoms	Liver Biopsy Findings	Prognosis
Alcoholic Fatty Liver	May occur in all drinkers after one to several weeks of heavy intake.	RUQ abdominal pain, tenderness and hepatomegaly. Liver function tests (LFTs) are mildly abnormal.	Accumulation of triglycerides in the hepatocytes.	Usually benign and fully reversible in weeks. Alcohol must be discontinued and a good diet ingested.
Alcoholic Hepatitis	Occurs in 15–35% of heavy drinkers. Onset is usually after 5–10 years of heavy consumption.	Fever, anorexia, nausea, vomiting, RUQ abdominal pain, jaundice. Lab data include leukocytosis, abnormal LFTs and prolonged PT.	Central parenchymal necrosis with inflammatory polymorphonuclear and lymphocytic infiltration. Alcoholic hyalin (Mallory bodies) may be present.	Variable. High mortality in patients presenting with severe liver impairment. Many patients recover; but if drinking is continued, they have an 80–90% chance of developing cirrhosis. Some patients have progressive liver disease despite abstinence and good nutrition.
Alcoholic Cirrhosis	Occurs in 10–25% of all heavy drinkers. Risk increases exponentially with amount and duration of consumption. Genetic factors such as HLA type also influence risk.	Weakness, anorexia, and weight loss. Stigmata include signs of hypogonadism and hyperestrogenization (testicular atrophy, gynecomastia, palmar erythema, spider telangiectasias). Lab values include hypoalbuminemia and prolonged PT. Other LFTs may be only minimally abnormal.	Distorted hepatic architecture and circulation due to ongoing necrosis, nodular regeneration and diffuse increase in fibrous connective tissue.	Poor. Complications include portal hypertension leading to ascites, edema, variceal hemorrhage, and splenomegaly; hepatic encephalopathy; hepatorenal syndrome; and an increased incidence of hepatocellular carcinoma.

brosis, Mallory bodies, and fatty changes which are not present in INH hepatitis. A strong argument can be made against a liver biopsy in this case since the treatment is the same with both diagnoses (see Questions 23–25) and her prothrombin time is increased by three seconds.

23. A diagnosis of alcoholic hepatitis is made based upon liver biopsy findings. How should M.W. be treated?

Treatment is nonspecific and supportive. Measures include bedrest, discontinuation of ethanol and any other hepatotoxic drugs such as INH, and a diet high in calories, vitamins, and as much protein as tolerable to promote liver regeneration. Supplementation with IV amino acids may improve hepatic function and survival as reported in a small group of patients (102). Every effort must be made to keep this patient off of alcohol after discharge from the hospital since she has a 80–90% chance of developing cirrhosis if she continues to drink.

24. Should this patient be given corticosteroids?

The use of corticosteroids in alcoholic hepatitis has been advocated to decrease inflammation and to suppress various immunological factors such as T-lymphocytes and immunoglobulins. These factors are thought to be mediators of liver damage and the subsequent progression to cirrhosis (103). However, controlled trials with corticosteroids consistently do not demonstrate any improvement in liver status, rate of clinical recovery, or mortality in patients like M.W. with mild to moderate disease (104–106). A few trials using prednisolone 40 mg orally per day demonstrated a decrease in early mortality in patients with severe disease and encephalopathy (104,106,107). However, no improvement in long-term survival or decreased incidence of cirrhosis occurred in these patients. Many other studies note a lack of benefit even in patients with severe alcoholic hepatitis (105,108–111). In summary, corticosteroids are not recommended at this time for treatment of alcoholic hepatitis.

25. Should this patient be restarted on INH after the alcoholic hepatitis has resolved?

No. Although a year of INH therapy clearly reduces the incidence of active TB in patients like M.W. (positive tuberculin reactor with chest x-ray findings consistent with previous tuberculosis infection), alcoholism is a relative contraindication to its use. The risk of INH hepatitis is high in this patient who is over 50 years of age, a heavy drinker, and who now has a history of liver disease. The risk of additional injury to the liver outweighs the benefit of INH prophylaxis. Because she has received four months of INH, her chance of TB activation has been lowered. One study clearly demonstrated a significant reduction in TB even with only 3–6 months of INH prophylaxis (112).

UPPER GI HEMORRHAGE

26. A.B., a 54-year-old male with alcoholic cirrhosis and ascites, is admitted for hematemesis, lightheadedness, and orthostatic hypotension. Medications prior to admission include spironolactone (Aldactone) 100 mg bid, folic acid 1 mg qd, thiamine 100 mg qd, and multivitamins 1 tablet qd. Pertinent laboratory studies on admission include: hemoglobin 9 gm/dl, hematocrit 27%, and prothrombin time (PT) 17 seconds. What are the possible causes of upper GI hemorrhage in this patient?

Possible causes for this patient's bleeding include gastroesophageal varices, erosive esophagitis or gastritis, a mucosal tear (Mallory-Weiss), peptic ulcer disease, and cancer of the esophagus or stomach (113).

27. Endoscopy confirmed bleeding esophageal varices. How should this patient be managed?

a. He should be stabilized hemodynamically. Spironolactone should be temporarily discontinued and intravascular volume should be replaced with packed red cells and saline. Monitoring of the central venous pressure is recommended to avoid volume overload and increases in portal pressure which might increase variceal bleeding (113). In restoring intravascular volume, the patient's ascites may be unavoidably worsened.

b. A nasogastric tube should be placed and gastric lavage be performed with iced water or saline to reduce bleeding and to remove the blood. Otherwise GI absorption of ammonia from blood proteins may precipitate hepatic encephalopathy in this patient.

c. The patient should be given phytonadione (vitamin K_1, AquaMephyton) 10 mg subcutaneously daily for 3 days to correct his prolonged PT. However, a response may not be seen since it is likely that the hepatic synthesis of clotting factors is impaired in this patient. Continued bleeding may necessitate administration of fresh frozen plasma.

d. Aqueous vasopressin (Pitressin) should be administered to stop the bleeding. This drug decreases portal blood flow and portal venous pressure by vasoconstriction of the splanchnic arteriolar bed. Blood flow through the bleeding varices is then reduced and clot formation is facilitated. Vasopressin should be administered as a continuous IV infusion at a dosage of 0.3–0.9 units/minute or approximately 5×10^{-3} units per kg of body weight per minute (113,114). Therapy should begin with a low dose and the dose may be gradually increased as needed. There are no advantages to selective intraarterial administration into the superior mesenteric artery. Changes in portal and systemic hemodynamics, control of bleeding, and side effects are comparable with intraarterial and intravenous administration (114,115).

e. If this patient continues to bleed significantly despite the above measures, balloon tamponade with the Minnesota tube or surgical decompression by a portal-systemic shunt may be necessary (113).

f. Injection sclerotherapy of varices has been used successfully to control acute bleeding (116–118). Utilizing a flexible fiberoptic endoscope, agents such as sodium morrhuate are injected directly into the varices to cause sclerosis and obliteration of these vessels. Early experience indicates that this technique is safe and effective for control of acute bleeding episodes. Also, recurrent variceal bleeding may be prevented by close endoscopic follow-up of patients and repeated injections of varices (118,119). The high early mortality associated with variceal hemorrhage and rebleeding may be lowered by this technique (120). More experience is needed to fully evaluate the efficacy and risks of this mode of therapy.

28. What are the side effects of vasopressin therapy?

This drug should be used cautiously in patients with heart disease and hypertension. Recent myocardial infarction and severe coronary artery disease are contraindications to its use. Increased coronary and systemic vascular resistance and decreased myocardial contractility and output are pharmacological effects of vasopressin (121). Myocardial ischemia and infarction and ventricular arrhythmias are reported side effects (122). Patients should be placed on a cardiac monitor and their blood pressure should be measured frequently. Dilutional hyponatremia and excess water retention due to the drug's antidiuretic effect have been reported (123). Abdominal cramping may occur due to stimulation of peristaltic activity. Severe vasoconstriction and local tissue necrosis may result if vasopressin is extravasated during IV infusion (124).

ALCOHOL-INDUCED CARDIOTOXICITY AND NEUROPATHY

29. The patient, a 40-year-old heavy drinker, comes to the Emergency Room complaining of palpitations of several hours duration. He admits to a bout of heavy drinking during the past two days. The patient's other complaint is tingling, pain, and weakness in his feet and legs of several months duration.

The patient's EKG indicates atrial fibrillation with a ventricular rate of 90–100 beats/minute. The physician diagnoses the problem as the "holiday heart" syndrome. Explain.

Acute arrhythmias may occur in patients after an intensive drinking bout, often after holidays and weekends (125). These patients usually have a background of greater than ten years of heavy ethanol use. Atrial fibrillation is most commonly seen; but atrial flutter, paroxysmal atrial tachycardia, atrial and ventricular premature beats, junctional tachycardia, and ventricular tachycardia have all been reported (125,126). These arrhythmias usually resolve within 48 hours and no other clinical evidence of heart disease can be found in these patients. Cardiac studies in some of these patients have demonstrated evidence of early left ventricular dysfunction (125,127). Abnormal systolic time intervals and depressed cardiac outputs can be documented.

Factors presumed to be responsible for the arrhythmias include hypoglycemia, abnormalities in serum electrolytes (potassium, magnesium, and phosphate), and ethanol's direct effects on the electrophysiology of the heart. Alterations in conduction velocity and action potential duration and changes in plasma catecholamine levels can be attributed to ethanol (125,128).

30. How should this patient be managed?

The patient should be monitored until the atrial fibrillation resolves. Serum glucose and electrolytes should be checked and corrected if abnormal. Digoxin (Lanoxin) may be given to control the ventricular rate and to convert the rhythm to normal sinus rhythm. Chronic antiarrhythmic therapy is not indicated. The patient should be counseled regarding alcoholism and treatment programs available.

Many episodes of alcohol-associated arrhythmias do not require treatment. Others may require cardioversion or acute and chronic treatment with digoxin and other antiarrhythmic drugs (125).

31. What is alcoholic cardiomyopathy? Should this patient be studied with echocardiography, systolic time intervals, or radionuclide exams to assess left ventricular function and to rule out this entity?

Cardiomyopathy is a second type of alcohol-induced cardiotoxicity. The diagnosis is made after excluding other causes of biventricular congestive heart failure (CHF) in young patients (20–50 years) with a long history of excessive alcohol consumption (more than ten years) (129,130). Factors responsible for this CHF are several; ethanol and acetaldehyde can cause cardiac muscle damage and fibrosis. They also impair contractility by interfering with calcium transport and binding in the heart muscle (131,132). Nutritional deficiencies may also impair myocardial function. Treatment consists of the usual measures for CHF. The early stages of alcoholic cardiomyopathy may be arrested or improved with abstinence. However, the overall prognosis once symptoms are present is poor.

This patient need not be studied since he has no clinical signs of CHF. Very likely he may have early subclinical evidence of left ventricular dysfunction (133,134). He should be encouraged to stop drinking since the early stages of alcoholic cardiomyopathy may be reversible.

32. How should this patient's peripheral neuropathy be treated?

Peripheral neuropathy is seen in a small percentage (10–20%) of alcoholic patients. The neuropathy consists of symmetrical sensory and motor deficits as well as paresthesias, burning pain, decreased or loss of deep tendon reflexes, muscle weakness and atrophy (46,51,135). The onset and progression are slow, and the neuropathy usually begins distally and progresses proximally. The feet and legs are usually affected first and often exclusively. Nerve biopsy findings include axonal degeneration thought to be caused by ethanol and acetaldehyde and demyelination which is a result of thiamine deficiency (136). Slow improvement over weeks to months can be expected with abstinence, nutritional therapy, and supplementation with thiamine 100 mg per day orally.

DRUG THERAPY CONSIDERATIONS IN THE ALCOHOLIC PATIENT

33. *Drug Interactions.* E.W., a known heavy drinker, comes into the community pharmacy to purchase two bottles of Extra-Strength Tylenol (acetaminophen, 500 mg per capsule). She states that she hopes this pain reliever will be effective for her chronic back pain which resulted from an automobile accident last year. What drug interaction should this patient be warned about?

Chronic heavy ethanol ingestion potentiates the hepatotoxicity of acetaminophen. Cases of liver damage have been reported in alcoholic patients ingesting the drug for therapeutic purposes at the recommended doses of 3–4 gm/day (137–139). This patient should be warned not to exceed 8 capsules or a total of 4 grams of acetaminophen per day. She should also check her other medications for their acetaminophen content.

At least two factors in alcoholic patients are responsible for this interaction. Protein malnutrition and fasting deplete hepatic stores of glutathione which is necessary to detoxify the reactive acetaminophen metabolite(s) responsible for hepatic injury (140). In addition, chronic alcohol intake increases the production of these toxic metabolite(s) by stimulation of hepatic microsomal enzymes (141).

34. What other ethanol-drug interactions should clinicians be aware of?

With the widespread use of alcohol in the general population, clinicians must always keep ethanol-drug interactions in mind. Alcohol intolerance may occur in patients on chlorpropamide (Diabinese) and other sulfonylureas, metronidazole (Flagyl), and procarbazine (Matulane) (73). Recently, a reaction similar to the disulfiram-ethanol interaction has been reported in patients who drank while receiving one of the newer, broader spectrum cephalosporins (cefamandole and cefoperazone) (142–145).

The hepatic metabolism of drugs is modified by ethanol intake. Acute ingestion of large amounts of ethanol significantly inhibits the microsomal oxidative enzyme systems. The metabolic clearance of benzodiazepines (146–148), mephenytoin (149), barbiturates, chloral hydrate, meprobamate, tolbutamide, and warfarin is decreased in acutely intoxicated patients (150,151). These patients may experience enhanced or prolonged drug activity. In contrast, chronic ethanol consumption accelerates the hepatic clearance of some drugs by stimulation of the microsomal enzyme system. This interaction has been demonstrated with barbiturates, meprobamate, phenytoin, tolbutamide, and warfarin (150,151). Larger doses of these drugs may be required in alcoholic patients. These interactions between alcohol consumption and drug metabolism must be considered when selecting drugs and determining their doses.

35. What are other drug therapy considerations in alcoholic patients?

Compliance. Compliance to prescribed medication regimens may be unreliable. During drinking bouts and blackout spells, patients may forget to take their medications or take more than the prescribed amount. Clinicians should keep this problem in mind when planning drug therapy regimens and assessing therapeutic response in these patients. Drugs with a low therapeutic index, such as oral anticoagulants, insulin, or cancer chemotherapeutic agents intended for outpatient use, may need to be withheld from these patients or administered only under supervision.

Pharmacodynamic Effects. The pharmacodynamics of drugs may be affected by alcohol (152). These effects must be considered when monitoring drug therapy. Alcohol may enhance the desired therapeutic or undesired side effects of medications. For example, the vasodilation occurring with ethanol ingestion may add to the effects of antihypertensive medications and nitrates. Orthostatic hypotension may occur in some patients. Another example of a pharmacodynamic alteration is the additive gastritis and GI bleeding seen in patients who drink and take aspirin.

Pharmacokinetic Effects. The pharmacokinetics of many drugs may also be affected by alcohol ingestion. Ethanol's effects on drug metabolism were discussed in Question 34. Other pharmacokinetic alterations have also been reported. Changes in bioavailability of drugs with a substantial first-pass hepatic clearance have been reported in cirrhotic patients. One study demonstrated a significant increase in the bioavailability of two such drugs, meperidine and pentazocine, when administered orally (153). Portal-systemic shunting due to cirrhosis is responsible for this increase. Oral dosages of drugs with a high first-pass clearance may need to be decreased in cirrhotic patients. Otherwise enhanced or prolonged pharmacological effects may be unexpectedly seen.

Hypoalbuminemia, which is common in alcoholic patients, may lower the protein binding of drugs. Changes in the volume of distribution and perhaps the amount of unbound, free drug may occur. These changes may in turn alter the intensity and duration of pharmacological effects. Specific examples of this pharmacokinetic alteration are cited in several review articles (154,155).

Drug metabolism may be altered in alcoholic liver disease (156). Unfortunately, there is no test of hepatic drug elimination presently available in clinical practice. It is difficult to predict in a given patient with alcoholic liver disease whether drug elimination will be retarded, unchanged, or accelerated. Many variables such as drug and patient characteristics as well as type of liver disease are important factors that determine whether significant alterations in drug metabolism will occur.

Clinicians must consider pharmacokinetic alterations when planning and assessing drug therapy in alcoholic patients. Specific examples reported in the literature would be helpful if a similar situation is encountered (153–156). Close monitoring of therapeutic and side effects and serum concentrations of drugs will provide guidelines for therapy.

References

1. U.S. Department of HEW: *Third Special Report to the U.S. Congress on Alcohol and Health from the Secretary of Health, Education, and Welfare,* Rockville, MD, 1978.
2. Smart RG: Some recent studies of teenage alcoholism and problem drinking. In *Phenomenology and Treatment of Alcoholism,* edited by WE Fann, I Karacan, AD Pokorny and RL Williams, Spectrum Publications, New York, 1980, p 127.
3. Schuckit MA: Phenomenology and treatment of alcoholism in the elderly. In *Phenomenology and Treatment of Alcoholism,* edited by WE Fann, I Karacan, AD Pokorny and RL Williams, Spectrum Publications, New York, 1980, p 167.
4. Mendelson JH et al: Biologic concomitants of alcoholism. N Engl J Med. 1979; 301:912.
5. Mendelson JH et al: Diagnostic criteria for alcoholism and alcohol abuse. In *The Diagnosis and Treatment of Alcoholism,* edited by JH Mendelson and NK Mello, McGraw-Hill, New York, 1979, p 2.
6. Criteria Committee, National Council on Alcoholism: Criteria for the diagnosis of alcoholism. Ann Intern Med. 1972; 77:249.
7. Pattison EM: The NCA diagnostic criteria: critique, assessment, alternatives. J Stud Alcohol. 1980; 41:965.
8. Jacobson GR: Comment on EM Pattison's "The NCA diagnostic criteria: critique, assessment, alternatives." J Stud Alcohol. 1980; 41:981.
9. Screening tests for alcoholism (editorial). Lancet. 1980; 2:1117.
10. Mezey E: Ratio of plasma ∝-amino-n-butyric acid to leucine in alcoholism (editorial). Gastroenterology. 1978; 75:742.
11. Pokorny AD et al: Stages in the development of alcoholism. In *Phenomenology and Treatment of Alcoholism,* edited by WE Fann, I Karacan, AD Pokorny and RL Williams, Spectrum Publications, New York, 1980, p 45.
12. Goodwin DW: The genetics of alcoholism. Substance Alcohol Actions/Misuse. 1980; 1:101.
13. Goodwin DW: Genetic component of alcoholism. Ann Rev Med. 1981; 32:93.
14. Goodwin DW et al: Alcohol problems in adoptees raised apart from alcoholic biologic parents. Arch Gen Psychiatry. 1973; 28:238.
15. Goodwin DW et al: Drinking problems in adopted and nonadopted sons of alcoholics. Arch Gen Psychiatry. 1974; 31:164.
16. Bohman M: Some genetic aspects of alcoholism and criminality. Arch Gen Psychiatry. 1978; 35:269.
17. Cadoret RJ et al: Inheritance of alcoholism in adoptees. Br J Psychiatry. 1978; 132:252.
18. Lieber CS: Metabolism and metabolic effects of alcohol. Semin Hematol. 1980; 17:85.
19. Weir DG: The pathophysiology of alcohol and acetaldehyde metabolism in the liver. Eur J Clin Invest. 1978; 8:263.
20. Thompson WL: Management of alcohol withdrawal syndromes. Arch Intern Med. 1978; 138:278.
21. Behnke RH: Recognition and management of alcohol withdrawal syndrome. Hosp Practice. 1976; 11:79.
22. Josephson GW et al: Rational management of alcohol withdrawal seizures. South Med J. 1978; 71:1095.
23. Gessner PK: Is diphenylhydantoin effective in treatment of alcohol withdrawal? (letter) JAMA. 1972; 219:1072.
24. Rothstein E: Prevention of alcohol withdrawal seizures: the roles of diphenylhydantoin and chlordiazepoxide. Am J Psychiatry. 1973; 130:1381.
25. Chu NS: Carbamazepine: prevention of alcohol withdrawal seizures. Neurol. 1979; 29:1397.
26. Sampliner R et al: Diphenylhydantoin control of alcohol withdrawal seizures. JAMA. 1974; 230:1430.
27. Knochel JP: Hypophosphatemia in the alcoholic (editorial). Arch Intern Med. 1980; 140:613.
28. Ryback RS et al: Clinical relationships between serum phosphorus and other blood chemistry values in alcoholics. Arch Intern Med. 1980; 140:673.
29. Mezey E: Alcohol and renal vitamin D metabolism (editorial). Gastroenterology. 1980; 78:651.
30. Lentz RD et al: Treatment of severe hypophosphatemia. Ann Intern Med. 1978; 89:941.
31. Knochel JP: Hypophosphatemia. West J Med. 1981; 134:15.
32. Flink EB: Nutritional aspects of magnesium metabolism. West J Med. 1980; 133:304.
33. Rude RK et al: Magnesium deficiency and excess. Ann Rev Med. 1981; 32:245.
34. Mezey E: Liver disease and nutrition. Gastroenterology. 1978; 74:770.
35. Thomson AD: Alcohol and nutrition. Clinics Endocrin Metab. 1978; 7:405.
36. Wilson FA et al: Ethanol and small intestinal transport. Gastroenterology. 1979; 76:388.
37. Green PHR et al: Drugs, alcohol and malabsorption. Am J Med. 1979; 67:1066.
38. Thompson WL et al: Diazepam and paraldehyde for treatment of severe delirium tremens. Ann Intern Med. 1975; 82:175.
39. Anthony RM et al: Paraldehyde pharmacokinetics in ethanol abusers (abstract). Fed Proc. 1977; 36:285.
40. Kaim SC et al: Treatment of the acute alcohol withdrawal state: a comparison of four drugs. Am J Psychiatry. 1969; 125:1640.
41. Sellers EM et al: Alcohol intoxication and withdrawal. N Engl J Med. 1976; 294:757.
42. Choice of benzodiazepines. Med Let Drugs Ther. 1981; 23:41.
43. Greenblatt DJ: Clinical pharmacokinetics of oxazepam and lorazepam. Clin Pharmacokinetics. 1981; 6:89.
44. Ameer B et al: Lorazepam: a review of its clinical pharmacological properties and therapeutic uses. Drugs. 1981; 21:161.

45. Schenker S et al: Hepatic and Wernicke's encephalo-pathies: current concepts of pathogenesis. Am J Clin Nutr. 1980; 33:2719.

46. Appel SH: Neurological syndromes associated with alcohol. In *Phenomenology and Treatment of Alcoholism,* edited by WE Fann, I Karacan, AD Pokorny and RL Williams, Spectrum Publications, New York, 1980, p 69.

47. Hoyumpa AM: Mechanisms of thiamine deficiency in chronic alcoholism. Am J Clin Nutr. 1980; 33:2750.

48. Wood B et al: Thiamine status in alcoholism. Aust NZ J Med. 1977; 7:475.

49. Thomson AD et al: Observations on the mechanism of thiamine hydrochloride absorption in man. Clin Sci. 1972; 43:153.

50. Butters N et al: Clinical symptoms, neuropathology, and etiology. In *Alcoholic Korsakoff's Syndrome,* Academic Press, New York, 1980, p 1.

51. Feuerlein W: Neuropsychiatric disorders of alcoholism. Nutr Metab. 1977; 21:163.

52. Robinson D: *Talking Out of Alcoholism. The Self-Help Process of Alcoholics Anonymous,* University Park Press, Baltimore, 1979.

53. Pattison EM: The selection of treatment modalities for the alcoholic patient. In *The Diagnosis and Treatment of Alcoholism,* edited by JH Mendelson and NK Mello, McGraw-Hill, New York, 1979, p 128.

54. Beckman LJ: An attributional analysis of Alcoholics Anonymous. J Stud Alcohol. 1980; 41:714.

55. Patek AJ et al: Recovery from alcoholism in cirrhotic patients. Am J Med. 1981; 70:782.

56. Armor DJ et al: *Alcoholism and Treatment.* National Institute on Alcohol Abuse and Alcoholism (NIAAA) Report, No. R-1739, 1976.

57. Miller WR et al: Abstinence and controlled drinking in the treatment of problem drinkers. J Stud Alcohol. 1977; 38:986.

58. Fried R: Biochemical actions of anti-alcoholic agents. Substance Alcohol Actions/Misuse. 1980; 1:5.

59. Kwentus J et al: Disulfiram in the treatment of alcoholism. J Stud Alcohol. 1979; 40:428.

60. Lundwall L et al: Disulfiram treatment of alcoholism. J Nerv Ment Dis. 1971; 153:381.

61. Eneanya DI et al: The actions and metabolic fate of disulfiram. Ann Rev Pharmacol Toxicol. 1981; 21:575.

62. Hald J et al: A drug sensitizing the organism to ethyl alcohol. Lancet. 1948; 2:1001.

63. Elenbaas RM: Drug therapy reviews: management of the disulfiram-alcohol reaction. Am J Hosp Pharm. 1977; 34:827.

64. Baekeland F et al: Correlates of outcome in disulfiram treatment of alcoholism. J Nerv Ment Dis. 1971; 153:1.

65. Fuller RK et al: Disulfiram for the treatment of alcoholism. Ann Intern Med. 1979; 90:901.

66. Stoll D et al: Disulfiram-alcohol skin reaction to beer-containing shampoo (letter). JAMA. 1980; 244:2045.

67. Haley TJ: Disulfiram: a reappraisal of its toxicity and therapeutic application. Drug Metab Rev. 1979; 9:319.

68. Eisen HJ et al: Disulfiram hepatotoxicity (letter). Ann Intern Med. 1975; 83:673.

69. Ranek L et al: Disulfiram hepatotoxicity. Br Med J. 1977; 2:94.

70. Keeffe EB et al: Disulfiram hypersensitivity hepatitis. JAMA. 1974; 230:435.

71. Goyer PF et al: Hepatotoxicity in disulfiram-treated patients. J Stud Alcohol. 1979; 40:133.

72. Taylor JW et al: Mathematical analysis of a phenytoin-disulfiram interaction. Am J Hosp Pharm. 1981; 38:93.

73. Hansten PD: *Drug Interactions,* 4th ed, Lea and Febiger, Philadelphia, 1979.

74. O'Reilly RA: Dynamic interaction between disulfiram and separated enantiomorphs of racemic warfarin. Clin Pharmacol Ther. 1981; 29:332.

75. Viamontes JA: Review of drug effectiveness in the treatment of alcoholism. Am J Psychiatry. 1972; 128:1570.

76. Mottin JL: Drug-induced attenuation of alcohol consumption. Quart J Stud Alcohol. 1973; 34:444.

77. Huey LY: Psychiatric problems of alcoholics. Postgrad Med. 1978; 64:123.

78. Schuckit MA: Alcoholism and affective disorder: diagnostic confusion. In *Alcoholism and Affective Disorders,* edited by DW Goodwin and CK Erickson, Spectrum Publications, New York, 1979, p 9.

79. Kline NS et al: Lithium therapy in alcoholism. In *Alcoholism and Affective Disorders,* edited by DW Goodwin and CK Erickson, Spectrum Publications, New York, 1979, p 21.

80. Reynolds CM et al: Prophylactic treatment of alcoholism by lithium carbonate: an initial report. In *Alcoholism and Affective Disorders,* edited by DW Goodwin and CK Erickson, Spectrum Publications, New York, 1979, p 31.

81. Lindenbaum J: Folate and vitamin B_{12} deficiencies in alcoholism. Semin Hematol. 1980; 17:119.

82. Lindenbaum J et al: Nutritional anemia in alcoholism. Am J Clin Nutr. 1980; 33:2727.

83. Eichner ER: The hematologic disorders of alcoholism. Am J Med. 1973; 54:621.

84. Romero JJ et al: Intestinal absorption of folic acid in the chronic alcoholic monkey. Gastroenterology. 1981; 80:99.

85. Mezey E: Effect of ethanol on folate transport by hepatocytes (editorial). Gastroenterology. 1980; 78:872.

86. Halsted CH: Folate deficiency in alcoholism. Am J Clin Nutr. 1980; 33:2736.

87. Cooper RA: Hemolytic syndromes and red cell membrane abnormalities in liver disease. Semin Hematol. 1980; 17:103.

88. Ibrahim NG et al: Ethanol inhibition of rabbit reticulocyte haem synthesis at the level of aminolaevulinic acid synthetase. Br J Haematol. 1979; 41:235.

89. Sullivan LW et al: Suppression of hematopoiesis by ethanol. J Clin Invest. 1964; 43:2048.

90. Liu YK: Effects of alcohol on granulocytes and lymphocytes. Semin Hematol. 1980; 17:130.

91. Bjorkholm M: Immunological and hematological abnormalities in chronic alcoholism. Acta Med Scand. 1980; 207:197.

92. Liu YK: Leukopenia in alcoholics. Am J Med. 1973; 54:605.

93. Cowan DH: Effect of alcoholism on hemostasis. Semin Hematol. 1980; 17:137.

94. Alcoholic liver disease: morphological manifestations. Lancet. 1981; 1:707.

95. Thaler H: Alcohol consumption and diseases of the liver. Nutr Metab. 1977; 21:186.

96. Lesesne HR et al: Alcoholic liver disease. Postgrad Med. 1973; 53:101.

97. Viteri AL et al: Alcohol and liver disease. Postgrad Med. 1977; 61:184.

98. Mitchell JR et al: Isoniazid liver injury: clinical spectrum, pathology, and probable pathogenesis. Ann Intern Med. 1976; 84:181.

99. Gronhagen-Riska C et al: Predisposing factors in hepatitis induced by isoniazid-rifampin treatment of tuberculosis. Am Rev Respir Dis. 1978; 118:461.

100. Kopanoff DE et al: Isoniazid-related hepatitis. Am Rev Respir Dis. 1978; 117:991.

101. Cross FS et al: Rifampin-isoniazid therapy of alcoholic and nonalcoholic tuberculosis patients in a U.S. Public Health Service cooperative therapy trial. Am Rev Respir Dis. 1980; 122:349.

102. Nasrallah SM et al: Aminoacid therapy of alcoholic hepatitis. Lancet. 1980; 2:1276.

103. Kawanishi H et al: Impaired concanavalin A-inducible suppressor T-cell activity in active alcoholic liver disease. Gastroenterology. 1981; 80:510.

104. Helman RA et al: Alcoholic hepatitis-natural history and evaluation of prednisolone therapy. Ann Intern Med. 1971; 74:311.

105. Blitzer BL et al: Adrenocorticosteroid therapy in alcoholic hepatitis. Am J Dig Dis. 1977; 22:477.

106. Maddrey WC et al: Corticosteroid therapy of alcoholic hepatitis. Gastroenterology. 1978; 75:193.

107. Lesesne HR et al: Treatment of alcoholic hepatitis with encephalopathy. Gastroenterology. 1978; 74:169.

108. Porter HP et al: Corticosteroid therapy in severe alcoholic hepatitis. N Engl J Med. 1971; 284:1350.

109. Campra JL et al: Prednisone therapy of acute alcoholic hepatitis. Ann Intern Med. 1973; 79:625.

110. Shumaker JB et al: A controlled trial of 6-methylprednisolone in acute alcoholic hepatitis. Am J Gastroenterol. 1978; 69:443.

111. Depew W et al: Double-blind controlled trial of prednisolone therapy in patients with severe acute alcoholic hepatitis and spontaneous encephalopathy. Gastroenterology. 1980; 78:524.

112. Iseman MD: Containment of tuberculosis—preventive therapy with isoniazid and contact investigation. Chest. 1979; 76:801 (suppl).

113. Cello JP: Gastroesophageal variceal hemorrhage. West J Med. 1979; 130:531.

114. Chojkier M et al: A controlled comparison of continuous intraarterial and intravenous infusions of vasopressin in hemorrhage from esophageal varices. Gastroenterology. 1979; 77:540.

115. Barr JW et al: Similarity of arterial and intravenous vasopressin on portal and systemic hemodynamics. Gastroenterology. 1975; 69:13.

116. Johnston GW et al: A review of 15 years' experience in the use of sclerotherapy in the control of acute haemorrhage from oesophageal varices. Br J Surg. 1973; 60:797.

117. Terblanche J et al: A prospective evaluation of injection sclerotherapy in the treatment of acute bleeding from esophageal varices. Surgery. 1979; 85:239.

118. Clark AW et al: Prospective controlled trial of injection sclerotherapy in patients with cirrhosis and recent variceal haemorrhage. Lancet. 1980; 2:552.

119. Johanson CA: Unpublished data. San Francisco, 1981.

120. Graham DY et al: The course of patients after variceal hemorrhage. Gastroenterology. 1981; 80:800.

121. Bosch J et al: Effects of somatostatin on hepatic and systemic hemodynamics in patients with cirrhosis of the liver: comparison with vasopressin. Gastroenterology. 1981; 80:518.

122. Kelly KJ et al: Vasopressin provocation of ventricular dysrhythmia. Ann Intern Med. 1980; 92:205.

123. Marubbio AT: Antidiuretic hormone effect of pitressin during continuous pitressin infusion (letter). Gastroenterology. 1972; 62:1103.

124. Crocker MC: Intravascular guanethidine in the treatment of extravasated vasopressin. N Engl J Med. 1981; 304:1430.

125. Ettinger PO et al: Arrhythmias and the "holiday heart": alcohol-associated cardiac rhythm disorders. Am Heart J. 1978; 95:555.

126. Greenspon AJ et al: Provocation of ventricular tachycardia after consumption of alcohol. N Engl J Med. 1979; 301:1049.

127. Regan TJ et al: Varied cardiac abnormalities in alcoholics. Alcoholism: Clin Exper Res. 1979; 3:40.

128. Regan TJ: Of beverages, cigarettes and cardiac arrhythmias (editorial). N Engl J Med. 1979; 301:1060.

129. Alcoholic heart disease (editorial). Lancet. 1980; 1:961.

130. Welch CC: Alcoholic heart disease. Postgrad Med. 1977; 61:138.

131. Rubin E: Alcoholic myopathy in heart and skeletal muscle. N Engl J Med. 1979; 301:28.

132. Bing RJ: Cardiac metabolism: its contributions to alcoholic heart disease and myocardial failure. Circulation. 1978; 58:965.

133. Askanas A et al: The heart in chronic alcoholism: a noninvasive study. Am Heart J. 1980; 99:9.

134. Steinberg JD et al: Prevalence of clinically occult cardiomyopathy in chronic alcoholism. Am Heart J. 1981; 101:461.

135. Follender AB: Neurologic problems prevalent in alcoholics. Postgrad Med. 1977; 61:166.

136. Behse F et al: Alcoholic neuropathy: clinical, electrophysiological, and biopsy findings. Ann Neurol. 1977; 2:95.

137. Licht H et al: Apparent potentiation of acetaminophen hepatotoxicity by alcohol. Ann Intern Med. 1980; 92:511.

138. LaBrecque DR et al: Increased hepatotoxicity of acetaminophen in the alcoholic (abstract). Gastroenterology. 1980; 78:1310.

139. McClain CJ et al: Potentiation of acetaminophen hepatotoxicity by alcohol. JAMA. 1980; 244:251.

140. Strubelt O: Interactions between ethanol and other hepatotoxic agents. Biochem Pharmacol. 1980; 29:1445.

141. Sato C et al: Increased hepatotoxicity of acetaminophen after chronic ethanol consumption in the rat. Gastroenterology. 1981; 80:140.

142. Drummer S et al: Antabuse-like effect of B-lactam antibiotics (letter). N Engl J Med. 1980; 303:1417.

143. Foster TS et al: Disulfiram-like reaction associated with a parenteral cephalosporin. Am J Hosp Pharm. 1980; 37:858.

144. Portier H et al: Interaction between cephalosporins and alcohol (letter). Lancet. 1980; 2:263.

145. Reeves DS et al: Antabuse effect with cephalosporins (letter). Lancet. 1980; 2:540.

146. Desmond PV et al: Short-term ethanol administration impairs the elimination of chlordiazepoxide (Librium) in man. Eur J Clin Pharmacol. 1980; 18:275.

147. Hoyumpa AM et al: Effect of ethanol on benzodiazepine disposition in dogs. J Lab Clin Med. 1980; 95:310.

148. Whiting B et al: Effect of acute alcohol intoxication on the metabolism and plasma kinetics of chlordiazepoxide. Br J Clin Pharmacol. 1979; 7:95.

149. Zysset T et al: Increased systemic availability of drugs during acute ethanol intoxication: studies with mephenytoin in the dog. J Pharmacol Exper Ther. 1980; 213:173.

150. Linnoila M et al: Drug interactions with alcohol. Drugs. 1979; 18:299.

151. Sellers EM et al: Drug kinetics and alcohol ingestion. Clin Pharmacokinetics. 1978; 3:440.

152. Vesell ES: Elucidation of the pharmacokinetic interaction between acutely administered ethanol and benzodiazepines (editorial). J Lab Clin Med. 1980; 95:305.

153. Neal EA et al: Enhanced bioavailability and decreased clearance of analgesics in patients with cirrhosis. Gastroenterology. 1979; 77:96.

154. Blaschke TF: Protein binding and kinetics of drugs in liver diseases. Clin Pharmacokinetics. 1977; 2:32.

155. Piafsky KM: Disease-induced changes in the plasma binding of basic drugs. Clin Pharmacokinetics. 1980; 5:246.

156. Williams RL et al: Hepatic disease and drug pharmacokinetics. Clin Pharmacokinetics. 1980; 5:528.

Chapter 48

Vascular Headache

Juan R. Robayo

The nature and severity of headache are not always reflective of the pathology which it represents; both benign and malignant conditions may be manifested with the same intensity. Fortunately, vascular headaches are descriptive enough to be diagnosed by the clinician, and drug therapy can be initiated to abort an attack or to prevent future episodes. However, etiologies of the various types of vascular headaches are not well understood; and as a result, therapy is empiric.

During a migraine attack, a number of vascular changes occur as a result of complex relationships among the prostaglandins (particularly prostaglandin E-1), serotonin, tyramine, renin, angiotensin, and estrogenic substances. Consequently, the patient may experience pulsation and tenderness of the temporal arteries and prominent veins of the forehead and temple, flushed skin, increased perspiration, intracerebral arterial constriction, extracerebral arterial dilatation, nausea, vomiting, diarrhea, visual disturbances, photophobia, lightheadedness, and vertigo (1,5,8–14).

Vascular headaches of the migrainous type (Table 1) affect prepubertal male and female children in about equal numbers, but affect two to three times more young women than men (2,5,14). Because these headaches affect young women more commonly, hormonal changes, either endogenous or exogenous, may play a significant role in their etiology (1,2,4–6,9).

During a vascular headache not all areas of the head are affected; in fact, the majority of the anatomical regions in the head are not sensitive to pain. Those which are pain-sensitive are the scalp, the intracranial venous sinuses, the dura at the base of the skull, the large arteries at the base of the brain and the cranial nerves V,VII,IX and X (1). These are all subject to various neuronal and hormonal controls. The site of pain is, however, unilateral in about 70% of the cases, and about 20% of patients will have pain on the same side during each episode (1,5,7).

There are many factors which may precipitate vascular headaches: stress or nervous tension, worry, alcohol, hormonal changes, glare, physical exertion, lack of sleep, noise, foods which contain nitrites, glutamates, tyramines, and drugs like nitroglycerin, hydralazine, oral contraceptives, reserpine and corticosteroid withdrawal. Other more severe medical causes such as brain tumors, abscesses, subdural hematomas, cerebral hemorrhages, glaucoma, and bacterial meningitis must be ruled out (15).

Innovative Therapies. While emphasis will be given in this chapter to currently accepted and approved therapies, other therapies will be presented (Tables 4,6). Drugs like heparin, reserpine, bromocriptine, dipyridamole, clonidine, prednisone and cyproheptadine, among others, merit consideration because in some respects these represent futuristic therapies and are in concert with current concepts (8,9).

1. *Classic Migraine.* **A 25-year-old woman comes to the hospital because of a right-sided, frontal-temporal, throbbing headache not relieved by 975 mg of aspirin. The headache was preceded by scotomas and numbness with tingling of the face and is accompanied by nausea, vomiting, and photophobia. Con-**

tributory history includes a hysterectomy several months earlier, after which she had been prescribed estrogen replacement therapy; since that time she has had several similar headaches of two days duration. The physical examination is unremarkable, and a careful neurologic examination is within normal limits. The admitting diagnosis is "Vascular Headache, Classic Migraine Type." What subjective and objective data from the above description are consistent with classic migraine, and what is the most likely etiology in this patient?

In view of this patient's non-remarkable findings on physical examination and negative neurologic work-up, it is highly unlikely that this headache is a symptom of a serious underlying disease. These examinations would have uncovered an underlying disease such as cranial arteritis, bacterial endocarditis, cervical disc disease, sinusitis, dental disease, glaucoma, subarachnoid hemorrhage (manifested by subhyaloid hemorrhage), or focal central nervous system dysfunction. In the face of this patient's negative neurological examination and normal physical examination, other diagnostic studies such as a cervical spine x-ray, computerized brain scanning, lumbar puncture, and isotopic brain scanning will probably not uncover a lesion. Therefore, at this point, this patient's history suggests a primary vascular headache of the classic type (Table 1). The visual manifestations or scotomas, numbness, tingling, lightheadedness, nausea, vomiting, and photophobia have been described by numerous authors to indicate a migrainous cephalgia (1,2,5,22–24). Although unilateral, throbbing headaches such as this are typical of classic migraine, some patients may present with bilateral frontal headache (24,28). Prodromal symptoms such as those experienced by this patient are seen in classic migraines, but they are absent in the more frequently occurring common type migraine. There is often a positive family history in classic migraine, whereas a genetic association is less clear in the common variety. In this case, the most likely etiology is hormonal imbalance, requiring an adjustment in her estrogen therapy. (Also see the chapter entitled Contraception.)

Table 1.

CLASSIFICATION OF HEADACHE[1,2,4,5,6,105]

I. VASCULAR
   A. Migraine Type
      1. Classic
      2. Common

   B. Non-Migraine Type
      1. Hemiplegic
      2. Ophthalmoplegic
      3. Lower-half (Facial)

   C. Cluster (histaminic or Horton's Cephalalgia)

II. MUSCLE CONTRACTION (PSYCHOGENIC)
   1. Tension
   2. Depression

III. COMBINED VASCULAR AND MUSCLE CONTRACTION

IV. TRACTION AND INFLAMMATORY
   1. Mass lesions (tumors, hematomas)
   2. Diseases of eyes, ears, nose, throat and teeth
   3. Cranial neuralgias
   4. Allergies
   5. Infections (meningitis)
   6. Arteritis, phlebitis
   7. Occlusive vascular disease

V. DELUSIONAL CONVERSION, OR HYPOCHONDRIACAL STATES

2. How should this patient's acute attack be treated?

The treatments for acute migraine attacks are

presented in Table 2. The fact that this patient's attack is unresponsive to aspirin and requires hospitalization indicates that aggressive therapy is necessary. In addition to rest in a quiet room (30), ergotamine tartrate 2 mg sublingually, rather than orally, should be given after the aura, when the vasoconstrictive phase is over. Additional doses of 1 mg should be given every one-half hour if no improvement occurs, to a maximum of 6 mg per attack. Most clinicians consider this to be the vasoconstrictor of choice (1,6,16,31,32). Other vasoconstrictors such as ergonovine maleate or isometheptene may be given if ergotamine tartrate is not tolerated; these are not more effective, but

Table 2.

ABORTIVE TREATMENT OF MIGRAINE ATTACK*

Drug	Dose/Day	Route	References
ANALGESICS			
Aspirin	325–975 mg qid	oral, rectal	30,35,111
Acetaminophen	325–975 mg qid	oral, rectal	30,35
Codeine	30–60 mg qid	oral, parenteral	35,79,111
Morphine	5–10 mg qid	parenteral	35,79,111
ANTIEMETICS			
Chlorpromazine	25–50 mg qid	parenteral, rectal	30,31,32,35
Prochlorperazine	5–25 mg tid-qid	parenteral, rectal	32
Thiethylperazine	10 mg tid	oral, rectal, parenteral	30,32
VASOCONSTRICTORS			
Ergotamine tartrate	1–2 mg "stat," repeat every ½ hr to a maximum of 6 mg per attack.	oral, sublingual, rectal	30,111,117,121
	0.25–0.5 mg "stat," repeat in 1–2 hours, if necessary	parenteral	4,30,111,117,121
	0.36 mg q 5 min, maximum of 6 inhalations in 24 hours	inhalation	4,111,117,121
Midrin	2 capsules "stat," followed by 1 capsule q 1 hr until relief, but not more than 5 capsules in 12 hr period	oral	4,32,33,120
Ergonovine maleate	0.2–0.4 mg q 1 hr, not to exceed 2 mg total	oral, parenteral	35
Dihydroergotamine mesylate	1 mg at first warning, repeat at 1 hr intervals up to 3 mg, if necessary	parenteral	4
SEDATIVES			
Diazepam	5–10 mg tid	oral	30
Sodium amobarbital	50–60 mg bid	oral	30
STEROIDS			
Prednisone (To be tapered over 3 to 4 days)	40–60 mg/day	oral	3,111

* "Why it is that patients with nearly identical clinical headache syndromes respond differently to (antimigraines) is puzzling and remains unexplained." Headache 1980: 20:336.

they are better tolerated by some patients (5,16, 32–35).

Should there be no improvement after the maximum dose of ergotamine, then a narcotic analgesic such as morphine sulfate 10 mg intramuscularly at six hour intervals is indicated since aspirin did not seem effective.

An antiemetic such as prochlorperazine (see Table 2) should be given for the patient's nausea and vomiting. Diazepam may be given for sedation, although it may not be necessary if a narcotic and a phenothiazine have already been used (16,30,31).

Earlier therapeutic interventions yield faster results and usually require lower doses of each drug (29). The type and amount of medication required to abort an attack will likely yield similar results in subsequent attacks (5,29).

3. One of the clinicians taking care of this patient has used Cafergot-PB (ergotamine tartrate, caffeine, Bellafoline, and pentobarbital) tablets with success in the past. What is the rationale for including caffeine in some antimigraine preparations?

Caffeine by itself may be contraindicated in migraine attacks because it is a stimulant and may prevent patients from sleeping or resting during an attack; however, it has been shown to enhance drug absorption and at the same time work as a vasoconstrictor by prolonging the action of norepinephrine (5,6,29,30,36,37). In general, fixed-dose drug combinations should not be used because flexibility of dosing and individualization of therapy are lost (38–40).

4. *Common Migraine with Concomitant Medical Problems.* A 45-year-old male comes to the clinic because of severe headaches associated with a persistent numbness in his left arm. The headaches are throbbing in nature, hemicranial, accompanied by abdominal cramps, nausea and vomiting, and without an aura or prodrome. He has had four episodes in the last three months. Other medical problems include hypertension, currently treated with hydrochlorothiazide, and congenital absence of the right kidney. After a complete physical and neurologic examination, it appears that the headaches are of a vascular migrainous type. What characteristics of this patient should be considered in planning therapy? Why is he a candidate for

migraine prophylaxis, and what drugs would be appropriate?

Avoidance of Vasoconstrictors. Although migraine can manifest at any age, it is infrequent after the fourth decade of life (24). Neurological manifestations (eg, this patient's arm numbness) in older patients are of significance because their occurrence precludes the use of vasoconstrictors (1). Therefore a prophylactic approach is recommended. The criteria for migraine prophylaxis are listed in Table 3. Other examples of relative contraindications to vasoconstrictors would be patients with ischemic heart disease and patients with prolonged prodromes (1,14,24).

Migraine Prophylaxis. A variety of drugs have been employed in migraine prophylaxis (see Table 4). *Methysergide maleate* is considered by many to be the drug of choice for this purpose, although it will not abort an acute attack and its precise mechanism of action is unclear. However, some clinicians would be reluctant to use methysergide in this patient with one kidney, because fibrotic changes, including retroperitoneal fibrosis, have been associated with prolonged use (2,35,43), and renal failure due to ureteral obstruction could be a consequence. When this drug is prescribed, it should not be used for more than four to five continuous months, at which time it should be slowly tapered over a couple of weeks to provide the patient with a one-month drug holiday; then therapy can be resumed as before. Patients should be asked to report symptoms indicative of toxicity such as cold, numb or painful extremities, flank or chest pain, or dysuria because these require drug discontinuation.

Table 3.

CRITERIA FOR MIGRAINOUS HEADACHE PROPHYLAXIS[4,5,22]

1. Patients who have headaches more than once a month.
2. Patients who cannot tolerate drugs used to abort an attack.
3. Patients with significant medical problems which present relative contraindications to vasoconstrictors.
4. Patients with predictable patterns of attacks.
5. Patients whose headaches are disabling and must remain headache-free in order to function in society.

Propranolol would be a reasonable choice for migraine prophylaxis in this patient and it would also be beneficial in the treatment of his hypertension (16,44–53). It is now considered the beta-blocker of choice for migraine prophylaxis; other beta-blockers do not appear to be as effective (16,54–59). *Amitriptyline* is also effective in migraine prophylaxis, and this effect is independent of its antidepressant properties (85,86).

Other, less established treatments for migraine prophylaxis are listed in Table 4. Of the other antihypertensive medications which have been employed in migraine prophylaxis, *clonidine* has been observed by some to be effective (60–62), but others have found it either less effective than propranolol or no better than placebo (63,64). *Reserpine* may be effective but requires more study (65,66). Neither of these drugs has FDA approval for this use. It should be pointed out that vasodilators like hydralazine should be avoided in the treatment of his hypertension, because they may precipitate migraine attacks in predisposed individuals.

5. *Cluster Headache.* A 50-year-old male is referred to the neurology service because of severe, right-sided headaches which have occurred nightly and wakened him from his sleep for the past several nights. The headaches are nonthrobbing and extremely painful. They are described by the patient as severe pain with burning behind the right eye; they are accompanied by tearing, blurred vision, nasal discharge, and a droopy right

Table 4.
DRUG THERAPY IN MIGRAINE PROPHYLAXIS

Drug	Dose/Day	Route	References
VASOCONSTRICTORS			
Ergonovine maleate	0.2 mg tid	oral	35
Ergotamine tartrate	1 mg bid May skip 1–2 days a week	oral	1,4,35
BETA-BLOCKERS			
Propranolol hydrochloride	40–100 mg tid-qid	oral	4,46,47,52,58
ANTISEROTONIN			
Methysergide maleate	2 mg tid-qid	oral	16,42,117,121
Cyproheptadine hydrochloride	12–24 mg/day	oral	4,16,32,42,112,121
OTHERS			
Amitriptyline	25–200 mg/day	oral	4,16,58,85
Aspirin	325 mg bid-tid	oral	71,73
Bromocriptine	1.25–5.0 mg/day	oral	58,80,81
Carbamazepine	100 mg bid-qid	oral	119
Clonazepam	1–2 mg bid	oral	109
Clonidine	0.1 mg bid-tid	oral	4,58,60,117
Dipyridamole	25–50 mg tid-qid	oral	16,58,72
Heparin	2,500–5000 units at weekly intervals	parenteral aereosol	107,108
Indomethacin	25–50 mg tid	oral	106,117
Phenelzine	15 mg tid	oral	24,58
Reserpine	0.2 mg qod for 6–8 weeks	parenteral	66
Sulfinpyrazone	200 mg bid-qid	oral	16

Table 5.

ABORTIVE TREATMENT OF CLUSTER HEADACHE

Drug	Dose/Day	Route	References
Ergotamine tartrate	1 mg "stat," may repeat every 30 minutes to a maximum of 6 mg per 24 hours	oral	4,5,29
	2 mg "stat," may repeat every 30 minutes to a maximum of 6 mg per 24 hours	sublingual	4,5
	0.36 mg "stat," one inhalation every 5 minutes to a maximum of 6 inhalations per day.	inhalation	4,5
	1 mg "stat," not to exceed 3 mg per week	intramuscular	4,5
Dihydroergotamine	0.5–1 mg "stat," may repeat every hour to a maximum of 3 mg	parenteral	1,32,35
Methoxyflurane	10–15 drops in a handkerchief and inhale for several seconds	inhalation	110
Methysergide maleate	2 mg qid	oral	121
Prednisone	20 mg bid-qid	oral	58,96,116
Indomethacin	25 mg tid-qid	oral	58
Chlorpromazine	75–700 mg/day	oral	115,121

Table 6.

DRUG THERAPY IN CLUSTER HEADACHE PROPHYLAXIS

Drug	Dose/Day	Route	References
Methysergide maleate	2 mg tid-qid	oral	1,4,32,118
Ergotamine tartrate	1 mg bid off one day each week	oral	4,32,118
Lithium carbonate	300 mg bid-qid	oral	32,58,90,91,94,113,118
Cyproheptadine	4 mg tid-qid	oral	4,121
Methylprednisolone	16 mg qod	oral	4,32
Prednisone	20 mg bid	oral	1,32,58,118

eyelid. The episodes begin abruptly and last about half an hour. There is no history of nausea, vomiting, photophobia, or tight neck muscles. The patient has a 30-year history of cigarette smoking, one pack per day, and admits to drinking socially. The physical and neurological examinations are within normal limits. What subjective and objective evidence in this case are suggestive of cluster headache and how is it treated?

Cluster headaches frequently occur at night without prodromal symptoms. The attacks generally occur nightly for weeks or months and then disappear for months or years (hence the term *cluster*). The pain is intense and steady in nature, frequently lasts 30 to 60 minutes (rarely more than two hours), and is characterized by a uni-

lateral, orbital localization. Rhinorrhea, burning, blurred vision, lacrimation, and ptosis, all evident in this patient, commonly accompany the pain. Vomiting is rare. Cluster headaches occur predominantly in males. During periods of clustering, patients will often report that headaches are induced by vasodilators such as nitroglycerine or ethanol. This patient should avoid alcoholic beverages until the cluster resolves. The treatment of cluster headaches (Tables 5 & 6) is similar to that for migraine, but response to treatment is less reliable. Abortive treatment is complicated by the fact that the headaches are extremely rapid in onset and without prodromal symptoms. However, the headaches tend to occur at the same time each day, and treatment can be planned for their anticipated occurrence.

References

1. Dalessio DJ (Ed): Wolff's Headache and other head pain, 4th Ed, Oxford University Press, 1980.
2. Ryan RE Sr. et al: *Headache and Head Pain*, C.V. Mosby Co, Saint Louis, 1978.
3. Friedman AP: Nature of headache. Headache. 1979; 19:163.
4. Diamond S and Dalessio DJ: *The Practicing Physician's Approach to Headache*, 2nd Ed. The Williams and Wilkins Co, Baltimore, 1978.
5. Raskin NH et al: Headache. In *Major Problems in Internal Medicine*. Vol. XIX, W. B. Saunders Co., Philadelphia, Pa. 1980.
6. Rosenberg RN (Ed): *The Treatment of Neurological Diseases*, SP Medical & Scientific Books, New York, 1979.
7. Appenzeller O (Ed): *Pathogenesis and Treatment of Headache*, Spectrum Publications, Inc, New York, 1976.
8. Bruyn GW: The biochemistry of migraine. Headache. 1980; 20:235.
9. Botney M: An inquiry into the genesis of migraine headache. Headache. 1981; 21:179.
10. Dalessio DJ: Classification and mechanism of migraine. Headache. 1979; 19:114.
11. Fanchamps A: Pharmacodynamic principles of antimigraine therapy. Headache. 1975; 15:79.
12. Horrobin DF: Prostaglandins and migraine. Headache. 1977; 17:113.
13. Brainard JB: Angiotensin and aldosterone elevation in salt-induced migraine. Headache. 1981; 21:222.
14. Robayo JR et al: Vascular headaches of the migrainous type: Current theories and therapies. Hosp Pharm. 1980; 15:244.
15. DeGowin EL et al: *Bedside Diagnostic Examination*, 4th Ed, Macmillan Publishing Co, New York, 1981, pp 69–79.
16. Diamond S et al: Review article: Current thoughts on migraine. Headache. 1980; 20:208.

17. Sommerville BW: Estrogen withdrawal migraine. Duration of exposure required and attempted prophylaxis by premenstrual estrogen administration. Neurology. 1975; 25:239.
18. Desrosiers JJJ: Headaches related to contraceptive therapy and their control. Headache. 1973; 13:117.
19. Saper JR: Migraine I: Classification and pathogenesis. II: Treatment. JAMA. 1978; 239:2380. and 239:2480.
20. Hanington E: Diet and migraine. J Hum Nutr. 1980; 34:175.
21. McCulloch J et al: Phenylethylamine and cerebral blood flow. Neurology. 1977; 27:817.
22. Hedges TR: An ophthalmologist's view of headache. Headache. 1979; 19:151.
23. Melen O et al: Visual disturbances in migraine. Postgrad Med. 1978; 64:139.
24. Lance JW: *Mechanism and Management of Headache*, 3rd Ed, Butterworth, London, 1978.
25. Dalton K: Migraine and oral contraceptives. Headache. 1976; 15:247.
26. Dennerstein L et al: Headache and sex hormone therapy. Headache. 1978; 18:146.
27. Kudrow L: The relationship of headache frequency to hormone use in migraine. Headache. 1975; 15:36.
28. Olesen J: Some clinical features of the acute migraine attack. An analysis of 750 patients. Headache. 1978; 18:268.
29. Rall TW et al: Drugs affecting uterine motility. Oxytocin, prostaglandins, ergot alkaloids, and other agents. In *The Pharmacological Basis of Therapeutics*, 6th Ed, Gilman AG, Goodman LS and Gilman A (Eds), Macmillan Publishing Co., New York, 1980, pp 939–947.
30. Wilkinson M: The treatment of acute migraine attacks. Headache. 1976; 15:291.
31. Graham JR: Migraine headache: Diagnosis and management. Headache. 1979; 19:133.

32. Napolitano LV et al: Treating headache: Matching therapy to headache type. Patient Care. 1980; 14:14.

33. Diamond S: Treatment of migraine with isometheptene, acetaminophen, and dichloralphenazone combination: A double-blind, crossover trial. Headache. 1976; 15:282.

34. Ryan RE: A study of Midrin in the symptomatic relief of migraine headache. Headache. 1974; 14:33.

35. Vick NA: Headache. In: *Grinker's Neurology*, 7th Ed, Charles C. Thomas, Springfield, 1976, pp 731–742.

36. Schmidt R et al: The effect of caffeine in the intestinal absorption of ergotamine in man. Eur J Clin Pharmacol. 1974; 7:213.

37. Friedman AP: Paroxysmal disorders. Migraine and other types of headache. In *Textbook of Neurology*, 6th Ed, Edited by Merritt HH, Lea & Febiger, Philadelphia, 1979 p 839.

38. Herxheimer H: The danger of fixed drug combinations. Int J Clin Pharmacol. 1975;12:70.

39. Crout JR: Fixed combinations prescription drugs: FDA policy. J Clin Pharmacol. 1974; 14:249.

40. Dengler HJ et al: Report of a workshop on fixed-ratio drug combinations. Europ J Clin Pharmacol. 1975; 8:149.

41. Sicuteri F: Prophylactic and therapeutic properties of 1-methyl-lysergic acid butanolamide in migraine: Preliminary report. Int Arch Allergy Appl Immunol. 1959; 15:300.

42. Lance JW et al: Comparative trial of serotonin antagonists in the management of migraine. Br Med J. 1970; 2:327.

43. McComb JE et al: Retroperitoneal fibrosis: Case presentation and review of the literature. Ariz Med. 1979; 36:63.

44. Rabkin R et al: The prophylactic value of propranolol in angina pectoris. Am J Cardiol. 1966; 18:370.

45. Wykes P: The treatment of angina pectoris with coexistent migraine. Practitioner. 1968; 200:702.

46. Borgesen SE et al: Prophylactic treatment of migraine with propranolol. Acta Neurol Scand. 1974; 50:651.

47. Wideroe TE et al: Propranolol in the treatment of migraine. Br Med J. 1974; 2:699.

48. Weber RB et al: The treatment of migraine with propranolol. Neurology. 1972; 22:366.

49. Malvea BP et al: Propranolol prophylaxis of migraine. Headache. 1973; 12:163.

50. Nair KG: A pilot study of the value of propranolol in migraine. J Postgrad Med. 1975; 21:111.

51. Ludvigsson J: Propranolol used in prophylaxis of migraine in children. Acta Neurol Scand. 1974; 50:109.

52. Forssman B et al: Propranolol for migraine prophylaxis. Headache. 1976; 16:238.

53. Borgesen SE: Propranolol for migraine. Compr Ther. 1977; 3:53.

54. Anthony M: Beta-blockers in migraine prophylaxis. Drugs. 1978; 15:249.

55. Ekbom K: Alprenolol for migraine prophylaxis. Headache. 1975; 15:129.

56. Briggs RS et al: Timolol in migraine prophylaxis. Headache. 1979; 19:379.

57. Stensrud P et al: Comparative trial of Tenormin (atenolol) and Inderal (propranolol) in migraine. Headache. 1980; 20:204.

58. Diamond S and Medina JL: Newer drug therapies for headache. Postgrad Med. 1980 (July); 68:125.

59. Mathew NT: Prophylaxis of migraine and mixed headache. A randomized controlled study. Headache. 1981; 21:105.

60. Kallanranta T et al: Clonidine in migraine prophylaxis. Headache. 1977; 17:169.

61. Heathfield KWG et al: The long-term management of migraine with clonidine. Practitioner. 1978; 208:644.

62. Sillanpaa M: Clonidine prophylaxis of childhood migraine and other vascular headache. A double-blind study of 57 children. Headache. 1977; 17:28.

63. Das SM et al: Clonidine in prophylaxis of migraine. Acta Neurol Scandinav. 1979; 60:214.

64. Boisen E et al: Clonidine in prophylaxis of migraine. Acta Neurol Scand. 1978; 58:288.

65. Fog-Moller F et al: Therapeutic effect of reserpine on migraine: Relationship to blood amine levels. Headache. 1976; 15:275.

66. Nattero G et al: Reserpine for migraine prophylaxis. Headache. 1976; 15:279.

67. Carroll JD et al: The effects of reserpine injection on methysergide treated control and migrainous subjects. Headache. 1974; 14:149.

68. Couch JR et al: Platelet aggregability in migraine. Neurology. 1977; 27:843.

69. Hanington E et al: Migraine: A platelet disorder. Lancet. 1981; 11:720.

70. Dalessio DJ: Use of platelet antagonists in the treatment of migraine. Headache. 1976; 16:129.

71. O'Neill BP et al: Aspirin prophylaxis in migraine. Lancet. 1978; 2:1179.

72. Masel BE et al: Platelet antagonists in migraine prophylaxis. A clinical trial using aspirin and dipyridamole. Headache. 1980; 20:13.

73. Ryan ER and Ryan ER: Migraine prophylaxis: A new approach. Laryngoscope. 1981; 91:1501.

74. Jick H: Effects of aspirin and acetaminophen in gastrointestinal hemorrhage. Results from the Boston Collaborative Drug Surveillance Program. Arch Intern Med. 1981; 141:316.

75. Kapplan NM: Cardiovascular complications of oral contraceptives. Ann Rev Med. 1978; 29:31.

76. Mann JI et al: Oral contraceptives and death from myocardial infarction. Br Med J. 1975; 2:245.

77. Pearce J: Migraine: A psychosomatic disorder. Headache. 1977; 17:125.

78. Diamond S et al: Panel discussion: The use of analgesics in headache. Headache. 1979; 19:185.

79. Parnell P: Tranquilizers and mood elevators in the treatment of migraine: An analysis of the Migraine foundation questionnaire. Headache. 1979; 19:78.

80. Hockaday JM et al: Bromocriptine in migraine. Headache. 1976; 16:109.

81. Graham JJ et al: Prolactin suppression in the treatment of premenstrual syndrome. Med J Austral. 1978; 2:18.

82. Couch JR: Evaluation of the relationship between migraine headache and depression. Headache. 1975; 15:41.

83. Friedman AP: Prophylaxis of migraine. Headache. 1973; 13:104.

84. Friedman AP: Migraine. Symposium on headache and related pain syndromes. Med Clin North Am. 1978; 62:481.

85. Couch JR et al: Amitriptyline in the prophylaxis of migraine. Neurology. 1976; 26:121.

86. Couch JR: Amitriptyline in migraine prophylaxis. Arch Neurol. 1979; 36:695.

87. Medina JL et al: The nature of cluster headache. Headache. 1979; 19:309.

88. Kutt H et al: Neurological diseases. In: *Drug Treatment. Principles and Practice of Clinical Pharmacology and Therapeutics,* 2nd ed., edited by Avery GS, Adis Press, Sydney, 1980, p 1034–1036.

89. Ekbom K: Lithium in the treatment of chronic cluster headache. Headache. 1977; 17:39.

90. Kudrow L: Lithium prophylaxis for chronic cluster headache. Headache. 1977: 17:15.

91. Mathew NT: Clinical subtypes of cluster headache and response to lithium therapy. Headache. 1978; 18:26.

92. Medina JL et al: Lithium carbonate therapy for cluster headache. Arch Neurol. 1980; 37:559.

93. Lieb J et al: Lithium treatment of chronic cluster headaches. Br J Psych. 1978: 133:556.

94. Ekbom K: Lithium for cluster headache: Review of the literature and preliminary results of long-term treatment. Headache. 1981; 21:132.

95. Amdisen A: Lithium. In: *Applied Pharmacokinetics: Principles of Therapeutic Drug Monitoring,* edited by Evans WE, Schentag JJ and Jusko WJ, Applied Therapeutics Inc., San Francisco, 1980, p 586–617.

96. Couch JR et al: Prednisone therapy for cluster headache. Headache. 1978; 18:219.

97. Kudrow L: Prevalence of migraine, peptic ulcer, coronary heart disease and hypertension in cluster headache. Headache. 1976;16:66.

98. Conn HO et al: Nonassociation of adrenocorticosteroid therapy and peptic ulcer. N Engl J Med. 1976; 294:473.

99. Andersson PG: Ergotamine headache. Headache. 1975; 15:118.

100. Medina JT et al: Drug dependency in patients with chronic headaches. Headache. 1977; 17:12.

101. Rowsell AR et al: Ergotamine-induced headaches in migrainous patients. Headache. 1973; 13:65.

102. Klimek A et al: The phenomenon of "drug dependency" in the treatment of migraine with propranolol. Headache. 1977; 17:75.

103. Euge I et al: Ergotism due to therapeutic doses of ergotamine tartrate. Am Heart J. 1965; 70:665.

104. Apesos J et al: Lower extremity arterial insufficiency after long-term methysergide maleate therapy. Arch Surg. 1979; 114:964.

105. Classification of Headache: Ad Hoc Committee on Classification of Headache. JAMA. 1962; 179;127.

106. Anthony M et al: Indomethacin in migraine. Med J Austral. 1968; 1:56.

107. Thonnard-Neumann E: Migraine therapy with heparin: Pathophysiologic basis. Headache. 1977; 16:284.

108. Thonnard-Neumann E: Heparin in migraine headache. Headache. 1973; 13:49.

109. Stensrud P et al: Clonazepam (Rivotril) in migraine prophylaxis. Headache. 1979; 19:333.

110. Kudrow L: Cluster headache: Diagnosis and management. Headache. 1979; 19:142.

111. Edmeads J: Management of the acute attack of migraine. Headache. 1973; 13:91.

112. Klimek A: Cyproheptadine in the treatment of migraine and related headache. Ther Hung. 1979; 27:93.

113. Klimek A et al: Lithium therapy in cluster headache. Eur Neurol. 1979; 18:267.

114. Raskin NH and Schwartz RK: Interval therapy of migraine: Long-term results. Headache. 1980; 20:336.

115. Caviness VS and O'Brien P: Cluster headache: Response to chlorpromazine. Headache. 1980; 20:128.

116. Jammes JL: The treatment of cluster headaches with prednisone. Dis Nerv Syst. 1975; 36:375.

117. Parkes JD: Diseases of the central nervous system. Relief of pain: headache, facial neuralgia, migraine, and phantom limb. Br Med J. 1975; 4:90.

118. Kudrow L: Cluster headache: Diagnosis and management. Headache. 1979; 19:142.

119. Murray TJ: Migraine: An overview. Can Pharm J. 1977; 110:150.

120. Popovich NG et al: Therapeutic management of migraine headache. U.S. Pharmacist. 1980; 5:37.

121. Diamond S and Baltes BJ: Chemotherapy of severe headache. Drug Ther. 1972; 2:28.

Chapter 49

Parkinson's Disease

Sam K. Shimomura

Clinical Presentation

Parkinsonism is a neurological disease characterized by tremor, akinesia, rigidity, and disorders of posture and equilibrium. The onset is slow and progressive, with symptoms manifesting themselves over several months to several years. The tremor of parkinsonism, which is probably the most obvious outward sign, is regular and rhythmic; it is most conspicuous when the patient is at rest, but is absent during sleep.

The rigidity, caused by the hypertonicity of the muscles acting against each other, may assume a characteristic "cogwheel" quality. Bradykinesia is the most incapacitating feature of the disease. Early signs of parkinsonism are usually unilateral and almost imperceptible at first and then slowly progress in severity and spread from one area of involvement to the whole body. Another sign of Parkinson's disease is a loss of facial movement resulting in a masklike face. Changes in handwriting are also one of the initial signs of parkinsonism; the script becomes small and illegible as the tremor worsens. Postural instability is one of the later findings in the disease and may progress to the characteristic festinating gait of parkinsonism. Other signs and symptoms are sialorrhea, seborrhea, constipation, and changes in speech and mentation (1,2).

An estimated 200,000 to 400,000 persons in the United States are afflicted with this neurological disorder, and an estimated 40,000 new cases become apparent each year (2,3,4). Parkinson's disease is slightly more common in men than in women (1). A detailed analysis of 672 cases of idiopathic parkinsonism by Hoehn et al (5) showed that the mean age of onset of the disease was 55.3 years, and two-thirds of these patients developed the disease between the ages of 50 and 69. The age of onset was the same for men as for women. The mortality rate was found to be nearly three times that of the general population of the same age, sex, and race. The mean duration of illness from diagnosis to death was 9.4 years for primary parkinsonism. The most common cause of death is not the disease itself, but arteriosclerotic heart disease, bronchopneumonia, and malignant neoplasms. The study by Hoehn was performed before the introduction of levodopa in 1967. Since then, long-term studies indicate that levodopa reduces the overall mortality by about 50% (6,7).

Pathogenesis

Although the biochemical basis of Parkinson's disease is complex, the primary defect appears to be a neurotransmitter imbalance (a relative excess of acetylcholine and an absolute deficiency of dopamine in the basal ganglia). Other neuroregulator substances such as norepinephrine, gamma aminobutyric acid, histamine and serotonin may have some modifying influence on the primary transmitters. Acetylcholine has an excitatory effect on the central nervous system and is responsible for the tremor associated with parkinsonism. This is supported by studies which demonstrate that centrally-acting cholinesterase inhibitors, such as physostigmine, aggravate parkinsonian tremor, while centrally-acting anticholinergics such as benztropine tend to diminish the tremor (8). Anticholinergics have been employed in the treatment of parkinsonism for over 100 years and were the mainstay of therapy until the introduction of levodopa.

The finding that reserpine produced a Parkinson-like syndrome by depleting the brain of dopamine provided insight into the biochemical basis of Parkinson's disease. Coupled with autopsy findings that showed an absence or deficiency of dopamine in the basal ganglia, the evidence is quite strong that dopamine deficiency is a central feature of the biochemical basis of parkinsonism. A number of drugs which act through the dopaminergic system have been shown to be effective to varying degrees in parkinsonism. Levodopa, the immediate precursor of dopamine, directly increases dopamine content in the brain and is currently the most effective treatment for parkinsonism. Several drugs eg, bromocriptine, piribedil, as well as apomorphine and its congener n-propylnoraporphine) directly stimulate dopamine receptors. Other drugs (eg, amphetamines and amantadine) may increase dopamine at the receptor either by releasing intact striatal dopamine stores or by blocking dopamine re-uptake (9,10,11).

Although this chapter emphasizes the drug therapy of idiopathic parkinsonism, drugs are only a part of an overall therapeutic regimen that also includes physiotherapy, exercise, psychological support, and occasional surgical intervention. Currently, there is no cure for this disease, and the goal of therapy is to provide maximum relief of symptoms and to maintain the independence and mobility of the patient.

Because Parkinson's disease is chronic, clinicians can come to know patients and their problems through frequent contact over many years. Careful monitoring of these patients' drug therapy is important. The drugs used for this disease require careful dose adjustment and have a high potential for adverse reactions and drug interactions. Therefore, a sympathetic and knowledgeable clinician can contribute to the education of the patient regarding his or her drug therapy, thus insuring greater compliance, fewer complications and a better prognosis.

Subjective and Objective Findings

1. A.M. is a 63-year-old female with complaints of anxiety, nervousness, tremors, and weakness of the right hand. She also has a five-year history of open-angle glaucoma that has been treated with pilocarpine 1% and a ten-year history of hypertension which has been untreated. She feels her complaints are exacerbated by stressful situations; her weakness and tremor were initially noted at the time of her husband's death three months ago. She also says that her symptoms are worsened by pressure at work and that she "feels all tied up." Her friends have told her that her voice is changing.

On physical examination, the patient is a well-developed, well-nourished, white female in no acute distress. She has noticible tremor in both hands and cogwheel rigidity of both arms. There is a slightly masklike face and sialorrhea. Her blood pressure is 190/112 mm Hg reclining and 188/105 mm Hg sitting. The rest of her history and physical examination are noncontributory. Her laboratory tests are normal except for a creatinine clearance of 50 ml per minute. What subjective and objec-

Table 1.

ANTI-PARKINSON DRUGS

Drug	Dose	Side Effects
Anticholinergics:		
Trihexyphenidyl (Artane) 2 and 5 mg tablets 5 mg time-released capsules 2 mg/5 ml elixir	1 to 5 mg tid, start with low doses. Doses over 20 mg a day are rarely tolerated.	Blurred vision, dry mouth, vertigo, drowsiness, muscle weakness, mild confusion. In toxic doses, tachycardia, hallucinations, agitation, elevation of body temperature. Contraindicated in narrow-angle glaucoma.
Biperiden (Akineton) 2 mg tablets	2 mg tid to qid.	See above.
Cycrimine (Pagitane) 1.25 and 2.5 mg tablets	Initially 1.25 mg bid to tid. Usual range 3.75 to 15 mg daily in divided doses.	See above.
Procyclidine (Kemadrin) 2 and 5 mg tablets	Initially 2.5 mg bid or tid. Usual dosage range 10 to 20 mg daily in three or four doses.	See above.
Benztropine (Cogentin) 0.5, 1.0 and 2.0 mg tablets	Initially 0.5 to 1 mg daily with slow increase to 1 to 2 mg per day. Maximum dose 6 mg in divided doses.	See above.
Diphenhydramine (Benadryl) 25 and 50 mg capsules 12.5 mg/5 ml elixir	Initially 25 mg at bedtime and 75 mg daily in divided doses. Usual range 75 to 150 mg daily with 300 mg per day maximum.	Drowsiness, confusion, dizziness, atropine-like effects.
Chlorphenoxamine (Phenoxene) 50 mg tablets	Initially 50 mg tid. May increase to 100 mg qid.	See above.
Dopaminergic Drugs:		
Levodopa (Larodopa, Dopar, Levopa, Bendopa) 100 mg, 250 mg and 500 mg	Initially 300 to 500 mg a day with slow increase to 2 to 8 grams per day.	Nausea, vomiting, anorexia, hypotension, abnormal movements, behavioral changes, cardiac arrhythmias.
Levodopa/Carbidopa (Sinemet) 100 mg/10 mg, 100 mg/25 mg and 250 mg/25 mg tablets	300/75 to 1500/150 mg per day. Maximum dose 2000/200 mg per day.	Same as above, except less nausea, vomiting, and cardiac arrhythmias.
Amantadine (Symmetrel) 100 mg capsules and syrup containing 50 mg/5 ml	100 mg with breakfast for 5 to 7 days and then 100 mg with breakfast and lunch.	Hyperexcitability, tremor, slurred speech, ataxia, depression, hallucinations, insomnia, livedo reticularis.
Bromocriptine (Parlodel) 2.5 mg tablet	Initially half of a 2.5 mg tablet twice daily with meals. Dosage may be increased by 2.5 mg per day with meals every 14–28 days. Maintenance doses averaging 15 mg a day have been effective. Maximum dose 100 mg/day.	Nausea, abnormal involuntary movements, confusion, hallucinations, dizziness, drowsiness, faintness/fainting, vomiting, asthenia, abdominal discomfort.

tive clinical data are compatible with a diagnosis of Parkinson's disease in this patient?

The subjective evidence for parkinsonism includes weakness, the feeling of being "all tied up," and the observations of friends that her voice is changing. Objective signs of her parkinsonism include tremors, cogwheel rigidity, sialorrhea, and a masklike face. Stress from her husband's death and pressures at work may have precipitated or exacerbated her disease. There are no laboratory tests to confirm a diagnosis of parkinsonism, and this diagnosis is based solely on signs, symptoms, and the exclusion of other possible neurological conditions.

Anticholinergics

2. When should anticholinergics be utilized in Parkinson's disease?

Anticholinergics are indicated in patients with relatively mild disease where tremor and sialorrhea are the most prominent features. Overall, anticholinergic drugs rarely produce more than a 20% improvement in tremor, rigidity and akinesia. They may also be used in conjunction with levodopa in those patients whose symptoms are not controlled by levodopa alone. In some patients, there may be a synergistic effect when these agents are given together (1,2,4).

3. Which is the preferred anticholinergic agent for this patient?

There are numerous, centrally-acting anticholinergic agents available on the market, but no one agent appears to be consistently superior to another or have a specific effect on a particular clinical feature of parkinsonism.

Since trihexyphenidyl is the most widely used agent, and therefore the one with the most accumulated clinical data, it would be a good choice for this patient. If a longer-acting agent is preferred, benztropine would be the drug of choice.

4. *Glaucoma.* **Are anticholinergic agents and levodopa contraindicated in this patient because of her glaucoma?**

One of the great myths concerning drugs is that systemic anticholinergics and sympathomimetic agents aggravate or even cause open-angle glaucoma. This misconception has arisen because of a lack of distinction between narrow-angle and open-angle glaucoma and topical versus sys-

temic therapy. Patients with an abnormally narrow angle between the iris and cornea may experience a dangerous rise in intraocular pressure with topical and, more rarely, with systemic anticholinergic or sympathomimetic agents. However, patients with open-angle glaucoma can safely use systemic anticholinergic drugs and levodopa in conjunction with their normal topical ophthalmic therapy (cholinergic eye drops that cause miosis). Before starting anticholinergic or sympathomimetic therapy, however, all patients should be screened for a narrow-angle anterior chamber to prevent precipitating a first attack of acute, angle-closure glaucoma (12,13). In conclusion, open-angle glaucoma is not a contraindication for using anticholinergic agents or levodopa.

5. *Adverse Effects.* **A.M. was begun on trihexyphenidyl 1 mg three times daily. What subjective and/or objective clinical data should be monitored in this patient in order to assess adverse effects from her anticholinergic therapy?**

Because of this patient's advanced age, diminished renal function, and history of psychological problems, she may be particularly sensitive to toxic effects from her anticholinergic therapy. Her intraocular pressure should be monitored, as well as such commonly seen anticholinergic effects as urinary retention, dry mouth, blurred vision, constipation, ataxia, somnolence, delusions, and hallucinations.

Amantadine

6. This patient's tremor and sialorrhea have improved, but her rigidity and ability to move freely have not improved despite increases of trihexyphenidyl to 3 mg three times daily. Due to her complaints of dry mouth, urinary retention, and drowsiness, her trihexyphenidyl dosage has been reduced, and amantadine (Symmetrel) 100 mg per day has been initiated. What might be a rationale for adding amantadine to this patient's regimen instead of levodopa? When should response to amantadine be expected?

Amantadine, originally introduced as an antiviral agent, has moderate anti-Parkinson effects. While it is not as effective as levodopa, it is also much less toxic. Amantadine should be tried in this patient before exposing her to the risks and demands of levodopa therapy. There is an almost immediate onset of action with amantadine, and if no significant improvement is seen in two weeks, the drug should be discontinued. If the patient responds to amantadine, chances are good she will also obtain good relief from levodopa (10).

7. Renal Disease. The usual adult dose of amantadine is 100 mg twice daily. Why is this dose inappropriate for this patient?

Approximately 90% of amantadine is excreted unchanged by the kidney, and it therefore quickly accumulates in patients with decreased renal function. Recommendations for dose reduction in patients with renal impairment are as follows: 100 mg bid for patients with normal renal function (Cl_{cr} 100 ml/min); 200 mg/100 mg on alternate days for Cl_{cr} of 60 ml/min; 100 mg daily for Cl_{cr} of 50 ml/min; 200 mg twice weekly for Cl_{cr} of 30 ml/min; 100 mg thrice weekly for Cl_{cr} of 20 ml/min; and 200 mg/100 mg alternating every seven days for Cl_{cr} or 10 ml/min (16). Therefore 100 mg daily would be an appropriate amantadine dose for this patient.

While there are no data which correlate plasma amantadine concentrations with therapeutic effectiveness, a dose of 200 mg per day in normal subjects usually produces steady-state plasma concentrations of 0.2 to 0.9 mcg/ml. If plasma levels are available, levels above 1.0 to 1.5 mcg/ml should be viewed with concern (16,17).

8. Adverse Effects. What subjective and/or objective clinical data should be monitored in this patient in order to detect adverse drug effects from amantadine?

In general, amantadine produces few significant adverse effects in the dosage range of 200 to 300 mg usually employed in parkinsonism. Most are mild, transient, and readily reversible upon discontinuation (eg, gastrointestinal complaints, edema, rash, and dryness of the mouth) (15). In higher doses, toxic effects such as confusion, dizziness, disorientation, depression, and hallucinations have been reported. In addition, patients taking anticholinergic agents along with amantadine are more likely to develop adverse central nervous system reactions.

9. Livedo Reticularis. A.M. has been taking amantadine 100 mg per day for five months with adequate response. She now appears in the clinic with edema of the lower legs and a faint lavender network which sometimes intensifies to an almost purplish-black color over a few minutes. This purplish mottling first appeard on the thighs and spread over the lower legs and later was found on the forearms. What is the relationship between this skin condition and A.M.'s amantadine therapy? How is this condition treated?

Amantadine has been reported to cause livedo reticularis, a condition characterized by a diffuse, rose-colored mottling of the skin; it is usually confined primarily to the lower extremities, but in some patients it also appears on the arms. A mild ankle edema commonly occurs in conjunction with the livedo reticularis, and the skin discoloration is most noticeable when the patient stands or is exposed to cold. The condition is reversible in two to six weeks upon discontinuation of the amantadine and is relatively benign clinically, even when the amantadine is continued.

The reported prevalence of amantadine-induced livedo reticularis has been quite high in several studies. In 1970, Shealy et al (18) first reported this adverse reaction in 10 of 18 female patients receiving 100 to 200 mg of amantadine for a period of a month or more. Shortly after this, Vollum et al (19) reported livedo reticularis in 21 of 21 women and 15 and 19 men who were receiving amantadine. However, Vollum also observed some degree of livedo reticularis in 32 of 51 untreated control patients who did not have Parkinson's disease. Silver and Sach (20) noted this adverse effect in 10 of 34 patients. Although livedo reticularis occurred in a high percentage of patients in these three studies, other studies of large groups of patients being treated with amantadine for parkinsonism did not mention this reaction. The only large study looking for this side effect reported a prevalence of only eight cases out of 430 patients studied (15).

Amantadine may produce this adverse effect by causing a release of norepinephrine from peripheral nerve terminals which, in turn, causes vasoconstriction. The impaired peripheral blood flow could result in the appearance of livedo reticularis and pedal edema (21).

In conclusion, the skin discoloration seen in A.M. appears to be a benign, reversible side effect that does not generally require discontinuation of amantadine.

Levodopa

10. *Early Versus Late Initiation.* A.M. is currently receiving trihexphenidyl 2.0 mg three times daily, and amantadine 100 mg per day. Her tremors are adequately controlled, but her rigidity and bradykinesia are becoming more troublesome. She is considering early retirement because of difficulty in performing job-related tasks. She lives alone with no one to help her with daily activities. Since the greatest benefit of levodopa is seen during the first few years of therapy, should levodopa be withheld until the parkinsonism causes a significant disruption in her life, or should it be started now in the hopes of returning her to a more normal lifestyle?

There has been a controversy among neurologists concerning when to start levodopa therapy. There is general agreement that after the first few years of dramatic relief from levodopa, there is a gradual fall-off in efficacy and an increase in troublesome adverse effects. Therefore, many neurologists reserve levodopa for patients with moderate to severe parkinsonism who are incapacitated by their disease (22,23). They feel by delaying the use of levodopa, or, if it is used, keeping the dosage as low as possible will help assure a longer useful period. On the other hand, some neurologists prefer to start levodopa in relatively mild cases of parkinsonism when levodopa can restore the patient to normal function. Advocates of early treatment feel that levodopa will not only confer nearly normal functioning early on in the disease, but also increase the lifespan of the patient.

A recent study looked at three groups of patients in order to determine whether duration of disease or duration of levodopa therapy was responsible for the fall-off in levodopa efficacy. Group I consisted of patients with symptoms for one to three years before beginning levodopa (N = 19); Group II patients had symptoms for four to six years (N = 16); and Group III patients, seven to nine years (N = 23). Each group had a dramatic decrease in disability in the first year followed by gradual worsening. When the total duration of disease was held constant, disability scores were similar for all three groups. For example, after six years of disease, Group I had received four years of levodopa therapy, and Group II had the drug for only one year, yet their disability scores

were similar. The data from this study suggest that duration of disease rather than duration of levodopa therapy is responsible for the gradual worsening of the disease, and delaying therapy only deprives the patient of years of improved disability and does not confer any benefits in later years (24). Based on these findings, A.M. should be started on levodopa immediately rather than waiting until she is severely disabled. Levodopa may allow her to continue working and to remain active and independent.

11. *Initiation of Therapy.* How should levodopa therapy be initiated in this patient?

Levodopa therapy is usually initiated concomitantly with the decarboxylase inhibitor, carbidopa. This combination is available in a 1:10 ratio of carbidopa to levodopa (Sinemet-10/100 and Sinemet-25/250) and in a 1:4 ratio (Sinemet-25/100). Peripheral dopa decarboxylase is saturated by a dose of 70 to 100 mg of carbidopa. Patients who are starting therapy with Sinemet-10/100 at a dose of one to two tablets three times a day may experience nausea and vomiting, because they are receiving doses of carbidopa insufficient to saturate dopa decarboxylase. For this reason, Sinemet-25/100 is the preferred tablet size for initiating therapy and for patients on low maintenance doses. It is reasonable to begin this patient on one tablet of Sinemet-25/100 three times a day and monitor her for beneficial effects on her tremor, rigidity, and bradykinesia. The dosage may be titrated upwards by 100 mg increments every day or every other day until adverse effects, such as nausea and vomiting or abnormal involuntary movements, become troublesome; an adequate therapeutic response is achieved; or a maximum dose of levodopa (2000 mg) is reached.

12. *Carbidopa.* What are the advantages and disadvantages of using carbidopa in combination with levodopa?

Levodopa is metabolized to dopamine by the enzyme, L-aromatic amino acid (dopa) decarboxylase. Since dopamine does not cross the blood-brain barrier, most of the levodopa administered orally is wasted by conversion to dopamine in the periphery. By combining levodopa with a decarboxylase inhibitor which does not cross the blood-brain barrier, a larger proportion of levodopa is available to enter the brain.

The advantages of combining a decarboxylase

inhibitor with levodopa are: (a) the dose of levodopa can be reduced about 75%; (b) a number of the peripheral side effects, such as nausea, vomiting and cardiac arrhythmias, are reduced since less levodopa metabolites are being formed; (c) the patient can be titrated to an optimal dose of levodopa in a matter of weeks rather than months, because the necessity for developing a tolerance to the peripheral side effects is diminished; (d) pyridoxine will not antagonize the therapeutic efficacy of levodopa when used with this combination; (e) fluctuations in control of the patient's symptoms are somewhat improved by the longer duration of action of the combination; and (f) the number of patients who improve and the degree of improvement are slightly greater, because peripheral side effects are minimized and relatively larger doses can be tolerated (24–26). Central nervous system side effects, such as abnormal involuntary movements and mental changes, tend to occur earlier and be more severe because more of the active drug crosses the blood-brain barrier.

13. *Adverse Effects*. What subjective or objective clinical data should be monitored in this patient to detect levodopa/carbidopa adverse effects?

Levodopa causes numerous adverse effects, most of which are more annoying than serious. The drug primarily affects the gastrointestinal, cardiovascular and central nervous systems (6,10).

Cardiac arrhythmias, such as sinus tachycardia and premature ventricular contractions, appear to be caused by dopamine, norepinephrine, and other metabolites of levodopa. Carbidopa decreases the peripheral metabolism of levodopa and decreases the prevalence of cardiac effects (26). Parkinson patients tend to have low blood pressure, and the addition of levodopa may aggravate the *hypotension,* especially early in therapy.

Levodopa causes *mental changes* manifested as depression, paranoia, agitation, delusions, hallucinations, insomnia, dementia, and loss of memory. Drug-induced mental changes are often difficult to distinguish from those caused by old age or the disease itself. These side effects can usually be controlled by a reduction of dose.

Abnormal involuntary movements occur in over half the patients taking levodopa for more than six months and present as grimacing, chewing movements, bobbing of the head and neck, rocking movements of the trunk, and active tongue movements.

14. *Hypertension in Parkinsonian Patients.* A.M.'s hypertension probably needs to be treated. How will her antihypertensive therapy be affected by her anti-Parkinson drug therapy?

Reserpine should be avoided in this patient, since it depletes CNS dopamine stores and, in high doses, may aggravate her Parkinson's disease (27). Methyldopa has been reported to both potentiate and antagonize the effects of levodopa. It may act as a "false" neurotransmitter, thus antagonizing the effect of levodopa, or it may act as a decarboxylase inhibitor, thus potentiating levodopa. Because of its unpredictable effects in patients on levodopa, it, too, should be avoided in this patient (28). (Other levodopa drug interactions are described in Table 2.)

If A.M.'s hypertension is to be treated, a thiazide diuretic would be the drug of choice, unless her renal function deteriorates to the point where thiazides are no longer effective. Uric acid levels may be elevated by thiazide diuretics. In parkinsonian patients, uric acid levels have been observed to increase, sometimes precipitously, for no apparent reason (29). When monitoring uric acid levels, it should be remembered that levodopa may cause a false elevation of serum and urinary uric acid when the colorimetric method is used, but not when the more specific uricase method is utilized. Levodopa has also been implicated in causing hyperuricemia and two cases of gout, but the validity of the report is open to question, because pretreatment evaluation of uric acid was not reported, and subsequent uric acid determinations were performed by the colorimetric method (34).

15. *"On-Off" Effect.* L.O. is a 66-year-old woman who first complained of stiffness and tremor six years ago. She was placed on trihexyphenidyl and obtained significant relief of her tremor initially. Her disease progressed with increasing rigidity and bradykinesia. Amantadine and then levodopa/carbidopa were added. She did well for the first two years of levodopa therapy but has markedly deteriorated over the past year.

She has frequent fluctuation in her response to levodopa, swinging from full-blown

Table 2.

DRUG INTERACTIONS WITH LEVODOPA

Drug	Adverse Effect	Probable Mechanism	Reference
Benzodiazepines, e.g., chlordiazepoxide and diazepam	Decreased anti-Parkinson effect in an occasional patient.	Unknown.	35
Methyldopa	May increase or decrease anti-Parkinson effect.	May increase effect because it is a decarboxylase inhibitor. The mechanism for inhibiting effect unknown, but may act as a false transmitter for dopamine in the brain.	34
Monoamine oxidase inhibitors, e.g., isocarboxazid, pargyline, phenelzine, tranylcypromine	Hypertensive crisis.	Increase in storage and release of dopamine, norepinephrine or both.	76
Neuroleptics, e.g., chlorpromazine, prochlorperazine, haloperidol	Decreased anti-Parkinson effect.	Inhibition of dopamine reuptake and blockade of dopamine receptors.	6,77
Pyridoxine	Decreased anti-Parkinson effect. Does not occur in patient receiving the combination of levodopa/ carbidopa.	Increased decarboxylation of levodopa in the periphery.	78
Phenytoin	Decreased anti-Parkinson effect.	Unknown.	79
Papaverine	Decreased anti-Parkinson effect.	Unknown.	74,75

parkinsonism to good periods when she can move and talk almost normally. More recently, the "free" periods have been getting shorter and are accompanied by severe dyskinesias. Most of the time, she is bed-bound and unable to sit or turn. She also has difficulty swallowing or speaking. The fluctuations in her status are unpredictable and are seen at various times through the day and during dosing intervals for levodopa/carbidopa.

What subjective and objective information concerning L.O. allows a distinction to be made between "on-off" phenomenon and "end-of-dose" deterioration? Why is this distinction important in terms of management of these effects in this patient?

The "on-off" effect has been described as "the sudden and abrupt onset of a marked inability to move (akinesia, "off" effect) that may last minutes to hours, followed by an equally abrupt return of the ability to move that is often accompanied by abnormal involuntary movements" (36). Dose, duration of levodopa therapy, and severity of disease may influence the frequency of this adverse effect. Sweet and McDowell reported that 50% of their patients developed the "on-off" effect over five years when the mean initial dose of levodopa was 5 gm (37). On the other hand, Shaw and associates (7) found only a 10% frequency when the mean initial dose was 3.2 gm. While the mechanism for this phenomenon has not been established, it does not appear to be correlated with blood levels of levodopa.

The "end-of-dose deterioration" or "wearing-off" subtype of the "on-off" effect is related to the blood level of levodopa. The "on" period correlates with the peak levodopa levels and the "off" period with

the trough levels. End-of-dose deterioration occurred in 65% of 178 patients in a long-term study
(7). This form of the "on-off" effect is treated by
giving more frequent, smaller doses of levodopa
to smooth out the blood level fluctuations or by
adding or switching to bromocriptine which has
a longer duration of therapy than levodopa.

It would appear, on the basis of the description
given, that L.O. suffers from classic "on-off" phenomena. Treatment of this problem is difficult.
Decreasing the dose of levodopa and imposition
of three- to seven-day drug holidays may be helpful (38,39). Administration of bromocriptine also
has been suggested as a possibly helpful measure
(37).

16. *Long-Term Efficacy.* What is the long term efficacy of levodopa? Is L.O.'s course typical?

Initially, about 75% of Parkinson patients respond favorably to levodopa therapy, but after a
period of two to three years, the response diminishes, becomes more uneven and is accompanied
by more side effects. Marsden et al report that
one-third of 400 patients followed over five years
continue to benefit from the drug; another third
have lost some of their initial response but are
still better than before treatment; and the remaining third lost all initial benefits and are worse
off than before therapy (40).

Delaney and Fermaglich report similar findings in their 70 Parkinson patients treated with
levodopa. They found that 63 patients (90%) were
improved during the first year. After five years,
only 37 patients (52.9%) remained improved, and
33 (47.1%) experienced a worsening of their condition (41).

The causes of this fall-off in efficacy in levodopa are unknown. Hypotheses include: (a) inadequate or diminished cerebral dopa decarboxylase leading to decreased conversion of levodopa
to dopamine; (b) loss of striatal dopamine receptors; and (c) loss of output pathways from the
striatum or loss of other motor pathways.

While levodopa does not appear to reverse or
even stop the progression of parkinsonism, the
improvement of mobility it affords delays the onset of fatal complications and allows a nearly normal lifespan (22,42).

17. *Alternate Modes of Therapy.* L.O. has become refractory to the therapeutic effects of levodopa; what alternate modes of therapy are being investigated?

No major advances in the drug treatment of
parkinsonism appear on the horizon. Much of the
current research is on adjuvant drugs which may
enhance the efficacy or reduce the toxicity of current agents. Development of drugs for parkinsonism is hindered by the lack of an animal model.
No animals develop this disease or anything
similar.

The *direct dopamine receptor agonists* are the
most promising group of new drugs for the treatment of parkinsonism. While levodopa requires
conversion in the brain to its active form, dopamine, this group of drugs acts directly to stimulate intact postsynaptic receptors, thereby bypassing the degenerated nigra. Several drugs in
this group (ie, apomorphine, n-propylnoraporphine, lisuride, piribedil, and lergotrile) have been
studied but largely abandoned due to lack of efficacy or intolerable side effects.

Bromocriptine appears to be nearly as effective
as levodopa and is occasionally useful in parkinsonian patients no longer responding to levodopa.
Other advantages of this direct-acting dopamine
agonist over levodopa include a longer half-life
(six to eight hours), greater efficacy against
tremors, and reduction of the "on-off" effect and
abnormal involuntary movements. On the other
hand, orthostatic hypotension and mental changes
are increased with bromocriptine. Because it is
only equal in efficacy to levodopa and higher in
central side effects and cost, bromocriptine may
not be a major advance in the treatment of parkinsonism as had earlier been expected. It is now
approved by the FDA for use in parkinsonism.

Domperidone, a specific dopamine antagonist,
has been suggested as an adjunct to bromocriptine, since it does not cross the blood-brain barrier. Thus, peripheral side effects could be reduced without interfering with the central therapeutic effects. Further studies are needed to assess the practicality of this approach (46).

The *monoamine oxidase inhibitors* are another
class of drugs currently being investigated. This
class of drugs was first tried in the early 1960's
but was too toxic and was quickly overshadowed
by the introduction of levodopa. Recently, monoamine oxidase has been found to have two forms
(MAO-A and MAO-B). MAO-B is the specific enzyme catalyzing the degradation of dopamine and
phenylethylamines. Deprenyl, an inhibitor of

MAO-B, is being studied as an adjunct to levo-dopa to enhance its effectiveness, reduce the maintenance dose, and control the wearing-off phenomenon. It has not been found to be effective in controlling the severe "yo-yo" type of the "on-off" effect. Deprenyl has little anti-Parkinson effect when given alone, and when combined with levodopa and carbidopa, will only offer a modest advantage in selected patients (27,43–45).

Another alternate mode of therapy for this patient is a *drug holiday.* Transient withdrawal (five to seven days) of levodopa may increase motor responsiveness and decrease the dyskinesias, "on-off" phenomena and psychiatric disorders associated with chronic levodopa. A study of 14 patients found that most patients required only half their previous dose of levodopa following a drug holiday and nearly all of their adverse effects, especially the psychiatric complications, disappeared. Drug holidays may help 70 to 80% of patients on chronic levodopa, and the beneficial effects last for 9 to 12 months. During the drug holiday, the patient should be hospitalized, because it is a dangerous procedure that leaves the patient frozen, akinetic, and unable to turn or swallow. In severely bed-ridden patients such as L.O., low-dose subcutaneous heparin and other precautions may be necessary to avoid pulmonary emboli, aspiration or infections. When levodopa is reinstituted, the dose should be reduced by at least 50% (47).

18. *Swallowing Difficulties.* What instructions might be useful to patient L.O., who is having difficulty in ingesting her levodopa/carbidopa because of swallowing difficulties?

Although only 15 to 20% of patients with Parkinson's disease complain of swallowing problems, a study using cinefluoroscopy showed that approximately 95% of the parkinsonism patients studied had swallowing disturbances (48). This difficulty in swallowing is partly responsible for the sialorrhea seen in advanced parkinsonism. The inability to cope with oral secretions may predispose the patient to pulmonary aspiration and pneumonia (49). Unfortunately, levodopa and levodopa/carbidopa (Sinemet) are not available as oral suspensions or in an injectable form. However, if a patient is unable to swallow the large levodopa capsules, the white, odorless, tasteless powder can be emptied and mixed with soft food or a liquid.

If a patient requires a liquid formulation for administration through a nasogastric tube, a suspension in cherry syrup or other vehicle can be prepared. The concentration of levodopa should not exceed one gram in 5 to 10 ml. The suspension should be buffered with citric acid and sodium citrate to a pH between four and five because an alkaline pH will enhance deterioration. The suspension is generally stable for 24 hours if it is stored in a dark, tightly-closed, refrigerated container. If the color of the suspension changes to a darker shade, it should be discarded because this indicates decomposition of the levodopa (50,51).

19. *Diet.* Should L.O. be placed on a special diet because of her dysphagia and drug therapy?

Parkinsonism patients should follow normal good eating habits. However, a number of years ago, a low-pyridoxine diet plan was developed, because excessive amounts of pyridoxine reportedly reversed the therapeutic effects of levodopa (52–54). Pyridoxal phosphate is a cofactor of the enzyme dopa decarboxylase, which converts levodopa to dopamine and thereby enhances the peripheral metabolism of levodopa. Since dopamine cannot cross the blood-brain barrier, peripheral metabolism of levodopa results in diminished amounts of levodopa that are available to enter the brain. The amount of pyridoxine found in the average diet is estimated to be less than 1 mg per day, which is much less than the 5 to 10 mg per day needed to nullify levodopa effects (52, 53). With the addition of carbidopa, a decarboxylase inhibitor, to levodopa (Sinemet), even large doses of pyridoxine will not adversely interact with levodopa. Therefore, restriction of pyridoxine is unnecessary in this patient on Sinemet (24).

High protein intake has been reported to neutralize the therapeutic effect of levodopa and sometimes precipitates an "on-off"phenomenon (see Question 15) (56). Since levodopa is absorbed and transported like other amino acids, it has been postulated that high protein diets interfere with the absorption of levodopa. However, diets that do not exceed the recommended dietary allowance of 0.8 gm/kg/day of protein (55–57) are probably of no concern.

Since constipation is often a problem in the elderly Parkinson patient, bran or other high fiber food may be included in the diet. If L.O.'s physical impairment is severe enough, her meat and other large foods may have to be cut up for her. In addition, a semi-soft diet may be advised if her dysphagia causes marked problems (57).

20. *Diabetes in Parkinsonian Patients.* D.B. is a 56-year-old female with a 10-year history of adult-onset diabetes and a five-year history of Parkinson's disease. Her diabetes has been well controlled on diet and tolbutamide 500 mg tid, and her parkinsonism was controlled with amantadine and trihexyphenidyl. However, she now requires the addition of levodopa/carbidopa. Does levodopa or amantadine alter glucose levels?

Oral administration of amantadine causes no significant changes in plasma insulin or blood sugar concentrations. Levodopa increases growth hormone and serum cholesterol (approximately 10%), and it has been shown to decrease glucose tolerance with a delayed and exaggerated insulin response in experimental studies (58,59). However, levodopa has not induced diabetes nor has it significantly altered the insulin requirement of a previously diagnosed diabetic (6).

21. Will levodopa interfere with urine testing for glucose and ketones in this patient?

Urine Glucose. Levodopa may cause a false negative reading in the presence of glycosuria when the glucose oxidase method (Clinistix) is used, and a false positive "trace" reading with the copper reduction method (Clinitest). In one study, six of 25 urine specimens taken from patients receiving 0.75 to 3 grams of levodopa daily and fortified with glucose to 1% produced a negative glucose oxidase test. In addition, the glucose oxidase reaction was inhibited in 13 of 17 specimens from patients receiving 3.5 to 5.0 grams of levodopa daily. Furthermore, 19 of 43 specimens obtained from patients receiving levodopa produced a trace reaction with the Clinitest copper reduction test in the absence of glycosuria (60).

The chemical responsible for the false negative glucose oxidase test and the false positive "trace" copper reduction test is 3,4, dihydroxyphenylacetic acid (DOPAC), a metabolite of levodopa. It is a potent reducing agent which keeps the indicator dye, orthotoluidine, used in Clinistix, in its reduced form, thus producing a false negative reaction for glucose.

In spite of this interference, Tes-Tape or Clinistix can still be used in testing for glucose in patients on levodopa. The Tes-Tape appears to act as a mini-ascending chromatography system which separates the glucose from the DOPAC. Since glucose migrates faster than DOPAC, it is present above the area where the tape is dipped, and a positive reaction can be read. Similarly, if only part of the test area of the Clinistix is dipped in the urine sample, a positive reaction can be observed above the immersed portion (60).

Urine Ketones. False positive readings for urinary ketones have been reported with Ketostix and Labstix in patients receiving 0.5 to 5.0 grams of levodopa daily. Most investigators report Acetest to be unaffected by levodopa (61–63). However, Dawson (64) reported one patient on 2.5 grams of levodopa who was noted to have a false positive reading to Acetest, as well as to Ketostix and Labstix. Levodopa and its metabolites, dopamine and 3,4, dihydroxyphenylacetic acid (DOPAC), have all produced a color reaction with Ketostix and Labstix, but not generally with Acetest tablets (62).

22. *Melanoma.* A 62-year-old male recently developed classic signs of Parkinson's disease (tremors, rigidity, and bradykinesia). In reviewing his past medical history, it was noted that he had a malignant melanoma removed three years ago. What effect, if any, will levodopa have on a patient with a history of cancer?

Levodopa may have a beneficial effect on certain types of cancers and may be contraindicated in others. Levodopa provided relief from bone pain caused by metastatic breast cancer in 10 of 30 women. These 10 patients also showed resolution of bone scan activity and roentgenographic evidence of bone recalcification (65).

The beneficial effects of levodopa in breast cancer may be related to its ability to suppress prolactin. However, the role of prolactin in mammary carcinogenesis is unclear (66); other mechanisms may be involved, since the bone pain from prostatic cancer and metastatic hypernephroma has also responded to levodopa (67).

A temporal relationship has been demonstrated between the administration of levodopa and the recurrence of melanoma in eight cases reported in the literature (68–72). Levodopa is a common intermediate in the biosynthesis of melanin, as well as catecholamines. Melanin synthesis begins with the hydroxylation of tyrosine to levodopa and levodopa to dopaquinone, followed by stepwise conversion to melanin. Levodopa may also influence melanomas indirectly by stimulating growth hormone, which may stimulate melanoma growth. On the other hand, a recent prospective study of 1,099 melanoma patients of the Melanoma Clinical Cooperative Group noted only one patient who had been taking levodopa (71). This indicates that levodopa probably plays an inconsequential role in the rapid increase in the incidence observed for melanoma. In fact, levodopa and its analogues have been shown to be preferentially taken up by human and murine melanoma cells and are toxic to them.

While the cause-and-effect relationship between levodopa and melanomas is at best tenuous, it still seems prudent to avoid levodopa in patients with a history of melanoma for medical-legal reasons. Alternate therapy such as bromocriptine has been suggested in these rare patients with both parkinsonism and a history of melanoma.

23. *Apparent Treatment Failure.* **An 82-year-old male patient in a nursing home is being treated with papaverine for cerebral arteriosclerosis. During the past three months, there has been a gradual onset of tremors without noticeable rigidity or bradykinesia. The patient was started on levodopa. After a month, the patient was receiving two grams of levodopa per day without any effect on his tremors. Why is this 82-year-old gentleman an apparent treatment failure?**

There are a number of possible causes for this patient's apparent failure to respond to levodopa. First, not every elderly patient with tremors is afflicted with parkinsonism. Silversides (73) studied 2,915 residence of eight Toronto Metropolitan Homes for the Aged and found that 133, or 4.5% had been diagnosed as suffering from parkinsonism. However, re-examination revealed that only 81 of the 133, or 61%, of these patients actually had Parkinson's disease. This patient should be examined by a neurologist to rule out other possible causes of tremor. Then, if the patient does have Parkinson's disease, his drug therapy should be re-examined. In general, anticholinergic agents are more effective in alleviating the tremor, while levodopa is more effective in reducing the akinesia and rigidity. It is also important to remember that levodopa has a very slow therapeutic onset when it is given without a decarboxylase inhibitor. Although some benefit would be expected within a month, some patients may require several months and a dose of 8 grams per day to achieve maximum effect. Also, at least a quarter of parkinsonism patients may not respond at all to levodopa (6).

Another important consideration in any instance of treatment failure is poor adherence to the dosage regimen by either the patient or the staff taking care of him.

Drug interactions are another cause of treatment failure (see Table 2). Clinicians should be aware that papaverine, pyridoxine, reserpine, and neuroleptics are notorious for negating the beneficial effects of levodopa.

Duvoisin (74) and Posner (75) report that papaverine in doses of 100 mg per day can reverse the beneficial effects of levodopa over a period of several weeks. Once the papaverine is discontinued, the expected response to levodopa reappears in five to seven days. The exact mechanism is unknown, but there is some evidence to suggest that papaverine may block the dopamine receptor in the striatum. Not only should papaverine be avoided in parkinsonism patients, but it should probably be avoided in all patients since there is no evidence to indicate that it is effective for cerebral arteriosclerosis.

In conclusion, in this patient the best course of action would be to discontinue papaverine and levodopa and to reassess the patient's diagnosis. If he does indeed have parkinsonism, he would probably do better on a trial of anticholinergic agents, since they appear to be more effective than levodopa against tremor. If this therapy is not sufficient, or his condition progresses, amantadine may be added.

References

1. Calne DB: *Parkinsonism: Physiology, Pharmacology and Treatment.* Edward Arnold Ltd., London, 1970.
2. Wagner SL: The management of Parkinson's syndrome. Med Clin North Am. 1972; 56:693.
3. Pollock M et al: The prevalence, natural history, and dementia of Parkinson's disease. Brain. 1966; 89:429.
4. Yahr MD: The treatment of parkinsonism. Med Clin North Am. 1972; 56:1377.
5. Hoehn MM et al: Parkinsonism; onset, progression and mortality. Neurol. 1967; 17:427.
6. Yahr MD: Levodopa. Ann Intern Med. 1975; 83:677.
7. Shaw KM et al: The impact of treatment with levodopa on Parkinson's disease. Q J Med. 1980; XLIX:283.
8. Duvoisin RC: Cholinergic-anticholinergic antagonism in parkinsonism. Arch Neurol. 1967; 17:124.
9. Moskowitz MA et al: Catecholamines and neurologic diseases. N Engl J Med. 1975; 293:332.
10. Cohen MM et al: Pharmacotherapy of Parkinson's disease. Am J Hosp Pharm. 1977; 34:531.
11. Hornykiewicz D: Parkinson's disease and its chemotherapy. Biochem Pharmacol. 1975; 24:1061.
12. Anon: Effects of systemic drugs with anticholinergic properties for glaucoma. Med Let Drugs Ther. 1974; 16:28.
13. Ignoffo R et al: Glaucoma. J Am Pharm Assoc. 1972; NS12:520.
14. Mawsdsley C et al: Treatment of parkinsonism by amantadine and levodopa. Clin Pharmacol Ther. 1972; 13:575.
15. Schwab RS et al: Amantadine in Parkinson's disease—review of more than two year's experience. JAMA. 1972; 222:792.
16. Horadam VW et al: Pharmacokinetics of amantadine hydrochloride in subjects with normal and impaired renal function. Ann Intern Med. 1981; 94:454.
17. Ing TS et al: Toxic effects of amantadine in patients with renal failure. CMAJ. 1979; 120:695.
18. Shealy CN et al: Livedo reticularis in patients with parkinsonism receiving amantadine. JAMA. 1970; 212:1522.
19. Vollum DI et al: Livedo reticularis during amantadine treatment. Br Med J 1971; 2:627.
20. Silver DE et al: Livedo reticularis in Parkinson's disease patients treated with amantadine hydrochloride. Neurol. 1972; 22:665.
21. Pearce LA et al: Amantadine hydrochloride: alteration in peripheral circulation. Neurol. 1974; 24:46.
22. Fahn S et al: Considerations in the management of parkinsonism. Neurol. 1978; 28:5.
23. Lesser RP et al: Analysis of the clinical problems in parkinsonism and the complications of long-term levodopa therapy. Neurol. 1979; 29:1253.
24. Markham CH et al: Evidence to support early levodopa therapy in Parkinson's disease. Neurol. 1981; 31:125.
25. Markham CH et al: Carbidopa in Parkinson's disease and in nausea and vomiting of levodopa. Arch Neurol. 1974; 31:128.
26. Boshes B: Sinemet and the treatment of parkinsonism. Ann Intern Med. 1981; 94:364.
27. Richman A et al: An extrapyramidal syndrome with reserpine. Can Med Assoc J. 1955; 72:457.
28. Sweet RD et al: Methyldopa as an adjunct to levodopa treatment of Parkinson's disease. Clin Pharmacol Ther. 1972; 13:23.
29. Eisler T: Parkinsonism—new drugs and new approaches. D M. 1979; 25:1.
30. Cawein MJ et al: False rise in serum uric acid after L-dopa. N Engl J Med. 1970; 283:659.
31. McDowell F: Clinical laboratory abnormalities. Clin Pharmacol Ther. 1971; 12(part 2):335.
32. Jonas S: Hyperuricemia and levodopa. N Engl J Med. 1971; 285:1488.
33. Paladine WJ: Gout and levodopa. N Engl J Med. 1972; 286:376.
34. Honda H et al: Gout while receiving levodopa for parkinsonism. JAMA. 1972; 219:55.
35. Hunter KR et al: Use of levodopa with other drugs. Lancet. 1970; 2:1283.
36. Lieberman AN et al: Treatment of Parkinson's disease with bromocriptine. N Engl J Med. 1976; 295:1400.
37. Sweet RD et al: Five years' treatment of Parkinson's disease with levodopa: therapeutic results and survival of 100 patients. Ann Intern Med. 1975; 83:456.
38. Weiner WJ et al: Drug holiday and management of Parkinson's disease. Neurol. 1980; 30:1257.
39. Check WA: Drug holidays for patients with parkinsonism. JAMA. 1979; 242:17.
40. Marsden CD et al: Success and problems of long-term levodopa therapy in Parkinson's disease. Lancet. 1975; 1:345.
41. Delaney P et al: Parkinsonism and levodopa: a five-year experience. J Clin Pharmacol. 1976; 16:652.
42. Anon: Levodopa: long-term impact on Parkinson's disease. Br Med J. 1981; 282:417.
43. Eisler T et al: Deprenyl in Parkinson's disease. Neurol. 1981; 31:19.
44. Schachter M et al: Deprenyl in the management of response fluctuations in patients with Parkinson's disease on levodopa. J Neurol Neurosurg and Psychiat. 1980; 43:1016.
45. Goldstein L: The "on-off" phenomena in Parkinson's disease—treatment and theoretical considerations. Mount Sinai J of Med. 1980; 47:80.
46. Agid et al: Bromocriptine associated with a peripheral dopamine blocking agent in treatment of Parkinson's disease. Lancet. 1979; 1:570.
47. Koller WC et al: Complications of chronic levodopa therapy: long-term efficacy of drug holiday. Neurol. 1981; 3:473.
48. Logemann JA et al: Dysphagia in parkinsonism. JAMA. 1975; 231:69.
49. Lieberman AN et al: Dysphagia in Parkinson's disease. Am J Gastroenterology. 1980; 74:157.
50. Blacow NW: *Martindale The Extra Pharmacopoeia.* The Pharmaceutical Press, London, 1977, p 846.
51. Williams FF: DISS—Drug Information Sharing Service. Hosp Pharm. 1973; 8:361.

52. Von Woert MH: Low pyridoxine diet in parkinsonism. JAMA. 1972; 219:1211.

53. Yahr MD et al: Pyridoxine and levodopa in treatment of parkinsonism. JAMA. 1972; 220:861.

54. Cabot EE: Physician's advice needed in diet for parkinsonism. Modern Hospital. 1971; 166:142.

55. Gillespie NG et al: Diets affecting treatment of parkinsonism with levodopa. J Am Diet Assoc. 1973; 62:525.

56. Mena I et al: Protein intake and treatment of Parkinson's disease with levodopa. N Engl J Med. 1975; 292:181.

57. Selvey NP: Diet for patients receiving levodopa therapy for parkinsonism. JAMA. 1976; 236:1169.

58. Kitomaki O et al: Effects of L-dopa on plasma growth hormone and insulin. Acta Neurol Scand. 1972;(supp) 51:125.

59. Sirtori CR et al: Metabolic responses to acute and chronic L-dopa administration in patients with parkinsonism. N Engl J Med. 1972; 287:729.

60. Feldman JM et al: Levodopa and tests for urinary glucose. N Engl J Med. 1970; 283:1053.

61. Pocelinko R et al: Doped dipsticks. N Engl J Med. 1969; 281:1075.

62. Cawein MJ et al: Levodopa and tests for ketonuria. N Engl J Med. 1970; 283:659.

63. Wolcott GT et al: Levodopa and tests for ketonuria. N Engl J Med. 1970; 283:1522.

64. Dawson WL: Levodopa and tests for ketonuria. N Engl J Med. 1970; 283:264.

65. Minton JP: The response of breast cancer with bone pain to L-dopa. Cancer. 1974; 33:358.

66. Buckman MT et al: Prolactin in clinical practice. JAMA. 1976; 236:871.

67. Nixon DW: Use of L-dopa to relive pain from bone metastases. N Engl J Med. 1975; 292:647.

68. Skibba JL et al: Multiple primary melanoma following administration of levodopa. Arch Pathol. 1972; 93:556.

69. Robinson E et al: Levodopa and malignant melanoma. Arch Pathol. 1973; 95:213.

70. Lieberman AN et al: Levodopa and melanoma. Neurol. 1974; 24:340.

71. Sober AJ et al: Levodopa therapy and malignant melanoma. JAMA. 1978; 240:554.

72. Bernstein JE et al: Levodopa administration and multiple primary cutaneous melanomas. Arch Dermatol. 1980; 116:1041.

73. Silversides JL: Parkinsonism may be diagnosed too freely in elderly patients. JAMA. 1976; 235:1091.

74. Duvoisin RC: Antagonism of levodopa by papaverine. JAMA. 1975; 231:845.

75. Posner DM: Antagonism of levodopa by papaverine. JAMA. 1975; 233:768.

76. Hunter KR et al: Monoamine oxidase inhibitors and L-dopa. Br Med J. 1970; 3:388.

77. Ayd FJ: A survey of drug-induced extrapyramidal reactions. JAMA. 1961; 175:1054.

78. Duvoisin RC et al: Pyridoxine reversal of L-dopa effects in parkinsonism. Trans Am Neurol Assoc. 1969; 94:81.

79. Mendez JS et al: Diphenylhydentoin blocking of levodopa effects. Arch Neurol. 1975; 32:44.

Chapter 50

Epilepsy

Rex S. Lott

Approximately 10% of the general population will experience a convulsion at some time, while epilepsy—a chronic condition characterized by recurrent seizures—affects 0.5–1.0%. Idiopathic epilepsy accounts for about 70% of cases; "symptomatic" epilepsy in the remainder of patients results from various central nervous system deficits caused by problems such as meningitis, trauma, tumors, or exposure to toxins. Isolated seizures are associated with alcohol withdrawal, fever, metabolic derangements, and other reversible insults (1,2).

Epilepsy is treated almost exclusively with pharmacotherapy. Educating patients regarding medications, consulting with other health care providers concerning techniques for optimal application of available anticonvulsants, and utilization and proper interpretation of serum drug concentrations are essential to patient care.

Adequate, early control of epileptic seizures is important. Optimal anticonvulsant therapy may completely control this condition in 60% of patients (3). Control of seizures allows normalization of patients' life styles and prevents physical harm associated with seizures. Optimum treatment depends upon accurate classification (diagnosis) of seizure type as well as upon appropriate choice and use of medications (Table 1) (4).

Diagnosis

Seizure diagnosis is usually straightforward if an adequate history and description of the clinical seizure are available. Physicians are not always able to directly observe patients' seizures; thus family, teachers, nurses, and others who have frequent direct contact with patients should learn to objectively observe and record these events. It

Table 1.

MAJOR ANTICONVULSANTS[a] USEFUL FOR VARIOUS SEIZURE TYPES[4]

	Generalized Tonic-Clonic	Simple Partial	Complex Partial	Absence
Most effective with least toxicity	Phenytoin Carbamazepine Valproate (?)	Phenytoin Carbamazepine Valproate	Carbamazepine Phenytoin Valproate (?)	Ethosuximide Valproate[b]
Some effectiveness and toxicity	Primidone Phenobarbital Clonazepam (?)	Primidone Phenobarbital	Primidone Phenobarbital Clonazepam (?)	Clonazepam Trimethadione Phenobarbital (?)
Of little value	Ethosuximide Trimethadione	Clonazepam Ethosuximide	Trimethadione Ethosuximide	Phenytoin Carbamazepine Primidone

[a] Drugs are listed in general order preference within each category.
[b] The place of valproate is uncertain because of the potential liver toxicity of this compound.

is important that the patient's behavior prior to the onset of the seizure is recorded (eg, did the patient complain of feeling ill or describe an unusual sensation?). The onset, duration, and characteristics of the seizure should also be described as completely as possible; observations such as deviation of the eyes to one side or localization of convulsive activity to one portion of the body are extremely helpful to the physician. In addition, the patient's behavior following the seizure should also be noted, because the presence or absence of postictal confusion may be extremely helpful in formulating a seizure diagnosis. Those who observe a seizure should be strongly discouraged from labeling rather than fully describing the event. Accurate seizure diagnosis is crucial to selecting the most appropriate pharmacotherapy for individual patients.

Terminology associated with epileptic seizures has undergone recent revision. However, older terminology (ie, grand mal, petit mal) is still commonly used. The newer International Classification of Epileptic Seizures is shown in Table 2.

Generalized tonic-clonic (grand mal) seizures are the most common type. The patient initially loses consciousness and falls. The onset of tonic muscle spasms is often accompanied by a cry which results from air being forced through the larynx. Following the tonic phase, there is a period of generalized, bilateral repetitive clonic movements. Patients are often incontinent of urine during these seizures. Upon cessation of clonic movements, the patient will regain consciousness but remain confused and lethargic for a period of time (postictal state). Simple or complex partial seizures may progress to generalized tonic-clonic episodes. The aura experienced by some patients is a manifestation of the partial seizure.

Absence (petit mal) seizures occur primarily in children and usually disappear at puberty, although the patient may develop a second type of seizure. Absence seizures consist of episodes of brief loss of consciousness which may be accompanied by mild clonic facial movements; falling does not occur. The patient is unaware of his surroundings and will have no memory of events occurring during the seizures. Consciousness returns rapidly and there is no postictal confusion.

Atonic or akinetic seizures ("drop attacks") are generally uncommon, although they are seen frequently in mentally retarded patients. They are often associated with myoclonic seizures charac-

Table 2.

INTERNATIONAL CLASSIFICATION OF EPILEPTIC SEIZURES[5]

I. Partial seizures (seizures beginning locally)
   A. Partial seizures with elementary symptomatology (generally without impairment of consciousness).
      1. With motor symptoms (e.g., Jacksonian, postural, aphasic)
      2. With special sensory or somato-sensory symptoms (e.g., visual, auditory, olfactory, vertiginous)
      3. With autonomic symptoms
      4. Compound forms (elementary or complex symptoms)
   B. Partial seizures with complex symptomatology (generally with impairment of consciousness). ("Complex" implies organized, high level cerebral activity.)
      1. With impaired consciousness alone
      2. With cognitive symptomatology (e.g., déjà vu, "dreamy" state)
      3. With affective symptomatology
      4. With psychosensory symptomatology (e.g., illusions, hallucinations)
      5. With "psychomotor symptomatology" (e.g., automatisms)
      6. Compound forms
II. Generalized seizures (bilateral symmetrical seizures or seizures without focal onset)
   A. Absence seizures (petit mal)
      1. Simple (impaired conscousness only)
      2. Complex (myoclonic, retropulsive, atonic, automatisms, autonomic or mixed forms)
   B. Bilateral massive epileptic myoclonus
   C. Infantile spasms
   D. Clonic seizures
   E. Tonic seizures
   F. Tonic-clonic seizures (grand mal)
   G. Atonic seizures
   H. Akinetic seizures
III. Unilateral (or predominantly unilateral) seizures
IV. Unclassified epileptic seizures

terized by severe, rapid muscular contraction. There is a sudden loss of consciousness and muscle tone which results in dramatic falls. Seated patients may violently slump forward. Attacks are of brief duration, but there is frequent morbidity from uncontrolled falls.

Elementary partial (focal motor or sensory) seizures are localized to a single cerebral hemisphere. They are usually brief and there is no loss of consciousness. A variety of motor and sensory manifestations are seen. A single limb or appendage may twitch or there may be an abnormal sensory experience such as an unusual smell.

Complex partial (psychomotor or temporal lobe) seizures result from spread of abnormal focal discharges to the other cerebral hemisphere. Consciousness is impaired and the patient may exhibit complex, but inappropriate, behavior such as lip smacking, clothes tearing or aimless wandering. There are often brief periods of postictal confusion.

ANTICONVULSANT THERAPY

Serum Drug Concentrations

The individual patient's clinical response in terms of seizure frequency and severity must be the major monitoring parameter for anticonvulsant therapy. However, wide availability of anticonvulsant serum level determinations has had a significant impact on the treatment of epilepsy (6–9). Serum levels of these drugs are useful for a number of reasons. First, there is a poor correlation between administered doses and resulting steady-state serum concentrations (10). Administration of "usual therapeutic doses," even on a mg/kg basis, may result in either subtherapeutic or potentially toxic serum concentrations. As most anticonvulsants are eliminated primarily by hepatic metabolism, a great deal of this observed variation probably results from interindividual variation in metabolic capacity. Second, there is an excellent correlation between brain tissue concentrations and serum levels of anticonvulsants (11). This is reflected in clinical observations of an excellent relationship between serum concentrations and clinical response. Therapeutic serum concentration ranges are well established for ethosuximide (Zarontin), carbamazepine (Tegretol), phenytoin (Dilantin), and phenobarbital (10,12). Serum drug levels within the therapeutic ranges for these drugs will produce maximum therapeutic response with minimal toxicity for most patients. Therapeutic serum concentrations have been proposed for valproate (Depakene), primidone (Mysoline), and clonazepam (Clonopin); however, more research is required before these serum concentration ranges can be considered as more than broad guidelines (10).

Indications for Use. Measurement of serum drug levels is likely to provide clinically useful information in the following situations:

Uncontrolled seizures despite administration of greater-than-average doses. Serum concentrations may help distinguish between lack of drug efficacy and either malabsorption, noncompliance, or rapid metabolism leading to subtherapeutic serum concentrations.

Recurrence of seizures in a previously controlled patient. This is often due to non-compliance with the medication regimen.

Documentation of intoxication. In patients who become clinically intoxicated, it is useful to document the dose and blood level responsible.

Assessment of patient compliance. Although this use for blood levels is recommended widely, it must be remembered that before a patient is labeled as non-compliant, the steady-state blood levels resulting from reliable intake of a given dose in that patient must be available for comparison.

Documentation of desired results from a dose change or other therapeutic maneuver (eg, administration of a loading dose). Additionally, when a patient is receiving multiple anticonvulsants, serum levels of all drugs should be determined following a change in the dose of one drug. Altered serum levels of one drug frequently produce changes in the metabolism of other drugs.

Assessment of therapy in patients with infrequent seizures. Usually, titration of anticonvulsant dosage on the basis of seizure frequency is appropriate. Under these conditions, serum anticonvulsant levels are much less important than seizure frequency as a monitoring parameter. However, in patients with infrequent seizures—especially when therapy is first begun—it may be desirable to administer maintenance doses of medication which are sufficient to produce steady-state serum concentrations well within the drug's therapeutic range. In this way, the likelihood of successful drug therapy is maximized, even though the dosage and resultant serum concentration may be higher than actually necessary.

When precise dosage changes are required. For example, depending on the serum concentration and the individual patient's metabolic capacity, very small phenytoin dose changes may result in large changes in serum concentration and clinical response. Knowledge of the serum drug concentration before the dosage change may allow the clinician to select a new maintenance dose most appropriate for the individual patient.

Routine repeated measurement of serum drug levels are probably unnecessary. If there is no change in the patient's clinical status, one may usually assume that the serum level remains unchanged. Frequent (eg, monthly) "routine" serum level determinations are expensive and, because of day-to-day laboratory variability, may lead to temptation to make unnecessary dose changes. Some clinicians feel that measurement of serum levels every 6–12 months is reasonable as a routine procedure.

Sample Timing. Blood samples for anticonvulsant serum levels should usually be drawn during the post-absorption phase after steady-state has been reached. A minimum of 4–5 half-lives should be allowed to pass after a dose change or initiation of therapy before serum levels are determined. For most situations, blood drawn in the morning before any medications are taken will provide a reproducible, post-absorption serum level. Table 3 lists pertinent pharmacokinetic properties for commonly-used anticonvulsants. This information can be used to aid in proper timing of serum level measurements.

Saliva Drug Concentrations. The monitoring of saliva levels of anticonvulsants may be a useful alternative or adjunct to the use of serum levels. Salivary epithelium acts as a dialysis membrane allowing non-protein-bound (free or pharmacologically active) drug to passively diffuse into saliva. Saliva anticonvulsant concentrations should more closely approximate levels of drug available for penetration into the central nervous system than do total serum concentrations. In addition, saliva can be collected noninvasively. This offers an advantage in situations where multiple or serial venipunctures would be required or where patients are uncooperative.

The relationship between saliva and plasma levels for several anticonvulsants has been studied (13–15). Saliva levels of phenytoin, carbamazepine and ethosuximide appear to correspond closely to plasma levels of free drug. Approximate saliva/plasma ratios are: phenytoin 0.10 (eg, desired saliva concentration range is 1.0–2.0 mcg/ml), carbamazepine 0.26 and ethosuximide 1.04. These ratios remain constant in most situations. However, under conditions which change protein binding of these drugs (eg, renal failure—see Question 22), the ratio will change. Nevertheless, saliva levels will continue to reflect the concentration of active drug and will therefore be useful in therapeutic monitoring.

There is greater variability in the saliva/plasma ratios for phenobarbital and primidone (13,14). Diffusion of phenobarbital into saliva is significantly affected by saliva pH, because the drug's pKa of 7.2 is very close to the middle of the range

Table 3.

PHARMACOKINETIC PROPERTIES OF MAJOR ANTICONVULSANTS

Drug	Half-Life	Time to Steady-State[a]	Usual Therapeutic Serum Concentration	Dosage Schedule
Phenytoin	Variable with dose	5–30 days	10–20 mcg/ml	qd (bid)
Phenobarbital	2–4 days	8–16 days	15–40 mcg/ml	qd
Primidone	3–12 hrs	12–48 hrs	5–15 mcg/ml (15–40 mcg/ml for derived phenobarbital)	bid-tid
Carbamazepine	8–12 hrs on chronic dosing	2–4 days	5–12 mcg/ml	bid-tid
Valproate	10–16 hrs	2–3 days	10–100 mcg/ml (?)	tid-qid
Clonazepam	20–40 hrs	3–7 days	5–70 ng/ml	bid-tid
Ethosuximide	30 hrs (Children) 60 hrs (Adults)	5–10 days	40–100 mcg/ml	qd (bid)

[a] Based on 4 half-lives. This lag time should allow determination of steady-state serum concentrations within limits of most assay sensitivities.

for normal saliva pH. Mathematical or graphical methods may be used to correct for the influence of pH (13). The saliva/plasma ratio for phenobarbital after pH correction is approximately 0.43. Primidone saliva levels are not influenced by pH; the reason for fluctuation in the saliva/plasma ratio for this drug is not completely understood. Bartels and associates (16) were able to show a relationship between salivary flow rate and saliva/serum ratio for primidone. They proposed that the rate of primidone's diffusion into saliva is limited by the drug's lipid solubility. They recommended using stimulated saliva samples which produced a concentration ratio of 0.7.

While it has been possible to demonstrate consistent anticonvulsant saliva/plasma level ratios in populations of patients, clinicians should use these established ratios cautiously. Individual patient variability in protein binding may alter these relationships and potentially lead to unnecessary or inappropriate dosage regimen changes. Ideally, the saliva/plasma ratio for the individual patient should be established before saliva levels are used for clinical monitoring purposes.

For some patients, particularly those who are receiving anticholinergic medications concomitantly, it may be necessary to stimulate saliva flow. This can be accomplished by having the patient chew on a piece of paraffin or by placing a citric acid crystal in his or her mouth. The laboratory should be contacted before samples are sent. Because anticonvulsant levels in saliva are much lower than in serum, it may be necessary to establish a separate standard curve using higher than usual drug dilutions. It is also necessary to measure the pH of the saliva sample to accurately interpret phenobarbital levels. As exposure to air may markedly alter pH, the sample should be immediately drawn up into a syringe, excess air expelled, and the syringe capped.

Polypharmacy

Traditionally, polypharmacy with anticonvulsants has been accepted. When seizures were incompletely controlled with a single medication, a second, third, or even a fourth drug was added. In some situations, therapy was initiated with two medications for a single seizure type (eg, phenytoin and phenobarbital for generalized tonic-clonic seizures). However, at present, there is no evidence that combination therapy in patients with a single seizure type offers any advantage over therapy with a single drug (17–19).

Shorvon and Reynolds (20) found retrospectively that seizure control improved significantly in only 36% of their patient sample during the six months following introduction of a second anticonvulsant. They also found a significant correlation between improved control and the presence of optimum blood levels of at least one medication. These results imply that administration of doses necessary to produce maximum effective serum levels should result in adequate seizure control with a single drug in many patients. Prospectively, Shorvon and Reynolds (17,18) were able to achieve satisfactory seizure control using a single drug (phenytoin or carbamazepine) in 90% of previously untreated patients. They estimated that without monitoring serum drug levels, 60–70% of their patients would have been treated with a second drug. In an additional study, these authors were able to eliminate multi-drug treatment and maintain monotherapy in 72% (29 of 40) of a series of outpatients with chronic epilepsy (21). Although some patients' seizures were exacerbated during drug withdrawal, both seizure control and subjectively assessed mental function improved in 55% of the patients switched to monotherapy. Thus, although "it is more difficult to reduce polypharmacy than to avoid it in the first place," there appear to be significant improvements in patient status to be gained through reduction in the number of anticonvulsants administered.

Some authors (22) now advocate discontinuation of the first drug which is tried if it produces no improvement in seizure frequency. Addition of a second drug is recommended only when doses of the first drug which produce optimum serum concentrations have caused partial improvement. Nevertheless, Reynolds et al (18) found that they were able to achieve reductions of 98% in the frequency of generalized tonic-clonic seizures and 92–93% for partial seizures using a single drug. Where two types of seizures occur in the same patient (eg, absence and generalized tonic-clonic), polypharmacy is often necessary because a single drug may not be effective for both types of seizures.

Duration of Therapy

1. T.N. is a 19-year-old male college freshman who first developed recurrent absence

spells accompanied by occasional (2–4 yearly) generalized tonic-clonic seizures at age 6. His seizures were subsequently controlled with ethosuximide and phenobarbital. He has had no seizures for six years and remains on both drugs. Serum levels are 85 mcg/ml for ethosuximide and 39 mcg/ml for phenobarbital. A recent electroencephalogram (EEG) was interpreted as "essentially normal with some minimal slowing and no paroxymsal features." What is the prognosis for successful discontinuation of this patient's anticonvulsant therapy?

Many experts advocate attempting to withdraw anticonvulsants after varying seizure-free periods (23,24). Discontinuation of medications is advantageous for economic, medical, and psychosocial reasons. Costs associated with physician visits, blood level determinations, and the medications themselves are eliminated. The risks of adverse effects from long-term medication are eliminated, and patients can expect fewer restrictions on their lifestyles.

Two studies (25,25a) examined prognosis following termination of anticonvulsant therapy; these studies have identified several patient-specific characteristics which allow assessment of the risk of relapse. In both studies, patients were seizure free for four years before medication withdrawal was attempted. Sex, race, and family history were not useful as predictors of outcome.

Holowach and associates (25) identified several features which characterized patients with a good prognosis. Those with onset of seizures before age eight and those in whom seizures were completely controlled within six years of onset were less likely to relapse. Complete seizure control within two years of onset was an especially favorable predictor. Recurrence was less likely in those with a single seizure type; this was especially true for grand mal, petit mal, and febrile multiple seizures. While patients with multiple seizure types relapsed more frequently, the prognosis was better if petit mal was one of the seizure types. Partial seizures (especially Jacksonian) carried a high risk of recurrence. Absence of organic brain damage as an etiologic factor implied a good prognosis. EEG's were of limited predictive value.

The study by Emerson and associates (25a) confirmed that early control of seizures (less than 7 years) and absence of organic etiologic factors predicted successful medication discontinuation. However, these investigator's findings conflicted with those of Holowach and associates in some areas. Emerson and associates found that onset of seizures after age 7 predicted a more favorable prognosis. They also found that the presence of definite EEG abnormalities predicted a high rate of recurrence. In addition, this study identified several other predictors of less favorable outcome: low anticonvulsant serum levels, more than 30 generalized tonic-clonic seizures before control, and I.Q. below 70. Overall, the two most useful predictive factors were the EEG and the number of generalized tonic-clonic seizures before control.

In patient T.N., the prognosis for successful withdrawal of medications appears good. There are no EEG abnormalities; apparently he has not had a large number of generalized tonic-clonic seizures; the age at onset implies a favorable prognosis by the criteria of both studies; his seizures were controlled relatively rapidly; and he is not mentally retarded. T.N.'s anticonvulsant serum levels are "high" by the criteria of Emerson and associates (25a); they defined high serum levels as 15 mcg/ml or more of phenytoin or phenobarbital and 60 mcg/ml or more of ethosuximide. However, serum anticonvulsant levels do not appear to be a major prognostic factor. Thus, attempting to discontinue T.N.'s medications would be reasonable at this time.

2. *Discontinuation of Therapy.* What procedure is recommended for discontinuation of T.N.'s medications?

Withdrawal of anticonvulsants in other than emergency situations should be done slowly. There is a significant risk that too rapid withdrawal may precipitate status epilepticus. The studies cited in the previous question (25,25a) employed a two to three month withdrawal period for each drug. Phenobarbital has a long half-life and one would expect it to be "self-tapering." Therefore, one would expect little difficulty with rapid withdrawal. Nevertheless, gradual reduction of phenobarbital would be more prudent. Should seizures recur during drug withdrawal, reinstitution of a therapeutic dose of the drug being withdrawn is recommended.

Absence spells frequently disappear before adulthood (26). On this basis, it may be best to withdraw T.N.'s ethosuximide first. Phenobarbital withdrawal could then be attempted following successful discontinuation of ethosuximide.

FEBRILE SEIZURES

3. A 9-month-old female infant is brought to the emergency room after having a generalized tonic-clonic convulsion lasting approximately 10 minutes. The episode occurred in association with an upper respiratory infection (URI). Upon arrival in the emergency room, her temperature was 39.5° C rectally. She was alert at this time; all laboratory and neurologic findings including lumbar puncture were normal. The patient has no history of neurologic abnormality, but her 7-year-old brother suffers from both absence spells and generalized tonic-clonic seizures. What is the relationship between febrile seizures and epilepsy? How may this patients' convulsion be classified on the basis of the data available?

Approximately 2–4% of children will have a febrile seizure between 6 months and 6 years of age (27–30). Febrile seizures are diagnosed when the patient's first convulsion is associated with a temperature above 38° C, the patient is less than 6 years old and there is no evidence of acute metabolic disorder or central nervous system infection or inflammation. *Simple febrile seizures* last less than 15 minutes, have no focal features, do not occur in a series, and have a total duration of less than 30 minutes. *Complex febrile seizures* are of long duration, show focal characteristics, and occur in series (30). Complex febrile seizures are considered by some as epileptic seizures precipitated by fever, especially if the child previously exhibited neurologic abnormality (28). Thus, all febrile seizures are not considered as epileptic seizures. There is however, a higher risk of subsequent epilepsy in children with febrile convulsions. Overall, 2–3% of these patients will develop afebrile seizures. Generally, repeated convulsions, occurrence of the first febrile seizure in the first year of life, family history of epilepsy, and complex febrile seizures predispose to subsequent epileptic seizures (30).

This patient's convulsion is typical of a simple febrile seizure. It is common for febrile seizures to occur in association with viral URI's. The lack of previous abnormality and negative findings on lumbar puncture and laboratory work-up help to confirm the diagnosis of simple febrile seizure.

4. How are febrile seizures treated during the acute episode?

Because this patient is stable at present, immediate anticonvulsant therapy is not required. Measures to reduce her elevated temperature should be initiated to reduce the risk of further seizures. Acetaminophen or aspirin and tepid sponge baths are useful. Should a second seizure occur, diazepam (Valium) 0.3 mg/kg by slow IV injection (1 mg/min) will usually terminate the episode (28).

Phenobarbital

5. On the basis of the subjective and objective data available for this patient, formulate a plan for treatment with anticonvulsant medication.

The need for prophylactic anticonvulsant treatment in children who have had febrile seizures is controversial. One-third of children will have a recurrence of febrile seizures (29), and multiple or severe febrile seizures may cause temporal lobe lesions resulting in complex partial (temporal lobe) epilepsy (28,30). Recurrence is more common (50%) if the first febrile seizure occurs before one year of age. Although prophylactic anticonvulsants would seem especially useful for afebrile seizures or epilepsy, the effect of such therapy has not been evaluated. (29).

This patient appears to be a candidate for anticonvulsant treatment on the basis of her age and the family history of epilepsy. Chronic phenobarbital therapy in doses sufficient to maintain serum concentrations of 15 mcg/ml or greater significantly reduces recurrence of febrile seizures (30). In this patient, phenobarbital should be initiated at 5 mg/kg/day and the dose should be titrated to achieve effective serum concentrations. Fishman (30) recommends continuous treatment for 30 months. Others recommend continuing therapy until age 5 or 6, as febrile seizures rarely occur after this age (27). Additionally, her parents should be instructed to institute antipyretic measures at the onset of any febrile illness.

Phenobarbital is commonly prescribed for "prn" use at the onset of febrile episodes to prevent development of febrile seizures (31). This practice should be strongly discouraged. Efficacy of this approach is questionable, because several days are required for phenobarbital to accumulate to therapeutic serum concentrations, and use of adequate loading doses may cause marked sedation. In addition, febrile seizures often occur either prior to recognition of febrile illness or during the first 24 hours (27).

6. Two years after initiation of phenobarbital in the above patient, her parents complain that she is hyperactive, she "races" around the house, has no attention span, has frequent tantrums, and seems generally irritable. She currently receives 60 mg/day of phenobarbital. The serum concentration is 21 mcg/ml. They question whether phenobarbital could be causing or aggravating this behavior. Discuss the relationship between phenobarbital and hyperactivity. How may this problem be managed?

Hyperactivity and other behavior disturbances are relatively common in children and adolescents treated with phenobarbital (32,33). Wolf and Forsythe (32) observed this response in 42% of 109 children; phenobarbital was discontinued in half of those affected. Behavior disturbances appeared during the first few months, were not correlated with serum drug concentrations, and were reversible in the majority of patients. Hyperactivity occurred in 18% of patients who had had febrile seizures and were not treated with phenobarbital. It is difficult to assess the contribution of phenobarbital to this patient's hyperactivity, as no baseline behavior information is available. Gradual discontinuation of phenobarbital would allow assessment of the drug's role; however, there is a risk of recurrence of febrile seizures with this maneuver.

Garrettson (34) recommends two approaches to this problem. First, changing the medication to mephobarbital may be helpful. Although mephobarbital is rapidly converted to phenobarbital *in vivo*, there are anecdotal reports that it causes less behavior disturbance. However, this may only reflect mephobarbital's lower rate of use. Mephobarbital doses of approximately twice those of phenobarbital are needed to produce equivalent phenobarbital serum levels (24). Second, methylphenidate (Ritalin) or dextroamphetamine may reduce hyperactive behavior. Garrettson recommends methylphenidate at doses up to 20 mg/day.

Other anticonvulsants have not been proven effective for prevention of febrile seizures. However, there is some evidence that primidone may be useful (30,35) at daily doses of 25 mg/kg. Primidone is also converted partially to phenobarbital. Thus, it may also cause behavior disturbances. This author has observed behavioral disturbances apparently due to primidone in adolescents. Valproic acid may also be of value. Two studies found 20–30 mg/kg of valproate to be as effective as 4–5 mg/kg of phenobarbital (35,36). Another study, however, found no benefit from valproate at 40 mg/kg (serum concentrations above 40 mcg/ml in 90% of the study group) (37). Even if valproate is found to be prophylactically effective for febrile seizures, the risk of potential liver toxicity (see Question 13) would appear to prohibit its routine use in a condition where the benefits of drug therapy are not proven.

Substitution of mephobarbital for phenobarbital is probably the most reasonable course in this patient. Addition of dextroamphetamine or methylphenidate would introduce the risk of side effects such as appetite suppression with temporary growth retardation. Phenobarbital can be discontinued and mephobarbital begun simultaneously at a dose of 100 mg daily. The serum concentration of phenobarbital should be determined after approximately two weeks to ensure that appropriate blood levels are being maintained. Given this patient's age, assessment of efficacy of the maneuver will depend on reports by the parents and others who have close contact with the child. Should this approach be unsuccessful, methylphenidate should be considered for addition to the regimen.

ABSENCE SEIZURES

Ethosuximide

7. T.D., a 7-year-old girl, is reported by her teacher to have 3–4 episodes of "staring" daily. The spells last a few seconds, there are no observable convulsive movements, and she is fully alert afterward. T.D.'s school performance is somewhat below average, despite an I.Q. of 125. EEG reveals a 3/second spike-wave pattern. Typical absence seizures are diagnosed. How is drug therapy for this form of epilepsy chosen, initiated, and monitored?

Ethosuximide is probably the drug of choice for absence seizures (4,24). Controlled trials have demonstrated its efficacy, and potential toxicity is less than that seen with trimethadione or valproate. Trimethadione is less effective and is associated with risks of blood dyscrasias and visual disturbances (2,24). Valproate is probably as effective as ethosuximide, but is associated with hepatotoxicity (see Question 13) and should be reserved for use in patients who do not respond to ethosuximide.

Ethosuximide therapy is begun at a dose of 20 mg/kg or 250 mg bid; the dose can be increased by 250 mg/day every 7–10 days as necessary to control seizures (22,24). The delay between dose increases is necessary to allow accumulation to new steady-state blood levels and to evaluate the effect of these blood levels on seizure frequency. As the average half-life of ethosuximide in children is 30 hours (38,39), this delay allows approximately 5–6 days for achievement of steady-state and 2–5 days for assessment of response. A therapeutic serum concentration range of 40–100 mcg/ml for ethosuximide is well established (24,39). However, as there is no clearly defined toxicity syndrome associated with high ethosuximide serum levels, cautious "pushing" of the dose and serum level may allow further response in resistant patients.

Although it is traditionally administered in divided doses, ethosuximide's long half-life indicates that a single daily dose is feasible and effective (38,40). Acute side effects, especially nausea and vomiting may occur with administration of large single doses, and in these situations, divided doses may be necessary.

8. What should T.D.'s parents be told concerning ethosuximide, its side effects, and their significance?

It is important to educate the parents, and the patient, regarding the importance of regular administration of the drug. Noncompliance is a common problem with anticonvulsants, and rapid discontinuation of these drugs (often secondary to noncompliance) is associated with precipitation of status epilepticus. The concept that the medication controls rather than cures the seizure disorder should be reinforced. It is also important to inform both the parents and the patient that a therapeutic response may not occur immediately and that dosage adjustments may be necessary.

The parents should also be informed of the common occurrence of nausea and sedation with initiation of ethosuximide (39). Tolerance to these effects does develop, although temporary dose reduction is sometimes necessary. Subtle degrees of sedation may persist throughout therapy and may not be noticed until the drug is discontinued (41).

GENERALIZED TONIC-CLONIC SEIZURES

9. Three months later, T.D.'s absence spells have been reduced to a frequency of one every two weeks with an ethosuximide dose of 750 mg/day. Initial drowsiness and nausea have decreased dramatically. However, she is brought to the emergency room by her parents because she suffered a 2 minute generalized tonic-clonic convulsion. What is the relationship between this patient's tonic-clonic seizure and ethosuximide therapy? How should this development be managed in T.D.?

It is commonly believed and often stated in the literature that ethosuximide (and trimethadione) may either precipitate or worsen tonic-clonic seizures; however, this effect has not been clearly demonstrated, and there is some evidence that both drugs may actually be beneficial in control of tonic-clonic seizures (42,43). A number of patients who initially present with absence seizures later develop tonic-clonic seizures. Some clinicians feel that phenobarbital or phenytoin should be initiated with ethosuximide to prevent this occurrence. Livingston et al (44) found that 80.5% of their patients treated with a drug specific for absence spells developed "grand mal" seizures, while only 36% did so while receiving combined therapy. On the other hand, Richens (11,24) feels that medication for tonic-clonic seizures should be initiated only after these seizures actually appear. He also raises the concern that routine use of drugs such as phenobarbital or phenytoin may unnecessarily aggravate absence spells.

In summary, the subsequent occurrence of generalized tonic-clonic seizures is common in patients who initially develop absence seizures. It is not possible to assess the possible causative role of ethosuximide for this development in this patient.

Drug therapy for prevention of further generalized tonic-clonic seizures is now indicated. In young children, especially females, many clinicians feel that phenobarbital is the drug of choice (45). Long-term phenytoin therapy is associated with several side effects which may become of major cosmetic importance: hirsutism (46–48), gingival hyperplasia (49,50), and coarsening of facial features (51,52). However, phenobarbital may cause either sedation or hyperactivity and behavior disturbances.

Phenobarbital should be initiated in T.D. at a dose of 3–5 mg/kg/day. The requirement for higher doses must be based on seizure frequency. If tonic-clonic seizures continue to occur after steady-state has been reached (approximately 1–2 weeks), the dosage should be gradually increased using serum concentrations as a guide. T.D. should be monitored for the development of either sedation or hyperactivity.

Valproate

10. Valproate is reported to be effective for treatment of both absence and generalized tonic-clonic seizures. Should patient T.D. be considered for therapy with this drug rather than a combination of ethosuximide and phenobarbital or phenytoin?

Valproate is very effective for the treatment of absence spells and also appears to be effective against tonic-clonic episodes in some patients (53–57). However, in most trials examining its effect on tonic-clonic seizures, valproate has been added to previous regimens of other drugs. Thus, its effect on tonic-clonic seizures may be adjunctive rather than primary. Valproate also tends to increase the serum concentration and clinical effect of preexisting doses of phenobarbital (see Question 12); this may play a role in its effect against tonic-clonic seizures for some patients. More study is required to establish the usefulness of valproate for tonic-clonic seizures.

Some authors (4) suggest that, since valproate appears to be effective for tonic-clonic seizures, it may be a preferred drug for those with combined absence-tonic-clonic seizures. There are advantages to using a single drug. However, given the present lack of documented efficacy of valproate for tonic-clonic seizures and the potential for hepatic damage, it may be best to reserve this drug for those patients who cannot be controlled on a combination of two primary agents.

11. R.V. is an 8-year-old, 35 kg patient who began to experience both absence and generalized tonic-clonic seizures at age 6. His current medications consist of phenobarbital 300 mg/day (serum level of 38 mcg/ml), phenytoin 400 mg/day (serum level of 18 mcg/ml), and ethosuximide 250 mg bid (serum level of 52 mcg/ml). His tonic-clonic seizures have been completely controlled for seven months. However, one month ago the frequency of his absence spells increased from one or two daily to 5–15 daily. Ethosuximide serum levels were consistent with previous determinations. An attempt to increase the ethosuximide dosage to 750 mg daily resulted in intractable nausea and vomiting. Valproate is to be substituted for ethosuximide. How should valproate therapy be initiated and monitored in patient R.V.?

Prior to beginning valproate, baseline liver function tests (SGOT, SGPT, alkaline phosphatase, and bilirubin) should be obtained (57). These tests should be repeated every one to two weeks during the first three months of therapy to allow early detection of biochemical changes suggesting hepatotoxicity. In addition, R.V. should be examined frequently for signs or symptoms of liver disease (eg, scleral icterus, abdominal pain, clay-colored stools).

A reasonable initial dose for R.V. would be 125 mg of valproate as syrup (2½ ml) bid. Most patients will tolerate starting doses of 7–10 mg/kg/day without the excessive nausea and sedation which are often seen when the higher doses recommended by the manufacturer are administered. Weekly dose increases of 5–10 mg/kg/day are usually tolerated well. R.V. should be given valproate capsules as soon as the daily dosage schedule permits. Currently, the maximum recommended dose of valproate is 60 mg/kg/day. Most patients respond to lower doses in this author's experience. The primary determinant of adequate valproate dosage is seizure frequency. A therapeutic serum concentration range of 50–150 mcg/ml is proposed (57). However, this range is based on preliminary studies, and there is no well-defined toxicity syndrome seen with valproate serum levels above this range. Many patients observed by the author have had marked responses to serum concentrations below the proposed therapeutic range.

Excessive sedation and nausea may occur during initiation of valproate therapy. These symptoms are usually transient and can usually be alleviated by either temporarily reducing the dose or administering valproate with food.

12. *Valproate Interactions.* Valproate is reported to interact with both phenytoin and phenobarbital. What are the mechanisms and likely consequences of these interactions in R.V.? How should this patient be monitored?

Phenobarbital. Valproate predictably alters the pharmacokinetics and clinical effect of phenobarbital. Steady-state phenobarbital serum levels may increase by 25–50% when valproate is added. These changes result from inhibition of phenobarbital metabolism; plasma clearance is thereby reduced and the half-life increases by approximately 50% (58). This interaction probably explains the excessive sedation that is seen in some patients when valproate is added to regimens containing phenobarbital (59). Many clinicians reduce the dose of phenobarbital by one-quarter to one-half when valproate is added. In this patient, a reduction to 200 mg/day will reduce the risk of excessive sedation while maintaining approximately the same serum concentration of phenobarbital.

Phenytoin. Valproate usually causes a decrease in phenytoin serum levels. This interaction appears to involve displacement of phenytoin from binding sites, but the exact mechanism is not well established (60). The reduction in total serum phenytoin is accompanied by increased levels of unbound drug and increased renal clearance of unchanged phenytoin (60,61). It is possible that valproate causes both protein binding displacement and inhibition of phenytoin metabolism. Alternatively, when phenytoin is displaced from serum proteins, one would expect free serum levels to increase as a result of further saturation of the capacity-limited enzyme system responsible for phenytoin metabolism. Thus, patients receiving both valproate and phenytoin might be expected to exhibit either increased therapeutic response or toxicity from lower serum levels of total phenytoin. While such clinical effects have not been observed, practitioners should interpret serum phenytoin levels cautiously when patients are also receiving valproate. Analysis of this drug interaction and its clinical significance is further complicated by the observation that total serum phenytoin may return to pre-valproate levels after 5–12 months of continuous therapy (62). When valproate and phenytoin are administered con-

comitantly, decisions concerning the phenytoin dosage regimen alteration should be based primarily on the patient's clinical status.

Other Interactions. In R.V., the addition of valproate may also elevate total phenytoin serum concentrations as a result of increased phenobarbital serum levels. Phenobarbital competes with phenytoin for hepatic metabolic enzymes. The impact of this interaction will be minimized by the recommended reduction in phenobarbital dosage. A further consideration is the stimulation of valproate metabolism by phenytoin and phenobarbital. The clinical significance of this interaction in R.V. is minor, because valproate is being added to his regimen. It is likely that R.V. will require somewhat higher doses of valproate to achieve therapeutic results than he might otherwise.

In summary, it would be prudent to reduce R.V.'s phenobarbital dose to 200 mg/day. This will prevent a dramatic increase in phenobarbital serum levels and may eliminate an increase in phenytoin serum concentration. No alteration in phenytoin dosage is necessary. R.V. should be monitored closely for clinical signs of phenytoin and/or phenobarbital intoxication. Serum levels of both phenytoin and phenobarbital should be determined frequently; however, phenytoin levels must be interpreted cautiously.

13. *Valproate Hepatotoxicity.* Five weeks later, R.V. is taking 500 mg of valproate tid. His serum valproate concentration is 57 mcg/ml. He has had no absence seizures for two and a half weeks. On a routine clinic visit, his SGOT is reported to be 37 IU/ml (normal 7–17) and SGPT is 31 IU/ml (normal 6–14). Baseline liver function tests were all normal in R.V. Alkaline phosphatase, bilirubin, prothrombin time, and serum albumin are all normal. Physical examination was negative for scleral icterus, abdominal pain or other signs of liver disease. Discuss valproate-related hepatotoxicity. How should R.V. be managed on the basis of these new findings?

Several deaths from hepatic failure have been associated with valproate therapy (57,63,64). Transient increases in liver enzymes (SGOT, SGPT) occur during the first two to three months of therapy; in some patients, this effect is dose-related and disappears with dose reduction or discontinuation (57,65). Sussman and McLain (66) found reversible decreases in plasma fibrinogen levels in nine patients receiving valproate; several of these patients had other liver function test abnormalities and thrombocytopenia, but none exhibited clinical bleeding manifestations. Browne (57) estimates a 15–30% incidence for all types of hepatic toxicity. However, on the basis of published reports and cases reported to the manufacturer, serious hepatotoxicity appears to be uncommon. The mechanism of valproate-associated liver damage is not established. There is some evidence that the drug causes direct hepatocellular damage and interferes with oxidation of fatty acids (63,64,67).

Browne (57) recommends discontinuation of valproate if: a) SGOT/SGPT levels increase to above three times the upper limit of normal, b) symptoms of hepatitis appear, or c) other laboratory tests of hepatic function (serum albumin concentration, alkaline phosphatase, coagulation studies, or bilirubin) become abnormal. When there are less dramatic elevations in SGOT/SGPT with no other abnormalities, it may be possible to continue valproate at lower doses with careful monitoring of liver function tests.

As R.V. presently exhibits only elevations in SGOT and SGPT, it is probably not necessary to discontinue valproate. The valproate dose should be reduced to 1250 mg/day; SGOT/SGPT, alkaline phosphatase, bilirubin, and coagulation tests should be monitored weekly. In addition R.V.'s parents should be instructed to observe the patient closely for signs or symptoms suggesting hepatic disease.

Phenytoin

14. An 18-year-old, 85 kg male college student recently suffered his first convulsion. His roommate witnessed the episode, and stated that, without warning, the patient fell to the floor with "a loud, moaning grunt." He became very rigid for a few seconds, and then began "thrashing around and foaming at the mouth" for "a couple of minutes." The patient was completely unconscious for 5–10 minutes after the convulsive movements ceased. During the convulsion, the patient was incontinent of urine. The roommate transported him to the hospital immediately after he regained consciousness. On arrival, the patient was groggy and mildly confused.

The patient denied any history of previous seizures, head trauma, or recent drug or alcohol ingestions. Complete physical examination was normal. Laboratory studies including glucose, electrolytes, drug screen, and lumbar puncture were normal except for a markedly elevated CPK. A complete neurologic examination was also normal. An EEG showed diffuse slowing with no focal abnormalities; it was interpreted as essentially normal.

The patient had a second seizure while hospitalized. The nursing staff described an episode identical to that related by the roommate. No localizing signs or aura were noted by the nursing staff or the patient. There was symmetric bilateral involvement of the extremities. The entire seizure lasted 85 seconds. How is the information available concerning this patient used to select drug therapy?

Selection of an appropriate anticonvulsant depends upon accurate seizure assessment and classification. In addition, commitment of a patient to drug therapy which may be life-long should be approached cautiously. Such therapy should be instituted only after it is established that the patient suffers from recurring rather than isolated seizures. Accurate classification of seizure type depends primarily on the patient's history and seizure descriptions by observers. Results of neurological examination and laboratory data are of only secondary usefulness.

In this patient, both seizures were described identically and were characteristic of classic generalized tonic-clonic seizures. The absence of localizing signs such as unilateral convulsion or head aversion and the absence of an aura indicate that the patient's seizures are primary rather than secondarily generalized. The primary nature of the generalized seizures is also supported by the lack of focal abnormalities in the EEG. Negative results of biochemical and physical examinations tend to reduce the likelihood that there is an underlying metabolic or physical etiology. The patient's elevated CPK is of no significance; it is an expected finding following extreme muscular exertion and muscle damage secondary to the fall accompanying the seizure. In summary, this patient appears to suffer from recurrent primary generalized tonic-clonic seizures, and prophylactic anticonvulsant therapy is indicated.

Based on the patient's seizure diagnosis, possible choices for anticonvulsant therapy would usually include phenobarbital, phenytoin, or carbamazepine. Carbamazepine is usually very effective for this seizure type, but many clinicians would not consider it a primary drug for this seizure type on the basis of its reputation for inducing toxic effects such as bone marrow suppression (see Question 39). Phenobarbital would be a less desirable choice for this patient, since it is more sedating than either phenytoin or carbamazepine. Sedation would be undesirable in this mentally-active student. Phenytoin is non-sedating for most patients. While its use is associated with a number of side effects, most clinicians still consider it to be the drug of first choice for this seizure type.

15. On the basis of the factors discussed above, phenytoin was selected for this patient. The initial dosage was 400 mg hs. The patient was to return to the clinic in two weeks for determination of a phenytoin serum level and evaluation of his response. Further dose adjustments were planned as indicated by clinical response and serum drug concentrations. It was felt that complete seizure control was a reasonable goal for drug therapy in this patient. Evaluate the choice of initial phenytoin dosage for this patient.

Selection of a nontoxic, therapeutic dose of any anticonvulsant is difficult in the absence of information regarding the drug's disposition in the individual patient being treated (eg, prior doses and resulting steady-state serum levels). Although average doses and average resulting serum levels are often quoted, there is significant interpatient variability. Phenytoin serum levels of 10 mcg/ml or greater will be achieved in a large proportion of adult patients receiving 4–5 mg/kg/day; however, either subtherapeutic or potentially toxic levels may occur in significant numbers (68–70). Thus, careful assessment of clinical response and use of serum level results are important to dosage individualization.

An initial dose of 400 mg/day would be appropriate for this patient. As an outpatient, he should be informed that symptoms such as blurred or double vision, difficult speech ("thick" tongue), dizziness or staggering may indicate that his dose is too high; he should be instructed to notify his physician, pharmacist, or other health care provider of these symptoms.

16. *Phenytoin Accumulation Kinetics.* What are the characteristics of phenytoin accumulation kinetics? When should phenytoin serum levels be measured in this patient?

Because phenytoin exhibits dose-dependent (Michaelis-Menten) pharmacokinetics, the usual concepts of "clearance" and "half-life" are meaningless. The apparent half-life of the drug changes with dose and serum level. Thus, it becomes difficult to predict the time required to reach steady-state after initiation of a new maintenance dose; the time required depends on both the dose and the individual patient's kinetic parameters, Vmax and Km (69). Vmax is a kinetic constant representing the maximum rate of phenytoin elimination from the body. Km is the Michaelis Constant; it is the serum phenytoin concentration at which the rate of elimination is one-half of Vmax. Many clinicians assume that phenytoin's apparent half-life is approximately 24 hours, and wait 5–7 days before assessing the patient's clinical response and measuring serum drug concentrations. Both clinical studies (69) and model simulations (70) using observed values for Vmax and Km indicate that up to 30 days may be required for serum levels to reach 90% of the steady-state resulting from a dose of 4 mg/kg/day. Occasionally, such a dose may exceed a patient's Vmax. Accumulation of extremely high serum phenytoin levels with probable intoxication will result. Similarly, if doses sufficient to produce steady-state serum levels of 10–15 mcg/ml are given, 5 to 30 days may be required to reach 90% of these levels (70). One should not assume that steady-state has been reached unless widely-spaced, serial serum concentrations indicate that accumulation has ceased. Alterations, especially increases, in phenytoin dosage before steady-state has been reached may result in marked fluctuation of serum levels and seizure control. In this author's experience, such situations occur frequently in practice and result in unnecessary confusion and expense.

Given the variability in phenytoin's accumulation kinetics, a reasonable approach to timing of blood level measurements would involve weekly serum level determinations during the first month of treatment to detect either excessive accumulation or subtherapeutic dosing. Even though serum levels appear stable and are in the usual therapeutic range after one month, continued slow accumulation may occur. Close monitoring of phenytoin levels is still advisable after this period. As always, the patient's clinical response must be correlated with serum levels.

17. *Oral Phenytoin Loading Doses.* **Considering the potential delay in accumulation of phenytoin, would a loading dose be of value for this patient? How should loading doses be administered?**

Administration of a loading dose would allow therapeutic serum concentrations of phenytoin to be achieved more rapidly. More rapid control of his seizure activity will also result. As he is apparently active and pursuing an education, more rapid seizure control may be a significant goal. Oral loading doses are often recommended in the literature and often utilized clinically. However, there is little documentation of the safety and efficacy of oral phenytoin loading in outpatients. Serum concentrations approximating the usual therapeutic range were achieved after 8 hours in 70% of a group of outpatients given 1000 mg (average 14.2 mg/kg) oral loading doses (71). Seizure control was adequate, and loading was well-tolerated when the total dose was given in increments over 4 hours; single 1 gm doses were associated with gastrointestinal upset. Sinus bradycardia and a shortened P-R interval occurred in two patients after single 900 mg doses of phenytoin. However, these changes were not associated with peak serum levels, and their overall significance is uncertain (72).

Oral phenytoin absorption is unpredictably slow. Peak serum levels following large oral doses are often not achieved for 6–14 hours (72). Record et al (73) estimated that 18 mg/kg given in 3 doses over 6 hours would produce serum levels of 13 to 20 mcg/ml 12 hours after completion of loading. No rigid evaluations of this recommendation are available, although they compare well with intravenous loading regimens. Intravenous loading doses of 18 mg/kg will maintain phenytoin serum levels above 10 mcg/ml for 24 hours (74).

While administration of an oral loading regimen to the patient is pharmacokinetically sound and has certain therapeutic advantages, lack of documented safety and difficulty of monitoring ambulatory patients for potential complications would indicate caution in recommending such a procedure. A reasonable approach to shortening the time required to achieve adequate serum concentrations with a lower risk of complications involves administration of 1½–2 times the prescribed maintenance dose for the first two or three days of treatment. Serum phenytoin levels should be checked on the day following completion of such a "mini-loading" and weekly thereafter.

18. *Phenytoin Intoxication.* **The patient was given phenytoin 200 mg in the morning and 400 mg at bedtime for three days. A phenytoin serum level drawn the morning of the fourth day was reported as 12 mcg/ml. No new seizures had occurred, and there were no side effects other than mild sedation in the morning. He was then instructed to take only 400 mg at bedtime. One week later, his phenytoin level was reported as 18 mcg/ml. Mild nystagmus on far, lateral gaze was noted, but the patient had no subjective complaints and remained free of seizures. At the end of three weeks the patient complained of some double vision and feeling "unsteady." Significant nystagmus was seen. The phenytoin level was 24 mcg/ml. How should this patient's phenytoin dosage regimen be altered?**

The signs and symptoms in conjunction with the serum levels indicate mild phenytoin intoxication. Reduction in phenytoin dosage is indicated. As there is no indication that steady-state has been achieved, techniques for estimating the patient's Vmax and Km cannot be readily employed, and the size of the dosage reduction must be determined empirically. A reduction of 40 to 70 mg in the daily dose would be reasonable. A larger reduction may result in a dramatic fall in serum levels. This dosage reduction can be accomplished by using 30 mg phenytoin capsules with the usual 100 mg capsules. Many clinicians would also have the patient omit one day's dose of phenytoin before beginning the new maintenance dose. This would accelerate the decrease in phenytoin serum levels. Following the dosage reduction, clinical response and serum levels should be assessed closely. It is possible that the new maintenance dose may still be excessive. If the patient's Vmax for phenytoin is low, continued accumulation of drug may occur, and serum levels may continue to increase following the dosage reduction (70).

19. *Phenytoin Oral Dosage Forms.* **S.K. is a 24-year-old state hospital patient with a history of complex partial seizures with secondarily generalized tonic-clonic seizures. On his present phenytoin dose of 300 mg every morning, reported serum levels have ranged**

from 3.2 to 13.5 mcg/ml. Control of his seizures also fluctuates widely. He is strongly suspected of "cheeking" his phenytoin capsules. The patient's phenytoin has been changed to a suspension form to reduce opportunities for this behavior. Discuss the differences in bioavailability and biopharmaceutics among phenytoin dosage forms. Based on these differences, determine an appropriate dose of phenytoin suspension for S.K. Are any special instructions necessary to ensure proper administration of this preparation?

Surreptitious refusal to take medications is a frequent problem in psychiatric patients. In addition, elderly, physically handicapped, or pediatric patients may have difficulty swallowing capsules. In these situations, phenytoin suspension may be useful.

There are no reported differences in bioavailability between phenytoin capsules and suspension; in addition, chewable phenytoin tablets (Dilantin Infatabs) are equally well absorbed (75–77). However, both the suspension and chewable tablets contain phenytoin acid rather than sodium phenytoin. Unlike many products, the label indicates the content in terms of either phenytoin acid or sodium phenytoin rather than in terms of active drug. Therefore, phenytoin capsules contain only 92% of the label content as phenytoin acid (eg, a 100 mg capsule contains 92 mg of phenytoin acid). Because small changes in dose may result in dramatic changes in serum phenytoin concentrations and clinical response, this difference in phenytoin content should be considered when the dosage form is changed.

If it is assumed that 300 mg of phenytoin capsules is a therapeutic dose for S.K., an appropriate dose of phenytoin suspension would be approximately 92% of 300 mg, or 275 mg of suspension. This would be 11 ml of suspension containing 125 mg/5 ml.

It is important to insure that the proper phenytoin suspension preparation is prescribed and dispensed for administration. Phenytoin suspension is available in two strengths; the pediatric suspension contains 30 mg/5 ml, and the adult suspension contains 125 mg/5 ml. Patients should be instructed carefully concerning proper use of phenytoin suspension. An accurate dosage measuring device should be provided. The person measuring the dose should be instructed to thoroughly shake the container before measuring each dose, because settling of phenytoin suspension occurs. As a result, when fresh bottles of suspension are inadequately shaken, patients may receive too low a dose. Later, patients may receive too high a dose with resulting toxicity.

20. Is there any need to alter frequency of phenytoin administration when phenytoin suspension is used for S.K.?

The F.D.A. has recently required that all phenytoin capsule preparations be re-labeled as either "prompt" or "extended." Clinicians have been cautioned that, because of its slow dissolution and absorption, Parke-Davis' Dilantin Sodium Kapseals are the only extended product and are the only phenytoin product suitable for once-a-day dosing (78). Presumably, if preparations which are absorbed rapidly are administered as a single daily dose, wide fluctuations in phenytoin serum levels may result in either loss of seizure control or intoxication.

Published documentation of significant differences in phenytoin serum levels resulting from use of rapidly absorbed versus slowly absorbed preparations is lacking. Most studies on the feasibility of single daily phenytoin doses have used Parke-Davis' Kapseals (79–81). The likely effects of absorption rate and dosing interval on steady-state phenytoin serum levels have been examined using a Michaelis-Menten pharmacokinetic model (82). Predicted fluctuations with rapidly absorbed products administered once daily are not likely to be clinically significant unless the patient requires a very high daily dose or has a low therapeutic index. Although the rate of phenytoin absorption does not appear to be of major clinical significance to therapy, extent of absorption (relative bioavailability) may dramatically affect steady-state serum levels and clinical response. Dose-dependency seen with phenytoin pharmacokinetics tends to magnify the effects of even minor changes in bioavailability. In conclusion, the clinical significance of differences in absorption rates for oral phenytoin preparations is yet to be determined, but appears minor at present (82,82a).

Patient S.K. can probably be adequately managed with administration of his phenytoin suspension as a single daily dose. His clinical response and serum levels should be monitored carefully to detect significant effects of the suspension or dosage schedule on seizure control.

21. *Intramuscular Phenytoin.* S.K. has been stabilized while receiving 275 mg of phenytoin daily as suspension. Serum drug concentrations are stable at 10–12 mcg/ml and he has had no seizures for two months. S.K. has been transferred to the acute medical unit following a two-day history of anorexia, nausea, occasional vomiting, and abdominal pain accompanied by diarrhea. He is now NPO. Intramuscular phenytoin has been ordered. Discuss the biopharmaceutic differences between oral and intramuscular phenytoin and devise a dosage regimen and plan for use of IM phenytoin in S.K.

Intramuscular administration of phenytoin is generally not recommended, especially in situations requiring either rapid onset of effect or long-term use of IM injections. Injectable phenytoin is highly alkaline (pH 12) and potentially very irritating to tissue. Following IM injection, the drug may precipitate at the injection site because of the change in pH. As a result, phenytoin crystals form a repository or depot from which the drug is very slowly absorbed (83–85). Absorption is approximately 93% complete from IM sites, but is prolonged for 3–5 days (83).

Changing from oral to IM phenytoin administration will result in a 40–60% fall in serum phenytoin levels (86) as a result of the extreme prolongation of absorption. This fall may be prevented by administering 1½ times the oral dose as IM medication (86) for the duration of IM therapy. After 7–10 days, especially in patients receiving the drug in divided doses, serum levels may begin to rise as a result of increased absorption from multiple depots. This may necessitate further dosage adjustments. When the patient is returned to oral therapy, the phenytoin dose should be 50% of the pre-IM oral dose for a time period equal to the duration of intramuscular therapy (86).

Intramuscular injections of phenytoin are painful, although severe muscle damage does not appear to occur (87). As parenteral phenytoin products contain only 50 mg/ml of sodium phenytoin, multiple injections of a maximum of 2–3 ml each will be required in many patients. If IM phenytoin is instituted for prolonged intervals, the nursing staff should be reminded to rotate injection sites. In this patient, 450 mg/day (9 ml, or 3–5 injections daily) of IM phenytoin will be required. This dosage will take into account the change from phenytoin acid to sodium phenytoin. Serum levels should be determined every 3–4 days, and the IM dose reduced if serum levels increase above 13–14 mcg/ml. When the patient is restarted on oral medication, he should receive 150 mg/day of phenytoin sodium capsules for a period of time equal to the duration of IM therapy.

As treatment with IM phenytoin requires careful dosage adjustment and is unpleasant for patients, this drug should be administered by IV rather than IM injection whenever feasible (see Questions 49 and 50 for discussion of intravenous administration of phenytoin).

22. *Renal Disease.* A patient with end-stage renal failure has recently developed recurring seizures for which phenytoin was prescribed. The patient is receiving hemodialysis three times weekly. The phenytoin dosage was increased to 260 mg/day three weeks ago. Over the past week, symptoms of phenytoin intoxication have slowly developed. Nystagmus, ataxia, slurred speech, and mild drowsiness are present. The serum phenytoin concentration is 13 mcg/ml. How does uremia alter phenytoin's pharmacokinetics, and how might these alterations explain this patient's apparent intoxication at serum levels which are usually well-tolerated?

Phenytoin is extensively metabolized by hepatic microsomal enzymes; less than 5% of the drug is excreted unchanged by the kidneys (68). Therefore, one might anticipate little effect of renal disease on the clearance of phenytoin. However, uremic patients consistently exhibit total phenytoin serum levels which are lower than those seen in non-uremic patients (88). Lowered serum levels result primarily from the effects of uremia on the binding of phenytoin to albumin. Decreased concentration of serum albumin may also play a role in some patients (89). Normally, phenytoin is approximately 85–90% protein-bound, while in uremic patients the fraction bound is reduced to 70–80%. Thus, for a given total phenytoin serum level, the level of free phenytoin will be higher in uremic patients. One would expect to see both therapeutic response and toxicity occurring at lower serum levels in such patients. Despite the higher concentration of unbound drug, hemodialysis does not appear to remove significant amounts of phenytoin from the body (90). However, hemodialysis does unpredictably alter the protein binding of the drug (91,92).

As a result of these effects of renal disease on phenytoin's kinetics, it has been recommended that free (unbound) rather than total phenytoin levels be monitored (91). This can be accomplished with reasonable accuracy by measurement of either erythrocyte phenytoin levels or saliva levels (91,93).

23. *Hepatic Disease.* **A patient who is receiving 390 mg of phenytoin daily has developed hepatitis-B antigen-positive hepatitis. There is marked jaundice and dramatic elevations in SGOT and SGPT. How may hepatitis alter this patient's phenytoin dosage requirements? What additional patient monitoring may be required?**

The effect of liver disease on phenytoin kinetics is not well studied. There are case reports of phenytoin intoxication in patients with liver disease, and presumably, reduced metabolism of phenytoin may have played some role (68,94). Blaschke and associates (95) found that acute viral hepatitis did not alter phenytoin clearance in five patients. There was an increase in the percentage of unbound drug possibly resulting from reduced serum albumin concentration and/or elevated bilirubin levels. Thus, as in uremic patients, patients with acute inflammatory hepatic disease may show an altered relationship between total phenytoin serum levels and clinical response. Careful monitoring of this patient's status possibly combined with assessment of free phenytoin (saliva or erythrocyte) levels may be necessary.

24. *Phenytoin Hypersensitivity.* **A 22-year-old female began taking phenytoin 300 mg/ day three weeks ago for control of generalized tonic-clonic seizures. She has now returned to the clinic complaining of a generalized pruritic skin rash, fever, and myalgias. She describes having a "cold" (fever and sore throat) for three days. The rash first appeared this morning and appears erythematous and scaly. The oral mucous membranes appear inflamed and swollen. Physical examination disclosed hepatosplenomegaly and generalized lymph node enlargement. Her sclera were mildly icteric. Temperature was 39°C, pulse was 115/minute, and blood pressure was 116/62 mm Hg. Laboratory studies revealed an elevated WBC count (12,400/mm³)**

with 18% eosinophils. The WBC differential was otherwise normal. Other laboratory results were normal with the following exceptions: total bilirubin was 3.0 mg/dl (normal 0.1 to 1.2); direct bilirubin was 1.6 mg/dl (normal 0 to 0.3); alkaline phosphatase was 245 mU/ml (normal 35–85); LDH was 640 mU/ml (normal 110–240); SGOT was 410 mU/ml (normal 25–55); SGPT was 90 mU/ml (normal 5–25). Serum phenytoin concentration was 11 mcg/ml. What subjective and objective findings in this patient provide evidence for a hypersensitivity reaction to phenytoin?

This patient's symptoms and laboratory findings are typical of reported cases of phenytoin hypersensitivity (96,97). Her "cold"-like symptoms, skin rash, lymphadenopathy, and hepatosplenomegaly are typical multisystemic manifestations of this reaction. The predominating clinical picture in reported cases may be one of erythema multiforme/Stevens-Johnson syndrome, hepatic necrosis, pseudolymphoma, or serum sickness. Nevertheless, many or all signs and symptoms may co-exist (97). This patient's laboratory results point to significant hepatic involvement. Marked eosinophilic leukocytosis is a common finding. The relatively low serum phenytoin concentration is not unusual, as these hypersensitivity reactions are not dose or serum level related.

Phenytoin hypersensitivity most commonly occurs during the first month of treatment. Although this reaction is uncommon, it causes significant morbidity, and approximately one-third of the cases involving hepatotoxicity are fatal (97). While the mechanism for these reactions has not been established, clinical features (eosinophilia, rash, lymphadenopathy) are characteristic of a delayed hypersensitivity type immune response.

Lymphadenopathy seen with phenytoin is particularly interesting since, in some patients, the condition may closely resemble lymphoid malignancy, hence, the term "pseudolymphoma." Patients with lymphadenopathy associated with phenytoin appear to fall into four groups: 1) Benign lymphoid hyperplasia which does not resemble lymphoma histologically and disappears following drug withdrawal; 2) Pseudolymphoma which is clinically similar to benign hyperplasia, but histologically is identical to a true lymphoma. Typical Reed-Sternberg cells may be seen. Pseudolymphoma also disappears after phenytoin is withdrawn; 3) True lymphoma has developed rarely in patients receiving phenytoin and does not regress when the drug is stopped; and 4) Pseudo-pseudolymphoma in which true malignant lymphoma develops later in a patient who has had a pseudolymphoma reaction (98). The last two groups seem to occur primarily after prolonged therapy. Retrospective epidemiologic studies have produced conflicting evidence relating phenytoin and other anticonvulsants to the occurrence of malignancy (99,100). It is believed that lymphoma may result from immunosuppressive effects of phenytoin (100) which are thought to allow development of malignant cell lines.

Monitoring for the development of phenytoin hypersensitivity is most important during the first few months of treatment. Laboratory indices of hepatic damage (SGOT/SGPT and bilirubin) should be evaluated monthly during the first six months of treatment. Patients should be instructed to report the development of skin rash, especially if accompanied by "flu"-like symptoms or fever, to their health care provider immediately.

25. How should this patient's hypersensitivity reaction be managed?

It is mandatory that phenytoin be discontinued immediately. In addition, many clinicians would administer systemic corticosteroids (eg, prednisone 60–120 mg/day) to this patient because of the severe multisystemic involvement. Because of the evidence for hepatic damage, this patient should be monitored closely for signs of hepatic failure such as changes in mental status, progression of jaundice, and hypoalbuminemia. Occurrence of these signs and symptoms may necessitate institution of measures such as "bowel sterilization" with non-absorbable antibiotics, lactulose therapy, and dietary protein restriction.

Improvement in symptoms and laboratory manifestations may be delayed for several days. Recovery usually occurs over a period of several weeks, although laboratory abnormalities may persist for several months (98a).

When phenytoin is discontinued, alternative anticonvulsant therapy should be instituted. Either phenobarbital or carbamazepine would appear to be reasonable alternative drugs for this patient.

26. *Phenytoin-Induced Gingival Hyperplasia.* A 10-year-old boy receiving 150 mg of phenytoin daily as chewable tablets is to be fitted with braces for his teeth. He currently exhibits moderate gingival hyperplasia which is associated with difficult maintenance of oral hygiene and resultant halitosis. Discuss phenytoin-induced gingival hyperplasia and possible management techniques which may be helpful for this patient.

Gum hyperplasia related to phenytoin is common and troublesome. Prevalence estimates range as high as 84% of treated patients (49), although the actual prevalence will vary according to the rating system used and the degree of gum change rated as hyperplastic. A realistic prevalence estimate is probably 40–50% of treated patients (101). However, prevalence or incidence rates are misleading, because the occurrence and severity of this adverse effect are related to the dose and serum level of phenytoin (102,103). In one study, no patient had normal gingiva if the phenytoin serum level exceeded 20 mcg/ml (102). Gingival hyperplasia is of obvious cosmetic importance. Also, as in this patient, formation of pockets of tissue leads to difficulties with oral hygiene. Severe halitosis (fetor oris) may result.

The mechanism of phenytoin-induced gingival hyperplasia is not well understood. The drug is excreted in saliva, and there is a correlation between saliva concentration and hyperplasia (104); however, this correlation may simply reflect higher serum levels producing greater pharmacologic effect. A likely mechanism involves stimulation of release of various mediators (eg, heparin) from gingival mast-cells (50). Released heparin may stimulate fibroblasts to synthesize excessive new connective tissue. Local irritation secondary to dental plaque and food particles may further stimulate this process. Thus, poor oral hygiene may also perpetuate gingival hyperplasia. Some patients may be especially predisposed to gum hyperplasia because they accumulate relatively higher levels of phenytoin in gingival tissue (105).

There are three approaches to treatment of existing gum hyperplasia (50): a) Dosage reduction or discontinuation of phenytoin, if possible, will permit reduction or complete reversal of hyperplasia. Substitution of an alternate anticonvulsant such as carbamazepine may be necessary. b) Surgical gingivectomy will correct the problem temporarily. In most patients, hyperplasia will eventually recur. c) Oral physiotherapy (periodontal treatment) eliminates local irritants and maintains oral hygiene. As this patient is to be fitted with braces, which will further complicate oral hygiene, institution of some form of treatment and prevention of further tissue enlargement are important. Assuming that phenytoin is producing adequate seizure control, a combination of gingivectomy followed by periodontal treatment may be the best approach.

Theoretically, use of chewable phenytoin tablets in this patient may aggravate hyperplasia. Exposure of gingiva to high local concentrations of drug may result from braces' holding fragments of tablets in close contact with tissue (106). There is some question as to the significance of this relationship; however, if the patient is able to swallow capsules, a change to this dosage form may be beneficial and will usually be less expensive. The most appropriate dose of phenytoin sodium capsules for this patient would be 160 mg/day. If chewable tablets are used, having the patient rinse and swallow after each dose may eliminate potential problems. Use of phenytoin suspension may also be a theoretically useful option. However, drug particles may still be retained by the braces, and maintenance of uniform dosage may be more difficult.

Oral hygiene programs appear to effectively reduce the degree and severity of gingival hyperplasia when they are initiated before phenytoin therapy (50). Patients who are beginning phenytoin therapy should be educated as to the role of oral hygiene in diminishing this side effect. The use of oral hygiene aids such as dental floss or Water-Pik type appliances may be beneficial.

27. Describe other effects of phenytoin on connective tissue growth.

There is some evidence that phenytoin, and possibly other anticonvulsants, may have a generalized stimulating effect on formation of connective tissue (107). Coarse facial features and calvarial thickening have been associated with prolonged, high-dose anticonvulsant therapy (51,52). Phenytoin was commonly used in these patients and there was a correlation between the presence of marked gingival hyperplasia and coarsening of features (51). This effect has also been observed in one member of each of two sets of identical twins (52). This syndrome consists of enlargement of the nose and lips, and thickening of subcutaneous tissue of the face and scalp. Patients' faces take on the appearance seen in those with acromegaly, but changes are not seen in other parts of the body (eg, the hands). Of 222 mentally retarded patients with seizure disorders, two-thirds were affected (51). Affected patients appear to have more severe seizure disorders and to receive higher

doses of drugs. Thus, it is possible that epilepsy itself or injury from seizures may influence this syndrome. Nevertheless, the risk of this reaction provides further impetus to reduce anticonvulsant doses to the lowest effective level.

28. Anticonvulsant-Related Anemia. B.N., a 32-year-old mentally retarded patient, receives phenytoin 260 mg/day and phenobarbital 100 mg/day. Tonic-clonic seizures occur 4–5 times yearly. Serum phenytoin concentration is 16 mcg/ml and serum phenobarbital concentration is 31 mcg/ml. A routine annual CBC revealed a hemoglobin of 10.8 gm/dl (normal 13.5–16) and a MCV of 108 cubic microns (normal 82–96). Serum folate concentration was 2.8 mcg/ml (normal 7–18); serum B_{12} was normal. Other laboratory results were normal. Physical examination was unremarkable except for mild pallor and a swollen "beefy red" tongue. B.N.'s diet is normal. What is the relationship between B.N.'s drug therapy and her clinical and laboratory manifestations?

On the basis of B.N.'s laboratory results and symptoms, she appears to have a folate-deficient megaloblastic anemia. Characteristically, this condition is manifested as a macrocytic anemia which may be accompanied by glossitis and skin pallor (see Anemias chapter). As her diet is normal and physical exam is negative, it appears likely that anticonvulsant treatment is responsible for this condition.

Altered folate metabolism commonly results from anticonvulsant therapy. Low serum folate levels occur in up to 91% of patients, and macrocytosis is seen in up to 50%. Actual megaloblastic anemia is very uncommon (less than 0.75%) (107–109). Phenytoin is most commonly associated with this effect, but other anticonvulsants have been implicated. In addition to anemia, altered folate metabolism is postulated to result in mental symptoms such as dementia in some patients (110,111).

The mechanism of anticonvulsant-related folate deficiency is not known. Possible mechanisms include: a) increased folate metabolism secondary to hepatic enzyme induction, b) inhibition of absorption of dietary folate, c) antagonism of folate coenzymes, and d) increased utilization of folic acid as a coenzyme for hepatic enzymes induced by drug therapy (including those enzymes which metabolize anticonvulsants) (111). Evidence that phenytoin inhibits folate absorption is inconclusive, and this mechanism is probably not important (112). Anticonvulsants may also directly interfere with DNA synthesis which would result in megaloblastic changes and a secondary folate deficiency (113,114).

The significance of anticonvulsant-related folate deficiency in non-anemic patients is unclear. The evidence that patients' mental status improves with folate replacement is conflicting, and there is no known clear relationship between anticonvulsant-associated teratogenesis (see below) and folate deficiency (108,115). Therefore, there seems to be little justification for folate replacement in asymptomatic patients with decreased serum folate levels since only a small fraction will develop anemia.

29. How should B.N.'s anemia be treated, and how should the effect of this treatment be monitored?

Anticonvulsant-related megaloblastic anemia responds readily to treatment with small oral doses of folic acid; 1 mg daily should be sufficient to correct B.N.'s anemia and secondary symptoms such as glossitis (111). Within one week of instituting folate therapy, there should be a reticulocytosis and a beginning elevation in hemoglobin and RBC count. Macrocytosis may require several weeks to disappear, as macrocytic RBC's must die and be removed by the reticuloendothelial system. Pallor should disappear as hemoglobin normalizes. B.N. should be observed over three to four weeks to insure that remission of signs occurs. CBC's should be repeated weekly during this time to monitor correction of anemia.

B.N.'s folic acid supplementation should probably be continued indefinitely. Although relapse of anemia occurs in only 10% of patients, long-term folate prophylaxis is inexpensive and usually harmless.

30. Are there any potential interactions between B.N.'s folic acid supplementation and her anticonvulsant therapy?

Folic acid replacement therapy may precipitate increased seizure activity in this patient, and her clinical status and serum drug concentrations should be monitored closely during initiation of therapy. While controlled studies have not shown consistent precipitation of seizures, occasional patients may rapidly exhibit this effect (108,115). Folate at doses of 5–30 mg/day may cause significant, although usually small, decreases in phenytoin serum levels (116,117). Folate appears to stimulate phenytoin metabolism and may increase urinary excretion (118). Similar effects may occur with phenobarbital and carbamazepine (119). In certain patients, the decrease in serum anticonvulsant concentration may be sufficient to precipitate seizures. Unfortunately, there is little information concerning the effects of smaller doses of folate on serum levels or seizure control.

31. *Phenytoin Encephalopathy and Neurologic Effects.* Ms. P. recently had her phenytoin dose increased from 300 mg daily to 400 mg daily in response to an apparent increase in seizure frequency. At 300 mg/day, the phenytoin serum level was 11 mcg/ml. After three weeks at the new dose, Ms. P. is brought to the physician by her sister who reports that the patient has become confused, staggers, and has developed "funny" movements of her face and arms. In addition, she has had several seizures over the past few days which consist of arching of her neck and back for 10–20 seconds with mild clonic movements of both arms. Abnormal facial and arm movements are noted to consist of rapid, jerky random movements of the arms and repetitive rolling tongue movements accompanied by facial grimacing. Ms. P. is disoriented to time and place. No nystagmus is seen. Discuss Ms. P.'s symptoms and their relationship to phenytoin therapy.

Ms. P. is probably exhibiting phenytoin encephalopathy, an acute change in mental status and seizure frequency which may accompany elevated phenytoin serum levels. In addition, her choreiform movements are also probably a result of phenytoin intoxication (107,120). Based on her previous serum level and the magnitude of the recent dose increase, intoxication with phenytoin is likely; a serum level should be determined immediately to confirm this. In addition, a complete neurologic examination should be performed to rule out other potential causes for Ms. P.'s sudden change in neurological status.

Increased seizure frequency and a change in seizure pattern to include manifestations of opisthotonos may accompany phenytoin encephalopathy. Confusion, delirium and other changes in mental status are also frequently associated (107). While this syndrome is probably much less common than classical phenytoin intoxication (nystagmus, ataxia, CNS depression), clinicians should be alert to the possibility of its occurrence. On clinical grounds, one may be tempted to further increase the phenytoin dosage in an effort to control the increased seizures, while dose reduction is actually the appropriate method of correcting such a situation. Nystagmus is absent in some cases, and this further complicates assessment. This sign often does not appear until phenytoin levels fall.

Choreiform movement disorders are an uncommon complication of phenytoin therapy. Affected patients are often mentally retarded or have functional or structural CNS impairment (121, 122). In addition to chorea, patients may also exhibit dystonia and asterixis. The movement disorders are usually reversible after discontinuation of the causative drug. Other anticonvulsants may also cause dyskinesias as a part of an intoxication syndrome (123).

32. Ms. P's serum phenytoin level was reported as 32 mcg/ml. The neurological workup was otherwise negative. After the daily dose was reduced to 360 mg, her mental symptoms cleared and the choreiform movements disappeared. No seizures were reported during the following eight weeks. However, she continued to complain of being mildly "unsteady" on her feet. Nystagmus on far, lateral gaze is not present. Serum phenytoin is reported as 24 mcg/ml. As Ms. P.'s seizures are now under apparently complete control, is there any problem maintaining her on mildly intoxicating doses of phenytoin? Does prolonged intoxication with phenytoin increase the likelihood of permanent cerebellar dysfunction or peripheral neuropathy?

Patients who are chronically maintained on intoxicating doses of phenytoin appear to be at some risk for developing irreversible neurologic damage. Cerebellar degeneration resulting in symptoms such as dysarthria, ataxic gait, intention tremor and muscular hypotonia is of particular concern (109,124). Generalized seizures may also cause cerebellar degeneration secondary to hypoxia. For this reason, there is some controversy concerning the relative importance of phenytoin in the development of this condition. However, a number of reported cases involved patients without hypoxic seizures (124,125). Animal studies also suggest that high serum levels of phenytoin cause

permanent cerebellar damage. It is possible that in some patients, cerebellar damage results from the effects of both phenytoin and seizure-related hypoxia.

Symptomatic phenytoin-related peripheral neuropathy is uncommon, although electrophysiologic evidence of impaired neuronal conduction may be found in a larger number of patients (126,127). Symptomatic patients may complain of paresthesias and muscle weakness; there may be occasional muscle wasting. Knee and ankle tendon reflexes are absent in 18% of patients on long-term phenytoin therapy; impairment of vibration and position sense may accompany areflexia. The upper limbs are affected rarely (126). Absence of tendon reflexes appears to correlate with a duration of phenytoin therapy greater than 15 years (126). Presence of sensory symptoms and electrophysiologic impairment appears to be associated with the presence of elevated serum phenytoin levels (127). There is little information as to the reversibility of phenytoin neuropathy. Areflexia may be irreversible (126), while electrophysiologic abnormalities may be closely related to excessive blood levels and therefore reversible following dosage reduction or discontinuation (127).

In this patient, the general discomfort of mild phenytoin intoxication and the potential for producing cerebellar degeneration would appear to dictate an alteration in therapy. Dosage reduction to 330 mg daily should be attempted first, as this dose may produce adequate seizure control without toxic symptoms. Should seizures recur at this lower dose, it may be advisable to attempt to treat her epilepsy with an alternate anticonvulsant such as carbamazepine. Some clinicians would advocate combination therapy with nonintoxicating doses of phenytoin and another anticonvulsant such as phenobarbital.

COMPLEX PARTIAL EPILEPSY

Primidone

33. A.R. is a 17-year-old female who experiences complex partial seizures characterized by dizziness and a "buzzing" sensation followed by unconsciousness. During these episodes she occasionally exhibits clonic movements of the left arm and purposeless picking at her clothes. Therapy was initiated with phenobarbital. She now takes 190 mg

daily. Despite a serum phenobarbital level of 43 mcg/ml she still experiences three or four "spells" monthly. Prior to treatment, she was having four to five seizures per month. She frequently complains of drowsiness, and during an interview her speech was noted to be thick and slightly slurred. There is nystagmus on lateral gaze and mild ataxia. Her physician is considering changing her medication to primidone. Is this contemplated medication change rational since primidone is metabolized to phenobarbital? What other alternate medications might be considered?

The rationality of substituting primidone for phenobarbital in this patient is questionable. Traditionally, primidone has been regarded as a drug of choice for treatment of complex partial (psychomotor) seizures. However, documentation of its superiority to other medications for this type of seizure is lacking. Both animal studies (128) and clinical trials (129–131) have failed to show that primidone is more effective than phenobarbital when doses are used which produce equal phenobarbital serum levels. However, tonic-clonic seizures may be more responsive to primidone than phenobarbital (128,131).

Primidone is metabolized to both phenobarbital and phenyl-ethyl-malonamide (PEMA) (132). All three compounds are thought to be active anticonvulsants (133), although primidone itself is not consistently active in animal models (129). Presumably, it is primidone and PEMA which make primidone different from phenobarbital.

As A.R.'s complex partial seizures have not responded well to maximal doses of phenobarbital, there is little likelihood that primidone will be effective. Either phenytoin or carbamazepine would be appropriate alternative medications (4). Many clinicians now consider carbamazepine to be the drug of first choice for this seizure type. This patient's age and sex and the potential adverse effects of phenytoin (hirsutism, gingival hypertrophy, etc.) might influence a decision in favor of carbamazepine.

34. *Primidone Dosage.* A.R. is to receive a therapeutic trial of primidone in an attempt to avoid the potential toxicities of phenytoin and carbamazepine. How can a maintenance dose be selected which will produce therapeutically effective drug serum levels while avoiding toxicity?

As a general rule of thumb, five-fold higher doses of primidone are required to produce equivalent phenobarbital serum levels, although there is considerable variation among individuals. As A.R. is intoxicated on her present phenobarbital dose, a lower equivalent primidone maintenance dose should be prescribed. Using a four-fold conversion factor, 750 mg of primidone daily should provide a nontoxic regimen. Primidone itself has a half-life of approximately 8 hours (132); this daily dose should therefore be divided and given tid to avoid wide fluctuations in primidone serum levels.

35. *Initiation of Primidone Therapy.* How should primidone therapy for A.R. be initiated? How do this drug's side effects or toxicities differ from those of phenobarbital?

Ordinarily, primidone therapy should not be initiated at full therapeutic doses, because many patients experience considerable drowsiness and ataxia during early therapy. These effects may be accompanied by nystagmus and nausea. Initial side effects are closely related to serum levels of primidone rather than phenobarbital or PEMA (134). However, patients who have previously received phenobarbital are often tolerant to these initial side effects. In addition to these side effects, occasional patients report psychological reactions to primidone including difficulty concentrating and personality changes (135).

In this patient, primidone can probably be abruptly substituted for her current phenobarbital regimen. Serum phenobarbital concentrations should decline to nontoxic levels if the primidone dosage conversion has been appropriate. Serum levels of both primidone and phenobarbital should be determined after one week of therapy to assess adequacy of dosage in terms of primidone. As phenobarbital will probably not be at steady-state, this serum level, in conjunction with the patient's clinical status, will serve only as a rough index of the accuracy of dose conversion.

36. *Primidone-Phenytoin Interaction.* A.R.'s primidone dose was eventually titrated to 1000 mg daily. At this dose she continued to have two to three "spells" per month. Serum primidone was 11 mcg/ml and serum phenobarbital was 36 mcg/ml. There were no signs of intoxication. On the basis of some improvement with primidone, her physician elected to add phenytoin 260 mg/day (5 mg/kg). Three weeks later, she was drowsy, ataxic, and dysarthric. Serum phenytoin was 14 mcg/ml, while primidone was 5 mcg/ml and phenobarbital was 45 mcg/ml. How can these laboratory findings and the patient's intoxicated state be explained?

A.R. appears to be suffering from phenobarbital intoxication resulting from a drug interaction between phenytoin and primidone. In patients receiving primidone, concomitant phenytoin therapy may cause a significant elevation in phenobarbital serum levels. Serum levels of primidone usually remain unchanged (136,137). This effect appears to result from competitive inhibition of metabolism between phenytoin and phenobarbital; induction of enzymes which convert primidone to phenobarbital has not been demonstrated (138).

The decline in A.R.'s primidone level is not consistent with the known characteristics of this interaction. She should be questioned about her compliance with her primidone regimen. If she has omitted this medication, primidone levels would fall more rapidly than phenobarbital levels and produce a pattern similar to the one seen here.

It is often difficult to achieve even minimally "therapeutic" serum primidone levels without producing phenobarbital intoxication when patients are also receiving phenytoin. In this type of situation, it is probably preferable to use phenobarbital alone, as the primidone component of therapy is not likely to be effective. A second option is treatment of the patient with an alternate single drug such as phenytoin or carbamazepine.

Carbamazepine

37. A.R.'s physician has decided to abandon primidone and phenytoin because of the difficulties encountered and her poor response to the regimen. He now wants to use carbamazepine. Since the patient's seizures have been only partly responsive to other drug treatment, is carbamazepine likely to be effective? How should therapy be initiated in this patient?

The decision to abandon phenytoin and primidone and avoid initiation of a polypharmacy regimen at this time is probably reasonable. Carbamazepine is equal in efficacy to phenytoin

(139,140) and primidone (141) in the treatment of complex partial (psychomotor) seizures. It is also effective for tonic-clonic and simple partial seizures (142). Because it differs chemically from other anticonvulsants, it is an excellent alternative for those patients who are not controlled by other medications. Some clinicians now consider carbamazepine a drug of first choice for generalized tonic-clonic and simple or complex partial seizures (4). Therefore, a trial with carbamazepine therapy seems justifiable for this patient even though her seizures were not well controlled by previous therapy.

Acute administration of full maintenance doses of carbamazepine often results in excessive side effects such as nausea and diplopia. Therapy should be initiated at relatively low doses and titrated against both therapeutic and toxic effects. For this reason, it may be advisable to delay discontinuing her current regimen or to slowly taper primidone and phenytoin as effective levels of carbamazepine are achieved. This will also help minimize any difficulties with increased seizures upon discontinuation of phenytoin and primidone. Therapy should be initiated at a dose of 200 mg bid. Dosage can be increased over one to two weeks until a minimally effective serum level of approximately 8 mcg/ml is achieved. Doses of 10–20 mg/kg/day will usually provide this serum level during long-term therapy (142).

38. Carbamazepine Pharmacokinetics. Over two weeks, A.R.'s carbamazepine dose was increased to 400 mg bid (15 mg/kg/day). Phenytoin and primidone were discontinued. After one week at 800 mg of carbamazepine daily, the serum level was 9 mcg/ml. No seizures occurred for four weeks, and A.R. tolerated the medication well. However, she then began to experience approximately one seizure weekly. A repeat carbamazepine level was 6 mcg/ml. What is the reason for the fall in her serum level and recurrence of seizures?

Two possibilities must be considered in this situation. As A.R. has previously been noncompliant with her medication regimen, she should be questioned concerning her actual intake of medication. If erratic drug intake is detected, efforts to educate her as to the need for regular medication intake and to help her remember to take the drug should be instituted.

These events are also consistent with the known kinetic behavior of carbamazepine (143). This drug exhibits time-dependent pharmacokinetics; the clearance changes over time, because carbamazepine stimulates its own metabolism and the metabolism of other drugs. The half-life following acute single doses is approximately 35 hours; on chronic dosing, the half-life decreases to 10–20 hours. Thus, with maintenance treatment, dosage requirements tend to increase. Up to one month may be required for this process to reach completion (144,145).

Assuming that compliance is not the main problem, A.R.'s carbamazepine dose should be increased. The drug's pharmacokinetics are linear with respect to acute dose changes (143). Thus, 50% increase in dose should re-establish a serum level of 9 mcg/ml. Therefore, a new dose of 1200 mg/day would be appropriate. Most patients can be adequately maintained on a bid dosage schedule. However, acute side effects such as nausea and dizziness are often associated with administration of large single doses. It may be desirable to prescribe 400 mg tid for this patient.

39. Carbamazepine Toxicities. Carbamazepine has a reputation for causing hematologic and hepatic toxicity. What is the significance of these toxicities? How should A.R. be monitored for their potential occurrence?

Hematologic. Aplastic anemia (146,147) and agranulocytosis (148) have occurred in association with carbamazepine therapy. A number of cases of aplastic anemia resulted in fatality. However, the majority of cases and fatalities were associated with treatment of older patients for trigeminal neuralgia (147). In addition, many patients were receiving other medications or were incompletely described. Pisciotta (147) assessed causal relationships as "probable" in only 4 of 18 cases of various hematologic reactions to the drug. Therefore, severe blood dyscrasias from carbamazepine appear to be quite rare and to have occurred most commonly in a population of nonepileptic patients. This conclusion is supported by the lack of reported hematologic toxicity in various series and clinical trials (139,149–151).

Transient leukopenia is seen in some patients taking carbamazepine. It is ususally mild and reversible despite continued administration of the drug (142,149,152,153). Total leukocyte counts may fall below 4,000 cells/mm^3 in some patients, but platelet and erythrocyte counts remain normal and there are no symptoms (eg, fever and sore throat) which might suggest onset of agranulo-

cytosis. Despite maintenance of therapy, leukocyte counts usually return toward normal.

Laboratory monitoring of patients' hematologic status is recommended during carbamazepine treatment. However, as Pisciotta points out (157), the likelihood of detecting cases of aplastic anemia or agranulocytosis through monitoring is very low. A reasonable monitoring program would consist of: a pre-therapy complete blood count (CBC) (including a platelet count), monthly repeat CBC's for the first 12–18 months, and CBC's every two to three months thereafter (146). There is no information to support a dosage relationship for carbamazepine-related hematologic disorders.

Hepatic. Carbamazepine-induced liver damage appears to be extremely rare despite frequent mention of this as a potential problem (146,154). Aggressive laboratory monitoring of liver function tests is probably not necessary. Alkaline phosphatase levels are often elevated in patients taking carbamazepine (and other anticonvulsants) (149). This is felt to result from enzyme induction and is not necessarily evidence for hepatic disease (142).

40. Carbamazepine Intoxication. A.R.'s seizure frequency was reduced to once monthly while she was receiving a regimen of carbamazepine 1400 mg/day which produced a steady-state serum level of 10.5 mcg/ml. Following a seizure, her physician decided to increase her carbamazepine to 1800 mg/day in an attempt to improve response. Two days after the dosage increase, A.R. began complaining of nausea, double vision, dizziness, and a mildly unsteady gait. Discuss A.R.'s symptoms in relation to those of carbamazepine intoxication.

Intoxication with carbamazepine is not as well-defined a syndrome as phenytoin intoxication. A.R.'s present complaints are commonly associated with higher serum drug levels, but they may occur at much lower levels. Gastrointestinal intolerance particularly may occur at low doses and limit therapy (154). The pattern of A.R.'s symptoms should be evaluated. If they occur in relation to drug administration, it may be possible to alleviate them by administering smaller doses more frequently (142). Reduction of her dosage to 1600 mg/day may be necessary.

A further manifestation of carbamazepine overdosage reported by Troupin (142) is "paradoxical intoxication" similar to that seen with phenytoin.

The condition is characterized by increased seizure frequency; it usually occurs with carbamazepine serum levels of 20 mcg/ml or greater.

41. Carbamazepine Psychotropic Effects. Carbamazepine is reported to have a "psychotropic" effect. What is the nature of this effect and its clinical significance?

Carbamazepine's chemical structure is similar to that of imipramine and other tricyclic antidepressants. On this basis, it is attractive to speculate that the drug possesses antidepressant or behavior altering properties. Several studies have reported that alertness and attentiveness improved when carbamazepine was substituted for traditional, sedating anticonvulsants such as phenytoin and phenobarbital (153,155). This author's experience with the use of carbamazepine in mentally retarded patients supports these observations. Improved mental performance and behavior have not been consistently reported, but the discrepancy may occur because in some studies, carbamazepine was added to previous medications (150) (negative results) while in others, it was substituted for previous drugs or directly compared with standard drugs (141,157) (positive results).

The exact nature of this psychotropic effect and its mechanism are not yet clear. One study (157) demonstrated that carbamazepine therapy was associated with a reduction in error rates for tasks involving complex skills and mental manipulation when compared with phenytoin therapy. This effect seemed mainly evident in patients with below average intelligence or emotional difficulty. The improved performance also correlated with patients' subjective reports of feeling more alert and less "drugged" while taking carbamazepine. Since most of the data supporting this psychotropic effect came from comparative studies, it is difficult to conclude that this drug has specific positive effects. It may be that it simply has fewer negative effects (eg, sedation) than other standard anticonvulsants. Several studies have documented psychomotor slowing, psychiatric side effects, and decreased motor performance associated with phenytoin and phenobarbital, and these effects have been correlated with serum levels (158–160).

42. Carbamazepine-Induced SIADH. A patient who recently began taking carbamazepine returns to the physician's office complaining of headache, vomiting, and dizziness. He is mildly confused. Upon admission to the hospital, examination was negative for neurologic findings. However, the patient gradually became more confused and stuporous. Laboratory results were: serum sodium 112 mEq/L, serum potassium 3.9 mEq/L, serum chloride 90 mEq/L, BUN 12 mg/dl, and albumin 3.2 gm/dl. Discuss the relationship between this patient's hyponatremia and carbamazepine. How is this condition managed?

Syndrome of inappropriate antidiuretic hormone (SIADH) is a well-documented reaction to carbamazepine (161,162). The drug appears to stimulate release of ADH from the pituitary. Although this effect is predictable enough for carbamazepine to be useful in the treatment of some forms of diabetes insipidus, water intoxication in patients treated with carbamazepine is uncommon (163). The effect is probably dependent on dose and blood level (161,162,164). SIADH may be more common in patients who receive carbamazepine alone; concomitant phenytoin therapy appears to counteract the antidiuretic effect of carbamazepine (162,165). It is not totally clear whether this is a result of phenytoin-induced inhibition of ADH release or reduction of carbamazepine serum levels by phenytoin.

In the present patient, dosage reduction may permit correction of water intoxication with continued maintenance of seizure control. If this is not possible, it will probably be necessary to discontinue carbamazepine and attempt to control seizures with alternate medications.

43. Anticonvulsant-Oral Contraceptive Interaction. A 26-year-old woman suffering from complex partial seizures with secondary generalization is receiving phenytoin 400 mg/day (serum level 11 mcg/ml) primidone 500 mg/day (primidone serum level 6 mcg/ml, phenobarbital serum level 31 mcg/ml) and carbamazepine 600 mg/day (serum level 5.3 mcg/ml). She currently reports having two or three partial seizures and one generalized seizure every three to four months. Despite treatment with Lo/Ovral (norgestrel 0.3 mg with ethinyl estradiol 30 mcg), she has learned that she is pregnant. Her last menstrual period was 1½ months ago. What is the relationship between this patient's apparent con-

traceptive failure and her anticonvulsant therapy?

There are several reports of reduced efficacy of oral contraceptives in patients receiving various anticonvulsants. A retrospective study indicates that the relative risk of pill failure is approximately 25 times higher in women taking anticonvulsants (166). Presumably, this interaction results when anticonvulsants induce hepatic enzymes, causing more rapid metabolism of contraceptive steroid hormones. There is not enough information to determine whether, in individual patients, use of higher dosage contraceptives can overcome this effect.

Assuming that this patient was taking her contraceptive on a regular basis, it is very likely that her anticonvulsants are responsible for the pill failure. Patients receiving anticonvulsants should be informed that this interaction may occur and be advised to use other methods of contraception.

44. *Teratogenicity.* What are the risks of teratogenic effects from this patient's medication regimen? What steps might be taken to minimize these risks?

This patient's child is at a relatively high risk of having congenital abnormalities. There has been exposure to two groups of drugs which are highly suspected of being teratogens in humans: estrogen/progestin combinations and anticonvulsants. Exposure to oral contraceptives is associated with limb reduction defects, cardiovascular abnormalities, skeletal malformations, and a variety of other abnormalities (167).

Various anticonvulsants—especially phenytoin, barbiturates, and oxazolidinediones—are now well accepted by most authorities as having teratogenic effects. However, there is some controversy regarding the relative contributions of drugs and parental epilepsy itself (168). Overall, the risk of major congenital malformations in children exposed to anticonvulsants *in utero* appears to be two to three times greater than the baseline risk in the general population (169).

Major congenital malformations associated with anticonvulsants include cleft lip, cleft palate, and cardiac septal defects (170,171), and it is the occurrence of these abnormalities which is used to estimate the relative risk noted above. However, there may be syndromes consisting of multiple abnormalities associated with prenatal exposure

to these drugs. Slightly different syndromes may be associated with individual drugs:

Fetal Hydantoin Syndrome (172–174) is characterized by pre- and post-natal growth and mental retardation, cranial and facial abnormalities (hyperplastic nasal bridge, inner epicanthal folds, hypertelorism), limb abnormalities, and cardiac defects.

Fetal Trimethadione Syndrome (175,176) is similar to fetal hydantoin syndrome. Characteristics include development delay (mental and physical), V-shaped eyebrows, low-set ears, palate abnormalities with speech difficulties, and irregular teeth.

Fetal hydantoin syndrome is fully expressed in at least 10% of the infants exposed. Some characteristics of the syndrome may be seen in an additional 30% (173,174). Similar syndromes have been reported in association with phenobarbital and primidone (169). Perhaps the most disturbing feature of these fetal anticonvulsant syndromes is the prevalence of mental and growth subnormalities, ranging from mild to severe, which appear to persist into at least the seventh year of life (173).

The mechanism of anticonvulsant-related teratogenesis is not known. There is a possibility that it is related to phenytoin-induced folate deficiency, but this is not supported by animal experiments (177,178). Similarities in physical appearance between affected infants (179) and adults with coarsened features (52) make it tempting to speculate that phenytoin's effects on collagen metabolism may play some role.

Minimization of teratogenic risks in pregnant epileptics may be possible. If feasible, prior to conception, seizure control should be optimized using the fewest medications possible. During pregnancy, serum drug levels should be monitored carefully, as the clearances of some drugs increase as pregnancy progresses (180). Careful monitoring, with dosage adjustment as necessary, may aid in preventing the increased seizure frequency seen in approximately 45% of pregnant epileptics (169). Falls and anoxia associated with uncontrolled seizure activity may increase the risk of congenital malformations.

In this patient, one can presume that significant exposure of the fetus to anticonvulsants has already occurred. The primary concern at this point would be optimization of seizure control. Any major alterations in the mother's anticonvulsant regimen should be attempted in such a way that risks of precipitating seizures are minimized. Based upon the seizure type and current serum levels of medications, increases in the dose of carbamazepine may be advisable. At this time, reduction or elimination of other medications should be attempted very cautiously if at all.

In addition to the risk of congenital malformations, *in utero* exposure to anticonvulsants has also been linked to severe neonatal hemorrhage (181). This bleeding disorder occurs most commonly within 24 hours of birth and is associated with a reduction in vitamin K-dependent clotting factors in the infant. Pre-delivery administration of phytonadione to the mother and intravenous administration of phytonadione to the infant immediately after delivery are recommended. If either prothrombin time or partial thromboplastin time is prolonged in the cord blood, the infant may require fresh frozen plasma. Although this hemorrhagic syndrome appears to be relatively uncommon, at-risk newborns should be monitored carefully for its occurrence.

45. *Anticonvulsant-Related Bone Disease.* C.D. is a 42-year-old, mildly retarded, black resident of a nursing home. She takes phenytoin 460 mg/day, phenobarbital 120 mg/day, and primidone 500 mg/day for control of tonic-clonic seizures. Her seizures are well controlled. Serum levels are phenytoin 11 mcg/ ml, phenobarbital 23 mcg/ml, and primidone 3 mcg/ml. She was diagnosed as epileptic at age 16 and has been treated since that time with various drugs. She spends the majority of her time indoors and participates in few activities. On annual physical examination, she is found to have a serum calcium of 8.8 mg/dl (normal is 9.2–11.1). Albumin and phosphorous are normal, but alkaline phosphatase is elevated to 245 IU/L (normal is 60-140). Her physical examination is normal with the exception of complaints of "aching in her bones" and radiologic evidence of a previously undetected, poorly healed rib fracture. What is the relationship between C.D.'s anticonvulsant therapy and her physical and laboratory findings?

The combination of symptoms, radiologic signs, and biochemical findings suggests the presence of osteomalacia related to C.D.'s anticonvulsant therapy. Decreased serum calcium, elevated alkaline phosphatase, and evidence of a possibly

spontaneous fracture are all consistent with the presence of this adverse drug effect. Affected patients will also have reduced serum levels of 25-hydroxycalciferol, and if the condition is severe, there may be myopathy, bone pain, or increased seizure frequency secondary to hypocalcemia (182). Serum phosphate is usually normal. Radiologic evidence of loss of bone mass is uncommon unless osteomalacia or rickets is severe; small reductions in bone mass (less than 30–50%) are only detectable by sophisticated techniques such as photon absorption densitometry (182).

Various studies have found biochemical and/or radiologic evidence of osteomalacia in 20–30% of treated epileptics (183,184); in one series, 75% of those treated with anticonvulsants for more than 10 years had osteomalacia (185). The exact prevalence in a particular population probably depends partially on the presence of predisposing factors such as reduced intake of dietary vitamin D, reduced sunlight exposure, recurrent infection, lack of physical activity, and dark skin pigmentation; nevertheless, duration and extent of exposure to anticonvulsants plays a major role (182–185). Patients receiving multiple anticonvulsants appear to be at higher risk (183,184). While increased duration of therapy probably increases the likelihood of the development of osteomalacia, significant biochemical changes may appear within six months of the initiation of treatment (182,186). Phenytoin alone appears to cause less disturbance in vitamin D and calcium metabolism than phenobarbital, primidone, or a combination of medications (187).

Osteomalacia is believed to result from anticonvulsant-induced reduction in effective vitamin D activity (188). The ultimate metabolically active form of vitamin D (1,25-dihydroxycalciferol) is formed through hydroxylation of calciferol by the liver (producing 25-hydroxycalciferol) and subsequently the kidney. Induction of hepatic enzymes by anticonvulsant drugs is thought to result in increased metabolism of 25-hydroxycalciferol (25-OHD) to inactive, polar metabolites. Thus, patients receiving anticonvulsants have significantly lower 25-OHD serum levels than do untreated patients (189,190). However, serum levels of 1,25-dihydroxycalciferol are apparently not reduced (191). Thus, anticonvulsants may alter responsiveness of target tissues (gut, kidney and bone) to vitamin D instead of or in addition to altering metabolism (188). The result of decreased vitamin D activity is a tendency for serum calcium to fall. Secondary hyperparathyroidism then develops, leading to increased bone resorption and eventual osteomalacia.

46. How should this patient's osteomalacia be treated?

Further laboratory investigation of C.D.'s status is necessary before one can decide how aggressively the apparent osteomalacia should be treated. Hahn (182) recommends multiple determinations of fasting serum levels of calcium, phosphorous, and alkaline phosphatase and use of the mean levels of these parameters. In addition, a 24-hour urinary calcium excretion rate should be determined as an aid in assessing calcium absorption; values below 8 mg/24 hours indicate reduced intestinal calcium absorption. Careful radiologic evaluation may allow the physician to detect demineralization and poorly healed old fractures. Tolman et al (185) based the diagnosis of osteomalacia on the presence of any 3 of 4 findings: hypocalcemia, hypophosphatemia, increased alkaline phosphatase, and radiologic findings such as reduced bone density, faulty calcification, and pseudofractures. If feasible, serum levels of 25-OHD should also be determined.

As C.D. appears to have signs and symptoms of significant bone disease, therapy with vitamin D and calcium is necessary. Dosage requirements for vitamin D appear to be highly variable (182). C.D. has several risk factors which predispose to vitamin D deficiency, and aggressive treatment is probably justified. Treatment should be started with 10,000 units/day (50,000–75,000/week) of vitamin D and 500 mg of elemental calcium daily (182). Treatment should be continued for four to six months or until biochemical and radiologic findings return to normal. Serum calcium should be monitored closely to ensure that vitamin D overdosage doesn't occur. Nursing staff should be alerted to observe her carefully for symptoms such as drowsiness, nausea, behavior changes, and muscle weakness. After C.D.'s biochemical and radiologic findings have normalized, 10,000 units/week of vitamin D alone should be given as maintenance therapy (182).

A further step in the treatment or prevention of osteomalacia for this patient would be to attempt to reduce the number of antiepileptic medications used. It may be possible to eliminate primidone and/or phenobarbital and control the patient's seizures with phenytoin alone.

47. What evidence exists that prophylactic vitamin D therapy is useful for patients receiving anticonvulsants?

The value of routinely administering large vitamin D supplements to such patients has not been demonstrated, and this practice remains controversial. It has been clearly demonstrated that vitamin D corrects biochemical and radiologic changes of existing anticonvulsant-related osteomalacia (182,187,192). In children receiving phenobarbital alone, 28,000 IU/week of vitamin D prevented the appearance of biochemical signs of osteomalacia (192). In children on combined phenobarbital and phenytoin therapy, it is estimated that at least 8000–10,000 IU/week of vitamin D (in addition to 3000–4000 IU/day from dietary sources) would be necessary to maintain normal serum levels of 25-OHD (190). Therefore, the dose of vitamin D necessary to prevent development of biochemical rickets or osteomalacia is not established, but an additional 5000–10,000 IU/week would probably be a reasonable prophylactic dose. In an individual patient, the actual dose requirement probably depends upon the presence of risk factors such as inactivity or reduced sun exposure.

A decision to administer prophylactic vitamin D to otherwise healthy patients who are taking anticonvulsants should probably be made on an individual basis. Hahn (182) recommends prophylactic vitamin D therapy (10,000 units/week) for patients with one or more risk factors who have received anticonvulsants for more than six months. Risk factors described by Hahn are multiple drug high-dose regimens, marginal vitamin D intake, limited sunlight exposure, limited physical activity, gastrointestinal malabsorption, renal disease, and severe recurrent infections. Patients receiving prophylactic vitamin D should be followed closely; serum and urinary calcium levels should be checked every two to three months to avoid development of hypervitaminosis D.

STATUS EPILEPTICUS

48. A 22-year-old, 85 kg male was recently diagnosed as having idiopathic epilepsy. For the past three months he has been treated with 400 mg/day of phenytoin which had completely eliminated his generalized tonic-clonic seizures. The steady-state serum phenytoin level was 12 mcg/ml. While at his

parents' home, he apparently had two tonic-clonic seizures, each lasting 3–4 minutes. During the ambulance ride to the hospital he had a third convulsion. On arrival at the hospital he was unconscious. Shortly afterward he began having another seizure. How should this patient's status epilepticus be treated?

Tonic-clonic status epilepticus exists when a patient has repeated seizures without recovery from the post-ictal state. This constitutes an emergency situation; up to 20% of such episodes result in fatal respiratory arrest. In addition, poorly-treated status epilepticus may result in CNS damage and worsening of the seizure disorder (193).

The immediate therapeutic concern in this patient is to ensure adequate ventilation and to terminate seizure activity. If possible, a plastic airway should be placed; however, this is often not possible while the patient is convulsing. Objects (eg, spoons, tongue blades, etc.) should never be forced into the mouth of a seizing patient. At the least, the patient should be positioned on his side to allow drainage of saliva and mucus from the mouth. Intravenous diazepam in a dose of 10 mg should be given immediately for termination of seizure activity. It is considered the agent of choice for rapid but temporary control of status epilepticus (194). The effectiveness of diazepam depends on rapidly achieving high serum concentrations. This can normally be accomplished by IV administration at a rate of 5 mg per minute or less. Intramuscular diazepam is absorbed too slowly to be effective in this situation (194,195). After IV administration, serum levels of diazepam fall rapidly as a result of rapid distribution; this short distribution (alpha phase) half-life correlates with the short duration of action and frequent recurrence of seizures when diazepam is used alone. For this reason, treatment with a long-acting anticonvulsant should also be initiated as soon as possible (194).

Intravenous diazepam has a relatively low toxicity profile. Cardiac or respiratory depression and hypotension may occur but are less likely with injection rates of 5 mg per minute or less. These toxic effects appear to be related partly to the propylene glycol solvent used in parenteral solutions of diazepam (194).

In addition to diazepam, many physicians administer a large dose of intravenous glucose as soon as blood samples for serum chemistry and anticonvulsant levels are drawn. This maneuver will correct any hypoglycemia which may be present as an underlying cause of status epilepticus.

49. What drug should be administered to this patient for prolonged control of seizures? What is an appropriate dose, route, and method of administration?

Phenytoin would be the anticonvulsant of choice for this patient. Maintenance therapy which produced moderate serum levels was previously effective. In the absence of obvious precipitating factors such as CNS infection or head trauma, one often finds that status epilepticus results from poor compliance with maintenance medications. Therefore, institution of adequate phenytoin therapy is the best first choice of treatment for this patient. Another advantage of using phenytoin is the lower level of sedation and respiratory depression produced by this drug in patients who are also treated with diazepam (194).

This patient's present phenytoin serum level is unknown, and compliance is uncertain. It is therefore not possible to accurately estimate a loading dose of phenytoin necessary to achieve a specific serum level. The best approach would be administration of a full therapeutic loading dose of 18 mg/kg (1500 mg) intravenously. Serum phenytoin levels should increase by approximately 23 mcg/ml (74,196). In patients not previously receiving phenytoin, this loading dose should maintain serum levels above 10 mcg/ml for 24 hours. Even if this patient has been compliant with his previous maintenance regimen, a level of approximately 35 mcg/ml would be expected. Most toxic effects from such a serum level should disappear over 24 hours, and any harmful effects of possible phenytoin intoxication are probably outweighed by the benefits of adequate seizure control (194,196).

Intravenous phenytoin is usually administered by direct injection into a running intravenous line. The rate of administration should be 50 mg/minute or less to minimize the risk of hypotension and cardiac arrhythmias. Cardiovascular status (blood pressure, EKG) should be monitored closely during administration. Hypotension or EKG abnormalities usually reverse if the injection is slowed or stopped temporarily (74).

50. The patient's physician is very reluctant to administer this dose of phenytoin by direct intravenous injection. Can phenytoin be administered by intravenous infusion through a volume control set?

The practical difficulties associated with direct intravenous push administration of phenytoin undoubtedly contribute to the low usage of this drug by this route. In many hospitals direct intravenous injections must be administered by a physician, and many physicians would be unwilling to commit the 30–45 minutes necessary to administer this patient's loading dose at a safe rate. In addition, the rate of direct intravenous injection is difficult to control and there is a potential risk of too rapid administration resulting in cardiac or respiratory toxicity.

There has been a great deal of controversy concerning the compatability of phenytoin injection with IV solutions for infusion. Phenytoin is a weak acid (pKa approximately 8), and its solubility in water is very low. The injectable dosage form consists of sodium phenytoin dissolved in a mixture of 40% propylene glycol and 10% alcohol; the pH is adjusted to approximately 12 with sodium hydroxide. Addition of the preparation to intravenous fluids results in dilution of the solvent system and some reduction in pH. A possible result would be precipitation of free phenytoin. However, a number of studies indicate that phenytoin may be diluted, preferably in small total volumes, with saline solutions (197–199). Despite formation of crystals in many solutions, measured phenytoin concentrations are essentially identical to those predicted. Thus, dilution of the required volume of phenytoin injection to a final volume of approximately 100 ml with 0.45 or 0.9 percent saline in a volume control set should provide an appropriate final solution for administration. An inline final filter of 0.45–0.22 micron pore size should be used to prevent the infusion of crystals (197). The administration rate should be limited to 50 mg per minute or less. Although there appear to be no published studies evaluating such phenytoin infusions, this method of administration has been successfully employed in a number of patients.

51. Following administration of phenytoin, no further seizures occurred. The laboratory reported that serum chemistries were all normal. Phenytoin serum levels were 5 mcg/ml on admission and 24 mcg/ml one hour after administration of the loading dose was completed. What maintenance dose of phenytoin should be administered, and when should this regimen be started?

Serum levels appear to confirm the role of noncompliance in this episode of status epilepticus. As the patient was apparently well-controlled on 400 mg/day previously, this would also be a reasonable maintenance dose at this time. Administration of maintenance doses should be resumed approximately 24 hours after administration of the loading dose. Initially, serum levels will be somewhat higher than necessary, but will approach the previous steady-state within a few days.

52. What other medications are useful for treatment of status epilepticus?

Phenobarbital may also be useful in the treatment of status epilepticus in patients who cannot tolerate phenytoin, or in whom phenytoin has previously proved ineffective. It is also recommended for patients who continue to seize following administration of appropriate loading doses of phenytoin (194). This drug must be administered cautiously to patients who have received diazepam since the cardiovascular and respiratory effects of these drugs may be addictive. As phenobarbital is absorbed slowly after intramuscular injections, it should be administered intravenously. A dosage of 8–20 mg/kg should be given at a rate no faster than 60 mg/minute. Blood pressure, respirations, and EKG should be monitored during administration (194).

Paraldehyde may also be useful for patients who do not respond to other anticonvulsants. However, the toxicity is high; pulmonary edema and hemorrhage may occur following IV administration, and IM or rectal paraldehyde can cause local tissue damage. The recommended dose is 0.1–0.15 ml/kg IV or IM. It is best to use glass syringes for injection because paraldehyde may dissolve plastic if contact is prolonged. Before intravenous administration, paraldehyde should be diluted 1:10 with normal saline.

Lidocaine has been used successfully for control of focal and tonic-clonic seizures (200,201). Various dosage schedules have been employed; however, in those situations where lidocaine serum levels were measured, it appears that therapeutic serum levels approximate those for control of cardiac dysrhythmias. Therefore, loading doses of 1.5–3.0 mg/kg followed by an infusion 30–60 mcg/kg/minute would seem to be appropriate. Much more study of the effect of lidocaine on seizures is required before this drug can be recommended in other than "last resort" situations.

References

1. Anon: Epilepsy: Medical aspects. Comprehensive Epilepsy Program, Minneapolis, 1978.

2. Tharp BR: Recent progress in epilepsy—diagnostic procedures and treatment. Calif Med. 1973; 119:19.

3. Bruni J: Recent advances in drug therapy for epilepsy. Can Med Assoc J. 1979; 120:817.

4. Porter RJ et al: Efficacy and choice of antiepileptic drugs. In *Advances in Epileptology—1977,* edited by H Meinardi and AJ Rowan, Swets & Zeitlinger B.V., Amsterdam, 1978, p 220.

5. Gastaut H: Clinical and electroencephalographic classification of epileptic seizures. Epilepsia. 1970; 11:102.

6. Eadie MJ: Plasma level monitoring of anticonvulsants. Clin Pharmacokinetics. 1976; 1:52.

7. Kutt H et al: Usefulness of blood levels of antiepileptic drugs. Arch Neurol. 1974; 31:283.

8. Lund L: Anticonvulsant effect of diphenylhydantoin relative to plasma levels. Arch Neurol. 1974; 31:289.

9. Sherwin AL et al: Improved control of epilepsy by monitoring plasma ethosuximide. Arch Neurol. 1973; 28:178.

10. Hvidberg EF et al: Clinical pharmacokinetics of anticonvulsants. Clin Pharmacokinetics. 1976; 1:161.

11. Richens A: *Drug Treatment of Epilepsy,* Henry Kimpton Publishers, London, 1976, p 14.

12. Troupin AS et al: Tegretol (carbamazepine)—a double-blind comparison with Dilantin (phenytoin). Neurology. 1977; 27:511.

13. McAuliffe JJ et al: Salivary levels of anticonvulsants: a practical approach to drug monitoring. Neurology. 1977; 27:409.

14. Cook CE et al: Phenytoin and phenobarbital concentrations in saliva and plasma measured by radioimmunoassay. Clin Pharmacol Ther. 1975; 18:742.

15. Horning MG et al: Use of saliva in therapeutic drug monitoring. Clin Chem. 1977; 23:157.

16. Bartels H et al: Flow-dependent salivary primidone levels in epileptic children. Epilepsia. 1979; 20:431.

17. Reynolds EH et al: One drug (phenytoin) in the treatment of epilepsy. Lancet. 1976; 1:923.

18. Shorvon SD et al: One drug for epilepsy. Br Med J. 1978; 1:474.

19. Shorvon SD et al: One drug in the treatment of epilepsy. In *Advances in Epileptology—1977,* edited by H Meinardi and AJ Rowan, Swets and Zeitlinger B.V., Amsterdam, 1978; p 300.

20. Shorvon SD et al: Unnecessary polypharmacy for epilepsy. Br Med J. 1977; 1:1635.

21. Shorvon SD et al: Reduction in polypharmacy for epilepsy. Br Med J. 1979; 2:1023.

22. Penry JK et al: The use of antiepileptic drugs. Ann Intern Med. 1979; 90:207.

23. Livingston S: Medical treatment of epilepsy: Part II. Southern Med J. 1978; 71:432.

24. Richens A: Clinical pharmacology and medical treatment. In *A Textbook of Epilepsy,* 1st ed, edited by J Laidlaw and A Richens, Churchill Livingstone, London, 1976, p 185.

25. Holowach J et al: Prognosis in childhood epilepsy: Follow-up study of 148 cases in which therapy had been suspended after prolonged anticonvulsant control. N Engl J Med. 1972; 286:169.

25a. Emerson R et al: Stopping medication in children with epilepsy: Predictors of outcome. N Engl J Med. 1981; 304:1125.

26. Marsden CD: Neurology. In *A Textbook of Epilepsy,* 1st ed, edited by J Laidlaw and A Richens, Churchill Livingstone, London, 1976, p 15.

27. Brown JK: Fits in childhood. In *A Textbook of Epilepsy,* 1st ed, edited by J Laidlaw and A Richens, Churchill Livingstone, London, 1976, p 66.

28. Ouellette EM: The child who convulses with fever. Pediatr Clin North Am. 1974; 21:467.

29. Nelson KB et al: Prognosis in children with febrile seizures. Pediatrics. 1978; 61:720.

30. Fishman MA: Febrile seizures: the treatment controversy. J Pediatr. 1979; 94:177.

31. Asnes RS et al: The first febrile seizure: a study of current pediatric practice. J Pediatr. 1975; 87:485.

32. Wolf SM et al: Behavior disturbance, phenobarbital and febrile seizures. Pediatrics. 1978; 61:728.

33. Camfield CS et al: Side effects of phenobarbital in toddlers; behavioral and cognitive aspects. J Pediatr. 1979; 95:361.

34. Garrettson LK: Using phenobarbital to prevent febrile seizures. Drug Therapy. 1975; November:64.

35. Cavazzuti GB: Prevention of febrile convulsions with dipropylacetate (Depakine). Epilepsia. 1975; 16:647.

36. Wallace SJ et al: Successful prophylaxis against febrile convulsions with valproic acid or phenobarbitone. Br Med J. 1980: 280:353.

37. Williams AJ et al: Sodium valproate in the prophylaxis of simple febrile convulsions. Clin Pediatr (Phila). 1979; 18:426.

38. Goulet JR et al: Metabolism of ethosuximide. Clin Pharmacol Ther. 1976; 20:213.

39. Browne TR et al: Ethosuximide in the treatment of absence (petit mal) seizures. Neurology. 1975; 25:515.

40. Buchanan RA et al: Ethosuximide dosage regimens. Clin Pharmacol Ther. 1976; 19:143.

41. Jeavons PM: Choice of drug therapy in epilepsy. Practitioner. 1977; 219:542.

42. Lorentz De Haas AM et al: Ethosuximide (alpha-ethyl-alpha-methylsuccinimide) and grand mal. Epilepsia. 1964; 5:90.

43. Mustard HS et al: Tridione therapy in epilepsy: a review of results in 156 patients with petit mal epilepsy with special reference to side reactions. J Pediatr. 1949; 35:540.

44. Livingston S et al: Petit mal epilepsy: results of a prolonged follow-up study of 117 patients. JAMA. 1965; 194:227.

45. Livingston S et al: Phenobarbital vs phenytoin for grand mal epilepsy. Am Fam Physician. 1980; 22:123.

46. Livingston S: Medical treatment of epilepsy: Part I. Southern Med J. 1978; 71:298.

47. Livingston S et al: Managing anticonvulsant side effects of the skin, hair and gums. Current Prescribing. 1978; August:54.

48. Reynolds EH: Chronic antiepileptic toxicity: a review. Epilepsia. 1975; 16:319.

49. Angelopoulos AP: Diphenylhydantoin gingival hyperplasia—a clinicopathological review: 1. Incidence clinical features and histopathology. J Can Dent Assoc. 1975; 41:103.

50. Angelopoulos AP: Diphenylhydantoin gingival hyperplasia—a clinicopathological review: 2. Aetiology pathogenesis differential diagnosis and treatment. J Can Dent Assoc. 1975; 41:275.

51. Lefebvre EB et al: Coarse facies calvarial thickening and hyperphosphatasia associated with long-term anticonvulsant therapy. N Engl J Med. 1972; 286:1301.

52. Falconer MA et al: Coarse features in epilepsy as a consequence of anticonvulsant therapy: report of cases in two pairs of identical twins. Lancet. 1973; 2:1112.

53. Pinder RM et al: Sodium valproate: a review of its pharmacologic properties and therapeutic efficacy in epilepsy. Drugs. 1977; 13:81.

54. Vining EPG et al: Valproate sodium in refractory seizures. Am J Dis Child. 1979; 133:274.

55. Adams DJ et al: Sodium valproate in the treatment of intractable seizure disorders: a clinical and electroencephalographic study. Neurology. 1978; 28:152.

56. Bruni J et al: Valproic acid: review of a new antiepileptic drug. Arch Neurol. 1979; 36:393.

57. Browne TR: Valproic acid. N Engl J Med. 1980; 302:662.

58. Patel IH et al: Phenobarbital—valproic acid interaction. Clin Pharmacol Ther. 1980; 27:515.

59. Sackellarea JC et al: Stupor following administration of valproic acid to patients receiving other antiepileptic drugs. Epilepsia. 1979; 20:697.

60. Perucca E et al: Drug interactions with phenytoin. Drugs. 1981; 21:120.

61. Mattson RH et al: Valproic acid in epilepsy: clinical and pharmacological effects. Ann Neurol. 1978; 3:20.

62. Bruni J et al: Valproic acid and plasma levels of phenytoin. Neurology. 1979; 29:904.

63. Suchy FJ et al: Acute hepatic failure associated with the use of sodium valproate: report of two fatal cases. N Engl J Med. 1979; 300:962.

64. Gerber N et al: Reye-like syndrome associated with valproic acid therapy. J Pediatr. 1979; 95:142.

65. Willmore LJ et al: Effect of valproic acid on hepatic function. Neurology. 1978; 28:961.

66. Sussman NM et al: A direct hepatotoxic effect of valproic acid. JAMA. 1979; 242:1173.

67. Mathis RK et al: Hepatic failure from valproic acid. N Engl J Med. 1979; 201:436.

68. Richens A: Clinical pharmacokinetics of phenytoin. Clin Pharmacokinetics. 1979; 26:153.

69. Allen JP et al: Phenytoin accumulation kinetics. Clin Pharmacol Ther. 1979; 26:445.

70. Ludden TM et al: Rate of phenytoin accumulation in man: a simulation study. J Pharmacokinetics Biopharm. 1978; 6:399.

71. Wilder BJ et al: Plasma diphenylhydantoin levels after loading and maintenance doses. Clin Pharmacol Ther. 1973; 5:268.

72. Evens RP et al: Phenytoin toxicity and blood levels after a large oral dose. Am J Hosp Pharm. 1980; 37:232.

73. Record KE et al: Oral phenytoin loading in adults: Rapid achievement of therapeutic plasma levels. Ann Neurol. 1979; 5:268.

74. Cranford RE et al: Intravenous phenytoin: Clinical and pharmacokinetic aspects. Neurology. 1978; 28:874.

75. Albert KS et al: Bioavailability of diphenylhydantoin. Clin Pharmacol Ther. 1974; 16:727.

76. Smith TC et al: Absorption and metabolism of phenytoin from tablets and capsules. Clin Pharmacol Ther. 1976; 20:738.

77. Neuvonen PJ: Bioavailability of phenytoin: clinical pharmacokinetic and therapeutic implications. Clin Pharmacokinetics. 1979; 4:91.

78. Kennedy D et al: New prescribing directions for phenytoin. FDA Drug Bull. 1978; 8:27.

79. Buchanan RA et al: The metabolism of diphenylhydantoin (Dilantin) following once-daily administration. Neurology. 1972; 22:126.

80. Haerer AF et al: Effectiveness of single daily doses of diphenylhydantoin. Neurology. 1972; 22:1021.

81. Cocks DA et al: Control of epilepsy with a single daily dose of phenytoin sodium. Br J Clin Pharmacol. 1975; 2:449.

82. Sawchuk RJ et al: Steady-state plasma concentrations as a function of the absorption rate and dosing interval for drugs exhibiting concentration-dependent clearance: consequences for phenytoin therapy. J Pharmacokinetics Biopharm. 1979; 7:543.

82a. Tindula PJ et al: Generic phenytoin versus Dilantin for once-a-day dosing. Am J Hosp Pharm. 1981; 38:1114.

83. Kostenbauder HB et al: Bioavailability and single-dose pharmacokinetics of intramuscular phenytoin. Clin Pharmacol Ther. 1975; 18:449.

84. Serrano EE et al: Plasma diphenylhydantoin values after oral and intramuscular administration of diphenylhydantoin. Neurology. 1973; 23:311.

85. Serrano EE et al: Intramuscular administration of diphenylhydantoin: Histologic follow-up studies. Arch Neurol. 1974; 31:276.

86. Wilder BJ et al: A method for shifting from oral to intramuscular diphenylhydantoin administration. Clin Pharmacol Ther. 1974; 16:507.

87. Wilder BJ et al: Oral and intramuscular phenytoin. Clin Pharmacol Ther. 1976; 19:360.

88. Letteri JM et al: Diphenylhydantoin metabolism in uremia. N Engl J Med. 1971; 285:648.

89. Odar-Cederlof I et al: Impaired plasma protein binding of phenytoin in uremia and displacement effect of salicylic acid. Clin Pharmacol Ther. 1976; 20:36.

90. Martin E et al: Removal of phenytoin by hemodialysis in uremic patients. JAMA. 1977; 238:1750.

91. Sherwin AL et al: Correlation between red cell and free plasma phenytoin levels in renal disease. Neurology. 1976; 26:874.

92. Steele WH et al: Alterations of phenytoin protein binding in vivo haemodialysis in dialysis encephalopathy. Europ J Clin Pharmacol. 1979; 15:69.

93. Reynolds F et al: Salivary phenytoin concentrations in epilepsy and in chronic renal failure. Lancet. 1976; 2:384.

94. Hull RL et al: Phenytoin toxicity due to severe liver disease. Drug Intell Clin Pharm. 1977; 11:57.

95. Blaschke TF et al: Influence of acute viral hepatitis on phenytoin kinetics and protein binding. Clin Pharmacol Ther. 1975; 17:685.

96. Haruda F: Phenytoin hypersensitivity: 38 cases. Neurology. 1979; 29:1480.

97. Parker WA et al: Phenytoin hepatotoxicity: a case report and review. Neurology. 1979; 29:175.

98. Sisca TS: An unusual dual hypersensitivity reaction induced by diphenylhydantoin. Am J Hosp Pharm. 1973; 30:446.

98a. Aeren JF et al: Phenytoin hypersensitivity reaction; hepatic necrosis. Drug Intell Clin Pharm. 1980; 14:252.

99. Clemmesen J et al: Are anticonvulsants oncogenic? Lancet. 1974; 1:705.

100. Li FP et al: Malignant lymphoma after diphenylhydantoin (Dilantin) therapy. Cancer. 1975; 36:1359.

101. Angelopoulos AP et al: Incidence of diphenylhydantoin gingival hyperplasia. Oral Surg Oral Med Oral Path. 1972; 34:898.

102. Kapur RN et al: Diphenylhydantoin-induced gingival hyperplasia: Its relationship to dose and serum level. Develop Med Child Neurol. 1973; 15:483.

103. Little TM et al: Diphenylhydantoin-induced gingival hyperplasia: Its response to changes in drug dosage. Develop Med Child Neurol. 1975; 17:421.

104. Babcock JR et al: Gingival hyperplasia and dilantin content of saliva: a pilot study. JAMA. 1964; 68:195.

105. Conard GJ et al: Levels of 5,5-diphenylhydantoin and its major metabolite in human serum saliva and hyperplastic gingiva. Am J Dental Res. 1974; 53:1323.

106. Livingston S et al: Gingival hypertrophy after diphenylhydantoin. N Engl J Med. 1972; 287:990.

107. Reynolds EH: Chronic antiepileptic toxicity: a review. Epilepsia. 1975; 16:319.

108. Norris JW et al: Folic acid deficiency and epilepsy. Drugs. 1974; 8:366.

109. Reynolds EH: Anticonvulsants, folic acid and epilepsy. Lancet. 1973; 1:1376.

110. Neubauer C: Mental deterioration in epilepsy due to folate deficiency. Br Med J. 1970; 2:759.

111. Reynolds EH: Neurological aspects of folate and vitamin B_{12} metabolism. Clinics Haematol. 1976; 5:661.

112. Rosenberg IH: Absorption and malabsorption of folate. Clinics Haematol. 1976; 5:589.

113. Wickramasinghe SN et al: Megaloblastic erythropoiesis and macrocytosis in patients on anticonvulsants. Br Med J. 1975; 4:136.

114. Taguchi H et al: The effect of anticonvulsant drugs on thymidine and deoxyribosenucleic acid synthesis by human marrow cells. Br J Haematol. 1977; 36:181.

115. Richens A: Drug Treatment of Epilepsy, Henry Kimpton Publishers, London, 1976, p 118.

116. Baylis EM et al: Influence of folic acid on blood-phenytoin levels. Lancet. 1971; 1:62.

117. Makki KA et al: Stimulation of drug metabolism by folate replacement in folate-deficient epileptic patients. Br J Clin Pharmacol. 1980; 9:304P.

118. Furlanut M et al: Effects of folic acid on phenytoin kinetics in healthy subjects. Clin Pharmacol Ther. 1978; 4:294.

119. O'Hare J et al: Increase in seizure frequency following folic acid. J Irish Med Assoc. 1979; 72:241.

120. Ahmad S et al: Involuntary movements caused by phenytoin intoxication in epileptic patients. J Neurol Neurosurg Psychiatry. 1975; 38:225.

121. Nausieda PA et al: Phenytoin and choreic movements. N Engl J Med. 1978; 298:1093.

122. Chalhub EG et al: Phenytoin-induced dystonia and choreoathetosis in two retarded epileptic children. Neurology. 1976; 26:494.

123. Chadwick D et al: Anticonvulsant-induced dyskinesias: a comparison with dyskinesias induced by neuroleptics. J Neurol Neurosurg Psychiatry. 1976; 39:1210.

124. McLain LW Jr et al: Cerebellar degeneration due to chronic phenytoin therapy. Ann Neurol. 1980; 7:18.

125. Rapport RL et al: Phenytoin-related cerebellar degeneration without seizures. Ann Neurol. 1977; 2:437.

126. Lovelace RE et al: Peripheral neuropathy in long-term diphenylhydantoin therapy. Arch Neurol. 1968; 18:69.

127. Eisen AA et al: Peripheral nerve function in long-term therapy with diphenylhydantoin. Neurology. 1974; 24:411.

128. Gallagher BB et al: Relationship of the anticonvulsant properties of primidone to phenobarbital. Epilepsia. 1970; 11:293.

129. Olesen OV et al: The metabolic conversion of primidone (Mysoline) to phenobarbitone in patients under long-term treatment. Acta Neurol Scand. 1967; 43:348.

130. White PT et al: Relative anticonvulsant potency of primidone: a double-blind comparison. Arch Neurol. 1966; 14:31.

131. Oxley J et al: A comparison of phenobarbitone and primidone in the control of seizures in chronic epilepsy. Br J Clin Pharmacol. 1979; 7:414P.

132. Gallagher BB et al: Metabolic disposition of primidone and its metabolites in epileptic subjects after single and repeated administration. Neurology. 1972; 22:1186.

133. Rall TW et al: Drugs effective in the therapy of the epilepsies. In The Pharmacological Basis of Therapeutics, 6th Ed., edited by LS Goodman, A Gilman and AG Gilman, McMillan Publishing Co., Inc., New York, 1980, p 448.

134. Gallagher BB et al: Primidone, diphenylhydantoin and phenobarbital: Aspects of acute toxicity. Neurology. 1973; 23:145.

135. Plaa GL: Acute toxicity of antiepileptic drugs. Epilepsia. 1975; 16:183.

136. Schmidt D: The effect of phenytoin and ethosuximide on primidone metabolism in patients with epilepsy. J Neurol. 1975; 209:115.

137. Reynolds EH et al: Interaction of phenytoin and primidone. Br Med J. 1975; 2:594.

138. Garrettson LK et al: Phenytoin-primidone interaction. Br J Clin Pharmacol. 1977; 4:693.

139. Troupin A et al: Carbamazepine—A double-blind comparison with phenytoin. Neurology. 1977; 27:511.

140. Simonsen N et al: A comparative controlled study between carbamazepine and diphenylhydantoin in psychomotor epilepsy. Epilepsia. 1976; 17:169.

141. Rodin EA et al: A comparison of the effectiveness of primidone versus carbamazepine in epileptic outpatients. J Nerv Ment Dis. 1976; 163:41.

142. Troupin AS: Carbamazepine: the evaluation of a new drug. Syva Monitor. 1981; 8:1.

143. Bertilsson L: Clinical pharmacokinetics of carbamazepine. Clin Pharmacokinetics. 1978; 3:128.

144. McNamara PJ et al: Time course of carbamazepine self-induction. J Pharmacokinetics Biopharm. 1979; 7:63.

145. Bertilsson L et al: Autoinduction of carbamazepine metabolism in children examined by stable isotope technique. Clin Pharmacol Ther. 1980; 27:83.

146. Troupin AS: The choice of anticonvulsants—a logical approach to sequential changes—a comment from an American neurologist. In A Textbook of Epilepsy, 1st Ed., edited by J Laidlaw and A Richens, Churchill Livingstone, London, 1976, p 248.

147. Pisciotta AV: Hematologic toxicity of carbamazepine. Adv Neurol. 1975; 11:355.

148. Hawson GAT et al: Agranulocytosis after administration of carbamazepine. Med J Aust. 1980; 1:82.

149. Livingston S et al: Carbamazepine (Tegretol) in epilepsy: Nine-year follow-up study with special emphasis on untoward reactions. Dis Nerv System. 1974; 35:103.

150. Rodin EA et al: The effects of carbamazepine on patients with psychomotor epilepsy: Results of a double-blind study. Epilepsia. 1974; 15:547.

151. Cereghino JJ et al: Carbamazepine for epilepsy: a controlled prospective evaluation. Neurology. 1974; 24:401.

152. Monaco F et al: Further observations on carbamazepine plasma levels in epileptic patients: Relationships with therapeutic and side effects. Neurology. 1976; 26:936.

153. Schain RJ et al: Carbamazepine as an anticonvulsant in children. Neurology. 1977; 27:476.

154. Huf RL et al: Liver functions in children receiving carbamazepine. J Pediatr. 1978; 93:884.

155. Troupin AS et al: The quantification of anticonvulsant side-effects as a guide to drug choice. In Advances in Epileptology—1977, edited by H Meinardi and AJ Rowan, Swets & Zeitlinger B.V., Amsterdam, 1978, p 370.

156. Stores G: Behavioural effects of antiepileptic drugs. Develop Med Child Neurol. 1975; 17:647.

157. Dodrill CB et al: Psychotropic effects of carbamazepine in epilepsy: a double-blind comparison with phenytoin. Neurology. 1977; 27:1023.

158. Hutt SJ et al: Perceptual-motor behaviour in relation to blood phenobarbitone level: A preliminary report. Develop Med Child Neurol. 1968; 10:626.

159. Reynolds EH et al: Serum anticonvulsant concentrations in epileptic patients with mental symptoms: a preliminary report. Br J Psychiatry. 1974; 124:440.

160. Dodrill CB: Diphenylhydantoin serum levels, toxicity and neuropsychological performance in patients with epilepsy. Epilepsia. 1975; 16:593.

161. Kato DB: Dilutional hyponatremia and water intoxication during carbamazepine therapy: a case report and review of the literature. Drug Intell Clin Pharm. 1978; 12:392.

162. Perucca E et al: Water intoxication produced by carbamazepine and its reversal by phenytoin. Br J Clin Pharmacol. 1980; 9:302P.

163. Helin I et al: Serum sodium and osmolality during carbamazepine treatment in children. Br Med J. 1977; 2:558.

164. Rado JP: Water intoxication during carbamazepine treatment. Br Med J. 1973; 3:479.

165. Sordillo P et al: Carbamazepine-induced syndrome of inappropriate antidiuretic hormone secretion: reversal by concomitant phenytoin therapy. Arch Intern Med. 1978; 138:299.

166. Coulam CB et al: Do anticonvulsants reduce the efficacy of oral contraceptives? Epilepsia. 1979; 20:519.

167. Nora JJ et al: Exogenous progestogen and estrogen implicated in birth defects. JAMA. 1978; 240:837.

168. Shapiro S et al: Anticonvulsants and parental epilepsy in the development of birth defects. Lancet. 1976; 1:272.

169. Montouris GD et al: The pregnant epileptic: a review and recommendations. Arch Neurol. 1979; 36:601.

170. Janz D: The teratogenic risk of antiepileptic drugs. Epilepsia. 1975; 16:159.

171. Monson RP et al: Diphenylhydantoin and selected congenital abnormalities. N Engl J Med. 1973; 289:1049.

172. Hanson JW et al: The fetal hydantoin syndrome. J Pediatr. 1975; 87:285.

173. Hanson JW et al: Risks to the offspring of women treated with hydantoin anticonvulsants, with special reference to the fetal hydantoin syndrome. J Pediatr. 1976; 89:662.

174. Hanson JW: Fetal hydantoin syndrome. Teratology. 1976; 89:662.

175. Zackai EH et al: The fetal trimethadione syndrome. J Pediatr. 1975; 87:280.

176. Goldman AS et al: Fetal trimethadione syndrome. Teratology. 1978; 17:103.

177. Speidel BD et al: Epilepsy anticonvulsants and congenital malformations. Drugs. 1974; 8:354.

178. Mercier-Parat L et al: The dysmorphogenic potential of phenytoin; experimental observations. Drugs. 1974; 8:340.

179. Hill RM et al: Infants exposed in utero to antiepileptic drugs: a prospective study. Am J Dis Child. 1974; 127:645.

180. Canafax DM et al: Phenytoin therapy in a pregnant epileptic: the role of pharmacokinetic monitoring. Drug Intell Clin Pharm. 1979; 13:534.

181. Bleyer WA et al: Fatal neonatal hemorrhage after maternal anticonvulsant therapy. JAMA. 1976; 235:626.

182. Hahn TJ: Bone complications of anticonvulsants. Drugs. 1976; 12:201.

183. Sotaniemi EA et al: Radiologic bone changes and hypocalcemia with anticonvulsant therapy in epilepsy. Ann Intern Med. 1972; 77:389.

184. Richens A et al: Disturbance of calcium metabolism by anticonvulsant drugs. Br Med J. 1970; 4:73.

185. Tolman KG et al: Osteomalacia associated with anticonvulsant drug therapy in mentally retarded children. Pediatrics. 1975; 56:45.

186. Reunanen MI et al: Serum calcium balance during early phase of diphenylhydantoin therapy. Int J Clin Pharmacol Biopharm. 1976; 14:15.

187. Offermann G et al: Antiepileptic drugs and vitamin D supplementation. Epilepsia. 1979; 20:3.

188. Habener JF et al: Osteomalacia and disorders of vitamin D metabolism. Ann Rev Med. 1978; 29:327.

189. Hahn TJ et al: Effect of chronic anticonvulsant therapy on serum 25-hydroxycalciferol levels in adults. N Engl J Med. 1972; 287:900.

190. Hahn TJ et al: Serum 25-hydroxycalciferol levels and bone mass in children on chronic anticonvulsant therapy. N Engl J Med. 1975; 292:550.

191. Jubiz W: Plasma 1,25-dihydroxyvitamin D levels in patients receiving anticonvulsant drugs. J Clin Endocrinol Metab. 1977; 44:617.

192. Liakakos D et al: Serum alkaline phosphatase and urinary hydroxyproline values in children receiving phenobarbital with and without vitamin D. J Pediatr. 1975; 87:291.

193. Celesia GG: Modern concepts of status epilepticus. JAMA. 1976; 235:1571.

194. Browne TR: Drug therapy of status epilepticus. Am J Hosp Pharm. 1978; 35:915.

195. Hillestad L et al: Diazepam metabolism in normal man. I. Serum concentration and clinical effects after intravenous, intramuscular and oral administration. Clin Pharmacol Ther. 1974; 16:479.

196. Cranford RE et al: Intravenous phenytoin in acute treatment of seizures. Neurology. 1979; 29:1474.

197. Cloyd JC et al: Concentration-time profile of phenytoin after admixture with small volumes of intravenous fluids. Am J Hosp Pharm. 1978; 35:45.

198. Bruman JL et al: Phenytoin crystallization in intravenous fluids. Drug Intell Clin Pharm. 1977; 11:646.

199. Salem RB et al: Investigation of the crystallization of phenytoin in normal saline. Drug Intell Clin Pharm. 1980; 14:605.

200. Lemmen LJ et al: Intravenous lidocaine in the treatment of convulsions. JAMA. 1978; 239:2025.

201. Reitscha WJ et al: Intravenous lidocaine in the treatment of seizures. Drug Intell Clin Pharm. 1980; 14:436.

Chapter 51

Skin Diseases

C. A. Bond

Types of Lesions

Acute Lesions. Acute lesions are character-ized by redness, swelling, heat, itching, and ooz-ing. Generally, the more severe the dermatitis, the milder the initial topical therapy should be. The initial treatment for acute lesions should be a wet dressing.

Subacute and Chronic Lesions. There are no absolute rules for treating subacute or chronic lesions. If the lesion is dry, an oleaginous or oc-clusive base should be used. If there are exten-sive, thick, or hyperkeratotic areas, a keratolytic may be incorporated into the vehicle or used separately.

Dermatologic Drug Delivery Systems

Wet Dressings. Wet dressings provide evapo-rative cooling which causes vasoconstriction and soothes and cools inflamed skin, dries oozing le-sions, softens crusts, aids in cleaning wounds, and assists the draining of purulent wounds. If the wet dressing is ice cold, it will help relieve pru-ritus; however, ice cold dressings should be re-served for small lesions, because cooling large parts of the body (with a bath) can be quite uncom-fortable. Wet dressings are most useful for acutely inflamed oozing lesions, erosions, and ulcers. In most instances, wet dressings should be the sole therapy until the oozing or weeping subsides. If other topical medications are applied to a oozing or weeping lesion, they will be washed away and will not provide the desired effect. The most fre-quently used wet dressings are normal saline and aluminum acetate 5% solution (Burow's solution) diluted 1:10 to 1:40 for use. Table 1 lists the so-lutions that are useful for wet dressings. Boric acid is of little use as a topical agent. It can be absorbed through the skin and cause systemic toxicity; thus, boric acid should not be used in wet dressings.

Depending on the affected area and its size, a patient utilizing a wet dressing may soak the af-fected area directly in the solution for 15 to 30 minute periods three to six times per day. If larger areas are involved or when the affected area can-not be easily soaked (eg, a shoulder) a clean towel or cloth soaked in the solution (lightly wrung out) may be directly applied to the lesion(s). The soaked cloth should be left in place for 10 to 15 minutes

Table 1.

WET DRESSINGS

Agent	Strength	Preparation	Germicidal Activity	Astringent Activity	Comments
Normal Saline	0.9%	1 tsp. to a pint of water	–	–	inexpensive, easy to prepare
Aluminum Acetate					
Burow's Solution	5%	Dilute to 1:10–1:40	mild	+	
Domeboro packets/ tablets	—	one packet/tablet to a pint of water yields a 1:40 solution; two yields a 1:20 solution	mild	+	
Potassium Permanganate	65 mg and 330 mg tablets	Dilute to 1:4000 to 1:16,000: 65 mg tablet to 250 cc to 1000 cc. 330 mg tablet to 1500 cc to 5000 cc	moderate	–	stains skin, clothing
Silver Nitrate	0.1–0.5%	1 tsp. of a 50% stock solution to 1000 cc will yield a 0.25% solution	good	+	stains everything it touches, can cause pain
Acetic Acid*	1%	Dilute 1:5 with standard 5% household vinegar	good	+	smells, can be irritating

*Used primarily for *Pseudomonas aeruginosa* infections.

and then resoaked in the solution and reapplied. The patient may repeat this procedure for 30 minutes to two hours three times daily. If large areas are involved, the patient may draw a bath, add appropriate amounts of medications, and soak for 15 to 30 minute periods three to six times per day. When using wet dressings, evaporation will cause a concentration of the solution which can make the solution too irritating to use. A 1:40 concentration of Burow's solution left standing at room temperature for 30 minutes will yield a 1:10 solution. Wet dressings are most comfortable if they are slightly cool to warm depending on the patient's preference. When drying the affected area after application of the wet dressing, care must be taken not to irritate the inflamed skin by rubbing it with a towel. The proper technique for drying the skin is to pat the area gently with a soft clean towel.

In addition to wet dressings (medicated or unmedicated) which may be applied to large areas of the body via a bath, other topical therapies may be particularly useful when applied by this route. Soothing and antipruritic colloidal bath additives may be useful in treatment of widespread eruptions such as lichen planus, pityriasis rosea, urticaria, and other weeping eczemas where there is crusting. Colloidal oatmeal utilizing one cup of oatmeal (Aveeno) shaken with two cups of cold tapwater and poured into six inches of a lukewarm bath produces a quite pleasing and soothing bath. Alternatively, a starch bath utilizing two cups of hydrolyzed starch (Linit) or cornstarch mixed with four cups of tap water and added to a bath may be used. A mixture of equal parts baking soda and starch may also be used. Epsom salts baths made by dissolving three cups of magnesium sulfate in six inches of a lukewarm tub are useful in treating pyoderms, furuncles, and necrotic acne, especially when the back, shoulders, and buttocks are affected. Occasionally, potassium permanganate baths (1:10,000) may be used in treating smelly bullous or ulcerating generalized lesions, such as seen with pemphigus or mycosis fungoides. Water-soluble coal tar preparations applied via a bath for the treatment of psoriasis may be the most acceptable way to apply this particular medication, because ointments or creams containing coal tar are smelly and have a tendency to stain materials they come in contact with.

A variety of bath oils are available: Alpha-Keri, Ar-Ex, Domol, Kauma, Lubath, Lubath-ML, Lubriderm, and Syntex. These are most useful in preventing and treating mild cases of dry skin. With moderate to severe cases of dry skin, additional topical oleaginous products are generally required to improve the condition. Patients may make their own bath oil by adding two ounces of olive oil or Nivea oil to a cup of milk and adding it to a bath.

The major problem associated with wet dressings or baths is the development of macerated skin from excessive exposure. Should maceration occur, this type of therapy should be temporarily discontinued. Closed wet dressings (occlusive covering over a wet dressing) are rarely used in treating dermatologic conditions because of the increased risk of maceration and heat retention, but they may occasionally be used with abscesses or cellulitis. Additionally, irritation may occur from medicated wet dressings if they become too concentrated.

Powders. Powders are drying, cooling, absorb moisture, and expose more surface area for quicker evaporation. They are used mainly in intertriginous areas to decrease friction which can cause mechanical irritation and are useful in the treatment of intertrigo, chafing, athlete's foot, jock itch, and diaper rash. Occasionally, powders are applied on top of ointments to prevent clothing from absorbing the ointment. The liberal use of powders is helpful in the prevention of bed sores or pressure sores.

Powders can be applied with a cotton puff or shaker. Care should be taken to minimize breathing of the powder, since this can lead to respiratory tract irritation, particularly in infants. Powders should not be applied to lesions where there is marked oozing or exudation, since the powders tend to cake into hard granules, making them difficult and painful to remove. The most commonly employed powders are talc or mixtures of talc and zinc oxide.

Lotions. Lotions are liquid vehicles for carrying medication. They may be lubricating, cooling, or drying depending on the formulation. Alcohol is frequently added to lotions to provide a cooling effect, and occasionally an astringent, such as aluminum, is added to precipitate protein and dry and help seal an oozing wound. Lotions are best for treating superficial dermatoses, especially if there is slight oozing. Lotions are particularly useful if large areas are affected or when applied to intertriginous areas. Generally, lotions are the least oleaginous and occlusive of the topical vehicles, and thus are not very useful in conditions where the skin is dry. Lotions should not be applied to hairy areas where they tend to get crumbly or to a markedly oozing dermatitis where they tend to cake and form hard, cement-like plaques under which infections can occur.

It is not necessary to remove lotions from the skin more than once daily. Generally, lotions are applied three or four times daily, applying fresh over old as long as possible. Since many lotions are suspensions, it is advisable to shake the lotion well prior to application. Six ounces of a lotion is generally adequate to cover the entire body of an average adult.

Emulsions. Emulsions may be divided into two classes, oil-in-water and water-in-oil, and appear in solid or liquid dosage forms. Most creams which are used clinically are oil-in-water emulsions, and many ointments are water-in-oil emulsions. The indications for liquid oil-in-water emulsions are similar to those for lotions except that this type of dosage form provides greater occlusion and would be more useful in conditions where dry skin predominates. Liquid water-in-oil emulsions have similar indications to ointments except that they can be applied more easily than ointments. Water-in-oil emulsions are most useful in conditions where dry skin predominates and should be avoided in hairy or intertriginous areas. As with lotions, six ounces of a liquid oil-in-water or a liquid water-in-oil emulsion are required for application to all exposed skin on an average adult.

With extemporaneously prepared emulsions, chemical compatibilities must be taken into consideration, because it is important that the drug be evenly distributed throughout the base and remain distributed. Accordingly, water soluble drugs should be dispersed in oil-in-water emulsions or other water miscible bases and not in oils, greases, waxes, fats, or petrolatum. Lipid soluble drugs should be dispersed in oils, greases, waxes, water-in-oil emulsions, petrolatum, and not in water miscible bases. Insoluble medications may be incorporated in any base in which they form a stable and even mixture. Table 2 lists some of the commercially available oil-in-water and water-in-oil emulsions. As the amount of oil increases, the viscosity of the emulsion will also increase. Because of this, emulsions containing more than

Table 2.

COMMERCIALLY AVAILABLE EMULSION BASES

Oil-in-Water	Water-in-Oil
Acid Mantle Cream	Aquaphor
Almay Emulsion Base	Eucerin (Aquaphor and
Cetaphil	Water)
Dermabase	Hydrophilic Petrolatum USP
Dermovan	
Hydrophilic Ointment USP	Hydrosorb
	Hydrous Lanolin
Keri	Lubriderm
Multibase	Nivea Cream
Neobase	Polysorb
Unibase	Qualatum
Vanibase	Velvachol

30% oil should be dispensed in wide mouth jars to aid the patient in application.

Gels. Gels are a form of ointment (semisolid emulsion) with propylene glycol and carboxypolymethylene that are clear, nongreasy, nonstaining, nonocclusive, and quick drying. They are thixotropic, becoming thinner with rubbing, and may sting on application. Gels are most useful when applied to hairy areas or when applied to the face (or other areas) where it may not be considered cosmetically acceptable to have the residue of a vehicle remaining on the skin.

Creams. Creams are the most commonly used vehicle in dermatology. Most are oil-in-water emulsions and are intended to be rubbed in well until they vanish (vanishing cream). Creams generally do not provide much occlusiveness and are best suited for application on nonirritable dermatoses (nonacute). The most common mistake made by patients applying creams is that they use too much and don't rub it in fully. Generally, if the cream can be seen on the skin after application, the patient has made one or both of these application mistakes and is wasting the preparation or not getting the full therapeutic benefits possible from the medication. One gram of cream should cover 100 sq cm of area. Table 3 lists the approximate amount of cream required for application to various parts of the body (1).

Ointments. Ointments are inert bases such as

petrolatum or consist of droplets of water suspended in a continuous phase of oleaginous material. Ointments may be either insoluble in water, soluble in water, or can be emulsified with water. Ointments are most useful in relieving dryness, brittleness, and treating fissures because of their occlusive properties. They are often used on chronic lesions and should not be used on acutely inflamed lesions. Because of their occlusive properties, ointments should not be applied to intertriginous areas where they will trap heat and sweat, or to hairy areas. Ointments may be cosmetically unacceptable to some patients. Since ointments generally spread more easily than creams, 5 to 10% less ointment is required to cover the same area that a cream will cover. (See Table 3 for amounts required to cover various areas of the body.)

Aerosols. Aerosols are the most expensive and inefficient way to apply dermatologicals. Their only advantage over other dosage forms is that they do not require direct mechanical contact with the skin and may be useful if mechanical application causes intolerable pain for the patient. If an aerosol is used, it should be shaken well prior to use, and the patient should be cautioned to not spray the product around the face where it could get into the eyes, nose, or could be inhaled. Generally, aerosols should be sprayed from about six inches above the skin in bursts of one to three seconds. Aerosols are also useful for application in hairy areas if a special applicator nozzle is used.

New Delivery Systems. With the possible addition of solvents such as dimethylsulfoxide, many drugs could potentially be administered directly through the skin. Additionally, other delivery systems such as CIBA's Transderm-V, which is a 2.5 sq cm adhesive tape designed to deliver 0.5 mg of scopolamine directly into the blood-stream via the skin over a 72-hour period to prevent motion sickness, are presently available. This system or similar ones offer great potential for sustained delivery of pharmaceuticals over extended periods of time.

Selection of a Delivery System. The major function of the dosage forms previously mentioned is to provide a vehicle for the delivery of medication to its site of action. Drugs cross epidermal cell membranes by a process of diffusion which can be facilitated by the following factors: pH gradient, concentration gradient, increased temperature, a thin stratum corneum, increased hydration, increased dermal circulation, and disruption of the integrity of the barrier function of the epidermis. It should be noted that the barrier function of the epidermis is present in all layers of the epidermis.

There is an old saying regarding dermatological therapy which may be particularly useful in selecting dosage forms. If a lesion is wet, dry it; if dry, wet it. With an acute inflamed lesion, wet dressings are most useful in drying the lesion. With chronically inflamed lesions, where dryness, lichenification, and scaling are often present, ointment bases are most useful. With chronic dermatological lesions, the choice of the vehicle may often be determined by the patient himself based upon what he has found to work best. It is also not uncommon for patients with chronic dermatologic condition to use several different types of vehicles at the same time (eg, cream bases during the day and ointment bases at night).

TOPICAL CORTICOSTEROIDS

1. *Atopic Eczema.* P.K., a 17 year-old-male, is currently being followed in the University Dermatology Clinic for his atopic eczema.

Table 3.
AVERAGE AMOUNTS OF CREAM NEEDED TO COVER VARIOUS PARTS OF THE BODY

Single Application	Area (For Each Part Listed)	Amount Needed For 7 Days
2 gm	Both hands, head, face, genital, anal	45 gm (1.5 oz)
3 gm	One arm, front or back of trunk	60 gm (2 oz)
4 gm	One leg	90 gm (3 oz)
30–60 gm	Whole body	1–2.5 kg (2.5–5 lbs)

Thirty percent of his body is covered by an eczematous rash, with extensive involvement of the popliteal and antecubital fossas. His chief complaint is extreme pruritus over the involved areas, as well as cosmetic disfiguration in the antecubital fossas, around the neck, and on the forehead.

Family History: The patient's mother and aunt have bronchial asthma; one sister (L.K.), age 15, has hay fever and atopic eczema; his father and younger brother, age 11, appear to have no atopic manifestations.

Past Medical History: An eczematous rash was first noted on P.K. one month after birth. The scalp, face, and neck were the only areas affected, and the rash continued with varying degrees of severity until age two and a half years when it spontaneously resolved. P.K. developed hay fever at age six with occasional attacks of asthma (last attack, age 15). An eczematous rash reappeared at age 12 and has not disappeared since that time. His skin has followed a variable course, clearing in the summer and during periods of little stress and worsening during the winter and periods of stress.

Physical Exam: The patient presented as a well nourished, well developed white male with no physical abnormalities noted except for his skin. Skin: oozing, crusted, erythematous, hyperkeratotic, hyperpigmented, maculopapular, and fine vesicular eruptions on face, neck, dorsal aspects of both arms and legs, hands, and chest. There is some evidence of secondary bacterial infection in both antecubital fossas and on portions of the left leg.

What are the relevant biopharmaceutical considerations for selecting a topical corticosteroid for P.K.?

A human bioassay procedure based on the intensity of blanching of the skin is useful in predicting the bioavailability and clinical effectiveness of various corticosteroid topical preparations (2). Clinical response is also evaluated by applying the agents to areas of experimentally produced irritation (3,4).

The various proprietary formulations of topical corticosteroids offer a wide range of potencies (Table 4). The relative potency assigned to a topical corticosteroid is determined by the ability of the preparation to penetrate the skin after re-

lease from the vehicle, the intrinsic activity of the corticosteroid at the receptor, and the rate of clearance from the receptor. It is believed that topical corticosteroids penetrate into the stratum corneum by passive diffusion which varies considerably depending on which part of the body a preparation is applied to. When a standard hydrocortisone preparation was applied to various parts of the body, absorption was found to be 0.14% on the plantar surface of the foot, 1% on the forearm, 4% on the scalp, 7% forehead, 13% on the cheeks, and 36% on the scrotum. Because of the high penetrability on the groin, axillae, and face, lower potency topical preparations (hydrocortisone 0.5%–1%) should be used on these areas. In areas where penetrability is poor, such as the elbows, knees, palms, or soles, higher strength preparations should be used (See Table 4.)

For P.K., a 1% hydrocortisone cream should be used on his face and other areas of high penetrability to reduce the possibility of complications. Since P.K. appears to be in considerable distress, a cream of high potency (moderately potent classification or higher strength from Table 4) should be used initially on the areas that are not infected or where high penetrability is not a problem (see below for further discussion) to "cool" down these lesions quickly.

If equal amounts of a corticosteroids are formulated in appropriate ointment, gel, cream, and lotion bases, the gel and ointment bases are generally more active (5,6,7). The addition of certain substances will enhance penetrability and potency. Adding urea to hydrocortisone will double the potency, while dimethylsulfoxide will increase the potency four-fold (8). Increasing the concentration of a corticosteroid in a preparation will also increase potency, but not in a linear fashion. Increasing the concentration of hydrocortisone by ten-fold only increased the potency of this preparation by a factor of four, resulting in considerable wastage (9). Since P.K. has a fine vesicular eruption, it would be more appropriate to use a cream vehicle initially. However, since patients often may express a preference (cream, gel, ointment, etc.), it would be appropriate to ask him if he has a preference.

2. Occlusive Dressing. Since it has been some time since P.K. has been aggressively treated for his atopic eczema and he has many hot inflamed lesions, should occlusion be

used? What complications could develop from occlusion? How would you occlude the lesions on P.K.'s chest?

Occlusion, which increases hydration of the skin, will also increase the penetration and thus the potency of a corticosteroid preparation. As a general rule, occlusion will enhance the potency of a corticosteroid by a factor of ten (8). Occlusion may be accomplished by selecting an ointment base, applying an ointment base (nonmedicated) over another corticosteroid preparation (gel, cream, lotion, or aerosol), by wrapping the area with plastic (such as Saran Wrap), or by wearing a plastic suit (space suit) over the affected area. Several hours of occlusion is all that is necessary to increase potency; thus relatively short periods of occlusion are clinically useful. Occlusion can be uncomfortable and can lead to sweat retention and an increased risk of bacterial and candida infections (see Question 8). To reduce these problems and also reduce the chances of systemic side

effects, occlusion should not be maintained for more than 12 hours in a 24 hour period. With P.K.'s atopic eczema, occlusion should/could be used on the "hottest" lesions only until they can be brought under control and then discontinued, because, as a general rule, patients with atopic eczema may not tolerate occlusion for prolonged periods because of their low itch threshold (due to the increased heat, sweat retention, and possible maceration). While occlusion is quite useful for cooling off hot, inflamed areas, the long-term benefit in a patient with atopic eczema is reduced by the increased pruritus which often leads to noncompliance. Once the lesions are controlled, the occlusion should be discontinued. With other chronic dermatologic conditions (eg, psoriasis) that are not associated with severe pruritus, occlusion could be used for prolonged periods of time if necessary.

When using occlusion in patients with atopic eczema, care should be taken to not occlude un-

Table 4.
POTENCIES OF TOPICAL CORTICOSTEROIDS

Most Potent:

Amcinonide (Cyclocort) cream	0.1%
Betamethasone dipropionate (Diprosone) lotion, ointment	0.05%
Halcinonide (Halog, Halciderm) cream	0.1%
Fluocinonide acetate (Lidex) cream, ointment	0.05%
Fluocinolone acetonide acetate (Topsyn) gel	0.05%

Very Potent:

Betamethasone dipropionate (Diprosone) cream	0.05%
Betamethasone-17-benzoate (Benisone, Uticort) gel	0.025%
Betamethasone-17-valerate (Valisone) lotion, ointment	0.1%
Triamcinolone acetonide (Aristocort, Kenalog) cream	0.5%

Moderately Potent:

Fluocinolone acetonide (Synalar) cream	0.2%
Triamcinolone acetonide (Aristocort, Kenalog) ointment	0.1%
Fluocinolone acetonide (Synalar) ointment	0.025%
Flurandrenolide (Cordran) ointment	0.05%

Potent:

Fluocinolone acetonide (Synalar) cream	0.025%
Triamcinolone acetonide (Kenalog) lotion	0.025%
Triamcinolone acetonide (Kenalog) cream	0.1%
Flurandrenolide (Cordran) cream	0.05%
Betamethasone-17-valerate (Valisone) cream	0.1%

Less Potent:

Flumethasone pivalate (Locorten) cream	0.03%
Desonide (Tridesilone) cream	0.05%
Hydrocortisone	1%

affected skin (because of the low itch threshold). Of the methods previously described, the best approach would be to apply a corticosteroid cream, *rub in thoroughly,* and apply an occlusive ointment base over the cream. The most severe lesions on P.K.'s chest should be treated in this manner.

3. P.K. was given a prescription for halcinonide (Halog) 0.1% cream 3 oz, apply once at h.s., refill 100 times. Why, based on biopharmaceutical consideration, is this prescription inappropriate? In general, how should topical corticosteroids be used?

Corticosteroids tend to penetrate human skin very slowly, leading to a reservoir effect. With low potency preparations, this reservoir effect will persist for several days, and with the most potent preparations under occlusion, the effects may persist for up to 14 days (11,12,13). The clinical implication of this reservoir effect on chronic conditions is that there is a cumulative effect with repeated application of topical corticosteroids, often allowing a reduction in the number of applications per day and the use of a less potent preparation after the acute inflammatory processes are brought under control. P.K.'s present regimen is inappropriate because multiple daily applications will be needed initially to control inflamed lesions. Subsequently, once control is achieved, less potent preparations with reduced frequency of applications should be attempted.

It should be pointed out that many (particularly the newer, more potent) corticosteroids are in specially formulated bases which maximize their release and potency. Mixing these preparations with other bases or vehicles may markedly reduce the potency far beyond that which would normally be expected from the dilution. It is recommended that before mixing commercially available products with other bases or vehicles the pharmacist check with the manufacturer to see if an incompatibility exists.

General Principles of Topical Corticosteroid Therapy

(a) Topical corticosteroids should be applied two to four times per day initially. Increasing the frequency of application from once a day to three times a day has been clearly shown to be superior. Increasing the frequency of application from three to six daily applications has not been shown to

be any more efficacious than three applications per day (10).

(b) Use an appropriate strength preparation to bring the condition under control. It should be pointed out that 33 to 50% of all dermatological conditions requiring topical corticosteroids can be managed with medium or low strength preparations (11).

(c) After initial control, maintenance therapy should be with the weakest strength preparation that will control the problem. Reductions in applications should also be attempted. It may be advisable to give two different strength preparations to the patient, a mild one for routine use and a more potent one for flairs or resistant lesions.

(d) Occluded areas and certain areas of the body such as the face and flexures are more prone to develop side effects. If corticosteroids have to be used on the face or flexures, hydrocortisone should be used to reduce the probability of side effects.

(e) Children and patients with liver failure are at risk for systemic toxicities.

(f) Preparations should be rubbed in thoroughly and where possible should be applied while the skin is moist (eg, after bathing) since this will enhance the effect.

(g) With chronic conditions such as atopic eczema, it is best to discontinue therapy gradually. This will reduce the chances of a flair developing in the underlying condition.

4. *Indications for Topical Corticosteroids.* How effective are topical corticosteroids in treating atopic eczema? In what other conditions are topical corticosteroids effective? Which conditions could be made worse?

Topical corticosteroids are the drugs of first choice in treating atopic eczema. Generally, treatment is initiated with a potent fluorinated steroid, with occlusion if tolerated, and after the lesions are controlled, maintenance therapy is provided by 1% hydrocortisone or a low strength flourinated corticosteroid such as triamcinolone acetonide 0.025%. With chronic maintenance therapy, frequency of applications and potency of the corticosteroid should be kept to a minimum.

Topical corticosteroids are also the drugs of choice for all inflammatory and pruritic eruptions, and are quite useful with hyperplastic disorders and infiltrative disorders. The following conditions generally respond well to topical corticosteroids: allergic contact dermatitis, alopecia areata, atopic eczema, discoid lupus erythematosus, granuloma annulare, hypertrophic scars and keloids, lichen planus, lichen simplex, lichen striatus, necrobiosis lipoidica, various nail disorders, pretibial myxoedema, primary irritant dermatitis, psoriasis, sarcoidosis, seborrheic dermatitis, and varicose eczema (14,11).

The following conditions are worsened by topical corticosteroids and they should not be applied to areas affected by these conditions (15): acne vulgaris, ulcers, scabies, warts, molluscum contagiosum, fungal infections, and balanitis.

5. *Side Effects.* What are the side effects that can be expected from topical corticosteroid therapy?

Side effects from topical corticosteroids are infrequent. When they do occur, they are related to the potency of the preparation used, frequency of use, duration of use, anatomical site of application, and individual patient factors. Any of the previously discussed factors which increase potency, such as occlusion, increase the chances of side effects occurring.

Local Effects. Epidermal and dermal atrophy, telangiectasia, localized fine hair growth, bruising, hypopigmentation, and striae may result from repeated application of topical corticosteroids. Epidermal changes consisting of a reduction in cell size may begin within several days of starting therapy; these changes are generally reversible after therapy is stopped (16). Exposed areas are most vulnerable to epidermal atrophy. Dermal atrophy generally takes several weeks to occur and may be irreversible, depending on how long the patient has used the corticosteroid and individual host factors such as the age of the skin (17). Inguinal, genital, and perianal areas are most vulnerable to dermal atrophy. Most cases of dermal atrophy are probably reversible within six to nine months after stopping the corticosteroid. Telangiectasia, which occurs most often on the face, neck, groin, and upper chest, may not be reversible after stopping corticosteroid therapy. Striae, which occur most commonly on the groin, axillary, and inner thigh areas, are usually permanent. Fine hair growth may be particularly bothersome to female patients using corticosteroid preparations on the face. This problem is generally reversible after stopping therapy. Hypopigmentation, predominantly a problem for dark skinned patients, is generally reversible after stopping therapy.

6. It is noted that P.K. has acne lesions on his face. Could this present a problem for topical corticosteroid therapy on the face?

The face is particularly vulnerable to corticosteroid side effects because of enhanced penetration. Acne, rosacea, and perioral dermatitis can be seen on the face secondary to corticosteroid application. It may take several weeks to months for these problems to develop, and they can be distinguished from naturally occurring disorders because the corticosteroid-induced lesions are generally at the same level of development, and they occur in areas where a history of corticosteroid application can be elicited. Generally, steroid acne, rosacea, and perioral dermatitis resolve after discontinuing the drug. Application of corticosteroid preparations (particularly the potent ones) to areas around the eye can lead to increased intraocular pressure, glaucoma, cataracts, an increased risk of ocular mycotic infections, and an exacerbation of preexisting herpes simplex infections (14).

P.K.'s acne lesions may get worse secondary to the application of topical corticosteroids. He should be warned to apply the corticosteroid preparation only to the atopic eczema and avoid areas where acne exists. If the atopic eczema and acne lesions are in the same area *and* his acne gets worse after using the topical corticosteroid, P.K. must make a decision as to which of these two dermatologic conditions bothers him more (probably the atopic eczema) and treat the condition which is most disturbing. Some improvement in corticosteroid-exacerbated acne may be seen by decreasing the strength of the topical product applied to the face and/or reducing the frequency of application. An alternative to this approach, if P.K.'s acne is severe, would be to continue topical corticosteroid therapy but treat the acne with systemic antibiotics (see Question 29).

7. P.K. states that L.K. (his sister), who also has atopic eczema, started using a new topical corticosteroid preparation (halcinonide) 10 days ago. She has complaints of burning lasting for one hour after every application of this product. The burning occurred after each application since the first day of application, and she stopped using the product two days ago because of this. He wonders if she may be allergic to the product.

Rarely will a patient become allergic to a topical corticosteroid preparation. When it does occur, it is generally not due to the corticosteroid but to a preservative or other ingredient in the formulation. Allergic sensitization may be seen within two weeks after starting therapy and may be difficult to diagnose since the corticosteroid may modify the allergic reaction. One should suspect an allergic reaction if lesions change appearance after starting therapy, when healing does not occur within an expected period of time, or when the condition improves and then abruptly gets worse.

Because of the time course of the burning in L.K. (starting the first day and lasting only one hour), it is doubtful that she is actually allergic to this product. However, atopic eczema patients often have "sensitive" skin and may have idiosyncratic reactions to a variety of topical preparations. To remedy this situation, L.K. should be given another topical corticosteroid preparation which has a different formulation (base and preservatives). If the reaction continues with a new product, an allergy workup may be necessary and patch testing may be considered.

8. *Systemic Effects*. P.K. also states that his sister was given hydrocortisone injections several months ago when she was hospitalized for knee surgery. He wonders if he will require such injections if he has to have an operation or if he should wear a Medi-Alert tag. P.K. also states that his sister received a lot of antibiotics and wonders if he is at risk for developing skin infections.

Systemic adrenal axis suppression from topically applied corticosteroids appears to be more of a theoretical risk than clinical entity in adults. While suppression has been reported, these cases can be attributed to excessive use by the patient or to application of corticosteroids to large areas of the body for prolonged periods under occlusion. Because young children have been shown to have significantly enhanced percutaneous absorption of corticosteroids, they have a greater risk of developing adrenal axis suppression and other systemic side effects. To reduce this risk, it is advisable to use hydrocortisone topical preparations in children and limit the use to short periods of time. Additionally, patients with impaired clearance of corticosteroids (liver failure) should also use hydrocortisone and be monitored closely for signs of systemic toxicity. The chances of developing an infection secondary to topical administration of

corticosteroids would appear to be more of a theoretical risk than a common occurrence. While anecdotal reports do appear in the literature documenting secondary bacterial infections, there is scant evidence to suggest that they occur with any reasonable frequency.

Although the risk of developing an Addisonian crisis in surgery secondary to topical steroids is extremely low, patients who have used potent topical corticosteroids over large areas of their bodies (> 30%), used occlusion, or are at greater risk (see above) are often given systemic hydrocortisone prophylactically prior to surgery. P.K. probably would not need such supplementation and he would not need to purchase a Medi-Alert tag.

9. *Topical Antibiotics*. Since P.K. appears to have a bacterial infection associated with his atopic eczema, could a corticosteroid and an antibiotic preparation be used together? What are the risks associated with topical antibiotics?

There is evidence to suggest that combination therapy with a corticosteroid-antibiotic preparation is more efficacious than either agent alone in treating impetiginized eczema (18,19). Presumably, the corticosteroid suppresses the clinical signs of infection and helps to reestablish the normal skin barrier function which allows the skin's normal defense mechanisms to ward off the infection. Other infections where this combination leads to an improved response rate are otitis externa, certain intertriginous eruptions, and possibly seborrheic eczema (14).

Since most commercially available antibiotics are combinations, it may be useful to look at the spectrum of individual antibiotics for pathogens on the skin. The following is a synopsis of common antibiotics used on the skin:

Bacitracin. Effective against all anaerobic cocci, most strains of *streptococci, staphylococci,* and *pneumococci.* Not effective against most gram negative organisms.

Gentamicin. Effective against most gram negative organisms (similar to neomycin) including *Pseudomonas* and many strains of *S. Aureus.*

Gramicidin. Effective against most gram positive organisms; not effective against most gram negative organisms.

Neomycin. Effective against most gram negative organisms (except *Pseudomonas*) and some gram positive organisms. Group A *streptococci* are resistant.

Polymixin B. Effective against most gram negative organisms (including *Pseudomonas*). Most strains of *Proteus, Serratia,* and gram positive organisms are resistant.

The rationale for combining several antibiotics is to cover a wide spectrum of potential infecting organisms; therefore a combination of at least two antibiotics is required. Dermatologic infections frequently are mixed, with cultures showing two or more organisms present in sufficient quantities to be responsible for the infection. Bacitracin is combined with neomycin and/or Polymixin B to treat superficial dermatologic infections. All three of these bactericidal agents are synergistic, resulting in increased efficacy and perhaps a broader spectrum of activity (11). Topically applied gentamicin should be avoided if possible because other agents are generally equally effective and there is a risk of developing gentamicin-resistant organisms.

Since P.K.'s secondarily infected lesions probably harbor a variety of organisms, a product containing bacitracin and/or neomycin and/or polymixin B should be used. Topical antibiotics should be used only with superficial infections. Systemic antibiotics should be employed for deep infections because of greater efficacy.

There have been many reports of contact dermatitis caused by topical antimicrobials. Neomycin sensitivity has been reported in 50% of patients with allergic eczematous contact dermatitis (20), 6% of patients patch tested with common allergens (21), and 8% of randomly chosen subjects tested with both patch and intradermal methods (22). In a study of 1158 patients, the incidence of sensitization to neomycin was 1.1% (23). This report is interesting because the population studied had no preexisting dermatologic problems, and it probably represents the true incidence of allergic sensitization to neomycin in the general population. Also, a high incidence of sensitization was reported when preparations containing neomycin were used in the long-term treatment of leg ulcers (24). The steroid contained in many neomycin preparations does not prevent these allergic reactions, although it may decrease the severity of the reaction. Additionally, ointment vehicles containing neomycin may have a higher rate of sensitization than creams; however, this is difficult to quantitate.

If the patient has been sensitized to neomycin, the incidence of cross-sensitization to gentamicin is 40% (25), to streptomycin 10–90% (25,26), and to kanamycin 56% (27).

Hypersensitivity reactions, usually manifested by a rash, have followed the topical use of nitrofurazone (Furacin). Because the overall incidence of sensitization is relatively high, nitrofurazone is not recommended for the treatment of bacterial infections complicating serious burns.

Ethylenediamine, employed as a stabilizer in ointment preparations such as Mycolog (neomycin, nystatin, gramicidin and triamcinolone acetonide), has been associated with contact dermatitis (28). Tetracycline and oxyquinoline (eg, Vioform) topical preparations can also cause sensitivity reactions.

If the skin infection is severe, deep, is associated with fever or other systemic manifestations, systemic antimicrobials should be used. If a topical antibiotic preparation is indicated, it should be employed with full awareness of its sensitizing properties (29,30,31).

10. *Pruritus.* **P.K.'s chief complaint is pruritus. How should pruritus be managed?**

Pruritus is the most common cutaneous symptom. It has many different causes and has been associated with many systemic diseases. Among these are obstructive biliary disease, anemia, hypertension, gout, various malignant diseases, thyroid disease (both hyper and hypo), diabetes mellitus, and pregnancy (usually the first trimester) (32). In the absence of a cutaneous dermatitis, a careful history and physical exam should be performed to rule out one of the systemic causes of pruritus.

Although often detrimental, scratching is the most common method of relieving pruritus, probably causing the receptor nerve endings to become damaged or fatigued. One would therefore expect topically applied local anesthetics or antihistamines to be effective in dulling the sensation, but this approach is often disappointing, probably because of the poor absorption of the salt forms of the drugs through the intact epidermis and the low concentrations used in many over-the-counter preparations. If adequate concentrations of local anesthetics are employed (benzocaine 20% or lidocaine 3–4%), pruritus or pain may be reduced for up to 45 minutes. If these agents are used, they are most useful for relieving pruritus or pain for short periods of time when the patient would require relief most (eg, when trying to go to sleep at night) (33). An additional drawback to the use of these agents is their ability to cause an allergic contact dermatitis (benzocaine 0.17% incidence; lidocaine, extremely rare) (23,33).

Cold water or ice cubes are effective in the relief of pruritus, as are products containing aluminium acetate (Burow's solution), tannic acid, or calamine. Additionally, since the nerves which mediate the itch response also mediate pain, analgesics theoretically may provide some limited benefits.

Moisturizing mixtures such as Keri Lotion, Lubriderm, or simply, mineral or baby oil are useful in the treatment of pruritus caused by dry skin, which is often encountered in the elderly or during the winter. Bathing should be restricted to avoid additional drying, the irritant effect of alkaline soaps, and the trauma of toweling.

Topical corticosteroid applications can be very effective. They reduce inflammation and are often contained in a cream base which helps to soothe the affected area.

Systemic antihistamines evoke a favorable response for many patients suffering from pruritus, although their major beneficial effect may be due to sedation. There is disagreement over which antihistamine or antiserotonin agent is more efficacious in the treatment of pruritus (34,35). There is evidence, based on clinical trials and the relative amounts of histamine required to produce itching, that hydroxyzine may be more effective than diphenhydramine or cyproheptadine (36,37). Many practitioners now consider hydroxyzine to be the antihistamine of choice for the treatment of pruritus; dosages of 10–25 mg tid to qid are commonly employed.

11. P.K. presents to the outpatient pharmacy with the following prescriptions: hydroxyzine 25 mg tid prn, #90, refill × 20; triamcinolone acetonide cream 0.1%, apply tid, 2 lbs, refill × 6; betamethasone valerate ointment 0.1%, 30 gm, apply prn flair, refill × 3; triple antibiotic ointment, apply qid to infected areas, 1 oz, NR. The patient has a return appointment in the Dermatology Clinic in three weeks. What suggestions might be made to P.K. at this time?

The general goals of therapy for atopic eczema

are to decrease pruritus, suppress inflammation, lubricate the skin, and reduce anxiety. Additionally, the following recommendations are useful for atopic ezcema or any other irritant dermatitis:

(a) Clothing should be soft and light. Cotton or corduroy are preferred. Wools and coarse heavy synthetics should be avoided.

(b) Heat should be avoided because it often makes the eczema worse. The environment should be well ventilated, cool, and have low humidity (30–50%). Rapid changes in ambient temperature should be avoided.

(c) Bathing should be kept to a minimum (no longer than 5 minutes) and the patient should use a non-irritating soap (eg, Basis soap). A colloid bath or the use of appropriate amounts of a bath oil may be useful.

(d) The skin should be kept moist with frequent applications of emollients (Keri, Lubriderm, Nivea, Aquaphor, Eucerin, or petrolatum).

(e) Primary irritants such as paints, cleansers, solvents, and chemical sprays should be avoided.

Additionally, smallpox vaccinations are contraindicated in patients with eczema and pemphigus, because they predispose the patient to severe disseminated vaccinia. Since the patient can also become infected through contact with a vaccinated person, none of the patient's family can be vaccinated unless they assume separate residence until the scab has fallen off (7). Also, the patient should be warned to avoid people with active herpes simplex infections since a severe disseminated infection which can be life-threatening may occur (15).

12. P.K. continued to do well and returned to the outpatient clinic pharmacy three months later to request refills of his topical corticosteroid prescriptions. He stated that the infected areas have cleared and his fingers are the only area that is not well controlled. He has applied the betamethasone valerate ointment to his hands five to six times per day for the last three weeks without any noticeable improvement. He used the triamcinolone cream according to directions on other areas of his body that were affected. He followed other recommendations faithfully and wonders if anything else could be done for his hands. He also states he occasionally is bothered by sedation from the hydroxyzine.

First, the patient is overusing the topical corticosteroid, and tachyphylaxis is probably occurring. Tachyphylaxis can occur within one week after starting therapy but generally takes several weeks to a month to occur (38–40). To treat this problem, P.K. should stop applying the bethamethasone valerate ointment for four to seven days and then restart therapy, applying the medication in the proper manner. It has been suggested by some that limited courses of treatment separated by short resting periods might be more effective than continuous treatment. However, documentation for this type of therapy is lacking at present.

A prescription might be requested from P.K.'s physician for flurandrenolide 4 mcg/sq cm tape (Cordran) after he stops the corticosteroids for four to seven days. While this product is expensive, it is very useful for small areas because it combines the protectant (bandage) effect of the tape with occlusion and a corticosteroid. It is very useful on the hands (particularly the fingers) because other vehicles are often quite messy when applied to the hands. When using Cordran tape, general principles previously outlined for occlusion should be followed.

Sedation from hydroxyzine is fairly common. The following are ways to minimize/reduce the sedation:

(a) Reduce the strength of hydroxyzine to 10 mg tablets.

(b) Have P.K. take the hydroxyzine on a scheduled basis since some tolerance to the sedative properties will probably develop.

(c) Switch to a less sedating antihistamine. However, part of the benefit derived from antihistamines is related to their sedative action; this property helps the patient sleep and decreases the anxiety which is common with persistent pruritus.

(d) If the above three measures have been tried and sedation is still a problem, P.K. must decide which is worse, the sedation or the pruritus, and make his own decision whether or not to use the antihistamine.

13. *Nonprescription Topical Hydrocortisone.* M.P. is a 29-year-old housewife who requests Rhulicort Cream (hydrocortisone 0.5%) for her hands, which are irritated from dishwater. Comment on this situation.

A 0.5% hydrocortisone preparation is indicated for temporary relief of minor skin irritations, itching and rash due to eczema, dermatitis, insect bites, poison ivy, poison oak, poison sumac, soaps, detergents, cosmetics, jewelry, and for itchy genital and anal areas. These preparations should not be used in children under two years of age without approval of the child's physician (33). At present it is difficult to evaluate whether higher strength corticosteroid preparations are more effective for these conditions than 0.5% hydrocortisone. The minimum concentration of hydrocortisone considered to be effective is 0.5%, although 0.25% concentrations have been found effective for certain dermatoses in some studies (33,40).

Before recommending a 0.5% over-the-counter (OTC) hydrocortisone product, an assessment should be made as to whether or not the use of such a preparation is warranted (see Question 14).

14. T.C. is a 26-year-old, 60 kg female who requests one of the "new" topical nonprescription hydrocortisone preparations for a rash on her face. T.C. states that the rash is on her cheeks and gets worse when she goes out into the sun. She also complains of feeling tired and would like a vitamin product. Additionally, she requests a bottle of 1000 five grain aspirin for her sore joints. The rash appears erythematous and covers both cheeks with a butterfly configuration. T.C. admits to using no other medications. Should a hydrocortisone preparation be recommended?

The symptoms that T.C. describes are consistent with systemic lupus erythematosus and she should be referred to her physician for an appropriate diagnostic work up. The following considerations are offered as an overall guide for assessing patients having conditions where the use of 0.5% hydrocortisone may be indicated:

(a) Does the patient have constitutional symptoms such as: fever, joint pains, muscle pains, headache, difficulty moving the affected area, or excessive swelling of the affected area?

(b) Does the patient have a history of a severe chronic disease process such as: anemia, malnutrition, lung disease, kidney disease, heart disease, diabetes mellitus, cancer, alcoholism, or a systemic infection? Is the patient being treated by a physician for a dermatologic condition?

(c) Does your drug history indicate a possible drug allergy to a prescription medication the patient is taking? (See Question 30.)

(d) Is the patient taking any medication which

may impair his immune system? This may include: systemically administered corticosteroid preparations, antimetabolites or other cancer chemotherapeutic agents, and radiation therapy.

(e) Does the area appear macerated, eroded, or infected? Is bleeding present? If infected, the area will generally appear red and swollen, and pus or drainage may be present.

(f) Does the affected area involve the eye or mucous membranes?

(g) For the patient having poison ivy, oak, or sumac, is there a possibility that the patient may have inhaled the smoke from the burning of one of these plants?

(h) For patients having rectal complaints, check for bleeding or hemorrhoids.

(i) For patients having genital complaints, check for venereal disease, lice, or scabies.

(j) Has the patient's problem worsened after starting to use a 0.5% hydrocortisone preparation or has the condition not improved significantly after one week of therapy?

(k) Did the patient's problem return after appearing to clear up with the use of a 0.5% hydrocortisone preparation?

Patient Considerations When 0.5% Hydrocortisone is Used

(a) Determine which product(s) the patient may have already used to treat this problem and if it is/was effective.

(b) A 0.5% hydrocortisone preparation should not be applied to areas of the skin that are infected, because it may permit some infections to spread and cause ulceration and scarring. This can be particularly dangerous since the anti-inflammatory effects of the 0.5% hydrocortisone preparation may allow the infection to worsen without the patient noticing it.

(c) The patient should note some improvement in two to three days after starting to use 0.5% hydrocortisone preparations. If not, consider referring the patient to his physician.

(d) A 0.5% hydrocortisone preparation should be applied to the affected area three to four times a day and *rubbed in thoroughly.* This is very important if the patient is to receive the full anti-inflammatory effects.

(e) Occlusion will enhance the effects of 0.5% hydrocortisone preparations. See the general guidelines for occlusion (Question 2) for further instructions.

(f) If pain is present, consider recommending aspirin or acetaminophen 650 mg qid.

(g) If itching is severe, consider recommending an over-the-counter sleep aid. Generally itching bothers people most when they are trying to go to sleep. If the area that itches is small, an ice cube or cold compress applied to the affected area will bring relief. If there are numerous scratch marks around the affected area, consider recommending that the patient wear cotton gloves at night to protect the area and reduce the chances of infection.

(h) If the patient has a contact/irritant dermatitis due to soaps, detergents, cosmetics, jewelry, etc., the condition will generally persist until the patient stops contact with the offending agent. Many times the patient's skin problem may be traced to recent use of a new cosmetic, cleaning agent, clothes, etc. Some detective work may be necessary to discover the cause of the problem. If the hands are affected (a common occurrence), recommend that the patient purchase rubber gloves and wear them while contacting the offending agent or when using irritating substances which will aggravate the underlying problem. Additionally, recommend applying the 0.5% hydrocortisone preparation before putting the gloves on as this will enhance the anti-inflammatory effect.

WOUND HEALING

15. T.T. is a 43-year-old male who underwent a laparotomy for staging of his Hodgkin's Disease three weeks ago. The patient has not received any chemotherapy or radiation because his surgical wound has been quite slow to heal. T.T. is eating well and has received multivitamins plus minerals for five weeks. His physician is considering adding zinc and vitamin A to his oral medications to improve the wound healing. Would zinc or vitamin A therapy be appropriate?

The evidence that oral zinc improves wound healing is unsatisfactory. Although oral zinc therapy may be useful in patients with dietary deficiency, zinc deficiency is probably only partially responsible for the delayed healing. A few studies indicate that oral zinc benefits wound healing, but other factors (eg, ascorbic acid deficiency) that could have been responsible for delayed wound healing were not considered (41,42,43).

While doses of zinc vary, it is generally thought that a 220 mg dose of zinc sulfate (equivalent to 50 mg elemental zinc) given orally three times a day for seven to eight weeks will improve wound healing in zinc-deficient patients. If no improvement is noted by this time, the delay in wound healing should not be ascribed to a zinc deficiency. The only reported side effect with this regimen is nausea which can be minimized by taking the zinc with meals (44).

Vitamin A reverses the inhibitory effect of cortisone on the healing of open wounds in man and animals (45). Apparently, topical and systemic vitamin A stimulates the healing of cortisone-retarded wounds but does not enhance wound healing in subjects not receiving cortisone. Presumably, vitamin A restores the inflammatory process suppressed by corticosteroids.

The normal healing process in rats can be accelerated by topical administration of vitamin A acid and its derivatives (46,47,48). More extensive research is needed to evaluate the effects of vitamin A on wound healing in normal human subjects, since most of the research to date has been in animals. Recommendations on doses for humans would be premature at this time.

It is doubtful that T.T.'s wound healing can be accelerated with zinc or vitamin A. Additionally, the F.D.A. has not recognized any claims that these substances will have a positive effect on wound healing (49). Any over-the-counter products making this claim are now considered misbranded.

SUNBURN

Sunlight is composed of light in wavelengths from 290 nm (near ultraviolet) to about 2500 nm (infrared). The visible region is between 290 nm and 700 nm. The portion of the spectrum which is important for sunburn and suntanning lies in the ultraviolet spectrum ranging from 290 to 400 nm (see Fig. 1). The ultraviolet light spectrum is subdivided into: UVA (longwave), 320–400 nm, which is useful for photochemotherapy (see Question 21) and is the range where most drug-induced photosensitivity reactions occur; UVB (middlewave), 290–320 nm, which is responsible for suntanning and burning; and UVC (shortwave), 100–290 nm, or germicidal region because of the ability of this wavelength to kill one-celled organisms. Within the sunburning region (UVB), about 10% of the ultraviolet light penetrates into the dermis at 290 nm; this increases as wavelengths increase toward 320 nm. Other wavelengths of light are also absorbed and, if intense enough, can produce burning. This type of burning is different from sunburn in that it is due to generated heat rather than a photochemical reaction.

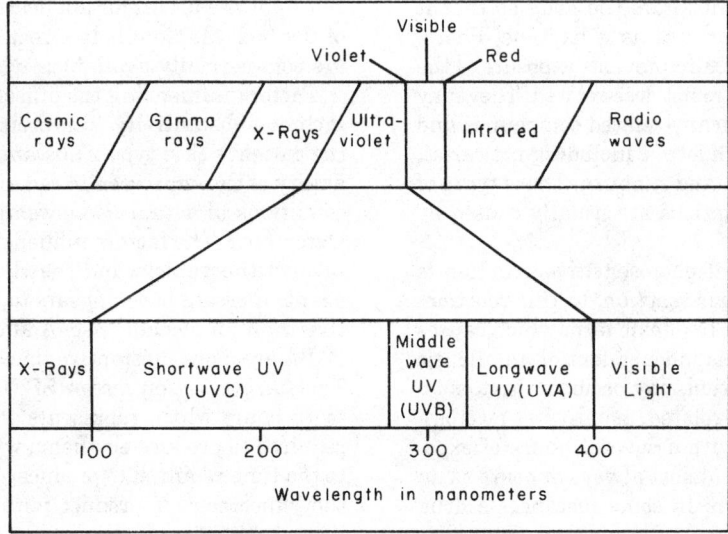

Figure 1. Electromagnetic Spectrum.

Pathogenesis of Sunburn. The vascular changes that occur secondary to exposure to sunlight are biphasic. An immediate, faint, transient reddening of the skin occurs shortly after exposure to ultraviolet light and fades within 30 minutes after stopping the exposure. A delayed erythema reaction occurs after a latent period of two to six hours and peaks at 10 to 24 hours after ultraviolet light exposure. This erythema gradually subsides over the next two to four days. Peeling follows four to seven days after a moderate to severe sunburn. The mechanisms by which these two types of erythema are produced are not completely understood. Kinins (50,51), histamine (52), prostaglandins (53–58), other vasoactive substances (59), hydrolytic enzymes (60), and free radicals (61) have all been implicated as mediators of the erythema caused by sunlight. While prostaglandins have received much attention in the scientific and lay press, none of these substances is universally accepted as the mediator (cause) of sunburn.

Photosensitization. In a patient who experiences a more severe sunburn than would be normally expected from the exposure to ultraviolet light, or who develops a rash in areas exposed to the sun, the clinician should suspect a photosensitivity reaction from ultraviolet light in the UVA band. Photosensitivity reactions can occur from topically applied or systemically administered compounds. There are two types of photosensitivity reactions, both of which require the presence of drug and light. The first is a *photoallergic reaction,* in which light alters the drug so that it becomes antigenic or acts as a hapten. Photoallergic eruptions require previous exposure to the offending drug and are not dose-related. They may be induced by chemically-related compounds and appear in a variety of forms, including urticarial, bullous, eczematous, and sunburn. These types of photosensitivity eruptions are usually caused by topical agents.

The second type of photosensitive eruption is known as a *phototoxic reaction.* In this reaction, light alters the drug to a toxic form which causes tissue damage that is independent of an allergic response. This eruption may occur on first exposure to drug, is dose-related, usually has no cross-sensitivity, occurs within several hours of exposure to the sun, and almost always appears as an exaggerated sunburn. In some instances a drug may produce both photoallergic and phototoxic

reactions (62,63). See the question on drug eruptions (Question 30) for a listing of drugs which cause photosensitivity reactions.

16. *Sunscreens.* **H.M. is a 16-year-old, blond, blue eyed male who requests advice on how he may be able to obtain a tan without burning. He can normally go out in the sun for only one to two hours before he starts to burn, and he almost never tans. Is there a way H.M. could obtain a tan without burning? How should sunscreens be employed?**

The same wavelengths of light which cause burning are responsible for melanocyte stimulation and increased skin pigmentation. The only satisfactory method of tanning without burning is short repetitive exposures to the sun. This stimulates melanocytes without exposing the skin to excessive radiation. Sunscreening agents block the penetration of ultraviolet light and should be used after limited exposure to the sun, before burning begins (7).

In general, prevention of sunburn by the use of sunscreens is easier than treatment once it occurs. Sunscreening products may be divided into two groups. Agents which are opaque and block out sunlight include titanium dioxide or zinc oxide. Agents which absorb ultraviolet light include para-aminobenzoic acid (PABA) and its esters, benzophenones, and anthranilates. The opaque sunscreens are very good for small areas (nose or lips) but are not practical for application to large areas of the body. Agents which absorb ultraviolet light are useful for application to large areas of the body. Table 5 lists screening agents which are commercially available.

Factors influencing the efficacy of a sunscreen include substantivity, sun protection factor, and the patient's skin type. *Substantivity* refers to the ability of the sunscreen to remain effective under conditions of actual use (sweating, contact with water, etc.). The factors influencing substantivity involve the vehicle and the chemical absorbing agent. A cream base appears to be more substantive than an alcohol base. Additionally, esters of PABA are more substantive than PABA (56,57,58). The *sun protection factor* (SPF) is a scale from 2 to 15 hours which represents a ratio of the time required to produce erythema with the sunscreen to the time required to produce erythema without the sunscreen. A product with a SPF of eight means that if a person applied this product and then sat out in the sun, they would have as much erythema at the end of eight hours as they would have had at one hour without applying the preparation. All sunscreening products now have SPF's on their labels.

Skin sensitivity to sunlight has been classified into four types: Type I: always burns, never tans; Type II: usually burns, sometimes tans; Type III: Occasionally burns, gradually tans; Type IV: minimally burns, readily tans. Persons with type I or II skin (H.M.), may begin to show erythema after only 10 to 20 minutes of noontime exposure (64).

In selecting a sunscreen, the person's skin type is the most important factor. People with skin Type I should use a product with a SPF in the 12–15 range, while those with skin Type IV require either no product at all or one with a SPF of 2–4. The sunscreen should be applied frequently because it can be washed away by sweat or water. Of the products available, it appears that Supershade is the most efficacious based on SPF, substantivity, and ability to block both UVA and UVB. Supershade is also unscented.

In H.M.'s case, he may approach suntanning in one of two ways: a) Spend one hour in the sun unprotected and apply a sunscreen to block all ultraviolet light (SPF 12–15) for the remainder of the time he is in the sun. Sun exposure may be gradually increased by 15 to 30 minute intervals (prior to application of the sunscreen) on a daily basis. b) Apply a sunscreen with a SPF of 8–12 prior to any sun exposure. The method chosen for H.M. to obtain a tan should be based on

Table 5.

COMPARATIVE TABLE FOR SUNSCREENING PRODUCTS

Product	Company	SPF					Adsorbs	
		2–4	4–6	6–12	12–15		UVA	UVB
Afil	Texas Pharmacol.		x				x	x
Blockout	Sea & Ski Corp.			x				x
Eclipse	Herbert Labs			x				x
Total Eclipse	Herbert Labs				x		x	x
Partial Eclipse	Herbert Labs		x					x
Maxafil	Texas Pharmacol.		x				x	x
Pabafilm	Owen		x					x
Pabagel	Owen		x					x
Pizbuin	Westwood			x			x	x
Presun 4	Westwood		x					x
8	Westwood			x				x
15	Westwood				x		x	x
Protan	Westwood	x						x
RVP	Elder	x					x	x
RV Paque	Elder		x				x	x
Sea & Ski	Sea & Ski Corp.			x				x
Solbar	Person & Corey		x				x	x
Sun Dare	Texas Pharmacol.	x						x
Sun Down	DOME		x				x	x
Supershade	Shering Plough				x		x	x
Uval	Dorsey			x			x	x

how long he will be in the sun and if sun exposure will be on a daily or intermittent basis. In general, the most effective way to achieve a lasting tan is with short exposures to sunlight (initial exposure would be based on skin type) repeated on a regular basis while gradually increasing sun exposure as tolerance permits.

17. *Protection Against Photosensitivity.* T.B. is a 18-year-old female who requests information about which sun tanning/burning product(s) she should purchase for her two-week trip to Florida. She is redheaded, has a very fair complexion, and states that she only gets a slight tan and usually gets sunburned after being in the sun for one to two hours. T.B. is currently taking tetracycline 250 mg bid for her acne (no visible acne lesions are present). How would the presence of this potentially photosensitizing drug affect your decision on selecting a sunscreen?

Although the SPF is of primary importance in selecting a product, patients like T.B. who are taking a potentially photosensitizing drug must consider the type of absorbing chemical. Since drug-induced photosensitivity reactions occur in the UVA range, a product containing a benzophenone or anthranilate which absorbs both UVA and UVB should be used. PABA and its derivatives block only UVB and would not be expected to provide protection against drug-induced photosensitivity reactions (64). Since T.B. is taking this medication primarily for cosmetic reasons, she should stop the tetracycline the day before exposure to the sun and during the two weeks while she is in Florida. Table 5 lists screening agents which are commercially available and would be useful for preventing potential photosensitivity reactions.

18. *Treatment of Sunburn.* M.K. is a 33-year-old female who requests something for sunburn relief. She fell asleep in the sun for about four hours and now has a rather painful sunburn over about 30% of her body. It has been two hours since she has come out of the sun and no blistering is apparent. How should M.K. be treated?

Based on the above history and type of burn present (first degree), M.K. probably could be managed with over-the-counter therapy. The following outline summarizes the therapy available for the treatment of sunburn.

General Treatment For Sunburn

(a) Wet dressings may provide some relief. A cool (not cold) bath may provide relief of pain and has a cooling and soothing effect.

(b) Topical corticosteroids (Potent, see Table 4) reduce inflammation and pain. To provide maximum benefit, these should be applied as soon as possible. Over-the-counter 0.5% hydrocortisone may provide some relief, but efficacy has not been established nor have there been comparative studies with the more potent topical corticosteroids.

(c) Emollients should be applied frequently to prevent dryness and reduce pain.

(d) If pain is severe, sedation may be useful to help the patient sleep.

(e) Analgesics such as aspirin or acetaminophen are valuable adjuvants in relieving burn pain. Many people prefer aspirin because it is a prostaglandin inhibitor and antiinflammatory agent in high doses and theoretically should provide greater benefit than acetaminophen. Since prostaglandins are believed to be involved in the delayed erythema reaction of sunburn, there is speculation that patients experiencing sunburn should take 1200 mg of aspirin every four hours for one day after the sunburn has begun in hopes of preventing or modifying this reaction. If gastrointestinal upset or tinnitus occurs, the high-dose aspirin therapy is discontinued. At the present time, there is no scientific evidence to support or refute high-dose aspirin therapy. Undoubtedly, high doses of aspirin provide more pain relief than standard doses, but whether this regimen modifies the sunburn reaction is unknown.

(f) Local anesthetics are rarely indicated because of the possibility of sensitization and their relatively short duration of action (30–45 minutes). They may be useful in helping a patient get to sleep however.

(g) For severe sunburn, in addition to the therapy for a mild sunburn, 40–60 mg of prednisone daily for three days will almost completely abate a potentially severe sunburn (11).

PSORIASIS

The basic pathological lesion of psoriasis is caused by a loss of control of the normal growth-regulating mechanisms in the epidermis (65). The normal turnover time for a cell to proceed from the generative layer of the skin to the point where it sloughs off is 27 days. In the psoriatic, the turn-over time is decreased to three to four days. Therefore, the cells do not mature, and keratinization fails to reach completion (7,66,67). The epidermis is thickened by the increase in mitotic activity of the generative layer. Along with the increased cell turnover, there is a corresponding increase in nucleo-protein synthesis as well as an increase in certain enzymes responsible for growth. Vascular changes are seen, with the blood vessels becoming dilated and tortuous. The blood vessels extend further up into the skin than normal, which allows bleeding to occur when the lesions are subjected to trauma. Inflammation with leukocyte infiltrates is also seen to varying degrees and is secondary to the underlying psoriatic lesion.

19. *Topical Therapy.* **Z.K. is a 16-year-old female who has developed erythematous scaly lesions on her knees, elbows, and scalp over the past three months. The lesions have become more diffuse over the last several weeks with many loosely attached silvery scales. Z.K.'s mother has psoriasis, and now Z.K. appears to have developed the disease. Approximately 20% of her body surface area is affected by these lesions. What topical therapies are available for psoriasis; which ones would be most appropriate for Z.K.?**

The Goeckerman and Ingram regimens are commonly employed treatment programs for inducing and prolonging remissions in patients with psoriasis. The Goeckerman regimen employs coal tar or its derivatives and ultraviolet light. A coal tar ointment (2–5% crude coal tar or its equivalent) is applied several times a day and removed 24 hours after the initial application; this is followed by exposure to ultraviolet light. In addition, a coal tar bath, using a water soluble preparation, is given at least once a day. With successive daily treatments, the exposure to ultraviolet light is gradually increased. This particular regimen produces a significant number of remissions which can last 6–18 months (68,69).

The Ingram regimen differs in that an anthralin paste is applied to each psoriatic plaque, and stockinet dressings are applied over the lesions. This regimen is very effective but requires close supervision because anthralin irritates normal skin (70).

Each of these regimens can be modified. Frequently, topical corticosteroids and occlusive dressings are used as adjuvants.

If the psoriatic lesions are not extensive, psoriasis should be treated conservatively with topical agents. Corticosteroid creams, the mainstays of topical therapy, are often used with occlusive dressings to increase their penetration into the skin. A variety of coal tar preparations are available and may be used by themselves or incorporated into corticosteroid creams. Ammoniated mercury is generally less effective than coal tar but can be substituted if necessary. Salicylic acid is sometimes incorporated into these preparations to help remove thick scales. Anthralin may be used, but it is usually reserved for more severe cases of psoriasis because of its harsh effects on uninvolved skin (66,71,72).

Because of Z.K.'s age, she should be initially managed with the least noxious therapy. This should include a moderately potent topical corticosteroid preparation (see Table 4) and a coal tar shampoo. If this proves ineffective, modified Goeckerman or Ingram regimens may be employed. Only after all forms of topical therapy have been employed and failed should systemic therapies be considered.

20. *Systemic Therapy.* **K.M. is a 26-year-old, 157 lb white male who was referred to the Dermatology Department in December of 1981 to initiate inpatient treatment for psoriasis. The patient's pertinent family history included a paternal grandfather with psoriasis, a maternal grandmother with a history of glaucoma and cataracts, and a mother with a history of glaucoma. The patient had psoriasis since age 14 and first sought medical treatment in 1973. At that time he received methotrexate in a regimen of 2.5 mg daily for six months, until mouth and stomach ulcers developed. The methotrexate was stopped and gentian violet oral swabs and antacids were prescribed for treatment. During methotrexate therapy, the patient's psoriasis had started to clear, but upon discontinuing methotrexate the condition slowly exacerbated. Spontaneous improvement occurred in the early summer of 1974, and the patient was lost to follow up until a fractured arm required hospitalization in December 1975. At this time he received topical treatment with coal tar, salicylic acid, and various corticosteroid creams. Upon removal of the cast, a clearing of the psoriasis in that area was discovered. The patient continued to use**

the above mentioned creams without occlusion and various home remedies (ie, mange baths, over-the-counter medications, and diets) until 1979. No improvement or adverse effects were noted over this period.

Physical examination revealed a young white male who was well nourished and healthy. The review of systems was within normal limits, with no symptoms of arthritis. The dermatological examination revealed guttate and small plaque psoriasis over the patient's arms and legs (approximately 25% of the body) and scalp (100%). The patient exhibited nail involvement manifested by brittle, pitting nails.

Complete blood count, serum glucose, blood urea nitrogen, serum creatinine, and urinalysis were all within normal limits. The SGOT was 25 U/ml (normal 10–40 U/ml), alkaline phosphatase was 86 IU/L (normal 13–39 IU/L), and LDH was 161 U/ml (normal 60–120 U/ml).

During this hospital admission (December 1981), which included the physical examination and laboratory data mentioned above, a diagnosis of psoriasis vulgaris was made, admitting topical medications were continued, and a complete visual examination was performed.

What systemic therapies would be appropriate for K.M., and how should they be administered? What side effects should be considered in monitoring systemic therapy?

Systemic therapy is reserved for moderate to severe forms of psoriasis when less toxic forms of therapy have failed. Methotrexate and methoxsalen with UVA light are used for systemic therapy. Methotrexate is the only systemic therapy that at present enjoys F.D.A. approval, but methoxsalen and UVA light (acronym PUVA) enjoy widespread usage. Because of the widespread success of PUVA therapy and the lower relative potential risks of PUVA, it will probably be approved by the F.D.A. and replace methotrexate in the treatment of psoriasis in the near future.

Methotrexate. Methotrexate (MTX) is not curative, but it suppresses psoriatic lesions and induces prolonged remissions in up to 75% of patients (73). The following are relative contraindications to the use of MTX in psoriasis: history of significant renal function abnormalities; liver impairment or history of hepatic disease; preg-

nancy; anemia; leukopenia; thrombocytopenia; active peptic ulcer disease; active infection; and an unreliable patient.

Three dosage schedules are commonly used in the treatment of psoriasis:

(a) Large doses (10–25 mg; occasionally as much as 37.5 mg) may be administered weekly by the oral, intramuscular, or intravenous route. As the dose is increased, more frequent blood counts are indicated.

(b) A large weekly dose may be administered over a 36-hour period. Usually, 2.5 to 5 mg is given orally every 12 hours for three doses or every 8 hours for four doses. The total dose should not exceed 37.5 mg/week.

(c) Low oral doses may be given daily with rest periods. Usually, 2.5 mg is given daily for five days, followed by a minimum two-day rest period; a second five-day course is followed by a rest period of at least seven days.

The three schedules are about equally effective; however, a given amount of MTX is less toxic when given as a single dose. Thus, dosage regimen "c" produces more toxicity than does "a" or "b." If the cellular kinetics of psoriatics are considered, schedule "b" appears to be the most appropriate (74). This regimen is probably also the least toxic (73,76).

Since K.M. has already been treated with what appears to be regimen "c" and developed toxicity, it would be appropriate to use regimen "b" if methotrexate were used. Whichever regimen is used (most people use regimen "b"), it is important to remember that all dosage regimens should be tailored to the individual patient. The goal of MTX therapy is not to cure psoriasis but to achieve a tolerable level of disease activity with the lowest possible dose (77).

The side effects encountered with MTX as used in psoriatics are essentially the same as those found in patients treated for cancer, but less severe. The most commonly reported adverse reactions are dose-related and include ulcerative stomatitis, leukopenia, abdominal distress, and nausea. If side effects occur, MTX therapy may be temporarily discontinued, or stopped altogether if they are severe. Irreversible and sometimes fatal hepatotoxicity (cirrhosis and fibrosis) is a common complication in patients taking MTX chronically. Serum enzymes and other liver function tests do not correlate with the severity of liver damage and are generally not predictive.

For this reason a liver biopsy is performed prior to the initiation of MTX and yearly thereafter in some institutions (78,79). Alcohol may increase the prevalence and severity of this adverse reaction. There is also a theoretical risk of oncogenicity with the use of methotrexate, and this must be taken into consideration before this type of therapy is considered.

21. K.M. is put on regimen "b." Two months later he complains of sores in his mouth and a persistent upset stomach. His psoriasis has improved (now only 15% of his body is affected), but it still is quite debilitating and he feels his current therapy is cosmetically unacceptable. A decision is made to stop methotrexate therapy because of toxicity and inadequate response. K.M.'s job will not allow a prolonged hospitalization, so modified Goeckerman or Ingram regimens cannot be used. What other therapy may be recommended at this time?

Photochemotherapy. Photochemotherapy, combining the use of chemicals and electromagnetic radiation to treat various skin disorders, represents one of the more promising advances in dermatologic therapy in recent years, and will probably replace methotrexate therapy for patients with severe psoriasis. Since the original report by Parrish et al in 1974 (80), numerous studies including two multicenter co-operative clinical trials (95,96) have appeared, indicating impressive effectiveness in treating psoriasis with a photoactive psoralen, methoxsalen (acronym 8 MOP) and ultraviolet radiation of wavelength A (acronym PUVA) (81–94). Since methoxsalen responds to a maximum absorptive spectrum of 365 nm (97,98), only longwave ultraviolet light (UVA) ranging from 320–400 nm is utilized as the light source.

PUVA therapy should be reserved for patients with moderate to severe psoriasis. Patients with debilitating involvement of the palms and soles of feet may also receive PUVA treatments. Methoxsalen dosage is determined on the basis of weight (0.6 mg/kg). The UVA exposure, measured in terms of Joules/cm^2, is initially determined by the patient's skin reaction to sunlight (See Question 16). The patient normally receives two to three treatments per week which are at least 48 hours apart. If no response is noted after 30 treatments, the patient is considered a treatment failure (99). With the onset of significant clearing, the exposure to the UVA and the dose of methoxsalen may remain constant until complete clearing is noted.

Nausea, pruritus, and erythema are the most commonly reported side effects to PUVA (95). Nausea, usually transient, may be minimized by having the patient take the methoxsalen with food or milk. If nausea still persists, antiemetic agents such as prochlorperazine may be tried. If still unrelieved, the dosage of methoxsalen may be decreased by 10 mg (93,100). Pruritus, quite common especially during the early stages of photochemotherapy, responds to frequent applications of bland emollients. If this is ineffective, antihistamines or sedatives are often effective (95). If pruritus continues, the affected areas may be shielded from UVA, or the patient may temporarily discontinue PUVA treatments until the symptoms subside.

Perhaps the greatest long-term risk associated with PUVA therapy involves the potential for oncogenicity. Stern et al (101), reporting on 1373 patients who received PUVA therapy, found that the risk of cutaneous carcinoma was 2.63 times the expected rate for age, sex, and geographically matched populations. However, Stern found that several factors correlated with increased risk of cutaneous carcinoma: skin type, history of exposure to ionizing radiation, or a previous history of cutaneous carcinoma. If patients with these factors were eliminated from those studied, the risk of developing carcinoma was not significantly higher than that for a normal population. Before the risks of carcinoma can be accurately assessed, further studies must be done, following patients for longer periods of time. Other risk factors associated with the development of carcinoma such as exposure to tar (102,103), arsenic (104), and immunosuppressive agents (105,106, 107) may influence the risk of developing carcinoma, since many patients have been exposed to these agents prior to receiving PUVA therapy.

While experimental and requiring a IND, PUVA therapy is effective and safe for short-term therapy of patients with moderate to severe forms of psoriasis. How this new therapy compares with other, traditional forms of therapy is not known with certainty. While other comparative studies need to be done, most of the patients utilized in the PUVA studies had been treated with other, generally more toxic forms of therapy for their psoriasis and failed to respond. Table 6 summa-

Table 6.

COMPARISONS OF THERAPIES FOR PSORIASIS

| | Goeckerman | Ingram | Cortisteroids | | Metho-trexate | Hydroxy-urea | PUVA |
			Topical	Systemic			
Response (%)	*	*	up to 100%	100%	67–78%	50–96%	90–100%
Relapse (%)	up to 100%	up to 100%	100%	100%	——	100%	95–90%
Average Length of Time Before Relapse	6–18 months	27–29 days	several wks	several wks	——	4 wks	?
Potential for Adverse Effects							
Short-Term	low	moderate	low	low-moderate	moderate	moderate	low
Long-Term	low	low	moderate	high	high	high	low (?)
Patient Acceptance	low	low	moderate	high	moderate	moderate	moderate to high
Hospitalization Required	yes (14–19 days)	yes (18–21 days)	no	no	no	no	no
Reference	138,139,141, 143,146,149	138,140,143, 144,145,147	139,140, 146	138,140,141, 142,143	138,143, 148	138,143	80–96

*Because of the extreme variability in regimens (corticosteroids and other therapies are often included) percent response is difficult to estimate.

This table is reproduced with permission of the American Society of Hospital Pharmacists.

rizes the results of psoriasis treatment with PUVA and other forms of therapy.

The F.D.A. Dermatology Advisory Committee reviewed PUVA therapy in December 1977 and April 1978 and agreed unanimously that it is effective. However, the F.D.A. has not approved methoxsalen for use in psoriasis because of unanswered questions concerning the long-term therapy required for maintained remission.

DANDRUFF/SEBORRHEIC DERMATITIS

22. P.P. is a 20 year-old-male who requests an OTC product for his persistent dandruff. The patient has noticeable white flakes on his shoulders and appears to have a moderate amount on certain hairy areas (neck, side burns, eyebrows, and the borders of his scalp). His scalp appears reddened at the hairline, and P.P. says it feels like his scalp is inflamed. He washes his hair twice per week with a nonmedicated shampoo. What should be recommended?

Using Table 7, which is offered to help distinguish dandruff, seborrheic dermatitis, and psoriasis, it appears that P.P. has seborrheic dermatitis. Both dandruff and seborrheic dermatitis are the result of increased cell turnover and retention of nucleated cells on the scalp (11). Neither microorganisms, increased sebum production, nor sebum composition appear to be causative factors. In general, OTC therapy adequately controls dandruff and many cases of seborrheic dermatitis. Patients who have seborrheic dermatitis like that illustrated in P.P. and whose condition has not improved within two weeks after starting appropriate OTC therapy, or whose condition worsens after starting OTC therapy, should consult their physician.

The following summarizes general therapy for dandruff and seborrheic dermatitis (108,11):

General Shampoo Instructions

(a) The scalp should be shampooed frequently: three times a week until the dandruff is under control, then twice a week thereafter.

(b) Agitation of the scalp while shampooing is

desirable. A rubber scalp agitator may be employed for those with short or fragile fingernails.

(c) If a medicated shampoo is employed, contact time should be as long as possible—at least five minutes. Also, it is desirable to shampoo at least twice, the first shampooing to remove oil and dirt and to wet the scalp and the second to allow the medicated shampoo to work on the scalp. A third shampooing can also be employed if results are inadequate (108).

Dandruff

(a) Follow general shampoo instructions.

(b) Both selenium sulfide 1–2% (Selsun, Exsel) and zinc pyrithione 1–2% (Head and Shoulders, Danex, Zincon) appear to be equally effective (109). Use of these agents should be discontinued if cutaneous irritation, conjunctivitis, or hair loss occurs. A selenium-containing shampoo may stain blond or white hair brown or orange, does not remove oil well, and may discolor nails.

(c) Salicylic acid (1–3%) with sulfur (4%) combinations (Sebulex, Ionil, Vanseb) are effective but less so than those preparations containing selenium or zinc pyrithione.

(d) Tar shampoos 1–4% (Sebutone, Zetar, Ionil T) have activity and make flaking less visible, but do not lower cell counts. Tar shampoos have an antipruritic effect and may be useful if there is pruritus associated with the dandruff.

Seborrheic Dermatitis

(a) Follow general shampooing instructions or, if not on the scalp, wash the area frequently.

(b) Use a hydrocortisone 1% preparation applied two to three times daily. The efficacy of 0.5% hydrocortisone is unknown at present but may be recommended with the caution that if the condition has not improved within seven days the patient should consult a physician.

(c) If hard to remove, thick crusts or scales are present, a warm mineral oil compress may be applied for 30 minutes prior to shampooing/washing. If this is ineffective, a Keralyt gel (3% salicylic acid, 3% sulfur) is quite effective when applied overnight with or without occlusion.

(d) If seborrheic blepharitis is present, a steroid/antibiotic/phenylephrine suspension (Blephamide, Cetapred) should be applied two or three times daily.

ACNE

Pathogenesis. The basic lesion of acne involves an inflammation of the pilosebaceous follicles of the skin. Only certain areas of the body are affected; the size of the sebaceous gland of most hair follicles is roughly proportional to the size of the hair (110), but areas of the body where acne occurs contain large sebaceous glands with small or rudimentary hairs. This combination is particularly favorable for the development of acne, which explains why it occurs on the face, neck, or upper trunk, and not on the scalp or other hairy parts of the body.

At puberty, under the influence of androgens, and perhaps other substances, the sebaceous glands increase in size and activity. In response, the follicular walls hypertrophy. When this in-

Table 7.
DIAGNOSTIC FEATURES OF DANDRUFF, SEBORRHEIC DERMATITIS, AND PSORIASIS

	Dandruff	Seborrheic Dermatitis	Psoriasis
Location	Scalp	Scalp, eyebrows, mustache, beard, groin, gluteal crease, ears, umbilicus	Scalp, elbows, knees, genitalia, upper gluteal fold
Characteristics	Does not fluctuate stable condition	Worsened by stress, environment	Influenced by stress, mechanical irritation
Appearance	White flakes	White flakes, mild erythema, may become thick and turn yellow and greasy	Red erythematous plaques with loosely adherent sliver scales. Early psoriasis may look like dandruff or seborrheic dermatitis
Treatment	Shampoo	Shampoo, corticosteroids	See question on psoriasis

crease in keratinization occurs, the flow of sebum to the outside skin becomes mechanically blocked (110,111). The pilosebaceous follicle starts to dilate and becomes filled with entrapped sebum and cellular debris. At this point the lesion is known as a comedo or whitehead. A blackhead occurs when the comedonal mass protrudes from the follicle, giving it a dark appearance.

When the comedo forms, bacteria which are normally present on the skin and in the follicular canal are especially favored in this nutrient-rich environment of the plugged pilosebaceous gland. Organisms most often found in the pilosebaceous follicle are the acid-producing bacteria *Corynebacterium acnes, Staphylococcus albus* and the fungus *Pityrosporon ovale* (111,112). Of these, *Corynebacterium acnes* and to a lesser extent, the other bacteria produce lipolytic enzymes (113). These enzymes are capable of converting the sebum, which is normally composed of esterified long-chain fatty acids, into short-chain free fatty acids. It has been shown that free fatty acids, especially those of 8 to 14 carbon chains, have the ability to provoke a nonspecific type of inflammatory response which results in the development of a "pimple" which may progress to a pustule, nodule, cyst, or abscess.

The role of diet as a means of acne therapy has been exaggerated, and opinions on the usefulness of diet vary greatly from practitioner to practitioner. There is no evidence to support the value of eliminating various dietary items in helping the course of the disease (7,68,111,114). Some patients, though, insist they have flareups from certain foods. In such cases, those foods should be avoided.

23. *General Recommendations.* **B.B. is a 16-year-old male who comes to the pharmacy requesting help for his acne. B.B. has many closed comedones (whiteheads) and some blackheads on his chin, cheeks, and forehead. He admits to no other areas that are affected at this time. B.B. washes his face once daily. What are the general goals of therapy for B.B.?**

The goal of acne therapy is to interrupt the degeneration of the pilosebaceous follicles so that cysts will not form and scarring will not occur. Treatment is directed toward keeping the skin clean and to the peeling of skin so that the follicular orifices are kept open and draining prop-

erly. The following is a list of general recommendations that should be given to the patient prior to starting therapy (115–116):

(a) Wash the face twice to three times daily with soap, water, and a washcloth. The goal of washing is to keep the face dry, slightly erythematous, and free of sebum. Medicated soaps or abrasive scrubs offer no advantage over ordinary soap, water, and a washcloth.

(b) Heat and humidity generally make acne worse. Sunlight is generally beneficial if exposure is not excessive.

(c) Oily or greasy cosmetics should be avoided. The use of cosmetics is not recommended, but if the patient insists, suggest a water-base cosmetic rather than an oil-base one.

(d) Shampoo frequently—many patients with acne also have dandruff.

(e) Mechanical irritation (eg, rubbing, picking, cradling of the chin, and athletic straps) should be avoided since it tends to make the acne worse.

(f) Stress or emotional upsets may make the acne worse.

24. *Benzoyl Peroxide.* **B.B. has used a topical acne product containing salicylic acid, sulfur, and resorcinol for the past six weeks, but he feels that it has not been very effective. In addition to the general recommendations described above, what should be recommended at this point?**

Benzoyl peroxide is now considered to be the most efficacious OTC product for the treatment of acne. It has antibacterial effects due to hydrogen peroxide liberated on the skin, and its use results in an 84% decrease in aerobic and 98% decrease in anaerobic bacteria on the skin after 14 days of treatment. Additionally, benzoyl peroxide reduces free fatty acids on the skin by 50 to 60% after 14 days of use (11). Eighty percent of patients treated with benzoyl peroxide will improve dramatically (117). Benzoyl peroxide is most useful for mild acne which consists primarily of comedones and very few pustules. Instructions for its use are as follows:

(a) Start treatment with a 5% preparation, applying after washing at bedtime. Gradually increase the application to twice daily treatment; the endpoint is mild dryness, slight erythema, and a decrease in the number and size of lesions. Have patient count the number and type of lesions on affected areas to get a rough idea of effectiveness. The patient should improve in three to four weeks. If not, try a 10% preparation and/or increase the frequency of application until the treatment end point has been reached.

(b) Creams and lotions are equally potent, and gels are much more potent. Lotions should be shaken well and all preparations should be stored in a cool place. Application may normally cause a feeling of warmth or slight stinging.

(c) Beneficial results may be delayed for two weeks.

(d) Avoid application to eyes, eyelids, lips, or mucuous membranes, because these areas are more susceptible to the irritant effects. Some tolerance to the irritant effects may be seen with repeated use. Benzoyl peroxide may lighten hair or clothing.

(e) Other medicated acne preparations should not be used unless directed by a dermatologist.

Sulfur, salicylic acid, and resorcinol are less efficacious than benzoyl peroxide and should be used only by patients who are allergic to benzoyl peroxide or by those in whom an intolerable level of irritation is produced.

25. Tretinoin. B.B. purchased a benzoyl peroxide 5% preparation. Six months later he returned and stated that initially the benzoyl peroxide worked very well, but now his acne has gotten worse. He now has many comedones and pustules, and some of the lesions looked inflamed. He also states he has applied the benzoyl peroxide up to four times a day and his acne has worsened. What type of therapy should be recommended at this point?

B.B. meets the criteria for moderate acne and should receive treatment with tretinoin or topical antibiotics at this time. Since he seems to have fairly tough skin (has been able to tolerate up to four daily applications of benzoyl peroxide) tretinoin therapy would be appropriate at this time.

The exact mechanism of action of tretinoin remains unknown at this time. Tretinoin increases epidermal cell turnover and decreases the cohesiveness of cells in the horny layer which inhibits the formation of comedones and helps expel and loosen existing comedones (11,121–124). There is considerable variation among patients in tolerance to tretinoin; some patients may be able to tolerate multiple daily applications and many other patients are not able to use it at all. The instructions for use are as follows:

(a) Start with 0.1% cream or solution (fair skinned people—0.05% cream or gel). Apply once a day as a light application at bedtime. Areas around the eyes and mouth should be avoided, because they are particularly sensitive to the effects of tretinoin.

(b) Since washing appears to increase its potency, tretinoin should be applied to dry skin at least 15 minutes after washing.

(c) No other acne preparations should be used unless initiated by the patient's physician, and the face should be washed no more than twice daily with a gentle soap.

(d) Increased effects from sunlight may be noted, and proper precautions should be taken. There is experimental evidence that animals treated with tretinoin and exposed to ultraviolet light had a higher incidence of skin cancers.

(e) The patient should expect redness and peeling within one week; this may persist for three to four weeks. A flare in the acne often occurs in the first four to six weeks of therapy. This can be explained as a surfacing of the lesions beneath the skin, an expected part of therapy. To fully evaluate tretinoin therapy, three months of continuous therapy are required.

(f) The patient should expect erythema, peeling, and a mild flush with mild dryness as a treatment endpoint. Because of variations in skin sensitivity, some patients may require multiple daily applications while others may require application as infrequently as every three days. This treatment endpoint may be reached by adjusting the frequency of applications, the strength of the preparation, or the vehicle.

26. B.B. received a prescription for tretinoin 0.1% solution, sig: apply h.s. While having his prescription filled, he asks what he should do with the large amount of benzoyl peroxide he has recently purchased. He can't remember if his physician told him not to use it.

At this point B.B. should probably use only the tretinoin (unless specifically told to use both by his physician). He should not throw the benzoyl peroxide away, because if the tretinoin proves to be ineffective, B.B.'s physician may wish to use combination tretinoin-benzoyl peroxide therapy. The rationale for this type of therapy is that the benzoyl peroxide lowers bacteria counts and free fatty acid levels while the tretinoin makes the skin more permeable and helps prevent and remove comedones. It is claimed that combination therapy is less irritating than tretinoin alone and may alleviate the need for systemic antibiotics in most patients with moderate to severe acne. However, tretinoin and benzoyl peroxide are chemically incompatible due to the oxidization potential of the benzoyl peroxide. When tretinoin is applied at bedtime and benzoyl peroxide in the morning, the therapeutic effect is greater than that achieved by either agent used alone (115,116, 125).

27. Two days after B.B. received his tretinoin 0.1% solution, he calls to report that he experiences extreme pain 15–20 minutes after application; this pain persists for about two hours. What is happening?

Most likely B.B. is applying the tretinoin to hydrated skin where there is a marked increase in its irritancy. He should be cautioned to wait at least 15 minutes after washing his face before applying the tretinoin. If he is currently waiting 15 minutes, he may wish to wait 30–45 minutes after washing his face before applying the tretinoin. If these measures prove to be unsuccessful, a reduction in the strength and/or a change to the cream or gel will reduce the likelihood of irritation.

28. Topical Antibiotics. A.K. is a 15-year-old female who has comedones and pustules over most of her face. There is some redness and irritation. She states that she has tried benzoyl peroxide products and found them too irritating and not that effective. What should be recommended at this time?

Since A.K. appears to have a moderately severe form of acne and she cannot use a benzoyl peroxide preparation, the recommendation of tretinoin would be inappropriate, because this product is usually more irritating than benzoyl peroxide. At this point, a trial of topical antibiotics would be appropriate.

See Table 8 for a comparison of topical antibiotics. Topical clindamycin has received the most study and use. Topical erythromycin and tetracycline are considered less effective than topical clindamycin and have very few indications (eg, allergy to clindamycin) (118,119). In one study, topical clindamycin was found to be equal in effectiveness to oral tetracycline 500 mg bid for inflammatory acne (120). However, most authorities consider topical antibiotics less efficacious than systemic antibiotics. While toxicity is low, one case of pseudomembranous colitis from topical application of clindamycin has been reported (119). The instructions for use are as follows:

(a) Apply twice daily with finger tips after cleansing the face. Most commercially available preparations have built-in applicators.

(b) The onset of beneficial effects is often delayed for three or four weeks.

(c) Watch for appearance of allergic sensitization or irritation.

(d) Other topical acne preparations should not be used unless directed by a dermatologist.

Table 8.
TOPICAL ANTIBIOTICS FOR ACNE

Drug	Strength	Commercially Available	Extemporaneous Preparation	Comments
Clindamycin (Cleocin T)	1–3%	yes	May use capsule (HCl) or ampule (phosphate). Vehicle: 80% isopropyl, 10% propylene glycol, 10% water. Stable 6 months. May put in Neutrogena's Vehicle N or C Solve.	May have residue from extemporaneously prepared preparation.
Tetracycline (Topicycline)	.22%	yes	Rarely done.	Will stain skin yellow. Will fluoresce under black light.
Erythromycin (Staticin)	2%	yes	Erythromycin base or sterate. Put in Neutrogena's Vehicle N or C Solve. Stable 3 months.	May cause burning or irritation.

29. Systemic Therapy. A.K. received a prescription for Cleocin T 1%, sig: apply twice daily. Three months later she returns with much worsened acne. There are more comedones and pustules, some abscesses, marked inflammation, and several apparent acne scars. How should A.K. be treated at this time?

A.K. has fairly severe acne and would be a candidate for systemic therapy. Both antibiotics and estrogens are used for the systemic treatment of acne.

Antibiotics. Systemically administered antibiotics suppress the growth of cutaneous flora and cause a decrease in free fatty acids within the pilosebaceous follicles. The antibiotics used in treating acne do not directly pass through the epithelial lining of the pilosebaceous follicle. Instead, they are sequestered in cells surrounding the sebaceous follicle and are then shed into the sebum. Sequestration explains why low doses of antibiotics are effective for maintenance therapy and also accounts for the lag time (typically two to six weeks) observed between administration of various drugs and onset of therapeutic effects (127).

It appears that tetracycline, erythromycin, clindamycin, minocycline, and trimethoprim-sulfamethoxazole are all equal in their effectiveness against acne (128,129). Tetracycline is considered the drug of first choice and is relatively safe when used in doses less than one gram per day (129). Erythromycin is probably the drug of second choice. Clindamycin, while quite effective, should not be used systemically to treat acne because of its ability to cause a potentially fatal pseudomembranous colitis. Minocycline, which is quite effective, is generally reserved for patients who do not respond to tetracycline or erythromycin because of its cost and its ability to cause gastrointestinal side effects and dizziness. Because of limited study, the place of trimethoprim-sulfamethoxazole in the treatment of acne remains unclear. The principles of use are as follows:

(a) Use appropriate topical therapy in addition to systemic antibiotics.

(b) Use full doses of tetracycline or erythromycin in divided dosages (one gram per day). Some improvement, noted by a decrease in new lesions, should be seen in two to six weeks. Eight weeks of therapy is required to fully evaluate antibiotic therapy.

(c) Once remission is achieved, the dose of the antibiotic should be reduced to the lowest effective dose. This is usually 250 mg to 500 mg per day.

Estrogen Therapy. High-dose estrogen birth control pills are generally effective in the treatment of acne (130–132). The estrogen in the birth control pills counteracts the effects of endogenous androgens and causes a decrease in sebaceous gland size and sebum production (132,133). Limitations to the use of birth control pills for acne are the age of the patient, potential complications, and the one to four month lag time seen when these agents are used (134). As one might expect, birth control pills with a high estrogen component (such as Enovid E or Ovulen) are more effective than those with a low estrogenic component. Unless the acne is quite severe and other measures fail, the risk is generally not worth the benefit. A.K.'s age would make estrogen therapy inappropriate. Also, acne may get worse after discontinuing birth control pills and may persist in severe form for as long as one year.

DRUG ERUPTIONS

30. D.Z. is a 42-year-old male who is currently taking penicillin V 250 mg qid, diazepam 5 mg tid prn, and Maalox 30 ml prn. He now complains of a red maculopapular rash that has recently appeared on his arms and chest. He has taken the penicillin V for eight days. Comment on the above situation.

Clinically recognizable adverse drug reactions are manifested more often on the skin than any other organ or organ system (135). It has been estimated that between 1% and 5% of hospitalized patients develop a drug eruption (15,126, 136,137). Outpatient statistics are much more difficult to obtain but probably are in the same range. There is no correlation of age, diagnosis, or severity of illness with the likelihood of developing a drug eruption (7). Women appear to be twice as likely to develop a drug eruption as men.

Penicillins are the most frequently implicated class of drugs causing eruptions. Drugs which are frequent offenders and the percentage of people given the drug who actually develop an eruption are: trimethoprim/sulfamethoxazole (5.9%), ampicillin (5.2%), semisynthetic penicillins (carbenicillin, cloxacillin, dicloxacillin, methicillin, nafcillin, oxacillin) (3.6%), corticotropin (2.8%), erythromycin (2.3%), sulfisoxazole (1.7%), gentamicin (1.6%), penicillin G (1.6%), practolol (1.6%), cephalosporins (1.3%), quinidine (1.2%), nitrofurantoin (0.91%), heparin (0.77%), trimethobenzamide (0.66%), barbiturates (0.5%), indomethacin (0.44%), chlordiazepoxide (0.42%), diazepam (0.38%), propoxyphene (0.34%), isoniazid (0.3%), guaifenesin (0.29%), chlorothiazide (0.28%), furosemide (0.26%), phenytoin (0.11%), flurazepam (0.05%) (126).

The most common type of eruption encountered in clinical practice, and probably the one most often overlooked, is the exanthematic eruption. This type of reaction comprises both morbilliform (measles-like) and scarlatiniform (scarlet fever-like) eruptions (7). Since drug eruptions often mimic other types of dermatitis, it is necessary to have a good understanding of the mimicked disease state to make the proper diagnosis. Table 9 lists drugs commonly associated with drug eruptions.

Treatment. Most drug eruptions occur within one week after starting therapy. The exception to this is the penicillins, which can have a more prolonged onset of up to several weeks. Generally, all that is needed to treat a drug eruption is to withdraw the offending agent. The lesions should clear completely within 7 to 14 days. Treatment is primarily supportive (see Introduction and Topical Steroids as outlined previously in sections of this chapter), and if the reaction is severe, a one to two week course of prednisone 40–60 mg/day will control symptoms within 48 hours (11).

ATHLETE'S FOOT

Athlete's foot is the most common type of fungal infection. It has been estimated that 30 to 70% of the population will at some time during their adolescent or adult lives have a fungal infection of the feet. More than 80% of patients who acquire a fungal infection of the feet will develop a protective cell-mediated immunity, and in 50% of these patients, circulating antibodies can be demonstrated (7,11,15). Chronic infections occur in 20% of those infected and are probably related to the fact that these patients have a less than adequate cell-mediated immune response.

The dermatophytes *Trichophyton rubrum* and *Trichophyton mentagrophytes* are responsible for most cases of athlete's foot. Dermatophyte fungi live in the superficial layers of the epidermis, toe-

nails, and in the hair. In order for these fungi to grow, keratin must be present; there are serum inhibitory factors which generally protect living tissues against deep penetration. Individual host factors are probably the most important determinants of susceptibility to dermatophyte infections. Other contributing factors are serious systemic diseases, hot and humid climate, tight fitting shoes, poor nutrition, and poor hygiene. There must also be trauma to the skin before an infection can occur. Despite the widely held opinion that transmission of the infection occurs between individuals, this has not been shown to be a major causative factor (15). The fungi may live for more than five months in contaminated shoes, socks, flooring, or clothes.

Preventative Measures

(a) Avoid public showers or wear sandals while showering.

(b) Keep feet clean and dry. Dry carefully between toes; dust with powder.

(c) Change shoes and socks frequently. Absorbent cotton socks are preferred.

(d) Shoes with good ventilation such as sandals are probably best. Avoid plastic shoes.

(e) If there are extensive callouses on the feet, a keratolylic should be used in conjunction with the antifungal agent (applied separately).

(f) Rotate shoe wear so shoes have an opportunity to dry out.

(g) Clothing and towels should be changed frequently and be well laundered in hot water.

31. *Treatment.* B.T. is a 16-year-old male who asks the pharmacist to recommend something for his itching, burning, and scaling feet. One foot has only scaly lesions around the toes, and the other foot has scaling and some weeping areas around the toes. He plays basketball and thinks he has his first case of athlete's foot. What products would be appropriate for B.T.?

Since this is the first infection for B.T., a product containing either undecylenic acid or tolnaftate should be employed. Since tolnaftate is fungicidal (vs fungistatic for undecylenic acid) and is more effective, it is generally preferred. Additionally, tolnaftate is less irritating than undecylenic acid. The cream preparations of either tolnaftate or undecylenic acid cream should be applied two to three times per day. In most cases,

Table 9.
DRUGS ASSOCIATED DRUG ERUPTIONS (150–162,7,11,15,135)

Drug	Epidermal necrolysis	Exfoliative dermatitis	Stevens–Johnson Sn.	Fixed drug	Urticarial	Photosensitive	Acneiform	Alopecia	Purpura	Maculopapular	Bullous	Erythema nodosum	Erythema multiforme	Eczematous
Allopurinol	x				o			o	o	x				
Anticoagulants			o	o				x						
Antimetabolites								x		x				o
Barbiturates	x	x	x	x	o	o	o		o	o		x	x	
Cephalorporins					o					x				x
Chlordiazepoxide				o	o	o				x				
Codeine					o	x							x	o
Corticosteroids							x		o					
Diazepam					o					x				
Erythromycin					o					x				
Gentamicin										x				x
Griseofulvin					o	o	x			o			x	
Gold		o			o	o		o	x	x			o	o
Indomethacin					o			o	o	x				
Iodides/Bromides					o		x			o	x	x		
Isoniazid		o			x		x			x				
Lithium					o		x	o		x				
Nitrofurantoin		o			x					x				o
Oral Contraceptives				x	o	x	x	o		o		x		
Penicillin	x	o	o	o	x				o	x	o	x	x	x
Phenophthalein	o			x	o					o	o			
Phenothiazines	o	o			o		x			o			x	
Phenylbutazone	x	o	x	x	o			o	x	x	o		o	
Phenytoin	x	x	x	o	o		o	o		o			x	
Practolol		o								x				x
Quinidine				o		o			x	x			o	
Salicylates				x	o				o	x		x		
Sulfonamides	x		o	x	x	x			o	x	x	x	x	
Sulfonylureas	x	o	x		o	x				o	o		o	
Tetracycline	x			x	x					x			x	
Thiazides					o	x			o	o			x	
Trimethoprim/Sulfamethoxazole	x	o			o					x	o			

More Frequently Reported = x   Reported = o

the lesions should clear in one to two weeks; treatment should continue for one to two weeks after the lesions clear completely. Some improvement should occur within five days; up to six weeks of treatment may be required in some cases. Table 10 summarizes the various products that show efficacy in treating athlete's foot (7,11,15,163–167).

B.T. has some weeping lesions on one foot. This foot should be treated with wet dressings to dry up the weeping areas before the topical medication is applied. (See the section on Wet Dressings in the beginning of this chapter.)

32. *Treatment Failure.* Two months later B.T. returns and states that his athletes foot seemed to have cleared up after six weeks of treatment with tolnaftate but now it has come back. He has the same symptoms as before, but now three toenails on his left foot have become very thick and brittle and look like they are infected. What are the possible explanations for B.T.'s apparent failure at this point? How should B.T.'s fungal infection be managed at this point?

The most common reasons for treatment failures are:

(a) Patient noncompliance with application of topical medication or failure to follow the preventative measures outlined above.

(b) Patients with thick hyperkeratotic involvement of the affected areas will harbor the fungi, because the topical medication will not penetrate into hyperkeratotic areas and eradicate the infection. If hyperkeratotic areas are present, they should be treated with a salicylic acid keratolytic (eg, Whitfield's ointment) applied twice or three times daily or with Keralyt gel applied under occlusion overnight or for two to three hours in the evening until the hyperkeratotic areas are dissolved. In either case, topical antifungal therapy should be applied at a different time.

(c) Topical therapy is ineffective for fungal infection of the nails (apparently a problem with this patient). When the nails are affected, it is extremely difficult to cure the infection. Nail involvement may be treated with application of 10% glutaraldehyde solution, buffered to a pH of 7.5, twice daily for one to four months. Fresh solutions must be prepared every two weeks. However, removal of the infected nail with concomitant systemic griseofulvin therapy (see Question 34) may be the most effective way to deal with recurrent nail infection. In either case, concomitant topical therapy should be employed.

(d) The patient may have an inadequate cell-mediated immunologic response. Patients with this problem generally require chronic topical therapy to suppress the infection and in many cases will require prolonged courses of systemic griseofulvin. (See Question 34.)

Table 10.

ANTIFUNGAL AGENTS (15,163–170)

	Effectiveness				
	Overall Fungal Effectiveness	Tinea Infections (Not Capitis)	Tinea Capitis	Tinea Versicolor	Candida
Miconazole 2%	75%–95%	+ + +	N O T E F F E C T I V E	+ + +	+ + +
Clotrimazole 1%	30%–88%	+ + +		+ + +	+ + +
Haloprogen 1%	60%–80%	+ +		+ + +	+ +
Tolnaftate 1%	60%–70%	+ +		+ +	– – –
Undecylenic Acid	27%–68%	+		– – –	– – –
Whitfield's Ointment (Salicylic Acid 3%) (Benzoic Acid 6%)	57%	+		– – –	– – –
Griseofulvin	up to 100%	+ + +	+ + +	– – –	– – –
Selenium		– – –	– – –	+ +	– – –

33. *Haloprogin, Clotrimazole, Miconazole.* **B.T. has heard that there are some newer, more potent topical antifungal agents. How do they compare to tolnaftate?**

Haloprogin is a very effective topical agent in the treatment of dermatophytoses (athlete's foot). In double-blind studies, haloprogin and tolnaftate were equally effective and significantly better than placebo (168). Clotrimazole and miconazole are considered by many to be more effective than tolnaftate or haloprogin, although this is difficult to document. Clotrimazole, miconazole, or haloprogin should be used with mixed fungal infections or when the causative agent is unknown, because these agents are effective against both dermatophytes and candida; tolnaftate is effective only against dermatophytes. In addition, these agents are also effective in the treatment of *T. cruris,* which often causes jock itch (169,170). In *T. versicolor* infections, these agents are more effective and have better patient acceptability than the selenium sulfide preparations which have been used in the past (170).

34. *Griseofulvin.* **P.Z. is a 25-year-old male who has suffered from athlete's foot for nine years. He has used every topical preparation available, both OTC and prescription. All his toenails are infected. A decision is made to treat him with griseofulvin. How does the drug work? What other fungal infections can be treated with griseofulvin, and how should treatment be employed?**

Griseofulvin is incorporated into the stratum corneum where it prevents further fungal invasion and reproduction. The drug is most useful in *Tinea* (ringworm) infections. Prior to the introduction of this drug, scalp ringworm could be treated only with x-ray. Although griseofulvin is effective in uncomplicated cases of scalp ringworm, it is only moderately effective against body ringworm and is least effective in ringworm affecting the hands, feet, or nails. In the latter case, prolonged treatment is required. Treatment is not justified unless there is severe discomfort or there is significant cosmetic disfigurement. A microsized griseofulvin preparation should be employed to aid absorption. The drug should be taken with milk or fatty foods, because absorption is increased. The patient should be aware that the effects of alcohol may be potentiated by griseofulvin.

Principles of Use

(a) For uncomplicated (no nail involvement) fungal infections where topical therapy was ineffective or where the infection is so large that topical therapy is not practical, one gram per day in divided doses should be given for three to four weeks.

(b) For *Tinea capitis* infections, the same dosage of griseofulvin is employed, but up to six weeks of treatment may be required. Therapy should be continued for at least two weeks after all lesions disappear.

(c) For nail involvement, treatment should begin with 1.5 to 2 gm/day in divided doses for the first month of therapy and then the dosage should be gradually reduced to 1 gm/day over the next several months. The duration of therapy for fingernails should be 5 or 6 months, for toenails 6 to 18 months. Often removal of the toenail(s) is necessary. The chances of total clearing of fungal infections where toenails are involved is estimated to be around 15%.

(d) In patients with chronic, recurrent infections the minimal effective suppressive dose of griseofulvin should be employed. Topical therapy should also be utilized. Generally, patients who are to receive chronic suppressive therapy with griseofulvin should have a documented failure with topical agents.

35. After one day of therapy with microsized griseofulvin, P.Z. developed a vesicular eruption on both hands and a headache. What is the most likely explanation for this reaction?

Most likely P.Z. is experiencing a dermatophytid or "Id" reaction which is an allergic reaction to products which are released from dying microorganisms. The lesions should be treated with wet soaks if they are weeping; topical corticosteroids are often beneficial for dry lesions. A similar type of reaction is seen in patients with syphillis, where nearly 50% of patients will experience malaise, fever, and an exacerbation of existing skin lesions within 8 to 24 hours after treatment with penicillin. This reaction is known as the Jarisch-Herxheimer reaction. The headache (a frequent side effect from griseofulvin) P.Z. is experiencing may be minimized by having P.Z. take the drug with food and/or split the daily dose into smaller, more frequent doses. For reasons that are unknown, the headache from griseofulvin abates on its own with continued therapy. If severe, the

headache can be treated with aspirin or acetaminophen.

CONTACT DERMATITIS:
POISON IVY, OAK, AND SUMAC

Poison Ivy (Rhus) dermatitis is the major cause
of allergic contact dermatitis in the United States,
exceeding all other causes combined. It is estimated that 50 to 95% of the population is sensitive to the plant to some degree. The severity of
the condition varies from mild discomfort to an
extremely painful and debilitating condition. Rhus
dermatitis is caused by sensitization to an allergic substance in the leaves, stems, and roots
of poison ivy, poison oak, and poison sumac plants.
All three plants contain the same sensitizing
oleoresin, urushiol oil, which contains pentade-
cacatechol, the actual sensitizing agent. Therefore the dermatitis caused by the three different
plants is identical.

Direct contact with the plant is not necessary
for the rash to occur. Highly susceptible individuals may develop severe dermatitis merely from
exposure to Rhus oleoresin carried by pollen or
by smoke from burning leaves. The oleoresin may
remain active for months on clothing, shoes, tools,
and sporting equipment. Once the toxic substance comes in contact with the skin, it can be
spread by the hands to other areas of the body
(genitals, eyes, etc.) or to people who may come
into close contact with the exposed person. Although washing with soap and water will not prevent the dermatitis unless done within fifteen
minutes of exposure, it will prevent spread of the
oleoresin to other parts of the body (7,15,171–
175).

Rhus dermatitis can be contracted throughout
the year, including the winter, when it results
from exposure to the roots of the plant. The virulence of the leaf sap varies little during the fo-
liage period. The incidence of poison ivy is higher
during the spring because the leaves are tender
and bruise easily and the call to the outdoors is
stronger.

After an initial incubation period of 5 to 21
days, a patient would be expected to react to the
exposure to the oleoresin in 12 to 48 hours. A mild
exposure to these plants in a sensitized person
results in an appearance of the typical erythematous, vesicular, and sometimes oozing rash in
two to three days with complete clearing in one
to two weeks. With a large area of exposure, the
lesions will appear within 6 to 12 hours and may
appear blistered, eroded, and in some cases ulcers
may appear. Healing will occur more slowly, often
requiring two to three weeks for complete resolution of symptoms. Factors which contribute to
the development of poison ivy/oak/sumac are the
concentration of the oleoresin exposed to the skin,
area of exposure, duration of exposure, site of exposure, genetic factors, and immune tolerance. It
is of primary importance to determine what areas
of the body are affected. If the eyes, genital areas,
mouth, respiratory tract, or more than 15% of the
body is affected, the patient should receive a course
of systemic corticosteroids.

Since different sites of the body differ in their
sensitivity to the oleoresin and because patients
will spread the Rhus oleoresin to different parts
of their body over a period of time, lesions will
often erupt over a period of several days. A common misconception many people have is that the
fluid from the Rhus-induced vesicles will spread
the disease to unaffected areas.

**36. K.P. is a 27-year-old female who has
recently returned from an outing in the woods.
She now has several linear, vesicular eruptions on one arm and hand. She believes she
has poison oak and requests recommendations for therapy. What should be recommended at this point? What should be recommended if the condition becomes more
severe?**

Weeping lesions should be treated with wet
dressings as outlined in the beginning of this
chapter. Lesions which are not wet or weeping
should be treated with calamine lotion applied
twice to four times daily. Alternatively, a topical
0.5% hydrocortisone preparation could be used.
More effective treatment would require prescription of a potent topical corticosteroid preparation.
If her poison oak becomes much more severe, additional treatment with prednisone 60 mg per day
for at least two or three weeks will be required;
such therapy should be withdrawn slowly (over
one to two weeks) to prevent a flare or rebound
reaction (171–175).

**37. Z.T. is a 19-year-old male who has just
returned from a fishing trip and now has an
erythematous, linear, dry eruption on his left
arm and a generalized eruption on his hands
and face. He states he had been in areas of**

dense poison ivy and that they may have burned some of this in their nightly campfire. Z.T. has washed himself and his clothes thoroughly. How should he be treated?

The fact that Z.T. has a rash on his face and it is not linear (as one would expect if he had just contacted the plant) suggests that he may have contacted the smoke of a burning poison ivy plant. This can be quite serious since the oleoresin can be carried in smoke and if inhaled can cause severe respiratory problems. Z.T. should be observed for signs of respiratory difficulties and should be referred to a physician for a course of systemic corticosteroids.

38. Z.T. was seen by his physician who prescribed prednisone (80 mg per day for 14 days, then decrease the dose by 5 mg per day each day thereafter) and calamine lotion (tid to affected areas). After 12 days Z.T. calls the pharmacy to say that the lesions seem to be getting worse. The lesions cleared after 8 days of treatment and he began rapidly tapering the prednisone at that time. Why is he experiencing a relapse?

Two weeks is the absolute minimum systemic corticosteroid therapy that would be required to treat severe cases of poison ivy/oak/sumac. The oleoresin remains fixed in the skin, and if the systemic corticosteroid is withdrawn too soon the lesions will return. This is probably the most common reason for treatment failure with systemic corticosteroids.

39. Z.T.'s corticosteroid therapy was reinstated, and after several weeks most of the lesions had disappeared and the prednisone therapy had been completed. However, he continued to have a rash on his hands. Upon further questioning, it became apparent that he was continuing to apply Caladryl lotion, which he had substituted for calamine lotion, to his hands. What is a likely cause of this persistent rash?

Caladryl contains diphenhydramine in addition to the usual constituents of calamine lotion, and topical application of this and other antihistamines may cause an allergic contact sensitivity reaction. He should stop using this product to see if this will cause the rash to clear. A list of common contact sensitizers is found in Table 11. The treatment for sensitivity reactions is basically the same as that outlined for poison oak/ivy/sumac.

Table 11.

FREQUENT CONTACT SENSITIZERS (172–174)

Substance	Found in
Ammonia	Soaps, Chemicals, Hairdyes
Balsam of Peru	Cosmetics
Benzyl Alcohol	Medications, Cosmetics
Caine Anesthetics	Medications
Carba	Rubber
Chromium	Jewelry
Epoxy Resin	Glue
Ethylenediamine	Stabilizer in many topical products
Formaldehyde	Shoes, Clothing, Soaps, Insulation
Mercaptobenzothiazol	Rubber
Napthyl	Rubber
Neomycin	Topical Medications
Nickel Sulfate	Jewelry, Fasteners
Parabens	Preservative in many topical products
Paraphenylenediamine	Hair dyes, Leather
Potassium Dichromate	Shoes, Leather
Thiomersal	Preservatives, contact lens products
Thiram	Rubber Products
Turpentine	Pain Products
Wool Alcohols	Lanolin containing products, Clothes

SCABIES/PEDICULOSIS

Scabies. Scabies is caused by the mite *Sarcoptes scabiei*. The 0.3 mm by 0.4 mm female mite, after being fertilized, burrows into the stratum corneum where she can lay up to 40 eggs. The mite can travel up to 5 mm per day and can live for one to two months. The burrows appear as irregular grayish-black lines which may be "s" shaped and generally have a papule at one end (indicating where the mite is). The most common sites for scabies are interdigital spaces, elbows, wrists, feet, buttocks, axillary folds, penis, and nipples in females. The severe pruritus, which occurs predominantly at bedtime, is generally not apparent for two to four weeks after infestation and probably represents a hypersensitivity reaction to the organism, eggs, and the feces of the mite that is deposited in the burrows. In subsequent infestations the pruritus may occur much earlier. Most infested adults harbor 10 to 12 mites which are capable of reproducing themselves in about three weeks. Transmission of scabies most frequently occurs by direct person to person contact but can be transmitted via infested clothing, linens, or towels. The female mite can survive away from the host for only two to three days.

Pediculosis. Pediculosis, or infestation with lice, is caused by the 1 to 4 mm-long blood-sucking louse, *Phthirus pubis* (crabs) or *Pediculus humanus*. *P. humanus* causes head and body infestation and can be transmitted through shared clothing, combs, brushes, or bedding. *P. pubis* is generally spread by direct person to person contact and is only rarely transmitted via shared clothing or bedding. Both species of louse are completely dependent on blood for survival and cannot survive away from their host for more than 24 hours. As the lice burrow their way through the skin, they inject their digestive juices and fecal material into the skin which contributes, along with the puncture wound, to the pruritus which the patient experiences. The pruritus caused by lice seems to bother patients more during the day than at night, whereas the pruritus associated with scabies generally bothers the patient more at night. Females, which can lay up to 10 eggs per day, attach their eggs (nits) to hair shafts. They hatch in seven to nine days and become adults in another week. The nits are quite useful to confirm the diagnosis. The adult louse lives about 30 days under ideal conditions. Head lice are mainly seen in children and can become epidemic in isolated communities. Body lice are rarely encountered in this country and the most common type of infestation is with the pubic louse.

Drug Therapy (7,11,15,176–182). Gamma benzene hexachloride (GBH) (Kwell, Lindane, Gamene) is the treatment of choice for pediculosis and scabies. It is available in a shampoo, cream, or lotion form and is generally quite effective. However, there have been cases of scabies that are resistant to GBH. Patients should bathe prior to application of GBH.

Head Lice. One ounce of GBH shampoo should be worked into a lather and left on the scalp for five minutes. The hair should be thoroughly rinsed, and a fine tooth comb used to remove nits. In rare cases a repeat shampoo may be necessary in 24 hours.

Body Lice. See treatment for scabies.

Pubic Lice. One ounce of cream or lotion should be applied to infested and adjacent areas, left in place for 24 hours, and then washed off. Alternatively, GBH shampoo may be used (see Head Lice). Treatment may be repeated in one week if necessary. Eye lash infestations can be treated by application of petrolatum two to three times per day for eight days.

Scabies. GBH cream or lotion should be applied to the entire body from the neck down. All exposed areas must be covered. Approximately 30–60 ml of GBH lotion is required for total body application and it should be left in place for 24 hours before washing it off. Transmission is unlikely after 24 hours. A second application may be employed one week later to destroy any recently hatched larvae or nymphs. Alternative treatment of scabies would include crotamiton applied twice during a 48 hour period, 6–10% precipitated sulfur in a water washable base applied nightly for three nights, or 20 to 25% benzyl benzoate in an alcoholic vehicle applied daily for two to three days.

Pruritus. Treat as previously outlined. Topical corticosteroids may also be used.

Preventive Measures. All close contacts/family members should be treated to avoid reinfestation. All recently worn clothing, bedding, towels, should be laundered in hot water. Ironing with a hot iron is also effective in destroying the lice and scabies. Alternatively, clothing that may be infested can be stored away from the human host for four to five days. Care should be taken not to share personal items. Good personal hygiene should be encouraged. Toilets should be cleaned with hot water and disinfected.

40. T.T. received the following prescription for scabies: GBH lotion 8 oz, sig: Apply as directed. After six days he returns to the pharmacy asking for a refill. He states that he has applied the GBH for five days in a row but still has symptoms. In addition, he asks if the medication could be responsible for the CNS stimulation and headaches he is experiencing. What is the most likely explanation for his complaints?

Even after effective treatment of scabies with GBH, it can take weeks for the pruritus and inflammation (hypersensitivity) to subside. Although it is unlikely that this patient is a treatment failure (more information is needed), failures do occur. Common causes of treatment failure include failure to apply GBH to *all* areas below the neck, re-infection, and scabies which may be resistant to GBH.

Up to 9% of topically applied GBH can be absorbed and may be contributing to this patient's complaints. Although rare, CNS stimulation, convulsions, nausea, vomiting, and headaches have been reported with the use of GBH (181,182).

Since patients tend to apply medication until it is gone, only the minimum amount necessary for one application should be dispensed. Obviously eight ounces was excessive and T.T. should stop using the GBH. Other factors that may enhance absorption are excoriated skin and hot or warm skin. Thus it is recommended that patients allow their skin to cool after bathing and before applying the GBH. There also is some evidence that children may absorb more GBH than adults (181,182).

References

1. Schlagel C et al: The weights of topical preparations required for total and partial body coverage. J Invest Dermatol. 1964; 42:253.

2. Stoughton RB: Bioassay system for formulations for topically applied glucocorticosteroids. Arch Derm. 1972; 106:825.

3. Gip L et al: The rapidity of effect of different types of topical corticosteroids: a double-blind comparison between diproderm ointment 0.05% and calmurihydrocortisone 1%. Curr Ther Res. 1974; 16:300.

4. Kaidbey KH et al: Assay of topical corticosteroids. Arch Derm. 1976; 112:808.

5. Barry BW et al: Comparative bioavailability of proprietary topical corticosteroid preparations: vasoconstrictor assays on thirty creams and gels. Br J Derm. 1974; 91:323.

6. Barry BW et al: Comparative bioavailability and activity of proprietary topical corticosteroid preparations: vasoconstrictor assays on thirty-one ointments. Br J Derm. 1975; 93:563.

7. Fitzpatrick TB et al: *Dermatology in General Medicine*, second edition, McGraw Hill, New York, 1979.

8. Maibach HI: In vivo percutaneous penetration of corticoids in man and unresolved problems in the efficacy. Dermatologia. 1976; 152 (suppl 1):11.

9. Maibach HI et al: Topical corticosteroids: in Azarnoff (editor) *Steroid Therapy*, W. B. Saunders, Philadelphia, 1975.

10. Kaidbey K et al: Assay of topical corticosteroids. Arch Derm. 1976; 112:808.

11. Arndt KA: *Manual of Dermatologic Therapies*, second edition, Little, Brown and Co., Boston, 1978.

12. Barry B et al: Comparative bioavailability of proprietary topical corticosteroid preparations; vasoconstrictor assays on thirty creams and gels. Br J Derm. 1974; 91:323.

13. Barry B et al: Comparative bioavailability and activity of proprietary topical corticosteroid preparations; vasoconstrictor assays on thirty-one ointments. Br J Derm. 1975; 93:563.

14. Miller JA et al: Topical corticosteroids—clinical pharmacology and therapeutic use. Drugs. 1980; 19:119.

15. Steward W et al: *Dermatology—Diagnosis and Treatment of Cutaneous Disorders,* Disorders, C.V. Mosby, St. Louis, 1978.

16. Delforno C et al: Corticosteroid effect on epidermal cell size. Br J Derm. 1978; 98:619.

17. Wilson Jones E: Steroid atrophy—a histological appraisal. Dermatologica. 1976; 152 (suppl 1):107.

18. Leyden JJ et al: The case for steroid-antibiotic combinations. Br J Derm. 1977; 91:179.

19. Wachs GW et al: Co-operative double blind trial of antibiotic corticoid combination in impetiginized atopic dermatitis. Br J Derm. 1976; 95:323.

20. Epstein E: Allergy to dermatologic agents. JAMA. 1966; 198:517.

21. Rudner ES et al: Epidemiology of contact dermatitis in North America 1972. Arch Derm. 1972; 108:537.

22. Patrick J et al: Neomycin sensitivity in the normal (nonatopic) individual. Arch Derm. 1970; 102:532.

23. Prystowsky S et al: Allergic contact hypersensitivity to nickel, neomycin, ethylenediamine, and benzocaine. Arch Derm. 1979; 115:959.

24. Kirton V et al: Contact dermatitis from neomycin and framycin. Lancet. 1965; 1:138.

25. Pirila V et al: The pattern of cross sensitivity to neomycin. Dermatol. 1968; 136:321.

26. Epstein S et al: Cross sensitivity to various "mycins." Arch Derm. 1962; 86:101.

27. Pirila V et al: On cross sensitization between neomycin, bacitracin, kanamycin and framycetin. Dermatol. 1960; 121:335.

28. Epstein E et al: Ethylenediamine-allergic contact dermatitis. Arch Derm. 1968; 98:476.

29. Anon: Hypersensitivity skin reactions due to neomycin. Medical Letter. 1967; 9:71.

30. Anon: Nitrofurazone—atopical antimicrobial drug. Medical Letter. 1967; 9:71.

31. Pirila V et al: Twelve years of sensitization to neomycin in Finland. Report of 1760 cases of sensitivity to neomycin and/or bacteracin. Acta Derm Vener. 1967; 47:419.

32. Hassar M et al: Treatment of pruritus. Rational Drug Therapy. 1975; 9:1.

33. FDA: Report on topical analgetics. Federal Register. 1979; 44:234.

34. Anon: Cyproheptadine (Periactin) for allergic and pruritic dermatoses. Medical Letter. 1967; 9:28.

35. Fischer RW: Comparison of antipruritic agents administered orally. A double-blind study. JAMA. 1968; 203:418.

36. Baraf CS: Treatment of pruritus in allergic dermatoses: An evaluation of the relative efficacy of cyproheptadine and hydroxyzine. Curr Ther Res. 1976; 19:32.

37. Rhoades RB et al: Suppression of histamine-induced pruritus by three antihistaminic drugs. J Clin Imm. 1975; 55:180.

38. Barry BW et al: Vasoconstrictor activities and bioavailabilities of seven proprietary corticosteroid creams assessed using non-occluded multiple dosage regimen; clinical implications. Br J Derm. 1977; 97:555.

39. DuVivier A et al: Acute tolerance to effects of topical glucocorticosteroids. Br J Derm. 1976; 94 (suppl. 12):25.

40. Anon: OTC topical hydrocortisone. Medical Letter. 1980; 22:37.

41. Editorial: Zinc sulfate administered orally: wounds reported to heal faster. JAMA. 1966; 196:33.

42. Greaves MW et al: Effects of long-continued ingestion of zinc sulfate in patients with venous leg ulceration. Lancet. 1970; 2:889.

43. Serjeant GR et al: Oral zinc sulfate in sickle cell ulcers. Lancet. 1970; 2:891.

44. Bailey G et al: Toxic epidermal necrolysis. JAMA. 1965; 191:979.

45. Hunt TK et al: Effect of Vitamin A on reversing the inhibitory effect of cortisone on healing of open wounds in animals and man. Ann Surg. 1969; 170:633.

46. Lee KH et al: Mechanism of action of salicylates VIII: Effect of topical application of retinoic acid on wound-healing retardation action of a few anti-inflammatory agents. J Pharm Sci. 1970; 59:1036.

47. Lee KH et al: Mechanism of action of retinyl compounds on wound healing: Structural relationship of retinyl compounds and wound healing retardation action of salicylic acids. J Pharm Sci. 1969; 58:773.

48. Lee KH et al: Studies on the mechanism of action of salicylates VI: Effect of topical application of retinoic acid on wound healing retardation action of salicylic acids. J Pharm Sci. 1969; 58:773.

49. FDA: Report on skin protectants. Federal Register. 1978; 4110:03.

50. Epstein J et al: Ultraviolet light-induced kinin formation in human skin. Arch Derm. 1967; 95:532.

51. Greves M et al: Pharmacologic agents released in ultraviolet inflammation studied by continuous skin perfusion. J Invest Derm. 1970; 54:365.

52. Valtonen E et al: The effect of the erythemal reaction caused by ultraviolet irradiation on mast cell degranulation in the skin. Acta Derm Vener. 1964; 44:269.

53. Logan P et al: Vascular permeability changes in inflammation. I. The role of endogenous permeability factors in ultraviolet injury. Br J Exp Path. 1966; 47:300.

54. Crunkhorn P et al: Interaction between prostaglandins E and F given intradermally in the rat. Br J Pharmacol. 1971; 41:507.

55. Goldyne M et al: Prostaglandins and cutaneous inflammation. J Invest Derm. 1975; 64:377.

56. Lord J et al: The effects of photosensitizers and UV radiation and the biosynthesis and metabolism of prostaglandins. Br J Derm. 1976; 95:397.

57. Kaidbey K et al: The influence of corticosteroids and topical indomethacin on sunburn erythema. J Invest Derm. 1976; 66:153.

58. Morrison W et al: The effects of indomethacin on long wave ultraviolet induced delayed erythema. J Invest Derm. 1977; 68:130.

59. Logan G et al: The inflammatory reaction in ultraviolet injury. Br J Exp Path. 1966; 47:286.

60. Johnson B et al: Lysosomes and the reactions of skin to ultraviolet radiation. J Invest Derm. 1969; 53:85.

61. Pathak M et al: Free radicals in human skin before and after exposure to light. Arch Biochem Biophys. 1961; 123:468.

62. Coleman WP: Unusual cutaneous manifestations of drug hypersensitivity. Med Clin N Am. 1967; 51:1073.

63. Epstein E: Photoallergy. Arch Derm. 1971; 106:741.

64. Anon: Sunscreening agents. Medical Letter. 1979; 21:46.

65. Anon: Topical sunscreening agents. Medical Letter. 1972; 14:27.

66. Faber EM et al: Studies on the nature and management of psoriasis. Calif Med. 1971; 114:1.

67. Sidi E et al: Psoriasis, Charles C. Thomas, Co., Springfield, IL, 1968.

68. Domonkos AN: Andrews' Diseases of the Skin, 6th ed, WB Saunders Co., Philadelphia, 1971.

69. Perry HO et al: The Goeckerman treatment of psoriasis. Arch Derm. 1968; 98:178.

70. Cormaish S: Ingram method of treating psoriasis. Arch Derm. 1965; 92:56.

71. Faber EM et al: A current review of psoriasis. Calif Med. 1968; 108:440.

72. Faber EM et al: Psoriasis—A questionnaire survey of 2,144 patients. Arch Derm. 1968; 98:248.

73. Anon: Methotrexate in the treatment of psoriasis. Medical Letter. 1972; 14:41.

74. Weinstein GD et al: Methotrexate for psoriasis. Arch Derm. 1971; 103:33.

75. Almeyda J et al: Drug reactions, XV Methotrexate, psoriasis, and the liver. Br J Derm. 1971; 85:302.

76. Dahl MD: Methotrexate hepatotoxicity in psoriasis, comparison of different dosage regimens. Br Med J. 1972; 1:654.

77. Sams WM et al: Use of methotrexate in psoriasis. Arch Derm. 1972; 105:383.

78. Griesman FA et al: Methotrexate-associated liver disease in psoriatic patients. Northwest Med. 1972; 71:609.

79. Tobias H et al: Hepatotoxicity of long-term Methotrexate therapy for psoriasis. Arch Int Med. 1973; 132:391.

80. Parrish JA et al: Photochemotherapy of psoriasis with oral methoxsalen and longwave ultraviolet light. N Engl J Med. 1974; 291:1207.

81. Swanbeck G et al: Treatment with psoralens and long-wave ultraviolet light. Acta Dermatovener. 1975; 55:367.

82. Weber G: Combined 8-methoxypsoralen and black light therapy of psoriasis. Br J Derm. 1974; 90:317.

83. Simipathi T et al: Photochemotherapy in the treatment of psoriasis. Br J Derm. 1977; 96:587.

84. Honigsmann H et al: Photochemotherapy for pustular psoriasis. Br J Derm. 1977; 97:119.

85. Weismann K et al: Treatment of resistant psoriasis with oral 8-methoxypsoralen and longwave ultraviolet light (PUVA). Acta Dermatovener. 1977; 57:73.

86. Wasserman G et al: Treatment of psoriasis with orally administered 8-methoxypsoralen and longwave length ultraviolet radiation. Can Med Assoc J. 1978; 118:1379.

87. Schaefer H et al: Simplification of local therapy of psoriasis with 8-methoxypsoralen. Br J Derm. 1976; 94:363.

88. Hanke C et al: Combination therapy for psoriasis. Arch Derm. 1979; 115:1074.

89. Petrozzi J et al: Photochemotherapy of psoriasis (PUVA) without specialized equipment. Arch Derm. 1978; 114:387.

90. Petrozzi J et al: Topical methoxsalen and blacklight in the treatment of psoriasis. Arch Derm. 1977; 113:292.

91. Parrish J et al: Photochemotherapy of psoriasis. Arch Derm. 1977; 113:1529.

92. Briffa D et al: A randomized, controlled clinical trial comparing photochemotherapy with dithranol in the initial treatment of chronic plaque psoriasis. Clin Exper Derm. 1978; 3:339.

93. Wolff K et al: Photochemotherapy for psoriasis with orally administered methoxsalen. Arch Derm. 1976; 112:943.

94. Roenigk H et al: Photochemotherapy for psoriasis. Arch Derm. 1977; 113:1667.

95. Melski J et al: Oral methoxsalen photochemotherapy for the treatment of psoriasis: A cooperative clinical trial. J Invest Derm. 1977; 68:328.

96. Roenigk H et al: Photochemotherapy for psoriasis. Arch Derm. 1979; 115:576.

97. Wolff K et al: Phototesting and dosimetry for photochemotherapy. Br J Derm. 1977; 96:1.

98. Pathak M et al: Photobiology and photochemistry of furocumarins (psoralens). In: Pathak M, Harber L and Seigi M, eds. Sunlight and Man. University of Tokyo Press; 1974; p 335.

99. Lynch W et al: Essentials of PUVA therapy-guidelines for photochemotherapy. Cutis. 1977; 20:494.

100. Polano MK et al: Difference in efficiency of two delivery forms of 8-methoxypsolarens. Dermatologica. 1977; 154:216.

101. Stern RS et al: Risk of cutaneous carcinoma in patients treated with oral methoxsalen photochemotherapy of psoriasis. N Engl J Med. 1979; 300:809.

102. Urbach F: Modification of ultraviolet carcinogenesis of photoactive agents: preliminary report. J Invest Dermatol. 1959; 32:373.

103. Rook AJ et al: Squamous epitheliema possibly induced by the therapeutic application of tar. Br J Cancer. 1956; 10:17.

104. Sommers SC et al: Multiple arsenicols cancers of skin and internal organs. Cancer. 1953; 6:347.

105. Walder BK et al: The skin and immunosuppression. Austral J Derm. 1976; 17:94.

106. Hoxtell EO et al. Incidence of skin carcinoma after renal transplantation. Arch Derm. 1977; 113:436.

107. Koranda FC et al: Cutaneous complications in immunosuppressed renal homograph recipients. JAMA. 1974; 229:419.

108. Sayre RM et al: Performance of six sunscreen formulations on human skin: A comparison. Arch Derm. 1979; 115:46.

109. Orentreich N et al: Comparative study of two antidandruff preparations. J Pharm Sci. 1969; 58:1279.

110. Freinkel RK: Pathogenesis of acne vulgaris. N Engl J Med. 1969; 280:1161.

111. Frank SB: Acne Vulgaris, Charles C. Thomas, Springfield, 1971.

112. Scehadeh NH et al: The bacteriology of acne. Arch Derm. 1963; 88:829.

113. Reisner RM et al: Lipolytic activity of corynebacterium acne. J Int Derm. 1968; 51:190.

114. Andrews CC: Acne vulgaris. Med Clin N Am. 1965; 49:737.

115. Melski J et al: Topical therapy for acne. N Engl J Med. 1980; 302:503.

116. Swinyer L: Topical agents alone in acne. JAMA. 1980; 243:1640.

117. Cotterill J: Benzyl peroxide. Acta Dermatovener. 1980; 89 (suppl):57.

118. Anon: Topical antibiotics. Medical Letter. 1980; 22:107.

119. Leyden J et al: Topical antibiotics and topical antimicrobial agents in acne therapy. Acta Dermatovener. 1980; 89 (suppl):75.

120. Stoughton RB et al: Topical antibiotic therapy for acne. Cutis. 1980; 26:424.

121. Logan WS: Vitamin A and keratinization. Arch Derm. 1972; 105:748.

122. Kalivas J: Acne vulgaris—Fact, fancy and in between. Rational Drug Ther. 1973; 7:1.

123. Mandy SH: The art of tretinoin therapy in acne. Cutis. 1975; 855.

124. Package insert: Retin-A. Johnson and Johnson, 1974.

125. Fulton JE et al: Benzoyl peroxide and vitamin-A acid in acne vulgaris. J Cutan Pathol. 1974; 1:191.

126. Arndt K et al: Rates of cutaneous reactions to drugs. JAMA. 1976; 235:918.

127. Freinkel RK et al: Effects of tetracyclines on the composition of sebum in acne vulgaris. N Engl J Med. 1965; 283:850.

128. Stewart WD et al: Therapeutic agents in acne vulgaris: II-D-alpha amino benzyl penicillin, erthromycin, and sulfadimetloxine. Can Med Assoc J. 1965; 92:1339.

129. Ad Hoc Committee on use of antibiotics in dermatology: Systemic antibiotics for treatment of acne vulgaris. Arch Derm. 1975; 111:1630.

130. Palitz LL: Abstract of a preliminary report on norethynodrel (Enovid) in the control of acne in females. Arch Derm. 1962; 86:237.

131. Palitz LL et al: Envoid for acne in the female skin. Skin. 1964; 3:243.

132. Strauss JS et al: Systemic estrogen therapy of acne. Prog Derm. 1967; 2:7.

133. Strauss JS et al: Effect of cyclic progestin estrogen therapy of sebum and acne in women. JAMA. 1964; 190:815.

134. Jelinek JE: Cutaneous side effects of oral contraceptives. Arch Derm. 1970; 101:181.

135. Baer RL et al: Types of cutaneous reactions to drugs. JAMA. 1967; 202:710.

136. Barr DP: Hazards of modern diagnosis and therapy— the price we pay. JAMA. 1955; 159:1452.

137. MacDonald MG et al: Adverse drug reactions, Experience of Mary Fletcher Hospital during 1962. JAMA. 1964; 190:1071.

138. Farber E et al: A current review of psoriasis. Calif Med. 1968; 108:440.

139. Perry H et al: The Goeckerman treatment of psoriasis. Arch Derm. 1968; 98:178.

140. Farber E et al: Psoriasis—a questionnaire survey of 2,144 patients. Arch Derm. 1968; 98:248.

141. VanScott E: Therapy of psoriasis—1975. JAMA. 1976; 235:197.

142. Baker H: Psoriasis: A review II. Dermatologica. 1975; 150:136.

143. VanScott E: Psoriasis: Practical therapeutic perspectives. Rational Drug Therapy. 1973; 7:1.

144. Seville RH: Simplified dithranol treatment for psoriasis. Br J Derm. 1975; 93:205.

145. Marriott P et al: Clobitasol propionate ointment compared with dithranol in Lassar's paste in the treatment of psoriasis. Br J Derm. 1976; 94 (suppl):101.

146. Weinstein G: Managing psoriasis. Postgrad Med. 1972; 93:191.

147. Gay M et al: Anthralin toxicity. Arch Derm. 1972; 105:213.

148. Weinstein G: Methotrexate. Ann Int Med. 1977; 86:199.

149. Farber E: Studies on the nature and management of psoriasis. Calif Med. 1971; 114:1.

150. Crounse RG et al: Changes in scalp hair roots as a measure of toxicity from cancer chemotherapeutic drugs. J Invest Derm. 1960; 35:83.

151. Schiff BL et al: Cutaneous reactions of anticoagulants. Arch Derm. 1968; 98:136.

152. Fisher AA: *Contact Dermatitis.* Lea and Febiger, Philadelphia, 1967, pp 82–90.

153. Coleman WP: Unusual cutaneous manifestations of drug hypersensitivity. Med Clin N Am. 1967; 51:1073.

154. Torok H: Dermatitis medicamentosa: A ten year study. Derm Int. 1969; 6:57.

155. Derbes V: The fixed eruption. JAMA. 1964; 190:765.

156. Savin J: Current causes of fixed drug eruptions. Br J Derm. 1970; 83:546.

157. Shapiro S et al: Drug rash with ampicillin and other penicillins. Lancet. 1969; 2:969.

158. Hitch JM: Acneiform eruptions induced by drugs and chemicals. JAMA. 1967; 200:879.

159. Weary P et al: Acneiform eruptions resulting from antibiotic administration. Arch Derm. 1969; 100:179.

160. Rostenberg A et al: Life threatening drug eruptions. JAMA. 1965; 194:660.

161. Shelley WB: *Consultations in Dermatology,* WB Saunders, Philadelphia, 1972.

162. Bianchine JR et al: Drugs as etiologic factors in the Stevens-Johnson syndrome. Am J Med. 1968; 44:390.

163. Epstein, et al: Dermatopharmacology of griseofulvin. Cutis 1971; 15:271.

164. Fulton JE: Miconazole therapy for endemic fungal disease. Arch Derm. 1975; 111:596.

165. Smith E: New topical agents for dermatophytosis. Cutis 1976; 17:54.

166. Grant L: A further look at the treatment of gynchomycosis with topical glutaraldehyde. J Am Pod Assoc. 1964; 64:158.

167. Clayton YM et al: A double blind trial of topical micronzole and clotrimazole against superficial fungal infections and erythrasma. Clin Exp Dermtol. 1976; 1:225.

168. Hermann H: Clinical efficacy studies of haloprogin, a new topical antimicrobial agent. Arch Derm. 1972; 106:839.

169. Anon: Newer antifungal preparations. Medical Letter 1976; 18:101.

170. Millikan LE: Superficial and cutaneous fungal infections. Postgrad Med. 1976; 60:52.

171. Epstein W: Poison oak hyposensitization. Arch Derm. 1974; 109:356.

172. Adams RM: *Occupational Contact Dermatitis,* Lippincot, Philadelphia, 1962.

173. Fisher A: *Contact Dermatitis,* 2nd ed., Lea and Febiger, Philadelphia, 1973.

174. Rodner EJ et al: The frequency of contact sensitivity in North America, 1972–1974. Contact Dermatitis 1975; 1:277.

175. Kligman AM: Poison Ivy (Rhus) dermatitis. Arch Derm. 1958; 77:149–180.

176. Orkin M et al: This scabies pandemic. N Engl J Med. 1978; 9:496.

177. Shaw P et al: Recent trends of scabies in the United States. J Infect Dis. 1976; 134:414.

178. Nienhuis M et al: Treatment of pediculosis and scabies. U.S. Pharm. 1980; 4:80.

179. Orkin M: Today's scabies. JAMA. 1975; 233:882.

180. Orkin M et al: Treatment of today's scabies and pediculosis. JAMA. 1976; 236:1136.

181. Feldmann RJ et al: Percutaneous penetration of some pesticides and herbicides in man. Toxicol Appl Pharmacol 1974; 28:126.

182. Lee B et al: Scabies: Transcutaneous poisoning during treatment. Pediatrics 1977; 59:643.

Chapter 52

Eye Diseases

Steven R. Abel and Dick R. Gourley

An understanding of primary ocular disorders requires some knowledge of ocular anatomy and physiology. Vaughan (1) provides a comprehensive discussion in his text. The following review will assist the practitioner in understanding conditions covered in this chapter.

OCULAR ANATOMY AND PHYSIOLOGY

The eyeball is approximately one inch in diameter and is highly complex. It is housed in the orbital cavity, formed by two bony orbits that serve as sockets which are lined with fat to protect the eyeball. Six ocular muscles allow for movement of the eyeball.

The outer coat of the eye is comprised of the sclera, conjunctiva and cornea. The sclera is the white, dense, fibrous protective coating. It is covered by a thin layer of loose, connective tissue, the episclera, which contains blood vessels to nourish the sclera. The conjunctiva is a mucous membrane that covers the anterior portion of the eye and lines the eyelids. The cornea is the transparent, avascular tissue which functions as a refractive and protective window membrane through which light rays pass en route to the retina. The corneal epithelium and endothelium are lipophilic and the centrally-located stroma is hydrophilic. These three corneal layers are particularly important in that they affect drug penetration through the cornea. The best penetration through the intact cornea is accomplished with biphasic preparations, or those that are both fat and water soluble.

The choroid, ciliary body and iris are known collectively as the uveal tract. The iris is a colored, circular membrane suspended between the cornea and the crystalline lens. It functions to control the amount of light that enters the eye. The choroid lies between the sclera and retina. It is largely comprised of blood vessels which nourish the retina. The ciliary body is adherent to the sclera and contains the ciliary muscle and ciliary processes. The ciliary muscle contracts and relaxes the zonular fibers which hold the crystalline lens in place. The ciliary processes are responsible for the secretion of aqueous humor, a clear liquid which occupies the anterior chamber. The anterior chamber is bounded anteriorly by the cornea and posteriorly by the iris, and the posterior chamber lies between the posterior iris and the crystalline lens.

The inner segment of the eye contains the retina with the optic nerve. The retina contains all sensory receptors for light transmission. The optic nerve transmits visual impulses from the retina to the brain.

The crystalline lens, aqueous humor and vitreous assist the cornea with the process of refraction. The lens has an inner nucleus surrounded by the cortex and enveloped by an outer capsule. The only lens-related disorder discussed in this review is drug-induced opacification (cataract formation). Disorders involving the aqueous humor will be discussed in the section on glaucoma. The primary function of the vitreous is to maintain the shape of the eye.

The eyelids and eyelashes are the outermost means of protection for the eye. The eyelids contain various sebaceous and sweat glands which may become infected or inflamed and contribute to various ocular disorders.

The eye is innervated by both the sympathetic and parasympathetic nervous systems. Parasympathetic fibers originating from the oculomotor nerve in the brain innervate the ciliary muscle and sphincter pupillae muscle which constricts the pupil. Parasympathomimetic (cholinergic) agents cause miosis. Parasympatholytic (anticholinergic) agents cause mydriasis and cycloplegia. Cycloplegia results in decreased accommodation from temporary paralysis of the ciliary muscle and zonules, and causes production of blurred images on the retina. Tear secretion by the lacrimal glands is also a parasympathetic function.

Sympathetic fibers from the superior cervical ganglion in the spinal cord innervate the dilator pupillae muscle, the blood vessels of the ciliary body, the episclera and the extraocular muscles. Sympathomimetics cause mydriasis without affecting accommodation. The exact role of the sympathetic nervous system in glaucoma and its treatment is not fully understood. Postulated adrenergic innervation is discussed in Question 6.

GLAUCOMA

Glaucoma, a disease characterized by an increase in *intraocular pressure (IOP)*, is primarily a disease of middle age; an estimated 2% of all individuals over the age of 40 have glaucoma. It may occur in other age groups as well. IOP relates to the production of aqueous humor by the ciliary processes and the outflow of aqueous humor through the trabecular meshwork. Applanation tonometry is used to measure IOP, based upon the pressure required to flatten a small area of the central cornea. Generally an IOP of between 10–20 mm Hg is considered normal. Measurement of an IOP of 22 mm Hg or greater should arouse suspicion of glaucoma, although a more rare form of glaucoma is associated with low IOP. Elevated IOP causes a pathologic cupping of the optic nerve such that glaucoma can often be diagnosed by inspection of the optic disc with an ophthalmoscope. Other provocative and confir-

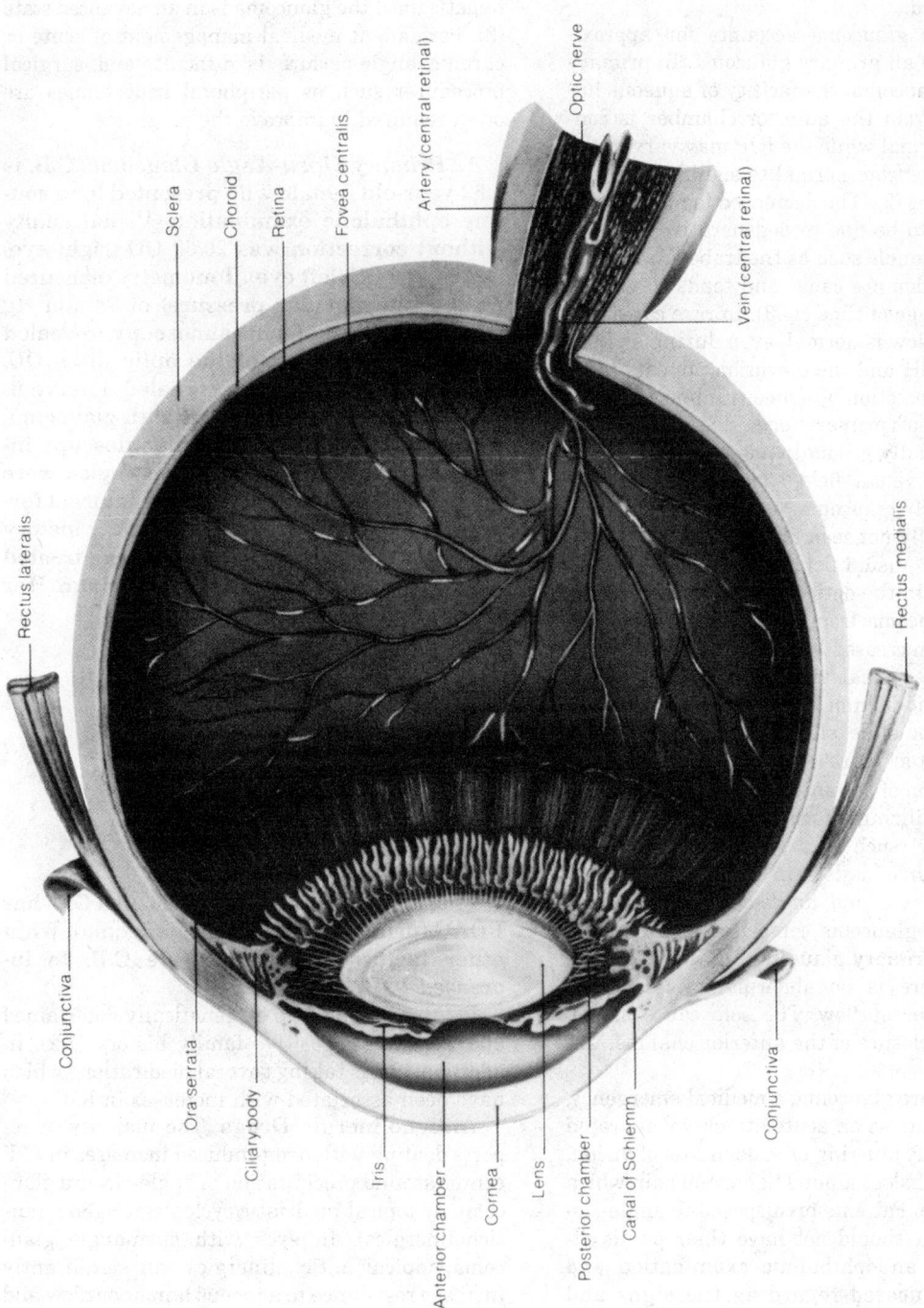

Optic nerve

Artery (central retinal)

Vein (central retinal)

Sclera

Choroid

Retina

Fovea centralis

Rectus lateralis

Rectus medialis

Conjunctiva

Ora serrata

Ciliary body

Iris

Anterior chamber

Cornea

Lens

Posterior chamber

Canal of Schlemm

Conjunctiva

Anatomy of the human eye. (Artwork courtesy of Burroughs Wellcome.)

Figure 1. Anatomy of the Eye.

matory tests for open-angle glaucoma include tonography and a water-drinking test, but these are rarely used.

Open-angle glaucoma accounts for approximately 90% of all primary glaucoma. In primary open-angle glaucoma, the facility of aqueous humor outflow from the anterior chamber is constantly subnormal while the IOP may vary in the course of a day from normal to significantly elevated pressures (2). The decreased facility of outflow appears to be due to degenerative changes in outflow channels such as the trabecular meshwork and Schlemm's canal and tends to worsen with the passage of time (1–3). In rare cases, the facility of outflow is normal, even during a phase of elevated IOP, and the elevation appears to be due to hypersecretion of aqueous humor (2).

The onset of primary open-angle glaucoma (POAG) is usually gradual and asymptomatic. A defect in the visual field examination may be present in early glaucoma, but loss of peripheral vision is usually not seen until late in the course of the disease. Visual field defects correlate well with changes in the optic disc and help in differentiating glaucoma from ocular hypertension in patients with increased IOP. Studies indicate that patients with normal visual fields and an IOP between 22 and 30 mm Hg have no greater than a 5% likelihood of developing visual field loss in periods up to ten years (4).

Examination of the anterior chamber angle by gonioscopy, utilizing a corneal contact lens, magnifying device (such as a slit-lamp microscope) and light source assists in differentiating between open-angle and *angle-closure glaucoma*. Angle-closure glaucoma comprises approximately 5% of all primary glaucoma. In angle-closure glaucoma there is no abnormal resistance to aqueous humor outflow. The sole cause of elevated IOP is closure of the anterior chamber angle (2).

Angle-closure glaucoma, a medical emergency, usually presents as an acute attack with a rapid increase of IOP, blurring or sudden loss of vision, appearance of haloes around lights and pain which is often severe. Patients predisposed to angle-closure glaucoma should not have their pupils dilated during an ophthalmic examination and should be educated regarding the signs and symptoms of angle closure. Acute attacks may terminate without treatment, but if the IOP remains high, irreparable damage to the optic nerve

may occur (1). In chronic angle-closure, the closure is gradual and the patient may be asymptomatic until the glaucoma is in an advanced state (2). Permanent medical management of acute or chronic angle-closure is difficult, and surgical procedures such as peripheral iridectomies are often required to improve the prognosis.

1. *Primary Open-Angle Glaucoma.* **C.B. is a 52-year-old female who presented for a routine ophthalmic examination. Visual acuity without correction was 20/60 OD (right eye) and 20/100 OS (left eye). Tonometry measured an IOP (intraocular pressure) of 38 mm Hg OU (both eyes). Ophthalmoscopy revealed physiologic cupping of the optic discs OU. Visual field examination revealed a nerve fiber bundle defect consistent with glaucoma. Pupils were normal OU, and gonioscopy indicated that anterior chamber angles were open OU. There were no signs of cataract formation. C.B. related a positive family history for glaucoma. She is presently being treated for hypertension, CHF, and asthma. Her medications include:**

> **Amitriptyline 75 mg hs**
> **Chlorpheniramine 4 mg q 6 h prn**
> **Digoxin 0.25 mg qd**
> **Furosemide 40 mg bid**
> **Methyldopa 500 mg qid**
> **NTG 1/150 gr SL prn**
> **Theophylline (sustained release) 300 mg q 12 h**

Findings on examination indicated C.B. has POAG (primary open-angle glaucoma). What other factors may predispose C.B. to increased IOP?

POAG is thought to be genetically determined and C.B. has a positive family history (1,2). In addition, she is taking several medications which have been associated with increases in IOP.

Anticholinergic Drugs. The majority of reports dealing with drug-induced increases in IOP center around precipitation of angle-closure glaucoma by topical mydriatic/cycloplegic agents (anticholinergics). In eyes with open-angle glaucoma, topical anticholinergics can significantly increase resistance to aqueous humor outflow and elevate IOP with the anterior chamber remaining grossly open (5). As part of any routine ophthalmic examination the pupils are dilated with a mydriatic/cycloplegic (unless otherwise contraindicated). Measurement of IOP is always done prior to this procedure, so use of these agents would not have influenced the IOP readings in C.B.

With systemic anticholinergic agents, if the quantity of drug administered is sufficient to cause pupillary dilatation, the risk of precipitating angle-closure increases. There appears to be no reason to fear aggravation of open-angle glaucoma unless the amount reaching the eye is sufficient to cause cycloplegia (5). Consideration must be given to medications with anticholinergic side effects (antihistamines, benzodiazepines, disopyramide, phenothiazines, tricyclic antidepressants) though literature documentation of glaucoma potentiation is scarce. C.B. is receiving chlorpheniramine prn and amitriptyline hs, but her pupil examination is normal, with no evidence of mydriasis or cycloplegia. In this case, it is highly unlikely that these medications contributed to her increased IOP.

Adrenergic Drugs. Adrenergic agents such as CNS stimulants, vasoconstrictors, appetite suppressants and bronchodilators may produce minimal pupillary dilatation. These have no proven adverse influence on IOP in either normal eyes or eyes with open-angle glaucoma, so the use of theophylline in C.B. would also be an unlikely source of increased IOP (6).

Other Drugs. No conclusive evidence proving production of angle-closure glaucoma by vasodilators, including administration in controlled studies, has ever been published, though slight increases in IOP have been reported (7). Use of nitroglycerin prn in C.B. is not a cause for concern. There have been isolated reports of other medications causing mydriasis in glaucoma patients. These include muscle relaxants (carisoprodol), monoamine oxidase inhibitors, fenfluramine, ganglionic blocking agents, salicylates, oral contraceptives and chlorpropamide (8). Succinylcholine, ketamine (9) and caffeine (7) have been associated with increases in IOP. Alpha-chymotrypsin has been reported to increase IOP in patients who have received the medication during operative procedures, and these patients probably have obstruction of outflow channels by debris generated from use of the enzyme (10). Corticosteroid-induced increase in IOP is discussed in Question 18. Should C.B. require administration of any other medications related to increases in

IOP, potential adverse effects may be avoided by proper, routine follow-up.

2. How should therapy for POAG be initiated in C.B.?

Table 1 outlines topical agents used in the treatment of glaucoma. Sugar (11) suggests that the practitioner has three options available as initial therapy in POAG: pilocarpine, epinephrine or timolol (Timoptic). *Pilocarpine* has historically been the initial treatment of choice. Therapy is usually begun using lower concentrations (0.5–1%), one drop administered qid. Pilocarpine is a direct-acting cholinergic (parasympathomimetic) that causes contraction of ciliary muscle fibers attached to the trabecular meshwork and scleral spur. This opens the trabecular meshwork to enhance aqueous humor outflow. There may also be a direct effect on the trabecular meshwork. Pilocarpine causes miosis by contraction of the iris sphincter muscle, but the miosis is not related to the decrease in IOP. The onset of miosis is rapid, occurring in 10 to 15 minutes, while IOP decreases within one hour, and the duration of action is four to eight hours. Melanin in the iris is a binding site for pilocarpine, and effects on IOP may be decreased in heavily pigmented eyes (4).

Epinephrine is a sympathomimetic agent that stimulates both alpha and beta receptors. It is thought that stimulation of alpha receptors causes an increase in aqueous humor outflow, while stimulation of beta receptors causes a decrease in the production of aqueous humor. The latter is the more important effect of epinephrine in treating open-angle glaucoma. The exact mechanism of action is currently under review (see Question 6). When used alone, epinephrine produces a 30–35% decrease in the rate of aqueous humor production, and use in conjunction with carbonic anhydrase inhibitors may produce a 65–70% decrease (4). Epinephrine is often used in younger patients or patients with cataracts where miosis and the resultant decreased vision from cholinergic agents is a problem. Epinephrine is a first-line drug in the therapy of POAG, but is most often used as a second agent in combination rather than as the initial single agent for therapy.

Timolol, a beta-adrenergic blocker, appears to lower IOP by causing a decrease in aqueous humor production. Some studies have demonstrated a slight effect on the facility of outflow, but this

Table 1.

TOPICAL AGENTS USED IN THE TREATMENT OF OPEN-ANGLE GLAUCOMA

Generic	Mechanism	Strength	Duration	Usual Dose	Trade	Manufact.	Comments
MIOTICS							
pilocarpine	parasympathomimetic	0.25–10%	4–6 hours	1–2 gtts tid-qid	Isopto Carpine Pilocar Pilocel	Alcon CooperVision Professional	Long-term proven effectiveness. Little rationale for use of concentrations exceeding 4% or administration more frequently than q 4 h. Side effects of miosis with decreased vision and brow ache are frequent sources of patient complaints.
carbachol	parasympathomimetic	0.75–3%	8 hours	1–2 gtts tid-qid	Carbacel Isopto Carbachol	Professional Alcon	Primarily used in patients allergic to or intolerant of other miotics. May be used as frequently as q 4 h. Corneal penetration is enhanced by benzalkonium chloride in commercial preparations. Side effects similar to pilocarpine.
physostigmine	anticholinesterase (reversible)	0.25–0.5%	12–36 hours	1 gtt qid (oint. hs)	Isopto Eserine Eserine Ointment	Alcon CooperVision	Rarely used. Solutions are unstable. Decomposition products are irritating to the eye. Side effects similar to pilocarpine.
neostigmine	anticholinesterase (reversible)	3–5%	4–6 hours	1 gtt qid	Prostigmin	Roche	Rarely used. Corneal penetration is poor. Side effects similar to pilocarpine.
demecarium	anticholinesterase (irreversible)	.125, .25%	days/wks.	1 gtt up to bid	Humorsol	MSD	Rarely used. Long duration. Less frequent administration enhances compliance. Side effects similar to pilocarpine.
echothiophate	anticholinesterase (irreversible)	.03, .06, .125, .25%	days/wks.	1 gtt bid	Echodide Phospholine Iodide	Alcon Ayerst	Most used anticholinesterase agent. Long duration, though usually dosed bid which enhances compliance. Solutions are relatively unstable. Side effects similar to pilocarpine, especially in concentrations exceeding 0.06%. Increased cataract formation has been associated with its use.
isoflurophate	anticholinesterase (irreversible)	0.025%	days/wks.	1/4" q 8–72 hours	Floropryl	MSD	Rarely used. Long duration. Less frequent administration enhances compliance. Side effects similar to pilocarpine.

MYDRIATICS						
epinephrine	sympathomimetic	0.25–2%	12 hrs.	Epinal (borate), Eppy-N, Epifrin (hydrochloride), Glaucon, Epitrate (bitartrate)	Alcon, Barnes Hind, Allergan, Alcon, Ayerst	Good response is often seen with use of lower concentrations (0.5–1%). Bitartrate salt contains one-half the labeled strength in epinephrine free base equivalent. bid dosage enhances compliance. Cosmetic complaints associated with use include hyperemia and pigment deposits on the cornea and conjunctiva. Not recommended for use in aphakic patients due to 20–30% incidence of cystoid macular edema.
dipivefrin	sympathomimetic	0.1%	12 hrs.	Propine	Allergan	Prodrug of epinephrine associated with decrease in systemic side effects if absorbed. bid dosage enhances compliance.
BETA-BLOCKERS						
timolol	beta-blocker (sympatholytic)	0.25–0.5%	12–24 hrs.	Timoptic	MSD	Effective with few associated ocular side effects. bid dosage enhances compliance. Use with caution in patients with preexisting CHF or pulmonary disease.

does not seem to be significant (12–14). Concentrations or dosages exceeding one drop of 0.5% timolol administered bid have not been shown to produce further significant decrease in IOP (15). Therapy is usually initiated with 0.25% administered as one drop bid. An escape phenomenon, or tachyphylaxis, has been seen with timolol. If a patient has a large initial decrease in IOP, the IOP will often stabilize at a lesser reduction in approximately four to six weeks (16–18). Timolol has been shown to be at least as effective as pilocarpine and epinephrine. Timolol may be more efficacious in diurnal IOP control (19–21).

C.B. has a history of CHF and asthma. Timolol has been associated with a reduction of resting pulse rate and worsening of CHF (22,23). Generally the change in pulse rate is slight, in the range of five to eight beats per minute. Pulmonary effects such as dyspnea, airway obstruction and pulmonary failure have also occurred (24–26).

Systemic absorption of timolol has been studied in the rabbit and human following topical administration (27,28). Affrime (28) found that plasma levels of timolol were not detected in most subjects following topical administration; however, a level of 9.6 ng/ml was detected in one subject. The beta-blocking plasma concentration of timolol has been estimated to be about 5–10 ng/ml (17). Though systemic absorption following topical administration does not appear to be significant in most cases, care should be taken when timolol is used in patients with sinus bradycardia, CHF and pulmonary disease.

Systemic effects, including tachycardia, hypertension and faintness, occur rarely with epinephrine (29). As with timolol, patients in whom systemic effects could potentiate preexisting problems should be closely monitored. For these reasons, pilocarpine 1%, administered one drop OU qid is the initial treatment of choice in this patient. In the uncomplicated patient, timolol may be a better choice, primarily due to a lower incidence of intolerable side effects and increased compliance with bid dosing.

3. *Patient Instructions.* **Pilocarpine 1%, one drop OU qid, is ordered for C.B. How should C.B. be instructed regarding proper use of her pilocarpine, compliance, and expected therapeutic and side effects?**

Merck, Sharp and Dohme suggest a method for administration of Timoptic that has proven effective with all types and sizes of plastic ophthalmic dropper bottles. C.B. should be instructed to hold the inverted pilocarpine bottle between her thumb and middle finger. The index finger is left free to depress the bottom of the container, releasing one drop for the dose. With a little practice, this technique is easy to master. The lower eyelid should be drawn downward with the index finger of the opposite hand, or pinched between the thumb and index finger to form a pouch. The patient should look up and administer the drug into the pouch.

Patients must be encouraged to continue regular use of their medications for effective treatment of their glaucoma. Since chronic glaucoma is a silent disease, like hypertension, there is little positive reinforcement to continue therapy; the only noticeable effects are side effects. It is best to administer the pilocarpine every six hours, a schedule consistent with its duration of action (see Table 1).

C.B. should be warned that pilocarpine (and other miotics) may cause ciliary spasm and may result in brow ache and myopia, characterized by blurred vision (30). Also, miosis causes decreased vision in poor light, so night driving may be hazardous for patients. Miotics have also been associated with retinal detachments, especially in aphakic eyes (eyes from which the crystalline lens has been removed) (31).

Systemic, cholinergic effects such as nausea, vomiting, sweating, salivation and diarrhea have been associated with use of all miotics, though most reports have been associated with use of anticholinesterase agents (32,33). C.B. should report any such effects to her physician. As is the case with any topical agent, occlusion of the puncta by applying slight pressure with the finger during administration may decrease the systemic absorption and incidence of side effects.

4. Two weeks after initiation of therapy, C.B. returns for follow-up. Her IOP measures 32 mm Hg OD and 30 mm Hg OS. She denies non-compliance (confirmed by miotic pupils). She has no complaints of intolerable side effects. How should therapy be altered?

The concentration of pilocarpine may be increased and the dosage schedule made more frequent to achieve continuous pressure-lowering effects. Concentrations in excess of four percent and dosage administration more frequently than every four hours have shown little advantage in controlling increased IOP (4). The *pilocarpine*

Ocusert, an elliptically-shaped unit designed to fit in the conjunctival cul-de-sac, is available in two strengths which release 20 mcg or 40 mcg per hour for one week. This dosage form increases compliance in some patients and provides better control of IOP. The Ocusert system may cause discomfort, however, and retention in the eye may be difficult in some patients.

If control of IOP is not achieved with optimal use of pilocarpine, another miotic may be substituted. *Carbachol* is used most frequently when resistance or intolerance to other miotics develop. In addition to having direct cholinergic effects, carbachol is more resistant to cholinesterase than is pilocarpine. Added benefits of increased release of acetylcholine from parasympathetic nerve terminals and a weak anticholinesterase effect may be beneficial. Carbachol preparations contain benzalkonium chloride as a preservative, which also enhances the otherwise very poor corneal penetration of the drug. Carbachol is usually administered bid to tid, though response varies and more frequent administration may be required.

Anticholinesterase agents inhibit the enzyme cholinesterase, thereby increasing the amounts of acetylcholine and its naturally occurring cholinergic effects. Physostigmine (Eserine) is a reversible cholinesterase inhibitor and was the first medication used in the treatment of glaucoma. It is rarely used at present because chronic use has been associated with allergic irritation and follicular hypertrophy of the palpebral conjunctiva (4). Physostigmine is sensitive to heat and light and oxidizes to a pink or rusty color indicating that it should be discarded. Other reversible cholinesterase inhibitors include neostigmine, 3 to 5%, administered every four to six hours, and demecarium (Humorsol), which has a much longer duration of action than physostigmine.

Echothiophate iodide (Phospholine Iodide) is an irreversible cholinesterase inhibitor which primarily inactivates pseudocholinesterase and secondarily inhibits true cholinesterase. Echothiophate iodide is the most widely used cholinesterase inhibitor in treating open-angle glaucoma and would be the best alternative to pilocarpine in treating C.B. It is marketed as a powder plus diluent because of product instability. Following reconstitution, the product is stable for 30 days at room temperature or six months under refrigeration. Echothiophate iodide has a long duration of action which affords better control of IOP; the side effects of miosis and myopia

are more constant. Concentrations higher than 0.06% are associated with a significant increase in subjective complaints such as the previously mentioned brow ache (34,35). Another irreversible cholinesterase inhibitor, isoflurophate (diisopropyl fluorophosphate, DFP) is occasionally used in open-angle glaucoma associated with aphakia. In general, anticholinesterase agents that are used in open-angle glaucoma have a long duration of action (see Table 1) but are dosed on a bid, q 12 h schedule (36).

Hazards in Use of Anticholinesterase Agents. Miotics, primarily cholinesterase inhibitors, have been associated with the formation of iris cysts. Formation of iris cysts may be prevented by the use of phenylephrine in combination with the cholinesterase inhibitor (37). Also, there is considerable clinical evidence that cataracts occur more frequently and progress more rapidly in patients over 50 years of age treated with echothiophate iodide. The initial changes consist of clusters of small vacuoles located in the anterior subcapsular region, giving a characteristic mossy appearance (4). Similar changes have been noted in patients treated with demecarium or isoflurophate. Such changes may occur in 8–10% of nonglaucomatous eyes and in a similar percentage of eyes treated with pilocarpine or carbachol, but they are seen in up to 60% of eyes treated with echothiophate iodide for more than six months (38–40). Following continuous therapy for three years, about 50% of treated eyes demonstrate a loss of visual acuity due to lens changes. Initially, visual acuity may not be affected, and most cases do not progress when therapy is stopped at the early stage (4). Based upon this, anticholinesterase agents are often reserved for use in aphakic glaucoma, with notable exceptions such as C.B.

C.B. should be managed with miotic therapy until IOP is proven unresponsive to maximal therapy with these agents. If response is unsatisfactory with the echothiophate iodide, or visual changes and intolerance occur, a trial of pilocarpine plus timolol or epinephrine along with careful monitoring in view of her other underlying disease states is warranted.

5. *Surgical Patients.* **J.W. has been treated for POAG with echothiophate iodide 0.06% and timolol 0.5%, one drop OU bid. He is to be admitted to the hospital in the near future for an exploratory laparotomy under general**

anesthesia. Should the glaucoma therapy be continued up to the time of surgery?

Cholinesterase inhibitors decrease levels of pseudocholinesterase, the enzyme responsible for the hydrolysis and metabolism of succinylcholine and procaine (41,42). Reports have appeared in the literature substantiating potentiation of these agents by concomitant use of cholinesterase inhibitors (43,44). The echothiophate therapy should be changed to pilocarpine two to four weeks prior to the surgical procedure. Patients receiving cholinesterase inhibitors who exhibit signs of overdose should be managed with pralidoxime and atropine (45).

6. *Combined Therapy with Timolol and Epinephrine.* **S.H. has been treated with timolol 0.5%, one drop OU bid for approximately eight weeks. IOP control has proven inadequate and epinephrine hydrochloride 1%, one drop OU bid, has been added to his regimen. Are these two agents synergistic in treatment of glaucoma?**

Pharmacologically, timolol and epinephrine should be antagonistic. Goldberg (46) demonstrated that patients pretreated with timolol had significantly reduced response to epinephrine; however, epinephrine pretreatment did not affect the IOP reduction of timolol. Thomas (47) has shown that patients treated with epinephrine alone for two weeks had a statistically significant increase in facility of outflow. One day after timolol was added to the regimen of these patients, no significant change in the facility of outflow was present, but two weeks of combined therapy resulted in a statistically significant decrease in outflow facility. Thomas further defines a model of ocular adrenergic receptor sites to explain the effects of timolol and epinephrine. According to this model, beta receptors involved with outflow are possibly located in the trabecular meshwork. Stimulating these receptors with epinephrine increases the outflow of aqueous humor, but the receptors maintain no tone on the outflow mechanism, so blocking them with timolol has no effect on outflow. Beta receptors mediating inflow are possibly located in the ciliary processes, and stimulating them with epinephrine increases aqueous humor production. It is postulated that these receptors provide a tone to the inflow mechanism and when blocked with timolol there is a resultant decrease in aqueous humor production. Ad-

ditionally, alpha receptors may play a role in the inflow mechanism. They may be located in the walls of blood vessels supplying the ciliary processes, and when stimulated with epinephrine, the vessels may constrict, leading to decreased blood flow and consequently decreased aqueous humor production. Following this model, timolol affects IOP by decreasing the rate of aqueous humor production without affecting outflow facility. The net effect of epinephrine reflects the balance of opposing beta and alpha effects on inflow and beta effects increasing outflow. The complete mechanism is not fully understood and studies are currently being done to determine whether chronic use of timolol and epinephrine may be additive based upon the presumably unblocked alpha agonist effect of epinephrine (46). Timolol has been shown to be additive with miotics and carbonic anhydrase inhibitors (48,49), though further research is being completed.

7. Following two weeks of therapy with timolol and epinephrine, S.H. complains of "red eyes." Could this be due to the medications? Have additional adverse effects been reported with these preparations? How may these be avoided?

Conjunctival hyperemia has been seen with timolol, although allergic conjunctivitis and conjunctival vessel vasoconstriction with rebound hyperemia have been more frequently associated with epinephrine therapy. Permanent corneal and conjunctival pigmentation may occur, especially in patients using epinephrine for longer than one year (50–53).

Hypersensitivity and supersensitivity with long-term use have also been reported with epinephrine (54,55). A burning sensation upon administration of epinephrine preparations may be minimized by use of the borate salt which has a pH more compatible with the eye (56). Discolored solutions of epinephrine should be discarded.

Other ocular side effects reported in conjunction with timolol include superficial punctate keratitis, corneal anesthesia, allergic blepharoconjunctivitis and dry-eye syndrome (57). Additional systemic side effects include palpitations, hypotension and syncope, as well as CNS effects such as lightheadedness, mental depression and disorientation (24). Dermatologic reactions (rash, alopecia) and GI upset have been reported. There has been one report of hypoglycemia (58), and timolol has been implicated in the worsening of myasthenia gravis in one patient (59). The puncta may be occluded with the finger during administration to decrease the possibility of systemic absorption. Although timolol has been used effectively in many patients without significant side effects, the clinician should realize that topical timolol is not free of adverse effects.

8. C.W. is a 66-year-old woman with a ten-year history of POAG who recently had cataract surgery. Prior to surgery she was treated with pilocarpine 4%, one drop OU qid and epinephrine hydrochloride 1%, one drop OU bid. Should this therapy be continued postoperatively?

Twenty to thirty percent of aphakic patients will develop macular edema when treated with epinephrine (4). Initial symptoms include blurring and distortion of vision which may occur within a few weeks to months. The maculopathy is reversible if therapy is stopped. Improvement is usually seen within one month, though it may take six or more weeks to recover maximum vision. Therapy should be reevaluated in C.W. with use of miotics and/or timolol.

9. *Epinephrine Products.* K.V. is a 58-year-old woman who presents with a prescription for Glaucon 2%. The pharmacist informs her that he only stocks Epitrate 2% and he would like to substitute that product. Are these two preparations therapeutically equivalent?

The two are not equivalent. Glaucon is the hydrochloride salt of epinephrine and Epitrate is the bitartrate salt. Also available is Eppy-N, epinephryl borate. The 2% bitartrate salt contains 1.1% epinephrine free base equivalent, while the 1% concentration of the borate or hydrochloride salt is equivalent to 1% epinephrine free base. The bitartrate salt of epinephrine is used in the various pilocarpine-epinephrine combination products. There have been no significant therapeutic or toxic differences between the salts when used in equivalent concentrations.

10. What is dipivefrin (Propine)?

Dipivefrin is a prodrug of epinephrine that is more lipophilic, thereby enhancing its corneal penetration. Dipivefrin is rapidly hydrolyzed to epinephrine upon administration. The rationale behind use of the prodrug is the production of the desired therapeutic effect with fewer side effects

than with conventional therapy. Dipivefrin, available as a 0.1% solution which is administered bid, produces reductions in IOP that are comparable to 1–2% epinephrine (60). Studies have shown dipivefrin to be better tolerated than epinephrine. However, reports of side effects similar to those occurring with epinephrine have been serious enough to require discontinuation of the dipivefrin in certain cases (61–64).

11. *Carbonic Anhydrase Inhibitors.* B.A. is a 59-year-old male with a six-year history of POAG which remained uncontrolled despite treatment with pilocarpine 4%, one drop OU q 4 h, epinephrine hydrochloride 2%, 1 drop OU bid, and timolol 0.5%, one drop OU bid. One month ago, echothiophate iodide 0.25%, one drop OU bid was prescribed in place of the pilocarpine. IOP remains 36 mm Hg OU. How should B.A. be managed?

Maximal medical therapy for POAG utilizes topical agents plus a carbonic anhydrase inhibitor. Table 2 lists available carbonic anhydrase inhibitors, their onset and duration of action and usual dosages. Acetazolamide is the carbonic anhydrase inhibitor that is most frequently used in the treatment of POAG; it is also used in acute angle-closure glaucoma (see Question 13). Dose-response curves are being studied for the carbonic anhydrase inhibitors (65). Carbonic anhydrase occurs in high concentrations in the ciliary processes and retina of the eye. The exact mechanism by which carbonic anhydrase inhibitors lower IOP is not understood, but it is felt that these agents act to buffer an acid residue which may be present in secretory cells as a result of production of alkaline aqueous humor. The net effect may be a 40–60% decrease in aqueous humor secretion, although it may be balanced by up to a 40% decrease of aqueous humor outflow (4,66). Carbonic anhydrase inhibitors are ineffective when administered topically (67).

Side effects commonly associated with carbonic anhydrase inhibitors are a frequent source of patient intolerance. Such effects include paresthesias (often transient) and GI intolerance (anorexia, weight loss). Drowsiness, malaise and depression may be overlooked and attributed to causes other than carbonic anhydrase inhibitor therapy. A metallic taste has been associated with carbonic anhydrase inhibitors, as have ureteral colic, hypokalemia, renal calculi formation, loss

Table 2.

CARBONIC ANHYDRASE INHIBITORS USED IN TREATMENT OF GLAUCOMA

Generic	Trade	Manufact.	Strength	Onset (Min.)	Peak (Hours)	Duration (Hours)	Usual Dose
Acetazolamide -Injection	Diamox	Lederle	500 mg	5–10		2	500 mg
Acetazolamide -Tablets	Diamox	Lederle	125 & 250 mg	120	4	6–8	250 mg qid
Acetazolamide -Sequels	Diamox	Lederle	500 mg	120	8–18	22–30	500 mg bid
Dichlorphenamide	Daranide Oratol	MSD Alcon	50 mg 50 mg	30	2–4	6–12	50 mg tid
Ethoxzolamide	Cardrase Ethamide	Upjohn Allergan	125 mg 125 mg	90	3–4	7	125 mg qid
Methazolamide	Neptazane	Lederle	50 mg	120	4–8	10–12	50 mg tid

of libido and systemic acidosis (68–70). Metabolic acidosis has been seen less frequently with dichlorphenamide, and formation of renal calculi is thought to be less with methazolamide because there is no interference with urinary citrate excretion (4).

Rarely, patients may develop dermatitis, myopia, agranulocytosis and aplastic anemia. These side effects may be related to the fact that carbonic anhydrase inhibitors are sulfonamides (71). Carbonic anhydrase inhibitors may cause alkalinization of the urine and complicate therapy with agents dependent upon urine pH for excretion or reabsorption. In patients treated with carbonic anhydrase inhibitors, the results of gonioscopy may be invalid, as these agents cause some widening of the anterior chamber angle (2).

12. *Other Drugs.* What other agents have been investigated for the management of open-angle glaucoma?

Ross (72) demonstrated that topical isoproterenol caused a decrease in IOP which was most likely related to a decreased production of aqueous humor. Krupin (73) has shown that topical prazosin lowers IOP in rabbit eyes, and this effect appears to be due to a decreased production of aqueous humor. Propranolol, in doses of 20–40 mg administered tid-qid, has been used in long-term management of glaucoma (74).

Research has been performed with pilocarpine gel administered bid to provide around-the-clock control of IOP with fewer side effects and improved compliance (75–77). Topical guanethidine has been shown to decrease IOP by decreasing aqueous humor production and has been used alone and in combination in the treatment of open-angle glaucoma (78–81).

13. *Angle-Closure Glaucoma.* D.H. is a 72-year-old male who presents to the emergency room with an intensely red right eye, a "steamy" appearing cornea, complaints of haloes around lights and extreme pain. A diagnosis of acute angle-closure glaucoma is made. How should the patient be managed?

The patient should be seen by an ophthalmologist since acute angle-closure glaucoma is a medical emergency. Medical treatment usually consists of administration of pilocarpine 2–4%, one drop every five minutes for four to six administrations. It is suggested that the puncta be covered during administration to decrease the possibility of systemic absorption. Stronger miotics are contraindicated as they may potentiate angle-closure (4).

Acetazolamide 500 mg IV is frequently administered in addition to hyperosmotic agents (see Table 3). Orally, 50% glycerin is the usual drug of choice; it is administered in dosages of 1–1.5 gm/kg (82,83). Isosorbide is an alternative, especially in diabetics since it is not metabolized to provide calories (84,85). Ethyl alcohol (2–3 ml/kg) has proven effective and may be helpful in emergency situations when other agents are unavailable (86). Parenterally, mannitol is the drug of choice. It is administered in doses of 1–2 gm/kg, is not metabolized to provide calories and may be used in patients with renal failure (87–89).

Hyperosmotic agents act by creating an osmotic gradient between the plasma and ocular fluids (90). Those agents which are confined to the extracellular fluid space, such as mannitol, produce greater effect on blood osmolality at the same dosage than do agents distributed in total body water (90). Hyperosmotic agents which rapidly penetrate the eye (eg, alcohol) have less effect than those which penetrate slowly or not at all (eg, mannitol) (90). Intravenously administered drugs produce a faster, somewhat greater effect than oral agents. Palatability may be a problem with oral agents and can be improved by serving these agents over crushed ice or with lemon juice or cola flavoring.

Primary side effects of hyperosmotic agents include headache, nausea, vomiting, diuresis and dehydration. It is important that the patient who complains of headache not be allowed to drink, as this will counteract the osmotic effects of these agents. Precipitation of pulmonary edema and CHF have been reported with hyperosmotic agents (91,92), and an allergic reaction has been reported with mannitol (93).

OCULAR SIDE EFFECTS OF SYSTEMIC MEDICATIONS

14. B.C., a 58-year-old male, has a two-year history of hypertension which has been managed with hydrochlorothiazide 50 mg and reserpine 0.25 mg daily. He takes chlorpheniramine 12 mg bid prn allergies. One week ago, chlorpromazine 25 mg tid was added to his medication regimen. He complains of occasional blurred vision and red eyes. Could these symptoms be related to his medications?

Thiazide diuretics have been associated with acute myopia that may last from 24 to 48 hours (94,95). However, hydrochlorothiazide should be considered an unlikely cause of B.C.'s blurred vision.

The primary ocular side effect associated with chlorpromazine is deposits on the lens. These deposits are rare when the total dose of chlorpromazine is less than 0.5 kg (94,95). During the past week of therapy, B.C. could have received a maximum of 525 mg, assuming the medication was taken as prescribed. When lens deposits occur, they often do not appreciably affect vision (94,95). This, along with the short duration of therapy, would suggest that chlorpromazine lens deposits are not a cause of B.C.'s visual complaints. However, phenothiazines have anticholinergic side ef-

Table 3.

HYPEROSMOTIC AGENTS

Generic	Mode of Admin.	Strength	Onset	Peak	Duration	Dose	Ocular Penetration	Distribution
Urea	IV	30%	30–45 min. (at 90–120 drops/min.)	1 hr.	5–6 hrs.	1–1.5 gm/kg	good	TBW*
Mannitol	IV	5, 10, 15% 20%	30–60 min.	1 hr.	6–8 hrs.	1–2 gm/kg	very poor	E+
Glycerin	PO	50%	10–30 min.	30 min.	4–5 hrs.	1–1.5 gm/kg	poor	E+
Isosorbide	PO	45%	10–30 min.	1 hr.	5 hrs.	1.5–2 gm/kg	good	TBW*
Sodium Ascorbate	IV	20%	70 min.	1–2 hrs.	12 hrs.	2–5 ml/kg	good	TBW*
Ethyl Alcohol	PO	50%				2–3 ml/kg	good	TBW*

*TBW = total body water
+E = extracellular water

Urea—(Ureaphil) Abbott, (Urevert) Travenol
Mannitol—(Osmitrol 5,10,15,20%), Travenol
Glycerin—(Glyrol 75%), CooperVision, (Osmoglyn 50%), Alcon
Isosorbide—(Ismotic 45%), Alcon

fects, and the blurred vision may be associated with mydriasis produced by the chlorpromazine.

B.C. may be one of the approximately 1% of the population that experiences blurred vision secondary to chlorpheniramine. This effect has been seen in patients receiving 12–14 mg/day (94,95). The redness is most likely due to the reserpine, which commonly causes flushing of the eyes secondary to dilation of conjunctival blood vessels (94,95).

Table 4 outlines some of the more common ocular side effects associated with systemic medications. Each case should be individually evaluated and alternative therapy considered in intolerant patients.

Table 4.

OCULAR SIDE EFFECTS OF SYSTEMIC MEDICATIONS

Drug Class	Effect(s)	Clinical Remarks	Reference

Analgesics
  narcotics, including
  pentazocine
	miosis	Miosis is seen most often with morphine in normal doses and is slight with other agents. The effect is secondary to CNS action on the pupilloconstrictor center.	94,95

	tearing irregular pupils paresis of accommodation diplopia	These effects are associated with narcotic withdrawal.	94,95

Anticholinergics
  atropine, dicyclomine, glycopyrrolate
  propantheline, trihexyphenidyl
	mydriasis
	cycloplegia
	decreased
	  accommodation
	photophobia
		Systemic anticholinergic agents may cause mydriasis, and less frequently cycloplegia. The mydriasis has been associated with precipitation of angle-closure glaucoma. Photophobia is related to the mydriasis. Patients may also complain of decreased accommodation for near objects.	94,95

Anticonvulsants phenytoin	nystagmus ataxia	Effects have been seen in patients with high blood levels (greater than 20 mcg/ml), and occur rarely with other hydantoins.	94,95
trimethadione	visual glare	A prolonged glare, or dazzle, occurs when eyes are exposed to light. The glare is reversible, occurs at the retinal level, and is more common in adolescents and adults while occurring rarely in young children.	94,95
Antihistamines chlorpheniramine	blurred vision	Blurred vision occurs rarely, in approximately one percent of patients taking 12–14 mg per day.	94,95

	mydriasis,
	  decreased
	  lacrimal secretions
		These effects occur rarely.	94,95

Table 4. (continued)

OCULAR SIDE EFFECTS OF SYSTEMIC MEDICATIONS

Drug Class	Effect(s)	Clinical Remarks	Reference
Antihypertensives			
clonidine	miosis	Miosis is seen in overdose.	96
	dry, itchy eyes	These effects occur rarely.	96
diazoxide	lacrimation	About 20% of patients treated with diazoxide experience lacrimation that may continue after the drug is discontinued.	94
guanethidine	miosis ptosis conjunctivitis blurred vision	These effects are sporadically documented. One study reported a 17% incidence of blurred vision in patients taking 70 mg guanethidine per day.	94,95
reserpine	miosis	Miosis is slight, but has been reported to last up to one week following administration of a single dose.	94,95
	conjunctivitis	Flushing of eyes is common, secondary to dilation of conjunctival blood vessels.	94,95
Anti-infectives			
chloramphenicol	optic neuritis	This effect is rare unless a total dose of 100 grams and duration of administration of six weeks are exceeded. Vision improves in most patients following discontinuation of the drug.	94,95
chloroquine	corneal deposits	Corneal deposits develop within a few months in a moderate proportion of patients receiving ordinary doses of the drug. The deposits are visible with use of a biomicroscope, appear as white-yellow in color, but are of no consequence.	94,95
	retinopathy (macular degeneration)	Serious retinopathy has been caused by taking greater than 250 mg chloroquine diphosphate or 200 mg chloroquine sulfate per day to an amount exceeding 100 grams. Usual development follows treatment for periods of one to three years, but may be seen in six months. Visual loss may be peripheral, with progression to central vision loss and disturbance of color vision. Rarely effects such as blurred vision are seen earlier in patients receiving larger doses (500–700 mg/day). Macular changes may progress following discontinuation because these agents concentrate in pigmented tissue.	94,95

Table 4. (continued)

OCULAR SIDE EFFECTS OF SYSTEMIC MEDICATIONS

Drug Class	Effect(s)	Clinical Remarks	Reference
ethambutol	retrobulbar neuritis	At doses of 15 mg/kg/day, ethambutol is virtually void of ocular side effects. Such effects are rare at doses of 25 mg/kg/day for a duration of a few months. Patients treated for prolonged periods should have routine visual examinations including visual fields. Most effects are reversible following discontinuation of the drug.	94,95
gentamicin	pseudotumor cerebri	Pseudotumor cerebri with secondary papilledema and visual loss appears to occur rarely, but has been well documented.	94,95
isoniazid	optic neuritis	Incidence is not well defined, but appears to be significantly less than peripheral neuritis. Evaluation is difficult since most patients are malnourished, chronic alcoholics or receiving multiple medications. Preexisting eye disease does not appear to be a disposing factor.	94,95
nalidixic acid	visual sensations	This is the most common ocular effect associated with nalidixic acid, and the main feature is a brightly colored appearance of objects. This occurs soon after the drug is taken.	94,95
	visual loss	A temporary effect, visual loss may last from one-half hour up to 72 hours.	94,95
	papilledema	This occurs primarily in infants and young children, and is secondary to increased intracranial pressure. The effects are reversible upon withdrawal of the drug.	94,95
sulfonamides	myopia	Myopia is acute and reversible, and is the most common ocular effect seen with systemic sulfonamides.	94,95
	conjunctivitis	Primarily seen with sulfathiazole, occurring in about 4% of patients between the fifth and ninth day of therapy.	94,95
	optic neuritis	Optic neuritis has been reported, even in low dosages. It is usually reversible with complete recovery of vision.	94,95
tetracyclines	myopia	Myopia appears to be acute, transient and rare.	94,95

Table 4. (continued)

Ocular Side Effects of Systemic Medications

Drug Class	Effect(s)	Clinical Remarks	Reference
	papilledema	Papilledema has been reported, more frequently in children and in infants than in adults, and is rare.	94,95
Anti-inflammatory agents			
ibuprofen	decreased vision	Decreased vision and changes in color vision have been rarely reported.	94
indomethacin	decreased vision	Decreased vision and changes in color vision have been rarely reported.	94,95
phenylbutazone	decreased vision	Decreased vision is the most common ocular side effect of phenylbutazone and may be due to increased lens hydration.	94,95
	conjunctivitis retinal hemorrhage	These effects occur less frequently. The conjunctivitis may be associated with development of Stevens-Johnson syndrome or an allergic reaction.	94,95
Anti-neoplastic agents			
busulfan	cataracts	Cataracts have been seen in patients treated with high doses of busulfan.	94,95
doxorubicin	conjunctivitis excessive tearing	These effects may last for several days following treatment.	94,95
fluorouracil	ocular irritation lacrimation	These are the most common ocular effects, which are reversible and seldom interfere with continued therapy.	94,95
vinca alkaloids (especially vincristine)	extraocular muscle paresis ptosis	The onset of extraocular muscle paresis or paralysis may be seen as early as two weeks after therapy is initiated. These effects are dose-related and most patients obtain full recovery following discontinuation of the agent.	94,95
Barbiturates	miosis mydriasis disturbances in ocular movement ptosis	Most significant ocular side effects of barbiturates are seen in chronic users or in toxic states. Pupillary responses are variable, with miosis seen most frequently except in toxicity when mydriasis predominates. Nystagmus and weakness in extraocular muscles may be seen. Chronic abusers have a characteristic ptosis.	94,95

Table 4. (continued)

OCULAR SIDE EFFECTS OF SYSTEMIC MEDICATIONS

Drug Class	Effect(s)	Clinical Remarks	Reference
Corticosteroids	cataracts	Development of posterior subcapsular cataract has been associated with systemic corticosteroid therapy. The incidence of cataract formation is increased in patients who have received greater than 15 mg prednisone or its equivalent daily for periods exceeding one year.	94,95
	increased intra-ocular pressure	Though this effect has been reported more extensively with topical corticosteroid preparations, it has been associated with systemic therapy. This appears to be of little consequence in patients without preexisting glaucoma and glaucoma patients should be routinely monitored if receiving systemic corticosteroids.	94,95
	papilledema	Intracranial hypertension or pseudotumor cerebri from systemic corticosteroids has been well reported. The incidence appears to be greater in children than in adults, and is primarily associated with chronic therapy.	94,95
Digitalis	altered color vision, visual acuity	Changes in color vision, a glare phenomenon and a snowy appearance in objects have been associated primarily with digitalis intoxication, with a small number of cases with reversible reductions in visual acuity being noted. Digitalis therapy has also been associated with changes in the visual fields.	94,95
	decreased intra-ocular pressure	Digitalis derivatives have been associated with decreases in intraocular pressure, but clinical use for glaucoma is not practical as the required therapeutic systemic dose for this effect is very near the toxic dose.	94,95
Diuretics carbonic anhydrase inhibitors thiazides	myopia	These diuretics have been associated with an acute myopia that may last from 24–48 hours. The myopia is probably caused by an increase in the anteroposterior diameter of the lens which may be reversible even if drug use is continued.	94,95

Table 4. (continued)

OCULAR SIDE EFFECTS OF SYSTEMIC MEDICATIONS

Drug Class	Effect(s)	Clinical Remarks	Reference
Estrogens clomiphene	blurred vision mydriasis visual sensations visual field changes	Five to 10% of patients taking clomiphene experience ocular side effects. Blurred vision is the most common effect, though visual sensations such as flashing lights, distortion of images and various colored lights (primarily silver) may occur.	94,95
oral contraceptives	optic neuritis pseudotumor cerebri retrobulbar neuritis	These effects have been reported in association with oral contraceptives, though the incidence appears to be quite rare. In patients with retinal vascular abnormalities, use of oral contraceptives is questionable. There are numerous other possible ocular side effects associated with these agents and further documentation of these effects is required.	94,95
Phenothiazines chlorpromazine	deposits on the lens	Lens deposits are rare when the total dose of chlorpromazine has been less than 0.5 kg. They become visible after a total dose of 1 kg in most cases and the incidence may increase to 90% after 2.5 kg or more. Usually the deposits do not appreciably affect vision. The cornea and conjunctiva may be affected after the lens shows pigment changes.	94,95
	retinal pigment deposits	Retinal pigment deposits have been reported in patients receiving chlorpromazine, but the number of cases is small and further documentation is necessary.	94,95
thioridazine	pigmentary retino- pathy	The incidence of pigmentary retinopathy is primarily associated with use of maximal daily dosages or average doses that have exceeded 1000 mg. It appears that daily dosages up to 600 mg are relatively safe, while the range between 600–800 mg is uncertain but rarely suspect. If over 800 mg daily are administered, periodic ophthalmoscopic examinations should be made, as changes may be discovered before visual acuity is compromised.	94,95

Table 4. (continued)

OCULAR SIDE EFFECTS OF SYSTEMIC MEDICATIONS

Drug Class	Effect(s)	Clinical Remarks	Reference
Tricyclic antidepressants	mydriasis cycloplegia	The most common ocular side effect of the tricyclic antidepressants is mydriasis. Cycloplegia may rarely occur. There have been reports of precipitation of angle-closure glaucoma.	94,95

OCULAR EMERGENCIES

15. *Chemical Burns.* **A 24-year-old construction worker has splashed an unidentified chemical in his eyes and enters a nearby pharmacy complaining of burning in both eyes. Should the pharmacist attempt to treat the patient or refer him to a hospital emergency room?**

Chemical burns require immediate attention. The immediate treatment is copious irrigation using the most accessible source of water (eg, shower, faucet, drinking fountain, hose, bathtub). After at least five minutes of initial irrigation, the patient should be taken immediately to the emergency room. A water-soaked towel or cloth should be kept on his eyes during transport.

Other Ocular Emergencies

Health care professionals are often approached by patients with acute ocular problems. Before briefly reviewing these conditions, it is necessary to stress that patients should be referred to an ophthalmologist if the practitioner has even the slightest doubt regarding proper therapy. It is generally difficult to effectively evaluate the severity of ocular disorders without the benefit of training or a thorough ophthalmologic work-up.

In addition to chemical burns, there are other cases which can be considered ocular emergencies requiring immediate treatment (1). Included in this listing is corneal trauma from abrasion or foreign bodies. Often the patient will complain of a gritty, scratchy feeling and will be aware of the presence of a foreign body. Patients with corneal ulcers should also immediately see an ophthalmologist. The corneal tissue is an excellent culture medium for bacteria such as *Pseudomonas*

aeruginosa, and therapy should be initiated as soon as possible to avoid corneal perforation and possible loss of the eye (1).

Generally, cases of conjunctivitis are not emergency situations with the exception of gonococcal conjunctivitis. In suspected cases, the patient should see an ophthalmologist to avoid potential corneal perforation (1). Patients with symptoms of red, tender, swollen eyelids with exophthalmos and mild pain may be suffering from orbital cellulitis or endophthalmitis which require immediate treatment with systemic antibiotics.

Signs and symptoms of acute angle-closure glaucoma, an ocular emergency, are reviewed in Question 13. Severe iritis causes extreme pain and photophobia and requires prompt treatment. Visual loss, whether sudden, complete or transient, or flashes of light may signify various potentially damaging ocular disorders including retinal artery occlusion, optic neuritis, amaurosis fugax or retinal detachment, and the patient should be evaluated by an ophthalmologist as soon as possible. Referral is also recommended for patients with pupil disorders, diplopia, nystagmus or ocular hemorrhage.

COMMON OCULAR DISORDERS

Stye (Hordeolum). Sties are infections of the hair follicles or sebaceous glands of the eyelids. The most common infecting organism is *Staphylococcus aureus.* Treatment consists of hot, moist compresses and topical antibiotics (eg, sulfacetamide). Over-the-counter products should not be recommended. Sties that do not respond to warm compresses within a few days should be evaluated by an ophthalmologist.

Conjunctivitis. Conjunctivitis is a common

external eye problem which involves inflammation of the conjunctiva. The symptoms are a diffusely reddened eye with a purulent or serous discharge accompanied by itching, smarting, stinging, or a scratching, "foreign body" sensation. Patients with pain, decreased vision, unequal distribution of redness, irregular pupils, or opacity should receive immediate referral to an ophthalmologist, as these are signs of more serious eye disease.

Conjunctivitis can be bacterial, fungal, parasitic, viral, or allergic in origin. Most cases of bacterial conjunctivitis are caused by *Staphylococcus aureus*, pneumococcus (in temperate climates), or *Haemophilus aegyptius* (in warm climates), although a number of other organisms may be responsible. The infection usually starts in one eye and is spread to the other by the hands. It may be spread to other persons. Unlike bacterial conjunctivitis, corneal infections can rapidly obliterate vision; therefore, accurate diagnosis is important.

16. *Acute Bacterial Conjunctivitis (Pinkeye).* **L.T. is a 6-year-old boy with diffuse bilateral conjunctival redness that has been present for two days. Crusting discharge is deposited on his lashes and the corners of his eyes. His vision is normal, and his pupils are round and equal. The diagnosis of acute bacterial conjunctivitis is made and sodium sulfacetamide 10% ophthalmic drops, two drops in each eye every two hours while awake, are prescribed. What other measures should be employed? What instructions should his parents receive?**

Although treatment of typical bacterial conjunctivitis such as this is empirical, a culture should be obtained. Other ophthalmic antibiotic drops or ointments, such as neomycin-polymixin-B-gramicidin combination (Neosporin), are also used in these situations. Proper management of this infection also includes mechanical cleaning of the eyelids and avoidance of spreading the infection to other children. The deposits should be removed as often as possible with moist cotton swabs or cotton-tipped applicators. A mild baby shampoo can be used to moisten the applicator. Firm adherent crusts may be softened with warm, moist compresses. Because this material is infectious, it should be disposed of in a sanitary fashion. The common use of washcloths by several individuals will spread the bacterial conjunctivitis.

17. *Allergic Conjunctivitis.* **A 10-year-old girl has had redness of both eyes accompanied by hay fever for the past two months (June and July). There is no crusting on her eyelids and her vision is normal; she rubs her eyes frequently. What treatments are available?**

Topical vasoconstrictors may be used to treat the hyperemia, but they should not be used excessively since rebound congestion may occur. Antihistamine tablets or syrup will give considerable but temporary relief. The ideal treatment would be removal of the allergen, but this is usually impossible with seasonal allergies. Topical corticosteroids provide dramatic relief, but their use must be limited because of potential adverse effects (see below). Sodium cromoglycate (2% drops) may be effective as an alternative for those who fail to respond to normal treatment for allergic conjunctivitis.

OPHTHALMIC CORTICOSTEROIDS

The various topical ophthalmic corticosteroid preparations are described in Table 5. The salt form affects the ability of the preparation to penetrate the cornea; biphasic salts penetrate the intact cornea better than water-soluble salts. However, ability to penetrate through the cornea does not indicate increased therapeutic effectiveness. Prednisolone acetate 1% has been shown to have the longest half-life in the cornea and aqueous humor and the best anti-inflammatory effect based upon a measured decrease in corneal infiltration of radiolabeled polymorphonuclear leukocytes (102–104).

18. *Increased IOP.* **L.P. has been treated with topical prednisolone acetate 1%, one drop OU qid for eight weeks. Prior to therapy, IOP measured 16 mm Hg OU, but on the last follow-up visit, readings were 26 mm Hg OD and 28 mm Hg OS. Comment.**

Armalay (105) and Becker (106) have shown that three genetically distinct subgroups of random populations respond with various increases in IOP associated with the administration of topical corticosteroid preparations (see Table 6). Although corticosteroid-induced increases in IOP are associated most frequently with topical preparations, systemic corticosteroids may cause a similar response, though somewhat lesser in magnitude (107). It appears that topical corticosteroids

Table 5.
CORTICOSTEROIDS FOR OPHTHALMIC USE

Generic	Salt form	Strength	Dosage Form	Trade Name	Mfg.	% decrease in corneal inflammation		half-life (min)	
						epithelium intact	epithelium absent	cornea	aqueous
Cortisone	acetate	0.5,1, 1.5%	suspension	none known	none				
	acetate	1.5%	ointment	none known	none				
Dexamethasone	alcohol	0.1%	suspension	Maxidex	Alcon	40	42	90	145
	Na phosphate	0.1%	solution	Decadron	MSD	19	22	60	89
	Na phosphate	0.05%	ointment	Maxidex	Alcon	12	unknown		
				Decadron	MSD				
Fluorometholone		0.1%	suspension	FML	Allergan	31	37		
Hydrocortisone		0.2%	solution	Optef	Upjohn				
	acetate	0.5%	solution	Eye-Cort	Mallard				
	acetate	1.5%	ointment	Hydrocortone	MSD				
Medrysone		1%	suspension	HMS	Allergan				
Prednisolone	acetate	0.12%	suspension	Econopred	Alcon	26	30	89	136
				Pred Mild	Allergan				
	acetate	0.25%	suspension	Predulose	Softcon				
	acetate	1%	suspension	Econopred Plus	Alcon	51	53	112	156
				Pred Forte	Allergan				
	Na phosphate	0.12%	solution	Inflamase	CooperVision	23	42	44	85
	Na phosphate	0.5%	solution	Hydeltrasol	MSD				
				Metreton	Schering				
	Na phosphate	1%	solution	Inflamase Forte	CooperVision	28	47	49	85
	Na phosphate	0.25%	ointment	Hydeltrasol	MSD				

Table 6.

IOP RESPONSE TO TOPICAL STEROIDS IN RANDOM POPULATION

Author	Parameter of Response	No. of Subjects	Low	Medium	High	Mean
Armalay (1965)	Increase of pressure in eye medicated with 0.1% dexamethasone	80	≤5 mm Hg	6–15 mm Hg	≥16 mm Hg	5.5 mm Hg
			66%	29%	5%	
Becker (1965)	Final pressure in eye medicated for 6 wks with 0.1% bethamethasone	50	≤19 mm Hg	20–30 mm Hg	≥32 mm Hg	17.0 mm Hg
			70%	26%	4%	
	Time to maximum response		2 wks.	4 wks.	4 wks.	

exert their effects by decreasing aqueous humor outflow, while systemic corticosteroids may increase aqueous humor production (107). The effects on IOP are apparently not related to the ability of the corticosteroid to penetrate the cornea. Dexamethasone has been associated with the greatest IOP increase (108). Fluorometholone and medrysone are less potent topical corticosteroids and have been associated with a lesser, though sometimes significant, increase in IOP (109). The pressure response is almost uniformly reversible upon discontinuation of the offending agent.

Cataracts

Both oral and topical corticosteroids may cause cataracts. Available data (110,111) show an approximate 23% incidence of posterior subcapsular cataract (PSC) formation in patients treated with 10–16 mg/day of prednisone orally or its equivalent for one year or more. There is an estimated 70% or greater occurrence of PSC in patients treated with dosages in excess of 16 mg/day over the same time period. Patients receiving less than 10 mg/day of prednisone or its equivalent are unlikely to develop PSC, although some contend that the concept of a "safe" dose should be abandoned because of variable patient sensitivity to this side effect (173). In most cases, the cataracts cause few subjective complaints and little measurable decrease in visual acuity. Though systemic corticosteroids are primarily implicated, use of topical corticosteroids has also been associated with the formation of PSC (112). Patients treated with every-other-day corticosteroid dosing may be at a lower risk for formation of PSC (113). Any patient receiving long-term corticosteroids should have routine ophthalmic follow-up.

SYSTEMIC SIDE EFFECTS FROM OPHTHALMIC MEDICATION

19. J.F. a 62-year-old female, received one drop of phenylephrine 10% in each eye, to dilate the pupils. Shortly after administration, her blood pressure increased to 210/130 mm Hg for five minutes and she became confused. Are reactions of this type common in patients receiving topical phenylephrine? Have other topical medications been associated with systemic effects?

One group of investigators (114) reported 33 cases of possible adverse effects associated with topical phenylephrine 10%. However, when phenylephrine 10% or tropicamide (Mydriacyl) 1% was administered to 150 patients in a double-blind study, no statistically significant difference between experimental and control groups with respect to blood pressure or pulse rate was observed (115). Care should be taken when phenylephrine 10% is administered in patients with hypertension or cardiac abnormalities, where systemic absorption could be hazardous. No similar reports have been associated with topical use of phenylephrine 2.5%.

In addition to the previously mentioned systemic effects of cholinergics (Question 3), epinephrine (Question 2) and timolol (Question 2), side effects such as psychosis have been associated with topical atropine (116), cyclopentolate (Cyclogyl) (117), and scopolamine (118). There have been reports of death in association with topical atropine (116). Ataxia has been seen with use of homatropine (119), while only a single report of unconsciousness has been associated with the use of tropicamide (120).

Topical chloramphenicol-polymyxin-B sulfate

ophthalmic ointment has been associated with bone marrow aplasia following intermittent use for four months (121). A Cushingoid reaction has been reported in a two and one-half year-old female treated with topical dexamethasone alcohol (Maxidex) qid, OU for a period of 14 months (122).

INTRAOCULAR PENETRATION OF ANTIBIOTICS

Topical antibiotics are used to control the majority of ocular infections. In intraocular infections, systemic antibiotics may be administered. Many studies dealing with intraocular penetration of antibiotics have been performed on rabbits, but little human data are available. Table 7 summarizes the penetration into the aqueous humor of several antibiotics. Subconjunctival administration achieved therapeutic levels with the greatest regularity. Ocular inflammation was reported to increase penetration in some instances. With rare exception, intravitreal penetration was insignificant or non-existent.

CONTACT LENS SOLUTIONS

The first contact lenses to be designed and prescribed were made of glass in 1888 by Eugene Fick. The corneal contact lens made of plastic (hard and soft) was first prepared by Kevin Touly in 1947 (138). Of the 100 million Americans who must wear corrective lenses, approximately 20% use contact lenses. There are over 70 products on the market for use with hard and soft contact lenses. The most comprehensive list of ingredients of products may be found in the *Handbook of Non-Prescription Drugs* (139) and in Krezanoski's review of soft lenses and their solutions (167).

Corneal lenses have a diameter of about 9 mm and float on the precorneal tear film. They are available in both hard and soft form, though the hard lenses are still the most commonly used. When properly fitted they may be worn all day, but should be removed before sleeping. Corneal contact lenses are used for cosmetic and occupational purposes (athletics, steamy work areas) and for the correction of refractive errors when spectacle lenses are not sufficient (cataracts). They are also used to correct unilateral aphakia where the greater discrepancy in image size created by

spectacle lenses interferes with binocular vision (139,140).

Hard Contact Lens Care

The majority of hard contact lenses are made of polymethylmethacrylate (PMMA). Another resin used is a polymerized product of acrylic acid esters (141). PMMA is not reactive to weak alkalis or acids but is reactive to strong acids and to some solvents, an important factor in the cleaning of contact lenses. The three most important physical properties of PMMA include its hardness, optical quality, and hydrophobic nature.

PMMA has a hardness of 3.0 compared to glass (4.5–6.5) and diamond (10.0). Hard contact lenses are more susceptible to scratching than even the poorest grade of glass lenses. Therefore, they require careful cleaning, storage, and handling. In terms of its optical characteristics, PMMA has outstanding clarity which allows for 90–92% light transmission. This is the same as untinted spectacle lenses. Because it is hydrophobic, only 0.4% water is absorbed over a 24-hour period at 20°C (138,139).

There are two other materials which are used for hard lenses. Cellulose acetate butyrate (CAB) has a light transmission of 88% and also has a higher gas permeability than PMMA lenses. The other type of material used is a combination of PMMA and silicone. The term "silicone lens" is a generic name for contact lenses containing an amount of polysiloxane. This combination produces a lens material which is more flexible and has a higher gas permeability. These two types of lenses are also referred to as HGP (hard gas permeable) lenses (142,143).

When patients receive their contact lenses, they are instucted by the ophthalmologist, optician or optometrist on the proper care of the lenses. Topics discussed with the patient include:

    a. Cleaning of the hard contact lenses;
    b. Proper storage and soaking;
    c. Method of wetting hard contact lenses;
    d. Differences in the solution types that coincide with the three above-mentioned functions.

The solutions used for these purposes are described in Table 9 and the questions which follow.

20. *Cleaning.* M.W. is wearing hard contact lenses for the first time. Is it necessary for him to clean the lenses daily?

Hard contact lenses should be cleaned with a cleaning solution at least once weekly, or more often depending upon the personal hygiene, occupation and rate of protein and contaminant production of the wearer. The purpose of the cleaning solution is to remove any mucus, lipid, or debris from the lens surface. The patient can detect the materials on the lens by visual inspection, touch and/or eye comfort. Cloudy vision would also indicate that the lenses need to be cleaned. The patient should begin by cleaning the hard lenses daily and adjusting the schedule based on the degree of contamination on the lens. If the patient is not sure, he should take the lenses in

Table 7.

INTRAOCULAR PENETRATION OF ANTIBIOTICS

Drug	Dose	Route	Subject	Concentration[1] Primary Aqueous	Secondary Aqueous	Ref.
Ampicillin	75 mg/kg	IV	Rabbit	4.75 mcg/ml (at 1 hour)	9.6 mcg/ml[2]	123
	100 mg	Subconj.	Rabbit	1000 mcg/ml (at 1 hour)		123
Methicillin	75 mg/kg	IV	Rabbit	0.63 mcg/ml	3.5 mcg/ml[2]	123
	various	IV	Human	not detected	not detected	124
	100 mg	Subconj.	Rabbit	166.5 mcg/ml (at 1 hour)		123
Oxacillin	75 mg/kg	IV	Rabbit	not detected		123
	100 mg	Subconj.	Rabbit	145 mcg/ml (at 1 hour)	70 mcg/ml (at 4 hours)	123
Dicloxacillin	50 mg	Subconj.	Rabbit	181 mcg/ml (at 1 hour)		125
Cloxacillin	50 mg/kg	IV	Rabbit	1.5 mcg/gm[3] (at 30 min.)		126
Cephalothin	1 gm	IV	Human		0.55 mcg/ml (at 15 min.)	127
	50 mg	Subconj.	Rabbit	54 mcg/ml (at 1 hour)		128
Cephaloridine	1 gm	IV	Human		28.4 mcg/ml, peak (at 1 hour) 7.31 mcg/ml (at 8 hours)	129
Cephalexin	2 gm	Oral	Human	1.5 mcg/ml (at 2 hours)		130
Cefazolin	25 mg	Subconj.	Rabbit	15.3 mcg/ml (at 1 hour)		131
Lincomycin	600 mg[4]	IM	Human	1–2 mcg/ml		132
Trimethoprim Sulfamethoxazole	160 mg 800 mg	Oral[5]	Human	0.19–0.4 mcg/ml 10–29 mcg/ml		133
Gentamicin	0.2 mg/lb	IM	Rabbit	not detected		134
	10 mg	Subconj.	Rabbit	4.5 mcg/ml (at 2 hours)	12.2 mcg/ml (at 2 hours)	135
Tobramycin	80 mg	IM	Human	0.3 mcg/ml (at 1 hour)		136
	10 mg	Subconj.	Human	18.9 mcg/ml (at 1 hour)		136
Chloramphenicol	50 mg/kg	IV	Rabbit	0.7 mcg/ml (at 1 hour)		137
	10 mg	Subconj.	Rabbit	28 mcg/ml (at 30 min.)		137

[1]Concentrations expressed are as averages unless indicated as a range
[2]Level following paracentesis of the anterior chamber
[3]Level achieved after injection of probenecid prior to the cloxacillin
[4]Total dose of 2.4 gm was administered as 600 mg IM q 4 h prior to sample determination
[5]One evening dose was administered with a second dose the following morning. Samples were drawn following the second dose.

to the optician for inspection at varying intervals of wear. Cleaning solutions contain detergents and preservatives which have surface cleansing action. Because of these detergent-like properties, the lenses should be rinsed thoroughly prior to storage or insertion in the eye. Abrasive cleaners are used by opticians for removing stains and other foreign particles from hard contact lenses. The four basic methods of cleaning hard contact lenses are described in Table 8 (139,141,144,145). Based on cost and efficacy, the hydraulic cleaning method is most often recommended.

21. M.J. is a new contact lens wearer who complains of a burning, stinging sensation when she inserts her lenses, and after 2–4 hours of wear she notices tearing. She also complains of glare and photophobia which occur more frequently than with her glasses. Could the contacts or the contact lens solutions cause this?

Both new lenses and cleaning solutions can cause ocular discomfort. Discomfort may indicate that the new lenses need further adjustment, or discomfort may occur from wearing the lenses too long at first (141). An example of an initial break-

in routine for hard lenses is illustrated in Table 9.

If the patient does not follow these directions, tearing, burning and stinging could result. If the cleaning solution is not rinsed off the lenses thoroughly after cleaning, corneal and lid irritation as well as visual disturbances may develop (146). After the lens has been cleaned, rinsed under the tap and a wetting solution applied, it should be held up to the light and inspected for oil, grease, other foreign material or dry spots. If any of these are observed, the cleaning and wetting process should be repeated (139,141,144,146). If the discomfort continues for several days despite adherence to the break-in schedule and proper care of the lenses, the optician, optometrist or ophthalmologist should be consulted. The tearing and burning sensations usually disappear after the patient has adapted to the hard lenses. Photophobia, which is normal in the initial wearing period, can be remedied by sunglasses (139).

22. *Wetting Solutions.* M.J. (from previous question) asks about the primary functions of a wetting solution and why she needs to use it.

Wetting solutions are used to cushion and lubricate the surfaces between the lens and the cornea as well as the lid. They also provide a viscous protective coating over the lens surface which prevents direct finger contact and the transfer of oily sebaceous deposits from the skin to the lens surface. They convert the hydrophobic lens surface to a hydrophilic surface which is more easily covered by the lacrimal fluid and provide a long-lasting wetted surface (139,144–146).

Table 8.

CLEANING HARD CONTACT LENSES

The four basic methods of cleaning contact lenses are:

Friction Rubbing—the application of a special cleaning solution to the surface of the lens followed by rubbing between the thumb and forefinger. This is the least efficient way to clean lenses, and can result in scratching or warping of the contact lenses.

Spray Cleaning—the contact lenses are placed in perforated unit which is held under a running faucet.

Hydraulic Cleaning—the lenses are placed in a special container which permits a back and forth pumping action through a liquid cleaner. Several studies demonstrated that this method is very efficient in cleaning lenses. However, if the mechanical agitation is performed too vigorously with thin lenses, warpage can result.

Ultrasonic Cleaning—the lenses are placed in a cleaning solution through which ultrasonic waves are passed. This is the most efficient cleaning method, but the cost of the unit makes it impractical for home use.

Reprinted from *U.S. Pharmacist,* February 1977, with permission.

Table 9.

TYPICAL BREAK-IN SCHEDULE FOR HARD CONTACT LENSES

Day	Schedule	Total Hrs
1	2 hr on/2 hr off/2 hr on	4
2	3 hr on/2 hr off/2 hr on	5
3	4 hr on/2 hr off/2 hr on	6
4	6 hr on/2 hr off/2 hr on	8
5	From Day 5 on, increase wear by one hour per day, with one hour rest periods as needed.	

23. M.J. wants to know what wetting solution you would recommend.

The ideal wetting solution should: spread over the entire surface of the lens; form a film that does not wash away easily; be non-irritating and non-sensitizing; not leave a residue on the lens after drying; have a cleansing and antiseptic action; be self-sterilizing; and have the proper degree of viscosity for efficient lubrication (139). All the wetting solutions that are presently available meet the above criteria to some degree. It is very difficult to objectively select a particular product. The different formulations make individual patient acceptance of the product a key factor. One point to be made is not to mix solutions from different manufacturers. The mixing of anionic and cationic agents could inactivate one or both agents and may cause a precipitate (139,146,148,149).

24. Because she was unable to obtain the wetting solution that she had used for four years, B.I. purchased a wetting solution made by another manufacturer. She now complains of ocular discomfort. Could this change in solutions be the cause?

Yes. Solutions from different companies vary in formulation, buffering systems, self-sterilizing capacities and compatibility with solutions from other manufacturers. A patient may experience a burning and stinging sensation when changing wetting solutions due to the differences in formulation (139,141,144–146). Patients should adapt to a new solution after a few days. If not, they should change solution. Initial comfort of a wetting solution depends upon the pH of the solution. The pH of tears is 7.3 and the comfort range of these solutions is between a pH of 6 and 8. The safety range lies between a pH of 4 and 10.

25. A 16-year-old female is seen in the opthalmology clinic with an infected right eye. The culture and sensitivity results indicate that she has a *Pseudomonas* infection. She wears hard contact lenses and other than being out of her wetting solution for several weeks, she has not noted any change in her habits that would cause the infection. What could cause this condition?

The patient has been wearing her contact lenses, but has not been using a wetting solution prior to insertion. It should be determined whether or not the patient has been using saliva as a wetting agent. This is often done by contact lens wearers for expediency, but because it contains many microorganisms transmittable to the eye, saliva should never be used as a wetting solution (it should be noted that 6.6% of the population has *Pseudomonas aeruginosa* as indigenous oral flora) (147). Another source of possible contamination is eye makeup.

26. *Soaking Solutions.* Why must soaking solutions be used in the care of hard contact lenses?

Hard contact lenses should be stored in an appropriate soaking solution whenever they are out of the eye. A soaking solution is used to maintain sterility of the contact lenses; maintain lens hydration and wetability; and leach out (in storage) ocular secretions from lenses and keep protein and mucous particles from drying on the lens surface.

Soaking solutions include bactericidal agents such as benzalkonium chloride and chlorobutanol. EDTA (ethylenediamine tetracetic acid) is added to enhance their effectiveness (148–150). Tests have shown that lenses contaminated with high concentrations of bacteria (*Staphylococcus albus* or *aureus*, *Proteus vulgaris* and *Pseudomonas aeruginosa*) are rendered free of viable bacteria after overnight storage in soaking solutions; lenses stored in tap water or dry storage remained contaminated (148–151). Tap water contains minerals which can deposit on lenses, and distilled water is an excellent medium for bacterial growth; therefore, they are not recommended as storage solutions.

27. How often should a soaking solution be changed? Is one solution better than another?

Soaking solutions should be changed daily. The storage unit used should not contain sponge rubber pads or be made of soft colored plastic, as these may compromise the pH and bactericidal activity of the soaking solution. The following procedures should be followed when using a soaking solution:

a. Fill the container daily
b. Allow the solution to remain for 15 minutes
c. Discard solution
d. Add new solution to container and store lenses (139).

Most commercial solutions are comparable, but solutions from different manufacturers should never be mixed.

Table 10.

Contact Lens Solutions

Hard Lens Products	Purpose	Instructions for Use	Cautions	Ingredients
1. Cleaning Solutions	Use to remove secretions, debris and other foreign bodies from hard contact lenses.	Use cleaning solutions daily or as needed by one of four methods: friction rubbing, hydraulic, spray, or ultrasonic cleaning. After cleaning, rinse lens thoroughly before placing lens in eye.	If lens is not rinsed after cleaning, irritation from the cleaning solution may result. Do not mix solutions from different manufacturers due to incompatabilities. DO NOT USE WITH SOFT LENSES.	Benzalkonium chloride, thimerosal, edetate disodium, chlorobutanol, boric acid, nonionic detergents, other cleaning agents which are not specified by manufacturer
2. Wetting Solutions	Used to convert hydrophobic lens surface to a hydrophilic one. Increase comfort by increasing lubrication, and cushioning effect between the corneal surface and the lens. Protect the lens.	After rinsing the lens, apply the wetting solution to the lens. Hold up to the light to check for complete wetting; rewet if necessary.	Do not use saliva as a wetting solution. Do not mix solutions from different companies. DO NOT USE WITH SOFT LENSES.	Methylcellulose, hydroxypropyl cellulose, polyvinyl alcohol, benzalkonium chloride, edetate disodium, sodium chloride, potassium chloride, chlorobutanol, lipiden polymeric system
3. Soaking Solutions	Used to store hard contact lens and to maintain lens hydration and sterility.	Lenses should be stored in a case with a soaking solution when not in use. Solutions should be changed daily and the lens case cleaned daily.	If tap water or agents other than soaking solutions are used, lens contamination may result. Lenses should be rinsed after taking them out of the soaking solution; otherwise irritation may result. DO NOT USE WITH SOFT LENSES.	Thimerosal, benzalkonium chloride, edetate disodium, polyvinyl alcohol, chlorobutanol
4. Multifunctional Solutions	Used as cleaning, wetting, and/or soaking solutions.	Directions are the same as above, but with modifications since these are combination products.	If possible, it is better to use individual solutions rather than a multifunctional solution. DO NOT USE WITH SOFT LENSES.	Includes all ingredients as listed above.

Soft Lens Products	Purpose	Instructions for Use	Cautions	Ingredients
1. Cleaning Products	Used to clean soft lenses by removal of protein deposits and other debris.	If using a prophylactic cleaner, place 2–3 drops to both the concave and convex lens surfaces and rub for 20–30 seconds between the index finger and thumb. If using papain enzyme cleaner, submerge the lens in the solution for a minimum of four hours. Ideally, should clean with prophylactic cleaner after enzyme cleaner. Rinse thoroughly after cleaning.	Rinse thoroughly after cleaning.	Papain, thimerosal, sorbic acid, edetate disodium, sodium phosphate, sodium chloride, tyloxapol, hydroxyethylcellulose, polyvinyl alcohol, potassium chloride, poloxamer 407
2. Thermal Disinfecting and Rinsing Products	Used to rinse soft lenses after cleaning. Solutions used with thermal disinfection units to disinfect soft lenses.	Use as a rinse after cleaning. Carefully inspect the lens against a light and dark background after rinsing. Allow to air dry for a minute or two after rinsing. Use as directed for thermal disinfection.	Do not use tap water instead of these solutions.	Thimerosal, sorbic acid, sodium chloride, boric acid, sodium borate, edetate disodium, sodium phosphate, poloxamer 407
3. Chemical Disinfecting Solutions	Used to chemically disinfect soft lenses.	Submerge cleaned and rinsed soft lenses in the solution for a minimum of four hours in a closed container. After disinfecting, rinse thoroughly.	Rinse thoroughly to protect lens and to prevent irritation to the eye. Do not use tap water instead of a sterile rinsing solution.	Thimerosal, chlorhexidine, tris (2-hydroxyethyl), tallow ammonium chloride, sodium bicarbonate, sodium phosphate, propylene glycol, polysorbate 80, soluble polylema, sodium chloride, boric acid, edetate disodium, sodium borate
4. Lubricating/ Rewetting Eye Drops	Used to relieve discomfort from prolonged wear and to rehydrate lens while it is in the eye.	Place 1–2 drops in the eye as needed.	Overuse can interfere with the oily layer of the tear film and accelerate lens drying.	Thimerosal, sorbic acid, povidone, polyoxyethylene, edetate disodium, sodium chloride, hydroxyethylcellulose, potassium chloride

28. *Multifunctional Solutions.* J.K. has heard that all-purpose solutions are just as good as the individual solutions and much cheaper. Is this true?

If cost or compliance is a problem, these solutions (also known as multi-purpose, combination or convenience solutions) are a viable alternative. The ideal solution should wet, clean and soak effectively. However, these solutions tend to compromise on one or more of these necessary functions and are not more effective than the individual solutions (151). If the patient will not or cannot afford individual solutions, the all-purpose solution is better than no solution at all.

29. *Cushioning Agents.* Will use of a cushioning agent decrease the discomfort of wearing hard contact lenses?

Cushioning or preinsertion solutions are very viscous (containing polyvinyl pyrollidone or polyvinyl alcohol), and provide a cushioning film over the lens and serve as a wetting solution as well. While the cushioning effect of these agents lasts longer than that of wetting solutions, they do leave a coat or film on the lens if allowed to dry. These agents may cause a blurring of vision for 5–10 minutes after insertion due to their extreme viscosity, but they will decrease discomfort during the breaking-in period with hard contact lenses (141).

30. B.W., who has been a hard contact lens wearer for six years, has been complaining of a burning sensation when she wears her contacts. When questioned it is found that she has not changed solutions, uses three separate solutions, and the contacts themselves are a perfect fit. Her only medication is pseudoephedrine 30 mg tid and chlorpheniramine 8 mg tid. Could these drugs cause this problem?

Yes. Antihistamines and decongestants will decrease lacrimal secretions. The best approach would be to discontinue the medications. However, if this cannot be done, a preinsertion agent (cushioning agent) should be utilized. In patients who have insufficient mucous due to hormonal disturbances or chronic antihistamine use, the use of a preinsertion agent is effective in relieving the burning sensation caused by the tear insufficiency (141).

Soft Contact Lens Care

Soft hydrophilic lenses have been used since they were first described by Wichterle and Lim in 1962. They were introduced in the United States in 1971, although they have been in use in other countries since the early 1960s. The U.S. Food and Drug Administration (FDA) ruled that soft contact lenses would be classified as drugs and require proof of safety and efficacy (hard contact lenses have been exempted from this due to their history of safe use) (152). Most soft contact lenses are made of hydroxymethyl methacrylate (HEMA) and newer soft lenses should be evaluated with reference to the standard material (153).

HEMA absorbs 37–60% of its own weight in water. The refractive index varies from 1.53 (in dry state) to 1.43 (fully hydrated in normal saline) (141). In terms of its optical characteristics, HEMA has a light transmission of 97%. Compared to hard contact lenses, soft lenses can absorb drugs and other ingredients such as buffers and preservatives. Some drugs may discolor the soft contact lens; patients should be warned not to instill ophthalmic medications and to be cautious of cosmetic and hair spray use while the contacts are in the eye. Other disadvantages of soft contact lenses as compared to hard contact lenses include: less clarity of vision, unstable vision when blinking due to the flexibility of the soft lenses, greater susceptibility to damage due to their ability to absorb drugs, problems with cleaning and storage, inability to correct astigmatism (139), greater expense (144,154), and less durability because of their physical properties (144).

Advantages of soft lenses compared to hard lenses are numerous. The soft lens is lost less frequently since it is flexible and adheres rather than "popping off" with impact as do hard lenses. Soft contact lenses closely follow the contour of the eye and provide for better patient comfort. Also, little adjustment is needed after fitting. They are particularly good for occasional wear because of their short break-in time. A typical break-in schedule is illustrated in Table 11.

In general, patients can wear hard contact lenses for up to 12 hours after the break-in period, and soft lenses for up to 18 hours. Since there are no standards for determining success rates for wearing contact lenses, the results of studies vary (155). The sensations produced by

Table 11.

Typical Break-in Schedule for Soft Contact Lenses

Day	Schedule	Total Hrs.
Day 1 & 2	3 hr on/1 hr off/3 hr on/1 hr off/3 hr on	Total 9 hr
Day 3 & 4	4 hr on/1 hr off/4 hr on/1 hr off/4 hr on	Total 12 hr
Day 5 & 6	6 hr on/1 hr off/6 hr on/1 hr off/4 hr on	Total 16 hr

From Day 7 on the patient may wear the lenses 8 hr at a time with 1 hr rest intervals as an optimal use pattern. Some optometrists recommend an even shorter break-in time or eliminate the break-in altogether. This is dependent upon the soft lens and the patient's experience with contacts in the past.

soft lenses are quite similar to those produced by normal eye tissue, thus contributing to the avoidance of the "contact lens look" (frequent blinking, holding the chin up, avoiding quick eye movement) produced by hard contact lenses (152).

The care of soft contact lenses is much different from that of hard contact lenses. Hard contact lens solutions cannot be used with soft lenses. The cleaning and storage of soft contacts will vary with manufacturer. One should ascertain which soft contact lens is being worn before recommending a product. The major considerations in caring for soft lenses concern the cleaning and "sterilizing" of the lenses. It is quite important to remove bacteria and fungi from soft lenses, because these organisms can cause infections and can cause degradation of the lens material through enzymatic processes. The removal of deposits of meibomian oils, mucoproteins, remnants of fungi and calciferous deposits is a particular problem and requires a cleaning process (152).

Soft Lens Cleaning. The major problem encountered by the soft lens wearer is keeping the lens clean. Rubbing and rinsing the lens with normal saline solution has been recommended as the procedure for cleaning soft lenses. However, there are several solutions now available for this purpose. These solutions offer several approaches to removal of protein and other deposits from the lenses. Surfactants and enzymes are two examples. Nonenzymatic cleaning solutions (surface active cleaners) should be used daily by most patients. The enzymatic cleaners may be used with other solutions or alone. If used alone, the enzymatic cleanser is normally used every three days; if used with other cleansers, it is only used once a week. The purpose of cleaning is to remove protein deposits prior to "sterilization" of the lens.

Since the buildup of protein deposits varies among soft lens users, the frequency of cleaning should be determined on an individual basis. Removal and prevention of deposit buildup will not only increase wearing comfort, but will also increase the efficiency of the "sterilization" process (152,157,158,160,161,166).

Soft Lens Sterilization. Since soft lenses must remain hydrated, there is always the possibility that they may furnish a medium that will support bacterial growth if not properly sterilized. Daily sterilization will reduce this possibility. Although "sterilization" may not be an exact description of what is done with the lens, it is the term in general use. It may be more accurate to say that the lens should be disinfected or "ascepticized" on a daily basis.

Heat Sterilization. An effective method for sterilization consists of putting the lens in normal saline in the carrying case and placing the case in boiling water for 15 minutes. Care must be taken to avoid completely boiling away all the water. This technique is somewhat inconvenient; however, there are special heat disinfecting units which allow the process to automatically shut itself off after adequate heat exposure has been accomplished. These units are somewhat cumbersome for travel. If the lens is not adequately cleaned before sterilization, the heat of the boiling water may leave a residue of denatured proteins on the lens. If this occurs repeatedly over a period of time, the useful life of the lens will be shortened. The major pathogens that are most troublesome are *Staphylococcus aureus, Pseudomonas aeruginosa, Bacillus subtilis, Candida albicans* and *Herpes simplex.* Boiling is usually adequate to destroy these organisms; however, spores will not be destroyed by boiling (152,157,166).

After the heat sterilization process has been completed, the lenses are ready to wear. However, they should be rinsed in normal saline prior to insertion.

Cold Sterilization. Cold sterilization relies on a chemical process. At the present time, all FDA approved soft contact lenses can be disinfected by chemicals (139,166). Chlorhexidine- and thiomersalate-preserved saline storage solutions have been used. Studies of the effectiveness of these solutions indicate that chlorhexidine is the more effective but has poor fungicidal activity (139,166). Because thiomersalate is slower acting but is a more effective antifungal, almost all of these products contain both chlorhexidine and thiomersalate. Another method utilizes an iodophore concentrate followed by treatment with thiosulfate neutralizing solution.

Cold sterilization is convenient and portable, initially inexpensive (although heat disinfection is less expensive in the long run), and causes less coagulation of mucoprotein left on the lens than does heat sterilization. However, there is a risk of ocular irritation by solution constituents, the solutions cannot cope with large influxes of microorganisms, the solution method is slow, and some solutions are appropriate only for specific lenses. Thus, each method offers its own advantages and disadvantages.

Soft Lens Storage and Soaking. The solution used for soaking and storage of the soft lens is normal saline. This is necessary to maintain the proper state of hydration and prevent the particular lens characteristics (size, light transmission) from changing. Normal saline solutions should be prepared daily to prevent the possibility of pathogen growth. Lens care kits provide sodium chloride tablets and instructions for solution preparation. Some prepackaged sodium chloride solutions contain thiomersol as a preservative to prevent bacterial growth. Sodium chloride tablets used for the preparation of soaking solutions should be free of additives, adhesives, lubricants or coatings, as these substances may adversely affect soft lenses. Manufactured injectable saline solutions should not be used as soaking solutions since they frequently contain benzalkonium chloride as a preservative (152,157, 166).

31. A patient who is switching from hard to soft contact lenses has several bottles of
solutions for hard lenses. Can he use these hard contact lens solutions with soft contact lenses?

No. All chemicals, including medications, preservatives and buffers tend to bind to the lens surface, causing film formation (157,158,160,166). For this reason, conventional solutions should never be used with soft lenses. Patients should be instructed to read all literature concerning the soft lenses they are purchasing, as various soft lenses require different systems.

32. The patient described above wore hard contact lenses for eight years before switching to soft contact lenses for comfort. He admits that he cared for his hard contact lenses in a somewhat haphazard manner. What points should be emphasized regarding the care of his new soft contact lenses?

Cleaning. A regular cleaning schedule is important. Daily cleaning (with normal saline or a surface active cleaner) prevents bacterial contamination and lens damage from mucous build-up, dirt, cosmetics and other environmental contaminants (161). It also aids in the sterilization process. Enzymatic cleaners can be used on a weekly basis in conjunction with other cleaning solutions. Some investigators feel that invisible as well as visible protein deposits may cause allergic reactions if enzymatic cleaners are not used (162). However, daily enzymatic cleaning is not recommended, because absorption into the lens may be enhanced and eye irritation may result. Furthermore, it has been postulated that enzyme cleaners may shorten lens life. There are many soft contact lens cleaning products, and some are intended for specific soft lenses. The manufacturer's recommendations should be followed.

Disinfection. Whether a heat sterilization process or a cold, chemical sterilization process is used, daily disinfection is essential to prevent microorganism growth within the soft contact lenses.

Storage. Soft contact lenses will dehydrate and become brittle if they are left exposed to the air. Thus, failure to store soft contact lenses in normal saline may result in ruined lenses. Hard contact lenses should also be stored in a soaking solution (as described in Questions 26 & 27), but if accidentally left on the counter overnight, they require only cleaning and rehydration. If soaking solution for hard lenses is not available, they can be stored in distilled water (as a short-term measure), but soft contact lenses will become sticky if stored in hypotonic solutions or water. Soft contact lenses are also more susceptible to contamination if not stored properly (139,144,156–158,162).

33. A patient falls asleep while wearing his soft contact lenses. When he awakes he cannot remove the soft lens. What can the patient do?

The soft contact lenses are hydrophilic and unless there is proper hydration they may adhere to the cornea. In this case, rehydration using artificial tears or normal saline will probably loosen the lens. If not, the patient should be referred to his optometrist, ophthalmologist or emergency room.

34. T.D. wants to know if there is a contact lens that can be worn for an extended period of time.

Yes. In January 1981 the FDA approved the marketing of extended wear soft lenses for general use. Prior to this, they had only been approved for use by patients who had undergone cataract surgery. The extended wear lenses are recommended for patients who cannot or don't want to remove, clean and disinfect soft lenses on a daily basis. These lenses have been approved only for nearsightedness due to the need for a thin, high water-content lens (farsightedness requires a thicker lens which would not have as high a water-content). The higher water-content lenses allow oxygen to reach the cornea which is essential for extended wear (167).

35. F.E. has been diagnosed as having bacterial conjunctivitis and sulfacetamide 10% drops have been prescribed. Will his use of soft contact lenses cause any problems? Can any medications be used with soft contact lenses in place?

Medication absorption may be hindered by contact lenses. Failure to remove the lenses may also produce a film of medication on the lenses which may cause blurred vision and damage the lenses.

An important exception is pilocarpine. Administration of pilocarpine to patients wearing soft contact lenses resulted in a prolongation of the drug's effect (159,165). Soft lenses soaked in pilocarpine have also been used effectively in the treatment of glaucoma. This form of treatment is not used for all patients due to cost and annoyance of the system. It is often used in glaucoma secondary to trauma, inflammation and related disorders (159,164,165).

References

1. Vaughan D et al: *General Ophthalmology,* 9th ed, Lange Medical Publications, Los Altos, 1980.
2. Chandler PA et al: *Glaucoma,* 2nd ed, Lea and Febiger, Philadelphia, 1979.
3. Scheie HG et al: *Adler's Textbook of Ophthalmology,* 8th ed, WB Saunders, Philadelphia, 1969.
4. Kolker AE et al: *Becker-Shaffer's Diagnosis and Therapy of the Glaucomas,* 4th ed, CV Mosby, St. Louis, 1976.
5. Grant WM: Action of drugs on movement of ocular fluids. In *Annual Review of Pharmacology,* 9th vol, Annual Reviews, Inc., Palo Alto, 1969, p 85.
6. Grant WM: Ocular complications of drugs. JAMA. 1969; 207:2089.
7. Grant WM: Systemic drugs and adverse influence on ocular pressure. In *Symposium on Ocular Therapy,* 3rd vol, CV Mosby, St. Louis, 1968, p 57.
8. Davies DM editor: *Textbook of Adverse Drug Reactions,* Oxford University Press, New York, 1977.
9. Dukes M: *Meyler's Side Effects of Drugs,* Annual 1, Excerpta Medica, Amsterdam, 1977, p 363.
10. Kirsch R: Glaucoma following cataract extraction associated with use of alpha-chymotrypsin. Arch Ophthalmol. 1964; 72:612.
11. Sugar S: The ten commandments for management of primary open-angle glaucoma. Ann Ophthalmol. 1979; 11:783.
12. Zimmerman T et al: Timolol and facility of outflow. Invest Ophthalmol Vis Sci. 1977; 16:623.
13. Sonntag JR et al: Effect of timolol therapy on outflow facility. Invest Ophthalmol Vis Sci. 1978; 17:293.
14. Yablonski ME et al: A fluorophotometric study of the effect of topical timolol on aqueous humor dynamics. Exper Eye Res. 1978; 27:135.
15. Zimmerman TJ et al: Timolol: dose response and duration of action. Arch Ophthalmol. 1977; 95:605.
16. Boger WP et al: Long-term experience with timolol ophthalmic solution in patients with open-angle glaucoma. Ophthalmology. 1978; 85:259.
17. Heel RC et al: Timolol: a review of its therapeutic efficacy in the topical treatment of glaucoma. Drugs. 1979; 17:38.
18. Boger WP: The treatment of glaucoma: role of beta-blocking agents. Drugs. 1979; 18:25.
19. Boger WP et al: Clinical trial comparing timolol ophthalmic solution to pilocarpine in open-angle glaucoma. Am J Ophthalmol. 1978; 86:8.

20. Moss AP et al: A comparison of the effects of timolol and epinephrine on intraocular pressure. Am J Ophthalmol. 1978; 86:489.

21. Hass I et al: Comparison between pilocarpine and timolol on diurnal pressure in open-angle glaucoma. Arch Ophthalmol. 1980; 98:480.

22. Britman NA: Cardiac effects of topical timolol. N Engl J Med. 1979; 300:566.

23. Kim JW et al: Timolol-induced bradycardia. Anesthesia and Analgesia. 1980; 59:301.

24. McMahon CD et al: Adverse effects experienced by patients taking timolol. Am J Ophthalmol. 1979; 88:736.

25. Guzman CA: Exacerbation of bronchorrhea induced by topical timolol. Am Rev Respir Dis. 1980; 121:899.

26. Jones FC et al: Exacerbation of asthma by timolol. N Engl J Med. 1979; 301:270.

27. Schmitt CJ et al: Penetration of timolol into the rabbit eye. Arch Ophthalmol. 1980; 98:547.

28. Affrime MB et al: Dynamics and kinetics of ophthalmic timolol. Clin Pharmacol Ther. 1980; 27:471.

29. Ballin N et al: Systemic effects of epinephrine applied topically to the eye. Invest Ophthalmol. 1966; 5:125.

30. Drance S: Comparison of action of cholinergic and anticholinesterase agents in glaucoma. Invest Ophthalmol. 1966; 5:130.

31. Alpar JJ: Miotics and retinal detachment. Ann Ophthalmol. 1979; 11:395.

32. Ellis PP: Systemic effects of locally applied anticholinesterase agents. Invest Ophthalmol. 1966; 5:146.

33. Hiscox PEA et al: Cardiac arrest occurring in a patient on echothiophate iodide therapy. Am J Ophthalmol. 1965; 60:425.

34. Harris LS: Dose response analysis of echothiophate iodide. Arch Ophthalmol. 1971; 86:502.

35. Kellerman L et al: Preliminary observations on the use of new concentrations of echothiophate iodide in the treatment of glaucoma. Am J Ophthalmol. 1966; 62:278.

36. Atchoo PD et al: Phospholine iodide (0.03%) in the therapy of glaucoma. Am J Ophthalmol. 1966; 62:1044.

37. Chin NB et al: Iris cysts and miotics. Arch Ophthalmol. 1964; 71:611.

38. Shaffer R et al: Anticholinesterase drugs and cataracts. Am J Ophthalmol. 1966; 62:613.

39. deRoetth A: Lens opacities in glaucoma patients on phospholine iodide therapy. Am J Ophthalmol. 1966; 62:619.

40. Axelsson U et al: The frequency of cataract after miotic therapy. Acta Ophthalmol. 1966; 44:421.

41. Wahl JW et al: Echothiophate iodide. Am J Ophthalmol. 1965; 60:419.

42. deRoetth A et al: Blood cholinesterase activity of glaucoma patients treated with phospholine iodide. Am J Ophthalmol. 1966; 62:834.

43. Pantuck EF: Echothiophate iodide eye drops and prolonged response to suxamethonium. Br J Anesthesia. 1966; 38:406.

44. Gesztes T: Prolonged apnoea after suxamethonium injection associated with the eye drops containing an anticholinesterase agent. Br J Anesthesia. 1966; 38:408.

45. Quinby G: Further therapeutic experience with pralidoximes in organic phosphorous poisoning. JAMA. 1964; 187:202.

46. Goldberg I et al: Timolol and epinephrine. A clinical study of ocular interactions. Arch Ophthalmol. 1980; 98:484.

47. Thomas JV: Ocular adrenergic receptor sites pertinent to aqueous humor dynamics. Ann Ophthalmol. 1980; 12:96.

48. Boger WP: Beta adrenergic blocking agents and glaucoma. J CE Ophthalmol. 1978; 40:14.

49. Smith R et al: Addition of timolol maleate to routine medical therapy: A clinical trial. Br J Ophthalmol. 1980; 64:779.

50. Corwin ME et al: Conjunctival melanin depositions. Arch Ophthalmol. 1963; 69:317.

51. Cleasby G et al: Epinephrine pigmentation of the cornea. Arch Ophthalmol. 1967; 78:74.

52. Reinecke RD et al: Corneal deposits secondary to topical epinephrine. Arch Ophthalmol. 1963; 70:170.

53. Mooney D: Pigmentation after long-term topical use of adrenaline compounds. Br J Ophthalmol. 1970; 54:823.

54. Aronson SB et al: Ocular hypersensitivity to epinephrine. Invest Ophthalmol. 1966; 5:75.

55. Flach A et al: Supersensitivity to topical epinephrine after long-term epinephrine therapy. Arch Ophthalmol. 1980; 98:482.

56. Vaughan D et al: A new stabilized form of epinephrine for the treatment of open-angle glaucoma. Arch Ophthalmol. 1961; 66:232.

57. VanBuskirk EM: Corneal anesthesia after timolol maleate thearpy. Am J Ophthalmol. 1979; 88:739.

58. Angelo-Nielsen K: Timolol topically and diabetes mellitus. JAMA. 1980; 244::2263.

59. Shavitz S: Timolol and myasthenia gravis. JAMA. 1979; 242:1611.

60. Theodore J et al: External ocular toxicity of dipivalyl epinephrine. Am J Ophthalmol. 1979; 88:1013.

61. Mandell AI et al: Dipivalyl epinephrine. A new prodrug in the treatment of glaucoma. Trans Am Acad Ophthalmol Otolaryngol. 1978; 85:268.

62. Kohn AN et al: Clinical comparison of dipivalyl epinephrine and epinephrine in the treatment of glaucoma. Am J Ophthalmol. 1979; 87:196.

63. Yablonski ME et al: Dipivefrin use in patients with intolerance to topically applied epinephrine. Arch Ophthalmol. 1977; 95:2157.

64. Kaback MB et al: The effects of dipivalyl epinephrine on the eye. Am J Ophthalmol. 1976; 81:768.

65. Stone RA et al: Low-dose methazolamide and intraocular pressure. Am J Ophthalmol. 1977; 83:674.

66. Galin MA et al: Acetazolamide and outflow facility. Arch Ophthalmol. 1966; 76:493.

67. Thomas RP et al: Acetazolamide and ocular tension. Am J Ophthalmol. 1965; 60:241.

68. Pepys MB: Acetazolamide and renal stone formation. Lancet. 1970; 1:837.

69. Parfitt AM: Acetazolamide and sodium bicarbonate-induced nephrocalcinosis and nephrolithiasis. Arch Intern Med. 1969; 124:736.

70. Wallace TR et al: Decreased libido-a side effect of carbonic anhydrase inhibitors. Ann Ophthalmol. 1979; 11:1563.

71. Werblin TP et al: Aplastic anemia and agranulocytosis in patients using methazolamide for glaucoma. JAMA. 1979; 241:2817.

72. Ross RA et al: Effects of topically applied isoproterenol on aqueous dynamics in man. Arch Ophthalmol. 1979; 83:39.

73. Krupin T et al: Effect of prazosin on aqueous humor dynamics in rabbits. Arch Ophthalmol. 1980; 98:1639.

74. Ohrstrom A et al: Long-term treatment of glaucoma with systemic propranolol. Am J Ophthalmol. 1978; 86:340.

75. Goldberg I et al: Efficacy and patient acceptance of pilocarpine gel. Am J Ophthalmol. 1979; 88:843.

76. Ticho U et al: Piloplex, a new long-acting pilocarpine polymer salt. A: long-term study. Br J Ophthalmol. 1979; 63:45.

77. Zeev M et al: Piloplex, a new long-acting pilocarpine polymer salt. B: comparative study of the visual effects of pilocarpine and piloplex drops. Br J Ophthalmol. 1979; 63:48.

78. Bonomi L et al: Effect of guanethidine and other sympatholytic drugs upon the pupillary response to electrical stimulation of the sympathetic system in rabbits. Am J Ophthalmol. 1965; 61:544.

79. Bonomi L et al: Outflow facility after guanethidine sulfate administration. Arch Ophthalmol. 1967; 78:337.

80. Romano J et al: Evaluation of a 5% guanethidine and 0.5% adrenaline mixture (Ganda 5·05) and of a 3% guanethidine and 0.5% adrenaline mixture (Ganda 3·05) in the treatment of open-angle glaucoma. Br J Ophthalmol. 1979; 63:52.

81. Hoyng FJ et al: The combination of guanethidine 3% and adrenaline 0.5% in 1 eyedrop (GA) in glaucoma treatment. Br J Ophthalmol. 1979; 63:56.

82. Casey TA et al: Oral glycerol in glaucoma. Br Med J. 1963; 2:851.

83. Drance SM: Effect of oral glycerol on intraocular pressure in normal and glaucomatous eyes. Arch Ophthalmol. 1964; 72:491.

84. Barry KG et al: Mannitol and isosorbide. Arch Ophthalmol. 1969; 81:695.

85. Becker B et al: Isosorbide: an oral hyperosmotic agent. Arch Ophthalmol. 1967; 78:147.

86. Obstbaum SA et al: Low-dose oral alcohol and intraocular pressure. Am J Ophthalmol. 1973; 76:926.

87. Adams RE et al: Ocular hypotensive effect of intravenously administered mannitol. Arch Ophthalmol. 1963; 69:55.

88. Smith EW et al: Reduction of human intraocular pressure with intravenous mannitol. Arch Ophthalmol. 1962; 68:734.

89. Hill K et al: Intravenous hypertonic urea in the management of acute angle-closure glaucoma. Arch Ophthalmol. 1961; 65:497.

90. Galin MA et al: Ophthalmological use of osmotic therapy. Am J Ophthalmol. 1966; 62:629.

91. D'Alena P et al: Adverse effects after glycerol orally and mannitol parenterally. Arch Ophthalmol. 1966; 75:201.

92. McCurdy DK et al: Oral glycerol: the mechanism of intraocular hypotension. Am J Ophthalmol. 1966; 61:1244.

93. Spaeth GL et al: Anaphylactic reaction to mannitol. Arch Ophthalmol. 1967; 78:583.

94. Fraunfelder FT: Drug-induced Ocular Side Effects and Drug Interactions, Lea and Febiger, Philadelphia, 1976.

95. Grant WM: Toxicology of the Eye, 2nd ed, Charles C Thomas, Springfield, 1974.

96. Fraunfelder FT executive director: National Registry of Possible Drug-Induced Ocular Side Effects, Annual Reports 1976–1977 and 1977–1978, Department of Ophthalmology, University of Oregon Health Science Center, Portland.

97. Smolin G: Staphylococcal blepharitis. In Current Ocular Therapy, edited by FT Fraunfelder and RF Hampton, WB Saunders, Philadelphia, 1980, p 434.

98. Stein HA et al: The Ophthalmic Assistant: Fundamentals and Clinical Practice, 3rd ed, CV Mosby, St. Louis, 1976.

99. Baum JF: Current concepts in ophthalmology: ocular infections. N Engl J Med. 1978; 299:28.

100. Sabiston DW: The use of antibiotics in ophthalmology. Drugs. 1977; 14:207.

101. Ganley JP: Uveitis. In Current Ocular Therapy, edited by FT Fraunfelder and RF Hampton, WB Saunders, Philadelphia, 1980, p 485.

102. Leibowitz H et al: Bioavailability and effectiveness of topically administered corticosteroids. Trans Am Acad Ophthalmol Otolaryngol. 1975; 79:78.

103. Leibowitz H et al: Anti-inflammatory effectiveness in the cornea of topically administered prednisolone. Invest Ophthalmol. 1974; 13:757.

104. Kupferman A et al: Therapeutic effectiveness of fluorometholone in inflammatory keratitis. Arch Ophthalmol. 1975; 93:1011.

105. Armalay MF: Statistical attributes of the steroid hypertensive response in the clinically normal eye. Invest Ophthalmol. 1965; 4:187.

106. Becker B et al: Glaucoma and corticosteroid provocative testing. Arch Ophthalmol. 1965; 74:621.

107. Godel V et al: Systemic steroids and ocular fluid dynamics II: Systemic versus topical steroids. Acta Ophthalmol. 1972; 50:664.

108. Cantrill HL et al: Comparison of in vitro potency of corticosteroids with ability to raise intraocular pressure. Am J Ophthalmol. 1975; 79:1012.

109. Stewart RH et al: Intraocular pressure response to topically administered fluorometholone. Arch Ophthalmol. 1979; 97:2139.

110. Oglesby RB et al: Cataracts in rheumatoid arthritis patients treated with corticosteroids: Description and differential diagnosis. Arch Ophthalmol. 1961; 66:519.

111. Oglesby RB et al: Cataracts in patients with rheumatic diseases treated with corticosteroids: further observations. Arch Ophthalmol. 1961; 66:625.

112. Yablonski MF et al: Cataracts induced by topical dexamethasone in diabetics. Arch Ophthalmol. 1975; 94:474.

113. Sevel D et al: Lenticular complications of long-term steroid therapy in children with asthma and eczema. J Allergy Clin Immunol. 1977; 60:215.

114. Fraunfelder FT et al: Possible adverse effects from topical ocular 10% phenylephrine. Am J Ophthalmol. 1978; 85:447.

115. Brown MN et al: Lack of side effects from topically administered 10% phenylephrine eye drops: A controlled study. Arch Ophthalmol. 1980; 98:487.

116. Morton HG: Atropine intoxication: its manifestations in infants and children. J Pediatr. 1939; 14:755.

117. Marks HH: Psychotogenic properties of cyclopentolate. JAMA. 1963; 186:430.

118. Freund M et al: Toxic effects of scopolamine eye drops. Am J Ophthalmol. 1970; 70:637.

119. Hoefnagel D: Toxic effects of atropine and homatropine eye drops in children. N Engl J Med. 1961; 264:168.

120. Wahl JW: Systemic reaction to tropicamide. Arch Ophthalmol. 1969; 82:320.

121. Abrams SM et al: Marrow aplasia following topical application of chloramphenicol eye ointment. Arch Int Med. 1980; 140:576.

122. Musson K: Cushingoid status: induced by topical steroid medication. J Pediatr Ophthalmol. 1968; 5:33.

123. Records RE et al: The intraocular penetration of ampicillin, methacillin and oxacillin. Am J Ophthalmol. 1967; 64:135.

124. Records RE: The human intraocular penetration of methicillin. Arch Ophthalmol. 1966; 76:720.

125. Records RE: Intraocular penetration of dicloxacillin in experimental animals. Invest Ophthalmol. 1968; 7:663.

126. Salminen L: Cloxacillin distribution in the rabbit eye after intravenous injection. Acta Ophthalmol. 1978; 56:11.

127. Records RE: Intraocular penetration of cephalothin II. Human Studies. Am J Ophthalmol. 1968; 66:441.

128. Records RE: The cephalosporins in ophthalmology. Survey Ophthalmol. 1969; 13:345.

129. Records RE: Intraocular penetration of cephaloridine: observations in experimental animal and human eyes. Arch Ophthalmol. 1969; 81:331.

130. Boyle GL et al: Intraocular penetration of cephalexin in man. Am J Ophthalmol. 1970; 69:868.

131. Abel R et al: Intraocular penetration of cefazolin sodium in rabbits. Am J Ophthalmol. 1974; 78:779.

132. Becker EF: The intraocular penetration of lincomycin. Am J Ophthalmol. 1969; 67:963.

133. Pohjanpelto PEJ et al: Penetration of trimethoprim and sulphamethoxazole into the aqueous humor. Br J Ophthalmol. 1974; 58:606.

134. Furgiuele FP: Ocular penetration and tolerance of gentamicin. Am J Ophthalmol. 1967; 64:421.

135. Litwack KD et al: Penetration of gentamicin. Arch Ophthalmol. 1969; 82:687.

136. Petounis A et al: Penetration of tobramycin sulphate into the human eye. Br J Ophthalmol. 1978; 62:660.

137. George FH et al: Ocular penetration of chloramphenicol: effects of route of administration. Arch Ophthalmol. 1977; 95:879.

138. Moore CD et al: Evolution of corneal contact lenses. In Corneal Contact Lenses, 2nd ed, edited by LJ Girard, CV Mosby Co, St. Louis, 1970, p 12.

139. Lamy PP et al: Contact lens products. In Handbook of Non-Prescription Products, 6th ed, edited by P Penna, American Pharmaceutical Association, Washington, 1977, p 293.

140. Girard LJ: Indications and contraindications of the use of corneal contact lenses. In Corneal Contact Lenses, 2nd ed, CV Mosby Co, St. Louis, 1970, p 93.

141. Hales RH: Contact Lenses: A Clinical Approach to Fitting. Williams and Wilkins Co, Baltimore, 1978, p 12.

142. Lee J: Contact lenses and care products. In Ophthalmology and Contact Lens Pharmaceutics, Allergan Pharmaceuticals, Inc, 1979.

143. Arons IJ: Contact lenses in the 80s: an international overview. Contact Lens Forum. 1981; 6:21.

144. Gourley DR: Contact lenses, contact lens solutions and the eye. US Pharm. 1977; 2:40.

145. Dabezies OH: Contact lens and their solutions: a review of basic principles. EENT Monthly. 1966; 45:39.

146. Camp RN et al: Handling of the lens—insertion, removal, cleaning and storage. In Corneal Contact Lenses, 2nd ed, edited by LJ Cirard, CV Mosby Co, St. Louis, 1970, p 205.

147. Hall NC: The story of saliva: why it should never be used as a wetting solution for contact lens wearers. Contact Lens Med Bull. 1974; 7:43.

148. Dabenzies OH: Contact lens hygiene: past, present and future. Contact Lens Med Bull. 1970; 3:3.

149. Dabezies OH: Wet vs dry storage of corneal contact lenses, a statistical evaluation. Am J. Ophthalmol. 1965; 59:684.

150. Bettman JW: Contact lens storage, wet or dry? A bacterial analysis. Am J Ophthalmol. 1963; 56:77.

151. Dabezies O: Convenience solutions: the great compromise. Contact Lens Med Bull. 1974; 7:45.

152. Gourley DR: The pharmacist and contact lenses. Pharmat. 1977; 4:1.

153. Bailey NJ: Making contact. Contact Lens Forum. 1981; 6:16.

154. Newell FW: What price contact lenses? JAMA. 1977; 238:627.

155. Atkinson KW and Port MJA: Patient management and instruction. In Contact Lenses: A Textbook for Practitioner and Student, 2nd ed, edited by J Stone and AJ Phillips, Butterworths, Boston, 1980, p 187–212.

156. Bitonte JL and RH Keates, eds: Symposium on the flexible lens. CV Mosby Co, St. Louis, 1972, p 30.

157. Cureton Gl et al: Soft contact lens solutions: past, present and future. J Am Optom Assoc. 1974; 45:123.

158. Lamy PP: Soft contact lenses: how to help customers who use them. Pharm Times. 1976; April: 70.

159. Stone J: Special types of contact lenses and their uses. In Contact Lenses: A Textbook for Practitioner and Student, 2nd ed, edited by J Stone and AJ Phillips, Butterworths, Boston, 1981, p 675.

160. Bailey NJ: The effect of contact lens solutions on the SOFLENS contact lens. Proceedings of the Second National Research Symposium of Soft Contact Lenses. Excerpta Medica. 1977: 23.

161. Shively CD: Accessory solutions utilized in contact lens care and practice. In Soft Contact Lenses: Clinical and Applied Technology, edited by M Ruben, John Wiley & Sons, New York, 1978, p 383.

162. Krezanoski J: Fenestrated lens hygiene. Contact Lens Soc Am J. 1973; 7:9.

163. Hales, RH: Contact Lenses: A Clinical Approach to Fitting, Williams & Wilkins Co, Baltimore, 1978, p 64.

164. Galin MA: Therapy of glaucoma with hydrophilic lenses. In Soft Contact Lenses: Clinical and Applied Technology, edited by M Rubin, John Wiley & Sons Co, New York, 1978, p 281.

165. Kaufman HE et al: The medical uses of soft contact lenses. Tran Am Acad Ophthal Otol. 1971; 75:361.

166. Stewart-Jones JH, Hopkins GA and Phillips AJ: Drugs and solutions in contact lens practice and related microbiology. In Contact Lenses: A Textbook for Practitioner and Student, 2nd ed, edited by J Stone and AJ Phillips, Butterworths, Boston, 1980, p 59.

167. Krezanoski JZ: A new look at soft lenses and their solutions. Am Pharm. 1981; 21:260.

168. Newell FW: *Ophthalmology: Principles and Concepts,* 4th ed, CV Mosby Co, St. Louis, 1978, p 377.

169. Fraunfelder FT: *Drug-Induced Ocular Side Effects and Drug Interactions,* Lea and Febiger, Philadelphia, 1976, p 180.

170. Gourley DR and Records RE: Cataracts: etiology and treatment. US Pharm. 1980; 5:37.

171. Bercher B: The side effects of corticosteroids. Invest Ophthal. 1964; 3:492.

172. David DS and Berkowitz JS: Ocular effects of topical and systemic corticosteroids. Lancet. 1969; 2:949.

173. Skalka HW and Prchal JT: Effect of corticosteroids on cataract formation. Arch Opthalmol. 1980; 98:1773.

Chapter 53

Contraception

— Betty J. Dong, James C. Eoff III, and Mary Anne Koda-Kimble —

The ideal contraceptive, one which is safe and completely reliable, still remains to be developed. Diaphragms, intrauterine devices, and oral contraceptives constitute the major forms of antifertility devices available for women today. Although numerous risks have been associated with their use, oral contraceptives continue to be the most effective method of fertility control with the exception of sterilization. The publicity regarding the adverse effects of oral contraceptives has caused many women to look at alternative methods of contraception. It is imperative that clinicians have a sound knowledge of the practical aspects of all types of contraceptives available to both men and women before advising patients on the use and choice of contraceptive methods. Table 1 compares the efficacy and relative risks of the various contraceptive methods.

FEMALE REPRODUCTIVE PHYSIOLOGY

The female reproductive cycle involves a complex interaction between the hypothalamus, anterior pituitary, ovary, and uterus. The average menstrual cycle is 28 days in duration and can be divided into phases, using events in the ovary or uterus as reference points. When the ovary is used as a reference point, the cycle can be divided into three phases: the follicular or pre-ovulatory phase, the ovulatory phase, and the luteal or postovulatory phase. When the uterus is used as a reference point, the cycle can also be divided into three phases: the menstrual, proliferative, and secretory phases. The menstrual and proliferative phases of the uterus occur during the follicular phase of the ovary, and the secretory phase of the uterus corresponds to the luteal phase of the ovary.

Follicular Phase. This phase of the cycle is dominated by estrogen, begins at the onset of menstruation (menstrual phase), and lasts approximately 14 days. The low estrogen levels which exist at the beginning of this phase stimulate the release of follicle stimulating hormone (FSH) from the anterior pituitary. FSH stimulates the development of several primordial follicles within the ovary. As these mature, they produce estrogen in increasing amounts. Estrogen is responsible for endometrial growth, an increase in the size and tortuosity of the uterine glands, and for increased thickness and hyperemia of the uterine mucosa (proliferative phase). At the same time, most of the follicles stimulated by FSH regress and the dominant follicle matures. The rise in estrogen levels also depresses FSH secretion through a negative feedback mechanism and stimulates the release of luteinizing hormone (LH) from the pituitary through a positive feedback mechanism.

Ovulatory Phase. Ovulation occurs on the 14th or 15th day of the cycle in response to an LH surge triggered by the elevated levels of estrogens. Luteinizing hormone stimulates the final stages of maturation of the ovum, causes its release (ovulation), and stimulates the formation of the corpus luteum from the ruptured follicle.

Luteal or Secretory Phase. During this phase, which is progestogen dominated, the corpus luteum produces progesterone and estrogen. Progesterone thickens the endometrium, increases the tortuosity of the uterine glands, and causes them to secrete a thick fluid in preparation for implantation of the ovum. As progesterone levels rise, the release of LH is suppressed by a negative feedback mechanism. If implantation has not occurred by the 25th day of the cycle, the corpus luteum begins to regress and the levels of estrogen and progesterone decline. When these hormone levels decrease, the endometrium cannot be maintained and is sloughed off (menstruation). At this point (approximately the 28th day of the cycle), a new follicular phase begins. If implantation (pregnancy) occurs, the corpus luteum is maintained by human chorionic gonadotropin (HCG), which is the luteotrophic hormone secreted by the placenta (1).

HORMONAL CONTRACEPTION

Alteration of the normal hormonal balances required for fertility can be achieved by a number of methods. The combination birth control pills (BCP) are the most widely used.

Combination BCPs

Conventional combination birth control pills contain both estrogen and progestin in constant amounts which are taken throughout the entire 21 days of the cycle. The theoretical pregnancy rate for women who take these agents appropriately is less than one per 100 women-years (1,2). However, the actual pregnancy rate is somewhat greater because of noncompliance. For example, the pregnancy rate among women taking BCPs during their first year of marriage was 2–2.5% (3,4). The low failure rate of the combination BCPs is attributed to their multiple mechanisms of action:

a. the estrogens suppress FSH secretion, blocking follicular development and ovulation;

Table 1.

EFFICACY OF VARIOUS CONTRACEPTIVE METHODS

Method	Efficacy[1]	Relative Risk[2]
Tubal Ligation	0.04	2
Vasectomy	0.15	1–2
Birth Control Pills		
Combination (> 50 mcg of estrogen)	< 1	4
Combination (50 mcg of estrogen)	< 1	3
Combination (< 35 mcg of estrogen)	1–2	2
Mini-Pills	1–2	2
Biphasic	1–2	2
Postcoital Estrogens	1–2	1
Intrauterine Devices	1.5–3	5
Diaphragm	2–13	1
Condoms	0.4–4.8	1
Spermicides (Foams and Suppositories more effective than Creams and Gels)	2.5–4	1
Rhythm Methods		
Basal Body Temperature	1–3	0
Calendar	14–20	0
Vaginal Mucus	20–25	0
No Contraception (Chance)	90	

[1]Efficacy is expressed in terms of the number of pregnancies which would occur if 100 women were to use the method for one year. When ranges are given, the lower number often represents the theoretical effectiveness of the method. The higher number represents actual user effectiveness and incorporates human error. Effectiveness is influenced greatly by user motivation and correct contraceptive use.

[2]Risk (on a scale of 0–5) is the likelihood of developing an acute or long-term complication with the use of this method relative to the use of other contraceptive methods. It does not incorporate the risk inherent in pregnancy should the method fail.

b. the estrogen and progestin suppress LH secretion so no ovulation can occur even if follicular development is attained;

c. presence of progestin early in the cycle thickens cervical mucus, which interferes with sperm migration;

d. the progestin causes a disturbance in the endometrium, making it unsuitable for implantation of the egg;

e. there may be alteration in tubal transport of the ova through the fallopian tubes (5,6).

The combination BCPs can be divided into several general types of formulations: those which contain more than 50 mcg of estrogen; those which contain 50 mcg of estrogen; and those which contain less than 50 mcg of estrogen (30–40 mcg in current commercial preparations). See Table 2. Products containing 50 mcg or less of estrogen may also have lower progestogen doses relative to those containing high doses of estrogen. BCPs containing 50 mcg or less of estrogen have the advantage of a lower incidence of cardiovascular side effects. However, combinations with very low doses of estrogen and/or progestogen are also associated with a greater incidence of spotting, breakthrough bleeding, and missed periods (7–9). They may also be less effective in malnourished women, who may malabsorb the estrogen component (10,11), or in women taking drugs which may interact with BCPs to decrease their effectiveness (12). Although they contain less estrogen, the low-dose formulations appear to be as effective as BCPs which contain 50 mcg or more of estrogen (13).

The combination BCP's also differ from one another with respect to their estrogen and progestogen dominance. Any given BCP's estrogenic activity is determined by the quantity of estrogen contained in that product as well as the specific progestogen which it contains, since the latter may possess independent estrogenic activity, anti-estrogenic activity or, in many cases, both types of activity. Furthermore, the various progestogens used in BCPs differ in their progestogenic potency and androgenic activity (14). (See Table 3.) It has been determined that, in humans, there is no difference between the two estrogens used in oral contraceptives; mestranol and ethinyl estradiol are essentially equipotent when doses of 50–100 mcg are compared (15).

Determination of a given contraceptive's estrogenic or progestogenic dominance is useful in evaluating hormone-related side effects and in the subsequent selection of an appropriate agent. (See Table 4.)

Biphasic and Triphasic Pills

Recently, a new type of combination BCP has been released in which the amount of estrogen and/or progestogen varies throughout the cycle to more closely mimic hormone levels during the normal menstrual cycle. The total amount of hormone ingested monthly is less than that contained in most combination products, but the break-through bleeding and spotting associated with the traditional very low-dose combinations is minimized (16,17). The amounts of hormone in these products are listed in Table 2. These agents are similar in effectiveness to other combination BCP products (17).

Progestogen-Only BCP's or Mini-Pills

The "mini-pills" are oral contraceptives which contain progestogen only, in a dose which is lower than that contained in the combination BCPs. The products which are available contain 0.075 mg of norgestrel (Ovrette) or 0.35 mg of norethindrone (Nor-Q.D.; Micronor). Unlike the combination products, which can be taken on an interrupted cycle (21 days on and 7 days off), the mini-pills must be taken daily to be effective. Because they lack the protective effects of estrogens and require a higher degree of patient compliance, their actual effectiveness is somewhat less than that of the combination BCPs. It has been estimated that the failure rate is 1.1–2.5 per 100 women-years (4,18–20). The mini-pills act by causing a thick, hostile cervical mucus which decreases sperm penetration; altering the endometrium so that it is unsuitable for implantation of the ovum; and producing subtle changes in the hypothalamic-pituitary-ovarian system which inhibit ovulation in 30–40% of women taking these agents (21,22).

Morning-After Pills

High doses of estrogen alone or in combination with progestogens may be given to women who have had unprotected mid-cycle intercourse. Intercourse at mid-cycle carries a 2–30% risk of pregnancy. When these women are given estrogens early in the post-coital period, the risk of

Table 2.

ORAL CONTRACEPTIVE INGREDIENTS

Brand Name (# Tabs/Pkt)	Estrogen Content (mcg/tab)		Progestogen Content (mg/tab)		
COMBINATION BCPs					
Enovid-E (20,21)	Mestranol	(100)	Norethynodrel	(2.5)	
Norinyl 2 mg (20)	Mestranol	(100)	Norethindrone	(2.0)	
Ortho-Novum 2 mg (21)	Mestranol	(100)	Norethindrone	(2.0)	
Ovulen (20,21,28)	Mestranol	(100)	Ethynodiol diacetate	(1.0)	
Norinyl 1+80 (21,28)	Mestranol	(80)	Norethindrone	(1.0)	
Ortho-Novum 1/80 (21,28)	Mestranol	(80)	Norethindrone	(1.0)	
Enovid 5 mg (20)	Mestranol	(75)	Norethynodrel	(1.0)	
Ortho-Novum 10 mg (21)	Mestranol	(60)	Norethindrone	(1.0)	
Norinyl 1+50 (21,28)	Mestranol	(50)	Norethindrone	(1.0)	
Ortho-Novum 1/50 (21,28)	Mestranol	(50)	Norethindrone	(1.0)	
Norlestrin 2.5/50 (21,Fe)	Ethinyl estradiol	(50)	Norethindrone acetate	(2.5)	
Demulen (21,28)	Ethinyl estradiol	(50)	Ethynodiol diacetate	(1.0)	
Norlestrin 1/50 (21,28,Fe)	Ethinyl estradiol	(50)	Norethindrone acetate	(1.0)	
Ovcon-50 (21,28)	Ethinyl estradiol	(50)	Norethindrone	(1.0)	
Ovral (21,28)	Ethinyl estradiol	(50)	dl-Norgestrel	(0.5)	
Norlestrin 1+35 (21,28)	Ethinyl estradiol	(35)	Norethindrone	(1.0)	
Ortho-Novum 1/35 (21,28)	Ethinyl estradiol	(35)	Norethindrone	(1.0)	
Brevicon (21,28)	Ethinyl estradiol	(35)	Norethindrone	(0.5)	
Modicon (21,28)	Ethinyl estradiol	(35)	Norethindrone	(0.5)	
Ovcon-35 (21,28)	Ethinyl estradiol	(35)	Norethindrone	(0.4)	
Loestrin 1.5/30 (21,Fe)	Ethinyl estradiol	(30)	Norethindrone acetate	(1.5)	
Lo/Ovral (21,28)	Ethinyl estradiol	(30)	dl-Norgestrel	(0.3)	
Nordette	Ethinyl estradiol	(30)	l-Norgestrel	(0.15)	
Loestrin 1/20 (21,Fe)	Ethinyl estradiol	(20)	Norethindrone acetate	(1.0)	
PROGESTOGEN-ONLY BCPs					
Micronor			Norethindrone	(0.35)	
Nor-Q.D.			Norethindrone	(0.35)	
Ovrette			dl-Norgestrel	(0.075)	
BIPHASIC COMBINATION BCPs					
Ortho-Novum 10/11	Ethinyl estradiol	(35)	Norethindrone	(0.05)	Days 1–10
	Ethinyl estradiol	(35)	Norethindrone	(1.0)	Days 11–21
TRIPHASIC COMBINATION BCPs					
Investigational	Ethinyl estradiol	(30)	l-norgestrel	(0.05)	Days 1–6
(Some contain dl-norgestrel at	Ethinyl estradiol	(40)	l-norgestrel	(0.075)	Days 7–11
twice the dose)	Ethinyl estradiol	(30)	l-norgestrel	(0.125)	Days 12–22

Table 3.

COMPARATIVE PHARMACOLOGY OF THE PROGESTOGENS

Progestogen	Progestogenic Activity (Equipotent Doses)	Antiestrogenic Activity	Estrogenic Activity[1]	Androgenic/ Anabolic Activity[2]	Product Examples
Norgestrel	0.5 mg	+ +	None	+ + +	Ovral Lo-Ovral
Norethindrone Acetate	1.0 mg	+ + +	None[3]	+ + +	Loestrin Norlestrin
Ethynodiol Diacetate	1.0 mg	+[3]	None[3]	+ (not anabolic)	Demulen Ovulen
Norethindrone	2.5 mg	+[4]	+[5]	+	See Footnotes 4,5
Norethynodrel	10 mg	None	+ +	None	Enovid Enovid E

References: 14,267,268

[1]Estrogenic activity is due to metabolism of the progestogen to an estrogenic substance.

[2]Androgenic effects are due to the progestogen's structural similarity to the androgen, testosterone.

[3]Norethindrone acetate and ethynodiol diacetate are partial agonists. They potentiate estrogen activity at low doses and antagonize at high doses. In the doses used in all BCPs, the predominant effect observed is the antiestrogenic activity.

[4]An estrogen antagonist when the estrogen:progestogen ratio contained in a BCP is ≥ 50:1. Product examples include Ortho-Novum; Norinyl 1 + 50.

[5]An estrogen agonist at a dose of less than 50 mcg. Product examples include: Brevicon; Micronor; Modicon; Nor-Q.D., Ovcon-35.

pregnancy is decreased substantially, to 0.16–1.6%, probably by preventing ovum implantation (23–25). Several regimens have been used.

Diethylstilbesterol (DES). The FDA has approved the use of high doses of DES as a "morning after" pill in emergency situations such as rape, incest, or when, in the physician's judgment, the patient's physical or mental well-being is in jeopardy. It is *not* to be used routinely as a contraceptive. DES (25 mg bid for 5 days) should be initiated within 24 hours and not later than 72 hours after exposure to be effective. Patients should be warned to take a full course despite the occurrence of nausea which can be minimized by concurrent use of an antiemetic. Although there is no evidence that this dose of DES is carcinogenic to the potential fetus, voluntary termination of the pregnancy by abortion should be seriously considered if such therapy fails (26–28).

Ovral (50 mcg ethinyl estradiol and 0.5 mg dl-norgestrel). High doses of post-coital Ovral have been used with a success rate similar to that obtained with DES but with less nausea. Two tablets are taken 24–72 hours after coitus and followed by another two tablets 12 hours later. If vomiting occurs within one hour after taking the pills, further treatment may be indicated. Menstruation should occur in 2–3 weeks (29–31).

High-Dose Estrogens. Several investigators have used conjugated or esterified estrogens, estrone, or ethinyl estradiol in a variety of doses and have observed a success rate similar to that observed with DES (1,4,25). Dosage regimens used include ethinyl estradiol 2.5 mg bid for 5 days, conjugated estrogens 20–30 mg/day for 5 days, and estrone 5 mg bid for 5 days. All regimens should be started within 24 hours of intercourse to achieve maximum effectiveness.

Table 4.

ESTROGENIC AND PROGESTOGENIC DOMINANCE OF ORAL CONTRACEPTIVES

Estrogenic Dominance	Degree	Progestogenic Dominance
Enovid 5 mg Enovid-E	VERY HIGH	Ortho-Novum 10 mg Ortho-Novum 5 mg Ortho-Novum 2.5 mg Norlestrin 2.5/50 Enovid 10 mg Micronor Nor-Q.D.
Ortho-Novum 1/80 Norinyl 1 + 80 Ortho-Novum 2 mg Ortho-Novum 0.5	HIGH	Ovulen Loestrin 1.5/30 Ovral Enovid 5 mg Demulen Loestrin 1/20 Norlestrin 1 mg
Ovcon-50 Ovulen Ovulen 0.5 Brevicon Modicon Ovcon-35 Norlestrin *Ortho-Novum 1/50 *Norinyl 1 + 50 *Demulen *Lo/Ovral *Ortho-Novum 1/35 *Norlestrin 1 + 35	INTERMEDIATE	Ovulen 0.5 Lo/Ovral Norinyl 1 + 50 Ortho-Novum 1/50 Ortho-Novum 1/35
Ovral Norlestrin 2.5 Loestrin 1.5/30 Loestrin 1/20 Ortho-Novum 10 mg Norinyl 10 mg	LOW TO VERY LOW	Ortho-Novum 2 mg Enovid E Othro-Novum 1/80 Norinyl 1 + 80 Brevicon Modicon Ovcon-35
Nor-Q.D. Micronor Ovrette	NONE	

*Relatively balanced with regard to estrogenic and progestogenic effects.

Long-Acting Progestogens

Injectable medroxyprogesterone acetate (Depo-Provera), a long-acting progestogen which is administered once every three months (150 mg/dose), has been used as a contraceptive in many underdeveloped countries. It is an effective form of contraception which has a failure rate of 0.25 pregnancies per 100 women-years; however, it is not approved for contraceptive use in the United States. The FDA's major concerns are the following: prolonged amenorrhea and/or uterine bleeding during and after its use; variable and unpredictable return of fertility; and development of mammary nodules in dogs (4,32,33).

USE OF ORAL CONTRACEPTIVES

1. *Risks vs. Benefits.* L.H., a 24-year-old, healthy, non-smoking female wishes to start BCPs. However, she has read a great deal in the lay literature about the adverse effects of these agents and is concerned about the risks and benefits associated with their use. Overall, do the benefits of the BCPs outweigh their risks?

There is now 20 years of experience with the BCPs, and the weight of evidence strongly suggests that the benefits associated with BCP use outweigh the risks if patients are selected carefully.

Benefits. The benefits associated with BCP use, in addition to protection from the risks of pregnancy, include:

a. Alleviation of dysmenorrhea (2,34–37), premenstrual tension (36,38–41), heavy menses (42–43) and irregular menses (2,44).

b. Protection against iron deficiency anemia because menstrual blood loss is decreased (2).

c. Protection from pelvic inflammatory disease (PID). BCP users are one-half as likely to develop PID as nonusers. This may be related to a thickening of the cervical mucus secretions, to stronger uterine contractions which prevent the ascension of bacteria into the uterus and fallopian tubes, or to prevention of pregnancies and abortions which are likely to be sources of infection. Progestogens may also inhibit gonococcal growth (2,45–47).

d. Lower incidence of ectopic pregnancy. BCP-users are one-tenth as likely to develop ectopic pregnancies as nonusers. This may be related to the decreased incidence of PID which can lead to blocked fallopian tubes and predispose to ectopic pregnancy (48,49).

e. Lower incidence of benign breast disease (BBD) or noncancerous breast lumps and cysts. BCP-users develop these lesions about one-half as often as nonusers (50–52). There is no increased incidence of breast cancer (53–55).

f. Risk of ovarian cancer decreased by one-third to one-half (56,57); lower incidence of noncancerous ovarian cysts (58).

g. Risk of endometrial cancer decreased by one-half to two-thirds (49,60–62).

h. Protection against toxic shock syndrome (4).

Risks. Beyond the relatively minor side effects associated with BCP use, which may diminish with continued use or which may be minimized through manipulation of the hormonal content of the BCP (see Questions 5–14), certain women are at increased risk for the cardiovascular complications of estrogen. These include venous thromboembolism, hypertension, cerebrovascular disease (stroke), and ischemic heart disease.

Women who are over the age of 45 or over the age of 35 and also smoke are at greatest risk (see Table 7). This risk is dose related. Therefore, BCPs containing estrogen should be avoided in women over the age of 35 who smoke or who already have evidence of or a predisposition to cardiovascular disease. BCPs should not be used in women over the age of 45 (also see Questions 15–17).

BCPs have no adverse effects on childbearing, although fertility may be delayed by several months (see Question 20). The relationship between BCP use and cervical cancer, pituitary cancer, or melanoma is unclear (4). Nonmalignant liver tumors may occur with an incidence of 1–2 cases/100,000 women-years. These may rupture and cause death by internal bleeding (64–67,226–229). Gall bladder disease is increased two-fold in BCP users (2,96,223). Also see Question 27 and 28.

2. What information should be obtained from L.H. before oral contraceptives are initiated?

Information regarding the date of L.H.'s last menstrual period, the regularity of her menses, and the amount of bleeding should be obtained. The possibility of pregnancy should be ruled out; if necessary, a pregnancy test should be ordered. A history of the patient's prior contraceptive experience (use, response, side effects, and compliance) can be useful in predicting her response to the agent selected. A routine physical examination which includes a blood pressure, breast examination, pelvic examination, PAP smear, and liver function evaluation should be performed and repeated annually since she is under the age of 35. The blood pressure of patients with a family history of hypertension should be checked every 3–6 months (see Question 18). The blood sugar of patients predisposed to diabetes should be evaluated six months after the initiation of therapy and annually thereafter (see Questions 22,23). After the age of 35, patients should be evaluated more frequently, perhaps at six-month intervals.

Before selecting a BCP, all contraindications to the use of BCPs should be considered and ruled out (see Table 5). Several diseases and/or conditions seem to predispose patients to an increased risk of mortality and morbidity. The most important and well-accepted risks associated with the development of BCP side effects include the age of the patient, a history of smoking, and the duration of contraceptive use (4,68–70). A family history of diabetes, hypertension, or cardiovascular disease must be weighed against the risks of pregnancy since patients with the aforementioned conditions are at greater risk for adverse effects.

3. Product Selection. L.H.'s history and physical examination revealed that she has not taken oral contraceptives previously. Her family history was negative for diabetes, hypertension and cardiovascular disease, and her physical examination was within normal limits. Her menstrual periods are regular and last 3–4 days. She has no history of dysmenorrhea. What criteria should be used to select a specific BCP for L.H.?

The selection of an oral contraceptive is often empiric and based upon the clinician's patient experience. Most prescribers initiate patients on combination oral contraceptives containing 50 mcg or less of estrogen to minimize estrogen-related complications (14,71). More specifically, a combination product, such as Ortho-Novum 1/50 or Lo/Ovral, which is balanced in terms of its progestational and estrogenic effects is selected. Combination products which contain 35 mcg or less of estrogen (eg, Lo/Ovral) are more likely to be associated with break-through bleeding, spotting, and missed periods during the first three

cycles than combination products containing 50 mcg of estrogen (7–9). Since break-through bleeding and spotting diminish with each successive cycle, no change should be considered before the third cycle is completed in a patient with these complaints. Also see Question 6.

Many prescribers still attempt to select a BCP based upon their assessment of the specific endocrinologic make-up of the patient as determined by body weight and/or menstrual characteristics (72). Proponents of this method claim that side effects of the BCP are thereby minimized. Women who have 2–4 days of light flow with little or no cramping are thought to do well on contraceptives which have the lowest doses of estrogen and progestogen (eg, Brevicon; Ovcon-35). Women with regular menses who have a moderate flow of 4–6 days duration and moderate cramping do well on a BCP with intermediate progestational potency (eg, Norinyl 1 + 50; Lo/Ovral). Finally, women with heavy menses of 6 days or more and moderate to severe cramping require a high progestogen contraceptive such as Ovral or Loestrin 1.5/30.

If body build is used as a guide to BCP selection, women with a slight build weighing less than 110 pounds benefit from a low estrogen-low progestogen contraceptive such as Lo/Ovral. Conversely, women with heavier builds weighing more than 160 pounds often respond well to a high progestogen pill such as Norlestrin 2.5 (72).

Others have suggested that the contraceptive should be selected to complement the patient's endocrinologic profile. On this basis, women with acne, oily skin, and hirsutism would be given a contraceptive with low androgenic properties such as Brevicon, while women with excessive nausea, bloating, and heavy menses would receive a contraceptive with low estrogen properties such as Ovral (14).

Since this patient has no critical findings to suggest that she would particularly benefit from a contraceptive with high or low progestogen or estrogen content, she should be initiated on a contraceptive such as Lo/Ovral which has balanced estrogenic and progestogenic activity and a low dose of estrogen. She should then be observed for three cycles before any change in the contraceptive is made.

The mini-pills, or progesterone-only pills, should be reserved for those patients who have contraindications to the use of estrogen since they are less

Table 5.

CONTRAINDICATIONS TO THE USE OF THE BIRTH CONTROL PILLS

Absolute Contraindications	Comments
Past or present history of thromboembolic disease	See Question 15.
Past or present history of cerebrovascular accidents	Increased risk of thrombotic and hemorrhagic stroke with BCP use occurs in older hypertensive women who also smoke (69, 104,129,269–272).
Past or present history of coronary artery disease and myocardial infarction.	See Question 17 and Table 7.
Past or present history of hepatic adenoma	See Question 28.
Age over 35 years, especially if the woman is a heavy smoker	See Questions 1,2,17 and Table 7. Mini-pill may be the BCP of choice if an oral contraceptive is required (4,63,68,69).
Markedly impaired liver function or history of chronic idiopathic jaundice, recurrent generalized jaundice, and pruritis of pregnancy	See Question 28. Liver disorders of pregnancy often recur with BCP use. The incidence of acute hepatitis may be increased in BCP users (273).
Pregnancy	See Question 21.
Past or present history or a strong family history of malignancy of the breast, reproductive system, or any estrogen-dependent tumors	See Questions 1 and 19. Although BCPs have *not* been shown to increase the risk of breast, ovarian, or endometrial cancer, a theoretical risk exists when women with these cancers ingest estrogen. Women with strong family histories of breast or reproductive organ malignancies should be strongly advised to use other means of contraception.

Relative Contraindications	Comments
Undiagnosed menstrual bleeding	Any abnormal bleeding may be indicative of uterine malignancy and should be investigated before BCP institution. The effects of BCPs on menstrual blood flow may confuse the diagnosis.
Undiagnosed breast lumps	See Question 19. If benign breast lumps grow, a BCP with a lower estrogen dose or a mini-pill may be required. If they continue to grow, BCPs should be discontinued.
Varicose veins	Varicosity is a risk factor for thromboembolic disease, and the BCP may have to be discontinued if varicosities worsen with its use. Mini-pills may be the BCPs of choice in women with this problem. Women with severe varicose veins should be strongly advised to use other forms of contraception.
Noncompliance or unreliability (eg, altered mentation; alcoholism; psychiatric disturbances)	These women should be strongly encouraged to use another form of contraception which does not require close follow-up for BCP toxicity and patient compliance for effectiveness.
Women under 30 years of age who smoke heavily	Although there is no evidence of increased risk of cardiovascular complications in such individuals, these women should be strongly advised to stop smoking. See Questions 1,2,17 and Table 7.
Headaches	See Questions 24 and 25. Worsening of headaches or the new onset of headaches, especially those associated with visual changes, should be considered a contraindication to the use of the pill. Cyclic headaches may be responsive to hormone manipulation. Low-dose combination BCPs or mini-pills may be the BCPs of choice.

Table 5. (continued)

CONTRAINDICATIONS TO THE USE OF THE BIRTH CONTROL PILLS

Relative Contraindications	Comments
Hypertension	See Question 18. The new onset of hypertension or any worsening of existing hypertension should be considered as indications for stopping the pill. Cyclic fluid retention which aggravates hypertension may be responsive to hormone manipulation. Low-dose combination BCPs or mini-pills may be the BCPs of choice.
Diabetes or strong family history thereof; gestational diabetes	See Questions 22 and 23. BCP-induced diabetes is a contraindication to further use since it is not always reversible.
Blood dyscrasias	Polycythemia, leukemia, and sickle cell anemia all carry the risk of increased thrombosis and their presence should be considered a strong relative contraindication to BCP use. See Question 15.
Gall bladder disease	See Question 27.
Major surgery with immobilization or casting of the lower extremities	This situation places the patient at risk for thromboembolism and the BCP should be discontinued, particularly if the patient has other risk factors for embolism. See Question 15 (109–111,285).
Depression, epilepsy, asthma, history of abnormal liver function, uterine fibromyoma	See Questions 26 and 28. May initiate BCPs with caution. Monitor for exacerbation of these problems and discontinue or change to low-dose combination or mini-pill.

effective and rely heavily on patient compliance (See Questions 31–32).

4. *Patient Instructions.* L.H. is placed on Ortho-Novum 1/50 with instructions to take "as directed." She is currently mid-cycle and plans to be married in one month. When should she begin taking her pills and how soon will they be effective? What general instructions should be given to L.H. regarding the use of this product?

Ortho-Novum is available in packets containing 21 or 28 tablets. For the 21-day packet, the first day of menstruation is considered "day one." L.H. should be instructed to begin taking her BCPs on the fifth day of her menstrual cycle and to take them every day thereafter at approximately the same time each day until the packet is completed. No pills are taken for the next seven days. Menstruation usually begins two or three days after the last pill. The 28-day packet includes 7 inert tablets, thereby eliminating the need to count days. When these tablets are prescribed, the patient simply takes one tablet daily.

L.H. could begin taking her BCPs immediately, but her body would have to become adjusted to a new hormone cycle and it would be impossible to predict where she would be in her cycle during her honeymoon. Beginning the BCPs during a menstrual cycle offers the added assurance that L.H. won't be pregnant when she begins her pills.

If L.H. is mid-cycle now, she is also likely to be mid-cycle and at high risk for becoming pregnant when she gets married next month. Even though the combination BCPs are said to be effective immediately, she should use an additional method of contraception during her first cycle in the event that escape ovulation occurs. Condoms, diaphragms, and spermicidal foams or suppositories should be considered. See Questions 36–38.

In addition to the general instructions for use, the patient should be taught signs and symptoms which may signal severe side effects of the pill. These should be brought to the attention of a health provider as soon as possible. Some prescribers use the mnemonic "ACHES" to help the patient remember key signs and symptoms (4):

A Abdominal pain (severe) may be indicative of gall bladder disease, hepatic adenoma, pancreatitis or a blood clot.

C Chest pain (severe) may be indicative of a pulmonary embolism or myocardial infarction.

H   Headaches (severe) may be a sign of a stroke or migraine headache.

E   Eye problems including blurred vision, flashing lights, or blindness may be indicative of hypertension or stroke.

S   Severe leg pain, especially in the thighs or calves, may be indicative of venous thromboembolism.

Side Effects

5. *Missed Menses.* L.H. calls after completing the first month (21 days) of her Ortho-Novum 1/50. She has waited seven days and menses has not started. Should she continue the pill or wait for her menses to begin?

L.H. should be questioned regarding her compliance with the new BCP prescription, her pattern of intercourse, her use of alternate methods of contraception, and the recent ingestion of drugs which may have decreased the effectiveness of her BCPs (see Questions 29 and 30). If there is no reason to believe that she is likely to be pregnant, she should begin a second packet at the regularly scheduled time (7 days after the last pill was ingested). This advice is reasonable since she just began taking the BCPs and missed periods are common during the first three cycles of use.

If, on the other hand, L.H. had been taking oral contraceptives for several months without such problems, she would be advised to stop taking the pill and to use another method of contraception until pregnancy is ruled out (see Questions 6 and 21).

Patients who continue to miss menses may require a change to a BCP with lower progestogenic activity, such as Norlestrin or Demulen. If this is not successful, a BCP with greater estrogenic activity should be tried.

6. *Break-through Bleeding and Spotting.* C.K., a 25-year-old woman who has been taking Norlestrin 1+50 (norethindrone acetate 1 mg; ethinyl estradiol 50 mcg) for the past 3 months, complains of irregular periods and spotting. Her specific history is as follows:

1st month: Spotting after the second week

2nd month: No unusual bleeding problems

3rd month: Spotting after the second week

What are the primary causes of break-through bleeding and spotting? How can they be managed?

Break-through bleeding (BTB) and spotting are bleeding episodes which occur at times other than during the normal menstrual cycle. BTB is more copious and similar to a menstrual discharge, whereas spotting consists of a minimal discharge or staining. BTB occurs in 5–8% of patients taking the pill and is most often associated with pills with low estrogenic activity (14,71,73). It is most likely to occur in association with BCPs which contain 50 mcg or less of estrogen or with those products which also contain a potent antiestrogenic progesterone such as norethindrone acetate (see Table 3). Since estrogens are responsible for maintaining an intact endometrium, degeneration or sloughing may occur in the presence of inadequate estrogenic activity. Other causes of spotting and BTB which must be considered include missed pills (see Question 8), drug interactions (see Questions 29 and 30), and uterine pathology.

BTB and spotting which occur early in the cycle such as that described by this patient or in association with a single missed pill are most often due to insufficient estrogen. These events most commonly occur in the first three months of the cycle and may diminish over time as the patient becomes adjusted to a new hormonal environment. Therefore, there is no need to change birth control pills prior to the completion of three cycles. Occasionally, spotting may occur when patients take their BCPs at a different time each day. This is a particular problem with the low-dose estrogen tablets or combinations with low estrogenic potency. This may be minimized by instructing the patient to take the pill at the same time each day in an attempt to maintain constant hormone levels in the body.

If C.K. continues to experience similar problems beyond the third cycle, one could consider changing her BCP to one with a less antiestrogenic progesterone such as Ortho-Novum 1/50, which contains norethindrone. Rarely, a more estrogenic BCP, containing 80 mcg of estrogen, may be needed (eg, Ortho-Novum 1/80). Spotting is not a serious problem, and if C.K. is not experiencing other troublesome side effects, she may continue taking Norlestrin 1 + 50 and consider it an acceptable consequence of BCP use.

BTB which primarily occurs late in the cycle is most likely due to insufficient progesterone. This may also be manifested as heavier, more prolonged menstrual cycles. In these instances, one may consider changing to a BCP with greater progestogenic activity.

Persistent or recurrent menstrual dysfunction requires a thorough search for underlying uterine pathologies such as polyps or an ectopic pregnancy.

7. How should C.K. be instructed to take her BCPs should spotting or BTB occur?

Patients who are initiated on BCPs which contain low doses of estrogen (50 mcg or less) should be informed that spotting and, less frequently, BTB are common during the first three cycles of use while the body becomes accustomed to the new hormonal milieu. Should these events occur, C.K. should continue taking the pill as usual to establish the new hormonal pattern. If BTB or spotting continue beyond three months, she should return for reevaluation, and another BCP should be considered. Some patients experience prolonged menstrual periods when they are taking BCPs with insufficient progestogenic activity. Should this occur, they should still resume their next BCP packet at the usual time, that is, seven days after the last pill of the previous cycle was ingested.

8. Missed Pills. C.K. experienced breakthrough bleeding (BTB) when she forgot to take her pills for 3–4 days. She calls and wants to know what she should do. What advice should to given to women who miss their pills?

In general, patients who miss their pills should be instructed to make-up their missed doses as soon as possible to maintain adequate suppression of follicular development and to prevent BTB and spotting. If one dose is missed, the patient should take the pill as soon as she remembers or double the next day's dose. Jackson (74) found no evidence of escape ovulation when one missed combination pill was taken 10–12 hours later. When 1–5 pills were missed, the pregnancy rate increased to 7.2%; and when 6–19 pills were missed, the pregnancy rate increased to 31.2%. Since the likelihood of becoming pregnant is also greater if a pill is missed early in the cycle (first two weeks) or if the patient is a relatively new user, an additional method of contraception should

be recommended for the remainder of the cycle if a pill is missed under either of these two circumstances. Patients who miss their pills mid-cycle may also take morning-after pills (see Introduction). If two pills are missed, the patient should double up the dose for the next two consecutive days and use an additional method of contraception for the remainder of the cycle.

Break-through bleeding is common when any number of pills is missed (287), as illustrated by C.K. If three or more pills are missed and BTB occurs, the patient should be instructed to discontinue the pills, consider this normal menses, and resume another cycle on the fifth day of "menses." She should begin using a secondary means of contraception such as a spermicidal foam or diaphragm immediately and continue through the second week of the following cycle.

If a patient continues to "miss" pills on a regular basis, an alternative method of contraception should be seriously considered.

9. Estrogen Excess. After two months, L.H. complains of intolerable morning nausea, bloating, and ankle edema. Her breasts are swollen and tender to the touch. Lately she has also noticed a "whitish" vaginal discharge with no other symptoms. What is the most probable cause of L.H.'s complaints and how should they be managed?

Since many articles on the adverse effects of contraceptives appear in the lay press, clinicians must be prepared to objectively evaluate any complaints which a patient may attribute to her BCPs. Adverse effects which are vague or vary monthly and which appear to parallel new information reported to the public may not actually be related to the patient's BCPs. In one study of 147 women, over 60% experienced various side effects from oral contraceptive placebos. Only one-third of these placebo-treated patients were totally asymptomatic (75).

However, this patient's symptoms are consistent with estrogen excess. Nausea tends to occur during the first month of use but usually disappears by the third or fourth cycle. The patient should be instructed to take the pill in the evening with dinner, since this seems to decrease the incidence of nausea. The bloating, swollen breasts, and ankle edema are explained by increased reabsorption of salt and water by the kidney. Salt restriction and intermittent use of diuretics can afford the patient relief. The whitish discharge, or leukorrhea, is a normal physiological reaction of the glands that line the inner portion of cervix to the estrogen component of the pill. However, bacterial and fungal infections should be ruled out. Other excess estrogen side effects not exhibited by this patient are described in Table 6 (1,14,73,76).

Symptoms of excess estrogen usually decrease with time; however, if they persist beyond three months, the patient should be switched to a less estrogenic pill. BCPs containing progestogens with estrogenic properties (eg, norethynodrel) should be avoided as well. The BCP of choice for this

patient would also contain less than 50 mcg of estrogen, such as Norlestrin 1 + 35 or Ortho-Novum 1/35. Ovral, which is strongly antiestrogenic, or a mini-pill (if the patient is very compliant) are alternatives.

If the patient is changed to a BCP with a lower estrogen content, some clinicians recommend the use of an additional contraceptive method during the first cycle of use. Theoretically, the pituitary can escape from the influence of estrogen suppression when a patient is switched to lower doses of estrogen, but this does not appear to occur clinically and is not a mandatory recommendation (77).

Table 6.

HORMONAL SIDE EFFECTS OF ORAL CONTRACEPTIVES

Side Effects Related to Estrogen Excess[1]	Comments

General: Occur during pill days
  Nausea and vomiting
  Dizziness
  Edema and fluid retention
  Irritability and bloating
  Cyclic headaches
  Cyclic weight gain
  Poor-fitting contact lenses
	See Question 9. Estrogen-induced fluid retention may aggravate hypertension, cardiac disease, seizures, headaches, and depression. Corneal edema may result in poor-fitting contact lenses (274–277).

Reproductive
  Cystic breast changes and tenderness
  Uterine enlargement
  Leukorrhea
  Hypermenorrhea
  Cervical extrophia
	Fibrocystic breast disease and uterine fibroids can enlarge with excessive estrogen stimulation. Management involves decreasing the dose of estrogen by changing to a pill with a potent antiestrogenic progestogen or switching to the mini-pill.

Suppression of lactation	See Question 33
Side Effects Related to Estrogen Deficiency[2]	**Comments**
Early spotting and break-through bleeding on days 1–7.	See Questions 3,6–8, and 10. Occurs most often when low-dose combinations are initiated. Often improves after the third cycle of use.
Amenorrhea or decreased menstrual flow	See Question 5. Worsens with time.

Other
  Irritability
  Nervousness
  Depression
  Decreased libido
  Hot flashes and other vasomotor symptoms
  Atrophic vaginitis
  Dyspareunia	

Table 6. (continued)

HORMONAL SIDE EFFECTS OF ORAL CONTRACEPTIVES

Side Effects Related to Progestogen Excess[3]	Comments

General
  Noncyclic weight gain and increased appetite
  Tiredness, fatigue, weakness
  Decreased menstrual flow
	See Question 11. Become worse over time and generally require a change to a BCP with a less potent progestogen.

Androgenic
  Oily skin and scalp
  Acne
  Hirsutism
  Depression
	Managed by changing to a less androgenic progestogen. Avoid norgestrel and norethindrone acetate-containing preparations.

Monilial vaginitis	Becomes worse over time. Most commonly associated with BCPs containing strong antiestrogenic progestogens (278–281).

Those occuring during pill-free days.
  Nausea and vomiting
  Dizziness
  Edema and bloating
  Cyclic weight gain
  Cyclic headaches
  Breast tenderness
	These symptoms resemble those of estrogen excess but occur *only* during pill-free days. They are presumably due to rebound water and sodium retention.

Side Effects Related to Progestogen Deficiency	Comments
Late break-through bleeding and spotting on days 8–21	See Questions 3 and 6–8.
Heavy menstrual flow and clotting	
Delayed withdrawal bleeding	
Weight loss	

[1]These symptoms may also be caused by progestogen deficiency. Some side effects related to estrogen excess may decrease over time. Unless they are intolerable, a 3-cycle trial is warranted.

[2]These side effects may be secondary to the potent antiestrogenic effect of progestogen which can be managed by manipulating the progestogen component.

[3]These side effects may also be due to estrogen deficiency secondary to a strong antiestrogenic progestogen in the BCP.

10. *Estrogen Deficiency.* **A 48-year-old postmenopausal woman with endometriosis has been taking Ovral for one month. She now complains of hot flashes at night, increased nervousness and irritability. How should she be managed?**

The symptoms described above are due to estrogen deficiency complicated by her postmenopausal state and the very potent antiestrogenic progestogen, norgestrel, which is contained in Ovral. The patient should be switched to a prod-

uct which contains a less antiestrogenic progestogen such as norethindrone 50 mcg. If the symptoms persist, a product which contains larger doses of estrogen, such as Ortho-Novum 1/80, should be considered. Other symptoms consistent with estrogen deficiency which are not manifested by this patient are listed in Table 6 (1,14,73,76).

11. *Progestogen Excess.* **A 22-year-old tall, slender, depressed woman is seen in the outpatient clinic with complaints of abnormal**

hair growth on her chin and breast which she has removed by electrolysis. Past drug history revealed the recent use of tetracycline 250 mg/day for acne. Physical examination was normal except for slight hair growth as noted above. She has also noticed increased perspiration, but no voice changes. She has been taking Norlestrin 2.5 mg for three years. How should this patient be managed?

The increased perspiration, acne, hirsutism, and depression in this patient could well be due to the androgenic effects of the progesterone, norethindrone acetate, contained in Norlestrin. However, other underlying endocrinologic disorders should be ruled out. A contraceptive containing a progestogen with less androgenic tendencies, such as ethynodiol diacetate (Demulen) or norethindrone (Brevicon), should be considered in this patient with masculine features. Norethindrone acetate (Norlestrin) and norgestrel (Ovral) should not be used in such patients because of their potent androgenic properties. Other symptoms of progestogen excess not manifested by this patient are listed in Table 6 (1,14,73,76).

12. *Weight Gain.* A 24-year-old woman who has been taking Norlestrin for one year complains of a ten-pound weight gain at her annual physical examination. Could the weight gain have been related to her BCP?

Weight gain can be caused by either the estrogen or progesterone component depending on the duration of pill usage. Estrogens can cause a transient or cyclic weight gain early in the cycle due to salt and water retaining effects (1,14,73,76). The patient may be switched to a lower estrogenic preparation or treated temporarily with diuretics. Progesterone can also cause weight gain with prolonged use due to its anabolic and appetite-stimulating properties (1,14,73,76). Usually the weight increases slowly and the gain is minor (5–10 lbs, although 30-lb gains have been reported), so that it is usually unnecessary to change pills.

13. *Chloasma.* A 30-year-old woman who has been taking Ortho-Novum 1/80 for 18 months is noted to have a brownish macular area of pigmentation on her forehead and malar regions. She indicates that this developed while she was vacationing in Florida last month. What is your assessment of this

patient's problem and how should it be managed?

This patient has a condition known as chloasma, melasma, or the "mask of pregnancy" which is a form of hyperpigmentation caused by the BCPs. Apparently, the estrogens stimulate the melanocytes while the progestogens cause their spread. As illustrated by this patient, these hyperpigmented areas present as symmetrically distributed, irregularly-shaped brown macules that most commonly occur on the forehead, malar eminences, lower cheeks and upper lip. The pigmentation, which is similar to that sometimes associated with pregnancy, tends to develop slowly and can appear from 1–20 months after starting therapy (78,79). BCP-induced melasma fades more slowly than that related to pregnancy and may be permanent (80,81). In seven patients, no improvement was noted 3½ years after the pill was discontinued (82).

Although hyperpigmentation is one of the most common cutaneous complications of oral contraceptives, the true incidence is difficult to assess. Carruthers observed an incidence of 4% after one year of BCP use; the incidence increased to 37% by the fifth year of use (79). Resnik reported an incidence of 29% (82). Chloasma appears to be more prevalent in women who live in geographical areas with more sunlight, in dark-skinned races, and in women with a history of melasma during pregnancy. One study determined that 87% of women with BCP-induced melasma had this condition during pregnancy (82).

The use of sunscreens may be useful in women who are predisposed to this side effect. Also, taking the BCPs at night may theoretically be helpful, because circulating hormone levels will be minimal during the day when the skin is exposed to the sun. As noted earlier, patients with chloasma may not experience reversal even if the BCPs are discontinued. One group used a skin-lightener (hydroquinone cream 2–5%) (Eldoquin) for one month and noted temporary improvement in 18/20 patients (83,84).

This patient's Ortho-Novum 1/80 should be discontinued and she should be given a low-dose estrogen and progestogen combination BCP or a mini-pill. The patient should be informed that chloasma is only of cosmetic significance and does not indicate cancerous changes.

14. *Acne.* A 24-year-old woman who discontinued her combination-type BCPs three months ago because she wanted to become pregnant complains of a severe case of acne. What is the association between BCPs and acne? How should this patient be managed?

Most women who have an acne problem when they begin taking BCPs experience an improvement in the lesions after 1–4 months of therapy (81). This is related to the estrogen component, which decreases the size of the sebaceous glands and decreases production of androgen by the ovaries and adrenal glands through inhibition of pituitary function. Estrogens also increase the synthesis of proteins which bind androgens (85,86).

A few women can develop acne in association with BCP use if they are taking a pill which contains an androgenic progestogen such as norgestrel (eg, Ovral) or norethindrone acetate (eg, Norlestrin). This form of acne responds when the patient is changed to a BCP with greater estrogenic dominance (87–89). See Table 4.

Post-contraceptive acne, which is illustrated by this patient, is a common complaint and is thought to be caused by a compensatory hypersecretion of gonadotropins (88–91). It is usually seen in women who have been on the pill for at least one year and occurs three to four months after the pill has been discontinued (88). These lesions are self-limiting and subside in 6–12 months without treatment. They are also responsive to conventional forms of acne therapy (88). See the chapter on Skin Diseases.

Complications

15. Thromboembolic Phenomena. A 24-year-old woman was hospitalized with shortness of breath, a slight fever, and a tender, swollen right calf. She has no history of smoking, hypertension, diabetes or hyperlipidemia, but she has been taking Norlestrin 1 mg for three years. A diagnosis of deep venous thrombosis and pulmonary embolism was made, and the patient was treated with heparin by infusion and warfarin 5 mg daily. Ten days later she was discharged on warfarin. Her prothrombin time on the day of discharge was 23 seconds. How could the patient's oral contraceptive use have contributed to the development of her deep venous thrombosis and pulmonary embolism? Which component was responsible?

Oral contraceptive use is a definite risk factor in the development of thromboembolism. The first case-report of deep vein thrombosis attributed to BCPs appeared in 1961 and was followed by several others. Major concern about this adverse effect occurred in the late sixties following the publication of several retrospective studies which suggested that the risk of death from thromboembolic disease was 4–8 times greater in women who used the pill than in those who did not (92–96). Although the results of these retrospective studies were challenged (97–102), they have since been supported by similar results derived from three, large-scale, prospective studies. These include two which were conducted in Britain (103–107) and one which was conducted in the United States, commonly known as the Walnut Creek Study (108). While each of these studies differs in its design, they all conclude that *women using oral contraceptives run a 2–4 times greater risk than nonusers of developing superficial or deep venous thrombosis and pulmonary embolism.* Furthermore, oral contraceptive users are more prone to the development of thromboembolism following major surgery than are nonusers (103, 109,110,285).

The overall excess mortality from venous thromboembolism attributed to the BCPs is about two to three per 100,000 women annually.

The positive clinical association between BCP use and venous thromboembolism is also supported by plasma fibrinogen chromatography studies which show that BCP users have 4–5 times more "silent" thrombi than do nonusers (111–113).

Unlike other cardiovascular problems associated with BCP use, the risk of thromboembolism is probably not increased in smokers nor is it related to the duration of BCP use (96,105,108,114–116).

Statistically, patients with blood type O appear to be protected against the formation of thromboemboli as compared to those with blood types A, B and AB (105,117). Blood type A is most common in patients with thromboembolic disease (117,118), and patients with blood group A antigen exhibit a greater "hypercoagulability" of blood while receiving BCPs (119). Interestingly, individuals with this blood type have slightly lower levels of antithrombin III (119). Similarly, White women users of BCPs are at greater risk for thromboembolic disease than are Black women taking oral contraceptives (117).

Because estrogen is the component in BCPs

which is primarily responsible for the "hypercoagulable" state, the risk of developing venous thromboembolic disease is lower with the low-dose estrogen BCPs (105,120,121,123). However, the progestogen component (eg, norethindrone acetate) has been linked with an increased risk of subclinical thrombosis (105,113,120).

Estrogens elevate levels of several clotting factors and increase the prothrombin time after one to three cycles of use (102,124,125); they also reduce the activity of the fibrinolytic system. This appears to be a dose-related effect. Factors VII, X, and XII are increased in all users, and Factors I, II, V, VIII, and IX are increased in most users. Estrogens may also reduce the activity of antithrombin II and decrease the inhibitory activity of activated Factor X (68,126–128). Finally, long-term BCP use is associated with an increased platelet count and platelet aggregation (68).

16. Three weeks later, the patient returns to clinic and her prothrombin time is 24 seconds. She wants to resume her oral contraceptive. How should this situation be managed?

There are two major reasons why Norlestrin should not be resumed in this patient. The first is the presumptive association between her BCP use and a thromboembolic event in a woman less than 30 years of age who had no other risk factors (129). See the previous question.

The second relates to the potential interaction between the BCP and warfarin. It is generally accepted that oral contraceptives can diminish the effects of anticoagulants by increasing the concentrations of clotting factors and depressing antithrombin III activity (130). However, enhancement of the anticoagulant effect has also been reported. de Teresa et al studied the prothrombin time in 12 patients taking anticoagulants alone and together with BCPs. The mean prothrombin time was significantly higher when patients took both drugs concurrently; however, it remained within the therapeutic range. The authors suggest that this effect could be due to inhibition of hepatic microsomal enzymes by estrogens (131). Although this interaction needs clarification, it is evident that an adjustment of anticoagulant therapy may be needed when BCPs are added or discontinued.

The mini-pill would not be an acceptable alternative since the progestogens in some oral contraceptives have been implicated as the cause of superficial leg vein thromboses (105,113,120). The patient should be counseled on other methods of contraception such as the diaphragm, IUD or the use of the condom by her partner (See Questions 35–37).

17. A.J. is a 25-year-old woman who wishes to begin taking BCPs. She does not smoke, she has no family history of diabetes, and she is nulliparous. A physical examination reveals that her blood pressure is 100/70 mm Hg and that her cholesterol levels are within normal limits. She has no family history of cardiovascular disease. What is the risk of myocardial infarction in this patient and others who use oral contraceptives?

Overall, the risk of myocardial infarction associated with BCP use is 2–4 times that observed in nonusers; however, the risk is primarily concentrated in women 35 years of age or older, in heavy smokers, and in women who possess a combination of risk factors for myocardial infarction (See Table 7) (69,132–142). The risk of MI associated with BCP use in A.J., who is less than 35 years of age and without other risk factors for MI, is extremely small, approximately 1–2/100,000 women (69,283).

Table 7 lists the various risk factors for myocardial infarction in women, as well as the effect of those factors on the development of an MI relative to women who neither smoke nor use BCPs. Of note is the fact that BCP use alone increases the risk of MI in older women; smoking (>15 cigarettes per day) is a major risk factor for MI in women of all ages; and the combination of BCP use and smoking appears to have a synergistic effect, especially in women over the age of 45. Heavy cigarette smoking (≥15/day) can increase the risk tremendously in older women taking BCPs.

The major risk factors, other than age, smoking and BCP-use, include hypertension, high levels of low-density cholesterol, diabetes, and a history of preeclampsia. Each of these factors increases the risk for an MI 3–4 times. The combined effects of any of these factors is synergistic, as illustrated by the fact that the presence of 3 or more of them increases the risk for the development of an MI 128-fold (132,133,136–138,142).

New evidence suggests that the risk of MI is related to both the estrogen and progestogen con-

Table 7.

THE RELATIVE RISK OF MYOCARDIAL INFARCTION (MI) ASSOCIATED
WITH BIRTH CONTROL PILLS (BCPs) AND OTHER FACTORS[4]

Risk Factors for MI[1]	Incidence[2]		Relative Risk of MI[3]
Age (Years)	Non-Users	BCP-Users	
<30	1.9	? ≈ Same	? minimal
30–39	4.0	11	2.7–3
40–44	22	89*	3–4
Smoking			
Age 30–39			
0–14 cigarettes/day	2	6	3
> 15 cigarettes/day	11	30	3.7–4
Age 40–44			
0–14 cigarettes/day	12	47	4
> 15 cigarettes/day	61	246	4
Hyperlipidemia			3–4
Hypertension			3–4
Diabetes			3–4

[1]The presence of any three risk factors increases the risk for MI to 128 (See Question 17)

[2]Incidence is expressed as # cases/100,000 non-users or 100,000 BCP-users

[3]Risk is expressed as the risk of developing an MI relative to women of the same age who do not use BCPs

[4]Adapted from reference 69

tent of the BCPs (120,123). Epidemiologically, a decrease in the incidence of BCP-related MIs has been associated with the use of low-dose estrogen BCPs. However, this observation may also be attributed to lower doses of progestogens. For example, women using oral contraceptives containing 3–4 mg of norethindrone acetate had a 1.5–2.0 times greater risk of developing an MI than women using otherwise similar estrogen-containing contraceptives containing only 1–2 mg of norethindrone acetate. A similar pattern was observed for women taking BCPs containing the progestogen, norgestrel (123). These progestogens may increase the risk of cardiovascular disease by decreasing high density lipoprotein cholesterol, which appears to be protective against heart disease (283,284).

On the basis of these observations, low-dose estrogen and progestogen BCPs should be used whenever feasible in the young (less than 35 years of age), nonsmoking woman with no cardiovascular risk factors. Nonsmoking women aged 35–45 years who have no other cardiovascular risk factors may decide that the benefits of BCP-use outweigh their limited risks. Women 35–45 years of age who smoke or have other cardiovascular risk factors and women over the age of 45 should not use oral contraceptives as a method of birth control.

18. Hypertension. S.W. is a 25-year-old, obese woman who has been taking Ovulen for the past two years. She smokes 1½ packs of cigarettes per day and has a strong history of cardiovascular disease. Two weeks ago, her blood pressure was noted to be 150/105 mm Hg and her BCPs were discontinued at that time. On this visit, her blood pressure remains the same. The plan is to institute hydrochlorothiazide 50 mg daily and resume her BCPs. What is the relationship between hypertension and BCPs? Is it reasonable to resume S.W.'s BCPs at this time?

Women who take BCPs are 2–3 times more likely to develop hypertension (blood pressure > 140/90) than nonusers (143–145). The incidence of hypertension was 4% in users versus 1.5% in nonusers in a prospective U.S study (143). In most White women, BCPs cause a minimal increase in blood pressure (4 mm Hg systolic and 1 mm Hg diastolic) which returns to baseline pressures or below after BCPs are discontinued. In a few women, major elevations of blood pressure have been reported (146–148). Similar observations have not been made in Black women. With the exception of age and race, no other factors which increase the risk of hypertension in women using BCPs have been identified. For example, women with a history of hypertension or preeclampsia during pregnancy are not predisposed to the hypertensive effects of BCPs (149).

Blood pressure may continue to rise with the duration of BCP use (2,150), but this is not a consistent finding (2). Since hypertension secondary to the pill may develop slowly over a period of 3–36 months (63,70,151) and may not decline for 3–6 months after the pill is discontinued (average 3 months), BCP-related hypertension cannot be ruled out in S.W. Her Ovulen should be discontinued for a minimum of 3 months before further evaluation is pursued. Since S.W. has other risk factors for myocardial infarction (obesity, smoking, and hypertension), she should be strongly advised to discontinue her BCPs permanently and use an alternative method of contraception.

BCP-induced hypertension is most likely related to both the estrogen and progestogen components. The underlying mechanisms are not known but may be related to the effects of these hormones on sodium and water retention and increased renin activity (59,152,153).

19. Breast Disease.
A 25-year-old woman with a history of chronic cystic disease of the breast wishes to use birth control pills. What is the relationship between BCPs and benign breast disease (BBD) and breast cancer? Is this woman a candidate for BCP use?

Oral contraceptive users are one-half as likely to develop benign breast disease (eg, fibroadenoma, chronic cystic disease, unbiopsied breast lumps) as those who do not use BCPs. This protective effect is most likely related to the progestogen component and may become less significant with the more extensive use of the low-dose combination BCPs (50–52).

Even though BBD is associated with an increased risk of breast cancer, oral contraceptives do not have the same protective effect against the latter. However, women taking the pill do not appear to be at greater risk for the development of breast cancer. This paradox may be explained by a differential effect of BCPs on the type of BBD which progresses to breast cancer and that which does not. The former can only be diagnosed by biopsy (53–55,59).

Because some forms of BBD may progress to breast cancer over a period of many years and because malignant breast cells may be hormone-sensitive, BCPs should be used cautiously in women with existing, undiagnosed breast lumps. Women with BBD who take BCPs should be monitored closely for any change in the size or character of their lumps.

Despite the lack of evidence linking BCPs to breast cancer, other means of contraception should be used in women with a strong family history of breast cancer, a history of cancer in one breast, abnormal mammograms, or recurrent chronic cystic mastitis.

20. Post-Pill Amenorrhea.
A 29-year-old woman who took BCPs for four years has not had a menstrual period since she discontinued their use two years ago. Her earlier history of irregular periods was improved when she took oral contraceptives. One year ago, a 3-month trial of clomiphene citrate (Clomid) induced spotting but was otherwise unsuccessful. How prevalent is post-pill amenorrhea and how should it be managed?

Post-pill amenorrhea and infecundity can be a major concern associated with the use of oral contraceptives (163,164). However, recent studies show that the rate of conception is decreased only for the first three months after the pill is discontinued. When amenorrhea does occur, 90–95% of patients resume menses 6–18 months after the pill has been discontinued (157,158). When delivery rates of former BCP users and former diaphragm users were compared, they were the same by 30 months in parous women and 42 months in nulliparous women (165).

This patient's prolonged amenorrhea and infecundity are probably related to a problem which existed prior to her use of BCPs, as noted by her past history of irregular periods. She should receive a complete infertility work-up. If galactorrhea is also present, a pituitary tumor should be excluded (159–162,282).

21. Teratogenicity.
D.A., a 32-year-old woman, has been taking Ovral for seven years. She missed her last period and was instructed to continue taking Ovral for one more

cycle. When she missed her second period, she had a pregnancy test which was positive. What are the effects of BCPs on miscarriage and fetal development? Was D.A. appropriately advised?

D.A. has been taking Ovral for seven years and assuming she has had no previous problems with missed periods, she was definitely misadvised. Such women should be advised to discontinue their BCPs immediately and to use another form of contraception until pregnancy is ruled out.

BCPs have no deleterious effects on the fetus nor do they increase the incidence of miscarriage in women who discontinue their use *prior to* conception (49,166,167). However, BCPs may have a teratogenic effect when women, such as D.A., inadvertently take these agents early in pregnancy (166,168). Investigators looking at this issue have come to conflicting conclusions. Some have found no relationship between the pill and birth defects (169–171), while others conclude the opposite. Although the teratogenic effects of BCPs have not been conclusively established, it is reasonable to avoid their use if at all possible in pregnant women.

D.A. should be advised of the possible teratogenic effects of the BCPs and an abortion should be considered.

22. Diabetes. **A 28-year-old mildly obese diabetic woman wishes to start BCPs. Her diabetes was first diagnosed when an abnormal fasting blood sugar noted during the third trimester of her second pregnancy failed to regress after delivery. Family history revealed a father and sister with diabetes. Presently her diabetes is controlled by diet alone and her urine sugars have been negative. How significant is the diabetogenic effect of oral contraceptives? Has one component been implicated? Which BCP would you recommend for this patient?**

Combination-type oral contraceptives do not alter the fasting blood sugar in the majority of healthy users and the use of the pill does not increase the risk of clinically apparent diabetes in otherwise healthy women (172,173). However, BCPs can definitely alter the oral and intravenous glucose tolerance test (GTT) and induce overt diabetes in predisposed individuals (174–176,182). The women at greatest risk include those with a family history of diabetes, those who have

had hyperglycemia during pregnancy (gestational diabetes), those who have borne infants greater than 8–9 pounds, obese women, women who have used BCPs for a prolonged period of time (more than 10 years), older women (>40 years), and women taking BCPs with higher estrogen and progestogen contents (173,174,177–182). These risk factors may be additive (175). Most studies indicate that the GTT returns to normal after discontinuation of the BCP (177–182); the notable exception is a woman such as this patient with a history of gestational diabetes (177–179).

It is not entirely clear how the oral contraceptives impair carbohydrate metabolism. Various metabolic alterations are probably contributory since elevated levels of pyruvate, lactate, growth hormone, cortisol, triglycerides, and cholesterol have been observed in BCP users (172,174,183–185). However, BCPs most likely affect insulin activity. Progressive deterioration of glucose tolerance has been observed in association with early hyperinsulism, and the development of insulin resistance has been associated with impaired insulin secretion relative to the glucose level. Alteration in insulin receptor affinity and the number of insulin receptors may also be responsible for the diabetogenic effect of BCPs (172–174,178, 186,187,189,191).

These effects appear to be dependent on both the dose and type of hormone ingested by the individual. Mestranol, for example, may be more diabetogenic than ethinyl estradiol, although this is not a consistent finding (188). Lowering the estrogen content without alteration of the progestogen has resulted in improved glucose tolerance and increased insulin secretion (172–174, 177,181,191).

The progestogen component has also been implicated in altering carbohydrate metabolism, presumably by lowering insulin receptor affinity and numbers. The worst offender is norgestrel, followed by ethynodiol diacetate. Norethindrone causes mild insulin and glucose alterations (173, 189,190,191).

Therefore, a low-dose estrogen combination pill containing norethindrone (eg, Brevicon) or a progestogen-only pill (eg, Micronor) may be tried in patients presdisposed to the diabetogenic effects of these agents. Norgestrel and ethynodiol diacetate combinations should be avoided. However, non-hormonal methods of contraception should be strongly considered in patients such as the one described above and in patients whose glucose intolerance persists, because none of the oral contraceptives are entirely free of diabetogenic potential.

23. A 22-year-old woman whose juvenile-onset diabetes is controlled with insulin would like to use a birth control pill. Are the diabetogenic and thromboembolic effects of the oral contraceptives contraindications to their use in this patient?

This patient is already diabetic, so the fear of inducing diabetes is irrelevant. However, BCPs may alter the patient's diabetic control and the insulin dose may have to be adjusted, but adequate control can be accomplished (178). Because the risks to the diabetic patient and her fetus should she become pregnant are far greater than the risk of BCP use per se, oral contraceptives are not absolutely contraindicated in this situation.

The effect of oral contraceptives on the progression of vascular complications associated with diabetes is not well-studied. Goldzieher et al found no significant increased risk for the development of diabetic vascular disease as assessed by electron microscopic examination of the capillary membrane (192). However, others have reported an increased incidence of cerebral thrombosis and myocardial infarction in diabetics taking oral contraceptives compared to control groups using other means of contraception (193). Since diabetes and oral contraceptive use are both risk factors for myocardial infarction, any diabetic patient taking BCPs should be warned of this and monitored carefully for evidence of retinal, renal, and cardiovascular disease as well as adequate control of blood sugar. The low-dose estrogen or progestogen-only oral contraceptives may expose the patient to less risk (see Question 17), but condoms and diaphragms should be offered as an alternative. Because diabetics are predisposed to risks associated with the IUDs, these devices should not be used in these individuals.

24. *Headache.* A 26-year-old woman who is taking Ovral presents with a recent onset of throbbing headaches which are preceded by blurred vision, nausea, and vomiting and are unrelieved by aspirin or acetaminophen; however, a dark room seems to help. Her sister and an aunt suffer from migraine headaches. What is the relationship between BCPs

and headache? How should this woman's headache be managed?

The relationship between BCPs and headaches is complex. Some women with a history of chronic headaches note a striking improvement in their symptoms while taking BCPs (194), while others note an exacerbation of existing headaches or an onset of new headaches (195–199).

Headaches associated with the pill present clinically in two basic ways: a tension-type headache which may occur at any time throughout the cycle and a migraine-type headache which predominantly occurs mid-cycle or during the 7-day period when the patient is "off" the pill (195–199). Thus, any patient complaining of headaches should be questioned about the relationship between her symptoms and her menstrual cycle to determine if there is a pattern of headache attacks. The new or recent onset of severe headaches associated with visual changes or blindness requires immediate evaluation for thrombosis. Discontinuation of the BCP is warranted since these symptoms may forewarn an impending stroke or cerebral thrombosis (200,201).

The etiology of BCP-related headaches is unknown, although they may be due to withdrawal of progesterone and, more likely, estrogens. In eight women with migraine, estradiol injections administered 3–6 days prior to the onset of menses delayed migraine headaches for 3–9 days. No delay was noted with the similar administration of progesterone injections (202,206). Other factors such as sodium and water retention secondary to the estrogen component and ordinary tension may be contributory factors.

Because good clinical studies are lacking, the incidence of BCP-related headaches is difficult to ascertain. Reported incidences of patients developing migraine headaches de novo while taking BCPs range from 11% (207) to 50% (195). The headaches encountered are typical of the classic migraine headache as illustrated by this patient (196,198,200).

Although it has been suggested that a combination of a weak progesterone and weak estrogen or a strong combination of both hormones results in the lowest incidence of headache attacks, clinical experience indicates that deterioration of migraine headaches is not likely to be improved by changing to a BCP with a different hormone balance (197,199).

Diuretics and conventional headache regimens

have been used to treat BCP-related headaches (197); however, these treatments are often ineffective until the BCP has been discontinued (196). Since this patient's symptoms are typical of migraine and since she has a family history of this problem, it is unlikely that any manipulation of her oral contraceptives will achieve freedom from this side effect. Thus, she should be advised to discontinue oral contraceptives and use another method of birth control.

25. Should a woman with a history of headaches or migraines use BCPs as a method of contraception?

As noted earlier, some women experience marked improvement of existing headaches when they begin taking birth control pills. However, it is also well documented that patients with a prior history of migraine are likely to note an increased incidence and severity of attacks while taking BCPs. These attacks are frequently refractory to conventional forms of treatment until the pill is discontinued (195–199). Several factors may be predictive of women who are likely to experience worsening of their migraines while taking the pill: age over 30 years, parity, prolonged menstrual cycles beyond the normal 27–30 days; migraines which occur at specific periods during the menstrual cycle; migraines relieved during the last trimester of pregnancy, and the onset of migraines after pregnancy (199). Some have suggested that any woman who experiences her headaches mid-cycle should use alternative methods of contraception.

In any case, any woman with a history of headaches prior to starting BCPs should be monitored closely for an increased incidence and severity of headaches. These symptoms may not be obvious to the patient nor may she relate them to her BCPs. Only through specific questioning of her symptoms or a drug history which indicates an increased intake of analgesics will this side effect of BCPs become apparent.

26. *Depression.* R.N., a 28-year-old woman with a history of depression, wishes to use BCPs. She currently takes amitriptyline (Elavil) 150 mg at bedtime. What is the relationship between BCPs and depression? Is this patient a candidate for BCPs?

The relationship between BCPs and depression is not clear. Some investigators have noted an increased incidence of depression (approxi-

mately 5–6%) in women taking BCPs (208–216), while others have been unable to detect a correlation (217–219). Clinically, depression may become more severe or improve in women taking the pill. Furthermore, depression may be insidious and undetectable by women taking BCPs; only after discontinuation of the BCPs will some women make the observation that they felt much more depressed while taking BCPs.

BCP-related depression has been attributed to estrogen excess, progestogen excess, estrogen deficiency, and pyridoxine deficiency (209,210,220–222). Thus, many clinicians would initiate patients such as R.N. on a low-dose estrogen and progestogen combination BCP such as Modicon or Brevicon (0.5 mg of norethindrone and 35 mcg of ethinyl estradiol) and monitor them closely for symptoms of worsening depression. Alternatively, a mini-pill could be used if depression worsens. Others have treated depressed women taking BCPs with vitamin B–6 or pyridoxine 25–50 mg daily. This practice is based on the theory that B–6 deficiency in these women causes abnormal tryptophan and, ultimately, brain amine metabolism which leads to depression (220–222).

All of the above may be attempted in this patient, but if her depression becomes severe, BCPs should be discontinued and she should use an alternative method of contraception.

27. *Cholecystitis.* A 34-year-old woman was admitted to the emergency room with an acute attack of severe epigastric and lower abdominal pain accompanied by nausea, vomiting, diarrhea, and low-grade fever. The patient has no history of peptic ulcer disease, but an oral cholecystogram last year revealed a large number of gall stones. The patient has been taking Ovulen for the past year. What gastrointestinal complications should be considered in this BCP-user?

Oral contraceptives appear to be associated with a two-fold increase in the incidence of cholecystitis and cholelithiasis, particularly during the first year of use (2,96,223). This represents a morbidity rate of 158 cases versus 79 cases per 100,000 women. The mechanism of this effect is unknown but may be related to an alteration of bile acid composition and cholesterol saturation by hormone components of the BCPs.

Mesenteric vascular disease with necrosis and infarction of the bowel should also be considered in BCP-users with acute gastrointestinal complaints. Since more than 20 such cases have been reported, the relationship between this condition and BCP use may not be fortuitous (224,225).

28. Describe liver complications related to BCP use.

Benign liver tumors (benign hepatoma, hepatic adenoma, focal nodular hyperplasia, rarely malignant forms) have been associated with the long-term (more than 5 years) use of high-dose estrogen BCPs. The incidence is extremely low (3/100,000 women per year). Although the tumors are generally benign, death can result from intrahepatic or extrahepatic tumor rupture and hemorrhagic shock. Patients who have been using high-dose estrogens for several years should be switched to low-dose preparations if at all feasible. Such women should be monitored regularly for liver enlargement, pain or tenderness (65–67,226–229).

Cholestatic Jaundice. Malaise, anorexia, nausea, and pruritus can occur 2 weeks to several months (usually less than 4 weeks) after beginning the pill. Later, dark urine and jaundice may appear. Discontinuation of BCPs results in complete clinical remission within a few weeks to a month (230). No specific hormonal component has been implicated, although anabolic steroids, estriol, estradiol, and C-17 alkylated steroids can produce cholestatic jaundice (231,232). Women with a history of jaundice during pregnancy are at particular risk (233). Laboratory abnormalities include an elevated indirect bilirubin (3–10 mg/dl), moderately elevated transaminase values (100–300 U), and mild increases in BSP retention. Alkaline phosphatase is rarely elevated and laboratory alterations may occur without other symptoms (230,234–236). Mild elevations may be well-tolerated, but such women should be warned of symptoms associated with cholestatic jaundice.

29. *Drug Interactions.* A.M., a 28-year-old woman with positive sputum cultures for *Mycobacterium tuberculosis,* was initiated on INH, ethambutol and rifampin. Six months later she discovered she was six weeks pregnant even though she had been taking Ovral for the entire time and denied missing any doses. Have any of the antitubercular drugs been implicated in reducing the effectiveness of oral contraceptives? How should such patients be managed?

There are numerous studies associating the combined use of rifampin and BCPs with pregnancy or menstrual abnormalities (237–240). In 1973, five cases of pregnancy occurred in women receiving both oral contraceptives and rifampin (240) and as early as 1971, menstrual disorders were reported in 70% of women receiving this same combination (238). By comparison, only 4% of women receiving BCPs and other antituberculous drugs experienced menstrual abnormalities (239). As a result, the following warning appears in rifampin package inserts: "It has been reported that the reliability of oral contraceptives may be affected in some patients being treated for tuberculosis with rifampin in combination with at least one other antituberculous drug. In such cases, alternative contraceptive measures may need to be considered; menstrual disturbances have also been noted."

Rifampin may decrease the effectiveness of BCPs by inducing the hepatic metabolism (hydroxylation) of estrogens, thereby decreasing estrogen levels below those needed for contraception (240–243). Patients using low-dose estrogen products, such as patient A.M., are more likely to experience menstrual irregularities and loss of contraception control than those using high-dose products (242,243).

Since the efficacy of oral contraceptives does not appear to be affected by PAS, INH, or streptomycin, these agents may be used instead to treat tuberculosis. In the alternative, another method of birth control could be used by the patient taking rifampin.

30. What other drugs interact with oral contraceptives?

Antibiotics. Intermenstrual bleeding and occasional pregnancies have been reported in oral contraceptive users also receiving the antibiotics ampicillin, tetracycline, sulfamethoxypyridazine, and chloramphenicol (244,245). Women receiving phenoxymethylpenicillin, neomycin, and nitrofurantoin have experienced intermenstrual bleeding while on oral contraceptives (243,245). The mechanism seems to be a reduction in the enterohepatic circulation of the sex hormones due to an inhibition of gut bacteria by the antibiotics. Hydrolytic enzymes produced by these bacteria release free steroids from their conjugated forms which are produced by the liver. Inhibition of this process may diminish the quantity of hormone reentering the circulation (246). Most clinicians do not consider the interaction between antibiotics and BCPs significant enough to avoid their combined use (247). Nevertheless, patients who are on low-dose BCPs should be warned of this potential interaction and advised to use additional forms of contraception during antibiotic administration.

Anticoagulants. See Question 16.

Anticonvulsants. Phenytoin, primidone, and carbamazepine may decrease the effectiveness of oral contraceptives by inducing enzymatic metabolism of the hormones. Increased spotting and three pregnancies have been observed in patients receiving BCPs together with antiepileptic drugs (243,245,248,249). Because of this interaction, many clinicians recommend other methods of contraception for patients receiving these drugs. Loss of seizure control may occur as a result of the fluid retention associated with the BCPs.

Barbiturates. Abundant animal data indicate that the barbiturates increase the metabolism of estrogens and decrease their half-lives (249). Of 51 oral contraceptive users who received phenobarbital, thirty experienced break-through bleeding (BTB) and one pregnancy was reported. It seems likely that BTB and spotting were the clinical correlates of the enzyme induction which occurred secondary to phenobarbital (249).

Mini-Pills

31. A 36-year-old woman who smokes two packs of cigarettes per day wishes to use BCPs. Which BCPs should be considered for this patient? What instructions should accompany their use?

The use of combination BCPs is contraindicated in this patient because she is at risk for the development of cardiovascular side effects associated with their use (see Question 17). One could consider the use of the mini-pills which contain progestogen only in lower doses than those contained in the combination tablets. However, the safety of the progestogen-only pills needs further study, since many of the complications associated with the oral contraceptives have been attributed to both the estrogen and progestogen component. The progestogen component appears to play a major role in the development of diabetes, hypertension, and cardiovascular complications when combined with estrogens (187,189,190,283,284). This is discussed in detail in the proceedings of a

special symposium which was held on the effects of progesterone in the oral contraceptives (250).

Because these agents are associated with a high incidence of irregular menses, it is imperative to first determine whether this patient currently has a history of abnormal genital bleeding to assure that any existing underlying pathology will not be attributed to the mini-pills. These pills should be avoided in women with a history of gestational diabetes, mononucleosis, or ectopic pregnancy (1,177,250).

Unlike the combination BCPs, the mini-pills must be taken every single day. If one pill is missed, it should be made up on the following days and an alternate form of contraception should be used until the next menstrual cycle. Patients taking the mini-pill may have regular menstrual cycles; however, many have scanty periods, spotting, and irregular cycles. This may cause a great deal of anxiety, because it is difficult to tell, in this situation, exactly where one is in a cycle. A patient who does not have a period for 45 days or more should have a pregnancy test. Some individuals have as few as two menstrual periods annually while taking the mini-pill (1).

Since 40% of women taking the mini-pill continue to ovulate, an additional method of contraception used during mid-cycle should improve the effectiveness of the mini-pill. Also, since pregnancy rates associated with the use of the mini-pill are highest during the first few months of use, a secondary method of contraception is advised for the first one to two cycles of use. Failure rates are lower for women who have switched from the combination BCP to the mini-pill (1,4).

32. What are some indications for use of the mini-pill?

In addition to women who may be at greater risk for the cardiovascular effects associated with the estrogen component of the combination BCPs, women who are experiencing intolerable side effects related to estrogen or progestogen excess may be successfully switched to the mini-pill.

Signs and symptoms related to estrogen excess which are alleviated by the mini-pill include headache, leg pain, hypertension, chloasma, and weight gain. Those related to progestogen excess include vaginitis, acne, and weight gain. Depression may be related to excess estrogen or progestogen.

Mini-pills have also been recommended for lactating women because the decreased milk production associated with the use of estrogens has not been observed with their use. See Question 33.

33. *Lactation.* **A 24-year-old woman gave birth to her second baby one week ago. She plans to breast feed. How soon after delivery should she resume her BCPs to assure adequate contraception?**

Postpartum amenorrhea lasts 2–3 months in the nonbreast-feeding mother and from 4–24 months in the breast-feeding mother (251). However, ovulation can occur 6–8 weeks after delivery and occurs in 80% of women prior to the onset of menstruation. Although breast-feeding is associated with prolonged postpartum amenorrhea and, perhaps, ovulation suppression, it is *not* a foolproof method of contraception and there is a 7–10% risk of conception during the postpartum amenorrheic period (252,253).

Therefore, contraception may be initiated immediately in the woman who does not plan to breast feed and 6 weeks postpartum in the woman who plans to breast feed. This delay allows for the establishment of milk flow so that it is less likely that BCPs will have any adverse effects on lactation.

Since estrogens may decrease milk flow, many clinicians prefer to use mini-pills in lactating women (256,257). However, low-dose combination products are not likely to have an adverse effect on milk flow once it is established and studies on infants breast-fed by mothers taking combination BCPs have shown no difference in weights when compared to infants breast-fed by mothers not taking BCPs (251,254,255). Furthermore, the Academy of Pediatrics has recently issued a statement approving the use of combination products in breast-feeding mothers once lactation has been established. Currently, there is no evidence that the amount of hormones excreted in breast milk is sufficient to cause ill effects in the infant.

OTHER BIRTH CONTROL METHODS

Sterilization

34. A 37-year-old female has taken oral contraceptives for the past 12 years. Her blood pressure is normal and she has no history of adverse effects to the BCPs. She smokes 1½

packs of cigarettes daily. What alternate forms of contraception are available to this woman?

Based on the current evidence which points to the importance of age and smoking as risk factors for cardiovascular disease, this woman should be strongly advised to use another form of contraception.

Her desire for a reversible or irreversible means of contraception should be determined. If she desires a reversible contraceptive method, an IUD, a diaphragm with spermicide, vaginal spermicide, or condom can be considered (See Questions 35–37).

However, if she does not plan on having children, sterilization would be the most effective and convenient method of contraception. Further, there is relatively little risk associated with these procedures on a short-term or long-term basis in the hands of experienced practitioners. Tubal ligation and vasectomy are the most common methods of contraception used in the United States by married couples over 30–35 years of age who desire no more children. For a detailed discussion of these procedures and their complications see references 1 and 258.

Intrauterine Devices

35. A 27-year-old female who has had two children wants to wait three to four years before she has another child. She cannot tolerate oral contraceptives and wishes to use an intrauterine device (IUD). Is an IUD a feasible method of contraception for this woman? How effective are these devices and what is their mechanism of action? What complications are associated with their use?

The intrauterine device (IUD) is the second most effective reversible method of contraception. Pregnancy rates vary from 2–5 per 100 women-years (1,70,259,260). There are two varieties of IUDs. Some are chemically inert devices which are made of a nonabsorbable material such as polyethylene impregnated with barium sulfate for radiopacity (eg, Lippes Loop; Saf-T-Coil). Others are impregnated with chemicals such as copper or progesterone that are continually eluted into the uterus (Copper T, Copper 7; Progestasert).

Mechanism of Action. IUDs produce a number of cellular and biochemical alterations in the endometrium which may be responsible for their contraceptive effect. All unmedicated and copper devices stimulate an inflammatory or foreign body reaction in the uterus, causing infiltration of the endometrium with numerous polymorphonuclear leukocytes, foreign body giant cells, mononuclear cells, plasma cells and macrophages. These cells probably engulf the spermatozoa or ovum, preventing fertilization and implantation. Increased production of prostaglandins may also play a role in their contraceptive efficacy.

Medicated IUDs also have local effects which add to their contraceptive efficacy. Copper interferes with enzyme systems, with cellular DNA content in the endometrium, with glycogen metabolism, and with estrogen uptake by the uterine mucosa. IUDs containing progesterone interfere with the normal hormone-stimulated cycle of the endometrium, making implantation unlikely. The small amounts of progesterone released by these devices do not appear to affect ovarian function and are not detectable in the blood stream (1,70,259–263).

Contraindications. This patient can be considered a candidate for IUD insertion if no contraindications exist. Absolute contraindications include pregnancy, active pelvic inflammatory disease (PID), and a very small uterus (less than 4.5 cm diameter). Relative contraindications include a history of recurrent PID, acute cervicitis, valvular heart disease, an abnormal pap smear, immunosuppression, abnormal menstrual bleeding, anemia, and copper allergy (259,260).

Selection. The most important factor to consider in selecting an IUD is the clinician's competence and familiarity with the IUD selected. Other patient-related factors include: reason for IUD use (termination of childbearing vs spacing of children); whether the patient is nulliparous or parous; menses characteristics; and history of previous IUD use and expulsion.

If the patient does not wish to have any more children, an IUD which may be inserted permanently (ie, has no requisite replacement interval) such as the Lippes Loop or Saf-T-Coil may be used. In women who plan to use the IUD for child-spacing, such as the patient described above, the copper IUDs which require replacement every 3–5 years or Progestasert, which must be replaced yearly, are viable alternatives. Progestasert may be the IUD of choice in women with painful, heavy menses or a history of IUD expulsion. The Cu-7 and small Saf-T-coil, which have small diameters, are the IUDs of choice in nulliparous women

with a small cervical os. However, if it appears unlikely that a woman will receive regular medical follow-up care, the medicated IUDs should not be used (1,70,259–263).

Complications. Major complications associated with IUD use include a 50–100% incidence of increased menstrual bleeding or spotting and anemia, with the exception of Progestasert; spontaneous expulsion and cramping soon after insertion; an increased risk (two-fold) of developing PID (261,262); uterine perforation; spontaneous abortions; and ectopic pregnancies. When pregnancy occurs while the IUD is in place, most authorities recommend immediate removal of the IUD. An abortion rate of 54% was noted when the device was left in place compared to 25% if it was promptly removed. There was also an increased frequency of low birth weights when the device was left in place.

Patient Instruction. Patients should be encouraged to check for string placement frequently during the first three months of use and following each menstrual period thereafter. Tampons and menstrual pads should be checked closely for the presence of the IUD since most expulsions occur during the menstrual period. Other forms of contraception should be used during the first three months of insertion, at least during mid-cycle. The patient should bring to the attention of the clinician any of the following: a misplaced string; signs of infection including fever, pelvic pain or tenderness, unusually severe cramping or bleeding, or a foul discharge; and missed periods or irregular bleeding. Women using medicated IUDs should be advised when replacement is necessary and all patients should be warned against any attempt to remove the IUD themselves (1,70,259–263).

Diaphragms

36. A 24-year-old female has been taking oral contraceptives for the past three years since the birth of her first child. She has discontinued the BCPs and wants to wait at least three months before conception. What contraceptive method would be most effective in the interim? How should it be used?

The most effective interim contraceptive method would be the diaphragm in combination with a spermicide (See Question 37). Although the IUD is more effective, this patient wants protection for a relatively short period of time and proper use of the diaphragm would achieve effectiveness approaching that of an IUD. The diaphragm is a soft rubber cup with a metal spring reinforcing the rim. The device is inserted vaginally and placed over the cervical os to block access of sperm to the cervix. It is held in place by the spring tension of the rim, the woman's vaginal muscle tone and the pubic bone. The diaphragm does not fit tightly enough to entirely prevent the passage of all sperm around the rim, so the manufacturers recommend that it be used with spermicidal cream or jelly (approximately one tablespoon in the dome and around the rim). Therefore, it serves as a container to hold the spermicide in place and as a mechanical barrier (1,264).

To be effective, the diaphragm must be properly fitted. Although there are some reports of a low effectiveness rate associated with their use, most failures are related to improper use, poor motivation, improper insertion, improper fit, displacement during intercourse, or a defect in the device (1). With proper instruction and appropriate use on a regular basis, the combination of the diaphragm with spermicide is a highly effective method of contraception. Vessey et al reported a pregnancy rate of 2.4 per 100 women-years for established users of the diaphragm (107).

The diaphragm can be inserted up to six hours or more before intercourse; however, if it has been inserted more than two hours before intercourse, application of additional spermicide is recommended. If more than one act of intercourse occurs with the diaphragm in place, a second application of spermicidal jelly or cream is desirable. The diaphragm must not be removed for six hours after intercourse to ensure activity of the spermicide. Douching is contraindicated while the device is in place since this may dilute or remove the spermicide. The diaphragm should not be left in place more than 24 hours because infection may result (1,264).

When properly cared for, a diaphragm may last up to two years, but most clinicians recommend that a new one be purchased each year or earlier if defects are noticed. Following removal, the diaphragm is washed with mild soap and warm water, then dried and dusted with cornstarch or unscented talcum and stored in its container.

The diaphragm is one of the safest methods of contraception. The most common side effects are minor allergic reactions and vaginal irritation

secondary to the spermicide. Switching brands of spermicides usually alleviates this problem. In the rare case of allergy to rubber, plastic diaphragms are available.

Diaphragms are particularly ideal for women who cannot tolerate oral contraceptives or IUDs, for those who need a short-term interim method of contraception, for women who are breast feeding and for women who engage in sexual intercourse infrequently and do not need continuous protection.

Condoms-Spermicides

37. A couple on a one-week vacation forgot to bring the woman's birth control pills. What is the most effective nonprescription method of contraception they can use in the interim?

The most effective nonprescription method of contraception is a combination of spermicidal agents and condoms. If this combination is used correctly, the contraceptive effectiveness equals the IUD and approaches that of the BCPs.

Condoms. Although condoms are not the most effective method of contraception when used alone, they are simple to use, inexpensive, easily obtainable, and do not require a physical examination or a physician's prescription. They offer the additional benefit of preventing sexually transmitted diseases. The failure rate associated with their correct and regular use is estimated to be less than 5 pregnancies per 100 couple-years (1).

Condoms are made of rubber (or latex) or a collagenous, "skin-type" tissue which is obtained from lamb cecum; the latter are expensive and used less extensively. The rubber condoms are available in a variety of sizes and types (opaque, transparent, colored, plain-ended, reservoir-ended, rippled, pagoda-shaped, strictured, contoured). They may be dry or lubricated with a water-soluble substance or silicone. Lubricated or "wet" condoms are frequently used because they facilitate insertion of the erect penis and are less likely to tear on insertion. However, the same effect may be achieved by lubricating a less-expensive dry condom with contraceptive cream or a water soluble jelly (eg, KY Jelly, Ortho Personal Lubricant). Petrolatum and other oils should not be used since these may cause deterioration of the rubber.

Tearing or rupture of the condom is the most common cause of contraceptive failure, although this occurs infrequently (1). As mentioned earlier, this may be minimized with lubrication or by use of the reservoir-ended condom which provides ample space for the ejaculated semen. If a plain condom is used, 1–2 cm of space should be left at the end of the penis to accommodate the ejaculate.

The condom should be placed on the penis before it comes in contact with the vagina since sperm may be present in the urethral secretions prior to ejaculation. Following intercourse, the penis should be withdrawn before the erection completely subsides to prevent leakage of sperm within the vagina. When removing the penis, the rim of the condom should be held firmly to further prevent loss of the condom and semen within the vagina.

Spermicides. There are three major forms of spermicides available without precription: creams, jellies, and gels; suppositories or vaginal tablets; and foams. Some of these preparations are designed to be used in conjunction with a diaphragm or other contraceptive method, while others can be used alone. The latter are generally more potent and have a different consistency than preparations intended for use with a diaphragm.

Both types of preparations contain two components: an inert base which serves as a mechanical barrier to the cervical os and a spermicidal chemical which actively immobilizes and kills sperm. The most frequently used spermicide is a poly oxyethylated alkylphenol (nonionic surfactant) commonly called nonoxynol-9.

The choice of a particular product largely depends upon patient preference. The foams are the most effective form because they are more likely to be distributed properly over the cervical os. The suppositories are convenient to carry, but should be inserted high into the vagina approximately 30 minutes prior to intercourse to allow time for dissolution and proper foam formation over the cervical os. The creams, jellies, and gels are water-soluble but they melt quickly and may not form as effective a barrier as the foam. Except for the tablets or suppositories, spermicidal agents should be applied just prior to intercourse and application should be repeated for each consequent intercourse. The patient should be warned against douching within six hours after intercourse to assure spermicidal effectiveness.

Failures related to the use of spermicides stem primarily from patient error which includes improper placement, inconsistent use, inadequate agitation of the bottle to properly disperse the spermicidal agent and produce adequate foam, douching too soon after intercourse, and the use of insufficient amounts of foam. Adverse effects associated with spermicidal use include only occasional allergic reactions (1,265).

Male Oral Contraception

38. Is there a male oral contraceptive available in the United States?

At this time, there are no commercially available or FDA-approved male oral contraceptives in the United States, although there are some clinical trials in progress testing a variety of investigational agents. Several compounds can arrest spermatogenesis, but most of these substances also have mutagenic or carcinogenic properties.

Gossypol. Gossypol is a compound which has been isolated in China from cotton seeds, roots, and stems. This compound does not appear to be carcinogenic and has reportedly been administered to several thousand men in the past decade with a high degree of success (up to 99% effective). Chinese investigators claim that gossypol "kills" spermatozoa in the epididymis and has no direct effect on spermatogenesis. The recommended dose is 12–20 mcg daily for 2½ months or until the infertile state is reached. A dose of 12½ mcg administered twice weekly thereafter maintains the infertile state. Fertility is reestablished several months after discontinuation of therapy. The major side effects of gossypol include a slight decrease in serum potassium concentrations and gastrointestinal complaints. More studies are needed to confirm the optimistic conclusions of the Chinese investigators (1,266).

Hormones. Estrogens, progestogens, and androgens suppress the production of gonadotropins and can induce azoospermia and oligospermia in males. Of these, androgens are the most desirable, because estrogens can cause feminization and other serious cardiovascular effects, and progestogens can produce impotence without the assurance of sterility.

Testosterone can induce azoospermia which can be maintained for substantial periods of time without toxicity. The combined use of steroids such as danazol or one of the synthetic progestogens (to suppress the pituitary gonadotropins) with testosterone (to maintain libido) has also been effective. Testosterone may also act synergistically with progestogens or danazol to induce azoospermia. These observations indicate that hormonal manipulation is a potentially effective form of male contraception, but more research is needed before definite conclusions can be reached (286).

References

1. Hatcher RA et al: *Contraceptive Technology 1982–1983,* 11th Ed, Irvington Publishers Inc., New York, 1982.
2. Royal College of General Practitioners' Oral Contraception Study: *Oral Contraceptives and Health,* Pitman, New York, 1974.
3. Vaughan B et al: Contraceptive efficacy among married women aged 15–44 years. Vital and Health Statistics. Series 23. Data from the National Survey of Family Growth. 1980; 5:1–62.
4. Kols A et al: Oral contraceptives in the 1980s. *Population Reports.* Series A. Number 6. Population Information Program, The Johns Hopkins University, Baltimore, 1982.
5. Balin H et al: Pharmacophysiologic and clinical aspects of oral contraceptives. Semin Drug Treat. 1973; 3:121.
6. Morris JM: Mechanisms involved in progesterone contraception and estrogen interception. Am J Obstet Gynecol. 1973; 117:167.
7. Roy S et al: Comparison of metabolic and clinical effects of four oral contraceptive formulations and a contraceptive vaginal ring. Am J Obstet Gynecol. 1980; 136:920.
8. Bergstein NAM: Clinical efficacy, acceptability and metabolic effects of new low dose combined oral contraceptives. Acta Obstet Gynecol Scand. 1976; Suppl 54:51.
9. James A et al: Experiences with the new oral contraceptive Ovysmen. J Intern Med Res. 1980; 8:86.
10. Krishnaswamy K: Drug metabolism and pharmacokinetics in malnutrition. Clin Pharmacokin. 1978; 3:216.
11. Prasad KV et al: Pharmacokinetics of norethindrone on Indian women. Contraception. 1979; 20:77.
12. Back DJ et al: Interindividual variation and drug interactions with hormonal steroid contraceptives. Drugs. 1981; 21:46.
13. Woutersz TB: A low-dose combination oral contraceptive: experience with 1,700 women treated for 22,489 cycles. J Reprod Med. 1981; 26:615.
14. Dickey RP: Initial pill selection and managing the contraceptive pill patient. J Gynaecol Obstet. 1979; 16:547.
15. Goldzieher JW: Comparative studies of the ethinyl estrogens used in oral contraceptives II: Antiovulatory response. Am J Obstet Gynecol. 1975; 122:619.
16. Ortho Pharmaceutical Corporation. *Ortho-Novum 10/11: A Biphasic Regimen* (Product Monograph). Omega Communications, Springfield, New Jersey, 1981.
17. Zador G: Fertility regulation using triphasic administration of ethinyl estradiol and levonorgestrel in comparison with the 30 plus 150 microgram fixed dose regime. Acta Obstet Gynecol Scand. 1979; Suppl 88:43.
18. Board JA: Continuous norethindrone 0.35 mg as an oral contraceptive agent. Am J Obstet Gynecol. 1971; 109:53.
19. Foley M et al: Clinical trial and laboratory investigation of a low-dose progestogen-only contraceptive, Exluton. Int J Fertil. 1973; 18:246.
20. Zanartu J et al: Low dose oral progesterones to control fertility. I: Clinical investigation. Obstet Gynecol. 1974; 43:87.
21. Moghissi KS et al: Effect of microdose norgestrel on endogenous gonadotrophic and steroid hormones, cervical mucus properties, vaginal cytology and endometrium. Fertil Steril. 1971; 22:424.
22. Moghissi KS et al: Contraceptive mechanism of microdose norethindrone. Obstet Gynecol. 1973; 41:585.
23. Rinehart W: Post-coital contraception—an appraisal. Population Reports. Series J. 1976; 9:J-141.
24. Blye RP: The use of estrogens as post-coital contraceptive agents. Am J Obstet Gynecol. 1973; 116:1004.
25. Dixon GW et al: Ethinyl estradiol and conjugated estrogens as postcoital contraceptives. JAMA. 1980; 244:1336.
26. Kuchera LK: Postcoital contraception with diesthlstilbestrol. JAMA. 1971; 218:562.
27. Haspels AA: The effect of large doses of estrogen post coitum in 2000 women. Eur J Obstet Gynecol Reprod Biol. 1973; 3:113.
28. Morris JM: Postcoital antifertility agents and their teratogenic effect. Contraception. 1970; 2:85.
29. Yuzpe AA et al: A multicenter clinical investigation employing ethinyl estradiol combined with dl-norgestrel as a postcoital contraceptive agent. Fertil Steril. 1982; 37:508.
30. Porter J et al: Postcoital contraception. Med J Aust. 1981; 1:85.
31. Schilling LH: An alternative to the use of high-dose estrogens for postcoital contraception. J Am Coll Health Assoc. 1979; 27:247.
32. Castle WM et al: Efficacy and acceptability of injectable medroxyprogesterone. S Afr Med J. 1978; 53:842.
33. Powell LC et al: Effect of depo-medroxyprogesterone acetate as a contraceptive agent. Am J Obstet Gynecol. 1971; 110:36.
34. Cullberg J: Mood changes and menstrual symptoms with different gestagen/estrogen combinations. Acta Psych Scand. 1972; Suppl 236:1.
35. Judd HL et al: Physiology and pathophysiology of menstruation and menopause. In: *Gynecology and Obstetrics: The Health Care of Women,* 2nd ed, Romney SL et al (eds), McGraw-Hill, New York, 1981, p 886.
36. Moos RH: Psychological aspects of oral contraceptives. Arch Gen Psych. 1968; 19:87.
37. Goodwin JH: Are combined oral contraceptives appropriate therapy for primary dysmenorrhea? J Nurse-Midwifery. 1980; 25:17.

38. Paige KE: Effects of oral contraceptives on affective fluctuations associated with the menstrual cycle. Psychosom Med. 1971; 33:515.

39. Silbergeld S et al: The menstrual cycle: a double-blind study of symptoms, mood and behavior, and biochemical variables using Enovid and placebo. Psychosom Med. 1971; 33:411.

40. Andersch B et al: Premenstrual complaints. 2. Influence of oral contraceptives. Acta Obstet Gynecol Scand. 1981; 60:579.

41. Kutner SJ et al: Types of oral contraceptives, depression, and premenstrual symptoms. J Nervous Mental Dis. 1972; 155:153.

42. Callard GV et al: Menstruation in women with normal or artificially controlled cycles. Fertil Steril. 1966; 17:684.

43. Nilsson L et al: Clinical studies on oral contraceptives—a randomized doubleblind, crossover study of 4 different preparations. (Anovlar Mite, Lyndiol Mite, Ovulen, and Volidan). Acta Obstet Gynecol Scand. 1967; 46 (Suppl 8):1.

44. Gray RH: Patterns of bleeding associated with the use of steroidal contraceptives. In: *Endometrial Bleeding and Steroidal Contraception: Proceedings of a Symposium on Steroid Contraception and Mechanisms of Endometrial Bleeding, Geneva, Sept 12–14, 1979,* Diczfalusy E et al (eds), Pitman Press, Bath, England, 1980. p 14.

45. Anon: Pill users protected against PID if they have used OCs for longer than one year. Family Planning Perspectives. 1982; 14:32.

46. Eschenbach DA et al: Pathogenesis of acute pelvic inflammatory disease: role of contraception and other risk factors. Am J Obstet Gynecol. 1977; 128:838.

47. Westrom L: Incidence, prevalence, and trends of acute pelvic inflammatory disease and its consequences in industrialized countries. Am J Obstet Gynecol. 1980; 138:880.

48. Ory HW and Women's Health Study: Ectopic pregnancy and intrauterine contraceptive devices: New perspectives. J Am Coll Obstet Gynecol. 1981; 57:137.

49. Vessey M et al: Outcome of pregnancy in women using different methods of contraception. Br J Obstet Gynaecol. 1979; 86:548.

50. Brinton LA et al: Risk factors for benign breast disease. Am J Epidemiol. 1981; 113:203.

51. Lees AW et al: Oral contraceptives and breast disease in premenopausal northern Albertan women. Int J Cancer. 1978; 22:700.

52. Ravnihar B et al: An epidemiologic study of breast cancer and benign breast neoplasias in relation to the oral contraceptive and estrogen use. Eur J Cancer. 1979; 15:395.

53. Vessey MP et al: Breast cancer and oral contraceptives: findings in Oxford-Family Planning Association Contraceptive Study. Br Med J. 1981; 282:2093.

54. Ramcharan S et al: Infective and parasitic diseases; malignant neoplasms; benign neoplasms. In *The Walnut Creek Contraceptive Drug Study: A Prospective Study of the Side Effects of Oral Contraceptives. Vol 3. An Interim Report: A Comparison of Disease Occurrence Leading to Hospitalization or Death in Users and Nonusers of Oral Contraceptives.* Ramcharan S et al, Center for Population Research, Bethesda, Maryland, 1981. p 43.

55. Royal College of General Pratitioners' Oral Contraception Study. Breast cancer and oral contraceptives: Findings in Royal College of General Practitioners' study. Br Med J. 1981; 282:2088.

56. Brinton LA et al: Breast cancer risk factors among screening program participants. J Nat Cancer Inst. 1979; 62:37.

57. Newhouse ML et al: A case control study of carcinoma of the ovary. Br J Preventative Social Med. 1977; 31:148.

58. Fathalla MF: Incessant ovulation—A factor in ovarian neoplasia? (Letter). Lancet. 1971; 2:163.

59. LiVolsi VA et al: Fibrocystic breast disease in oral contraceptive users: A histophathological evaluation of epithelial atypia. N Engl J Med. 1978; 299:381.

60. Hulka BS et al: Protection against endometrial carcinoma by combination product oral contraceptives. JAMA. 1982; 247:745.

61. Kaufman DW et al: Decreased risk of endometrial cancer among oral contraceptive users. N Engl J Med. 1980; 303:1045.

62. Salmi T: Risk factors in endometrial carcinoma with special reference to the use of estrogens. Acta Obstet Gynecol Scand. 1979; Suppl 86:1.

63. Rinehart W et al: OCs—Update on usage, safety, and side effects. *Population Reports.* Series A. Number 5. Population Information Program. The Johns Hopkins University, Baltimore, 1979.

64. Vessey MP et al: Oral contraceptives and benign liver tumours. Br Med J. 1977; 2:1064.

65. Jick H et al: Oral contraceptives—induced benign liver tumors—the magnitude of the problem (Letter). JAMA. 1978; 240:828.

66. Ansari AH et al: Liver tumors and oral contraceptives. Fertil Steril. 1978; 29:643.

67. Keifer WS Jr et al: Liver neoplasms and the oral contraceptives. Am J Obstet Gynecol. 1977; 128:448.

68. Stadel BV: Oral contraceptives and cardiovascular disease. First of two parts. N Engl J Med. 1981; 305:612.

69. Stadel BV: Oral contraceptives and cardiovascular disease. Second of two parts. N Engl J Med. 1981; 305:672.

70. Rosenfield A: Oral and intrauterine contraception: A 1978 risk assessment. Am J Obstet Gynecol. 1978; 132:92.

71. Dickey RP et al: Oral contraceptives: selection of the proper pill. Obstet Gynecol. 1969; 33:273.

72. Talwar PP et al: Side effects of drugs: The relation of body weight to side effects associated with oral contraceptives. Br Med J. 1977; 1:1637.

73. Neslon J: Clinical evaluation of side effects of current oral contraceptives. J Reprod Med. 1971; 6:50.

74. Jackson JL: The missed pill: Preliminary report. In: *Progress in Conception Control.* Moyer DL (ed), Lippincott & Co, Philadelphia, 1968.

75. Aznar R et al: Incidence of side effects with contraceptive placebo. Am J Obstet Gynecol. 1969; 105:1144.

76. Carey HM: Principles of oral contraceptives. Part II: Side effects of oral contraceptives. Med J Aust. 1971; 2:1242.

77. Briggs M et al: Changing from a high to low dose contraceptive. Br Med J. 1975; 1:575.

78. Carruthers R: Chloasma and the pill. Br Med J. 1967; 3:307.

79. Carruthers R: Chloasma and the pill. Med J Aust. 1966; 2:17.

80. Anon: Drug reaction VII: Adverse cutaneous effects to oral contraceptives. Br J Derm. 1969; 81:946.

81. Jelinek JE: Cutaneous side effects of oral contraceptives. Arch Derm. 1970; 101:181.

82. Resnik S: Melasma induced by oral contraceptive drugs. JAMA. 1967; 199:601.

83. Arndt KA et al: Topical use of hydroquinone as a depigmenting agent. JAMA. 1965; 194:965.

84. Spencer MC: Topical use of hydroquinone for depigmentation. JAMA. 1965; 194:962.

85. Strauss JS et al: Effect of cyclic progestin-estrogen therapy on sebum and acne in women. JAMA. 1964; 190:815.

86. Palitz LL et al: Enovid for acne in the female skin. 1964; 3:243.

87. Gibbs WP: Acne and Ovral (Letter). Arch Derm. 1974; 109:912.

88. Kligman AM: Pimples following the pill. Arch Derm. 1972; 105:298.

89. Woodward RK: Acne stimulation by Ovral (Letter). Arch Derm. 1974; 110:812.

90. Olson RL et al: Postcontraceptive acne (Letter). Arch Derm. 1972; 105:928.

91. Weigland D et al: *Cutaneous Medicine Case Studies.* Medical Examination Publishing Co, New York, 1971. p 60.

92. Boston Collaborative Drug Surveillance Program: Surgically confirmed gallbladder disease, venous thromboembolism and breast tumors in relation to postmenopausal estrogen therapy. N Engl J Med. 1974; 290:15.

93. Inman WHW et al: Investigation of deaths from pulmonary, coronary, and cerebral thrombosis and embolism in women of childbearing age. Br Med J. 1968; 2:193.

94. Vessey MP et al: Investigation of the relation between use of oral contraceptives and thromboembolic disease. Br Med J. 1968; 2:199.

95. Vessey MP et al: Investigation of the relation between use of oral contraceptives and thromboembolic disease. A further report. Br Med J. 1969; 2:651.

96. Boston Collaborative Drug Surveillance Programme: Oral contraceptives and venous thromboembolic disease, surgically confirmed gall-bladder disease, and breast tumours. Lancet. 1973; 1:1399.

97. Drill VA et al: Oral contraceptives and thromboembolic disease. JAMA. 1968; 206:77.

98. Drill VA et al: Thromboembolic disorders and oral contraceptives. JAMA. 1969; 207:1151.

99. Drill VA: Oral contraceptives and thromboembolic disease I. Prospective and retrospective studies. JAMA. 1972; 219:593.

100. Royal Australian College of General Practitioners: Anovulants: Thrombosis and other associated changes. Med J Aust. 1974; 2:440.

101. Fuertes-De La Haba A et al: Thrombophlebitis among oral and nonoral contraceptive users. Obstet Gynecol. 1971; 38:259.

102. Goldzieher JW et al: Oral contraceptives and thromboembolism: A reassessment. Am J Obstet Gynecol. 1975; 123:878.

103. Vessey MP: Female hormones and vascular disease: An epidemiological overview. Br J Family Planning. 1980; 6(Suppl 3):1.

104. Royal College of General Practitioners' Oral Contraception Study. Further analyses of mortality in oral contraceptive users. Lancet. 1981; 1:541.

105. Royal College of General Practitioners' Oral Contraception Study. Oral contraceptives, venous thrombosis, and varicose veins. J Roy Coll Gen Pract. 1978; 28:393.

106. Vessey MP et al: Mortality in oral contraceptive users (Letter). Lancet. 1981; 1:549.

107. Vessey MP et al: A long-term follow-up study of women using different methods of contraception: An interim report. J Biosocial Sci. 1976; 8:375.

108. Petitti DB et al: Risk of vascular disease in women: Smoking, oral contraceptives, noncontraceptive estrogens, and other factors. JAMA. 1979; 242:1150.

109. Vessey MP et al: Postoperative thromboembolism and the use of oral contraceptives. Br Med J. 1970; 3:123.

110. Greene GR et al: Oral contraceptive use in patients with thromboembolism following surgery, trauma, or infection. Am J Public Health. 1972; 62:680.

111. Sagar S et al: Oral contraceptives, antithrombin III activity, and postoperative deep-vein thrombosis. Lancet. 1976; 1:509.

112. Stamatakis JD et al: Surgery, venous thrombosis and anti-Xa. Br J Surg. 1977; 64:709.

113. Alkjaersig N et al: Association between oral contraceptive use and thromboembolism: A new approach to its investigation based on plasma fibrinogen chromatography. Am J Obstet Gynecol. 1975; 122:199.

114. Lawson DH et al: Oral contraceptive use and venous thromboembolism: Absence of an effect of smoking. Br Med J. 1977; 2:729.

115. Maguire MG et al: Increased risk of thrombosis due to oral contraceptives: A further report. Am J Epidemiol. 1979; 110:188.

116. Vessey MP et al: Investigation of relation between use of oral contraceptives and thromboembolic disease. A further report. Br Med J. 1969; 2:651.

117. Jick H et al: Venous thromboembolic disease and 'A', 'B', 'O' blood type. Lancet. 1972; 2:123.

118. Mourant AE et al: Blood groups and blood clotting. Lancet. 1971; 1:223.

119. Fagerhol MK et al: Antithrombin III concentration and ABO blood groups. Lancet. 1971; 2:664.

120. Inman WH et al: Thromboembolic disease and the steroidal content of oral contraceptives. A report to the Committee on Safety of Drugs. Br Med J. 1970; 2:203.

121. Stolley PD et al: Thrombosis with low-estrogen oral contraceptives. Am J Epidemiol. 1975; 102:197.

122. Bottiger LE et al: Oral contraceptives and thromboembolic disease: Effects of lowering oestrogen content. Lancet. 1980; 1:1097.

123. Meade TW et al: Progestogens and cardiovascular reactions associated with oral contraceptives and a comparison of the safety of 50- and 30-mcg preparations. Br Med J. 1980; 280:1157.

124. Dugdale M et al: Hormonal contraception and thromboembolic disease, effects of the oral contraceptives on hemostatic mechanisms. J Chron Dis. 1971; 23:775.

125. Mink IB et al: Progestational agents and blood coagulation. V. Changes induced by sequential oral contraceptive therapy. Am J Obstet Gynecol. 1974; 119:401.

126. Wessler S et al: Estrogen-containing oral contraceptive agents: A basis for their thrombogenicity. JAMA. 1976; 236:2179.

127. Petersen C et al: Antithrombin III: Comparison of functional and immunologic assays. Am J Clin Pathol. 1978; 69:500.

128. von Kaulla E et al: Antithrombin III depression and thrombin generation acceleration in women taking oral contraceptives. Am J Obstet Gynecol. 1971; 109:868.

129. Porter JB et al: Oral contraceptives and nonfatal vascular disease—recent experience. Obstet Gynecol. 1982; 59:299.

130. Schrogie JJ et al: Effect of oral contraceptives on vitamin K-dependent clotting activity. Clin Pharmacol Ther. 1967; 8:670.

131. de Teresa E et al: Interaction between anticoagulants and contraceptives: An unsuspected finding. Br Med J. 1979; 2:1260.

132. Mann JI et al: Myocardial infarction in young women with special reference to oral contraceptive practice. Br Med J. 1975; 2:241.

133. Mann JI et al: Risk factors for myocardial infarction in young women. Br Prev Soc Med. 1976; 30:94.

134. Mann JI et al: Oral contraceptives and death from myocardial infarction. Br Med J. 1975; 2:245.

135. Mann JI et al: Oral contraceptive use in older women and fatal myocardial infarction. Br Med J. 1976; 2:445.

136. Jick H et al: Oral contraceptives and nonfatal myocardial infarction. JAMA. 1978; 239:1403.

137. Shapiro S et al: Oral contraceptive use in relation to myocardial infarction. Lancet. 1979; 1:743.

138. Rosenberg L et al: Oral contraceptive use in relation to nonfatal myocardial infarction. Am J Epidemiol. 1980; 111:59.

139. Collaborative Group for the Study of Stroke in Young Women: Oral contraceptives and stroke in young women: Associated risk factors. JAMA. 1975; 231:718.

140. Petitti DB et al: Use of oral contraceptives, cigarette smoking, and risk of subarachnoid haemorrhage. Lancet. 1978; 2:234.

141. Jick J et al: Oral contraceptives and nonfatal stroke in healthy young women. Ann Intern Med. 1978; 89:58.

142. Slone D et al: Relation of cigarette smoking to myocardial infarction in young women. N Engl J Med. 1978; 298:1273.

143. Fisch TR et al: Oral contraceptives and blood pressure. JAMA. 1977; 237:2499.

144. Fisch TR et al: Oral contraceptives, pregnancy and blood pressure. In: Ramcharan S, ed. *The Walnut Creek Contraceptive Drug Study: A Prospective Study of the Side Effects of Oral Contraceptives.* Vol. 1. Washington, D.C.: Government Printing Office, 1974; 105 [DHEW publication no. (NIH) 74-562].

145. Ramcharan S et al: The occurrence and course of hypertensive disease in users and nonusers of oral contraceptive drugs. In: Ramcharan S, ed. *The Walnut Creek Contraceptive Drug Study: A Prospective Study of the Side Effects of Oral Contraceptives.* Vol 2. Washington, D.C.: Government Printing Office, 1976:1 [DHEW publication no. (NIH) 76-563].

146. Weir RJ et al: Contraceptive steroids and hypertension. J Steroid Biochem. 1975; 6:961.

147. Harris PWR: Malignant hypertension associated with oral contraceptives. Lancet. 1969; 2:466.

148. Tobon H: Maglignant hypertension, uremia and hemolytic anemia in a patient on oral contraceptives. Obstet Gynecol. 1972; 40:681.

149. Pritchard JA et al: Blood pressure response to estrogen-progestin oral contraceptive after pregnancy-induced hypertension. Am J Obstet Gynecol. 1977; 129:733.

150. Hoover R et al: Oral contraceptive use: Association with frequency of hospitalization and chronic disease risk indicators. Am J Public Health. 1978; 91:266.

151. Crane MG et al: Hypertension, oral contraceptive agents and conjugated estrogens. Ann Intern Med. 1971; 74:13.

152. Royal College of General Practitioners' Oral Contraception Study: Oral contraceptives, venous thrombosis, and varicose veins. J Roy Coll Gen Pract. 1978; 28:393.

153. Tapla HR et al: Effect of oral contraceptive therapy on the renin angiotensin system in normotensive and hypertensive women. Obstet Gynecol. 1973; 41:643.

154. Linn S et al: Delay in conception for former "pill" users. JAMA. 1982; 247:629.

155. Pardthaisong T et al: The return of fertility following discontinuation of oral contraceptives in Thailand. Fertil Steril. 1981; 25:532.

156. Vessey MP et al: Fertility after stopping different methods of contraception. Br Med J. 1978; 1:265.

157. Tyson JE et al: Neuroendocrine dysfunction in galactorrhea-amenorrhea after oral contraceptive use. Obstet Gynecol. 1975; 46:1.

158. Rice-Wray et al: Return of ovulation after discontinuance of oral contraceptives. Fertil Steril. 1967; 18:212.

159. Terperman L et al: Oral contraceptive history as a risk indicator in patients with pituitary tumors with hyperprolactinemia: a case comparison study of twenty patients. Neurosurg. 1980; 7:571.

160. Wingrave SJ et al: Oral contraceptives and pituitary adenomas. Br Med J. 1980; 280:685.

161. Gomez F et al: Nonpuerperal galactorrhea and hyperprolactinemia: Clinical findings, endocrine features and therapeutic responses in 56 cases. Am J Med. 1977; 62:648.

162. Kleinberg DL et al: Galactorrhea: A study of 235 cases, including 48 with pituitary tumors. N Engl J Med. 1977; 296:589.

163. Tolis G et al: Prolonged amenorrhea and oral contraceptives. Fertil Steril. 1979; 32:265.

164. Hull MGR et al: Post-pill amenorrhea: A causal study. Fertil Steril. 1981; 36:472.

165. Vessey MP et al: Fertility after stopping different methods of contraception. Br Med J. 1978; 1:265.

166. Janerich DT et al: Oral contraceptives and birth defects. Am J Epidemiol. 1980; 112:73.

167. Rothman KJ et al: Oral contraceptives and birth defects. N Engl J Med. 1978; 299:522.

168. Kasan PN et al: Oral contraception and congenital abnormalities. Br J Obstet Gynecol. 1980; 87:545.

169. Harlap S et al: Births following oral contraceptive failures. Obstet Gynecol. 1980; 55:447.

170. Savolainen E et al: Teratogenic hazards of oral contraceptives analyzed in a national malformation register. Am J Obstet Gynecol. 1981; 140:521.

171. Ferencz C et al: Maternal hormone therapy and congenital heart disease. Teratology. 1980; 21:225.

172. Briggs M: Biochemical effects of oral contraceptives. Adv Steroid Biochem Pharmacol. 1976; 5:65.

173. Wynn V et al: Comparison of effects of different combined oral contraceptive formulations on carbohydrate and lipid metabolism. Lancet. 1979; 1:1045.

174. Briggs MH et al: Randomized prospective studies on metabolic effects of oral contraceptives. Acta Obstet Gynecol Scand Suppl. 1982; 105:25.

175. Wingerd J et al: Oral contraceptive use and other factors in the standard glucose tolerance test. 1977; 26:1024.

176. Spellacy WN et al: Glucose, insulin and growth hormone studies in long term users of oral contraceptives. Am J Obstet Gynecol. 1970; 106:173.

177. Spellacy WN: Carbohydrate metabolism in male infertility and female fertility-control patients. Fertil Steril. 1976; 27:185.

178. Kalkhoff RK: Effects of oral contraceptive agents on carbohydrate metabolism. J Steroid Biochem. 1975; 6:949.

179. Szabo AJ et al: Glucose tolerance in gestational diabetic women during and after treatment with a combination-type oral contraceptive. N Engl J Med. 1970; 282:646.

180. Much BR: Effect of long term use of oral contraceptives on glucose tolerance. Arch Gynaekol. 1976; 220:185.

181. Spellacy WN et al: The effects of a "low-estrogen" oral contraceptive on carbohydrate metabolism during six months of treatment: A preliminary report of blood glucose and plasma insulin values. Fertil Steril. 1977; 28:885.

182. Wynn V: Effect of duration of low dose oral contraceptives administration on carbohydrate metabolism. Am J Obstet Gynecol. 1982; 142:739.

183. Doar JWH et al: Effects of obesity, glucocorticoids and oral contraceptive therapy on plasma glucose and blood pyruvate levels. Br Med J. 1970; 1:149.

184. Wynn V et al: Some effects of oral contraceptives on carbohydrate metabolism. Lancet. 1966; 2:715.

185. Spellacy WN et al: Human growth hormone levels in normal subjects receiving an oral contraceptive. JAMA. 1967; 202:451.

186. Srivastava MC et al: Insulin metabolism, insulin sensitivity, and hormonal responses to insulin infusion in patients taking oral contraceptive steroids. Eur J Clin Invest. 1975; 5:425.

187. Kalkhoff RK: Metabolic effects of progesterone. Am J Obstet Gynecol. 1982; 142:735.

188. Leis D et al: Comparison of ethinyl estradiol and mestranol in sequential type oral contraceptives in their effects on blood glucose and serum insulin in oral glucose tolerance tests. Fertil Steril. 1977; 28:737.

189. Spellacy WN: Carbohydrate metabolism during treatment with estrogen, progestogen, and low dose oral contraceptives. Am J Obstet Gynecol. 1982; 142:732.

190. Spellacy WN et al: Effects of norethindrone on carbohydrate and lipid metabolism. Obstet Gynecol. 1975; 46:560.

191. Spellacy WN et al: Carbohydrate metabolism prospectively studied in women using a low estrogen oral contraceptive for six months. Contraception. 1979; 20:137.

192. Goldzieher JW et al: Absence of capillary microangiopathy in oral contraceptive users with glucose intolerance. Obstet Gynecol. 1978; 51:89.

193. Garcia MJ et al: Morbidity and mortality in diabetics in the Framingham population: Sixteen year follow-up study. Diabetes. 1974; 23:105.

194. Whitty CWM et al: Effect of oral contraceptives on migraine. Lancet. 1966; 1:856.

195. Phillips BM: Oral contraceptives and migraine. Br Med J. 1968; 2:99.

196. Shafey S et al: Vascular headaches and oral contraceptives. Ann Intern Med. 1966; 65:863.

197. Desrosiers HH: Headaches related to contraceptive therapy and their control. Headache. 1973; 13:117.

198. Diddle AW et al: Oral contraceptives, medication and headaches. Am J Obstet Gynecol. 1969; 105:507.

199. Dalton K: Migraine and oral contraceptives. Headache. 1976; 15:247.

200. Shafey S et al: Neurologic syndromes occurring in patients receiving synthetic steroids (oral contraceptives). Neurol. 1966; 16:205.

201. Walsh FB et al: Oral contraceptives and neuro-ophthalmologic interest. Arch Ophthal. 1965; 74:628.

202. Kudrow L: The relationship of headache frequency to hormone use in migraine. Headache. 1975; 15:36.

203. Utian WH: Estrogen, headache and oral contraceptives. S Afr Med J. 1974; 48:2105.

204. Eicher E: Estrogen deprivation headaches. Obstet Gynecol. 1968; 32:294.

205. Grant E: Relation between headaches from oral contraceptives and development of endometrial arterioles. Br Med J. 1968; 2:402.

206. Somerville BW: The role of estradiol withdrawal in the etiology of menstrual migraine. Neurol. 1972; 22:355.

207. Grant E: Relationship of arterioles in the endometrium to headache from oral contraceptives. Lancet. 1965; 1:1143.

208. Herzberg BN et al: Depressive symptoms and oral contraceptives. Br Med J. 1970; 4:142.

209. Leeton J: Depression induced by oral contraception and the role of vitamin B6 in its management. Aust NZ J Psychiat. 1974; 8:85.

210. Lewis A et al: An evaluation of depression as a side effect of oral contraceptives. Br J Psychiat. 1969; 115:697.

211. Glick ID: Mood and behavioral changes associated with the use of the oral contraceptive agents. Psychopharmacol. 1967; 10:363.

212. Herzberg BN et al: Depressive symptoms and oral contraceptives. Br Med J. 1971; 3:495.

213. Marcotte DB et al: Psychophysiologic changes accompanying oral contraceptive use. Br J Psychiat. 1970; 116:165.

214. Herzbert BN et al: Oral contraceptives, depression and libido. Br Med J. 1970; 4:142.

215. Kutner SJ et al: Types of oral contraceptives, depression, and premenstrual symptoms. J Nerv Ment Dis. 1972; 155.

216. Fortin JN et al: Side effects of oral contraceptive medication; a psychosomatic problem. Can Psychiat Assoc J. 1972; 17:3.

217. Leeton J et al: The relationship of oral contraceptives to depression. Aust NZ J Obstet Gynecol. 1971; 11:237.

218. Goldzieher JW et al: Nervousness and depression attributed to oral contraceptives: a double blind placebo controlled study. Am J Obstet Gynecol. 1971; 111:1013.

219. Murawski BJ et al: An investigation of mood states in women taking oral contraceptives. Fertil Steril. 1968; 19:50.

220. Grant E et al: Effect of oral contraceptives on depressive mood changes and on endometrial monoamine oxidase and phosphatases. Br Med J. 1968; 3:777.

221. Winston F: Oral contraceptives, pyridoxine and depression. Am J Pysch. 1973; 130:1217.

222. Adams PW et al: Effects of pyridoxine HCl (vitamin B-6) upon depression associated with oral contraception. Lancet. 1973; 1:897.

223. Ramcharan S et al: An interim report—A comparison of disease occurrence leading to hospitalization or death in users and nonusers of oral contraceptives. In: *The Walnut Creek Contraceptive Drug Study: A Prospective Study of the Side Effects of Oral Contraceptives. Vol. 3.* Center for Population Research, Bethesda MA, 1981. (NIH Pub. No. 81-564)

224. Egger G et al: Ischaemic colitis and oral contraceptives; case report and brief review of the literature. Acta Hepatogastroenterol (Stuutg). 1974; 21:221.

225. Vessey MP: Thromboembolism, cancer and oral contraceptives. Clin Obstet Gynecol. 1974; 17:65.

226. Rooks JB et al and Cooperative Liver Tumor Study Group: Epidemiology of hepatocellular adenoma: The role of oral contraceptive use. JAMA. 1979; 242:664.

227. Klatskin G: Hepatic tumors: possible relationship to use of oral contraceptives. Gastroenterol. 1977; 73:386.

228. Bein NN et al: Recurrent massive haemorrhage from benign hepatic tumours secondary to oral contraceptives. Br J Surg. 1977; 64:433.

229. Nime F et al: The histology of liver tumors in oral contraceptive users observed during a national survey by the American College of Surgeons Commission on Cancer. Cancer. 1979; 44:1481.

230. Ockner R et al: Hepatic effects of oral contraceptives. N Engl J Med. 1967; 276:331.

231. Medline A et al: Pruritus of pregnancy and jaundice induced by oral contraceptives. Am J Gastroent. 1976; 65:156.

232. Kappas A: Estrogens and liver. Gastroent. 1967; 52:113.

233. Haemmerli P et al: Recurrent intrahepatic cholestasis of pregnancy. Medicine. 1967; 46:299.

234. Harley RA et al: Topics in clinical medicine: the liver and oral contraceptives. Johns Hopkins Med J. 1969; 124:112.

235. Miale JB et al: The effects of oral contraceptives on the results of laboratory tests. Am J Obstet Gynecol. 1974; 120:264.

236. Larsson-Cohn U et al: Oral contraception and liver function tests. Br Med J. 1965; 1:1414.

237. Skolnick JL et al: Rifampin, oral contraceptives and pregnancy. JAMA. 1976; 236:1381.

238. Relmers D: Simultaneous use of rifampin and other antituberculous agents with oral contraceptives. Prax Pneumol. 1971; 25:255.

239. Cohn HD: Rifampin and the pill. JAMA. 1974; 228:828.

240. Nocke-Finck L et al: Effects of antibiotics on estrogen excretion in women taking oral contraceptives. Acta Endocrinol. 1973; 177(Suppl):136.

241. Syvalahti EK et al: Rifampin and drug metabolism. Lancet. 1974; 2:232.

242. Bolt HM et al: Interaction of rifampin treatment with pharmacokinetics and metabolism of ethinyloestradiol in man. Acta Endocrinol. 1977; 85:189.

243. Hempel E et al: Drug stimulated biotransformation of hormonal steroid contraceptives: Clinical implications. Drugs. 1976; 12:442.

244. Bacon JF et al: Pregnancy attibutable to interactions between tetracycline and oral contraceptives. Br Med J. 1980; 280:292.

245. Back DJ et al: Drug interactions with oral contraceptives. Int Planned Parenthood Federation Med Bull. 1978; 12:4.

246. Back DJ et al: The effect of antibiotics on the enterohepatic circulation of ethinylestradiol and norethisterone in the rat. J Steroid Biochem. 1978; 9:527.

247. Joshi JV et al: A study of interaction of low dose combination oral contraceptives with ampicillin and metronidzaole. Contraception. 1980; 22:643.

248. Laenger H et al: Epileptic drugs and failure of oral contraceptives. Lancet. 1974; 2:600.

249. Hansten PD: Drug interactions that inhibit oral contraceptive efficacy. Drug Interactions Newsletter. 1981; 1:9.

250. Anon: The minipill—A limited alternative for certain women. Population Reports. Series A. Number 3. Population Information Program. The Johns Hopkins University. Baltimore, 1979.

251. Chopra JG: Effect of steroid contraceptive on lactation. Am J Clin Nutr. 1972; 25:1202.

252. Das SK et al: A clinico-pathological study of lactational amenorrhea. J Obstet Gynecol (India). 1966; 16:156.

253. Janerich DT et al: Fertility patterns after discontinuation of use of oral contraceptives. Lancet. 1976; 1:1051.

254. Campodonico I et al: Effect of a low-dose contraceptive (150 mcg levonorgestrel and 30 mcg ethinylestradiol) on lactation. Clin Therap. 1978; 1:454.

255. Kamal I et al: Clinical, biochemical and experimental studies on lactation. 2. Clinical effects of gestagens on lactation. Am J Obstet Gynecol. 1980; 136:159.

256. Badraqui MHH et al: Effects of some progestational steroids on lactation. J Biosoc Sci. 1977; Suppl 4:135.

257. Guiloff E et al: Effect of contraception on lactation. Am J Obstet Gynecol. 1974; 118:42.

258. Henry A et al: Reversing female sterilization. Population Reports, Series C, 1980; No 8.

259. Piotrow P et al: IUDs—Update on safety, effectiveness and research. Population Reports, Series B. 1979; No 3.

260. Liskin L et al: IUDs: An appropriate contraceptive for many women. Population Reports, Series B. 1982; No 4.

261. Burkman RT and Women's Health Study: Association between intrauterine devices and pelvic inflammatory disease. Obstet Gynecol. 1981; 57:269.

262. Westrom L: Incidence, prevalence and trends of acute pelvic inflammatory disease and its consequences in industrialized countries. Am J Obstet Gynecol. 1980; 138:880.

263. Perlmutter JF: Pregnancy and the IUD. J Reprod Med. 1978; 21:133.

264. Hatcher R et al: Contraception: Part I: Foams, mechanical devices. Perinatal Care. 1978; 2:21.

265. Coleman S et al: Spermicides—Simplicity and safety are major assets. Population Reports, Series H. 1979; No 5.

266. National Coordinating Committee on Male Antifertility Agents. Gossypol—a new antifertility agent for males. China Med J (New Series). 1978; 4:6.

267. Chihal HJ et al: Estrogen potency of oral contraceptive pills. Am J Obstet Gynecol. 1975; 121:75.

268. Dickey RP et al: Potency of three new low estrogen pills. Am J Obstet Gynecol. 1976; 125:976.

269. Collaborative Group for the Study of Stroke in Young Women: Oral contraception and increased risk of cerebral ischemia or thrombosis. N Engl J Med. 1973; 288:871.

270. Collaborative Group for the Study of Stroke in Young Women: Oral contraceptives and stroke in young women: Associated risk factors. JAMA. 1975; 231:718.

271. Jick H et al: Oral contraceptives and nonfatal stroke in healthy young women. Ann Intern Med. 1978; 89:58.

272. Inman WH: Oral contraceptives and fatal subarachnoid haemorrhage. Br Med J. 1979; 2:1468.

273. Morrison AS et al: Oral contraceptives and hepatitis. A report from the Boston Collaborative Drug Surveillance Program, Boston University Medical Center. Lancet. 1977; 1:965.

274. Caron GA: Contact lenses and oral contraceptives. Br Med J. 1966; 1:980.

275. Chihal HJ et al: Estrogen potency of oral contraceptive pills. Am J Obstet Gynecol. 1975; 121:75.

276. Ruben M: Contact lenses and oral contraceptives. Br Med J. 1966; 1:1110.

277. Sabell A: Oral contraceptives and the contact lens wearer. Br J Physiol Optom. 1970; 25:127.

278. Walsh H et al: Candida vaginitis associated with use of oral progestational agents. Am J Obstet Gynecol. 1965; 93:904.

279. Walsh H et al: Oral progestational agents as a cause of candida vaginitis. Am J Obstet Gynecol. 1968; 101:991.

280. Spellacy WN et al: Vaginal yeast growth and contraceptive practices. Obstet Gynecol. 1971; 38:343.

281. Catterall RD: Candida albicans and the contraceptive pill. Lancet. 1966; 2:830.

282. Maheux R et al: Oral contraceptives and prolactinomas. A case control study. Am J Obstet Gynecol. 1982; 143:134.

283. Plunkett ER: Contraceptive steroids, age, and the cardiovascular system. Am J Obstet Gynecol. 1982; 142:747.

284. Wynn V et al: The effect of progestins in combined oral contraceptives on serum lipids with special respect to high density lipoproteins. Am J Obstet Gynecol. 1982; 142:766.

285. DeStefano F et al: Oral contraceptives and postoperative venous thrombosis. Am J Obstet Gynecol. 1982; 143:227.

286. Bremner WJ et al: The prospects for new, reversible male contraceptives. N Engl J Med. 1976; 295:1111.

287. Talwar PP et al: Increased risk of breakthrough bleeding when one oral contraceptive tablet is missed. N Engl J Med. 1977; 296:1236.

Chapter 54

Disorders of the Adrenals

Donald T. Kishi

This chapter will focus upon the potential morbidity of glucocorticoids and the development of strategies to minimize adverse effects which are associated with their use. Specific uses of the glucocorticoids are described in other chapters of this book. Problems arising from the use of glucocorticoids occur as a result of suppression of normal regulation and production of cortisol (hydrocortisone, HC) or as a direct consequence of supraphysiologic doses.

HYPOTHALAMIC-PITUITARY-ADRENOCORTICAL REGULATION

The biosynthesis and secretion of hydrocortisone (HC) is regulated by the hypothalamic-pi-

tuitary-adrenocortical (HPA) axis. The hypothalamus secretes corticotrophin releasing factor (CRF) which travels to the anterior pituitary via the hypophyseal portal system. The CRF then stimulates the anterior pituitary secretion of adrenocorticotrophic hormone (ACTH). ACTH enters the general circulation and stimulates the zonae reticularis and fasciculata of the adrenal cortices to synthesize and secrete HC.

The serum concentrations of ACTH and HC follow a diurnal or circadian rhythm. In the normal individual, the HC concentration begins to increase between 2 a.m. and 6 a.m.; peak levels occur between 6 a.m. and 8 a.m. The serum levels of HC decrease throughout the day until approximately midnight when the nadir is reached. HC serum concentrations do not rise or fall smoothly;

rather, there are multiple minor peaks and valleys throughout the day (1). These minor peaks and valleys can be partially explained by the release of CRF in response to stressful stimuli. Furthermore, variations of plasma ACTH and HC levels are under negative feedback control by the HPA axis; that is, as HC or synthetic glucocorticoid levels increase, ACTH secretion decreases. Whether this feedback inhibition is exerted at the level of the hypothalamus or the anterior pituitary is not known. This negative feedback inhibition can be overcome by physical or emotional stress which can stimulate the HPA axis to produce hydrocortisone. This effect of stress is abrogated when the HPA axis is suppressed secondary to chronic exogenous glucocorticoid therapy (2,3).

The diurnal rhythm of the HPA axis may not be found in patients who have impaired consciousness (4), temporal lobe or other forebrain disease (5), Cushing's syndrome, or anorexia nervosa (6). Since the diurnal rhythm is in a part a function of the awake-sleep or activity-inactivity cycle, individuals who work at night would be expected to have an inverted diurnal rhythm. Induction of inversion of the diurnal cycle requires one or two weeks. The average amount of HC secreted daily varies with the age, sex, and size of the individual: adult males - 20.4 mg; adult females - 17.4 mg; and children 12 mg/m^2. In stress situations, the adrenal cortices can secrete up to 400 mg/24 hours (7,8).

Malfunctions of the HPA Axis

Derangements in the HPA axis can be broadly categorized into those resulting in hypercortisolism and those resulting in hypocortisolism. Chronic hypercortisolism results in a condition known as *Cushing's syndrome*. This syndrome can result from an overproduction of ACTH by the pituitary gland (Cushing's disease) and resultant overproduction of cortisol; or from an overproduction of cortisol by an adrenocortical tumor. Cushing's syndrome is characterized by the Cushing habitus—moon facies, centripetal obesity, thin extremities, buffalo hump, striae, easy bruisability, and hypertension. Laboratory data consistent with Cushing's syndrome include hyperglycemia, hypernatremia, hypokalemia, polycythemia, eosinopenia, lymphopenia, and elevated serum cortisol levels. This syndrome can also result from chronic use of supraphysiologic doses of exogenous glucocorticoids.

Addison's disease is the result of hypocortisolism which can be absolute or relative to the body's need. The hypocortisol condition can result from surgical or chemical adrenalectomy or hypophysectomy, trauma to the adrenals or pituitary, sudden discontinuation of exogenous glucocorticoids in adrenally suppressed patients, or from stressful conditions in patients unable to increase endogenous cortisol release. The signs and symptoms of this condition are as described for Addison's disease.

Pharmacokinetic Considerations

Total plasma HC levels range from 7–20 mcg/dl. In this range, approximately 90% of the HC is bound to plasma protein. HC is metabolized by the liver to dihydro and tetrahydro metabolites which are conjugated to glucuronides and sulfates. This is the rate-limiting step in HC clearance. Approximately 1% of the usual daily production of HC, or about 200 mcg of unaltered HC, is excreted in the urine each day (9). This low fraction of HC renal excretion in normal patients can be attributed to the high degree of protein binding and passive tubular reabsorption of HC (11). Renal clearance is increased when plasma HC levels are increased (10,11). The metabolism and excretion of the synthetic glucocorticoids parallel that of HC. For example, prednisolone is cleared predominantly via hepatic metabolism with 7–15% of a dose excreted unchanged in urine (12). Phenytoin and phenobarbital can induce hepatic enzymes which increase the metabolic clearance of HC and synthetic glucocorticoids. Similarly, increased clearance is found in hyperthyroid patients (13).

HC is reversibly bound to corticosteroid binding globulin (CBG or transcortin), corticosteroid binding albumin (CBA) and minimally to erythrocytes and leukocytes. At normal levels, CBG binds the majority of circulating HC. As the concentration of HC is increased, the CBG sites become saturated; consequently, the CBA-bound and the free fractions increase. Exogenous glucocorticoids are bound to CBG and CBA but to a significantly lesser degree. For example, prednisolone is 65% bound in patients with normal albumin levels. Prednisolone or HC protein binding is non-linear; that is, as the plasma level and/or dose is increased, the fraction bound decreases (12).

In hypo- or dysproteinemic states, the total endogenous HC levels are decreased. Conversely, in conditions associated with increased CBG (pregnancy, estrogen therapy), the total plasma HC levels are elevated. These alterations in total endogenous HC levels are not of clinical significance because it is the unbound fraction of HC which is metabolically active (10,14,15) and the HPA axis apparently regulates the free HC level (10). However, the administration of exogenous glucocorticoids to patients with altered protein binding capacities will result in significant differences in glucocorticoid pharmacological effects (12). See Question 18 and Table 3 of this chapter.

Synthetic Glucocorticoids

Comparisons of Glucocorticoids. Most standard pharmacology texts and articles which review the clinical use of glucocorticoids contain tables similar to Tables 1 and 2. These tables have been accepted and utilized as the basis for determining equipotent doses, relative mineralocorticoid potency, and durations of action. However, the data upon which these tables are based are limited.

The relative anti-inflammatory potencies of the glucocorticoids were determined by comparing the subjective relief of rheumatoid arthritis symptoms, or by comparing the degree of absolute eosinopenia induced by various doses of a glucocorticoid relative to a given dose of hydrocortisone. Consequently, if a series of patients experienced comparable relief of arthritic symptoms with 5 mg of prednisone and 20 mg of hydrocortisone, the relative anti-inflammatory potency was reported as 4 times that of hydrocortisone. In addition to the subjective nature of this rating system, the values for relative potency can be further challenged because little or no consideration was given to the time when the responses were measured relative to when the dose was given.

Meikle and Tyler (16) monitored plasma cortisone suppression to determine the potencies of prednisolone and dexamethasone relative to hydrocortisone. Plasma levels of cortisone were measured at fixed time intervals of 8 and 14 hours following a glucocorticoid dose and the intrinsic potencies of the agents were determined by back extrapolation to zero time. Based on their work, the following values were obtained for prednisone: relative intrinsic potency 1.05; relative potencies at 8 and 14 hours were 3.0 and 5.2 times hydrocortisone, respectively. For dexamethasone, the intrinsic potency was 17 relative to hydrocortisone; at 8 and 14 hours the relative potencies were 52 and 154 times that of hydrocortisone, respectively.

Comparisons of the relative potencies of the glucocorticoids are further complicated by the results of the studies by Kowozer et al (17) and Gambertoglio et al (18). These investigators noted

Table 1.

COMPARISON OF VARIOUS GLUCOCORTICOIDS WITH HYDROCORTISONE

Glucocorticoid	Anti-inflammatory Potency	Equivalent Potency (mg)	Sodium Retaining Potency
Hydrocortisone	1.0	20	2
Cortisone	0.8	25	2
Prednisolone	4.0	5	1
Prednisone	3.5	5	1
Methylprednisolone	5.0	4	0
Triamcinolone	5.0	4	0
Paramethasone	10.0	2	0
Betamethasone	25.0	0.60	0
Dexamethasone	30.0	0.75	0

that some patients are more susceptible to glucocorticoid effects because of differences in the glucocorticoid rate of metabolism. Since the clinical effects of glucocorticoids are proportional to the tissue concentrations of glucocorticoids, differences in the metabolic clearance rates will significantly influence calculations of comparative potencies. Therefore, the relative potencies as they are currently defined in these tables need to be re-evaluated.

The glucocorticoids also are categorized as being either short, intermediate, or long-acting according to the duration of clinical effects. The basis for this categorization is the result of a study which measured the duration of HPA axis suppression after 50 mg of prednisone was administered to a single patient (19). Following suitable recovery periods, the study was repeated in the same patient with "equipotent" doses of the other glucocorticoids. While this categorization appears to be generally correct, the studies by Kowozer et al and Gambertoglio et al cited above indicate that these categories could be further subdivided according to the rate of glucocorticoid metabolic clearance. Furthermore, the assumption that the duration of HPA axis suppression is identical to the duration of anti-inflammatory activity needs to be affirmed.

Uses. The uses of the glucocorticoids can be divided into two broad categories: replacement therapy and anti-inflammatory/immunosuppressive therapy. Replacement therapy is indicated when the endogenous production of hydrocortisone is absent or deficient. As such, replacement therapy represents the only instance when glucocorticoid use is essential. Nevertheless, the glucocorticoids are predominantly used for their anti-inflammatory/immunosuppressive activity. The glucocorticoids will exert nonspecific anti-inflammatory effects regardless of the etiology of the inflammation. Although the glucocorticoids modify the inflammatory response, they are not curative and do not correct the underlying cause of the inflammation.

The decision to use glucocorticoids must be based upon an appropriate balance of the risks against the benefits of their use. Because these agents are not curative, nonacute and chronic inflammatory conditions should be treated with small doses which can be slowly increased if necessary. The goal of glucocorticoid therapy of chronic inflammatory diseases is to achieve functional but not complete symptomatic relief with the lowest possible dose. Generally in these situations, the glucocorticoids are adjunctive and not the primary treatment modality. For acute, self-limited conditions such as a bad case of poison oak, large doses of glucocorticoids can be initiated and subsequently tapered rapidly. For acute, life-threatening conditions, large doses of glucocorticoids are utilized until control is achieved. Subsequently, in an effort to control the disease and minimize glucocorticoid toxicity, the dose is tapered slowly, if possible. Patients receiving glucocorticoids should be monitored for both therapeutic benefits as well as for signs of toxicity.

Table 2.

HALF-LIVES AND DURATIONS OF ACTION
OF VARIOUS SYSTEMIC GLUCOCORTICOIDS

Glucocorticoid	Half-life (minutes)	Duration HPA Suppression (hours)
Hydrocortisone	80–118	12
Cortisone	30	12
Prednisolone	115–212	24–36
Prednisone	60	24–36
Methylprednisolone	78–188	24–36
Triamcinolone		24–36
Paramethasone		24–36
Dexamethasone	110–210	more than 48
Betamethasone		more than 48

ADRENOCORTICAL INSUFFICIENCY

1. L.P. is a 60-year-old woman who enters the hospital with a five-day history of progressively increasing back pain, malaise, weakness, anorexia, worsening of her arthritis, and arthralgias in previously unaffected joints. She consulted her gynecologist when her rheumatologist could not be contacted. Her gynecologist recommended hospitalization to rule out pyelonephritis. Physical examination revealed a temperature of 38° C, a pulse rate of 100 beats/minute, and a respiratory rate of 16 breaths/minute. She has a 15-year history of rheumatoid arthritis and a one-month history of low back pain caused by osteoporosis which was documented by spinal x-rays. She is currently taking aspirin 900 mg qid for her arthritis, and she occasionally uses antacids as needed. For the past six years, she has been taking prednisone 5 mg tid until it was gradually discontinued over the past 10 days. One day prior to admission she took her last dose of prednisone 5.0 mg. She denies taking any other medications and does not smoke cigarettes or drink alcoholic beverages.

Laboratory tests which were obtained upon admission were reported as follows: hematocrit 38%; white blood cells 11,000/mm³, neutrophils 60%, lymphocytes 25%, eosinophils 10%, monocytes 5%, serum sodium 135 mEq/Liter, potassium 5.8 mEq/Liter; blood glucose 70 mg/dl; creatinine 1.5 mg/dl; blood urea nitrogen 28 mg/dl; serum glutamic oxaloacetic transaminase (SGOT) 15 IU/Liter; lactic dehydrogenase (LDH) 80 IU/Liter (nl 52–149 IU/Liter); alkaline phosphatase 200 IU/Liter (nl 23–71 IU/Liter); and total bilirubin was 1.0 mg/dl. Urinalysis noted a dark yellow color, 2–5 white blood cells/high power field, and no other pertinent findings.

The assessment at this time is adrenocortical insufficiency secondary to the discontinuation of glucocorticoid therapy.

What evidence in this patient's presentation is compatible with hypocortisolism?

Patient L.P.'s malaise, arthralgias anorexia, fever, recent history of discontinuation of glucocorticoid therapy, hypoglycemia, eosinophilia, hyperkalemia, and hyponatremia are compatible with hypocortisolism. The assessment of hypocortisolism probably is reasonable despite the fact that L.P.'s last dose of prednisone was one day prior to admission.

2. What screening tests would be of benefit in substantiating the assessment of hypocortisolism in this patient?

Two or more serum cortisol levels which are subnormal would be diagnostic of hypocortisolism in this patient.

Two rapid screening tests can be used to establish adrenocortical insufficiency. The basis for both these tests is that ACTH stimulates the adrenal cortex to produce hydrocortisone.

Table 3.

DRUGS WHICH ALTER CORTISOL LEVEL

Drug	Effect on Plasma Cortisol Level	Ref
Alcohol	Increased in nonalcoholics; no change in alcoholics	132,133
Amphetamines	Increases	134
Carbenoxolone	Increases	135
Estrogens	Increases	131
Heparin	Increases—False evaluation with fluorometric assay	136
Lysine Vasopressin	Increases	137
Methoxamine	Increase	138
Nicotine	Increases	139

Cosyntropin Test. Cosyntropin (Cortrosyn) is a synthetic peptide unit of natural ACTH which retains full ACTH activity. It differs from the natural product in that it is less allergenic. One-tenth (0.1) mg of cosyntropin is approximately equivalent to 10 units of natural ACTH. After a baseline plasma cortisol level is drawn, 0.25 mg of cosyntropin is administered intramuscularly. One-half to one hour after the injection, a second plasma cortisol level is drawn. If the patient has adrenocortical insufficiency, the plasma cortisol level will not be elevated to greater than twice the baseline value. This test does not distinguish between adrenocortical and pituitary etiologies of adrenocortical insufficiency (20).

ACTH Screening Test. After a baseline plasma cortisol level is drawn, 25 U of ACTH is administered intramuscularly. One hour after injection a plasma cortisol level is drawn. If the patient has normal adrenocortical function, the plasma cortisol will increase by 25 mcg/dl (range 11.3–47.8 mcg/dl). If the patient has adrenocortical insufficiency (Addison's disease), the plasma cortisol will increase by 1.5–2.5 mcg/dl. This test also does not distinguish between adrenocortical and pituitary etiologies of hypocortisolism (21).

3. What are the different types of glucocorticoid withdrawal syndromes?

Rapid tapering and/or discontinuation of therapy can trigger a variety of glucocorticoid withdrawal syndromes:

Type 1 - Glucocorticoid Insufficiency. The patient has symptoms of glucocorticoid insufficiency, has no evidence of flare-up of the condition being treated, and has objective evidence of HPA axis suppression.

Type 2 - Flare-up of The Condition Being Treated. The patient with this withdrawal syndrome has reactivation of the inflammatory condition which is being treated, has symptoms of glucocorticoid deficiency, and has no objective evidence of HPA axis suppression.

Type 3 - Dependence. A patient who has no objective evidence of HPA suppression and no evidence of reactivation of the condition being treated but who is symptomatic of glucocorticoid insufficiency would fall into this category.

Type 4 - Asymptomatic. This type of patient has objective evidence of HPA axis suppression, no evidence or symptoms of a flare-up of the conditions for which steroids were used, and no symptoms of glucocorticoid insufficiency.

Dixon and Christy (22) have described patients who fit into the various categories and note that combinations of Types 1, 2 and/or 3 withdrawal syndromes can occur. According to the above classifications, objective evidence of HPA axis suppression consists of low serum cortisol levels, absence of diurnal variation in serum cortisol levels, and subnormal response to ACTH stimulation tests. Amatruda et al (23) noted that patients who were being withdrawn from glucocorticoids developed a syndrome which was characterized by fever, anorexia, nausea, lethargy, arthralgias, desquamation of the skin, weakness and weight loss. These patients had normal HPA axis function and were not adrenally suppressed.

Knowledge of the types of glucocorticoid withdrawal syndromes is of value when doses of glucocorticoids are being reduced. Similarly, the possibility of the existence of the patient who may be asymptomatic in the face of hypocortisolism and subnormal HPA axis function should be considered when discontinuing glucocorticoids.

4. What factors influence the suppression of the HPA axis by exogenous glucocorticoids?

Sustained supraphysiologic tissue levels of cortisol or other glucocorticoids can suppress the HPA axis. This HPA axis suppression is based on negative feedback inhibition of ACTH release from the anterior pituitary gland; that is, elevated glucocorticoid levels inhibit the pituitary secretion of ACTH. The resultant decrease in ACTH minimizes stimulation of the adrenal cortex to synthesize and release cortisol. If pituitary secretion of ACTH is inhibited for a long period of time, adrenocortical atrophy and unresponsiveness may be followed by pituitary unresponsiveness as well. Factors which influence HPA axis suppression include the dosing regimen, duration of therapy, dose, glucocorticoid, as well as the tissue and serum concentrations of the glucocorticoid.

Dosing Regimen. A daily divided dose of glucocorticoid suppresses the HPA axis more than the same dose administered once a day. Similarly, a single daily dose regimen is more suppressive than an alternate-day dosing regimen. When the dosing interval is increased, the decreased concentration of glucocorticoid minimizes the exposure of the HPA axis to negative feedback inhibition. (See Question 9.)

Dose and Individual Variation. The specific dose of a particular glucocorticoid which will suppress the HPA axis varies and is influenced both by the dosing regimen and the patient's ability to metabolically clear the drug. In one study (24), single morning doses of prednisone 5.0–7.5 mg for at least one year did not suppress adrenal function as evidenced by normal* responsiveness to the cosyntropin test. Prednisone doses of 10.0–12.5 mg and 15 mg resulted in blunted** responses to cosyntropin testing in 33% and 47% respectively; 20 mg doses of prednisone resulted in blunted responses in 20% and complete adrenal suppression in 44%. Therefore, suppression of the HPA axis is more likely with increasingly larger doses of exogenous glucocorticoids, and is substantially affected by inter-individual differences.

Agent Used. At equivalent doses, a long-acting glucocorticoid will cause more adrenal suppression than an intermediate-acting agent, which in turn will be more suppressive than a short-acting agent. HPA axis suppression has been associated with topical (25), inhalation (26), ophthalmic (28), rectal (29) and systemic glucocorticoid therapy.

5. Following the discontinuation of L.P.'s chronic prednisone therapy, when would her HPA axis begin to recover?

Plasma ACTH and 17-OHCS levels were monitored in 6 patients following the gradual withdrawal of supraphysiologic glucocorticoid doses (30). The duration of glucocorticoid therapy in these patients ranged from 1–10 years. Patient L.P. received prednisone therapy for the past 6 years and should recover in a manner similar to these six patients.

Phase I. During the first month following the discontinuation of their glucocorticoids, these patients had low plasma ACTH and 17-OHCS levels. Plasma and urine 17-OHCS levels were low in response to 50 U ACTH infused over an 8-hour period. Subjectively, the patients complained of weakness, malaise, anorexia, nausea, arthralgias, myalgias, and despondency.

Phase II. During the second through the fifth months, the patients' plasma ACTH concentrations were either normal or supranormal; however, plasma 17-OHCS and adrenal responsiveness to ACTH infusion remained low. The diurnal rhythm of ACTH secretion returned during this phase.

Phase III. During the sixth through the ninth months, both plasma ACTH and 17-OHCS returned to normal levels; however, adrenal responsiveness to ACTH infusions remained subnormal.

Phase IV. Following the ninth month, the patients had normal plasma ACTH and 17-OHCS levels and normal responses to ACTH infusion and metyrapone testing.

The following can be concluded based upon these data: pituitary function recovers before adrenocortical function, and patients who are stressed can be at risk to develop adrenal insufficiency for up to nine months after discontinuation of long-term glucocorticoid therapy.

6. Would ACTH administration hasten the recovery of L.P.'s HPA axis following the discontinuation of her prednisone?

Administration of ACTH gel or zinc ACTH every 2 to 3 days to patients who had just been withdrawn from chronic glucocorticoid therapy did not hasten adrenal responsiveness. Monthly plasma cortisol and ACTH levels during the first nine months following withdrawal were similar to those of patients who did not receive ACTH injections (31). This lack of effect of exogenous ACTH perhaps is due to ACTH-binding antibodies and/or the possible suppression of a non-ACTH pituitary factor that is important to the recovery of atrophied adrenal cortices. This explanation is consistent with the finding that serum levels of ACTH can be supranormal and persist for several months before adrenocortical responsiveness returns following the cessation of chronic glucocorticoid therapy (30). Therefore, ACTH administration probably would not hasten the recovery of patient L.P.'s HPA axis.

7. How should L.P. be tapered off her glucocorticoid?

Gradual discontinuation of glucocorticoid therapy is usually indicated after attenuation of an acute self-limited condition (eg, poison oak—Question 13), when the patient is experiencing a severe glucocorticoid adverse reaction (eg, psychosis), or after control of a chronic condition (eg, SLE) has been achieved. In the latter instance, the objectives of gradually reducing the glucocorticoid dose would be to achieve the minimal ef-

---

*Normal—a greater than 7 mcg/dl increase in serum cortisol level over baseline one hour after 250 mcg of cosyntropin.

**Blunted—an increase of less than 7 mcg/dl in serum cortisol levels over baseline one hour after 250 mcg of cosyntropin.

fective dose and to minimize or prevent glucocorticoid adverse reactions.

The gradual withdrawal of glucocorticoid therapy is not without risk. Two major concerns are loss of control, or reactivation of the condition being treated, and the precipitation of adrenal insufficiency in a patient whose HPA axis is suppressed.

Patient acceptance and education are essential when discontinuing long-term glucocorticoid therapy. If the patient is unwilling to accept the minor discomforts associated with weaning of the glucocorticoid, any attempt to taper the glucocorticoid will probably be met with noncompliance. The patient also must be made aware of the benefits and the risks associated with tapering glucocorticoids. When the gradual dosage reductions are initiated, the patient should be knowledgeable about the signs and symptoms of adrenal insufficiency and when to contact her physician. There are no standard protocols for glucocorticoid withdrawal, but the following approach has been suggested (32):

(a) Decrease the dose of prednisone by 2.5 to 5.0 mg every three to seven days. If the disease flares up, increase the dose and then taper more gradually, switch to alternate day therapy, or add adjunctive therapy.

(b) Once the patient is at the physiologic dose of glucocorticoid, she should be switched to hydrocortisone 20 mg every morning. At this point, the patient should receive instructions and an identification card and/or bracelet. The patient can also be given a preloaded dexamethasone syringe with instructions on how and when to administer the drug.

(c) After two to four weeks of hydrocortisone 20 mg every morning, a morning dose is withheld and a plasma cortisol level is drawn. The patient is instructed to taper the morning dose by 2.5 mg weekly until she achieves a morning dose of 10 mg per day. At this point, the patient's plasma cortisol level should be evaluated every four weeks as described above. Once her morning plasma level is greater than 10 mcg/dl, the morning dose may be discontinued; however, hydrocortisone 50 mg bid may be needed during stressful situations such as dental work, minor surgical procedures, or minor infections (32). For major stress such as trauma or operative procedures, the dose of hydrocortisone should be increased to 100 mg every 6 to 8 hours during, and for three to four days following,

the stress. The dose should then be tapered until the physiologic range is reached.

(d) The patient should be seen monthly until her cosyntropin screening test is normal.

8. Following the discontinuation of L.P.'s prednisone, her rheumatoid arthritis has been poorly controlled despite other anti-arthritic medications. Chronic ACTH therapy is being considered for this patient. Why are the advantages of chronic ACTH therapy outweighed by the disadvantages?

The major advantage of ACTH over glucocorticoids is that the adrenal cortex is stimulated rather than suppressed. The remainder of the HPA axis can be suppressed, however, with long-term ACTH administration. Abrupt discontinuation of ACTH therapy can cause adrenocortical insufficiency, especially if the patient is under stress. Although patients in one study who received chronic daily ACTH injections for a period of one month to ten years did not develop overt signs of adrenocortical insufficiency after withdrawal of ACTH therapy (33), metyrapone testing of these individuals did reveal some degree of pituitary unresponsiveness. Thus, withdrawal symptoms following ACTH therapy develop much less frequently than with glucocorticoid therapy. Furthermore, ACTH therapy is associated with fewer catabolic effects because ACTH also stimulates adrenal androgen secretion (34).

The disadvantages of ACTH as compared to glucocorticoids limit its usefulness. ACTH must be administered parenterally at least once daily. The serum half-life of ACTH is only 15 minutes and the stimulatory action on the adrenal cortex is dependent on ACTH serum concentrations (34). Severe allergic reactions such as anaphylaxis are another major disadvantage of ACTH. The synthetic corticotrophin, cosyntropin generally is not considered to be antigenic. Furthermore, the amount of cortisol secreted by the adrenal cortex is not consistent and refractory states can occur with time. Finally, sodium retention may prove to be a significant disadvantage in cardiac or hypertensive patients because ACTH stimulates both glucocorticoid and mineralocorticoid secretion (34).

In conclusion, the usefulness of chronic ACTH therapy is extremely limited and would not be applicable to this patient.

9. As an alternative to chronic ACTH therapy, alternate-day dosing with a synthetic

glucocorticoid agent has been selected for this patient. What is the rationale for this dosing regimen?

The objective of the alternate-day dosing regimen is to minimize suppression of the HPA axis and the adverse effects associated with chronic glucocorticoid therapy while maintaining the desired therapeutic effect. When glucocorticoids are administered on an alternate-day schedule, the patient's 48-hour requirement for steroids is administered as a single dose every other morning.

Administration of the glucocorticoid in the morning mimics the normal diurnal variation of plasma hydrocortisone (high levels in the morning and low levels at night). Administration of the glucocorticoid on alternate days provides a rest period from elevated plasma glucocorticoid levels. This rest period allows the HPA axis time to recover from the suppressive effects and other tissues to recover from the metabolic effects of the exogenous glucocorticoids.

Alternate-day therapy can be used whenever chronic or long-term glucocorticoid therapy is anticipated. However, as a general rule it should be instituted only after the condition being treated has been controlled with divided daily or single daily dose therapy. The alternate-day dosing regimen should not be used for replacement glucocorticoid therapy since it does not supply sufficient hormone during the "off" day.

The major limitation to the use of this dosing regimen is the loss in control of the disease state being treated. If the disease process cannot be controlled on this dosing regimen, it should not be utilized (35–39).

10. What glucocorticoids can be used in the alternate-day regimen?

The use of paramethasone, dexamethasone, or betamethasone in alternate-day dosing regimens is undesirable because these glucocorticoids have metabolic effects and suppressive effects on the HPA axis in excess of 48 hours following a single dose. The value of alternate-day dosing would thereby be negated. The tissue and HPA suppressive effects of prednisone, prednisolone, methylprednisolone and triamcinolone last 24 to 36 hours following a single dose. Triamcinolone has the longest biological half-life of the intermediate-acting steroids. Although all of these intermediate-acting glucocorticoids theoretically can be used for alternate-day therapy, the mass of accumulated clinical experience has been with prednisone.

Hydrocortisone and cortisone are short-acting (less than 12 hours) and are considered unsuitable for use with the alternate-day dosing regimen (19,40).

11. Patient L.P. will be treated with alternate-day prednisone if possible, but therapy is to be initiated with prednisone 5 mg daily in the morning. The prednisone dose will be increased by 5 mg increments until the desired degree of control is obtained or until her previously adequate dose of prednisone 5 mg tid is reached. At that time how should patient L.P. be switched to an alternate-day prednisone regimen?

The total dose of prednisone per day should gradually be consolidated into a single morning dose. In this patient, the prednisone 5 mg tid dosing schedule might be consolidated as follows:

	6 AM	12 N	6 PM
	5.0 mg	5.0 mg	5.0 mg
Day 1	10.0 mg	0	5.0 mg
Day 2	12.5 mg	0	2.5 mg
Day 3	15.0 mg	0	0

This conversion to a single morning dose was rapidly achieved with patient L.P. because of previous dosage alterations which began about 10 days prior to her hospitalization. The majority of patients will require a slower transition period. During the transition, the patient should be monitored for withdrawal symptoms and the control of the condition being treated.

On alternating days, the dose should be incrementally decreased and increased until the total 48 hour dose is given on alternate mornings. On the "off" mornings, no glucocorticoid is given. For example, if the daily morning dose is 15 mg of prednisone, then a typical dosing schedule would be represented by the following:

Day 4	15 mg
Day 5	20 mg
Day 6	10 mg
Day 7	25 mg
Day 8	5 mg
Day 9	30 mg
Day 10	0 mg
Day 11	30 mg
Day 12	0 mg

In this example, the patient changed to an alternate-day dosing regimen by 5 mg/day increments. However, a slower rate of change may be required by some. If the patient becomes symptomatic on the "off" days, a single, small dose of glucocorticoid should be given on the "off" days and gradually reduced.

The rationale for switching to an alternate-day regimen must be explained to the patient in order to gain acceptance of and compliance with the regimen. During the initial phases of dose consolidation and transition to alternate-day dosing, the patient should be made aware of the mild, transient withdrawal symptoms which may occur. Once the alternate-day dosing pattern is established, the "on" day dose should be gradually tapered to the lowest tolerated level (40). Control of the condition being treated should be monitored closely. Should an acute flare occur, abandonment of the regimen should be evaluated against the risks associated with its continued use.

If the patient is in a stress situation, abandonment of the alternate-day regimen may be necessary. The need to abandon or modify the dosing regimen will be dependent on the amount and type of stress being experienced by the patient. For example, a patient scheduled for major surgery should have the regimen modified to provide maximal stress coverage.

12. L.P.'s arthritis is not being adequately controlled on prednisone 30 mg every other morning. How can her dosing regimen be modified to gain control and yet maintain some of the benefits of an alternate-day dosing regimen?

First, factors which might be decreasing the effect of prednisone should be excluded (see Table 4), as should the question of patient compliance to the therapeutic plan. Secondly, the arthritic complaints should be assessed more rigorously. If control is poor during the "off" day, then it would be reasonable to increase the "off" day's dose from 0 to 5 mg and decrease the "on" day's dose from 30 mg to 25 mg. L.P.'s regimen then will be 25 mg every other day, alternating with 5 mg every other day. If this regimen is still ineffective, then the process could be repeated, although the advantage over daily dosing certainly is debatable at this point.

13. An acute case of poison oak dermatitis has been successfully treated with prednisone 20 mg tablets tid for five days. Why should this patient's prednisone be gradually discontinued?

Table 4.

FACTORS WHICH ALTER GLUCOCORTICOID RESPONSE

Factor	Mechanism	Glucocorticoid	Glucocorticoid Response	Reference
Aminophylline	↑ Absorption	Prednisone	Decreased	125
Antacids	—	Prednisone	No Effect	124
Barbiturates	↑ Metabolism	Prednisone	Decreased	47
Barbiturates	↑ Metabolism	Methyl-Prednisolone	Decreased	129
Ephedrine	↑ Metabolism	Dexamethasone	Decreased	130
Estrogen	↑ CBG, ↓ Metabolism	Hydrocortisone	Increased	131
Estrogen	↑ CBG, ↓ Metabolism	Prednisolone	Increased	17,131
Liver Disease	↓ Protein Bind-	Prednisone	Increased	See Question 18
Phenytoin	↑ Metabolism	Dexamethasone	Decreased	128,129
Rifampin	↑ Metabolism	Prednisone	Decreased	125
Tablet Formulation	Alters Bio-availability	Prednisone	Varied	123

Abrupt discontinuation of prednisone can cause a flare-up of the condition under treatment, precipitate acute adrenocortical insufficiency, or induce glucocorticoid withdrawal symptoms even with short-courses of therapy. Good and associates (43) reported the appearance of withdrawal symptoms in one patient who received a single 40 mg dose of prednisone. Others (44) reported impaired responsiveness to the cosyntropin stimulation test for up to five days following prednisone 25 mg bid for five days. In contrast to these two reports, patients who received four to six grams of hydrocortisone over 24 to 48 hours for septic shock did not manifest adrenal insufficiency following abrupt cessation of therapy (42). Apparently, inter-individual differences are substantial.

There are no established guidelines for discontinuing short-course glucocorticoid therapy. In this particular situation, this patient's dosing regimen could be decreased from 20 mg tid to 60 mg each morning. Subsequent daily doses could be halved on each succeeding day such that the daily regimen would be gradually tapered from 60 mg to 30 mg to 15 mg to 7.5 mg and to 5.0 mg before it is discontinued on the next day. However, it is highly unlikely that acute adrenocortical insufficiency would be precipitated following the abrupt discontinuation of a five day course of high-dose prednisone. Although abrupt prednisone discontinuation could theoretically result in the reappearance of this patient's dermatitis and could cause mild symptoms of glucocorticoid withdrawal, it seems rather excessive to supply the patient with another prescription for 5.0 mg tablets accompanied by elaborate tapering instructions. Practically, it would seem more reasonable to modify the above schedule for short-course glucocorticoid discontinuation.

EXCESS GLUCOCORTICOID EFFECTS

14. C.H., a 30-year-old woman, is seen in clinic for a 10-year history of obesity. On physical examination, blood pressure is 160/95 mm Hg, pulse rate is 88 beats/minute, and respiratory rate is 17 breaths/minute. The patient is afebrile and her obesity is especially noticeable on her trunk, face, and back. Striae are present on her abdomen and breasts, and her menstrual periods have been either irregular or absent for several years. She takes no medications, does not smoke cigarettes, and does not consume alcoholic beverages. The results of C.H.'s laboratory tests were as follows: hematocrit 52%; white blood cells 12,000/mm³, neutrophils 87%, lymphocytes 8%, monocytes 5%; serum sodium 148 mEq/Liter; potassium 3.0 mEq/Liter; blood glucose 285 mg/dl; and the urinalysis was within normal limits except for 4+ glucosuria. The liver and renal function tests were within normal limits. The assessment at this time is Cushing's syndrome. What subjective or objective data in this patient are compatible with this assessment?

Patient C.H.'s centripetal obesity, striae, hypertension, irregular menstrual periods, polycythemia, hypernatremia,, hypokalemia, hyperglycemia, and glucosuria are compatible with Cushing's syndrome.

15. What tests would be of benefit in substantiating the assessment of Cushing's syndrome in this patient?

Elevated serum concentrations of cortisol in both the morning and afternoon suggest chronic hypercortisolism and lack of the usual diurnal pattern of cortisol secretion. Therefore, this patient's concentration of cortisol in the serum should be evaluated. The overnight *dexamethasone suppression test* also is useful in assessing the possibility of Cushing's syndrome. In this test, 1.0 mg of dexamethasone is administered orally between 11:00 p.m. and 12:00 a.m. and the serum concentration of cortisol is measured at 8:00 a.m. the following morning. In normal patients, the dexamethasone should suppress the hypothalmic-anterior pituitary-adrenal axis and the plasma 17-OHCS level to less than 5 mcg/dl. The plasma 17-OHCS concentration, however, may not be depressed to this level in patients who are under physical or emotional stress. Patients who are receiving phenytoin or phenobarbital may also have higher than expected plasma concentrations of 17-OHCS (46–47).

Dexamethasone is the glucocorticoid of choice for testing the suppressibility of the HPA axis. The amount of this glucocorticoid required to suppress the HPA axis will not significantly increase the plasma or urinary 17-OHCS concentrations because it is so potent on a milligram basis.

16. The assessment of Cushing's syndrome was confirmed in this patient and a

bilateral adrenalectomy was performed. During the operation and the subsequent 24-hour period, hydrocortisone 100 mg every 8 hours was administered. The postoperative course was uncomplicated and the hydrocortisone dose was rapidly tapered to 10 mg tid. What other adrenal corticosteroid should be prescribed for this patient?

This patient had a bilateral adrenalectomy. Therefore, replacement therapy with a mineralocorticoid must be prescribed for her in addition to her glucocorticoid. Fludrocortisone and desoxycorticosterone are the commercially available mineralocorticoids. Fludrocortisone is the 9-alpha derivative of hydrocortisone and possesses 125 times the mineralocorticoid and 12–15 times the anti-inflammatory potency of hydrocortisone. Although fludrocortisone is a glucocorticoid, it possesses mineralocorticoid effects that are comparable to those of aldosterone. This synthetic adrenocortical steroid is available for oral administration as tablets providing 0.1 mg of fludrocortisone acetate (Florinef) per tablet. The usual dose is 0.1 mg daily, although doses ranging from 0.1 mg three times weekly to 0.2 mg daily have been used.

Desoxycorticosterone is a precursor of aldosterone and possesses $1/30$ the mineralocorticoid potency. Like aldosterone, desoxycorticosterone is essentially devoid of anti-inflammatory effects. Unlike fludrocortisone, it is available in parenteral and sublingual tablet dosage forms (47a,48).

17. Patient C.H. is hospitalized about one year later because of an automobile accident. Physical examination and radiological evaluations are unremarkable except for a concussion and a brief period of unconsciousness. During the ensuing 24 hours the patient's blood pressure drops to 90/65 mm Hg and treatment with normal saline and serum albumin is initiated. Laboratory tests at this time are as follows: hematocrit 46%; white blood cells 8,000/mm³, neutrophils 60%, lymphocytes 25%, eosinophils 10%; blood glucose 70 mg/dl; creatinine 2.0 mg/dl; blood urea nitrogen 40 mg/dl; serum sodium 145 mEq/Liter; and serum potassium 5.5 mEq/Liter. What would be a reasonable assessment of this patient's condition in light of these clinical data?

These clinical data suggest acute adrenal insufficiency. This patient, with a history of bilat-

eral adrenalectomy, cannot increase the secretion of glucocorticoids to meet the increased stress requirements of her traumatic injury. Whenever this condition is suspected, a baseline serum cortisol should be obtained and 100 mg of hydrocorticosone should be administered intravenously immediately. This initial dose should be followed by 100 mg of the hydrocortisone every 8 hours for 36 to 48 hours. The patient's fluid, electrolyte, and glucose balance should be maintained and other supportive therapy given as the need arises. Once the patient's condition has stabilized, the intravenous administration of hydrocortisone can be replaced with 50 mg oral doses of hydrocortisone every six hours. This can be tapered by 20–30% per day until the maintenance dose is reached. Fludrocortisone should be added once the daily maintenance dose of hydrocortisone reaches about 25 mg every 6 hours (49).

18. A 28-year-old woman with systemic lupus erythematosus (SLE) is receiving prednisone 60 mg/day. She has a past history of alcohol abuse and her laboratory tests are compatible with hepatocellular injury. What published evidence supports an alteration in this patient's prednisone dose?

Prednisone and cortisone are biologically inactive until biotransformed by the enzymatic action of hepatic 11-beta-hydroxydehydrogenase to prednisolone and hydrocortisone, respectively. The efficiency of this biotransformation for prednisone is 100% and for cortisone 50–70% (9,48,50). Powell et al (51) noted a significant difference in plasma prednisolone levels when 20 mg of prednisone and 20 mg of prednisolone were administered to patients with acute hepatitis or active chronic hepatocellular disease. Apparently, hepatic dysfunction decreases the efficiency of the biotransformation of prednisone to prednisolone. In contrast, other studies noted that hepatic disease had minimal effect on the conversion of prednisone to prednisolone (19,52,54).

Powell et al (51) also compared the half-lives of intravenous prednisolone in three control patients and in three patients with liver disease (two inactive and one active). The half-lives in the control patients were 150, 180, and 195 minutes. The half-lives in the patients with liver disease were 195, 220, and 250 minutes. Similarly, Araki et al (52) noted that the half-life of intravenous prednisolone was 157 minutes in cirrhotic patients and 115 minutes in healthy patients. Similar increases in prednisolone half-lives were reported in patients with chronic active liver disease with hepatic necrosis (53,54). However, the significance of these observed increases in the plasma half-life of prednisone is unclear because the correlation between plasma half-life of glucocorticoids and the pharmacological duration of action is unclear.

Liver disease often is associated with increased serum bilirubin concentrations and decreased albumin synthesis. The lower the serum albumin concentration, the lower the percentage of glucocorticoid binding. For example, at serum albumin concentrations of 4.0 gm/dl prednisolone is 65% bound; at 3.5 gm/dl it is 55% bound; and at 2.5 gm/dl it is 45% bound (12,51). Additionally, hypoalbuminemia has been correlated with an increased risk of glucocorticoid side effects. The frequency of adverse reactions (facial plethora, hemorrhage, psychosis, hyperglycemia, myopathy) at albumin levels of 2.5 gm/dl and 4.0 gm/dl were 37% and 15% respectively (12).

Hyperbilirubinemia also increases the percentage of unbound prednisolone. This increased free fraction of prednisolone is attributed to a competition between prednisolone and bilirubin for albumin binding sites (55).

This patient's compromised liver function results in two counterbalancing effects. The biotransformation of prednisone (inactive) to prednisolone (active) can be impaired and result in a decrease in available active drug. This effect might be counterbalanced by the decreased albumin, elevated bilirubin, and decreased metabolic clearance of prednisolone. If the patient's prednisone medication could be switched to prednisolone, part of the problem would be obviated. The other variables which may increase prednisolone effects, however, remain. Therefore, either prednisolone or prednisone 60 mg/day may be prescribed because in either case the patient's clinical response needs to be closely monitored.

19. An afebrile patient with obstructive pulmonary disease is receiving prednisone 10 mg qid. Culture and sensitivity tests of the patient's sputum, urine, and blood are negative, but a complete blood count indicates a white blood cell count of 20,000/mm³, with neutrophils 85%, lymphocytes 10%, and monocytes 5%. How might this lymphocytopenia and neutrophilia be explained on the basis of the glucocorticoid therapy?

Lymphocytopenia. In animal studies, glucocorticoids decrease lymphocytes in the circulation by redistributing them into other body compartments such as the bone marrow (51,58). Moreover, circulating T-lymphocytes are decreased to a greater extent than B-lymphocytes (59,60). Much of the data concerning lymphoid depletion following glucocorticoid administration are based upon animal studies. Because of marked differences in lymphocyte kinetics between various animal species, extrapolation of these data to man must be done with caution (56).

In man, lymphocyte counts decreased to 25–50% of baseline values following a single dose of hydrocortisone 400 mg IV (59), prednisolone 1.0 gm IV (61), methylprednisolone 1.0 gm IV (62) or prednisone 50 mg orally (60). The nadir in the lymphocyte count occurred 4–6 hours after the dose and reverted to baseline values within 24 hours after the dose, with one exception. Following methylprednisolone, the lymphocytopenia persisted for 48 hours. Patients receiving alternate day prednisone had no lymphocytopenia on the "off" day (63).

The glucocorticoids also affect lymphocyte function. They decrease the blastogenic response of T-lymphocytes to mitogens (63) and antigens (64), and inhibit ongoing antibody synthesis. Glucocorticoids do not interfere with the induction of antibody response if the antigen is introduced just prior to or during glucocorticoid therapy. IgA levels are decreased by glucocorticoids, and IgG levels begin to decrease 2–6 days after institution of glucocorticoids. Following a 5-day course of methylprednisolone 16 mg every 4 hours, IgG levels were depressed by 50% and remained depressed for 3 months.

Human leukemic lymphocytes are more sensitive to glucocorticoids than normal lymphocytes (56).

Neutrophilia. Glucocorticoids increase the number of circulating neutrophils by stimulating their release from the bone marrow (66), mobilizing them from the margins of blood vessel walls (67), inhibiting their migration out of the circulation in response to macrophage aggregation factor (62), and by prolonging their half-life (68).

Although the number of circulating white blood cells may be increased by glucocorticoids, intracellular killing of bacteria may be impaired (66). This inability to destroy phagocytized bacteria is secondary to lysosomal stabilization and failure of lysosomes to fuse with phagocytic vacuoles. The glucocorticoid preparation used may also be of importance. In mice, succinate-linked hydrocortisone and methylprednisolone did not enhance local infection in contrast to the phosphate-linked hydrocortisone preparations (69). In a similar study, acetate- and phosphate-linked steroids potentiated infections; however, succinate-linked glucocorticoids did not (70).

Adverse Glucocorticoid Effects

20. *In Pregnancy.* A 25-year-old asthmatic patient, who has been receiving prednisolone 15 mg daily, is now pregnant. The activity of her disease does not allow for discontinuation of the prednisolone. What potential complications should be anticipated because of her pregnancy?

Teratogenesis. In a review article concerning the effects of maternal medications on the fetus and the newborn, Adamson and Joelsson (75) cite a 10% incidence of cleft palate in association with the use of cortisone during the first ten weeks of gestation. The authors also noted that it is during the tenth week of gestation that the palate closes. Warrell and Taylor (76) reported 8 still births and 9 infants at risk (placental insufficiency and acute fetal distress) during 34 pregnancies in which the mothers received prednisolone (2.5 to 30 mg daily) before and throughout their pregnancy. The patients were receiving prednisolone for eczema, ulcerative colitis, urticaria, asthma, rheumatoid arthritis, or lupus erythematosus. In a control group of women with similar diseases, there were no still births, three premature births and one death secondary to status asthmaticus during labor. Although no specific data were presented, the authors state that none of the infants had clinical evidence of adrenal insufficiency. Although teratogenesis may be a problem with glucocorticoid administration, discontinuation of medications which are essential to maternal well-being may pose a greater hazard to the fetus.

Neonatal Adrenocortical Insufficiency. Although this complication of glucocorticoid therapy is a possibility, there are no reported cases. One case of fetal adrenocortical necrosis was noted on post-mortem examination (75).

Maternal Adrenocortical Insufficiency. During the stress of parturition and during the post-partum stage, the patient who has been receiving glucocorticoids during pregnancy should receive supplemental glucocorticoids to prevent acute adrenal insufficiency.

21. *In Surgical Patients.* A 28-year-old woman with ulcerative colitis has been treated with prednisone 20 mg bid, hydrocortisone 100 mg enema at bedtime, and sulfasalazine. The oral prednisone was discontinued about six months prior to admission. The patient is now hospitalized for a major surgical procedure. What are some of the consequences of this patient's history of glucocorticoid therapy that must be considered at this time?

Although the patient has not received oral prednisone for about six months, she has been receiving hydrocortisone enemas which are absorbed to a significant degree (80–82). Therefore, the possibility of HPA axis suppression should be considered, especially because the night-time administration of these glucocorticoid enemas enhances adrenal insufficiency. Consequently, this patient should receive preoperative, intraoperative, and postoperative glucocorticoid therapy because of the potential inability of the adrenals to respond to the stress of major surgery. For major surgical procedures, hydrocortisone 100 mg should be given by continuous infusion every 6 hours at the beginning of anesthesia and continued for 72 hours following the procedure. The duration of therapy should be extended if postoperative complications were to develop. If no complications develop, the hydrocortisone dose can be changed to the previous glucocorticoid maintenance level (49). Similar glucocorticoid coverage has been recommended for minor operative procedures or invasive studies, except coverage may be discontinued 24 hours after the procedure (49). For some very minor procedures, a single 100 mg dose of hydrocortisone immediately preceding the stress would suffice.

This patient's wounds also may not heal as quickly as might be expected. The glucocorticoids impair wound healing as a result of their anti-inflammatory and catabolic properties. Inhibition of vascularization and collagen deposition as well as the stabilization of lysosomal membranes may also contribute to delayed wound healing.

In wounds sutured together (closed wound), the tensile strength of the wound is decreased if steroids are administered within three days of surgery (74). In open wounds, the rate of epithelialization is decreased and contraction delayed. This effect is seen even if steroids are not initiated until after the inflammatory process has been established and contraction has begun (77).

22. Gastrointestinal Effects. A patient with arthritis has been receiving prednisone 5 mg tid for approximately one year. He now complains of non-specific upper abdominal pain. What are two major gastrointestinal adverse effects of prednisone?

Ulcer. In the early 1950's, the glucocorticoids were still considered the "silver bullet" of rheumatoid arthritis therapy. It was also during this time that the glucocorticoids acquired their reputation of being ulcerogenic. A number of mechanisms for glucocorticoid-induced ulceration have been proposed: thinning of gastric mucus, decreased regeneration of gastric mucosal cells secondary to a slowing down of the mitotic process, and an increase in acid production. The majority of the evidence for these effects is based on animal data (82–88).

The initial reports of glucocorticoid-induced gastric ulceration were in patients with rheumatoid arthritis. Up to 31% of this patient population reportedly developed this adverse effect (89,90). However, in other conditions such as asthma (91,92), ulcerative colitis (93), allergic disorders (94) and dermatologic disorders (95) in which glucocorticoids were used, the incidence of ulceration did not exceed the 5–10% range which is found in the general population (96). This difference in the incidence of glucocorticoid associated ulceration in arthritics vs. non-arthritics can be explained on the following basis. Patients with rheumatoid arthritis usually receive other antiinflammatory agents (aspirin, phenylbutazone, or indomethacin) in addition to their glucocorticoid therapy. These other anti-inflammatory agents are well known gastric irritants and are capable of inducing ulcers when used without glucocorticoids. One study (97) noted no difference in the incidence of ulcer in arthritics receiving glucocorticoids and those who did not.

The precise relationship between peptic ulceration and glucocorticoid therapy, therefore, is unclear. Patients who appear to be at risk are those who are being treated for nephrotic syndrome or liver disease, or who are comatose post-craniotomy. Other predisposing factors include a total prednisone intake exceeding 1000 mg, a history of ulcer disease, concomitant use of known gastric irritants, and stress (98,99). It may be desirable to use prophylactic antacids pending clarification of the relationship of glucocorticoids and ulcers.

Pancreatitis. Early post-mortem examinations of this pathologic entity noted a 40% incidence of glucocorticoid-induced pancreatitis in nephrotic children (100) and a 28.5% incidence in rheumatoid arthritics (101). Nevertheless, this adverse effect is not well-established.

The mechanism for glucocorticoid-induced pancreatitis also is not clear. Nelp (102) suggested that glucocorticoids induce hyperlipidemia and fatty necrosis of the pancreas. Alternatively, glucocorticoids may alter the electrolyte content of pancreatic juices, resulting in inspissation and consequent pancreatic duct obstruction. Perforation of an ulcer and leakage of gastric juices onto the pancreas has also been suggested as a mechanism.

The clinical presentation of glucocorticoid-induced pancreatitis is similar to that of peptic ulcer disease, and complaints of epigastric upper abdominal pain should not be attributed solely to peptic ulceration (103).

23. Intracranial Hypertension. An acute episode of ulcerative colitis has been successfully managed with prednisone 40 mg per day. The dose was gradually reduced in increments of 5 mg per day. Three days after the medication had been discontinued, the patient became irritable and complained of headache and visual disturbances. Papilledema is noted on ophthalmologic exam. What might be a reasonable assessment of this patient's clinical situation?

This patient's symptoms are compatible with intracranial hypertension, which has been associated with too rapid discontinuation of glucocorticoid or ACTH therapy. When these medications have been administered chronically, doses should be tapered over a one month period, and abrupt decreases in dose of 50% or more should be avoided (104).

Post-glucocorticoid benign intracranial hypertension has been reported primarily in pediatric patients. The pathogenesis of the syndrome is unclear. Objective findings include an enlarged subarachnoid space and ventricular enlargement in long-standing cases. Severe visual loss may also occur if the condition persists.

The syndrome is treated by reinstituting glucocorticoid therapy at one-half to one-third the original dose. The dose is then slowly tapered over a two to three month period. If visual deterioration is marked, high-dose hydrocortisone (up to 400 mg/day) or operative decompression is recommended.

24. Osteoporosis. A 60-year-old post-menopausal female is seen by her private physician for low back pain. On x-ray, a compression fracture of one of her vertebrae is noted. She has been taking prednisone 10 mg/day for chronic asthmatic conditions for "years." Why does prednisone predispose this patient to this fracture?

Post-menopausal females, men older than 60 years of age, rheumatoid arthritic patients, diabetic patients, and immobilized patients appear to be predisposed to the development of osteoporosis. Chronic glucocorticoid therapy in these patients, therefore, increases the risk of this potential complication.

The osteoporosis occurs primarily in the axial skeleton: vertebral column and pelvic girdle. Spontaneous compression fractures of the lumbar vertebrae are most common. Fractures of the ribs and other bones can occur following minor trauma (105). Osteoporotic changes are not noted radiologically until they are far advanced and usually are asymptomatic until a bone is fractured.

It is not known how glucocorticoids induce osteoporosis; however, the following might account for this adverse effect. The glucocorticoids inhibit calcium absorption from the intestine and decrease calcium reabsorption by the renal tubules (106,107). They also may inhibit production of osteoblasts (108) and thereby inhibit new bone formation, as in Cushing's syndrome (109,110). Furthermore, glucocorticoids may decrease collagen formation or increase collagen catabolism in bone matrix. The evidence for increased bone resorption is conflicting (74). Finally, glucocorticoids may increase parathyroid hormone levels. The PTH levels of patients receiving chronic glucocorticoid therapy were approximately double that of a control group (109). In another group of patients who received a four hour 200 mg infusion of hydrocortisone, PTH levels were increased within 15 minutes of the initiation of the infusion. At one hour, the average PTH serum concentration was 152% of baseline values; and at three hours, the PTH levels peaked at 172% of baseline (109). Of

note is that parathyroid hyperplasia has been described in rats treated with glucocorticoids and in patients with Cushing's syndrome.

25. Hyperglycemia. A patient has been receiving prednisone 60 mg daily for systemic lupus erythematosus. She now presents with complaints of polydipsia, polyuria, and a blood sugar of 395 mg/dl. Why might this problem be attributable to the glucocorticoid therapy?

Glucocorticoids cause hyperglycemia by stimulating gluconeogenesis and by inhibiting the peripheral utilization of glucose.

Glucocorticoids are catabolic and cause a dose-related hyperaminoacidemia. This increase in amino acid levels results in pancreatic alpha-cell stimulation and hyperglucagonemia which stimulates glycogenolysis (111). Hyperaminoacidemia also increases enzymes such as glucose-6-phosphatase, fructose-6-phosphatase, and phosphoenolpyruvate carboxykinase which are involved in gluconeogenesis. Glucocorticoids also decrease glucose utilization by interfering with glucose entry into the cell and by inhibiting phosphorylation.

Maximal hyperglycemia occurs eight hours after a dose of glucocorticoid, and the duration of hyperglycemia is related to the glucocorticoid dose. Following 15 mg, 45 mg, and 90 mg of prednisone, hyperglycemia persisted for 10–12 hours, 12–16 hours, and 18–24 hours, respectively (113).

Glucocorticoid therapy can either aggravate pre-existing diabetes or precipitate it de novo. The hyperglycemia is usually mild; however, diabetic coma and acidosis have been associated with glucocorticoid therapy (114). Although continuation of the glucocorticoid usually reverses the hyperglycemia, several months may elapse before the reversal is complete (115).

Dietary restriction and/or oral hypoglycemic agents or insulin can control glucocorticoid-induced hyperglycemia. Large insulin doses are sometimes required (116,117). Decreasing the glucocorticoid dose might help to decrease the degree of hyperglycemia (115), although this effect of dosage reduction is conflicting (113). Alternate-day glucocorticoid dosing has also been reported to decrease glucose intolerance (118).

26. Electrolyte Effects. A 50-year-old patient with congestive heart failure is being treated with digoxin 0.25 mg daily, hydrochlorothiazide 50 mg twice daily, and a low sodium, high potassium diet. The patient has developed polyarteritis which requires therapy with a corticosteroid. Which glucocorticoid would be best for this patient?

Depending on the specific agent used, the dose and the physiologic status of the patient, glucocorticoids can either induce sodium retention by increasing tubular cation exchange (an aldosterone-like effect), or can cause a sodium diuresis by increasing the glomerular filtration rate (GFR) and by correcting the pathological stimulus to hypersecretion of aldosterone. The net effect of the glucocorticoid depends on which of the two actions (sodium diuresis or retention) predominates. For example, in a normal patient, the aldosterone-like effect of hydrocortisone predominates over its effect on the GFR. However, in diseases with high aldosterone levels, the anti-inflammatory action of the glucocorticoid may alleviate the underlying stimulus for aldosterone production. The net effect in the latter instance may be sodium diuresis (119).

The dose of glucocorticoids also affects sodium metabolism. For example, small doses of prednisolone can induce an increase in GFR which predominates over its aldosterone-like effect, and large doses predominantly increase the aldosterone-like action (119). Large doses of hydrocortisone usually increase sodium retention only for a few days, after which the sodium retention decreases in spite of continued therapy. Small hydrocortisone doses, however, are associated with persistent sodium retention and potassium loss (71). It should be noted that all the glucocorticoids induce potassium loss regardless of mineralocorticoid activity, secondary to their protein wasting effects.

Thus, in patients who have conditions such as CHF, in which sodium retention can be an aggravating factor, glucocorticoids associated with a lesser degree of mineralocorticoid effects should be used. Digitalis glycosides should be administered with the awareness that all glucocorticoids cause potassium wasting. (See Congestive Heart Failure chapter and Table 5.)

27. Hypersensitivity. A patient claims to have suffered an asthmatic attack immediately after receiving hydrocortisone intravenously. She noted that her physician cautioned her not to use or have hydrocortisone prescribed for her. Can systemic glucocorticoids cause hypersensitivity reactions?

Hypersensitivity reactions to systemically administered glucocorticoids have been reported. Mendalson et al (120) reported a case in which an asthmatic patient developed generalized urticaria, angioedema and severe bronchospasm following an intravenous dose of methylprednisolone. Challenge of the patient with the diluent in the intravenous methylprednisolone preparation did not cause a similar reaction, but an oral dose of methylprednisolone did elicit identical symptoms. Anaphylactoid types of reaction have also been reported following the use of intra-articular hydrocortisone therapy (121,122).

28. Psychiatric Effects. Hydrocortisone 100 mg every 6 hours IV was prescribed for an acute flare of inflammatory bowel disease. One hour after the first dose, the patient became agitated and paranoid. The patient has no

Table 5.

EFFECTS OF GLUCOCORTICOIDS
ON OTHER DRUG THERAPY

Drug	Effect of Glucocorticoid	Reference
Amphotericin	Potentiates Hypokalemia	140
Diuretics	Potentiates Hypokalemia	See Question 26
GI Irritants	Potentiates GI Ulceration	See Question 22
Hypoglycemic Agents	Antagonizes Hypoglycemia	See Question 25
Salicylates	Increases Salicylate Clearance	141

history of mental illness but was depressed due to the reactivation of her bowel disease. Glucocorticoids were discontinued about six months ago because her disease had become quiescent. Why can this patient's agitation and paranoia be attributable to her glucocorticoid therapy?

Psychiatric reactions to glucocorticoids may be mild and involve simple insomnia or a general sense of well being, or may be severe and involve acute psychotic reactions such as schizophrenia and paranoia. (One of my patients claimed that 10 milligrams of prednisone instilled a sense of euphoria comparable to two marijuana cigarettes.) Patients with a past or present history of psychiatric illness may be predisposed to the mental effects of prednisone; however, these reactions can occur in patients without any psychiatric history. These mind-altering adverse glucocorticoid effects increase in frequency with larger doses, but they have been reported to occur at any dose (126,127). Psychiatric reactions should be treated by rapidly tapering the patient off glucocorticoid therapy. However, this may not be possible without losing control of the condition being treated. Antipsychotic medications can be tried but results are inconsistent.

This patient was predisposed to this adverse glucocorticoid effect because of her state of mental depression. Nevertheless, a direct cause and effect cannot be established between this patient's acute psychotic reaction and her hydrocortisone therapy although the setting and timing are compatible. This patient's hydrocortisone dose probably cannot be tapered immediately because of her acute bowel disease. A phenothiazine or butyrophenone may be tried and perhaps another glucocorticoid, if substituted for the hydrocortisone, might be worthwhile.

References

1. Krieger DT et al: Circadian variation of the plasma 17-hydroxycorticosteroids in central nervous system disease. J Clin Endocrinol. 1966; 26:929.
2. Estep HL: Neuroendocrine aspects of surgical stress. In *An Introduction to Clinical Neuroendocrinology,* Bajusz E (Ed), S Karger, Basel, 1967, p 106.
3. Estep HL et al: Pituitary-adrenal dynamics during surgical stress. J Clin Endocrinol. 1963; 23:419.
4. Eik-Nes KB et al: Diurnal variation of plasma 17-OHCS in subjects suffering from severe brain damage. J Clin Endocrinol. 1958; 18:764.
5. Krieger DT et al: Characterization of the normal temporal pattern of plasma corticoid levels. J Clin Endocrinol. 1971; 32:266.
6. Bliss EL et al: Endocrinology of anorexia nervosa. J Clin Endocrinol. 1957; 17:766.
7. Kenny FM et al: Cortisol production rates II: Normal infants, children and adults. Pediatrics. 1966; 37:34.
8. Bayliss RI: Surgical collapse during and after corticosteroid therapy. Br Med J. 1958; 2:935.
9. Peterson RE et al: The physiological disposition and metabolic fate of cortisone in man. J Clin Invest. 1957; 36:1301.
10. Beisel WR et al: Cortisol transport and disappearance. Ann Intern Med. 1964; 60:641.
11. Hellman L et al: Tracer studies of the absorption and fate of steroid hormones in man. J Clin Invest. 1956; 35:1033.
12. Lewis GP et al: Prednisone side effects and serum protein levels. Lancet. 1971; 2:778.
13. Martin MM et al: Effect of altered thyroid function upon adrenocortical ACTH and methopyrapone (SU 4885) responsiveness in man. J Clin Endocrinol. 1965; 25:20.
14. Mills IH et al: The effect of estrogen administration on the metabolism and protein binding of hydrocortisone. J Clin Endocrinol. 1960; 20:515.
15. Pincus G et al: In *Steroid Dynamics,* Academic Press, New York, 1966, p 13.
16. Meikle AW and Tyler FH: Potency and duration of action of glucocorticoids. Effects of hydrocortisone, prednisone, and dexamethasone and human pituitary-adrenal function. Am J Med. 1977; 63:200.
17. Kowozer M et al: Decreased clearance of prednisolone, a factor in the development of corticosteroid side effects. J Clin Endocrinol Metab. 1974; 38:407.
18. Gambertoglio J et al: The pharmacokinetics in cushingnoid and non-cushingnoid transplant patients. Clin Res. 1979; 27:231A.
19. Harter JG: Corticosteroids, their physiologic use in allergic disease. NY J Med. 1966; 66:827.
20. Cosyntropin. Medical Letter. 1971; 13:33.
21. Maynard DE et al: A rapid test for adrenocortical insufficiency. Ann Intern Med. 1965; 64:552.
22. Dixon RB and Christy NP: On the various forms of corticosteroid withdrawal syndrome. Am J Med. 1980; 68:224.
23. Amatruda TT Jr et al: Certain endocrine and metabolic facets of the steroid withdrawal syndrome. J Clin Endocrinol Metab. 1965; 25:1207.
24. Klinefelter HF et al: Single daily dose prednisone therapy. JAMA. 1979; 241:2721.
25. Scoggins RB et al: Percutaneous absorption of corticosteroids. N Engl J Med. 1965; 273:831.
26. Lindner WR: Adrenal suppression by aerosol steroid inhalation. Arch Intern Med. 1964; 113:665.

27. Lindner WR: Adrenal suppression by ophthalmic steroids. Arch Ophthalmol. 1968; 79:174.

28. Ibid.

29. Matts SGF et al: Adrenocortical and pituitary function after intrarectal steroid therapy. Br Med J. 1963; 2:24.

30. Graber AL et al: Natural history of pituitary-adrenal recovery following long-term suppression with corticosteroids. J Clin Endocrinol. 1965; 25:11.

31. Gleischer NK et al: ACTH antibodies in patients receiving depot ACTH to hasten recovery from pituitary-adrenal suppression. J Clin Invest. 1967; 46:196.

32. Byyny RL: Withdrawal from glucocorticoid therapy. N Engl J Med. 1976; 295:30.

33. Reed PL et al: Adrenocortical and pituitary responsiveness following long-term high-dosage corticotrophin administration. Ann Intern Med. 1964; 61:1.

34. Singer B: Adrenal corticosteroid-physiological considerations. Br Med J. 1972; 1:36.

35. Adams DA et al: Adrenocortical function during intermittent corticosteroid therapy. Ann Intern Med. 1966; 64:542.

36. Harter JG et al: Studies on an intermittent corticosteroid dosage regimen. N Engl J Med. 1963; 269:591.

37. MacGregor RR et al: Alternate-day prednisone therapy. N Engl J Med. 1969; 280:427.

38. Martin MM et al: Intermittent steroid therapy. N Engl J Med. 1968; 279:273.

39. Walton J et al: Alternate-day vs shorter interval steroid administration. Arch Intern Med. 1970; 126:601.

40. Dluhy RG et al: Pharmacology and chemistry of adrenal glucocorticoids. Med Clin North Am. 1973; 57:1155.

41. Nichols T et al: Diurnal variation in suppression of adrenal functions by glucocorticoids. J Clin Endocrinol. 1965; 25:343.

42. Christy JH: Treatment of gram negative shock. Am J Med. 1971; 50:77.

43. Good TA et al: Symptomatology resulting from withdrawal of steroid hormone therapy. Arthritis Rheum. 1959; 2:299.

44. Streck WF and Lockwood DH: Pituitary adrenal recovery following short term suppression with corticosteroids. Am J Med. 1979; 66:910.

45. Ziff M et al: The effects in rheumatoid arthritis of hydrocortisone and cortisone injected intra-articularly. Arch Intern Med. 1952; 90:774.

46. Buchanan RA et al: Diphenylhydantoin: Interactions with other drugs in man (continued). In *Antiepileptic Drugs,* Ed by DM Woodbury et al: Raven Press, New York, 1972, p 181.

47. Burstein S et al: Phenobarbital-induced increases in 6-beta-hydroxycortisol excretion. Clue to its significance in human urine. J Clin Endocrinol Metab. 1965; 25:293.

47a. Haynes RC Jr and Murad F: Adrenocorticotrophic hormone; adrenocortical steroids and their synthetic analogs; inhibitors of adrenocortical steroid biosynthesis. In *The Pharmacological Basis of Therapeutics,* 6th edition, edited by AG Gilman, LS Goodman, and A Gilman, The MacMillan Co, New York, 1980, p 1466.

48. Thomas P: Withdrawal of corticosteroid therapy. In *Guide to Steroid Therapy,* JB Lippincott Co, Philadelphia, 1968, p 195.

49. Plumptom FS et al: Corticosteroid treatment and surgery: The management of steroid cover. Anesthesia. 1969; 24:12.

50. Jenkins JS et al: The conversion of cortisone to cortisol and prednisone to prednisolone in man. Br Med J. 1967; 2:205.

51. Powell LW et al: Corticosteroids in liver disease. Studies on the biological conversion to prednisone to prednisolone and plasma protein binding. Gut. 1972; 13:690.

52. Araki Y et al: Dynamics of corticosteroids in man. In *Steroid Dynamics,* Pincus G et al (Eds), Academic Press, New York, 1966, p 463.

53. Uribe M et al: Oral prednisone for chronic active liver disease. Dose responses and bioavailability studies. Gut. 1978; 19:1131.

54. Uribe M et al: Kinetics and interconversion of prednisone and prednisolone in chronic active liver disease (CALD) after oral doses. Gastroenterology. 1976; 71:932.

55. Uribe M et al: Why hyperbilirubinemia and hypoalbuminemia predispose to steroid side effects during treatment of chronic active liver disease (CALD). Gastroenterology. 1977; 72:1143.

56. Claman HN: Corticosteroids and lymphoid cells. N Engl J Med. 1972; 287:388.

57. Cohen JJ: Thymus derived lymphocytes sequestered in the bone marrow of hydrocortisone treated mice. J Immunol. 1972; 107:841.

58. Fauci AS et al: Effect of hydrocortisone on guinea pig peripheral blood lymphocyte subpopulations. Fed Proc. 1974; 33:750.

59. Fauci AS et al: The effect of in vivo hydrocortisone on subpopulations of human lymphocytes. J Clin Invest. 1974; 54:240.

60. Yu DTY et al: Human lymphocyte subpopulations. Effect of corticosteroids. J Clin Invest. 1974; 53:565.

61. Coberg AJ et al: Disappearance rates and immunosuppression of intermittent intravenously administered prednisolone in rabbits and human beings. Surg Gynecol Obstet. 1970; 131:933.

62. Western WL et al: Communications: Site of action of cortisol in cellular immunity. J Immunol. 1973; 110:880.

63. Caron GA: Prednisolone inhibition of DNA synthesis by human lymphocytes induced in vitro by phytohaemaglutinin. Int Arch Allergy Appl Immunol. 1967; 32:191.

64. Hellman DH et al: Effect of cortisol on the transformation of human blood lymphocytes by antigens and allogenic leucocytes. In *Proceedings of Sixth Leucocyte Culture Conference,* Schwarz MR (Ed), New York, Academic Press, 1972, p 581.

65. Balow JE et al: Glucocorticoid suppression of macrophage migration inhibitory factor. J Exp Med. 1973; 137:1031.

66. Biship CR et al: Leukokinetic study. A nonsteady state kinetic evaluation of the mechanism of cortisone-induced granulocytosis. J Clin Invest. 1968; 47:249.

67. Vincent PC et al: The intravascular survival of neutrophils labeled in vivo. Blood. 1974; 43:371.

68. Dale DC et al: Alternate day prednisone. Leukocyte kinetics and susceptibility to infections. N Engl J Med. 1974; 291:1154.

69. Brothers JR et al: Enhancement of infections by corticosteroids: Experimental clarification. Surg Forum. 1973; 24:30.

70. Fauvre RM et al: Comparative effects on corticosteroids on host resistance to infection in relation to chemical structure. J Exp Med. 1967; 125:807.

71. David DS et al: Adrenal glucocorticoids after twenty years. A review of their clinically relevant consequences. J Chron Dis. 1970; 22:637.

72. Van Metre TE et al: Growth suppression in asthmatic children receiving prolonged therapy with prednisone and methylprednisolone. J Allergy. 1959; 30:103.

73. Falliers CH et al: Childhood asthma and steroid therapy as influence on growth. Am J Dis Child. 1963; 105:127.

74. Soyka LF: The treatment of nephrotic syndrome in childhood: Use of alternate-day prednisone regimen. Am J Dis Child. 1967; 113:693.

75. Adamsons K Jr et al: The effect of maternal medications on the fetus and the newborn infant. Am J Gynecol. 1966; 96:437.

76. Warrell DW et al: Outcome for the fetus of mothers receiving prednisolone during pregnancy. Lancet. 1968; 1:117.

77. Stephens FO et al: Effect of delayed administration of corticosteroids on wound contraction. Ann Surg. 1971; 173:214.

78. Stephens FD et al: Effect of cortisone and vitamin A on wound infection. Am J Surg. 1971; 121:567.

79. Hunt TK et al: Effect of vitamin A on reversing the inhibitory effect of cortisone on healing of open wounds in animals and man. Ann Surg. 1969; 170:663.

80. Farmer RG et al: Treatment of ulcerative colitis with hydrocortisone enemas: Relationship of hydrocortisone absorption, adrenal suppression, and clinical response. Dis Col Rect. 1970; 13:355.

81. Nabarro JDN et al: Rectal hydrocortisone. Br Med J. 1957; 2:272.

82. Spencer JA et al: The rectal absorption of 6-alpha C-14 H-3 prednisolone. Proc Soc Exp Biol Med. 1960; 103:74.

83. Dyre JC et al: Studies on the mechanism of the activation of peptic ulcer after nonspecific trauma. Effect of cortisone on gastric secretion. Am Surg. 1958; 147:738.

84. Garb AE et al: Steroid-induced gastric ulcer. Arch Intern Med. 1965; 116:899.

85. Menguy R et al: Effect of cortisone on mucoprotein secretions by the gastric antrum in dogs. Pathogenesis of steroid ulcers. Surg. 1963; 54:19.

86. Rasanan T: Fluctuations in the mitotic frequency of the glandular stomach and intestine under the influence of ACTH, glucocorticoids, stress, and heparin. Acta Physiol Scand. 1963; 58:201.

87. Skoryna SG et al: A new method of producing experimental gastric ulcers. The effects of hormonal factors on healing. Gastroenterology. 1958; 34:1.

88. Smith AT et al: The acute effects of prednisone on the gastric mucosa. Am J Dig Dis. 1968; 13:79.

89. DuBois EL et al: The corticosteroid-induced peptic ulcer: a serial roentgenological survey of patients receiving high doses. Am J Gastroent. 1960; 33:435.

90. Kemmerer WH et al: Peptic ulcer in rheumatoid arthritis patients on corticosteroid therapy. Arthritis Rheum. 1958; 1:122.

91. Rees HA et al: Long-term steroid therapy in chronic intractable asthma. Br Med J. 1962; 1:1575.

92. Siegel SC: Corticosteroids and ACTH in the management of the atopic child. Ped Clin North Am. 1969; 16:287.

93. Zetzel L et al: ACTH and adrenal-corticosteroids in the treatment of ulcerative colitis. Am J Dig Dis (New Series). 1958; 3:916.

94. Baldwin HS et al: Evaluation of steroid treatment in asthma. Allergy. 1950; 32:109.

95. Sanders SL et al: Corticosteroid therapy of pemphigus. Arch Derm Syph. 1960; 82:717.

96. Ivy AC: The problem of peptic ulcer. JAMA. 1946; 132:1053.

97. Atwater EC et al: Peptic ulcer in rheumatoid arthritis. Arch Intern Med. 1965; 115:184.

98. Cantu RC et al: Evaluation of the increased risk of gastrointestinal bleeding following intracranial surgery in patients receiving high steroid dosages in the immediate postoperative period. Int Surg. 1960; 50:325.

99. Conn HO et al: The nonassociation of adrenocortical steroid therapy and peptic ulcer. N Engl J Med. 1976; 294:473.

100. Riemenschneider TA et al: Corticosteroid-induced pancreatitis in children. Pediatrics. 1968; 41:428.

101. Carone FA et al: Acute pancreatic lesions in patients treated with ACTH and adrenal corticoids. N Engl J Med. 1957; 257:690.

102. Nelp NB: Acute pancreatitis associated with steroid therapy. Arch Intern Med. 1961; 108:702.

103. Schreier RW et al: Steroid-induced pancreatitis. JAMA. 1965; 194:564.

104. Neville BGR et al: Benign intracranial hypertension following corticosteroid withdrawal in childhood. Br Med J. 1970; 3:554.

105. Rosenberg EF: Rheumatoid arthritis. Osteoporosis and fractures related to steroid therapy. Acta Med Scand. 1958; 162 (Suppl):211.

106. Harrison HE et al: Transfer of 45-Ca across intestinal wall in vitro in relationship to action of vitamin D and cortisol. Am J Physiol. 1960; 199:265.

107. Laake H: The action of corticosteroids on the renal reabsorption of calcium. Acta Endocrinol. 1960; 34:60.

108. Duncan H: Bone dynamics of rheumatoid arthritis patients treated with adrenal corticosteroids. Arthritis Rheum. 1967; 10:216.

109. Fucik RF et al: Effects of glucocorticoids on functions of the parathyroids in man. J Clin Endocrinol Metab. 1975; 40:152.

110. Krane SM: Metabolic bone disease. In Harrison's Principles of Internal Medicine, Eighth Ed., McGraw-Hill Book Co., New York, 1977, p 2031.

111. Marco J et al: Hyperglucagonism induced by glucocorticoid treatment in man. N Engl J Med. 1973; 288:128.

112. Perley M et al: Effects of glucocorticoids on plasma insulin. N Engl J Med. 1966; 274:1235.

113. Walton J et al: Alternate day vs shorter interval steroid administration. Arch Intern Med. 1970; 126:601.

114. Pierce LE et al: Hyperglycemic coma associated with corticosteroid therapy. NY State J Med. 1969; 69:1785.

115. Miller SE et al: Clinical features of the diabetic syndrome appearing after steroid therapy. Postgrad Med J. 1964; 40:660.

116. Debosa RC et al: Insulin hypersensitivity and physiologic insulin antagonists. Physiol Review. 1958; 38:389.

117. Perley M et al: Plasma insulin responses to glucose and tolbutamide of normal weight and obese diabetic subject. Diabetes. 1966; 15:867.

118. Siegel RR et al: Reduction of toxicity of corticosteroid therapy after renal transplantation. Am J Med. 1972; 53:159.

119. Liddle GW: Effect of the anti-inflammatory steroids on electrolyte metabolism. Ann NY Acad Sci. 1959; 82:854.

120. Mendalson LM et al: Anaphylaxis-like reactions to corticosteroid therapy. J Allergy and Clin Immunol. 1974; 54/3:125.

121. O'Garra JA: Anaphylactoid reactions to hydrocortisone injections. Br Med J. 1962; 1:615.

122. King RA: A severe anaphylactoid reaction to hydrocortisone. Lancet. 1968; 2:1093.

123. Levy G et al: Studies on inactive prednisone tablets USP XVI. Am J Hosp Pharm. 1964; 21:402.

124. Tanner AR et al: Concurrent administration of antacids and prednisone. Effect on serum levels of prednisone. Br J Clin Pharmacol. 1979; 7:397.

125. Ayers JW et al: A clinically significant adverse drug interaction: Prednisone and aminophylline. APHA Acad Pharm Sci. (Abstr) 1978; 8:133.

126. Glasser GH: Psychotic reactions induced by corticotrophin (ACTH) and cortisone. Psychosomatic Medicine. 1953; 15:280.

127. Kimball CP: Psychological dependency on steroids. Ann Intern Med. 1971; 75:111.

128. Buffington GA et al: Interaction of rifampin and glucocorticoids. Adverse effect on renal allograft function. JAMA. 1976; 236:1958.

129. Stjernhol MR and Katz FH: Effects of diphenylhydantoin, phenobarbital and diazepam on the metabolism of methylprednisolone and its sodium succinate. J Clin Endocrinol Metab. 1975; 41:887.

130. Brooks SM et al: The effects of ephedrine and theophylline on dexamethasone metabolism in bronchial asthma. J Clin Pharmacol. 1977; 17:308.

131. Spangler AS et al: Enhancement of the antiinflammatory action of hydrocortisone by estrogen. J Clin Endocrinol. 1969; 29:650.

132. Merry J et al: Plasma hydrocortisone response to ethanol in chronic alcoholics. Lancet. 1969; 1:921.

133. Merry J et al: The effect of alcohol, barbiturate, and diazepam on hypothalamic/pituitary/adrenal function in chronic alcoholics. Lancet. 1972; 2:990.

134. Besser GM et al: Influence of amphetamines on plasma corticosteroid and growth hormone levels in man. Br Med J. 1969; 4:528.

135. Gollan JL et al: The effect of carbenozolone sodium on the plasma 11-hydroxycorticoid levels in chronic gastric ulceration. Aust NZ J Med. 1975; 5:231.

136. Kendall JW et al: Flurometric determination of corticosteroids: An interfering substance in impure dichloromethane which fluoresces with benzyl alcohol preservative in heparin. J Clin Endocrinol. 1968; 28:1373.

137. Tucci JR et al: Vasopressin in the evaluation of pituitary adrenal function. Ann Intern Med. 1968; 69:191.

138. Nakai Y et al: Adrenergic control mechanism for ACTH secretion in man. Acta Endocrinol. 1973; 74:263.

139. Kershbaum A et al: Effect of smoking and nicotine on adrenocortical secretion. JAMA. 1968; 203:275.

140. Chunk D-K et al: Reversible cardiac enlargement during treatment with amphotericin B and hydrocortisone. Report of 3 cases. Am Rev Resp Dis. 1971; 103:831.

141. Graham GG et al: Patterns of plasma concentrations and urinary excretion of salicylate in rheumatoid arthritis. Clin Pharmacol Ther. 1977; 22:410.

Chapter 55

Thyroid Diseases

Betty J. Dong

The emphasis of this chapter is on the rational use, clinical application, and risks and benefits of the various pharmacologic agents used in the treatment of hypo- and hyperthyroidism. The reader is referred to standard medical textbooks for more detailed diagnostic information.

HORMONE SYNTHESIS AND REGULATION

Triiodothyronine (T_3) and *thyroxine (T_4)* are the two biologically active thyroid hormones produced by the thyroid gland, and their production is under negative feedback control by the pituitary and hypothalamus. Thyroid stimulating hormone (TSH), which is released from the pituitary in response to low circulating levels of thyroid hormone, promotes hormone synthesis and release by increasing glandular activity. When sufficient synthesis has occurred, high circulating hormone levels block further production by inhibiting TSH release. As the levels of hormone drop, the hypothalamic-pituitary centers again become responsive by releasing TSH (1).

Of the two active thyroid hormones, T_3 is more potent than T_4, but its serum concentration is lower. Formerly, all T_3 was thought to have been produced intrathyroidally, but recent findings indicate that about 80% of the total daily T_3 production results from the peripheral conversion of T_4 to T_3 through monodeiodination of T_4 (2–5). T_4 also has intrinsic biological activity and does not function solely as a prohormone; approximately 35–40% of secreted T_4 is converted to T_3. Certain chronic and acute diseases can modify the rate of conversion of T_4 to T_3 and the serum level of T_3 (5). (See Question 2.)

T_3 and T_4 exist in the circulation in the free (active) and protein-bound (inactive) forms. Nearly 100% of T_4 is bound: 80% to thyroxine binding globulin (TBG), 15% to thyroxine binding prealbumin (TBPA) and 4–5% to albumin while only 0.02% is free (5,6). This affinity for plasma proteins accounts for its slow metabolic degradation and long half-life of 7 days. In contrast, T_3 is considerably less strongly bound to plasma proteins and about 0.2% exists as free hormone. Its lesser protein-binding affinity accounts for its three-fold greater metabolic potency and its shorter half-life of 1.5 days (3,5,6).

THYROID FUNCTION TESTS

The basic tests that should be used in the initial evaluation of thyroid status include the TT_4 by Murphy Pattee, the resin T_3 uptake (RT_3U), and the free thyroxine index (FTI). The protein bound iodine (PBI) has mostly been replaced by more specific tests but is included here for completeness. Further assessment of thyroid status should include a thyroid uptake (RAIU), scan, and antibodies. The plasma thyroid stimulating hormone (TSH) is most useful in confirming the diagnosis of hypothyroidism; the T_3 suppression test, the T_3 by radioimmune assay (T_3-RIA), and the thyrotrophin releasing hormone test (TRH) aid in the diagnosis of T_3 toxicosis and hyperthyroidism.

Adjuncts to the above tests may include use of the photomotogram and cholesterol values.

PBI. The *PBI (Protein Bound Iodine)* is a measure of the iodine content of precipitated plasma protein and provides an indirect estimate of the circulating levels of thyroxine (T_4). Both inorganic compounds, such as SSKI, and organic iodine, such as that in IVP dyes, will falsely elevate the PBI (7–9). Although the PBI is still used as a measure of the iodoproteins in certain thyroid disorders, it has largely been replaced by more specific tests. Likewise, the *BEI (Butanol Extractable Iodine)* and the T_4 *by column (Thyroxine by Column Chromatography)*, which also depend on iodometry, have been superseded by the iodine-independent TT_4 by Murphy Pattee (7).

TT_4. The TT_4 *by Murphy Pattee* utilizes a displacement technique to measure the amount of thyroxine bound to a specific binding protein in the patient's serum. Since the size, shape, and charge of the T_4 molecule rather than iodine content determine the results of this test, the TT_4 is not affected by iodides or organic dyes (7,8). Since thyroxine is 65% iodine by weight, the following conversion can be used to express the results of the TT_4 in terms that correspond to PBI or iodine content:

$$T_4I\ (T_4\ iodine) = TT_4 \times 0.65$$

RT_3U. The *Resin T_3 Uptake (RT_3U)* approximates the binding capacity of TBG (Thyroxine Binding Globulin). Radioactive labeled triiodothyronine (T_3) is added to the patient's serum and given time to equilibrate. Since T_3 has less affinity for TBG than T_4, it will not displace T_4 from the protein and will only bind to available sites. Following equilibration, a resin is added to absorb the unbound T_3. In hyperthyroidism, most binding sites on the TBG are occupied and the RT_3U is high; the converse is true in hypothyroidism. Thus, the RT_3U has a direct relationship to the serum thyroxine and an inverse relationship to the levels of circulating TBG. It is not a very sensitive indicator of thyroid function and should be interpreted in conjunction with the TT_4 (7,8).

FTI. Since all of these tests (PBI, BEI, T_4 by Column, TT_4 by Murphy Pattee, and RT_3U) are indirect measures of protein-bound thyroxine, alterations in the serum concentration of TBG by drugs, by disease states, or through genetic abnormalities of TBG synthesis will influence their results. The *Free Thyroxine Index (FTI)* is of value in correct interpretation of the total T_4 when TBG is abnormal and relates quite favorably with thyroid status as derived from the more accurate measurement of free T_4 concentration by equilibrium dialysis. (7,8)

RAIU. The *RAIU (Radioactive Iodine Uptake)* is a measure of iodine utilization by the gland. A tracer dose of I^{131} is administered, and the radioactivity of the gland is measured at 5 and 24 hours after ingestion. The normal values of this test vary and depend to a large extent on the sufficiency of dietary iodine in various geographical areas (16). Some hyperthyroid patients will have peak uptake values within the first few hours after the tracer dose is administered and the uptake will then fall progressively to lower, even subnormal levels. Therefore, the uptake of the RAI should be measured at 5 and 24 hours after the tracer dose. The RAIU indirectly reflects both the need for iodine and the thyroid function. As a measurement of thyroid activity, the test is said to have a clinical accuracy of 70 to 90% and gives much better results in the hyperthyroid than in the hypothyroid ranges. Any condition which affects the thyroid requirement for iodine will alter the RAI uptake (7). Therefore, iodine deficiency resulting from rigorous diuretic therapy or from iodine deficient diets will cause a falsely increased RAIU due to depletion of total iodide pools. Likewise, dilution of total iodide pools from excessive iodide ingestion (eg, contrast dyes) will result in a falsely low RAIU.

Scan. A *scan* of the gland is performed simultaneously with the I^{131} uptake or after ingestion of 99^m Tc per technetate. The scan allows an estimate of gland size, outlines the radioactivity of the gland, and exposes hypermetabolic (hot) areas and hypometabolic (cold) areas. The possibility of carcinoma must be considered if cold areas are present. Therefore, a scan is of utmost importance in the assessment of thyroid disease (7,8).

TgAb; Anti-M Antibodies. The *antithyroglobulin (TgAb)* and *antimicrosomal (Anti-M) antibodies* to the thyroid gland are detected by radioimmune assay and by the tanned red cell (TRC) agglutination method respectively. The presence of these antibodies indicates an autoimmune process, although it does not determine the nature of the problem. About 95% of patients with Graves' disease and 80% of patients with Hashimoto's thyroiditis will have positive antibodies (17). The presence of positive antibodies alone does not indicate thyroid disease, since 5–10% of asymptomatic individuals, as well as individuals with other nonthyroidal autoimmune disorders, will have positive antibodies (17,18).

Clinically, the anti-M antibodies seem to be more specific than TgAb in assessing disease activity. Although both antibodies are elevated during acute flares of the disease, lower titers of anti-M remain positive during quiescent periods of the disease while antithyroglobulin levels are negative.

TSH. The plasma *TSH (Thyroid Stimulating Hormone)* level is determined by radioimmune assay and is one of the most sensitive tests used in the diagnosis of hypothyroidism (10). It is used to detect early mild or borderline hypothyroidism, where TSH levels may be clearly elevated while thyroxine levels are normal, and to assess adequate T_4 or T_3 replacement therapy for hypothyroidism. It can also be used to distinguish between primary and secondary hypothyroidism. The latter is characterized by undetectable or minimal TSH levels (7). Since TSH has a chemical structure similar to HCG, LH, and FSH, false elevations may be reported in pregnant or postmenopausal women (11).

T_3(RIA). The *T_3 (RIA)* is the measurement of total T_3 (bound and free) by radioimmune assay. Since T_3, like T_4, is protein bound, adjustments in T_3 levels need to be made for proper interpretation of the test when there are alterations in protein binding. The *free T_3 index (FT$_3$I)* corrects for this variation in protein binding and allows a reasonable estimate of free T_3 as measured by equilibrium dialysis (12). The free T_3 index is simply the product of free T_3 by radioimmune assay and resin T_3 uptake $[FT_3I = T_3(RIA) \times RT_3U]$.

The T_3 (RIA) is of value in diagnosis of hyperthyroid states (7,8) and may be decreased by certain disease states.

TRH. The *TRH (Thyrotropin-Releasing Hormone Test)* is a very useful test to measure pituitary TSH responsiveness (7). A test dose of 400 mcg TRH is given as an IV bolus and samples of serum are taken at 0, 15, 30, 60, 90, and 120 minutes for determination of TSH. In euthyroid patients, a prompt increase in TSH is observed, with peak levels in 20–30 minutes. In hypothalamic hypothyroidism, the pituitary responds sluggishly to exogenous TRH and produces a slow but continuous rise in TSH. In patients with pri-

Table 1.

COMMON THYROID FUNCTION TESTS

Test	Measure	Normals (for UC Laboratories)	Comments
PBI	Iodine of precipitated proteins—approximates thyroxine iodine.	4.0–8.0 mcg/dl	Organic and inorganic iodides cause false elevation. Influenced by alterations of protein or protein binding.
BEI	Iodine of precipitated proteins—butanol extraction	3.5–7.5 mcg/dl	No interference with inorganic iodides. Organic iodides will cause false elevation. Influenced by alterations of protein or protein binding.
T$_4$I (by column)	Thyroxine iodine of precipitated proteins, utilizing anion exchange resin and column chromatography.	3.0–7.5 mcg/dl	Inorganic and many organic iodides do not interfere. May see false elevation with some radiocontrast dyes. Influenced by alterations of protein binding.
TT$_4$ by Murphy Pattee	Displacement of thyroxine by competitive protein binding. Measured as total thyroxine.	5.0–12 mcg/dl	Specific for thyroxine. No interference by iodides. Influenced by alterations of protein or protein binding.
RT$_3$U	Labeled T$_3$ remaining on resin after saturation of binding sites. Indirect measure of binding sites.	25–35%	Influenced by alterations in protein or protein binding sites.
FTI	The product of the TT$_4$ × RT$_3$U gives the free thyroxine serum level as if measured by dialysis.	1.3–4.2	Compensates for alterations in protein binding.
RAIU	Radioactivity of the thyroid after a trace dose of I^{131}.	1 hr = 0–5% 5 hr = 5–15% 24 hr = 15–35%	Lowered by dietary or medicinal iodide intake.
TSH	TSH by radioimmune assay.	Less than 10 μIU/ml	Most sensitive index of hypothyroidism. FSH, LH and HCG may cause false elevations.
T$_3$ by RIA (radioimmune assay)	T$_3$ levels. Directly related to TBG concentrations.	100–180 ng/dl	Also influenced by alterations in protein binding.
TGAB	Antibodies to thyroglobulin by radioimmune assay.	0–8%	Elevated in Graves' and Hashimoto's; may be undetectable with remission.
Antimicrosomal by TRC	Antibodies to microsomal antigen by tanned red cell technique.	Titers 1:00	More sensitive of the two antibody techniques. Titers will be detectable even after remission.
T$_3$ Suppression Test	Measures hypothalamic-pituitary-thyroid negative feedback axis.	Suppression of RAI to 50% of baseline RAIU after T$_3$ therapy.	Lack of suppression is seen in Graves' disease and indicates autonomous functioning of the gland.

mary hypothyroidism, the basal levels of TSH are elevated and the pituitary is hyper-responsive; TSH levels often reach 100–200 μIU/ml 30 minutes after TRH administration. In hypothyroid patients with hypopituitarism, no response of TSH to TRH would be expected (10). Thus, the TRH test not only differentiates primary from secondary hypothyroidism; it also differentiates hypopituitary from hypothalamic hypothyroidism. Hyperthyroid patients do not respond to TRH, or else they show only a blunted response. Patients receiving adequate T₄ replacement treatment, chronic cortisone, or L-dopa treatment may have a blunted response to the TRH test (13–15).

Origin of Deficiency	Basal TSH Level	TSH Levels After TRH Stimulation
Thyroid	High	Exaggerated
Pituitary	Low	No Response
Hypothalamic	High	Sluggish Response
Hyperthyroid	Suppressed	No Response/Blunted

T₃ Suppression Test. The *T₃ suppression test* (7) is used to determine whether the thyroid gland is functioning under normal TSH-dependent negative feedback mechanisms or whether the gland is functioning autonomously (independent of TSH) as with Graves' disease. The administration of a 5 to 7 day course of triiodothyronine (T₃) 75–100 mcg daily will suppress TSH secretion (decrease RAIU) of a gland operating under normal feedback control, while an autonomously functioning gland will not be suppressed. Therefore, by comparing the RAIU before and after T₃ administration it is possible to determine whether the gland is TSH-dependent or autonomous. A fall from the baseline RAIU to 50% or less is indicative of suppression.

Cholesterol. *Cholesterol levels* may be used as an adjunct to confirm thyroid dysfunction but are not diagnostic in themselves. In hypothyroidism, the cholesterol level is elevated since its rate of degradation is decreased in relation to its synthesis (7,8). Conversely, cholesterol levels may be decreased in hyperthyroidism. However, many extrathyroidal factors influence the plasma cholesterol, so that this test is not an accurate reflection of thyroid status.

Photomotogram. A *photomotogram* is a device with an electric eye that measures the speed of the ankle jerk. The time from the beginning of the hammer tap to half relaxation is measured by interruption of a light beam which is directed on a photocell. Normal values are 250 to 350 mil-

liseconds; lower values are seen in hyperthyroidism and higher values in hypothyroidism. This test is not diagnostic in itself but is useful in the confirmation of a diagnosis (8).

1. **R.K. is a 42-year-old obese female who was admitted to the hospital because of increasing fatigue, sluggishness, shortness of breath, and pitting edema of the legs over the past three weeks. Bilateral pleural effusions on chest x-ray documented worsening of her congestive heart failure (CHF). Her other medical problems included cirrhosis of the liver, diabetes, and chronic bronchitis for which she takes tolbutamide and Lugol's solution three times a day.**

Pertinent physical findings included a palpable thyroid, bibasilar rales, an enlarged heart and liver, 4+ pitting edema, and normal deep tendon reflexes. The diagnosis of worsening CHF secondary to hypothyroidism was entertained based on the following laboratory findings:

PBI 13 mcg/dl; Cholesterol 385 mg/dl; Photomotogram 300 millisec; RAIU 24hr = 13%; SCAN: Normal sized gland with homogenous uptake; TT₄ 1.4 mcg/dl; RT₃U 35%; T₃ (RIA) 22 ng/dl; TSH 4 μIU/ml; FTI 0.5; Anti-M = negative; TgAb 3%; TRH test results:

$$
\begin{aligned}
0 \text{ min} &= 4 \text{ μIU/ml} \\
15 \text{ min} &= 13 \text{ μIU/ml} \\
30 \text{ min} &= 18 \text{ μIU/ml} \\
60 \text{ min} &= 14 \text{ μIU/ml} \\
120 \text{ min} &= 5 \text{ μIU/ml}
\end{aligned}
$$

Evaluate and explain R.K.'s thyroid status based on her clinical and laboratory findings.

Although low output failure can be a presenting sign of hypothyroidism, the normal TSH and TRH stimulation test definitely establish euthyroidism despite the confusing results of her other thyroid function tests. The elevated PBI and depressed RAIU are consistent with her history of iodide ingestion and dilution of total iodide pools. The low TT₄, T₃ (RIA), and FTI may be explained by her cirrhosis and co-existing medical problems (see Question 2). The absence of thyroid antibodies, the normal scan, and the presence of normal deep tendon reflexes as measured by the photomotogram further substantiate the diagnosis of euthyroidism. In this case, the elevated cholesterol level is not the result of hypothyroidism.

2. Explain the results of the TT_4, FTI, and T_3 (RIA) seen in R.K.

R.K.'s thyroid function results are consistent with the euthyroid sick syndrome. Abnormal thyroid function values have been widely described in euthyroid patients with a wide variety of systemic diseases, including acute and chronic starvation, acute infections, and chronic cardiac, pulmonary, renal, hepatic, and neoplastic diseases (5,19,20–26). This euthyroid sick syndrome occurs in 37 to 70% of hospitalized inpatients (20) and requires appropriate recognition to eliminate unnecessary and dangerous hormone intervention. The changes consist of normal or low total T_4, a normal or low calculated FTI, although measured free T_4 is actually normal or high, a normal or borderline high TSH, a normal or low free T_3 and total T_3 (approximately 15–20 ng/100 ml), and a high reverse $T_3(rT_3)$. Normal TSH and TRH tests are paramount in establishing the existence of the euthyroid sick syndrome. These changes have been attributed to complex abnormalities in hypothalamic-pituitary-thyroid relationships and to an alteration in extra-thyroidal metabolism of T_4 whereby its hepatic conversion to active T_3 is reduced while that to inactive reverse T_3 is increased (19). The high concentration of measured free T_4 found in these patients may be a compensatory response to the decreased peripheral conversion of T_4 to T_3 and may be responsible for maintaining their euthyroid state.

No thyroid hormone treatment is indicated in patients like R.K. The abnormal laboratory findings reverse with correction of the nonthyroidal illness.

3. A 45-year-old male complains of fatigue, dry skin, and constipation. His other medical problems include alcoholism for 10 years, cirrhosis, grand mal seizures treated with phenytoin 300 mg daily and phenobarbital 30 mg tid, and rheumatoid arthritis for which he takes aspirin 5 gr, 20 tablets daily. The results of his thyroid function tests were: TT_4 4.2 mcg/dl; RT_3U 40%; and TSH 6 μIU/ml. How should these laboratory findings be interpreted?

He is not hypothyroid as evidenced by the normal TSH level. A number of factors could account for the decreased TT_4 and increased RT_3U. Phenytoin can displace T_4 from its binding sites, causing spuriously low values for TT_4 and high values

for RT_3U (27,28). Anti-inflammatory doses of salicylates can displace thyroxine from both TBG and TBPA, causing lowered values for TT_4 and no change in or increased RT_3U values (27,29). Furthermore, this patient may have decreased TBG production because of his cirrhosis. Other factors which have been reported to lower TT_4 and increase RT_3U by decreasing TBG and TBPA are stress, severe infections, and a hereditary decrease in TBG.

Thus, this patient is taking several drugs which can displace thyroxine from its plasma protein binding sites, and he may have decreased plasma proteins available for binding because of his liver disease. In order to correct for these alterations in protein binding, the FTI (Free Thyroxine Index) should be calculated as described previously. FTI = 4.2 × .40 = 1.68. Therefore, R.C. is euthyroid.

4. A 23-year-old sexually active female who is taking birth control pills comes to clinic for evaluation of extreme nervousness, diaphoresis, and scanty menstrual periods. Although she appears healthy, the possibility of hyperthyroidism is entertained on the basis of a TT_4 of 14 mcg/dl and an RT_3U of 23%. Based upon this information, what would be a reasonable assessment of this patient's thyroid status?

She is not hyperthyroid as evidenced by calculation of a normal FTI. The elevated TT_4 and the depressed RT_3U are consistent with the increased TBG levels observed in pregnancy and oral contraceptive users (30). Since TBG and therefore bound T_4 levels are increased by estrogens, values for PBI, T_4 by column and BEI will be elevated. Conversely, since there is an absolute increase in the amount of protein, the RT_3U will be decreased. However, thyroid function tests should return to normal 2–4 weeks after discontinuation of oral contraceptives, although some investigators report 2–4 months may be required (30). Progesterone-only oral contraceptives do not appear to affect protein binding; consequently they do not alter thyroid function tests.

5. A 45-year-old teacher presents with symptoms suggestive of hypothyroidism along with complaints of a headache. A diagnosis of hypothyroidism is confirmed by low TT_4, RT_3U, and FTI values. Skull x-rays reveal an

enlarged sella turcica and the possibility of secondary hypothyroidism is entertained. What laboratory tests help to differentiate primary from secondary hypothyroidism?

Primary hypothyroidism results from a disturbance within the thyroid gland; secondary hypothyroidism is caused by pituitary or hypothalamic disturbances. TSH levels are elevated in primary hypothyroidism, and minimal or undetectable TSH levels are present in secondary hypothyroidism.

With the availability of the TSH level, there is little justification for the TSH stimulation test which has also been used to differentiate primary from secondary hypothyroidism. In primary hypothyroidism, exogenous TSH will cause a rise in thyroid activity. The response is measured by comparing the RAI uptake before and after the administration of 10 IU of bovine TSH (Thytropar). In primary hypothyroidism there is no rise

in RAI uptake; in secondary hypothyroidism RAI increases by 10% (7).

HYPOTHYROIDISM

The signs and symptoms of hypothyroidism are summarized in Table 2. Since thyroid hormone is essential for function and maintenance of all body systems, symptoms attributed to slowing down of all normal body processes and mental faculties would be expected. The causes of hypothyroidism are listed in Table 3.'

Hashimoto's thyroiditis, an autoimmune disorder, is the most common cause of hypothyroidism other than iatrogenic destruction of the gland (32). It is associated with an underlying defect or block in intrathyroidal organo-binding of iodide so that inactive or insufficient amounts of active hormones are made, producing hypothyroidism.

Table 2.

SIGNS AND SYMPTOMS OF HYPER- AND HYPOTHYROIDISM

Body Systems	Hypothyroidism	Hyperthyroidism
General	Cold intolerance, hoarseness, weight gain despite decreased appetite, and sweating	Heat intolerance, weight loss with increased appetite, increased sweating
Eyes	Edematous eyelids, ptosis	Prominence of the eyes, puffiness of lids, lid lag, lid retraction, pain, irritation, loss of visual acuity
Neck	Goiter in primary hypothyroidism, none in pituitary or hypothalamic disorder	Goiter
Respiratory	Dyspnea, CO_2 retention	Dyspnea
Cardiac	Cardiac enlargement, poor heart sounds, precordial pain, low-output failure	Palpitations, high output failure, angina-like pains, atrial fibrillation
Gastrointestinal	Constipation	Diarrhea; increased frequency of bowel movements
Genitourinary	Menorrhagia, dysmenorrhea	Polyuria, decrease in menstrual flow, amenorrhea
Neuromuscular	Muscle weakness, muscle pain, joint pain, paresthesias, delayed DTR's	Fatigue, weakness, tremors, rapid DTR's
Emotional	Emotional instability, depression, lethargy	Nervousness, irritability, insomnia, emotional lability
Dermatological	Pale facies with yellowish tint; large tongue; dry, brittle, sparse hair, especially on the eyebrows; cool and dry skin, brittle nails	Thinning of hair, fine texture; hot, moist skin; flushing; onycholyis of the nails; pretibial myxedema

Table 3.

CLASSIFICATION OF HYPOTHYROIDISM

I. Nongoitrous (no gland enlargement)

 A. Primary hypothyroidism (dysfunction of the gland)
  1. Idiopathic atrophy
  2. Iatrogenic destruction of the thyroid
   a) Surgery
   b) Radioactive iodine therapy
   c) X-ray therapy
  3. Post-inflammatory thyroiditis
  4. Cretinism (congenital hypothyroidism)

 B. Secondary hypothyroidism: Deficiency of TSH due to pituitary dysfunction

 C. Tertiary hypothyroidism: Deficiency of TRH due to hypothalamic dysfunction

II. Goitrous hypothyroidism (enlargement of the thyroid gland)

 A. Dyshormonogenesis: Defect in hormone synthesis, transport or action
 B. Hashimoto's thyroiditis
 C. Drug-induced: Iodides, lithium, thiocyanates, phenylbutazone, sulfonylureas
 D. Congenital cretinism: Maternally-induced
 E. Iodide deficiency
 F. Natural goitrogens: Rutabagas, turnips, cabbage

Hashimoto's thyroiditis may be related to *Graves' disease,* a frequent cause of hyperthyroidism. Both diseases share some common clinical features: positive antibody titers, lymphocytic infiltration causing an enlarged thyroid gland (goiter), a familial tendency, and a predilection for women. In fact, both diseases may coexist in the same gland, and thyrotoxicosis can precede the onset of Hashimoto's thyroiditis, suggesting that Graves' disease and Hashimoto's thyroiditis may be the same disease manifesting in differing ways (17,32).

6. *Hypothyroidism.* M.W. is a 23-year-old music student who thinks that her neck has become increasingly "fatter" over the past three to four months. She describes herself as gaining weight (70 kg), feeling mentally sluggish, tiring easily, and finds that she is unable to hit the high notes like she used to. On physical examination a puffy facies, yellowish skin, delayed DTR's (deep tendon reflexes), and a firm, enlarged thyroid are noted. Laboratory data included TT_4 4mcg/dl, RT_3U 25%, TSH 20 µIU, TgAb 55%, antimicrosomal by TRC 1:2500, Hct (Hematocrit) 33%, Hgb (Hemoglobin) 12 gm/dl, RBC 3,500/mm³, MCV 104, and a RAIU at 24 hours was 7%. What would be a reasonable assessment of this patient's thyroid status based upon her clinical and laboratory findings?

M.W. presents with many of the clinical features of hypothyroidism as presented in Table 2. These include weight gain, mental sluggishness, easy fatigability, lowering of the voice pitch, a puffy facies, a yellowish tint of the skin, delayed DTR's, and an enlarged thyroid. The diagnosis of hypothyroidism is substantiated by her laboratory findings of a borderline low TT_4 and RT_3U, a low FTI, an elevated TSH value, positive antibodies, and a low radioactive iodine uptake (17,31).

The presence of a firm goiter and thyroid antibodies, as well as clinical symptoms of hypothyroidism, strongly suggest Hashimoto's thyroiditis. She has no history of prior antithyroid drug usage, surgery, or radioactive iodine treatment, which are the most common forms of iatrogenic hypothyroidism.

M.W. also appears to have a macrocytic anemia. Anemia can be expected in hypothyroidism because thyroid hormones stimulate erythropoiesis. Three major types of anemia (33) have been observed in hypothyroidism: a) A mild normochromic normocytic anemia is found in 25% of hypothyroid patients. It is unresponsive to iron therapy but is easily reversed by thyroid administration. b) Hypochromic microcytic anemia appears in 4 to 15% of hypothyroid patients. Contributing factors may include achlorhydria and menorrhagia. This anemia will respond to iron therapy without correction of the hypothyroidism. c) A macrocytic anemia, as observed in this patient, may also appear in hypothyroidism. Folate deficiency (34) and pernicious anemia have been implicated (17,33); treatment with folate and B-12, respectively, corrects the anemia.

7. *Treatment with Thyroid Hormone.* What thyroid preparation should be used to treat M.W.'s hypothyroidism? Are there significant differences, advantages, or disadvantages among the various generic and brand formulations of thyroid hormones?

The principal objective of thyroid hormone therapy is attainment and maintenance of a euthyroid state. Any of the commercially available preparations can accomplish these goals, although there may be significant bioequivalence differences between brand and generic preparations. These thyroid preparations can be classified as either synthetic (levothyroxine, L-triiodothyronine, liotrix) or naturally from animal tissues (desiccated thyroid, thyroglobulin) (1,35).

Desiccated thyroid (USP) is derived from pork thyroid glands, although beef and sheep are also used. The USP requires only that desiccated thyroid contain between 0.17% and 0.23% organic iodine by weight. These requirements do not seem stringent enough because potency may vary with changes in the proportion of the two active hormones (T_3 and T_4) or with changes in the amount of organic iodine present. This variable potency seems to be particularly true of generic formulations as compared to the biologically standardized Armour brand of desiccated thyroid (36,37). Inactive desiccated thyroid preparations which contain small amounts of T_3 and T_4 or even iodinated casein instead of hormone have been identified (37–39). Likewise, preparations of greater than expected activity resulting from abnormally high content of T_3 have caused thyrotoxicosis (40,41). Prolonged storage of desiccated thyroid preparations may result in loss of potency, but it probably is not as important as once thought (37). In addition to its variable potency,

Table 4.

THYROID PREPARATIONS

Drug/Dosage Forms	Composition	Grain Equivalent	Comments
Thyroid USP (Armour) (TAB ¼ gr, ½ gr, 1 gr, 1½ gr, 2 gr, 3 gr, 4 gr, 5 gr	Desiccated hog, beef, or sheep thyroid gland. Standardized by iodine content.	1 grain[1]	Unpredictable T_4:T_3 ratio; unstable, deteriorates upon prolonged storage. Produces abnormal laboratory function tests. Generic brands may not be bioequivalent. Armour brand preferred.
Thyroglobulin (Proloid) TAB, ½ gr, 1 gr, 1½ gr, 2 gr, 3 gr	Thyroglobulin extract. Standardized biologically to give a T_4:T_3 ratio of 2.5:1.	1 grain	No advantage over thyroid extract but more expensive.
L-thyroxine (Levothroid, Synthroid) TAB 0.025 mg, 0.050 mg, 0.1 mg, 0.15 mg, 0.175 mg, 0.2 mg, 0.3 mg, INJ 500 mcg	Synthetic T_4	100 mcg[1]	Stable, predictable potency but variable absorption. May be more potent than desiccated thyroid because of its stability. When changing from greater than 2 gr desiccated thyroid to synthetic T_4, may want to lower the T_4 dose by ½ grain to avoid toxicity. Generic may not be bioequivalent.
L-triiodothyronine (Cytomel) TAB 5 mcg, 25 mcg	Synthetic T_3	25 mcg	Need to use TSH levels to monitor therapeutic response. Requires multiple daily dosing schedule. Complete absorption.
Liotrix (Euthroid) (Thyrolar) TAB −½, −1, −2, −3	T_4:T_3 in 4:1 ratio 60 mcg T_4:15 mcg T_3 50 mcg T_4:12.5 mcg T_3	Euthyroid-1 Thyrolar-1	No real need for liotrix since T_4 is converted to T_3 peripherally. Expensive, stable, and predictable content. Euthroid is 20% more potent than Thyrolar. This should be considered when changing from one preparation to the other.

[1]60 mg (1 gr) of desiccated thyroid was equal to 60 mcg of T_4 (42).

allergic reactions to the animal protein may occur. The only apparent advantage of desiccated thyroid appears to be its low cost. Desiccated thyroid should not be considered the drug of choice for replacement therapy (41). Patients already maintained on desiccated thyroid products may consider switching to L-thyroxine (T_4) or using the Armour brand of desiccated thyroid. When changing therapy from desiccated thyroid to T_4, it should be remembered that 60 mg (1 gr) of desiccated thyroid may not be equal in potency to 100 mcg of T_4 (42).

Thyroglobulin (Proloid) is a purified extract of hog gland standardized biologically to give a T_4:T_3 ratio of 2.5:1. It has no advantages over desiccated thyroid and is more expensive.

The synthetic thyroid preparations differ from one another in their relative potency, onset of action, and biological half-life. *L-thyroxine (Synthroid, Letter), or T_4,* is one of the most commonly used thyroid preparations. Its advantages include stability, uniform potency, relatively low cost, and lack of allergenic foreign protein. The long half-life of five to seven days makes once-a-day dosing possible and allows the creation of special convenience schedules such as omission of medication on weekends. Although most patients absorb 60 to 65%, absorption may vary considerably (43). Various generic preparations of L-thyroxine may not be bioequivalent (37,44–46) to brand products (47,48) and have resulted in inadequate replacement therapy. Until such time that levothyroxine products become more uniform, generic substitution for brand products should not be encouraged. Therapy can be easily monitored by use of TT_4 and RT_3U.

L-triiodothyronine (Cytomel), or T_3, has a relatively short half-life of 1.5 days, and multiple daily dosing is needed to insure a uniform response. Other disadvantages include a higher incidence of cardiac effects, difficulty in monitoring therapeutic/toxic effects with conventional TT_4/RT_3U laboratory tests, and its high cost. For these reasons, L-triiodothyronine is not recommended for routine thyroid hormone replacement. It is widely used as a diagnostic agent in the T_3 suppression test and in patients in whom short-term TSH suppression is necessary. Therapy should be monitored by TSH and T_3 (RIA).

Liotrix (Euthroid, Thyrolar) is a combination of synthetic T_4 and T_3 in a ratio of 4:1. It is stable and has predictable potency but is relatively more expensive than the other thyroid preparations. It is important to note that Euthroid is 20% more potent than Thyrolar when corresponding grain equivalents are compared. This preparation was once recommended as the drug of choice for thyroid replacement because it approximates the normal secretion of the human thyroid gland. However, since a significant amount of T_4 (30–40%) is converted peripherally to T_3 there is no rationale or need for such an expensive preparation (2–5,35).

8. *Thyroxine Therapy.* What would be an appropriate starting and maintenance dose of thyroxine for M.W.? When and how should her therapy be monitored?

Dosage. Many textbooks formerly recommended thyroxine replacement doses of 200 to 300 mcg per day because the thyroid gland normally secretes 100 to 300 mcg per day. Also, it had been suggested that TT_4 laboratory values be maintained in the high upper limits of normal to make up for lack of T_3 administration. It is now known that T_4 is converted peripherally to T_3 (2–5), and that 89% of hypothyroid patients are euthyroid on 100–200 mcg per day of thyroxine (49). A dose of 200 mcg or less per day normalizes TSH levels (50) and doses of 300 mcg per day may be excessive and result in hyperthyroidism (51). These lower replacement doses correlate well with body weight (approx. 2.25 mcg/kg) (49), although elderly patients may require less than their younger counterparts. In the elderly, the smaller requirements (approx. 2.0 mcg/kg) may reflect the progressive decrease in thyroxine degradation rate that occurs with age (271).

In the absence of risk factors necessitating small dose increments (old age, cardiac disease, and long duration of hypothyroidism), M.W. can be started with the full replacement dose of thyroxine (1,35). This 70 kg patient should be treated with 0.15 mg of thyroxine daily (70 kg × 2.25 mcg/kg = .157 mg) and monitored both for toxicity and therapeutic response. An alternate and more conservative dosing schedule would be to initiate 0.1 mg daily of T_4 for one or two weeks and then to increase the dose if there is no evidence of toxicity (hyperthyroidism). Small incremental increases in doses can be achieved when needed by varying the dosing schedule (eg, take 0.15 mg every day except weekends).

Monitoring. TT_4, RT_3U, and FTI should be obtained about six weeks after the initiation of therapy because T_4 has a half-life of seven days, and three or four half-lives are needed to reach steady state. Patients with hypothyroidism of greater than one year's duration may need six months or longer to achieve steady state levels after initiation of T_4 therapy. In addition, T_4 concentrations obtained at six weeks may be transiently elevated due to a decrease in the metabolic clearance caused by the hypometabolic state of hypothyroidism (52). These laboratory data, in combination with her subjective and objective symptoms provide appropriate monitoring parameters. TSH levels may also be monitored and should be normal in 10 to 14 days (50).

With the correct dose, reversal of symptoms should occur within one to two weeks. Some symptoms such as anemia and hair and skin changes may take several weeks to be corrected (17).

9. *Triiodothyronine Therapy.* A 45-year-old school teacher complains of fatigue and vague muscular aches and pains which she attributes to insufficient thyroid medication. On physical examination the gland was palpable but not enlarged, and deep tendon reflexes were 2+ and brisk. Her dose of triiodothyronine (Cytomel) was increased to 25 mcg three times per day about 2 weeks ago based upon the results of a recent TT_4 which was 1.4 mg/dl. She denies taking any other medications. Why might this dose of T_3 be inappropriate for her?

This low TT_4 value does not provide adequate justification for increasing the dose of this patient's medication. Since she is receiving T_3, the TT_4, which is a measure of bound T_4, will always be low and will never reach normal levels. In fact, her vague complaints may be related to hyperthyroidism since she is receiving the equivalent of 0.3 mg of thyroxine (T_4) daily. Either TSH or $T_3(RIA)$ is more appropriate in monitoring patients receiving T_3 therapy. A $T_3(RIA)$ should be obtained to rule out hyperthyroidism in this patient. Furthermore, her medication should be changed to thyroxine 0.15 mg per day to facilitate monitoring and to simplify her dosing regimen. This empirical dose can then be adjusted as needed.

10. *Parenteral Dosing.* A 70-year-old male with long-standing hypothyroidism has been receiving L-thyroxine 0.2 mg daily. He is currently in the hospital with a stroke, and paralysis has left him unable to swallow oral medications. What would be a reasonable method of administering thyroid hormone to this man?

L-thyroxine has a long serum half-life of 5 to 7 days, and thyroxine administration can be delayed for up to a week if this patient is able to take oral medications at that time (53). However, if parenteral administration is required, L-thyroxine is available as an IM or IV injection. The IV route is preferred because intramuscular absorption may be slow and unpredictable, particularly in the presence of compromised circulation. One should be aware that oral absorption of T_4 is incomplete (usually 60 to 65%) and can vary from 30 to 90% (43), and that parenteral doses should be adjusted as a result.

11. *Pregnancy.* P.K. is a 35-year-old female who receives L-thyroxine 0.15 mg daily for Hashimoto's thyroiditis. Laboratory assessments of her thyroid status show a TT_4 of 5 mcg/dl and a RT_3U of 25%. She is 6 weeks pregnant. What dosing adjustments will be required because of her pregnancy?

Whether the added demands and stress of pregnancy require an increase in maternal thyroid supplementation is unclear. Theoretically, the increase in thyroid hormone bound to TBG as a result of pregnancy is balanced initially by a decrease in thyroxine elimination so that the amount of free, active T_4 remains the same. When a new steady state is reached, however, the absolute rate of thyroid elimination should remain unchanged (54,55). Therefore, no real adjustment upward in dosing should be required. Clinically, this theory appears to be true. Patients should be maintained on their usual thyroid replacement dose during pregnancy and evaluated closely with TT_4 and FTI every 3 weeks for the first few months. Laboratory values of TT_4 and FTI should be in the upper limits of normal to insure adequate replacement, and dosage should be increased, if needed, to prevent hypothyroidism. TSH levels are not helpful and will be misleading during pregnancy because human chorionic gonadotropin interferes with the assay of TSH.

It is unclear if inadequately treated maternal hypothyroidism poses any risk to the developing fetus; normal children have been born to myxedematous mothers (55,56). On the other hand, abnormal fetal development secondary to poor placental maturation, spontaneous abortions, congenital defects, mental retardation and an increased rate of still births have been associated with maternal hypothyroidism (57–60). Since thyroid hormone does not cross the placenta in significant amounts, maternal hypothyroidism, if it affects the fetus at all, must do so indirectly in ways that have yet to be shown. A small risk of congenital hypothyroidism can result if maternal antibodies from Hashimoto's thyroiditis cross over into the fetal circulation (61–64). The infant's cord blood at birth should be assayed for TSH to insure euthyroidism.

This pregnant patient's low TT_4 and RT_3U are of concern. The TT_4 should be much higher and the RT_3U lower due to pregnancy-associated increases in TBG. The calculated FTI of 1.25 is also somewhat low. The dose of T_4 should be increased to 0.2 mg after ruling out the possibility of patient noncompliance. The TT_4, RT_3U, and FTI should be repeated in 6 weeks, and the dosage should be adjusted as needed to keep thyroid function tests in the upper limits of normal.

12. *Neonatal Hypothyroidism.* The above patient, P.K., delivered a healthy baby at term without difficulty. The baby's postpartum serum T_4 level was 5 mcg/dl. At home he became lethargic, had a weak cry, sucked poorly, and failed to thrive. What is your assessment of the situation? (Include treatment plan and prognosis.)

The symptoms are suggestive of hypothyroidism. The early clinical findings of congenital hypothyroidism include dry skin, lethargy, poor feeding, hoarse voice, delayed development, constipation, large tongue, neonatal jaundice, and piglike facies. Respiratory difficulties, delayed skeletal maturation, and choking are common findings (65–67).

The postpartum serum concentration of T_4 is low in this patient and should be verified by further diagnostic procedures. Normal T_4 levels postpartum are 6–14 mcg/dl, rising to 10–20 mcg/dl in the next few days and returning to the normal range of 4–10 mcg/dl by two months of age. Values for the FTI are also elevated in normal infants and do not decrease to adult levels before 12 months of age. T_3 levels are less than adult serum concentrations at birth but increase to adult levels within a few days. TSH serum concentrations are useful in documenting hypothyroidism because TSH concentrations should surge on the first day or two of life (68).

An x-ray examination of the knee, revealing a moth-eaten appearance termed epiphyseal dysgenesis is virtually pathognomonic of early hypothyroidism (66). Therefore, an x-ray of the knee, several measurements of TT_4, and TSH levels should confirm the diagnosis of congenital hypothyroidism.

If this infant is hypothyroid, his normal development will be determined by the age at which treatment is started, the adequacy with which it is maintained, and the degree of initial athyreosis. The replacement dose of T_4 or T_3 varies according to the age of the infant (65–67) as follows: infants 0–12 months of age require 50–75 mcg of T_4; children 12–24 months of age require 75–125 mcg of T_4; children 2–4 years of age require 100–150 mcg of T_4; and those 4–12 years of age require 100–300 mcg of T_4. Equivalent doses of T_3 can be used (see Table 4). If the infant is extremely sensitive to the effects of thyroid hormone, small initial doses of T_4 can be increased gradually by 12½ mcg every one to two weeks as tolerated until the therapeutic dose is achieved. If vigorous treatment is needed, intravenous 100 mcg doses of T_4 can be given and then followed by daily maintenance doses. One should take care to watch for symptoms of excessive doses of thyroid hormone, such as hyperactivity and irritability. The dosage of thyroid replacement can be monitored by the TSH level, which provides the most reliable index of therapeutic efficacy.

Mental development and physical growth of infants do not seem to be affected if treatment is initiated prior to 3 months of age (67,68). When treatment is delayed until 6 months to one year of age, normal mental development is impaired despite subsequent treatment (69).

13. *Unresponsiveness to Thyroid Hormone.* R.T. is a 45-year-old female who complains of sluggishness and cold intolerance. Her present medical problems include Hashimoto's thyroiditis treated with dessicated thyroid 4 grains daily, hypercholesterolemia treated with cholestyramine 4 gm four times daily, and arteriosclerotic heart disease which has resulted in decreased mental acuity. Her laboratory data include a cholesterol level of 280 mg/dl, a TSH of 15 µU/ml, an FTI of 1.0, and positive antithyroglobulin and antimicrosomal antibodies. She admits that she has increased her dose of thyroid because she feels better on the higher dose. Why is this

patient seemingly unresponsive to thyroid therapy?

This patient's complaints and laboratory values confirm hypothyroidism which has been inadequately treated despite thyroid therapy. Possible causes of therapeutic failure usually include noncompliance, error in diagnosis, poor absorption, inactive preparation, rapid metabolism, and tissue resistance (43,70). The last two factors are extremely rare, and noncompliance and error in diagnosis do not appear to be reasonable explanations in this case. The possibilities of poor absorption and an inactive product should be examined further. Since cholestyramine binds thyroxine and delays its absorption (71), R.T. should be questioned as to the time of administration of her thyroid and cholestyramine; these two medications should be administered at least one hour apart. Evidence for incomplete or malabsorption of the hormone may be obtained by comparing the patient's response to the oral and parenteral thyroxine. Gastrointestinal disorders such as steatorrhea may also interfere with the enterohepatic circulation of orally administered thyroid and lead to excessive fecal loss (72). After instructions regarding the proper spacing of her thyroid medication and cholestyramine, the thyroid medication should be changed to an equivalent dose of L-thyroxine, and therapeutic response should be re-evaluated in one month.

14. *Hypercholesterolemia.* Could R.T.'s hypothyroidism be responsible for her hypercholesterolemia?

Hypercholesterolemia has been associated with hypothyroidism (17). Although the rate of cholesterol synthesis is normal in hypothyroidism, the rate of cholesterol clearance is decreased. Similarly, slow removal of triglycerides may result in hyperlipidemia. Hypercholesterolemia is frequently observed before the appearance of clinical hypothyroidism. Treatment with thyroxine alone should lower the cholesterol levels provided there are no other contributing etiologies. In fact D-thyroxine (Choloxin) has been recommended as an agent for the treatment of hyperlipidemia.

Severe Myxedema

15. *Impending Myxedema Coma.* R.B. is a 65-year-old alcoholic who arrived at the emergency room in acute agitation and complaining of chest pain unrelieved by nitro-

glycerin. His medical problems include alcoholic cardiomyopathy, angina, and hypothyroidism. Although he has been repeatedly advised to take his thyroxine regularly, he continues to take it sporadically. An FTI drawn 4 months ago was 1.0. He was given chlorpromazine 25 mg IM along with morphine sulfate 10 mg IM. After the injection, the nurse noticed increased mental depression, lethargy, and shallow breathing. His oral temperature was 34.5°C, and he exhibited chills and shakes. What is your assessment of this patient's subjective and objective data?

R.B. has several symptoms consistent with impending myxedema coma. Myxedema coma is the end stage of long-standing, uncorrected hypothyroidism. The classic features are hypothermia, delayed deep tendon reflexes, and an altered sensorium which may range from stupor to coma. Other predominant features may include carbon dioxide retention, severe hypoglycemia, hyponatremia, and paranoid psychosis (76). Since myxedema coma frequently occurs in the elderly, it is often difficult to distinguish the signs and symptoms from senility or from other disease states, as in this elderly alcoholic patient.

Precipitating factors include cold weather or hypothermia; stressful situations such as surgery, infection, or trauma; coexisting disease states such as myocardial infarction, diabetes, hypoglycemia, or fluid and electrolyte abnormalities (especially hyponatremia); and medications such as respiratory depressants and diuretics (77). Chlorpromazine and morphine may be responsible for what appears to be impending myxedema coma in this patient. In severely myxedematous patients, respiratory depressants (anesthetics, narcotic analgesics, phenothiazines, sedative-hypnotics) alone or in combination with the hypothermic effects of the phenothiazines can aggravate the pre-existing hypothermia and carbon dioxide retention of hypothyroidism and precipitate myxedema coma (35,73–75). Tranquilizers such as chlorpromazine should not be given; small doses of less depressive sedative-hypnotics such as the benzodiazepines should be used only when absolutely necessary. Myxedematous patients are inherently sensitive to the respiratory depressant effects of narcotic analgesics, especially morphine. A dose as small as 10 mg may induce coma in a hypothyroid patient or cause death in a patient who is already comatose. If morphine is required, the dose should be decreased to ⅓ to ½ the usual analgesic dose and the respiratory rate should be closely monitored (17).

16. What would be a reasonable therapeutic plan for the management of this patient's myxedema coma?

Emergency treatment of myxedema coma is directed toward thyroid replacement, maintenance of vital function and elimination of precipitating factors. Immediate and aggressive therapy with large replacement doses of thyroxine are necessary because myxedema coma is associated with a mortality rate of 60 to 70% (78,79). L-thyroxine 500 mcg IV should be given initially to saturate the TBG (76,78,80). This initial dose can be either increased or decreased depending on the patient's size and presence of restrictive factors. The initial dose in this patient may be adjusted downward to 200 mcg because of his cardiac disease. If the proper therapy has been instituted, consciousness and decreased TSH levels are achieved within 24 hours along with restoration of normal vital signs (80). Maintenance doses should be regulated by the patient's response; however, minimal maintenance doses in the absense of untoward effects should be about 50 mcg of T_4 daily or about 5 mcg of T_3 every six hours (81).

Supportive measures include assisted ventilation, glucose for hypoglycemia, restriction of fluids for hyponatremia, and the use of blood or plasma expanders to prevent circulatory collapse and maintain blood pressure. The use of blankets to treat the hypothermia is not advised since vasodilation will occur and further compromise the cardiovascular components of shock. Although steroids have not been shown to be clearly beneficial in primary myxedema, they may be life saving in patients with hypopituitarism presenting as myxedema coma. Since it is difficult to distinguish between primary and secondary myxedema, the use of hydrocortisone 50 to 100 mg every six hours is recommended (76,81).

Appropriate measures should be taken to relieve his chest pain while the possibility of a myocardial infarction is ruled out. The use of a narcotic antagonist such as naloxone may also be beneficial in this particular instance because it can reverse the effects of the morphine. Naloxone has also been known to be capable of arousing comatose patients in alcoholic intoxication (268).

17. *Hypothyroidism with CHF.* E.B. is a 45-year-old male admitted with complaints of

substernal chest pain with pressure, shortness of breath, dyspnea on exertion, and orthopnea. Other subjective and objective data suggest an assessment of congestive heart failure (CHF) complicated by myocardial infarction. Significant past medical history revealed Graves' disease treated with radioactive iodine (RAI) ablation three years ago without recurrence of symptoms. On physical examination cardiomegaly, obesity, facial edema and puffiness, delayed DTR's, and pretibial edema were noted. Pertinent laboratory findings included a TT_4 of 1.8 mcg/dl; RT_3U of 15%; CPK of 150; SGOT of 80; and an LDH of 250. Chest x-ray revealed cardiomegaly and pleural effusions, and an ECG showed bradycardia and flattened T-waves with ST depression. Diuretics and digitalis were instituted without reversal of the cardiac abnormalities. Why do these clinical findings suggest hypothyroidism?

E.B.'s history of RAI therapy, abnormal thyroid function tests, symptoms, and physical findings confirm the presence of severe hypothyroidism. "Myxedema heart" is often suggestive of low output CHF since the symptoms are similar: cardiomegaly, dyspnea, edema, pleural effusions, and abnormal cardiogram (17). The cardiac damage results from deposition of mucopolysaccharides in the myocardium.

Although E.B.'s enzyme elevations (SGOT, CPK, and LDH) are suggestive of an MI, they may be due to the altered metabolism, and liver and cardiac status may be normal. The enzymes can be fractionated to determine their origin.

18. What might be the effect of thyroid therapy on the cardiac status of this patient?

If E.B.'s cardiac abnormalities are caused by hypothyroidism rather than organic disease, treatment with adequate thyroxine will restore the heart size, reverse the ECG findings, and normalize the serum enzyme elevations within 2 to 4 weeks. Angina may develop or worsen with thyroxine therapy (17,82,82a), so treatment should be carefully instituted. In the absence of organic disease, digitalis is not effective and may even be harmful. Hypothyroid patients have an increased sensitivity to digitalis, and digitalis toxicity is a possibility unless the maintenance dose is decreased (83,84).

19. How aggressively should thyroid hormone therapy be initiated in patient E.B.?

What is the hormone replacement of choice in patients with cardiac disease?

Patients with long-standing hypothyroidism, cardiac disease, or advanced age tend to be extremely sensitive to the cardiac effects of thyroid hormone. Normal therapeutic doses in these individuals may result in severe angina, myocardial infarction, cardiac failure, or tachycardia (17,82).

Treatment should, therefore, be cautiously initiated with minute amounts (0.0125–0.025 mg) of T$_4$ and increased by increments of 0.0125–0.025 mg of T$_4$ or its equivalent every 2 to 4 weeks. The rapidity with which the increments can proceed is determined by how well each increased dose is tolerated. If cardiac toxicity occurs with increased dosage, a longer interval or smaller increments can be employed. In some patients with severe cardiac sensitivity, complete euthyroidism may never be achieved. The correct dose appears to be a compromise between prevention of myxedema and induction of cardiac toxicity (82a).

Triiodothyronine (Cytomel) has been suggested by some to be the agent of choice in patients with cardiac abnormalities. The onset of action of T$_3$ is 1–3 days as compared to 3–5 days for T$_4$. After therapy is withdrawn, the effects of T$_3$ are dissipated in 3–5 days, while 7–10 days are needed for T$_4$. Thus, if toxicity occurs, the effects of T$_3$ will rapidly disappear upon cessation of therapy, an advantage in the cardiac patient. Nevertheless, T$_3$ is not recommended for therapy here since it is biologically more potent and requires finer, more difficult regulation of dosage to insure smooth and uniform blood levels. Furthermore, it appears to cause a higher incidence of cardiac toxicity, especially the aggravation of angina (17,35).

HYPERTHYROIDISM

The signs and symptoms of hyperthyroidism are summarized in Table 2. Although various thyroid abnormalities as listed in Table 5 can cause hyperthyroidism, the most common is Graves' disease.

Thyrotoxicosis and diffuse goiter occurring along with any one or all of the following manifestations: exophthalmopathies, pretibial myxedema, and acropachy comprise the syndrome of Graves' disease. This autoimmune disorder is characterized by positive antibodies, nonsuppres-

sibility and circulating immunoglobulins that have the ability like TSH to stimulate the thyroid gland (85). LATS (long acting thyroid-stimulator), previously thought to be the IgG immunoglobulin responsible for Graves' disease, is found via the McKenzie mouse assay in only 50–70% of patients with active disease and therefore is probably not the causative agent of Graves' (86). Other thyroid stimulators such as TSI (thyroid stimulating immunoglobulin) and TDI (thyroid displacing immunoglobulin), which are specific for human thyroid, have been identified in virtually 100% of patients with Graves (87,88).

20. *Graves' Disease.* S.K. is a 38-year-old female physician who is admitted for a possible myocardial infarction. Her complaints include chest pain unrelieved by nitroglycerin, nervousness, palpitations, muscle weakness, weight loss despite increased appetite, epistaxis, and easy bruisability. Her other medical problems include: deep venous thrombosis treated with warfarin (Coumadin) 5 mg daily—last prothrombin time (PT) was 26 seconds; angina treated with nitroglycerin 0.4 mg; and atrial fibrillation (AF) treated with digoxin 0.375 mg daily. Physical examination of this patient reveals a thin, flushed, hyperkinetic, and nervous female. Blood pressure is 180/90 mm Hg; pulse is 102 beats/min; respiratory rate is 30 breaths/min; temperature is 37.5°C. Other findings include lid lag with stare, minimal proptosis with tearing, decreased visual acuity, a diffusely enlarged thyroid gland without nodules, a bruit

Table 5.

CAUSES OF HYPERTHYROIDISM

Graves' disease (toxic diffuse goiter)

Toxic uninodular goiter (Plummer's disease)

Toxic multinodular goiter

Nodular goiter with hyperthyroidism due to exogenous iodine (Jod-Basedow)

Exogenous thyroid excess through self-administration (Factitious hyperthyroidism)

Tumors (thyroid adenoma, follicular carcinoma, thyrotropin secreting tumor of the pituitary, and hydatiform mole with secretion of a thyroid stimulating substance) in the left lobe of the thyroid, warm moist skin with multiple bruises, tachycardia, slight diarrhea, acropachy, 2+ pitting edema, a fine tremor, proximal muscle weakness, and irregular menses. Laboratory data include TT$_4$ 30 mcg/dl; RT$_3$U 45%; RAIU at 24 hr 80%; PT 40 sec; anti-M 1:6400; TgAb 65%; Scan: Diffusely enlarged gland, 3–4 times normal size. What subjective and objective data are suggestive of hyperthyroidism in this patient?

S.K. presents with many of the clinical and laboratory features associated with an increased metabolic state resulting from excessive thyroxine (see Table 2). Her symptoms include lid lag (lid falls behind movement of the eye and narrow white rim of sclera becomes visible between the upper lid and cornea), a hyperactive gland as evidenced by a bruit, stare, proptosis, palpitations, tachycardia, diarrhea, irregular menses, nervousness, tremor, muscle weakness, weight loss despite increased appetite, increased perspiration, and flushing of the skin (17,85). The symptoms are confirmed by an elevated TT$_4$, RT$_3$U, FTI, RAIU and a goiter on scan.

Her elevated laboratory findings, clinical features, and presence of positive antibodies suggest Graves' disease which is aggravating her cardiac status and other medical problems.

21. Hypoprothrombinemia. Could patient S.K.'s hypoprothrombinemia be related to her thyrotoxicosis? What effect could this have on her subsequent drug treatment?

Warfarin Metabolism. Net circulating levels of vitamin K-dependent clotting factors generally are not altered in hyperthyroid patients because both the synthesis and catabolism of these clotting factors are increased. However, an enhanced anticoagulant response occurs when the warfarin-induced decrease in clotting factor synthesis is combined with the hyperthyroidism-induced increase in clotting factor catabolism (89–91,94). The opposite is true in hypothyroidism, where there is a decrease in both metabolism and synthesis of clotting factors. In hypothyroid patients, the response to oral anticoagulants is delayed due to slower catabolism of clotting factors (92,94,95). Therefore, thyrotoxic patients will need less warfarin, while myxedematous patients will require more warfarin to achieve the same hypoprothrombinemic response. The anticoagulant response to warfarin should be monitored carefully

in patients with thyroid abnormalities and the dose adjusted as the thyroid status changes with therapy.

Thioamide Effects. Treatment of hyperthyroid patients with thioamides, especially propylthiouracil has been associated with hypoprothrombinemia, thrombocytopenia, and bleeding (96–99). These drugs depress the bone marrow as well as clotting factors II, VII, III, IX, X, and XIII, and vitamin K. The effects of these drugs on the clotting factors and vitamin K appear to be due to a subclinical hepatic alteration in the synthesis of the clotting factors (96), although toxic hepatitis has also been reported (100–105) with both PTU and methimazole. The duration of therapy before the onset of symptoms has been two weeks to 18 months. The bleeding is responsive to vitamin K or blood transfusions. Prothrombin times may remain depressed for up to two months after discontinuation of therapy (97).

22. Response to Digoxin. After treatment with radioactive iodine (RAI), patient S.K.'s daily dose of digoxin was increased to 0.5 mg because of persistent atrial fibrillation. After 3 months she returns with complaints of nausea and vomiting; the gland was palpable and considerably decreased in size. The ECG showed ST depression, AV block, and occasional bigeminy. What is the assessment of these subjective and objective data?

The gastrointestinal symptoms of nausea and vomiting, together with the ECG changes of block and bigeminy strongly suggest digitalis toxicity. Continuation of the high dose of digoxin which was required initially during her thyrotoxicosis after apparent resolution of her hyperthyroidism increases the likelihood of digitalis toxicity.

23. Why was such a large dose of digoxin required initially?

The atrial fibrillation (AF) of hyperthyroidism is often resistant to digitalis. A comparison of the response to digitalis in euthyroid patients with AF before and after exogenous T$_3$ administration demonstrated that the daily digoxin requirement of 0.2 mg for a ventricular rate of 70 was increased to 0.8 mg (106). Higher doses of digoxin without side effects are better tolerated by the hyperthyroid individual (106,107).

This apparent resistance of thyrotoxic patients to digitalis has been attributed to changes in intrinsic myocardial function, to an increased volume of distribution (Vd), and to increased glomerular filtration (83,84). Conversely, hypothyroid patients are inordinately sensitive to the effects of digitalis and require smaller doses for a therapeutic response.

Regardless of the mechanism of the altered sensitivity to digitalis, one should be aware that higher than normal doses may be required in thyrotoxicosis, and that the initial dose will need reduction as euthyroidism or hypothyroidism results.

24. T_3-Toxicosis. C.R. is a 27-year-old female with a three-month history of intermittent heat intolerance, sweats, tremor, and severe muscle weakness which has limited her ability to climb stairs. Her appetite has increased remarkably despite weight loss, and she is bothered by the pounding of her heart and some minor difficulty in swallowing. There is a positive family history of thyroid disease and she denies taking any thyroid medications or having had any radiation to her neck. She has previously received iodide drops with improvement in her symptomatology, but exacerbation of her disease occurred despite continued administration of iodides. Her other medical problems include diabetes which is controlled with diet, arthritis which is treated with aspirin 5.4 grams/day, and a history of noncompliance with clinic visits.

Pertinent physical findings include a blood pressure of 180/90 mm Hg, a pulse of 110 beats/minute, hyper-reflexia, lid lag, and a diffusely enlarged thyroid gland which is about four times normal (about 100 grams). Available laboratory data included the following: TT_4 15 mcg/dl, RT_3U 40%, RAIU at 5 hours: 45% and at 24 hours: 85%, Anti-M: 1:3200, TgAb = 25%, and blood glucose 350 mg/dl.

What is a reasonable assessment of these subjective and objective data?

C.R.'s clinical findings verify the presence of an autoimmune hyperthyroid state. However, the serum TT_4, RT_3U, and FTI are only at the upper limits of normal and are out of proportion to the severity of her disease state and her other laboratory findings. The possibility of a variant type of hyperthyroidism known as T_3-toxicosis (108) should be considered. The clinical features include signs and symptoms of thyrotoxicosis, normal or borderline levels of TT_4, FTI, an elevated

RAIU, and elevated T_3 levels through preferential secretion and peripheral conversion of T_4 to T_3. A T_3 (RIA) should be obtained to establish the diagnosis.

Elevation of T_3 levels may precede elevation of T_4 levels and the development of overt hyperthyroidism. It has been suggested that T_3-toxicosis represents a preliminary stage of classical T_4-toxicosis and may be useful for early diagnosis or as an indication of relapse following withdrawal of thioamide therapy (109–111). The decreased TT_4 could also be explained by displacement of T_4 from TBG by aspirin.

25. Iodides. Why were the iodide drops initially effective in improving this patient's symptomatology, but later unable to prevent an exacerbation of her disease?

Iodides inhibit thyroid hormone release, block iodotyrosine and iodothyronine synthesis, and decrease the vascularity of the thyroid gland (112, 115). However, large doses may accentuate hyperthyroidism because of a marked increase in available substrate for hormone synthesis (See Question 52).

The inhibitory effect of iodides on iodotyrosine and iodothyronine organification, known as the Wolff-Chaikoff effect, is similar to that of the thioamides. (112,115–117). The Wolff-Chaikoff effect depends on the establishment of high intrathyroidal concentrations of iodides and is not overcome by TSH stimulation. However, the normal gland can "escape" from this block even with continued iodide use (112,115–117). The gland "escapes" by decreasing iodide transport or by "leaking" iodide (112); both of these mechanism serve to decrease intrathyroidal iodide and thereby decrease the block to organification. Patients who already have high intrathyroidal iodine (i.e., Graves' Disease), patients with underlying defects in organic binding mechanisms (i.e., Hashimoto's), or euthyroid patients previously treated with RAI or surgery for Graves' disease seem to be unduly sensitive to this effect of iodides so that smaller doses can elicit the Wolff-Chaikoff effect resulting in, respectively, amelioration of symptoms or precipitation of hypothyroidism (118–120). "Escape" may also occur (113), as seen with this patient.

The most important effect of iodides is their ability to promptly inhibit thyroid hormone release when doses of 6 mg or more per day are given. The mechanism is unknown, although this effect can be partially overcome by an increase in TSH secretion. Thus the normal gland can escape in 7–14 days because inhibition of thyroid hormone release stimulates reflex increases in TSH secretion. Nevertheless, this early inhibitory effect is responsible for the improvement in symptoms within 2–7 days of initiation of therapy for hyperthyroidism. This rapid onset of effect constitutes the rationale for its use in thyroid storm and as an ameliorative measure while awaiting the onset of the therapeutic effects of thioamide or RAI (17,112).

Large doses of iodides are also used two weeks prior to thyroid surgery to increase the firmness of the thyroid gland by decreasing its size, vascularity, and friability. Not only does iodide facilitate a smoother and less complicated surgery (112), but also the induction of a euthyroid state by iodides decreases postoperative complications.

Stable iodine can be administered orally either as an unpleasant tasting Lugol's solution (5% iodine and 10% potassium iodide), containing 8 mg of iodide per drop, or as the more palatable saturated solution of potassium iodide (SSKI), containing 50 mg of iodide per drop. The minimum effective daily dose is 6 mg, although larger doses (eg, 5 to 10 drops four times a day of SSKI) are frequently administered (121).

The advantages of iodide therapy are that it is simple, inexpensive, relatively nontoxic, and there is no glandular destruction. Disadvantages include "escape," accentuation of thyrotoxicosis, allergic reactions, relapse after discontinuation of treatment, and subsequent interference with RAI if used prior to therapy (122–124).

26. Treatment Modalities for Hyperthyroidism. What are the advantages and disadvantages of the different treatment modalities which may be applicable to the above case?

The three major modalities for the treatment of hyperthyroidism are the thioamides, radioactive iodine (RAI), and surgery (122–124), although iodides and propranolol alone have been advocated. In most cases any of these three modalities may be employed, and it is controversial which is the optimal means of therapy. Often the final decision is empiric, depending on the physician's available resources and the patient's desires.

Thioamides. The thioamides are the preferred treatment for children, pregnant women, and young adults (122). Since thyrotoxicosis is considered a self-limiting disease, the thioamides can control symptoms until spontaneous remission of the disease occurs, without the added risk of hypothyroidism often associated with RAI and surgery. Disadvantages of thioamide therapy include the large number of tablets required, possible drug toxicity, the long duration of treatment, and the low incidence of remission after discontinuation of therapy. This patient's relatively large gland and severe disease make the prognosis for remission somewhat less favorable. A delay in onset of thioamide therapy may be expected if intraglandular stores of thyroid were increased by her prior iodide therapy. Furthermore, her noncompliance and difficulty in swallowing may necessitate another means of treatment.

Surgery. Surgery is considered the treatment of choice when there is suspicion of malignancy, esophageal obstruction with difficulty in swallowing, a large goiter which regresses poorly on RAI or drug therapy, or contraindications to drug (eg, toxicity) or RAI therapy (eg, pregnancy) (125–127). If patient C.R.'s minor difficulty in swallowing persists due to poor regression of goiter size with drug therapy, surgery is a viable alternative. If surgery is contemplated, it is imperative that the patient be brought to surgery in a euthyroid state to prevent rapid postoperative rises in T_4 and subsequent thyroid storm (127,128).

Subtotal thyroid surgery has been successful in 90% of patients, and both subtotal and total thyroidectomies have been advocated (125,127 129). Subtotal thyroidectomy potentially avoids the predictable hypothyroidism of total thyroidectomy; however, the residual thyroid tissue is a potential site for recurrent hyperthyroid disease. Return of thyrotoxicosis after subtotal thyroidectomy should be treated with RAI because the incidence of surgical complications is increased ten-fold with a second surgery (126). Surgical treatment of hyperthyroidism is safe and effective. The disadvantages to the surgical approach are the patient's fear of surgery, expense, hospitalization, and the small risk of postoperative complications.

RAI. RAI is the preferred treatment for debilitated, cardiac, or elderly patients who are poor surgical candidates. It is also preferred for patients who failed to respond to drug therapy or who experienced adverse drug reactions, as well as for those with recurrent hyperthyroidism after surgery (130,130a). The use of RAI is restricted to adults over some arbitrary age, such as 20–35 years old (17) because of fears of inducing genetic damage or neoplasia. However, after more than 25 years of clinical experience with RAI, it is generally accepted that it is a safe and effective treatment modality. There is no reported evidence of genetic damage after ingestion of I^{131}; the dose of radiation to the gonads is less than 3 rads, which is comparable to other radiographic diagnostic tests such as barium enemas (17,124). The incidence of leukemia or malignancy is no higher in recipients of I^{131} than in those receiving medical or surgical treatments of hyperthyroidism (131,132). RAI is painless, effective, economical, and quick, but fear of radiation and the high incidence of hypothyroidism may deter usage. In this young patient, the prior use of iodides probably has diluted total iodide pools, making effective thyroid concentration of radioactive iodine more difficult (124,130).

Thioamide Therapy

27. C.R. is started on treatment with propylthiouracil 200 mg every six hours after obtaining a baseline TT_4 and RT_3U. After one week she complains angrily that her symptoms are worse and the medication is not working. She reluctantly admits missing doses because of difficulty in swallowing, cough, and a sore throat. What is one theoretical advantage of PTU over methimazole in the treatment of hyperthyroidism?

The thioamides act by blocking the organification of thyroid hormone synthesis (133) and perhaps by an immunosuppressive effect on thyroid autoantibody synthesis (135a). Propylthiouracil (PTU), but not methimazole, also blocks the peripheral conversion of thyroxine (T_4) to triiodothyronine (T_3) and this may play a significant role in its therapeutic effectiveness (134). A significantly greater fall in the T_3 concentration and the T_3/T_4 ratio can be demonstrated in hyperthyroid patients treated acutely with PTU and iodide than with methimazole and iodide (135).

28. Was this patient receiving an appropriate dose of PTU?

Initially, high blocking doses of PTU (400 to 800 mg daily, depending on the degree of toxi-

cosis) should be given in four divided doses, as in this patient. Equipotent doses of methimazole, which is ten times more potent than PTU on a milligram per milligram basis, can also be used (133). On rare occasions, doses of 1200 mg daily of PTU or its equivalent may be required in patients with large goiter (four times normal size) or with severe disease. Because of its short half-life, PTU must be dosed every six hours, or every four hours in severe hyperthyroidism; methimazole can be given every eight hours. After the initial period of high-dose therapy the daily dose can be gradually reduced to that which maintains the patient at an euthyroid state, generally 100 to 300 mg PTU daily or its equivalent.

29. What additional objective baseline data should be obtained to monitor both the efficacy and toxicity of PTU?

Prior to the administration of thioamides such as PTU, a baseline TT_4, RT_3U, and white blood cell count (WBC) with differential should be obtained. The thyroid function tests are useful in monitoring the efficacy of therapy and the WBC with differential can detect the development of agranulocytosis. The baseline WBC with differential is helpful because hyperthyroidism per se may be associated with a relative reduction in the neutrophil count. Routine serial determinations of the WBC are not helpful in monitoring the development of agranulocytosis because the onset of symptoms are so abrupt. All patients should be told to report rash, fever, sore throat, or any type of flu-like symptoms which may be signs of agranulocytosis (see Question 36). A repeat TT_4 and RT_3U should be obtained after one month of therapy and again one month after any change in the dosing regimen of thioamides.

30. What would be an optimal period of thioamide treatment for patient C.R.?

Thioamide therapy of one to two years duration has been the usual standard of practice (122,124) despite the lack of good data regarding the optimal treatment period. Short-term therapy (mean 4.7 months, given till the patient is euthyroid) has been advocated as a means to save time, money, and improve compliance without sacrificing therapeutic outcome. One such short-term therapy has been associated with a remission rate of about 39%, which is comparable to that obtained with conventional long-term treatment (136). However, much lower rates of remis-

Table 6.
TREATMENT OF HYPERTHYROIDISM

Modality	Drug	Dose	Mechanism of Action	Toxicity	Indications
THIOAMIDES	Propylthiouracil 50 mg tablets	400–800 mg/d (maximum 1200 mg/d) initially; maintenance of 100–300 mg daily.	Blocks organification of hormone synthesis, Blocks peripheral conversion of T_4 to T_3 (PTU only), immunosuppressive.	Skin rashes, gastrointestinal symptoms, arthralgias, hepatitis, blood dyscrasias, hypoprothrombinemia.	Children, young adults, pregnancy. Contraindication to surgery or RAI therapy.
	Methimazole (Tapazole) 5 and 10 mg tablets	40–80 mg/d (maximum 120 mg/d) initially; maintenance of 10 to 30 mg daily.			
IODIDES	Lugol's Solution 8 mg/drop (5% Iodine, 10% Potassium iodide) Saturated Potassium Iodide (SSKI) 50 mg iodide per drop.	Only 6 mg/day is effective although 5–10 drops tid orally are usually given for 10 to 14 days prior to surgery.	Decreases the vascularity of gland and increased firmness; blocks release of thyroid hormone.	Hypersensitivity reactions: skin rashes, mucous membrane ulcers, anaphylaxis, metallic taste, rhinorrhea, parotid and submaxillary swelling.	Preoperative preparation prior to surgery; can be used long-term for patients with mild disease and small goiters.
	Sodium iodide (NaI) USP 1 gm/10 cc 2 gm/20 cc	0.5–2 gm IV over 24 hr.			Thyroid storm.
ADRENERGIC ANTAGONISTS	Propranolol (Inderal) 10, 40, 80 mg tablets, 1 mg/cc IV (or equivalent beta blocker)	10 to 40 mg orally every six hours. 0.5–1 mg IV slow.	Blocks the effects of thyroid hormone peripherally, no effect on the underlying disease. Blocks peripheral conversion of T_4 to T_3.	Related to symptoms of beta blockade: bradycardia, CHF, blocks hyperglycemic response to hypoglycemia, CNS symptoms at high doses.	Symptomatic relief while awaiting onset of action of thioamides, RAI; preoperative preparation for surgery; thyroid storm.
	Reserpine 0.1, 0.25 mg tablets, 2.5 mg/cc per 2 cc ampules.	1–3 mg IV every 8 hrs.	Catecholamine depletion.	Effects of sympathetic blockade: nasal congestion, hypotension; CNS effects.	Thyroid Storm (Propranolol is drug of choice).

Category	Drug/Preparation	Dose	Action	Side Effects	Indications/Contraindications
	Guanethidine (Ismelin) 10, 25 mg tablets	20–50 mg orally every 8 hours.	Catecholamine depletion.	Severe postural hypotension, effects of sympathetic blockade.	
SURGERY	Preoperative preparation with iodides, thioamides, or propranolol prior to surgery.		Subtotal, total thyroidectomy.	Cosmetic scarring, hypothyroidism, hypoparathyroidism, risks of surgery: vocal cord damage, poor wound healing, infection, risks of anesthesia.	Obstruction, choking, malignancy, pregnancy in 2nd trimester. Contraindication to RAI or thioamides.
RADIOACTIVE IODINE	I^{131} radioactive isotope.	80 to 100 microcurie per gram of thyroid tissue.	Destruction of the gland.	Hypothyroidism; fear of radiation-induced leukemia, genetic damage, and malignancy; rarely, radiation sickness.	Adults, elderly patients who are poor surgical risks, cardiac disease, patients with a history of prior thyroid surgery, contraindications to thioamide usage.
MISCELLANEOUS AGENTS	Prednisone or equivalent corticosteroid	50–140 mg daily in divided doses.	Decrease LATS, decreased T_4 levels, suppression of inflammatory processes; blocks conversion T_4 to T_3.	Complications of steroid therapy.	Ophthalmopathy, Thyroid Storm (Use IV steroid).
	Lithium (Eskalith) 300 mg capsules	600–1200 mg daily in divided doses.	Similar to the effects of iodides in blocking hormone release.	Increased incidence of toxicity with serum levels above 1.5 mEq per liter; toxicity increased with hyponatremia, diuretics; gastrointestinal disturbances, tremor, confusion, slurred speech, seizures, coma.	Alternative to iodides and thioamides as a last resort when other modalities are contraindicated.

sion have also been noted with conventional therapy, and many caution against overenthusiastic adoption of such short-term therapy (137–139). When antithyroid thioamide treatment was extended over the empirical two year interval, a remission rate of 75–85% was obtained (135). Thus, longer treatment periods are justifiable in compliant patients and can be reinstituted if hyperthyroidism reappears shortly after therapy has been discontinued (139). In C.R., this goal may not be achievable, given her history of noncompliance.

31. Can thioamide therapy affect any of her preexisting medical conditions?

Thyrotoxicosis can activate or intensify diabetes by increasing the metabolism of insulin (17). Therefore, effective therapy with thioamides may restore control of this patient's diabetes.

Her arthritis should not be affected by the PTU, although both PTU and methimazole have been associated with the development of lupus and lupus-like syndromes. This adverse drug reaction is rare; the incidence is less than 0.1% (140–142). Lupus-like syndromes include skin ulcers (143), splenomegaly (143,144), migratory polyarthritis (145), pleuritis and pericarditis (141,146), periarteritis (147), and renal abnormalities (140,146). Serological abnormalities may also occur and include hyperglobulinemia (140,146), positive LE preparations (140), and antinuclear antibodies (ANA) (140,145,148). Recovery occurs after adequate steroid therapy and withdrawal of the thioamides. Since cross-reaction between methimazole and PTU is likely to occur for these adverse effects, these patients should be treated with surgery or RAI. C.R.'s treatment should be monitored with this side effect in mind, but the occurrence of this syndrome is infrequent enough that a trouble-free course of therapy can be anticipated.

32. Why was the thioamide therapy ineffective in C.R.?

The onset of action of the thioamides is slow because they block the synthesis rather than the release of thyroid hormone (122,124). Therefore, hormone secretion will continue until the large stores are depleted, and this may take four to ten weeks, especially since this patient received prior iodide therapy. However, some improvement should have been noted after one week. This inadequate response may be due to patient noncompliance since the dose and dosing interval seem appropriate. If patient C.R. had been taking her medications as directed, an increase in dose may be justified and therapy can be guided by the patient's symptoms, gland size, and laboratory values. The RAIU should be low if iodide trapping has been blocked by sufficient doses of thioamides.

33. What adjunctive therapy might help to alleviate some of this patient's symptoms while awaiting the apparent onset of PTU effects?

While awaiting the "effects" of the thioamides, iodides and/or propranolol can be used to ameliorate some of her symptoms. Since iodides previously have been ineffective in this patient, propranolol should be instituted in the interim. Propranolol will decrease nervousness, palpitations, fatigue, weight loss, diaphoresis, heat intolerance and tremor since many of the signs and symptoms of thyrotoxicosis are mediated by sympathetic overactivity (156–158). It is also of surprising value in improving many of the neuromuscular manifestations of hyperthyroidism (159–161). Patients generally remain mildly symptomatic and fail to regain weight. Thyroid function tests are not affected, although propranolol inhibits peripheral conversion of T_4 to T_3 (162).

Remission of the disease has occurred on propranolol alone, and propranolol has been used as the only treatment for thyrotoxicosis (163,164). It also is effective in the management of thyroid storm (128), as a pre-operative preparation for surgery (165–168) and in the management of thyrotoxicosis during pregnancy (54,56,169,170). It should be recalled that this patient is diabetic by history and the effects of beta-adrenergic blocking drugs in diabetic patients must be considered (also see the Diabetes chapter).

34. Propranolol 40 mg twice daily is prescribed for C.R. Why might this dose be inappropriate for this patient?

The effects of thyrotoxicosis in propranolol kinetics and plasma levels require more study. The elimination half-life ($t\frac{1}{2}$) and volume of distribution (Vd) of propranolol did not change when hyperthyroid patients became euthyroid (171a, 172,175a). However, the systemic clearance of total and free propranolol was significantly greater when patients were hyperthyroid than when they had become euthyroid (172,175a). Plasma protein binding of propranolol was reduced when patients were thyrotoxic (175a). In another study (173), the metabolic clearance rates and Vd of propranolol were higher in 15 thyrotoxic patients than in matched euthyroid controls. Furthermore, plasma propranolol levels were lower in thyrotoxic patients and these levels increase once euthyroidism is achieved (171,174,175a). Others have noted no significant differences in propranolol levels between thyrotoxic and euthyroid patients (172). Large variations in propranolol levels (175–177) exist between individuals who receive identical doses of propranolol and these large intraindividual variations probably account for some of the discrepancies in these studies (17,163).

With such conflicting data the appropriate dose should be based on a reduction in heart rate and other objective improvements resulting from beta-adrenergic blockade.

35. A pruritic area over the pretibial aspects of both legs as well as several maculopapular erythematous patches were noticed during the physical examination of this patient. Do these dermatological reactions require the discontinuation of her PTU?

Although C.R. may be experiencing a drug rash from PTU, pretibial myxedema or the dermopathy of Graves' disease may also be possible due to the location of the pruritic area. About 4% of patients with Graves' disease exhibit dermatological changes which are associated with infiltrative exophthalmos. It appears as thickening of the skin due to mucopolysaccharide infiltration, accentuation of hair follicles, and erythema with pruritus and is responsive to topical corticosteroids (149).

PTU and methimazole have both been associated with the production of a maculopapular pruritic rash in 5–6% of patients (122). If the rash is mild, drug therapy can be continued while the symptoms are treated with an antihistamine and a topical steroid; such rashes generally subside spontaneously. Alternatively, another thioamide can be substituted because cross-sensitivity to this side effect is not likely. If the rash is associated with other systemic manifestation of a drug reaction (eg, fever, arthralgias), other treatment should be selected.

36. Why should C.R.'s complaints of a sore throat and cough not be casually dismissed without further consideration?

Agranulocytosis or granulocytopenia (defined as less than 250/mm³ and 1500/mm³ respectively of neutrophils and granulocytes) is one of the most severe adverse hematological reactions associated with the thioamides (150). A more precise history should be obtained from this patient and the clinician should be particularly alert for a temperature 101°F or greater for two or more days and malaise or other flu-like findings which appeared temporally with her sore throat. If subjective or objective data are compatible with agranulocytosis, the PTU should be discontinued pending laboratory results of a WBC with a differential. Continuous serial monitoring of WBC counts are not of value in preventing agranulocytosis because symptoms may occur abruptly.

The incidence of agranulocytosis or granulocytopenia ranges from 0.5 to 6% (150–153). There is no predilection for age or sex, and the risk of this hypersensitivity reaction may be either idiosyncratic or dose-related (153,154). McGavack et al (153) found no reactions in 900 patients receiving less than 25 mg of methimazole daily but a 5.4% incidence of granulocytopenia including one death in patients receiving more than 30 mg daily. Likewise, in 931 patients taking PTU, a 2.8% incidence of decreased granulocytes was seen with doses less than 150 mg daily and a 4.5% incidence was noted in those taking more than 250 mg daily (153). Wibert et al reported two cases of agranulocytosis among 25 patients receiving 120 mg methimazole daily (154).

Agranulocytosis usually occurs within the first few months of therapy, although it can occur later (153). Fatality may result from overwhelming infection. The drug should be discontinued and the patient monitored for signs of infection and antibiotics should be instituted if necessary. If the patient recovers, granulocytes will begin to reappear in the peripheral blood within a few days to three weeks; a normal granulocyte count occurs shortly thereafter (153,155).

Although it would be best to proceed with another form of treatment, rechallenge with the same drug may or may not produce a similar reaction. Some cases of granulocytopenia have resolved despite continuation of thioamides (140,152). Very little information is available regarding cross-sensitivity between agents; instances of both cross-sensitivity and the lack thereof have been reported (155).

37. PTU is discontinued due to agranulocytosis in C.R. and surgery is scheduled for

when her granulocytes are normal. What pre-operative thyroid preparation is needed for C.R. prior to surgery? What postoperative complications are associated with thyroi-dectomy?

The patient should be in a euthyroid state at time of surgery to avoid precipitation of thyroid storm and enhanced morbidity. Generally, iodides (see Question 25), thioamides (127), or propran-olol can be used. The combination of iodides and propranolol may be more effective than either used alone (166–168). Propranolol used alone has been associated with thyroid crises postoperatively (165,178) and may be less effective than iodides in decreasing gland friability and vascularity. Since C.R. received only one week of thioamide therapy, her gland probably still contains large stores of hormone and pretreatment probably is necessary.

Postoperative complications include hypopar-athyroidism, adhesions, laryngeal nerve damage, infection, poor wound healing, and the risks of anesthesia and surgery itself (125). The risks of hypothyroidism are higher the first year after surgery, although there is an insidious rise in in-cidence over the following 10 years (179). The incidence of hypothyroidism ranges from 4 to 42%.

38. A 23-year-old male with Graves' dis-ease has been euthyroid for three months while taking methimazole 10 mg tid. Never-theless, he has trouble remembering to take it three times a day and desires a more sim-plified regimen. Could this patient be placed on a single daily dose of methimazole 30 mg?

Several clinical studies have demonstrated that single daily doses of methimazole or PTU are therapeutically effective, particularly in patients who are initially made euthyroid with multiple dosing (180,180a–182). Some patients may be ef-fectively treated with a single dose regimen throughout therapy (136,183,184). The success rate of this approach depends upon the size of the gland and severity of the disease. According to various studies, euthyroid states were achieved in 39% (136), 68% (181), 83% (183), and 93% (182) of hy-perthyroid patients.

Methimazole has been suggested as the pre-ferred agent for once-a-day dosing because of its longer duration of action (181,183), but PTU may be more rapidly effective due to its ability to block extrathyroidal conversion of T_4 to T_3 (184). In spite

of its short plasma half-life, a single 30 mg dose of methimazole has a duration of action of 24 hours (185). Apparently, the duration of action of the antithyroid agents is not correlated with the plasma half-life but rather with the size of the dose and the intrathyroidal concentration of the drug (70).

Since this patient is now euthyroid as a result of treatment with a divided daily dosage sched-ule, he could be tried on a single daily dosing regimen and observed for exacerbation of his Graves' disease. A single daily dose regimen as the initial therapy may be tried in selected pa-tients as a means to increase patient acceptance and compliance.

39. B.D. is a 35-year-old female who has been taking PTU 100 mg daily for over two years. Although she has been clinically eu-thyroid, her goiter never appeared to shrink in size. After the following laboratory values were obtained, thyroxine 0.1 mg daily was in-itiated. A TT_4 was 6 mcg/dl and a RT_3U was 23%. A T_3 suppression test showed the follow-ing results:

	Baseline RAIU	After T_3 100 mcg Daily for 7 Days
2 hr	6%	8%
5 hr	15%	14%
24 hr	33%	25%

After two months, the thyroxine and the PTU were discontinued, and she again became thyrotoxic four months later. What might have been the rationale for the addition of thyrox-ine to this patient's PTU therapy?

Thyroxine was added as an attempt to decrease the size of the goiter which was assumed to be a result of excess TSH production due to suppres-sive doses of PTU. The reported TT_4 and RT_3U are normal and thus of no value in supporting this assumption. However, an elevated TSH level would help ascertain if this was the primary rea-son for the goiter. If so, the easiest solution to this problem would be to decrease the dose of PTU; in cases where titration of the proper dose of PTU is difficult, the combination of T_4 and PTU can be used.

40. What are the prognostic implications of the T_3 suppression test in this patient?

The T_3 suppression test, as described earlier in this chapter, can determine whether the thyroid gland is functioning under normal TSH-dependent negative feedback mechanisms or whether the gland is functioning independently of TSH. The administration of T_3 should suppress TSH secretion and decrease subsequent measure of radioactive iodine uptake (RAIU). Therefore, comparisons of RAIU before and after T_3 administration can determine whether the thyroid gland is TSH-dependent or autonomous. In B.D.'s case, the results of the T_3 suppression test indicate that the gland is not suppressed and is functioning independently of TSH. The results of this test suggest a poor prognosis for permanent remission of the disease, especially in view of the fact that this patient has been receiving PTU for over two years.

The suppressibility of the thyroid has been correlated with the potential for remission of hyperthyroidism after discontinuation of antithyroid drug therapy (85,139,186–189). McKenzie and associates found that suppressibility at the end of a course of antithyroid drug treatment was associated with a relapse of 50%, while the relapse rate was 78% among those with nonsuppressible thyroid function (85). Although Alexander et al found a lower relapse rate (26%) among those with suppressible thyroid function (186,187), only 10% of their patients with nonsuppressible results remained euthyroid upon discontinuation of drug therapy. Cassidy found that remission could be predicted with 96% accuracy when the RAIU was 30% of baseline or less, and the likelihood of relapse could be predicted with 89% accuracy when the uptake was 50% or more; uptakes of 30 to 59% did not allow a reliable prediction (188). Slingerland et al (139) have recommended continuous therapy with thioamides until such time the suppression test is less than 20% in order to achieve a high rate of remission.

In B.D. the results of the suppression test indicate autonomous function and nonsuppressibility. This indicates a poor prognosis for remission, and re-exacerbation of the disease should have been expected.

41. What subjective or objective data in patient B.D. would justify a longer course of thioamide therapy?

It is not clear why some patients remain in permanent remission while others relapse upon discontinuation of thioamides, because these drugs do not change the basic abnormality of Graves' disease. However, patients with clinical characteristics which have been correlated with disease remissions may deserve a longer trial of antithyroid agents before changing to RAI or surgery.

Permanent remission usually is expected in 50 to 60% of the patients treated with antithyroid drugs (190,191), although permanent remission after drug treatment is probably less than 40% (136,192–194). Relapse rates as high as 80% (192) have been reported.

A number of clinical features are associated with a higher rate of permanent remission and may be predictive of patients who are good candidates for drug treatment. These include small goiters, mild and short duration of symptoms and disease, reduction in goiter size during treatment, lack of thyroid-stimulating antibodies, and return of thyroid suppressibility with treatment (187,189,191,195,196).

Although further study is needed, the initial absence of HLA-B8 antigen may be an indication that drug treatment will be ultimately successful; the presence of HLA-B8 antigen in thyrotoxic patients is associated with a 1.8 times greater probability of relapse after thioamide therapy (197). Others have noted that status of HLA D_RW_3 and level of TSH receptor antibody was predictive of remission or relapse (198).

Excess dietary iodide has been reported to increase the likelihood of relapse (193,199), but others (200) have been unable to confirm these findings. More study is needed to determine the relationship between iodide intake and the rate of relapse.

B.D.'s poor regression of goiter and nonsuppressibility decrease her chance for remission with longer term therapy. Although thioamide therapy can be continued indefinitely to control the thyrotoxicosis if there is no evidence of toxicity, surgery or radioactive iodine therapy should be seriously considered for this patient who has already received PTU for over two years.

42. A 32-year-old woman who is 3 months pregnant is referred for management of her Graves' disease. What are the therapeutic ramifications of managing thyrotoxicosis during pregnancy?

Hyperthyroidism has been estimated to occur in 0.02 to 1.4% of the pregnant population (201).

Pregnancy may ameliorate the symptoms of thyrotoxicosis, but typically the disease warrants therapy. The use of radioactive iodine and the chronic administration of iodides during pregnancy are contraindicated since these will cross the placenta to produce fetal goiter (202,203) and athyreosis (204); as little as 12 mg of iodide daily has produced neonatal goiters (203) and neonatal death (202,203). Also, long-term use of propranolol should be avoided because it has been associated with fetal respiratory depression, a small placenta, intrauterine growth retardation, impaired response to anoxia, and postnatal bradycardia and hypoglycemia (54,205). However, if rapid control of hyperthyroidism is required, short-term use for less than one week of either propranolol or iodides may be instituted.

Either surgery or the thioamides can be used. Surgery should only be performed during the second trimester to avoid spontaneous abortion (54,201,206). Iodides and propranolol can be used preoperatively without adverse effects on the fetus. PTU may be the thioamide of choice, because maternal ingestion of methimazole has produced scalp defects (207) and aplasia cutis (208).

The thioamides such as PTU cross the placenta and are active against the fetal thyroid. In contrast, neither exogenous nor maternal thyroid hormone reach the fetal circulation except when maternal thyroid concentrations are extremely high. Therefore, fetal hypothyroidism and goiter may develop when large doses of PTU are administered to the mother, even if the mother is hyperthyroid. In order to avoid goiter and suppression of the fetal thyroid, which begins to function at about 12 to 14 weeks of gestation, PTU is usually prescribed in doses of 300 mg or less during pregnancy (206). Such modest doses of PTU are thought to provide satisfactory control of maternal hyperthyroidism and are not believed to cause clinically evident thyroid dysfunction in the neonate. However, the use of PTU in pregnancy is being more critically evaluated in light of the findings by Cheron and associates (269). These investigators demonstrated that a small but significant reduction in neonatal serum thyroxine occurs even when small, 100–200 mg, doses of PTU are administered during pregnancy to mothers with Graves' disease. It is not known at this time whether a mild transient reduction in serum thyroxine of the magnitude noted in Cheron's study causes long-term impairment of mental development or is otherwise detrimental to the newborn. The present concensus seems to be that transient fetal or neonatal hypothyroidism do not appear to be a major threat to the baby (270). Nevertheless, it is advisable to maintain the mother in a mildly hyperthyroid state. Mild maternal hyperthyroidism seems to be well tolerated, but maternal hypothyroidism is poorly tolerated by both the mother and fetus (also see Question 11). Laboratory indices should also be in the upper ranges of normal.

There is no rationale to adding thyroid hormone to the mother's regimen to avoid fetal hypothyroidism because thyroid hormones do not cross the placenta. Such thyroid supplementation can only increase the maternal requirement for PTU and decrease fetal thyroid hormone production (206,209). If the mother has not been thyrotoxic throughout pregnancy, a normal infant can be expected. It is also prudent to recall that PTU, propranolol, and iodides are secreted in breast milk (206,210).

If Graves' disease in the mother is associated with high maternal serum levels of thyroid-stimulating immunoglobulin (TSI), an IgG that readily crosses the placenta, the possibility of neonatal hyperthyroidism should be considered. In such a situation, the mother can be given small doses of PTU in order to reach and treat the fetal thyroid because neonatal hyperthyroidism is critical. Perhaps an even better alternative would be to closely observe the newborns at risk and to administer PTU only to these with demonstrable hyperthyroidism (270).

RAI Therapy

43. B.J. is a 35-year-old female with newly diagnosed Graves' disease complicated by CHF and angina. Thioamide therapy was discontinued after one week of PTU because of severe granulocytopenia. After a few days treatment with Lugol's solution, 5 drops daily, she received RAI therapy. Three months later, she is still symptomatic. Why was it necessary to treat this patient prior to RAI therapy and why was the choice of Lugol's solution inappropriate?

Severely hyperthyroid patients, hyperthyroid patients with cardiac disease, and those who are debilitated or elderly should receive antithyroid treatment prior to RAI therapy. The goal of such pretreatment is to deplete stored thyroid hormone and to minimize post-RAI hyperthyroidism or thyroid storm caused by leakage of hormones from the damaged thyroid gland (130,211). RAI therapy can be initiated in other hyperthyroid patients safely without pretherapy (194,212).

The use of iodides prior to RAI therapy decreases the uptake of RAI by the thyroid gland. This effect of iodides persists for a few days to a week. Iodides can be instituted one day after RAI therapy if needed to control symptoms of hyperthyroidism. The thioamides can be used prior to RAI therapy to achieve a euthyroid state, but they should be discontinued one week before and for one to seven days after treatment to facilitate optimum uptake and retention of I^{131} by the gland. Pretreatment with thioamides may lower the cure rate and increase the need for subsequent doses of RAI (194,213). Propranolol can be used before, during, and after RAI therapy without interfering with its uptake. In B.J., the iodides should have been discontinued before RAI therapy and propranolol should have been instituted before RAI therapy since a short course of thioamide was received. Iodides might be preferable to propranolol if this patient's CHF worsens after RAI therapy.

44. Patient B.J. is still symptomatic three months after RAI therapy. When should this patient begin to experience subjective and objective benefits from the RAI therapy?

Although benefits from RAI therapy can be evident within one month, three to six months are required for attainment of the euthyroid state in approximately 60% of patients treated with a single nonablative dose of RAI. The remaining 40% of patients become euthyroid over one year after two or more doses. This slow onset is a disadvantage, but symptomatic control can be obtained quickly by administration of a thioamide, propranolol, or iodide 1 to 14 days after the I^{131} dose.

At least six months should elapse before a second radioactive dose of iodide is administered, and most recommend a full year's wait before repeating I^{131} administration. It is inadvisable to give a second dose before the major effects of the first dose have become apparent. Although the use of iodides prior to RAI in patient B.J. may have decreased the amount of I^{131} taken up by this patient's thyroid, it would still be advisable to wait at least six months before a second dose is given (130,194).

45. A 54-year-old female returns to thyroid clinic after being lost for follow-up for 6 months. She was initially treated with RAI three years ago but required a repeat dose of RAI 6 months ago for recurrence of hyperthyroidism. She currently has no other medical problems and is on no medications. She is a mildly obese, puffy-faced female wrapped in several layers of clothing. She complains of fatigue and lack of energy. Her reflexes are delayed and her skin is cool and dry. What is a likely explanation for her symptoms?

This patient should be evaluated for hypothyroidism secondary to RAI therapy; TT_4, RT_3U, and a TSH level would aid in the diagnosis. Iatrogenic hypothyroidism is the major complication of I^{131} therapy, although the hypothyroidism may only be transient in some cases (214,215). The incidence of iatrogenic myxedema after RAI is often reported as 7 to 8% but it increases at a constant rate of 2.5% per year. Various studies have noted the incidence to be 26% after 7 years, 28.8% after 10 years (179), 70% after 10 years (217), and 45% after 14 years (216).

Prevention of iatrogenic hypothyroidism has been directed toward calculation of a dose that will produce neither recurrent hyperthyroidism nor hypothyroidism. Unfortunately, the results of studies employing lower doses of I^{131} to avoid hypothyroidism have not been encouraging (218–221). Thus, the appearance of iatrogenic hypothyroidism may be inevitable with time. However, hypothyroidism is easily managed and is an acceptable therapeutic endpoint. Since hypothyroidism after RAI therapy is latent and often insidious, patients should be made aware of and closely monitored for subsequent hypothyroidism. Awareness of the possibility of transient hypothyroidism early after RAI therapy may prevent unnecessary replacements.

Ophthalmopathy of Graves' Disease

46. A 50-year-old lady first developed "large eyes with stare," weakness, diaphoresis, and thyroid enlargement in 1970. She was diagnosed as having Graves' disease and treated with RAI with some regression of eye symptoms. She is clinically euthyroid, although physical examination revealed severe bilateral conjunctival edema and injection, proptosis of the right eye, incomplete lid

**closure, and decreased visual acuity. She
complains of photophobia, tearing, and extreme irritation. What is the association of
this patient's ocular changes to Grave's
disease?**

This patient presents with symptoms consistent with the infiltrative ophthalmopathy of
Graves' disease. The eye signs of Graves' disease
are the most striking abnormality of this disorder. Fortunately, no more than 1 to 2% of patients
are affected. The eye involvement can occur at
any time and is usually bilateral, although unilateral involvement may occur. Following I^{131} or
surgery the ocular symptoms usually subside or
remain stable; some cases will progress during
the euthyroid period (222).

It is unknown why the eye and its muscles are
attacked in Graves' disease. Histologic examination reveal lymphocytic infiltration, increased
mucopolysaccaride content, fat, and water in all
retrobulbar tissue. Ocular symptoms include
edema, chemosis, excessive lacrimation, photophobia, corneal protrusion (proptosis), scarring,
ulceration, extraocular muscle paralysis with loss
of eye movements, and blindness from retinal and
optic nerve damage (17,222).

**47. What considerations and recommen-
dations do you have regarding the management of her ocular symptoms?**

Since the pathophysiology of the ocular symptoms is not well understood, treatment is limited
to symptomatic and empiric measures once the
euthyroid state is achieved. Periorbital edema and
chemosis are worse in the morning after being in
the horizontal position; elevation of the head while
in bed and treatment with diuretics and salt restriction may be helpful. Protective glasses are
useful in decreasing photophobia and external irritation. Topical corticosteroid drops are effective
in decreasing local irritation, but they should be
used cautiously since they increase the risk of
infection. Ocular irritants such as smoke and dust
should be avoided. Incomplete lid closure predisposes to corneal scarring and ulceration, so lubricant eyedrops containing methylcellulose
should be applied several times daily and at night
to keep the bulbs moist. Taping the eyelids shut
at night may prevent drying and scarring. Lateral surgical closure of the lids (tarsorrhapy) may
be required to improve lid closure.

When the ophthalmopathy is severe and progressive, a more aggressive approach should be
taken. Systemic corticosteroids have been used
with both dramatic effect and marginal results in
the emergency treatment of progressive exophthalmos with decreasing visual acuity. Prednisone doses of 35 to 80 mg daily have been effective, but doses as large as 100 to 140 mg daily
may be required (223). X-ray therapy to the pituitary and to the orbit have shown both beneficial and nonbeneficial results (17). Some have
recommended x-ray therapy to the orbit in conjunction with systemic steroids as the initial
treatment of choice.

When the above measures and thyroid ablation fail to arrest the progression of visual loss
and exophthalmos, then surgical decompression
should be considered.

Thyroid Storm

**48. H.L., a 48-year-old woman, was admit-
ted to the hospital with a three-week history
of fatigability, weakness, dyspnea on exertion, shortness of breath, and palpitations.
One year prior to admission she began noticing a preference for cold weather and an increase in nervousness and emotional lability.
After her husband died a few days ago, she
experienced increased irritability, insomnia,
tremor, and a 104°F fever which she attributed to an upper respiratory tract infection.
She denies any current medication. Review
of her laboratory data, which were obtained
on admission, noted a TT_4 of 30 mcg/dl. What
is the assessment based upon this patient's
subjective and objective data?**

It appears that the patient is experiencing thyroid storm, which is a life-threatening medical
emergency (128,224). The clinical manifestations
of thyroid storm (128,224,225) are the acute onset
of high fever (sine qua non), tachycardia, tachypnea, and the following organ systems involvement: cardiovascular—tachycardia, pulmonary
edema, hypertension, and shock; central nervous
system—tremor, emotional lability, confusion,
psychosis, apathy, stupor, and coma; gastrointestinal—diarrhea, abdominal pain, nausea and
vomiting; and liver—enlargement, jaundice, and
nonspecific elevations of bilirubin and prothrombin time. Hyperglycemia was a clinical finding in
12 out of 18 episodes.

Thyroid storm may develop in about 2 to 8%
of hyperthyroid patients. The pathogenesis of
thyroid storm is not well understood, but the con-

dition can be described as an "exaggerated" or decompensated form of thyrotoxicosis. The term "decompensated" implies failure of body systems to adequately resist the effects of thyrotoxicosis. It cannot be completely attributed solely to the release of massive quantities of hormones which may occur after surgery or following RAI therapy. Catecholamines also have an important role; the increased quantities of thyroid hormone in conjunction with increased sympathetic and adrenal output contribute to many of the manifestations of thyroid storm. Although thyroid hormones seem to have an independent action, amelioration of many of the symptoms of hyperthyroidism may be accomplished by catecholamine blocking agents such as reserpine and guanethidine.

49. What treatment plan should be initiated promptly in patient H.L.?

Accurate, continuous, and immediate treatment of storm may significantly decrease the mortality of thyroid storm. Mortality rates as low as 7% and survival rates as high as 50% have been reported. Treatment of thyroid storm should be directed against four major areas (128,224–226):

Decrease in Synthesis and Release of Hormones. Large doses of thioamides, either PTU 600 to 1200 mg daily or methimazole 60 to 120 mg daily, should be given in divided doses. Theoretically, PTU may act more rapidly since it can prevent the peripheral conversion of T_4 to T_3, a dominant source of the hormone. Iodides, which rapidly block further secretion of thyroxine, should be given at least one hour after thioamide administration so as to avoid blocking the latter's therapeutic effect. Iodides can be administered as an intravenous drip of sodium iodide (NaI) 1 to 3 gm over 24 hours or orally as Lugol's solution 30 drops daily. Such a combination may ameliorate symptoms within one day.

Reversal of the Peripheral Effects of Hormones and Catecholamines. Depleting agents such as reserpine and guanethidine are effective in decreasing tachycardia, agitation, and tremulousness. Reserpine in doses of 1 to 3 mg IM/IV every 8 hours (128,227) or guanethidine 20 to 50 mg orally every eight hours can be tried (225). Intravenous administration of reserpine is preferred over intramuscular injection since absorption from IM sites is poor if circulatory collapse is present. Propranolol has been used with success in decreasing the tachycardia and other symptoms of

thyrotoxicosis. It is the agent of choice and is effective in patients refractory to reserpine and guanethidine (128).

Supportive Treatment of Vital Functions. This may include sedation, oxygen, intravenous glucose, vitamins, treatment of infections with antibiotics, digitalization to maintain the cardiac status, rehydration, and treatment of hyperpyrexia with cooling blankets, sponge baths and the judicious use of antipyretics. If hypoadrenalism is suspected, hydrocortisone 100 to 200 mg every six hours intravenously should be given. Pharmacologic doses of steroids acutely depress serum T_3 levels and may be beneficial in storm (228–230).

Elimination of Precipitating Causes of Storm. Factors which have been associated with the induction of thyroid storm include infection (most common), trauma, inadequate preparation prior to thyroidectomies, surgical operations, stress, diabetic acidosis, pregnancy, emboli, abrupt discontinuation of antithyroid medications, drug therapy, and RAI therapy.

DRUG-INDUCED THYROID DISEASE

50. *Lithium and Antidepressants.* A 56-year-old male complains of sluggishness, cold intolerance, fatigue, and a "rundown" feeling which doctors have attributed to the depressive phase of his bipolar affective illness. He had previously been well controlled on imipramine 300 mg daily, but lithium carbonate 900 mg daily was added four months ago because of unreasonable mirthfullness and uncontrollable gift buying tendencies. On physical examination, a puffy face and a large goiter were prominent. What is a reasonable assessment of these subjective and objective data?

Although the incidence of goiter and hypothyroidism in the manic depressive population is not known, the possibility of lithium- and possibly imipramine-induced hypothyroidism should be considered. Thyroid function tests should be obtained to rule out these suspicions.

The antithyroid effects of lithium were first demonstrated in the management of manic depressive patients. Lithium acts like the iodides in inhibiting the release of hormonal and nonhormonal iodine from the gland (231–233). It may also affect the pituitary-thyroid axis (234). The exact mechanism of lithium's effect on the gland has not been clarified, although it is known that lithium is highly concentrated by the gland. The effects of lithium on indices of thyroid function include a low PBI and TT_4, elevated TSH levels, and an increased RAIU (235).

Lithium-induced goiter with (236–239), or without (240) hypothyroidism appears in a small percentage of the population after five months to two years of therapy. The goiters respond to discontinuation of lithium or to suppression with thyroid hormone despite continuation of lithium therapy. In two patients the goiter had to be surgically removed due to pressure symptoms (240).

In this case, imipramine may be exerting an additive or a synergistic antithyroid effect. Antithyroid effects have also been attributed to imipramine (241,242).

In most cases of lithium-induced thyroid abnormality a prior history of compromised thyroid function, such as thyroiditis or strong family history of compromised thyroid function, such as thyroiditis or strong family history of thyroid disease, was present (238,239). Therefore, baseline TT_4, RT_3U, antibodies, RAIU, and scan should be obtained prior to the initiation of lithium therapy. Patients should also be questioned regarding a family history of thyroid disease, and the concurrent use of tricyclic antidepressants should be noted.

51. A 46-year-old male is admitted for evaluation of atrial fibrillation. Laboratory studies are within normal limits, although the results of thyroid function tests were abnormally high. This patient's concurrent manic illness had been treated with lithium up to one month prior to this hospitalization. At that time, he discontinued the lithium therapy without the knowledge of his physician. Why might this patient's atrial fibrillation be attributable to the discontinuation of lithium therapy?

Thyrotoxicosis has been reported after lithium withdrawal (243–245) and this patient's atrial fibrillation may be a result of excess thyroid hormone activity. Lithium's antithyroid action is substantial and may be comparable to that of the thioamides; T_4 levels may decline by 20 to 35% (246,247,232,233). Therefore, this patient's underlying hyperthyroidism was probably unmasked by the discontinuation of the lithium.

Lithium even has been recommended as an adjunct to RAI therapy, because it does not interfere with RAI uptake and increases the retention of RAI by the thyrotoxic gland by inhibiting its rate of disappearance (235,248,249). Burrow et al found that the thyroidal half-life of I^{131} is increased by lithium (235). This would be beneficial in localizing the dose of radiation to the gland.

Because of the limited clinical experience with lithium in thyrotoxicosis, its use should be restricted to situations where rapid suppression of thyroid hormone secretion is needed and where iodides are contraindicated. It should not be considered as an alternative to thioamides but rather as an adjunct.

52. _Iodides._ A 54-year-old Vietnamese male presents with a six-month history of weakness, fatigue, tremor, heat intolerance, and palpitations. On physical examination a 40 gram multinodular gland was noted. He denies any family history of thyroid disease or ingestion of any thyroid medication. The only interesting finding was that the onset of his complaints occurred after an intravenous pyelogram (IVP). Could the iodine from the IVP be responsible for his symptoms? Have iodides produced hyperthyroidism?

Iodide-induced hyperthyroidism, known as Jod-Basedow phenomenon, was first described in the 1800's when patients residing in iodide-deficient areas became toxic upon adequate iodide supplementation (250). Other reports have appeared since (251–253). Both T_3 toxicosis and classical T_4 toxicosis have occurred following iodide ingestion (254,255) or injection of roentgenographic contrast media (256–258).

Although it has been presumed that both iodide deficiency and large multinodular goiter are essential for the production of Jod-Basedow phenomenon, it has also been reported among patients residing in iodine sufficient areas (112,112a) and in patients with normal glands (259) following the administration of iodide. Large doses of iodides should be avoided in patients with nontoxic multinodular goiter.

53. _Sulfonylureas._ A 37-year-old male returns to the clinic after ten weeks of treatment with PTU 300 mg every six hours. He expresses concern about the size of his goiter, which seems larger to him. He also complains of extreme fatigue, sweating, dizzi-

ness, and depression which he attributes to his personal problems. His only other medication is tolbutamide (Orinase) 500 qid for diabetes. Laboratory values show an FTI of 0.8, a TSH of 22 microIU, and an FBS of 50 mg/dl. What is your assessment of his complaints and laboratory findings?

This patient is hypothyroid according to the present subjective and objective findings. The thyroid function probably was suppressed excessively because the large initial dose of PTU was not decreased after 4 to 6 weeks. Furthermore, large doses of sulfonylureas, such as tolbutamide, inhibit thyroid hormone formation. This effect has been observed with large doses of chlorpropramide but not with tolbutamide in daily doses of 1 to 2 gm (260). Hypothyroidism appears to be more common among diabetics treated with sulfonylureas than those treated by diet or insulin (261).

This patient's complaints of dizziness, sweating, and fatigue suggest a hypoglycemic reaction which is confirmed by a low blood sugar. Hypoglycemia may occur in hypothyroid patients treated with insulin or hypoglycemic agents because hypothyroidism delays the metabolism of insulin (17). The tolbutamide should be discontinued and his diabetes should be re-evaluated after correction of his hypothyroid state.

NODULES

54. A 20-year-old female noted a lump in the right side of her neck. There is no history of radiation, no family history of thyroid disease, no local symptoms, and no symptoms suggestive of hypo- or hyperthyroidism. The right lobe of the thyroid is occupied by a 3 × 3 cm firm, immovable nodule, while the left lobe is barely palpable. All thyroid function tests are within normal limits although the gland is not suppressible. A scan shows a large "hot" nodule occupying the right lobe and a nonexistent left lobe. How should this patient's "hot nodule" be managed?"

"Hot" nodule is a term used to describe an area of the thyroid which is concentrating iodine or "hyperfunctioning" as shown on scan. It appears as an area of greater density than the rest of the gland. The hyperfunctioning autonomous nodule typically suppresses activity in the remainder of the gland, but it need not produce clinical or chemical evidence of hyperthyroidism and may

remain unchanged for years. Some nodules may develop into toxic goiters, causing overt symptoms of toxicosis. Most "hot" nodules are benign, although malignancies have been reported (262, 263).

Treatment of the "hot" nodule will depend upon the existing clinical situation. If the "hot" nodule has suppressed the other lobe of the thyroid, is not causing toxic symptoms, and is the only source of thyroid production, the patient should be left alone and closely monitored for signs of toxicity (263). If the other parts of the gland have not been suppressed by the functioning "hot" nodule, thyroid suppression therapy may be tried to shrink the nodule. A toxic "hot" nodule is treated either by surgery or radioactive iodine ablation. Since the normal thyroid tissue is suppressed, the RAI will be concentrated only by the "hot" nodule, sparing the suppressed tissue. After treatment, the suppressed tissue should begin functioning again (264).

55. A 29-year-old female is found to have a left thyroid nodule on routine physical examination. She has no history of neck radiation, a negative family history of thyroid disease and no symptoms suggestive of hypo- or hyperthyroidism. A hard, non-tender 3 × 4 cm nodule occupies the left lobe of the gland. Thyroid function tests are within normal limits. The scan shows a cold nodule; the echo reveals a solid mass ruling out the possibility of a cyst. Antibodies are negative. How should this patient's "cold nodule" be managed?

A "cold" nodule is a "hypofunctioning" area of the thyroid which fails to collect radioiodine. It is depicted on the scan as a lighter or less dense area as compared to the rest of the gland. The possible considerations include Hashimoto's thyroiditis, benign adenomas, cysts, and malignant tumors. The absence of antibodies and solidarity of the mass by echo rules out the possibility of cyst or Hashimoto's thyroiditis. Most "cold" nodules turn out to be benign adenomas rather than cancers. The incidence of malignancy in a cold nodule varies between 10 and 20% (265). A history of irradiation increases the likelihood of cancer in a nodule and favors surgery (266). The nature of the nodule is important. Fixation of the nodule to the strap muscles or trachea, a hard bulging characteristic, any pain or tenderness, or voice hoarseness may indicate malignancy (264).

The appropriate treatment depends on a number of judgmental factors made by the physician and the patient. Absolute guidelines are not available, although the following indicators can be used (264,267). Recent growth of a solid nodule, presence of disturbing symptoms such as a choking sensation, a history of irradiation to the neck and upper head as a child, males, young age (under 30), a negative family history of thyroid disease, or failure of regression of the nodule on thyroxine therapy for 6 months are all signs which favor surgery (264). Nodules in women over 30 without disturbing local signs, with no recent growth, or of a long standing nature are more likely to be benign and can be followed or excised surgically. Suppression therapy with thyroxine to decrease TSH secretion may shrink the nodule. However, the decrease in size does not eliminate the possibility of malignancy. A positive response (shrinkage of the nodule) should be seen after a trial of thyroxine 0.2 mg daily for 3 to 6 months; otherwise, surgery should be strongly considered.

56. A 25-year-old female had thymic radiation at age 7. She is asymptomatic, has no family history of thyroid disease, and has never taken thyroid. On physical examination the thyroid was palpable and no nodules were found. What is the significance of irradiation to the thyroid at a young age? How should this patient be managed?

It is now known that there is an association between external radiation administered to the head, neck, and upper thorax of infants, children, and adolescents and the subsequent development of abnormal and neoplastic changes in the thyroid gland. Any irradiation above 50 rads to the area of the thyroid during childhood should be of concern. Numerous articles report a 1 to 7% incidence of neoplastic changes occurring 10 to 30 years after the initial irradiation (124,266). Other abnormalities found include Hashimoto's thyroiditis, benign adenomas, and Graves' disease. All patients with a history of thyroidal irradiation during childhood should be evaluated for thyroid abnormalities. Examination of the thyroid gland manually, as well as a thyroid scan, antibodies, TT_4, RT_3U, and RAIU should be performed. In the absence of any abnormality the patient should be re-evaluated yearly.

References

1. Brennan M: Clinical pharmacology series on pharmacology in practice 5. thyroid hormones. Mayo Clin Proc. 1980; 55:33.

2. Braverman LE et al: Conversion of thyroxine (T_4) to triiodothyronine (T_3) in athyreotic human subjects. J Clin Invest. 1970; 49:855.

3. Pittman CS et al: The extra thyroidal conversion rate of thyroxine to triiodothyronine in normal man. J Clin Invest. 1971; 50:1187.

4. Surks MI et al: Determination of iodothyronine absorption and conversion of L-thyroxine (T_4) to L-triiodothyronine (T_3) using turnover rate techniques. J Clin Invest. 1973; 52:805.

5. Schimmel M et al: Thyroidal and peripheral production of thyroid hormones. Ann Intern Med. 1977; 87:760.

6. Oppenheimer JH: Role of plasma proteins in the binding, distribution and metabolism of the thyroid hormone. N Engl J Med. 1968; 278:1153.

7. Lizarralde G: Function tests and the physiology of thyroid homeostasis. Cont Educ for Family Physicians. 1977; 7:70.

8. Larsen PR: Tests of thyroid function. Med Clin North Am. 1975; 59:1063.

9. Davis PJ: Factors affecting the determination of the serum protein bound iodine. Am J Med. 1966; 40:98.

10. Hershman JM et al: Control of thyrotrophin secretion in man. N Engl J Med. 1971; 285:997.

11. Odell W et al: Radioimmunoassay of thyrotropin in human serum. J Clin Endocrinol Metab. 1965; 25:1179.

12. Sawin CT et al: The free triiodothyronine (T_3) index. Ann Intern Med. 1978; 88:474.

13. Patel YC et al: Serum thyrotropin (TSH) in pituitary and hypothalmic hypothyroidism normal or elevated basal levels and paradoxical responses for thyrotropin releasing hormone. J Clin Endocrinol Metab. 1973; 37:190.

14. Otsuki M et al: Influence of glucocorticoids on the TRF-induced TSH response in man. J Clin Endocrinol Metab. 1973; 36:95.

15. Spaulding SW et al: L-dopa suppression of thyrotropin releasing hormone response in man. J Clin Endocrinol Metab. 1972; 35:182.

16. Pittman JA et al: Changing normal values for thyroidal radioactive uptake. N Engl J Med. 1969; 280:1431.

17. Degroot L J et al: *The Thyroid and Its Diseases*, 4th ed, J Wiley & Sons, New York, 1975.

18. Dingle PR et al: The incidence of thyroglobulin antibodies and thyroid enlargement in a general practice in north east England. Clin Exp Immunol. 1966; 1:277.

19. Chopra IJ et al: Misleadingly low free thyroxine index and usefulness of reverse triiodothyronine measurement in nonthyroidal illnesses. Ann Intern Med. 1979; 90:905.

20. Bermudez F et al: High incidence of decreased serum triiodothyronine concentration in patients with non-thyroidal disease. J Clin Endocrinol Metab. 1975; 41:27.

21. Carter JN et al: Effect of severe, chronic illness on thyroid function. Lancet. 1974; 2:971.

22. Chopra IJ et al: Reciprocal changes in serum concentrations of 3,3',5'-triiodothyronine (Reverse T_3) and 3,3',5'-triiodothyronine (T_3) in systemic illness. J Clin Endocrinol Metab. 1975; 41:1043.

23. Burger A et al: Reduced active hormone levels in acute illness. Lancet. 1976; 1:653.

24. Spector DA et al: Thyroid function and metabolic state in chronic renal failure. Ann Intern Med. 1976; 85:724.

25. Talwar KK et al: Serum levels of thyrotropin, thyroid hormone, and their response to thyrotrophin releasing hormone in infective febrile illness. J Clin Endocrinol Metab. 1977; 44:398.

26. Walfish PG et al: Serum triiodothyronine and other clinical and laboratory indices of alcoholic liver disease. Ann Intern Med. 1979; 91:13.

27. Hansten PD: *Drug Interactions,* 4th Ed, Lea & Febiger, Philadelphia, 1979.

28. Molholm HJ et al: The effect of diphenylhydantoin on thyroid function. J Clin Endocrinol Metab. 1974; 39:785.

29. Good BF et al: The effect of salicylate and related drugs on thyroxine binding in man. Aust J Exp Biol Med Sci. 1965; 43:291.

30. Heath H et al: Conjugated estrogen therapy and tests of thyroid function. Ann Intern Med. 1974; 81:351.

31. Hall R et al: Hypothyroidism: clinical features and complications. Clin Endocrinol Metab. 1979; 8:29.

32. Doniach D et al: Goitrous autoimmune thyroiditis (Hashimoto's disease). Clin Endocrinol Metab. 1979; 8:63.

33. Fein HG et al: Anemia in thyroid disease. Med Clin North Am. 1975; 59:1133.

34. Hines JD et al: Megaloblastic anemia secondary to folate deficiency associated with hypothyroidism. Ann Intern Med. 1968; 68:792.

35. Cobb WE et al: Drug therapy reviews: management of hypothyroidism. Am J Hosp Pharm. 1978; 35:51.

36. Rees-Jones RW et al: Triiodothyronine and thyroxine content of dessicated thyroid tablets. Metabolism. 1977; 26:1213.

37. Rees-Jones RW et al: Hormonal content of thyroid replacement preparations. JAMA. 1980; 243:549.

38. Braverman LE et al: Anomalous effects of certain preparations of dessicated thyroid on serum protein-bound iodine. N Engl J Med. 1964; 270:439.

39. Mangieri CN et al: Potency of United States pharmacopeia dessicated thyroid tablets as determined by the antigoitrogenic assay in rats. J Clin Endocrinol Metab. 1970; 30:102.

40. Pileggi VJ et al: Determination of thyroxine and triiodothyronine in commercial preparations of dessicated thyroid and thyroid extract. J Clin Endocrinol Metab. 1965; 25:949.

41. Jackson IMD et al: Why does anyone still use dessicated thyroid USP? Am J Med. 1978; 64:284.

42. Sawin CT et al: A comparison of thyroxine and dessicated thyroid in patients with primary hypothyroidism. Metabolism. 1978; 27:1518.

43. Hays MT: Absorption of oral thyroxine in man. J Clin Endocrinol Metab. 1968; 28:749.

44. Stoeffer SS et al: Potency of brand name and generic levothyroxine products. JAMA. 1980; 244:1704.

45. Stoeffer SS: Substitution of levothyronine products. JAMA. 1979; 241:1229.

46. Shroff AP et al: Standards for levothyronine preparations. JAMA. 1980; 244:658.

47. Ingbar JC et al: Equivalence of thyroid preparations. JAMA. 1980; 244:1095.

48. Jacobson JM et al: Nonequality of brand name thyroxine preparations. JAMA. 1980; 243:733.

49. Stock JM et al: Replacement dosage of L-thyroxine in hypothyroidism. N Engl J Med. 1974; 290:529.

50. Cotton GE et al: Suppression of thyrotropin (TSH) in serum of patients with myxedema of varying etiology treated with thyroid hormones. N Engl J Med. 1971; 285:529.

51. Braverman LE et al: Effects of replacement doses of sodium L-thyroxine on the peripheral metabolism of thyroxine and triiodothyronine in man. J Clin Invest. 1973; 52:1010.

52. Brown ME et al: Transient elevation of serum thyroid hormone concentration after initiation of replacement therapy in myxedema. Ann Intern Med. 1980; 92:491.

53. Bernstein RS et al: Intermittent therapy with L-thyroxine. N Engl J Med. 1969; 281:1444.

54. Burrow GN: Hyperthyroidism during pregnancy. N Engl J Med. 1978; 298:150.

55. Montoro M et al: Successful outcome of pregnancy with hypothyroidism. Ann Intern Med. 1981; 94:31.

56. Burrow GN: The thyroid in pregnancy. Med Clin North Am. 1975; 59:1089.

57. Greenman GW et al: Thyroid dysfunction in pregnancy, fetal loss and follow-up evaluation of surviving infants. N Engl J Med. 1962; 267:426.

58. Man EB et al: Thyroid function in human pregnancy—development and retardation of a 4-year-old progeny of euthyroid and of hypothyroxinemic women. Am J Obstet Gynecol. 1971; 109:12.

59. Man EB et al: Thyroid function in human pregnancy. Am J Obstet Gynecol. 1976; 125:949.

60. Potter JD: Hypothyroidism and reproductive failure. Surg Gynecol Obstet. 1980; 150:251.

61. Blizzard RM et al: Maternal autoimmunization to thyroid as a probable cause of athyreotic cretinism. N Engl J Med. 1960; 263:327.

62. Parker RH et al: Thyroid antibodies during pregnancy and in the newborn. J Clin Endocrinol Metab. 1960; 21:792.

63. Goldsmith RE et al: Familial autoimmune thyroiditis maternal fetal relationship and the role of generalized autoimmunity. J Clin Endocrinol Metab. 1973; 37:265.

64. Sutherland JM et al: Familial non goitrous cretinism apparently due to maternal antithyroid antibody. N Engl J Med. 1960; 263:336.

65. Illig R: Congenital hypothyroidism. Clin Endocrinol Metab. 1979; 8:49.

66. Lightner ES: Congenital hypothyroidism—clues to an early clinical diagnosis. J Fam Prac. 1977; 5:527.

67. Maerpaa J: Congenital hypothyroidism—aetiological and clinical aspects. Arch Dis Child. 1972; 47:256.

68. Raiti S et al: Cretinism—early diagnosis and its relation to mental prognosis. Arch Dis Child. 1971; 46:692.

69. Smith DW et al: Mental attainments of hypothyroid children—review of 128 cases. Pediatrics. 1957; 19:1011.

70. Refetoff I: Thyroid hormone therapy. Med Clin North Am. 1975; 59:1147.

71. Northcutt RC et al: The influence of cholestyramine on thyroxine absorption. JAMA. 1969; 208:1857.

72. Hiss JM et al: Thyroxine metabolism in untreated and treated pancreatic steatorrhea. J Clin Invest. 1962; 41:988.

73. Weg JG et al: Hypothyroidism and alveolar hypoventilation. Arch Intern Med. 1965; 115:302.

74. Nordqvist P et al: Myxoedema coma and CO_2 retention. Acta Med Scand. 1960; 166:189.

75. Mitchell JRA et al: Hypothermia after chlorpromazine in myxoedematous psychosis. Br Med J. 1959; 2:932.

76. Blum M: Myxedema coma. Am J Med Sci. 1972; 264:433.

77. Menedez CE et al: Thyrotoxic crisis and myxedema coma. Med Clin North Am. 1973; 57:1463.

78. Holvey D et al: Treatment of myxedema with intravenous thyroxine. Arch Intern Med. 1964; 113:89.

79. Nicoloff JT: Treatment of hypothyroidism and myxedema coma. Mod Treat. 1969; 6:465.

80. Ridgway EC et al: Acute metabolic responses in myxedema to large doses of intravenous L-thyroxine. Ann Intern Med. 1972; 77:549.

81. Green WL: Guidelines for treatment of myxedema. Med Clin North Am. 1968; 52:43.

82. Keating FR et al: Treatment of heart disease associated with myxedema. Progr Cardiovasc Dis. 1961; 3:364.

82a. Levine HD: Compromise therapy in the patient with angina pectoris and hypothyroidism. Am J Med. 1980; 69:411.

83. Croxson MS et al: Serum digoxin in patients with thyroid disease. Br Med J. 1975; 3:566.

84. Doherty JE et al: Digoxin metabolism in hypo- and hyperthyroidism. Ann Intern Med. 1966; 64:489.

85. McKenzie JM: Graves' disease. Med Clin North Am. 1975; 59:1177.

86. Kriss J: The long acting thyroid stimulator. Calif Med. 1968; 109:203.

87. Knox AJS et al: Circulating lymphocytes from patients with Graves disease to produce thyroid stimulating immunoglobulin (TSI). J Clin Endocrinol Metab. 1976; 43:330.

88. McKenzie JM et al: Reconsideration of thyroid stimulating immunoglobulin as cause of hyperthyroidism in Graves disease. J Clin Endocrinol Metab. 1976; 42:778.

89. McIntosh TJ et al: Increased sensitivity to warfarin in thyrotoxicosis. J Clin Invest. 1970; 49:63a.

90. Self T et al: Warfarin-induced hypoprothrombinemia potentiation by hyperthyroidism. JAMA. 1975; 231:1165.

91. Vagenakis AG et al: Enhancement of warfarin induced hypoprothrombinemia by thyrotoxicosis. John Hopkins Med J. 1972; 131:69.

92. Loeliger EA et al: The biological disappearance rate of prothrombin factors VII IX X from plasma in hypo- hyper- and during fever. Thromb Diath Haemorrh. 1964; 10:267.

93. Ikkala E et al: Plasma coagulation factors in thyrotoxicosis. Acta Endocrinol. 1962; 40:307.

94. Hansten PD: Oral anticoagulants and drugs which alter thyroid function. Drug Intell Clin Pharm. 1980; 14:331.

95. Rice AJ et al: Decreased sensitivity to warfarin in patients with myxedema. Am J Med Sci. 1971; 262:211.

96. Gilbert DK: Hypoprothrombinemia as a complication of propylthiouracil. JAMA. 1964; 189:855.

97. Gotta AW et al: Prolonged intraoperative bleeding caused by propylthiouracil induced hypoprothrombinemia. Anesthesiology. 1972; 37:562.

98. Greenstein R: Hypoprothrombinemia due to propylthiouracil therapy. JAMA. 1960; 173:1014.

99. Naeye RL et al: Hemorrhagic state after propylthiouracil treatment. Am J Clin Path. 1960; 34:254.

100. Becker CE et al: Hepatitis from methimazole during adrenal steroid treatment for malignant exophthalmos. JAMA. 1968; 206:1787.

101. Fedotin MS: Liver disease caused by propylthiouracil. Arch Intern Med. 1975; 135:319.

102. Martinez-Lopez JI et al: Drug-induced hepatic injury during methimazole therapy. Gastroenterology. 1962; 43:84.

103. Mikas AA et al: Fulminant hepatitis and lymphocyte sensitization due to propylthiouracil. Gastroenterology. 1976; 70:770.

104. Parker LN: Hepatitis and propylthiouracil. Ann Intern Med. 1975; 82:228.

105. Fischer MG: Methimazole-induced jaundice. JAMA. 1973; 223:1028.

106. Frye RL et al: Studies on digitalis—the influence of triiodothyronine on digitalis requirement. Circulation. 1961; 23:376.

107. Morrow DH et al: Studies on digitalis—influence of hyper- and hypothyroidism on the myocardial response to ouabain. J Pharmacol Exper Ther. 1963; 140:324.

108. Ivy HK et al: Triiodothyronine (T_3) toxicosis. Arch Intern Med. 1971; 128:529.

109. Hollander CS et al: Hypertriiodothyroninemia as a premonitory manifestation of thyrotoxicosis. Lancet. 1971; 2:731.

110. Marsden P et al: Hormonal pattern of relapse in hyperthyroidism. Lancet. 1975; 1:944.

111. Shenkman L et al: Recurrent hyperthyroidism presenting as triiodothyronine toxicosis. Ann Intern Med. 1972; 77:410.

112. Vagenakis AG et al: Adverse effects of iodides on thyroid function. Med Clin North Am. 1975; 59:1075.

112a. Vagenakis AG et al: Iodide induced thyrotoxicosis in Boston. N Engl J Med. 1972; 287:524.

113. Nagataki S et al: Effects of iodides on thyroidal iodine turnover in hyperthyroid subjects. J Clin Endocrinol Metab. 1970; 30:469.

114. Hamburger JI: *Clinical Thyroidology,* 2nd printing, Northland Thyroid Lab, Southfield, Michigan, 1974, p 206.

115. Wolff J: Iodide goiter and the pharmacological effects of excess iodide. Am J Med. 1969; 47:101.

116. Braverman LE et al: Changes in thyroidal function during adaptation to large doses of iodides. J Clin Invest. 1963; 42:1216.

117. Begg TB et al: Iodide goiter and hypothyroidism. Quart J Med. 1963; 32:251.

118. Boyle JA et al: Phenomenon of iodide inhibition in various states of thyroid function with observations on one mechanism of its occurrence. J Clin Endocrinol Metab. 1965; 25:1255.

119. Braverman LE et al: Enhanced susceptibility to iodide myxedema in Hashimoto's. J Clin Endocrinol Metab. 1971; 32:515.

120. Braverman LE et al: Induction of myxedema by iodide in patients euthyroid after radioactive or surgical treatment of diffuse toxic goiter. N Engl J Med. 1969; 281:816.

121. Friend DG: Iodide therapy and the importance of quantitating the dose. N Engl J Med. 1960; 263:1358.

122. Jackson IMD: Management of thyrotoxicosis. Am J Hosp Pharm. 1975; 32:933.

123. Thomas ID: Hyperthyroidism—diagnosis and treatment. Drugs. 1976; 11:119.

124. McClung MR et al: Treatment of hyperthyroidism. Ann Rev Med. 1980; 31:385.

125. Black BM: Surgery for Graves' disease. Mayo Clin Proc. 1972; 47:966.

126. Hardin WJ et al: Indications for thyroid surgery. Postgrad Med. 1975; 57:121.

127. Heiman P et al: Surgical treatment of thyrotoxicosis—results of 272 operations with special reference to preoperative treatment with antithyroid drugs and L-thyroxine. Br J Surg. 1975; 62:683.

128. Raber JH: The pharmacotherapy of thyroid storm. Drug Intell Clin Pharm. 1980; 14:344.

129. Perzik SL: Total thyroidectomy in the management of Graves' disease. Am J Surg. 1976; 131:284.

130. Sterling K: Radioactive iodide therapy. Med Clin North Am. 1975; 59:1217.

130a. McDougall IR et al: Radioactive iodine (I[131]) therapy for thyrotoxicosis. N Engl J Med. 1971; 285:1099.

131. Dobyns BM et al: Malignant and benign neoplasms of the thyroid in patients treated for hyperthyroidism—a report of the cooperative thyrotoxicosis therapy follow-up study. J Clin Endocrinol Metab. 1974; 38:976.

132. Saenger EL et al: Incidence of leukemia following treatment of hyperthyroidism. JAMA. 1968; 205:855.

133. Marchant B et al: Antithyroid drugs. Pharmacol Ther [B]. 1978; 3:305.

134. Geffner DL et al: Propylthiouracil blocks extrathyroidal conversion of T_4 to triiodothyronine and augments thyrotropin secretion in man. J Clin Invest. 1975; 55:224.

135. Abuid J et al: Triiodothyronine and thyroxine in hyperthyroidism—comparison of the acute changes during therapy with antithyroid agents. J Clin Invest. 1974; 54:201.

135a. McGregor AM et al: Carbimazole and the autoimmune response in Graves' disease. N Engl J Med. 1980; 303:302.

136. Greer MA et al: Short-term antithyroid drug therapy for the thyrotoxicosis of Graves' disease. N Engl J Med. 1977; 297:173.

137. Burr WA et al: Relapse after short-term antithyroid therapy of Graves' disease. N Engl J Med. 1979; 300:200.

138. Tamai H et al: Thionamide therapy in Graves' disease: relation of relapse rate to duration of therapy. Ann Intern Med. 1980; 92:488.

139. Slingerland DW: Long-term antithyroid treatment in hyperthyroidism. JAMA. 1979; 242:2408.

140. Amrhein JA et al: Granulocytopenia lupus-like syndrome and other complications of propylthiouracil therapy. J Pediatr. 1970; 76:54.

141. Best MM et al: A lupus-like syndrome following propylthiouracil administration. J Ky Med Assoc. 1964; 62:47.

142. Librick L et al: Thyrotoxicosis and collagen-like disease in three sisters of American Indian extraction. J Pediatr. 1970; 76:64.

143. Walzer RA et al: Immunolukopenia as an aspect of hypersensitivity to propylthiouracil. JAMA. 1963; 184:743.

144. Sammon TJ et al: Disseminated intravascular coagulation complicating propylthiouracil therapy. Clin Pediatr. 1972; 10:739.

145. Hung W et al: A collagen-like syndrome associated with antithyroid therapy. J Pediatr. 1973; 82:852.

146. Wing ES et al: Observations on the use of propylthiouracil in hyperthyroidism. Bull John Hopkins Hosp. 1952; 90:201.

147. McCormick RV: Polyarteritis occurring during propylthiouracil therapy. JAMA. 1950; 144:1453.

148. Cetina JA et al: Antinuclear antibodies and propylthiouracil therapy. JAMA. 1972; 220:1012.

149. Kriss J et al: Therapy with occlusive dressings of pretibial myxedema with fluocinolone acetonide. J Clin Endocrinol Metab. 1967; 27:595.

150. Rosove MH: Agranulocytosis and antithyroid drugs. West J Med. 1977; 126:339.

151. Chevalley J et al: A four-year study of the treatment of hyperthyroidism with methimazole. J Clin Endocrinol Metab. 1954; 14:948.

152. Van Winkle W Jr et al: Clinical toxicity of thiouracil survey of 5745 cases. JAMA. 1946; 130:343.

153. McGavack TH et al: Untoward hematologic responses to the antithyroid compounds. Am J Med. 1954; 17:36.

154. Wiberg JJ: Methimazole toxicity from high doses. Ann Intern Med. 1972; 77:414.

155. Bartels EC: Agranulocytosis during propylthiouracil therapy. Am J Med. 1948; 5:48.

156. Becker FO et al: Sympathetic blockade in hyperthyroidism. Arch Intern Med. 1974; 129:967.

157. Grossman WM et al: Effects of B-blockade on peripheral manifestations of thyrotoxicosis. Ann Intern Med. 1971; 74:875.

158. Robayo JR: Pharmacokinetics in drug therapy—propranolol hydrochloride as adjunct therapy in the treatment of thyrotoxicosis. Am J Hosp Pharm. 1976; 33:169.

159. Kammer GM et al: Acute bulbar muscle dysfunction and hyperthyroidism—a study of 4 cases and review of the literature. Am J Med. 1974; 56:464.

160. Rothberg MP et al: Propranolol and hyperthyroidism—reversal of upper motor neuron signs. JAMA. 1974; 230:1017.

161. Weinstein R et al: Propranolol reversal of bulbar dysfunction and proximal myopathy in hyperthyroidism. Ann Intern Med. 1975; 82:540.

162. Feely J et al: Propranolol, triiodothyronine, reverse triiodothyronine and thyroid disease. Clin Endocrinol. 1979; 10:531.

163. Mazzaferri EL et al: Propranolol as primary therapy for thyrotoxicosis. Arch Intern Med. 1976; 136:50.

164. McLarty DG et al: Remission of thyrotoxicosis during treatment with propranolol. Br Med J. 1973; 2:332.

165. Ljunggren JG et al: Preop treatment of thyrotoxicosis with a B-adrenergic blocking agent. Acta Chir Scand. 1975; 141:715.

166. Feek CM et al: Combination of potassium iodide and propranolol in preparation of patients with Graves' disease for thyroid surgery. N Engl J Med. 1980; 302:883.

167. Michie W et al: Beta blockage and partial thyroidectomy for thyrotoxicosis. Lancet. 1974; 1:1009.

168. Lee TC et al: Use of propranolol in surgical treatment of thyrotoxic patients. Ann Surg. 1973; 177:643.

169. Bullock JL et al: Treatment of thyrotoxicosis during pregnancy with propranolol. Am J Obstet Gynecol. 1975; 121:242.

170. Langer A et al: Adrenergic blockage—a new approach to hyperthyroidism during pregnancy. Obstet Gynecol. 1974; 44:181.

171. Nies AS et al: Clinical pharmacology of propranolol. Circulation. 1975; 52:6.

171a. Bell JM et al: Studies on the effect of thyroid dysfunction on the elimination of B-adrenoreceptor blocking drugs. Br J Clin Pharmacol. 1977; 4:79.

172. Riddell JG: Effect of thyroid dysfunction on propranolol kinetics. Clin Pharmacol Ther. 1980; 28:565.

173. Rubenfeld S et al: Propranolol pharmacokinetics in thyrotoxicosis. Clin Res. 1978; 26:295A.

174. Feely J et al: The effect of age and hyperthyroidism on plasma propranolol steady state concentrations. Br J Clin Pharmacol. 1978; 6:446.

175. Feely J et al: Propranolol dynamics in thyrotoxicosis. Clin Pharmacol Ther. 1980; 28:40.

175a. Feely J et al: Increased clearance of propranolol in thyrotoxicosis. Ann Intern Med. 1981; 94:472.

176. Rubenfeld S et al: Variable plasma propranolol levels in thyrotoxicosis. N Engl J Med. 1979; 300:353.

177. Feely J et al: Beta blocking drugs and thyroid function. Br Med J. 1977; 4:1352.

178. Eriksson M et al: Propranolol does not prevent thyroid storm. N Engl J Med. 1977; 296:263.

179. Green M et al: Thyrotoxicosis treated by surgery or iodine[131] with special reference to development of hypothyroidism. Br Med J. 1964; 1:1005.

180. Wise PH et al: Single-dose block replace regimen in treatment hyperthyroidism. Am Heart J. 1975; 90:273.

180a. Wise PH et al: Single-dose block replace drug treatment in hyperthyroidism. Br J Med. 1973; 4:143.

181. Barnes HV et al: A simple test for selecting the thioamide schedule in thyrotoxicosis. J Clin Endocrinol Metab. 1972; 35:250.

182. Greer MA et al: Treatment of hyperthyroidism with single daily dose of PTU. N Engl J Med. 1965; 272:888.

183. Kammer H et al: Use of antithyroid drugs in a single daily dose. JAMA. 1969; 209:1325.

184. Bouma DJ et al: Single daily dose methimazole treatment of hyperthyroidism. West J Med. 1980; 132:13.

185. Vesell ES et al: Altered plasma half-lives of antipyrine, propylthiouracil, and methimazole in thyroid dysfunction. Clin Pharmacol Ther. 1975; 17:48.

186. Alexander WD et al: Thyroidal suppressibility after stopping long term treatment of thyrotoxicosis with antithyroid drugs. Metabolism. 1968; 18:58.

187. Alexander WD et al: Prediction of the long term results of antithyroid drug therapy for thyrotoxicosis. J Clin Endocrinol Metab. 1970; 30:540.

188. Cassidy CE: Use of a thyroid suppression test as a guide to prognosis of hyperthyroidism treated with antithyroid drugs. J Clin Endocrinol Metab. 1965; 25:155.

189. Yamato M et al: Thyroid suppression test and outcome of hyperthyroidism treated with antithyroid drugs and triiodothyronine. J Clin Endocrinol Metab. 1979; 48:72.

190. Solomon DH et al: Prognosis of hyperthyroidism treated by antithyroid drugs. JAMA. 1953; 152:201.

191. Hershman JM et al: Long-term outcome of hyperthyroidism treated with antithyroid drugs. J Clin Endocrinol Metab. 1966; 26:803.

192. Thalassinos NC et al: Five-year follow-up of thyrotoxicosis treated with antithyroid drugs. Endokrinologie. 1974; 63:325.

193. Wartofsky L: Low remission after therapy for Graves' disease—possible relation of dietary iodine with antithyroid therapy results. JAMA. 1973; 226:1083.

194. Reynolds LR et al: Antithyroid drugs and radioactive iodine. Fifteen years experience with Graves' disease. Arch Intern Med. 1979; 139:651.

195. Shizume K et al: Long-term results of antithyroid drug therapy for Graves' disease—follow-up for more than five years. Endocrinol Jap. 1970; 17:327.

196. Teng CS et al: Changes in thyroid—stimulating antibody activity in Graves' disease treated with antithyroid drugs and its relationship to relapse: A prospective study. J Clin Endocrinol Metab. 1980; 50:144.

197. Irvine WJ et al: Correlation of HLA and thyroid antibodies with clinical course of thyrotoxicosis treated with antithyroid drugs. Lancet. 1977; 2:898.

198. McGregor AM et al: Prediction of relapse in hyperthyroid Graves' disease. Lancet. 1980; 1:1101.

199. Alexander WD et al: Influence of iodine intake after treatment with antithyroid drugs. Lancet. 1965; 2:866.

200. Siersbaek-Nielson K et al: Low remission after long-term antithyroid treatment of Graves' disease in relation to iodine intake. Acta Endocrinol (Kbh) Supp. 1975; 199:170.

201. Goluboff LG et al: Hyperthyroidism associated with pregnancy. Obstet Gynecol. 1974; 44:107.

202. Carswell F et al: Congenital goiter and hypothyroidism produced by maternal ingestion of iodides. Lancet. 1970; 1:1241.

203. Galina MP et al: Iodide during pregnancy—an apparent cause of neonatal death. N Engl J Med. 1962; 267:1124.

204. Green H et al: Cretinism associated with maternal sodium iodide I[131] therapy during pregnancy. Am J Dis Child. 1971; 122:247.

205. Pruyn SC et al: Long-term propranolol therapy in pregnancy: maternal and fetal outcome. Am J Obstet Gynecol. 1979; 135:485.

206. Burrows GN: Maternal-fetal considerations in hyperthyroidism. Clinics Endocrinol Metab. 1978; 7:115.

207. Milham S Jr et al: Maternal methimazole and congenital defects in children. Teratology. 1972; 5:125.

208. Muytaba Q et al: Treatment hyperthyroidism in pregnancy with propylthiouracil and methimazole. Obstet Gynecol. 1975; 46:282.

209. Selenkow HA: Antithyroid-thyroid therapy of thyrotoxicosis during pregnancy. Obstet Gynecol. 1972; 40:117.

210. Bauer JH: Propranolol in human plasma and breast milk. Am J Cardiol. 1979; 43:860.

211. Becker DV et al: Complications of radioactive treatment of hyperthyroidism. Semin Nucl Med. 1971; 1:433.

212. Beierwaltes WH: The treatment of hyperthyroidism with [131]I. Semin Nucl Med. 1978; 8:95.

213. Goolder AWG et al: Treatment of thyrotoxicosis with low doses of radioactive iodine. Br Med J. 1969; 3:442.

214. Sawers JSA et al: Transient hypothyroidism after iodine-131 treatment of thyrotoxicosis. J Clin Endocrinol Metab. 1980; 50:226.

215. Macfarlane IA et al: Transient hypothyroidism after iodine-131 treatment for thyrotoxicosis. Br Med J. 1979; 2:421.

216. Dunn JT et al: Rising incidence of hypothyroidism after radioactive iodine therapy of thyrotoxicosis. N Engl J Med. 1964; 271:1037.

217. Nofal MM et al: Treatment of hyperthyroidism with sodium iodide [131]I. JAMA. 1966; 197:605.

218. Hagan GA et al: Comparison of high and low dosage levels of ^{131}I in the treatment of thyrotoxicosis. N Engl J Med. 1967; 277:559.

219. Cevallos JL et al: Low-dosage ^{131}I therapy of thyrotoxicosis (diffuse goiters). N Engl J Med. 1974; 290:141.

220. Rapoport B et al: Low-dose sodium iodide ^{131}I therapy in Graves' disease. JAMA. 1973; 224:1610.

221. Roudebush CP et al: Compensated low-dose ^{131}I therapy of Graves' disease. Ann Intern Med. 1977; 87:441.

222. Werner SC: Eye changes of Graves' disease—medical aspects. Mod Probl Ophthal. 1975; 14:409.

223. Apers RC et al: Prednisone treatment in endocrine ophthalmopathy. Mod Probl Ophthal. 1975; 14:414.

224. Rosenberg I: Thyroid storm. N Engl J Med. 1970; 283:1052.

225. Mazzaferri EL et al: Thyroid storm—a review of 22 episodes with special emphasis on the use of guanethidine. Arch Intern Med. 1969; 124:684.

226. Mackin JF et al: Thyroid storm and its management. N Engl J Med. 1974; 291:1396.

227. Dillon PT et al: Reserpine in thyrotoxic crisis. N Engl J Med. 1970; 283:1020.

228. Degroot L J et al: Dexamethasone suppression of serum T_3 and T_4. J Clin Endocrinol Metab. 1976; 42:976.

229. Duick DS et al: Effect of single-dose dexamethasone on the concentration of serum triiodothyroxine in man. J Clin Endocrinol Metab. 1974; 39:1151.

230. Williams DE et al: Acute effects of corticosteroids on thyroid activity in Graves' disease. J Clin Endocrinol Metab. 1975; 41:354.

231. Spaulding SW et al: The inhibiting effect of lithium on thyroid hormone release in both euthyroid and thyrotoxic patients. J Clin Endocrinol Metab. 1972; 35:905.

232. Temple R et al: The use of lithium in Graves' disease. Mayo Clin Proc. 1971; 47:872.

233. Temple R et al: The use of lithium in the treatment of thyrotoxicosis. J Clin Invest. 1972; 51:2746.

234. Lauridsen UB et al: Lithium and the pituitary—thyroid axis in normal subjects. J Clin Endocrinol Metab. 1974; 39:383.

235. Burrow GN et al: Effect of lithium on thyroid function. J Clin Endocrinol Metab. 1971; 32:647.

236. Candy J: Severe hypothyroidism—an early complication of lithium therapy. Br Med J. 1972; 3:277.

237. Luby ED et al: Lithium carbonate-induced myxedema. JAMA. 1971; 218:1298.

238. Rogers MP et al: Clinical hypothyroidism occurring during lithium treatment—two case histories and a review of thyroid function in 19 patients. Am J Psych. 1971; 128:158.

239. Shopsin B: Effect of lithium on thyroid function. Dis Ner Syst. 1970; 31:237.

240. Schou M et al: Occurrence of goiter during lithium treatment. Br Med J. 1968; 3:710.

241. Prange AJ Jr et al: Enhancement of imipramine by thyroid stimulating hormone—clinical and theoretical implications. Am J Psych. 1970; 127:191.

242. Prange AJ Jr et al: Enhancement of imipramine antidepressant activity by thyroid hormone. Am J Psych. 1969; 126:457.

243. Bafaqueen HH et al: Lithium and thyrotoxicosis. Lancet. 1976; 1:1409.

244. Cubitt T; Lithium and thyrotoxicosis. Lancet. 1976; 1:1247.

245. Rosser R: Thyrotoxicosis and lithium. Br J Psychiat. 1976; 128:61.

246. Kristensen O et al: Lithium carbonate in the treatment of thyrotoxicosis. Lancet. 1976; 1:603.

247. Lazarus JH et al: Treatment of thyrotoxicosis with lithium carbonate. Lancet. 1974; 2:1160.

248. Gershengorn MC et al: Use of lithium as an adjunct to radioiodine therapy of thyroid carcinoma. J Clin Endocrinol Metab. 1976; 42:105.

249. Turner JG et al: Lithium as an adjunct to radioiodine therapy for thyrotoxicosis. Lancet. 1976; 1:614.

250. Erman AM et al: Modification of thyroid function induced by chronic administration of I_2—in presence of autonomous thyroid tissue. Acta Endocrinol. 1972; 70:463.

251. Connolly RJ et al: Increase in thyrotoxicosis in endemic goiter area after iodination of bread. Lancet. 1970; 1:500.

252. Stewart JC et al: Thyrotoxicosis induced by iodine contamination of food—a common unrecognized condition. Br Med J. 1976; 1:372.

253. Vidor GI et al: Pathogenesis of iodine induced thyrotoxicosis—studies in northern Tasmania. J Clin Endocrinol Metab. 1973; 37:901.

254. Ahmed M et al: Triiodothyroxine thyrotoxicosis following iodide ingestion. J Clin Endocrinol Metab. 1974; 38:574.

255. Nilsson G: Self-limiting episodes of JODBASEDOW. Acta Endocrinologia. 1973; 74:475.

256. Blum M et al: Hyperthyroidism after iodinated contrast medium. N Engl J Med. 1974; 291:24.

257. Silas AM et al: Hyperthyroidism after use of contrast medium. Br Med J. 1975; 4:162.

258. Fairhurst BJ et al: Hyperthyroidism after cholecystography. Br Med J. 1975; 3:630.

259. Savoie JC et al: Iodine-induced thyrotoxicosis in apparently normal thyroid glands. J Clin Endocrinol Metab. 1975; 41:685.

260. Skinner NS Jr et al: Studies on the use of chlorpropamide in patients with diabetes mellitus. Ann N Y Acad Sci. 1959; 74:830.

261. Hunton RB et al: Hypothyroidism in diabetics treated with sulfonylurea. Lancet. 1965; 2:449.

262. Degroot L J et al: Thyroid carcinoma and radiation—a Chicago epidemic. JAMA. 1973; 225:487.

263. Horst W et al: 306 cases of toxic adenoma—clinical aspects findings in radioiodine diagnostics radiochromatography and history—results of I^{131} and surgical treatments. J Nucl Med. 1967; 8:515.

264. Greenspan FS: Thyroid nodules and thyroid cancer. West J Med. 1974; 121:359.

265. Messaris G et al: Incidence of carcinoma in cold nodules of the thyroid gland. Surgery. 1973; 74:447.

266. Refetoff S et al: Continuing occurrence of thyroid carcinoma after irradiation to the neck in infancy and childhood. N Engl J Med. 1975; 292:171.

267. Wright HK et al: Current therapy of thyroid nodules. Surg Clin North Am. 1974; 54:277.

268. Lyon LJ et al: Reversal of alcoholic coma by naloxone. Ann Intern Med. 1982; 96:464.

269. Cheron RG et al: Neonatal thyroid function after propylthiouracil therapy for maternal Graves' disease. N Engl J Med. 1981; 304:525.

270. Solomon DH: Pregnancy and PTU. N Engl J Med. 1981; 304:538.

271. Rosenbaum RL et al: Levothyroxine replacement doses for primary hypothyroidism decreases with age. Am Intern Med. 1982; 96:53.

Chapter 56

Diabetes Mellitus

Mary Anne Koda-Kimble and Michael D. Rotblatt

DEFINITION AND CLASSIFICATION

Diabetes is a term which is used to describe a metabolic syndrome characterized by symptomatic glucose intolerance. There is a considerable amount of evidence to support the notion that, clinically and genetically, diabetes is a heterogeneous group of disorders (1–8).

It is currently estimated that there are 4 to 5 million diabetics in the United States of whom approximately ⅓ are males and ⅔ are females. By the year 2000, it is estimated that there will be 20 million diabetics in the United States. This prediction is based on the observation that approximately 600,000 new cases of diabetes are diagnosed annually and that 50,000 to 100,000 diabetics die each year (2).

On the basis of new information relating to the pathogenesis of diabetes and the plethora of terminology used to characterize diabetic subjects in the literature, the American Diabetes Association rejected its former classification of diabetes based upon age of onset (ie, juvenile-onset diabetes and adult-onset diabetes) in favor of a new classification suggested by the National Diabetes Data Group (8). Because the precise pathophysiologic mechanisms remain poorly understood, this group recommended a classification based primarily on clinical presentation.

Type I Diabetes (IDDM)

Approximately 5–10% of the diabetic population has Type I diabetes (Insulin Dependent Diabetes Mellitus—IDDM). These patients have no pancreatic reserve, have a tendency to develop ketoacidosis and are dependent upon exogenous insulin to sustain life. The onset of the disease may occur over 1–2 months or abruptly over a few days (4). The mean age of onset is 12 years, although it is also observed in adults. This form of diabetes is closely associated with certain histocompatibility antigens (HLA) on the sixth chromosome (B8, Bw15, Dw3, Dw4) and the presence of circulating islet cell antibodies early in the disease. It has been postulated that in genetically predisposed individuals, autoimmune destruction of the islet cells is triggered by viruses, chemicals and other unknown environmental factors. There is growing evidence that further genetic heterogeneity exists within IDDM (3–5,8).

Within days or weeks following the initial diagnosis, many Type I diabetics experience an apparent remission or alleviation of their hyperglycemia which is reflected in markedly decreased insulin requirements. This is called the "honeymoon" period because it only lasts for a few months. During this period, patients should be maintained on insulin even if the dose is very low, since interrupted treatment is associated with a greater incidence of resistance and allergy to insulin. See Question 20.

Type II Diabetes (NIDDM)

Type II diabetics comprise approximately 90% of the diabetic population. Also known as Non-Insulin Dependent Diabetes Mellitus (NIDDM), it is characterized by the presence of endogenous insulin, an absence of ketosis, an absence of circulating islet cell antibodies and a lack of association with certain histocompatibility antigens. Unlike IDDM, symptoms are relatively mild and gradual in onset and are generally easily controlled with diet, oral sulfonylureas or insulin. The diagnosis is generally made after the age of 40, but can occur during childhood and young adulthood as discussed below. There is also a stronger family history of diabetes in this group of diabetics than in Type I, insulin dependent diabetics.

Like IDDM, there is a growing body of evidence which suggests that this class of diabetes includes a heterogeneous group of disorders. For example, diabetics classified as Type II may release high (insulinplethoric), low (insulinopenic), or normal amounts of insulin in response to a glucose challenge and exhibit varying degrees of tissue insulin resistance. They may also exhibit altered or delayed patterns of insulin release characterized by an absence of the initial rapid release of insulin in response to glucose. Subclassifications of these patients have been suggested based upon weight (1,5,8), age of onset (9–11), insulin levels (7,10,11), and the presence or absence of a chlorpropamide-alcohol flush (CPAF) (12,13). Karam (1) and the National Data Group (8) suggest a division of this class of diabetics based on weight.

Non-obese NIDDM. Approximately 10% of the diabetic population are non-obese, Type II diabetics. These individuals generally have low insulin levels in response to glucose (1,10,11), although this is not always the case (9–11). Included in this group are the *Maturity Onset Diabetes of the Young (MODY)* or *"Mason-Type" diabetics* who develop a mild form of diabetes during childhood, adolescence or as young adults (usually less than 25 years of age). This form of diabetes is associated with a strong family history which suggests autosomal dominant transmission. Unlike Type I diabetes, the disease is generally mild and controlled over long periods of time (20-year follow-ups) with diet and oral agents (9–11). A few of these individuals may be treated with insulin but there is no history of ketosis. Some investigators have observed that this form of diabetes appears to be associated with a low incidence of diabetic complications (10,14), but this has not been a consistent finding (11). Others have suggested that the presence of a chlorpropamide-alcohol flush (see Questions 30–32) may serve as a genetic marker for this type of diabetes (12,13) and that this form of diabetes may not be limited to NIDDMs who develop diabetes at a relatively young age (13). The prevalence of MODY is unknown, but many investigators suspect that it may be more common than once thought since many individuals with this form of diabetes may have been diagnosed as having juvenile onset or Type I diabetes based upon age of onset. A mild form of the disease which is easily controlled, together with a lack of history of ketoacidosis and a strong family history of diabetes, is strongly suggestive of MODY.

Obese NIDDM. Obese non-insulin dependent diabetics constitute the majority of the diabetic population and 60–90% of the Type II diabetics (9). The predominant defect in these individuals appears to be tissue resistance to the effect of insulin as reflected by high levels of insulin in response to a glucose challenge. Theoretically, overeating stimulates the secretion of large amounts of insulin which in turn "down regulate" or decrease the number of insulin receptors on the cellular surface of the target organ. In addition, high insulin levels promote lipogenesis and the production of distended adipocytes which have fewer insulin receptors per cell surface area. Thus, the obese diabetic is the product of a vicious cycle which may be broken through decreased caloric intake and weight loss (1,2,8).

Others have suggested that the model of hyperalimentation → hyperinsulinism → down-regulation of insulin receptors → insulin resistance may account for the decreased glucose tolerance in Type II diabetics with mild postprandial hyperglycemia. However, in more severe Type II diabetics with fasting plasma glucose levels ≥ 200 mg/dl, a postreceptor defect as a cause of insulin resistance in combination with inadequate insulin responses to glucose may predominate as underlying causes of glucose intolerance (15–18). In other words, these two patterns—(1.) high insulin levels in combination with low numbers of insulin receptors and (2.) low insulin levels in combination with post-receptor insulin resistance—may be a continuum of a common underlying defect or two heterogeneous disorders (17).

A low calorie diet and a program of physical exercise are the primary forms of therapy for obese, Type II diabetics. In patients who are symptomatic, oral hypoglycemic agents or insulin are used. See Questions 23, 26–28.

CARBOHYDRATE METABOLISM

An understanding of the signs and symptoms associated with diabetes is based upon a knowledge of the multiple metabolic effects of insulin as well as glucose metabolism and homeostasis in diabetic and nondiabetic subjects during the fed (postprandial) and fasting states.

The homeostatic mechanisms in the body are aimed at maintaining a blood glucose concentration within a range of 40–160 mg/dl. A minimum concentration of 40 mg/dl is required to provide adequate fuel for the brain which is heavily reliant on glucose as an energy source and is not dependent upon the presence of insulin for its utilization. When blood glucose concentrations exceed the reabsorptive capacity of the kidneys (approximately 180 mg/dl), glucose spills into the urine, resulting in energy and water loss. Muscle and fat also use glucose as a major energy source but require the presence of insulin. If glucose is not available, these tissues are able to use other substrates such as amino acids and fatty acids for fuel.

Postprandial Glucose Metabolism in the Nondiabetic (Fig. 1)

Following the ingestion of food, blood glucose concentrations rise and stimulate the release of insulin. Insulin is key to efficient glucose utilization. It promotes the uptake of glucose, fatty acids and amino acids and their conversion to storage forms in most tissues. As a result, it also decreases the blood sugar so that none will be unnecessarily wasted in the urine. In muscle, insulin promotes the uptake of glucose and its storage as glycogen (A). It also stimulates the uptake of amino acids and their conversion to protein (B). In adipose tissue, glucose is converted to free fatty acids and stored as triglycerides (C). The presence of insulin also prevents the breakdown of these triglycerides to free fatty acids, a form which may be transported to other tissues for utilization (D). The liver does not require insulin for glucose transport, but the presence of insulin does facilitate the conversion of glucose to glycogen (E). Glycogenolysis (the breakdown of liver glycogen) is the major source of glucose during the fasting state.

Fasting Glucose Metabolism in the Nondiabetic (Fig 1.)

In the fasting individual, hypoglycemia inhibits the release of insulin. Additionally, a number of hormones (eg, glucagon, epinephrine, growth hormone, and glucocorticoids) are released which oppose the effect of insulin and promote an increase in blood sugar. As a result of this lack of insulin, several processes occur which maintain and conserve a minimum blood glucose level for the central nervous system. Glycogen in the liver is broken down to glucose (glycogenolysis) (F); amino acids are converted to glucose through gluconeogenesis (G); there is a diminished uptake of glucose by insulin dependent tissues to conserve glucose for the brain; and finally, triglycerides are broken down to free fatty acids which are used as fuel by those tissues (primarily muscle and fat) which are unable to use glucose in the absence of insulin.

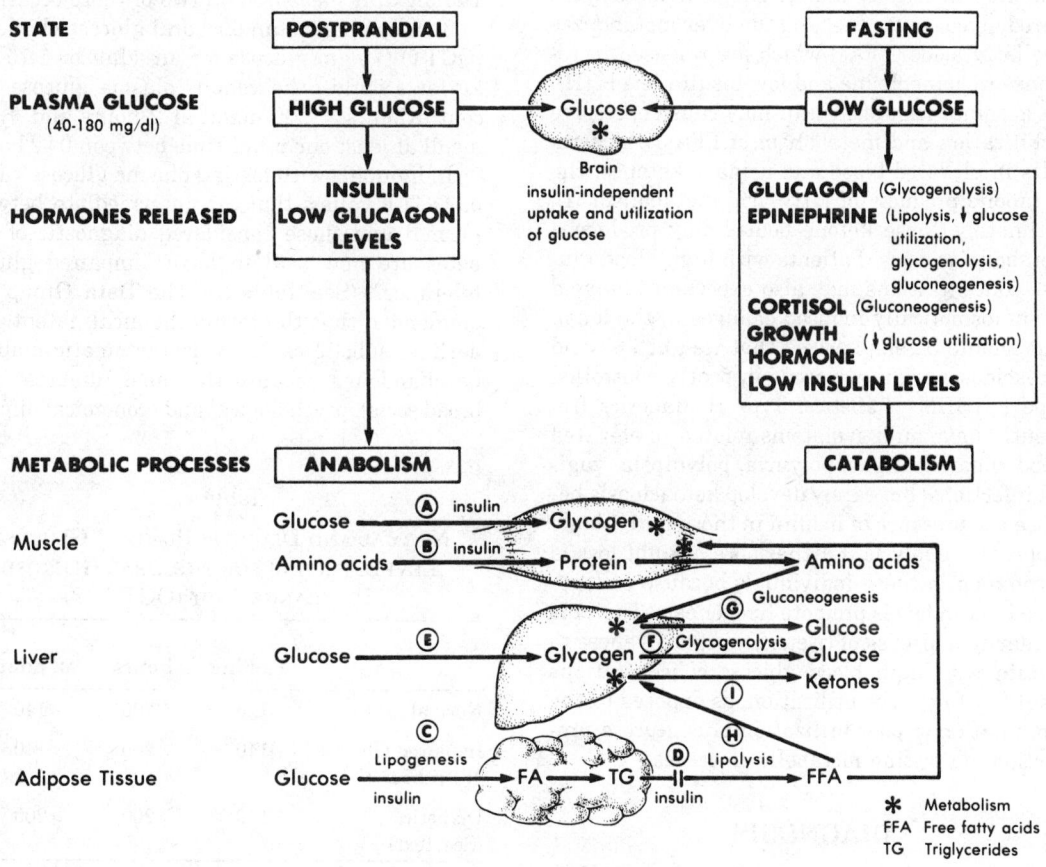

Figure 1. Glucose Metabolism.

SIGNS AND SYMPTOMS

In a diabetic, blood glucose concentrations remain high after a meal because the uptake, utilization and storage of glucose by adipose tissue and muscle are diminished secondary to an absence of insulin or tissue resistance to insulin's effects. Because glucose is inaccessible to the cells (even though glucose concentrations are high), fasting metabolism which further increases the plasma glucose concentrations through glycogenolysis and gluconeogenesis is triggered. If glucose concentrations exceed the renal threshold, glucose spills into the urine, taking water with it by the process of osmotic diuresis. As a result of the loss of calories and water, patients experience symptoms of polyuria, polydipsia, fatigue and weight loss despite normal or excessive food intake. Since high glucose levels provide an excellent medium for bacterial growth, diabetics may also present with recurrent respiratory, vaginal and other infections. Muscle begins to metabolize stored glycogen for fuel and the liver metabolizes free fatty acids (FFAs) which are released in response to epinephrine and low insulin levels (H). An absolute lack of insulin may cause excessive mobilization and metabolism of FFAs which results in elevated blood and urinary ketones, the metabolic products of fatty acid metabolism (I). Ultimately, these ketone bodies may produce a metabolic acidosis. Patients with high blood glucose concentrations may also experience blurred vision (osmotically-induced changes in the lens).

It should be emphasized that weight loss and ketoacidosis primarily occur in poorly controlled Type I (IDDM) diabetics. Type II diabetics frequently have mild symptoms related to elevated blood sugars (fatigue, polyuria, polydipsia, vaginal infections) but rarely develop ketoacidosis because the presence of insulin in these individuals suppresses lipolysis. Furthermore, weight loss is uncommon in these individuals because endogenous insulin levels promote lipogenesis. Theirs is primarily a disease of tissue unresponsiveness to insulin with high blood glucose concentrations resulting from poor utilization, as opposed to the combination of poor utilization plus glucose production via fasting metabolic processes.

DIAGNOSIS

The diagnosis of diabetes is relatively simple in those individuals who present with the clas-sical signs and symptoms of diabetes in association with unequivocal hyperglycemia (≥ 200 mg/dl). The diagnosis is more confusing in those individuals who are asymptomatic but have glycosuria or hyperglycemia on routine examination. The interpretation of oral glucose tolerance tests (OGTT) in these individuals has varied from clinician to clinician based upon which of the numerous criteria for normal vs abnormal were accepted. In view of this confusion, the National Diabetes Data Group (8) developed criteria for the diagnosis of diabetes which have been adopted by the American Diabetes Association. See Table 1. For nonpregnant individuals of any age, a diagnosis of diabetes can be made if:

1. the patient presents with the classical signs and symptoms of diabetes (polyuria, polydipsia, ketonuria, rapid weight loss) and has an unequivocally high fasting (≥ 140 mg/dl) or random (≥ 200 mg/dl) venous plasma glucose concentration.

2. a fasting plasma concentration of ≥ 140 mg/dl is measured on two or more occasions.

3. following a standard oral glucose challenge (OGTT) (75 gm glucose for an adult or 1.75 gm/kg for a child), the venous plasma glucose concentration is ≥ 200 mg/dl at 2 hours and ≥ 200 mg/dl at least one other time between 0–2 hours.

Individuals with fasting plasma glucose values or OGTT values that are intermediate between normal and those considered diagnostic of diabetes are now said to have "impaired glucose tolerance." (See Table 1.) The Data Group recommended that the terms chemical, latent, borderline, subclinical, and asymptomatic diabetes be abandoned because the label "diabetes" has broad social, psychological and economical impacts.

Table 1.

NORMAL AND DIABETIC PLASMA* GLUCOSE
LEVELS (MG/DL) FOR THE ORAL GLUCOSE
TOLERANCE TEST (OGTT) (8)

	Fasting	½, 1, 1½ hours	2 hours
Normal	<115	<200	<140
Impaired Glucose Tolerance	<140	≥200	140–200
Diabetic (See Text)	≥140	≥200	≥200

*Equivalent capillary or *blood* glucose concentrations are approximately 10% less.

Numerous factors, including infections, pregnancies and other forms of stress, metabolic imbalances, lack of physical activity, diet and drugs (see Tables 16 and 17) may impair glucose tolerance or increase plasma glucose, and these must be eliminated as a source of abnormal results before a firm diagnosis of diabetes is made (see ref 8 for an extensive list of these factors). For example, an individual who has not fasted for a minimum of 10 hours may have an elevated fasting plasma glucose; one who has fasted too long (> 16 hours) or has not ingested sufficient carbohydrate prior to testing may have an impaired glucose tolerance. Patients who are tested for glucose tolerance during or soon after an acute illness such as a myocardial infarction, when glucose counterregulatory hormone levels are high, are often diagnosed as diabetic. Subsequent to this acute stimulus, glucose tolerance returns to normal and the patient becomes asymptomatic. The Data Group recommends that these individuals be classified as having a "previous abnormality of glucose tolerance" (8). Numerous drugs may alter glucose tolerance through their effects on insulin release, tissue response to insulin and through direct cytotoxic effects on the pancreas. These are discussed in more detail in Questions 45–52 and Tables 16 and 17. Drugs and other chemicals may also falsely elevate plasma glucose levels through interference with specific analytical methods (8).

Other tests in addition to the plasma glucose concentrations may be abnormal in the diabetic, but they are not necessarily diagnostic. These include elevated serum triglycerides and ketones; the presence of glucose and ketones in the urine; elevated glycosylated hemoglobin; and high, low or normal insulin and C-peptide levels. Some of these are discussed below and others are discussed in the introductory section on monitoring.

Urine Glucose. The presence or absence of glycosuria may be used as a screening method for the detection of diabetes (19), but its presence is not diagnostic because glycosuria may occur when the renal threshold for glucose is decreased (eg, pregnancy) or when there are other sugars and interfering substances in the urine. See Table 14 for a list of drugs which cause false positive tests for glycosuria. The use of urine glucose as a monitoring tool for diabetics is discussed later in this introduction and in Questions 6–8, 24, 25.

Glycosylated Hemoglobin (Hb A_{1c}). Also see section on monitoring methods later in this introduction for a more complete discussion of Hb A_{1c}. Glycosylated hemoglobin levels generally reflect the mean blood glucose concentrations over 4–6 weeks and are almost always elevated in diabetics; however, preliminary data indicate that elevated glycosylated hemoglobin levels are not as sensitive as the OGTT in detecting individuals with impaired glucose tolerance. A major reason why glycosylated hemoglobin levels cannot be used as a criterion for diagnosing diabetes at this time is that there is little standardization of the testing procedure from one laboratory to the next and therefore "normal" values vary with the institution. Eventually, Hb A_{1c} assays may be used for the screening and diagnosis of diabetics (22–24).

Insulin Levels. Immunoreactive insulin concentrations which are measured *before* a patient receives insulin may be useful in determining whether the symptoms of diabetes are primarily related to insulin deficiency or tissue resistance. Normal fasting insulin concentrations are 10–25 μU/ml. They range from 50–130 μU/ml 1 hour after a standard glucose challenge and return to concentrations of ≤ 100 μU/ml after 2 hours. Concentrations of < 50 μU/ml at 1 hour and < 100 μU at 2 hours in the presence of elevated plasma glucose concentrations strongly suggest insulinopenia. Conversely, concentrations much greater than 100 μU/ml under these same circumstances suggest hyperinsulinemia and tissue resistance. The absence of insulin even in response to a stimulus such as IV tolbutamide is consistent with Type I diabetes. Immunoreactive insulin concentrations cannot be accurately interpreted in patients who have received exogenous insulin because insulin antibodies develop in virtually all of these patients. The measurement of insulin concentrations remains experimental at this time and is primarily used in the context of research (1).

C-Peptide Levels. Proinsulin is cleaved in the β cells of the pancreas to form equimolar amounts of C-peptide and insulin. The measurement of C-peptide is not confounded by the administration of exogenous insulin; its presence reflects the presence of endogenous insulin and, therefore, a functioning pancreas. C-peptide concentrations have been used to diagnose insulinomas (high C-peptide despite attempted suppression with exogenous insulin); hypoglycemia secondary to the surreptitious administration of exogenous insulin (low C-peptide concentrations in the presence of high insulin concentrations and hypoglycemia);

and non-insulin dependent diabetics who are being treated with exogenous insulin. However, the measurement of C-peptide is technically complex and its primary value is in clinical research where it is used to follow β cell function in diabetic subjects (25).

LONG-TERM COMPLICATIONS

Long-term sequelae account for the majority of the morbidity and mortality in the diabetic population (26). In one study, 56% of the diabetic population had died 40 years after diabetes had been diagnosed as compared to a 10% mortality in a nondiabetic control group. Approximately 33% died of uremia and 25% died of a cardiovascular complication. Diabetes is also the leading cause of new blindness in the United States.

Currently there is considerable debate regarding the relationship of hyperglycemia per se to the pathogenesis of these complications; nevertheless, most diabetologists acknowledge that the prevalence of at least some of these complications correlates with the duration of disease and the degree of glycemic control (27,28). In Type I diabetics, long-term complications are rarely observed in individuals who have had the disease for less than ten years (26); however, by the third decade of the disease, 50–70% have complications of varying degrees of severity. It has been estimated that clinically important complications are present in 20–40% of Type I diabetics (29,30).

At the present time, it is impossible to predict which diabetics will develop long-term complications. Some Type I and Type II diabetics progress through the disease for 30–40 years without major complications while others proceed through an apparently inexorable course of widespread sequelae (31). This observation is further evidence of the heterogeneous nature of the disease and has led to the theory that a predisposition to these complications may be genetically linked (but not consistently) to diabetes (31). It is also unlikely that a single pathogenic event underlies the development of all diabetic complications, although widespread irreversible glycosylation of proteins, similar to that which is observed in Hb A_{1c}, has been postulated as that event (32). Neuropathy, macrovascular and microvascular disease, and chronic hyperglycemia account for the majority of diabetic complications discussed below.

Cardiovascular Disease. Although the pathogenesis of cardiovascular disease does not differ in diabetics, these individuals do appear to have a more widespread and rapid progression of this disease as well as a greater disposition to hypertension, congestive heart failure and perhaps coronary artery disease (33). One prospective study showed that 55% of diabetics were hypertensive (34). Another showed that diabetic men are two times more likely to develop atherosclerotic disease when compared with nondiabetic men matched for age and presence of other risk factors (35). Diabetes affects young and premenopausal women to an even greater extent; these women have 3–4 times the risk of developing cardiovascular disease when compared to their nondiabetic counterparts (35). This increased prevalence of macrovascular disease is reflected in the mortality rates caused by this disease. In the North American population generally, 33% will die of atherosclerotic disease. In contrast, it has been estimated that 75% of North American diabetics will die of atherosclerotic disease, making it the major cause of death in this population (26,36). These sobering figures point to the importance of minimizing or eliminating all other preventable risk factors for cardiovascular disease in diabetics such as smoking, hypertension, hyperlipidemias, and obesity through the prescription of exercise, diet, and appropriate medications.

Peripheral Vascular Disease. Peripheral vascular disease in the diabetic is an extension of the atherosclerotic process and to some extent is also the result of microvascular disease and neuropathy found in these individuals. Clinically, it presents as an absence of pulses, coolness in one extremity but not the other and, in its worst form, gangrene or slow healing skin ulcerations which may ultimately lead to systemic infection or amputation. Prevention through proper foot care is the primary focus of treatment (1). The possible prophylactic role of antiplatelet agents such as salicylates is currently under evaluation (Question 53).

Ocular Complications. Diabetics may experience refractive changes associated with poor diabetic control. They may also develop senile-type cataracts early in age and a type of glaucoma which is relatively resistant to treatment. The most common ocular complication, however, is diabetic retinopathy which usually appears after 15–20 years and may occur in up to 80% of diabetics (37). Microvascular disease characterized by thickening of the capillary membrane may be the underlying lesion for two forms of retinopathy. The first and most common presentation is a background retinopathy characterized by microaneurisms which may progress to hard, yellow exudates signifying chronic leakage; retinal edema; and punctate hemorrhage. "Cotton wool" patches may appear and subside over a period of several weeks. This form of retinopathy may be associated with loss of central vision but is generally associated with an excellent visual prognosis (2,38,39).

Proliferative retinopathy which is characterized by neovascularization (presumably due to retinal hypoxia) is much rarer, but is, nevertheless, the leading major cause of new blindness in the United States (40). Neovascularization ultimately leads to fibrosis, adhesions, vitreous hemorrhage and retinal detachment (2,38,39). Recent evidence suggests that photocoagulation therapy may arrest progression and decrease loss of vision associated with neovascularization (39,40). Since hypertension (37,41,42), smoking (41), uremia (41) and, perhaps, hyperglycemia (42) predispose diabetics to more rapid progression of retinopathy, every effort should be made to treat these disorders vigorously. Men (42) and non-white women (41) may also be at greater risk for proliferative retinopathy.

Nephropathy. End-stage renal disease characterized by nephrotic syndrome and azotemia is a major cause of death in Type I diabetics. Diabetic glomerulosclerosis caused by thickening of capillary basement membranes is first signaled by proteinuria which generally has an onset 10–15 years after the diagnosis of diabetes (2,43). Approximately 40% of juvenile onset diabetics who survived for 40 years had some evidence of renal disease (44). Treatment consists of early detection through annual urinalysis for protein, correction of existing hypertension, and low sodium diets. The management of end stage renal disease is discussed elsewhere (44,45) and in the Kidney Diseases chapter of this text. The management of diabetes in a patient with renal disease is considered in Questions 21 and 38.

Neuropathy. Neuropathy, which may be a consequence of metabolic disturbances in the neurons or secondary to microangiopathy affecting capillaries supplying the neurons, is a common complication of diabetes. Clinically, the neuropathy presents as a peripheral neuritis or autonomic insufficiency. Symptomatic peripheral neuropathy may occur in 25% of diabetics and is characterized by paresthesias and pain in the lower extremities which may be mild or severe and unrelenting; decreased vibration sense; decreased ankle and knee jerks; and decreased conduction velocity. The decreased sensation associated with peripheral neuropathy contributes to the progression of foot injuries and infections which may go unnoticed by the patient until they are severe (1,45). The treatment of painful peripheral neuropathy is considered in Questions 40–41.

Autonomic neuropathy may present as gastroparesis with a feeling of fullness and nausea (see Question 42); urinary retention; impotence in males (manifested as retrograde ejaculation or an inability to attain an erection); and, rarely, postural hypotension, diarrhea (nocturnal; incontinence), and other signs and symptoms characteristic of a lumbar sympathectomy. The presence of autonomic insufficiency may have profound effects on the diabetic's reaction to drugs such as nitroglycerin and various antihypertensives. These are considered throughout the chapter (1,46).

TREATMENT

There are three major components to the treatment of diabetes: diet; drugs (insulin and oral hypoglycemic agents); and exercise. Each of these components interacts with the other to the extent that no assessment and modification of one can be made without a knowledge of the other two.

Diet

Diet plays a primary and crucial role in the therapy of all diabetics. In 1979, the American Diabetes Association modified its recommendations for a diabetic diet to reflect new knowledge relating to nutrition generally and to the effect of diet on cardiovascular disease (48). The goals of a diabetic diet are:

1. To provide adequate calories to maintain normal growth and development of a young diabetic and ideal body weight in other diabetics. For obese, Type II diabetics this generally means a calorie restricted diet.

2. To provide adequate carbohydrates for exogenously administered insulin. Regularly scheduled meals and snacks which provide consistent amounts of carbohydrate, protein and fat are essential to the prevention of hypoglycemic reactions in insulin dependent diabetics.

3. To minimize acute excursions in blood glucose levels through the restriction of simple sugars (glucose, sucrose, lactose). The inclusion of complex carbohydrates and high fiber carbohydrates is not discouraged in that these food sources provide 50–60% of the caloric intake. Chronic low-calorie, low-carbohydrate diets (< 80 gm/day) should be discouraged, especially in Type I diabetics, since they may lead to ketosis.

4. To minimize dietary contributions to cardiovascular disease by restricting the intake of saturated fats to 10% of the total calories and encouraging patients to decrease their sodium intake. Ten percent of the caloric intake may be provided by polyunsaturated fats.

5. To provide adequate protein (12–20%) to assure adequate growth and nutrition. The amount of protein provided depends on the nutritional state of the patient. For example, the protein content may be liberalized for pregnant women and children and restricted in patients with uremia or hepatic encephalopathy.

Other dietary recommendations which have been made relate to the use of artificial sweeteners, foods high in fiber, and alcohol.

Artificial Sweeteners. When the FDA was considering banning saccharin because of evidence linking this artificial sweetener to bladder cancer in rats, the ADA took the official stand that such sweeteners should be used "prudently" in young children and pregnant women, but that the benefits of their use outweighed the risks in diabetics and obese persons who had the need to include sweet foods in their diets (49). Fructose, xylitol, mannitol and sorbitol are caloric sweeteners used in many "dietetic" foods. Although some of these sugars are metabolized to glucose, they do produce less postprandial hyperglycemia than glucose in individuals who are not severely insulin deficient (50) and moderate use of these sweeteners will probably have little effect on diabetic control. However, they are caloric and therefore have no value in low-calorie diets; furthermore, the excessive intake of sorbitol sweetened foods (30–50 gm/day) may produce an osmotically-induced diarrhea (50). Because the long-term effects of these agents on diabetes is not well-studied, the ADA neither accepts or rejects their use (48). A new artificial, noncaloric sweetener, aspartane, which apparently has no unpleasant aftertaste may become the artificial sweetener most used by diabetics in the near future.

Fiber. High fiber diets are recommended by some clinicians on the basis that fiber slows the absorption of carbohydrates and minimizes blood glucose excursions postprandially. The ADA encourages the substitution of unrefined carbohydrates with fiber for refined carbohydrates when this is acceptable to the patient (48,51).

Alcohol. The ADA does not prohibit the inclusion of small amounts of alcohol in the diabetic diet, although the caloric contribution to diet must be considered. See Question 54.

Finally, the ADA stressed the importance of patient education regarding fundamental nutritional concepts and emphasized the need for flexibility and choice within a diabetic's diet. They even acknowledge that, for some patients, the adjustment of insulin dose may be preferable to alteration of the dietary plan (48).

Exercise

In the nondiabetic, a variety of homeostatic mechanisms maintain plasma glucose within a normal range. In the fasting state, muscle primarily utilizes FFA for fuel; however, with exercise there is increased utilization of glucose which is provided initially from the breakdown of muscle glycogen and subsequently from hepatic glycogenolysis and gluconeogenesis. These effects are mediated through suppression of insulin secretion and the release of norepinephrine, epinephrine, growth hormone, cortisol and glucagon. In insulin dependent diabetics, hyperglycemia, normoglycemia or hypoglycemia can occur secondary to exercise depending on the degree of control, recent administration of insulin, and food intake (See Question 22). In the non-insulin dependent diabetic, there is generally a decrease in the plasma glucose concentration, although symptomatic hypoglycemia is uncommon. With the knowledge that diabetics are predisposed to cardiovascular disease, along with the renewed interest of Americans in physical exercise, more attention has been paid to the metabolic response to exercise in the diabetic patient. In general, moderate, regular exercise is highly recommended for non-insulin dependent diabetics and encouraged in insulin dependent diabetics if special precautions are taken (See Question 22). Exercise in the latter group must be tempered by increased food intake, delayed administration of insulin, a decreased dose of insulin, or a combination of these maneuvers (53,54).

Drugs

Insulin, along with diet, is crucial to the survival of Type I, insulin dependent diabetics and plays a major role in the therapy of Type II diabetics when their symptoms cannot be controlled with diet alone or together with oral antidiabetic agents. It is also used in Type II diabetics during periods of intercurrent illness or stress (eg, surgery or pregnancy). The use of oral sulfonylureas is reserved for the treatment of symptomatic Type II diabetics whose symptoms cannot be controlled with diet and exercise alone. The clinical use of these agents and the complications associated with their use are discussed in the pages which follow.

Overall Goals of Therapy

For each therapeutic modality there is considerable debate with regard to specific therapeutic endpoints, which vary with the different viewpoints on diabetic control and the methods used to monitor diabetic therapy (ie, urine glucose, blood glucose, Hb A_{1c}). These will be discussed in appropriate sections of this chapter. However, there are some overall goals with which most all diabetologists agree. Since there is presently no cure for diabetes, the overall goals of therapy are:

1. Try to keep the patient free of symptoms relating to hyperglycemia (polyuria, polydipsia, weight loss, fatigue, recurrent infection, ketoacidosis) or hypoglycemia.

2. Try to maintain the patient as close to euglycemia as possible without exposing him/her to undue risk for hypoglycemia. This effort at maintaining euglycemia is aimed toward slowing the progression of the chronic complications associated with diabetes.

3. In children, normal growth and development should be attained.

4. Try to integrate the patient into the health care team through intensive education. Many studies have demonstrated that the diabetic patient's knowledge and understanding of his disease can have a tremendous positive influence on diabetic control.

METHODS OF MONITORING GLYCEMIC CONTROL

In addition to monitoring signs and symptoms associated with hyperglycemia, hypoglycemia, and long-term complications of diabetes, several chemical measurements may be used by the patient and clinician to directly or indirectly assess glycemic control.

Urine Glucose Tests

Correlation with Plasma Glucose. Urine glucose concentrations indirectly reflect blood glucose levels and rely on normal renal thresholds for glucose, complete bladder emptying, and accurate testing of an appropriate urine sample. Changes in urine glucose lag behind changes in blood glucose and the testing methods used are at best semi-quantitative. Figure 2 (55) clearly illustrates the poor correlation between urine glucose test results and simultaneous measurements of plasma glucose concentrations which has been confirmed by numerous investigators (56–58). Of note is that in patients with normal renal thresholds for glucose, a "negative" reading for urine glucose may correspond to a blood glucose ranging from hypoglycemia ($\leq$ 60 mg/dl) to hyperglycemia (180 mg/dl). In patients with elevated thresholds for glucose (such as the elderly), this range becomes an even more significant problem in interpreting urine test results.

Indications. Diabetic control is more accurately reflected and affected by blood glucose monitoring. However, home blood glucose monitoring is relatively new and may not be acceptable to many patients or clinicians. Accurate monitoring is not critical for some patients (mainly non-insulin dependent diabetics who are well controlled) and many others simply cannot or will not utilize the more invasive blood glucose monitoring techniques (especially the very young or elderly). For these diabetics, urine glucose testing is a convenient, practical, inexpensive and painless (albeit less accurate) means to monitor diabetic control.

Comparison of Methods. The two methods of testing for urine glucose are the glucose oxidase method (Diastix, Tes-Tape, Clinistix) which is specific for glucose, and the copper reduction method (Clinitest, Benedict's solution) which may detect the presence of other reducing substances in the urine as well as glucose.

Copper Reduction Method. Of the two, the copper reduction method (Clinitest) is more quantitative, especially for larger amounts (≥ 1%) of glucose in the urine (59). This is an important advantage for insulin dependent diabetics who more frequently spill large amounts of glucose in the urine, who may adjust their insulin dosage in accordance with urinary glucose results, and who thus require more quantitative data. (Clinitest tablets have replaced the older Benedict's solution, which is no longer available.)

Because urine tests give no clue to impending hypoglycemia, many clinicians using this method to monitor day to day diabetic control recommend that insulin-requiring patients "aim" for trace amounts of glucose in their urines at all times.

Glucose Oxidase Methods. The glucose oxidase methods are generally considered more qualitative; that is, they are very sensitive to glucose at low concentrations but often give false low readings in the presence of high concentrations of glucose (as well as in the presence of ketones) (60). Large amounts of glucose (2, 3, and 4%) were interpreted as 0.5% or less in 502 of 804 urines tested with Tes-Tape (61). Diastix also tends to measure too low in the high range, but has a color chart that is more quantitative than Tes-Tape. The color reactions for both Tes-Tape and Diastix are difficult to read in the higher concentrations (Diastix tends to speckle). Also, Tes-Tape may be too sensitive at times, resulting in positive reactions to negative or negligible glycosuria (59).

Nevertheless, for non-insulin dependent diabetics who rarely spill sugar into the urine if

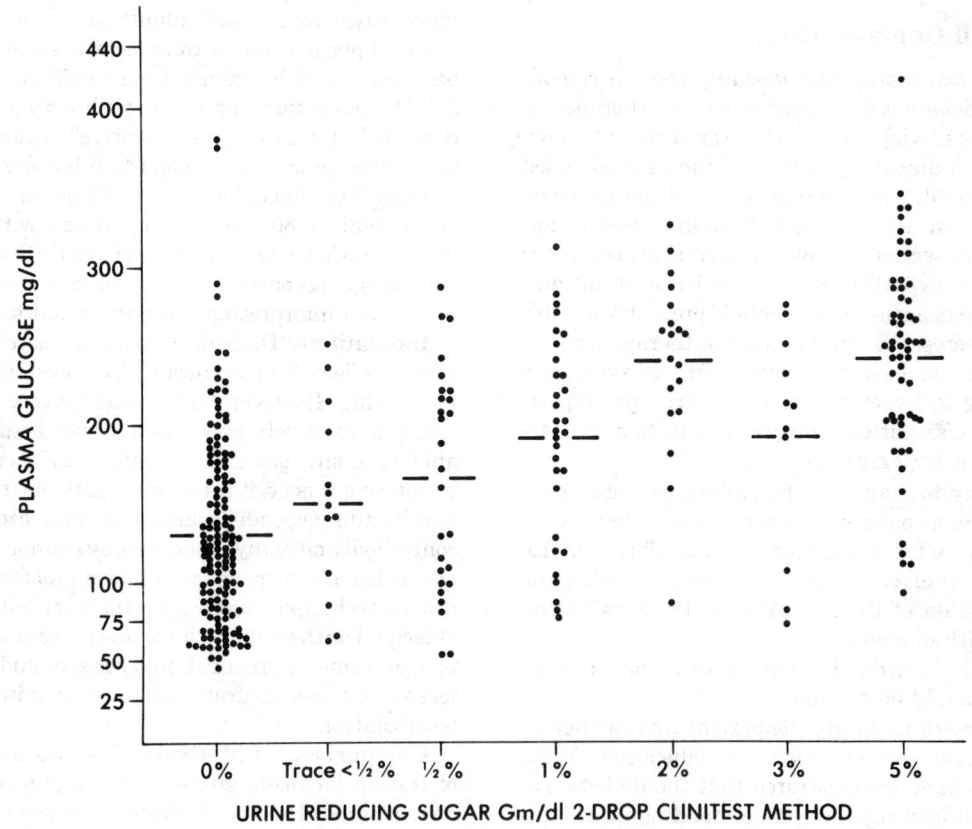

Modified from Malone et al. (55).

Figure 2. Poor Correlation Between Urine Glucose Test Results and Simultaneous Plasma Glucose Determinations.

properly controlled, a glucose oxidase test is the method of choice because of its simplicity, sensitivity, and specificity for glucose. Diastix (or Keto-Diastix which can also test for ketones) is often the glucose oxidase test of choice since it is somewhat more quantitative than Tes-Tape. Clinistix is the least quantitative of all the glucose oxidase products and is now rarely used.

Since acute hypoglycemia is not a significant problem in Type II diabetics, a goal of negative urine glucose results at all times is reasonable in this group.

"Plus" System. Prior to 1980, each urine test had its own "+" value attributed to individual urine concentrations and color blocks. This system created confusion in evaluating results because there was a lack of uniformity among products. Fortunately, the plus system was eliminated voluntarily but is still often referred to in the literature (see Table 2).

Other Issues. The instructions for use (Questions 6–8, 24), drug interference (Question 25) and interpretation of results (Question 9) are discussed in other sections of this chapter.

Fasting Blood or Plasma Glucose
(Normal FPG = 70–110 mg/dl)

Fasting plasma or blood glucose concentrations remain the most commonly used means of assessing diabetic control primarily because of their theoretical reproducibility. Prior to the advent of home blood glucose monitoring, clinicians generally extrapolated the serial results of these concentrations to overall diabetic control. Two-hour postprandial (2HPP) blood glucose concentrations have also been used to assess the degree of diabetic control when fasting glucose concentrations were within normal limits. The inherent disadvantage of this method (even in conjunction with urine test results) is that diabetic control is based upon a plasma glucose concentration measured at a single point in time and which is subject to alteration by a myriad of factors including diet, drugs, and stress.

Many laboratories now measure glucose concentrations in *plasma* rather than whole blood because they are not subject to changes in the hematocrit. Corresponding *blood* glucose concentrations are approximately 10% lower.

Home Blood Glucose Monitoring (HBGM)

The advent of home blood glucose monitoring has made the ideal goal of achieving euglycemia (70–140 mg/dl) pre- and postprandially a realistic and achievable one. For the first time, patients and their physicians are able to directly assess the effects of drug doses, dietary patterns, exercise and illness on their blood glucose concentrations. Home blood glucose tests are particularly valuable in patients with uninterpretable negative urine glucose results. In the ideal world, they would replace urine glucose tests as the day-to-day monitoring test of choice in insulin-requiring diabetics. Practically, however, they are expensive, invasive and complex. Further, to achieve maximum benefit from HBGM both the clinician and patient must be tremendously motivated and willing to spend the time required to understand its use in achieving glycemic control. Selection

Table 2.

GLUCOSE CONCENTRATIONS AND OLDER PLUS SYSTEM OF URINE
GLUCOSE TESTING PRODUCTS

Test	Glucose Concentration/(Plus Values)							
Clinitest (5-drop)	0%	*	¼% (tr)	½% (+)	¾% (++)	1% (+++)	≥2% (++++)	*	*
Clinitest (2-drop)	0%	*	tr(<½%)	½%	*	1%	2%	3%	5%
Diastix	0%	1/10% (tr)	¼% (+)	½% (++)	*	1% (+++)	≥2% (++++)	*	*
Tes-Tape	0%	1/10% (+)	¼% (++)	½% (+++)	*	*	≥2% (++++)	*	*

*No such reading.

and use of home blood glucose testing materials are discussed in Question 13. Patients in whom home blood glucose monitoring is particularly valuable are discussed below (62):

Unstable Type I diabetics. HBGM provides the unstable insulin dependent diabetic with several benefits. Instant feedback provides an increased sense of control and motivation for the new diabetic, and frequent blood glucose checking helps the patient correlate diet, exercise, and insulin with blood glucose concentrations. Most importantly, HBGM can tighten control in unstable patients.

Pregnant diabetics. Infant morbidity and mortality are closely associated with maternal hyperglycemia. With tight control, utilizing HBGM, the diabetic mother can expect to deliver a live, healthy infant.

Patients having difficulty recognizing true hypoglycemia. Acute anxiety attacks or rapidly dropping blood sugar may mimic a true hypoglycemic attack. This can easily be evaluated by a finger-prick at the time the "reaction" occurs.

Patients with an abnormal or unstable renal threshold. Although the average renal threshold for glucose is approximately 180 mg/dl, the thresholds between individual patients may vary greatly. Urine glucose testing is only useful if the renal threshold is known. HBGM can be used to determine that threshold. In addition, urine testing is of less value and can be frustrating when a patient has an abnormally high threshold or a threshold for glucose which may change over time. HBGM can be used in any patient to provide more accurate information when urine testing is inadequate.

Anuria. Patients who are anuric secondary to renal failure, or have difficulty urinating normally due to a diabetes-induced neurogenic bladder, may not be able to use a urine test. HBGM is a viable alternative.

Impaired color vision. For color blind patients who cannot distinguish colors on the urine test (or HBGM) charts, a reflectance colorimeter with a digital readout is useful.

Glycosylated Hemoglobin (Hemoglobin A_{1c})

Hemoglobin A, which constitutes 90% of hemoglobin in adults, is slowly and irreversibly glycosylated at the N terminal of the beta chain.

This reaction is nonenzymatic and the extent to which it occurs is dependent on the mean plasma glucose concentration. Since glycosylation is an irreversible process, the concentrations of hemoglobin A_{1c} reflect the mean serum plasma glucose concentrations over the approximate life of the red cell. In nondiabetics, the Hb A_{1c} level (expressed as % of total hemoglobin) is less than 6%. It may be present in three times this amount in diabetics. In addition to Hb A_{1c}, very small amounts of negatively charged minor hemoglobin components are formed by the addition of other sugars or sugar phosphates to the N terminal of the beta chain (Hb A_{1a} – 1% and Hb A_{1b} – 1%). These components do not increase in parallel with plasma glucose concentrations but their amounts are fairly constant. Because these components move rapidly with Hb A_{1c} when subjected to electrophoresis or chromatography, they are often included in glycosylated hemoglobin values reported by the laboratory. Analytical methods which are not specific for Hb A_{1c} measure total glycosylated hemoglobins or total fast hemoglobins, which is the total of Hb A_{1a+b+c}. Approximately 2–3% is added to the value for Hb A_{1c} so that nondiabetics generally have a Hb A_1 value $\leqslant$ 8%. Clinically, there is a high degree of correlation between Hb A_{1c} levels and total glycosylated hemoglobin (Hb A_1) levels (20,21).

The measurement of glycosylated hemoglobin enables the clinician to evaluate the mean plasma glucose concentration over the past 4–6 weeks, and studies show that glycosylated hemoglobin levels correlate closely with many parameters of diabetic control including fasting, random and 2-hour postprandial glucose levels, clinical assessment, insulin dose/kg and duration of diabetes. Its advantages are that it may be measured without any special patient preparation (eg, fasting) and that its levels are generally not subject to acute changes in insulin dosing, exercise, or diet. Normalization of glycosylated hemoglobin may be the simplest way for a clinician to evaluate the achievement of relative euglycemia. However, Hb A_{1c} does not replace the use of urine or home blood glucose monitoring which must be used to evaluate acute changes in blood glucose concentrations and to make acute changes in insulin doses.

In the unstable, uncontrolled diabetic, measurements of total glycosylated hemoglobin (Hb A_1) may be elevated by an intermediate, labile form of glycosylated hemoglobin (preA$_{1c}$) unless samples are subjected to certain precautionary procedures. Elevations also occur in the presence of HbF (eg, pregnancy) or other unusual hemoglobins which are not separable from Hb A_{1c} (thalassemia, sickle cell). Because the clearance of Hb A_{1c} is tied to the red blood cell life span, levels are low in patients with hemolysis and uremia (20,21).

INSULIN

Clinicians and patients are currently confronted with a confusing array of insulin products which vary with regard to onset and duration of action, insulin concentration, animal source, and purity. This confusion has been exacerbated by the fact that two new manufacturers of insulin (Nordisk and Novo) have entered the U.S. market and each uses different terms and brandnames for its products. Further, this increased competition has resulted in a "war" among manufacturers to produce purer and purer products which have questionable clinical benefits. Table 6 displays insulin products which are currently available in the USA.

Onset and Duration of Action

All manufacturers of insulin produce products which are short-acting, intermediate-acting and long-acting. The onset of action, peak effect and duration of action of each of these insulins is discussed below and displayed in Table 3. However, in applying these data the clinician must realize that most of them were obtained through the measurement of insulin levels and glycemic response of normal, healthy volunteers to phar-

macologic doses of insulin in the fasting state or in well-controlled diabetics stabilized in a metabolic ward. In actuality, there is tremendous intersubject and intrasubject variation in response to insulin (63); there are numerous factors including the formation of blocking antibodies, exercise, site of injection, massage of the injection site, ambient temperature, and interactions between mixtures of insulin which may alter an individual patient's time pattern of insulin response (See Table 4). A knowledge of when one might expect the various insulins to exert their effects, however, is absolutely essential to the rational manipulation of insulin doses (see Questions 9,12,14).

Short-acting Insulins. *Regular Insulin* [Lilly, Squibb, Nordisk (Velosulin), Novo (Actrapid)] and *Semilente Insulin* [Lilly, Squibb, Novo (Semitard)] are the rapid-onset, short-acting insulins which are available. Regular insulin has an onset of action between 15–60 minutes, a peak action of 2–4 hours and a duration of action of 5–7 hours. Semilente insulin has a somewhat delayed onset and peak action relative to regular insulin (1–2 hours and 4–6 hours, respectively) and a considerably longer duration of action (12–16 hours) (2). Because Semilente is not as rapid-acting as regular insulin, the latter is the most commonly used short-acting insulin. In Type I diabetics who have used regular insulin for 2 or more years, it may have a delayed peak effect which can occur as late as 4–10 hours following the injection, and its quick action may be diminished by mixture with NPH or Lente insulins (see Question 11) (64,65). Regular insulin is the only form of insulin which may be administered intravenously, since all other insulin products are suspensions.

Table 3.

COMPARISON OF VARIOUS INSULIN PREPARATIONS

Insulin	Onset (hrs)	Peak (hrs)	Duration (hrs)	Appearance
Regular	½–1	2–4	5–7	clear
Semilente	1–2	4–6	12–16	cloudy
NPH	1–1½	6–14	24+	cloudy
Lente	1–2½	6–14	24+	cloudy
PZI	6–8	14–24	36+	cloudy
Ultralente	6	18–24	36+	cloudy

Intermediate-acting Insulins. *NPH or Isophane Insulin* [Lilly, Squibb, Nordisk (Insulatard), Novo (Protaphane)] and *Lente Insulin* [Lilly, Squibb (Zinc Suspension), Novo (Monotard and Lentard)] are the intermediate-acting insulins. Both have an onset of action of approximately 2 hours, a peak action of approximately 6–14 hours and a duration of approximately 24 hours. See Table 3. The onset and peak action of Lente insulin may be slightly delayed relative to NPH (2,66). Again, it must be emphasized that this pattern of response is at best a generalization. Several investigators have noted that patients may have a rapid or delayed pattern of response to both NPH and lente insulins and that patients change their patterns of response to these insulins over the course of the disease (64,65,67). See Question 3.

Long-acting Insulins. *Protamine Zinc Insulin-PZI* [Lilly, Squibb] and *Ultralente* [Lilly, Squibb, Novo (Ultratard)] are the long-acting insulins. These insulins have a slow onset of activity (6–8 hours), a delayed peak action (14-26 hours) and a prolonged duration of action (36 hours). In the recent past they have been used infrequently because they provided insulin concentrations too low to handle acute glucose challenges related to meals but relatively high concentrations of insulin at night when the patient was not taking any food. Recently, however, with the new interest in mimicking the physiologic release of insulin, the long-acting insulins have been used in the morning to supply low "basal" levels of insulin in an attempt to suppress glycogenolysis and gluconeogenesis (89,100). Excess amounts of Protamine in PZI bind regular insulin, thereby abolishing its rapid onset of action; Ultralente may be mixed with regular insulin and Lente-type insulin with no effect on the time-action curve.

Insulin Concentration

Most all diabetics taking insulin are now using U-100 insulin (100 units/cc). U-80 insulin has been

Table 4.

FACTORS AFFECTING INSULIN ABSORPTION

Factors	Comment	Refs.

Site of injection	The rate of absorption of insulin is:
	   Fastest from the abdomen
	   Intermediate from the arm
	   Slowest from the thigh
		104,151

Exercise of the injected area	Controversial. The absorption of regular insulin is increased if injected just prior to exercise.	151,152,104
Ambient temperature	Heat (eg, hot weather, sauna, hot bath) increases the absorption. Cold (cold weather, water sports) has the opposite effect.	104
Local massage	Markedly increases rate of absorption. This may last for 2½ hours for intermediate preparations.	104
Insulin mixtures	Excess protamine in NPH may bind regular insulin within 5 minutes, thus delaying its onset. This is most significant with NPH:Reg mixtures >1:1. When regular exceeds NPH, this reaction becomes less significant. The amount of excess protamine varies from manufacturer to manufacturer. Excess zinc in lente preparations also binds regular insulin and blunts its onset of action. See Question 11.	63,114
Insulin antibodies	Blocking antibodies may bind insulin as it is absorbed and release it slowly, thus altering the time course of response.	68,69,436
Insulin degrading enzymes	Rare cases have been reported in which the presence of subcutaneous enzymes degrade insulin prior to absorption. These patients respond to IV or IM insulin.	143

discontinued; U-40 insulin is still occasionally used by a few older Type I diabetics who are unwilling to change concentrations. U-40 may also be used in diabetics taking very low doses of insulin since it is more dilute and can be more accurately measured. This problem can also be averted by diluting U-100 insulin with Insulin Diluting Solution which is available on special request from Lilly. The standard use of U-100 insulin has virtually eliminated insulin dosing errors which resulted from the use of an insulin syringe calibrated for a differing concentration of insulin.

Antigenicity

The various insulin products available on the market differ significantly with respect to their ability to stimulate insulin antibody formation. Virtually all diabetics taking insulin eventually form insulin blocking antibodies (IgG) six weeks to three months after treatment is initiated (68). These antibodies can combine with and delay the activity of exogenous insulin, but in most diabetics the total binding capacity is fairly low (10–20%) (65,69,70).

Before purified forms of insulin were available, it was theorized that the impurities present in insulin were the primary source of immunologic reactions to insulin. Although more purified insulins *are* less antigenic than their less pure counterparts (71), the primary determinant of insulin antigenicity is the animal source from which it is derived (72). Pure pork insulin, which differs structurally from human insulin by only one amino acid, is less immunogenic than insulin derived from beef, which differs from human insulin by 3 amino acids (73,74). Human insulin is expected to be less antigenic than pork insulin. Dealanated and sulfated insulins are experimental modifications which are said to be less antigenic and less neutralizable than other insulins (75). Occasionally, a patient who is resistant to all mammalian sources of insulin will respond favorably to fish insulin, probably because its structure differs so drastically from human insulin that there is little cross reaction with circulating antibodies (76,77). The immunologic complications of insulin therapy are discussed in Questions 18–20.

Purity

Since the introduction of "conventional" insulin (which contained greater than 10,000 ppm

proinsulin) by Eli Lilly and Co. in 1923, little was done to improve insulin purity until the last decade when technological advancements enabled insulin manufacturers to purify insulin to a high degree. Insulin purity is inversely proportional to proinsulin contamination (the b fraction of gel chromatography) which also reflects relative concentrations of other noninsulin materials such as glucagon, somatostatin, and pancreatic polypeptide. Gel filtration chromatography in 1972, and the addition of ion-exchange chromatography most recently, have produced insulins with less than $\frac{1}{1000}$ of the proinsulin contamination of the original "conventional" insulins that were manufactured for over 50 years.

In 1980, two Danish firms, Novo and Nordisk, introduced highly purified pure pork insulins with ⩽10 ppm proinsulin content into the U.S. market. Subsequently, Lilly and Squibb introduced similar products in addition to their other "less-purified" products which were beef/pork or predominantly beef insulins. These new pure pork, highly purified insulins were originally called "monocomponent," "rarely immunogenic," and "single component" by Novo, Nordisk and Lilly, respectively, but these names were superseded in 1980 by the FDA's term "purified" insulin. Unfortunately, this led to some confusion over the use of the term "purified." Prior to this time, Lilly had progressively purified insulin from "conventional" insulin(⩾10,000 ppm proinsulin) to "single peak" insulin (300-3,000 ppm proinsulin) in 1972, and again to "improved single peak" insulin (⩽50 ppm proinsulin) in 1980. Squibb was still marketing "conventional" insulin (>10,000 ppm proinsulin). By 1982 Lilly and Squibb had improved their non-"purified" (ie, >10 ppm proinsulin) insulin products to contain very nearly the same proinsulin content as "purified" insulins: ⩽20 ppm and ⩽25 ppm proinsulin, respectively. Yet, according to the FDA, only those products with ⩽10 ppm proinsulin could be labeled "purified".

The clinical importance of the "purified" insulins which contain ⩽10 ppm proinsulin versus the other available products is unknown, although it hardly seems significant in light of the vast differences in contamination prior to 1980. Currently, all insulins available in the United States contain no more than 25 ppm proinsulin (see Tables 5 and 6).

Because all insulins are now similar with respect to purification, animal source is the most important difference among the insulin products. Most of the "purified" insulins manufactured by Novo, Nordisk, and Lilly are of pure pork source, and may be intrinsically beneficial for this reason alone. Lilly also produces a standard line of beef/pork (70%/30%) mixtures (Iletin I), while Squibb's products are mostly pure beef (with the exception of their regular insulins, which are pure pork). Lilly's mixed beef/pork insulins are no less antigenic than pure beef insulins (81). However, there are no specific indications for pure beef insulins with the exception of the rare individual who is allergic to pork insulins but not to beef, or those individuals who avoid pork insulins for religious reasons.

Throughout this chapter, the term "purified" will refer to the FDA-designated highly purified insulins ($\leq$ 10 ppm proinsulin), most of which are also pure pork insulins.

Human Insulin

Lilly and Novo, the current manufacturers of biosynthetic human insulin (BHI)(to be released in late 1982 or early 1983), utilize different manufacturing processes to produce an insulin with an amino acid sequence identical to that of human pancreatic insulin. Lilly, through recent advances in recombinant DNA technology, manufactures A- and B-chains of human insulin cloned

by *Escherichia coli* from chemically synthesized genes. The two chains are then purified by high-performance liquid chromatography and linked together by disulfide bonds to form their BHI product. Conversely, Novo utilizes enzymatic conversion techniques to substitute alanine for threonine at the terminal end of pork insulin, and after similar purification, a corresponding biosynthetic human insulin is produced.

So far, BHI has proved to be similar, if not identical, to purified pork insulin with respect to almost all properties studied (82,83). Subtle differences in potency and pharmacokinetics found by a few investigators may or may not prove to be clinically significant. A slight increase in potency and the possibility that BHI is absorbed more rapidly than pork insulin may be advantageous by producing a more normalized plasma insulin profile and thus improving glycemic control (84). This awaits further investigation.

In theory, BHI might be expected to be less immunogenic than purified pork insulin, and certainly less than beef insulin, since the human amino acid sequence should be non-antigenic. On the other hand, there may be differences in tertiary folding of BHI, or trace contamination by E. coli or enzymatic products, which could produce an immune response similar to that of purified pork insulin (small, but detectable in many patients). Immunologic questions concerning BHI also await the results of current clinical trials

Table 5.

A HISTORY OF INSULIN PURIFICATION IN THE U.S.

	DISCONTINUED PRODUCTS			CURRENTLY AVAILABLE PRODUCTS*		
	"Conventional" Insulin	"Single Peak" Insulin	"Improved Single Peak" Insulin	"Improved Single Peak" Insulin	Squibbs "New" Insulin	"Purified" Insulin
PROINSULIN CONTENT (PPM):**	10,000–50,000	300–3,000	$\leq$50	$\leq$20	$\leq$25	$\leq$10**
Lilly	1923–1972	1972–1979	1980–1982 (Iletin I)	1982 (Iletin I)	—	1980 (Iletin II)
Nordisk	—	—	—	—	—	1980
Novo	—	—	—	—	—	1980
Squibb	1936–1981	—	—	—	1982	1982

*As of August 1982.

**Internal specifications for manufacturers vary. Novo insulins claim <1 ppm proinsulin.

comparing the use of BHI to purified pork insulin in diabetics. If BHI is shown to be less immunogenic than pork insulins, it may become another important advance in the treatment and prophylaxis of local and systemic allergy, immunologic resistance, and subcutaneous lipoatrophy. That these complications are already quite rare with the use of purified pork insulins somewhat mollifies this potential advantage of BHI.

Whether or not differences in potency, pharmacokinetics, or immunogenicity prove to be significant, the principal advantage of BHI at the present time appears to be its potential value as an unlimited supply of insulin. The availability of insulin derived from recombinant DNA should help to prevent the world-wide shortage of insulin which had been previously projected for the next decade.

Table 6.

INSULINS CURRENTLY AVAILABLE IN THE U.S.

Product (manufacturer)[1]	Type	Species Source[2]	Purity[3] (ppm proinsulin)
Rapid Acting			
Iletin I (Ly)	Regular	Beef-Pork	<20
Iletin II (Ly)	Regular	Pork or Beef	<10
Actrapid (Novo)	Regular	Pork	<10
Velosulin (Nord)	Regular	Pork	<10
"New" Insulin Inj. (Sq)	Regular	Pork	<25
"Purified" Insulin Inj. (Sq)	Regular	Pork	<10
Semilente Iletin I (Ly)	Semilente	Beef-Pork	<20
Semitard (Novo)	Semilente	Pork	<10
"New" Semilente Insulin (Sq)	Semilente	Beef	<25
Intermediate Acting			
NPH Iletin I (Ly)	NPH	Beef-Pork	<20
NPH Iletin II (Ly)	NPH	Pork or Beef	<10
Protaphane NPH (Novo)	NPH	Pork	<10
Insulatard NPH (Nord)	NPH	Pork	<10
"New" Isophane Insulin (Sq)	NPH	Beef	<25
"Purified" Isophane Insulin (Sq)	NPH	Beef	<10
Lente Iletin I (Ly)	Lente	Beef-Pork	<20
Lente Iletin II (Ly)	Lente	Pork or Beef	<10
Monotard (Novo)	Lente	Pork	<10
Lentard (Novo)	Lente	Beef-Pork	<10
"New" Insulin Zn Susp. (Sq)	Lente	Beef	<25
"Purified" Insulin Zn Susp. (Sq)	Lente	Beef	<10
Long Acting			
Protamine, Zn, & Iletin I (Ly)	PZI	Beef-Pork	<20
Protamine, Zn, & Iletin II (Ly)	PZI	Pork or Beef	<10
"New" Protamine Zn Insulin (Sq)	PZI	Beef	<25
Ultralente Iletin I (Ly)	Ultralente	Beef-Pork	<20
Ultratard (Novo)	Ultralente	Beef	<10
"New" Ultralente Insulin (Sq)	Ultralente	Beef	<25
Mixed			
Mixtard (Nord)	70% NPH, 30% Reg.	Pork	<10

1 — Ly = Lilly, Novo = Novo, Nord = Nordisk, Sq = Squibb.

2 — Mixed species sources are approximately 70% beef, 30% pork.

3 — Insulins with <10 ppm proinsulin are labeled "purified." Internal specifications of proinsulin content may vary with "purified" insulins. Novo claims the least contamination with <1 ppm proinsulin.

Insulin Storage

Room Temperature. All insulins currently available are stable for several months at room temperature (68–75°F). Modified insulins (Lente insulins, NPH, and PZI) maintain their potency for a period of at least 24 months at room temperature. During this time the fine precipitates may aggregate, making withdrawal of a uniform dose difficult. Color changes may be associated with a denaturation of protein and should be interpreted as consistent with loss of potency (85). Regular insulin is stable for 18 months at room temperature (86).

Temperatures >75°F. No one has studied the stability of insulins at temperatures of 75-100°F. At 100°F all insulins lose a significant amount of potency within 1–2 months. Deterioration occurs extremely rapidly at temperatures of 122°F (85). Lilly states that a "brief" exposure of NPH and PZI to 100°F may not result in significant loss of potency (2); however, aggregation of particles may occur at a much more rapid rate and insulins should be checked for this if they are delivered under improper storage conditions.

Refrigeration/Freezing. All insulins maintain their potency and physical properties for 36 months if stored in the refrigerator (85). Freezing apparently does not affect the potency of insulin but may cause aggregation of the precipitate (2).

These data have several implications. Many patients prefer injecting insulin which has been warmed to room temperature. This may be more than a comfort measure since the injection of cold insulin has been considered a contributing factor in the formation of lipodystrophies. The patient may keep the vials of insulin currently in use out of the refrigerator; nevertheless, they should be stored in a cool area, not near the radiator or on a sunny window-sill. Insulin dispensed within a hospital need not be refrigerated. Finally, unless the weather is unusually warm, patients who are traveling generally do not have to purchase special paraphernalia to keep their insulin refrigerated. Insulation of the insulin between several layers of clothing should be sufficient.

Goals of Insulin Therapy

There is growing evidence that the progression and clinical development of longterm complications may be delayed or minimized through close control of blood glucose levels (28,87,88). (See the section on Long-Term Complications.) However, prior to the advent of home blood glucose monitoring and glycosylated hemoglobin there was no easy method of objectively achieving and assessing euglycemia. Because of the limitations inherent in monitoring diabetic control with single blood glucose levels in conjunction with urine glucose tests, most physicians were pleased if they could achieve trace amounts of glucose in the urine (to avoid hypoglycemia), relief of clinical signs and symptoms related to hyperglycemia, and a fasting blood glucose below 180 mg/dl (renal threshold). Realistically, these goals may still be valid in the majority of insulin-requiring diabetics who continue to monitor their disease with urine glucose tests. The only addition to these goals would be "normalization" of HB A_{1c} values (see below).

In patients who are highly motivated, educable, and willing to test their blood glucose on a regular basis the following goals may be used:

1. A fasting blood glucose of ≤130 mg/dl and a postprandial blood glucose of ≤180 mg/dl. (These are criteria which are consistent with a nondiabetic OGTT.) Several diabetologists advocate strict euglycemia, ie, a blood glucose of 70–140 mg/dl at all times (87,89–90). However, there is growing evidence that severe, and perhaps fatal, hypoglycemia may be associated with this goal (92,93). Therefore, any clinician who establishes euglycemia as a goal must be assured that the patient can competently interpret the significance of blood glucose concentrations measured at various times in the day and make appropriate adjustments in diet or insulin doses.

2. A blood glucose of no less than 60 mg/dl at any time (avoid hypoglycemia).

3. A normal Hb A_{1c} (<6%) or Hb A_{1a+b+c} (<8%). Normal values vary with each laboratory. Goldstein et al (21) suggest that normalization may not be a realistically achievable goal because in their experience patients who achieve a normal level have a higher incidence of hypoglycemic reactions. In accordance with the growing concern of some diabetologists with hypoglycemia, he suggests a more realistic goal of a Hb A_{1c} of <9%.

4. Negative urine glucose tests at all times.

New Methods of Insulin Delivery

In accordance with new treatment goals which include attainment of more physiologic blood glucose concentrations, new methods of delivering insulin in ways which mimic pancreatic release of the hormone have been explored and advocated. In the nondiabetic, the pancreas secretes a basal level of insulin throughout the day and boluses of insulin in response to snacks and meals. Two methods have been used to achieve a similar pattern of insulin release: insulin infusion pumps and intensive, split-dose insulin administration.

Insulin Infusion Pumps. Insulin pumps are available in open-loop and closed-loop (artificial pancreas) systems. The *closed-loop system* (Biostator) consists of three components: a battery-operated pump, a computer which controls the rate of insulin delivery, and a glucose sensor which feeds back into the computer. Thus, like the pancreas, the amount of insulin released is determined by the blood glucose concentration. The system is not portable (about the size of a television set) and has the capability of delivering glucose as well as insulin. It is used in clinical research and in the management of hospitalized diabetics who are in ketoacidosis, undergoing surgery, or are acutely ill. It is also used in complicated pregnant diabetics during the last trimester of pregnancy and especially during labor and delivery. In all of these situations, insulin requirements may fluctuate drastically (94,95). Insulin is usually delivered intravenously, but may also be delivered subcutaneously or intraperitoneally.

The *open-loop system* is composed of a battery-operated pump and a computer which can be programmed to deliver pre-determined amounts of insulin subcutaneously. These systems are portable and designed to deliver basal amounts of insulin throughout the day as well as meal-related boluses which are initiated by the patient 30 minutes prior to food ingestion. Although these systems are gaining popularity, the American Diabetes Association currently recommends that the use of these devices be limited to certain Type I diabetics who are unable to attain acceptable control using intensive dietary and insulin therapy (95) (see below). They should only be used in highly-motivated, compliant individuals under the guidance of a health care team trained and knowledgeable in their use. This is underscored by the reports of deaths (92,93), dermatologic complications (94,96,97) and mechanical complications (94,98) associated with their use. Currently, there is no evidence that insulin pumps

achieve better control than more intensive, split-dose insulin regimens (98–100,105). In summary, the cost ($1200-$2000 for pumps alone); complications associated with their use; lack of evidence that these devices achieve superior control to multiple insulin injections; and technical complexity of their effective operation limit the use of these devices to a very small percentage of insulin-requiring diabetics at this time. The establishment and alteration of insulin doses in patients using the insulin pump have been described by others (90,91).

Intensive, Split-Dose Insulin Administration. As the notion of glycemic control became widely accepted as a therapeutic goal, it became clear that the conventional method of dosing insulin once daily in the morning was not optimal. To remedy this situation, diabetologists began experimenting with various split dose regimens as outlined in Table 7 (64,89,90,101). A total daily dose of insulin is estimated empirically or according to guidelines similar to those listed in Table 8. The total daily dose of insulin is then split into several doses.

All patients who are initiated and wish to be optimally maintained on such regimens should initially test their blood glucose 4–8 times daily (before meals, after meals, bedtime and occasionally at 2–3 a.m. in the morning) to evaluate the effect of each insulin component. Once controlled, they may decrease testing to four times daily (before meals and at bedtime). Blood glucose should also be measured whenever the patient is unsure of whether or not he is hypoglycemic.

Several studies show that euglycemia equivalent to that attained with the use of an insulin pump can be achieved through administration of multiple daily doses of insulin (98–100,105).

Method 1 is probably the regimen most commonly used at this time (64,89,90,101). The patient injects a mixture of intermediate-acting and regular insulin twice daily. The morning regular insulin takes care of breakfast and its activity is primarily reflected by pre-lunch glucose levels. The morning dose of NPH takes care of the noon meal and its effectiveness is reflected by the pre-dinner glucose concentrations. The evening dose of regular insulin takes care of the evening meal and its effects are reflected by the bedtime glucose. The evening dose of NPH provides basal insulin levels during the night and takes care of any evening snack which is ingested. Its peak

Table 7.

INTENSIVE, SPLIT-DOSE INSULIN REGIMENS*

Time of Insulin Administration**	7 a.m. Before Breakfast	11 a.m. Before Lunch	6 p.m. Before Dinner	11 p.m. Bedtime	Comments
Method 1	NPH:Reg (⅔) 2:1–1:1	——	NPH:Reg (⅓) 1:1	——	Lente can be substituted for NPH. The 2:1 ratio of NPH:Reg is commonly recommended but clinically, a ratio approaching 1:1 may be needed to control mid-morning hyperglycemia. This ratio may also be needed to retain the fast action of regular insulin.
Method 2	NPH:Reg (⅔) 2:1–1:1	——	Reg (⅙)	NPH (⅙)	When NPH administration is delayed until bedtime, the peak effect occurs around breakfast time rather than 2–3 a.m. when its maximal effect on glucose is unlikely to be measured. Further, some residual action remains which can minimize the mid-morning hyperglycemia associated with breakfast.
Method 3	Reg (¼)	Reg (¼)	Reg (¼)	Reg (¼)	This corresponds to pre-meal boluses of insulin. The evening dose of regular is used to suppress glycogenolysis and lipolysis which occur during the fasting state.
Method 4	Reg (⅕) Ultralente or PZI (⅖)	Reg (⅕) ——	Reg (⅕) ——	—— ——	Some authors recommend against the use of PZI because it peaks during the middle of the night, thereby predisposing patients to nocturnal hypoglycemia. If PZI is used, it should be given as a separate injection, since excess protamine will bind regular when the ratio of PZI:Reg is greater than 1:1.

*Fractions in parentheses represent fraction of total daily dose (see Table 8) administered at that time of day. Mixtures of regular and NPH include the approximate ratios of those two insulins which have been recommended.

**The division of doses listed in this table should be used as a *guide* to the initiation of intensive split-dose insulin therapy. Each patient must closely monitor blood glucose concentrations, and doses of the appropriate insulin must be adjusted accordingly. See Questions 9, 12, 14.

effectiveness is reflected by a blood glucose concentration at 2–3 a.m.; however, since most diabetics do not test their glucose at that time, its effects can be evaluated to some extent by the pre-breakfast fasting blood glucose (see Questions 9,12,14). Both injections are administered 30 minutes prior to meals and should be mixed just prior to injection (See Question 11).

Method 2 is a variation of Method 1. It is the same except for the fact that the evening dose of NPH is given as a third injection at bedtime. This delays the peak effect so that it occurs at approximately 7 a.m. when the patient tests his first glucose of the day. An additional advantage of this method is that it theoretically minimizes nocturnal hypoglycemia which may be caused by the evening dose of NPH and provides some residual insulin activity in the morning for patients in whom mid-morning hyperglycemia is particularly troublesome (56,64).

Method 3 simply consists of the administration of four equal doses of regular insulin before meals and at bedtime. It is a regimen which was frequently used following the discovery of insulin but which was subsequently discarded when long-acting insulins were introduced. Its potential disadvantage is that it does not supply constant basal insulin levels which are necessary to suppress excessive glycogenolysis and gluconeogenesis during fasting periods (89).

Method 4 is an attempt to improve Method 3 through the addition of a long-acting insulin in the morning to provide basal insulin levels throughout the day. It theoretically provides insulin in exactly the same way the insulin pump does (basal levels plus pre-meal boluses). In doing so, it offers some of the same advantages of the pump in that it permits some degree of flexibility in the patient's lifestyle. For example, if a diabetic chooses to skip a meal, he omits a pre-meal bolus; conversely, if he chooses to eat a larger meal than usual, he increases his pre-meal bolus. Similar dose adjustments based upon blood glucose concentrations can be made to accomodate exercise patterns and the presence of acute illness. Both Ultralente (99) and PZI (100) have been used, although one author recommends against the use of PZI because its peak activity occurs during the night, thus exposing the patient to potential nocturnal hypoglycemia. Another disadvantage of PZI is that its excess protamine content makes it unsuitable for mixture with regular insulin in ratios of PZI:Regular which exceed 1:1 (2). Thus, it must be injected separately, if the rapid-acting effects of regular insulin are to be retained. See Question 11 and Table 9.

TREATMENT OF TYPE I DIABETICS
CLINICAL USE OF INSULIN

1. A.H., a slender 18-year-old female, is referred to the diabetic clinic by the University Student Health Service because a routine physical examination revealed glycosuria and a random plasma glucose ordered subsequently was 250 mg/dl. Approximately 4 weeks prior to this visit, A.H. moved cross country to attend college (this is the first time she has lived away from home). In retrospect, she has noted polydipsia, nocturia times 3, fatigue, and a 12-pound weight loss over this period, but she attributed this to the anxiety associated with her move away from home and the excitement with her new environment. Her past medical history is unremarkable with the exception of a long history of recurrent upper respiratory infections and three cases of vaginal monilia over the past six months. Her family history is negative for diabetes and she takes no medications.

Physical examination is within normal limits. Her weight is 50 kg.

Laboratory results are as follows: fasting plasma glucose 280 mg/dl (normal <115 mg/

Table 8.

USUAL TOTAL DAILY DOSE OF INSULIN*
(89,101)

Type of Diabetic	Dose
Type I —Initial dose	0.5–0.6 U/kg
Type I —Honeymoon phase	0.1–0.4 U/kg
Type I —With ketosis; during illness; in growth phase	0.5–1.0 U/kg
Type I —Pregnant	0.7 U/kg
Type II—With insulin resistance	0.7–2.5 U/kg

*This is an initial dose. Many patients on split dose therapy often require up to 1.2 U/kg. Insulin doses may change over time.

dl); **Hb A₁ 14% (normal 6–8%); urine glucose and ketones as measured by Keto-Diastix— ≥2% and trace, respectively.**

On the basis of the above history and laboratory findings, a presumptive diagnosis of Type I Diabetes is made. Which findings are consistent with this diagnosis?

A.H. meets several of the criteria which must be met for the diagnosis of diabetes. She has the classical symptoms of the disease (polyuria, polydipsia, weight loss, glucosuria, fatigue, recurrent infections) and a random blood glucose which is clearly greater than 200 mg/dl as well as a fasting plasma glucose which exceeds 140 mg/dl. The elevated glycosylated hemoglobin level is also consistent with the diagnosis.

Features of A.H.'s history which are consistent with Type I diabetes in particular include the relatively acute onset of symptoms in association with a major life event (moving away from home); the presence of ketones in the urine; the negative family history; a history of viral infections; and a relatively young age of onset. See Introduction.

2. How should A.H. be managed at this time?

The primary components of therapy for Type I diabetes are diet and insulin. As discussed earlier, the ideal management of this patient would include divided doses of insulin in conjunction with home blood glucose monitoring and a stable diet and exercise pattern. However, this is not a realistic goal in a patient who has initially been given the diagnosis of diabetes. In these patients, all forms of therapy must be initiated slowly along with careful patient education. Inundating A.H. with all of the complex details of diet, insulin administration, urine testing, home blood glucose monitoring, etc. at this time would be senseless and insensitive. The most important aspect of initial management includes answering A.H.'s immediate concerns about diabetes and explaining the disease in the simplest terms to minimize the anxiety which accompanies news of such a diagnosis.

Insulin should be initiated at this clinic visit to alleviate hyperglycemia, its attendant symptoms and to prevent the development of ketoacidosis. Even though the ultimate goal is to place the patient on split doses of insulin, initial therapy should be kept as simple as possible with a single morning dose of an intermediate-acting insulin (NPH or Lente). The initial dose used in

patients with moderate symptoms is empiric (10–20 units) or based upon guidelines such as those provided in Table 8. Based on the latter, A.H. would receive an initial dose of 0.5 U/kg or 25 units in the morning. The patient should be instructed with regard to insulin measurement and injection (Question 5) and urine testing (Questions 6–8) and an appointment should be made for the following week. Arrangements should also be made for individualized patient education over the course of the next several months.

3. Should NPH or Lente insulin be prescribed? Should the patient be initiated on a "purified" pork form of insulin?

Most clinicians use NPH and Lente interchangeably. Some have supported the use of Lente because it does not contain protamine, a foreign protein which is rarely antigenic (28,102). However, this theoretical increase in immunogenicity of NPH has not been established (80). Furthermore, Lente contains excess amounts of zinc and cases of "insulin allergy" secondary to the zinc content of the product have also been reported (103).

The onset of action, maximum effect and duration of these two insulins is basically the same, although Lente may be slightly slower in onset and have a slightly longer effect than NPH (66).

Recent evidence suggests that the rapid effects of regular insulin are more likely to be retained when mixed with NPH as opposed to Lente insulin (63,104) (Question 11). Since it is highly likely that this patient will eventually be administering a mixture of regular insulin and intermediate-acting insulin, these authors favor the initial use of NPH insulin.

Whether the patient should be initiated on a "purified" pork insulin is debatable. Some clinicians would argue that a highly purified, pure pork insulin such as NPH Iletin II (Lilly), Protaphane NPH (Novo) or Insulatard NPH (Nordisk) be prescribed to minimize insulin antibody formation in newly diagnosed diabetics. They argue that insulin antibodies may cross react with the patient's endogenous insulin (if present) or that insulin antibody-insulin complexes may play some pathogenic role in diabetic nephropathy (105). Minimizing antibody formation may also decrease the risk of immunologic complications of insulin (see Introduction, Questions 18–20, & Table 11). Others believe that low insulin antibody levels can be correlated with longer periods of remission (honeymoon period) or mild disease in newly diagnosed individuals.

Although these reasons are theoretically sound, they are clinically untested (78). Further, the cost of diabetic care must be considered. Except in unusual circumstances where competitive bidding takes place, the cost per vial of "purified" insulins is 1.5–2 times greater than the "less purified" forms of insulin such as Lilly's "Improved Single Peak" Iletin I or Squibb's "New" insulin. If the patient is financially able, a "purified" pork form of U-100 NPH insulin should be strongly considered (Iletin II, Insulatard, Protaphane). Otherwise, it is likely that she will achieve equal clinical control with the less purified beef/pork forms of insulin.

4. What kind of insulin syringe should be prescribed for A.H.?

Virtually all diabetics now use plastic disposable insulin syringes which do not require repeated sterilization before use. In the United States there are two major manufacturers of disposable insulin syringes suitable for injecting U-100 insulin: Becton-Dickinson (B-D) and Sherwood (Monoject syringes).

Both manufacturers have made tremendous improvements in their needles and syringes to the extent that insulin injections are relatively painless if proper technique is used. Generally speaking, the needles are finer (25,26,27 and 28 gauge), sharper, and lubricated for ease of insertion. Less pain is associated with the smaller, 27 gauge needles (106,107). The "dead space" (unmeasurable space at the hub of the needle) has been virtually eliminated so that mixing problems previously associated with its presence are no longer of concern. The length of the needle is ½" or ⅝"; the longer needle is used when back leakage of insulin occurs, and in obese diabetics. A ½", 27 gauge needle is suitable for AH.

Both manufacturers produce a 1 cc and ½ cc syringe which may be used for U-100 insulin. For patients such as A.H. who are using less than 40 units of insulin per injection, the ½ cc syringe is preferred (B-D Lo-Dose Syringe or Monoject Mini Syringe). These syringes have a smaller caliber barrel which allows for more accurate measurement of the highly-concentrated U-100 insulin. They also provide scales which allow the patient to measure insulin in 1-unit increments.

The 1cc, U-100 insulin syringes produced by these manufacturers differ with respect to the scales used on the barrel to mark insulin units. The B-D syringe uses an easily read single scale. Each mark or line is equivalent to 2 units and scale numbers are provided in 10 unit increments (ie, 10,20,30. . . . 100). In contrast, the Monoject syringe is labeled with two sets of scales. One set of markings corresponds to the even numbered units of insulin and one set corresponds to the odd numbers. The two parallel scales are marked in 10 unit increments beginning at 5 units (ie, 5,15,25. . . .95) and 10 units (ie, 10,20,30. . . .100). These scales were provided to allow the patient to more accurately measure odd numbers of insulin units; however, the adjacent markings are visually confusing which lead the ADA to recommend single-scale syringes. When patients such as A.H. are measuring very low doses of insulin, accuracy is critical. Both the B-D and Monoject ½ cc syringes use single-scales and each mark corresponds to *one* unit of insulin. This is a critical piece of information to a diabetic who is switched from a 1 cc B-D syringe (1 mark = 2 units) to a ½ cc syringe or vice versa.

A ½ cc U-100 insulin syringe with a ½", 27 G needle should be prescribed for A.H. Since both manufacturers use a single scale on their ½ cc syringe, cost and patient preference will govern the ultimate choice. Subjectively, patients will "feel" the difference between different brands or may prefer the "ease of bubble removal," physical characteristics or packaging of one syringe over another (107).

5. How should A.H. be instructed to measure and inject her NPH insulin?

Various maneuvers have been used to assist patients who are anxious about self-injection. These include the application of ice cubes to the site and the use of spring loaded devices which quickly inject insulin with light pressure application. However, these "tricks" are generally unnecessary, once the patient realizes that the injections are pain-free with the improved needles and proper technique.

Agitation. All insulins, with the exception of regular, are suspensions and must be agitated prior to withdrawal from the vial. A new, unused vial of NPH or Lente may require vigorous agitation to loosen the sediment which may have packed with storage. Otherwise, gentle agitation to minimize foaming is recommended.

Measurement. The patient should first withdraw the plunger to the level of insulin she intends to inject (25 units); she should then insert the needle into the vial and inject 25 units of air to prevent creation of a vacuum within the vial. The vial should then be inverted with the syringe and 25 units of NPH should be withdrawn. The bevel of the needle should be well below the surface of the insulin to avoid withdrawing air or bubbles into the syringe.

The barrel of the syringe should be held at eye level to check for the presence of air bubbles and to allow for accurate placement of the plunger tip at the 25-unit mark. If bubbles are present, they should be removed by tapping the syringe to coax the bubbles to the top of the barrel where they can be injected back into the insulin vial. Practically, it is easier to withdraw more than the amount to be injected and then move the plunger up to the prescribed amount.

Injection. After the insulin is measured, the syringe is placed on a flat surface to prepare an area for injection. Alcohol swabs may be used to clean the area of injection as well as the rubber stopper on the insulin vial, but their actual antiseptic value is questionable.

To inject the insulin subcutaneously, A.H. should be instructed to firmly pinch up the area to be injected (this creates a firm surface for injection), and to quickly insert the needle perpendicularly into the center of this area. The syringe should be held toward the middle or back of the barrel (like a pencil) with the bevel pointed upwards. Anxious patients have a tendency to "choke" the hub of the syringe to the extent that their fingers prevent proper insertion. A 45° angle of injection may be used for thin, emaciated individuals who have little subcutaneous fat.

Before injecting the insulin, the plunger should be pulled out to determine whether the needle has been inserted into a vein or artery. (Patients report that this occurs rarely.) If no blood appears in the barrel, the insulin may be injected. The skin should be released before the insulin syringe is withdrawn and pressure should be applied to the site of injection with an alcohol swab or a piece of cotton to prevent back leakage of the insulin as the needle is removed. The site should not be massaged, as this may accelerate the absorption and onset of action of the insulin (Table 4).

Reuse of Disposable Syringes. The insulin needle may be capped, refrigerated, and reused until it becomes dulled by repeated insertion into the rubber tip of the vial. Although the thought of reusing disposable syringes has been anathema to clinicians, resourceful diabetics who must minimize costs have consistently reused their syringes. Recent studies indicate that infections resulting from this practice are rare (108,109).

Rotation of Injection Sites. It is current practice to recommend that a patient rotate sites of injection between the arms, thighs, abdomen and buttocks. However, this practice has been questioned by Koivisto and Felig (110) who noted that the differences in rates of insulin absorption from these sites resulted in alterations in blood glucose control. They recommend that insulin injection sites be rotated within the same anatomical region to avoid this effect. (See Table 4.)

Rotating the site of injection was originally recommended to avoid the lipodystrophic effects of insulin; however, since insulin has been purified, these complications are less frequent and the importance of rotation less critical. Repetitive use of the same site of injection, however, may result in lipohypertrophy (Question 18) and does toughen the skin, thereby decreasing the ease of needle penetration.

6. *Clinitest Instructions.* Because urine test results will be used to modify A.H.'s insulin dose, it is decided that she should test her urine glucose with Clinitest (see Introduction). Review all the instructions which should eventually be discussed with A.H. with regard to the correct and optimal use of Clinitest.

The following are basic issues which should be included in discussions regarding the use of Clinitest.

Frequency. The frequency of urine testing is primarily governed by the degree of diabetic control. If the patient is labile or if insulin doses require adjustment (as in A.H.'s case), the urine glucose should be measured 3–4 times daily, usually before meals and at bedtime. In addition, she may wish to test her urine at an hour when a specific insulin is exerting its maximum and/or minimum effect. If her diabetes has been well-controlled on the same dose of insulin for some time, she may test her urine once or twice daily. The urine should be tested more frequently at the first sign of infection or with the occurrence of any change in activity or dietary patterns or emotional stress.

Double-voiding. The patient should be taught when to test double-voided specimens (see Question 7). Drinking a glass of water after first voiding the bladder will make production of a second urine specimen easier. For a newly-diagnosed diabetic such as A.H., it may prevent confusion to instruct the patient to test only double-voided specimens until she has become more familiar with her disease and therapy.

Procedure. A Clinitest tablet is dropped into a test tube containing 10 drops of water with 5 drops of urine for the 5-drop method, or with 2 drops of urine for the 2-drop Clinitest method (see Question 8). The tablet generates its own heat and anaerobic environment with the production of foam. For this reason the tube should not be agitated during the reaction.

Pass-through Phenomenon. The patient should observe the reaction while it is occurring since a very high glucose content results in the so-called "pass-through" phenomenon. This is demonstrated by a fleeting, bright orange color which occurs during the "boiling" and which fades to a greenish brown when the reaction ceases. The latter color may be misinterpreted as 0.75–1%, when there is actually more than 2% glucose in the urine (5-drop method).

Timing. Because the color may fade with time, it must be read precisely 15 seconds after the "boiling" has ceased. The time dependence of this color reaction should be stressed upon persons who might leave to do other chores while the reaction is taking place.

Testing for Urine Ketones. A patient who spills 2% or more glucose into her urine should also test her urine for acetone. Persistence of large amounts of glucose or ketones in the urine should be called to the physician's attention.

Drug Interference. Several drugs may interfere with the test to cause a false positive reaction. A properly used Tes-Tape strip may be used to help test for the presence of interacting substances (see Question 25).

Stability/Storage. Because Clinitest tablets disintegrate rapidly in the presence of moisture and light, they should not be stored in the bathroom medicine cabinet (the most logical location from the patient's viewpoint). The disintegration is easily detected since the appearance of the tablet changes from the normal speckled robin's egg blue to white with splotches of dark blue.

Toxicity. The tablets are poisonous and caustic. They should be manipulated with the lid of the container and kept out of the reach of small children. Should ingestion occur, do not induce vomiting.

7. Must A.H. check only double-voided urine specimens? Discuss the considerations for testing first- versus second-voided urine samples.

Diabetologists have traditionally instructed patients to test only second-voided urine specimens (a specimen collected 30 min after previously voiding the bladder); however, the first-voided urine sample is in many cases more useful as well as practical. This subject has been recently reviewed by Davidson (111), although there is still a divergence of opinions.

The argument for testing only second-voided specimens is that this sample more accurately reflects the degree of hyperglycemia at the time of testing. The urine is not "contaminated" with glucose that may have been excreted into the bladder several hours previously. This is particularly meaningful for the morning test, when urine has had time to accumulate in the bladder over a period of 8–10 hours. Since the preprandial urine tests usually occur at times of peak insulin action, the second-voided specimen more accurately reflects the effect of insulin at that particular time.

On the other hand, arguments for testing the first-voided urine are equally compelling. Firstly, double-voided urine specimens can be very inconvenient. Even when patients are instructed to double-void, many (understandably) do not or will not take the time to urinate twice before every meal to produce a second-voided sample. Secondly, postprandial glycosuria (or spills occurring several hours prior to the test) may be missed when the second-voided specimens are the only ones tested, thereby producing a false sense of security that control is better than it actually is. Thirdly, four separate studies have confirmed that roughly ⅔ to ¾ of paired first- and second-voided urine specimens yield identical results when tested with Diastix, Tes-Tape, or Clinitest (55,111). Higher levels of glycosuria are found in approximately 25% of the first-voided specimens and in only 5–6% of the second-voided samples. On the basis of these arguments, recommendations can be made for the appropriate use of first- and second-voided urine specimens.

Second-voided Specimens. Basically, second-voided specimens are needed only when urine glucose concentrations will be used to indirectly evaluate the plasma glucose concentrations at the specific time the test is performed. This is more critical in insulin dependent diabetics such as A.H. who will rely on urine test results to adjust insulin doses. Second-voiding is particularly important for the first morning test since the first-voided specimen is more likely to be elevated from glucose excursions during the night. Second-voided samples are also important prior to taking supplemental insulin during acute illnesses or stress or during the process of attempting to determine a patient's renal threshold for glucose. If A.H. is found to be a brittle diabetic who requires frequent insulin adjustments and is prone to both hyper- and hypoglycemia, second-voided specimens should be tested to continually adjust insulin doses.

First-voided specimens. If and when A.H. achieves good control of her diabetes, it may be reasonable to use first-voided specimens for testing before lunch, dinner, or the evening snack. This approach should increase compliance with urine testing and may even result in better control since the first-voided specimen generally shows a greater degree of glycosuria than the second-voided one. First-voided specimens are also appropriately used for routine urine testing in non-insulin dependent diabetics, since the actual time that glycosuria has occurred is less important than the total amount of glucose that has been spilled.

8. Should A.H. use the 5-drop or the 2-drop Clinitest method of testing for urine glucose?

Although the most popular method of using Clinitest has formerly been with the 5-drop method, the 2-drop Clinitest method is now recommended by the American Diabetes Association for use by insulin-dependent diabetics such as A.H. (60). The test simply uses 2 drops of urine mixed with the same amount of water and can quantitate higher levels of glycosuria (3% and 5%) compared to the 5-drop method (up to 2% only). See Table 2. Data concerning sensitivity of the test are contradictory. The 2-drop method has been demonstrated to be both less sensitive (59) and more sensitive (112) than the 5-drop method at low concentrations of glucose. Because the urine is more dilute, the "pass-through" phenomenon does not occur as frequently with the 2-drop method. Separate color charts are available for interpretation of the two tests.

9. A.H. was instructed to test a double-voided urine sample with Clinitest four times daily before meals and at bedtime; to record her results and any other unusual events or symptoms during each day; and to bring her records to clinic. One week later, trends in her urine test results were as follows:

7 a.m.	12 p.m.	5 p.m.	11 p.m.
1–2%	≥2%	1%	1%

Her fasting plasma glucose on this visit is 190 mg/dl and her urine sugar and acetone, as tested with Keto-Diastix, are 1% and negative. Subjectively, she feels a bit better but still urinates 2–3 times nightly. Her weight has remained stable over the past week. How should these results be interpreted? How should the insulin dose be altered?

Before attempting to adjust A.H.'s insulin dose based on her urine glucose test results, her compliance with testing double-voided samples must be ascertained, and it must be determined if there were any unusual circumstances in her life, diet or exercise patterns over the past week which might be affecting her response to insulin. Once these have been ruled out as confounding factors, one can begin to make gross adjustments in her insulin dose, realizing that "fine tuning" will be impossible until a consistent diet has been instituted.

Two principles must be kept in mind whenever urine tests are used to adjust insulin doses. First, do not change insulin doses based on a single urine measurement. Urine glucose testing is not accurate or reproducible enough to adjust insulin doses unless several tests have confirmed each other. Therefore, look for trends in urine test results over several days. (The only exception to this rule would be if supplemental insulin doses need to be given during periods of illness or stress.) Second, remember that all urine test procedures are only semi-quantitative, and that small differences in results may not, in fact, be real. At best, test results indicate small (negative to ½%), moderate (≤1 to 2%), or large (≥2%) amounts of glycosuria. See Fig 2.

The single dose of 25 units NPH is apparently inadequate to control A.H.'s symptoms. She is achieving some response in the late afternoon and evening (lunch and supper), but the delayed onset of NPH action and inadequate total daily dose has resulted in poor control of A.H.'s fasting and mid-morning hyperglycemia. It is unlikely that rebound hyperglycemia in response to nocturnal hypoglycemia caused by too much insulin (Questions 14 & 15) is a cause of the morning hyperglycemia in view of the fact that she remains hyperglycemic at bedtime.

As a first step toward better control, one could add a dose of rapid-acting regular insulin to her morning dose of NPH. This may improve the mid-morning hyperglycemia and thereby improve glucose levels for the remainder of the day. A dose of regular insulin which approximates one-half the dose of the morning NPH could be used to achieve the recommended NPH:Reg ratio of 2:1. See Table 7. However, this would mean adding 12 units of regular insulin to the total daily dose, which is a large increment clinically. Alternatively, one could increase the total daily dose to 30 units (0.6 units/kg) and administer 20 units as NPH and 10 units as regular insulin.

10. *Mixing Insulins.* A mixture of 20 units NPH and 10 units of regular insulin (Lilly Iletin II) was prescribed for A.H. How should she be instructed to measure and withdraw this insulin mixture?

The procedure used to mix and withdraw NPH and regular insulins is basically the same as that described for NPH in Question 5. The major difference is that air must be injected into the NPH vial *before* the regular insulin is measured and withdrawn. Also, regular insulin is measured and withdrawn into the insulin syringe *first* to avoid contamination of the regular vial of insulin with NPH which may ultimately alter the onset and duration of action of the regular insulin. When patients withdraw NPH or Lente insulin first, their vial of regular insulin eventually becomes cloudy. Contamination of the NPH insulin with regular insulin is probably insignificant because the excess protamine contained in NPH will bind the regular insulin (Question 11). Also, by first withdrawing regular insulin which is clear, A.H. will know if she has also withdrawn NPH insulin into the same syringe if she is interrupted, since the mixture should become somewhat cloudy from the NPH suspension. The procedure which A.H. should follow in mixing her insulins is as follows:

a. After dispersing the suspension of insulin, inject 20 units of air into the NPH vial and withdraw the needle.

b. Inject 10 units of air into the regular vial and withdraw 10 units of insulin as described in Question 5.

c. Insert the needle into the NPH vial and pull the plunger down to the 30 unit mark (20 units of NPH + 10 units of regular).

d. Inject immediately as directed in Question 5.

11. *Stability of Insulin Mixtures.* What are the chemical and clinical consequences of mixing regular insulin with NPH or Lente insulin?

In Vitro Interactions (Lilly Brands). When regular insulin is mixed with NPH or Lente insulins *in vitro,* regular insulin binds with the excess protamine present in NPH and, presumably, the excess zinc present in Lente. The binding is proportional to the ratio of regular to intermediate-acting insulin present in the mixure. Substantial binding of the regular insulin occurs in mixtures which contain a greater proportion of intermediate-acting insulin. However, as the amount of regular in the mixture approaches and exceeds that of the intermediate-acting insulins, more free regular insulin can be detected in the supernatant.

With NPH, the reaction occurs quickly and is complete in 15 minutes, but with Lente, the reaction does not reach equilibrium for 24 hours. Once the reaction is complete, the mixtures are stable for one month at room temperature or 3 months under refrigeration (2,114).

Clinical Response to Insulin Mixtures. In general, the clinical response to mixtures of regular insulin with Lente or NPH insulin corresponds well to the *in vitro* observations. Insulin mixtures in which the amount of intermediate acting insulin exceeds the amount of regular insulin are generally devoid of the rapid hypoglycemic effect of regular insulin. This is particularly true of the Regular/Lente mixtures. The rapid hypoglycemic effects of regular insulin become more apparent in 1:1 mixtures and are clearly present when the amount of regular insulin begins to exceed that of NPH or Lente (63,104).

However, *in vivo* studies demonstrate that an appreciable interaction occurs between intermediate-acting and regular insulin well before the *in vitro* equilibrium has been reached (63). Clinically, most of the rapid hypoglycemic effect of regular insulin is lost even 5 minutes after mixing regular with NPH or Lente insulins in a syringe (63).

Also, the clinical data observed for NPH insulin are valid only for the particular brand of NPH tested since products from various manufacturers contain different amounts of excess protamine. This may also hold true for the Lente mixtures. Nordisk NPH insulin (Insulatard NPH) contains less protamine than Lilly's NPH and it appears as though this is clinically significant (63,113,114). Even though *in vitro* binding can be detected chemically, there are no apparent differences between the glycemic response produced by a premixed NPH and regular product, Mixtard (70% NPH and 30% Regular), and two equivalent amounts of NPH and Regular insulins administered separately (113).

Recommendations. These new observations have important implications for diabetics who have difficulty achieving rapid hypoglycemic activity with regular/NPH or regular/Lente mixtures. These patients may need to increase the proportion of regular insulin beyond the usual recommended ratio (ie, may need proportions of regular insulin which exceed that of intermediate-acting insulin). Alternatively, using Nordisk brand insulins or injecting each insulin separately may help to retain the rapid-acting activity of regular insulin.

All patients administering mixtures of regular insulin with NPH or Lente should be instructed to mix the insulins just prior to injection. For diabetics using premixed Lilly insulins (prepared ahead of time by a visiting nurse, family member, etc.), the mixture should not be used before the reaction has reached equilibrium (15 minutes with NPH, 24 hours with Lente).

The stability and characteristics of other insulin combinations are tabulated in Table 9.

12. *Evaluating Fasting and Mid-Morning Hyperglycemia.* One week later, A.H. returns to the clinic with urine records which appear as follows:

7 a.m.	11:30 a.m.	5 p.m.	11 p.m.
1%	1–2%	0–¼%	½%

Subjectively, she feels substantially better. Her energy level is beginning to return to normal and her nocturia has diminished (1–2 times

nightly). Her weight remains the same and she has begun to develop some consistency in her dietary patterns with the help of a dietician. The fasting plasma glucose concentration is 190 mg/dl. Interpret A.H.'s urine pattern. How should she be managed at this point in time?

A.H.'s pre-dinner and bedtime urine tests have improved considerably, but her morning and pre-lunch tests remain elevated.

Fasting Hyperglycemia. The presence of moderate amounts of glucose in the urine at 7 a.m. suggests that A.H.'s fasting plasma glucose concentrations are high. This is corroborated by the level drawn in clinic. Morning hyperglycemia in A.H. may be the result of several factors:

a. An insufficient dose of NPH.
b. An insufficient duration of action of the morning dose of NPH.
c. The "dawn" phenomenon (126).
d. Reactive hyperglycemia in response to a nocturnal hypoglycemic episode (Somogyi effect).
e. A high carbohydrate bedtime snack.

The presence of glycosuria at bedtime and in the morning is consistent with the possibility that the morning NPH dose of insulin has a duration of action in A.H. which is too short to cover the glycemic excursions related to dinner. It may also be related to fasting glycogenolysis and gluconeogenesis which occur during the night and the *dawn phenomenon.* The latter consists of an early morning surge in the blood glucose which occurs between 5 a.m. and 8 a.m. and which follows a blood glucose nadir that occurs between 2:30 and 5 a.m. This phenomenon is observed in diabetics but not in nondiabetics and is associated with the presence of high free insulin concentrations during the nadir and low free insulin concentrations during the surge. The cause of this surge is unknown, although counterregulatory hormones have been implicated (126). Reactive hyperglycemia as a cause of the morning glycosuria in A.H. seems unlikely in view of the presence of glucose in her urine at bedtime. An insufficient morning dose of NPH is also an unlikely explanation since the afternoon urine glucose concentrations have improved tremendously. Increasing the dose of this insulin may result in a late afternoon hypoglycemic episode.

Morning Hyperglycemia. The presence of moderate to large amounts of glucose in A.H.'s

Table 9.

COMPATIBILITY OF INSULIN MIXTURES (2)

Mixture	Proportion	Comments
Regular + PZI	1:1 = PZI 2:1 = NPH 3:1 = NPH + Regular	The excess protamine in PZI combines with regular insulin and prolongs its action. PZI should not be mixed with regular insulin, but should be given as a separate injection.
Regular + NPH	Various	See text (Question 11). New evidence suggests that excess protamine in NPH products may also bind regular insulin and delay its onset and duration of action. This is particularly true of mixtures which contain a greater proportion of NPH. The clinical significance varies with different brands of NPH, which have different protamine contents. Advise the patient to mix insulins just prior to injection to retain as much of the rapid action as possible. Premixed combinations are stable for 1 month at room temperature and 2–3 months under refrigeration, but they may not retain the qualities of regular insulin.
Regular + Lente	Various	See text (Question 11). Regular insulin apparently binds with excess zinc in the Lente preparations and the rapid acting effects are lost in mixtures which contain a greater proportion of Lente insulin. The interaction can be detected clinically. Premixed combinations have the same stability characteristics as Regular:NPH mixtures described above.
Semilente + Lente or Ultralente	Any proportion	No incompatibilities.
Regular + Normal Saline	Any Proportion	Use within 2–3 hours of preparation.
Regular + Insulin Diluting Fluid	Any Proportion	Stable indefinitely.

urine at 11:30 a.m. is suggestive of mid-morning hyperglycemia. Mid-morning hyperglycemia frequently represents the maximum daily blood glucose excursion in diabetics and is the most difficult to manage (101,126). The following are possible explanations for mid-morning hyperglycemia:

a. An insufficient dose of regular insulin.
b. Delayed onset of action of regular insulin due to binding with NPH (likely in A.H.) or the presence of insulin-blocking antibodies (unlikely in A.H. who is a newly-diagnosed diabetic).
c. An insufficient dose of evening insulin to cover fasting glycogenolysis, gluconeogenesis, and the dawn phenomenon.

d. Excessive carbohydrate ingestion at breakfast.

When evaluating mid-morning hyperglycemia, it is important to remember that fasting hyperglycemia can contribute up to 50% of this plasma glucose excursion (126). Therefore, the primary mode of controlling hyperglycemia at this time of day may rely on initial control of the fasting plasma glucose level.

There are several possible solutions to A.H.'s pattern of glycosuria. These include increasing the dose of regular insulin to cover carbohydrate intake during breakfast; adding an evening dose of NPH insulin before dinner or at bedtime; injecting the morning dose of regular insulin separately and 1–2 hours prior to breakfast to minimize the dawn phenomenon and provide reasonable insulin levels to cover breakfast; and decreasing the carbohydrate content of breakfast. These authors favor a combination of these maneuvers.

1. Increase the total dose of insulin slightly, since the patient continues to spill glucose into the urine throughout the day (0.7 U/kg × 50 kg = 35 units).

2. Split the dose of insulin so that approximately ⅔ (24 units) is administered in the morning and ⅓ (12 units) is administered in the evening.

3. Provide a 1:1 ratio of NPH:Reg (12 units of each) in the morning in an attempt to retain the rapid action of regular insulin. Even though the total morning dose of insulin has been increased, this maneuver also lowers A.H.'s dose of NPH, thus minimizing possible afternoon hypoglycemia when the effect of NPH is at its peak.

4. The evening dose of insulin is traditionally given before dinner. At this point, the patient could be initiated on a 1:1 mixture of regular insulin and NPH. When NPH is added to the evening regimen, it is essential that, at least initially, the patient incorporate a bedtime snack into her diet.

13. *Home Blood Glucose Monitoring.* **A.H. is highly motivated to correct her hyperglycemia and agrees to a split dose of insulin. She is anxious to begin testing her blood glucose and wants to learn to adjust her own insulin doses. What products are available for home blood glucose monitoring (HBGM) and how are they used? Which one would be suitable for A.H.?**

Home blood glucose monitoring can be effectively achieved with one of several HBGM reagent strips which may be read with or without the aid of a reflectance colorimeter. See Table 10. Blood glucose reagent strips include Dextrostix (Ames), Visidex (Ames), and Chemstrip bG (Bio-Dynamics), none of which require a prescription. These products are slender plastic strips, similar to a Diastix urine test strip, with a glucose oxidase/peroxidase reagent pad on one end.

Method. A small finger prick is made with a sterile needle, lance or spring-loaded device (Autolet; Autoclix) on the side of a fingertip. An ample drop of blood is then milked from the finger and applied so that it completely covers the reagent pad. Smearing results in uneven coloration and difficult interpretation. After exactly one minute of contact time, the blood should be wiped off with a cotton ball or tissue (Chemstrip bG), or washed off the strip with a stream of water (Dextrostix or Visidex). After 1–2 minutes with Chemstrip bG or immediately with Dextrostix or Visidex, the colors that form on the reagent pad are compared to a color chart (much like urine tests) in which a particular color represents a blood glucose value. If the colors on the strip are in between two colors on the chart, a blood glucose estimate should be interpolated between these two values.

Table 10.
BLOOD GLUCOSE REAGENT STRIPS

Product	Range* (mg/dl)	Comments
Chemstrip bG (Bio-dynamics)	40–800	Reliable with or without a colorimeter. Several other advantages (see text). Compatible only with Accu-check bG colorimeter.
Dextrostix (Ames)	0–250	Unreliable if read visually. Compatible with Dextrometer, Glucometer, and Glucoscan colorimeters.
Visidex (Ames)	20–800	Cannot be used with colorimeters.

*without colorimeter

Chemstrip bG has an added advantage over the other products. After the blood has been wiped off the pad and left for 1–2 min, the color reaction will not change appreciably for several hours in open air, or up to 7 days if the strip is kept in the original container with its dessicator lid (115,116). Reagent strips which are not used in a colorimeter may also be cut lengthwise as a cost-savings measure.

Dextrostix are not recommended for visual use without a reflectance colorimeter for two reasons. First, they have a narrower range than Chemstrip bG or Visidex: 0–250 mg/dl compared to 40–800 mg/dl or 20–800 mg/dl, respectively. Second, and most importantly, Dextrostix do not reliably reflect accurate blood glucose values when read visually; they are comparable to the other products only when used with a colorimeter (116–118).

Colorimeters. The available reflectance colorimeters include the Dextrometer and Glucometer by Ames, the Glucoscan by Lifescan (all three of which use the Dextrostix reagent strips), and the Accu-Chek bG by Biodynamics (which uses the Chemstrip bG strips). The Glucometer, Ames' newest machine, has several advantages over their older model, the Dextrometer. However, all of the newer models are small, lightweight, easy to use and calibrate, are battery-operated, contain digital read-out displays, and have built-in buzzers to facilitate timing. Other than cost, selection of one meter over another depends on individual patient preference since each model has slightly different features (119).

The use of a reflectance colorimeter has the advantage of a large digital display which is easy to read and also obviates the need to interpolate or "estimate" the color match from the reagent strips themselves, which some patients may find difficult (especially those who are visually impaired). However, the colorimeter is an added initial expense and is not necessarily more accurate than properly used HBGM reagent strips designed for visual inspection (Chemstrip bG, Visidex). It is also cumbersome to carry when testing is not done at one location. Fortunately, the technology of reflectance colorimeters is experiencing a growth phase similar to that of electronic calculators. As a result, more simplified and compact colorimeters are being introduced on the market and it is anticipated that prices will decline.

Accuracy. Although quantitative results are achieved when reagent strips are used with or without a colorimeter (except Dextrostix alone), an error of ±10–20% is not uncommon and larger errors may be observed (116–118,120,121). Most diabetologists, however, contend that the accuracy is well within the range of clinical utility. Clinicians utilizing these products in the hospital or clinic should keep in mind that blood glucose concentrations determined by these methods are approximately 10% less (depending on the patient's hematocrit) than plasma glucose concentrations reported by the laboratory.

A.H.'s home blood glucose monitoring program can be initiated with Chemstrips bG because they do not require the use of a colorimeter and are procedurally more convenient than Visidex which must be rinsed with water. Furthermore, each strip can be marked with a date and time and brought back to clinic the following week to validate the patient's interpretation of the color changes. Some patients prefer to use the colorimeter at home and the Chemstrips during work or travel.

14. *Reactive Hyperglycemia.* A.H. was given a split dose of insulin: 12 U NPH and 12 U Regular 30–60 minutes before breakfast and 6 U NPH and 6 U Regular 30–60 minutes before dinner. She was instructed to test both her urine and home blood glucose before meals and at bedtime and to bring her results to clinic the following week. She was also instructed to call if she noted blood glucose levels below 60 mg/dl. The following week her overall urine and blood glucose results appeared as follows:

	7 a.m.	11 a.m.	6 p.m.	11 p.m.
Blood	220 mg/dl	190 mg/dl	130 mg/dl	70 mg/dl
Urine	¼–1%	neg	neg	neg

Overall, she is feeling much better. Her only complaint is that she awoke twice last week with nightsweats and nightmares. Assess A.H.'s blood and urine glucose results at this time. How should she be managed?

A.H.'s blood glucose results indicate that she remains hyperglycemic early in the morning and mid-morning. This time, however, rebound hyperglycemia secondary to nocturnal hypoglycemia (Somogyi effect) must be considered. Evidence which suggests that this may be occurring includes the patient's complaints of nightsweats and nightmares as well as a low bedtime blood glucose. This is an ominous sign since A.H. has already received an evening injection of NPH which will have peak effects at approximately 3 a.m. when the glucose nadir of the "dawn" phenomenon occurs (Question 12). When patients observe low bedtime blood glucose concentrations in association with high morning blood glucose concentrations, they should be instructed to test a blood glucose at 3 a.m. in the morning. (When A.H. did this she measured a blood glucose concentration of 40 mg/dl.) Hypoglycemia with rebound hyperglycemia may be managed by decreasing A.H.'s evening dose of NPH, by moving the evening dose of NPH to bedtime so that its peak effects occur during the glucose surge associated with the dawn phenomenon; or by splitting the dose of NPH so that ½ is administered with regular insulin before dinner and ½ is administered at bedtime.

Galloway recommends that the Somogyi effect be managed by decreasing the total dose of insulin by approximately 10% in Type I diabetics such as A.H. (74). Since the evening dose of regular insulin is adequately controlling glycemia related to the evening meal, its dose should remain the same; the evening dose of NPH can be decreased to 3 units and administered at bedtime. Thus, A.H.'s morning hyperglycemia will be managed with a *decreased* insulin dose. The importance of an evening snack should be re-emphasized, and A.H. should be encouraged to check another 3 a.m. blood glucose sample to assess the effect of this dose alteration.

In view of the hyperglycemia observed at 11 a.m., it would also be tempting to increase A.H.'s morning dose of regular insulin. However, when the 11 a.m. glucose concentration of 190 mg/dl is viewed in relationship to the fasting blood glucose of 220 mg/dl and the fact that glucose concentrations must have been considerably higher than this level following the breakfast meal, it would appear that the regular insulin is exerting considerable effect. Furthermore, increasing the total daily dose of insulin at this time could expose A.H. to more hypoglycemic episodes. Therefore, the a.m. dose of regular insulin should be kept the same at this time and reassessed following the institution of bedtime NPH.

A.H.'s urine test results indicate that her renal threshold for glucose is somewhat elevated and is between 190 and 220 mg/dl. They also illustrate the fact that negative urine glucose tests can occur in the presence of hyperglycemia as well as hypoglycemia and are of questionable value in monitoring a patient who wishes to achieve some degree of euglycemia. Further, the semi-quantitative qualities of urine glucose tests are illustrated by the fact that A.H.'s blood glucose concentration of 220 mg/dl was associated with a broad range of urine glucose test results (¼–1%).

15. *Hypoglycemia Management.* How should A.H. be taught to assess and manage any hypoglycemic reactions which may occur?

Hypoglycemia is defined as a blood glucose concentration of less than 50–60 mg/dl, and its occurrence is potentially fatal if it is not recognized and promptly treated.

The signs and symptoms associated with hypoglycemia include (in order of general appearance) those related to the parasympathetic nervous system (hunger, nausea); diminished cerebral function (lethargy, yawning, confusion, agitation, nervousness); increased sympathetic activity (tachycardia, sweating, tremor) and ultimately convulsions, stupor and coma. Tingling of the lips and tongue are common early symptoms, and drenching nightsweats and nightmares are common complaints of patients who develop insulin reactions at night. The degree to which many of these signs and symptoms occur often varies with the patient and rate of fall in the blood glucose concentration. Thus, A.H. must be taught to recognize those signs and symptoms which serve as early warning symptoms for her. Since signs and symptoms related to hypoglycemia may also occur when there is a rapid fall in blood glucose (even if it is in the hyperglycemic range), A.H. should be encouraged to test her blood glucose when she suspects a reaction and to treat the symptoms only if she is truly hypoglycemic.

Most hypoglycemic reactions are readily managed with the equivalent of 10 grams of glucose, which should raise the blood glucose approximately 40–50 mg/dl within 10–15 minutes. This amount of carbohydrate is provided by 4 ounces of a sweetened juice or nondiet soda, 1 tablespoonful of jelly, two packets of sugar, 5–6 lifesavers, or 4 sugar cubes. This "quick" source of sugar should be followed by small amounts of starch and protein to provide a continual source of glucose if a meal is not scheduled within the next half hour. Most diabetics have a tendency to overtreat hypoglycemic reactions with large quantities of juice or several candy bars, and this should be discouraged. One major advantage of home blood glucose monitoring is that the patient does not have to rely on subjective signs and symptoms to evaluate the effects of treatment.

A.H.'s friends should also be made aware of this potential complication of her insulin therapy and should be taught how to recognize the symptoms of hypoglycemia. Often, diabetics ignore early warning symptoms of hypoglycemia and progress to a point where they lose the judgment needed to treat the condition and become combative. A vial of glucagon should be kept on hand for management of A.H. should she lose consciousness.

Each time A.H. has a hypoglycemic reaction, she must determine its cause and take preventative corrective action. This entails assessment of her diet (did she skip or delay a meal or change its content?); exercise pattern; and insulin administration and dose. If hypoglycemic reactions consistently occur at a certain time of the day, she should determine whether this corresponds to the maximum effect of one of her insulins and reduce the dose of that insulin by 1–2 units (122) or add a supplemental snack to that part of the day.

16. Sick-Day Management. A.H.'s evening dose of NPH was decreased to 3 units and she was instructed to administer this insulin at bedtime instead of 6 p.m. She responded well to this regimen with pre- and postprandial blood glucose levels ranging from 80–150 mg/dl. Signs and symptoms of hypoglycemia have also disappeared, and occasional testing of her blood glucose at 3 a.m. reveals levels of 80–100 mg/dl. She has also gained 10 pounds and has been asymptomatic with regard to her diabetes. However, two days ago she began to develop signs and symptoms consistent with the flu. She has been anorexic and nauseated and now has begun to vomit. Her food intake is minimal. Should A.H. discontinue her insulin in view of the fact that she cannot eat at this time?

Insulin requirements always increase in the presence of infection and acute illness, even if food intake is diminished. Insulin dependent diabetics such as A.H. commonly decrease or eliminate insulin doses under these circumstances and it is just in this setting that ketoacidosis occurs.

Therefore, A.H. should be instructed to maintain her usual dose of insulin and to resume testing her blood glucose four times daily before meals (if she has since become less compliant in that regard). If blood glucose concentrations are above the usual range, *supplemental* doses of regular insulin should be administered in doses of 1 unit for each 30–40 mg/dl increment above the target goal up to a maximum of 4 units (122) (See section on Goals of Insulin Therapy) If the blood glucose is unresponsive to this dose, she should call her physician. For those testing urine only, 4 units of supplemental regular insulin are given before meals and at bedtime each time a double voided urine sample contains 1–2% glucose (123).

A.H. should also be instructed to test her urine for the presence of ketones if blood or urine glucose tests are consistently high and to watch for signs and symptoms related to hyperglycemia (polyuria, polydipsia) and ketoacidosis. (Diabetic ketoacidosis is presented on pages 313–319 of this text.) She should also attempt to maintain her fluid, mineral, and carbohydrate intake with easily digested foods and fluids.

17. Insulin Dosing in a Hospitalized Patient. A.G. is a 13½-year-old female who is admitted to the hospital with symptoms of polydipsia, polyuria, weight loss, easy fatigability, and a recent history of multiple upper respiratory tract infections. Her temperature was 39°C and her chest was congested. A urinalysis revealed 4+ glucose by the Clinitest method with no ketones. Her blood glucose at this time was 400 mg/dl. A diagnosis of juvenile-onset diabetes and pneumonia was made. The physician ordered appropriate fluids, and insulin "to be given according to the rainbow schedule." What is meant by the "rainbow" or "sliding scale" method for insulin dosing?

These terms refer to a method of adjusting dosages of subcutaneous *regular insulin* according to urine glucose readings obtained by the *copper reduction method*. The presence of acetone also influences the dose. Because there is no standard schedule, the physician must specifically indicate the number of units (s)he desires for each reading. Generally, insulin doses are in the range of 5 units for each "plus" sign (see Table 2). For example:

0–1+	(<½%)	0–5U
2+	(¾%)	5–10U
3+	(1%)	10–15U
4+	(≥2%)	15–20U

Mod. acetone—An additional 5U

Such a schedule is used for the hospitalized diabetic whose insulin requirements may vary with stress (eg, infections, surgery or any acute illness) or to determine the initial insulin requirements of a newly diagnosed diabetic. Generally the urine is tested every four hours and insulin administered accordingly. However, some have recommended that a six-hour interval be used in view of the fact that the peak effect and duration of action of regular insulin may be considerably delayed and prolonged in some individuals (2,124).

Now that blood glucose concentrations can be measured quickly and easily with test strips (see Question 13), it is more reasonable to dose insulin in an acute hospital situation on the basis of these values rather than the indirect urine values.

An important concept to keep in mind when using any form of rainbow schedule is that the blood or urine glucose value measured at a particular point in time should be used as the determinant of the *previous* dose of regular insulin rather than the current dose. In acknowledgement of this, many clinicians manage inpatient diabetics the same way they would manage an outpatient diabetic, except that more intensive, split-dose insulin therapy can be initiated immediately. For example, a total daily dose based upon previous doses of insulin, weight (see Table 8), or empirical clinical experience is calculated and split into two doses of NPH in the morning and afternoon (eg, ⅔ and ⅓ respectively). These basal doses are *supplemented* with regular insulin based upon guidelines discussed in Question 16. Ultimately, the blood or urine glucose concentration results are used to adjust insulin doses in a manner similar to those discussed previously (see Questions 9, 12 and 14). For example, the fasting blood glucose is used to adjust the evening dose of NPH, and the blood glucose concentration measured in the late afternoon is used to adjust the following day's dose of morning NPH. As an alternative, some would add the morning supplemental insulin doses to the *next* day's evening dose of intermediate-acting insulin and the afternoon and evening supplemental doses to the *next* day's morning dose of intermediate-acting insulin. The basis for this adjustment is that the morning supplemental doses reflect the inadequacy of the previous night's dose of NPH and the afternoon and evening supplemental doses represent the inadequacy of the previous morning's dose of NPH. Therefore, the next day's doses of NPH are increased by these amounts (64).

18. ***Dermatologic Complications of Insulin.*** R.C. is a 22-year-old female whose Type I diabetes was diagnosed four years ago. She is currently well-controlled on split doses of insulin (Squibb Brand). Her primary concerns on this visit are the unsightly indentations present on the anterior aspects of her thighs where she injects her insulin. On physical examination extensive areas of lipoatrophy as well as mild lipohypertrophy are noted on both the anterior, lateral and posterior aspects of her thighs. On history, the patient recalls that when she first began using insulin she developed "red, itchy" spots at the sites of insulin injection which have since disapppeared. What are the causes of R.C.'s dermatologic history and findings? How can they be managed?

Lipodystrophy secondary to the use of insulin may present in two ways and both are evident in R.C.: as atrophy (subcutaneous concavities caused by wasting of fat tissue) and as hypertrophy (tumorous-like fat pads at the site of injection).

Lipoatrophy. Lipoatrophy occurs most commonly in young women (as illustrated by R.C.) and children. Although its cause is unknown, the presence of lipolytic and immunogenic impurities in insulin are thought to be important. Prior to the purification of insulin, the reported incidence of this reaction was quite high (10–50%) (74,125); however, its occurrence should diminish considerably with the use of purer products (80,81). The lipolytic and immunogenic theories of lipoatrophy are consistent with R.C.'s current use of a beef-source insulin which is probably the most antigenic product currently available. Also, Squibb insulin previously had a very high proinsulin content which has recently been corrected. (See Table 5.)

Lipoatrophy most commonly appears 2 months to several years after use and may be related to the patient's failure to adequately rotate her injections. In Lilly's series of patients, 25% had a history of a local reaction to insulin (as did R.C.) and a similar number had co-existing hypertrophy. Like, R.C., 30% of their patients developed lipoatrophy at sites which had never been injected with insulin (2,74).

Management. The primary form of treatment of lipoatrophy is the injection of "purified" pork insulin directly into the lipoatrophic site. (See Table 11.) Using this method, improvement begins to occur in 2–4 weeks and complete recovery should be attained in 6 months. After one site has been restored to normal, the patient begins repeated injections into another lipoatrophic site. This form of therapy has been found to be 90–100% effective, but atrophy may recur unless insulin is injected into the same site every 3–4 weeks (74,81,123,127–129). If R.C. is unresponsive to "purified" insulin, one could try adding small amounts of dexamethasone (4 mcg/unit) to her insulin. This was reportedly successful in six out of nine patients after 6 months (130).

Lipohypertrophy. R.C. also exhibits mild areas of lipohypertrophy which are probably caused by the lipogenic effects of insulin. Most cases occur after many months or years of repeated injections into the same site. It is said to occur more frequently in young patients (36.5%) than adults (3%) (125) and may be self-perpetuating because the site of injection becomes anesthetized. Proper rotation of the injection sites may result in spontaneous regression of these lipomas (123). As expected, the injection of "purified" insulins into the affected site does not appear to improve this form of lipodystrophy and, in fact, cases of lipohypertrophy have been associated with their use (131, 132). (See Table 11.)

Local Skin Reactions. R.C. also has a history of local skin reactions to insulin. Before insulin was purified, erythema, pain, swelling and itching was reported to occur in up to 50% of patients initiated on insulin. The reactions may be immediate (onset 20–40 minutes and lasting 2–6 hours) or delayed (onset up to 12 hours after injection, peaking at 6–12 hours, and taking 1–7 days to subside). Frequently, as illustrated by R.C., spontaneous desensitization to insulin occurs by the time the first vial of insulin is completed (3 weeks to 3 months) and the local reaction subsides. If the reaction persists or is particularly bothersome, the patient may be switched to pure pork insulin. The incidence of local reactions has decreased considerably with the use of the more purified insulins (74,80,123).

19. *Dose Change with Switch to More Purified Insulin.* R.C. agrees to use a "purified" pork insulin in an attempt to resolve the disfiguring lipoatrophy of both legs. Will a reduction of insulin dose be necessary in this patient?

Varying reductions of dose requirements were originally reported in Europe when patients were changed from a conventional beef or beef/pork insulin to a "purified" pure pork insulin. These ranged from an immediate and dramatic decrease in insulin requirements to gradual reductions over many months (132–139). The immediate reduction in insulin requirement prompted the European manufacturers to warn clinicians of an initial 20% reduction in dose requirements, especially

Table 11.

INDICATIONS FOR "PURIFIED" PORK INSULIN (80,131,440)

Indications for Patients Who Have:	Comment
Local or Systemic Insulin Allergies	Some cases of systemic allergy resolve when patients are switched to a "purified" pork insulin. There is a decreased prevalence of local allergic reactions to these insulins (2,80). However, occasional systemic allergic reactions to "purified" insulins may occur as well, indicating that they also have some inherent antigenicity (437,438).
Immunologically-Based Insulin Resistance	When insulin resistance is due to the presence of excessive circulating insulin antibodies, the use of a "purified" pork insulin may be beneficial (2).
Lipodystrophies	Lipoatrophy often responds to a more purified product (80,133). Conversely, lipohypertrophy does not respond well to the "purified" insulins and, in fact, has been reported to develop during their use (132).
Temporary Requirements for Insulin	Because interrupted insulin therapy is more frequently associated with the development of local or systemic allergy and immunologic resistance (1,142), many diabetologists recommend the use of the "purified" pork insulins for patients who will require insulin only temporarily. These situations include gestational diabetes, insulin requirements during hyperalimentation, and in Type II diabetics requiring insulin during surgery or major stress.

when doses of over 40 units were used. Subsequent investigators, particularly in the U.S. where the change in insulin purity was less radical (Lilly's "single peak" insulin had been available for years), have not observed predictable changes in requirements (80,131,140,141). In one report, 211 insulin dependent diabetics were followed for three months on beef/pork "single peak" insulin and then for four months on pure pork "purified" insulin. Dosage requirements were both increased and decreased, and no consistent change in insulin requirement was found (80). A specific dosage reduction should not be made initially in R.C.'s regimen. However, she should be instructed to monitor her diabetic control as closely as possible for the first few weeks after changing products since a modification in insulin requirement may become apparent.

20. Insulin Allergy and Resistance. Discuss other immunologically-based adverse reactions to insulin and their treatment.

In addition to the dermatologic effects of insulin, there are at least two other adverse effects which have an immune basis: systemic insulin allergy and insulin resistance.

Systemic Allergic Reactions. Fortunately, systemic allergic reactions to insulin, which may present as urticaria, angioedema, laryngospasm, and hypotension, are very rare. A large percentage of the patients who present with this complication have had a history of interrupted insulin therapy and local reactions to insulin. The acute management of these individuals includes epinephrine, antihistamines and glucocorticoids as needed. The long-term treatment includes switching to the more purified pork insulins (although systemic allergic reactions to these insulins have also been reported) and desensitization if this maneuver is unsuccessful. (See Table 11.) The precise protocol for desensitization is described elsewhere (2,142).

Insulin Resistance. Insulin resistance is defined as a daily insulin requirement of 200 U or more for more than one week (> 2.5 U/kg for a child) in the absence of ketoacidosis, coma, or infection. It is a rare phenomenon which can be caused by high titers of circulating insulin-blocking antibody, decreased tissue responsiveness to insulin and, rarely, increased degradation of insulin in the subcutaneous tissue (143). Insulin resistance most often occurs in Type II diabetics

who have had a history of interrupted insulin therapy and allergic reactions to insulin (75% of cases) (74,142). It is a temporary condition which reverses spontaneously in 60% of patients within six months.

There are two primary forms of therapy for patients with immunologically based insulin resistance. The first revolves around switching the patient to the least antigenic form of insulin commercially available ("purified" pork insulins), which decreases insulin requirements in approximately 50% of patients (74,142). (See Table 11.) Investigational insulins such as sulfated insulin, dealanated insulin and fish insulins have been used successfully in the management of insulin resistance, but these are not available commercially (77,144).

The second form of therapy involves the administration of a short course of high dose glucocorticoids (eg, 40–80 mg prednisone daily for 10 days). Approximately 75% of patients given this therapy will have marked reductions in their insulin requirements 3–6 days after therapy is initiated. Since glucocorticoids are diabetogenic and inherently toxic, their use should be discontinued as quickly as possible (74,144).

Other less popular methods of treating insulin resistance in Type II diabetics include the administration of sulfonylureas, on the theory that insulin antibodies are less likely to cross react with endogenous insulin, and temporary discontinuation of insulin therapy may allow antibody titers to decline (145,146).

21. Insulin Requirements in Renal Failure. M.B. is a 32-year-old Type I diabetic who has been taking insulin for 15 years. Over the past year a gradual deterioration of her renal function, as reflected by urine protein, serum creatinine and blood urea nitrogen values, has been observed. What are the anticipated effects of decreased renal function on M.B.'s insulin requirements?

There are two major effects of decreased renal function on insulin requirement. In the early stages, a decrease in insulin requirements predominates; however, as the patient becomes progressively uremic, insulin requirements may increase or become extremely variable.

The kidney is the most important site of extrahepatic insulin metabolism and excretion (147, 148). Therefore, diminished kidney function is accompanied by a decreased clearance of endogenous or exogenous insulin, resulting in increased plasma concentrations of insulin. The nausea and anorexia which characterize uremia may lead to decreased carbohydrate intake and hypoglycemia in these individuals (149).

As renal function worsens, various factors which decrease glucose tolerance begin to predominate. These include increased hepatic gluconeogenesis, tissue resistance to the effects of insulin, elevated concentrations of counterregulatory hormones such as glucagon, and the presence of an unknown "hyperglycemic factor" which can be removed by dialysis (149).

As M.B.'s renal failure progresses through various stages of severity, many alterations of insulin dose can be anticipated. As in all other diabetics, activity and appetite must be closely monitored.

22. *Exercise and Insulin Requirements.* J.S. **is a 17-year-old, non-obese, Type I diabetic who was diagnosed at the age of 12. He is currently moderately well controlled on two daily doses of insulin (7 U regular/14 U NPH in the morning and 7 U regular/7 U NPH in the evening). His Hb A_{1c} is 10% and his blood glucose levels before meals range from 150–190 mg/dl. Fasting blood glucose concentrations in the clinic range from 130–170 mg/dl. He has rare hypoglycemic reactions which are associated with skipped meals, and he is generally compliant with his prescribed diet. What effect is jogging likely to have on his diabetic control? What precautions, if any, should he take?**

Exercise has varying effects on plasma glucose levels in insulin dependent diabetics such as J.S. In patients who are poorly controlled and insulin deficient (random blood glucose concentrations $\geq$ 300 mg/dl with or without ketones), exercise may actually raise glucose concentrations and induce ketosis. A combination of very low insulin levels in combination with an exaggerated release of epinephrine, glucagon and other counterregulatory hormones in these patients result in a combination of decreased glucose utilization by muscle along with excessive glucose production through hepatic glycogenolysis and gluconeogenesis. At least some insulin is required for glucose uptake and utilization during exercise (53,54).

Exercise may have minimal effects on J.S.'s plasma glucose, as in a nondiabetic (see Introduction); however, the predominant effect observed in IDDM diabetics who are moderately well controlled is a decrease in the blood glucose level during exercise as well as several hours after exercise (53,54,150,152). Caron and associates (150) found that 45 minutes of moderate exercise (bicycle ergometer) 30 minutes after breakfast reduced the peak glycemia for breakfast from 270 mg/dl on the nonexercise day to 203 mg/dl on the day of exercise and the peak glycemia following lunch from 270 mg/dl to 170 mg/dl. Usual doses of insulin were injected into the abdomen on the morning of exercise 30 minutes before breakfast. This study illustrates the prolonged effects of exercise on plasma glucose levels. The decreased glucose excursion following breakfast was probably related to the diversion of blood flow from the splanchnic area to the musculature, resulting in delayed absorption of nutrients, as well as the increased glucose utilization of exercising muscle. The decreased glucose excursion following lunch was presumably due to the effect of exercise on increased insulin receptor binding and to the continued uptake of glucose by muscle to replenish glycogen stores.

Hypoglycemia secondary to exercise has also been reported in patients such as J.S. (53,54). This may occur if insulin levels are too high, resulting in suppression of glycogenolysis and gluconeogenesis in the liver in the face of increased glucose utilization by muscle. High insulin levels may be the result of increased absorption of insulin from subcutaneous sites which can occur during exercise. The absorption of regular insulin is increased when it is administered just prior to exercise (5 minutes) (151) but does not appear to be affected if injected 30–40 minutes prior to exercise (104). Some have suggested that injection of insulin at a site which is not exercised (eg, the abdomen) may minimize this effect (151); however, the value of this maneuver has been questioned by others (54,104,152). The effect of exercise on the absorption of intermediate-acting insulins has been less well studied. One study shows that the absorption of intermediate-acting insulins is not augmented when exercise is performed 2½ hours after injection; however, its effect on absorption after shorter intervals was not studied (104). No alterations in insulin absorption (regular and intermediate-acting) were observed by Caron and associates when these mixtures were injected one hour prior to exercise (150).

In view of these findings, J.S. should be encouraged to exercise at least 30–40 minutes after an insulin injection and relatively soon after a meal or a snack. Exercise in the fasting state and evening exercise should be avoided due to the acute and prolonged effects of exercise on blood glucose. Because he is "moderately" well controlled, he may start his exercise without initially altering his dose of insulin, site of insulin injection, or diet. However, he should be made aware of the potential hypoglycemic effects of exercise and should increase his food intake prior to and *following* exercise as needed. An insulin dependent diabetic who is tightly controlled and has frequent hypoglycemic reactions should definitely increase his food intake prior to and following exercise. If hypoglycemic reactions persist, insulin doses should be decreased. Chronic physical training through regular exercise may eventually diminish J.S.'s insulin requirements (54).

If J.S. exercises on a regular basis, he should avoid drugs which may predispose him to hypoglycemic reactions such as alcohol, propranolol, and others listed in Table 18. If he participates in any exercise which may cause foot injury, the importance of appropriate foot care and regular inspection of the feet should be strongly reinforced.

ORAL HYPOGLYCEMIC AGENTS

Phenformin

Prior to 1977, when its general use was banned by the Food and Drug Administration, phenformin, a biguanide hypoglycemic agent, was available for the treatment of Type II diabetics. The withdrawal of this agent from the U.S. market was primarily based upon its association with fatal lactic acidosis (158,159). Phenformin and another biguanide, metformin, are still used in European countries. For those rare symptomatic Type II diabetics who are allergic to sulfonylureas; cannot use insulin (allergy; mental or physical disability); cannot be controlled on diet; and who have no predisposing factors to the development of lactic acidosis, phenformin can be obtained through an investigational new drug (IND) application issued by the U.S. Food and Drug Administration. Complete information regarding the use of phenformin and application forms may be requested from:

Division of Metabolism and
 Endocrine Drug Products (HFD-130)
Food and Drug Administration
5800 Fishers Lane
Rockville, Maryland 20857
(301) 443-3490

Sulfonylureas

The only oral hypoglycemic agents currently available in the United States are the sulfonylureas.

Mechanism of Action. Sulfonylureas stimulate the release of insulin from pancreatic beta cells initially; however, insulin levels tend to return to baseline values after a few (6–16) months of continued use. Because the sulfonylureas continue to exert a beneficial effect on glucose tolerance after their effects on insulin levels are no longer detectable, "extrapancreatic" effects of the sulfonylureas have been studied and proposed. These include an alteration in the pattern of insulin release so that the initial rapid release of insulin is restored; an increase in the number of insulin receptors at the cell surface; and a modulation of the effect of insulin on its own receptors (eg, decreasing the down-regulating effect of insulin). The extent to which any of these and many other proposed effects of sulfonylureas play a role in improved glucose tolerance remains to be resolved (153–157).

Sulfonylureas have no beneficial effects on the glucose tolerance of pancreatectomized individuals or Type I diabetics who have no pancreatic reserve. Their use, therefore, should be reserved for symptomatic Type II diabetics who are unable to achieve control on diet alone. (See Questions 23,24,26–28).

Second Generation Sulfonylureas. There are currently four "first generation" sulfonylureas available on the U.S. market (acetohexamide, chlorpropamide, tolazamide, and tolbutamide).

The "second generation" sulfonylureas (glyburide, glipizide, glibornuride, and others), though not yet available for general use at the time of this writing, have been widely used in Europe and elsewhere for years and will soon be introduced in the United States. The three second-generation agents discussed herein all share two basic properties: (1) primary metabolism in the liver to inactive compounds, and (2) duration of activity which requires no more than 1 or 2 daily doses.

Though these properties are desirable for general use as well as in the elderly or patients with renal impairment, they offer little in the way of advantages which are not already covered by at least one of the traditional first generation agents.

Care must be taken to ensure that these drugs are dosed properly since they are at least 50–200 times more potent than the first generation drugs, though the efficacy of all the sulfonylureas is generally considered comparable.

It has been suggested that the second generation sulfonylureas may be less susceptible than the older agents to displacement by other acidic, highly protein-bound drugs (160). This is primarily based on the data of Brown et al, who found that phenylbutazone and warfarin markedly affect the protein binding of tolbutamide and chlorpropamide, but not that of glyburide *in vitro* (161). Side effects of the second generation drugs are similar and probably occur with the same frequency, though this awaits post-marketing surveillance in this country.

Pharmacokinetics of Sulfonylureas

The biopharmaceutic and pharmacokinetic parameters of the individual agents have been reviewed extensively (162,163) and are summarized in the following text and in Table 12. It should be emphasized that the duration of hypoglycemic activity is related to the half-life of these compounds only in very general terms, and may correlate poorly in some cases. All of the sulfonylureas are highly protein bound (80–100%), mainly to albumin, though various binding characteristics have been demonstrated as previously mentioned. Food does not impair the extent of drug absorption, but may delay the peak effect of some agents.

Tolbutamide is the sulfonylurea with the shortest duration of action (6–12 hours). It is rapidly and totally metabolized in the liver to very weakly active or inactive compounds (carboxytolbutamide and hydroxytolbutamide) which are in turn excreted in the urine (164). The average half-life of tolbutamide is about 7 hours but has been demonstrated to vary considerably from this mean (range 4–25 hours) (165). Multiple daily dosing (2–3 times a day) is usually necessary.

Chlorpropamide, the longest acting sulfonylurea (24–72 hours), is (on the average) about 80% metabolized in the liver to compounds of unknown activity; about 20% is excreted unchanged by the kidneys (166,167). The metabolites appear to have much shorter elimination half-lives than the parent drug (166). For many years this drug was thought to be excreted totally unchanged in the urine, but studies using more sophisticated analytical techniques have shown otherwise. The average half-life of chlorpropamide is approximately 36 hours, though values have been shown to vary widely from subject to subject (25–60 hours) (162). It should be emphasized that the average amount of active drug that is reported to be excreted unchanged (20%) actually varies considerably (range 10–60%) and this, plus the long serum half-life and duration of hypoglycemic activity, should preclude the use of chlorpropamide in the elderly or in patients with renal impairment. Omitting a dose or two during temporary periods of decreased food intake (eg, surgery) will not result in cessation of hypoglycemic activity until several days have passed.

Acetohexamide is an intermediate-acting (12–18 hours) sulfonylurea which is principally metabolized and eliminated as L-hydroxyhexamide, a compound with greater activity than that of the parent drug (162). About 50% of this active metabolite is excreted in the urine; the rest is presumably metabolized further to an inactive compound. While the mean half-life of the parent drug is 1.3 hours, the mean half-life of L-hydroxyhexamide is about 5 hours. Thus, the hypoglycemic activity of acetohexamide is mainly due to its active metabolite. Like chlorpropamide, it is a poor choice for patients with renal impairment.

Tolazamide is the newest of the first generation sulfonylureas and shares an intermediate duration of activity (12–16 hours) with acetohexamide. Due to delayed absorption, its peak concentration and hypoglycemic effect is 4–8 hours vs 2–4 hours with most other sulfonylureas. Tolazamide is metabolized to six compounds; three of these are inactive and the other three retain partial activity. The half-life of the active drug is about 7 hours.

Although both tolazamide and acetohexamide share an intermediate duration of activity, clinical experience has shown that some patients respond well to a single daily dose (162). Compliance may be greatly increased if control is effected with this dosing schedule. However, usual clinical dosing is twice daily for both drugs.

Glyburide, or glybenclamide (the generic name

Table 12.

PHARMACOKINETICS OF THE ORAL HYPOGLYCEMICS

Drug	Equivalent Therapeutic Dose (mg)	Usual Minimum and Maximum Daily Dose	Mean Half-Life	Duration of Activity	Metabolism and Excretion	Comments
First-Generation Sulfonylureas						
Acetohexamide (Dymelor)	500	0.25–1.5 gm single or divided doses	6 hrs	12–18+ hr duration	Metabolite's activity greater than parent drug. Metabolite excreted, in part, via kidney.	Caution in elderly and patients with renal impairment. Significant uricosuric effects.
Chlorpropamide (Diabinese)	250	0.1–0.5 gm single dose	35 hrs	24–72 hr duration	Extensive metabolism to compounds with unknown activity. 20% excreted unchanged, which may vary widely.	Caution in elderly and patients with renal impairment. Higher frequency of alcohol-flushing, hyponatremia and perhaps other side effects.
Tolazamide (Tolinase)	250	0.1–1.0 gm single or divided doses	7 hrs	12–16+ hr duration	Some metabolites have weak activity excreted via kidney.	Like acetohexamine, some patients are controlled on a single daily dose.
Tolbutamide (Orinase)	1000	0.5–3.0 gm divided doses	7 hrs	6–12 hr duration	Totally metabolized to compounds with negligible activity.	Useful in patients with renal impairment.
Second-Generation Sulfonylureas						
Glyburide (Micronase)	5	1.25–30 mg single (or divided) dose	10 hrs	24 hr duration	Metabolized to compounds one of which may be weakly active.	Possible drug accumulation.
Glipizide (Glucotrol)	5	2.5–40 mg single or divided doses	4 hrs	≤24 hr duration	Metabolized to inactive compounds.	No special precautions.
Glibornuride	12.5	12.5–75 mg single or divided doses	8 hrs	≤24 hr duration	Metabolized to compounds which may be weakly active.	No special precautions.

in other countries), is totally metabolized in the liver to two major metabolites, one of which may have weak hypoglycemic activity (163). These metabolites are then excreted in the bile as well as in the urine. The mean half-life of glyburide has been variably reported at 2–12 hours (162, 168); some of this discrepancy may be due to multiphasic elimination kinetics. In fact, drug accumulation may occur on repeated dosing due to a slowly equilibrating "deep" compartment (169). The duration of activity is usually long enough to permit single daily doses. Most patients require 5–10 mg/day.

Glipizide is also primarily metabolized in the liver to two major compounds which are devoid of activity. Like glyburide, its half-life is relatively short (3–7 hours in various studies) (162), but it is capable of prolonged hypoglycemic activity (for 24 hours) in many patients.

Glibornuride is also totally metabolized to a number of compounds, only one of which has weak hypoglycemic activity. It has a half-life of approximately 8–10 hours, and also requires only 1–2 doses per day.

Plasma Concentrations. There is generally a very poor relationship between plasma concentrations of the sulfonylureas and fasting blood glucose or hypoglycemic activity (162,163). Not only is there a large patient-to-patient variation of concentrations with similar doses, there is little to no correlation between serum drug concentration and fasting blood glucose after prolonged administration. Serum drug concentrations thus offer us little help in dosing these drugs at the present time.

Dosing. Although some diabetologists advocate initiating patients on maximum doses of sulfonylureas (123) (See Table 12 for maximum doses), most recommend beginning the patient on low or moderate doses and gradually increasing the dose weekly (or less often) until the desired response is achieved. It is especially important to begin elderly patients on low doses since they are particularly susceptible to the hypoglycemic effects of these agents (see Question 37 and the section on Drug-Induced Hypoglycemia). Increasing the doses of sulfonylureas beyond the maximum amount usually results in a greater incidence of adverse effects without an increase in hypoglycemic effect.

Based on the delayed peak concentrations (2–4 hours) and similar peak effects seen with most of the sulfonylureas, some investigators have demonstrated, in single dose studies, that postprandial hyperglycemia is better controlled when sulfonylureas are dosed an hour or two prior to mealtime (162,170). However, it is difficult to relate these data to multiple dose administration, particularly for drugs with prolonged half-lives or long durations of activity. Although individualization of sulfonylurea administration for drugs with brief hypoglycemic activity (ie, tolbutamide) may be useful in some patients, more practical considerations such as compliance and gastrointestinal tolerance often require that the drugs be taken with or soon after a meal.

Pharmacokinetic Drug Interactions

Drug interactions with sulfonylurea therapy can be classified as (1) pharmacodynamic interactions (intrinsic drug effects altering insulin secretion, glucose production, peripheral glucose utilization, etc.), or (2) pharmacokinetic interactions (alterations in protein binding, liver metabolism, or renal excretion). Pharmacodynamic interactions will be discussed further in the sections on Drug-Induced Hypo- and Hyperglycemia.

Although chlorpropamide and tolbutamide are the sulfonylureas which are most commonly reported to interact with other drugs, this does not imply that other sulfonylureas cannot interact similarly. On the other hand, differences in the metabolism, excretion, protein binding or other characteristics of each sulfonylurea can markedly enhance or lessen its interacting potential. The second generation sulfonylureas, dosed in milligram rather than gram quantities, may be less likely to interact on a pharmacokinetic basis. This has yet to be established.

Hansten (171) and Jackson et al (172) have reviewed and listed the many potential pharmacokinetic interactions that have been reported with the sulfonylureas. Only the clinically significant interactions, or those that are often considered clinically significant, are discussed below. Table 13 lists these drugs and their proposed mechanisms.

Chloramphenicol. Two separate studies have similarly demonstrated that chloramphenicol, 2 gm daily for several days, nearly doubles the half-life of tolbutamide (173,174). Tolbutamide concentrations increase and blood glucose concentrations fall as a result. However, only one case of an actual hypoglycemic episode was reported. A group of patients on concomitant chloramphenicol therapy had prolonged half-lives (40–146 hours) of chlorpropamide; however, the cause and effect relationship is unclear (175).

Clofibrate. An increased hypoglycemic effect was suggested to be secondary to a clofibrate interaction in one semi-controlled study of 13 patients taking various sulfonylureas (176). Some hypoglycemic episodes were also noted and it was postulated that an interaction might be due to competition for protein binding sites on serum albumin. Lower serum albumin levels were found in the patients with enhanced diabetic control. Ferrari et al found a lower plasma glucose response to IV tolbutamide after 7 days of clofibrate administration (177). They suggested that clofibrate may have intrinsic hypoglycemic properties of its own. The clinical significance of this potential interaction is unclear and requires further substantiation.

Dicumarol (Bishydroxycoumarin). In a well-designed study of 16 patients, Skovsted et al found that the mean half-life of tolbutamide markedly increased from 4.9 hrs to 17.5 hrs after pretreatment with dicumarol (178). Serum tolbutamide concentrations also increased from an average of 0.4 mg/dl to 7.0 mg/dl after one week of dicumarol treatment in 4 subjects. However, tolbutamide kinetics were *not* affected by the other two coumarin derivatives (warfarin and phenprocoumon), nor were they affected by phenindione (an indandione derivative).

Chlorpropamide metabolism has also been reported to be affected by dicumarol in 3 diabetic subjects (179). The half-lives were measured in two patients and found to have increased 2–3 fold. One case of a hypoglycemic reaction due to concurrent dicumarol and chlorpropamide therapy was noted by these investigators.

Phenylbutazone, Oxyphenbutazone. Results from a well-designed study with 8 subjects clearly demonstrate that tolbutamide half-life is prolonged at least 2–3 fold after chronic treatment with phenylbutazone or its metabolite, oxyphenbutazone. This is due to an inhibitory effect on hepatic enzyme activity (180). A case of phenylbutazone-associated severe hypoglycemia (9 mg/dl) with acetohexamide was thought to be due to decreased renal excretion of the active metabolite, L-hydroxyhexamide (181). Protein binding displacement has also been suggested as a mechanism for phenylbutazone interactions (182).

Salicylates. Besides their intrinsic hypoglycemic effect (see Question 53), salicylates have been demonstrated to inhibit protein (primarily

Table 13.

POTENTIAL PHARMACOKINETIC INTERACTIONS WITH SULFONYLUREAS

	Significance*	↑ Sulfonylurea Effect			↓Effect
		Protein Binding Alteration	Hepatic Enzyme Inhibition	Decreased Renal Excretion	Enzyme Induction
Chloramphenicol	+ + +		X		
Clofibrate	+	?	?		
Dicumarol	+ + +		X		
Phenylbutazone	+ + +	X	X	X?	
Salicylates	+	X		X?	
Sulfonamide antimicrobials (some)	+ +	?	?		
Ethanol, chronic abuse	+ + +				X
Rifampin	+ + +				X

*   +—Possible interaction; needs substantiation.
  + +—Only certain drugs may interact. See text.
 + + +—Clinically significant interaction.

albumin) binding of chlorpropamide, acetohexamide, and tolbutamide *in vitro* (182). Salicylate interference with renal tubular secretion of chlorpropamide has also been suggested, but this is unclear (183). There are a few case reports associating enhanced blood levels or prolonged recovery from hypoglycemia with concomitant salicylate and sulfonylurea administration, but the majority of the evidence is extremely weak (183–185). Although this interaction is often accepted as fact, it clearly requires further study.

Sulfonamides. Numerous case reports and several studies have demonstrated that some sulfonamide antimicrobials can substantially interact with sulfonylureas (which are actually sulfonamide derivatives). However, most of the well-documented interactions have occurred with sulfonamides that are no longer available in the United States. This somewhat qualifies the clinical importance of this interaction.

Sulphaphenazole (not available in the U.S.) has caused the majority of severe, irrefutable, hypoglycemic episodes in patients on tolbutamide (180,186). Pharmacokinetic studies clearly demonstrate a 3–4 fold increase in tolbutamide half-life, effective within hours. Protein binding displacement and/or enzyme induction are the proposed mechanisms. Sulfamethazine (not available in the U.S.) and sulfamethizole (available in oral form, but rarely used) have produced a severe case of hypoglycemia (with chlorpropamide) (187) and an increase in tolbutamide half-life of about 60% in 6 patients (188), respectively.

Sulfisoxazole (Gantrisin) has been associated with a potential interaction (severe hypoglycemia) in 3 patients—one with chlorpropamide and phenformin after a large dose of sulfisoxazole (8 gm load, 1 gm qid × 24 hours) (189), one in an elderly patient on tolbutamide who was also taking chloramphenicol (190), and one with tolbutamide in a patient who also had renal failure (190). Although ⅔ of these patients have predisposing factors, it is interesting to note that sulfisoxazole has been shown to increase free tolbutamide concentrations *in vitro* (186).

Rifampin, Chronic Alcohol Use. Both rifampin and chronic alcohol use have been clearly demonstrated to influence the metabolism of tolbutamide in man due to hepatic enzyme induction (171). Impaired hypoglycemic response to tolbutamide would be expected (although the opposite may occur if alcohol abuse led to cirrhosis);

interactions with other sulfonylureas are unknown.

TREATMENT OF TYPE II DIABETICS
CLINICAL USE OF SULFONYLUREAS

23. L.H. is a 60-year-old moderately obese female (5′5″ and 160 lb) who was referred to the Diabetic Clinic when her gynecologist, who had been treating her for recurrent monilial infections, noted the presence of glucose on routine urinalysis. The patient was subsequently found to have fasting plasma glucose concentrations of 150 mg/dl and 167 mg/dl on two separate occasions. L.H. denies having any symptoms of polyphagia or polyuria, although she has been more thirsty than usual. She does complain of lethargy and often takes afternoon naps. Over the past year she has gained 10 pounds.

L.H.'s other medical problems include rheumatoid arthritis which is well-controlled on 3.6 gm aspirin daily and mild hypertension which has been corrected with hydrochlorothiazide 50 mg daily and methyldopa 500 mg twice daily. She also takes 1 gm of vitamin C daily which she increases to 5 gm daily at the first sign of a cold.

L.H.'s family history is significant for the fact that she has a sister (also overweight), aunt, and grandmother with diabetes.

Laboratory assessment reveals a fasting plasma glucose concentration of 147 mg/dl; aglycosuria (Diastix); and a Hb A$_{1c}$ of 11% (normal: 6–8%). All other values are within normal limits.

L.H. is given the diagnosis of Type II, non-insulin dependent diabetes of the obese. What features of L.H.'s history and physical examination are consistent with this diagnosis? How should she be managed at this time?

The features of L.H.'s history which are consistent with the diagnosis of Type II diabetes include a fasting plasma glucose ≥ 140 mg/dl on more than one occasion; obesity; age over 40; family history of diabetes; elevated Hb A$_{1c}$; and mild signs and symptoms related to hyperglycemia: increased thirst, lethargy, and recurrent monilial infection.

Since L.H.'s symptoms are mild, she should be managed with a low calorie diet that is consistent with the principles and goals of a diabetic diet (see Introduction). Since obesity and overeating are associated with increased resistance to endogenous insulin, L.H. should be strongly encouraged to lose weight. Many patients who lose weight are able to reduce their glucose intolerance. Since both insulin and sulfonylureas (which increase the release of and potentiate the action of insulin) increase insulin levels in a patient who is potentially insulinplethoric, their use is reserved for Type II patients who are poorly controlled (FPS $\geq$ 200 mg/dl) and severely symptomatic. Some diabetologists feel that the lipogenic and hypoglycemic effects of insulin make weight loss difficult for obese patients and that they should be avoided for this reason (1); this has been refuted by others, however (164).

24. What are the goals of L.H.'s diabetic therapy? Which urine test should be recommended for L.H. and how frequently should she test her urine?

Goals. The ultimate goal of dietary therapy is to achieve ideal body weight and thereby reverse carbohydrate intolerance and signs and symptoms related to hyperglycemia. Hypoglycemia is rarely a problem in these patients unless they are on high doses of insulin. Therefore, one should aim for normal fasting and postprandial blood glucose concentrations (see Table 1), a normal Hb A_{1c}, and consistently negative tests for urine glucose.

Urine Tests. Since the objective of the urine glucose test in a Type II diabetic is to simply determine whether or not glucose is present in the urine, a semi-quantitative test such as Clinitest is unnecessary. Instead, L.H. can use one of the more convenient glucose oxidase methods for testing urine (Diastix, Tes-Tape). (See the Introduction for further discussion of these products.) She should initially be instructed to test a first-voided urine four times daily (eg, before breakfast and 1–2 hours postprandially). Assuming that her renal threshold for glucose is normal, the presence of glucose would indicate that plasma glucose levels exceeded 180 mg/dl at some time following a meal. Once all urine samples are negative, she may decrease the frequency of her testing to once or twice daily; for example, before breakfast and 1–2 hours after breakfast when the plasma glucose is most likely to be maximally elevated for the day. Second-voided urines are un-

necessary in these patients because they are not being used to dose insulin.

25. *Drug Interference with Urine Tests.* L.H. will be using a glucose oxidase test to evaluate glycosuria. Which drugs can interfere with these urine tests and what is the chemical basis of their interference? Is L.H. taking any drugs which can interfere with the interpretation of her urine glucose tests? How can misleading interpretations secondary to drug interference be avoided?

There are many sources which list drugs that reportedly cause false-positive copper reduction tests and false-negative glucose oxidase tests for urine glucose, and L.H. is taking three drugs (salicylates, methyldopa, and ascorbic acid) which have been included on such lists. However, the significance of many of these drug-induced false-positive or false-negative reactions is poorly substantiated. In many cases drugs are added to the list on the basis of case reports or on the basis of *in vitro* data which may or may not reflect *in vivo* effects of these agents. (For most of these studies, specific quantities of a drug or its metabolite are added to a urine specimen spiked with a known amount of glucose.) Drugs have even been added to such lists on the basis of anecdotal reports of unknown origin which have become imbedded in the literature. For many of the drugs included in such lists, the literature is confusing and conflicting. A summary of the literature relating to drug interference with urine glucose testing is provided in Table 14. Those drugs for which there is substantial or controversial literature (including those being taken by L.H.) are discussed below.

Chemical Basis of Drug Interference. The following series of reactions from the basis of the glucose oxidase tests:

$$\underset{\text{in urine}}{\beta\ \text{D-glucose}} + \underset{\text{in air}}{\text{Oxygen}} \xrightarrow[\text{oxidase}]{\text{glucose}} \underset{\text{Acid}}{\text{Gluconic}} + H_2O_2$$

$$H_2O_2 \xrightarrow{\text{peroxidase}} \text{nascent oxygen}$$

$$\text{nascent oxygen} + \underset{\text{(pink)}}{\text{o-tolidine}} \xrightarrow{\quad * \quad} \underset{\text{(blue)}}{\text{o-tolidine}}$$

reduced   oxidized

*site of drug inhibition

oxidized   tartrazine   pale green
o-tolidine +   dye   ⟶   to
(blue)   (yellow)   deep blue

Strong reducing substances prevent the oxidation of o-tolidine, the indicator for glucose oxidase tests, and may thereby produce a false negative reaction (191). Substances strong enough to prevent this reaction may cause a false positive copper reduction test (Clinitest) as well:

$$Cu^{++}SO_4^= \xrightarrow[\substack{\text{reducing} \\ \text{substance}}]{\text{Glucose or any}} Cu_2^{+++}O_3^=$$

cupric sulfate   Glucose or any   cuprous oxide
                     reducing   (reduced)
                    substance

Salicylates. Salicylates may inhibit the glucose oxidase test or produce a false-positive Clinitest reaction through a reducing metabolite, gentisic acid. Fifty percent or $^5/_{10}$ urine specimens from patients ingesting 2.4 to 2.7 gm of aspirin daily caused false negative glucose oxidase readings, whereas $^5/_7$ readings were false-negative in patients ingesting 3.6 to 5.6 gm of aspirin daily (192). In most cases, those urines which inhibited the glucose oxidase test also caused false-positive Clinitest results. Thus, aspirin in arthritic doses (such as those taken by L.H.) or chronic aspirin ingestion may significantly affect urinary glucose determinations; however, occasional use of aspirin is unlikely to cause a problem.

Ascorbic Acid (Vitamin C). Ascorbic acid is a reducing agent which has long been suspected of producing false-negative glucose oxidase readings and false-positive copper reduction reactions. Ascorbic acid added to glucose-spiked urine in increasing concentrations was demonstrated to proportionately inhibit glucose oxidase tests and, to a lesser extent, cause false-positive copper reduction reactions (193,194). Feldman et al attributed 16–25% of 120 false-low glucose oxidase readings to significant ascorbic acid concentrations ($\geq$ 9 mg/dl) in the urine of patients tested (191). Brandt studied two subjects who received 2–3 gm of ascorbic acid daily and reportedly developed false-negative glucose oxidase tests (Tes-Tape) and false-positive copper reduction reactions (Benedict's test) (194). These false results were reversed after ion exchange treatment of the urine specimens to remove ascorbic acid (concentrations as high as 200 mg/dl). In contrast, three recent, well-designed studies have demonstrated

that nondiabetic patients without glycosuria ingesting up to 9 gm of ascorbic acid daily do not have false-positive copper reduction results using the two-drop Clinitest method (195–197). Although much of the literature on ascorbic acid is contradictory and difficult to interpret, it would be wise to assume that L.H.'s ascorbic acid may interact with urine test results unless proven otherwise and to take precautionary measures.

Methyldopa. A single case report of a false-positive Clinitest reaction from a patient ingesting 2 gm daily of methyldopa prompted concern that this drug, like levodopa (see below) may interact with urine testing (192). However, subsequent studies with large numbers of patients have demonstrated that methyldopa does not interact with either glucose oxidase or copper reduction tests (198,199).

Levodopa. Levodopa in high doses is also capable of affecting urine glucose tests through a metabolite thought to be 3,4-dihydroxyphenylacetic acid (DOPAC). Six of 25 urine specimens produced false-positive Clinitest reactions and false-negative Clinistix reactions in patients ingesting 0.75 to 3.0 gm of L-dopa. The ratio of false readings increased to $^{13}/_{17}$ samples in patients taking 3.5 to 5.0 gm of L-dopa (192). Levodopa may also cause false positive reactions for ketones with Ketostix or Keto-Diastix (171).

Avoiding Drug Interference. Fortunately, patients such as L.H. who are taking drugs which may potentially interfere with urine glucose readings may use Tes-Tape to ascertain the presence of true glucosuria despite the presence of an interfering substance. Once the tape has been dipped in urine and the alloted waiting time (60 seconds) has passed, an accurate glucose reading can be taken at the wet and dry border. The tape apparently acts as a mini-chromatography system which separates the inhibitor (which moves slowly) from the glucose which moves up the tape more quickly to react with the reagent at the diffusion front (192).

26. Despite several attempts at diet management, L.H. failed to lose substantial amounts of weight, and her fasting blood glucose concentrations began to rise over a period of one year to 225–250 mg/dl. Urine testing revealed the presence of glucose in 75% of the urines tested and a repeat Hb A_{1c} was 14.5%. L.H. has also begun to notice noc-

Table 14.

DRUGS OFTEN CONSIDERED TO INTERACT WITH GLUCOSE OXIDASE
OR COPPER REDUCTION URINE GLUCOSE TESTS

Drug (Ref)	Significance**	Interaction and Comments*
Antimicrobials		
Aminoglycosides (200)	0	No interaction in vitro with CRT or GOT.
Cephalosporins (201)	+ + +	False positive or misinterpretation of CRT. Does not affect GOT.
Chloramphenicol (171)	+	May cause false positive CRT. Unsubstantiated.
Isoniazid (171,202)	+	No interaction with Clinitest. False positive Benedict's is unsubstantiated.
Methenamine, formaldehyde, hippuric acid (197)	0	No interaction with Clinitest in vivo. Not tested with GOT.
Nalidixic acid (171,203)	+ +	False positive CRT. May not affect GOT.
Nitrofurantoin (171)	+	May cause false positive CRT. Unsubstantiated.
Para-aminosalicylic acid (171)	+	False positive Benedict's but no interaction with Clinitest or GOT. Unsubstantiated.
Penicillins (200)	+/+ +	Questionable interaction with CRT. Does not affect GOT.
Sulfonamides (171)	+	Large doses may cause false positive CRT. Unsubstantiated.
Tetracyclines (204)	0	No interaction with Clinitest.
Ascorbic Acid (192–197)	+ +	See text. Probable false negative GOT. Doubtful interaction with CRT.
Chloral Hydrate (171)	+	May cause false positive CRT. Unsubstantiated.
Levodopa (192)	+ +	See text. Dose-dependent interactions with both CRT and GOT.
Metaxalone (171)	+	May cause false positive CRT, no effect on GOT. Unsubstantiated.
Methyldopa (198,199)	0	See text. No interactions with CRT or GOT.
Morphine (171)	+	May cause false positive Benedict's. Unsubstantiated.
Phenacetin (171)	+	May cause false positive Benedict's. Unsubstantiated.
Phenazopyridine (205)	+ +	May cause false negative GOT, no effect on CRT. Needs substantiation.
Probenecid (171)	+	May cause false positive CRT, no effect on GOT. Unsubstantiated.
Salicylates (191,192)	+ +	See text. Dose-dependent interaction with both CRT and GOT.

*   CRT = Copper reduction tests (Clinitest, Benedict's) GOT = Glucose oxidase tests (Diastix, Tes-Tape, Clinistix)
**   0   = Does not interact with urine test.
      +   = Interaction reported or postulated but not substantiated. Unknown clinical significance.
    + +   = Suspected significant clinical interaction. Limited *in vivo* or *in vitro* data which may need corroboration.
  + + +   = Significant clinical interaction.

turia and a definite increase in fluid intake. She feels extremely fatigued and "doesn't have the energy to do anything." Are sulfonylureas or insulin indicated at this time? Is L.H. likely to respond to the sulfonylureas?

Although the use of sulfonylureas and insulin in obese, Type II diabetics is arguable (see Question 23), these agents are the only treatment forms available for patients such as L.H. who become significantly symptomatic and are not well-controlled on diet. Some clinicians would opt to use insulin at this point based upon the findings of the University Group Diabetes Program (UGDP) study, in which a higher incidence of cardiovascular deaths in diabetics was associated with the use of fixed doses of tolbutamide (See Question 36). Others would use insulin on the theory that as Type II diabetes progresses, insulinopenia associated with post-receptor defects in insulin activity become operative in the pathogenic process (16,17). Intensive insulin therapy in poorly-controlled Type II diabetics (FPG $\geq$ 200 mg/dl) reverses this post-receptor defect, improves endogenous insulin release in response to glucose, decreases mean fasting plasma glucose concentrations and Hb A_1, and improves glucose tolerance (16).

Another group of diabetologists would initiate oral sulfonylurea therapy to stimulate endogenous insulin release and potentiate its activity (206). Patients who are most likely to respond favorably to oral sulfonylureas are nonobese Type II diabetics (non-ketotic with pancreatic reserve) who have had diabetes for less than 10 years, have a fasting blood glucose of less than 200 mg/dl and an insulin requirement of < 40–50 units. L.H. fulfills many of these criteria, but she is overweight and has a fasting blood glucose concentration which is greater than 200 mg/dl. Thus, her initial response to oral agents cannot be predicted. Approximately ⅔–¾ of those patients who meet all of the criteria specified above will achieve satisfactory control with these agents initially (fasting and postprandial blood glucose concentrations of < 200 mg/dl). The remainder (16–36%) fail to respond to a one-month trial of maximum therapeutic doses (primary failure) (207–210).

27. The pros and cons of the oral sulfonylureas and insulin were discussed with L.H. and at this point in time she refuses insulin therapy, but is willing to try an oral agent in an attempt to alleviate her symptoms. Of the four agents available in the U.S., which is the drug of choice? How should L.H. be dosed?

Although there is certainly no unanimity or concensus, it is the opinion of these authors that the initial (first generation) sulfonylurea of choice for most patients is tolazamide. It has the advantage of an intermediate activity so that control can usually be achieved with no more than two doses per day. However, its duration of action is not so prolonged that accumulation is likely to result in extended hypoglycemic episodes which are difficult to manage (eg, as with chlorpropamide). The newer intermediate-acting second generation sulfonylureas seem equally promising, but offer no real advantage over tolazamide unless patients respond more frequently to a single daily dose.

It should be emphasized that, in clinical practice, a patient may not respond to maximal doses of one sulfonylurea and is then quite reasonably changed to another agent and so on until a response is seen. However, initial therapy should always begin with the drug most compatible with the individual patient, and some agents are simply contraindicated. Sulfonylureas of choice in special circumstances are discussed in questions which follow.

28. *Secondary Failure.* L.H. was encouraged to maintain her diet and was placed on 250 mg tolazamide daily. She did well for approximately two years (fasting plasma glucoses of 150–170 mg/dl; consistently negative urine tests; Hb A_{1c} 9–10%; asymptomatic) until eight months ago when she was hospitalized for pneumonia. During her hospitalization, fasting and random plasma glucose concentrations ranged from 370–450 mg/dl and she was managed with insulin. L.H. was discharged on 500 mg tolazamide daily and most recently (past three months) she has been taking 500 mg twice daily. Following her hospitalization, L.H. began to spill glucose into her urine and her fasting plasma glucose concentrations began to rise gradually (250–300 mg/dl) despite increasing doses of tolazamide. On this clinic visit, the fasting plasma glucose is 335 mg/dl and she again complains of extreme fatigue, polyuria, polydipsia and recurrent vaginal infections. She agrees to begin insulin. How should she be converted

from sulfonylureas to insulin therapy? Assess L.H.'s recent and past diabetic history and therapy.

L.H.'s history is consistent with *secondary failure* to treatment with sulfonylureas, which is characterized by progressively poor diabetic control that occurs following a one-month to several-year period of good diabetic control. This phenomenon is fairly common, and over a period of 1–9 years occurs in 25–29% of those patients who are initially well controlled on oral agents (145,210–213).

The etiology of secondary failure is unknown but may be related to increasing severity of the disease; exogenous diabetogenic factors such as obesity, illness, or drugs (see Tables 16 & 17); or inherent failure of the oral sulfonylurea.

Treatment includes identification and elimination of diabetogenic factors; switching the patient to another sulfonylurea (25–60% of patients reportedly respond to other sulfonylureas—chlorpropamide, which apparently has more potent hypoglycemic effects at maximum doses, is most commonly used) (212–214); or switching the patient to insulin. This switch to insulin may be temporary; 50% of such patients can be returned with success to oral therapy following acute control (2,123).

Since tolazamide has an intermediate duration of action, it is unlikely that any residual effects will remain beyond one day, and even if they do, L.H. is in such poor control that they are unlikely to be clinically significant. Therefore, L.H. can be instructed to discontinue her tolazamide and immediately begin insulin therapy. Insulin dosing procedures are exactly the same as those described in Questions 9, 12 and 14 except that her initial total daily dose of insulin is likely to be higher secondary to the presence of insulin tissue resistance. See Table 8 for dose.

ADVERSE EFFECTS OF THE SULFONYLUREAS

Adverse effects attributed to the sulfonylureas are infrequent (overall incidence is approximately 5%) and mild. Allergic skin reactions (approximately 1%) and gastrointestinal effects manifested as nausea, fullness and heartburn (approximately 1.5%) account for the majority of reported adverse effects. The gastrointestinal reactions appear to be dose-related and, in the ma-

jority of cases, they can be relieved by reducing the dose or instructing the patient to take the drug with meals. In many cases, these complaints resolve with continued use of the same dose of sulfonylurea (123,215).

In general, the incidence and severity of reported side effects for each individual sulfonylurea is directly related to its half-life. The incidence data for tolazamide and acetohexamide, which were introduced several years after tolbutamide and chlorpropamide, are based on relatively small patient populations. The available data indicate that tolbutamide, which is the shortest acting of all the agents, has the lowest incidence of side effects: 1–3% (209). In contrast, chlorpropamide, which is the longest-acting of the sulfonylureas, has the highest incidence of side effects: 5–8% (213,216). Acetohexamide and tolazamide have an intermediate incidence of side effects: 5% (212,214). The most frequently reported adverse reactions to the sulfonylureas include:

1. Gastrointestinal symptoms (discussed above)
2. Skin reactions—Question 29
3. Alcohol intolerance—Questions 30–32
4. Hepatotoxicity—Question 33
5. Hypothyroidism—Question 34
6. Blood dyscrasias—See Table 15
7. Hyponatremia (Syndrome of Inappropriate ADH)—Question 35
8. Cardiovascular effects (UGDP)—Question 36
9. Hypoglycemia—Question 37

Skin Reactions

29. An adult-onset diabetic who gives a history of allergy to sulfisoxazole develops a mild pruritic, maculopapular rash 3 weeks following the initiation of tolbutamide. What kinds of skin reactions have been attributed to the sulfonylureas? Was the use of a sulfonylurea contraindicated in this patient? Can she be treated with another sulfonylurea?

Pruritus and/or rash are among the most commonly reported side effects attributed to the sulfonylureas. The majority are minor and reversible (within 2 to 14 days if the offending drug is discontinued) (217). Although there have been occasional reports of spontaneous clearing despite continuation of therapy, the rash has also been noted to increase in severity following discontinuation of the drug (217,218).

Table 15.

EXAMPLES OF SULFONYLUREA-INDUCED BLOOD DYSCRASIAS

Blood Dyscrasia	Drug	Comments	Reference
Thrombocytopenia	Tolbutamide	2 patients with petechiae and hepatosplenomegaly	(209)
	Chlorpropamide	250 mg qd; 15 days onset; 3 cases	(323,324)
Leukopenia	Tolbutamide	1 patient	(209)
Neutropenia	Chlorpropamide	—	(325)
Agranulocytosis	Chlorpropamide	3 fatal cases; all taking less than 500 mg daily	(325–327)
Pancytopenia	Tolbutamide	Fatal	(328)
Pure Red Cell Aplasia	Chlorpropamide	1.125 gm daily × 3 mos. Reversible	(329)
Immune Hemolysis	Chlorpropamide	1 patient with "innocent bystander" reaction	(330)
	Tolbutamide/Phenacetin	0.5 gm tid × 3 mos.	
	Tolbutamide	1 gm daily × 1 year	(331)
Hemolysis in G6PD deficiency	Tolbutamide	1 gm daily × 12 days. Presence of acidosis and urinary tract infection may also have been contributing factors.	(332)

The rash, which usually is maculopapular, erythematous and discrete in nature, generally involves the face, neck, upper trunk and proximal portion of the arms. It may or may not be preceded or accompanied by pruritus (217). Baker reviewed the literature for cutaneous reactions to the sulfonylureas (218). Infrequently, patients may develop erythema multiforme, exfoliative dermatitis, photosensitivity reactions and lichenoid eruptions.

Because sulfonylureas have a sulfa-like structure, many authors have suggested that their use be avoided in those patients who are allergic to sulfonamides. Unless a severe reaction is documented, there is probably not a contraindication to the use of sulfonylureas in this situation. Dowling et al (219) demonstrated that the incidence of cross-sensitivity among various sulfonamides was 17%. One would expect that the incidence between two classes of drugs with sulfa-like structures would be considerably less. Some patients who have developed rash to one sulfonylurea may be managed successfully with another sulfonylurea (218,220,221). However, cross-sensitivity among the sulfonylureas has also been documented (216,218) and is said to be common.

Because this patient's reaction is mild, a trial of another sulfonylurea can be considered.

Chlorpropamide-Alcohol Flush

30. Police authorities at the county jail have called you with an interesting problem. A new inmate, prior to incarceration, had been treated for an unknown condition with a medication taken each morning. Unfortunately, all records have been lost and the inmate cannot remember the exact name of the drug. He believes that it starts with a "d" and from this and other sources the medication has been narrowed down to either disulfiram (Antabuse) or Diabinese (chlorpropamide). The only other apparent clue is that the patient experiences a flushing sensation of his face whenever he indulges in even a small amount of alcoholic beverage. No other symptoms accompany this sensation, which he describes as being not particularly unpleasant. Since the authorities at the jail are familiar with the Antabuse-like reaction that the inmate has described, they suspect the medicine in question to be disulfiram. You have been called as a consultant to verify their suspicion. Can chlorpropamide cause an Antabuse-like reaction?

An Antabuse-like reaction is known to occur in patients taking oral sulfonylurea drugs but is most frequently associated with chlorpropamide. The exact prevalence of this side effect is difficult to determine, but it may occur in approximately one-quarter to one-third of all patients receiving chlorpropamide (see Question 32).

Description. Within 10–20 minutes of even a small drink of alcohol, a facial flush occurs that is associated with a warmth or tingling sensation and may extend down to the neck or extensor surfaces of the arms. Conjunctival injection is often present and gives the patient a bull's-eyed appearance. The flush usually lasts about 30–60 minutes, although in severe cases it may be of several hours duration. Other mild reactions such as headache, light-headedness or breathlessness occasionally may occur, but the flush is rarely accompanied by vomiting, hypotension or other severe symptoms often associated with a true disulfiram-alcohol reaction (12,222,223). In fact, the reaction is now often referred to as the chlorpropamide-alcohol flush (CPAF) to distinguish it from Antabuse-like reactions caused by other drugs. The difference between CPAF and the disulfiram reaction is mainly that of intensity, the latter usually being much more severe and not simply confined to a flush. The drug in question may very well be chlorpropamide, especially since the patient does not consider the reaction to be particularly unpleasant.

31. Does this side effect occur with other sulfonylureas? How should patients complaining of CPAF be managed? What is the mechanism of the chlorpropamide-alcohol flush (CPAF)?

The flushing reaction seen so often with chlorpropamide is rare with other sulfonylureas. Less than 5% of diabetics treated with tolbutamide report a flushing reaction with alcohol (224,225); the prevalence for other sulfonylureas is probably similar. The fact that some individuals experience a flushing reaction from alcohol alone (without pretreatment of sulfonylureas or other drugs) (226,227) makes interpretation of uncontrolled reports almost impossible. In addition, many patients do not mention the reaction spontaneously, feeling that as diabetics they are transgressing in drinking alcoholic beverages.

Management. Patients initiating chlorpropamide therapy should always be informed of this potential side effect, as it may be particularly embarrassing or unpleasant if the reaction occurs without prior knowledge. If CPAF is a particular problem for a diabetic on chlorpropamide, changing to a different oral hypoglycemic agent will almost always eliminate the reaction.

Mechanism. The mechanism of CPAF has been continuously debated since the reaction was first reported in 1957, soon after the drug was introduced; there still is no unanimity of opinion. It was initially hypothesized that chlorpropamide, like disulfiram, blocked aldehyde dehydrogenase (the enzyme responsible for metabolizing acetaldehyde), thus increasing acetaldehyde concentrations after alcohol ingestion. Unfortunately, this could not be substantiated by early *in vivo* and later *in vitro* experiments (222,228). Recently, however, with the help of more sensitive assays, an increase in acetaldehyde concentration has been demonstrated in CPAF-positive patients pretreated with chlorpropamide and this theory is again in vogue with some investigators (229,230).

Nevertheless, elevated acetaldehyde concentrations cannot solely explain the mechanism of the CPAF reaction since endogenous opiates and prostaglandins have been found to be contributing factors. Naloxone, a specific opiate antagonist, blocked the flushing reaction in three CPAF-positive patients (231). This reaction was reproducible by the administration of an enkephalin analogue with opiate-like activity. In a separate study, met-enkephalin concentrations rose after alcohol administration in patients pretreated with chlorpropamide (232). Furthermore, it has been demonstrated that *in vitro*, acetaldehyde rapidly combines with both enkephalins and endorphins to form stable adducts with altered biological activities (233). Perhaps these adducts play a role in causing CPAF reactions in susceptible individuals. To further complicate the mechanism, prostaglandin inhibitors such as aspirin and indomethacin have been found to block the flushing reaction in many, but not all, patients studied (234,235). It is clear that the mechanism of CPAF in its entirety is not yet fully understood and, in fact, is probably due to a combination of several factors.

32. Chlorpropamide-alcohol flushing has been suggested to be an inherited trait with significant genetic implications. Is this true? What are these implications and are they, in fact, significant?

In 1978, Pyke and coworkers postulated that

CPAF is a dominantly inherited trait and is distinctly related to non-insulin dependent (type II) diabetes, especially when a strong family history of the disease is present (12,13). In this study, 51% of 234 type II diabetics were CPAF-positive, as compared to only 10% of type I diabetics and 10% of non-diabetic controls. Of those with type II diabetes, 81% with a first-degree family history were CPAF-positive, compared to 31% without a first-degree family history. Other data confirmed the inherited nature of the reaction, such as 12 pairs of identical twins, one or both of whom were diabetic, who reacted identically to the chlorpropamide-alcohol test.

Subsequent reports, however, have not confirmed these initial findings (226,236–239). Most other studies have found from 23% to 33% of type II diabetics to be CPAF-positive and were unable to correlate a family history of diabetes to the reaction (222,226,236,238,239). The apparent discrepancies between these results and those of Pyke's initial study may in part be due to methodologic problems (227,238,239). Most researchers rely on minute changes in facial temperature to define the CPAF-reaction, which is measured by a thermocouple applied to the cheek or forehead. This has led to some confusion in defining a positive or negative CPAF since a simple "on-off" flushing reaction has been replaced by a rather perplexing array of temperature changes. In addition, most investigators have used only one or two doses of chlorpropamide prior to alcohol ingestion to define a CPAF-reactor. It was recently demonstrated that pretreatment with chlorpropamide for several days will increase chlorpropamide concentrations (not unexpected, due to its long half-life) and will also increase the proportion of positive reactors (229,239,240). The "true" prevalence of CPAF awaits proper standardization of methods and a precise definition of the phenomenon.

Pyke and coworkers, utilizing the patient population from their initial study, also concluded that susceptibility to microvascular and, to a lesser extent, macrovascular disease are not only inherited traits, but that CPAF-positive diabetics are protected from these complications to some degree (241,242). Of 291 type II diabetics, 25% of CPAF-positive subjects had retinopathy compared to 54% of CPAF-negative subjects. Severe retinopathy was found in 4% vs 28%, respectively. Of 9 diabetics who were blind, only one was CPAF-positive. Similar but less convincing evidence was demonstrated for macrovascular complications such as myocardial infarction and peripheral vascular disease (but not for hypertension, cerebrovascular accidents and certain other large vessel complications). These results should not be considered conclusive until the methodologic problems discussed above have been solved.

A variety of discordant results and opinions have been issued on the subject of CPAF and diabetes. Partially because of this, an international workshop on Chlorpropamide-Alcohol Flushing and Diabetes was held in June of 1980. It was concluded that CPAF is most probably an inherited phenomenon, but its relationships to (type II or other) diabetes and susceptibility of microvascular or other complications are still unclear and require further investigation (243).

Hepatotoxicity

33. Four weeks following the initiation of chlorpropamide therapy (750 mg daily), E.T., a 56-year-old male, develops a fever and complains of nausea, vomiting and a pruritic rash. His urine has turned dark and his stools are clay colored. He seeks medical advice at the urging of friends who have noted his yellowed complexion. Initial laboratory tests indicate that he has an elevated serum bilirubin, alkaline phosphatase and eosinophil count. Could the patient's signs and symptoms be related to his chlorpropamide therapy? If so, could they be alleviated by decreasing the dose or changing to another sulfonylurea?

Mildly elevated liver function tests (alkaline phosphatase, cephalin flocculation, SGPT) have been associated with the ingestion of most all of the sulfonylureas (209,215,244–246); however, clinical jaundice is relatively rare. Of the commercially available preparations, chlorpropamide has been most frequently implicated (246,247), but few cases of chlorpropamide-induced jaundice have been reported since 1960 when the doses routinely used were lowered considerably from 1–3 gm to 250–500 mg. (E.T. is taking 750 mg daily.) Jaundice has also been associated with the ingestion of tolbutamide (244,245,248) and acetohexamide (249,250). No reports of tolazamide-induced jaundice were documented; however, it is the most recently marketed sulfonylurea and its literature is not extensive.

Early reports of chlorpropamide-induced cholestatic jaundice were associated with a rash and eosinophilia, suggesting that this may be a hypersensitivity-type reaction. Liver biopsies generally reveal intrahepatic cholestasis with minimal cellular damage (focal necrosis) (221).

In most cases symptoms develop within 6 weeks of therapy, as illustrated by E.T. (221), although a latent period of up to 24 months has been reported (248). Most cases are reversible within 1–2 months if the sulfonylurea is discontinued soon after the onset of symptoms. Although there have been reports of patients who have responded favorably when switched to a different sulfonylurea (221), others treated similarly have experienced recurrence of the jaundice (251). Therefore, a two-month trial off chlorpropamide is warranted in E.T. to see if the symptoms subside. If E.T. becomes symptomatic, he should be treated with insulin.

Hypothyroidism

34. A 55-year-old female with a 5-year history of diabetes mellitus, which has been well controlled with tolbutamide 0.5 gm tid, complains of weight gain, cold intolerance and fatigue. She is found to have a T3 resin uptake of 15.5% (normal: 25–35%), a low basal metabolic rate, and depressed tendon reflexes. A diagnosis of hypothyroidism is made. Could tolbutamide have induced these symptoms?

Although the antithyroid effects of carbutamide (a sulfonylurea which has been removed from the market) have been well documented in man and animals (251), it remains unclear whether any of the sulfonylureas currently used share these effects.

Hanno et al (252) demonstrated that tolbutamide reversibly inhibits the organic binding of I^{131} in man following a minimum of six months of therapy. The degree of this inhibition may be correlated with the total dose and duration of therapy. None of those patients in which inhibition was significant exhibited clinical signs or symptoms of hypothyroidism.

Portioli et al (253) and Hunton et al (254) screened patients who had been taking sulfonylureas for coexisting hypothyroidism. Both found

that the incidence of hypothyroidism (based on diminished T3 resin uptake and/or PBI) was higher in these patients than in those diabetics treated with diet and/or insulin or in non-diabetics. Hunton et al (254), who used a low PBI as the basis of their diagnosis, stated that 20% of those patients taking sulfonylureas would develop hypothyroidism. One should also consider that tolbutamide and chlorpropamide *may* have decreased the binding of T3 and T4 to thyroid binding globulin and could have thereby induced a false low PBI (255). None of the patients in these two studies exhibited overt signs and symptoms of hypothyroidism.

Burke et al (256) attempted, but were unable to confirm the findings of Hunton et al. They found no evidence of hypothyroidism in patients who had been on long-term sulfonylurea therapy.

Only four cases of symptomatic hypothyroidism, which clearly improved following discontinuation of sulfonylurea, have been reported. Tolbutamide 0.5 gm daily for a period of 6 weeks to 5 years was responsible for all of these (257–260). Until a well-controlled prospective study is done, it must be concluded that although sulfonylureas may occasionally induce mild abnormalities of thyroid function (decreased I^{131} uptake, decreased PBI, decreased T3 resin uptake) (217,261), clinically significant hypothyroidism is very rare. Since in all of these cases, symptomatic improvement and normalization of laboratory tests was noted as soon as four weeks following discontinuation of the medication, a trial withdrawal of tolbutamide may be warranted in this patient.

SIADH

35. A 65-year-old female has been receiving chlorothiazide, digoxin and chlorpropamide 500 mg daily. On examination, her blood sugar is found to be higher than usual, so her chlorpropamide is increased to 750 mg/day. Her renal function is within normal limits. Three months later she complains of progressive weakness, anorexia, nausea and dizzy spells. Laboratory examination reveals a serum sodium of 120 mEq/L, a serum osmolality of 320 mOsm/L and a urine osmolality of 600 mOsm/L. Can you attribute her condition to any of her drugs?

Chlorpropamide, and to a much lesser extent, tolbutamide (262) may enhance the effect of antidiuretic hormone (ADH) on the kidney, enhance the release of ADH centrally, and override the inhibitory effects of waterloading on ADH release (263). This effect has been used clinically in the treatment of diabetes insipidus.

Occasionally (approximately 4%), chlorpropamide induces a syndrome of inappropriate ADH in patients receiving the drug for diabetes mellitus (264–266). Elderly individuals, patients with congestive heart failure, and those taking diuretics are particularly predisposed to this effect of chlorpropamide. Thiazides may predispose patients because they induce the secretion of ADH by causing a negative sodium balance and by contracting extracellular volume. Some investigators have theorized that the syndrome of inappropriate ADH occurs in individuals who have a pre-existing defect in the feedback mechanism. That is, serum hypo-osmolality fails to turn ADH completely off. Even though the basal secretions which result from this effect may be minimal, potentiation of their effects by chlorpropamide may induce water intoxication with its attendant hyponatremia and progressive symptoms of headache, lethargy and, eventually, stupor and coma. Therapeutic waterloads for urinary tract infections and cancer chemotherapy should be used cautiously in patients taking chlorpropamide.

Tolazamide, acetohexamide and glyburide may actually have a diuretic effect in contrast to chlorpropamide and tolbutamide (262–265,267). Therefore, chlorpropamide should be discontinued in this patient who is predisposed to its effects on ADH activity and tolazamide or acetohexamide should be used instead.

UGDP

36. What is the University Group Diabetic Program (UGDP) study? Discuss the objectives, conclusions and criticism of the study and its impact on the current use of oral hypoglycemic agents.

In 1961, a cooperative, prospective study was initiated to evaluate the effectiveness of antidiabetic therapy in preventing vascular and late complications of diabetes. Eight hundred patients from 12 different diabetic clinics were included. All of these patients were recently diagnosed maturity onset diabetics of the nonketotic type who had a life expectancy of five years or more and who could be maintained free of symptoms on diet

alone. The patients were then randomly assigned to one of five treatment programs: (a) tolbutamide in a fixed dose of 1.5 grams, (b) placebo or diet alone, (c) insulin in a fixed dose, (d) insulin in variable doses, and (e) phenformin in fixed doses. An unexpected finding of a higher incidence of cardiovascular deaths in the tolbutamide and phenformin treated groups resulted in early termination of the study. After eight years, 26 cardiovascular deaths occurred in the tolbutamide group as opposed to 10–13 similar deaths in each of the other groups. Similar results were reported for the phenformin group (268–271).

Following publication of the UGDP results in both the professional and lay press, a great controversy regarding the study's validity and clinical implications appeared in the literature and this controversy persists today. The criticisms of the study, primarily relating to design and analysis, are voluminous and are well summarized elsewhere (123,210,272). Responses to these criticisms are also summarized elsewhere (273,274). In an effort to resolve this controversy, two outside groups of experts reviewed the data and its analysis (275,276). Despite this, there have been criticisms of the conclusions of these two groups and so the debate continues. The American Diabetes Association, which originally accepted the UGPD conclusions, more recently withdrew its support of the study in view of new data relating poor metabolic control to cardiovascular and other long-term diabetic complications and changes in diabetic therapy since 1961 (277,278). At the same time, it rejected formal governmental restrictions on the use of these agents and recommended that the decision to use sulfonylureas remain with the patient and physician.

In conclusion, although the cardiovascular effects of sulfonylureas are still debatable, a major impact of the study was to cause the medical community to reappraise a form of therapy which they had begun to take for granted. As a result, physicians who had been using these agents rather freely in "borderline" and asymptomatic diabetics began to reserve their use for symptomatic Type II diabetics who could not be controlled on diet and who would not or could not take insulin. At the same time, much greater emphasis was placed on diet therapy, exercise and the elimination of existing cardiovascular risk factors. These changes in therapeutic emphasis are reflected in the discussions on cardiovascular complications, diet and sulfonylurea therapy elsewhere in this chapter.

Hypoglycemia

37. C.A., a 68-year-old female who has had a 10-year history of Type II (NIDDM) diabetes and a 5-year history of mild renal failure (creatinine 1.5 mg/dl; BUN 30 mg/dl), is admitted to the hospital in coma. According to her daughter, her diabetes has been well controlled over the past several months with acetohexamide 1000 mg daily (she took her last dose approximately 9 hours prior to admission). Three days prior to admission she developed anorexia, nausea and vomiting in association with the flu and became progressively lethargic. Laboratory results on admission are as follows: plasma glucose 40 mg/dl; serum creatinine 3.0 mg/dl; blood urea nitrogen 80 mg/dl. What is this woman's diagnosis? Were there any predisposing factors?

C.A. has developed a case of severe hypoglycemia secondary to acetohexamide. As discussed in the section on Drug-induced Hypoglycemia later in this chapter, sulfonylureas account for almost all cases of drug-induced hypoglycemia in individuals over 60 years of age. All sulfonylureas in use worldwide have been implicated; however chlorpropamide, which is the oldest sulfonylurea on the market and has the longest duration of action, accounts for nearly 50% of all sulfonylurea-related hypoglycemic episodes. Glyburide, a long-acting second generation sulfonylurea is also commonly implicated.

Almost all cases of sulfonylurea-induced hypoglycemia occur in patients who are predisposed in some way and C.A. is no exception. She is an elderly woman with renal impairment who was on relatively high doses of an agent which is metabolized to an active product. Even in the face of decreased carbohydrate intake (anorexia and vomiting), she continued to take her usual dose of acetohexamide. The decreased intake and vomiting probably lead to dehydration and further compromise of her renal function. The accumulation of L-hydroxyhexamide (acetohexamide's active metabolite), which is excreted renally, no doubt contributed to her hypoglycemic episode.

Refractory hypoglycemia secondary to sulfonylureas is extremely lethal. Ten percent of all patients with this complication die and 2.7% suffer irreversible neurological sequelae (279).

SULFONYLUREA USE IN SPECIAL SITUATIONS

Renal Dysfunction

38. Acetohexamide has been withheld and C.A.'s kidney function is stabilized (Cl$_{cr}$ = 35 ml/min). Because she lives alone, has impaired eyesight secondary to cataracts and a severe case of arthritis, the institution of insulin for the treatment of her diabetes is impractical. Oral hypoglycemics are to be continued. What is the agent of choice?

Once C.A.'s plasma glucose concentrations and renal function have been stabilized, one must consider reinstitution of antidiabetic therapy. Sulfonylureas which depend on the kidney for elimination of active parent compounds or their metabolites should be avoided in elderly individuals and patients with decreased renal function (see Table 12). Sulfonylureas which are completely metabolized to inactive or weakly-active products may be considered, but long-acting agents should probably be avoided in the event that C.A. again becomes acutely ill or decreases her carbohydrate intake and becomes hypoglycemic. One is then left with tolbutamide which has the shortest duration of action and the inconvenience of multiple daily dosing. However, that inconvenience is probably outweighed by its safety advantages in this patient. It should be noted that tolbutamide has also caused prolonged hypoglycemic episodes in patients like C.A. so that it too should be used with caution.

Hepatic Dysfunction

39. A 60-year-old male with cirrhosis of the liver is found to have diabetes mellitus. Tolbutamide 0.5 gm tid is initiated. How will the patient's liver function affect the disposition of tolbutamide and the patient's response to this agent?

Since metabolism by the liver is the primary route of elimination of most sulfonylureas, patients with hepatic disease might be expected to have an exaggerated response to these drugs. Tolbutamide is the sulfonylurea which has been studied most extensively with respect to liver disease.

Tolbutamide elimination half-life in cirrhotics has been reported to be both increased (280) and unaltered (162). However, half-life alone is not a very useful parameter under these circumstances since it does not clearly indicate changes in clearance of the drug unless volume of distribution changes are also known. Decreased serum albumin concentrations in cirrhotics may increase the amount of free drug available for metabolism.

Nevertheless, patients with cirrhosis are indeed at increased risk for sulfonylurea-induced hypoglycemia. Gulati et al, in a double-blind placebo-controlled trial of 50 cirrhotic patients, found hypoglycemia to be a complication of 20% of the tolbutamide-treated group (281). It should be noted that the degree to which tolbutamide elimination is delayed cannot be predicted based on the degree of alteration of liver function tests (280).

A complicating factor in some cirrhotics is the induction of hepatic enzymes by alcohol, which may markedly increase tolbutamide metabolism and thereby decrease its effect (see Question 54).

Because liver disease may be a predisposing factor to severe, prolonged hypoglycemia induced by the sulfonylureas, these drugs should be avoided in cirrhotic patients. The rare occurrence of cholestatic jaundice secondary to the sulfonylureas may confuse the diagnostic picture in these patients and should be considered if signs and symptoms of obstruction progress during their use (see Question 33).

TREATMENT OF SPECIAL CONDITIONS IN DIABETICS

Peripheral Neuropathy

40. A.D., a 58-year-old man with diabetes of 6 years' duration, has been controlled with diet and tolazamide therapy. Glucose control has not changed over the last few years as measured by daily urine tests. However, over the past 6 months he has complained of increasing bilateral foot and leg pain, described as a burning or aching sensation, which has become so severe that he is unable to work. The pain is intensified at night, especially during sleep, and has become so sensitive to touch that he cannot tolerate bedcovers on his feet or legs. Non-narcotic analgesics, acetaminophen with codeine and percodan have not sufficiently alleviated the pain. Within the past two months, A.D. has become severely depressed over his pain and diabetes, with somatic complaints of early

morning awakening, weight loss, constipation, and generalized fatigue. How should A.D.'s painful neuropathy be managed?

Painful diabetic peripheral neuropathy (DPN) is a common complication of diabetes which usually involves the lower extremities. It ranges from mild paresthesias to severe pain that can become incapacitating and refractory to analgesic therapy. Although a multitude of drugs have been recommended for the treatment of DPN, few have been proven to be clinically effective.

Psychotropic Drugs. Since A.D.'s neuropathy has become incapacitating and is not relieved by narcotic analgesics, serious consideration should be given to the use of tricyclic antidepressants, phenothiazines or a combination of these two agents.

A typical regimen of amitriptyline 75 mg at bedtime and fluphenazine 1 mg tid was begun in A.D. with relief of pain within 48 hours. Both psychologic and somatic complaints of depression lessened dramatically. Over the next few weeks, amitriptyline was tapered to 25 mg at bedtime and fluphenazine to 1 mg bid, but further attempts to reduce dosage resulted in a flare-up of leg pain. Therapy should be tapered on an individual basis so that the least amount of drug needed is used to control symptoms. Most of the adverse effects of psychotropic drug therapy (sedation, anticholinergic effects, extrapyramidal reactions, cardiovascular effects, etc.) are dose-related, except for tardive dyskinesia, and the benefits of therapy should always be weighed against these risks. The risks and adverse effects of each class of psychotropic drugs (antidepressants and antipsychotics) must be assessed for the individual patient to determine if combination therapy can be utilized or if one class should be excluded due to patient-related contraindications. Although combination therapy with a drug from each psychotropic class is thought to be more effective than either agent alone, there are no controlled studies which have confirmed this observation. A.D. should continue treatment for as long as necessary to control pain, but periodic attempts should be made to reduce dosage and discontinue drug therapy.

Phenothiazines and tricyclic antidepressants have been used to manage chronic severe pain of various types including post-herpetic neuralgia, trigeminal neuralgia, lesions of the brachial and lumbosacral plexus and cancer (282,283). Although the actual mechanism of action for pain relief has not been well defined, it has been suggested that these drugs enhance the central inhibition of sensory input. A central mechanism of action is most likely since peripheral nerve conduction does not seem to be affected (284–286).

Although a well-designed, placebo-controlled study has yet to be done, numerous case reports and open trials have demonstrated the effectiveness of low dose psychotropic drugs, singly or in combination, to relieve the pain of DPN that is refractory to other treatment (284,285,287,288). In the only double-blind controlled study assessing the use of tricyclic antidepressant therapy, all 59 patients with DPN were also found to have substantial degrees of depression (286). After randomization and treatment with imipramine 100 mg hs, amitriptyline 100 mg hs, or diazepam 5 mg tid for 3 months, the painful neuropathies as well as the somatic and psychologic complaints of depression were strikingly reduced by antidepressant therapy. Both the neuropathy and the depression were closely associated in the presenting diagnosis as well as in response to treatment. Thus, antidepressant therapy may interfere centrally in a pain → depression → pain cycle. Although the mean period for complete relief of pain was 10 weeks in this study, remission of pain in several patients and in the few uncontrolled reports in the literature occurred within 48–72 hours. This is much shorter than the time usually needed to alleviate depression with tricyclic antidepressants; thus, there may be more than one mechanism for analgesic activity.

41. If A.D. had been unresponsive to psychotropic therapy, what other drugs could have been used to treat his painful diabetic neuropathy? How effective are they?

Carbamazepine. Case reports (289), open trials (290,291), and two placebo-controlled crossover studies (292,293) have demonstrated that carbamazepine is effective in relieving the paresthesias, and particularly the pain, of some patients with severe DPN. Dosages have varied from 100 mg tid to 200 mg qid. Dizziness and drowsiness are common but often transient, and gastrointestinal disturbances or dermatologic reactions are observed in 5–10% of patients. However, many diabetics do not respond to therapy and because of the small but very grave risk of blood dyscrasias, carbamazepine should be reserved for cases of painful DPN resistant to other measures. An

appropriate initial trial would be 100 mg tid for several weeks. If needed, the dose may be increased slowly as tolerated.

Phenytoin. Phenytoin was found to be effective in an uncontrolled trial of 60 patients with DPN (294). Forty-one patients (68%) were considered to have a good to excellent response to phenytoin 100 mg po tid-qid, and only 9 patients (15%) showed no improvement. Of those who benefited, initial improvement was always noted within 48–96 hours. A well-designed placebo-controlled trial in 38 diabetics confirmed the efficacy of phenytoin for the treatment of painful DPN (295). Phenytoin 100 mg tid for 2 weeks was statistically superior to a placebo regimen, and most patients who responded did so within 96 hours. Conversely, a separate double-blind placebo-controlled crossover study of 12 insulin dependent diabetics found phenytoin to be of no benefit in the treatment of DPN (296). Side effects such as ataxia, blurred vision, dizziness, and rash were reported in the treatment group. Patients in this group also had an impaired glucose tolerance to a standard meal (unexpected in Type I diabetics; see Question 51). Because of the results of this latter study, the known potential for impairment of diabetic control with phenytoin, and the numerous long-term adverse effects of this drug, phenytoin should not be used routinely for the treatment of DPN. A short trial may be warranted for severe cases resistant to other treatments.

Aldose Reductase Inhibitors. The use of aldose reductase inhibitors is also currently being investigated. Peripheral nerves, among certain other tissues, do not require insulin for glucose uptake. Excess glucose in these nerves is metabolized to sorbitol through a reaction catalyzed by the enzyme aldose reductase. One hypothesis for the pathogenesis of DPN (and perhaps of retinopathy as well) is that sorbitol and an additional metabolite, fructose, accumulate intracellularly and lead to nerve injury. The aldose reductase inhibitors, sorbinil and alrestatin, have been studied in the prevention of DPN in both animals and humans (297,298). Currently, they are valuable only as research tools and require further clinical study before their therapeutic role can be assessed.

Diabetic peripheral neuropathy, although mild in most patients, at times becomes so painful and incapacitating that it has led more than one diabetic to attempt suicide. It is no wonder that a plethora of therapies have been tested on these patients. Some of these drugs or chemicals, which have not been mentioned previously, include vitamins (either singly or in combination, especially the B vitamins) (299), clofibrate (300), thioctic acid (301), myo-inositol (302), hypertonic saline, and parenteral procaine. None of these therapies have been proven to be consistently efficacious, although some warrant further study. If simple analgesics are not effective, psychotropic drugs remain the treatment of choice for diabetics like A.D. with severe painful DPN. If A.D. had not responded within a few days, a longer trial with an antidepressant alone would be considered, especially since a component of depression was apparent. Carbamazepine and, secondly, phenytoin may be considered as alternatives for patients who are refractory to psychotropic therapy, have intolerable side effects to those agents, or have contraindications to the use of psychotropic medications.

Gastroparesis

42. H.D. is a 36-year-old man with a history of insulin dependent diabetes since the age of 12. He is currently in poor control with a fasting blood glucose this morning of 267 mg/dl. H.D. presents to the diabetes clinic with a two-month history of nausea, gas, constipation, and a bloating feeling in his stomach which occur at night and in the morning and are unrelieved by antacids. He also has peripheral neuropathy involving both hands and feet and some evidence of an autonomic neuropathy. An upper gastrointestinal series was ordered to rule out peptic ulcer disease and reflux esophagitis, but a preliminary diagnosis of diabetic gastroparesis was made. What is diabetic gastroparesis and how should H.D. be treated?

Gastroparesis is a diabetic disorder associated with symptoms that can cause mild discomfort to severe disability. Nausea, vomiting, early satiety, abdominal distension, and occasional bezoar formation are a result of delayed evacuation of solids and liquids from the stomach. Impaired diabetic control may also result from the disrupted delivery of food to the intestine. Abnormal motility of the gastric fundus or antrum is generally considered to be the mechanism which results in a prolongation of gastric emptying time. An alternative explanation is a reduction or absence of cyclic motor complex activity in the intestine, termed "housekeeper" activity, which normally clears the gut of residual material between meals (303–305). Many patients with diabetic gastroparesis, like H.D., also have evidence of neuropathy, particularly of the autonomic variety, although a direct cause and effect relationship has not been demonstrated.

Metoclopramide. If therapy is indicated, H.D. should receive a trial of metoclopramide, 10 mg po qid, before meals and at bedtime. Although treatment may not eliminate all symptoms, it should minimize most of his complaints. Metoclopramide is the first satisfactory treatment available for diabetic gastroparesis. Although the number of diabetics in controlled studies are sparse, case reports (306–313) and four double-blind placebo-controlled studies (304,314–316) have demonstrated that metoclopramide is an effective drug for this diabetic complication. In fact, metoclopramide seems to be effective in relieving symptoms of gastroparesis irrespective of the cause (diabetes, vagotomy, gastric surgery, idiopathic) (304,314–316). Past treatment of diabetic gastroparesis with pyloroplasty, partial gastrectomy, and cholinergic or cholinesterase inhibitor drugs was disappointing.

Metoclopramide improves gastric emptying time in most patients with diabetic gastroparesis and may also increase "intestinal housekeeper" activity to correct gastric stasis (304,316). Effects on gut motility are due to direct and/or indirect cholinergic properties of the drug on the gut muscle. Part of its effect on nausea and vomiting seems to be due to dopamine antagonism of the central vomiting center (316).

If H.D.'s poor diabetic control is due in part to abnormal carbohydrate digestion, metoclopramide may improve diabetic control as well as reduce the more obvious symptoms of gastroparesis.

43. Three weeks after initiating metoclopramide therapy (which reduced gastroparetic symptoms dramatically), H.D. complains of involuntary spasms of his neck and facial muscles and has noticed a need to pace the floor. Could this be due to metoclopramide treatment? What are the side effects and precautions for use of metoclopramide?

H.D. appears to have a dystonic reaction and akathesia which may be secondary to metoclopramide. Like the antipsychotic drugs, metoclopramide inhibits dopamine activity in the central nervous system and thus has the potential to generate similar adverse effects. Reversible extrapyramidal side effects such as akinesias, akathesias, and dystonic reactions have been estimated to occur in about 1% of patients (317). Potentially irreversible tardive dyskinesia may also occur after chronic metoclopramide therapy (318,319). If long-term therapy is considered, the potential for tardive dyskinesia warrants drug-free periods to determine if therapy is still necessary.

The side effects of metoclopramide are usually mild and reversible and, for the most part, are a result of central nervous system activity (320,321). Drowsiness and lassitude are not uncommon and gastrointestinal disturbances may occur due to the drug's effect on gut motility (although usually not reported as an adverse effect in patients with gastroparesis). Galactorrhea and menstrual disorders are caused by prolactin release which is a result of dopamine receptor blockade in the CNS (322). Special caution should be exercised when initiating metoclopramide therapy in a patient taking phenothiazines or other antipsychotic medications since concurrent use of these medications could potentiate metoclopramide's extrapyramidal side effects or vice versa. Patients with Parkinson's disease would also be poor candidates for metoclopramide therapy since their condition may be exacerbated by this drug.

If H.D.'s dystonic reaction does not reverse by itself, an anticholinergic drug such as benztropine or diphenhydramine would effectively alleviate this adverse effect.

Hypertension in the Diabetic

44. L.S. is a 49-year-old obese male with an 8-year history of Type II diabetes and a 9-year history of angina. He had a myocardial infarction 7 years ago. L.S.'s current problems include a blood pressure which has become increasingly elevated over the last three clinic visits and the recent onset of sexual impotence. Physical examination on this visit reveals a blood pressure of 185/110 mm Hg with no orthostatic changes. The fasting plasma glucose concentration is 120 mg/dl. L.S. has no evidence of diabetic nephropathy. Current medications include: tolbutamide 1 gm twice daily, propranolol 40 mg three times daily, nitroglycerin ointment 1″ every 8 hours, and nitroglycerin sublingually as needed for pain.

How should hypertension be managed in this obese, Type II diabetic? Are there any special considerations or cautions for treating hypertensive diabetics?

Both hypertension and diabetes are well known risk factors of morbidity and mortality from major cardiovascular events. The two diseases superimposed on an individual patient produce an additive risk of complications such as coronary heart disease, stroke, peripheral vascular disease, and congestive heart failure. Microvascular complications may also be accelerated. Consequently, hypertensive diabetics should benefit more from aggressive antihypertensive therapy than non-diabetics (333).

Does this imply that all diabetics with hypertension should be treated aggressively and in a similar fashion? Not necessarily. Many of the antihypertensive medications have adverse effects which are more serious or occur more frequently in the diabetic population. Thus, the drug therapy of hypertension in the diabetic must be approached cautiously and should be accompanied by frequent monitoring.

The benefits of thiazide diuretics and beta-blockers usually outweigh the risks involved (see Questions 45 and 46) unless specific contraindications are present. When choosing a sympatholytic agent for a diabetic, two side effects in particular must be remembered: sexual impotence and orthostatic hypotension. L.S. already complains of some degree of sexual impotence (possibly due to diabetic autonomic neuropathy); thus, methyldopa and guanethidine, which cause a higher prevalence of impotence, are relatively contraindicated and clonidine may be a more appropriate choice. While L.S. does not have orthostatic hypotension on physical examination, both nitroglycerin ointment and a potential autonomic neuropathy may predispose him to an orthostatic response so that even clonidine should be used carefully. The vasodilators, hydralazine and minoxidil, should also be used cautiously in L.S. since they may exacerbate his coronary artery disease. The presence of a beta-blocker in his regimen does, however, minimize this risk. (Also see the Essential Hypertension chapter.)

45. Diuretic-Induced Hyperglycemia. L.S. is to be treated with hydrochlorothiazide 50

mg daily. Is the diabetogenic effect of hydrochlorothiazide and other diuretics significant? Is their use contraindicated in L.S.?

The diabetogenic effect of thiazides and other diuretics is well recognized and accepted by the medical profession. However, the significance of this effect is not as well defined and has placed the use of diuretics in an uncertain light when used in the diabetic population. Furman has recently reviewed the literature on this subject and the reader is referred to this well-referenced article for a more detailed discussion (334). According to this author, much of the literature relating to diuretic-induced hyperglycemia was difficult to interpret due to the lack of parallel control studies. However, the following information may be used to place diuretic use in the proper perspective.

(a) Patients who are diabetic or are predisposed to diabetes have a higher risk of diuretic-induced hyperglycemia or impaired glucose tolerance than nondiabetics (335,336). Clinical diabetes may be precipitated in a small number of nondiabetics (337), but these individuals are probably predisposed to diabetes in some way.

(b) The impairment of diabetic control or magnitude of impaired glucose tolerance produced by diuretics is generally reported to be small and does not usually present a therapeutic problem (336,338). Serious hyperglycemic reactions do occur in a small percentage of patients, however, and diabetic coma with or without ketosis has been induced by a number of diuretics including thiazides, (339,340), chlorthalidone (341,342), furosemide (343–345), and ethacrynic acid (346).

(c) Duration of diuretic use is still an unknown factor in the impairment of glucose tolerance. While several studies demonstrate an effect on blood glucose or glucose tolerance within a few days of initiating diuretic therapy (335,337), other studies have found a diabetogenic effect only after years of diuretic treatment (347,348).

(d) The mechanisms of diuretic-induced hyperglycemia are still obscure. Hypokalemia is thought by some investigators to be an important contributory factor. Hypokalemia may inhibit peripheral utilization of glucose or inhibit insulin secretion at the pancreatic level. Hypokalemia itself, however, is probably not the primary factor in the development of abnormal glucose tolerance since it is not consistently found in diuretic-induced hyperglycemia (335,347,349,350); hyperglycemia has also followed the use of potassium-sparing diuretics (350). Insulin secretion or utilization may be inhibited by factors unrelated to potassium depletion. Nevertheless, potassium supplementation has been shown to reverse, at least partly, changes in blood glucose induced by diuretics in hypokalemic patients (350–352).

(e) Diuretic-induced hyperglycemia is reversible (335–337) in most cases, but in some cases may persist following discontinuation of the drug.

(f) Hyperglycemia and glucose intolerance have been reported to occur with thiazide and non-thiazide diuretics alike. Although the thiazides and chlorthalidone are most frequently implicated, this probably reflects the relative popularity of these drugs. Case reports or studies of diuretic-induced hyperglycemia in man exist for the following drugs: Thiazides (334–337,347–349,352), Bumetanide (353), Chlorthalidone (336,341,342, 354), Clopamide (355), Clorexolone (355), Ethacrynic acid (346,356), Furosemide (343,344,346, 357,358), Metolazone (359,360), and Triamterene (350).

To summarize, diuretic-induced hyperglycemia seems to occur frequently and, though usually mild, may sometimes precipitate severe reactions. Unfortunately, a diuretic is generally considered the initial drug of choice in most antihypertensive regimens. Because the demonstrable benefit of effectively controlling essential hypertension probably far outweighs the risks of drug-induced hyperglycemia, we feel that diuretics are not contraindicated in most diabetic patients.

During therapy, potassium concentrations should be monitored and potassium supplementation or potassium-sparing drugs should be utilized if needed. If impairment of diabetic control occurs which does not respond to potassium, a logical course of action may be taken depending on the circumstance of the patient. In an insulin dependent diabetic, an adjustment of insulin dose is usually all that is necessary. Similarly, a diabetic treated with an oral agent will respond to a slight dosage increase of the sulfonylurea, or a dosage decrease of the diuretic. If the reaction is severe, of course, the diuretic should be discontinued, although it is often difficult to identify that a reaction is clearly drug-induced. The main contraindication to diuretic therapy is in a diabetic previously controlled on diet alone who subsequently must choose between the addition of antidiabetic drug therapy (sulfonylureas or insulin) or discontinuation of diuretic therapy. In this case, every effort should be made to substitute a different antihypertensive regimen for the diuretic so that multiple drug therapy can be avoided.

46. *Beta-blocker Therapy.* Discuss the controversy surrounding the use of beta-blockers in diabetics. Should L.S. be switched from propranolol to a cardioselective beta-blocker?

Diabetics have a high prevalence of cardiovascular diseases such as hypertension and angina, which are commonly treated with beta blockers. Unfortunately, many of the glucodynamic and hemodynamic responses in diabetics are directly or indirectly mediated by beta-receptors, and thus may be significantly altered by this class of drugs. Beta-blocking drugs are relatively contraindicated in certain high-risk patients. Evidence is accumulating that many of the unwanted effects of these drugs may be attenuated with the use of the more cardioselective blockers. The use of beta-blocking drugs has evoked the following areas of concern for diabetics:

(a) *Beta-blockers may increase the frequency or severity of hypoglycemia or block the warning signals of a hypoglycemic episode.* Several cases of severe hypoglycemia associated with propranolol have been reported in both diabetic and non-diabetic patients (361–365). Patients who were not diabetic were generally predisposed to hypoglycemia. However, in a prospective study of 50 insulin-treated diabetics taking beta-blockers and 100 matched diabetic controls, the incidence of loss of consciousness (severe hypoglycemia) was the same in both groups (366). A number of smaller controlled studies have demonstrated that prior beta-blockade does not accelerate or potentiate the hypoglycemic response to insulin (367–370). Nevertheless, hypoglycemia may occur in a rare individual. Hypoglycemic reactions are thought to be due to blockade of glycogenolysis in a diabetic with already poor glycogen stores; they may also mask the initial warning signals of a hypoglycemic attack.

Diabetics have different signs and symptoms of hypoglycemia which tend to be consistent within the same individual. It is not surprising, then, that beta-blockers may modify the warning signs of some patients but not of others. Most of the warning signs are the result of a hypoglycemic-induced catecholamine response. Hypoglycemic tachycardia or palpitations are suppressed in a significant proportion of patients taking beta-blockers (368,371,372). Severe bradycardia re-

sulted in hypotension and seizures in one hypoglycemic patient who had been administered propranolol (373). Hunger, irritability, confusion, tremor and other signs or symptoms of hypoglycemia are variably affected by beta-blocker administration, and may be blunted in an occasional patient. Hypoglycemic sweating is not reduced and is often even enhanced by beta-blocker therapy (362,366,372–374). This can be an important warning signal in patients taking beta-blockers whose other signs of hypoglycemia have been attenuated. Although the cardioselective beta-blockers may not mask the tachycardia and associated warning signs as much as non-selective blockers (367,373), it is important to note that a diabetic placed on any beta-blocking agent may experience a change in his hypoglycemic warning signs.

(b) *Beta-blockers may delay the rate of recovery from hypoglycemia.* Diabetics in general have a sluggish counterregulatory response to hypoglycemia compared to healthy subjects. Beta-blocking agents have been demonstrated to further attenuate this rate of recovery in insulin-dependent diabetics, although cardioselective agents may impair recovery to a lesser extent (369,370,373). The mechanisms by which beta-blockers impair hypoglycemic recovery is still not clear, although they may oppose the effects of epinephrine, which is the primary counterregulatory hormone in diabetics. Impaired recovery may be associated with diminished availability of glycerol (through inhibition of lipolysis) and lactate, which are substrates for gluconeogenesis (368,369,373). Cardioselective beta-blockers do not affect lipolysis and lactate concentrations to the same extent as non-selective blockers (368,373).

(c) *Beta-blockers may alter the hemodynamic response to hypoglycemia, resulting in exaggerated hypertension.* During hypoglycemia, high levels of circulating epinephrine normally produce a rise in heart rate and systolic blood pressure and a fall in diastolic pressure. Non-selective beta-blockers, via unopposed alpha-mediated vasoconstriction, cause a rise in both systolic and diastolic pressures with reflex bradycardia or little change in heart rate (368,373). Conversely, a cardioselective beta-blocker such as metoprolol usually produces an increase in systolic pressure but only a slight increase or unchanged diastolic pressure and heart rate (367,368,373). Theoretically then, propranolol might be expected to produce an exaggerated hypertensive response, and a more selective beta-blocker would be preferred in a patient prone to hypoglycemia. However, hypertensive episodes during hypoglycemia have been associated with both non-selective (propranolol) and cardioselective (metoprolol) beta-blockers (364,375). As previously noted, a severe hypotensive episode has also been associated with propranolol in a hypoglycemic diabetic (373).

(d) *Beta-blockers may impair carbohydrate tolerance and worsen diabetic control.* Stimulation of beta receptors leads to insulin release in man (376); thus, it has been proposed that beta-blockers may impair insulin release in type II diabetics. Preliminary evidence has demonstrated that beta-blockers may impair diabetic control. Non-selective, but not cardioselective, beta-blockers have impaired glucose tolerance or increased blood glucose in several studies (377–379). An improvement in glucose tolerance and increased insulin concentrations were shown in some diabetics when switched from a non-selective beta-blocker to metoprolol (380). In other studies, an impairment was seen with both cardioselective and non-selective blockers (381,382). All patients studied were type II diabetics, most of whom were taking oral hypoglycemic agents. Although a reduction of insulin release has been hypothesized to be responsible for the impaired response, it is unclear whether insulin is actually reduced (377,379,382). Many diabetics do not have a hyperglycemic response to beta-blockers, and most of those who have this response undergo only slight elevations of glucose which may not be clinically significant. A few cases of severe acute hyperglycemia associated with beta-blocker therapy have occurred (383,384).

(e) *Beta-blockers may impair peripheral circulation.* Several cases of gangrene in the extremities of patients receiving propranolol have been reported (385). Diabetic patients who may have impaired peripheral circulation are already predisposed. Theoretically, the cardioselective beta-blockers would be less likely to compromise blood flow to the extremities since they have less effect on beta$_2$-mediated vasodilation.

Conclusion. In conclusion, beta-adrenergic blockers have the potential to affect diabetics in a variety of ways. Patients at particular risk for developing complications are (1) those who have frequent or severe hypoglycemic attacks (unstable type I diabetics), and (2) those with compromised hemodynamic function (patients with autonomic neuropathy or vascular insufficiency).

In these high-risk patients, beta-blocker therapy is relatively contraindicated. A cardioselective blocker is preferred if beta-blocker therapy is clearly necessary. It is the opinion of these authors that all diabetics should be maintained on the safest drug possible; L.S. should therefore be switched to a cardioselective agent. However, one should be aware that cardioselective beta-blockers lose their selectivity at higher doses.

47. Do any other antihypertensive medications affect diabetic control?

Clonidine. Clonidine has been demonstrated to produce hyperglycemia in animals, *in vitro* and, to a limited extent, in man. By acting on alpha$_2$ adrenergic receptors in the pancreas, clonidine is a powerful inhibitor of insulin release *in vitro* (386,387). A single 0.5 mg oral dose of clonidine increased plasma glucose by 12 mg/dl in 20 nondiabetic subjects. After four days of multiple dose treatment, a similar effect on plasma glucose, but no change in insulin concentrations was seen (388). A separate study could not corroborate the hyperglycemic effect of clonidine in man, but both studies found that clonidine depressed insulin response (334). A single case report of improved diabetic control after clonidine withdrawal suggests that this effect may be clinically important (386), but the actual clinical significance of this effect is still very limited. Clonidine, in oral doses of 0.45–0.9 mg/day, has also been shown to suppress the catecholamine response following insulin hypoglycemia and to reduce the signs and symptoms of the hypoglycemic episode.

Prazosin. Acute administration of prazosin has been shown to produce marked hyperglycemia in both normal and diabetic subjects (334). Although the mechanism has yet to be elucidated, it is suggested that the acute hypotensive effect of the drug may result in reflex hyperglycemia. If true, prazosin use should not pose a clinical problem since the acute hypotensive episode (and hyperglycemic effect) does not occur with chronic dosing.

Diazoxide. See Table 16.

DRUG-INDUCED HYPERGLYCEMIA

Important drugs which may produce hyperglycemia in normal patients or further impair carbohydrate tolerance in a diabetic are discussed in Questions 45, 46, 48–52 and summarized in Table 16. Drugs which have been reported to produce hyperglycemia but are clinically less significant are summarized in Table 17. Drugs inducing hyperglycemia in poisoning or overdose situations are not included in these tables.

Sympathomimetics

48. R.C., a 41-year-old insulin dependent diabetic, is well controlled on split doses of regular and NPH insulin and has been taking pseudoephedrine 30 mg qid × 7 days for a head cold. His other medications include nifedipine 10 mg tid and acetaminophen prn. Urine monitoring with Clinitest has shown more glucose (often ¾–1%) than usual (0–¼%). Can pseudoephedrine be the cause of his poor control? Discuss the use of adrenergic agents and sympathomimetics in general for diabetics.

Although over-the-counter drug products containing sympathomimetics (eg, cold products and diet aids) carry warning labels which caution against their use in diabetics, there is surprisingly little evidence that documents this as a clinically significant problem. It is well established that parenterally administered epinephrine increases blood glucose concentrations secondary to increased glycogenolysis, gluconeogenesis, and other catecholamine-induced mechanisms. Other sympathomimetics generally do not have as potent an effect on blood glucose as epinephrine and their use usually does not pose a practical problem in diabetics.

Salbutamol has been shown to produce rapid increases in plasma ketones, free fatty acids and insulin in normal subjects. In diabetics in which insulin secretion is impaired or absent, ketosis may result (389). The intravenous use of salbutamol or *ritodrine* has been associated with several cases of ketoacidosis, all but one of which occurred in diabetics (389–393). Hyperglycemia, acetonuria and glucosuria were also reported in three nondiabetic children who received therapeutic to high oral doses of *phenylephrine* (394–396).

Pseudophedrine may be aggravating R.C.'s diabetic control, though at this low to normal therapeutic dose it is quite unlikely. His underlying cold is much more likely to have produced hyperglycemia.

Calcium Antagonists

49. Is it likely that nifedipine is responsible for the increased glycosuria and hyperglycemia observed in R.C.? If so, by what mechanism?

The hypothesis that nifedipine and other calcium antagonists (eg, verapamil and diltiazem) might be diabetogenic through impairment of insulin secretion was based upon *in vitro* pharmacologic studies of their action and the knowledge that glucose-induced insulin release was dependent upon extracellular calcium ions (334). Results of clinical investigations in man, however, are conflicting.

Table 16.

IMPORTANT DIABETOGENIC DRUGS

Drug	Significance*	Mechanism/Comments	Selected References
Diazoxide	+ + +	↓ insulin secretion, ↓ peripheral glucose utilization, and others.	(334)
Diuretics	+ + +	Unclear. See text Question 45.	(334)
Glucocorticoids	+ + +	↑ gluconeogenesis. See text Question 52.	(402)
Oral contraceptives	+ +	Unclear. See text Question 50.	(334,404)
Phenytoin	+ +	↓ insulin secretion. See text Question 51.	(409)
Beta-adrenergic blockers	+/+ +	↓ insulin release? See text Question 46.	text

* +—Possibly important; limited reports or studies; needs substantiation
+ +—Clinically significant
+ + +—Clinically significant effect of substantial prevalence and/or magnitude

Verapamil. In one study, an infusion of verapamil did not affect glucose or insulin concentrations in normal subjects. However, verapamil has been demonstrated to reduce insulin's hypoglycemic response through a direct effect on the liver (397,398).

Nifedipine. Contradictory evidence also exists for nifedipine. Donnelly et al found that oral nifedipine (10 mg tid for one month) had no effect on the glucose tolerance of 8 diabetics and 8 nondiabetics (399). In contrast, another group studying nifedipine in similar doses (10 mg tid for 10 days) noted an improved glucose tolerance in healthy individuals and impaired glucose tolerance in 10 subjects with already impaired glucose tolerance (400). To make matters more confusing, Charles et al found that nifedipine induced distinct glucose intolerance in 6 healthy subjects (401). Basal insulin concentrations in these individuals were reduced by 26%, and fasting plasma glucose concentrations rose by 10%.

Although the data related to calcium antagonist-induced hyperglycemia is equivocal at best, preliminary data suggest that diabetics with existing pancreatic function (Type II, NIDDM) should be made aware that the use of these agents may

Table 17.

OTHER* DRUGS REPORTED TO CAUSE HYPERGLYCEMIA OR IMPAIR GLUCOSE TOLERANCE

Drug	Significance**	Proposed Mechanism/Comments	Selected References
Adrenergic agents/ sympathomimetics	+/+ +	↑ glycogenolysis, gluconeogenesis. See text Question 48.	text
L-Asparaginase	+ +	Unclear.	(427)
Calcitonin (synthetic salmon)	+	Obscure.	(428,429)
Calcium antagonists	+	↓ insulin secretion. See text Question 49.	(401)
Cimetidine	±	Obscure.	(430)
Caffeine	+	Obscure. Impairs glucose tolerance test in diabetics.	***
Clonidine	+	↓ insulin secretion. See text Question 47.	(386)
Colchicine	+	↓ insulin secretion.	(334)
Dextrothyroxine	+	Unclear.	***
Levodopa	+	Unclear. May ↓ insulin secretion.	***
Lithium	±	Obscure.	(431)
Morphine	±	Obscure.	***
Nicotinic acid	+	Obscure.	***
Phenothiazines/related drugs	±	↓ insulin secretion, hyperprolactinemia.	(334)
Pentamidine	+ +	Toxic to beta cells. May cause hypoglycemia initially.	(432)
Prazosin	±	Hyperglycemic reflex. See text Question 47.	(334)

*See Table 16.

** ±—Case reports only or contradictory studies.

+—Possibly important; limited reports or studies; needs substantiation.

+ +—Clinically significant.

+ + +—Clinically significant effect of substantial prevalence and/or magnitude.

***Reviewed with references in Hansten (171)

be associated with diminished diabetic control. However, in insulin dependent diabetics such as R.C., nifedipine is unlikely to have any effect on diabetic control.

Oral Contraceptives

50. K.W. is a 22-year-old insulin dependent diabetic who wishes to use an oral contraceptive (OC). Discuss the use of oral contraceptives for diabetics. What roles do estrogens and progestogens play in OC-induced diabetes? Are OCs contraindicated? If not, what type of OC can be recommended?

An association between oral contraceptive use and glucose intolerance was first reported in 1963. Since that time, numerous investigations have attempted to clarify the relative biochemical effects of the estrogen vs progestogen components, the risk factors of developing impaired glucose tolerance or overt diabetes, and the practical implications of OC use in the diabetic and nondiabetic populations. These subjects have been extensively reviewed (334,402–405) and though some important differences of opinion still exist, the prevailing views are summarized as follows:

Clinical Significance and Predisposing Factors. Although the incidence is difficult to determine, many women who use oral contraceptives have some elevation of plasma glucose concentrations, impaired glucose tolerance, and/or abnormal insulin concentrations. The effects are usually negligible and rarely produce clinical diabetes unless patients have the following risk factors: family history or other predisposition to diabetes (disputable); past history of hyperglycemia (particularly gestational diabetes in which OC-induced diabetes has been reported to be irreversible in several cases) (406); and existing glucose intolerance or clinical diabetes which may be aggravated by OC use (though diabetic control is rarely affected appreciably).

Mechanism. The mechanism of impaired carbohydrate metabolism from OC use is still obscure, but several theories have been proposed. These include: tissue insulin resistance, an elevation of free cortisol concentrations, an elevation of growth hormone concentrations, and altered tryptophan and pyridoxine metabolism. Each of these theories has been individually substantiated to some degree, but interrelating factors have yet to be determined. The first two theories

parallel the mechanism of action of glucocorticoid-induced diabetes. It is interesting to note that the clinical syndrome of the contraceptive/steroid abnormality is also similar to glucocorticoid-induced "steroid diabetes."

Effects of Estrogens and Progestogens. The use of mestranol or ethinyl estradiol alone do not significantly alter carbohydrate metabolism. Progestogens do alter carbohydrate metabolism and it is this component of oral contraceptives which is now thought to impair glucose tolerance. Of the 19-nortestosterone derivatives, norgestrel affects glucose tolerance to the greatest degree, followed by ethynodiol diacetate which may in turn have more effect than norethindrone (least effect) (404). The 17-acetoxyprogesterone derivatives (megestrol, medroxyprogesterone), which are not used in OC products, have the least effect on carbohydrate metabolism.

For unknown reasons, the combination OCs affect glucose tolerance to a greater degree than a progestogen alone, and the effect is more pronounced as the estrogen content increases (407). Combination products containing less than 50 mcg of estrogen may have the least effect on glucose tolerance (404). Ethinyl estradiol 35 mcg with norethindrone 0.4 mg (but not with norgestrel) had negligible effects on glucose tolerance in nondiabetic women followed for up to 6 months (408).

Cardiovascular Risks. Oral contraceptive use in women over 35 years of age significantly increases the risk of cardiovascular disease (see the chapter on Contraception). Since diabetics also have an increased cardiovascular complication rate, older diabetic OC users are doubly predisposed.

Duration of Effect. Carbohydrate abnormalities due to oral contraceptives are usually sustained for the duration of treatment; however, they may be transient in some patients, disappearing after a few months to years of continued treatment.

Recommendations. Oral contraceptive use in diabetics is relatively contraindicated only in women over 35 years of age, or if other risk factors are present (see the chapter on Contraception). In nondiabetic women with a history of gestational diabetes, the use of a different form of contraception is also recommended. K.W., who is already diabetic, should be placed on a low-dose, estrogen/norethindrone combination product or a progestogen-only pill, containing norethindrone. This also applies to nondiabetic women with risk factors for diabetes.

Phenytoin

51. R.D., a 53-year-old male with a family history of diabetes mellitus develops grand mal seizures following head trauma. He is to be treated with phenytoin. What is the effect of phenytoin on blood glucose and plasma insulin levels? Is the use of phenytoin contraindicated in this patient?

Several reports of phenytoin-induced glycosuria, hyperglycemia, diminished glucose tolerance results, and even hyperosmolar non-ketotic coma have appeared in the literature (409–415). The abnormalities are almost always associated with large doses or toxic concentrations of phenytoin, though mild carbohydrate abnormalities have also been found in some subjects with plasma concentrations in the therapeutic range. Hyperglycemia was directly related to dose and serum concentrations in one reported case in which glucose tolerance was normal with doses of 100, 200, and 300 mg/day of phenytoin, but abnormal with a dose of 400 mg/day (411). Since phenytoin undergoes dose-dependent kinetics, small increments in dosing may cause large increases in drug concentrations. It should be noted that some investigators have found no effect of phenytoin on carbohydrate metabolism, even in toxic doses (334).

Phenytoin-induced hyperglycemia seems to be due to decreased pancreatic insulin secretion (409). Pretreatment with therapeutic doses of phenytoin for as little as three days diminished insulin in response to glucose in nondiabetic patients (411,416). It is postulated that phenytoin affects passive or active diffusion of sodium and other electrolytes across the beta cell membrane to depress cell excitability (409,417).

Because phenytoin does not affect the peripheral utilization of insulin, it should have little, if any, effect on type I diabetics dependent on exogenous insulin. However, phenytoin has been demonstrated to alter or reverse tolbutamide-induced hypoglycemia and to increase insulin secretion *in vitro* (334). This may have implications for sulfonylurea-treated diabetics.

Clinically, hyperglycemia does not appear to be a significant problem in patients who are taking chronic, non-toxic doses of phenytoin. Nevertheless, close monitoring is warranted in those patients who are (a) receiving high doses of phenytoin or increasing their dose; (b) taking other diabetogenic medications or have a predisposition to diabetes such as R.D.; and (c) type II diabetics on sulfonylurea drugs. The use of phenytoin is not contraindicated in this patient.

Glucocorticoids

52. A.L., a 37-year-old obese female with SLE, has been taking 80 mg of prednisone daily for 6 months. During this period her weight has increased by 30 lb and she has developed glycosuria. She was referred to a diabetic clinic where a fasting plasma glucose was found to be 190 mg/dl with 1% glucose in her urine and no ketones. Physical examination shows an obese, 5′2″, 150 lb, depressed female with trunkal obesity and an acneiform rash. Her mother and one sister have diabetes. How could glucocorticoids contribute to diabetes mellitus? How should this patient be treated?

The term "steroid diabetes" was first used to describe hyperglycemia and glycosuria as seen in Cushing's Syndrome. It is now more commonly associated with exogenously administered glucocorticoids and has been associated with parenteral, oral, and even topical therapy (418). Glucocorticoids are one of the most common drug groups that unmask latent diabetes or aggravate preexisting disease, and they may produce hyperglycemia and overt diabetes in otherwise nonpredisposed individuals (402).

Steroid-induced diabetes is mainly due to the pharmacologic activity of the glucocorticoid on carbohydrate, protein, and lipid metabolism resulting in an increase in hepatic gluconeogenesis. Glucocorticoids also seem to cause a peripheral insensitivity to insulin at the site of the insulin receptor (419). Though steroid-induced diabetes is often mild and rarely associated with ketonemia, a wide spectrum of severity may be encountered from asymptomatic abnormal glucose tolerance tests to difficult-to-control insulin dependent disease (402,420). The onset of steroid diabetes or glucose intolerance can follow the administration of glucocorticoids within hours to days, or may only appear months to years after chronic therapy, if at all. The effect is generally considered to be dose-dependent and is usually, though not always, reversible upon discontinuation of the drug (402). Reversal may take several months after withdrawal of therapy.

Patients such as A.L. on chronic glucocorticoid therapy require frequent urinary or blood glucose monitoring. Mild diabetes in obese individuals, as in this case, can often be controlled by diet, but may require exogenous insulin supplementation or sulfonylurea therapy. A known diabetic whose condition is aggravated by glucocorticoids should modify treatment accordingly to restore control. Increasing the dose of insulin or oral agents may be sufficient, but some patients need to be changed from diet or oral therapy to insulin supplementation. Once the patient is on the least possible steroid dose, control is similar to that of any type II diabetic (see Question 23).

DRUG-INDUCED HYPOGLYCEMIA

Hypoglycemia occurs when insulin activity is inappropriately high relative to plasma glucose concentrations and/or when normal counterregulatory mechanisms for hypoglycemia (glycogenolysis and gluconeogenesis) are absent, compromised or suppressed.

Seltzer (279) comprehensively reviewed all cases of drug-induced hypoglycemia in 1979 and found that over 90% of those reported since 1970 were caused by the sulfonylureas. Salicylate toxicity accounts for many of the cases in young children, and alcohol is a major cause of hypoglycemia during the third, fourth and fifth decades of life. Sulfonylurea-induced hypoglycemia is also common during the fourth and fifth decades of life and becomes the leading cause of drug-induced hypoglycemia in individuals over 60 years of age. Over 10% of all cases of drug-induced hypoglycemia were associated with combinations of agents known to cause or predispose to hypoglycemia (eg, alcohol plus insulin; sulfonylurea plus insulin).

Several factors predispose individuals to drug-induced hypoglycemia and it is the unusual case which is not associated with one or more of these.

Decreased Carbohydrate Intake. Decreased carbohydrate intake ultimately results in depletion of liver glycogen and since hepatic glycogenolysis is essential to the maintenance of plasma glucose concentrations in the fasting state, its depletion can compromise a patient taking a hypoglycemic agent. Acute decreases in carbohydrate intake (eg, secondary to nausea and vomiting) are most important in individuals who have marginal glycogen stores due to irregular eating habits (eg, alcoholics; elderly individuals).

Age. The number of cases of drug-induced hypoglycemia per decade appears to be approximately the same between the ages of 30 and 60 and increases markedly thereafter. The elderly are most likely predisposed because their renal function is physiologically diminished (see below) and they have a greater tendency toward irregular eating patterns.

Renal Failure. Renal impairment may predispose individuals to drug-induced hypoglycemia by several mechanisms. First, endogenous and exogenous insulin clearance is impaired because the kidney is responsible for metabolic degradation of approximately 50% of insulin. Thus, insulin concentrations are elevated in individuals with renal failure (149). Second, many of the drugs which cause hypoglycemia rely on the kidney for elimination of unchanged drug or their active metabolites. Therefore, patients with renal failure may accumulate these active substances and thereby enhance or prolong their activity. Patients who are uremic often become nauseated and anorexic and may voluntarily decrease their carbohydrate intake. Nevertheless, the effects of different degrees of renal failure on carbohydrate metabolism are complex. See Question 21.

Hepatic Dysfunction. The liver is the primary source of plasma glucose during a fasting state: first, through glycogenolysis and second, through gluconeogenesis. Impairment of liver function may therefore alter these counterregulatory effects. The liver is also responsible for the metabolism and, in some cases, the inactivation of drugs which induce hypoglycemia. If this function is impaired, active drug or metabolite may accumulate, thereby exaggerating the drug effect on plasma glucose.

Drugs which have been reported to cause hypoglycemia are discussed in Questions 37, 46, 53 and 54 and summarized in Table 18.

Salicylates

53. M.C. is a 52-year-old, Type II diabetic controlled on diet and chlorpropamide 250 mg daily. She has evidence of diabetic nephropathy with a creatinine of 2.2 mg/dl. Her complaints of joint pain, early morning fatigue and joint stiffness of both hands are diagnosed as rheumatoid arthritis. She is to start on aspirin 3.9 gm daily. Will aspirin therapy affect this patient's diabetic control? Is there an interaction between aspirin and oral sulfonylureas? Discuss the implications of salicylate use in diabetics.

Table 18.

DRUGS WHICH MAY PRODUCE HYPOGLYCEMIA*

Drug	Significance**	Mechanism/Comments	Selected References
Anabolic steroids	+ +	Complex metabolic effects. More significant in diabetics.	***
Beta-adrenergic blockers	+ +	↓ glycogenolysis, ↓ warning signs. See text Question 46.	text
Clofibrate	+	Unclear. May improve glucose tolerance in diabetics.	***
Disopyramide	±	Unclear. Case reports only.	(433)
Ethanol	+ + +	↓ gluconeogenesis. See text Question 54.	(425)
Fenfluramine	+/+ +	↑ peripheral glucose utilization.	(434)
Guanethidine	+	Unclear.	(435)
MAO inhibitors	+ +	Unclear. Can potentiate insulin or sulfonylurea therapy.	***
Oxytetracycline	+	Obscure.	***
Pentamidine	+ +	↑ insulin release via toxic effect.	(432)
Salicylates	+ +	↑ insulin secretion among others. High doses only. See text Question 53.	(421)
Sulfonylureas	+ + +	↑ insulin secretion, insulin receptor effect. See text Question 37.	(279)

*See Table 13 for pharmacokinetic drug interactions enhancing sulfonylurea activity.

** ±—Case reports only or contradictory studies.
+—Possibly important; limited reports or studies; needs substantiation.
+ +—Clinically significant.
+ + +—Clinically significant effect of substantial prevalence and/or magnitude.

***Reviewed with references in Hansten (171).

Hypoglycemic Effects. One of the least appreciated pharmacologic effects of salicylates is their ability to decrease blood glucose. At high doses (about 4–6 gm/day) salicylates can produce at least some degree of blood glucose lowering in both diabetics and nondiabetics (421). The effect may be enhanced in diabetics with elevated blood glucose, and aspirin has even been used in the past as a hypoglycemic agent to replace or allow dosage reductions of insulin or the sulfonylureas (421). In 6 diabetic subjects, 6 gm of aspirin daily caused a decrease in mean fasting blood glucose from 371 mg/dl to 128 mg/dl after 10 days of therapy (422).

A number of studies have demonstrated that salicylates improve glucose tolerance, enhance insulin release in response to glucose, and restore the acute insulin response in Type II diabetics. Salicylates enhance insulin secretion through their effects on prostaglandins and may increase the peripheral uptake of glucose (421,423). The main limitation to further study of salicylates as potential hypoglycemic agents is the high and often toxic doses which are needed to achieve this effect. Salicylate-induced hypoglycemic reactions have been reported in both children and adults in acute poisoning cases. Conversely, hyperglycemia has also occasionally been associated with salicylate toxicity.

Interaction with Sulfonylureas. *In vitro* studies and a few poorly substantiated case reports have suggested that high dose salicylates may also potentiate the hypoglycemic effect of sulfonylureas by a pharmacokinetic interaction (see section on Oral Sulfonylureas).

Antiplatelet Effects. Recently, evidence has accumulated that the progression of diabetic vascular complications and retinopathy in particular may be related to the increased platelet aggregation observed in diabetics. On the basis of this observation, it has been postulated that aspirin or other prostaglandin inhibitors which inhibit platelet aggregation may halt or slow the progression of vascular complications. Although there is only limited clinical evidence for the routine use of these agents at this time, two large multicenter trials are currently investigating this hypothesis (424).

Because M.C. is predisposed to the hypoglycemic effects of salicylates by several mechanisms, she should be initiated on a lower dose or another antirheumatic agent should be considered. Mechanisms for the potential development of hypoglycemia in M.C. include: (a) the intrinsic hypoglycemic effect of aspirin (though the dose is not exceptionally high, concomitant renal impairment may increase serum concentrations); (b) a potential pharmacokinetic drug interaction with a sulfonylurea. Furthermore, one should strongly consider discontinuing chlorpropamide in M.C. in favor of tolbutamide or insulin. See Question 38.

Alcohol

54. C.F., a 22-year-old newly diagnosed insulin dependent diabetic, enjoys a glass or two of wine with her evening meal. Discuss the use and considerations of alcohol consumption in relation to diabetes. What effects does alcohol have on a diabetic patient, particularly a diabetic using insulin? Is alcohol contraindicated in this, or any, diabetic?

Clinicians and diabetics alike tend to be reluctant about permitting the use of alcoholic beverages in the diets of diabetic patients. However, barring contraindications which are similar in the nondiabetic and diabetic alike (eg, hypertriglyceridemia, gastritis, pancreatitis), a diabetic can safely enjoy a moderate alcohol intake as long as she is cognizant of its limitation. For an in-depth discussion, the reader is referred to a comprehensive and practical review of alcohol and diabetes by McDonald (425), part of which is summarized below.

Although excessive and chronic use of alcohol, such as in alcoholics, can produce hyperglycemia and impair glucose tolerance, this is of limited clinical significance outside of this particular population. It should be emphasized, though, that chronic heavy intake of ethanol has been demonstrated to markedly decrease the half-life of tolbutamide, probably through enzyme induction (171). Also, patients receiving chlorpropamide may suffer from the chlorpropamide-alcohol flush reaction (see Questions 30–32).

The vast majority of alcohol-related problems are due to a hypoglycemic effect of ethanol which is primarily caused by a depression of gluconeogenesis. Along with diabetics, the risk of hypoglycemia is increased in normal subjects who are fasting or who otherwise have depleted glycogen stores. Obese individuals are, on the other hand, unusually resistant to the hypoglycemic effects of alcohol. The fasting diabetic is a special hypoglycemic risk when alcohol is ingested. Fortunately, as long as ethanol is consumed with, shortly before, or after a meal (which slows absorption and provides a glucose source), the magnitude of alcohol that must be ingested to produce hypoglycemia is such that moderate amounts of ethanol intake are thought to be quite safe. A moderate amount is considered to be no more than 2 oz of ethanol per day, or two 4 oz glasses of wine. Although this same alcohol intake is associated with increased HDL-cholesterol and a decreased incidence of coronary artery disease in nondiabetics, it is not yet known if diabetics will benefit from this fortuitous association.

The effect of alcohol in diabetics on insulin or sulfonylurea treatment is of greater concern. Ingestion of alcohol is by far the most common cause of profound and lethal hypoglycemic coma in adults and children in the United States (279). The concomitant use of insulin or a sulfonylurea with alcohol greatly increases this risk of hypoglycemic coma in diabetics, especially if they are malnourished, chronic alcoholics. In one report, 5 insulin dependent alcoholics were discovered in severe hypoglycemic coma after binge drinking; 2 patients died and the other 3 suffered irreparable brain damage (426). Other case reports have associated sulfonylurea-alcohol combinations with severe hypoglycemia or coma (279). It should be emphasized that children are particularly sensitive to the hypoglycemic effects of alcohol; this is especially true for diabetic children, who should not receive alcoholic beverages. Also, even small amounts of ethanol may produce intoxication in susceptible individuals. This is especially undesirable in diabetics who must inject themselves with insulin.

Many diabetics also find the nutritional effect of ethanol somewhat confusing. Alcoholic beverages contain mainly ethanol and carbohydrates, both of which contribute to calories. Beverages with high carbohydrate contents, such as sweet dessert wines and liqueurs, should be avoided. Acceptable beverages with low or negligible carbohydrate contents include distilled spirits (whiskey, gin, vodka, rum) and dry table wines. Ethanol provides 7 Cal/gm. The number of calories from a particular non-carbohydrate alcoholic beverage can be determined using the following formula:

$$0.8 \times \text{proof} \times \text{ounces} = \text{Cal.}$$

In summary, alcohol can be included in the diet of diabetics (even those on insulin or oral agents) who understand that mild to moderate intake should not be exceeded and that ingestion in association with meals is least likely to produce hypoglycemia. Special considerations include (a) chronic alcoholics and enzyme-induction of tolbutamide; (b) the chlorpropamide-alcohol flush reaction; and (c) labile diabetics who are prone to hypoglycemia. Even though C.F. fits into the latter category, daily wine with dinner is perfectly acceptable as long as she understands the limitations.

References

1. Karam JH: Diabetes mellitus, hypoglycemia and lipoprotein disorders. In *Current Medical Diagnosis and Treatment 1982,* edited by M A Krupp and M J Chatton, Lange Medical Publications, Los Altos, California, 1982, p 741.
2. Diabetes Mellitus, 8th ed, Waife SO (ed): Lilly Research Laboratories, Indianapolis, Indiana, 1980.
3. Rotter JI et al: Heterogeneity in diabetes mellitus-Update, 1978. Evidence for further genetic heterogeneity within juvenile-onset insulin-dependent diabetes mellitus. Diabetes. 1978; 27:599.
4. Cahill GF et al: Insulin-dependent diabetes mellitus: The initial lesion. N Engl J Med. 1981; 304:1454.
5. Rotter JI et al: The genetics of the glucose intolerance disorders. Am J Med. 1981; 70:116.
6. Skyler JS et al: Diabetes mellitus: Progress and directions. Am J Med. 1981; 70:101.
7. Ginsberg H et al: Effect of insulin therapy on insulin resistance in Type II diabetic subjects. Diabetes. 1981; 30:739.
8. National Diabetes Data Group. Classification and diagnosis of diabetes mellitus and other categories of glucose intolerance. Diabetes. 1979; 28:1039.
9. Tattersal RB et al: A difference between the inheritance of classical juvenile-onset and maturity-onset type diabetes of young people. Diabetes. 1975; 24:44.
10. Barbosa J et al: Plasma glucose, insulin, glucagon and growth hormone in kindreds with maturity-onset type of hyperglycemia in young people. Ann Intern Med. 1978; 88:595.
11. Fajans S et al: Clinical and etiologic heterogeneity of idiopathic diabetes mellitus. Diabetes. 1978; 27:1112.
12. Leslie RDG et al: Chlorpropamide-alcohol flushing: A dominantly inherited trait associated with diabetes. Br Med J. 1978; 2:1519.

13. Pyke DA et al: Chlorpropamide-alcohol flushing: A definition of its relation to non-insulin-dependent diabetes. Br Med J. 1978; 2:1521.
14. Tattersal RB et al: Mild familial diabetes with dominant inheritance. Q J Med. 1974; 43:339.
15. Olefsky JM et al: Mechanisms of insulin resistance in obesity and noninsulin-dependent (Type II) diabetes. Am J Med. 1981; 70:151.
16. Scarlett JA et al: Insulin treatment reverses the insulin resistance of type II diabetes mellitus. Diabetes Care. 1982; 5:353.
17. Skyler J: Editorial: Type II diabetes: Toward improved understanding and rational therapy. Diabetes Care. 1982; 5:447.
18. Genuth SM: Insulin secretion in obesity and diabetes: An illustrative case. Ann Intern Med. 1977; 87:71.
19. Davidson JK et al: Diabetes screening using a quantitative urine glucose method. Diabetes. 1978; 27:810.
20. Bunn HF: Review. Evaluation of glycosylated hemoglobin in diabetic patients. Diabetes. 1981; 30:613.
21. Goldstein DE et al: Clinical application of glycosylated hemoglobin measurements. Diabetes. 1982; 31 (Suppl 3):70.
22. Bolli G et al: Hb A_1 in subjects with abnormal glucose tolerance but normal fasting plasma glucose. Diabetes. 1980; 29:272.
23. Santiago JV et al: Hemoglobin A_{1c} levels in a diabetes detection program. J Clin Endocrinol Metab. 1978; 47:578.
24. Kesson CM et al: Glycosylated hemoglobin in the diagnosis of non-insulin-dependent diabetes mellitus. Diabetes Care. 1982; 5:395.
25. Hoekstra JBL et al: Review. C-Peptide. Diabetes Care. 1982; 5:438.

26. Marks HH et al: Onset, course, prognosis, and mortality in diabetes mellitus. In *Joslin's Diabetes Mellitus, 11th Edition,* edited by A Marble et al, eds. Lea & Febiger, Philadelphia 1971, p 209.

27. Pirart J: Diabetes mellitus and its degenerative complications: A prospective study of 4,400 patients observed between 1947 and 1973. Diabetes Care. 1978; 1:168 and 252.

28. Skyler JS: "Control" and diabetic complications. Diabetes Care. 1978; 1:204.

29. Anon: Prolonged disease-free survival in diabetics. Br Med J. 1981; 282:1339.

30. Oakly WG et al: Long-term diabetes: A clinical study of 92 patients after 40 years. Q J Med. 1974; 43:145.

31. Winegrad AI et al: The complications of diabetes mellitus. N Engl J Med. 1978; 298:1250.

32. Williamson JR et al: Vascular complications of diabetes mellitus. N Engl J Med. 1980; 302:399.

33. Colwell JA et al: Pathogenesis of atherosclerosis in diabetes mellitus. Diabetes Care. 1981; 4:121.

34. Knowles HC et al: The course of juvenile diabetes treated with unmeasured diet. Diabetes. 1965; 14:239.

35. Garcia MJ et al: Morbidity and mortality in diabetes in the Framingham population. Six year follow-up. Diabetes. 1974; 23:105.

36. Steiner G: Diabetes and atherosclerosis—An overview. Diabetes. 1981; 30 (suppl 2):1.

37. Palmberg PF: Diabetic retinopathy. Diabetes. 1977; 26:703.

38. Morse PH et al: Ophthalmologic management of diabetic retinopathy. N Engl J Med. 1976; 295:87.

39. Rand L: Recent advances in diabetic retinopathy. Am J Med. 1981; 70:595.

40. Diabetic Retinopathy Study Research Group: Photocoagulation treatment of proliferative diabetic retinopathy. The second report of Diabetic Retinopathy Study finding. Ophthalmology. 1978; 85:82.

41. Knowler WC et al: Increased incidence of retinopathy in diabetes with elevated blood pressure. N Engl J Med. 1980; 302:645.

42. Bodansky HJ et al: Risk factors associated with severe proliferative retinopathy in insulin-dependent diabetes mellitus. Diabetes Care. 1982; 5:97.

43. Mauer S et al: The kidney in diabetes. Am J Med. 1981; 70:603.

44. Paz-Guevara AT et al: Juvenile diabetes mellitus after forty years. Diabetes. 1975; 24:559.

45. Goetz FD et al: The treatment of diabetic kidney disease. Diabetologia. 1970; 17:267.

46. Clements RS: Review. Diabetic neuropathy—New concepts of its etiology. Diabetes. 1979; 28:604.

47. Hilsted J: Review: Pathophysiology in diabetic autonomic neuropathy: Cardiovascular, hormonal, and metabolic studies. Diabetes. 1982; 31:730.

48. American Diabetes Association: Principles of nutrition and dietary recommendations for individuals with diabetes mellitus:1979. Diabetes Care. 1979; 2:520.

49. American Diabetes Association: Policy statement: Saccharin. Diabetes Care. 1979; 2:380.

50. Olefsky JM et al: Fructose, xylitol and sorbitol. Diabetes Care. 1980; 3:390.

51. Anderson JW et al: Fiber and diabetes. Diabetes Care. 1979; 2:369.

52. McDonald J: Alcohol and diabetes. Diabetes Care. 1980; 3:629.

53. Skyler JS: Diabetes and exercise: Clinical implications. Diabetes Care. 1979; 2:307.

54. Richter EA et al: Diabetes and exercise. Am J Med. 1981; 70:201.

55. Malone JI et al: The role of urine sugar in diabetic management. Am J Dis Child. 1976; 130:1324.

56. Tattersall R et al: Patient self-monitoring of blood glucose and refinements of conventional insulin treatment. Am J Med 1981; 70:177.

57. McCarter D et al: Self-monitoring of blood glucose by diabetic patients. Calif Pharmacy. 1982; 29:22.

58. Ohlsen P et al: Discrepancies between glycosuria and home estimate of blood glucose in insulin-treated diabetes mellitus. Diabetes Care. 1980; 3:178.

59. James RC et al: Evaluation of some commonly used semiquantitative methods for urinary glucose and ketone determinations. Diabetes. 1974; 23:474.

60. Kohler E: On materials for testing glucose in the urine. Diabetes Care. 1978; 1:64.

61. Leonards JR: Evaluation of enzyme tests for urinary glucose. JAMA. 1957; 163:260.

62. Christiansen C et al: Home blood glucose monitoring: Benefits for the patient and educator. Diabetes Educator. 1980; 6:13.

63. Galloway JA et al: Factors influencing the absorption, serum insulin concentration, and blood glucose responses after injections of regular insulin and various insulin mixtures. Diabetes Care. 1981; 4:367.

64. Bressler R: Insulin Therapy. In *Management of Diabetes Mellitus,* edited by R Bressler and DG Johnson, John Wright-PSG Inc, Boston, 1982, p 51–89.

65. Podolsky S et al: Treatment of diabetes with insulin. In *Clinical Diabetes: Modern Management,* edited by S Podolsky, Appleton-Century-Crofts, New York 1980, p 91.

66. Deckert T: Intermediate-acting insulin preparations: NPH and lente. Diabetes Care. 1980; 3:623.

67. Hallas-Moller K: The lente insulins. Diabetes. 1956; 5:7.

68. Berson SA et at: Insulin I^{131} metabolism in human subjects: Demonstration of insulin binding globulin in circulation of insulin treated subjects. J Clin Invest. 1956; 35:170.

69. Bolinger RE et al: Disappearance of I^{131}-labeled insulin from plasma as a guide to management of diabetes. N Engl J Med. 1964; 270:767.

70. Faulk WP et al: Human anti-insulin antibodies. J Immnunol. 1971; 106:1112.

71. Root MA et al: Immunogenicity of insulin. Diabetes. 1972; 21(Suppl 2):657.

72. Tantillo JJ et al: Immunogenicity of "single peak" beef-pork insulin in diabetic subjects. Diabetes. 1974; 23:276.

73. Feldman R et al: Immunologic studies in a diabetic subject resistant to bovine insulin but sensitive to porcine insulin. Am J Med. 1963; 35:411.

74. Galloway JA: The complications of insulin therapy. In *Management of Diabetes Mellitus,* edited by R Bressler and DG Johnson, John Wright-PSG Inc, 1982, p 91–114.

75. Davidson JK et al: Immunologic insulin resistance. Diabetes. 1978; 27:307.

76. Yalow R et al: Reaction of fish insulins with human insulin antiserums. N Engl J Med. 1964; 270:1171.

77. Burrill K et al: The use of fish (bonito) insulin: A simple test to evaluate the role of insulin antibodies in insulin resistance. Diabetes 1971; 20:344.

78. Shore PN et al: Chronic urticaria from isophane insulin therapy. Arch Dermatol. 1975; 111:94.

79. Caplan SN et al: Protamine sulfate and fish allergy (letter). N Engl J Med. 1976; 295:172.

80. Galloway JA: Insulin treatment for the early 80s: Facts and questions about old and new insulins and their usage. Diabetes Care. 1980; 3:615.

81. Galloway JA et al: Insulin treatment in diabetes. Med Clin North Am. 1978; 62:663.

82. Skyler JS et al: Biosynthetic human insulin: Progress and prospects. Diabetes Care. 1981; 4:140.

83. De Meyts P et al: In vitro studies on biosynthetic human insulin: an overview. Diabetes Care. 1981; 4:144.

84. Gerich JE: An appraisal of the role of biosynthetic human insulin in the future treatment of diabetes mellitus. Diabetes Care. 1981; 4:262.

85. Storvick W et al: Effect of storage temperature on stability of commercial insulin preparations. Diabetes. 1968; 17:499.

86. Galloway JA et al: A comparison of acid regular and neutral regular insulin. Diabetes 1973; 22:471.

87. Kaplan SA et al: Diabetes mellitus. Ann Intern Med. 1982; 96:635.

88. Brownlee M et al: Diabetic control and vascular complications. In *Atherosclerosis Reviews,* edited by R Paoletti and AM Gotto Jr, Raven Press, New York 1979, p 29.

89. Skyler JS et al: Algorithms for adjustment of insulin dosage by patients who monitor blood glucose. Diabetes Care. 1981; 4:311.

90. Jovanovic L et al: Current concepts in insulin delivery. Drug Therapy (Hosp). 1980; Feb:9.

91. Skyler JS et al: Optimizing pumped insulin delivery. Diabetes Care. 1982; 5:135.

92. Unger RH: Meticulous control of diabetes: Benefits, risks, and precautions. Diabetes. 1982; 31:479.

93. Centers for Disease Control: Deaths among patients using continuous subcutaneous insulin infusion pumps. Morbidity & Mortality Weekly Report. 1982; No.31:80.

94. Santiago JV: Improved metabolic control in diabetes: New tools and old techniques revisited. Diabetes Care. 1979; 2:312.

95. American Diabetes Association: Indications for use of continuous insulin delivery systems and self-measurements of blood glucose. Diabetes Care. 1982; 5:140.

96. Pietri A et al: Cutaneous complications of chronic continuous subcutaneous insulin infusion therapy. Diabetes Care. 1981; 4:624.

97. Levandoski LA et al: Localized skin reactions to insulin: Insulin lipodystrophies and skin reactions to pumped subcutaneous insulin therapy. Diabetes Care. 1982; 5(Suppl 1):6.

98. Marliss EB et al: Present and future expectations regarding insulin infusion systems. Diabetes Care. 1981; 4:325.

99. Nelson JD et al: Role of continuous component in subcutaneous "open-loop" insulin delivery. Lancet. 1980; 1:1383.

100. Rizza RA et at: Control of blood sugar in insulin-dependent diabetes: Comparison of an artificial endocrine pancreas, continuous subcutaneous insulin infusion, and intensified conventional insulin therapy. N Engl J Med. 1980; 303:1313.

101. Lambert AE et al: Use of an artificial pancreas as a tool to determine subcutaneous insulin doses in juvenile diabetes. Diabetes Care. 1979; 2:256.

102. Donaldson JB: Current concepts in the treatment of diabetes mellitus. Med Clin N Am. 1965; 49:1349.

103. Feinglos MN et al: "Insulin" allergy due to zinc. Lancet. 1979; 1:122.

104. Berger M et al: Absorption kinetics and biologic effects of subcutaneously injected insulin preparations. Diabetes Care. 1982; 5:77.

105. Skyler JS et al: A comparison of insulin regimens in insulin-dependent diabetes mellitus. Diabetes Care. 1982; 5(Suppl 1):11.

106. Campbell RK: Diabetes care products. In *Handbook of Nonprescription Drugs, 6th ed,* American Pharmaceutical Association, Washington DC 1979, p 175.

107. Caswell M et al: Disposable insulin syringe preference of children and youth. Diabetes Care. 1978; 5:330.

108. Crouch M et al: Reuse of disposable syringe-needle units in the diabetic patient. Diabetes Care. 1979; 2:418.

109. Greenough A et al: Disposable syringes for insulin injection. Br Med J. 1979; 2:1467.

110. Koivisto VA et al: Alterations in insulin absorption and in blood glucose control associated with varying insulin injection sites in diabetic patients. Ann Intern Med. 1980; 92:59.

111. Davidson MB: The case for routinely testing the first-voided urine specimen. Diabetes Care. 1981; 4:443.

112. Paysinger AL et al: Accuracy of copper-reduction and glucose-oxidase tests for various glucose concentrations. Am J Hosp Pharm. 1981; 38:1493.

113. Kolendorf K et al: Absorption, effectiveness and side effects of highly purified porcine NPH-insulin preparation (Leo). Eur J Clin Pharmacol. 1978; 14:117.

114. Lilly Research Laboratories, Personal Communication with Dr. SM Chernish, Clinical Investigation Division, Feb 11, 1982 and June 9, 1982.

115. Kubilis P et al: Stability of reacted reagent strips (Chemstrips) for blood glucose determinations. Diabetes Care. 1981; 4:412.

116. Shapiro B et al: A comparison of accuracy and estimated cost of methods for home blood glucose monitoring. Diabetes Care. 1981; 4:396.

117. Clements Jr RS et al: Comparison of various methods for rapid glucose estimation. Diabetes Care. 1981; 4:392.

118. Kubilis P et al: Comparison of blood glucose testing using reagent strips with and without a meter (Chemstrips bG and Dextrostix/Dextrometer). Diabetes Care. 1981; 4:417.

119. McCarter D et al: Self-monitoring of blood glucose by diabetic patients. Calif Pharmacist. 1982; 29:22.

120. Reeves ML et al: Comparison of methods for blood glucose monitoring. Diabetes Care. 1981; 4:404.

121. Birch K et al: Self-monitoring of blood glucose without a meter. Diabetes Care. 1981; 4:414.

122. Skyler JS et al: Algorithms for adjustment of insulin dosage by patients who monitor blood glucose. Diabetes Care. 1981; 4:311.

123. Davidson MB: *Diabetes Mellitus: Diagnosis and Treatment. Vol 1.* John Wiley and Sons, New York, 1982.

124. Bressler R et al: Insulin treatment of diabetes mellitus. Med Clin North Am. 1971; 55:861.

125. Fabrykant M et al: Nature and prevention of local skin lesions from insulin administration. Metab. 1954; 3:1.

126. Schmidt MI et al: The dawn phenomenon, an early morning glucose rise: Implications for diabetic intraday blood glucose variation. Diabetes Care. 1981; 4:579.

127. Watson BM et al: A treatment for insulin induced atrophy. Diabetes. 1971; 20:628.

128. Teuscher A: Treatment of insulin lipoatrophy with monocomponent insulin. Diabetologia. 1974; 10:211.

129. Wentworth SM et al: The use of purified insulins in the treatment of patients with insulin lipoatrophy. Diabetes. 1973; 22(Suppl 1):290.

130. Kumar D et al: Use of dexamethasone in treatment of insulin atrophy. Diabetes. 1977; 26:296.

131. Yue DK et al: New forms of insulin and their use in the treatment of diabetes. Diabetes. 1977; 26:341.

132. Wright AD et al: Very pure porcine insulin in clinical practice. Br Med J. 1979; 1:25.

133. Deckert T et al: The clinical significance of highly purified pig-insulin preparations. Diabetologia. 1974; 10:703.

134. Andreani D et al: Comparative trials with monocomponent (MC) and monospecies (MS) pork insulins in the treatment of diabetes mellitus. Horm Metab Res. 1974; 6:447.

135. Oakley NW: Effect of "fractionated" insulins on total plasma insulin binding capacity and insulin requirements in severe diabetes. Lancet. 1976; 1:994.

136. Evans DR et al: Hazards of monocomponent insulins (letter). Br Med J. 1976; 1:1146.

137. Asplin CM et al: Change of insulin dosage, circulating free and bound insulin and insulin antibodies on transferring diabetics from conventional to highly purified procine insulin. Diabetologia. 1978; 14:99.

138. Griffin NK et al: Reduction of insulin dose on changing diabetic children fron standard to monocomponent insulins. Arch Dis Child. 1979; 54:123.

139. Gray RS et al: Diabetic control in patients treated with once or twice-daily insulin injections, including a comparison of conventional beef and highly purified pork insulins. Diabetologia. 1981; 21:206.

140. Klaff LJ et al: Circulating antibodies in diabetics treated with conventional and purified insulins. South Afr. Med J. 1978; July 22:149.

141. Wentworth SM: Insulin dose change with increased purity (letter) Diabetes Care. 1981; 4:504.

142. Kahn CR et al: Immunologic reactions to insulin: Insulin allergy, insulin resistance, and the autoimmune insulin syndrome. Diabetes Care. 1979; 2:283.

143. Paulsen EP et al: Insulin resistance caused by massive degradation of subcutaneous insulin. Diabetes. 1979; 28:640.

144. Davidson JK et al: Immunologic insulin resistance. Diabetes. 1978; 27:307.

145. Barrett JC et al: Tolbutamide in the therapy of insulin resistance. Diabetes. 1962; 2(Suppl):35.

146. Karam JH et al: Insulin resistant diabetics with autoantibodies induced by exogenous insulin. Diabetes. 1969; 18:445.

147. Rabkin R et al: Effect of renal disease on renal uptake and excretion of insulin. N Engl J Med. 1970; 282:182.

148. Rubenstein AH et al: Role of the kidney in insulin metabolism and excretion. Diabetes. 1968; 17:161.

149. Amico JA et al: Diabetic managment in patients with renal failure. Diabetes Care. 1981; 4:430.

150. Caron D et al: the effect of postprandial exercise on meal-related glucose intolerance in insulin-dependent diabetic individuals. Diabetes Care. 1982; 5:364.

151. Koivisto VA et al: Effect of leg exercise of insulin absorption in diabetic patients. N Engl J Med. 1978; 1:479.

152. Kemmer FW et al: Exercise-induced fall of blood glucose unrelated to alteration of insulin mobilization. Diabetes. 1980; 28:1131.

153. Duckworth WC et al: Effect of chronic sulfonylurea therapy on plasma insulin and proinsulin levels. J Clin Endocrinol. 1972; 35:585.

154. Reaven G et al: Effect of chlorpropamide on serum glucose and immunoreactive insulin concentrations in patients with maturity-onset diabetes mellitus. Diabetes. 1967; 16:487.

155. Madsen J: Extrapancreatic and intrapancreatic action of antidiabetic sulfonylureas. A review. Acta Med Scand. 1967; 476(Suppl):109.

156. Feinglos MN et al: Sulfonylureas increase the number of insulin receptors. Nature. 1978; 276:184.

157. Prince MJ et al: Direct in vitro effect of a sulfonylurea to increase human fibroblast insulin receptors. J Clin Invest. 1980; 66:608.

158. Anonymous: Phenformin: Removal fron the general market. FDA Drug Bull. Aug 1977; 7:14.

159. Anonymous: Status of withdrawal of phenformin. FDA Drug Bull. Sept-Oct 1977; 7:19.

160. Skillman TG et al: The pharmacology of sulfonylureas. Am J Med. 1981; 70:361.

161. Brown KF et al: Displacement of tolbutamide, glibenclamide, and chlorpropamide from serum albumin by anionic drugs. Biochem Pharmacol. 1976; 25:1175.

162. Jackson JE et al: Clinical pharmacology of sulfonylurea hypoglycemic agents: part 1. Drugs. 1981; 22:211.

163. Balant L: Clinical pharmacokinetics of sulphonylurea hypoglycemic drugs. Clin Pharmacokin. 1981; 6:215.

164. Thomas RC et al: The metabolic fate of tolbutamide in man and in the rat. J Med Chem. 1966; 9:507.

165. Scott J et al: Pharmacogenetics of tolbutamide metabolism in humans. Diabetes. 1979; 28:41.

166. Taylor JA: Pharmacokinetics and biotransformation of chlorpropamide in man. Clin Pharmacol Ther. 1972; 13:710.

167. Campbell RK: Metabolism of chlorpropamide. Diabetes Care. 1981; 4:332.

168. Sartor G et al: Comparative single-dose kinetics and effects of four sulfonylureas in healthy volunteers. Acta Med Scand. 1980; 208:301.

169. Balant L et al: Behaviour of glibenclamide on repeated administration to diabetic patients. Eur J Clin Pharmacol. 1977; 11:19.

170. Sartor G et al: Effects of glipizide and food intake on the blood levels of glucose and insulin in diabetic patients. Acta Med Scand. 1978; 203:211.

171. Hansten PD: *Drug Interactions*, 4th ed. Lea and Febiger, Philadelphia 1979.

172. Jackson JE et al: Clinical pharmacology of sulfonyl-urea hypoglycemic agents: part 2. Drugs. 1981; 22:295.

173. Christensen LK et al: Inhibition of drug metabolism by chloramphenicol. Lancet. 1969; 2:1397.

174. Brunova E: Interaction of tolbutamide and chloramphenicol in diabetic patients. Int J Clin Pharmacol. 1977; 15:7.

175. Petitpierre B et al; Chlorpropamide and chloramphenicol (letter). Lancet. 1970; 1:789.

176. Daubresse JC et al: Potentiation of hypoglycemic effect of sulfonylureas by clofibrate (letter). N Engl J Med. 1976; 294:613.

177. Ferrari C et al: Potentiation of hypoglycemic response to intravenous tolbutamide by clofibrate (letter). N Engl J Med. 1976; 294:1184.

178. Skovsted L et al: The effect of different oral anticoagulants on diphenylhydantoin (DPH) and tolbutamide metabolism. Acta Med Scand. 1976; 199:513.

179. Kirstensen M et al: Accumulation of chlorpropamide caused by dicoumarol. Acta Med Scand. 1968; 183:83.

180. Pond SM et al: Mechanisms of inhibition of tolbutamide metabolism: phenylbutazone, oxyphenbutazone, sulphenzole. Clin Pharmacol Ther. 1977; 22:573.

181. Field JB et al: Potentiation of acetohexamide hypoglycemia by phenylbutazone. N Engl J Med. 1967; 277:889.

182. Judis J: Binding of sulfonylureas to serum proteins. J Pharm Sci. 1972; 61:89.

183. Stowers JM et al: A clinical and pharmacological comparison of chlorpropamide and other sulfonylureas. Ann N Y Acad Sci. 1959; 74:689.

184. Peaston MJT et al: A case of combined poisoning with chlorpropamide, acetylsalicylic acid, and paracetamol. Br J Clin Pract. 1968; 22:30.

185. Cherner R et al: Prolonged tolbutamide-induced hypoglycemia. JAMA. 1963; 185:883.

186. Christensen LK et al: Sulphaphenazole-induced hypoglycemic attacks in tolbutamide-treated diabetics. Lancet. 1963; 2:1298.

187. Dall JLC: Hypoglycemia due to chlorpropamide. Scott Med J. 1967; 12:403.

188. Lumholtz B et al: Sulfamethizole-induced inhibition of diphenylhydantoin, tolbutamide, and warfarin metabolism. Clin Pharmacol Ther. 1975; 17:731.

189. Tucker HStG, Jr., et al: Sulfonamide-sulfonylurea interaction (letter). N Engl Med J. 1972; 286:110.

190. Soeldner JS: Hypoglycemia in tolbutamide-treated diabetes. JAMA. 1965; 193:148.

191. Feldman JM et al: Tests for glucosuria: An analysis of factors that cause misleading results. Diabetes. 1973; 22:115.

192. Feldman JM et al: Inhibition of glucose oxidase paper tests by reducing metabolites. Diabetes. 1970; 19:337.

193. Mayson JS et al: False negative tests for urinary glucose in the presence of ascorbic acid. Am J Clin Pathol. 1972; 58:297.

194. Brandt R et al: Urinary glucose and Vitamin C. Am J Clin Pathol. 1977; 68:592.

195. Smith D et al: Effect of large-dose ascorbic acid on the two-drop clinitest determination. Am J Hosp Pharm. 1977; 34:1347.

196. Nahata MC et al: Noneffect of oral ascorbic acid on urinary copper reduction glucose test. Diabetes Care. 1978; 1:34.

197. Nahata MC et al: Lack of effect of ascorbic acid, hippuric acid, and methenamine (urinary formaldehyde) on the copper-reduction glucose test in geriatric patients. J Am Geriatr Soc. 1980; 28:230.

198. Bowers C et al: Noneffect of methyldopa on urine glucose tests. Diabetes Care. 1978; 1:36.

199. Ives TJ et al: Effect of methyldopa on urine glucose test methods. Am J Hosp Pharm. 1980; 37:683.

200. MacCara ME et al: In vitro effect of penicillins and aminoglycosides on commonly used tests for glycosuria. Am J Hosp Pharm. 1981; 38:1340.

201. MacCara ME et al: Cephalosporin-Clinitest interaction: comparison of cephalothin, cefazolin, and cephradine. Am J Hosp Pharm. 1978; 35:1064.

202. Self TH et al: Noneffect of isoniazid on urine glucose tests. Diabetes Care. 1980; 3:44.

203. Klumpp TG: Nalidixic acid . . . false positive glycosuria and hyperglycemia (letter). JAMA. 1965; 193:746.

204. Wester VL et al: Noneffect of oral tetracycline on urine glucose determination by the copper reduction method. Diabetes Care. 1980; 3:567.

205. Naumann HN: Prevention of pyridium interference in urinalysis by dithionite reduction or butanol extraction. Am J Clin Pathol. 1967; 48:337.

206. Davidson MB: *Diabetes Mellitus: Diagnosis and Treatment*. Vol 2. John Wiley and Sons, New York 1982.

207. Singer DL et al: Long-term experience with sulfonylureas and placebo. N Engl J Med. 1967; 277:450.

208. Jackson JE et al: Clinical pharmacology of sulfonylurea hypoglycemic agents: Part 1. Drugs. 1981; 22:211.

209. Balodimos MC et al: Nine years' experience with tolbutamide in the treatment of diabetes. Metab. 1966; 15:957.

210. Seltzer HS: Efficacy and safety of oral hypoglycemic agents. Annual Review Med. 1980; 31:261.

211. Boyden et al: Oral hypoglycemic agents. Adv Intern Med. 1979; 24:53.

212. Balodimos MC et al: Tolazamide in the treatment of diabetes mellitus: Clinical experience and review of the literature. Curr Ther Res. 1971; 13:6.

213. Cervantes-Amezeula A et al: Long term use of chlorpropamide in diabetes. JAMA. 1965; 193:759.

214. Balodimos MC et al: Acetohexamide therapy of diabetes mellitus. Metab. 1968; 17:669.

215. Jackson JE et al: Clinical pharmacology of sulfonylurea hypoglycemic agents: Part 2. Drugs. 1981; 22:295.

216. Powell T et al: Diabetes mellitus treated with chlorpropamide and tolbutamide. Diabetes. 1966; 15:269.

217. Skinner NS Jr et al: Studies on the use of chlorpropamide in patients with diabetes mellitus. Ann NY Acad Sci. 1959; 74:830.

218. Baker H: Drug reactions X: Adverse cutaneous reactions to oral hypoglycemic agents. Br J Derm. 1970; 82:634.

219. Dowling HF et al: Toxic reactions accompanying second courses of sulfonamides in patients developing toxic reactions during a previous course. Ann Intern Med. 1946; 24:629.

220. Bressler R et al: Evaluation of tolazamide in the treatment of diabetes mellitus. Curr Ther Res. 1965; 7:219.

221. Hamff H et al: Effects of tolbutamide and chlorpropamide on patients exhibiting jaundice as a result of chlorpropamide therapy. Ann NY Acad Sci. 1959; 74:820.

222. FitzGerald MG et al: Alcohol sensitivity in diabetics receiving chlorpropamide. Diabetes. 1962; 11:40.

223. Anon: Alcohol sensitivity to sulphonylureas. Br Med J. 1964; 3:586.

224. Capretti L et al: Chlorpropamide- and tolbutamide-alcohol flushing in non-insulin-dependent diabetes. Br Med J. 1981; 283:1361.

225. Dolgar H: Experience with the tolbutamide treatment of five hundred cases of diabetes on an ambulatory basis. Ann N Y Acad Sci. 1957; 71:275.

226. Micossi P: The prevalence of chlorpropamide alcohol flushing in non-insulin dependent diabetics (letter). Diabetologia. 1981; 20:510.

227. Wilkin JK: Flushing reactions: Consequences and mechanisms. Ann Intern Med. 1981; 95:468.

228. Asaad MM et al: Studies on the biochemical aspects of the "disulfiram-like" reaction induced by oral hypoglycemics. Eur J Pharmacol. 1976; 35:301.

229. Jerntorp P et al: Increase of plasma acetaldehyde: An objective indicator of the chlorpropamide alcohol flush. Diabetes. 1981; 30:788.

230. Barnett AH et al: Blood concentrations of acetaldehyde during chlorpropamide-alcohol flush. Br Med J. 1981; 283:939.

231. Leslie RDG et al: Sensitivity to enkephalin as a cause of non-insulin dependent diabetes. Lancet. 1979; 1:341.

232. Medbak S et al: Chlorpropamide alcohol flush and circulating met-enkephalin: A positive link. Br Med J. 1981; 283:937.

233. Lightman SL et al: Alterations in the activities of endogenous opiates by a metabolite of alcohol. J Endocrinol. 1980; 87:38P.

234. Strakosch CR et al: Blockade of chlorpropamide alcohol flush by aspirin. Lancet. 1980; 1:394.

235. Barnett AH et al: Blockade of chlorpropamide-alcohol flushing by indomethacin suggests an association between prostaglandins and diabetic vascular complications. Lancet. 1980; 2:164.

236. Köbberling J et al: The chlorpropamide alcohol flush. Lack of specificity for familial non-insulin dependent diabetes. Diabetologia. 1980; 19:359.

237. DeSilva NE et al: Low incidence of chlorpropamide-alcohol flushing in diet-treated, non-insulin-dependent diabetes. Lancet. 1981; 1:128.

238. Rodder JK et al: Facial skin temperature and the chlorpropamide/alcohol flush in diabetics (letter). Lancet. 1980; 2:1037.

239. Jefferys DB et al: Chlorpropamide alcohol flush (letter). Lancet. 1981; 1:440.

240. Jerntorp P et al: Is the blood chlorpropamide concentration critical in chlorpropamide alcohol flush? (letter) Lancet. 1981; 1:165.

241. Leslie RDG et al: Chlorpropamide alcohol flushing and diabetic retinopathy. Lancet. 1979; 1:997.

242. Barnett AH et al: Chlorpropamide-alcohol flushing and large-vessel disease in non-insulin-dependent diabetes. Br Med J. 1980; 281:261.

243. Harris M et al: Chlorpropamide alcohol flushing and diabetes. Diabetologia. 1981; 21:422.

244. Baird WR et al: Cholestatic jaundice from tolbutamide. Ann Intern Med. 1960; 53:194.

245. Camerini-Davelos R et al: Clinical experiences with tolbutamide. Five years' experience with tolbutamide. Diabetes. 1962; 11(Suppl):74.

246. Haunz EA et al: Liver function in chlorpropamide therapy. JAMA. 1964; 188:237.

247. Reichel J et al: Intrahepatic stasis following administration of chlorpropamide. Am J Med. 1960; 38:654.

248. Gregory DH et al: Chronic cholestasis following prolonged tolbutamide administration. Arch Path. 1967; 84:194.

249. Duncan TG et al: The comparative clinical effectiveness of tolbutamide and acetohexamide. Metab. 1968; 17:218.

250. Goldstein MJ et al: Jaundice in a patient receiving acetohexamide. N Engl J Med. 1966; 275:97.

251. Collens WS et al: Cholestatic jaundice following use of sulfonylurea drugs. NY State J Med. 1965; 65:907.

252. McGavack TH et al: Some clinical experiences with the arylsulfonylureas in the management of diabetes mellitus. Metab. 1953; 5:919.

253. Portioli I et al: Sulfonylureas and hypothyroidism (letter). Lancet. 1969; 1:681.

254. Hunton RB et al: Hypothyroidism in diabetics treated with sulfonylureas. Lancet. 1965; 2:449.

255. Hershman JM et al: Effect of sulfonylurea drugs on the binding of tri-iodothyronine and thyroxine to thyronine binding globulin. J Clin Endocrin Metab. 1968; 28:1605.

256. Burke G et al: Effect of long term sulfonylurea therapy on thyroid treatment in man. Metab. 1967; 16:651.

257. Burda CD: Sulfonylurea hypothyroidism in diabetics. Lancet. 1965; 2:1016.

258. Roberts HJ: Diabetogenic hyperinsulinism: pathogenesis and implications of sulfonylurea induced hypothyroidism. J Am Geriat Soc. 1967; 15:674.

259. Scharf J et al: Tolbutamide and hypothyroidism. Lancet. 1968; 1:250.

260. Schless GL et al: Oral hypoglycemic therapy associated with hypothyroidism. Ann NY Acad Sci. 1968; 148:813.

261. Hamwi GJ et al: The effects of chlorpropamide on endocrine function in patients with diabetes mellitus and its effects in other endocrine disorders. Ann NY Acad Sci. 1959; 74:820.

262. Hagan GA et al: Hyponatremia due to sulfonylurea compounds. J Clin Endocrin Metab. 1970; 31:570.

263. Early LE: Chlorpropamide antidiuresis. N Engl J Med. 1971; 284:103.

264. Fine D et al: Hyponatremia due to chlorpropamide. Ann Intern Med. 1970; 72:83.

265. Weismann PN: Chlorpropamide hyponatremia. N Engl J Med. 1971; 284:65.

266. Garcia M et al: Chlorpropamide-induced water retention in patients with diabetes mellitus. Ann Intern Med. 1971; 75:549.

267. Moses AM et al: Diuretic action of three sulfonylurea drugs. Ann Intern Med. 1973; 78:541.

268. Klimt Cr et al: The University Group Diabetes Program. A study of the effect of hypoglycemic agents on vascular complications in patients with adult-onset diabetes. 1. Design, methods and baseline characteristics. II. Mortality results. Diabetes. 1970; 19(Suppl 2):474.

269. University Group Diabetes Program. Effects of hypoglycemic agents on vascular complications in patients with adult-onset diabetes. III. Clinical implications of UGDP results. JAMA. 1971; 218:1400.

270. Knatterud GD et al: Effects of hypoglycemic agents on vascular complications in patients with adult-onset diabetes. V. Evaluation of phenformin therapy. Diabetes. 1975; 24(Suppl 1):65.

271. Knatterud GL et al: University Group Diabetes Program. Effects of hypoglycemic agents on vascular complications in patients with adult-onset diabetes. VII. Mortality and selected non-fatal events with insulin treatment. JAMA. 1978; 240:37.

272. Seltzer HS: A summary of criticisms of the findings and conclusions of the University Group Diabetes Program (UGDP). Diabetes. 1972; 21:976.

273. Prout TE et al: The UGDP controversy: Clinical trials versus clinical impressions. Diabetes. 1972; 21:1035.

274. Boyden TW: The oral hypoglycemic agents. In *Management of Diabetes Mellitus*, edited by R Bressler and DG Johnson, John Wright PSC Inc, Boston, 1982, p 115.

275. Report of the Committee for the Assessment of Biometric Aspects of Controlled Trials of Hypoglycemic Agents. JAMA. 1975; 231:583.

276. Food and Drug Administration (FDA) analysis of UGDP study. Fed Reg. Nov 14 1978; 48(220):52732.

277. American Diabetes Association. Policy Statement: Treatment of diabetes. Diabetes. 1970; 19:527.

278. American Diabetes Association. Policy Statement: The UGDP controversy. Diabetes. 1979; 28:168.

279. Seltzer HS: Severe drug-induced hypoglycemia: A review. Comprehensive Ther. 1979; 5(4):21.

280. Ueda H et al: Disappearance rate of tolbutamide in normal subjects and in diabetes mellitus, liver cirrhosis, and renal disease. Diabetes. 1963; 12:414.

281. Gulati PD et al: A double blind trial of tolbutamide in cirrhosis of the liver. Am J Dig Dis. 1967; 12:42.

282. Kocher R: The use of psychotropic drugs in the treatment of chronic, severe pains. Eur Neurol. 1976; 14:458.

283. Shimm DS et al: Medical management of chronic cancer pain. JAMA. 1979; 241:2408.

284. Davis JL et al: Peripheral diabetic neuropathy treated with amitriptyline and fluphenazine. JAMA. 1977; 238:2291.

285. Gade GN et al: Diabetic neuropathic cachexia. Beneficial response to combination therapy with amitriptyline and fluphenazine. JAMA. 1980; 243:1160.

286. Turkington RW: Depression masquerading as diabetic neuropathy. JAMA. 1980; 243:1147.

287. Romain LF: Treatment of peripheral diabetic neuropathy (letter). JAMA. 1978; 239:1037.

288. Battla H et al: Clinical trial of amitriptyline and fluphenazine in diabetic peripheral neuropathy. Southern Med J. 1981; 74:417.

289. Wilton TD: Diabetic neuropathy (letter). South Afr Med J. 1972; 46:1757.

290. Chakrabarti AK et al: Diabetic peripheral neuropathy: Nerve conduction studies before, during and after carbamazepine therapy. Aust N Z J Med. 1976; 6:565.

291. Badran AM et al: A clinical trial of carbamazepine in the symptomatic treatment of diabetic peripheral neuropathy. J Egypt Med Assoc. 1975; 58:627.

292. Rull JA et al: Symptomatic treatment of peripheral diabetic neuropathy with carbamazepine (Tegretol): Double blind crossover trial. Diabetologia. 1969; 5:215.

293. Wilton TD: Tegretol in the treatment of diabetic neuropathy. South Afr Med J. 1974; 48:869.

294. Ellenberg M: Treatment of diabetic neuropathy with diphenylhydantoin. N Y State J Med. 1968; 68:2653.

295. Chadda VS et al: Double blind study of the effects of diphenylhydantoin sodium on diabetic neuropathy. J Assoc Phys Ind. 1978; 26:403.

296. Saudek CD et al: Phenytoin in the treatment of diabetic symmetrical polyneuropathy. Clin Pharmacol Ther. 1977; 22:196.

297. Gonzalez ER: Medical News: Can aldose reductase inhibition ameliorate diabetic neuropathy? JAMA. 1981; 246:1169.

298. Culebras A et al: Effect of an aldose reductase inhibitor on diabetic peripheral neuropathy: preliminary report. Arch Neurol. 1981; 38:133.

299. Collens WS et al: The treatment of peripheral neuropathy in diabetes mellitus. Am J Med Sci. 1950; 219:482.

300. Berenyi MR et al: Treatment of diabetic neuropathy with clofibrate. J Am Geriatr Soc. 1971; 19:763.

301. Sachse G et al: Efficacy of thioctic acid in the therapy of peripheral diabetic neuropathy. Horm Metab. Res. 1980; Suppl 9: 105.

302. Salway JG et al: Effect of myo-inositol on peripheral-nerve function in diabetes. Lancet. 1978; 2:1282.

303. Schulze-Delrieu K: The study of gastric stasis: Static no longer. (Editorial) Gastroenterology. 1980; 78:867.

304. Malagelada JR et al: Gastric motor abnormalities in diabetic and post vagotomy gastroparesis: Effect of metoclopramide and bethanechol. Gastroenterology. 1980; 78:286.

305. Fox S et al: Pathogenesis of diabetic gastroparesis: A pharmacologic study. Gastroenterology. 1980; 78:757.

306. Brownlee M et al: Metoclopramide for gastroparesis diabeticorum. N Engl J Med. 1974; 291:1257.

307. Campbell IW et al: Gastric emptying in diabetic autonomic neuropathy. Gut. 1977; 18:462.

308. Longstreth GF et al: Metoclopramide stimulation of gastric motility and emptying in diabetic gastroparesis (Letter). Ann Intern Med. 1977; 86:195.

309. Hartong WA et al: Metoclopramide in diabetic gastroparesis (Letter). Ann Intern Med. 1977; 86:826.

310. Brady PG et al: Gastric bezoar formation secondary to gastroparesis diabeticorum. Arch Intern Med. 1977; 137:1729.

311. Braverman D et al: Metoclopramide for gastroparesis diabeticorum. Diabetes Care. 1978; 1:356.

312. Soler NG: Diabetic gastroparesis without autonomic neuropathy (Letter). Diabetes Care. 1980; 3:200.

313. Muls EE et al: Uncontrolled diabetes mellitus due to gastroparesis diabeticorum: Treatment with metoclopramide. Postgrad Med J. 1981; 57:185.

314. Berkowitz DM et al: Oral metoclopramide in diabetic gastroparesis and in chronic gastric retention after gastric surgery (Abstract). Gastroenterology. 1976; 70:A-5/863.

315. Perkel MS et al: Metoclopramide therapy in fifty-five patients with delayed gastric emptying. Amer J Gastroenterology. 1980; 74:231.

316. Snape WT et al: Metoclopramide to treat gastroparesis due to diabetes mellitus: A double-blind, controlled trial. Ann Intern Med. 1982; 96:444.

317. Pinder RM et al: Metoclopramide: A review of its pharmacological properties and clinical use. Drugs. 1976; 12:81.

318. Grimes JD et al: Adverse neurologic effects of metoclopramide. Can Med Assoc J. 1982; 126:23.

319. Grimes JD: Parkinsonism and tardive dyskinesia associated with long-term metoclopramide therapy (Letter). N Engl J Med. 1982; 305:1417.

320. Ponte CD et al: Review of a new gastrointestinal drug—Metoclopramide. Am J. Hosp Pharm. 1981; 38:829.

321. Schulze-Delrieu K: Metoclopramide. N Engl J Med. 1981; 305:28.

322. Aono T et al: Clinical and endocrinological analyses of patients with galactorrhea and menstrual disorders due to sulpiride or metoclopramide. J Clin Endocrinol Metab. 1978; 47:675.

323. Fitzpatrick WJ: Thrombocytopenia occurring during chlorpropamide therapy. Diabetes. 1963; 12:457.

324. Morley A et al: A case of thrombocytopenia associated with chlorpropamide therapy. Med J Aust. 1964; 2:988.

325. Stein JH et al: Agranulocytosis caused by chlorpropamide. Arch Intern Med. 1964; 113:186.

326. Karlin H: Fatal agranulocytosis following chlorpropamide treatment of diabetes. N Engl J Med. 1960; 262:1077.

327. White LLR: Fatal marrow aplasia during chlorpropamide therapy. Br Med J. 1962; 1:691.

328. Chapman I et al: Pancytopenia associated with tolbutamide therapy. JAMA. 1963; 186:595.

329. Recker RR et al: Pure red blood cell aplasia with chlorpropamide (review). Arch Intern Med. 1969; 123:445.

330. Logue GL et al: Chlorpropamide-induced immune hemolytic anemia. N Engl J Med. 1970; 283:17.

331. Malacarne P et al: Tolbutamide-induced hemolytic anemia. Diabetes. 1977; 26:156.

332. Bird GWG et al: Haemolytic anemia associated with antibodies to tolbutamide and phenacetin. Br Med J. 1972; 1:728.

333. Christlieb AR: The hypertensions of diabetes. Diabetes Care. 1982; 5:50.

334. Furman BL: Impairment of glucose tolerance produced by diuretics and other drugs. Pharmacol Ther. 1981; 12:613.

335. Goldner MG et al: Hyperglycemia and glycosuria due to thiazide derivatives administered in diabetes mellitus. N Engl J Med. 1960; 262:403.

336. Carliner NH et al: Thiazide- and phthalimidine-induced hyperglycemia in hypertensive patients. JAMA. 1965; 191:535.

337. Wolff FW et al: Drug-induced diabetes. JAMA. 1963; 185:568.

338. Bengtsson C: Impairment of glucose metabolism during treatment with antihypertensive drugs. Acta Med Scand. 1979; Suppl 628:63.

339. Gerich JE et al: Clinical and metabolic characteristics of hyperosmolar nonketotic coma. Diabetes. 1971; 20:228.

340. Diamond MT: Hyperglycemic hyperosmolar coma associated with hydrochlorothiazide and pancreatitis, N Y State J Med. 1972; 72:1741.

341. Cranston WI et al: Effects of oral diuretics on raised arterial pressure. Lancet. 1963; 2:966.

342. Curtis J et al: Chlorthalidone-induced hyperosmolar hyperglycemic nonketotic coma. JAMA. 1972; 220:1592.

343. Lavender S et al: Nonketotic hyperosmolar coma and frosemide therapy. Diabetes. 1974; 23:247.

344. Tasker PRW et al: Non-ketotic diabetic precoma associated with high-dose frosemide therapy. Br Med J. 1976; 1:626.

345. Khaleeli AA et al: Hyperosmolar non-ketotic diabetic coma induced by furosemide in modest dosage. Postgrad Med J. 1978; 54:43.

346. Cowley AJ et al: Diabetes and therapy with potent diuretics (letter). Lancet. 1978; 1:154.

347. Lewis PJ et al: Deterioration of glucose tolerance in hypertensive patients on prolonged diuretic treatment. Lancet. 1976; 1:564.

348. Amery A et al: Glucose intolerance during diuretic therapy. Lancet. 1978; 1:681.

349. Chazen JA et al: Etiological factors in thiazide-induced or aggravated diabetes mellitus. Diabetes. 1965; 14:132.

350. Walker BR et al: Hyperkalemia after triamterene in diabetic patients. Clin Pharmacol Ther. 1972; 13:643.

351. Rapaport MI et al: Thiazide-induced glucose intolerance treated with potassium. Arch Intern Med. 1964; 113:405.

352. McFarland KF et al: Changes in the fasting blood sugar after hydrochlorothiazide and potassium supplementation. J Clin Pharmacol. 1977; 17:13.

353. Olesen KH et al: Diuretic action of bumetanide in congestive heart failure. Postgr Med J. 1975; 51 (Suppl 6):54.

354. Anderson OO et al: Carbohydrate metabolism during treatment with chlorthalidone and ethacrynic acid. Br Med J. 1968; 2:798.

355. Hicks BH et al: A controlled study of clopamide, clorexolone, and hydrochlorothiazide in diabetics. Metabolism. 1973; 22:101.

356. Diamond S: Ethacrynic acid and diabetes (letter). JAMA. 1968; 206:1793.

357. Jones IG et al: Diabetes mellitus following oral diuretics. Practitioner. 1967; 199:209.

358. Breckenridge A et al: Glucose tolerance in hypertensive patients on long-term diuretic therapy. Lancet. 1967; 1:61.

359. Bennett WM et al: Efficacy and safety of metolazone in renal failure and the nephrotic syndrome. J Clin Pharmacol. 1973; 13:357.

360. Levey BA et al: Biochemical and clinical effects of metolazone in congestive heart failure. Curr Therap Res. 1975; 18:641.

361. Weled BJ et al: The hypoglycemic hazards of propranolol in diabetic patients: Case reports. Milit Med. 1980; 145:705.

362. Skinner DJ et al: Uses of propranolol (letter). N Engl J Med. 1975; 293:1205.

363. Kotler MN et al: Hypoglycemia precipitated by propranolol. Lancet. 1966; 2:1389.

364. McMurtry RJ: Propranolol, hypoglycemia and hypertensive crisis (letter). Ann Intern Med. 1974; 80:669.

365. Reveno WS et al: Propranolol and hypoglycemia. Lancet. 1968; 1:920.

366. Barnett AH et al: Can insulin-treated diabetics be given beta-adrenergic blocking drugs? Br Med J. 1980; 280:976.

367. Ostman J et al: A cardio-selective beta-blocker (metoprolol) in hypertensive, insulin-dependent diabetics. Acta Med Scand. 1980; Suppl.639:29.

368. Viberti GC et al: Beta blockade and diabetes mellitus: Effect of oxprenolol and metoprolol on the metabolic, cardiovascular, and hormonal response to insulin-induced hypoglycemia in insulin-dependent diabetics. Metabolism. 1980; 29:873.

369. Lager I et al: Beta-adrenergic blockade and recovery from hypoglycaemia in diabetic subjects: Normalization after lactate and glycerol infusions. Clinical Science. 1982; 62:131.

370. Lager I et al: Effect of beta-blockade on hormonal release during hypoglycaemia in insulin-dependent diabetics. Acta Endocrinol 1980; 95:364.

371. Deacon SP et al: Acebutolol, atenolol and propranolol and metabolic responses to acute hypoglycaemia in diabetics. Br Med J. 1977; 2:1255.

372. Strom L: Propranolol in insulin-dependent diabetes (letter). N Engl J Med. 1978; 299:487.

373. Lager I et al: Effect of cardioselective and non-selective beta-blockade on the hypoglycaemic response in insulin-dependent diabetics. Lancet. 1979; 458.

374. Wright AD et al: Beta blockers and hypoglycaemia. Diabetes Care. 1980; 3:204.

375. Shepherd AMM et al: Hypoglycemia-induced hypertension in a diabetic patient on metoprolol. Ann Intern Med. 1981; 94:357.

376. William-Olsson T et al: Differences in metabolic responses to beta-adrenergic stimulation after propranolol or metoprolol administration. Acta Med Scand. 1979; 205:201.

377. Holm G et al: The effect of beta-blockade on glucose tolerance and insulin release in adult diabetes. Acta Med Scand. 1980; 208:187.

378. Garrett BN et al: Metoprolol in diabetes mellitus: effect on glucose homeostasis. Clinical Science. 1980; 59:469s.

379. Groop L et al: Influence of beta-blocking drugs on glucose metabolism in patients with non-insulin dependent diabetes mellitus. Acta Med Scand. 1982; 211:7.

380. Waal-Manning HJ: Metabolic effects of beta-adrenergic blockers. Drugs 1976; (Suppl.1) 11:121.

381. Zaman R et al: The effect of acebutolol and propranolol on the hypoglycemic action of glibenclamide. Br J Clin Pharmacol. 1982; 13:507.

382. Wright AD et al: Beta-adrenergic-blocking drugs and blood sugar control in diabetes mellitus. Br Med J. 1979; 1:159.

383. Podolsky S et al: Hyperosmolar non-ketotic diabetic coma: A complication of propranolol therapy. Metabolism. 1973; 22:685.

384. Gold DD: Propranolol-associated hyperglycemia: A case report. Hosp Formulary. 1982; 17:92.

385. Hansten PD: Beta-blocking agents and antidiabetic drugs. Drug Intell Clin Pharm. 1980; 14:46.

386. Webster WB Jr et al: Clonidine and glucose intolerance. Drug Intell Clin Pharm. 1982; 16:325.

387. Leclercq-Meyer V et al: Mode of action of clonidine upon islet function. Diabetes. 1980; 29:193.

388. Metz S et al: Induction of defective insulin secretion and impaired glucose tolerance by clonidine. Diabetes. 1978; 27:554.

389. Gündoğdu AS et al: Comparison of hormonal and metabolic effects of salbutamol infusion in normal subjects and insulin-requiring diabetics. Lancet. 1979; 2:1317.

390. Thomas DJB et al: Salbutamol-induced diabetic ketoacidosis. Br Med J. 1977; 2:438.

391. Leslie D et al: Salbutamol-induced diabetic ketoacidosis (letter). Br Med J. 1977; 2:768.

392. Leopold D et al: Salbutamol-induced ketoacidosis. Br Med J. 1977; 2:1152.

393. Schilthuis MS et al: Fetal death associated with severe ritodrine-induced ketoacidosis. Lancet. 1980; 1:1145.

394. Baker L et al: Hyperglycemia and acetonuria simulating diabetes. Am J Dis Child. 1966; 3:59.

395. Inoue S: Effects of epinephrine on asthmatic children. J Alter. 1967; 40:337.

396. Porte D Jr: Sympathomimetic regulation of insulin secretion. Its relation to diabetes mellitus. Arch Intern Med. 1969; 123:253.

397. Andersson DEH et al: Effect of verapamil on blood glucose and serum insulin in patients with hyper- and hypothyroidism. Acta Med Scand. 1980; 208:375.

398. Andersson DEH et al: Effect of verapamil on glucose response to glucagon during intravenous infusion of somatostatin. Horm Metab Res. 1980; 12:554.

399. Donnelly T et al: Effect of nifedipine on glucose tolerance and insulin secretion in diabetic and non-diabetic patients. Curr Med Res Opin. 1980; 6:690.

400. Giugliano D et al: Impairment of insulin secretion in man by nifedipine. Eur J Clin Pharmacol. 1980; 18:395.

401. Charles S et al: Hyperglycaemic effect of nifedipine. Br Med J. 1981; 283:19.

402. Davies DM ed: Textbook of Adverse Drug Reactions, 2nd ed. Univ Press, Oxford, 1981.

403. Sondheimer S: Metabolic effects of the birth control pill. Clin Obstet Gynecol. 1981; 24:927.

404. Spellacy WN: Carbohydrate metabolism during treatment with estrogen, progestogen and low-dose oral contraceptives. Am J Obstet Gynecol. 1982; 142:732.

405. Steel JM et al: Contraception for the insulin-dependent diabetic women: The view from one clinic. Diabetes Care. 1980; 3:557.

406. Szabo AJ et al: Glucose tolerance in gestational diabetic women during and after treatment with a combination-type oral contraceptive. N Engl J Med. 1970; 282:646.

407. Wynn V et al: Comparison of effects of different combined oral-contraceptive formulations on carbohydrate and lipid metabolism. Lancet. 1979; 1:1045.

408. Spellacy WN: Carbohydrate metabolism prospectively studied in women using a low-estrogen oral contraceptive for six months. Contraception. 1979; 20:137.

409. Carter BL et al: Phenytoin-induced hyperglycemia. Am J Hosp Pharm. 1981; 38:1508.

410. Dahl JR: Diphenylhydantoin toxic psychosis with associated hyperglycemia. Calif Med. 1967; 107:345.

411. Furiss BL et al: Diphenylhydantoin induced hyperglycemia and impaired insulin release. Diabetes. 1971; 20:177.

412. Peters BH et al: Hyperglycemia with relative insulinemia in diphenylhydantoin. N Engl J Med. 1969; 281:91.

413. Treasure T et al: Hyperglycemia due to phenytoin toxicity. Arch Dis Child. 1971; Aug:563.

414. Klein JP: Diphenylhydantoin intoxication associated with hyperglycemia. J Pediatr. 1966; 69:463.

415. Goldberg EM et al: Hyperglycemic nonketotic coma following administration of dilantin. Diabetes. 1969; 18:101.

416. Malherbe C et al: Effect of diphenylhydantoin on insulin secretion. N Engl J Med. 1972; 286:339.

417. Pace CS et al: Ionic basis of phenytoin sodium inhibition of insulin secretion in pancreatic islets. Diabetes. 1979; 28:1077.

418. Gomez EC et al: Induction of glycosuria and hyperglycemia by topical corticosteroid therapy. Arch Dermatol. 1976; 112:1559.

419. Swartz SL et al: Corticosteroids: Clinical pharmacology and therapeutic use. Drugs. 1978; 16:238.

420. Perlman K et al: Steroid diabetes in childhood. Am J Dis Child. 1982; 136:64.

421. Baron SH: Salicylates as hypoglycemic agents. Diabetes Care. 1982; 5:64.

422. Gilgore SG: The influence of salicylate on hyperglycemia. Diabetes. 1960; 9:392.

423. Robertson RP: Prostaglandins as modulators of pancreatic islet function. Diabetes. 1979; 28:943.

424. Colwell JA: Pathogenesis of atherosclerosis in diabetes mellitus. Diabetes Care. 1981; 4:121.

425. McDonald J: Alcohol and diabetes. Diabetes Care. 1980; 3:629.

426. Arky et al: Irreversible hypoglycemia: A complication of alcohol and insulin. JAMA. 1968; 206:575.

427. Hui C-H et al: Risk factors for hyperglycemia in children with leukemia receiving L-asparaginase and prednisone. J Pediatr. 1981; 99:46.

428. Gattereau A et al: Hyperglycaemic effect of synthetic salmon calcitonin (letter). Lancet. 1977; 2:1076.

429. Evans IMA et al: Hyperglycaemic effect of synthetic salmon calcitonin (letter). Lancet. 1978; 1:280.

430. Jefferys DB: Effect of cimetidine on glucose handling (letter). Lancet. 1978; 1:383.

431. Waziri R: Lithium in diabetes mellitus: A paradoxical response. J Clin Psychiatry. 1978; 39:623.

432. Bouchard PH et al: Diabetes mellitus following pentamidine-induced hypoglycemia in humans. Diabetes. 1982; 31:40.

433. Goldberg IJ: Disopyramide (Norpace)-induced hypoglycemia. Am J Med. 1980; 69:463.

434. Turtle JR et al: Hypoglycemic action of fenfluramine in diabetes mellitus. Diabetes. 1973; 22:858.

435. Gupta KK: Guanethidine and glucose tolerance in diabetes (letter). Br Med J. 1968; 3:679.

436. Gibson RC et al: Duration and magnitude of insulin effect in juvenile-onset diabetics. Clin Res. 1966; 14:63.

437. Leslie D: Generalized allergic reaction to monocomponent insulin. Br Med J. 1977; 2:736.

438. Simmonds JP et al: Generalized allergy to porcine and bovine monocomponent insulins. Br Med J. 1980; 281:355.

439. Goldman JM et al: Generalized allergy to porcine and bovine monocomponent insulins (letter). Br Med J. 1980; 281:1494.

440. Skyler JS: A plethora of insulins (editorial). Diabetes Care, 1980; 3:638.

Chapter 57

Rheumatic Diseases

Stephen L. Dahl and Brian S. Katcher

RHEUMATOID ARTHRITIS

In the United States, arthritis affects about 20 million persons; one in four families is affected. Although rheumatoid arthritis occurs less frequently than osteoarthritis, which is a disease primarily of age, it is more serious because it is potentially crippling and extra-articular complications occasionally may be life-threatening. About one-fourth of those with arthritis have rheumatoid arthritis. Women are affected about three times more often than men. The disease occurs most frequently after the third decade of life but may occur at any age and children are frequently affected (1,2).

Rheumatoid arthritis is a chronic systemic disease of unknown etiology which primarily affects the joints. Exacerbations and remissions occur throughout the course of this disease, which tends to be progressive. The goals of therapy are to reduce pain and inflammation of the involved joints and preserve joint function. In addition, some forms of drug therapy may delay the progression of the disease.

1. *Early Acute Rheumatoid Arthritis.* **T.W. is a previously healthy 42-year-old, 60 kg, woman who has been suffering from morning stiffness which persists for several hours, anorexia, fatigue, and generalized muscle and joint pain during the past four months. Her symptoms have been much worse during the past month and a half, and she has been forced to limit her physical activities. She also notes that she is no longer able to wear her wedding ring due to swelling of her hands. Physical examination revealed bilaterally symmetrical swelling, tenderness, and heat of the metacarpophalangeal and proximal interphalangeal joints of the hands and the metatarsophalangeal joints of the feet. Pertinent laboratory findings included: erythrocyte sedimentation rate (ESR) by the Westergren method 52 mm/hr (normal less than 15 mm/hr); hemoglobin 10.6 gm/dl (normal 12 to 16 gm/dl); hematocrit 35% (normal 36 to 47%); platelets 480,000 (normal 140,000–400,000); albumin 3.8 gm/dl (normal 4.3 to 5.6 gm/dl); serum uric acid 3.0 mg/dl (normal 2–8 mg/dl); serum iron 40 mg/dl (normal 60–180 mg/dl); iron binding capacity 275 mg/dl, (normal 200–400 mg/dl), and rheumatoid factor performed by latex fixation method was pos-**itive in a dilution of 1:320. Tests for lupus erythematosus (LE), antinuclear antibodies (ANA), and tuberculin sensitivity were negative. X-ray films of the hands and feet showed soft tissue swelling with no evidence of tophi or calcification. Other routine laboratory data and physical findings were normal.**

What signs and symptoms of rheumatoid arthritis are manifested by this patient?

The presentation of rheumatoid arthritis is quite variable and may be difficult to differentiate from a variety of other rheumatoid and non-rheumatoid diseases (2,3). Signs and symptoms which are prominent features of rheumatoid arthritis in this patient are fatigue, anorexia, and morning stiffness which may precede localized joint involvement (1,2). About half of the patients with rheumatoid arthritis initially experience fatigue which later in the disease serves as a reliable index of disease activity (4). Duration of morning stiffness may also be useful as an index of disease activity. Characteristically, morning stiffness usually lasts more than an hour before the patient "limbers up" and may last most of the day. Stiffness may also occur after any prolonged period of inactivity such as sitting in a chair (2).

Bilaterally symmetrical joint swelling and pain, as illustrated by T.W., are characteristic of rheumatoid arthritis. Hand and feet involvement usually manifest as swelling and tenderness of the metacarpophalangeal, proximal interphalangeal, and metatarsophalangeal joints. The wrists, elbows, shoulders, hips, knees, ankles, and cervical spine are also frequently affected. As a consequence of prolonged, uncontrolled disease activity, irreversible changes such as subluxation, ulnar deviation, swan neck deformities, and boutonniere deformities may arise. Extra-articular manifestations are frequently observed in rheumatoid arthritis and range from harmless dermatological changes such as subcutaneous rheumatoid nodules which may appear on extensor surfaces such as the elbow in 25% of patients to rare, life-threatening complications such as rheumatoid vasculitis (1,2).

The laboratory findings in rheumatoid arthritis are characteristic of a chronic inflammatory disease. There is no specific test for the disease. T.W.'s elevated erythrocyte sedimentation rate (ESR) is a nonspecific indication of inflammation. Her hematologic findings are consistent with a mild anemia of chronic disease. The serum iron concentration is decreased, but the iron binding capacity is normal; binding capacity will be increased if she should subsequently develop an iron-deficiency anemia due to drug therapy or other causes. The degree of anemia correlates with the activity of the disease. Because the anemia arises secondary to a failure of iron release from the reticuloendothelial tissues, iron therapy will not correct it (1,2,5).

Serum albumin is often low, as illustrated by this patient. Although low serum albumin could theoretically result in decreased protein binding of salicylates and other highly protein bound non-steroidal anti-inflammatory drugs (NSAIDs) and yield higher free (and therefore active) drug serum levels, this does not usually occur possibly because the degree of hypoalbuminemia is generally mild and/or because the increase in free drug is offset by increased metabolism (6).

Rheumatoid factor, a macroglobulin (usually IgM) which reacts with IgG to form an immune complex, is found in the sera of up to 80% of patients with rheumatoid arthritis. However, the presence of rheumatoid factor is not pathognomonic, because it is not found in some patients with rheumatoid arthritis. In addition, rheumatoid factor may be found in high titers in other disease states, and some healthy individuals may have rheumatoid factor in their sera (7). Rheumatoid factor does not parallel disease activity, but high titers early in the course of the disease may indicate a graver prognosis (2,5,8–10). The LE preparation and test for antinuclear antibodies were performed to rule out systemic lupus erythematosus. However, both of these tests may be positive in as many as 15% of patients with rheumatoid arthritis (2).

Many of these clinical and laboratory features of rheumatoid arthritis are useful parameters for monitoring disease activity and its response to therapy. These and others are listed in Table 1.

2. *Treatment.* A diagnosis of rheumatoid arthritis is made. How should T.W. be treated?

The primary treatment objectives in rheumatoid arthritis are reduction of joint pain and inflammation, preservation of joint function, and prevention of deformity. A conservative approach combining drug therapy, rest, and physical therapy is the safest and most effective means of achieving these objectives (11,12).

Aspirin given in large doses, as discussed in

Table 1.

PARAMETERS USED FOR ASSESSING DISEASE
ACTIVITY AND DRUG RESPONSE IN
RHEUMATOID ARTHRITIS

Proximal Interphalangeal Joint Circumference

Number of Painful and Tender Joints

Number of Swollen Joints

Grip Strength

Duration of Morning Stiffness

Time to Onset of Fatigue

Time to Walk 50 Feet

Erythrocyte Sedimentation Rate

subsequent questions, is considered the mainstay of drug therapy by most clinicians. Systemic rest reduces inflammation, and articular rest achieved by splinting the affected joints may produce dramatic results (4). A comparison of complete bed confinement with ad lib activity in hospitalized patients demonstrated that absolute bed rest is unnecessary, but most of the patients in this study benefited from hospitalization, probably due to reduction of physical and emotional stresses and regular physical and salicylate therapy (13). Therefore, a liberal rest program should be prescribed for T.W. If an adequate rest program cannot be carried out at home, hospitalization should be considered.

Since active exercise increases inflammation, passive exercise should be utilized for T.W. until the acute inflammation subsides; this will prevent muscle atrophy, flexion contractures, and maintain joint function. The external application of heat, by soaking her hands and feet in warm water, hot baths, or hot paraffin treatments may reduce joint stiffness and allow greater benefit from passive exercise programs. Several heat applications per day may be more effective than a single longer treatment. An effective approach would be to prescribe heat and exercise treatments three times a day after meals and at bedtime after taking the prescribed doses of aspirin (14).

Finally, emotional support is very important. As many as 50% of patients experience their first symptoms following an emotional stress such as the death of a loved one, sickness in the family, divorce, or change in jobs (2). Disability from the disease may cause further emotional problems (15). Therefore, it is important that some time be spent with the patient and her family to insure that the treatment will have an optimal effect.

Aspirin

3. *Aspirin Dosage.* **T.W., who weighs 60 kg, is to begin taking aspirin, 975 mg four times daily (3.9 grams daily) in conjunction with an appropriate program of physical therapy and rest. Is this an appropriate dose of aspirin?**

Serum salicylate concentrations of 15 to 30 mg/ dl are considered necessary to achieve optimal anti-inflammatory responses with aspirin. Thus, large doses of aspirin must be ingested each day. For example, two studies demonstrated a daily aspirin dose of 5.2 grams to be more effective than either 2.6 grams or placebo in reduction of the duration of morning stiffness, delay in onset of fatigue, increase in grip strength, decrease in ESR, decrease in joint swelling and tenderness, and patient preference (16,17). The groups receiving 2.6 grams daily and placebo did not differ significantly from each other. In another trial, a daily aspirin dose of 3.6 grams was more effective than placebo when similar criteria were utilized to assess anti-inflammatory effect (18). However, the dose required to achieve optimal anti-inflammatory responses varies widely among individuals and appears to result from individual variation in metabolic capacity (19–22). Following administration of 65 mg/kg/day of aspirin, the dose that has been prescribed for T.W., plasma salicylate levels ranging from 5 to 28 mg/dl were observed among nine patients with rheumatoid arthritis after three days of therapy (23). Similarly, a range of 12 to 35 mg/dl was observed among 26 healthy individuals after three days of this regimen in another study (20). When a group of patients with backache or rheumatoid arthritis were given this dosage, a similar range of values, from 13 to 29 mg/dl, was reported (24).

These findings suggest that T.W. is taking a dosage of aspirin which is likely to achieve anti-inflammatory blood levels. However, this dose may also prove to be either insufficient or produce signs and symptoms of salicylate toxicity (see Questions 5 and 6). Because it is not possible to predict the optimal anti-inflammatory dosage for an individual, aspirin therapy is usually initiated at 2.6 to 3.9 grams daily in divided doses and slowly

increased, if necessary, to achieve an optimal anti-inflammatory response.

4. *Patient Information.* **What instructions should accompany this patient's aspirin prescription?**

First, this patient should appreciate the important role that large, regularly taken doses of aspirin play in the treatment of rheumatoid arthritis. In addition to providing substantial analgesia, large doses of aspirin are anti-inflammatory. When anti-inflammatory doses of aspirin are replaced with large oral doses of meperidine, codeine, or propoxyphene, patients experience a marked increase in symptoms. Fatigue and stiffness become severe, finger joint size is increased, range of motion is decreased, and grip strength is decreased (25). The daily ingestion of large amounts of aspirin is commonly approached with considerable skepticism unless the patient receives some explanation and encouragement.

Gastric intolerance is the major limitation to the successful use of large doses of aspirin and may take the form of epigastric distress or painless gastrointestinal bleeding (26). Small amounts of blood loss (microbleeding) occur with each aspirin dose, but individuals vary as to the amount of blood which is lost (27). Although continual aspirin ingestion may lead to iron-deficiency anemia in some patients, major gastrointestinal bleeding from aspirin appears to be a rare occurrence (28–31). The microbleeding caused by aspirin can be minimized by concurrent ingestion of food or antacids in sufficient amounts (32–35). By increasing the pH of the stomach, the amount of aspirin that exists in the absorbable unionized state is decreased and gastrointestinal microbleeding is reduced (33,36–39). However, if repeated therapeutic quantities of antacids are used, their effect on urinary pH must be considered (see Question 7). Ingesting aspirin with generous quantities of liquids such as a full glass of water or a warm, nonirritating beverage is advocated (40).

Aspirin is hydrolyzed to salicylic acid and acetic acid in the presence of moisture, so the container should be closed tightly and not stored in the bathroom. Although childproof safety closures are required on aspirin containers and are effective in reducing accidental ingestion (41), many arthritic patients are unable to cope with these safety closures due to diminished grip strength and hand deformities that arise from rheumatoid arthritis.

If aspirin is dispensed in a conventional closure container, it is necessary to explain the hazards of accidental ingestion by children and to obtain a signed release form (see chapter on Poisonings).

5. *Adjustment of Aspirin Dosage.* Five days later, T.W.'s serum salicylate level was 17 mg/dl and her symptoms were marginally improved. How rapidly can the aspirin dose be increased? Will capacity-limited salicylate metabolism cause any difficulties as her aspirin dosage is increased?

With small analgesic doses of aspirin, the elimination half-life of salicylate is about 2.5 hours (42). However, when aspirin is taken in large daily doses for anti-inflammatory effects, two of the five major pathways of salicylate elimination become saturated and the elimination half-life is prolonged up to 18 to 24 hours (43–46). Thus, several days of therapy are needed before steady state serum levels are attained. Presently, T.W.'s salicylate level has approached steady state, but another four or five days will be required before a new steady state plateau is reached following an additional increase in dose. Consequently, dosage should be changed only after intervals of several days.

After ingestion, aspirin is rapidly hydrolyzed to salicylate. Salicylate is eliminated from the body via direct renal excretion of unchanged drug and via biotransformation to salicyluric acid (capacity limited), salicyl phenolic glucuronide (capacity limited), salicyl acyl glucuronide, and gentisic acid with subsequent renal excretion (45). In addition, gentisic acid and salicyluric acid may be further metabolized to gentisuric acid which is eliminated renally (47). This is depicted in Figure 1. Salicylate pharmacokinetics are therefore complex and follow both first order and Michaelis-Menten elimination processes. Moreover, elimination of unchanged salicylate is highly pH-dependent (44), and the apparent volume of distribution increases with increasing doses (48). All of these factors must be considered when aspirin dosages are altered.

Small doses of salicylate are eliminated by apparent first order processes. As the salicylate dosage is increased, two pathways responsible for salicylate biotransformation become saturated, leading to disproportionate increases in serum salicylate levels. Still higher doses of salicylate lead to an increase in the apparent volume of distribution, apparently as a consequence of plasma protein binding site saturation. Thus, subsequent dosage increases are once again accompanied by proportionate increases in serum salicylate levels as the increase in the apparent volume of distribution and enhanced salicylate metabolism via the non-saturable pathways offset the effects of saturation kinetics on salicylate metabolism.

Total salicylate clearance decreases initially when salicylate dosage is increased but then stabilizes in the therapeutic range of 15 to 30 mg/100 ml (43). These findings are supported by observations of serum salicylate level increases that were roughly proportional to dosage increases in four patients whose initial salicylate levels were within the range of 15 to 30 mg/100 ml (24). Disproportionately large increases in serum salicylate concentrations were attained with small increases in daily dose in two patients who experienced a 300% increase in salicylate levels three days after their daily dose was increased from 65 mg/kg to 100 mg/kg (23). In both of these patients the initial serum concentration was below 15 mg/dl. Thus, enzyme saturation and the subsequent two- or three-fold decrease in clearance which occurs with higher doses may not yet have occurred. Also, urinary pH shifts during the interim may have contributed to the serum levels eventually attained in these patients (see Question 7). These reports support the concept that after an initial decrease in clearance due to saturable metabolism, total clearance stabilizes and remains constant as the effect of dose-dependent

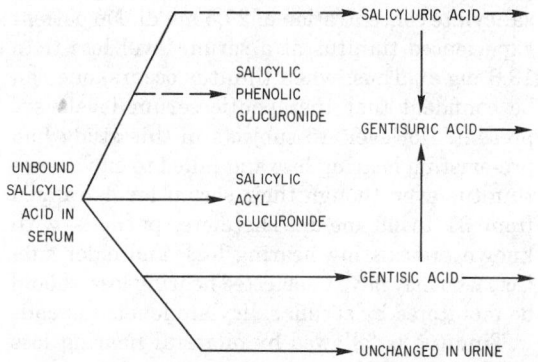

ELIMINATION PATHWAYS OF SALICYLIC ACID

Figure 1. Elimination Pathways of Salicylic Acid. The dotted lines indicate saturable pathways. With anti-inflammatory doses, elimination via the non-saturable metabolic pathways and urinary excretion become relatively more important as routes of elimination.

metabolism is offset by the combined effects of a dose-dependent increase in volume of distribution and enhanced salicylate metabolism and excretion via non-saturable pathways.

Therefore, if T.W.'s dose is increased from three tablets four times daily (3.9 grams or 65/mg/kg daily) to four tablets four times daily (5.2 grams or 87 mg/kg daily), the steady state level will probably increase proportionately, and a level of approximately 23 mg/dl can be anticipated. Although these dosage increments can be calculated, application of these findings to the general population should be performed cautiously until they are confirmed in a large number of patients. Slowly increasing the salicylate dose until the desired anti-inflammatory response is obtained remains a safe and effective method of salicylate dosing.

6. Could tinnitus, rather than blood levels, be used as an endpoint for salicylate dosing for T.W.? What are the relative merits of each approach?

Gradually increasing the daily dose of aspirin to the point of tinnitus, a ringing or high-pitched buzzing sensation in the head, and then reducing the dose by a couple of tablets a day is a time-honored technique which clinically results in anti-inflammatory activity (25). Tinnitus is dose-dependent (49). A study of salicylate-induced tinnitus in 67 patients and seven healthy volunteers demonstrated that this symptom may be a useful therapeutic endpoint in those with normal hearing (50). As might be expected (see Question 3), the number of tablets required per day varied widely, but tinnitus developed at an average serum salicylate concentration of 29.5 mg/dl. No patient experienced tinnitus at a serum level less than 19.6 mg/dl. Thus, when tinnitus occurs, one can be confident that therapeutic serum levels are present. However, 15 subjects in this study had pre-existing hearing loss and failed to experience tinnitus even though their serum levels ranged from 31 to 68 mg/dl. Therefore, patients with known pre-existing hearing loss, and older subjects who may have undetected hearing loss, should be monitored by serum salicylate levels instead.

Tinnitus is followed by bilateral hearing loss as serum levels approach 30 mg/dl, and this hearing loss becomes progressively greater with higher levels until it plateaus at serum levels of about 50 mg/dl (49). Both symptoms are completely reversible.

Therefore, if T.W. has good hearing, tinnitus can be used as a therapeutic endpoint. However, serum salicylate levels may be preferable where noncompliance is a concern or where other factors may influence serum salicylate levels (see Question 7).

7. Alteration in Salicylate Excretion. After several weeks of treatment with excellent results, T.W. experienced tinnitus on the day of a scheduled clinic visit. A serum salicylate was ordered and reported as 32 mg/dl. Previously, her serum salicylate levels were about 25 mg/dl. The only change in her treatment had been a recent discontinuation of the antacid (Maalox) she was taking with each aspirin dose. Explain this increase in her serum salicylate. How can this problem be avoided in the future?

When aspirin is used in anti-inflammatory doses, the renal excretion of unchanged salicylate becomes an important elimination pathway (see Question 5 and Figure 1); and the renal excretion of salicylate is highly pH-dependent (44,51). Both sodium bicarbonate and the "nonsystemic" antacids are capable of increasing urinary pH and increasing salicylate excretion. When sodium bicarbonate 4 gm daily was administered to 13 subjects, urinary pH increased from a range of 5.6 to 6.1 to a range of 6.2 to 6.9 and the average serum salicylate level fell from 27 mg/dl to 15 mg/dl (44). Similarly, regular therapeutic doses of magnesium and aluminum hydroxides (Maalox) resulted in appreciable increases in urinary pH and decreases in serum salicylate concentrations ranging from 30 to 70% in a group of pediatric patients (52). Daily administration of Maalox, 15 ml qid, increases average urinary pH approximately 0.7 to 0.9 units after several days of therapy; an equivalent fall in urinary pH is noted within two days after discontinuation of the antacid (53–55). A decrease in urinary pH from 6.5 to 5.5 in a patient whose serum salicylate level is within the therapeutic range of 20 to 30 mg/dl could double the serum salicylate concentration (44). Thus, T.W.'s discontinuation of her Maalox may have resulted in a more acidic urine, tinnitus, and elevated serum salicylate concentrations.

If T.W. is able to tolerate aspirin without an antacid, the aspirin dosage can be decreased. She should be encouraged to take her aspirin with meals to prevent epigastric discomfort and reduce gastrointestinal blood loss. Smaller doses of Maalox will not substantially alter urinary pH but may fail to raise gastric pH sufficiently to reduce gastrointestinal microbleeding (see Question 4).

Because urinary pH is such an important determinant of salicylate blood levels, these patients should monitor their urine acidity with pH paper (44). If this is attempted, pH determinations should be performed at approximately the same time each day because urinary pH follows a circadian pattern (53).

8. History of Aspirin Allergy. Aspirin is ordered for a patient who was recently hospitalized for evaluation and treatment of his rheumatoid arthritis. The patient's medical chart indicates allergy to aspirin. Is aspirin contraindicated for this patient?

The patient should be asked to describe his reaction to aspirin. If this patient is truly allergic to aspirin, then this medication is contraindicated. However, most patients who claim to be allergic to aspirin merely suffer from gastrointestinal distress which is not an allergic reaction. In these patients aspirin may be tolerated if administered with food, antacids, or large quantities of fluids. If aspirin is still not tolerated, a trial with one of the other NSAIDs may prove beneficial.

Aspirin intolerance (allergy) in association with asthma is cause for serious concern. Challenge with aspirin in these patients can initiate an explosive asthmatic reaction which may be fatal (56). Asthma, rhinorrhea, and nasal polyps usually accompany this type of aspirin intolerance, and about 2 to 4% of asthmatics will exhibit aspirin intolerance (56,57). These patients appear to experience a high degree of cross-reactivity to other chemicals, including indomethacin, naproxen, ibuprofen, fenoprofen, mefenamic acid, sodium benzoate (a widely used preservative), tartrazine (a dye, FD&C No. 5, which is used in foods and some drugs), and other substances (57–60). These substances are structurally dissimilar, but most of them are inhibitors of prostaglandin synthesis. Therefore, this reaction may result from an abnormal response to a common pharmacologic effect (61). Although sodium and choline salicylate have been administered to such aspirin-sensitive patients without untoward reactions, this should be attempted with great caution (56).

Some patients develop urticaria upon exposure to aspirin. This reaction is believed to be immunologically mediated, because there is no cross-reactivity with structurally dissimilar prostaglandin synthesis inhibitors (61). Cross-reactivity with sodium salicylate has been reported, indicating that the salicylate radical or a metabolite is responsible for inducing the immunologic reaction (57).

9. Alternative Salicylate Formulations. The patient with the alleged aspirin-allergy described above avoids aspirin because it has upset his stomach in the past. However, he is able to take high doses of Ecotrin, an enteric coated aspirin formulation, without experiencing GI intolerance. Is this a rational alternative to regular aspirin? What are appropriate alternatives for patients who do not tolerate therapeutic doses of aspirin?

Because aspirin is effective, well tolerated by many patients and inexpensive, it is considered by most practitioners to be the drug of choice for the initial management of rheumatoid arthritis. Each dose of aspirin should be taken with a full glass of water or with meals to reduce problems of gastrointestinal intolerance. If needed, antacids may be useful, but their effects on urinary pH, and therefore on blood levels, must be considered (see Question 7). Preparations which contain buffering agents such as Alka-Seltzer, Ascriptin, and Bufferin are frequently used by patients who do not otherwise tolerate aspirin. The antacid content in Alka-Seltzer may be sufficient to raise gastric pH and reduce gastrointestinal microbleeding, but this product contains more than a gram of sodium for each 10 grains of aspirin, making it undesirable for chronic use (35,62). Ascriptin and Bufferin probably contain too little antacid to appreciably reduce gastric microbleeding (32,63) but are occasionally better tolerated than regular aspirin. All of these preparations are more expensive than regular aspirin.

Enteric coated aspirin preparations reduce the gastrointestinal complications associated with regular aspirin therapy (63,64) but at the risk of incomplete absorption (65–68). Two preparations, Enseals and Ecotrin, were demonstrated to be reliably absorbed in one study involving small numbers of patients (69). Furthermore, other studies have demonstrated that enteric coated preparations may be reliably absorbed (70–73). Thus, enteric coated preparations may prove to be a useful alternative in some patients intolerant to regular aspirin. However, if arthritis suddenly flairs in a patient taking one of these preparations, incomplete absorption of the drug should be suspected.

In addition to altered formulations of aspirin, a number of salts of salicylic acid have been marketed as alternatives to aspirin. Products such as sodium salicylate, magnesium salicylate (Magan, Mobidin), choline salicylate (Arthropan), choline magnesium trisalicylate (Trilisate), and salicylsalicylic acid (Disalcid) may produce less gastrointestinal intolerance and microbleeding than aspirin (74,75) but are apparently not as potent anti-inflammatory agents (62,76,77). Salicylates probably exert their anti-inflammatory effects by a number of mechanisms and inhibition of prostaglandin synthesis may be an important factor in their action. Aspirin irreversibly inactivates an enzyme, cyclooxygenase, via acetylation of the enzyme (78). This enzyme is necessary for the synthesis of a number of prostaglandins, some of which possess inflammatory properties. Salicylic acid and other non-steroidal anti-inflammatory drugs (NSAIDs) also appear to inhibit the action of this enzyme (78). Although aspirin is rapidly hydrolyzed in the blood stream to salicylate, the anti-inflammatory effects of this metabolite alone cannot explain aspirin's potency. Aspirin appears to be more potent than other salicylates as an anti-inflammatory agent (77). In addition, the concentration of aspirin may persist for a somewhat longer period of time in joint fluid than in the blood (79). A salicylate salt may be tried as an alternative to aspirin but there is no evidence that the more expensive salicylate salts are superior to sodium salicylate.

Finally, a number of structurally different NSAIDs are available as alternatives to aspirin but are significantly more expensive (see Question 12).

Because enteric coated aspirin preparations are less expensive than the newer NSAIDs, this form of therapy may prove to be an appropriate alternative to regular aspirin in this patient. However, incomplete absorption of the preparation may precede a flare of arthritis.

10. Prolongation of Bleeding Time. T.W. is scheduled to have an impacted wisdom tooth removed. Will her aspirin therapy interfere with this procedure?

Aspirin prolongs bleeding time and should, therefore, be discontinued several days prior to the procedure. Several mechanisms may be responsible for the prolonged bleeding time. First

and most important, low doses of aspirin impair platelet aggregation. This effect on platelets is irreversible. Therefore, new platelets must be released into the circulation before the bleeding time will normalize. Thus, the bleeding time may be prolonged for several days following a single dose of aspirin (26,116). Secondly, aspirin and sodium salicylate appear to enhance blood fibrinolytic activity (117). Thirdly, near toxic doses of salicylates may induce a hypoprothombinemia which is reversible by vitamin K (26). Salicylate-induced hypoprothrombinemia is usually not clinically significant, but on rare occasions it can be the cause of bleeding when associated with severe liver dysfunction or malnutrition (118).

A study comparing the effects of aspirin and acetaminophen on the post-operative course after extraction of impacted wisdom teeth demonstrated significantly more bleeding with aspirin. This study involved 32 subjects, each of whom had bilaterally impacted wisdom teeth that were removed separately so each patient received aspirin once and acetaminophen once (323). Furthermore, bleeding that could not be completely arrested after dental surgery has been attributed to aspirin (324). T.W.'s aspirin therapy should be discontinued and she should not resume taking aspirin until her gums have begun to heal.

The time required for bleeding time to normalize varies from individual to individual, but bleeding times generally normalize in about 72 hours following discontinuation of aspirin (116). Currently, monitoring bleeding time is the most objective method for determining when patients are no longer at risk for aspirin-induced bleeding.

Choosing another NSAID for patients where prolonged bleeding times are of concern might be considered. The NSAIDs also prolong bleeding times via inhibition of platelet aggregation, although the inhibition is reversible (88–92). Some investigators have demonstrated no effect, or minimal effect, on platelets by sodium salicylate (119,120). Others have demonstrated an effect on platelets similar to other NSAIDs (121). Discontinuation of the NSAID drug results in normalization of platelet function in conjunction with drug elimination from the body. Thus, a NSAID with a short elimination half-life might be considered for such patients.

11. Pregnancy. A 28-year-old woman with rheumatoid arthritis has recently become pregnant and is concerned about the possi-

ble effects of aspirin on her baby. Will uninterrupted consumption of aspirin since conception placed the fetus at risk? How should her rheumatoid arthritis be managed during her pregnancy?

A prospective study of more than 50,000 pregnancies revealed similar malformation rates among children whose mothers had been moderately or heavily exposed to aspirin and those whose mothers had not been exposed to aspirin during the first four months of pregnancy (122). Lack of teratogenicity was also noted in the babies of 144 mothers who had used salicylates heavily throughout pregnancy (123). Therefore, aspirin probably is not teratogenic.

A prospective study of 41,000 pregnancies did not reveal any effect of maternal aspirin consumption on perinatal mortality or birthweight (124). However, conflicting results have been reported by other investigators (122). These positive findings may have been due to more careful patient selection utilizing maternal urine screens for salicylate and the fact that all of these women continued to take aspirin every week until delivery.

The exact mechanism by which aspirin may cause a greater incidence of stillbirths is unknown, but it may be related to inhibition of prostaglandin synthesis and subsequent premature closure of the ductus arteriosus in utero. The ductus arteriosus is normally open in utero and allows the contents of the right ventricle to bypass the high resistance pulmonary vascular bed and empty directly into the aorta. Closure in utero results in pulmonary hypertension with poor perfusion to the brain, liver, kidney, and other areas. Aspirin-induced premature closure of the ductus arteriosus in utero has been produced experimentally in lambs (125) and has been implicated in at least one human birth (126). This effect has been utilized therapeutically to close the ductus arteriosus in premature infants.

Aspirin-induced coagulation defects may also contribute to a higher mortality rate and also place the mother at greater risk of hemorrhage (see Question 10).

Finally, fetal and neonatal salicylate pharmacokinetics may be important. Because of greater protein binding in the fetus, neonatal salicylate concentrations are about 1.5 times higher than those in the mother (127,128), and newborns eliminate salicylates more slowly than adults (127).

About three-quarters of women with rheumatoid arthritis undergo a temporary remission during pregnancy (129). Relief generally occurs during the first trimester and persists for more than one month into the postpartum period. Thus, aspirin therapy may be successfully terminated in many women during pregnancy. If this woman's drug therapy cannot be terminated, she may safely continue taking aspirin during the first and second trimesters, but she should avoid aspirin, if possible, during the final stages of pregnancy. The effects of other anti-inflammatory drugs on the fetus are either unknown or adverse.

NSAIDs

12. A 58-year-old man with rheumatoid arthritis has been taking 4.6 gm of aspirin daily for 18 months with good control of his symptoms. He recently read about a new drug called piroxicam which is supposedly as effective as aspirin, less irritating to the stomach than aspirin, and more convenient since fewer tablets are needed. Describe the effectiveness, mechanism of action, side effects, and metabolism of the NSAIDs. Is this patient a candidate for piroxicam or any of the other non-steroidal anti-inflammatory drugs (NSAIDs)?

Piroxicam is one of a large number of NSAIDs that are currently marketed in the United States. The currently available NSAIDs consist of the propionic acid derivatives, ibuprofen (Motrin), fenoprofen (Nalfon), and naproxen (Naprosyn); the heterocyclic acetic acids, indomethacin (Indocin), tolmetin (Tolectin), and sulindac (Clinoril); the fenamic acids, mefenamic acid (Ponstel) and meclofenamic acid (Meclomen); the pyrazolones, phenylbutazone (Butazolidin) and oxyphenbutazone (Tandearil); and the oxicams which are represented by piroxicam (Feldene) in this country.

In clinical studies, all of these agents are superior to placebo, equally effective as aspirin in the treatment of rheumatoid arthritis, and possibly cause fewer side effects (80–87). However, these studies usually failed to adequately regulate aspirin dosage. For example, after a multicenter double-blind study in 80 patients, it was concluded that naproxen was as effective as aspirin and associated with fewer side effects (80). However, many of the side effects observed with aspirin were consistent with salicylism; salicylate levels were not monitored because titration of aspirin would have unblinded the study. Other studies used fixed dosages of aspirin that were probably inadequate for some patients.

While these NSAIDs may be structurally different, they possess similar pharmacologic properties and all inhibit prostaglandin synthesis (88–93). Not surprisingly, these drugs produce similar adverse effects, and gastrointestinal intolerance is the most common adverse effect observed, despite claims that they are better tolerated than aspirin. They do cause less gastrointestinal microbleeding than aspirin and are better tolerated than aspirin by some patients (94–102). The ulcerogenic potential of these drugs has yet to be clearly defined. The incidence of central nervous system side-effects such as frontal headaches and dizziness is significant with indomethacin, and the incidence increases significantly with daily doses exceeding 100 mg (103). Toxic amblyopia is rarely reported with ibuprofen therapy, and diarrhea may be more common with meclofenamate therapy (103).

These drugs are primarily metabolized in the liver to inactive metabolites which are subsequently eliminated in the urine (88–93,104–106).

Oxyphenbutazone is an active metabolite of phenylbutazone (26), and sulindac is a pro-drug which is metabolized in the liver to the active entity (104). The active metabolite undergoes significant enterohepatic circulation which accounts, in part, for sulindac's prolonged elimination half-life. Naproxen serum levels do not increase significantly with doses above 1000 mg daily. Apparently a renal threshold exists, and following large doses, naproxen is simply excreted unchanged in the urine (106). The elimination half-lives for these drugs vary from 2 hours for indomethacin to 38 hours for piroxicam (see Table 2). Thus, dosing frequencies vary from one to four times daily.

In summary, these drugs approach aspirin in effectiveness, but none is superior to aspirin. These NSAIDs induce less gastrointestinal intolerance and produce less gastric microbleeding than aspirin. However, the cost of therapy with these agents is significantly higher than treatment with aspirin. Thus, these drugs are effective alternates for patients who do not otherwise tolerate aspirin. This patient tolerates aspirin and it is producing the desired results. Therefore, switching

Table 2.

NSAIDs UTILIZED IN RHEUMATOID ARTHRITIS

Drug	Dosage Forms	Half-life (hrs)	Regimen	Usual Daily Doses	Maximum Daily Dose	Average* Wholesale Cost/Month ($)
Ibuprofen	300, 400, 600 mg tablets	1–3	qid	2400	3200	23.70
Fenoprofen	300, 600 mg capsules	2.5	qid	2400	3200	26.30
Naproxen	250, 375 mg tablets	13	bid	750	1000	25.60
Indomethacin	25, 50 mg capsules	2	qid	100	200	18.95
Tolmetin	200, 400 mg tablets	1	qid	1200	1600	23.00
Sulindac	150, 200 mg tablets	18	bid	300	400	18.62
Piroxicam	10 mg capsules	38	qd	10	20	**
Meclofenamate	50, 100 mg capsules	2	qid	300	400	17.10

*Wholesale cost based on usual daily doses. Actual patient cost will vary based upon dosage form, total daily dose and pharmacy mark-up.

**Had not been released at time of publication.

to piroxicam or another NSAID is not indicated for this patient.

13. A patient with rheumatoid arthritis has been placed on an aspirin regimen of three tablets four times daily. After three days of therapy, the patient has discontinued treatment due to severe abdominal pain. Her physician wishes to try her on one of the NSAIDs. Which one should be used?

The NSAID of choice would be an agent that is effective, well tolerated, unlikely to produce serious toxicity, and inexpensive. Because of potential for serious toxicity, phenylbutazone, oxyphenbutazone, and mefenamic acid are usually avoided where chronic treatment is indicated (26,107). The incidence of central nervous system side-effects precludes the use of optimal anti-inflammatory doses of indomethacin in many patients (103). Some have even questioned the efficacy of indomethacin in the management of rheumatoid arthritis (108). Trials comparing NSAIDs with each other in the management of rheumatoid arthritis are few, and the conclusions reached in these studies are subject to the same limitations that apply to studies comparing aspirin to various NSAIDs. Several double-blind crossover trials comparing indomethacin with naproxen noted that the two drugs were equally effective, but naproxen caused fewer side effects (109–112). Two crossover trials have compared ibuprofen, fenoprofen, and naproxen in patients with rheumatoid arthritis (113,114). In these studies, naproxen was most effective and ibuprofen was least effective. Naproxen was also tolerated the best. Despite the results of these trials, individuals vary both in their response and their ability to tolerate these drugs (113,115). Cost and convenience of administration are also considerations in the selection of a NSAID. (See Table 2.) A NSAID which can be administered only once or twice daily may enhance compliance.

In this patient, Naproxen, which may be dosed twice daily, can be tried first. Naproxen is well-tolerated and effective. It has another advantage of a possible enhanced effect with aspirin in patients who can tolerate this drug (See Question 21). Sulindac and meclofenamate are less expensive, but both drugs bear structural similarities to NSAIDs with more toxic effects. If this patient is unresponsive to naproxen, another NSAID may be tried because, as noted previously, patients vary in their response to these agents.

14. *Fluid Retention.* A patient with congestive heart failure treated with digitoxin 0.1 mg/day, furosemide 40 mg/day, and supplemental potassium presents with a prescription for a week of treatment of phenylbutazone following an acute flare-up of her arthritis. What information should be provided to this patient?

Phenylbutazone should be used with great caution in this patient because cardiac decompensation and pulmonary edema are recognized adverse reactions to phenylbutazone therapy (26). Frank edema may occur during the first two weeks of therapy in 10% of patients and is generally more likely in those with preexisting cardiac disease (6). In some cases, plasma volume may increase by up to 50%. The mechanism by which edema formation occurs is unknown. Local prostaglandin synthesis in the kidney may play a prominent role in regulating renal blood flow, especially in patients with lupus renal disease, congestive heart failure, or liver disease with ascites (130–132). Thus, when a prostaglandin inhibitor such as phenylbutazone is administered, renal blood flow is decreased and renal tubular reabsorption of sodium is increased. Not surprisingly, other NSAIDs also decrease renal function and increase fluid retention in these patients (133–135).

An additional factor to consider in this patient is that phenylbutzaone is a potent inducer of hepatic microsomal enzymes. A significant fall in digitoxin blood levels may occur with concomitant administration of phenylbutazone (136). Although not well documented, the possibility of this drug interaction should be considered. Thus, this patient should be advised to contact her physician if she notes swelling in her ankles, increasing shortness of breath, or increased dyspnea on exertion. The patient should weigh herself daily to detect any fluid retention before it becomes clinically apparent.

15. Why is treatment with phenylbutazone limited to short-term management of acute inflammatory disorders?

Serious hematological adverse reactions appear to occur more frequently with phenylbutazone and its active metabolite, oxyphenbutazone, than with other NSAIDs. Of 1,276 adverse reactions to phenylbutazone which were reported to the United Kingdom Committee on Safety of Medicines, 398 involved blood disorders and 205 of these were fatal (107). Although leukopenia and thrombocytopenia have been observed, most fatalities resulted from aplastic anemia or agranulocytosis (137–139). Because of the potential for severe hematological complications, in addition to an increased risk of edema formation, toxic hepatitis, and frequent gastrointestinal complications, phenylbutazone and oxyphenbutazone should be limited to short-term therapy of not more than one week during any one treatment period (26).

Gold

16. *Progressive Rheumatoid Arthritis.* **A 52-year-old woman with rheumatoid arthritis has been treated with a conservative program of rest, physical therapy, and anti-inflammatory doses of aspirin for eight months. Despite good compliance to her treatment, her disease has continued to progress as evidenced by more intensive joint involvement and worsening of her constitutional symptoms. Increasing ankle pain and swelling have forced her to consider seeking employment which would require her to spend less time on her feet. Inflammation and tenderness in her hands are particularly severe and are approaching the same levels experienced prior to treatment. Additionally, she is now complaining of dry eyes and mouth.**

X-ray examination revealed soft tissue swelling of the feet and hands, narrowing of the joint spaces, and erosions of the second and third metacarpophalangeal joints bilaterally. Abnormal laboratory data included a positive rheumatoid factor in a dilution of 1:1280, a Westergren erythrocyte sedimentation rate of 65 mm/hr, a hemoglobin of 9.8 gm/dl, hematocrit of 31%, and a serum ablumin of 3.8 gm/dl. Her salicylate level was 22 mg/dl.

At this point, it is decided to begin her on gold while continuing her basic conservative management. Why was gold prescribed for this patient's rheumatoid arthritis? What other drugs might be considered for this patient?

The majority of patients with rheumatoid arthritis can be controlled with conservative management consisting of physical therapy, adequate rest, and appropriate use of salicylates or NSAIDs. However, many patients who have progressive disease that remains uncontrolled despite optimal management with these measures may benefit from more aggressive treatment. The choice of therapy is determined by assessing the relative risk versus benefit ratio of the treatment alternatives. For example, glucocorticoids are the most potent anti-inflammatory drugs currently available, but chronic therapy is associated with serious long term adverse effects (140). In addition, glucocorticoids do not seem to alter the natural history of rheumatoid arthritis (141). Gold is an effective anti-inflammatory agent in the management of rheumatoid arthritis and may significantly slow or halt the progression of joint disease (142–147). Potentially serious adverse effects are associated with gold therapy but are usually reversible and seldom lead to complications if the patient is monitored appropriately.

Gold is most likely to be effective when employed early in the course of progressive disease (145). In one study of 57 gold-treated patients who were followed for 5 to 6 years, early initiation of gold therapy was clearly correlated with arrest of joint erosions. The greatest success was obtained in those in whom gold was initiated within 10 months after the onset of rheumatoid arthritis (147). However, gold is not employed in mild disease because of its potential for adverse drug reactions (152).

Gold therapy is a rational choice in this patient because of the progressive nature of her disease despite conservative management and anti-inflammatory doses of aspirin. The gold should be added to her present therapeutic plan (25) because its effectiveness is additive to that obtained from salicylates or non-steroidal anti-inflammatory drugs (153). Several months will pass before this patient begins to benefit from the gold (143).

Antimalarials, azathioprine, penicillamine, chlorambucil, and cyclophosphamide are reasonable alternatives to gold therapy in this patient. Weekly 50 mg injections of gold or daily oral doses of azathioprine 1.0 to 2.0 mg/kg were slightly more effective than 250 mg/day of chloroquine in a study of 33 patients after 24 weeks of treatment. Although gold and azathioprine produced comparable results in this study, the investigators considered gold to be the treatment of first choice in progressive disease unresponsive to salicylates alone (148). In another six month study (149), gold and penicillamine were equally effective in 86 patients, but more side effects were noted in the latter treatment group (149). In yet another study of 171 patients, complete remissions were more commonly associated with gold than with penicillamine or cyclophosphamide. Excellent responses were obtained with cyclophosphamide, but fears of malignancy limited its use early in the course of this disease (150). Cyclophosphamide 1.5 mg/kg/day also was noted to be marginally more effective than gold or azathioprine in the early treatment of progressive rheumatoid arthritis (151). In conclusion, comparative clinical trials suggest that gold is more effective than antimalarials, equal to penicillamine and azathioprine, but less effective than cyclophosphamide. Nevertheless, gold, penicillamine, and/or antimalarials are preferred by most practitioners over cyclophosphamide and other immunosuppressive agents, because this latter group of drugs are associated with increased risks of malignancy and devastating opportunistic infections. Furthermore, cytotoxic therapy should be avoided by young patients who are in the childbearing periods of their lives.

17. Comment on this woman's complaint of dry eyes and dry mouth. Will this alter her response to gold?

These symptoms are suggestive of Sjögren's syndrome, a chronic inflammatory disease of the salivary, lacrimal, and other glands. It is associated with a variety of connective tissure diseases and occurs in about 10 to 15% of those with rheumatoid arthritis. The treatment is usually symptomatic. The presence of these symptoms has been considered by some to be a contraindication to gold therapy (154). Evidently, this recommendation was based on a widely quoted but poorly controlled study which demonstrated a high incidence of gold toxicity in a small number of patients with Sjögren's syndrome. However, a review of 101 gold-treated patients, 41 of whom had Sjögren's syndrome, failed to demonstrate an association between Sjögren's syndrome and an increased risk of gold toxicity (155). In this review, patients with Sjögren's syndrome appeared to tolerate gold therapy better than those without the syndrome.

18. Gold Preparations. Which gold preparation should be used in this patient?

Two gold preparations are in wide use: gold sodium thiomalate (Myochrysine), an aqueous so-lution, and aurothioglucose (Solganol), an oil suspension. Each contains approximately 50% gold and dosages are expressed as milligrams of the salt. Both compounds are equally efficacious (152). Findings that aurothioglucose is superior in efficacy to gold sodium thiomalate are not supported by appropriate statistical analysis (156).

A vasomotor reaction (also termed nitritoid reaction), which frequently manifests as nausea, weakness, flushing, tachycardia, and/or syncope, may occur in up to 5% of patients receiving gold sodium thiomalate. These reactions are generally mild, transient, and frequently can be alleviated by having the patient lie down. Rarely, severe myocardial ischemia or infarction may result (157,158). The etiology of this reaction is unknown but may be related to the vehicle or preservative in the thiomalate preparation. It has not been reported to occur with aurothioglucose.

Non-vasomotor reactions, consisting of transient stiffness, arthralgias and myalgias, also developed in 15 of 100 patients following initiation of gold sodium thiomalate therapy in one retrospective study (159). The gold sodium thiomalate was replaced with aurothioglucose, and in six of these patients, the reactions decreased in severity after five injections of aurothioglucose. Although these reactions may have been related to chrysotherapy, they are also consistent with active rheumatoid arthritis that was subsequently controlled with continued therapy. In another series of 125 patients receiving either aqueous suspension or oil suspension of gold salts, a higher incidence of skin eruptions, stomatitis, and albuminuria was reported among these patients receiving the aqueous gold sodium thiomalate preparation (160). However, weekly doses ranged from 50 to 200 mg and may have have contributed to the differences in observed toxicity. Moreover, certain individuals may be predisposed to the nephrotoxicity of gold (161). Thus, dosing techniques and diffferences in patient population are important in evaluating adverse gold reactions.

In summary, both preparations probably are equally effective; however, the nitritoid reactions appear to be a unique side effect associated with gold sodium thiomalate. Therefore, patients with concomitant cardiovascular disease or patients who experience a nitritoid reaction following an injection of gold sodium thiomalate can be safely managed with aurothioglucose. In this patient, therapy can be initiated with either preparation.

19. *Dosage of Gold Salts.* What would be appropriate initial doses of gold for this patient and should her serum gold levels be monitored?

The standard treatment schedule for gold therapy consists of weekly intramuscular injections of 50 mg after initial 10 and 25 mg test doses. Treatment is continued until the total dose reaches one gram, or until toxicity occurs. If a satisfactory response has been achieved after one gram, maintenance doses of 50 mg every other week are administered. The interval between injections is gradually increased until 50 mg injections are administered monthly. These monthly injections continue for as long as the patient continues to respond (152,162).

Variations of this standard treatment regimen, such as increasing the weekly dose by 25% (156) or to 1 mg/kg (163), are not advantageous, and toxicity increases with these larger doses. The minimally effective dose for gold therapy has yet to be defined. A preliminary double-blind trial comparing a 10 mg weekly dose with a 50 mg weekly dose suggested that the smaller dose may be equally effective (165). Additional evidence is needed to confirm the efficacy of these smaller doses of gold.

Serum concentrations of gold have been measured by atomic absorption spectroscopy to assess if therapeutic response is related to "optimal" serum concentrations (166–167). Although some believe that clinical response is related to optimal serum gold concentrations (167–169), this has not been confirmed by retrospective and prospective studies (164,170–175). Furthermore, toxicity has not been correlated with serum gold concentrations (170,171,175).

Thus, the standard treatment schedule described above should be used for this patient.

20. *Monitoring for Adverse Reactions to Gold.* What subjective or objective patient data should be monitored to detect gold adverse reactions?

Patients receiving weekly gold injections should have a urinalysis and complete blood counts evaluated at least every other week. In addition, the patient should be interviewed each week prior to the gold injection to detect the occurrence of pruritus, skin eruptions, purpura, sore throat, and other symptoms of gold toxicity (162).

Cutaneous reactions are by far the most common manifestations of gold toxicity. Pruritus, erythema, or a fine morbilliform rash on the neck or extremities may develop after the first few injections. This reaction usually subsides within several days and does not seem to be affected by subsequent injections. Other dermatological reactions frequently appear as oral ulcerations or as various pruritic rashes at a cumulative dose of 300 to 800 mg (176). Although a highly pruritic localized eruption resembling pityriasis rosea is common, gold dermatitis may assume many different forms. Rarely, exfoliative dermatitis may occur (162,177). Therapy should be discontinued if dermatitis develops, but gold may be reintroduced in a reduced dosage schedule when the rash has cleared (see Question 23).

Mild and transient *proteinuria* during gold treatment does not mandate a discontinuation of therapy; however, gold treatments should stop when proteinuria is in excess of 1,000 mg/24hours. Nephrotic syndrome may occur, but it is reversible when gold therapy is stopped (177). A membranous glomerulopathy with immune complex deposition and vacuolar degeneration of epithelial cells in proximal tubules (176) is commonly noted upon renal biopsy in patients with gold nephropathy.

Blood count. Less than 3500 WBC/mm^3, a rapid reduction of hemoglobin, or less than 100,000 platelets are indications to stop gold therapy (152,176). Although eosinophilia is commonly associated with toxic reactions (178), it is not a reliable predictor of gold toxicity (176) and does not represent a need to discontinue gold therapy. In addition, eosinophilia merely may be a manifestation of rheumatoid arthritis.

Thrombocytopenia may be life-threatening and is sometimes difficult to treat because of the long half-life of gold (179). A number of cases have responded to cessation of gold therapy and the administration of steroids (180). Platelet transfusion may be necessary if hemorrhage is a problem (176,180). Other unusual but serious complications of gold therapy include colitis, pneumonitis, and hepatitis (184–187).

Chelating agents, such as dimercaprol (BAL) and penicillamine are of unproven benefit in the treatment of gold toxicity (176,181,182). Substantial removal of gold by peritoneal dialysis has been reported but more study of this technique is needed (183).

21. *Combination Therapy.* Several months usually elapse before therapeutic benefits can

be expected from gold therapy. Can a NSAID or glucocorticoid be added to this patient's aspirin therapy to control the pain and inflammation in the meantime? Will these drugs interact with aspirin in an adverse way?

This patient should continue aspirin therapy because she is tolerating it well and currently has optimal anti-inflammatory salicylate levels. An appropriate regimen of physical therapy and rest should be continued. Another drug may be added to provide symptomatic relief until she begins to respond to gold.

The addition of another *NSAID* to aspirin therapy has been utilized to achieve a greater anti-inflammatory response. However, the efficacy of adding another NSAID to optimal anti-inflammatory doses of aspirin remains to be demonstrated by controlled trials. Furthermore, the possibility of drug interactions must be considered when combining aspirin with other drugs. Finally, the risk of increased toxicity, particularly to the gastrointestinal tract must be considered. In an eight-week double-blind crossover study involving 36 patients with rheumatoid arthritis, aspirin plus placebo was compared to aspirin plus naproxen (188). In this study, the aspirin-naproxen combination was more effective and as well tolerated as aspirin alone. However, all patients were not receiving optimal anti-inflammatory doses of aspirin. Patients who were receiving larger aspirin doses were less likely to benefit from the addition of naproxen. Thus, the question of whether addition of another NSAID to optimal doses of aspirin is of benefit remains unanswered and additional studies are necessary.

Drug interactions between aspirin and some of the NSAIDs need to be clarified. Some investigators have found that aspirin impairs the absorption of indomethacin (189–190), while others have been unable to confirm this effect (191–193). All of the NSAIDs are highly protein bound and drug displacement from protein by either aspirin or another NSAID might enhance metabolism of the displaced drug (196). Concomitant aspirin administration lowers the average blood levels of ibuprofen, naproxen, and, most dramatically, fenoprofen (190,197). However, the clinical significance of these reports awaits additional studies.

The toxicity associated with aspirin-NSAID combinations has not been adequately assessed. However, if additive beneficial pharmacologic effects of these combinations are anticipated, additive toxicities also should be expected. Until appropriate studies appear, a NSAID may be empirically added to this patient's therapy.

Glucocorticoids usually are beneficial when added to aspirin therapy in the treatment of inflammatory manifestations of rheumatoid arthritis (140). However, they have no effect on the factors that initiate inflammation. Patients with rheumatoid arthritis who have been treated with glucocorticoids for two to five years display laboratory abnormalities, joint symptoms, and progression of disease similar to those treated with aspirin alone (140,141,198–200). In addition, chronic steroid therapy is associated with a wide spectrum of adverse effects in these patients: osteoporosis, aseptic necrosis of bone, and steroid myopathy may be particularly pronounced (140). Consequently, glucocorticoids are usually withheld until a good basic program has failed or extra-articular manifestations develop. In the latter instance glucocorticoids may be life-saving.

The possibility of an aspirin-glucocorticoid interaction also should be considered. Glucocorticoids decrease serum salicylate concentrations by inducing the hepatic metabolism of salicylate and/or by increasing its renal excretion. Dosage adjustments may be necessary following addition of a steroid (21,201).

Small doses of an intermediate acting glucocorticoid such as prednisone may be justified in this patient until a response from gold is achieved because her arthritis is disabling despite a comprehensive treatment program (176). This therapy may allow her continued employment. As soon as the beneficial effects of gold become apparent, the glucocorticoid should then be slowly tapered and discontinued. Unfortunately, this is not always possible, and the glucocorticoid dosage is then tapered to the lowest possible maintenance level.

22. *Adverse Reactions to Gold Salts.* After 10 weeks of treatment with aurothioglucose (total 435 mg), this patient developed pruritus and a rash on her abdomen. Gold was withheld and she was given a prescription for triamcinolone cream. Should this patient's gold therapy be discontinued?

Dermatological reactions to gold occur in 15 to 20% of patients (202). The mechanism is unknown. Because of fears of subsequent exfoliative dermatitis, many clinicians have abandoned gold therapy after the appearance of dermatitis or stomatitis. However, Klinefelter has described successful reinstitution of gold in 28 of 30 patients who developed dermatological reactions (202). Interestingly, one of these patients presented initially with severe exfoliative dermatitis. Many years had elapsed before she was rechallenged with gold, but it ultimately brought her arthritis under control. The approach that was used for reinstitution of gold therapy was as follows: After waiting at least six weeks after the lesions had healed completely, a 1 mg test dose was given intramuscularly. At intervals of two to four weeks the dose was increased from 1 to 2 mg, then from 2 to 5 mg, then to 10 mg. Thereafter, 5 mg increments were added until a dose of 50 mg weekly was attained. There was no additional gold toxicity in any of the 28 patients whose gold was reinstituted in this manner. Because of the potential benefit of subsequent treatment, gold therapy need not be abandoned in this patient.

23. Duration of Gold Therapy. This patient responded well to gold therapy and now, one year later, her rheumatoid arthritis is in remission. She is currently receiving monthly gold shots. How long should treatment be continued?

Treatment should continue indefinitely to sustain the remission because progression of the disease can be slowed. Seventy-three percent of patients who continued chrysotherapy for three years continued to experience excellent responses (203). Only 6% of patients who had received chrysotherapy for less than 18 months in this study were in "spontaneous" remission at the end of three years. Moreover, patients who initially responded during the first 20 weeks of gold treatments achieved better responses if maintenance therapy was continued. Other patients have been maintained in remission for many years with continued gold injections (204–206).

24. Poor Response to Gold Therapy. A 60-year-old man with rheumatoid arthritis of three years' duration has been receiving weekly gold injections for 20 weeks with neither toxicity nor therapeutic benefit. He has now received a cumulative dosage of 1 gram. Should this patient's gold therapy be discontinued?

This patient has received an adequate trial of gold therapy and should be considered a therapeutic failure. However, one prospective study

suggested that continuing gold therapy might prove beneficial in some patients (156). As part of this study, patients who failed to improve after 20 weeks of therapy were given weekly injections of 150% of the initial dose for eight additional weeks; if no response was noted, the dose was then increased to twice the original dose for four additional weeks. Nearly half of the non-responders subsequently achieved a satisfactory clinical response without an increase in toxicity. Although these findings are promising, this patient should be treated with another slow-acting antirheumatic drug such as penicillamine or an antimalarial.

Antimalarial Drugs

25. Dose. A middle-aged, 75 kg woman who had been treated with aspirin for approximately three years, is to receive hydroxychloroquine treatment for her rheumatoid arthritis. What doses would be appropriate and when should patient improvement be expected?

Chloroquine and hydroxychloroquine dosages have ranged from 250 to 800 mg daily. More recently, hydroxychloroquine has been employed at dosages of 2 to 4 mg/kg/day (176), although an upper limit of 3.5 mg/kg/day of hydroxychloroquine may be prudent (207). About two-thirds of patients who tolerate these antimalarial drugs will respond favorably; however, 6 to 12 weeks usually elapse before improvement is apparent (208). These antimalarials slow the rate of deterioration of functional capacity, induce a decline in rheumatoid factor, and lower serum globulin levels (148,209–212).

26. Risk of Antimalarial-Induced Retinopathy. How great is the risk of retinopathy from antimalarials when used for the treatment of rheumatoid arthritis? What monitoring procedures are appropriate?

All of the 4-amino-quinolines are capable of causing permanent and sometimes progressive loss of vision from retinopathy. This retinopathy appears to be dose-related; hydroxychloroquine, which became available after chloroquine had been in wide use, appears to be no safer than chloroquine in this regard (208,215). Hydroxychloroquine 200 mg, is approximately equivalent to chloroquine 250 mg.

Retinal lesions were noted in 8 of 45 patients who had been taking 250 to 750 mg of chloroquine daily for more than one year (216). In contrast, only two cases of retinal changes (without visual impairment) developed in 408 patients taking no more than 250 mg of chloroquine and 400 mg of hydroxychloroquine daily for one to nine years (217). One case of chloroquine-induced retinopathy was noted among 270 consecutive patients treated with 250 mg per day, 10 months annually for up to 15 years (218). In yet another report, only 6 of 2000 patients had retinal changes (207). Sixty-five of the patients in this report had consumed more than a kilogram of chloroquine, and none of the 2000 patients had experienced any loss of vision due to the drug.

Symptoms of chloroquine retinopathy are blurred vision, night blindness, and, eventually, scotomas (176). The fully developed lesion of chloroquine retinopathy is seen on ophthalmoscopy as a pigmentary disturbance with a characteristic "bulls eye" appearance in the macular region (176,208). Because chloroquines bind to melanin, they concentrate in the uveal tract and retinal pigment epithelium. Thus, chloroquines are retained for years in the retina, and retinopathy may be progressive even after stopping the drug. In two instances visual disturbances from chloroquine retinopathy did not occur until several years after the therapy had been discontinued (219).

Currently, eye examinations at six month intervals are recommended in order to detect a "premaculopathy" stage which is reversible when the drug is discontinued (208,220,221). Baseline patient studies should include an ophthalmologic examination and testing of paracentral visual fields to red test objects (176).

Benign corneal deposits of antimalarial drug also may occur in about 10% of patients (217). If this keratopathy is not annoying, therapy may be continued. This is a harmless side effect which can be reversed by withdrawal of the drug and is not related to the more serious and less frequent retinopathy.

This risk of drug-induced retinopathy must be weighed against the satisfactory, although not spectacular, benefits achievable with these antimalarials (223). Regular ophthalmologic examinations and conservative dosing can minimize this risk. The use of dark sunglasses in bright sunlight might also be helpful, because deposits of drug in the eye seem to impair the normal retinal defense mechanisms against light (207). Likewise, discontinuation of these antimalarials during two of the brightest summer months also has been recommended (218).

Penicillamine

27. M.M. is a 55-year-old man with progressive rheumatoid arthritis which has not been responsive to gold. Salicylates and other nonsteroidal anti-inflammatory drugs do not provide adequate control of his arthritis. Would penicillamine therapy be indicated for this patient? How should it be dosed and when is a response expected?

Penicillamine is effective for the treatment of rheumatoid arthritis (224–227). The initial British Multicentre Trial demonstrated that penicillamine at doses of 1.5 gms per day was effective, but adverse reactions occurred in 40% of these patients (226). Since then, smaller doses have been utilized successfully with fewer side effects (224,225). Currently, a "go low, go slow" approach is recommended (228). Most practitioners initiate penicillamine at 250 mg per day and increase the dosage after a minimum of four weeks to 500 mg day. If no response is observed after an additional four to eight weeks, the dosage is increased to 750 mg daily. Increasing the dosage to 1000 mg rarely is attempted in patients who are refractory to doses of 750 mg daily (176,228). As with gold and the antimalarials, two to three months of therapy are usually necessary before a response becomes apparent. Failure to respond to previous gold therapy does not appear to lessen the likelihood of a response to penicillamine (229,230). However, previous toxicity to gold therapy has been associated with an increased likelihood of toxicity to penicillamine therapy (231). Others have disputed this association (229,230).

28. *Adverse Reaction from Penicillamine.* M.M. has been receiving penicillamine for three months and is currently taking 750 mg daily. A routine urinalysis reveals 4+ proteinuria and a 24 hour quantitative urine reveals 2.3 grams of protein. Should future treatment with penicillamine be abandoned?

Proteinuria occurs in 5 to 26% of patients receiving penicillamine and primarily occurs between the sixth and twelfth month of therapy

(231–238). It appears to be related both to the duration of therapy and to the rate at which the penicillamine dosage is increased. Increasing the dosage slowly during initiation of therapy (222,228,229), or a small reduction in the daily dosage may reverse mild proteinuria (234). However, the appearance of more than two grams of protein in the urine is an indication to stop therapy (234). Although penicillamine-induced proteinuria is reversible, resolution may be slow (228,235). Proteinuria also may be accompanied by hematuria which seems to be related to the severity of renal involvement.

Reintroduction of penicillamine in patients who previously developed proteinuria usually is followed by a return of proteinuria at about the same time and at about the same cumulative dose as on the first occasion (239). Nevertheless, penicillamine was reinitiated successfully in five patients when 50 mg daily doses were increased at monthly intervals until a maintenance dose of 150 mg daily was achieved. After four months, incremental 50 mg doses were added at three month intervals if necessary (240). Thus, rechallenging M.M. with penicillamine is likely to result in recurrent proteinuria unless the penicillamine is reinitiated in very low doses over a prolonged period of time. However, most clinicians would prefer another antirheumatic drug in this situation.

29. What other side effects may occur during therapy with penicillamine?

A number of other adverse effects are associated with penicillamine therapy. *Rashes* are the most frequent complications and may present as scaly, maculopapular eruptions, diffuse erythrodermas, pruritus without rash, or lichenoid eruptions (235,237). "Early" rashes are generally erythematous eruptions resembling ampicillin rashes, and "late" rashes are generally intensely pruritic, discrete, and appear as scaly macules with reddish edges after five to twelve months of therapy (234).

Hematologic toxicities include leukopenia, agranulocytosis, aplastic anemia, and thrombocytopenia (234–237,241,242). Thrombocytopenia is the most common and frequently appears between the sixth and twelfth months of therapy (234,235,237).

Nausea, vomiting, and alterations in the sense of taste also occur early in the course of therapy.

Abnormalities of taste usually resolve with continued therapy and are not an indication to discontinue therapy (234). Finally, obliterative bronchiolitis, which was irreversible in some cases, has been reported in association with penicillamine treatment (236,237).

30. After one year of successful therapy with penicillamine, 750 mg per day, a patient complains of increasing weakness that is worse in the afternoon than in the morning. In addition, several of his friends have observed that his eyelids are drooping. Are these symptoms related to his therapy or to systemic manifestations of his arthritis?

Lupus erythematosus, myasthenia gravis, Goodpasture's syndrome, and dermatomyositis are rare but potentially serious toxicities that have been reported following long-term penicillamine therapy (243–247). Because all of these disorders are associated with immunological abnormalities, penicillamine may alter the immunologic response of some individuals. This patient's complaints are consistent with penicillamine-induced myasthenia gravis, and therapy should be withheld until this possibility has been evaluated.

Cytotoxic Drugs

31. This patient proved to have myasthenia gravis which was believed to be related to penicillamine therapy. Following discontinuation of the drug, his symptoms resolved. However, his rheumatoid arthritis has become increasingly active despite optimal aspirin therapy and the addition of prednisone 7.5 mg daily to his treatment regimen. Immunosuppressive agents are being considered. Which ones are most commonly used? What are their doses and toxicities? Which one is indicated for this patient?

The immunosuppressive agents azathioprine, cyclosphosphamide, or chlorambucil are effective in the treatment of severe progressive cases of rheumatoid arthritis, but they are also more toxic (151,248–258). Although daily *cyclophosphamide* 1.7 mg/kg was proven effective, it also was associated with a high degree of toxicity (250,252). As a result smaller doses are commonly used in order to reduce toxicity (257,258). Despite continuing controversy as to the efficacy of these smaller cyclophosphamide doses (252,257), some data suggest that low-dose cyclophosphamide therapy (1 mg/kg) is effective, and therefore, treatment should be initiated at this lower dose. Serious toxicities associated with cyclophosphamide therapy include leukopenia, alopecia, hemorrhagic cystitis, infections, herpes zoster, sterility, and bladder cancer (250,252,254,257–265).

Azathioprine is administered in doses of 0.75 to 2.5 mg/kg/day in the management of rheumatoid arthritis (255,266,267). In order to reduce the incidence of toxicity, therapy is usually initiated with small doses which are subsequently increased if needed after several months of therapy. Serious toxicities associated with azathioprine therapy include leukopenia, thrombocytopenia, macrocytic anemia, pancreatitis, liver damage, and rashes (251,256,268,269). Because azathioprine is relatively less toxic than cyclophosphamide, it is often preferred.

Chlorambucil is sometimes used in doses of 0.01 to 0.02 mg/kg/day initially. Subsequent doses are adjusted according to the leukocyte count (248). Leukopenia is the predominant toxicity with this drug and it must be monitored carefully. As with cyclophosphamide and azathioprine, a lag period of at least two to three months occurs prior to objective improvement of the arthritis (248).

The potential dangers of malignancy as a result of long-term therapy with immunosuppressive drugs is of considerable concern (270). Malignancy among immunosuppressed renal transplant patients is well documented, although some have attributed this increased malignancy to the possible oncogenic effects of foreign graft tissue or uremia in combination with immunosuppressive therapy (271). When the causes of death among rheumatoid arthritics who were treated with cytotoxic drugs were compared to the causes of death among rheumatoid arthritics who were treated without these drugs, neoplasia, particularly lymphoproliferative disease, was substantially more frequent in those treated with cytotoxic drugs (272). Although the oncogenic potential of immunosuppressive drugs in patients with rheumatoid arthritis is only suggestive, the risk of malignancy should always be considered. Nevertheless, these agents have a definite place in the management of severe systemic manifestations of rheumatoid arthritis.

Of these three agents, azathioprine is probably the agent of choice for this patient based on its relative safety as compared to the other two agents.

SYSTEMIC LUPUS ERYTHEMATOSUS

Systemic lupus erythematosus (SLE) is a chronic inflammatory disorder of unknown etiology. It can affect various organs including the skin, kidneys, nervous system, serous membranes, and joints. Like rheumatoid arthritis, it also is characterized by remissions and exacerbations.

SLE appears to be distributed throughout the world's population, but females far outnumber males in the development of this disorder. The female:male ratio is approximately 5:1 (273,274). Blacks may have a higher incidence of SLE and may have more serious disease.

Pathophysiology, Signs and Symptoms

32. *SLE*. J.D. is a 23-year-old black woman who was in good health until six months prior to admission when she saw her physician because of a low grade fever, inflammation and pain of the hands, increasing fatigue, and headaches. At that time, her birth control pills were discontinued because they were a possible cause of her headaches. The pain and inflammation in the hands eventually resolved, but her feet subsequently became painful and swollen. Approximately two months ago she experienced an erythematous, macular rash that involved her arms and face. Since then she has had to avoid direct sunlight. On physical examination she had some mild swelling and pain in the knees and mild alopecia.

Laboratory studies revealed an erythrocyte sedimentation rate by the Westergren method of 35 mm/hr (normal less than 15 mm/hr); hemoglobin 10.6 grams/dl (normal 12 to 16 grams/dl); hematocrit 35.5% (normal 36 to 47%); WBC 7500 (normal 4000 to 10,000); platelets 250,000 (normal 140,000 to 400,000); BUN 50 mg/dl (normal 8 to 25 mg/dl); and creatinine 2.5 mg/dl (normal 0.6 to 1.5 mg/dl). A prothrombin time was 14.5 seconds (control 13.0) and partial thromboplastin time was 37.0 seconds (normal 33.5). A urinalysis revealed 3+ proteinuria and 5–10 RBCs per high field microscopically. A rheumatoid factor (RF) performed by latex fixation was negative; antinuclear antibody (ANA) was positive with a titer of 1:320, and a positive lupus erythe-

matosus (LE) prep was found. The patient was diagnosed as having systemic lupus erythematosus.

Following admission, a renal biopsy was performed which revealed diffuse proliferative glomerular nephritis. Treatment with 60 mg of prednisone daily was initiated.

What are the signs and symptoms of SLE?

The manifestations of SLE are protean, and individuals may present with a wide variety of signs and symptoms. The American Rheumatism Association (ARA) has developed and tested a set of classification criteria for identifying individuals with SLE. These are listed in Table 3. An individual who is positive for any four of these 14 criteria without another known explanation has greater than a 90% likelihood of having SLE (273).

Migratory polyarthralgias or arthritis are cardinal symptoms of SLE, occurring in more than 90% of patients and presenting as the first symptoms in approximately two-thirds of patients (274). These attacks may occur in any diarthrodal joint and are most frequently experienced in the knees, proximal interphalangeal joints, and metacarpophalangeal joints. Unlike rheumatoid arthritis, joint deformities are uncommon; when they do occur, erosive bone changes that typify the joint involvement in rheumatoid arthritis are not observed (274).

Dermatologic involvement is a major clinical feature in SLE. Most often observed is an erythematous, often symmetrical rash located on the face, neck, or extremities. The classic "butterfly rash" observed in some patients is characterized by distribution over the bridge of the nose and malar eminences of the face (273,274). Sometimes the rash takes the form of discoid lupus, which begins as erythematous patches and progresses into elevated, edematous plaques which are covered with grayish scales. Additionally, painless ulcerations involving mucous membranes of the mouth, pharynx, or vagina may occur. Alopecia is a characteristic finding.

In addition to the articular and dermatologic manifestations, a number of other organ systems may become involved. Pleuritis, pericarditis, and Raynaud's phenomenon are commonly reported. However, the most serious complications of SLE are nephritis and/or neurologic complications.

33. What laboratory abnormalities present in J.D. are typical of SLE? What other

Table 3.

PRELIMINARY CRITERIA FOR DIAGNOSIS
OF SYSTEMIC LUPUS ERYTHEMATOSUS

1. Facial Erythema (butterfly rash)

2. Discoid Lupus

3. Raynaud's Phenomenon

4. Alopecia

5. Photosensitivity

6. Oral or Nasopharyngeal Ulceration

7. Arthritis Without Deformity

8. LE Cells

9. Chronic False-Positive Serologic Test for Syphilis

10. Profuse Proteinuria (greater than 3.5 gm/day)

11. Cellular Casts in Urine

12. One or Both of the Following:
    Pleuritis
    Pericarditis

13. One or Both of the Following:
    Psychosis
    Convulsions

14. One or More of the Following:
    Hemolytic Anemia
    Leukopenia
    Thrombocytopenia

laboratory abnormalities are frequently encountered in patients suffering from SLE?

Some of the laboratory findings in SLE are similar to those of any chronic inflammatory disease. Other findings are relatively specific for SLE and aid in the diagnosis of this disorder. J.D.'s elevated ESR is a non-specific indication of inflammation. Her anemia is also typical for SLE. Like rheumatoid arthritis, the anemia is most frequently due to chronic inflammation (275). However, some individuals may develop an autoimmune hemolytic anemia. In addition, renal disease may contribute to the development of anemia in some patients, and occasionally iron-deficiency anemia may arise as a result of gastrointestinal blood loss secondary to drugs or chronic renal failure.

Leukopenia has been reported in almost half of patients with SLE (275). Although circulating granulocytes, lymphocytes, or both may be depressed, lymphopenia in active lupus erythematosus is common and may have pathogenic significance. Despite the reduction in absolute numbers of lymphocytes, the production of immunoglobulins is increased, and circulating antibodies to a number of "self antigens," including native DNA, are found. It is the circulating antibodies that are responsible for the positive ANA and LE prep found in J.D. The presence of a "circulating anticoagulant" which is believed to be an immunoglobulin that blocks activation of prothrombin to thrombin may lead to prolongation of the partial thromboplastin time and prothrombin time (275) which was observed in J.D. Significant bleeding is uncommon unless the circulating anticoagulant is accompanied by thrombocytopenia or an actual decrease in prothrombin. Thrombocytopenia has been reported in 14% to 26% of patients (275).

The presence of proteinuria, hematuria, and red blood cell casts in J.D.'s urine indicates active renal involvement. During active disease, the serum complement may also be depressed.

34. What types of renal complications are found in SLE?

The renal lesions of SLE can be categorized into three major histological types. These types correlate somewhat with clinical features and prognosis (276–279).

Focal proliferative lupus nephritis may be found in up to a third of the patients in whom biopsies are performed and is characterized by incomplete glomerular damage in less than 50% of the glomeruli. Histologically, the involved glomeruli reveal mesangial and segmental endothelial-cell proliferation and irregular thickening of capillary loops (274,276,278). Renal involvement is characterized clinically by microscopic hematuria, pyuria, and mild proteinuria. Patients with this type of renal disease rarely develop nephrotic syndrome, hypertension, or end stage renal disease (277,278).

Diffuse proliferative lupus nephritis differs from focal proliferative nephritis primarily by extent of involvement. More than 50% of glomeruli show changes of mesangial and segmental endothelial cell proliferation and irregular thickening of capillary loops. In addition, a broader spectrum of active lesions is found, including tubular and interstitial damage (247). Unlike focal proliferative lupus nephritis, nephrotic syndrome, hypertension, and renal insufficiency are frequent complications of diffuse proliferative lupus nephritis (276–278).

Membranous lupus nephritis is the least common of the lupus nephropathies. It is characterized by uniform thickening of the glomerular basement membrane of the capillary loops with little or no hypercellularity. On immunofluorescence, immune complexes are distributed in a fine granular pattern along the epithelial side of the glomerular basement membrane of all loops. Although hematuria, pyuria, and proteinuria may be observed, persistent proteinuria is more common, and most patients develop nephrotic syndrome sometime during the course of the disease (277). Although renal failure may develop in a large proportion of these patient after a number of years, the long-term prognosis remains relatively good.

This classification system is useful in that each group seems to have its own natural history and transitions from one group to another are considered rare (276). However, certain problems remain. First, it lacks the means to indicate the degree or extent of activity and chronicity of histologic lesions. Second, it provides no criteria to define changes in renal histology over time other than by change in class. Third, tubular, interstitial, and vascular changes are not sufficiently described. Finally, it becomes difficult to classify a biopsy into one of the three groups when patients have had lupus nephritis for long periods, particularly after immunosuppressive drugs have been administered (274).

Glucocorticoids

35. How should J.D. be managed? What is her prognosis?

Treatment for SLE is primarily suppressive, and the specific therapy depends upon the type and degree of involvement. Bedrest and avoidance of emotional stress are helpful (273). If articular manifestations are the primary problem, these can be managed with *aspirin* administered in anti-inflammatory doses as described earlier (273). *Antimalarials* are sometimes employed for generalized rashes or discoid lupus (273). The principles for use are the same as described for rheumatoid arthritis. Topical steroids may be used for localized skin involvement. Systemic *gluco-*

corticoids are required in varying doses to control other systemic manifestations of the disease.

Because of the serious nature of diffuse proliferative lupus nephritis, aggressive therapy utilizing glucocorticoids is indicated for J.D. Treatment is frequently initiated with 1 mg/kg/day of prednisone (273,280). Subsequent alterations in the dosage are based upon changes in renal status. If her renal function improves, the dosage can be tapered to the smallest dose that maintains a stable renal function. If no response is observed or her renal function continues to deteriorate, the dose of prednisone may be increased to 2 mg/kg/day (273). Eventually more than 50% of the patients treated will experience a partial or complete remission of renal abnormalities and can be controlled on maintenance steroids. In general, these maintenance doses are higher than those required to control other systemic manifestations of SLE. Alternate-day steroids are not effective in this form of lupus nephritis (281).

Despite aggressive therapy, the relapse rate is high (greater than 50%), and the prognosis is grave. Five-year survival rates for steroid-treated patients are only 20 to 25% (278,279,282,312). A majority of these deaths are related to renal disease. High-dose steroids have improved the overall survival rate for patients with serious kidney disease, but many patients with severe renal disease and extensive glomerular involvement remain refractory to steroids (283). Because of inadequate response to steroids administered in this manner and the fact that prolonged high-dose steroid therapy is associated with numerous side effects, other treatment regimens are being investigated. One such regimen involves giving an intravenous "pulse" of one gram of methylprednisolone daily for three days in an attempt to induce a rapid halt in the inflammatory response and thereby allow lower maintenance doses of prednisone to be used to control the disease and ultimately reduce the rate of renal deterioration (284–286). This approach is still investigational and controlled studies are necessary to determine if this approach is either more efficacious or less toxic than the traditional dosing regimens.

36. How are other forms of lupus nephritis managed?

Because of the relatively good prognosis for patients with focal proliferative nephritis, aggressive therapy is not indicated. Prednisone or an equivalent intermediate acting glucocorticoid can be initiated in low doses and titrated upward if necessary to control the renal manifestations of the disease (276). Alternate day steroid therapy is successful in this form of lupus nephritis (281). Many of these patients may not need medications (278).

For membranous lupus nephritis, steroid therapy is indicated, and the dose is titrated to control proteinuria.

Cytotoxic Drugs

37. J.D.'s renal function continued to deteriorate and her prednisone was increased to 120 mg daily. Four days later, her renal status had not improved. Would a cytotoxic agent be a useful addition to the treatment of her diffuse proliferative lupus nephritis?

Although cytotoxic drugs such as azathioprine, cyclophosphamide, and chlorambucil have been used in the treatment of diffuse proliferative lupus nephritis for over fifteen years, questions concerning efficacy, cytotoxic drug of choice, indications, and appropriate dosing methods still remain unanswered.

Azathioprine. Early uncontrolled observations suggested that azathioprine used alone or added to steroids in patients with lupus nephritis improved creatinine clearance, reduced proteinuria and hematuria, and normalized serum complement levels (287–294). However, the progression of diffuse proliferative lupus nephritis varies markedly, and the results of controlled clinical investigations are equivocal. In one of the earliest studies, the addition of azathioprine 2.5 mg/kg/day to prednisone therapy in 16 lupus patients reduced morbidity and mortality and improved renal function when compared to 19 control patients receiving prednisone alone (295). In addition, a steroid sparing effect was noted in the patients taking azathioprine. This study has been criticized for lack of renal biopsy information and because seven patients originally randomized to one of the treatment groups died during the initial hospitalization. Five of these patients were receiving azathioprine. In a follow-up report on the patients who had received azathioprine for at least 18 months, 7 of 9 experienced acute exacerbations of their lupus and required hospitalization within one to six months after discontinuation of azathioprine (296). Only one of the patients continued on azathioprine experienced an acute exacerbation. However, in only one patient was the acute exacerbation associated with reduced renal function. Exacerbations occurred in the form of cerebritis, pleuritis, arthritis, and rash in the other patients.

In another controlled trial, 50 patients with moderate to severe diffuse proliferative lupus nephritis were allocated to four treatment groups: high-dose steroids, azathioprine alone, azathioprine plus steroids, or azathioprine plus heparin (297). All regimens containing azathioprine improved renal function and survival significantly more than the regimen of high dose steroids alone. These impressive results have not been confirmed in other controlled studies (298–300). In one study, 16 patients with active lupus glomerulonephritis were prospectively and randomly assigned to receive azathioprine plus large doses of prednisone or large doses of prednisone alone for six months (298). Outcomes in both groups were similar. After three years, three patients in each group had experienced renal flares (299). No deaths occurred in either group, and azathioprine did not significantly reduce the daily steroid requirement. In another prospective, randomized trial, high-dose prednisone (60 mg/day initially) was compared to azathioprine 3–4 mg/kg/day plus high-dose prednisone in 24 patients with life-threatening SLE (300). During a mean follow-up of 18 to 24 months, no differences between the two groups were observed with respect to mortality, renal, or extrarenal manifestations of the disease. No steroid sparing effect was noted in the group receiving azathioprine.

In summary, the exact role of azathioprine in the treatment of diffuse proliferative lupus nephritis is unclear. Azathioprine alone or in combination with steroids may not be useful in treating acute renal flare-ups or in improving short-term survival. It remains to be demonstrated whether the addition of azathioprine to the treatment regimen of patients with diffuse proliferative lupus nephritis will be of any long-term benefit.

Cyclophosphamide. The role of cyclophosphamide in the treatment of diffuse proliferative lupus nephritis is also unclear. In one study, all five patients who received cyclophosphamide for lupus nephritis were treatment failures; all were then given prednisone and three responded (301). Subsequent short-term, double-blind studies in patients with diffuse proliferative lupus nephritis

indicated that cyclophosphamide 3–4 mg/kg/day in combination with prednisone produced greater improvement than azathioprine plus prednisone or prednisone plus placebo (302,303). In a two and a half year follow-up report of thirty-eight patients with diffuse proliferative glomerulonephritis who had been treated with either cyclophosphamide or azathioprine (up to 4.0 mg/kg/day), low dose corticosteroids, or nothing at all, the fewest unfavorable outcomes were observed in the cyclophosphamide group (304). However, the advantages of this regimen were minimal. Other studies (305,306) were equally non-conclusive.

Chlorambucil. In uncontrolled studies, chlorambucil therapy has also been associated with improved renal function in patients with lupus nephritis (307,308). Chlorambucil was used in these two studies because patients were steroid-toxic and chlorambucil was thought to be less toxic than other cytotoxic drugs.

In conclusion, the use of these drugs should still be considered investigational and reserved for steroid-resistant cases of diffuse proliferative lupus nephritis (309). The potential benefits from these agents must be balanced against the potential for severe drug toxicity. Complications of cytotoxic therapy include bone marrow suppression, increased incidence of opportunistic infections, and the possibility of increased risk of malignancies.

38. *CNS symptoms.* **Five days after her prednisone dosage was increased to 120 mg daily, J.D. became disoriented and began experiencing auditory hallucinations and paranoia. Are these central nervous system (CNS) manifestations of her disease? Should her prednisone be increased still further?**

Neuropsychiatric complications are second only to renal disease as a cause of death in lupus erythematosus (273). Organic mental syndromes and central neurologic involvement, excluding seizures, have the most unfavorable prognosis. In order of decreasing frequency, the neuropsychiatric complications include: (a) alterations in mental function, including organic brain syndrome, affective illnesses, and schizophrenia-like disorders; (b) transient or recurrent seizure disorders, mostly of the generalized motor type; (c) paralytic disease resulting from either ischemic or hemorrhagic events; (d) tremor, choreoathetoid, and ataxic disorders; (e) facial sensory, extraocular movements, and pupillary abnormalities; (f) peripheral neuropathies (274). Therefore, J.D.'s deteriorating mental status is consistent with the CNS manifestations of SLE, and her symptoms are of a type associated with a poorer prognosis. However, high-dose steroid therapy may also produce CNS adverse effects similar to J.D.'s symptoms (310). Thus, a dilemma arises as to whether the steroid dosage should be increased or decreased in this situation. Because of the time course for the onset of CNS symptoms following the increase in prednisone dosage, the decision was made to increase the dose still further to 150 mg daily. Her hallucinations gradually resolved over the next several days, and she became increasingly more oriented.

Drug-Induced SLE

39. Could J.D.'s birth control pills have caused her SLE? What other drugs have been implicated in causing SLE and how does drug-induced lupus differ from the idiopathic form?

A number of drugs, including oral contraceptives, have been implicated in the development of lupus syndrome (311–314). Of the drugs implicated, hydralazine, procainamide, and isoniazid appear to have the most pronounced capacity to induce an SLE syndrome (315). Of the other drugs that have been implicated in inducing syndromes, prospective data to support these claims are lacking (see Table 4).

Drug-induced lupus differs from idiopathic SLE in a number of respects. The incidence of drug-induced lupus is not higher in blacks, and there is less female preponderance (315). Arthralgias, myalgias, and polyarthritis are the most common manifestations of both drug-induced lupus and idiopathic SLE. However, malar rashes, oral ulcers, and alopecia are less common in the drug-induced lupus syndrome (315). Pulmonary involvement is common with procainamide and isoniazid (315). The most important difference between drug-induced lupus and idiopathic SLE is the rarity of renal involvement in drug-induced lupus (311,315). Finally, central nervous system complications appear to be less common in drug-induced SLE. Drug-induced lupus usually resolves following discontinuation of the drug, although serologic abnormalities such as anti-nuclear antibodies may remain positive for years.

A genetically controlled polymorphism of the hepatic acetyltransferase enzymes is responsible for different rates of inactivation of drugs such as hydralazine, procainamide, and isoniazid. People

Table 4.

DRUGS IMPLICATED
IN LUPUS SYNDROME

Anticonvulsants	Oral Contraceptives
Chlorpromazine	Penicillamine
Gold Salts	Penicillin
Griseofulvin	Practolol
Hydralazine	Procainamide
Isoniazid	Propylthiouracil
Lithium Carbonate	Quinidine
Methyldopa	Sulfonamides
Nitrofurantoin	

who metabolize these drugs slowly may be more susceptible to drug-induced lupus. For example, slow acetylators are more prone to develop anti-nuclear antibodies to hydralazine and presumably are more likely to develop hydralazine-induced lupus. In one study, a positive ANA developed in 60% of the slow acetylators who had taken less than 400 grams of hydralazine; whereas none of the rapid acelytators who had taken a similar total dose had detectable ANA (316). Moreover, almost all patients who develop clinical symptoms of hydralazine-induced lupus are slow acetylators (315,317). Although procainamide-induced lupus develops in both slow and rapid acetylators (318), slow acetylators who receive procainamide develop a positive ANA more quickly than rapid acetylators and may develop procainamide-induced lupus syndrome after a shorter duration of therapy (319). To date, acetylator phenotype has not been demonstrated to play a role in the development of anti-nuclear antibodies or symptoms of SLE in patients taking INH (315).

Although oral contraceptives have been implicated in inducing SLE-like syndromes, controlled data to support these findings are still lacking (314,315). In addition, the renal involvement exhibited by J.D. is not consistent with a drug-induced lupus syndrome. However, estrogens may exacerbate idiopathic SLE. Therefore, discontinuation of J.D.'s birth control pills was prudent.

DEGENERATIVE JOINT DISEASE

Degenerative joint disease is an extremely common, progressive disorder of movable joints, particularly weight-bearing joints (320). Degenerative joint disease occurs in all mammalian species, and more than 80% of all people over 55 years of age have radiological evidence of this disease (320,321).

Although equal numbers of males and females develop this disease, males are more likely to become afflicted prior to the age of 45 (320). However, females may suffer more severe disease such as primary generalized hypertrophic osteoarthritis, erosive osteoarthritis, and Heberden's nodes (320–321).

Degenerative joint disease is also termed osteoarthritis; the two terms are frequently used interchangeably. However, the term osteoarthritis incorrectly implies that this disease is an inherently inflammatory process.

40. *Degenerative Joint Disease.* G.R. is a 190-pound, 60-year-old school teacher who developed painful, tender swelling in the right knee approximately one year ago. Since then she has experienced intermittent pain in the right knee and hip. She now has moderate morning stiffness in the hip and knee and some joint stiffness after inactivity. Her pain is significantly increased by ambulation. Examination of her joints revealed the presence of Heberden's nodes in both hands, limitation of flexion of the right hip to 90°, no synovial thickening, patellar crepitus (grating of the joint), and some tenderness at the joint margin of the right knee. Laboratory studies were all normal and a rheumatoid factor was negative. What signs and symptoms of degenerative joint disease are manifested in G.R.?

Symptoms of degenerative joint disease are usually referable to the particular joint or joints involved. Common complaints include joint pain, particularly on motion and weight bearing joints, stiffness after periods of rest, and aching at times of inclement weather. Crepitation on joint motion, limitation of motion, and changes in the shape of the joint may be detected on physical examination. The joint(s) may be tender to palpation, but signs of inflammation are relatively uncommon, except for effusion, which may be noted following trauma or vigorous use of the involved joint (320). The Heberden's nodes observed in G.R.'s hands are bony protuberances at the margins on the dorsal surfaces of the distal interphalangeal joints. These nodes are more common in women, tend to occur in families, and are often associated with other joint involvement (320). Degenerative disease of the hip generally becomes progressively more severe and eventually range of motion is lost. Degenerative disease of the knee is frequently observed in older women and is associated with crepitus, loss of motion, and flexion deformities. Softening of the posterior surface of the patellar may also occur when the knee is involved (320).

In addition to the above characteristics, most of which were observed in G.R., other manifestations frequently observed are vertebral column involvement and the presence of Bouchard's nodes on the proximal interphalangeal joints.

Results of laboratory studies are usually normal unless an underlying disease co-exists. Rheumatoid factor is negative (320).

41. *Treatment.* How should G.R. be treated?

Because the etiology and much of the pathophysiology pertaining to degenerative joint disease remains unexplained, drug therapy is empiric and is directed toward providing symptomatic relief. A number of theories have tried to explain the pathogenesis of pain, because degenerating cartilage is devoid of pain receptors. The possibility of a prostaglandin-mediated pain mechanism has been suggested based upon observations that prostaglandins may sensitize tissue to pain (321). This would provide a rationale for the use of prostaglandin-synthetase inhibitors.

In addition, intermittent inflammation contributes to the symptoms of degenerative joint disease in some cases. In these patients, swelling, warmth, or signs of effusion are notable in the afflicted joints (322). This inflammatory reaction may be important in the genesis of symptoms, but a role in the pathogenesis of cartilage breakdown or osteophyte proliferation remains to be demonstrated.

Traditionally, aspirin has been considered the drug of choice for symptomatic relief of pain and inflammation in degenerative joint disease (320). When aspirin is not tolerated, one of the NSAIDs is indicated for symptomatic relief (322). Theoretically, an analgesic such as acetaminophen may prove to be useful in cases where inflammation is not contributing to the patient's symptoms.

References

1. American Rheumatism Association: Primer on the rheumatic diseases. JAMA. 1973; 224:687 (suppl). Also available for a modest charge as a reprint from The Arthritis Foundation, 3400 Peachtree Road, N.E., Atlanta, Georgia 30326.
2. Katz WA: Rheumatoid arthritis. *In Rheumatic Diseases: Diagnosis and Management,* edited by WA Katz, JB Lippincott Co. Philadelphia, 1977.
3. Hollander JL: *The Arthritis Handbook,* Merck Sharpe and Dohme, West Point, Pa., 1974.
4. Smith RD et al: Rest therapy for rheumatoid arthritis. Mayo Clin Proc. 1978; 53:141.
5. Baum J et al: Laboratory findings in rheumatoid arthritis. In *Arthritis and Allied Conditions,* 9th ed., edited by DJ McCarty, Lea and Febiger, Philadelphia, 1979, p 493.
6. Miller RL et al: Inflammatory disorders. In *Clinical Pharmacology,* 2nd ed, edited by K Melmon and H Morrelli, MacMillian, New York, 1978, p 678.
7. Silverberg J et al: Rheumatoid factors in Graves' disease. Ann Intern Med. 1978; 88:216.
8. Epstein WV: Laboratory tests in rheumatic diseases. Med Clin North Am. 1977; 61:377.
9. McDuffie FC et al: Immunological tests in the diagnosis of rheumatic diseases. Bull Rheum Dis. 1977; 27:900 and 27:906.
10. Ragan C et al: The clinical features of rheumatoid arthritis: prognostic indices. JAMA. 1962; 181:663.
11. Engleman EP: Conservative management of rheumatoid arthritis. Med Clin North Am. 1968; 52:669.
12. Engleman EP: Conservative management of rheumatoid arthritis. In *Arthritis and Allied Conditions,* 8th ed., edited by JF Hollander and DJ McCarty, Lea & Febiger, Philadelphia, 1972; p 441.
13. Mills JA et al: Value of bedrest in patients with rheumatoid arthritis. N Engl J Med. 1971; 284:453.
14. Fye KH: Rheumatoid arthritis. Medical Staff Conference Presentation, Univ Calif San Francisco, March 15, 1978.
15. Zeitlin DJ: Psychological issues in the management of rheumatoid arthritis. Psychosomatics. 1977; 18:7.
16. Boardman PL et al: Clinical measurement of the anti-inflammatory effects of salicylates in rheumatoid arthritis. Br Med J. 1967; 4:264.
17. Calabro JJ, et al: Anti-inflammatory effect of acetylsalicylic acid in rheumatoid arthritis. Clin Orth Rel Res. 1970; 17:124.
18. Multz CV et al: A comparison of intermediate-dose aspirin and placebo in rheumatoid arthritis. Clin Pharmacol Ther. 1974; 15:310.
19. Dromgoogle SH et al: Correlation of plateau serum salicylate with rate of salicylate metabolism. Clin Pharmacol Ther. 1976; 20:120.
20. Furst DE et al: Salicylate metabolism in twins: evidence suggesting a genetic influence and induction of salicylurate formation. J Clin Invest. 1977; 60:32.
21. Graham GG et al: Patterns of plasma concentrations and urinary excretion of salicylate in rheumatoid arthritis. Clin Pharmacol Ther. 1977; 22:410.
22. Gupta N et al: Correlation of plateau serum salicylate level with rate of salicylate metabolism. Clin Pharmacol Ther. 1975; 18:350.
23. Paulus HE et al: Variations of serum concentrations and half-life of salicylate in patients with rheumatoid arthritis. Arthritis Rheum. 1971; 14:527.
24. Gibson T et al: Kinetics of salicylate metabolism. Br J Clin Pharmacol. 1975; 2:233.
25. Fremont-Smith K et al: Salicylate therapy in rheumatoid arthritis. JAMA. 1965; 192:1133.
26. Flower RJ et al: Analgesic-antipyretics and anti-inflammatory agents; drugs employed in the treatment of gout. In *The Pharmacological Basis of Therapeutics,* 6th ed. edited by AG Gilman, L Goodman and A Gilman, MacMillan Co, New York, 1980, p 682.
27. Leonards JR et al: Gastrointestinal blood loss during prolonged aspirin administration. N Engl J Med. 1973; 289:1020.
28. Ingelfinger FJ: Aspirin and the stomach. In *Controversy in Internal Medicine II,* edited by FJ Ingelfinger, RV Ebert, M Finland, and AS Relman, WB Saunders Co., Philadelphia, 1974, p 509.
29. Ingelfinger FJ: The side effects of aspirin. N Engl J Med. 1974; 290:1196.
30. Langman MJS: Aspirin is not a major cause of acute gastrointestinal bleeding. In *Controversy in Internal Medicine II,* edited by FJ Ingelfinger, RV Ebert, M Finland, PAS Relman, WB Sanders Co., Philadelphia, 1974, p 493.
31. Levy M: Aspirin use in patients with major upper gastrointestinal bleeding and peptic ulcer disease. N Engl J Med. 1974; 290:1158.
32. Bowen BK et al: Effect of sodium bicarbonate on aspirin-induced damage and potential difference changes in human gastric mucosa. Br Med J. 1977; 2:1052.
33. Cooke AR: The role of the mucosal barrier in drug-induced gastric ulceration and erosions. Digestive Diseases. 1976; 21:155.
34. MacKercher et al: Protective effect of cimetadine on aspirin-induced gastric mucosal damage. Ann Intern Med. 1977; 87:676.
35. Wood PHN et al: Salicylates and gastrointestinal bleeding: acetylsalicylic acid and aspirin derivatives. Br Med J. 1962; 1:669.
36. Baskin WN et al: Aspirin-induced ultrastructural changes in human gastric mucosa. Ann Intern Med. 1976; 85:299.
37. Brodie DA et al: Role of gastric acid in aspirin-induced gastric irritation in the rat. Gastroenterology. 1967; 53:604.
38. Cooke AR: Aspirin and the transmucosal potential difference. Ann Intern Med. 1976; 85:286.
39. Kivilausko I et al: Pathogenesis of experimental gastric mucosal injury. N Engl J Med. 1979; 301:374.
40. Leonards JR et al: Effect of pharmaceutical formulation on gastric-intestinal bleeding from aspirin tablets. Arch Intern Med. 1972; 29:457.
41. Sibert JR: Child resistant packaging and accidental child poisoning. Lancet. 1977; 2:289.

42. Rowland M et al: The clinical pharmacology of salicylates. Calif Med. 1969; 110:410.

43. Furst DE, et al: Salicylate clearance: the consequence of saturability in plasma protein binding and metabolism. Clin Pharmacol Ther (abstract). 1978; 23:113.

44. Levy G et al: Limited capacity for salicylphenolic glucuronide formation and its effect on the kinetics of salicylate elimination in man. Clin Pharmacol Ther. 1972; 13:258.

45. Levy G et al: Salicylate accumulation kinetics in man. N Engl J Med. 1972; 287:430.

46. Levy G: Clinical pharmacokinetics of aspirin. Pediatrics. 1978; 62:867.

47. Wilson JJ et al: Gentisuric acid: metabolic formation in animals and identification as a metabolite of aspirin in man. Clin Pharmacol Ther. 1978; 23:635.

48. Levy G et al: Relationship between dose and apparent volume of distribution of salicylate in children. Pediatrics. 1974; 54:713.

49. Myers EN et al: Salicylate ototoxicity: a clinical study. N Engl J Med. 1965; 273:587.

50. Morgan E et al: Tinnitus as an indication of therapeutic serum salicylate levels. JAMA. 1973; 226:142.

51. Levy G et al: Urine pH and salicylate therapy. JAMA (letter). 1971; 217:81.

52. Levy G et al: Decreased serum salicylate concentrations in children with rheumatic fever treated with antacid. N Engl J Med. 1975; 293:323.

53. Ayers JW et al: Circadian rhythm of urinary pH in man with and without chronic antacid administration. Eur J Clin Pharmacol. 1977; 12:415.

54. Gibaldi M et al: Effects of antacids on pH of urine. Clin Pharmacol Ther. 1974; 16:520.

55. Gibaldi M et al: Time course and dose dependence of antacid effect on urine pH. J Pharm Sci. 1975; 64:2003.

56. Abrishami MA et al: Aspirin intolerance—a review. Ann Allergy. 1977; 39:28.

57. Samter M et al: Intolerance to aspirin: clinical studies and consideration of its pathogenesis. Ann Intern Med. 1968; 68:975.

58. Prince HE: Aspirin and cross reactivity. Ann Allergy. 1977; 39:47.

59. Stenius BSM et al: Hypersensitivity to acetylsalicylic acid (ASA) and tartrazine in patients with asthma. Clin Allergy. 1976; 6:119.

60. Szceklik A et al: Asthmatic attacks induced in aspirin-sensitive patients by diclofenac and naproxen. Br Med J. 1977; 2:231.

61. de Weck AL: Immunologic and non-immunological mechanisms of intolerance to aspirin. Adv Clin Pharmacol. 1974; 6:31.

62. Anon: Is all aspirin alike? Med Let Drugs Ther. 1974; 16:57.

63. Lanza FL et al: Endoscopic evaluation of the effects of aspirin, buffered aspirin, and enteric coated aspirin on the gastric and duodenal mucosa. N Engl J Med. 1980; 303:136.

64. Mielants H et al: Salicylate-induced gastrointestinal bleeding: comparison between soluble buffered, enteric coated, and intravenous administration. J Rheumatol. 1979; 6:210.

65. Hollister LE et al: Studies of delayed-action medication—IV salicylates. Clin Pharmacol Ther. 1965; 6:5.

66. Lasagna L et al: How reliable are enteric-coated aspirin preparations? Clin Pharmacol Ther. 1965; 6:568.

67. Leonards JR et al: Absorption and metabolism of aspirin administered in enteric coated tablets. JAMA. 1965; 193:99.

68. Levy G et al: Failure of USP disintegration test to assess physiological availability of enteric coated tablets. NY State J Med. 1964; 64:3002.

69. Orozco-Alcalca JJ et al: Regular and enteric coated aspirin: a re-evaluation. Arthritis Rheum. 1979; 22:1034.

70. Baum J: Blood salicylate levels and clinical trials with a new form of enteric coated aspirin: studies in rheumatoid arthritis and degenerative joint disease. J Clin Pharmacol. 1970; 10:132.

71. Canada AT et al: The bioavailability of enteric-coated acetylsalicylic acid: a comparative study in rheumatoid arthritis I. Curr Ther Res. 1975; 18:727.

72. Canada AT et al: The bioavailability of enteric-coated acetylsalicylic acid: a comparison with buffered ASA in rheumatoid arthritis II. Curr Ther Res. 1969; 19:554.

73. Wiseman EH: Plasma salicylate concentrations following chronic administration of aspirin as conventional and sustained-release tablets. Curr Ther Res. 1969; 11:681.

74. Leonards JR: Absence of gastrointestinal bleeding following administration of salicylsalicylic acid. J Lab Clin Med. 1969; 74:911.

75. Leonards JR et al: Gastrointestinal blood loss from aspirin and sodium salicylate tablets in man. Clin Pharmacol Ther. 1973; 14:62.

76. Anon: Arthropan liquid and other salicylates for arthritis. Med Let Drugs Ther. 1976; 18:119.

77. Collier HOJ: A pharmacological analysis of aspirin. Adv Pharmacol Chemother. 1969; 7:333.

78. Moncada S et al: Mode of action of aspirin-like drugs. Adv Intern Med. 1978; 24:1.

79. Soren A: Transport of salicylates from blood to joint fluid. Arch Intern Med. 1973; 132:668.

80. Bowers DE et al: Naproxen in rheumatoid arthritis: a controlled trial. Ann Intern Med. (letter). 1975; 83:470.

81. Dornan J et al: Comparison of ibuprofen and acetylsalicylic acid in the treatment of rheumatoid arthritis. Can Med Assoc J. 1974; 110:1370.

82. Fries JR et al: Fenoprofen calcium in rheumatoid arthritis: a controlled double-blind crossover evaluation. Arthritis Rheum. 1973; 16:629.

83. Hill HFH et al: Multi-center double-blind crossover trial comparing naproxen and aspirin in rheumatoid arthritis. Scand J Rheumatol (suppl). 1973; 2:176.

84. Huskisson EC et al: Treatment of rheumatoid arthritis with fenoprofen: comparison with aspirin. Br Med J. 1974; 1:176.

85. Weintraub M et al: Piroxicam (CP16171) in rheumatoid arthritis: a controlled clinical trial with novel assessment techniques. J Rheumatol. 1977; 4:393.

86. Ward JR et al: Piroxicam and rheumatoid arthritis: a multi-center 14-week controlled double-blind study comparing piroxicam and aspirin. Royal Soc Med International Congress and Symposium Series. 1978; 1:31.

87. Diamond H et al: Naproxen and aspirin in rheumatoid arthritis: A multi-center double-blind crossover comparison study. J Clin Pharmacol. 1975; 15:335.

88. Brogden RN et al: Naproxen: a review of its pharmacological properties and therapeutic efficacy and use. Drugs. 1975; 9:326.

89. Brogden RN et al: Fenoprofen: review of its pharmacological properties and therapeutic efficacy in rheumatic diseases. Drugs. 1977; 13:241.

90. Brogden RN et al: Sulindac: a review of its pharmacological properties and therapeutic efficacy in rheumatic diseases. Drugs. 1978; 16:97.

91. Brogden RN et al: Tolmetin: a review of its pharmacological properties and therapeutic efficacy in rheumatic diseases. Drugs. 1978; 15:429.

92. Davies EF et al: Ibuprofen: a review of its pharmacological properties and therapeutic efficacy in rheumatic disorders. Drugs. 1971; 2:416.

93. Carty TJ et al: Piroxicam, a potent inhibitor of prostaglandin production in cell culture, structure-activity study. Prostaglandins. 1980; 19:51.

94. Arsenault A et al: Effect of naproxen on gastrointestinal microbleeding following acetylsalicylate medication, J Clin Pharmacol. 1975; 15:340.

95. Beirne JA et al: Gastrointestinal blood loss caused by tolmetin, aspirin and indomethacin, Clin Pharmacol Ther. 1974; 16:821.

96. Chernish SM et al: Comparison of gastrointestinal effects of aspirin and fenoprofen. Arthritis Rheum. 1979; 22:376.

97. Curtarelli G et al: Gastrointestinal bleeding under treatment with naproxen. Scand J Rheumatol (suppl). 1973; 2:48.

98. Halvorsen L et al: Comparative effects of aspirin and naproxen on gastric mucosa. Scand J Rheumatol (suppl). 1973; 2:43.

99. Loebl DH et al: Gastrointestinal blood loss, effect of aspirin, fenoprofen, and acetaminophen in rheumatoid arthritis as determined by sequential gastroscopy and radioactive fecal marker. JAMA. 1977; 237:976.

100. Lussier A et al: Gastrointestinal microbleeding after aspirin and naproxen. Clin Pharmacol Ther. 1978; 23:402.

101. Ridolpho AS et al: Effects of fenoprofen and aspirin on gastrointestinal microbleeding in man. Clin Pharmacol Ther. 1973; 14:226.

102. Schmid FR et al: Anti-inflammatory drugs and gastrointestinal bleeding: a comparison of aspirin and ibuprofen. J Clin Pharmacol. 1976; 16:418.

103. Simon LS et al: Non-steroidal anti-inflammatory drugs. N Engl J Med. 1980; 302:1179 & 1237.

104. Duggan DE et al: The disposition of sulindac. Clin Pharmacol Ther. 1977; 21:326.

105. Rubin A et al: Physiologic disposition of fenoprofen in man. III metabolism and protein binding of fenoprofen. J Pharmacol Exper Ther. 1972; 183:449.

106. Segre EJ: Naproxen metabolism in man. J Clin Pharmacol. 1975; 15:316.

107. Cuthbert MF: Adverse reactions to non-steroidal antirheumatic drugs. Curr Med Res Opin. 1974; 2:600.

108. O'Brien WM: Indomethacin: a survey of clinical trials. Clin Pharmacol Ther. 1968; 9:94.

109. Castles JJ et al: Multicenter comparison of naproxen and indomethacin in rheumatoid arthritis. Arch Intern Med. 1978; 138:362.

110. Kogstad O: A double-blind crossover study of naproxen and indomethacin in patients with rheumatoid arthritis. Scand J Rheumatol (suppl). 1973; 21:159.

111. Szanto E: A double-blind comparison of naproxen and indomethacin in rheumatoid arthritis. Scand J Rheumatol. 174; 3:118.

112. Hernandez LA et al: Clinical evaluation of two daily doses of naproxen and indomethacin: result of a double-blind crossover trial. Curr Med Res Opin. 1975; 3:359.

113. Huskisson EC et al: Four new anti-inflammatory drugs: responses and variations. Br Med J. 1976; 1:1048.

114. Reynolds PMG et al: A single-blind crossover comparison of fenoprofen, ibuprofen, and naproxen in rheumatoid arthritis. Curr Med Res Opin. 1974; 2:461.

115. Lewis JR: New anti-rheumatic agents: fenoprofen calcium (Nalfon), naproxen (Naprosyn), and tolmetin sodium (Tolectin). JAMA. 1977; 237:1260.

116. Stuart MJ et al: Platelet function in recipients of platelets from donors ingesting aspirin. N Engl J Med. 1972; 287:1105.

117. Moroz LA: Increased fibrinolytic activity after aspirin ingestion. N Engl J Med. 1977; 296:525.

118. Goldsweig HG et al: Bleeding, salicylates, and prolonged prothrombin time; three case reports and a review of the literature. J Rheumatol. 1976; 3:37.

119. O'Brien JR: Effects of salicylates on human platelets. Lancet. 1968; 2:779.

120. Sutor AH et al: Effect of aspirin, sodium salicylate, and acetaminophen on bleeding. Mayo Clin Proc. 1976; 46:178.

121. Evans G et al: The effect of acetylsalicylic acid on platelet function. J Exp Med. 1968; 128:877.

122. Slone D et al: Aspirin and congenital malformations. Lancet. 1976; 1:1373.

123. Turner G et al: Fetal effects of regular aspirin ingestion in pregnancy. Lancet. 1975; 2:338.

124. Shapiro S et al: Perinatal mortality and birth-weight relation to aspirin taken during pregnancy. Lancet. 1976; 1:1375.

125. Heyman MA et al: Effects of acetylsalicylic acid on the ductus arteriosus and circulation in fetal lambs in utero. Circ Res. 1976; 38:418.

126. Arcilla RA et al: Congestive heart failure from suspected ductal closures in utero. J Pediatr. 1969; 75:74.

127. Garretson LK et al: Fetal acquisition and neonatal elimination of a large amount of salicylate. Clin Pharmacol Ther. 1975; 17:98.

128. Levy G et al: Distribution of salicylate between neonatal and maternal serum at diffusion equilibrium. Clin Pharmacol Ther. 1975; 18:210.

129. Persellin RH: The effect of pregnancy on rheumatoid arthritis. Bull Rheum Dis. 1977; 27:922.

130. Dunn MJ et al: Prostaglandins and the kidney. Am J Physiol. 1977; 233:F169.

131. Kimberly RP et al: Urinary prostaglandins and the effects of aspirin on renal function in lupus erythematosus. Ann Intern Med. 1978; 89:336.

132. Kimberly RP et al: Aspirin-induced depression of renal function. N Engl J Med. 1977; 296:418.

133. Kimberly RP et al: Apparent acute renal failure associated with therapeutic aspirin and ibuprofen administration. Arthritis Rheum. 1979; 22:281.

134. Kimberly RP et al: Reduction in renal function by newer non-steroidal anti-inflammatory drugs. Am J Med. 1978; 64:804.

135. Walske JJ et al: Acute oliguric renal failure induced by indomethacin: possible mechanism. Ann Intern Med. 1979; 91:47.

136. Solomon HE et al: Interaction between digitoxin and other drugs in man. Am Heart J. 1972; 83:277.

137. Maurer EF: The toxic effects of phenylbutazone. N Engl J Med. 1955; 253:404.

138. McCarthy DD et al: Hematologic complication of phenylbutazone therapy. Can Med Assoc J. 1964; 90:1061.

139. Pretty HM et al: Agranulocytosis: a report of 30 cases. Can Med Assoc J. 1965; 93:1058.

140. Nelson AM et al: Glucocorticoids in rheumatic disease. Mayo Clin Proc. 1980; 55:758.

141. Bernstein CA et al: Rheumatoid patients after five or more years of corticosteroid treatment: a comparative analysis of 1983 cases. Ann Intern Med. 1961; 54:938.

142. Empire Rheumatism Council: Gold therapy in rheumatoid arthritis. Ann Rheum Dis. 1960; 19:95.

143. Empire Rheumatism Council: Gold therapy in rheumatoid arthritis: final report of a multi-center controlled trial. Ann Rheum Dis. 1961; 20:315.

144. Sigler JW et al: Gold salts in the treatment of rheumatoid arthritis: a double-blind study. Ann Intern Med. 1974; 80:21.

145. Cooperating Clinics Committee of the American Rheumatism Association: A controlled trial of gold salt therapy in rheumatoid arthritis. Arthritis Rheum. 1973; 16:353.

146. Luukhainen R et al: Effect of gold treatment on the progression of erosions in rheumatoid arthritis patients. Scand J Rheumatol. 1977; 6:123.

147. Luukhainen R et al: Effect of gold on progression of erosions in rheumatoid arthritis: better results with earlier treatment. Scand J Rheumatol. 1977; 6:189.

148. Dwosh IL et al: Azathioprine in early rheumatoid arthritis: comparison with gold and chloroquine. Arthritis Rheum. 1977; 20:685.

149. Huskisson EC et al: Trial comparing d-penicillamine and gold in rheumatoid arthritis. Ann Rheum Dis. 1974; 33:532.

150. Gumpel JM: Cyclophosphamide, gold and penicillamine-disease modifying drugs in rheumatoid arthritis-tailored dosage and ultimate success. Rheumatol Rehab. 1976; 15:217.

151. Currey HLF et al: Comparison of azathioprine, cyclophosphamide, and gold in the treatment of rheumatoid arthritis. Br Med J. 1974; 3:763.

152. Gottlieb NL: Chrysotherapy. Bull Rheum Dis. 1977; 27:912.

153. Davis JD: Fenoprofen, aspirin, and gold-induction in rheumatoid arthritis. Clin Pharmacol Ther. 1977; 21:52.

154. Freyberg RH et al: Gold therapy for rheumatoid arthritis. In Arthritis and Allied Conditions, 8th ed. edited by JL Hollander and DJ McCarty, Philadelphia 1972, p 455.

155. Gordon MH et al: Gold reactions are not more common in Sjogren's syndrome. Ann Intern Med. 1975; 82:47.

156. Rothermich NO et al: Chrysotherapy: a prospective study. Arthritis Rheum. 1976; 19:1321.

157. Gottlieb NL et al: Acute myocardial infarction following gold sodium thiomalate induced vasomotor (nitroid) reaction. Arthritis Rheum. 1977; 20:1026.

158. Harris BK: Myocardial infarction after a gold-induced nitroid reaction (letter). Arthritis Rheum. 1977; 20:1561.

159. Halla JT et al: Postinjection nonvasomotor reactions during chrysotherapy. Arthritis Rheum. 1977; 20:1188.

160. Lawrence JS: Comparative toxicity of gold preparations in treatment of rheumatoid arthritis. Ann Rheum Dis. 1976; 35:171.

161. Wooley PH et al: HLA-DR antigens and toxic reaction to sodium aurothiomalate and d-penicillamine in patients with rheumatoid arthritis. N Engl J Med. 1980; 303:300.

162. Zvaifler NJ: Gold and antimalarial therapy. In Arthritis and Allied Conditions, 9th ed., edited by DJ McCarty, Lea and Febiger, Philadelphia 1979, p 355.

163. Cats A: A multi-center controlled trial of the effects of different dosages of gold therapy, followed by a maintenance dosage. Agents Actions. 1976; 6:355.

164. Sharp JT: Comparison of two dosage schedules of gold salts in the treatment of rheumatoid arthritis. Arthritis Rheum. 1977; 20:1179.

165. McKenzie MJJ: An initial report on a double-blind trial comparing small and large doses of gold in the treatment of rheumatoid disease. Rheumatol Rehab. 1977; 16:78.

166. Dietz AA et al: Serum gold: 1. estimation by atomic absorption spectroscopy. Ann Rheum Dis. 1973; 32:124.

167. Krusius FE et al: Plasma levels and urinary excretion of gold during routine treatment of rheumatoid arthritis. Ann Rheum Dis. 1970; 29:230.

168. Lorber A et al: Gold determination in biological fluids by atomic absorption spectroscopy: application to chrysotherapy in rheumatoid arthritis patients. Arthritis Rheum. 1968; 11:170.

169. Lorber A et al: Monitoring serum gold values to improve chrysotherapy in rheumatoid arthritis. Ann Rheum Dis. 1973; 32:133.

170. Jessop JD et al: Serum gold determinations in patients with rheumatoid arthritis receiving sodium aurothiomalate. Ann Rheum Dis. 1973; 32:228.

171. Rubinstein HM et al: Serum gold II. levels in rheumatoid arthritis. Ann Rheum Dis. 1973; 32:128.

172. Gerber RC et al: Clinical response and serum gold levels in chrysotherapy: lack of correlation. Ann Rheum Dis. 1972; 31:308.

173. Gottlieb NL et al: Gold excretion correlated with clinical course during chrysotherapy in rheumatoid arthritis. Arthritis Rheum. 1972; 15:582.

174. Gottlieb NL: Serum gold levels. Arthritis Rheum. 1975; 18:626.

175. Mascarenhas BR et al: Gold metabolism in patients with rheumatoid arthritis treated with gold compounds—reinvestigated. Arthritis Rheum. 1972; 15:391.

176. Bunch TW et al: Disease modifying drugs for progressive rheumatoid arthritis. Mayo Clin Proc. 1979; 55:161.

177. Gerber RC et al: Gold therapy. Clin Rheum Dis. 1975; 1:307.

178. David P et al: Significance of eosinophilia during gold therapy. Arthritis Rheum. 1974; 17:1964.

179. Levin HA et al: Thrombocytopenia associated with gold therapy: observations on the mechanism of platelet destruction. Am J Med. 1975; 59:274.

180. Canada AT: Gold-induced thrombocytopenia. Am J Hosp Pharm. 1973; 30:340.

181. Davis P et al: Interaction of D-penicillamine with gold salts. Arthritis Rheum. 1977; 20:1413.

182. England JM et al: Gold-induced thrombocytopenia and response to dimercaprol. Br Med J. 1972; 2:748.

183. Combs RJ et al: Gold toxicity and peritoneal dialysis. Arthritis Rheum. 1976; 19:936.

184. Podell TE et al: Pulmonary toxicity with gold therapy. Arthritis Rheum. 1980; 23:347.

185. Smith W et al: Lung injury due to gold treatment. Arthritis Rheum. 1980; 23:351.

186. Stein HB et al: Gold-induced enterocolitis: case report and literature review. J Rheumatol. 1976; 3:21.

187. Winterbauer RH et al: Diffuse pulmonary injury associated with gold treatment. N Engl J Med. 1976; 294:919.

188. Wilkins RF et al: Combination therapy with naproxen and aspirin in rheumatoid arthritis. Arthritis Rheum. 1976; 19:677.

189. Jeremy R et al: Interaction between aspirin and indomethacin in the treatment of rheumatoid arthritis. Med J Aust. 1970; 2:127.

190. Rubin A et al: Interactions of aspirin with non-steroidal anti-inflammatory drugs in man. Arthritis Rheum. 1973; 16:635.

191. Brooks PM et al: Indomethacin—aspirin interactions: a clinical appraisal. Br Med J. 1975; 3:69.

192. Champion DG et al: The effect of aspirin on serum indomethacin. Clin Pharmacol Ther. 1972; 13:239.

193. Kaldestad E et al: Interactions of indomethacin and acetylsalicylic acid as shown by the serum concentrations of indomethacin and salicylate. Europ J Clin Pharmacol. 1975; 9:199.

194. Mainland DM and Cooperating Clinics Committee of the American Rheumatism Association: A three-month trial of indomethacin in rheumatoid arthritis, with special reference to analysis inference. Clin Pharmacol Ther. 1967; 8:11.

195. Pinals RS et al: Relative efficacy of indomethacin and acetylsalicylic acid in rheumatoid arthritis. N Engl J Med. 1967; 276:512.

196. Koch-Weser J et al: Binding of drugs to serum albumin. N Engl J Med. 1976; 294:311 and 1976; 294:526.

197. Grennan DM et al: The aspirin-ibuprofen interaction in rheumatoid arthritis. Br J Clin Pharmacol. 1970; 8:423.

198. Empire Rheumatism Council: Multi-center controlled trial comparing cortisone acetate and acetylsalicylic acid in the long-term treatment of rheumatoid arthritis: results of three years' treatment. Ann Rheum Dis. 1957; 16:277.

199. Joint Committee of the Medical Research Council and Nuffield Foundation on Clinical Trials of Cortisone, ACTH, and Other Therapeutic Measures in Chronic Rheumatic Diseases: A comparison of cortisone and aspirin in the treatment of early cases of rheumatoid arthritis. Br Med J. 1955; 2:695.

200. Rasher JJ et al: Radiological study of cervical spine and hands in patients with rheumatoid arthritis of 15 years' duration: an assessment of the effects of corticosteroid treatment. Ann Rheum Dis. 1978; 37:529.

201. Klinenberg JR et al: Effect of corticosteroids on blood salicylate concentration. JAMA. 1965; 194:131.

202. Klinefelter HF: Reinstitution of gold therapy in rheumatoid arthritis after mucocutaneous reactions. J Rheumatol. 1975; 2:21.

203. Srinivason R et al: Long-term chrysotherapy in rheumatoid arthritis. Arthritis Rheum. 1979; 22:105.

204. Marshall CM: Gold therapy in rheumatoid arthritis: a review of ten years' treatment. Med J Aust. 1965; 2:239.

205. Soler-Bechera J et al: Maintenance gold therapy for rheumatoid arthritis—analysis in 167 patients. Arthritis Rheum. 1965; 8:469.

206. Kean W et al: Long-term chrysotherapy. Arthritis Rheum. 1979; 22:495.

207. Mackenzie AH: An appraisal of chloroquine. Arthritis Rheum. 1970; 13:280.

208. Mackenzie AH et al: Chloroquine and hydroxychloroquine in rheumatological therapy. Clin Rheumat Dis. 1980; 6:3.

209. Cohen AS et al: A controlled study of chloroquine as an antirheumatic agent. Arthritis Rheum. 1958; 1:207.

210. Freedman A et al: Chloroquine in rheumatoid arthritis: a double-blindfold trial of treatment for one year. Ann Rheum Dis. 1960; 19:243.

211. Hamilton EBD et al: Hydroxychloroquine sulfate (plaquenil) in the treatment of rheumatoid arthritis. Arthritis Rheum. 1962; 5:502.

212. Popert AJ et al: Chloroquine diphosphate in rheumatoid arthritis. Ann Rheum Dis. 1961; 20:18.

213. Cann HM et al: Fatal acute chloroquine poisoning in children. Pediatrics. 1961; 27:95.

214. Markowitz JA et al: Chloroquine poisoning in a girl. JAMA, 1964; 189:950.

215. Anon: Chloroquine retinopathy. N Engl J Med. 1966; 275:730.

216. Henkind P et al: Ocular abnormalities in patients treated with synthetic antimalarial drugs. N Engl J Med. 1963; 269:433.

217. Scherbel AL et al: Ocular lesions in rheumatoid arthritis and related disorders with particular reference to retinopathy. N Engl J Med. 1965; 237:36.

218. Elman E et al: Chloroquine retinopathy in patients with rheumatoid arthritis. Scand J Rheumatol. 1976; 5:161.

219. Burns RP: Delayed onset of chloroquine retinopathy. N Engl J Med. 1966; 275:693.

220. Percival SP et al: Chloroquine ophthalmologic safety and clinical assessment in rheumatoid arthritis. Br Med J. 1968; 3:579.

221. Percival SP et al: Ophthalmologic safety of chloroquine. Br J Ophth. 1969; 53:101.

222. Rothermich NO: Coming catastrophies with chloroquine? Ann Intern Med. 1964; 61:203.

223. Hollander JL: The calculated risk of arthritis treatment. Ann Intern Med. 1965; 62:1062.

224. Dixon ASJ et al: Synthetic D-penicillamine in rheumatoid arthritis: double-blind controlled study of a high and low dosage regimen. Ann Rheum Dis. 1975; 34:416.

225. Mery C et al: Controlled trial of d-penicillamine in rheumatoid arthritis: dose effect and the role of zinc. Scand J Rheumatol. 1976; 5:241.

226. Multicentre Trial Group: Controlled trial of D-penicillamine in severe rheumatoid arthritis. Lancet. 1973; 1:275–280.

227. Shikawa Y et al: Clinical evaluation of D-penicillamine by multicentric double-blind comparative study in chronic rheumatoid arthritis. Arthritis Rheum. 1977; 20:1464.

228. Jaffe IA: The technique of penicillamine administration in rheumatoid arthritis. Arthritis Rheum. 1976; 18:513.

229. Multicentre Trial Group: Absence of toxic or therapeutic interaction between penicillamine and previously administered gold in a trial of penicillamine in rheumatoid disease. Postgrad Med J. 1974; 50:77 (Suppl 2).

230. Tsang IK et al: D-penicillamine in the treatment of rheumatoid arthritis. Arthritis Rheum. 1977; 20:666.

231. Webley M et al: Is penicillamine therapy in rheumatoid arthritis influenced by previous treatment with gold? Br Med J. 1978; 3:91.

232. Hill HFH: Penicillamine in rheumatoid arthritis: adverse effects. Scand J Rheumatol. 1979; 28:94.

233. Bacon PA et al: Penicillamine nephropathy in rheumatoid arthritis. Quart J Med. 1976; 45:661.

234. Hill HFH: Treatment of rheumatoid arthritis with penicillamine. Arthritis Rheum. 1977; 6:361.

235. Kean WF et al: The toxicity pattern of D-penicillamine therapy. Arthritis Rheum. 1980; 23:158.

236. O'Brien WM: Toxicity of D-penicillamine in rheumatoid arthritis. Ann Intern Med. 1980; 92:120.

237. Stein HB et al: Adverse effects of D-penicillamine in rheumatoid arthritis. Ann Intern Med. 1980; 92:24.

238. Dische FE: Immunopathology of penicillamine-induced glomerular disease. J Rheumatol. 1976; 3:145.

239. Jaffe IA: D-penicillamine. Bull Rheum Dis. 1977; 28:948.

240. Hill H et al: Resumption of treatment with penicillamine after proteinuria. Ann Rheum Dis. 1979; 38:229.

241. Kay AGL: Myelotoxicity of D-penicillamine. Ann Rheum Dis. 1979; 38:232.

242. Weiss AS et al: Toxicity of D-penicillamine in rheumatoid arthritis. Am J Med. 1970; 44:114.

243. Atcheson SG et al: Ptosisi and weakness after start of D-penicillamine therapy. Ann Intern Med. 1978; 89:939.

244. Cucher BG et al: D-penicillamine-induced polymyositis in rheumatoid arthritis. Ann Intern Med. 1976; 85:615.

245. Gordon RA et al: D-penicillamine-induced myasthenia gravis in rheumatoid arthritis. Ann Intern Med. 1977; 87:578.

246. Harpey JP et al: Lupus-like syndrome induced by D-penicillamine in Wilson's disease. Lancet. 1971; 1:292.

247. Sternlieb I et al: D-penicillamine induced Goodpasture's syndrome in Wilson's disease. Ann Intern Med. 1975; 82:673.

248. Amor B et al: Chlorambucil in rheumatoid arthritis. Clin Rheum Dis. 1980; 6:567.

249. Berry H et al: Trial comparing azathioprine and penicillamine in treatment of rheumatoid arthritis. Ann Rheum Dis. 1976; 35:542.

250. Cooperating Clinics Committee of the ARA: A controlled trial of cyclophosphamide in rheumatoid arthritis. N Engl J Med. 1970; 283:883.

251. Hunter T et al: Azathioprine in rheumatoid arthritis: a long-term follow-up study. Arthritis Rheum. 1975; 18:15.

252. Lidsky MD et al: Double-blind study of cyclophosphamide in rheumatoid arthritis. Arthritis Rheum. 1973; 16:148.

253. Thorpe P et al: Rheumatoid arthritis treated with chlorambucil. Med J Aust. 1976; 2:197.

254. Townes AS et al: Controlled trial of cyclophosphamide in rheumatoid arthritis. Arthritis Rheum. 1976; 19:563.

255. Urowitz MB et al: Azathioprine in rheumatoid arthritis: a double-blind study comparing full-dose to half-dose. J Rheumatol. 1974; 1:274.

256. Urowitz MB et al: Azathioprine in rheumatoid arthritis: a double-blind cross-over study. Arthritis Rheum. 1973; 16:411.

257. Williams HJ et al: Comparison of high-and low-dose cyclophosphamide therapy in rheumatoid arthritis. Arthritis Rheum. 1980; 23:521.

258. Symth CJ et al: Cyclophosphamide therapy of rheumatoid arthritis. Arch Intern Med. 1975; 135:789.

259. Aptchar RG et al: Bladder toxicity with chronic oral cyclophosphamide therapy in nonmalignant disease. Arthritis Rheum. 1973; 16:46.

260. Armstrong B et al: Delayed cystitis due to cyclophosphamide. N Engl J Med. 1979; 300:451 (letter).

261. Fairley KF et al: Sterility and testicular atrophy related to cyclophosphamide therapy. Lancet. 1970; 1:568.

262. Johnson WW et al: Urinary-bladder fibrosis and telangiectasia associated with long-term cyclophosphamide therapy. N Engl J Med. 1971; 284:290.

263. Miller JJ et al: Multiple late complications of therapy with cyclophosphamide including ovarian destruction. Am J Med. 1971; 50:530.

264. Plotz PH et al: Bladder complications in patients receiving cyclophosphamide for systemic lupus erythematosus or rheumatoid arthritis. Ann Intern Med. 1979; 91:221.

265. Wall RL et al: Carcinoma of the urinary bladder in patients receiving cyclophosphamide. N Engl J Med. 1975; 293:271.

266. Cade R et al: Low dose, long-term treatment of rheumatoid arthritis with azathioprine. South Med J. 1976; 69:388.

267. Pinals RS: Azathioprine in the treatment of chronic polyarthritis: long term results and adverse effects in 25 patients. J Rheumatol. 1976; 3:140.

268. Kawaniski H et al: Azathioprine-induced acute pancreatitis. N Engl J Med. 1973; 289:357.

269. Zarday Z et al: Irreversible liver damage after azathioprine. JAMA. 1972; 226:690.

270. Alexson E et al: Acute leukemia after azathioprine treatment of connective tissue disease. Am J Med Sci. 1977; 273:335.

271. Pirofsky B et al: Immunosuppressive therapy in rheumatic disease. Med Clin North Am. 1977; 61:419.

272. Parsons JL et al: The causes of death in patients with rheumatoid arthritis treated with cytotoxic agents. J Rheumatol (Abstract). 1974; 1:75 (suppl).

273. American Rheumatism Association: Primer on the rheumatic diseases. JAMA. 1973; 224:701 (suppl).

274. Decker JL et al: Systemic lupus erythematosus: contrasts and comparisons. Ann Intern Med. 1975; 82:391.

275. Budman DR et al: Hematologic aspects of systemic lupus erythematosus: current concepts. Ann Intern Med. 1977; 86:220.

276. Baldwin DS et al: Lupus nephritis: clinical course as related to morphologic forms and their transition. Am J Med. 1977; 62:12.

277. Baldwin DS et al: Lupus nephritis. Clin Rheum Dis. 1975; 1:639.

278. Baldwin DS et al: The clinical course of the proliferative and membranous forms of lupus nephritis. Ann Intern Med. 1970; 73:929.

279. Estes D et al: The natural history of systemic lupus erythematosus by prospective analysis. Medicine. 1971; 50:85.

280. Yount WJ et al: Corticosteroid therapy of collagen vascular disorders. Med Clin North Am. 1973; 57:1843.

281. Ackerman GL: Alternate day steroid therapy in lupus nephritis. Ann Intern Med. 1970; 72:511.

282. Pollack VE et al: Clinical and experimental natural history of the renal manifestations of systemic lupus erythematosus. J Lab Clin Med. 1964; 63:537.

283. Albert DA et al: Does corticosteroid therapy affect the survival of patients with systemic lupus erythematosus? Arthritis Rheum. 1970; 22:945.

284. Kimberly R et al: Clinical efficacy of high-dose intravenous methylprednisolone pulse therapy in systemic lupus erythematosus. Arthritis Rheum. 1979; 22:629.

285. Ponticelli C et al: High-dose methylprednisolone in active lupus nephritis. Lancet 1977; 1:1063 (letter).

286. Nebout T et al: Intravenous methylprednisolone pulses in diffuse proliferative lupus nephritis. Lancet. 1977; 1:909.

287. Adams DA et al: Azathioprine treatment of immunological renal disease. JAMA. 1967; 199:459.

288. Bardana EJ et al: Azathioprine in steroid insensitive nephropathy. Am J Med. 1970; 49:789.

289. Drinkard JP et al: Azathioprine and prednisone in the treatment of adults with lupus nephritis. Clinical, histological, and immunological changes with therapy. Medicine. 1970; 49:411.

290. Hayslett JP et al: The effect of azathioprine on lupus glomerulonephritis. Medicine. 1972; 51:393.

291. Lindeman RD et al: Long-term azathioprine-corticosteroid therapy in lupus nephritis and idiopathic nephrotic syndrome. J Chron Dis. 1975; 29:189.

292. Maher JF et al: Treatment of lupus nephritis with azathioprine. Arch Intern Med. 1970; 125:293.

293. Michael AF et al: Immunosuppressive therapy of chronic renal disease. N Engl J Med. 1967; 276:817.

294. Shelp WD et al: Effect of azathioprine on renal histology and function in lupus nephritis. Arch Intern Med. 1971; 128:566.

295. Sztennbok M et al: Azathioprine in the treatment of systemic lupus erythematosus: a controlled study. Arthritis Rheum. 1971; 14:639.

296. Sharon E et al: Exacerbation of systemic lupus erythematosus after withdrawal of azathioprine therapy. N Engl J Med. 1973; 288:122.

297. Case R et al: Comparison of azathioprine, prednisone, and heparin alone or combined in treating lupus nephritis. Nephron. 1973; 10:37.

298. Donadio JV et al: Treatment of lupus nephritis with prednisone and combined prednisone and azathioprine. Ann Intern Med. 1972; 77:829.

299. Donadio JV et al: Further observations on the treatment of lupus nephritis with prednisone and combined prednisone and azathioprine. Arthritis Rheum. 1974; 17:573.

300. Hahn BH et al: Azathioprine plus prednisone compared with prednisone alone in the treatment of systemic lupus erythematosus. Ann Intern Med. 1975; 83:597.

301. Fries JF et al: Cyclophosphamide therapy in systemic lupus erythematosus and polymyositis. Arthritis Rheum. 1973; 16:154.

302. Steinberg AD et al: Cyclophosphamide in lupus nephritis: a controlled trial. Ann Intern Med. 1971; 75:165.

303. Steinberg AD et al: A double-blind controlled trial comparing cyclophosphamide, azathioprine, and placebo in the treatment of lupus glomerulonephritis. Arthritis Rheum. 1974; 17:923.

304. Decker JL et al: Cyclophosphamide or azathioprine in lupus glomerulonephritis: a controlled trial: result at 28 months. Ann Intern Med. 1975; 83:606.

305. Donadio JV et al: progressive lupus glomerulonephritis. Treatment with prednisone and combined prednisone and cyclophosphamide. Mayo Clin Proc. 1976; 51:484.

306. Donadio JV et al: Treatment of diffuse proliferative lupus nephritis with prednisone and combined prednisone and cyclophosphamide. N Engl J Med. 1978; 299:1151.

307. Sabboer MS et al: Comparison of chlorambucil, azathioprine or cyclophosphamide combined with corticosteroids in the treatment of lupus nephritis. Br J Dermatol. 1979; 100:113.

308. Snaith MC et al: Treatment of patients with systemic lupus erythematosus including nephritis with chlorambucil. Br Med J. 1973; 2:197.

309. Wagner L: Immunosuppressive agents in lupus nephritis: a critical analysis. Medicine. 1976; 55:239.

310. Sergent JS et al: Central nervous system disease in systemic lupus erythematosus. Am J Med. 1975; 58:644.

311. Lee SL et al: Drug-induced systemic lupus erythematosus: a critical review. Sem Arthritis Rheum. 1975; 5:83.

312. Harpey JP: Lupus-like syndromes induced by drugs. Ann Allergy. 1974; 33:256.

313. Lee SL et al: Activation of systemic lupus erythematosus by drugs. Arch Intern Med. 1966; 117:620.

314. Garovich M et al: Oral contraceptives and systemic lupus erythematosus. Arthritis Rheum. 1980; 23:1396.

315. Weinstein A: Drug-induced systemic lupus erythematosus. Prog Clin Immunol. 1980; 4:1.

316. Perry HMJ et al: Relationship of acetyl transferase activity to anti-nuclear antibodies and toxic symptoms in hypertensive patients treated with hydralazine. J Lab Clin Med. 1970; 76:114.

317. Perry HMJ et al: Late toxicity to hydralazine resembling systemic lupus erythematosus or rheumatoid arthritis. Am J Med. 1973; 54:58.

318. Davies DM et al: Anti-nuclear antibodies during procainamide treatment and drug acetylation. Br Med J. 1975; 3:682.

319. Woolsey RL et al: Effect of acetylator phenotype on the rate at which procainamide induces anti-nuclear antibodies and the lupus syndrome. N Engl J Med. 1978; 198:1157.

320. American Rheumatism Association: Primer on the rheumatic disease. JAMA. 1973; 229:740 (suppl).

321. Lee P et al: The etiology and pathogenesis of osteoarthrosis: a review. Sem Arthritis Rheum. 1974; 3:189.

322. Bollet AJ: Analgesic and anti-inflammatory drugs in the therapy of osteoarthritis. Sem Arthritis Rheum. 1980; 11:130.

323. Skjelbred P et al: Acetylsalicylic acid vs paracetamol: effects on post-operative course. Eur J Clin Pharmacol. 1977; 12:257.

324. Davis MJ: Aspirin-induced prolonged bleeding: report of case. J Dent Child. 1976; 43:350.

Chapter 58

Gout and Hyperuricemia

Lloyd Yee Young

The disease of gout is due to a disorder of uric acid metabolism. It is manifested by hyperuricemia, acute or chronic recurrent arthritis, and deposits of monosodium urates. *Gout* should be considered as a clinical diagnosis and *hyperuricemia* as a biochemical one. These two terms are not synonymous and not interchangeable.

Uric acid serves no biological function; it is merely the end-product of purine metabolism. Unlike other animals, man lacks the enzyme, uricase, which degrades uric acid into more soluble products for excretion. As a consequence, uric acid is not metabolized in man and must be excreted renally. Therefore, elevated serum uric acid lev-

els can result from an increase in the production of uric acid; a decrease in the renal excretion; or a combination of these two mechanisms.

Overproduction of uric acid may result from excessive de novo purine synthesis, excessive nucleoprotein turnover, or excessive dietary purines. **Excessive de novo purine synthesis** is primarily associated with rare enzyme mutation defects. For example, a deficiency of hypoxanthine-guanine phosphoribosyl transferase (HG-PRTase) is associated not only with hyperuricemia and gout, but also with mental retardation, choreoathetosis, and self-mutilation by biting. This phenomenon has been named the Lesch-Nyhan syndrome (64). Excessive dietary ingestion of yeast or liver tablets, which are high in purines, also has caused hyperuricemia in health food faddists.

Excessive nucleoprotein turnover from neoplastic diseases such as multiple myeloma, leukemias, lymphomas, and Hodgkin's disease as well as from myeloproliferative disorders such as myeloid metaplasia or polycythemia vera, have all been associated with gout and hyperuricemia.

Underexcretion of uric acid results from a defect in renal excretion. Uric acid is completely filtered at the renal glomerulus and subsequently reabsorbed in the proximal tubule. Of the uric acid appearing in the urine, approximately 80–86% is a result of active tubular secretion in the distal end of the proximal tubule. The filtered urate which escapes reabsorption constitutes only about 14 to 20% of the excreted uric acid load. Therefore, excreted uric acid is almost entirely attributable to the tubular secretory process.

When large urate loads are filtered during hyperuricemia, urate reabsorption increases to avoid the dumping of large amounts of poorly soluble urate into the urinary tract. Simultaneously, the hyperuricemia somewhat stimulates tubular secretion in an effort to remove the excess urate. Thus, the kidney is capable of responding to fluctuations in the concentration of urate in the serum. The renal excretion of uric acid is complex and involves other variables including a postsecretory distal tubular reabsorptive process (65,66).

ACUTE GOUT

1. W.S., a 46-year-old male professor of religion, is seen by his physician because of a chief complaint of severe pain at the base of his left great toe and around the forward portion of his arch. This pain was first noted about two days ago a few hours after an uneventful four mile run. While asleep that evening, the patient experienced pain severe enough to awaken him. The pain was more constant the next morning, and for the remainder of the day the patient walked with a significant limp. He was still unconcerned as he attributed the pain to a sprain from his jogging. Last night, while asleep, the patient was awakened several times with episodes of pain around the base of his left great toe and around the instep of his left foot. The pain, which was at first moderate, became more

intense. The pain was not sharp or knife-like, but rather it was a constant gnawing pain which did not abate with time. His foot felt like it was being slowly tightened in a vise and the pain was more of a constant squeezing pressure sensation than an acute transient phenomenon. By this morning, his foot was so exquisitely painful that he could not even tolerate the weight of the bedcovers.

Pertinent past medical history includes left foot trauma during a motorcycle accident about 10 years ago and essential hypertension of about five years duration. The systolic blood pressure is generally about 140–145 mm Hg and the diastolic pressure about 90–95 mm Hg during treatment. The patient is currently receiving hydrochlorothiazide 50 mg bid and propranolol 40 mg bid. This happily married patient's social history is noncontributory except for a nightly bedtime glass of wine.

On physical examination the first metatarsal phalangeal joint was warm and tender to touch. The entire periarticular area was erythematous and swollen to such an extent that it was difficult to determine which joint was the focus of the inflammation.

What subjective or objective data in this patient history are compatible with the clinical features of gout?

Epidemiology. The risk of gouty arthritis is about the same for both men and women at any given serum uric acid concentration; however, many more men are hyperuricemic. There are six men for every woman with serum uric acid levels greater than 7.0 mg/dl and about six times as many men for every woman with gout at this level of serum uric acid. Overall, only about 5% of gouty arthritis cases occur in women. Thus, the disease of gout is primarily a disease of adult men (1–4).

The onset of gout is rare in prepubertal children and is uncommon before the age of thirty. The onset is classically during middle age; in one study, the average individual age at the time of the first attack was 48 years (2). Thus, the age and sex of patient W.S. are compatible with the typical profile of a gouty patient. Other epidemiological associations dealing with race, intelligence, geographical locale, genetic disposition, coronary artery disease, or hypertension probably contribute more confusion than clarity. The only epidemiological association of true importance is that of gouty arthritis with hyperuricemia (see later presentation in this chapter).

Number of Joints. Patient W.S. seems to be experiencing polyarticular gout as both his great toe and instep appear to be afflicted. Although initial gout attacks have traditionally been recognized as being primarily monoarticular (1), as many as 39% of the patients in one study experienced polyarticular involvement as their first manifestation of gout (4). In another study, 27% of the first 30 patients with gout had crystal-proven polyarticular onset and 60% subsequently experienced polyarticular symptoms (5). Radionuclide imaging has demonstrated that multiple joints may be undergoing low-grade inflammatory reactions while medical attention is being focused only on the one clinically affected joint (6). Thus, patient W.S.'s polyarticular gout is not as unusual as once thought, and is compatible with cases of gouty arthritis which presented as polyarticular disease (4–7). Nevertheless, this patient may in fact have only single joint involvement because the area around the base of his left great toe is too inflamed to attribute the inflammatory process to one or to multiple contiguous joints.

Podagra. An acute attack of the great toe (podagra) is the most frequent manifestation of acute gouty arthritis. Approximately 50% of patients with gout have the initial attack in either great toe and about 84% will have at least one attack of podagra sometime during the course of this disease (2). If the great toe is not affected, the acute attacks almost always affect other peripheral joints in the feet and ankles. The small joints in the hands are usually affected next, then the knees and elbows. While acute gouty arthritis may occur in other joints such as the shoulder, hips, and vertebrae, occurrence in these sites is extremely rare except in patients with established severe disease. Thus, the involvement of the great toe of patient W.S. is typical of the usual acute attack of gout.

A hypothesis as to why gout preferentially affects the great toe is based upon the concept of transient local increases in the concentration of monosodium urate (9). According to this explanation, urate diffuses more slowly across a synovial membrane than does water (10,11). Thus, when the patient is in a recumbent position, the reabsorption of synovial effusion from traumatic joints produces a transiently high intra-articular

urate concentration that is conducive to crystal precipitation. Synovial effusions are increased in the great toe during the day because of degenerative changes in that joint: the first metatarsophalangeal joint is the most common and often the only joint affected in degenerative joint disease of the foot. According to radiographic surveys and surgical dissections, the frequency of degenerative joint disease at the base of the great toe far exceeds that in any other weight-bearing joint (9). Although this concept explains why the great toe is most commonly affected by gouty attacks, additional studies are needed to explain why hyperuricemic individuals with presumably similar degenerative joint changes do not experience acute gouty arthritis. The genesis of acute gouty attacks probably involves a multitude of other variables (12).

It probably is not coincidental that the left foot of patient W.S. is afflicted because it was this foot which was traumatized in the motorcycle accident ten years ago.

Physical Stress. Gouty attacks also seem to be more common during episodes of increased physical exercise. Long walks, hikes, golf games or tight new shoes have historically been associated with the subsequent onset of podagra (9). Thus, this painful episode of foot pain experienced by patient W.S. after a four mile run also is compatible with these clinical observations.

Nocturnal Occurrence. Acute gouty arthritis commonly begins at night. Even Thomas Sydenham's 18th century classic description of an acute gouty attack begins: "The victim goes to bed and sleeps in good health. About two o'clock in the morning he is awakened by a severe pain in the great toe; more rarely in the heel, ankle, or instep." According to the Simkin hypothesis (9), small amounts of effusion fluid gravitationally enters into degenerative joints of the feet during the day when most people are busily walking about, and is reabsorbed during the night when the lower extremities are elevated. Thus, the onset of foot pain in patient W.S. during the night also is typical of gout.

Pain. Thomas Sydenham continues his classical description of an acute gouty attack as follows. "This pain is like that of a dislocation . . . . The pain, which was at first moderate, becomes more intense . . . . After a time this comes to a height . . . Now it is a violent stretching and tearing of the ligaments—now it is a gnawing pain and now a pressure and tightening. So exquisite and lively meanwhile is the feeling of the part affected, that it cannot bear the weight of bedclothes nor the jar of a person walking in the room. The night is spent in torture, sleeplessness, turning of the part affected, and perpetual change of posture . . . ." This description of the affected part is remarkably similar to the description presented by patient W.S.

2. What laboratory data should be obtained at this time if the clinical assessment is gout?

The cardiovascular and renal systems of all patients with gout should be examined because hypertension or impaired renal function are common in many gouty patients. It would be especially prudent to monitor the blood pressure of patient W.S. because of his history of hypertension. Preliminary laboratory investigations should include a complete blood count, urinalysis, BUN or serum creatinine, and a serum uric acid (13).

The sudden appearance of acute swelling and tenderness of a joint without a background of arthritis, such as in this patient, can be attributed not only to gout, but also to infection. If the patient is a young single man, the possibility of an infectious etiology for the acute inflammation would be more seriously considered. Furthermore, the infectious organism may be presumed to be gonococcus unless another organism is suspected (14). Although febrile reactions, leukocytosis, and elevation of the erythrocyte sedimentation rate generally are attributed to infectious disease, such symptoms also are common to acute gouty arthritis (4). In view of this patient's age, social history, and classic clinical features, acute gouty arthritis would be the most likely cause of his pain.

The diagnosis of acute gouty arthritis is confirmed only when large numbers of polymorphonuclear leukocytes and monosodium urate crystals are demonstrated in synovial fluid aspirated from the inflamed joint (15). Hyperuricemia by itself is not diagnostic of gout because many hyperuricemic individuals never develop symptomatic gout, and acute gout may be present in some patients with normal serum uric acid concentrations. The monosodium urate crystals from the synovial fluid are seen through a microscope with normal illumination as being long and needle-shaped. However, a polarizing microscope with a first-order red compensator usually is needed to demonstrate the presence of these negatively birefringent urate crystals (16).

In an occasional patient with acute gout, urate crystals cannot be found in aspirated fluid from the inflamed joint (17–19). Therefore, a diagnosis of acute gouty arthritis cannot be entirely ruled out when urate crystals are not present in the initial synovial aspirate. Repeated search of other involved joints (18), or even of the same joint a few hours later (17,19) may demonstrate the diagnostic urate crystals. In selected cases, electron microscopic examination of synovial fluid may be needed for the initial documentation of urate crystal-induced synovitis when polarizing microscopy has failed to identify these crystals (20). Patient W.S. should have his first metatarsophalangeal joint aspirated to confirm the clinical assessment of gout. Although his instep might be the primary focus of his acute attack, the first metatarsophalangeal joint is by far the most commonly affected. Aspiration of this joint even if asymptomatic and even if never previously involved clinically can be recommended as an aid in establishing a definitive diagnosis of gout (21,22).

Treatment

3. Acute gouty arthritis can be effectively treated in most instances by colchicine, indomethacin, phenylbutazone, oxyphenbutazone, corticosteroids, or the nonsteroidal anti-inflammatory drugs such as naproxen, fenoprofen, or piroxicam. What are two reasons why colchicine might be the agent of choice for patient W.S. at this time?

Colchicine is not a general anti-inflammatory drug and, unlike indomethacin, phenylbutazone, and the nonsteroidal anti-inflammatory drugs (NSAIDs), is relatively specific for relieving the symptoms of acute gout (23). Therefore, a positive therapeutic response to colchicine is considered as supportive evidence for a diagnosis of gout. Such supportive diagnostic evidence is of importance when synovial fluid cannot be obtained from small joints for inspection of urate crystals and when one considers the fact that even well-qualified clinicians fail to find urate crystals in as many as 15% of acute gouty effusions (24). As a result, colchicine is the agent of choice for the first acute attack of gout because it not only provides symptomatic relief to greater than 95% of patients when administered early in the course of an attack, but it also is a useful diagnostic tool. However, the response to colchicine must be interpreted with some caution in a few unusual instances. The arthritis which accompanies psoriasis and sarcoidosis sometimes responds somewhat to colchicine (23). Likewise, colchicine also can prevent acute attacks of familial Mediterranean fever (25,26) and perhaps even alleviate amyloidosis (27).

The case for colchicine in patient W.S. would not be as strong if urate crystals are found in the aspirate of synovial fluid. Nevertheless, Talbott (8) suggests that every gouty patient's response to colchicine should be assessed at least once. After a patient's response to colchicine for the first gouty attack has been documented, subsequent gouty attacks should be treated with the NSAIDs such as indomethacin or naproxen because these agents are better tolerated by the patient and have both analgesic and anti-inflammatory effects.

Patient W.S. also has a long history of hypertension which is now reasonably controlled with propranolol and hydrochlorothiazide. Indomethacin reportedly antagonizes the diuretic effects of furosemide. Whether indomethacin antagonizes the antihypertensive effect of hydrochlorothiazide and whether other prostaglandin-inhibiting anti-inflammatory agents have the same magnitude of effect are not known at this time. Prostaglandins do affect both sodium and water balance as well as blood pressure regulation. Therefore, prostaglandin inhibitors such as indomethacin and other nonsteroidal anti-inflammatory drugs should affect these processes as well. However, these precise interactions still need to be clearly established because of the opposing effects of different prostaglandins and because reports are still in preliminary stages.

Studies have consistently demonstrated that indomethacin can inhibit furosemide-induced increases of renal sodium excretion in both normal subjects and hypertensive patients (29–32). Indomethacin has reduced the hypotensive effect of furosemide as well (29). Furthermore, indomethacin 100 mg daily inhibited the antihypertensive response of seven patients to propranolol (33). Based on these data, antihypertensive patients should have their blood pressure frequently monitored if indomethacin is prescribed because alterations in antihypertensive doses may be necessary. It is not known whether gouty hypertensive patients will experience similar problems with indomethacin, or with the other general anti-inflammatory agents, since treatment of acute gouty attacks is only for a few days. Nevertheless, it is always best to be prudent and to monitor patients closely as short-term indomethacin use has induced hyperkalemia and renal insufficiency in three patients with gouty arthritis (34).

4. The plan is to treat this first attack of gout with colchicine, two 0.5 mg tablets initially, followed by one tablet every other hour until relief of joint pain or onset of gastrointestinal adverse affects. Why is this colchicine dosing interval being utilized?

For the fully developed acute attack, the traditional dose of colchicine has been one or two 0.5 to 0.6 mg tablets initially, followed by 0.5 to 0.6 mg hourly until there is relief of joint pain or development of gastrointestinal side effects such as diarrhea, nausea, or vomiting. Colchicine is administered hourly to minimize gastrointestinal toxicity because patients vary considerably with respect to the amount of colchicine they can tolerate. However, even with hourly colchicine, titration of dose to a maximal therapeutic response with gastrointestinal toxicity is difficult. Therefore, a longer dosing interval of 0.5 mg every other hour following the initial 1.0 mg dose should significantly decrease gastrointestinal problems and still not compromise the therapeutic response (35). If, through past experience, the approximate therapeutic or toxic dose of colchicine is known for a particular patient, one-half to two-thirds of this dose can be administered at once with the remainder given as 0.5 to 0.6 mg every other hour. This method of administration saves the patient much suffering since delays in treatment may result in greater failure rates as well as increased severity and duration of attacks.

5. Why do colchicine prescriptions usually limit the number of doses or number of tablets for each acute gouty attack?

The number of colchicine doses should be limited because an occasional patient may not develop florid gastrointestinal distress or simply may not have gout. Therefore, a maximum of 10 to 15 tablets generally is recommended. Although the lethal dose is estimated to be about 65 mg (37), serious toxicity may occur with much smaller doses; fatality has resulted from as little as 7.0 mg (36). Adverse effects from colchicine are usually reversible and consist most commonly of nausea, diarrhea, abdominal pain, and vomiting. More severe toxic effects from therapeutic doses of colchicine affect the hepatic, hematopoietic, and nervous systems, but usually occur only in elderly patients (36) or those with prior cardiac, hepatic, or renal disease (38). Reports of a toxic effect of colchicine on sperm production (39) have been refuted (40).

6. When should the therapeutic effects of colchicine begin to become apparent in patient W.S.?

The pain of acute gouty arthritis still is intense three to four hours after initiating colchicine therapy, but usually it is very apparent to patients that the pain no longer is increasing in severity. The pain begins to recede within four to eight hours and is generally quiescent within 12 to 16 hours. Generally, the pain, redness and swelling are completely resolved within 48 to 72 hours after the initiation of colchicine therapy. Nevertheless, there is considerable interpatient variation to this time-frame.

7. Patient W.S. is in excruciating pain and requests an analgesic to supplement his gout medication. Why might a narcotic analgesic be appropriate?

A dose or two of a narcotic analgesic may be reasonable to blunt the pain of acute gouty arthritis while awaiting the apparent benefits of colchicine action. Additionally, the narcotic analgesics have the added advantage of decreasing the troublesome diarrhea which accompanies colchicine use.

8. If intravenous colchicine were to be used for patient W.S., how would it be administered?

Intravenous colchicine solutions are extremely irritating and care must be taken to prevent extravasation during administration. The needle which is used to aspirate the colchicine solution into the syringe should be discarded, and a new needle used for the actual venopuncture.

The entire two to three milligram dose of colchicine should be diluted to 30 ml with normal saline and administered slowly over a period of five minutes. This dose may be repeated in 6 to 8 hours if needed, but the total intravenous amount of colchicine should not exceed 5.0 mg for a given attack of gouty arthritis (41). This latter point is underscored by a fatal case report of a 70-year-old man with apparently normal renal and hepatic function who developed marrow aplasia and pancytopenia after receiving 10 mg of colchicine intravenously over a period of five days for acute gouty arthritis (42).

9. Patient W.S. experienced dramatic relief of pain from his oral colchicine therapy. In fact his response was much better than expected. After receiving 1.5 mg of colchicine the patient could feel that the pain at the base of his great toe was no longer accelerating in intensity. About five hours after initiating colchicine the pain began to abate and the patient had a loose bowel movement. At about seven hours after initiating therapy, the pain was about 50% improved. After about 12 hours and a total dose of 4.0 mg of colchicine, the pain was about 80% improved and the patient had mild diarrhea.

The hydrochlorothiazide was discontinued on the following day and the serum uric acid concentration was 11.2 mg/dl according to the laboratory report. A synovial aspirate of the inflamed joint was not obtained, nor was a 24-hour urine sample for uric acid quantification. Other laboratory tests were within normal limits and the patient was instructed to monitor his blood pressure daily. The patient also was instructed to initiate therapy with the remainder of his colchicine prescription and to call his physician should another similar attack develop.

Why should (or should not) patient W.S. receive hypouricemic therapy at this time?

After the initial attack of acute gout, the interval between subsequent attacks varies from a few days to several years. No specific therapy is required during this interval, although it often is tempting to initiate hypouricemic therapy because of the clear association of hyperuricemia with gout and because urate-lowering medications are relatively safe. Nevertheless, antihyperuricemic drugs should not be prescribed indiscriminately. Once started, such therapy usually is continued indefinitely. Hypouricemic therapy should be initiated only when gouty patients have frequent acute attacks, urate tophi, or evidence of renal damage. If these indications are absent, hypouricemic drug therapy should await the natural course of events because nothing is lost by waiting. The acute attack always can be treated when it appears and it usually is resolved within days.

In particular, long-term hypouricemic medications should not be started for patient W.S. at this time because the above criteria for therapy are not met and, more importantly, the diagnosis of gout has not been firmly established by the demonstration of urate crystals in the synovial fluid of an inflamed joint. In today's era of routine laboratory tests, there is the tendency to overdiagnose gout in hyperuricemic individuals. It is not uncommon to find a hyperuricemic patient with a musculoskeletal problem inappropriately treated with urate lowering drugs. Therefore, patient W.S. should not be treated with hypouricemic drugs at this time.

Finally, antihyperuricemic drugs may not be needed in patient W.S. because his hyperuricemia and presumed acute gouty attack may have been the result of the hydrochlorothiazide. Hyperuricemia is a commonly encountered adverse effect of thiazide and other diuretics including furosemide, ethacrynic acid, chlorthalidone, and acetazolamide (43,44). These diuretics indirectly increase urate serum concentrations during extracellular fluid volume contraction. The volume depletion may enhance urate retention because of altered renal blood flow or changes in intra-renally generated angiotensin (45). The volume contraction also could cause hyperuricemia by inducing a generalized reabsorption of all solutes (46). Replacement of urinary salt and water losses prevents diuretic-induced hyperuricemia (44). Therefore, discontinuation of hydrochlorothiazide may be all that is needed to lower the serum urate concentration of patient W.S. Initiation of hypouricemic medications such as allopurinol or probenecid at this time would be premature.

10. After being relatively symptom-free since his first acute gouty attack eight months ago, patient W.S. now complains of pain around the base of his left great toe similar to that experienced in the past. This apparent gouty attack began last night after a late evening lecture. He was awakened by acute pain and took his last remaining colchicine tablet which seemed to be beneficial. About three months prior to this episode he had taken two doses of colchicine because of some vague pain in the same region; and about one month ago, similar vague discomfort responded to three tablets of colchicine.

On physical examination the first metatarsophalangeal joint of his left foot is markedly inflamed, tender, and brightly erythematous in appearance. Other findings are non-remarkable and his blood pressure of 135/85 mm Hg continues to be well-controlled on propranolol 20 mg bid. Examination of synovial fluid obtained from his first metatarsophalangeal joint noted a poor mucin clot, numerous polymorphonuclear leukocytes, and the diagnostic monosodium urate crystals. A blood sample also was obtained to measure the concentration of uric acid and creatinine.

What therapeutic intervention would be the most appropriate for patient W.S. at this time?

There are many well-established drugs available for the management of acute gout. Drugs such as indomethacin, phenylbutazone, colchicine, corticosteroids, and the nonsteroidal anti-inflammatory drugs are all highly effective, and disadvantages amongst these agents are relatively minor because these drugs are used for only a few days at a time. Therefore, the selection of the most appropriate drug for an acute attack of gout depends primarily upon physician and patient preferences.

Indomethacin has become the drug most frequently prescribed for the treatment of acute attacks of gouty arthritis and many consider it to be the drug of choice (47). When used in doses of 50 mg three times daily for two to three days followed by gradually tapering doses, this nonsteroidal anti-inflammatory agent is very effective. Adverse effects are minimal when used in this manner, although gastrointestinal disturbances, mental changes, headaches, rash, and leukopenia have been reported. The earlier use of indomethacin was associated with a high incidence of dose-related adverse effects because large doses of 100 to 200 mg four times daily were used at that time.

Phenylbutazone (Butazolidin) and its metabolite, *oxyphenbutazone* (Tandearil) can control 85 to 95% of acute attacks of gout within 24 to 36 hours. Therefore, phenylbutazone and oxyphenbutazone were the drugs of choice for patients unable to tolerate colchicine, prior to the recommendation that lower doses of indomethacin be used. In 1965, Gutman (48) suggested that the time had come for oxyphenbutazone (or phenylbutazone) to replace colchicine as the drug of choice for acute gout; however, he continued to use oral colchicine (49).

Phenylbutazone doses of 200 mg four times daily for the first day, followed by 200 mg three times daily for two additional days, are then rapidly tapered and discontinued over the next two days. Yu recommends administering 200 mg of phenylbutazone four times daily together with colchicine 1.0 to 2.0 mg daily (35,50).

The potential hematological toxicities of phenylbutazone are well documented but rare with short-term therapy. Thrombocytopenia (51) and acute gastrointestinal hemorrhages (52) have occurred after a single day of phenylbutazone therapy, but rare individual cases of toxicity to any drug are not unusual.

The new analgesic, nonsteroidal anti-inflammatory drugs (NSAIDs) such as ibuprofen, naproxen, and piroxicam are widely utilized in the management of numerous inflammatory diseases because they are highly effective and have minimal gastrointestinal toxicities. As a result, these agents increasingly are used in the treatment of acute gout.

In a multicenter study, *naproxen* 750 mg as a single dose followed by 250 mg three times daily was as effective as phenylbutazone 200 mg four times daily for 48 hours followed by 200 mg three times daily in 41 patients with acute gout (53). Another investigation compared two dosage regimens of naproxen and favored the regimen which used the higher loading dose (54). In this latter study, the regimen consisting of 750 mg of naproxen initially, followed in 8 hours with a 500 mg dose and 250 mg every 8 hours thereafter for 48 to 72 hours was better than a regimen of 600 mg initially, followed by 300 mg at 8 hour intervals. This author has been successful with 500 mg of naproxen for the first two doses with subsequent 250 mg doses three times daily. *Ibuprofen* 2400 mg/day in one patient (55) and in 10 other patients (56) resulted in rapid improvement and complete resolution of gouty arthritis within 72 hours. Variable *fenoprofen* doses not exceeding 3.2 gm/day were effective in 27 patients with 36 joints affected with acute gouty arthritis (57). In another double-blind comparison of fenoprofen

versus phenylbutazone, both drugs were highly effective in relieving acute gouty arthritis (58). Other new nonsteroidal anti-inflammatory drugs such as piroxicam in a dose of 40 mg once a day (59,60) and sulindac (61) also have been proven effective in the treatment of acute gouty arthritis. Adverse effects to these agents have been modest. (The NSAIDs are discussed further in the chapter entitled Rheumatic Diseases.)

This patient's first gouty attack responded well to colchicine and this positive response was useful in providing supportive evidence for a diagnosis of gout. However, the predictable diarrhea which accompanies this drug is especially disturbing to patients with podagra who must hobble to the bathroom on injured joints. Thus, one of the newer NSAIDs such as naproxen should be prescribed for patient W.S. for this acute attack of gout. Indomethacin and phenylbutazone are especially potent inhibitors of prostaglandin synthetase and indomethacin might be more undesirable than the newer NSAIDs in this hypertensive patient (see Question 3). The sodium and fluid retention properties of phenylbutazone also may be undesirable in this patient, and its mild uricosuric properties may complicate the scheduling of urinary uric acid excretion studies.

11. Patient W.S. responded well to naproxen. Within 72 hours of initiating therapy, his first metatarsophalangeal joint no longer was inflamed. The clinical laboratory noted that his serum uric acid concentration was 8.4 mg/dl, and he was provided with instructions for a 24-hour urine collection. Why is it important to assess the 24-hour urine for uric acid?

Some believe that urinary uric acid should be measured in every hyperuricemic patient (62), while other practitioners are unsure as to the benefit of such studies for all patients. Nevertheless, there is no question that quantification of urinary uric acid excretion is important, at least for some patients, because it is of diagnostic benefit in defining the cause of hyperuricemia and in determining the choice of the most appropriate hypouricemic agent.

Urinary uric acid excretion is usually measured in a 24-hour specimen to ascertain whether the patient overexcretes or underexcretes uric acid. Patients excreting less than 750 mg/day of uric acid into the urine generally are underexcretors, and those excreting more than 800 mg/day are categorized as overexcretors. A few overexcretors of uric acid suffer from genetic defects in enzymes such as hypoxanthine-guanine phosphoribosyl transferase (HGPRTase), or from disorders such as leukemias which are associated with increased turnover of cells. Moreover, overexcretors are probably best treated with the hypouricemic drug allopurinol, which inhibits the formation of uric acid, as opposed to a hypouricemic agent such as probenecid which increases urate excretion.

Predictions of urinary uric acid overexcretors by use of uric acid to creatinine (or creatinine clearance) ratios based upon spot mid-morning serum and urine samples (62) have been advocated because of the inherent difficulties in 24-hour urine collections. Unfortunately, diurnal variations in uric acid excretion often invalidate 24-hour excretion predictions based upon spot urine samples (63).

HYPERURICEMIA

12. Patient W.S. apparently has experienced at least two, and perhaps four, attacks of gout within the past 8 months. His thiazide diuretic was discontinued at the time of his first attack; however, he is still hyperuricemic with a serum uric acid concentration of 8.4 mg/dl. The uric acid excretion study noted that 690 mg of uric acid was excreted over the course of the 24-hour collection. What hypouricemic medication should this patient receive?

Two types of hypouricemic drugs have withstood the test of time and are commonly utilized in the management of hyperuricemia. Uricosuric drugs reduce the serum urate concentration by increasing the renal excretion of uric acid; and xanthine oxidase-inhibiting drugs decrease serum uric acid by inhibiting uric acid synthesis. The uricosuric drugs, probenecid and sulfinpyrazone, are the most logical hypouricemic agents for the management of patients who are underexcretors of uric acid; and the uric acid synthesis inhibitors such as allopurinol are the most logical for the overproducers of uric acid. Although this strategy for managing hyperuricemia certainly seems attractive, an inhibitor of uric acid synthesis should be effective in both underexcretors and overproducers. Because allopurinol is an effective hy-

pouricemic drug in all patients, and because comparisons of the relative propensity for adverse effects of uricosurics and allopurinol are non-definitive, allopurinol is most commonly prescribed for the management of hyperuricemia.

The uric acid excretion test result of patient W.S. was inconclusive. Patients excreting less than 750 mg/day of uric acid generally are considered to be underexcretors; however, 24-hour urine collections are notoriously difficult (67) and to conclude that patient W.S., who excretes 690 mg/day, is an underexcretor is too categorical. This patient does not have evidence of myeloproliferative disease, tophaceous deposits, or renal insufficiency and neither allopurinol nor the uricosuric drug, probenecid, are better than the other in this situation. Likewise, neither probenecid nor allopurinol is effective for the acute gouty attack, and either is effective only in the long-term management of hyperuricemia.

Allopurinol

13. The hyperuricemia of patient W.S. is to be treated with allopurinol. What would be an appropriate dose of this drug to initiate therapy?

The ability of allopurinol to lower serum uric acid is a dose-related phenomenon. The higher the dose of allopurinol, the greater the fall in serum uric acid levels. Generally, the dose required to normalize hyperuricemia in patients with mild disease is 200 to 300 mg/day and 400 to 600 mg/day in those with moderate or severe disease (68). Allopurinol doses of 300 mg/day in one study reduced the serum urate concentration to less than 7 mg/dl and halved the urinary uric acid excretion in about 70% of patients. The remaining patients needed 400 to 600 mg/day, although 200 mg/day sufficed in some (69). Therefore, it would be reasonable to expect that 300 mg/day of allopurinol would be appropriate for patient W.S. However, anecdotal data suggest that symptoms of acute gout may be slightly exacerbated during the first six weeks of allopurinol therapy because of uric acid mobilization from tissues. Although these data are merely suggestive, allopurinol therapy should be initiated slowly simply because nothing is lost by so doing. Patients generally have been hyperuricemic for a good many years and the extra week or two required to reach usual therapeutic doses should not make a difference. Thus, patient W.S. should receive 100 mg/day of allopurinol for the first two weeks of therapy. Thereafter, the dose should be increased to whatever is needed to reduce the urate serum concentration to less than 6.5 mg/dl. This gradual approach to initiating allopurinol in this situation is admittedly conservative and usually unnecessary.

14. When should the hypouricemic effect from allopurinol become apparent?

Serum uric acid levels usually begin to fall within one to two days after initiation of allopurinol therapy; maximal uric acid suppression usually requires seven to ten days (68,69). Clinical improvement takes longer. After approximately six months, one should observe a gradual decrease in size of established tophi and the absence of new tophaceous deposits if these were present in patient W.S.

15. If the half-life of allopurinol is less than two hours why is this drug commonly administered once a day?

Approximately 80% of an oral dose of allopurinol is rapidly absorbed when administered by the oral route. Once absorbed (30 minutes to two hours), allopurinol is rapidly cleared from plasma with a probable plasma half-life of less than two hours (70). A small portion of allopurinol is excreted in the urine unchanged but the remainder is rapidly oxidized to alloxanthine (oxypurinol). Oxypurinol is slowly eliminated from the blood by renal excretion, and has a prolonged plasma half-life of 18 to 44 hours in man. Neither oxypurinol nor allopurinol is bound to plasma proteins and both are filtered at the glomerulus. However, oxypurinol, unlike allopurinol, then undergoes proximal tubular reabsorption (71).

Oxypurinol also is a potent inhibitor of xanthine oxidase, but is one-fifth to one-tenth as potent as allopurinol *in vitro. In vivo,* however, it accounts for much of allopurinol's xanthine oxidase inhibitory effects because of its longer half-life.

Due to oxypurinol's long half-life and its acknowledged xanthine oxidase inhibitory effects, allopurinol can be administered on a once daily basis. In fact, dosing with allopurinol on any dosing schedule results in the same steady effect within a few days (71). The daily administration of a single 300 mg tablet of allopurinol gives results identical in all parameters to 100 mg three

times daily (72). Smaller doses should be used in patients with renal failure.

16. What subjective or objective clinical parameters should be evaluated to monitor for adverse effects to allopurinol?

The overall physical appearance, temperature, creatinine or BUN, SGOT, and eosinophil count of the patient should be evaluated for hypersensitivity-type reactions to allopurinol.

Allopurinol is exceptionally well tolerated with no severe dose-related adverse reactions of any major magnitude. Doses up to 1200 mg have been administered without untoward effects. Of the adverse drug reactions that are sometimes encountered with allopurinol, hypersensitivity-type reactions have been the most notorious. These generally present as mildly erythematous, purpuric, or maculopapular skin rashes which subside within a few days after the medication is discontinued. The rash most commonly occurs in patients with impaired renal function and is generally accompanied by fever, malaise, and aching. It often appears within one to five weeks of therapy and is frequently preceded by pruritus. However, the rash has appeared as part of a delayed hypersensitivity reaction as late as three months in one case and twenty-five months in another (73).

More severe hypersensitivity reactions have also been associated with allopurinol. One fatal case of generalized maculopapular exfoliative dermatitis with severe systemic allergic vasculitis has been reported (74). Another allopurinol-induced fatality has been attributed to toxic epidermal necrolysis with oliguria, sepsis and pneumonia (75). Two non-fatal cases of allopurinol hypersensitivity angiitis were characterized by pruritic dermatitis and renal failure 3 to 5 weeks after initiation of therapy (76), and at least five additional cases have been reported (77,78).

These cases shared similar characteristics. The onset of illness occurred about four weeks after initiation of therapy, and began with fever and pruritus or dermatitis. Variable hepatic impairment was present in all cases, although the predominant features were exfoliating dermatitis and renal failure. The dermatitis and renal failure were attributed to a systemic vasculitis and the non-fatal cases did not improve until large steroid doses were instituted, despite immediate discontinuation of allopurinol. Furthermore, it has been hypothesized that the variable nature of the liver toxicity may indicate that it is not part of the picture of systemic vasculitis, but may well represent a separate immunological reaction to allopurinol (78). Seven of the above nine cases of allopurinol vasculitis were accompanied by eosinophilia and all exhibited fever, dermatitis, and renal impairment. Severe hypersensitivity reactions to allopurinol may also occur more commonly in patients with renal impairment, although in the majority of cases, renal dysfunction is the result of, rather than the cause of, these reactions.

Periodic evaluation of liver function tests also would be helpful in detecting adverse effects of allopurinol. A recent literature review has uncovered 20 instances of presumed allopurinol hepatotoxicity (79). All of these cases met accepted criteria for hypersensitivity reactions including fever, rash, eosinophilia and non-caseating granulomas on liver biopsy. Most of these patients had compromised renal function or were treated with concomitant diuretics. The major metabolite of allopurinol, oxypurinol, is excreted renally and it has been suggested that this metabolite might be an intrinsic hepatotoxin at high blood levels (79).

Concomitant drug therapy also should be evaluated. For example, the Boston Collaborative Drug Surveillance Group (90) reported that dermatological reactions were observed in 22.4% of 67 patients receiving concomitant allopurinol and ampicillin, as compared to 7.5% of patients receiving only ampicillin, and 2.1% receiving only allopurinol. Allopurinol also significantly enhances the anticoagulant effects of bishydroxycoumarin, and less commonly, of warfarin. The dosages of mercaptopurine or azathioprine, which are metabolized by xanthine oxidase, should be decreased by one-third or one-fourth when the xanthine oxidase inhibitor, allopurinol, is administered concomitantly. Allopurinol also enhances the bone marrow toxicity which sometimes accompanies cyclophosphamide treatment.

Uricosuric Therapy

17. Patient W.S. has not experienced any gouty attacks since the initiation of allopurinol about 10 months ago. During a routine yearly physical examination, the SGOT was noted to be slightly increased to 90 units. All other liver function tests were within normal limits. The patient stated that he did develop a localized rash which later subsided without discontinuing any of his medications. Although these findings may not represent allopurinol hypersensitivity, the allopurinol is to be discontinued and probenecid started. How should uricosuric therapy be initiated?

Probenecid is well absorbed orally, and peak plasma concentrations occur within two to four hours. Its biological half-life is six to twelve hours and its active metabolites help to prolong the uricosuria. The dose of probenecid should be 250 mg twice daily for the first week of therapy; thereafter 500 mg may be given twice a day. If necessary, the dose may be increased to 2.0 gm daily. Initiation of uricosuric therapy must begin slowly because excretion of large amounts of uric acid increases the risk of urate stone formation in the kidney. This risk can be minimized by starting with small doses of uricosurics so that the kidney is not overwhelmed with a flood of uric acid; and maintenance of a high fluid intake to maintain urine flow of at least two liters per day also minimizes renal stone formation. Such a gradual approach to initiation of therapy also decreases the likelihood of precipitating an acute attack of gout.

Sulfinpyrazone (Anturane) is a phenylbutazone analogue that is also a very effective uricosuric agent. Like all uricosurics, it inhibits tubular secretion of uric acid at low doses; but at normal therapeutic doses, it inhibits the tubular reabsorption of uric acid. As with probenecid, therapy should be initiated slowly and doses increased gradually.

18. How soon after initiation of probenecid should the serum uric acid be decreased?

When therapy is begun, a prompt fall in plasma urate concentrations is usually seen and is accompanied by rapid urinary excretion of uric acid. After the first day or two, the urinary uric acid excess disappears in normal man; but in hyperuricemic individuals, the excess uric acid is continually mobilized until the body pool of urate is reduced to normal levels (80).

In patient W.S., probably no change in the serum uric acid concentration will be noted because he has been receiving allopurinol.

19. Does patient W.S. have any contraindications to the use of probenecid uricosuric therapy?

The fact that uricosuric drugs do not affect the production of uric acid, but merely increase its excretion, places limitations on their use. Probenecid cannot be used in patients with a glomerular filtration rate (GFR) less than 20 to 30 ml/min or a BUN greater than 40 mg/dl. If the GFR is 40 to 50 ml/min, the dose of probenecid needs to be increased. Patients with a history of frequent renal stones and patients who are gross over-excretors (more than 1000 mg/day) of uric acid should not be treated with uricosurics. Additionally, these agents should not be used in patients suffering an acute attack of gout. None of these contraindications are applicable to patient W.S. and probenecid can be safely prescribed for him.

20. Why is aspirin now contraindicated in patient W.S.?

Two tablets of aspirin 300 mg every six hours can completely antagonize the uricosuric effects of two grams of probenecid. This drug interaction probably involves several mechanisms including competition for renal tubular transport (81). Doses of salicylate which do not produce serum salicylate levels of at least 5 mg/dl do not significantly affect probenecid uricosuria. Interestingly, salicylates do not affect the ability of probenecid to inhibit the tubular secretion of penicillin. Acetaminophen (Tylenol) does not interfere with probenecid and is a reliable alternative for antipyresis and mild analgesia in these patients.

Asymptomatic Hyperuricemia

21. A 50-year-old man is seen by his physician for a routine evaluation. His physical examination is unremarkable and his laboratory evaluations are all within normal limits except for a serum uric acid concentration of 9.5 mg/dl which was noted on an SMA-12 panel. What is the clinical significance of this hyperuricemia?

There are several methods for the analysis of uric acid and each method and laboratory has different standard normal values for the same sample. The phosphotungstate or colorimetric method, commonly utilized in automated laboratory screening panels, is not as specific as the uricase method of uric acid analysis and generally provides values that are about 1 mg/dl higher.

In normal subjects, plasma becomes saturated with sodium urate at a concentration of 7 mg/dl.

However, supersaturated solutions of sodium urate form readily, and serum urate concentrations as high as 40 to 60 mg/dl are not uncommon in untreated nongouty patients with myeloproliferative disorders (82). It is not clear how uric acid can remain in a supersaturated solution and then, suddenly, under certain conditions, begin to precipitate out. However, it is known that plasma urate-binding protein deficiency, urate affinity for chondroitin sulfate, local pH changes, cold, trauma, and stress can cause seeding of urate crystals.

When maximum serum uric acid values from the Framingham Heart Study (2) were analyzed, gouty arthritis was noted to occur in 1.8% of those patients with levels between 6.0 to 6.9 mg/dl and in 11.8% of those with levels between 7.0 to 7.9 mg/dl. On the other hand, 15% of the men who had actually developed gouty arthritis did not have a serum uric acid value above 6.9 mg/dl and 81% of subjects with serum uric acid values of greater than 7.0 mg/dl did not develop gouty arthritis. Thus, the higher the serum concentration of uric acid, the greater the risk of developing gouty arthritis.

22. Should asymptomatic hyperuricemia, such as noted in this patient, be treated?

Individuals with high serum uric acid levels are more likely to develop acute gouty arthritis than normouricemic individuals, and the magnitude of the risk increases with increasing degrees of hyperuricemia. However, it would be excessive to treat all hyperuricemic individuals with uric acid lowering medications for a lifetime solely for the prevention of acute attacks of *gouty arthritis*. A large percentage of hyperuricemic patients may never experience an acute attack of gout. If an attack should occur, it can easily be treated within 48–72 hours, and after the acute episode has subsided, uric acid lowering medications can then be considered.

The key issue in the treatment of hyperuricemia concerns the effect of uric acid on renal function. *Renal disease* was commonly associated with gout, and renal failure was thought to be the eventual cause of death in as many as 25% of gouty patients. Thus, treatment of hyperuricemia is justifiable if renal disease is prevented. This renal damage, however, was noted to occur in a setting that included either hypertension, diabetes, renal vascular disease, glomerulonephritis, pyelonephritis, renal calculi, or some other cause of primary nephropathy independent of gout (83).

In fact, the coexistence of gout and renal insufficiency without hypertension is so rare that its presence should raise the suspicion of chronic lead toxicity (91,92). Therefore, the consensus now seems to be that hyperuricemia or uncomplicated gout by itself has no deleterious effect on renal function (84,85). When one considers the financial costs, risks of adverse drug reactions, and practical considerations such as patient compliance, drug treatment of asymptomatic hyperuricemia is difficult to justify (86).

Hyperuricemia with Renal Failure

23. A 54-year-old male with a history of congestive heart failure is hospitalized with a diagnosis of acute myelogenous leukemia. On admission the BUN was 49 mg/dl, serum creatinine was 2.1 mg/dl, and the serum uric acid was 16.2 mg/dl. On the following hospital day, chemotherapy was begun. His white blood cell count decreased within a week from 90,000/mm^3 on admission to 7,500/mm^3 as a result of the cytotoxic treatment. On the 7th day he complained of nausea, and his urine volume decreased to 35 ml/24 hours. At this time, the BUN increased to 115 mg/dl, serum creatinine increased to 10.6 mg/dl, and his serum uric acid increased to 22.6 mg/dl. Intravenous furosemide and urine alkalinization had no effect on his clinical condition, and hemodialysis was started because of continued clinical deterioration. During the ensuing two days, the urine output increased and then gradually returned to normal. His renal function continued to improve, and 16 days after hemodialysis was initiated, the serum creatinine was again 2.1 mg/dl.

What was the probable cause for the elevated serum uric acid level noted upon this patient's admission?

Upon superficial review, it would appear that the hyperuricemia in this patient is a result of both overproduction and underexcretion of uric acid. However, the major cause of hyperuricemia in this case is probably due to the overproduction of nucleic acids because of the leukemia. Mild to moderate renal failure is not usually a cause of hyperuricemia as long as the creatinine clearance is greater than 15 ml/minute. Apparently, renal urate secretory mechanisms remain functional and do not become defective until the glomerular filtration rate falls below 10 ml/minute. At this level of renal function, the defective secretory mechanism is unable to entirely compensate for the decrease in urate reabsorption, and hyperuricemia occurs (87).

24. Why was urine alkalinization tried in this patient?

Urine alkalinization was instituted because the serum uric acid was 22.6 mg/dl in the presence of oliguria. Uric acid is poorly soluble in water, but a pK$_a$ of 5.75 allows for greater solubility of the ionized form in alkaline environments. At a urine pH of 5, only 6 to 8 mg of uric acid are soluble per deciliter of urine. However, when urine is alkalinized to pH 7, the solubility of uric acid increases twenty-fold to 120–160 mg per deciliter. Although asymptomatic hyperuricemia is not associated with renal impairment, unusually high blood uric acid levels in the presence of oliguria and undue acidity may result in the intrarenal and urinary precipitation of urate (85). Thus, the desire to alkalinize the urine can be appreciated.

Urine can be alkalinized using *sodium* or *potassium bicarbonate* in an initial oral dose of four grams followed by one to two grams every four hours. Intravenous sodium bicarbonate can also be used, as it was in this patient. The pH should be tested (eg, nitrazine paper) at intervals throughout the day and the dose of bicarbonate should be adjusted accordingly. *Potassium* or *sodium citrate* can also be used in doses of one gram three to six times daily. The citrates have the same urine alkalinizing properties of sodium bicarbonate without neutralizing gastric secretions and without promoting a dumping syndrome. The bicarbonate and citrate doses should be evenly divided throughout the day and night. During the night, the urine becomes the most concentrated and acidic; thus it may be necessary to add an intravenous dose to the IV solution during the night in hospitalized patients. *Acetazolamide* (Diamox) is also capable of alkalinizing urine, but it can produce a mild metabolic acidosis which is undesirable in a patient with renal decompensation.

Although an alkaline urine is theoretically desirable to increase the solubility of uric acid, it is often difficult to achieve clinically without affecting other organ systems. In this patient with congestive heart failure, sodium intake is a problem and the benefits from alkalinization probably are not worth the effort. The ability of the kidneys to excrete potassium may also be of critical importance. The cation content of various alkalinizing agents is listed as follows:

Product	mEq/gram
Na HCO$_3$	11.9
Na Citrate · 2H$_2$O	8.4
K HCO$_3$	9.9
K Citrate · H$_2$O	9.3

25. Hemodialysis was initiated in this patient. How well is uric acid dialyzed and would prophylaxis against an acute attack be needed?

Uric acid is readily dialyzable despite the finding that uric acid is bound to plasma proteins (88). Apparently, this urate-albumin bond is weak and influenced by many factors. In fact, hemodialysis is so efficient in removing uric acid that each six-hour dialysis can reduce the uric acid level by 50%. In 16 patients with hyperuricemia and renal failure, each six-hour dialysis removed 1.5 to 13.4 grams of uric acid. Although 3.4 to 4.8 grams of uric acid can be removed by peritoneal dialysis, hemodialysis is estimated to be between 10 to 20 times more efficient in eliminating uric acid (89). Disequilibrium does not occur even with rapid hemodialysis and prophylaxis against an acute gouty attack is unnecessary.

References

1. Kelley WN: Gout and other disorders of purine metabolism. In Harrison's *Principles of Internal Medicine,* 9th ed, edited by KJ Isselbacher et al, McGraw-Hill, New York, 1980, p 479–487.
2. Hall AP et al: Epidemiology of gout and hyperuricemia; a long-term population study. Am J Med. 1967; 42:27.
3. Grahame R et al: Clinical survey of 354 patients with gout. Ann Rheum Dis. 1970; 29:461.
4. Hadler NM et al: Acute polyarticular gout. Am J Med. 1974; 56:715.
5. Baraf HSB et al: Gouty arthritis: prevalence of chronic synovitis, polyarticular attacks, and positive serological tests for rheumatoid factor. Arthritis Rheum. 1978; 21:544.
6. Rosenthall L et al: Radionuclide joint imaging in the diagnosis of synovial disease. Semin Arthritis Rheum. 1977; 7:49.
7. Lipsmeier EA: Acute gouty arthritis presenting as polyarticular disease. South Med J. 1982; 75:82.
8. Talbott JH: Gouty arthritis: a disease for all ages. Geriatrics. 1980; 35:71.
9. Simkin PA: The pathogenesis of podagra. Ann Intern Med. 1977; 86:230.
10. Simkin PA et al: Transsynovial exchange of small molecules in normal human subjects. J Appl Physiol. 1974; 36:581.
11. Simkin PA: Synovial permeability in rheumatoid arthritis. Arthritis Rheum. 1979; 22:689.
12. McCarty DJ: The gouty toe—a multifactorial condition. Ann Intern Med. 1977; 86:234.
13. Scott JT: Long-term management of gout and hyperuricemia. Br Med J. 1980; 281:1164.
14. Fessel WJ: Distinguishing gout from other types of arthritis. Postgrad Med. 1978; 63:134.
15. McCarty DJ et al: Identification of urate crystals in gouty synovial fluid. Ann Intern Med. 1961; 54:452.
16. Fox IH et al: Management of gout. JAMA. 1979; 242:361.
17. Schumacher HR et al: Acute gouty arthritis without urate crystals identified on initial examination of synovial fluid. Arthritis Rheum. 1975; 18:603.
18. Abeles M et al: Acute gouty arthritis. The diagnostic importance of aspirating more than one involved joint. JAMA. 1977; 238:2526.
19. Romanoff NR et al: Gout without crystals on initial synovial fluid analysis. Postgrad Med J. 1978; 54:95.
20. Honig S et al: Crystal deposition disease. Diagnosis by electron microscopy. Am J Med. 1977; 63:161.
21. Agudelo CA et al: Definitive diagnosis of gout by identification of urate crystals in asymptomatic metatarsophalangeal joints. Arthritis Rheum. 1979; 22:559.
22. Weinberger A et al: Urate crystals in asymptomatic metatarsophalangeal joints. Ann Intern Med. 1979; 91:56.
23. Wallace SL et al: Diagnostic value of the colchicine therapeutic trial. JAMA. 1967; 199:525.
24. Wallace SL et al: Preliminary criteria for the classification of the acute arthritis of primary gout. Arthritis Rheum. 1977; 20:895.
25. Dinarello CA et al: Colchicine therapy for familial Mediterranean fever. N Engl J Med. 1974; 294:934.
26. Zemer D et al: A controlled trial of colchicine in preventing attacks of familial Mediterranean fever. N Engl J Med. 1974; 294:932.
27. Rubinow A et al: Amyloidosis secondary to polyarticular gout. Arthritis Rheum. 1981; 24:1425.
28. Hansten PD: Furosemide and indomethacin. Drug Interactions Newsletter. 1981; 1:1.
29. Patak RV et al: Antagonism of the effects of furosemide by indomethacin in normal and hypertensive man. Prostaglandin. 1975; 10:649.
30. Frolich JC et al: Suppression of plasma renin activity by indomethacin in man. Circ Res. 1976; 39:447.
31. Smith DE et al: Attenuation of furosemide's diuretic effect by indomethacin: pharmacokinetic evaluation. J Pharmacokinetics Biopharm. 1974; 7:265.
32. Brater DC: Analysis of the effect of indomethacin on the response to furosemide in man: effect of dose of furosemide. J Pharmacol Exper Ther. 1979; 210:386.
33. Durao V et al: Modification of antihypertensive effect of beta-adrenoceptor blocking agents by inhibition of endogenous prostaglandin synthesis. Lancet. 1977; 1:1005.

34. Findling JW et al: Indomethacin-induced hyperkalemia in three patients with gouty arthritis. JAMA. 1980; 244:1127.

35. Yu TF: Milestones in the treatment of gout. Am J Med. 1974; 56:676.

36. Flower RJ et al: Analgesics-antipyretics and anti-inflammatory agents; drugs employed in the treatment of gout. In *The Pharmacological Basis of Therapeutics*, 6th ed, edited by AG Gilman, LS Goodman, and A Gilman, MacMillan, New York, 1980.

37. Osol A et al: *The United States Dispensatory,* 27th ed, JB Lippincott Co., Philadelphia, 1973, p 33.

38. Naidus RM et al: Colchicine toxicity. Arch Intern Med. 1977; 137:394.

39. Merlin HE: Azoospermia caused by colchicine: a case report. Fertil Steril. 1972; 23:180.

40. Bremner WF et al: Colchicine and testicular function in man. N Engl J Med. 1976; 294:1384.

41. Malawista SE: Discussion of a case report. Arthritis Rheum. 1978; 21:735.

42. Liu YK et al: Marrow aplasia induced by colchicine: a case report. Arthritis Rheum. 1978; 21:731.

43. Demartini FE: Hyperuricemia induced by drugs. Arthritis Rheum. 1965; 8:823.

44. Steele TH et al: Factors affecting urate excretion following diuretic administration in man. Am J Med. 1969; 47:564.

45. Manuel MA et al: Changes in urate handling after prolonged thiazide treatment. Am J Med. 1974; 57:741.

46. Wyngaarden JB: Diuretics and hyperuricemia. N Engl J Med. 1970; 283:1170.

47. Anon: Drugs for gout. Met Let Drugs Ther. 1976; 18:49.

48. Gutman AB: Treatment of primary gout: the present status. Arthritis Rheum. 1965; 8:911.

49. Gutman AB: The past four decades of progress in the knowledge of gout, with an assessment of the present status. Arthritis Rheum. 1973; 16:431.

50. Yu TF: Efficacy of colchicine prophylaxis in gout. Ann Intern Med. 1961; 55:179.

51. Seegmiller JE: The acute attack of gouty arthritis. Arthritis Rheum. 1965; 8:714.

52. Meyler L et al: *Side Effects of Drugs.* Williams and Wilkins, Baltimore, 1968, pp 116, 449, 500.

53. Sturge RA et al: Multicentre trial of naproxen and phenylbutazone in acute gout. Ann Rheum Dis. 1977; 36:80.

54. Wilkens RF et al: The treatment of acute gout with naproxen. J Clin Pharmacol. 1975; 15:363.

55. Franck WA et al: Ibuprofen in acute polyarticular gout. Arthritis Rheum. 1976; 19:269.

56. Schweitz MC et al: Ibuprofen in the treatment of acute gouty arthritis. JAMA. 1978; 239:34.

57. Wanasukapunt S et al: Effect of fenoprofen calcium on acute gouty arthritis. JAMA. 1978; 239:34.

58. Weiner GI et al: Double-blind study of fenoprofen versus phenylbutazone in acute gouty arthritis. Arthritis Rheum. 1979; 22:425.

59. Widmark PH: Piroxicam: its safety and efficacy in the treatment of acute gout. Am J Med. Supplement February 16, 1982; pages 63–65.

60. Bluestone RH: Safety and efficacy of piroxicam in the treatment of gout. Am J Med. Supplement Feb 16, 1982; pages 66–69.

61. Calabro JJ et al: Clinoril in acute gout. Acta Rheum Port. 1974; 8:163.

62. Simkin PA et al: Uric acid excretion: quantitative assessment from spot, midmorning serum and urine samples. Ann Intern Med. 1979; 91:44.

63. Wortmann RL et al: Limited value of uric acid to creatinine ratios in estimating uric acid excretion. Ann Intern Med. 1980; 93:822.

64. Lesch M et al: Familial disorder of uric acid metabolism and central nervous system function. Am J Med. 1964; 36:561.

65. Steele TH: Control of uric acid excretion. N Engl J Med. 1971; 284:1193.

66. Steele TH: Renal excretion of uric acid. Arthritis Rheum. 1975; 18(suppl):793.

67. Turner WJ et al: Vicissitudes in research: the twenty-four hour urine collection. Clin Pharmacol Ther. 1971; 12:163.

68. Rundles RW et al: Allopurinol in the treatment of gout. Ann Intern Med. 1966; 64:229.

69. Yu TF et al: Effect of allopurinol (4-hydroxypyrazolo-3 (4-d) pyrimidine) on serum and urinary uric acid in primary and secondary gout. Am J Med. 1964; 37:885.

70. Elion GB: Enzymatic and metabolic studies with allopurinol. Ann Rheum Dis. 1966; 25:608.

71. Hitchings GH: Pharmacology of allopurinol. Arthritis Rheum. 1975; 18(suppl):863.

72. Rodnan GP et al: Allopurinol and gouty hyperuricemia. JAMA. 1975; 231:1143.

73. Rundles RW et al: Metabolic effects of allopurinol and alloxanthine. Ann Rheum Dis. 1966; 25:615.

74. Jarzobski J et al: Vasculitis with allopurinol therapy. Am Heart J. 1970; 79:116.

75. Kantor GL: Toxic epidermal necrolysis, azotemia, and death after allopurinol therapy. JAMA. 1970; 212:478.

76. Mills RM: Severe hypersensitivity reactions associated with allopurinol. JAMA. 1971; 216:799.

77. Young JL Jr et al: Severe allopurinol hypersensitivity. Arch Intern Med. 1974; 134:553.

78. Boyer TD et al: Allopurinol-hypersensitivity vasculitis and liver damage. West J Med. 1977; 126:143.

79. Al-Kawas FH et al: Allopurinol hepatotoxicity: report of two cases and review of the literature. Ann Intern Med. 1981; 95:588.

80. Gutman AB: Uricosuric drugs with special reference to probenecid and sulfinpyrazone. Adv Pharmacol. 1966; 4:91.

81. Yu TF et al: Mutual suppression of the uricosuric effects of sulfinpyrazone and salicylate: a study in interactions between drugs. J Clin Invest. 1963; 42:1330.

82. Smyth CJ: Disorders associated with hyperuricemia. Arthritis Rheum. 1975; 18(suppl):713.

83. Berger L et al: Renal function in gout. Am J Med. 1975; 59:605.

84. Yu TF et al: Renal function in gout. (Part V). Factors influencing the renal hemodynamics. Am J Med. 1979; 67:766.

85. Yu TF et al: Impaired renal function in gout. Its association with hypertensive vascular disease and intrinsic renal disease. Am J Med. 1982; 72:95.

86. Liang MH et al: Asymptomatic hyperuricemia: the case for conservative management. Ann Intern Med. 1978; 88:666.

87. Rastegar A et al: The physiologic approach to hyperuricemia. N Engl J Med. 1972; 286:470.

88. Campion DS et al: Binding of urate by serum proteins. Arthritis Rheum. 1975; 18(suppl):747.

89. Kjelstrand CM et al: Hyperuricemic acute renal failure. Arch Intern Med. 1974; 133:349.

90. Boston Collaborative Drug Surveillance Program: Excess of ampicillin rashes associated with allopurinol or hyperuricemia. N Engl J Med. 1972; 286:505.

91. Batuman V et al: The role of lead in gout nephropathy. N Engl J Med. 1981; 304:520.

92. Reif MC et al: Chronic gouty nephropathy: a vanishing syndrome? N Engl J Med. 1981; 304:535.

Chapter 59

Pediatric Therapy

Gary C. Cupit and Victoria A. Serrano

Only 25% of all U.S. Food and Drug Administration (FDA) approved drugs are labeled as safe and effective in children (1). For the remaining 75%, there are insufficient data available for FDA approval, despite the therapeutic potential of these drugs for the pediatric population. As a result, children are often referred to as "therapeutic orphans."

Establishing safe and efficacious therapeutic regimens for children is challenging. From birth through adolescence the pediatric patient is continually changing with respect to growth, psychosocial development, and pharmacodynamic response. Therapeutic actions and adverse effects of many drugs may be quite different in neonates, infants, or older children than in adults. Proper application of pharmacokinetic principles to pediatric prescribing will minimize these age-related variations.

PEDIATRIC PHARMACOKINETICS

Information on the disposition of drugs in newborns and infants has increased considerably in the last ten years. For several classes of drugs, it is now possible to describe their pharmacokinetic profiles in various age groups. Important differences in absorption, distribution, metabolism, and excretion have been observed among premature neonates, full term newborns, and older children. Variables such as gestational and postnatal age have to be considered when designing a therapeutic schedule. Previous (eg, prenatal) or concomitant exposure to drugs, as well as the relative hypoxemia or severity of the pathologic status of the infant, must always be taken into account.

Since the maturational process is not fully predictable, it is becoming increasingly important to monitor therapeutic drug concentrations in the perinatal period. The immaturity of organs involved in drug metabolism and excretion may alter not only the pharmacokinetics but also the toxicity of many drugs. Furthermore, great variability exists in absorption, protein binding, distribution, metabolism, and excretion according to the gestational age and birth weight. The complexity of variabilities increases with common congenital anomalies and pathologic syndromes. It is important, however, to focus on the known consequences of the altered kinetic pattern.

Absorption. *Gastrointestinal Tract.* The absorption of drugs from the gastrointestinal tract is often regulated by pH-dependent diffusion and gastric emptying time. At birth, gastric pH is between 6–8 but falls to a pH of 1–3 in the first 24 hours. This decrease is not present in premature neonates because of an immature acid secreting mechanism. The pH then returns close to neutrality, and there is no further acid secretion until the tenth to fifteenth day of life. This period of relative achlorhydria gradually resolves, and adult values for gastric acidity are reached by two years of age (2).

The relatively alkaline pH of the stomach contents may partially explain the higher bioavailability reported in the newborn for several penicillins, as well as the reduced absorption of acid compounds such as phenobarbital and phenytoin.

In the newborn infant, gastric emptying time may be as long as six to eight hours and does not approach adult values until six months of age. Recent studies have shown that the rate of gastric emptying is a function of gestational maturity, postnatal age, and the type of the feeding (human milk or infant formula) (3). The gastric emptying rate, which is irregular because of unpredictable peristalsis and which can be greatly modified by the diet and feeding pattern, may have an important influence on the absorption rate of orally administered drugs.

Intramuscular Sites. The absorption rate of drugs following intramuscular administration is also altered in the newborn infant. The marked peripheral vasomotor instability of the newborn, the changes and variation in the relative blood flow to various muscles due to maturation adaptation, and the relative insufficiency of muscular contractions are all factors which may cause marked variations in the absorption rate of drugs.

Circulatory insufficiency and/or respiratory distress may lead to hypoxemia and further complicate this situation by resulting in vasoconstriction. Specific drug characteristics also influence this relative variability of intramuscular absorption. For example, phenobarbital (4) is rapidly absorbed from IM injections, while the IM absorption of diazepam (5) is delayed. Other agents such as gentamicin (6) and digoxin (7) exhibit an overall decrease in the total amount absorbed from IM sites.

Skin. Percutaneous absorption is greatly increased in newborn and young infants who have thin, well-hydrated skin. Drug absorption through the skin is inversely related to the thickness of the stratum corneum and directly related to skin hydration. This increased permeability is illustrated by the toxic effects associated with the topical use of hexachlorophene soaps and powders (8), salicylic acid ointments, and rubbing alcohol (9).

Protein Binding. Several factors significantly reduced the plasma protein binding of various drugs in the premature and full-term newborn. These include a reduced plasma protein concentration, a qualitatively different serum albumin (fetal albumin has a lower binding capacity for drugs), and a lower blood pH. Other endogenous substrates of maternal or neonatal origin such as unconjugated bilirubin may compete with acidic drugs at albumin binding sites (10). These factors have a variable influence on the binding of drugs and may lead to drug or endogenous substrate toxicity. Furthermore, various factors may potentiate each other. A rise in free fatty acid concentrations, due to intravenous fat emulsion or theophylline administration (11), may lead to a higher level of unconjugated bilirubin which may displace highly protein bound acidic drugs from albumin binding sites.

The protein binding of non-acidic compounds is also affected by gamma-globulin (12,13). In premature and full-term newborns, insufficient dietary protein or a gastrointestinal disturbance may contribute to the already low levels of gamma-globulin. Adult values are not reached until 7 to 12 years of age (14).

Another important factor which could have a significant effect on drug distribution in the newborn is the diminished concentration of a Y protein in the neonatal liver. The Y protein is a major hepatic anion binding protein to which several antibiotics bind (2).

In addition, the dose of digoxin required in infants is high when compared to adults. While an average maintenance digoxin dose for adults is 3–5 mcg/kg/day, it is 10–25 mcg/kg/day for infants. This decreased sensitivity to digoxin is the result of a lower binding affinity for digoxin receptors in the myocardium. Furthermore, 2½ times more digoxin binding sites occur on neonatal erythrocytes when compared to adult erythrocytes (16).

Volume of Distribution (Vd). The volume of distribution (Vd) of many drugs is different in infants as compared to adults because of decreased plasma protein binding and increased extracellular fluid volume per kilogram of body weight. Extracellular fluid volume decreases from 50% of body weight in premature infants to 35% in 4–6 month-old infants, to 25% in one-year-olds, and 20% in adults. Total body water changes from 86% in premature infants to 70% in full term infants and to 55% in adults (17).

In terms of drug dosing, this means that the loading dose (on a mg/kg basis) of a relatively water soluble drug would decrease as the child's age and weight increased. As a result of this ex-

panded apparent volume of distribution, a given plasma concentration in the newborn may correlate with higher total amounts of drug in the body than is reflected by the same plasma concentration in adults. Examples of drugs with larger apparent volumes of distribution in infants are phenobarbital (18), phenytoin (19), theophylline (20), and gentamicin (21).

Hepatic Metabolism. The development and activity of drug metabolizing enzymes in humans is a poorly defined area. Several specific compounds have been studied to develop an understanding of this field.

In newborns, a prolonged half-life for acetaminophen has been observed which is apparently due to decreased hepatic glucuronidation (22). This limited capacity for acetaminophen conjugation with glucuronic acid is partially compensated for by a well-developed capacity for sulfate conjugation.

Diazepam also has an increased plasma half-life in newborns because of decreased metabolism. Hydroxylation of the active demethylated metabolite of diazepam is minimal in the newborn and increases with maturation of the infant (23,24). In the full-term neonate, the apparent plasma half-life of diazepam ranges from 20–45 hours. The half-life in premature neonates is 40–100 hours (24).

Exposure of the infant in utero or in the first few days of life to compounds that increase the enzymatic activity of the liver may increase the elimination of diazepam. A prime example of such an induction is exposure of the fetus or the newborn to phenobarbital. After brief exposure to phenobarbital, the premature or full-term newborn infant has an apparent half-life for diazepam of 12–16 hours. This decreased half-life is paralleled by an increase in the hydroxylating and conjugating capacity of the liver as documented by urinary measurement of metabolites.

Other drugs which have a prolonged apparent half-life in infants because of decreased metabolism are listed in Table 1.

Renal Elimination. The kidneys play a vital role in drug elimination. At birth, all aspects of renal function in premature and full-term infants are diminished. Glomerular function at birth is more advanced than tubular function (14). Renal function comparable to that of adults is not achieved until the child is between six months and one year of age (10). Furthermore, glomeru-

Table 1.

PHARMACOKINETICS OF SELECTED
DRUGS IN NEONATES AND ADULTS[14]

Drug	Plasma Half-Life (hr)		Volume of Distribution (L/kg)	
	Neonates	Adults	Neonates	Adults
Indomethacin	20	6–7	0.35	–
Diazepam	25–100	15–25	1.8–2.1	1.6–3.2
Theophylline	18–26	3–9	1.0	0.45
Phenytoin	15–105	10–20	1.0	0.7
Phenobarbital	45–500	60–180	1.0	0.7
Digoxin	20–80	15–60	5–10	7
Meperidine	22	3–4	–	–

Table 2.

ANTIBIOTIC DOSAGE SCHEDULES IN
NEWBORN INFANTS

Drug	Infants Less Than One Week	Infants One to Four Weeks
Ampicillin	50–100 mg/kg (2)*	100–200 mg/kg (3)*
Gentamicin	5 mg/kg (2)	7.5 mg/kg (3)
Tobramycin	4 mg/kg (2)	6 mg/kg (3)
Kanamycin	15–20 mg/kg (2)	20–30 mg/kg (3)
Aqueous Penicillin G	50–100,000 U/kg (2)	50–100,000 U/kg (3)
Amikacin	15 mg/kg (2)	15 mg/kg (2)
Methicillin	50 mg/kg (2)	50–100 mg/kg (3–4)
Oxacillin	50 mg/kg (2)	50–100 mg/kg (3–4)
Nafcillin	40 mg/kg (2)	60 mg/kg (3)

*Number in parentheses is number of doses into which
the total daily dosage should be equally divided.

lar filtration, tubular secretion, and tubular reabsorption do not mature at the same rate, and urinary pH is lower in newborns than in children and adults. Evaluations of renal function in preterm and full-term infants have shown great differences in both the baseline level of renal function and the rate of maturation (25). Full-term infants have an initial creatinine clearance of 20 ml/1.73 m^2/min that rapidly increases by one month of age to 60 ml/1.73 m^2/min. Preterm infants, born prior to 34 weeks gestation, have initial creatinine clearances of 16 ml/1.73 m^2/min that only increase to 40 ml/1.73 m^2/min by the first month of life. These data, combined with measurements of the fractional excretion of beta-two microglobulins, demonstrate that the functional development of the glomerulus precedes the functional development of the proximal tubule until the thirty-fourth to the thirty-ninth week of gestation. Preterm infants have been noted to have a relative renal vasoconstriction to allow this tubular maturation and to protect the proximal tubules from an overload and prevent urinary losses of electrolytes, glucose, and amino acids.

Compounds which are not extensively metabolized and are primarily dependent on renal function for excretion are eliminated more slowly in neonates. Therefore, the maintenance doses of these drugs must be adjusted on the basis of the child's kidney function. Examples of these dose adjustments are listed in Table 2.

In contrast, the dose of drugs which depend upon the glomerular filtration rate (GFR) for efficacy (eg, diuretics) may have to be increased. Neonates have a diminished response to thiazide diuretics because of their lesser GFR and immature tubular function. Furosemide is usually the agent of choice in newborns since it is less dependent on GFR (26). Infants who do not respond to furosemide should be checked for the presence of proteinuria, since proteins may bind furosemide in the urine or ultrafiltrate, thereby lowering free or active drug concentrations (14).

APNEA

Apnea in the newborn period is a life-threatening condition. This condition is one of the most common abnormalities of the premature infant. Apnea has been defined as: 1) a given time period with complete cessation of respiration (15–30 seconds); or 2) the time without respiration after which functional changes are noted in the infant, such as cyanosis, hypotonia, or metabolic acidosis (27).

Apnea is thought to be a defect of central nervous system control of respiration. In addition to a central cause of apnea, an obstructive component of apnea has been identified. Current treatment modalities are summarized in Table 3.

1. *Aminophylline in an Apneic Patient.* E.H. is a one-day-old 2,500 gram premature male

Table 3.

NEONATAL APNEA THERAPY[27]

Treatment of Hypoxemia
- inspired oxygen

Treat pneumonia, RDS, etc.

Treat CHF or PDA

Transfuse

Apply continuous positive airway pressure

Avoidance of Triggering Reflexes

Avoid suction catheters

Avoid cold stimulus to face

Avoid hyperinflation during bagging

Increase of Afferent Input
- environmental temperature

Administer cutaneous stimulation

Avoid hyperoxia

Treatment of Primary Depression of Respiratory Center

Treat sepsis

Treat metabolic disorders

Administer CNS stimulants (eg, theophylline)

Administer narcotic antagonists (eg, naloxone)

---

infant born to a para 1 gravida 1 Caucasian mother. At birth, the child showed appropriate development for a gestational age of 32 weeks. The infant was admitted to the newborn intensive care unit so that he could be observed closely. After approximately 24 hours, the child had episodes of apnea followed by bradycardia which occurred 12 to 15 times daily. The infant was evaluated and begun on intravenous theophylline.

How is theophylline used in newborn infants to treat apnea? What dosing considerations must be undertaken?

The pharmacologic management of apnea has been undertaken in the last few years with the use of methylxanthines. Two of these agents, theophylline and caffeine, have received widespread acceptance in the treatment of this disorder, based on their success in decreasing the frequency of apneic episodes (28). To date, controlled comparisons between these two agents for efficacy and toxicity have not been completed.

Premature and full-term infants, as well as older children, have been evaluated pharmacokinetically to determine theophylline disposition (26,29,30). The two-fold increase in the volume of distribution for theophylline in newborns reflects

the greater tissue distribution of theophylline when compared to adults. In addition, an explanation for the altered volume of distribution may be the decreased protein binding observed in newborns. Theophylline is 56% protein bound in adults but only 36% protein bound in full-term infants (31).

While the elimination rates for theophylline in newborns are slower than those observed in older children, there does not appear to be a measureable difference in interpatient elimination in neonates 24–36 weeks of gestational age. Theophylline is metabolized in adult man via N-demethylation and C-oxidation to monomethylxanthines and methyluric acid (32). Premature infants do not completely utilize these demethylation pathways; instead, theophylline is N-methylated to caffeine by the premature and full-term infant (33,34,35). (In adults, this pathway has not been identified.) Therefore, the administration of theophylline to newborns may result in measureable serum concentrations of both methylxanthines. Caffeine, when administered to premature infants is excreted 85% unchanged in the urine, compared to less than 2% of caffeine excreted unchanged in the urine of adults. Adult patterns of excretion of theophylline are obtained by 7–9 months of age (34).

Theophylline may be administered orally, as a theophylline elixir and solution or other theophylline salts, and intravenously as aminophylline. Theophylline administered via the oral route in adult man is 100% bioavailable. Clinical observations in premature infants suggest that oral bioavailability of theophylline approaches 100%. Serum theophylline concentrations associated with successful management of apnea are 6–13 mcg/ml (36). This corresponds to approximately 10–20 mcg/ml in adults when adjusted for protein binding differences. Therapeutic serum concentrations may be obtained with 5–6 mg/kg of theophylline as a loading dose followed by 3–6 mg/kg/day as a total dose administered in two to three divided doses. A lower than usual plasma concentration of theophylline may be effective in the management of apnea. This approach should incur less risk of toxicity while maintaining therapeutic efficacy (37). Known pharmacokinetic data on theophylline and caffeine are shown in Table 4. From the data presented, a loading dose of 5 mg/kg followed by 2 mg every 12 hours should maintain a therapeutic concentration of theophylline in this patient. To avoid toxicity, confirmation with a trough concentration should be determined 24 to 48 hours after the institution of therapy.

Theophylline may be administered either orally or intravenously. Since many neonates initially have feeding problems when apnea and bradycardia are present, therapy is usually instituted intravenously and then switched to the oral route with one of the available non-alcoholic solutions.

2. The infant described previously was given theophylline 5 mg/kg as an intravenous loading dose over 20 minutes followed by 2 mg every 12 hours orally. The apneic and bradycardic episodes improved. How is theophylline therapy monitored? How long should therapy be continued? What toxicities may occur?

Monitoring theophylline therapy for apnea and bradycardia begins by observing a reduction in the number of apneic episodes. If an apneic episode occurs, documentation of time of episode and activity of the infant should be recorded. Is there a correlation between the dosage schedule of theophylline and an apneic episode, eg, at a trough period? Is an apneic episode produced by improper feeding schedules or volumes?

The duration of therapy for apnea is constantly under evaluation. Therapy with theophylline is usually continued for an initial period of one week longer than the last observed episode of apnea and bradycardia. If a neonate is then withdrawn from the drug and another episode occurs, therapy may then be instituted for another two to three weeks. Many infants have this problem persisting into the first few months of life. Therapy for as long as six months has been observed.

Toxicities noted in these neonates include tachycardia, agitation, irritability, and occasional spitting up of food. Tachycardia is the most frequently observed toxicity. This reaction usually responds to adjustment of the theophylline dosage based on pharmacokinetic monitoring. It should be noted, however, that the tachycardia may persist for 24 to 36 hours after dosage adjustments of theophylline since interconversion of theophylline to caffeine occurs in the neonate. Caffeine has a more delayed elimination rate and may prolong the tachycardia. Theophylline-induced seizures from accidental overdoses have been reported (41). Toxicity can be minimized with careful dosing and pharmacokinetic monitoring.

3. What benefits/toxicities does caffeine exhibit when compared to theophylline?

Orally administered caffeine citrate (50% caffeine base) is rapidly absorbed. A 10 mg/kg dose of caffeine citrate produces peak plasma caffeine concentrations of 6–10 mcg/ml 30 minutes to two hours following administration (38). The control of apnea is associated with plasma concentrations of 5–20 mcg/ml (39). Toxicity has not been observed in infants with plasma concentrations as high as 50 mcg/ml. As noted in Table 4, the clearance of caffeine in infants is considerably less than that of theophylline (40). Current dosage recommendations are 10 mg/kg of caffeine base initially with a maintenance dose of 2.5 mg/kg/day. Thus, this patient would receive 25 mg of caffeine citrate orally followed by 6.25 mg administered once daily. The wide range of safe caffeine serum concentrations has led some investigators to con-

Table 4.

PHARMACOKINETICS OF THEOPHYLLINE AND CAFFEINE IN NEONATES

Number of Neonates	Gestational Age	Vd (L/kg)	Cl (ml/hr/kg)	t½ (hr)	Ref
		Theophylline			
8	26–32	0.887 ± 0.21	39.0 ± 15.3	18.6 ± 6.5	29
6	26–32	0.690 ± 0.09	17.6 ± 2.3	30.2 ± 6.5	31
33	26–33	1.03 ± 0.2	23.9 ± 5.1	30.4	25
		Caffeine			
12	25–34	0.916 ± 0.07	8.9 ± 1.5	102.9 ± 17.9	38
18	26–33	0.83 ± 0.02	8.6 ± 0.36	68.5	25

sider this agent the preferred methylxanthine in neonates. However, the lack of availability of an intravenous caffeine preparation which does not displace bilirubin from binding sites, as does caffeine and sodium benzoate, is a disadvantage. Furthermore, the lack of availability of routine determinations for serum caffeine concentrations, makes the monitoring of therapy difficult.

4. How are severe intoxications of theophylline managed in the neonate? What factors must be considered?

Since the metabolism and elimination of theophylline and caffeine are widely variable in the pediatric age group, it is advisable to monitor these patients with frequent determinations of plasma concentrations of these compounds. Inadvertent overdosage and accumulation of methylxanthines in infants has been well documented (41–43). In addition, the elimination rate of theophylline is dose dependent and follows zero order processes above therapeutic serum concentrations in all age groups (44). Exchange transfusion has not been found to be effective in removing theophylline from plasma (43). A promising new technique for the treatment of the overdosed infant is charcoal hemoperfusion (45). Other prenatal and postnatal sources of theophylline that clinicians should consider are placental transfer in theophylline-treated asthmatic mothers (46) and the secretion of theophylline in breast milk. Under normal circumstances, the plasma concentrations attained prenatally in the fetus equal maternal theophylline plasma concentrations. Concentrations of theophylline in breast milk are approximately 70% of maternal serum concentrations (47,48).

ASTHMA

The management of the pediatric asthmatic patient is similar to the management of the adult. Major differences in pharmacotherapy will be emphasized at this time. (For a more complete discussion, see the chapter on Asthma.)

Prognostic factors associated with a favorable disease course outcome include prolonged breast feeding, avoidance of allergens in early infancy, persistently negative skin tests, and a negative family history of atopy.

Factors associated with a poor asthmatic prognosis are artificial feeding, severe symptoms at presentation, history of an atopic condition such as eczema, and nasal polyps (49).

5. *Acute Asthma.* H.W. is a 12-year-old 35 kg asthmatic patient who presents in status asthmaticus. Unresponsive to three courses of epinephrine 0.01 mg/kg administered 20 minutes apart, the child was begun on an aminophylline infusion of 6 mg/kg followed by 0.7 mg/kg/hr maintenance.

How does one manage the pediatric asthmatic patient acutely?

Acute management of the pediatric asthmatic patient has traditionally been subcutaneous epinephrine followed by intravenous aminophylline. This is supplemented with inhaled beta-2 sympathomimetics. In severe, uncontrolled cases or in patients previously maintained on prednisone, short courses of high dose corticosteroids such as dexamethasone or hydrocortisone have been administered parenterally. For example, a hydrocortisone dose of 7 mg/kg bolus followed by 2 mg/kg every six hours may be given for three days (50).

Administration of theophylline to pediatric patients is complicated by increased rates of elimination (51,52) and dose-dependent kinetics (53). An evaluation of continuous infusion versus bolus infusion of theophylline has shown sustained increases in bronchodilation with continuous infusion in children (54). The total daily dose of theophylline is higher on a mg/kg basis than it is for adults due to an increased clearance. General guidelines are: children 1–9 years—24 mg/kg/day; 9–12 years—20 mg/kg/day; 12–16 years—18 mg/kg/day; greater than 16 years—13 mg/kg/day or 900 mg/day (whichever is less) (55).

Recent studies have questioned the necessity for the parenteral administration of sympathomimetics. While parenteral beta-2 sympathomimetics offer no advantage over parenteral epinephrine (56), the inhalation of these agents produces a therapeutic effect equivalent to parenteral epinephrine (57). Since parenteral administration creates unnecessary anxiety in children, inhalation may become the preferred method of administering sympathomimetics.

6. *Chronic Asthma.* H.W. is now ready for discharge. During his hospital stay, it was noted in reviewing his records that this was his fifth hospital admission in less than a year. Although this patient responded well to ther-

apy with theophylline, corticosteroids acutely, and hydration, an allergy consult was obtained. The consultant's recommendations included allergy screening to be completed as an outpatient with the possibility of instituting hyposensitization therapy. Institution of a sustained release theophylline preparation was also recommended.

How does the management of the chronic pediatric asthmatic patient differ from adult management?

Chronic care of the pediatric asthmatic patient presents problems which are not encountered in adult asthmatics (58). A primary example is the use of immunotherapy to prevent asthmatic attacks. Children, unlike adults, present almost exclusively with a reversible extrinsic-type of bronchial asthma. To date, numerous studies have shown the value of adjunctive hyposensitization therapy in the management of pediatric extrinsic asthma (59,60). In adults, the effects of smoking, degenerative pulmonary disease, and industrial pollution lead to the development of nonspecific, ie, non-atopic, bronchial irritability.

If a patient is not adequately controlled with bronchodilators, consideration is given to adding either cromolyn sodium or corticosteroids. Cromolyn has been established as a potent inhibitor of mast cell release (61) and a useful agent for chronic asthma (62). The use of this agent, however, is difficult for children less than five because their inspiratory flow rate may not result in adequate inhalation of the powder from a spinhaler. Due to questionable bioavailability, lack of dose response data in children, expense, and inconvenience of administration, cromolyn is considered a second line drug in antiasthmatic therapy. Cromolyn may be useful, however, in those patients sensitive to CNS side effects from chronic administration of adrenergic agents (eg, hyperactivity).

Pediatric corticosteroid usage is limited by their effects on linear growth. The introduction of an inhaled corticosteroid, beclomethasone dipropionate, offers the advantage of local pulmonary action with minimal systemic toxicity (63,64). Although beclomethasone is preferable to daily oral steroid therapy, the use of alternate day oral steroid administration (65) is equally efficacious.

Expectorant drugs have historically been used in the treatment of chronic asthma. Recent recommendations, however, have eliminated agents such as potassium iodide from therapy (66).

COLD/COUGH/OTITIS MEDIA

7. *Common Cold.* D.S. is a three-year-old girl who has had a cold with a fever for two days. Her mother has given the child aspirin and nonprescription decongestants intermittently but wonders if an antibiotic is indicated, since the child's symptoms have not improved.

How should the common cold be managed in children?

The common cold is an acute viral illness which affects the upper respiratory tract and usually lasts seven days. Acute nasopharyngitis, as it is sometimes called, most frequently presents with symptoms of rhinorrhea, headache, malaise, cough, and arthralgias. In children, colds are usually accompanied by irritability and a fever in the range of 102–104°F. Allergic rhinitis, on the other hand, has a more abrupt onset and usually develops immediately after exposure to an allergen, such as pollen or animal dander. Initially, it is manifested by paroxysmal repetitive sneezing.

There is no known cure for the common cold. Antibiotics are not indicated as treatment for viral infections unless a secondary bacterial infection is suspected. Simple, symptomatic supportive measures are the mainstay of therapy.

A variety of agents, classified pharmacologically as sympathomimetics or decongestants (ephedrine, pseudoephedrine, phenylpropanolamine), antihistamines (chlorpheniramine, brompheniramine, triprolidine), and anticholinergics (belladonna, atropine, scopolamine) are available, usually in various combinations, as prescription and non-prescription nasal decongestant products. For example, Dimetapp is a popular prescription-only product containing (per 5 ml syrup) phenylephrine HCl 5 mg, phenylpropanolamine 5 mg, and brompheniramine 4 mg. Expectorants, antipyretic-analgesics, and cough suppressants are frequently included in these products (see Table 5). Oral decongestants are generally effective in recommended doses for opening nasal passages. Topical decongestants, though effective, may result in rebound congestion. Antihistamines are effective in allergic rhinitis, but only exhibit mild anticholinergic drying effects when used adjunctively in the management of the common cold (69). The treatment of fever in children is discussed in Questions 27–29 of this chapter and in the chapter on Fever.

Children less than six months of age are obligate nose breathers; thus it is vital to maintain nasal passageway patency. Some topical decongestant preparations contain antihistamines and should not be used in this age group. Absorption of these agents is enhanced, thus predisposing the child to systemic toxicity. As an alternative for nasal stuffiness, extemporaneously prepared normal saline nose drops may be used. Good technique must be used to avoid nasal solution contamination. Nasal drainage may be enhanced by propping up the infant's head. For example, having the child sleep in an infant carrier is often recommended. Other nondrug measures such as humidification of inspired air (vaporizers), in-

creased fluid intake, and local heat may be recommended and should be started early in the course of a cold and/or cough.

Otitis Media

Otitis media is one of the most common infectious diseases of childhood. In a study of 722 children followed from infancy through 7.5 to 13.5 years of age, 84% had at least one episode of otitis media and 40% had four or more episodes (70).

Diagnosis of otitis media depends predominantly on otoscopic findings and nonspecific symptomatology. Symptoms include earache, rubbing or tugging of the earlobes, otorrhea,

Table 5.

TREATMENT OF THE COMMON COLD IN CHILDREN[67,68,69]

Drug Class	Example Agent[A,B]	Recommended Dosage (mg/kg/dose)	Example Doses/Age Group		
			6–12 years	2–6 years	≤2 years
Nasal Decongestants (Sympathomimetics)					
Topical	Oxymetazoline HCl (Afrin®, Duration®)	—	2–3 drops or sprays (0.05%) twice daily	2–3 drops or sprays (0.025%) twice daily	C
Oral	Pseudoephedrine HCl (Sudafed®)	1 Q 4–6 hours	30 mg/dose (MAX 180 mg/day)	15 mg/dose (MAX 90 mg/day)	C
Antitussives	Codeine Phosphate[D]	0.2 Q 4–6 hours	5–10 mg/dose (MAX 60 mg/day)	2.5–5 mg/dose (MAX 30 mg/day)	C
	Dextromethorphan HBr (Romilar®)	0.2 Q 4–6 hours	5–10 mg/dose (MAX 60 mg/day)	2.5–5 mg/dose (MAX 30 mg/day)	C
Antihistamines	Chlorpheniramine Maleate (Chlortrimeton®)	0.1 Q 6 hours	2 mg/dose (MAX 12 mg/day)	1 mg/dose (MAX 6 mg/day)	C
Analgesics	Aspirin	10 (or 65 mg/yr of age/dose)	240 mg/dose	60–120 mg/dose	60 mg/dose
	Acetaminophen	10	240 mg/dose	60–120 mg/dose	60 mg/dose

A—Nonprescription single ingredient product given as example.

B—The FDA OTC Panel on Cold, Cough, Allergy, Bronchodilator, and Antiasthmatic Products has recommended all of these agents as safe and effective (Category I).

C—No recommendations on dosage except under the advice and supervision of a physician.

D—Requires a prescription in some states.

hearing impairment, vertigo, and balance disturbances. Only an earache and otorrhea indicate an active infection (71). Tympanometry, an extremely sensitive test of middle ear function, may be useful. In certain circumstances, tympanocentesis, needle aspiration of the middle ear, or myringotomy may be used to identify the type of middle ear effusion and to determine the infecting organism, if any (72).

Acute suppurative otitis media, as illustrated in the following example case, is distinguished from secretory (serous) otitis media by the presence of purulent fluid in the middle ear. In secretory otitis media, few polymorphonuclear cells are present in the aspirate, which may be serous or mucoid.

Chronic otitis media may go undetected or have an insidious and persistent presentation, both of which can result in serious sequelae. Chronic middle ear problems may result in hearing loss and thus play a role in the etiology of some school learning disabilities (73). Otitis media is frequently associated with eustachian tube dysfunction resulting in obstruction and/or abnormal reflux of nasopharyngeal secretions into the middle ear (74,75).

Table 6.

FACTORS AFFECTING THE OCCURRENCE OF OTITIS MEDIA[71]

Factor	Association With:
I. Infancy, Early Childhood	Tubal Obstruction Secondary to: A. high susceptibility to infection B. increased nasopharyngeal lymphoid tissue C. feeding with cow's milk D. supine posture when feeding E. shorter, wider, and less well-angulated tubes resulting in reflux
II. Race	American Indians, Eskimos
III. Sex	Males > Females
IV. Genetic	Down's Syndrome
V. Socioeconomic	–
VI. Season	Winter

Infecting Organisms. Rational treatment of otitis media is dependent upon the bacterial organism involved. *Streptococcus pneumoniae* and *Haemophilus influenza* are the most common agents isolated from middle ear exudates. *S. pneumoniae* is recovered in 25 to 50% of patients over six weeks of age (76,77) and 12 to 14% of those over seven years of age (78). The overall incidence of *H. influenza* otitis media is 14 to 27% (79); it is more likely to occur in children less than three years of age. Bilateral ear involvement appears to be more common when *H. influenza* is the causative organism.

Other organisms less frequently causing acute otitis media include Group A beta-hemolytic *Streptococcus, Neisseria catarrhalis, Staphylococcus aureus* and Gram-negative coliforms including *Escherichia coli, Klebsiella pneumoniae, Pseudomonas aeruginosa* and some *Proteus* species (71). In a study of neonatal otitis media, coliforms and *Staphylococcus aureus* were the most common organisms cultured (81).

Eight types of *S. pneumoniae* (types 1, 3, 6, 7, 14, 18, 19 and 23) account for approximately 75% of the cases of pneumococcal otitis media. These eight types are all represented in a multivalent pneumococcal vaccine. Clinical trials of the protective efficacy of this vaccine show that some protection against pneumococcal otitis media, especially type 19, is achieved (80).

8. *Otitis Media.* D.S., the three-year-old child described in the previous question, was given palliative treatment for her cold, and her symptoms subsided over the next four days. She then, however, became increasingly irritable, anorexic, and febrile. In addition, she occasionally tugged on her right earlobe. Her mother subsequently brought her to the University Family Practice Clinic.

On physical exam, she was observed to be a 14 kg, well developed, well nourished female in moderate distress. Her blood pressure was 100/70 mm Hg, pulse was 120/minute, temperature was 39.6°C, and respiratory rate was 30/minute. Otoscopic examination showed the right tympanic membrane to be red, bulging, non-mobile, and with drainage. The left tympanic membrane was red. Her throat was slightly injected. Her lungs were clear. A complete blood count was ordered, as were culture and sensitivity of the purulent right ear exudate. Otitis media was suspected, and ampicillin oral suspension (200 mg every 6 hours for ten days) was prescribed empirically.

Why was ampicillin prescribed? Should an oral decongestant and antihistamine be given as well?

Ampicillin. Despite the bacterial etiology of acute suppurative otitis media, the infection is frequently self-limiting in children (78). However, considering the complications of untreated otitis media, such as hearing loss and intracranial extension of the infection, antibiotics are indicated. Culture and sensitivity will ultimately determine the correct antibiotic choice, but ampicillin was empirically selected because of the high incidence of *H. influenza* in this age group. *S. pneumoniae* is also a likely cause. Both of these organisms are sensitive to ampicillin, and ampicillin achieves bactericidal concentrations in the middle ear. Some children cannot tolerate ampicillin because of severe diarrhea. Amoxicillin, a congener of ampicillin, is an effective alternative and reportedly causes less diarrhea.

Sympathomimetics and Antihistamines. Oral decongestants and antihistamines are frequently prescribed on the basis that prevention of eustachian tube obstruction, one of the factors that may be involved in the pathogenesis of otitis media, might be prevented. Nevertheless, the value of such treatment in acute otitis media remains unproven (71,78).

9. After two days of therapy with ampicillin, D.S. developed an erythematous, mildly pruritic, maculopapular rash over the majority of her body. Should her antibiotic therapy be changed?

Skin rashes of all types have been observed with sensitization to various penicillin derivatives. However, ampicillin causes the highest incidence of skin rashes (about 9%), and not all of the rashes caused by ampicillin are necessarily allergic in origin (82a,82b). Impurities in commercial ampicillin preparations can be a cause of rash (82c). Also, patients receiving concurrent allopurinol therapy and patients with infectious mononucleosis are extremely likely to develop ampicillin-induced rashes which may represent a toxic rather than an allergic reaction (82). Thus, it has been argued that ampicillin rash is not an absolute contraindication to subsequent treatment with ampicillin or any other penicillin (82d).

Nevertheless, allergy in this patient cannot be ruled out, and since there are several other antibiotics which are equally effective in the treatment of otitis media, D.S.'s antibiotic therapy should be changed.

10. What alternative antibiotic therapy could be used for D.S.?

Erythromycin is an acceptable alternative to penicillin in the treatment of *S. pneumoniae* in penicillin-allergic patients, and when given in combination with a sulfa drug, erythromycin is also effective against *H. influenza* (see Table 7). Erythromycin is considered one of the least toxic antibiotics used in children (83).

Cefaclor is an oral cephalosporin antibiotic with *in vitro* activity against a number of organisms including *S. pneumoniae* and *H. influenza* (84).

Table 7.

ANTIBIOTICS FOR OTITIS MEDIA

Drug	Dose	Schedule
Benzathine Penicillin G (intramuscular)	0.6–1.2 million units	single dose
Phenoxymethyl Penicillin (oral)	50 mg/kg/day (MAX 2 gm/day)	Q 6 h
Benzyl Penicillin (oral)	50,000 U/kg/day	Q 6 h
Ampicillin (oral)	50–75 mg/kg/day	Q 6 h
Amoxicillin (oral)	20–40 mg/kg/day	Q 8 h
Erythromycin Ethylsuccinate* (oral) PLUS	40–50 mg/kg/day	Q 6 h
Sulfisoxazole (oral)	100–150 mg/kg/day	Q 6 h
Cefaclor (oral)	20 mg/kg/day	Q 8 h
Trimethoprim with Sulfamethoxazole (oral)	8 mg/kg/day with 40 mg/kg/day	Q 12 h

*A combination of erythromycin ethylsuccinate (40 mg/ml) and sulfisoxazole acetyl (120 mg/ml) in an oral suspension is available.

Because of the recent occurrence of cases of otitis media caused by ampicillin-resistant strains of *H. influenza,* cefaclor has been recommended as a safe and effective alternative to ampicillin. About 5 to 10% of those who are allergic to penicillins will manifest cross-reactivity to cephalosporins (82). Trimethoprim-sulfamethoxazole is also effective in these cases and is useful in penicillin-allergic patients. See Table 7 for all antibiotic dosage recommendations.

CROUP AND EPIGLOTTITIS

Croup

Croup is a term used to identify several different respiratory illnesses. It is characterized by varying degrees of inspiratory stridor, cough, and hoarseness resulting from obstruction in the region of the larynx. Under the heading of croup, there are three decidedly different clinical and pathological categories: acute laryngotracheitis, laryngotracheobronchitis, and spasmodic croup.

Acute laryngotracheitis is an illness of variable severity which is caused by many viruses. This disease usually begins with cough, coryza, and fever and is followed within 12–48 hours by the gradual onset of upper airway obstructive signs and symptoms. The cough becomes "croupy" with gradual but progressive inspiratory stridor. Fever is nearly always present. The speed of progression and the final degree of upper airway obstruction are quite variable. Many children may manifest only hoarseness, stridor, and a barking cough, whereas others experience progressive obstruction with severe respiratory distress.

Laryngotracheobronchitis is seldom seen today but was commonly described in the 1920's and 1930's. Laryngotracheobronchitis implies an illness with both upper and lower airway disease. The onset of laryngotracheobronchitis is similar to that of present day acute laryngotracheitis, but the illness is complicated by progression down the trachea with frequent bronchial and pneumonic involvement. Superinfection with streptococcus or other pathogens is responsible for this severe illness (85).

Spasmodic croup is illustrated below.

11. *Spasmodic Croup.* **Mrs. G. calls one evening and states that her 4-year-old daughter awoke last night with a barking cough and seemed to have some difficulty in breathing. The symptoms subsided after she stayed with her daughter for about two hours. Tonight the same symptoms have begun. What recommendations for therapy can be made?**

Spasmodic croup has been incorporated in the overall clinical entity of croup. The onset always occurs at night in a child who was thought to be well or only have a mild cold. As the respiratory rate slows, the child awakens with sudden dyspnea, croupy cough, and inspiratory stridor. There is little or no fever, and relief is easily achieved by reassurance of the child and exposure to moist air.

Croup may be managed on an outpatient basis. Therapy first calls for assuring the parent that the child will recover through appropriate monitoring. If humidity is less than 80% in the patient's room, therapy with cool mist may be of value. If cool mist is unavailable, the patient may be placed in a bathroom where moisture from a hot shower will raise the humidity to a sufficient concentration.

If mist is being used in the management of croup, specific instructions should be given to the parents. First, cool mist is recommended. Heated mist offers no advantage over cool and can cause burns if one touches the heated mist vaporizer. Second, the mist should be directed into the room and away from the child. Frequently, cool mist will lower body temperature when directed at an infant. Finally, medications, such as liniments and other petroleum products, should not be added to the cool mist.

Although racemic epinephrine has not been found to be useful in long-term therapy, it does have benefits in the acute stages (86,87). More data have been developed on the inpatient use of this agent than in outpatient management.

Controversy exists over the use of corticosteroids in the management of croup (88,89). Because of unclear diagnostic criteria, the selection of patients who can be managed with corticosteroids is difficult (85). Patients who have true spasmodic croup (versus patients with acute laryngotracheobronchitis) may show a response to corticosteroids. Until this distinction is made in future studies, and dosages of corticosteroids are standardized, recommendations cannot be made.

Epiglottitis

Epiglottitis is a severe infection of the epiglottis. The epiglottis helps coordinate the functions of respiration and swallowing. When a substance is swallowed into the gastrointestinal tract, the epiglottis closes the upper airway to prevent aspiration. When the epiglottis becomes red and inflamed, it can swell to the point of occluding the airway and result in asphyxiation (90).

Epiglottitis has very few prodrums. The patient usually has a higher fever than in croup and has difficulty swallowing, as evidenced by drooling. A more complete differentiation of croup and epiglottitis is shown in Table 8.

The organism most frequently responsible for epiglottitis is *Haemophilus influenza* type B (91). Patients with epiglottitis should be hospitalized immediately, receive appropriate intravenous antibiotics and be monitored for respiratory occlusion. Of concern is the increasing frequency of *H. influenza* type B strains which are resistant to ampicillin and chloramphenicol. Many institutions, for this reason, initiate therapy with both drugs and await sensitivity test results before discontinuing one of these agents. Newer antibiotics have been developed which show great promise in the treatment of resistant strains.

Table 8.

DIFFERENTIATION OF CROUP AND EPIGLOTTITIS

	Croup	Epiglottitis
Etiologic Agent	Parainfluenza virus	Haemophilus influenzae
Age	< 3 years	3–7 years
Clinical Onset	Preceded by cough and rhinitis for several days	Rapidly (12–24 hrs), acutely ill
Dysphagia	None	Marked, occasional drooling
Fever	Variable, usually < 39.4°C (103°F)	> 39.4°C (103°F)
WBC	Normal	> 18,000 mm^3
Diagnostic Criteria	Clinical presentation and exclusion of other diseases	"Cherry-red" epiglottis on direct visualization
Treatment	Cool mist; racemic epinephrine	Ampicillin and/or chloramphenicol; possible intubation

CYSTIC FIBROSIS

Cystic fibrosis (CF) is a clinical syndrome which may directly or indirectly involve every organ system. This heterogeneous disorder is transmitted at birth as a Mendelian recessive trait (92), but may also involve other chromosomal alleles (93). To date, it is the most frequently encountered lethal genetic syndrome and is responsible for much of the chronic progressive pulmonary disease seen in children.

Originally a disease of infants and young children, CF today has become a disease of adolescents and young adults. With improved diagnosis and treatment, the median life expectancy of all CF patients nationwide has increased from four years of age to greater than 19 years (94).

The actual biochemical defect or defects of CF are as yet unknown. Diagnosis is, therefore, based upon clinical presentation. Almost all patients will have elevated concentrations of eccrine sweat electrolytes, and often parents will indicate that their child "tastes salty." There are several diagnostic tests for the measurement of electrolyte concentrations in sweat. The quantitative pilocarpine iontophoretic test (QPIT) and two newer and more rapid methods, the Orion skin electrode and the Medtherm conductivity apparatus, are used to screen for cystic fibrosis (95). The QPIT test involves stimulation of sweat with pilocarpine ionotophoresis. This test is technically the most difficult, but is quantitatively the most accurate. The Orion and Medtherm methods are less accurate and more expensive. It should be noted that an alarming number of false-positives and false-negatives do occur, especially with the newer tests. An abnormal sweat test with at least one additional diagnostic criterion such as obstructive lung disease or exocrine pancreatic insufficiency establishes the diagnosis of cystic fibrosis. See Table 9.

Pulmonary involvement is responsible for at least 95% of the morbidity and mortality associated with this disorder. Obstructive and progressive in nature, the first pulmonary lesions are dilation and hypertrophy of bronchial glands followed shortly by mucous plugging of peripheral airways. Infection soon results, and patients frequently suffer from chronic and recurrent bronchitis and bronchopneumonia (93). The two organisms most frequently implicated in the respiratory infections and resultant pulmonary tissue injury of CF are *Pseudomonas aeruginosa* and *Staphylococcus aureus.* Other bacteria, viruses, mycoplasmas and fungi may also be cultured from these patients (96).

P. aeruginosa can directly injure pulmonary tissue via toxins and enzymes. A humoral and cellular host immune response to the organism may also be responsible for the local inflammatory reaction. There is a certain strain of *P. aeruginosa* unique to CF patients. This strain, called mucoid *P. aeruginosa,* produces an extracellular polysaccharide material which may form a protective envelope that prevents antibody, antibiotic, and phagocyte penetration (97). The virulence of *S. aureus* in CF pulmonary infection may be due to a variety of toxins or to the organism's resistance to host defenses by virtue of its cellular structure.

With chronic and recurrent infections, continued tissue damage results. Progressive loss of pulmonary function is observed. In addition, minor trauma or infection can result in varying degrees of hemoptysis (93).

12. ***Cystic Fibrosis.*** **W.P. is an eleven-year-old white male with cystic fibrosis diagnosed at nine months of age. He has had a troublesome history of CF and is seen frequently in Children's Hospital Clinic. He has had thirteen hospitalizations for complications from his disease, three within the last year. These three have been associated with pneumonia, and sputum cultures were positive for *Pseudomonas aeruginosa,* alpha-hemolytic *Streptococcus,* and *Neisseria pharyngitis.* His infancy was complicated by failure to thrive,**

Table 9.

DIAGNOSTIC CRITERIA FOR CYSTIC FIBROSIS[94]

Criteria	Methodology	Positive Result	Comment
Sweat Test	As stated in text	Electrolyte concentration: Children and adolescents—> 60 mEq/L; adults—> 80 mEq/L	Many false positives
Pancreatic Function	Stool Content	↓ trypsin and/or chymotrypsin ↑ fat	
	Serum carotene concentration	↓	Nonspecific test
	Serum pancreatic isoamylase fraction	↑	May be normal or increased with partial pancreatic function
	Pancreatic output—direct measure	↓ enzymes, water, and electrolytes (especially bicarbonate)	
Pulmonary Function	Symptomatology	Cough, wheezing, dyspnea	
	Chest X-ray	Hyperinflation, infiltrates, bronchial thickening	Usually normal
	PFT's	↓	More often used as a monitoring parameter
Heredity	Family history	Parent or sibling with CF or suspected carrier state	
Fertility	Azoospermia	Present in 97% of males with CF	
	Anovulation	Present in females with CF	Often may be fertile and bear children

and currently he experiences poor weight gain secondary to pancreatic insufficiency and malabsorption. W.P. now presents in the Emergency Room with increased sputum production tinged with bright red blood for the past 24 hours. On physical exam, W.P. is febrile (T 39°C), mildly cachectic, and in moderate respiratory distress. Rales and rhonchi are present at both lung bases. Sputum is obtained for culture and sensitivity. W.P.'s medications on admission include: Keflex, Theodur, Pancrease (with meals), and a multivitamin supplement.

What is the rationale for prophylactic outpatient antibiotic therapy, Keflex in this case, and how should W.P.'s current pulmonary exacerbation be managed?

The prophylactic and therapeutic use of antibiotics in CF is a source of considerable disagreement among clinicians. Some clinicians treat patients continuously with antistaphylococcal drugs, while others treat intermittently on the basis of clinical features and sputum bacteriology. Prolonged therapy with cephalexin, which is effective against *S. aureus,* has been shown to decrease the frequency of respiratory illness, but as might be expected, the rate of infections with mucoid strains of *P. aeruginosa* increases (99).

It is common practice to treat acute illnesses, such as evidenced by this patient, with parenteral antibiotics for 10 to 21 days. Because of the likelihood of *P. aeruginosa* as the causative agent, most clinicians would initiate therapy with carbenicillin or ticarcillin plus gentamicin or tobramycin. Treatment is often difficult; *P. aeruginosa* is seldom eradicated from the sputum (96). Furthermore, there is even some evidence that seemingly inappropriate antibiotic therapy (on the basis of sputum culture) may be effective (97,98). When an antistaphylococcal regimen (cloxacillin) was compared with a regimen effective against both *S. aureus* and *P. aeruginosa* (carbenicillin with gentamicin) in acutely ill CF patients who were assigned treatment randomly without regard for sputum bacteriology, clinical and microbiological outcome were the same for both treatments (98). Cloxacillin was effective despite the fact that *P. aeruginosa* was the predominant sputum pathogen in most patients. This study needs confirmation, but it illustrates the fact that choice of antimicrobials in CF is often arbitrary.

In addition to antibiotic therapy, intermittent aerosol therapy is often used in conjunction with chest physiotherapy. Hydration, bronchodilators, alpha-adrenergic agents, and mucolytics are incorporated into individualized programs of intense pulmonary therapy, aimed at preventing disease progression and the development of irreversible pulmonary changes.

13. A second CF problem exhibited by W.P. is poor weight gain secondary to malabsorption and pancreatic insufficiency despite an excellent appetite. W.P. suffers from frequent bouts of diarrhea, especially after the evening meal and when he forgets to take his Pancrease capsules. These diarrheal stools are bulky and loose but not watery, and are associated with abdominal cramps, flatus, and bloating. His mother also notes that W.P.'s stools float in water. She is very concerned about his nutritional status, delayed maturation, and gastrointestinal problems.

How are malabsorption and pancreatic insufficiency managed in cystic fibrosis patients?

Most patients require supplemental pancreatic enzymes to achieve adequate digestion and absorption. Many patients continue to have significant steatorrhea and azotorrhea, however, despite large doses of oral supplements. The enzymes should be taken with meals, except those meals comprised of pure carbohydrate, and the dose should correlate with total caloric and fat content of the ingested food (96). See Table 10. The enzymes are inactivated by acid (pH < 4), and recent studies have suggested that acid neutralization with antacids or suppression of gastric acid secretion with cimetidine may significantly improve fat absorption (96,100).

Diet is another vital component in the management of cystic fibrosis gastrointestinal complications. Caloric requirements are usually doubled compared to normals of the same age, weight, and sex because of poor bioavailability of oral intake. Fat soluble vitamins (A, D, E, and K) are routinely supplemented, since their absorption is diminished in CF.

IMMUNIZATIONS

Many viral and bacterial diseases can be prevented through the use of immunizations. Some of the more common childhood diseases and in-

Table 10.

PANCREATIC ENZYME SUPPLEMENTS

Agent	Product Example	Usual Dose	Comment
Pancrelipase (porcine source)	Cotazym	1 to 3 capsules before meals or snacks OR 1 to 2 powder packets before meals or snacks	Adverse reactions include nausea, diarrhea, and hyperuricosuria (high doses)
	Pancrease	1 to 3 capsules before meals or snacks	
Pancreatin (porcine or bovine source)	Viokase (325 mg/tablet)	325 mg to 1 gm pancreatin NF with meals	Adverse reactions: same as above
	Elzyme 303 (300 mg/tablet)	same	Nonprescription drug; enteric coated
Miscellaneous Combination products*	Cotazym-B	1 to 2 tablets with or after meals	Nonprescription drug; contains bile salts
	Festal	same	Nonprescription drug; contains bile salts; enteric coated

*Contain other agents to promote digestion or minimize enzyme inactivation, ie, bile salts (emulsification of fats), calcium carbonate (antacid), simethicone (antiflatulent).

formation regarding their communicability are listed in Table 11. Vaccines are available for all the diseases listed in Table 11 with the exception of chicken pox (varicella-zoster) which is under investigation. The chicken pox vaccine, which consists of a live attenuated virus, has had limited use, but initial trials have been successful (102).

14. M.K., a two-month-old infant, returns to the clinic for his first scheduled well baby visit. The mother inquires about immunizations for her baby. What is the present status of immunizations in pediatrics, and when should some of these immunizations be given?

The schedule for routine active immunization of normal infants and children given in Table 12 can be adjusted to meet individual needs. It may also begin at any time of the year. An interruption in the recommended schedule does not interfere with the final immunity gained with completion, regardless of the delay between doses. When a child has an acute febrile illness, immunization should be delayed until the infection is controlled. Generally, contraindications for vaccination include: 1) immunosuppressive therapy; 2) recent (within 8 weeks) gamma globulin

(ISG), plasma, or blood transfusions; 3) pregnancy; 4) immunodeficiency disorders; 5) leukemia, lymphoma, or generalized malignancies; and 6) prior allergic reactions to the same or related vaccine. Minor, non-febrile illnesses such as the common cold are not contraindications (101).

Hypersensitivity reactions to vaccine are rare. An allergic reaction may occur as a result of a specific allergy to the vaccine itself or to trace components in the vaccine (eg, egg protein, preservatives, or antibiotics). Children who have manifested allergies to eggs can receive vaccines grown in chick or duck fibroblast tissue culture, eg, measles, rubella or mumps. Egg albumin yolk components are essentially absent from the fibroblast cultures.

Diphtheria

This disease occurs primarily in children and is associated with a high mortality rate in this age group. Toxicity related to this vaccine is extremely low (see Table 13).

Diphtheria toxoid is available in combination with tetanus toxoid and pertussis adsorbed vaccines DPT, and with tetanus toxoid (DT). A combination of tetanus and adult diphtheria (Td) is

Table 11.
COMMON CHILDHOOD COMMUNICABLE DISEASES[101]

Disease	Organism	Incubation Period	Communicability	Patient Treatment	Immunization	Contact Treatment
Chickenpox	Varicella-Zoster virus	10–21 days	1–2 days before and 5–6 days after rash	Adenine Arabinoside	Active: None *Passive: ZIG, ISG, or ZIP	ISG: 0.6 to 1.2 ml/kg
Diphtheria	Corynebacterium diphtheria	2–6 days	2–4 weeks untreated 1–2 days after antibiotics initiated	Diphtheria antitoxin: 20,000 to 120,000 U combined with penicillin or erythromycin	Active: Diphtheria toxoids Passive: Diphtheria toxoids/antitoxin	1) oral erythromycin 250 mg qid for 7 days or benzathine penicillin 1.2 million units 2) diphtheria toxoid immunization
Measles (Rubeola)	Measles virus	10–12 days	Beginning 5th day of incubation through 1st few days of rash	None	Active: measles virus vaccine Passive: unvaccinated normal children—0.25 ml/kg IM of ISG Unvaccinated immunosuppressed children—0.5 ml/kg (max 15 ml) of ISG IM	As under immunizations
Mumps	Mumps virus	14–21 days	7 days before and 9 days after parotid swelling	None	Active: mumps virus vaccine Passive: mumps immune globulin	Mumps hyperimmune serum globulin
Pertussis	Bordetella pertussis	5–21 days	Greatest during disease, ranges include 4 weeks; lessened with antibiotics	Erythromycin 50–100 mg/kg/day in 4 divided doses for 5–10 days	Active: pertussis vaccine Passive: none	Administer erythromycin or ampicillin for 10 days after contact or duration of cough in contacted patient
Polio	Polio viruses, Type 1,2,3	7–14 days	Virus persists in throat 1 week after onset of symptoms, may also be excreted in feces 4–6 weeks	None	Active: TOPV or IPV Passive: None	Administer TOPV
Rubella (German measles)	Rubella virus	14–21 days	7 days prior to and 5 days post appearance of rash	None	Active: Rubella virus vaccine Passive: ISG	See Text
Tetanus (Lock jaw)	Clostridium tetani	3 days–3 wks Average–8 days	None	Tetanus Immune Globulin (Human) 3000–6000 U IM Pen G or tetracycline for 10–14 days	Active: Tetanus toxoid Passive: Tetanus immune globulin (Human)	None required

*ZIG—Zoster Immune Globulin
ISG—Immune Serum Globulin
ZIP—Zoster Immune Plasma

Table 12.

RECOMMENDED SCHEDULE FOR ACTIVE
IMMUNIZATION OF NORMAL
INFANTS AND CHILDREN

2 months	DPT, TOPV
4 months	DPT, TOPV
6 months	DPT, TOPV
1 year	Tuberculin Test
15 months	Measles, Rubella, Mumps
18 months	DPT, TOPV
4–6 years	DPT, TOPV
14–16 years	Td—repeat every 10 years

Key: DPT: Diphtheria-Pertussis-Tetanus
TOPV: Trivalent Oral Polio Vaccine
Td: Combined tetanus and diphtheria (adult type)

also available. The antigenicity of the adult diphtheria vaccine is approximately 20–30% of the antigenicity of the pediatric strain. It should be noted that patients who acquire diphtheria naturally and recover from the disease do not acquire immunity. A booster immunization with diphtheria toxoid should be repeated in one year (101). The diphtheria carrier state is not prevented by immunization.

Tetanus

Tetanus is a noncommunicable childhood disease. It results from puncture wounds caused by contaminated articles, and it is associated with a very high mortality rate. The etiologic agent, *Clostridium tetani,* an anaerobic, spore-forming, Gram-positive rod, exists in nature as an extremely resistant spore. All the clinical features of tetanus are produced by an exotoxin; the organism itself causes no disease (104).

There is no natural immunity to tetanus. Prophylaxis can be achieved with active stimulation of antibody (tetanus toxoid), passive antibody transfer (tetanus immunoglobulin), or a combination of both. Immunization affords extremely high protection with minimal risk. Controversy exists concerning when to administer this vaccine to patients who cannot recall their last immunization or who have not received an immunization in quite some time. Recommendations for the use of tetanus toxoid and tetanus immunoglobulin (TIG) and other management are

presented in Table 14. It should be noted that too frequent administration of tetanus toxoid can result in a serum reaction and a qualitative change in the spectrum of antibodies produced (104,105).

Pertussis

No other vaccine has generated as much controversy as pertussis. Although this immunization has been responsible for decreasing the incidence of pertussis in children, it is also the cause of many side effects and reactions. *Bordatella pertussis* is the causative agent, and while much is known about its antigenic composition, little is known about specific antibody responses.

A significant number of adverse reactions are caused by pertussis immunization. When DPT and DT were compared, it was found that redness, swelling, and pain occurred in 50% of DPT recipients as compared to 18% of DT recipients. Fever was seen in 48% of those given DPT and 10% of those given DT. "Drowsiness" and "fretfulness" occurred twice as frequently in DPT recipients. Furthermore, four neurologic reactions to pertussis vaccination have been identified: prolonged, uncontrollable crying beginning a few hours after the injection and lasting at least one hour; excessive somnolence which begins several hours after the injection; febrile convulsions (0.2% risk); and gross encephalopathy. Thus, pertussis immunization is not without risk (106).

15. At 4 months of age, M.K. received her DPT (0.5 ml) immunization, and subsequently became febrile and experienced a generalized seizure. Should M.K.'s DPT series be continued?

As stated above, most authorities consider the pertussis component of DPT responsible for such a severe reaction. Infants experiencing a temperature of 105°F or higher after the administration of pertussis-containing vaccines should not receive additional doses. Convulsions, severe changes in consciousness, or focal neurological signs are also contraindications to further pertussis immunization. Static neurological conditions prior to immunization do not constitute a contraindication, and immunization should not be deferred. An evolving neurological disease, however, is a contraindication for pertussis immunization since evaluation of the disease may be obscured. Pertussis is still an integral part of a pediatric immunization program, and the elimination of per-

Table 13.

BENEFIT AND REACTIONS FROM IMMUNIZATIONS[103]

Disease	Vaccine
Diphtheria	**Tetanus Diphtheria Toxoid (Td)**
• occurs primarily in children • attacks throat and nasal passages • toxin damages heart, kidney, and nerves • 10% case fatality	• almost 100% protection from primary series plus booster • sore arm or bump at injection site and possible fever for 12 to 24 hours after injection • severe reactions very rare and usually occur in adults
Tetanus ("Lock jaw")	**Diphtheria/Pertussis/Tetanus Toxoids (DPT)**
• caused by contaminated dirt entering wounds • causes painful muscular contractions • 50% case fatality	• administered to children under 6 years old • almost all children protected after completing a primary series and booster • sore arm or bump at injection site and fever 12 to 24 hours after injection • very rarely causes brain disorder
Pertussis ("Whooping cough")	
• most severe in young infants • can cause ear infections, pneumonia and convulsions; rare, but most serious, is a brain disorder	
Polio	**Oral Polio Vaccine (OPV, Live, Sabin)**
• attacks the nervous system • causes muscular and/or respiratory paralysis • 10% case fatality	• 90% receiving primary series plus booster are protected • given by oral drops • no common reactions • a paralytic reaction to the vaccine occurs in person vaccinated or a close contact once in 3,000,000 doses
	Inactivated Polio Vaccine (IPV, Killed, Salk)
	• 90% protected after receiving a primary series plus booster • administered by injection • no common reactions
Measles	**Measles Vaccine**
• most serious common childhood disease • causes high fever (103°–105°F) and rash • may cause pneumonia or ear infection • causes deafness, blindness, convulsions, brain disorders in 1 of every 1000 children contracting the disease • those children who develop a brain disorder from measles have a 10% fatality rate	• 95% protection after one dose of vaccine • 10%–20% of immunized children may have a mild fever and rash within 10 days • 1 person in 1,000,000 vaccinated may develop a brain disorder
Rubella	**Rubella Vaccine**
• when contracted by pregnant women can cause miscarriage, stillbirth, or multiple birth defects including blindness, deafness and heart disease • usually mild disease with mild fever, rash and swollen glands • can cause joint pains, more frequently in teenagers	• 90% of persons receiving 1 dose will be protected • approximately 1% of young children and 5%–10% of teenagers may develop temporary arm, leg or joint pains • very rarely vaccine may cause a rash • children of pregnant women can be vaccinated
Mumps	**Mumps Vaccine**
• usually causes fever and swelling of salivary glands • may cause inflammation of testicles in adolescent and adult males • may cause pancreatitis • may cause a temporary brain disorder • can result in permanent deafness	• 90% of persons immunized will be protected • very rarely fever and swelling of salivary glands may occur after vaccination

Table 14.

RECOMMENDATIONS FOR TETANUS TOXOID AND
TETANUS IMMUNE GLOBULIN (TIG) (HUMAN)
IN WOUND MANAGEMENT

Type of Wound	Immunization Status
Unimmunized or Incomplete (One or Two Doses of Toxoid)	
Low-risk wound	One dose of Td[1] or DT[2] followed by completion of immunization; booster every 10 years afterward
Tetanus-prone wounds and wounds neglected over 24 hours	One dose of Td[1] or DT[2] plus 250–500 U TIG followed by completion of immunization.
Full Primary Immunization With Booster Dose Within 10 Years of Wound	
Low-risk wounds	No toxoid necessary
Tetanus-prone wounds	If more than 5 years since last dose, one dose of Td[1]. If less than 5 years, no toxoid necessary.
Wound neglected over 24 hours	One dose of Td plus 250–500 U TIG.
Full Primary Immunization With No Booster Doses Or Last Booster Dose Over 10 Years	
Low-risk wounds	One dose of Td
Tetanus-prone wounds	One dose of Td
Wounds neglected over 24 hours	One dose of Td plus 250–500 U TIG

[1]Td—(adult) should be used in patients over six years of age.

[2]DT—(pediatric) should be used in patients less than six years of age.

tussis immunization in pediatric practice is not recommended; rather, efforts should be made to "improve" the vaccine.

In M.K.'s case, the adult-type diphtheria-tetanus toxoid (Td) or DT should be substituted for the DPT vaccine, and the series should be continued. If M.K. had only become febrile, low dose DPT (0.1 to 0.25 ml) and/or intensive antipyretic therapy with each immunization might have been indicated. Reducing the DPT inoculum does not significantly affect the immunogenicity of the diphtheria and tetanus components of the vaccine, but it does reduce the degree of response to the pertussis component (107).

Polio Virus Vaccine

Since the advent of oral polio vaccine (OPV) and inactivated polio vaccine (IPV), the number of reports of paralytic polio has been reduced to fewer than a dozen cases annually. Debate continues over which immunization, OPV or IPV, should be recommended and utilized in pediatric immunization programs (103).

Present evidence shows that OPV provides more immediate and longer lasting protection than IPV. The use of OPV decreases the incidence of disease in nonimmunized persons when greater than 65–70% of the population is immunized. In addition, OPV does not require "booster" doses to convey immunity throughout life as does IPV.

There are several important limitations to the use of OPV. Persons over 18 years of age are apparently more susceptible to OPV-associated polio. Persons planning to travel in a polio endemic area should be given IPV, assuming sufficient time is available. If travel must be taken on a short notice, the patient and physician must weigh the risk of OPV use to the risk of infection abroad. In domestic outbreaks of polio, OPV is routinely given to adult contacts since the risk of natural disease is much greater than the risk from OPV. A second area of concern involves non-immunized parents of an infant scheduled to receive OPV as part of an immunization program. Some experts have recommended that the parents should receive IPV monthly for three doses, and at the third visit, OPV is given to the infant. The virus is excreted in the stool, and there have been reports of non-immunized adults contracting polio from children begun on polio immunization programs. The continued use of OPV vaccine in large scale immunization programs is recommended (109).

Pregnancy is not a contraindication to OPV immunization when protection is needed, as during an epidemic. OPV also appears suitable for breast-fed children. The passive transfer of antibodies from the mother through the breast milk does not seem to interfere with the vaccine-induced antigen-antibody response. Studies have shown similar antibody titers in both bottle-fed and breast-fed infants.

Measles/Mumps/Rubella

Measles. Attenuated live virus measles vaccine produces a benign infection that provides long standing immunity. Measles virus is extremely sensitive to small amounts of antibodies. Since antibodies which have been passed transplacentally persist during the first year of life, it is appropriate to defer immunization until 15 months of age when all maternal antibodies disappear (110,111).

Mumps. Mumps immunization remains controversial in childhood since mumps illness in children rarely produces complications. The CNS symptoms often reported as meningoencephalitis usually consist only of benign meningitis. Postinfectious encephalitis, a serious disease, is extremely rare (1/6,000). Deafness, frequently stated as a risk of mumps, occurs rarely (1/15,000) and is usually unilateral. Orchitis generally occurs only in adults. Controversy exists because vaccination at fifteen months of age may not protect children into their adult years. Some authors have advocated immunization during early puberty to insure protection into adulthood. Current immunization practices, however, still provide vaccination at fifteen months of age in combination with measles and rubella vaccines (105).

It should be noted that mumps virus vaccine temporarily suppresses the reaction to tuberculin skin tests. Therefore, tuberculin skin testing should be performed prior to, simultaneously with, or six weeks after administration of the vaccine.

Rubella. Rubella virus live is a preparation that was reformulated in 1979. This vaccine contains the RA27/3 strain of rubella virus (112). Compared to previously available vaccine strains of rubella virus (Cendehill, HPV-77), the RA27/3 strain induces a greater variety of antibodies and thus produces immunological response which more closely resembles that induced by natural rubella infection. Approximately 10 to 20% of women of childbearing age have not acquired natural immunity, and infection in this group carries a high risk of fetal abnormalities. Preventing infection of the fetus and the congenital rubella syndrome is a major objective of rubella immunization programs.

Previous concern existed when rubella immunization was administered to women who were unknowingly pregnant. Previous surveys estimate that approximately 10% of fetuses would acquire congenital rubella infection as a result of maternal immunization. The new RA27/3 vaccine dramatically reduces this risk of fetal infection (113); however, further studies are required before the recommendations can be made with regard to administration during pregnancy.

Present immunization recommendations for rubella vaccine include an immunization program at 15 months of age, designed to protect women by exposure to these immunized children. Immunization and/or rubella antibody titer screening at premarital examinations and postpartum prior to mothers leaving the hospital is also recommended. Antibody titers are also measured to evaluate antibody response 6–8 weeks after immunization in women who have received blood products or immunoglobulin within 8 weeks of immunization, which may inhibit antibody stimulation (114). In addition, these women should use some form of contraception for at least two months after immunization.

CHILDHOOD SOCIAL DISEASES
(Pinworms/Scabies/Lice)

Pinworms

Man is the only host for *Enterobius vermicularis*, commonly known as pinworms, and it is estimated that 10% of the total United States population is infected (115). Pinworm infestation is most common in residential areas with temperate climates. Infection is not limited to impoverished communities and is more often seen in whites than in blacks. In addition, pinworm infections exhibit a familial tendency (115), secondary to contamination of clothing and the home environment (116).

Enterobius vermicularis is a ubiquitous intestinal parasite in man. The adult worms, both male and female, inhabit the large bowel (cecum) where they are superficially attached to the cecal mucosa and adjacent areas. At night, the gravid female worm seeks oxygen and migrates out of the anus and deposits her eggs in the perianal skin region. The gravid worm can literally explode, laying as many as 17,000 eggs, or may deposit some and return to the colon (117). This causes intense anal pruritus and scratching. The child may appear tired and irritable because insomnia can result from nocturnal itching. Intestinal blockage can occur with a heavy infection, and obstruction of the appendix leading to appendicitis has been reported (116). Ulceration and colicky symptoms are uncommon but a low level of eosinophilia can occur (118). In young girls, a potential complication of enterobiasis is cystitis (119,120,121). Presumably, the female worms, during their nocturnal migration, enter and ascend the host's urethra, carrying enteric bacteria to her bladder. In addition, vaginitis, endometritis, and salpingitis can result via this mechanism (118).

Transmission of the disease occurs readily from person to person by hand-to-mouth contamination and by inhalation of air-borne eggs (122). The eggs are infective within two hours. The eggs are transferred to the mouth by the fingers or other contaminated objects, and the thin egg shells protect the worms from the acidic environment of the stomach. In the intestines, enzymes and bile acids dissolve the shells. After mating, the females then begin their anal migrations which can continue for up to four weeks.

Diagnosis is not made by examination of stool for ova (eggs) and parasites as with most intestinal parasitic infections. Diagnosis is made readily by the Scotch Tape method (123). A transparent plastic adhesive tape strip is applied to the perianal skin and is examined microscopically for the presence of eggs. It is best to collect the sample first thing in the morning (122). In addition, parents are instructed to examine the child's anal area for worms with a flashlight at night. When signs and symptoms strongly suggest pinworm infestation, as in the case below, three consecu-

tive early morning Scotch Tape testings are recommended since the female does not lay her eggs nightly (120).

16. *Pinworms*. K.K. is a 6-year-old white female who is brought to her pediatrician with a chief complaint of nocturnal rectal itching which causes insomnia. Her past medical history is significant for recurrent urinary tract infections. A physical examination reveals an irritable child with painful excoriations in the anal region and positive Scotch Tape tests. K.K. is worried that she may have "worms" like some of her classmates. How should K.K. be managed?

Pyrantel pamoate or mebendazole are the drugs of choice (124,125). These drugs are equally effective and usually safe. Hygienic measures should be instituted and the patient's family should be treated to prevent reinfection (see Table 15). In addition, follow-up Scotch Tape swab examination is recommended and should be negative for seven consecutive days before the patient is considered free from infection (118).

Scabies/Lice

Scabies. Scabies, due to *Sacroptes scabiei*, is another common, extremely contagious disorder

Table 15.

TREATMENT OF ENTEROBIUS VERMICULARIS

Drug of Choice	Dosage[124,125]	Comments[116,123,126]
Pyrantel pamoate (Antiminth®) 250 mg/5 ml oral suspension OR	A single dose of 11 mg/kg (max 1 gm); repeat after 2 weeks.	Side effects are mild and include occasional headache, nausea, vomiting, diarrhea. Infrequent dizziness, rash, fever, transient ◆ SGOT.
Mebendazole (Vermox®) 100 mg/tablet	A single dose of 100 mg (if > 2 yr); repeat after 2 weeks.	Chew tablets for best effect; contraindicated in pregnancy. No side effects reported.
Alternatives:		
Piperazine citrate (Antepar®) 500 mg/tablet 100 mg/ml syrup	65 mg/kg (max 2.5 gm/day) × 7 days; repeat after 2 weeks.	Side effects include nausea, vomiting, diarrhea, headache. Infrequent dizziness, rash, fever, rare visual disturbance, ataxia, ◆ SGOT. Safe to use during the last trimester of pregnancy.
Pyrvinium pamoate (Povan®) 500 mg/tablet 10 mg base/ml	5 mg/kg single dose (max 350 mg); repeat after 2 weeks.	Swallow tablets whole; discolors stool bright red; contraindicated in ASA-allergic patients. Side effects include vomiting, diarrhea, dizziness.

affecting infants and children as well as adults. The female scabies mite, when stimulated by warmth, burrows into the skin progressing at the rate of 2 to 3 mm per day (123). Its entire life cycle of 8 to 15 days appears to be complete in man, and no animal reservoir is known.

The diagnosis is based on the typical clinical picture of red papular tracts in the skin and excoriations of webs of fingers, wrists, elbows, areolar areas, genitalia, knees and ankles and is often overlooked in infants and children. Frequently, there is a lack of these pathognomic burrows, and what is observed is an atypical lesion distribution including the head, neck, palms, and soles with secondary eczematous changes which often suggest other diagnoses (127,128). When infestation is suspected, confirmation of the diagnosis must be made by microscopic identification of the mite and ova in skin scrapings from the involved area.

Scabies infestation has a cosmopolitan distribution, especially among poorer classes (123). Transmission of this mite is by personal contact, including neonatal hospital personnel, babysitters, and parents. Less frequently, transmission occurs through contact with inanimate objects such as clothing, towels, and bed linen.

Lice. The parasitic lice of man comprise three varieties: 1) *Pediculus capitis*, head louse; 2) *Pediculus humanus*, body louse, and 3) *Phthiris pubis*, crab louse (123). The head louse is most prevalent in school-aged children. It is an obligatory blood-sucking ectoparasite which is reaching near epidemic proportions throughout the country. The incidence, however, among American blacks is quite low. It is postulated that this is due to differences in hair shaft configuration, texture, grooming practices, or sebum composition (129,130).

Transmission occurs readily through the sharing of brushes, combs, and head wear, or from person to person contact, and is not the result of poor grooming or bad habits. Unlike body lice, the head louse is not a carrier of disease. On occasion, head louse infestation may be complicated by a secondary bacterial infection.

The louse attaches itself to the hair shaft close to the scalp and then lays its eggs, also known as nits. The nits are cemented in place by a secretion and incubate for approximately one week (131). Diagnosis is made by visual inspection of the hair.

Positive identification of both nits and lice can be made by microscopic examination.

17. *Scabies*. J.B. is an eighteen-month-old white male who was seen by his pediatrician for a rash that has been present for one month. Examination revealed an irritable child with generalized excoriated papulovesicular eruptions on his face, trunk, and extremities, including the palms and soles. Because of the suspicious nature of the eruptions, a history and physical examination of the mother was done. Similar lesions on her trunk, arms and legs, and webs of her fingers were seen. In addition, she gave a history of intense itching, especially at night. Microscopic examination of skin scrapings of lesions from both the mother and child confirmed the suspected diagnosis of scabies infestation.

How should the mother and child be treated? What instructions and special precautions should be given in the use of these medications?

Gamma benzene hexachloride (Kwell) was considered, until recently, to be the most effective and convenient agent for the treatment of scabies. It is available as a cream, lotion, and shampoo. However, the absorption of Kwell through the skin, especially excoriated skin, is significant and associated with both acute and chronic adverse effects (132). Infants absorb more drug percutaneously and are at additional risk. Crotamiton (Eurax) is the drug of choice because of its low incidence of side effects and its proven efficacy (see Table 16). It is available as a cream which is applied to the entire body.

The mother should be instructed to bathe the child and herself initially. Extremely hot water and scrubbing do not appear to be necessary. To minimize percutaneous absorption, the skin should then be allowed to dry and cool. The lotion or cream should be applied to the entire body, avoiding the eyes and mucous membranes. The scabies mite does not live in areas of sebaceous gland activity, therefore, the face and scalp are spared in adults (133). The minimum contact time per application which results in a reasonable cure rate is unknown. Recommended times vary from four to forty-eight hours (127,133,134). For infants and children, it should not be left on the skin for more than eight hours. The cream or lotion should be massaged into the skin. The child should then be dressed to cover the treated skin to avoid accidental ingestion through thumbsucking, etc. After the prescribed amount of time, a second bath should be taken. Symptomatic relief will be apparent within twenty-four hours.

18. How can reinfestation be prevented?

First, the remainder of the family should be examined and treated to avoid reinfestation by personal contact. All clothing and linen should be freshly laundered and the patients reexamined in one week. Occasionally, a second treatment course may be required. Symptoms of intense itching may persist. This can be due to active infestation or to irritant properties of the dead mites and their byproducts. Resistance of the scabies mite to Kwell has not been reported, and treatment failure appears to be due to poor compliance. Off the host, the mites only survive for two to three days at room temperature; therefore, room and house fumigation or spraying is not necessary (123).

19. Upon examination of the other family members, J.B.'s two sisters, ages five and eight, were found to be infested with both scabies and head lice. No secondary bacterial infections were noted. How should this problem be managed?

In addition to their scabicidal therapy and preventive measures, the parent should wash the girls' hair with Kwell shampoo and leave it on the scalp for four minutes. This procedure may be repeated the following day or after a seven day interval (124). Some advocate a repeat application on the following day (129). The child's hair should be thoroughly brushed after each application to facilitate nit and lice removal. Since the girls are of school age, they should be instructed not to share their brushes and combs with their classmates.

FLUIDS AND ELECTROLYTES

It is critical to avoid dehydration and maintain electrolyte balance in pediatric patients with diarrhea. Children, especially infants, are more susceptible to dehydration because of the greater rate of water turnover in relation to their body size. The first consideration to be made is whether

Table 16.
TREATMENT OF SCABIES AND LICE[124]

Scabies:	Drug of Choice		Comments
	10% Crotamiton (Eurax)	Topically (reapply 24 hours later)	Adverse reactions are minimal and include hypersensitivity and primary skin irritation.
	Alternatives		
	1% Gamma benzene hexachloride (Lindane, Kwell)	Apply topically once	Not recommended in pregnant women, infants, and people with massively excoriated skin. Acute Kwell toxicity includes: muscle spasm, confusion, blindness, and convulsions.
	Benzyl benzoate 12–25%	Topically	
	Sulfur in petrolatum	Topically	
Lice:	Drug of Choice		
	1% Gamma benzene hexachloride (Lindane, Kwell)	Apply topically once (reapply 5 to 7 days later)	Use of Kwell shampoo in children safe if contact time is brief
	Alternatives		
	Pyrethrins with piperonyl butoxide	Topically	
	0.03% Copper oleate	Topically	

the child should be referred for treatment or can be managed with oral fluid replacement as an outpatient.

In making this decision, consider the following questions: Does the child have any of the following signs and symptoms of dehydration?

    a. a depressed fontanel (useful up to six-months-of-age)
    b. sunken eyes
    c. dry mucus membranes around the eyes and mouth
    d. a diminished urine output
    e. a fever without perspiration

Are a large number of copious stools still being produced? Is there a risk of dehydration from inadequate monitoring or inability of the parent to take care of the child? Specific inquiries should be made about the number and consistency of stools in children with diarrhea. If the child is vomiting, oral replacement is extremely difficult. Are other signs and symptoms present, such as lethargy, severe emesis, or a history of convulsions, that preclude management at home? It is particularly valuable in assessing the patient with diarrhea to estimate the degree of dehydration. Most outpatient classifications consider weight loss to be a good criterion. Dehydration can be determined to be mild, moderate, or severe by estimating the percent of the weight loss. A 5% weight loss is considered mild dehydration, 10% is considered moderate and, greater than 10% is severe.

Mild to moderate diarrhea *without dehydration* is generally managed at home with oral hypotonic electrolyte solutions containing glucose (135,136,137). Glucose provides a caloric source and enhances the absorption of salt and water in the small intestine by mechanisms that are usually unimpaired in many toxin-induced diarrheas. Previously, parents were instructed to prepare salt and sugar solutions at home, but this is no longer recommended (138). Frequent errors in preparing the solutions led to problems in fluid and electrolyte balance. Skim milk and bouillon are similarly not recommended because of the high salt load and the danger of hypernatremia. Ready to feed commercial solutions containing glucose and electrolytes, such as Pedialyte and Lytren, are available. Other liquids used at home include "decarbonated" beverages, flavored gelatin products mixed at half the strength recommended on the package, or fruit juices. Kool-Aid and unflavored gelatin offer no advantage over water because they are low in potassium and sodium. The electrolyte content of commonly used solutions is listed in Table 17. In many situations, solutions may substitute sucrose for glucose, since little evidence exists to support either agent preferentially (139,140).

General recommendations for fluid maintenance in children are as follows: for the first 10 kg of body weight, administer 100 ml/kg/day to a maximum of 1000 ml; for children weighing 10–20 kg, give an additional 50 ml/kg/day for each kg over 10 kg; for children weighing more than 20 kg, give previous amount plus an additional 20 ml/kg/day for each kg over 20 kg. General recommendations for sodium and potassium maintenance are 3 mEq/kg/day and 2 mEq/kg/day respectively (141).

Febrile infants and children have increased losses of body water. Generally, maintenance fluid requirements are increased by 10% for each degree of Celsius increase of body temperature above normal. Increased loss of body water is also noted in infants who are receiving light phototherapy for hyperbilirubinemia or having their body temperature maintained with external warming lamps (142).

The refeeding of children after a bout of diarrhea may present some problems. Occasionally, infants with diarrhea have transient intolerance to lactose containing formulas; therefore, they are given a soy milk formula for two to six weeks until normal function of the gastrointestinal mucosal enzyme lactase returns. Proprietary milk base formulas may be reintroduced after an ini-

Table 17.

SODIUM, POTASSIUM, AND CALORIC CONTENT OF SOME COMMON COMMERCIAL PRODUCTS

Product	Sodium	Potassium	
	mEq/L	mEq/L	Calories/L
Coca-Cola	1.93	0.08	400
Pepsi-Cola	2.75	1.30	400
Seven-Up	4.15	0.10	400
Dr. Pepper	4.53	0.20	400
Gelatin (full-strength)	15.18	0.28	590
Pedialyte	30	20	200
Nutramigen	14	17	660

tial trial of lactose-containing formula to be sure of the infant's tolerance.

Antidiarrheal preparations, including anticholinergics and adsorbents, are not indicated in children under two years of age (143). Deaths have been reported in infants who received anticholinergics and continued accumulating fluid in the gastrointestinal tract without passing this fluid rectally. Stool volume is a valuable means of monitoring diarrhea, because many children can "third space" large amounts of fluids into their gastrointestinal tracts. Other supportive therapies with agents such as lactobacillus preparations have not been found to be of value in pediatric patients (144).

20. A 15-month-old infant was brought to the pediatric clinic with a history of a cold and diarrhea. The patient had been well until two days previously when nasal stuffiness and mild fever were noted. On the second day of illness, diarrhea that increased in frequency and water content was noted. The infant's weight was 12 kg, 1 kg less than his usual weight of 13 kg. The skin and mouth appeared dry. The child had not urinated in five hours. Temperature was 38.5° C, respiratory rate was 25/min, blood pressure was 98/58 mm Hg, and pulse was 100/min. Serum electrolytes were as follows: Sodium 132 mEq/L (nl: 135–145 mEq/L), Potassium 3.4 mEq/L (nl: 3.5–5.0 mEq/L), Chloride 98 mEq/L (nl: 100–106 mEq/L), and Bicarbonate 15 mEq/L (nl: 20–26 mEq/L).

What recommendations can be made for fluid and electrolyte replacement in this infant?

The amount of weight lost should be replaced as fluid in addition to the fluid required for maintenance. Also, calculations should be performed to determine the amount of electrolytes that must be replaced in addition to the maintenance electrolytes. In this case, the calculations are as follows:

a) The infant's well weight by history is 13 kg. Coupled with the clinical signs of dry skin in the axilla (with fever), dry mouth, and no urine in the last five hours, this amounts to an estimated dehydration of 8%.

b) *Fluid requirements* for the first 24 hours are:

Maintenance:

$$
\begin{aligned}
10 \text{ kg} \times 100 \text{ ml/kg} &= 1000 \text{ ml} \\
+ \ 3 \text{ kg} \times \ 50 \text{ ml/kg} &= \underline{\ 150 \text{ ml}} \\
& 1150 \text{ ml}
\end{aligned}
$$

Replacement:

$$
\begin{aligned}
1 \text{ kg weight loss} &= \underline{1000 \text{ ml}} \\
\text{Total} &= 2150 \text{ ml}
\end{aligned}
$$

c) *Electrolyte requirements* for the first 24 hours are maintenance requirements plus replacement of losses. Using the general guidelines for sodium and potassium maintenance cited previously, sodium maintenance requirements would be 39 mEq (3 mEq/kg × 13 kg), and potassium maintenance requirements would be 26 mEq (2 mEq/kg × 13 kg).

Sodium Replacement. In order to calculate the amount of sodium needed for replacement, the current amount of sodium in the body is estimated and subtracted from the normal amount of sodium in the body:

$$
\begin{aligned}
\text{normal} &= (\text{desired serum sodium}) \ (Vd \text{ of} \\
& \text{sodium}) \ (\text{well weight in kg}) \\
&= (140 \text{ mEq/L}) \ (0.6 \text{ L/kg}) \ (13 \text{ kg}) \\
&= 1092 \text{ mEq} \\
\text{observed} &= (\text{observed serum sodium} \ (Vd \text{ of} \\
& \text{sodium}) \ (\text{observed weight in kg}) \\
&= (132 \text{ mEq/L}) \ (0.6 \text{ L/kg}) \ (12 \text{ kg}) \\
&= \text{approximately 950 mEq}
\end{aligned}
$$

Therefore, sodium replacement for losses would be 142 mEq (1092 mEq minus 950 mEq). Added to the sodium maintenance requirement of 39 mEq calculated above, it can be seen that 181 mEq of sodium (142 mEq plus 39 mEq) will be required during the first 24 hours.

Potassium Replacement. The determination of potassium replacement is difficult since serum levels of potassium are not a reflection of total body stores. General guidelines are: if the serum potassium is equal to or greater than 3 mEq/L, supply maintenance only; if serum potassium is less than 3 mEq/L, twice the usual maintenance amount should be given. Exceptions would be severe ongoing losses from diarrhea secondary to diabetes or other diseases.

d) *Administration*: 50% should be administered in the first 8 hours and the remaining 50% over the next 16 hours. In addition, any ongoing losses from diarrhea should be replaced, every 6 hours for example. Replacement for diarrheal losses can either be estimated by replacing with one-third to one-half normal saline in equal volumes to the diarrheal fluid or the diarrheal fluid can be analyzed for sodium and potassium concentration and replacement made accordingly.

For example, fluid orders for this patient could be written as D5W with NaCl 85 mEq/L, add KCl 13 mEq/L only after patient voids; run fluids at 135 ml/hr for the first eight hours, then run fluids at 65 ml/hr for the next 16 hours. After the first 24 hours, the patient should be reassessed and maintenance fluid and electrolytes begun.

21. How should this patient's acidosis be corrected?

In those children who present with acidosis, it may be necessary to administer some alkali. Bicarbonate is the most frequently used agent and is distributed in the same extracellular fluid space as sodium. Therefore, when calculating bicarbonate requirements, the general recommendations are as follows:

[(desired HCO_3) (Vd HCO_3) (well weight in kg)] −
[(observed HCO_3) (Vd HCO_3) (observed weight in kg)] =
mEq HCO_3 required

Therefore,

[(25 mEq/L) (0.6 L/kg) (13 kg)] −
[(15 mEq/L) (0.6 L/kg) (12 kg)] = 87 mEq

However, only *one-half* this amount is replaced since the renal and compensatory mechanisms for bicarbonate must be recognized as being active in acidotic patients. Therefore, only 44 mEq would be replaced, with 22 mEq administered as sodium bicarbonate during the first eight hours and the remaining 22 mEq during the next 16 hours. The sodium content of sodium bicarbonate must be subtracted from the sodium chloride being administered to prevent hypernatremia.

INFANT NUTRITION

During the first year of life, growth is greater than in any other time period. An infant doubles his birth weight between 4 and 6 months of age and triples it by one year of age. The recommended daily dietary allowance (RDDA) for total caloric intake is approximately 120 Cal/kg of body weight/day for infants in the first six months, and approximately 105 Cal/kg/day in infants 6 months to one year of age. As would be expected, the pre-

mature or low birth weight infant has a greater caloric need than the full term infant and requires as much as 130 Cal/kg/day (145). Adult caloric requirements are 40 Cal/kg/day.

Of the total caloric intake, provision must be made for adequate intake of protein, carbohydrates, and fats. Protein intake should be approximately 2–3 gm/kg/day, or 7–16% of the total intake/day. (Adult protein requirements are approximately 1 gm/kg/day.) Carbohydrates should comprise 35–65% of the caloric intake, and fats should comprise 30–50% of the caloric intake. Of particular importance is the provision of essential fatty acids, linoleic and arachidonic acids, in the fat intake (146).

All commercial formulas are patterned after the nutrient qualities of breast milk. Cow's milk is used as the base in many of the formulas because it is safe, inexpensive, and convenient. Any formula that is selected should have an adequate distribution of protein, carbohydrates, and fat, and provide all the essential vitamins and minerals. Human milk contains 7% protein, 55% fat, and 38% carbohydrate. Milk contains two different types of protein: casein (the protein in the curd) and whey. The predominant protein in cow's milk is casein, while in human milk it is whey. Since the high casein content of cow's milk may produce a hard rubbery mass in the infant's stomach, cow's milk formulas are usually heat or acid treated to prevent curd formation. The fat in cow's milk differs from that found in human milk in two ways: the triglycerides of cow's milk consist of short and long chain fatty acids, while human milk contains primarily medium chain fatty acids. Also, human milk is composed of unsaturated fatty acids, while cow's milk primarily contains saturated fatty acids. Commercial formulas attempt to duplicate human milk by utilizing vegetable oils and medium chain triglyceride (MCT) oils (147). Table 18 shows a breakdown in the composition of many infant formulas.

Readily digestible carbohydrates are an important component of an infant's formula. Both human milk and cow's milk contain lactose as a predominant carbohydrate. Sucrose, glucose, dextrose, and fructose are present in commercially prepared formulas.

An important difference in human milk is that it contains immunoglobulins. The immunoglobulins of human milk are qualitatively and quantitatively different from those present in serum.

Table 18.

INFANT FORMULAS (ABBREVIATED CONTENTS)

	Cal/100 ml	Protein gm/100 ml	Fat gm/100 ml	CHO gm/100 ml	Na mEq/100 ml	K mEq/100 ml	Type CHO	Source Protein	Type Fat
STANDARD FORMULAS									
Breast Milk	75	1.1	4.5	6.8	0.7	1.3	Lactose	Human Milk	Human Milk Fat
Whole Cow's Milk	69	3.5	3.5	4.9	2.5	3.6	Lactose	Cow's Milk	Butterfat
Enfamil	66	1.5	3.7	7.0	1.1	1.8	Lactose	Cow's Milk	Corn, Oleo, Coconut Oil
Similac	66	1.8	3.6	7.0	1.3	2.3	Lactose	Cow's Milk	Coconut, Corn Oil
SMA Improved	66	1.5	3.5	6.8	0.7	1.4	Lactose	Demineralized Whey	Safflower Oil
THERAPEUTIC FORMULAS									
Milk Allergy									
Isomil	66	2.0	3.6	6.8	1.4	1.8	Sucrose Maltodextrins	Soy Isolate	Corn, Coconut Oil
Mull-Soy	66	3.1	3.6	5.2	1.6	4.0	Sucrose Invert Sugar	Soy	Soy Oil
Neo-Mull-Soy	66	1.8	3.5	6.4	1.7	2.5	Sucrose	Soy Isolate	Soy Oil
Nutramigen	66	2.2	2.6	8.6	1.3	2.6	Sucrose Arrowroot Starch	Hydrolyzed Casein	MCT Oil
Pro-Sobee	66	2.5	3.4	6.8	2.1	2.2	Corn syrup solids	Soy Isolate	Soy Oil
Medium-Chain Triglyceride (MCT) Formula									
Portagen	66	2.3	3.1	7.4	1.7	2.6	Sucrose Maltodextrins	Casein	MCT Oil
Carbohydrate (CHO) or Fat Restriction									
Formula 3232A	66	2.2	2.8	2.3	0.9	1.7	Tapioca Starch	Hydrolyzed Casein	MCT Oil, Corn Oil (fractionated coconut oil)
Pregestimil	66	2.2	2.8	8.8	1.9	2.3	Glucose	Hydrolyzed Casein	MCT Oil
Skim Milk	36	3.6	Trace	5.3	2.3	3.6	Lactose	Cow's Milk	None
Renal Solute Restriction									
PM 60/40	66	1.5	3.4	7.2	0.6	1.4	Lactose	Cow's Milk	Corn, Coconut Oil
Sodium Restriction									
Lonalac	66	3.4	3.5	4.8	0.1	2.6	Lactose	Casein	Coconut Oil

Adapted from McKenzie, 1979 (145)

The dominant immunoglobulin in human milk is IgA, which mainly occurs as secretory IgA. Secretory IgA (SIgA) is stable at low pH and comparatively resistant to proteolytic enzymes. It is present in the intestines of breast fed infants and defends them against infection by binding viruses and bacteria, thereby preventing them from invading the mucosa (148).

22. A three-month-old infant has been "spitting up" after his feedings for one week. He has been fed with Enfamil (a cow's milk based formula). Should he be given a soy based formula or other nutritional substitutes? What are the indications for therapeutic formulas?

This infant appears to have *milk intolerance* to lactose which generally presents as abdominal discomfort, "spitting up," and poor feeding habits. It can usually be managed by diluting the formula or slowing the feeding rate. Indications for therapeutic formulas include low-birth weight, milk allergy, fat restriction, congenital heart disease, and caloric and carbohydrate restrictions. See Table 18.

Low-birth weight infants require a higher caloric content for growth than full-term infants because of an increased caloric need and a decreased ability for an adequate volume intake of formula. Examples of commercial formulas with higher caloric concentrations are premature formula and specially formulated SMA-improved and Similac PM 60/40 (80 Cal/100 ml). In addition to a higher caloric content, these contain a greater concentration of protein.

Milk allergy is a disorder that must be differentiated from milk intolerance. Milk allergy is the commonest food allergy in young infants; prevalence of this condition ranges from 0.4 to 7.5% of infants in this country. The main allergens appear to include beta-lactalbumin, present in cow's milk but not in human milk, casein, alpha-lactalbumin, and bovine serum albumin (149). Since it is an allergic condition, it is manifested by rash, wheezing, and other allergic symptoms. All forms of milk protein must be eliminated from the diet and substituted with either soy or casein formulas. In "true" milk allergy, soy protein formulas are frequently cross-allergenic with cow's milk protein. If infants continue with protracted diarrhea after the usual formula manipulations, recent reformulation of the elemental diet should

be ruled out as an etiologic factor. Some "elemental" formulas now utilize glucose polymers rather than glucose as the major source of carbohydrates and these may produce an osmotic diarrhea (150).

Infants with *congenital heart disease* (CHD) usually require a concentrated formula with a low sodium content. The formula must be concentrated because many CHD infants tire easily during feedings. Formulas such as SMA improved, PM 60/40 or Lonalac may be concentrated to 100 Cal/100 ml without creating an excessive intake of solute.

Disaccharidase deficiency may occur as a result of a congenital defect, cystic fibrosis, or severe diarrhea. As a result of disaccharidase deficiency, the infant's ability to hydrolyze disaccharides is impaired, and increased quantities of undigested disaccharides in the colon create an osmotically-induced diarrhea. In these cases, a formula such as 3232A may be given to eliminate carbohydrates from the diet. Supplementation with glucose is recommended.

Infants with *galactosemia* resulting from deficiency of the enzyme galactose-1-phosphate uridyl transferase, must have galactose eliminated from their diet. Formulas such as Nutramigen would be acceptable. It should also be remembered that galactose is a component of breast milk as well. Therefore, infants with galactosemia must also have breast milk eliminated from their diet and switched to a commercially prepared formula (151).

Vitamins and Minerals

Vitamin and mineral requirements for infants are higher than those for adults. Vitamin and mineral recommendations for infants are listed in Table 19 (147,152). In breast fed infants, supplementation with vitamins C and D is recommended by American Academy of Pediatrics (152). A daily supplement of Vitamin C is recommended for infants who are formula fed unless this is specifically added by the manufacturer. Preterm infants, whether they are breast fed or formula fed, should receive a multivitamin, multimineral supplement in addition to vitamins D, E, and folic acid.

Iron. Iron supplementation should be instituted no later than 2 months of age in preterm infants and should continue through the first year of life. Preterm infants have smaller iron stores since their liver has not matured during the last trimester. The dosage of supplemental iron should not exceed 1 mg/kg/day for term infants and 2 mg/kg/day for preterm infants, up to a maximum of 15 mg/day. The best supplementation of iron is by formulas fortified with iron or with a liquid iron preparation diluted with 2–3 ml of liquid. Supplementation should continue at least to one year of age. Iron can be extremely poisonous in children, and no more than a one month supply should be dispensed at any one time. Since iron deficiency is the most common cause of anemia in infancy, screening for anemia should be performed at six months of age in preterm infants and nine months of age in term infants (153).

Fluoride. Recommendations for fluoride supplementation are listed in Table 20. These recommendations incorporate both the age of the patient and the fluoride content of the water supply. A fluoride solution may be prescribed for infants who are unable to chew or swallow a tablet.

Table 19.

VITAMIN AND MINERAL RECOMMENDATIONS
IN INFANCY/100 KCAL[147,152]

Vitamins		Minerals		
A	250.0 IU	Calcium	50.0	mg
D	40.0 IU	Phosphorus	25.0	mg
E	0.3 IU	Magnesium	6.0	mg
K	4.0 IU	Iron	0.15	mg
Ascorbic				
Acid	8.1 mg	Zinc	0.5	mg
Thiamine	40.0 mcg	Copper	60.0	mcg
Riboflavin	60.0 mcg	Manganese	5.0	mcg
Pyridoxine	35.0 mcg	Iodine	5.0	mcg
B_{12}	0.15 mcg			
Folic Acid	4.0 mcg			

Table 20.

RECOMMENDATIONS FOR FLUORIDE
SUPPLEMENTATION[154–156]

Age	Fluoride Water Concentration (ppm)		
	< 0.3	0.3–0.7	> 0.7
2 wk–2 yr	0.25 mg/day	0	0
2–3 yr	0.50 mg/day	0.25 mg/day	0
3–16 yr	1.00 mg/day	0.50 mg/day	0

NAUSEA AND VOMITING

Epidemics of nausea and vomiting, thought to be due to a viral infection, affect children as well as adults. The specific diagnosis and the organism responsible are usually not established. Most cases of nausea and vomiting are self-limiting and should be managed symptomatically. The ingestion of solids should be restricted for at least 8–10 hours after symptoms of nausea and vomiting have subsided. Small amounts (1 oz/hr) of "decarbonated" beverages, Pedialyte, or cracked ice and fruit punch should be administered as tolerated. Coke syrup is often useful; its high sugar content suppresses nausea and vomiting. Small amounts of carbohydrate, in the form of crackers, are administered to older children for this reason.

Pharmacologic treatment should be limited to infants with protracted vomiting. The phenothiazine derivatives are useful in vomiting but must be prescribed with caution because of their serious side effects, such as extra-pyramidal manifestations. Many clinicians still question the value of antiemetics in treating children who have an acute, self-limiting disorder. Some authorities have suggested that vomiting in gastroenteritis is a defense mechanism to shed pathogens and should not be suppressed (157).

DIAPER RASH

Dermatitis limited to the diaper area is a frequent problem in pediatric practice. Most authorities believe these rashes represent an irritant contact dermatitis caused by prolonged contact with urine or stool. Although various components of urine and stool have been implicated, including ammonia, bacteria and bacterial byproducts, urine and fecal pH, *Candida albicans*, and water, no single cause can be isolated. The theory of ammonia-induced rashes has been challenged by studies which demonstrated similar ammonia concentrations among infants with and without diaper rash (160); a strong ammonia odor has not been correlated with the genesis of diaper dermatitis. Moisture alone may alter the epidermal barrier, and old urine is a good culture medium for bacterial overgrowth. Direct irritation by an alkaline urine (pH 8 to 9) or the alkalinity of the stool may be responsible (158). A persistent rash may represent infection with *Candida albicans*.

Other irritants which should be suspected include residual chemicals or laundry detergents in the diaper (cloth or disposable), or a soap, medication, or lotion applied directly to the infant's skin. Factors which may exacerbate any rash in this area include a warm, moist environment which macerates the skin and facilitates fungal or bacterial invasion, local irritants, local infection, and mechanical irritation (159).

There are four clinical presentations of dermatitis associated with diaper wear: a) a mild and scaling rash in the perianal area; b) a sharply demarcated confluent erythema; c) ulceration distributed through the diaper area; and d) a beefy red confluent erythema with satellite lesions, vesiculopustular lesions and diffuse involvement of the genitalia.

23. R.S. is a 3-month-old infant who has had a severe "diaper rash" for the past four days. It is confined to the diaper area which is very inflamed and tender. There are vesicular satellite lesions on the periphery of the main erythematous area. The mother uses only cloth diapers and has not changed soap or her normal pattern of diaper care since the infant was born. Based on the clinical appearance of the rash and its long duration, the resident prescribed nystatin ointment and gave the mother detailed instructions for treatment. Why was nystatin prescribed, and how should diaper rash be treated generally?

Since R.S.'s rash is very inflamed with the presence of vesicular satellite lesions, and has been present for more than three days, local candidal infection is likely. Typically, a clinical presentation like type d, described previously, is seen when the dermatitis becomes secondarily invaded with *Candida albicans*. Diffuse involvement of the genitalia in the inguinal folds is also characteristic of this form. Therefore, the use of nystatin powder or ointment applied to the rash four times daily until the rash is gone, is recommended for R.S.

Treatment first involves removal of the primary irritant. Gentle rinsing of the skin with clear water is recommended; excessive cleansing should be discouraged. Talcum powder should be avoided or used with caution to avoid aspiration of talc particles by the infant. Cornstarch, although an effective drying agent, is contraindicated because it serves as a culture media for *C. albicans*. Some studies have implicated the use of plastic pants

or waterproof disposable diapers with a higher incidence of diaper rashes (161,162). A moisture proof barrier, however, will not result in more favorable growth conditions for skin bacteria if the wet diaper is changed promptly.

A stepwise approach should include the following (158,163): 1) change the diaper as soon as it is wet or at least every two to four hours, including a change at night; 2) avoid overnight use of plastic pants or disposable diapers; "triple diaper" with cotton diapers, and use a rubber pad; 3) expose the diaper area to air as frequently as possible; 4) if cotton diapers are used, rinse with diluted vinegar, (ie, one cup of vinegar in half a washing machine full of water for one-half hour) to reduce the alkalinity of the diaper; 5) *C. albicans* infection should be suspected if the rash is present for more than three days; it can be treated with an anticandidal agent such as nystatin powder or ointment four times daily or with every other diaper change; 6) 0.5–1% hydrocortisone ointment may be applied twice daily for up to one week for severe inflammation.

TEETHING

24. B.W., a 3-day-old baby boy and his mother are being discharged from the hospital. While obtaining discharge medications, the mother expresses some concern about the baby's dental care. The obstetrician informed her that B.W. was born with two teeth which were removed postpartum. She is now concerned that he will not develop baby teeth normally. What information should she receive?

Occasionally, infants may be born with teeth, and usually there are two in the position of the mandibular central incisors. Due to the danger of tongue laceration and aspiration of these natal teeth if they become loose, and the pain they can cause the nursing mother, these rudiments should be extracted. The mother should be told that the presence and removal of natal teeth does not interfere with the normal eruption of primary teeth.

Normal eruption of primary teeth rarely begins before four to five months of age, and is usually uneventful and often asymptomatic; see Table 21.

A significant number of infants erupt no teeth until the end of the first year. Delayed eruption of all teeth, however, may indicate systemic or

Table 21.

AGE OF ERUPTION OF THE PRIMARY TEETH[164]

	Age (Months)	
	Lower	*Upper*
Central Incisor	4–8	5.5–9.5
Lateral Incisor	5–9	7–11
Cuspid	14–18	16–20
First Molar	8–16	10–18
Second Molar	16–24	20–28

nutritional disturbances such as hypothyroidism, hypopituitarism, and rickets, or a prenatal event (164).

25. Five months later, B.W. has become increasingly irritable and has been waking up five or six times per night. He also seems to be drooling excessively. A brief examination of the child's mouth shows red and tender gums. No teeth are present and B.W. is afebrile. The mother is concerned that B.W. is teething and, therefore, has a secondary systemic illness. Are these symptoms unusual?

B.W.'s regular sleeping pattern has been disturbed by symptomatic teething. As the teeth penetrate the gums, the site may become tender and there will be increased salivation. Bacterial invasion through a break in the tissue or under a gingival flap covering the teeth may cause inflammation and edema, but "teething" does not cause systemic disturbances (165). In general, tooth eruption bears no relationship to the incidence of pediatric infections, diarrhea, fever, rashes, or convulsions. Teething, however, has been associated with restlessness, increased salivation, thumb-sucking, gum rubbing, and sometimes decreased appetite (166).

26. What course of treatment can be suggested for B.W.?

Gentle irrigation with water often relieves the inflammation around a gum flap. A topical anesthetic applied with a cotton-tipped applicator may be rubbed gently on the mucous membranes overlying the erupting tooth (167). A number of nonprescription products are available for this purpose (see Table 22). Long-term use of local anesthetics, however, is not recommended. Mucosal absorption of these agents can sensitize the patient to local anesthetics and can lead to severe

allergic reactions if future use becomes necessary (166).

Other palliative measures include having the child chew on a blunt, firm object or cracked ice wrapped in a soft cloth to hasten tooth eruption and thus relieve pain. Rubber teething rings of various shapes may be beneficial (169). Water-containing rings should be avoided since they can become infected with bacteria. Gingival incision for teething is rarely indicated. Proprietary teething aids which contain mercurial compounds should not be used because of possible systemic toxicity (167).

Aspirin and Acetaminophen. Both agents are commonly prescribed for younger children for the relief of pain associated with the eruption of primary dentition. Aspirin alleviates pain by two mechanisms, peripheral and central. Peripherally, aspirin inhibits prostaglandin synthesis, thereby preventing pain receptor sensitization to mechanical stimulation or to chemicals, such as bradykinin, that appear to mediate pain. Centrally, aspirin acts directly at a hypothalamic site for both its analgesic and antipyretic effects. The mechanism of acetaminophen's analgesic effect is uncertain. Both drugs may have serious side effects; therefore, dosage recommendations should be strictly followed (see Table 5). Finally, aspirin should *never* be used topically. The topical use of aspirin is responsible for the majority of oral chemical burns (166).

FEVER

Considerations for the management of fever include the magnitude of the temperature elevation, the etiology of fever, the duration of the febrile episode, and the age and general condition of the child. Temperatures of 38.9° C (102° F) or greater should be treated.

Prolonged fevers may be associated with serious disorders such as autoimmune collagen-vascular diseases, or malignancy. Most fevers in infants and children, however, are viral in origin, are of short duration, and have limited consequences (170,171). Proponents of conservative management believe that fever in children is rarely a serious problem; the treatment of fever may obliterate a clinical sign which is of value in monitoring the course of the disease and effectiveness of primary therapy; fever may enhance the body's defenses and/or reduce the viability of

Table 22.

TOPICAL TEETHING ANESTHETICS [166,168]

Product (Manufacturer)	Benzocaine	Other Active	Miscellaneous
		Ingredients	
Anbesol (Whitehall)	yes	Phenol Iodine	Glycerin; Alcohol
Baby Oragel (Commerce)	yes	—	Viscous water-soluble base
Benzodent (Vick)	yes	Eugenol 8-hydroxyquinoline sulfate	Denture adhesivelike base
Butyn (Abbott)	—	Butacaine Benzyl alcohol	Not stated
Dalidyne (Dalin)	yes	Methylbenzethonium Cl Tannic acid Camphor Menthol Chlorothymol Benzyl alcohol	Alcohol; aromatic base
Dr. Hands Teething Gel and Lotion (Roberts)	—	Tincture of pellitory Clove oil Menthol	Hamamelis water; Alcohol
Jiffy (Block)	yes	Eugenol	Alcohol
Numzident (Pure Pac)	yes	Eugenol Peppermint oil	Polyethylene glycol-like base
Numzit (Pure Pac)	—	—	Glycerin; Alcohol; gel vehicle
Orabase (Hoyt)	Available with or without	—	Pectin; Gelatin; Carboxymethylcellulose sodium; Polyethylene glycol; Mineral oil
Orajel (Commerce)	yes	—	Polyethylene glycol-like base
Teething Lotion (DeWitt)	yes	Benzyl alcohol Tincture of myrrh	Propylene glycerol; Glycerin; Alcohol

infecting organisms; and treatment with antipyretics carries the risk of adverse reactions. Those who would argue for vigorous management of fever would list their points as follows: the possibility of febrile convulsions, particularly during the first three years of life, can be diminished by the lowering of body temperature; the relief of patient discomfort resulting from fever is an important aspect of patient management; high fevers may produce CNS damage and should be treated vigorously; and while fever may be useful in the clinical management of an underlying disease, the availability of cultures and other laboratory techniques have reduced its importance (172).

Many parents have a serious misunderstanding about the role of fever in the etiology of many diseases (173). This misunderstanding has been termed "fever phobia" in the pediatric community (174). The only serious complications of fever are febrile status epilepticus and heat stroke, both of which are rare. Generally, fevers lower than 40° C are not associated with any harmful effects.

27. H.W. is concerned about the recent onset of fever in his two-year-old daughter who has had a temperature of 38.5° C for the past 12 hours. She has also had a mild cough and runny nose. H.W. is interested in obtaining an antipyretic and asks your advice. He is concerned that children have been poisoned with both aspirin and acetaminophen. Which antipyretic would you select for H.W. based on the therapeutic, pharmacokinetic, and toxicity information available?

Both aspirin and acetaminophen lower temperature by altering the response of the hypothalamus. Most investigations have found aspirin and acetaminophen to be similar in antipyretic effectiveness. Although both drugs exert their maximum effect within a similar amount of time, there seems to be a slightly greater maximum temperature change with acetaminophen, but aspirin appears to have a somewhat longer duration of effect (175). Dosages are presented in Table 5.

In both children and adults the clinical pharmacokinetic profile of aspirin is relatively complex and subject to wide interpatient variability (176). Orally administered aspirin is absorbed and hydrolyzed to salicylic acid. The biologic elimination half-life for salicylate varies between 2–8 hours. It is dose and patient dependent. The elimination of aspirin is complicated by saturation of two of its metabolic pathways at subtherapeutic dosage levels. Additionally, free salicylate is excreted in the urine and is dependent on urinary blood flow and pH. Other factors such as acidosis, age, and dehydration all contribute to the complex kinetics of this drug.

The clinical pharmacokinetic profile of acetaminophen is less complex (176). Following oral administration in children, the plasma half-life is 1–4 hours, and somewhat longer in neonates. While the glucuronide metabolite predominates in adults and the sulfate metabolite is more prominent in infants and children, there appears to be no difference in total elimination rate in all age groups (179).

Aspirin remains a leading cause of childhood poisoning and death (178). It also has a number of additional side effects including effects on the hemostatic system and the potential for producing gastric mucosal injury. This does not negate the efficacy of aspirin as an antipyretic. It does emphasize, however, the need for parents and physicians to be aware of the potential for salicylate toxicity.

Acetaminophen has an extremely low toxic potential. Adverse effects at therapeutic doses are reported rarely. The risk of serious hepatic injury following massive overdosage of acetaminophen is real and should be of some concern, although children appear to be less vulnerable to the effects of an acetaminophen overdose (175,180). To date, there is only one documented pediatric fatality due to acetaminophen overdosage in the United States (181).

28. Is it advantageous to administer aspirin and acetaminophen in combination?

Parents frequently inquire about the combination of aspirin and acetaminophen in the treatment of febrile children. In one study, concurrent administration of full doses of aspirin and acetaminophen resulted in a more sustained but not greater reduction in temperature (182). Another study showed that the combination of aspirin and acetaminophen was more effective than either drug alone (175). Alternate dosing with aspirin and acetaminophen has not been documented as being more efficacious. While there is a rational basis for the use of this approach, parent confusion and resulting dosing errors pose a practical problem for this regimen.

29. What alternatives to drug therapy are available to lower fever?

In addition to the pharmacologic control of fever, environmental methods of lowering body temperature have been used. These methods are based on loss of body heat through the principles of conduction, convection, radiation, and evaporation. Sponging with tepid water has been found to be more effective than exposure alone but less effective than drug treatment with antipyretics (183). It has also been found that tepid sponging only resulted in a lowering of body temperature to about 39° C. Sponging with ice water or alcohol/water mixtures (1:4 ratio) is more effective, but considerable discomfort is associated with these treatments (184). Also, acute alcohol poisoning is possible when ventilation is inadequate and concentrated solutions of alcohol are utilized (185). Shivering may also result from cold applications and will contribute to a rise in body core temperature from increased muscle activity. Therefore, immersion of patients in ice water baths is not recommended.

Additional information on the treatment of fever in children is presented in the chapter on Fever.

FEBRILE SEIZURES

Febrile seizures usually occur in children between six months and five years of age. Thirty to forty percent of those who have a febrile seizure and who do not receive prophylactic therapy will experience a second. Children who have had a febrile seizure may subsequently develop epilepsy. The presence of at least two of the following risk factors is accompanied by a high risk of epilepsy: a family history of nonfebrile seizures; abnormal neurological or developmental status prior to a febrile seizure; or an atypical febrile seizure, such as a prolonged or focal seizure (186). Of those children who have none of the above risk factors, only 2 or 3% subsequently develop epilepsy following a febrile seizure. In children with febrile seizures, a neurological deficit such as mental retardation or sensory and perceptual abnormalities may be present prior to the seizure episode. There is no evidence that these deficits reflect neurologic injury occurring at the time of the febrile seizure.

30. J.G.'s daughter had a "convulsion" that lasted for about 20 minutes when she had a fever of 40°C. The family history is remarkable for the mother having a seizure disorder. J.G. asks what drug therapy is used to treat this condition and for how long? What side effects might occur?

Anticonvulsant prophylaxis in therapeutic dosages may be considered under any of the following conditions: a) in the presence of abnormal neurological development; b) when a febrile seizure is longer than 15 minutes, focal, or followed by transient or persistent neurological abnormalities; or c) a history of nonfebrile seizures of genetic origin is present in a parent or sibling. Anticonvulsant prophylaxis is instituted for at least two years or for one year after the last seizure, whichever is the longer period of time. Discontinuation of therapy should be done slowly over a one to two month period.

Numerous studies show the risk of recurrence of febrile seizures can be reduced by the continuous daily administration of phenobarbital in dosages (3–5 mg/kg/day) sufficient to attain a minimum therapeutic concentration of 15 mcg/ml. Present evidence does not show that phenytoin is effective in the prophylaxis of febrile seizures. Experimental evidence suggests that the duration of febrile seizures can be reduced by the prompt administration of diazepam rectally in suppository form (186). Valproic acid is also effective in preventing recurrences of febrile seizures (187). However, this agent carries a greater risk of toxicity, especially for the liver, than does phenobarbital prophylaxis for children with febrile seizures. Also, the cost of treatment with valproic acid may be 5–6 fold greater than that with phenobarbital.

The use of phenobarbital is associated with side effects and toxic reactions in up to 40% of infants and children receiving this medication (188). These reactions are usually of the following types: a) behavioral changes—hyperactivity and rarely somnolence; b) sleep pattern disturbances—prolonged nocturnal wakening; c) interference with higher cortical or cognitive functions, eg, short term memory. Disturbances of behavior and patterns of sleep are not predictable but are the cause for discontinuation of therapy in up to 25% of patients.

REYE'S SYNDROME

Reye's syndrome is a neurological disorder of children which is characterized by encephalopathy and fatty infiltration of the viscera and which usually occurs five to seven days after an upper respiratory tract viral infection (189). Affected children suddenly exhibit central nervous system symptoms which begin with vomiting and are rapidly followed by agitation and delirium. The syndrome may progress to a brain stem dysfunction characterized by hyperpnea, increased pulse rate, and coma. In its most severe form, increased intracranial pressure and cerebral edema develop rapidly and result in brain stem compression. The etiology of Reye's syndrome remains unknown. A number of viruses have been isolated from patients with the syndrome, including varicella zoster, influenza type B, coxsackie A, and others (190). Toxins and drugs, including aspirin, have also been implicated in the pathogenesis of Reye's syndrome (191,192). It is a multifactorial disease and may require synergistic agents acting on susceptible individuals.

The Center for Disease Control criteria for the diagnosis of Reye's syndrome are as follows: a patient must have an acute noninflammatory encephalopathy and microvesicular fatty metamorphosis of the liver confirmed by biopsy or autopsy or a serum glutamic oxaloacetic transaminase (SGOT), serum glutamic pyruvic transaminase (SGPT), or serum ammonia greater than three times normal. If cerebrospinal fluid is obtained, the leukocyte count must be no greater than 8 per mm³. In addition, there should be no other explanation for the neurologic or hepatic abnormalities (193,194).

Staging. Staging is utilized to define severity of the illness and to allow rational therapeutic intervention (195). Staging is as follows: Stage 1—vomiting, lethargy, laboratory evidence of liver dysfunction; Stage 2—disorientation, combativeness, hyperactive reflexes; Stage 3—coma, decorticate rigidity, continued laboratory evidence of liver dysfunction; Stage 4—deepening coma, minimal liver dysfunction; Stage 5—seizures, loss of deep tendon reflexes, respiratory arrest, flaccidity. An additional component of this staging is classification of electroencephalogram results. These progress from a rhythmic slowing with dominant theta waves and rare delta waves in the earliest form of the disease to an isoelectric EEG in the most severe forms.

Cerebral Edema. One of the most lethal aspects of the disease is increased intracranial pressure (196,197). The cause of the increased intracranial pressure is thought to be cytotoxic edema. The edema in this process is diffuse since all cells undergo swelling caused by failure of the ATP-dependent sodium pump within cell membranes. Endothelial cells may swell and narrow the capillary lumen, while capillary permeability is not usually affected. The cerebral edema of Reye's syndrome usually shows an onset within 24 hours of presentation of neurological signs.

Management. Therapy of Reye's syndrome can range from mild to more aggressive forms (198). Endotracheal intubation with hyperventilation is one of the basic management techniques for these patients. With hyperventilation, PCO_2 is lowered in the plasma, resulting in a decreased cerebral blood flow and diminished pressure in the brain. Fluid restriction serves a dual purpose in preventing fluid overloading and in treating the syndrome of inappropriate secretion of antidiuretic hormone which may occur with cerebral edema. Much attention has been focused on the role of hypoglycemia in the pathophysiology of this disease. Blood sugar should be maintained at near normal or slightly elevated levels. Hyperosmolar agents such as mannitol and glycerol are utilized in combination with diuretics to maintain a serum osmolarity between 290–340 mOsm/kg. The use of potent diuretics such as furosemide may have effects other than diuresis (199). Furosemide blocks sodium uptake into the cerebrospinal fluid and brain tissue. While corticosteroids are often used in the management of cerebral edema of head trauma, their role in the management of cerebral edema of Reye's syndrome is less defined.

Hypothermia has been advocated as a means of decreasing the metabolic needs of the brain and reducing systemic blood pressure. While this is a valuable adjunct to the treatment of increased intracranial pressure, metabolic and technical problems have precluded its use on a wide scale basis. An adjunctive agent used with both hyperventilation and hypothermia of patients is the neuromuscular blocker pancuronium. By decreasing muscle tone, it is thought to decrease the transient elevation of intracranial pressure seen with movement or exertion on the part of the patient. Additionally, with hypothermia therapy it blocks the shivering response of the patient, which can result in an increase in body temperature during cooling. Other investigational agents that have been used to control intracranial pressure include barbiturates (eg, pentobarbital administered in doses efficient to produce coma), intravenous glycerol, and lidocaine (200–202).

Other therapeutic modalities that have been utilized in the management of this disorder include exchange transfusions (203), dialysis, hypothermic total body washout, and bowel sterilization. None of these measures have resulted in a decreased mortality when compared to standard intensive care monitoring (204,205). Presently, intensive care support constitutes the mainstay of therapy in Reye's syndrome.

ATTENTION DEFICIT DISORDERS

Attention Deficit Disorders (ADD), formerly referred to as Minimal Brain Dysfunction (MBD), have been defined as "a descriptive and diagnostic category which refers to children of near average, average, or above average general intelligence with certain learning or behavioral disabilities, ranging from mild to severe, which are associated with deviations of function of the central nervous system (CNS)" (206). ADD is further subdivided into categories of ADD with and without hyperactivity. Specific clinical characteristics for diagnosis of ADD are provided by the American Psychiatric Association Diagnostic and Statistical Manual (DSM III); see Table 23. The onset of the condition is generally before age 7, and the condition must be present for at least six months to support its diagnosis (207). Attention deficit disorders affect an estimated 5–20% of all elementary school age children (208). The incidence varies with the ambiguity of diagnostic criteria and declines markedly in children above ten years of age. Estimates indicate that approximately 2% of all elementary school children are receiving CNS stimulant medication for hyperactivity (209). In addition, there appears to be a striking preponderance of males to females with this condition.

Table 23.

CLINICAL CHARACTERISTICS OF ADD WITH HYPERACTIVITY[207]

A. Hyperactivity

At least two of the following:
1. Runs or climbs excessively
2. Unable to sit still or fidgets excessively
3. Difficulty staying seated
4. Motor restlessness during sleep
5. On the go continuously

B. Inattention*

At least three of the following:
1. Often fails to finish projects started
2. Often doesn't seem to listen
3. Distracted easily
4. Unable to concentrate on school work or other tasks requiring sustained attention
5. Sustained participation in a play activity difficult

C. Impulsivity*

At least three of the following:
1. Often acts before thinking
2. Shifts from one activity to another excessively
3. Despite normal cognitive skills, has difficulty organizing work
4. Requires a lot of supervision
5. Frequently disrupts class
6. Unable to wait for turn in games or group situations

*ADD without Hyperactivity would include those characteristics itemized in B and C.

Diagnosis. Individual traits commonly described in these children are: specific learning disabilities, a delay in the development of gross and/or fine motor skills, soft neurological signs, social incompetence, and secondary emotional effects (210). Certain organic and psychogenic states have been described with hyperactivity and must first be ruled out. These include mental retardation, neurologic injury or deterioration, hyperthyroidism, cerebral palsy, epilepsy, and maternal or sensory deprivation (211).

Behavioral, intelligence, and cognitive skills should be evaluated. A detailed history identifying key temperamental traits such as attentiveness, distractability, impulsivity, and excitability is required. Both parents and children should be questioned. Behavior rating scales, such as Connors' Teachers' Rating Scale (212) and Davids' Hyperkinetic Rating Scale (213) are helpful in this regard. Many children will have a significant history dating back to infancy (214). Observation of the child performing the task by the physician is especially relevant. It is often useful to measure the child's academic achievement, in addition to their I.Q. An EEG is generally not necessary unless a seizure disorder or degenerative process is suspected (214).

Treatment. Management of the child with ADD includes counseling of parents, teachers, and the child, behavior modification programs, remedial education, tutoring, and pharmacotherapy (215). All of these treatments are aimed at reducing abnormal behavior and correcting learning deficiencies.

Pharmacotherapy is used as adjunctive treatment in the school-age child with ADD. Drugs are used to alleviate or reduce hyperactivity and impulsive behavior, increase attention span, and improve motor coordination. Approximately 50 to 80% improve on short-term drug therapy regimens (216). Drugs which have been utilized include CNS stimulants, antidepressants, anticonvulsants, and antianxiety and antipsychotic agents; see Table 24. CNS stimulants, however, comprise the mainstay of pharmacotherapy.

The mechanism of action of CNS stimulants in ADD is not clearly understood. Amphetamine and methylphenidate are known to increase CNS catecholamine release from sympathetic nerve terminals and inhibit reuptake in the brain. If ADD is the result of decreased catecholamine levels centrally, primarily involving the reticular acti-

Table 24.

DRUGS COMMONLY USED IN THE TREATMENT OF ADD IN CHILDREN [208,215,216]

Class	Drug	Product Example	Average Daily Dose	Precautions/ Comments
CNS Stimulants	Methylphenidate	Ritalin	0.3–2 mg/kg	Many increase seizure activity in patients with epilepsy.
	Pemoline	Cylert	56.25–75 mg	Avoid in children < 6 years old. Monitor liver function tests.
	Dextroamphetamine	Dexedrine	0.5–2 mg/kg	Contraindicated in hypertension, hyper-thyroidism, and glaucoma.
	Deanol	Deaner	250–500 mg	Relative contraindica-tion in generalized seizure disorders. Side effects are minimal.
Antianxiety and Antipsychotic Agents	Chlordiazepoxide	Librium	10–50 mg	These agents lessen hyperactive behavior but do not decrease distractability or in-crease attention span.
	Chlorpromazine	Thorazine	10–30 mg	
	Thioridazine	Mellaril	20–75 mg	
Antidepressants	Imipramine	Tofranil	1–5 mg	Lowers seizure threshold—caution in patients with epi-lepsy. Agent of choice in the enuretic pa-tient with ADD.
Anticonvulsants	Phenytoin	Dilantin	50–200 mg	Used in children whose behavior and learning problems are complicated by seizures.
	Primidone	Mysoline	100–500 mg	

vating system, administration of CNS stimulants may correct the deficiency. Pemoline appears to enhance dopamine and RNA synthesis in the brain, and deanol is felt to be an acetylcholine precursor, which is converted intracerebrally. Recent studies of deanol in animals, however, have failed to confirm this mechanism (215).

Anorexia and insomnia are common dose-related side effects from CNS stimulants. Both usually diminish with time. Anorexia can be min-imized by administering the drugs after meals, and insomnia can be avoided by not dosing the child in the evening.

31. G.W. is a 7-year-old white male who was brought to his pediatrician because of dete-riorating scholastic performance that was noted by both his teacher and his parents. The pediatrician found G.W. to be neurolog-ically intact and of normal intelligence. He seemed somewhat uncoordinated and his at-tention span was short. After an extensive

evaluation, the pediatrician initiated therapy with methylphenidate 5 mg every morning. Within one month, G.W. was stabilized on doses of 10 mg in the morning and 5 mg at noon. G.W. remained on this dosage for seven months until summer vacation. The medication was then stopped for three months and restarted when school resumed.

Why was methylphenidate prescribed rather than dextroamphetamine? How was the dosage determined?

Methylphenidate, which lacks the social stigma of amphetamine, is considered the drug of first choice. Amphetamine, however, offers several advantages over methylphenidate: 1) lower cost; 2) oral absorption unaffected by food; and 3) it is available in a long-acting form, so the child will not have to take medicine at school, which may increase compliance (214).

Dosage recommendations for methylphenidate vary widely. Optimum doses for learning (0.3 mg/kg) may differ from those for behavior control (1.0 mg/kg) (217). However, others have suggested that 0.3 mg/kg per day is required for both optimal learning performance and minimized impulsivity (218). Since methylphenidate blood levels and improved performance disappear after about four hours, twice-daily dosage given four hours apart may be required (0.32 mg/kg/dose) (219). In this case, a commonly used low dose of 5 mg daily was used to initiate therapy. This schedule was then increased in increments of 2.5 mg based on therapeutic and toxic response.

32. Why was G.W.'s medication discontinued during the summer months?

All patients should have drug-free periods, for example, during summer vacation, to evaluate the underlying disease state. These drug holidays are of value in determining when to discontinue therapy.

33. G.W.'s mother has noticed that the intake of certain foods makes him worse. Is this likely, and is there a special diet G.W. should adhere to for better control of his ADD? Is diet an important component of ADD management?

In 1973, Feingold proposed that salicylate compounds, which are present naturally in many fruits and vegetables, and artificial colors and flavors can cause or worsen hyperkinesis and learning disabilities (225,226). Feingold therefore formu-

lated a diet free of these agents. His hypothesis suggests that hyperactivity is due to a nonimmunologic response to these substances in genetically susceptible children (227). Feingold reported improvement in 40 to 70% of hyperactive children who strictly adhered to the diet. More recent well-controlled studies, however, have failed to document any behavioral improvement, and the earlier positive results may be a result of psychological or placebo factors (228). If these foods or others seem to exacerbate the child's condition, they should be restricted unless the child's nutritional status is compromised.

Other nonstandard therapies related to diet include megavitamins, orthmolecular mineral therapy, and inducement of hypoglycemia (227,229). The efficacy of these methods, however, is questionable. Further documentation with well-controlled studies is required.

34. G.W.'s treatment schedule was continued for three years until it was noted that he did not appear to be growing at the same rate as the other boys his age. Is this an adverse effect of methylphenidate therapy?

Early reports suggested that methylphenidate or amphetamine treatment was associated with growth suppression as compared with controls (220). Tolerance to this effect appears to develop with chronic use, and catch-up growth seems to occur upon discontinuation of the drug. A more recent study found no correlation between dose and changes in height and weight percentiles (221). The authors concluded that any slowing of growth noted with initial treatment is compensated for later in life, both during and after treatment.

Chronic pemoline therapy may cause growth suppression by a direct effect on cartilage metabolism (224).

ENURESIS

Enuresis is one of the most common chronic conditions seen in pediatric practice, affecting up to 10% of school age children (230). Enuresis is defined as involuntary voiding of urine in the absence of any organic lesion after the age of five to six years (230,232). Most children become dry at night between the ages of 18 months and 4 years, usually after daytime control is achieved (233). Enuresis is a benign condition which is encountered 1.5 to 2 times more frequently in males than in females and may persist through puberty (231).

Somatic and psychogenic causes have been proposed. The somatic etiologies include a reduced functional bladder capacity, sleep pattern disturbances, urinary tract infections, abnormal or inadequate toilet training techniques, organic neurologic defects or immaturity, inherited predisposition to the condition, or, although not well documented, allergic cystitis due to various foods or chemicals with resultant urgency (230,234,235).

Environmental stress, revenge, nocturnal fear, and Oedipal complexes are examples of psychogenic etiologies. There is also an association with behavioral disturbances (Attention Deficit Disorders) and developmental delay (235).

35. S.N. is a 6-year-old male who is brought to his pediatrician. His mother complains that "he still wets the bed," and punishing the boy only seems to worsen the situation. Within the past year, S.N. achieved daytime bladder control, but now continues to wet his bed at least once or twice a week. How should this problem be evaluated and classified?

A thorough medical history is required including: a) a detailed family history, b) a review of the psychosocial aspects of the child's family life, and c) information concerning day and night wetting patterns and fluid intake. In one study, when both parents were enuretic, 77% of children were also enuretic; with only one enuretic parent, 44% were enuretic; and when the family history was negative, 15% of the children were enuretic (232). The child's evaluation should also include a general physical examination, emphasizing the rectal exam, to rule out any urologic abnormality or spinal cord lesion, and a neurological assessment, for muscle tone, reflexes, and sensory response (230,232). A urinalysis should be performed to rule out organic causes such as diabetes insipidus, diabetes mellitus, or urinary tract infections.

Once the diagnosis of enuresis is made, classification of the condition is based on onset and occurrence of the symptom; see Table 25. S.N. has primary nocturnal enuresis, which is the most common presentation.

36. What are the current modes of therapy available for enuresis?

Conditioning therapy is generally the first form of treatment initiated for enuretic patients in ad-

Table 25.

CLASSIFICATION OF ENURESIS [231,236]

	Percent of Enuretic Children
I. Onset of Symptom	
Primary—bladder control never achieved	66–75
Secondary/Acquired—relapse after at least 6 to 12 months of bladder control.	25–33
II. Occurrence of Symptom	
Nocturnal—night time only	85
Diurnal—daytime only	–
Nocturnal/Diurnal—night and day	–

dition to patient and family counseling for emotional problems. This method of behavior modification is based on arousing the child whenever urine moistens special electrically-wired bedsheets, thereby triggering a buzzer. It is effective in 30 to 50% of enuretic patients and should be continued for several weeks after the child has stopped wetting. Success rates as high as 75% have been reported (235). Approximately 30% of the patients may relapse after therapy is discontinued, but they frequently will respond to retreatment. The use of electrical sheets is relatively safe, but rashes from urinary sodium chloride electrolysis and electrical burns from faulty apparati have been reported (236).

Bladder training consists of stretching exercises to increase functional bladder capacity. Enuretic children appear to have a small functional bladder capacity for their age and therefore tend to void more frequently during the day (237). Their total daily volume, however, is equivalent to that of children with normal functional bladder capacities (238). Forced fluids are retained for as long as possible and then urine is expelled and measured. In a controlled study, these stretching exercises resulted in a larger bladder capacity and a cure in bedwetting in one third of the cases (237,238).

Drug therapy is frequently used in the management of enuresis. Anticholinergic agents such as propantheline were originally used as primary or adjunctive therapy to induce urinary retention. These agents were effective in some cases but only when used in conjunction with conditioning therapy (230).

Amphetamines taken at bedtime have been used with varying success. While no serious toxicities have been reported, nervousness and insomnia do occur with increasing dosage (230).

Tricyclic antidepressants, specifically imipramine, are frequently used for the treatment of enuresis. The basis for the antienuretic action of tricyclics is unknown, but, in contrast to the drug's delayed antidepressant effect, the onset of the antienuretic effect tends to be immediate (235). The effective plasma concentration in enuresis is 25–30% of the plasma concentration required for antidepressive therapy (239). Kales et al have suggested that early in the night, when sleep is deepest, imipramine decreases bladder excitability and/or increases its capacity. The child is thus permitted to sleep without wetting until later in the night when sleep is lighter and the child is more responsive to bladder stimuli (240).

The response to imipramine varies from 5–80%. The low response rates correspond to long-term follow up studies of patients who have been withdrawn from the drug (238). The average dose of imipramine used is 75 to 100 mg nightly, but the Food and Drug Administration (FDA) suggests that the dose should not exceed 2.5 mg/kg/day (235).

37. S.N. was given bladder training exercises and begun on imipramine therapy. What information about imipramine's efficacy and side effects should the parents receive?

Although the drug is usually effective, there are some who don't respond or who develop an apparent tolerance to the antienuretic effect of imipramine (235). Side effects are generally mild and dose-related. However, these drugs are potentially lethal in overdose and are now the commonest cause of fatal poisoning in children under the age of five years (241). When dispensing imipramine, the total amount should be limited, and syrup of ipecac should be dispensed as well. If an overdose occurs, the parents should be instructed to induce vomiting after contacting their physician or poison control center.

38. Are there any new agents used for antienuresis which might offer S.N. a safe and effective alternative to imipramine?

Recently, studies have indicated that nocturnal bedwetting can be reduced by decreasing urine output with desmopressin (DDAVP) (242). DDAVP is a synthetic long-acting analogue of vasopressin. Evening doses of 10 mcg of DDAVP were administered intranasally to 20 persistently enuretic children in a pilot study. A statistically significant positive response was elicited (243). Antidiuretic doses of DDAVP lack the adverse effects (cardiac arrhythmias, coronary vasoconstriction) of the older vasopressin analogues. Antienuresis is not a FDA approved indication for DDAVP, and additional more comprehensive studies are required concerning dosing, efficacy, and drug safety, both short and long term.

DRUG ADMINISTRATION

The administration of drugs to children requires special knowledge and technique primarily because dosages for children are often prescribed in amounts which are not commercially available. Drugs are almost universally compounded, tested, and marketed in adult dosage forms. Guidelines or recipes are available for the extemporaneous preparation of medications only available in adult strengths or dosage forms. Caution, however, must be used, since stability and bioavailability data are unavailable for many medications.

The administration of oral medicines to an infant is not difficult as long as caution is exercised not to choke the patient. Liquid medications should be placed on the middle of the tongue in the buccal cavity, preferably through a dropper. Oral syringes are also available for drug administration. These syringes are designed to prevent the attachment of intravenous needles and to prevent the inadvertent parenteral administration of an oral medication. They must be used with care since too rapid administration or squirting of the drug can result in aspiration of the liquid.

In pediatrics, it is common practice to disguise the taste of some medications in Karo syrup, applesauce, ice cream, or other palatable vehicle to increase compliance. Children should always be encouraged and praised for their cooperation in taking their medicine.

For pediatric patients, the placement of medications in the outer ear, and ear irrigation are the same as for adults with one exception. The auricle of the ear in older patients and adults is held up and back to straighten the canal. For children up to two or three years of age, however, the auricle is held down and out. This facilitates delivery of the medication to the middle ear.

Administration of nose drops in children varies from nasal instillation in adults. The child is placed on his back, across the bed, with his shoulders projecting over the edge so that his head is lower than his body. The prescribed number of drops are instilled and the patient is kept in this position for 2 to 5 minutes. Afterwards the patient is placed on his abdomen facing directly down toward the mattress.

Eye drops must be administered with extreme caution to children. Positioning and proper restraint of the child are necessary to prevent injury to the eye. The child's neck should be hyperextended with support provided under the shoulders. By having the head lower than the rest of the body, gravity will help to disperse the medication over the cornea. First, the lower lid must be gently retracted by using the thumb to pull down on the skin beneath the lower eyelid. In older children, a small pouch may be formed by gently holding both sides of the lower lid in a pinched fashion, forming a cup with the lower eyelid. The medication is then instilled with the prescribed number of drops into the eye, using caution to place the hand, with the dropper, balanced on the head of the patient. In this manner, any inadvertent turning or jumping of the patient would result in the hand moving with the head of the patient. This would prevent any injuries to the eye from a dropper being placed in close proximity and the patient turning into its direction. Using the same position technique, ophthalmic ointments can be applied. A thin line of ointment is then placed in the culdesac of the lower lid and the lid margin closed. The child should remain in this position for several minutes.

References

1. Howry LB et al: Physiologic considerations and patient medication administration. In *Pediatric Medications*, edited by LB Howry, RM Bindler and Y Tse, J.B. Lippincott Company Publishers, Philadelphia, 1981, p 3.
2. Yaffe SJ et al: Perinatal pharmacology. Annual Rev Pharmacol. 1974; 14:219.
3. Cavell B: Gastric emptying in preterm infants. Acta Paediatr Scand. 1979; 68:725.
4. Boreus IO et al: Plasma concentrations of phenobarbital in mother and child after combined prenatal and postnatal administration for prophylaxis of hyperbilirubinemia. J Pediatr. 1978; 93:695.
5. Morselli PL et al: Serum levels and pharmacokinetics of anticonvulsants in the management of siezure disorders. In *Clinical Pharmacology*, edited by Merkin, Year Book Medical Publishers, Chicago and London, 1978, p 89.
6. Assael BM et al: Gentamicin dosage in preterm and term neonates. Arch Dis Child. 1977; 52:883.
7. Szefler SJ et al: Paradoxal behavior of serum digoxin concentrations in an anuric neonate. J Pediatr. 1977; 91:487.
8. Tyrala FF et al: Clinical pharmacology of hexachlorophene in newborn infants. J Pediatr. 1977; 91:481.
9. McFadden S et al: Coma produced by topical application of isopropanol. Pediatrics. 1969; 43:622.
10. Morselli PL: Clinical pharmacokinetics in neonates. Clinical Pharmacokinetics. 1976; 1:81.
11. Cathcart-Rake WF et al: Metabolic responses to plasma concentrations of theophylline. Clin Pharmacol Ther. 1979; 26:89.
12. Kurz H et al: Differences in the binding of drugs to plasma proteins from newborn and adult man I. Eur J Clin Pharmacol. 1977; 11:469.
13. Kurz H et al: Differences in the binding of drugs to plasma proteins from newborn and adult man II. Eur J Clin Pharmacol. 1977; 11:469.
14. Morselli PL et al: Clinical pharmacokinetics in newborns and infants—age related differences and therapeutic implications. Clin Pharmacokinetics. 1980; 5:485.
15. Hamar C et al: Serum protein binding of drugs and bilirubin in newborn infants and their mothers. Clin Pharmacol Ther. 1980; 28:58.
16. Kearin M et al: Digoxin "receptors" in neonates: An explanation of less sensitivity to digoxin than in adults. Clin Pharmacol Ther. 1980; 28:346.
17. Friis-Hausen B: Body water compartments in children: Changes during growth and related changes in body composition. Pediatrics. 1961; 28:169.
18. Pitlick W et al: Phenobarbital pharmacokinetics in neonates. Clin Pharmacol Ther. 1978; 23:346.
19. Painter MJ et al: Phenobarbital and diphenylhydantoin levels in neonates with seizures. J Pediatr. 1978; 92:315.
20. Giacoia G et al: Theophylline pharmacokinetics in premature infants with apnea. J Pediatr. 1976; 89:829.
21. McCracken GH et al: Pharmacologic evaluation of gentamicin in newborn infants. J Infect Dis. 1971; 124:5214.
22. Miller RP et al: Kinetics of acetaminophen elimination in newborns, children, and adults. Clin Pharmacol Ther. 1976; 19:284.
23. Mandelli M et al: Placental transfer of diazepam and its disposition in the newborn. Clin Pharmacol Ther. 1975; 17:564.
24. Morselli PL et al: Diazepam elimination in premature and full term infants. J Perinatal Med. 1973; 1:133.
25. Aperia A et al: Postnatal development of renal function in preterm and full-term infants. Acta Paediatr Scand. 1981; 70:183.

26. Aranda JV et al: Pharmacokinetics of diuretics and methylxanthines in the neonate. Eur J Clin Pharmacol. 1980; 18:55.

27. Kattwinkel J: Neonatal apnea: Pathogenesis and therapy. J Pediatr. 1977; 90:342.

28. Aranda JV et al: Methylxanthines in apnea of prematurity. Clin Perinatal. 1979; 6:87.

29. Giacoia G et al: Theophylline pharmacokinetics in premature infants with apnea. J Pediatr. 1976; 89:829.

30. Aranda JV et al: Pharmacokinetic aspects of theophylline in premature infants. N Engl J Med. 1976; 295:413.

31. Aranda JV: Pharmacokinetic profiles of theophylline and caffeine in premature infants. In *Apnea of Prematurity*, Report of the Seventy-first Ross Conference on Pediatric Research, edited by JF Lucey, DC Shannon, and LF Soyka, Ross Laboratories, Columbus, OH, 1977, p 57.

32. Cornish HH et al: A study of the metabolism of theobromine, theophylline and caffeine in man. J Biol Chem. 1957; 228:315.

33. Bada HS et al: Interconversion of theophylline and caffeine in newborn infants. J Pediatr. 1979; 94:993.

34. Aldridge A et al: Caffeine metabolism in the newborn. Clin Pharmacol Ther. 1979; 25:447.

35. Bory C et al: Metabolism of theophylline to caffeine in premature newborn infants. J Pediatr. 1979; 94:988.

36. Langercrantz H et al: Plasma concentration—effect relationship of theophylline in treatment of apnea in preterm infants. Eur J Clin Pharmacol. 1980; 18:65.

37. Myers TF et al: Low dose theophylline therapy in idiopathic apnea of prematurity. J Pediatr. 1980; 96:99.

38. Aranda JV et al: Pharmacokinetic profile of caffeine in the premature newborn infant with apnea. J Pediatr. 1979; 94:663.

39. Aranda JV et al: Efficacy of caffeine in treatment of apnea in the low-birth weight infant. J Pediatr. 1977; 90:467.

40. Aranda JV et al: Maturation of caffeine elimination in infancy. Arch Dis Child. 1979; 54:946.

41. Gal P et al: Theophylline-induced seizures in accidentally overdosed neonates. Pediatrics. 1980; 65:547.

42. Simons FER et al: Theophylline toxicity in term infants. Am J Dis Child. 1980; 134:39.

43. Wells DH et al: Survival after massive aminophylline overdose in a premature infant. Pediatrics. 1979; 64:252.

44. Lesko LJ: Dose-dependent elimination kinetics of theophylline. Clin Pharmacokinetics. 1979; 4:449.

45. Chang TMS et al: Albumin-collodion activated charcoal hemoperfusion in the treatment of severe theophylline intoxication in a 3-year-old patient. Pediatrics. 1980; 65:811.

46. Arwood LL et al: Placental transfer of theophylline: Two case reports. Pediatrics. 1979; 63:844.

47. Yurchak AM et al: Theophylline secretion into breast milk. Pediatrics. 1976; 57:518.

48. Stec GP et al: Kinetics of theophylline transfer to breast milk. Clin Pharmacol Ther. 1980; 28:404.

49. Kuzemko JA: Natural history of childhood asthma. J Pediatr. 1980; 97:886.

50. Bierman CW et al: The pharmacologic management of status asthmaticus in children. Pediatrics. 1974; 54:282.

51. Weinberger M: Theophylline for treatment of asthma. J Pediatr. 1978; 92:1.

52. Ginschansky E et al: Relationship of theophylline clearance to oral dosage in children with chronic asthma. J Pediatr. 1977; 91:655.

53. Sarrazin E et al: Dose-dependent kinetics for theophylline: Observations among ambulatory asthmatic children. J Pediatr. 1980; 97:825.

54. Goldberg P et al: Intravenous aminophylline therapy for asthma: A comparison of two methods of administration in children. Am J Dis Child. 1980; 134:596.

55. Wyatt R et al: Oral theophylline dosage for the management of chronic asthma. J Pediatr. 1978; 92:125.

56. Sly MR et al: Comparison of subcutaneous terbutaline with epinephrine in the treatment of asthma in children. J Allergy Clin Immunol. 1977; 59:128.

57. Schwartz AL et al: Management of acute asthma in childhood: A randomized evaluation of β-adrenergic agents. Am J Dis Child. 1980; 134:474.

58. Leffert FL: The management of chronic asthma. J Pediatr. 1980; 97:875.

59. Johnston DE: Immunotherapy in children: Past, present, and future, Part I. Ann Allergy. 1981; 46:1.

60. Johnston DE: Immunotherapy in children: Past, present, and future, Part II. Ann Allergy. 1981; 46:59.

61. Cox JSG: Disodium cromoglycate. Br J Dis Chest. 1971; 65:189.

62. Bernstein IL et al: A controlled study of cromolyn sodium sponsored by the Drug Committee of the American Academy of Allergy. J Allergy Clin Immunol. 1972; 50:235.

63. Klein R et al: Treatment of chronic childhood asthma with beclomethasone dipropionate aerosol, Part I: A double-blind crossover trial in nonsteroid dependent patients. Pediatrics. 1977; 60:7.

64. Kershnar H et al: Treatment of chronic childhood asthma with beclomethasone dipropionate aerosol, Part II: Effect on pituitary-adrenal function after substitution for oral corticosteroids. Pediatrics. 1978; 62:189.

65. Wyatt R et al: Effects of inhaled beclomethasone dipropionate and alternate day prednisone on pituitary-adrenal function in children with chronic asthma. N Engl J Med. 1978; 299:1387.

66. American Academy of Pediatrics: Adverse reaction to iodide therapy of asthma and other pulmonary diseases. Pediatrics. 1976; 57:272.

67. Silver H et al: Drug therapy. In *Current Pediatric Diagnosis and Treatment*, 5th edition, edited by C Kempe, H Silver and D O'Brien, Lange Publications, Palo Alto, CA, 1978, p 1016.

68. Korberly BH: The treatment of the common cold with over-the-counter medication. Am Druggist. 1979; 179:17.

69. Cormier JF et al: Cold and allergy products. In *Handbook of Nonprescription Drugs*, 6th edition, American Pharmaceutical Association, Washington, DC, 1979, p 73.

70. Brownlee RC et al: Otitis media in children: Incidence, treatment and progress in pediatric practice. J Pediatr. 1969; 75:636.

71. Paradise JL: Otitis media in infants and children. Pediatrics. 1980; 65:917.

72. Brook I: A practical technique for typanocentesis for culturing aerobic and anaerobic bacteria. Pediatrics. 1980; 65:626.

73. Bennett FC et al: Middle ear function in learning-disabled children. Pediatrics. 1980; 66:254.

74. Halbrow C: Eustachian tubal function: Changes in anatomy and function with age and the relationship of these changes to aural pathology. Arch Otolarynol. 1970; 92:624.

75. Bluestone CD et al: Middle ear disease in children—pathogenesis, diagnosis and management. Pediatr Clin North Am. 1974; 21:379.

76. Howie VM et al: Otitis media: A clinical and bacteriological correlation. Pediatrics. 1970; 45:29.

77. Nilson BW et al: Acute otitis media: Treatment results in relation to bacterial etiology. Pediatrics. 1969; 45:351.

78. Rowe DS: Acute suppurative otitis media. Pediatrics. 1975; 56:285.

79. Feigin RD et al: Treatment of otitis media. Drug Ther. 1974; 4(9):116.

80. Makela PH et al: Pneumococcal vaccine and otitis media. Lancet. 1980; 8194:547.

81. Bland RD: Otitis media in the first six weeks of life: Diagnostic bacteriology and management. Pediatrics. 1972; 49:187.

82. Mandell GL and Sande MA: Antimicrobial agents: Penicillins and cephalosporins. In *The Pharmacological Basis of Therapeutics*, 6th edition, edited by LS Goodman and A Gilman, Macmillan Publishing Company, Inc., New York, 1980, p 1126.

82a. Bierman CW et al: Reactions associated with ampicillin therapy. JAMA. 1972; 220:1098.

82b. Corless JD et al: The rash associated with ampicillin therapy. So Med J. 1970; 63:1341.

82c. Knudsen ET et al: Reduction in incidence of ampicillin rash by purification of ampicillin. Br Med J. 1970; 1:469.

82d. Collaborative Study Group: Prospective study of ampicillin rash. Br Med J. 1973; 1:7.

83. Ginsburg CM et al: Erythromycin: A review of its uses in pediatric practice. J Pediatr. 1976; 89:872.

84. McLinn SE: Cefaclor in the treatment of otitis media and pharyngitis in children. Am J Dis Child. 1980; 134:560.

85. Cherry JD: The treatment of croup: Continued controversy due to failure of recognition of historic, ecologic, etiologic and clinical perspectives. J Pediatr. 1979; 94:352.

86. Westley CR et al: Nebulized racemic epinephrine by IPPB for the treatment of croup. Am J Dis Child. 1978; 132:484.

87. Taussig LM et al: Treatment of laryngotracheobronchitis (croup): Use of intermittent positive pressure breathing and racemic epinephrine. Am J Dis Child. 1975; 129:790.

88. Shaw EB: Corticosteroids and croup: Comments from a grass-rooted ivory tower. Pediatrics. 1972; 49:312.

89. Leipzig B et al: A prospective randomized study to determine the efficacy of steroids in treatment of croup. J Pediatr. 1979; 94:194.

90. Lewis JK et al: Occurrence of Haemophilus epiglottitis. Am J Dis Child. 1978; 132:424.

91. Faden HS: Treatment of Haemophilus influenzae type B epiglottitis. Pediatrics. 1979; 63:402.

92. Crozier DN: Cystic fibrosis: A not-so-fatal disease. Pediatr Clin North Am. 1974; 21:935.

93. Wood RE et al: Cystic fibrosis. Amer Rev Resp Dis. 1976; 113:833.

94. Wood RE: Cystic fibrosis: Diagnosis, treatment and prognosis. So Med J. 1979; 72:189.

95. Denning CR et al: Cooperative study comparing three months of performing sweat tests to diagnose cystic fibrosis. Pediatrics. 1980; 66:752.

96. Marks MI: The pathogenesis and treatment of pulmonary infections in patients with cystic fibrosis. J Pediatr. 1981; 98:173.

97. Pennington JE et al: Summary of a workshop on infections in patients with cystic fibrosis. J Infect Dis. 1979; 140:252.

98. Beaudry PH et al: Is anti-pseudomonas therapy warranted in acute respiratory exacerbations in children with cystic fibrosis? J Pediatr. 1980; 97:144.

99. Loening-Baucke VA et al: A placebo-controlled trial of cephalexin therapy in the ambulatory management of patients with cystic fibrosis. J Pediatr. 1979; 95:630.

100. Nassif EG et al: Comparative effects of antacids, enteric coating, and bile salts on the efficacy of oral pancreatic enzyme therapy in cystic fibrosis. J Pediatr. 1981; 98:320.

101. Committee on Infectious Disease: Tetanus. In *American Academy of Pediatrics*, Report of the Committee on Infectious Disease, 18th edition, Redbook, Evanston, IL, 1977, p 1.

102. Mufson MA: The new vaccines. Drug Ther. 1980; 10:39.

103. Marcuse EK: Pediatricians' immunization consent practice, Washington State. Pediatrics. 1979; 63:420.

104. Harrison HR and Fulginiti VA: Bacterial immunizations. Am J Dis Child. 1980; 134:184.

105. Shaw EB: Commentary on immunization. Am J Dis Child. 1980; 134:130.

106. Mortimer EA: Pertussis immunization: Problems, perspectives, prospects. Hosp Pract. 1980; 15:130.

107. Krugman RD: Pediatrics—immunization, 20 common questions and answers. Postgrad Med. 1976; 59:216.

108. Fulginiti VA: The problems of poliovirus immunization. Hosp Pract. 1980; 15:61.

109. Boffey PP: Polio: Salk challenges safety of Sabin's live-virus vaccine. Science. 1977; 196:35.

110. Shelton JE et al: Measles vaccine efficacy: Influence of age at vaccination vs duration of time since vaccination. Pediatrics. 1978; 62:961.

111. Marks JS et al: Measles vaccine efficacy in children previously vaccinated at 12 months of age. Pediatrics. 1978; 62:955.

112. Balfour HH et al: RA27/3 rubella vaccine: A four-year follow up. Am J Dis Child. 1980; 134:350.

113. Bernstein DI et al: Fetomaternal aspects of immunization with RA27/3 live attenuated rubella virus vaccine during pregnancy. J Pediatr. 1980; 97:467.

114. Landes RD et al: Neonatal rubella following postpartum maternal immunization. J Pediatr. 1980; 97:465.

115. Welch NM: Recent insights into the childhood "social diseases"—gonorrhea, scabies, pediculosis, and pinworms. Clin Pediatr. 1978; 17:320.

116. Tudor RB: Ridding children of common worm infections. Postgrad Med. 1975; 58:115.

117. Jones JE: Office parasitology. Am Fam Physician. 1980; 22:86.

118. Wolfe MS: Oxyuris trichostrongylus and trichuris. Clinics in Gastroenter. 1978; 7:201.

119. Blumenthal DS: Intestinal nematodes in the United States. N Engl J Med. 1977; 297:1437.

120. Kropp KA et al: Enterobius vermicularis (pinworms), introital bacteriology and recurrent urinary tract infection in children. J Urol. 1978; 120:480.

121. Welch TR: Pinworm infestation and urinary tract infection in young girls. Am J Dis Child. 1974; 128:887.

122. Katz M: Parasitic infections. J Pediatr. 1975; 87:165.

123. Brown HW: Intestinal nematodes of man; Class insecta. In *Basic Clinical Parasitiology*, 4th edition, edited by DL Belding, Appleton-Century-Crofts, New York, 1975, pp 105, 258.

124. Anon: Drugs for parasitic infections. Med Let Drugs Ther. 1979; 547:105.

125. Jones MJ et al: Infectious diseases of Indochinese refugees. Mayo Clin Proc. 1980; 55:482.

126. Johnston TS: Diagnosis and treatment of five parasites. DICP. 1981; 15:103.

127. Hurwitz S: Scabies in babies. Am J Dis Child. 1973; 126:226.

128. Fernandez N et al: Pathologic findings in human scabies. Arch Dermatol. 1977; 113:320.

129. Parish LC et al: Head lice: Epidemic in the schoolroom. Drug Ther. 1980; 10 (10):145.

130. Slonka GF et al: An epidemic of pediculus capitis. J Parasit. 1977; 63:377.

131. Anon: Treatment of head lice. Med Let Drugs Ther. 1980; 22:66.

132. Solomon LM et al: Gamma benzene hexachloride toxicity: A review. Arch Dermatol. 1977; 113:353.

133. Parish LC et al: Guide to the management of scabies. Drug Ther. 1978; 8(6):134.

134. Weston WL: Skin. In *Current Pediatric Diagnosis and Treatment*, edited by C Kempe, H Silver and D O'Brien, Lange Medical Publications, Palo Alto, CA, 1978, p 204.

135. Finberg L: The role of oral electrolyte-glucose solutions in hydration for children—international and domestic aspects. J Pediatr. 1980; 96:51.

136. Nalin DR et al: Comparison of low and high sodium and potassium content in oral rehydration solutions. J Pediatr. 1980; 97:848.

137. MacLean WE et al: Nutritional management of chronic diarrhea and malnutrition: Primary reliance on oral feeding. J Pediatr. 1980; 97:316.

138. Levine MM et al: Variability of sodium and sucrose levels of simple sugar/salt oral rehydration solutions prepared under optimal and field conditions. J Pediatr. 1980; 97:324.

139. Sack DA et al: Oral therapy in children with cholera: A comparison of sucrose and glucose electrolyte solutions. J Pediatr. 1980; 96:20.

140. Black RE et al: Glucose vs sucrose in oral rehydration solutions for infants and young children with rotavirus associated diarrhea. Pediatrics. 1981; 67:78.

141. Holliday MA et al: The maintenance need for water in parenteral fluid therapy. Pediatrics. 1957; 19:823.

142. Bell EF et al: The effects of thermal environment on heat balance and insensible water loss in low-birth weight infants. J Pediatr. 1980; 96:452.

143. Randall DL: Therapy of acute diarrheal diseases in children. Drug Ther. 1973; 5 (3):77.

144. Pearce JL et al: Controlled trial of orally administered lactobacilli in acute infantile diarrhea. J Pediatr. 1974; 84:261.

145. McKenzie MW et al: Infant formula products. In *Handbook of Nonprescription Drugs*, American Pharmaceutical Association, 6th edition, Washington, D.C., 1979; p 205.

146. Committee on Nutrition: Normal nutrition in infancy and childhood. In *Pediatric Nutrition Handbook*, American Academy of Pediatrics, Evanston, IL, 1979, p 92.

147. Woodruff CW: The science of infant nutrition and the art of infant feeding. JAMA. 1978; 240:657.

148. Hambreus L: Proprietary milk versus human breast milk in infant feeding: A critical appraisal from the nutritional point of view. Pediatr Clin North Am. 1977; 24:17.

149. Jelliffe EF: Infant feeding practices: Associated iatrogenic and comerciogenic diseases. Pediatr Clin North Am. 1977; 24:49.

150. Fisher SE et al: Chronic protracted diarrhea: Intolerance to dietary glucose polymers. Pediatrics. 1981; 67:271.

151. Ament ME: Therapeutic use of infant formulas. Drug Ther. 1972; 2 (7):14.

152. Committee on Nutrition: Vitamin and mineral supplement needs in normal children in the United States. Pediatrics. 1980; 66:1015.

153. Committee on Nutrition: Iron supplementation for infants. Pediatrics. 1976; 58:765.

154. Singer L et al: Total fluoride intake of infants. Pediatrics. 1979; 63:460.

155. Committee on Nutrition: Fluoride supplementation: Revised dosage schedule. Pediatrics. 1979; 63:150.

156. Driscoll WS: Dosage recommendation for dietary fluoride supplements. Am J Dis Child. 1979; 133:683.

157. Davidson M: Vomiting. In *Pediatrics*, 16th edition, edited by AM Rudolf, HL Barnett and AH Einhorn, Appleton-Century-Crofts, New York, 1977, p 983.

158. Weston WL et al: Diaper dermatitis: Current concepts. Pediatrics. 1980; 66:532.

159. Lipp JP et al: Health problems with specific concerns in infancy. In *Nursing Care of Children*, edited by E Waechter and F Blake, JB Lippincott, Philadelphia, 1976, p 320.

160. Leyden JJ et al: Urinary ammonia and ammonia-producing microorganisms in infants with and without diaper dermatitis. Arch Dermatol. 1977; 113:1673.

161. Wiener F: The relationship of diapers to diaper rashes in the one-month-old infant. J Pediatr. 1979; 95:422.

162. Jordan WE: Relationship of diapers to diaper rashes. J Pediatr. 1980; 96:957.

163. Jacobs AH: Eruptions in the diaper area. Pediatr Clin North Am. 1978; 25:209.

164. Anon: Developmental abnormalities in jaws and teeth. In *Nelson's Textbook of Pediatrics*, 11th edition, edited by V Vaughan, R McKay and R Behrman, W.B. Saunders, Philadelphia, 1979, p 1020.

165. Jacobson O: Teeth. In *Current Pediatric Diagnosis and Treatment*, 5th edition, edited by C Kempe, H Silver and D O'Brien, Lange Publications, Palo Alto, CA, 1978, p 234.

166. Cain CM and Rowles B: Infant teething: A review. U.S. Pharmacist. 1980; 5:33.

167. Anon: Management of selected clinical problems of the head and neck. In *Accepted Dental Therapeutics*, 38th edition, American Dental Association Publication, Chicago, 1979, p 299.

168. Oksas R: Dental products. In *Handbook of Nonprescription Drugs*, 6th edition, American Pharmaceutical Association, Washington, D.C., 1979, p 320.

169. Spock B: Teething. In *Baby and Child Care*, Pocket Books, New York, 1976, p 278.

170. Stern RC: Pathophysiologic basis for symptomatic treatment of fever. Pediatrics. 1977; 59:92.

171. Kluger MJ: Fever. Pediatrics. 1980; 66:720.

172. Yaffe SJ: Management of fever in infants and children. In *Fever*, edited by JM Lipton, Raven Press, New York, 1980, p 225.

173. Kapasi AA et al: Parents' knowledge and sources of knowledge about antipyretic drugs. J Pediatr. 1980; 97:1035.

174. Schmitt BD: Fever phobia. Am J Dis Child. 1980; 134:176.

175. Yaffe SJ: Comparative efficacy of aspirin and acetaminophen in the reduction of fever in children. Arch Intern Med. 1981; 141:286.

176. Levy G: Comparative pharmacokinetics of aspirin and acetaminophen. Arch Intern Med. 1981; 141:279.

177. Mielke CH: Comparative effects of aspirin and acetaminophen on hemostasis. Arch Intern Med. 1981; 141:305.

178. Temple AR: Acute and chronic effects of aspirin toxicity and their treatment. Arch Intern Med. 1981; 141:364.

179. Peterson RG et al: Pharmacokinetics of acetaminophen in children. Pediatrics. 1978; 62:877.

180. Peterson RG et al: Age as a variable in acetaminophen overdose. Arch Intern Med. 1981; 141:390.

181. Nogen AG et al: Fatal acetaminophen overdosage in a young child. J Pediatr. 1978; 92:832.

182. Steele RW et al: Oral antipyretic therapy: Evaluation of aspirin-acetaminophen combination. Am J Dis Child. 1972; 123:204.

183. Hunter J: Study of antipyretic therapy in current use. Arch Dis Child. 1973; 48:313.

184. Steele RW et al: Evaluation of sponging and of oral antipyretic therapy to reduce fever. J Pediatr. 1970; 77:824.

185. Moss MH: Alcohol-induced hypoglycemia and coma caused by alcohol sponging. Pediatrics. 1970; 46:445.

186. Freeman JM: Febrile seizures: A consensus of their significance, evaluation, and treatment. Pediatrics. 1980; 66:1009.

187. Wallace SJ et al: Successful prophylaxis against febrile convulsions with valproic acid or phenobarbitone. Br Med J. 1980; 1:353.

188. Consensus Development Panel: Febrile seizures: Long-term management of children with fever-associated seizures. Pediatrics. 1980; 66:1009.

189. Reye RD et al: Encephalopathy and fatty degeneration of the viscera. Lancet. 1963; 2:749.

190. Boutros AR et al: Reye syndrome: A predictably curable disease. Pediatr Clin North Am. 1980; 27:539.

191. MMWR. 1980; 29:532.

192. Starko KM et al: Reye's syndrome and salicylate use. Pediatrics. 1980; 66:859.

193. MMWR. 1980; 29:321.

194. Bore KE et al: The hepatic lesion in Reye's syndrome. Gastroenterology. 1975; 69:685.

195. Lovejoy FH et al: Clinical staging in Reye syndrome. Am J Dis Child. 1974; 128:36.

196. Shaywitz BA et al: Prolonged continuous monitoring of intracranial pressure in severe Reye's syndrome. Pediatrics. 1977; 59:595.

197. Shaywitz BA et al: Monitoring and management of increased intracranial pressure in Reye syndrome: Results in 29 children. Pediatrics. 1980; 66:198.

198. Mutchie KD: Drug therapy of Reye's syndrome. Am J Hosp Pharm. 1979; 36:767.

199. Cottrell J et al: Furosemide and mannitol-induced changes in intracranial pressure and serum osmolality and electrolytes. Anesthesiology. 1977; 47:28.

200. Cupit GC et al: High dose pentobarbital pharmacokinetics in children with elevated ICP. Pediatr Res. 1980; 14:466.

201. Swedlow DB et al: Pentobarbital pharmacokinetics in brain-injured children. Crit Care Med. 1980; 8:227.

202. Bobo RC et al: Reye syndrome: Treatment by exchange transfusion with special reference to the 1974 epidemic in Cincinnati, Ohio. J Pediatr. 1975; 87:881.

203. Bedford RF et al: Lidocaine or thiopental for rapid control of intracranial hypertension? Anesth Analg. 1980; 59:435.

204. Devivo DC et al: Reye syndrome: Results of intensive supportive care. J Pediatr. 1975; 87:875.

205. Corey L et al: Reye's syndrome: Clinical progression and evaluation of therapy. Pediatrics. 1977; 60:708.

206. Clements SD: Minimal brain dysfunction in children. HEW Public Health Service Publication. 1966.

207. Shaywitz BA et al: New diagnostic terminology for minimal brain dysfunction, Part I. J Pediatr. 1979; 95:734.

208. Saccar CL et al: Current status of drug therapy for minimal brain dysfuntion. Pediatr Alert. 1979; 4:81.

209. O'Leary SG et al: Behavior therapy and withdrawal of stimulant medication in hyperactive children. Pediatrics. 1978; 61:211.

210. Levine MD et al: Hyperactivity. Am J Dis Child. 1980; 134:409.

211. Schmitt BC et al: The hyperactive child. Clin Pediatr. 1973; 12:154.

212. Conners CK: A teacher rating scale for use in drug studies with children. Am J Psychiatry. 1969; 126:884.

213. Davids A: An objective instrument for assessing hyperkinesis in children. J Learn Disabil. 1971; 4:499.

214. Varga J: The hyperactive child—Should we be paying more attention? Am J Dis Child. 1979; 133:413.

215. Saccar CL: Drug therapy in the treatment of minimal brain dysfunction. Am J Hosp Pharm. 1978; 35:544.

216. Millichap JG: Drugs in management of minimal brain dysfunction. Ann NY Acad Sci. 1973; 205:321.

217. Sprague RL et al: Methylphenidate in hyperkinetic children: Differences in dose effects on learning and social behavior. Science. 1977; 198:1274.

218. Brown RT et al: Methylphenidate in hyperkinetic children: Differences in dose effects on impulsive behavior. Pediatrics. 1979; 64:408.

219. Satterfield JH et al: Multimodality treatment—A two-year evaluation of 61 hyperactive boys. Arch Gen Psychiatry. 1980; 37:915.

220. Safer DJ et al: Factors influencing the suppressant effect of two stimulant drugs on the growth of hyperactive children. Pediatrics. 1973; 51:660.

221. Gross MD: Growth of hyperkinetic children taking methylphenidate, dextroamphetamine, or imipramine/desipramine. Pediatrics. 1976; 58:423.

222. Anon: Pemoline (Cylert) for minimal brain dysfunction. Med Let Drug Ther. 1976; 18:5.

223. Conners CK et al: Magnesium pemoline and dextroamphetamine: A controlled study in children with minimal brain dysfunction. Psychopharmacologia. 1972; 26:321.

224. Dickinson LC et al: Impaired growth in hyperkinetic children receiving pemoline. J Pediatr. 1979; 94:538.

225. Beall JG: Food additives and hyperactivity in children. Congressional Record. 1973; p 519736.

226. Stare FJ et al: Diet and hyperactivity: Is there a relationship? Pediatrics. 1980; 66:521.

227. Golden GS: Nonstandard therapies in the developmental disabilities. Am J Child Dis. 1980; 134:487.

228. Conners CK: Food additives and hyperkinesis: A controlled double-blind experiment. Pediatrics. 1976; 58:154.

229. Arnold LE et al: Megavitamins for minimal brain dysfunction. JAMA. 1978; 240:2642.

230. Palmisano PA: Enuresis: Causes, cures and cautions. West J Med. 1976; 125:347.

231. Burke EC et al: Enuresis—Is it being overtreated? Mayo Clin Proc. 1980; 55:118.

232. McLain LG: Childhood enuresis. Current Problems in Pediatrics. 1979; 9:1.

233. Dische S: Childhood enuresis—A family problem. Practitioner. 1978; 221:323.

234. Simonds JF: Enuresis: A brief survey of current thinking with respect to pathogenesis and management. Clin Pediatr. 1977; 16:79.

235. Mikkelsen EJ et al: Enuresis: Psychopathology, sleep stage, and drug response. Urol Clin North Am. 1980; 7:361.

236. Kass EJ et al: Enuresis: Principles of management and result of treatment. J Urol. 1979; 121:794.

237. Forsythe W et al: Enuresis and the electric alarm: Study of 200 cases. Br Med J. 1970; 1:211.

238. Starfield B: Functional bladder capacity in enuretic and nonenuretic children. J Pediatr. 1967; 70:777.

239. Starfield B: Enuresis: Its pathogenesis and management. Clin Pediatr. 1972; 11:343.

240. Jorgensen OS et al: Plasma concentration and clinical effect in imipramine treatment of childhood enuresis. Clin Pharmacokinetics. 1980; 5:386.

241. Kales A et al: Effects of imipramine on enuretic frequency and sleep stages. Pediatrics. 1971; 60:431.

242. Cronin AJ et al: Poisoning with tricyclic antidepressants: An avoidable cause of childhood deaths. Br Med J. 1979; 1:722.

243. Birkasova M et al: Desmopressin in the management of nocturnal enuresis in children: A double-blind study. Pediatrics. 1978; 62:970.

244. Dimson FB: Desmopressin as a treatment of enuresis. Lancet. 1977; 1:1260.

Chapter 60

Geriatric Therapy

Martin J. Jinks

A revolution is taking place in America, a shift from a youthful society to one with significantly more older adults. Every day 5000 Americans turn 65 years old and by 1985, half the population will be over 50 years old (1,2). Of all individuals who have ever lived to age 65 years or older, more than half are alive today (3). Since 1900, 25 years have been added to the average lifespan, and in 1980, for the first time the number of adults over 60 years old surpassed the number of children under 10 years old (1). Today, individuals over 65 years of age comprise 11% of the population, and by 2025, older adults will comprise up to 23% of the population (4). Most importantly, the number of frail-old persons, those over 85 years, is increasing faster than any other age category, over

200% in the last 25 years, which is more than double the rate of the next fastest growing category (5).

Older adults have a higher rate of drug use compared to the general population. In 1980, persons over 65 years of age made up 11% of the population but were prescribed 25% of prescription drugs (4,5,6). This disproportionately high rate may actually be an underestimate since it excludes drugs provided to hospital patients and to patients during physician office visits. Eighty-five percent of aged ambulatory and 95% of nursing home patients receive prescription drugs, and those over 65 years of age refill prescriptions at a rate three times those under 65 years of age. The estimated annual prescription demand for aged patients is over 13 prescriptions per year (7). Additionally, 70% of aged patients self-medicate with non-prescription drugs without consulting with their physician or pharmacist (8). Out-of-pocket expenses for drugs are three times that of the general population and comprise the second highest out-of-pocket expense for all needs in the aged (9,10).

The adverse drug reaction rate in the aged is higher than that of young adults, and the aged are more frequently hospitalized due to adverse drug reactions (11,12). Many factors place geriatric patients at high risk for adverse drug reactions. A key determinant is the high rate of drug use discussed above. Physical factors also play an important role in increasing susceptibility to drug reactions. Fifty percent of the long-term care patients cannot hear ordinary conversation, and 24% suffer from speech impediments (13). Twenty-five percent of older adults living in the community have uncorrectable visual and auditory impairment (14). Many have chronic diseases which impair normal functioning, such as arthritis or Parkinsonism. Physical impairments coupled with the high rate of drug use in older adults inevitably cause errors in medication taking. Fifty-nine percent of one geriatric outpatient population committed errors in administration, and 25% of these errors were serious (15). In another study, misuse of medications was judged to be the cause of two-thirds of the community hospital admissions of geriatric patients with adverse drug reactions (12).

Finally, a most important determinant of the high adverse drug reaction rate in the aged is their increased physiological vulnerability to medication and impaired recovery from such drug insults. Homeostatic mechanisms in the cardiovascular and nervous systems are less efficient, drug metabolism and excretion decline, body tissue composition and drug volume of distribution change, and drug receptor sensitivity may be altered.

Drug Disposition

Absorption. Changes in the gastrointestinal tract during aging may influence drug absorption. Gastric pH increases, intestinal blood flow diminishes, and some impairment of both active and passive transport mechanisms occurs (16). These changes primarily affect dietary nutrients, and few drugs have been shown to be substantially affected. Based on the limited evidence available, no generalizations are possible.

Distribution. Cardiac output decreases about 1% per year from age 19 to 86 years (17). As a result of aging, a smaller amount of blood flow enters important target organs, such as liver, kidney and brain. Body composition is another important determinant of drug distribution which is altered during normal aging. Total body water and lean body mass both decline with age, and total fat content increases between ages 18 and 35 years from 18 to 36% in males and from 33 to 48% in females (18,19,20). Thus, the volume of distribution of drugs which are mainly distributed in body water or lean body mass, such as lithium or digoxin, is decreased in older adults and unadjusted dosing can result in higher blood levels. Conversely, the volume of distribution of highly lipid soluble drugs may be increased, thereby prolonging the half-life so that maximum effects are delayed. Long-acting benzodiazepines are examples of highly lipid-soluble drugs which take many days to achieve steady state and which can accumulate to toxic levels in aged patients after the initial monitoring period has ended (21). Finally, debilitated older adults may have decreased serum albumin levels so that drugs which are highly bound to albumin, such as diazepam, warfarin or phenytoin, may have elevated free concentrations and enhanced effects. In one large study of hospitalized geriatric patients, the serum albumin concentration was reported to fall progressively for each decade past 40 years of age, reaching a mean of 3.58 gm/dl (normal ≥ 4 gm/dl) in those older than 80 years of age (22).

Metabolism and Excretion. Animal studies indicate that the activity of liver microsomal drug metabolizing enzymes declines with age, but the clinical significance of this in aged humans is controversial. Large interindividual variation in liver metabolism exists for any given drug and in most cases may be more important than aging changes (16,18,23–26). Nevertheless, age-related changes in liver metabolism of specific drugs, such as phenylbutazone, warfarin and long-acting benzodiazepines, have been suggested (27–30). The matter is further complicated because liver mass declines and hepatic blood flow decreases 45% between ages 25 and 65 years (31). Drugs with high hepatic extraction ratios, such as barbiturates, lidocaine and propranolol, may have reduced hepatic metabolism in older adults as a secondary consequence of diminished hepatic blood flow and hepatic cell mass (32).

Age-related changes in renal function are probably the single most important physiological factor resulting in adverse drug reactions (33). The kidney is foremost among the body organs to lose functioning cells during aging, and histological studies reveal a decline in the absolute number of nephrons (34). In addition, arteriosclerotic changes and a declining cardiac output result in decreased renal perfusion by 40 to 50% between ages 25 and 65 years and a corresponding drop in glomerular filtration and urea clearance (33,35). Urine concentrating ability declines with aging as does renal sodium conservation (36,37). Tubular excretory capacity and creatinine clearance may also be reduced in aging (38,39).

Prolongation of plasma half-lives of a number of renally excreted drugs has been consistently shown in healthy older adults. The highest risk drugs are those that depend entirely on the kidney for elimination. Examples of these are listed in Table 1. Dosage decrements with these drugs are not routinely required in older adults with GFRs over 50 but close attention to drug monitoring is necessary, especially when high doses are contemplated or intercurrent illness is present. More problematical are the many drugs which are excreted partially by the kidney and partially by extrarenal mechanisms. Patient susceptibility to these drugs is difficult to predict clinically because of compensatory elimination pathways and confounding active metabolites. A recent review of the literature summarizes the major excretion routes of commonly prescribed drugs, both renal

Table 1.
DRUGS HIGHLY DEPENDENT ON RENAL FUNCTION FOR ELIMINATION[*]

acetazolamide	ibuprofen
allopurinol	lithium
amantadine	methenamine
aminoglycosides	methotrexate
amoxicillin	mithramycin
bleomycin	naproxen
cephalosporins (most)	nitrofurantoin
chlorpropamide	nitrosourea
cimetidine	pentamidine
clonidine	phenazopyridine
colistimethate	pyridostigmine
digoxin	sulfamethoxazole-
ethambutol	trimethoprim
flucytosine	sulfisoxazole
furosemide	thiazides
gallamine	ticarcillin
gold sodium thiomalate	vancomycin

[*]Reference 40.

and extrarenal, and provides the basis for the information in Table 1 (40).

As with younger patients, creatinine clearance is the most useful indicator of renal function in older adults. Changes in BUN are subject to many extrarenal variables, and BUN is often spuriously elevated. On the other hand, serum creatinine levels in older adults may persist in the normal range despite reduced creatinine clearance. This occurs because of the decrease in daily creatinine production which accompanies the decline in lean body mass associated with aging (41,42).

Drug Response

Homeostasis. Drug side effects which are mild or non-existent in younger patients may be a significant problem in older adults because of less efficient homeostatic adjustments. Orthostatic hypotension is an example of a common drug-induced disorder of homeostasis in aged; it results from impaired baroreceptor function and leads to inadequate adjustment of peripheral resistance and failure of autoregulation of cerebral blood flow (16,43). It is most often associated with agents that interfere with peripheral sympathetic nervous system activity, such as guanethidine, reserpine, phenothiazines, and tricyclic antidepressants (44). In one study of 100 geriatric psychiatric outpatients, almost 40% complained of dizziness and falling which was attributed to psychiatric medication (45). Those patients with conditions associated with impaired cardiac output and patients taking concurrent diuretic therapy were especially vulnerable. Also, aging impairs posture maintenance, and the effects of drugs on posture control may be contributory to drug-induced falls in older adults (46).

Target Organ Sensitivity. Exaggerated response to some drugs in older adults may reflect intrinsic change in receptor or organ sensitivity due to aging. Evidence of receptor alterations exist for nitrazepam, heparin (in females) and warfarin (47,48). The aging central nervous system is particularly vulnerable to qualitative as well as quantitative alterations in drug response. This occurs because the aging brain, like the aging kidney, loses a significant number of active cells during later life and some brain atrophy is a common, although not necessarily pathological, finding in older adults. Normal aging also involves a reduction in cerebral blood flow and oxygen consumption, and an increased cerebrovascular resistance (49). Older persons often have cerebral blood flows as much as 20% less than younger persons (17). In addition, inhibitory and excitatory pathways in the central nervous system are delicately balanced to modulate cognitive functions and behavior. With aging, there is a selective decline in some pathways and the preservation of others. For example, cholinergic neurons in the neocortex and hippocampal areas of the brain normally decrease with age. Pathological cholinergic deficits are associated with memory loss, confusion and other cognitive impairments (50). Indeed, drugs with anticholinergic properties are particularly notorious for inducing mental fuzziness and confusion in older patients. Finally, monoamine oxidase activity increases with normal aging and is reflected by a decline in norepinephrine and dopamine in aging brains (51). Since these neurological and biochemical reserves are reduced as a normal consequence of aging, it is not surprising that iatrogenic behavioral disorders are relatively common in older adults, and that drugs are one of the most common causes of sudden, unexplained mental impairment in the older adult. For example, one study found that 16% of 236 patients over 65 years old were hospitalized for behavioral disturbances directly attributable to drugs (52).

Polypharmacy in Older Adults

1. As the new consultant to a 60-bed skilled nursing facility, you are confronted with many examples of polypharmacy and drug use problems during your initial chart reviews. A typical case is B.J., an 80-year-old male who has resided there for the past ten months. A synopsis of B.J.'s chart is as follows:

Problem List:
  cardiomegaly
  hypertension
  rheumatoid arthritis
  organic brain syndrome
  constipation
  depression
  dizziness

Laboratory Information: Admission SMA-6: Na^+, K^+, Cl^-, CO_2, glucose, and BUN all within normal limits. Admission weight 70 kg, BP 105/60 mm Hg, and pulse 80/min. Subsequent measurements of vital signs are not systematically charted but occasional recordings in the nurses' notes indicate little change from admission values. No blood work or urinalysis have been done.

Current Medications:
  Lanoxin 0.125 mg qd
  Aldoril-15 tid
  Tolectin 200 mg tid
  ASA 10 gr tid
  Mellaril 25 mg tid
  Haldol 0.5 mg bid
  Cogentin 1 mg bid
  Elavil 25 mg hs
  Metamucil ii packets qd
  MOM 30 cc qd
  Dulcolax i pr qd prn if MOM ineffective
  Lomotil i qid prn
  Ferrous Sulfate 300 mg tid
  Dalmane 15 mg hs
  Zomax 100 mg tid prn pain
  2 gm sodium diet

Status: B.J. is ambulatory and receives meals in the facility cafeteria. Although he is in no acute distress, the nurses' notes indicate that B.J. is often confused and complains of dizziness and arthritic pain.

What basic questions must be asked in the evaluation of this patient's drug therapy? Make specific recommendations.

Assessment of B.J.'s complex medication profile involves the following considerations: Is each drug clearly indicated? If indicated, are dosing and administration appropriate? Are the lab work and vital signs appropriate and available to adequately evaluate therapy? Are there existing or potential problems with side effects, drug interactions or adverse reactions? What specific recommendations can be made to optimize this patient's drug therapy—are there any unnecessary drugs? Several examples of undesirable polypharmacy can be illustrated in reviewing B.J.'s medication profile:

Digoxin. B.J. has been treated for years for a "history" of heart disease. Cardiomegaly is itself not a sufficient indication for digitalization if the patient is asymptomatic and in sinus rhythm (53,54). Routine recording of vital signs and an ECG would be very helpful in assessing B.J.'s requirement for digitalis, but systematic documentation is unavailable in his chart. This is not unusual in nursing home patients as indicated by one study in which 93% of patients on digitalis lacked recorded monitoring of these basic parameters (55). Recommendation: Obtain ECG and physical examination for evidence of rhythm disturbances or congestive failure. If B.J. is asymptomatic, cautious discontinuation over several weeks should be attempted.

Antihypertensives. B.J.'s hypertension is possibly overtreated as evidenced by the low admission blood pressure and the presence of dizziness, probably a symptom of hypotension. Serial blood pressure measurements over time are not being done or are not being recorded and would be necessary to document iatrogenic hypotension. The indication for Aldoril-15 (a methyldopa/hydrochlorothiazide combination) is questionable. Methyldopa can aggravate B.J.'s depression and confusion. A logical goal is to discontinue it if possible. Hydrochlorothiazide is not present in full therapeutic doses in Aldoril-15, but the hazard of hypokalemia should be considered, especially because of his concurrent digitalis therapy. As many as 81% of nursing home patients receiving a thiazide/digitalis combination do not receive routine potassium monitoring (55). Recommendation: Monitor weekly blood pressures. If values remain low, discontinue Aldoril-15 and observe. If hypertension recurs, reinstitute therapy with hydrochlorothiazide alone. Measure potassium levels periodically and give potassium supplements if necessary.

Antiarthritics. B.J.'s rheumatoid arthritis is a proper indication for either aspirin or Tolectin (tolmetin) but their simultaneous use represents polypharmacy. Both act by the same mechanism, the inhibition of cyclo-oxygenase (i.e., prostaglandin synthesis). Also, aspirin has been reported to decrease Tolectin blood levels (56). The doses being used are subtherapeutic and this may explain the unsatisfactory antiinflammatory response, as well as the adjunctive use of Zomax. The latter drug is also a cyclo-oxygenase inhibitor and would therefore be redundant if effective doses of aspirin or Tolectin were employed. Besides having undesirable sedative properties, Zomax is also a chemical cousin to Tolectin. Recommendation: Discontinue Zomax and either aspirin or Tolectin. Administer the remaining drug in full antiinflammatory doses.

Psychotropics. B.J.'s history of "organic brain disease" was described as long-standing and mild in the admission workup, but subsequent nursing notes suggest that the symptoms of confusion and disorientation noticeably worsened soon after admission. Rapid deterioration is atypical of chronic dementing disease (see next section, senile dementia), and raises the suspicion that a reversible factor precipitated this decline. Psychotropic drugs, especially drugs with sedating and anticholinergic properties, are notorious for inducing mental fuzziness and confusion in older adults. The cognitive impairment of senile dementia can be greatly exaggerated by drugs like Dalmane, Mellaril, Haldol, Cogentin, and Elavil, all of which B.J. receives.

Neuroleptics are some of the most commonly prescribed drugs in nursing home patients. They are best reserved for geriatric patients with psychotic behavioral disturbances associated with functional or organic disorders, including senile dementia. Too often, however, neuroleptics are prescribed trivially for anxiety, insomnia, confusion, "senility" (a nonspecific term) and nonconformity to institutional life-style. In one typical drug utilization study, 86% of nursing home patients received at least one neuroleptic agent and 46% received two or more simultaneously (57). Even when a neuroleptic agent is indicated, the use of two or more, as seen in this patient, is irrational. Also, B.J.'s Cogentin therapy represents unnecessary polypharmacy unless extrapyramidal symptoms are clearly documented. Extrapyramidal symptoms are not likely to occur as long as the strongly anticholinergic Elavil continues to be administered, or if Haldol is discontinued.

The antidepressant Elavil may or may not be indicated. B.J. is taking many sedating drugs, such as methyldopa, Dalmane, Mellaril, Zomax and Elavil itself, and these may induce a pseudodepression which will resolve with a reduction in the number of sedating drugs. Even if B.J. suffers from true depression, the use of low bedtime doses, a common practice in nursing homes, is irrational if response is not carefully monitored and an attempt is made to titrate the dose to a reasonable therapeutic range. Most prescribers using antidepressants in this manner probably recognize they are achieving little antidepressant effect but don't have the time or interest to individualize the dose as they should. The sleep-inducing effect of the sedating tricyclics is used as a rationalization for this improper prescribing pattern.

Recommendation: In view of the atypical deterioration of B.J.'s cognitive function, all psychotropic medication should be tapered and discontinued. Obtain a baseline assessment of cognitive function and psychiatric status by a gerontologist or psychiatrist to competently establish the presence or absence of psychotic behavioral disturbances and/or depression. Manage each disorder with a single drug in full therapeutic doses.

Laxatives. It is not uncommon to see nursing home patients receiving one to three laxative drugs simultaneously in conjunction with an antidiarrheal. B.J. is not an exception. Constipation is predominantly the result of immobility, poor dietary intake and drugs, such as Mellaril, Elavil, Cogentin and ferrous sulfate. A problem with chemical bowel regulation is that it can mask symptoms of underlying organic diseases or drug reactions. Diarrhea, for example, is an early symptom of digitalis intoxication. Another hazard is the unwitting introduction of unwanted ingredients into the patient's regimen. Metamucil Packets contain 250 mg of sodium per packet and represent a significant increment to B.J.'s 2 gm. daily restriction. Recommendation: Encourage ambulation and dietary measures. If the elimination of constipating drugs is not feasible, limit laxative use to a bulk-forming agent or possibly

a stool softener. Replace Metamucil Packets with Effersyllium (7 gm Na/packet) or with psyllium powder. Avoid continuous use of stimulant laxatives.

Iron. A review of B.J.'s chart discloses that ferrous sulfate has been given continuously without written evidence of an indication and without hemoglobin levels or any other recorded blood work. Recommendation: Obtain hemoglobin and other iron indices and discontinue iron if deficiency cannot be documented.

2. B.J.'s regimen was evaluated and revised over several weeks. The medication list was reduced to hydrochlorothiazide, a potassium supplement, Tolectin, Metamucil powder and Dalmane as needed. On these drugs, B.J. was much less confused and his dizziness disappeared. The elimination of drugs was thought to be responsible for improvement of his disabling symptoms. Why is polypharmacy so prevalent in institutionalized geriatric patients?

The practice of gerontology has been described as the art of taking aged patients off of their unnecessary medications. Polypharmacy thrives under conditions where multiple chronic diseases coexist in patients with communication problems. These factors lead to imperfect diagnoses and unclear drug indications. Failure to document indications for drugs is as high as 60% in skilled nursing facility patients (57). Monitoring drug therapy in these patients is especially vexating. Busy physicians assign a low priority to nursing home patients in terms of individual attention, and much of the prescribing and follow-up is done by telephone. Duplication of drug classes often result, or unrecognized drug side effects are treated with more drugs. With little actual patient contact, prescribers often continue drugs in stabilized patients long after the benefit is clearly evident to avoid the inconvenience of meticulous dose adjustments and follow-up monitoring.

Underlying the difficult task of caring for institutionalized geriatric patients is the problem of gerontophobia. A common attitude among health professionals is that the old patient is less deserving than the young patient since he is closer to death and has no distant future. Gerontophobiacs feel little can be done for the institutionalized old, and that benign neglect is acceptable. One recent survey of physicians disclosed that 40%

believe the nursing home is where old people go to die, and only 21% feel that they are actually in charge of their nursing home patients (58). Gerontophobia includes indifference to the finer details of medication management.

Pseudodementia

3. Several months later, B.J. begins to show noticeable mental deterioration following the death of his best friend in the nursing home. He bitterly complains of poor memory and expresses anxiety about increasing disorientation to his surroundings. Valium is prescribed but it only serves to increase confusion and induce lethargy. B.J. becomes more withdrawn, unsociable and cognitively impaired. Symptoms of paranoia emerge, including suspicion, fear, agitation and refusal to eat. A trial of thioridazine suppresses the undesirable behavior but results in extreme lethargy and confusion. What do these signs and symptoms suggest?

The problem is whether B.J.'s deterioration represents progressive senile dementia or pseudodementia. The latter is a syndrome which mimicks a functional psychiatric illness or psychoses caused by sensory deprivation, medications or underlying organic diseases. The most common cause of pseudodementia in older adults is depression (59–61). It is likely the cause of B.J.'s symptoms and may have been precipitated by the recent loss of his best friend. Pseudodementia resulting from depression is often recognized only after the patient unexpectedly recovers or is serendipitously given a trial of antidepressants. The danger of misapplying the diagnosis of senile dementia to a depression of the aged is unnecessary institutionalization or, if already institutionalized, therapeutic neglect.

The differentiation of depression from senile dementia is difficult. The symptoms of depression in the older adult masquerade quite effectively as dementia. Often depression overlays preexisting senile dementia, as with B.J. However, subtle clinical differences do exist, and some are exhibited by B.J. The onset of his symptomatology is abrupt rather than insidious. He has insight into his distress and has strong emotions. This contrasts to a lack of insight and shallow emotions in patients with senile dementia. Pseudodementia patients complain vigorously of memory def-

icits as opposed to their chronically demented counterparts who are relatively oblivious to memory deficits. B.J. also exhibits a loss of social skills, and this is different from senile dementia where there may be a marked retention of social skills until late in the disease. In addition, memory and intelligence testing would most likely engender "don't know" responses by B.J. compared to the typical "near miss" answers by senile dementia patients. B.J. would exhibit inconsistencies in cognitive performance testing compared to the global impairment observed in senile dementia (3,61,62). Despite these clinical differences, the difficulty in distinguishing pseudodementia due to depression from true irreversible dementia is illustrated by several studies in which the diagnosis of dementia was incorrectly applied to a large percentage of patients (63–65).

4. How should B.J.'s pseudodementia be treated?

A trial of antidepressants is indicated in older adults whenever the diagnosis of senile dementia is uncertain or when atypical affective features persist in conjunction with senile dementia. Conservative antidepressant therapy under these conditions is reported to benefit a significant number of cognitively impaired geriatric patients (66).

Because older adults are more sensitive to the sedative, anticholinergic and cardiovascular side effects of tricyclic (and tetracyclic) antidepressants, conservative dosing and management is appropriate. Starting doses should be low and small increments should be made at a slow rate. An initial dose of 10 mg (amitriptyline equivalents) twice daily with slow increases over one to two weeks to 50 mg twice daily will disclose patients with exceptional sensitivity to side effects. This daily dose should be maintained for at least two weeks and the patient should be observed for a response. If no response is obtained and side effects do not preclude higher doses, further increments can be made. As with younger patients, there is considerable individual variability in antidepressant dosage requirements in geriatric patients. Some geriatric patients appear to respond to doses of 100 mg/day or less while others may require full therapeutic doses of 200 mg/day or more before reduction to maintenance levels can be achieved. Monitoring of antidepressant blood levels is very useful when feasible. As with younger patients, the duration of therapy is dependent on the premorbid history and severity of the depressive episode, but probably ranges from 3 to 12 months for a first episode. Unfortunately, many of the specific parameters for dosing and duration of therapy have not been well quantified in the geriatric literature.

Senile Dementia (Alzheimer's Disease)

5. P.D.H. is a retired author and teacher who is admitted to the hospital because of delusions and inappropriate behavior. Friends describe the patient as being bright, methodical and meticulous until six years ago when he began to experience memory lapses and easy irritability. Students and colleagues recall about this time P.D.H. began to miss appointments and lectures on occasion, and over the next few years he became dependent on notes, guides and calendars to meet obligations. His mental status apparently deteriorated steadily over the next six-year period but was largely overlooked until very serious problems began about one year ago. At that time he became overtly anxious and irritable and began to have delusions. Recently he expressed the belief that his publisher was "out to get him," and he armed himself with two pistols. He discharged several rounds into the bedroom wall late one night after hearing voices unconnected to bodies, and was brought to the hospital by police. After a careful history and workup was obtained, the mental deterioration was diagnosed as Alzheimer's Disease. What signs and symptoms of senile dementia (Alzheimer's Disease) are manifested by P.D.H.?

The clinical findings for P.D.H. typify senile dementia of the Alzheimer's type. This disease has a progressive, indolent course over several years and memory loss is usually the earliest sign. Initially, the condition does not severely interfere with employment or daily performance, but the individual often struggles to perform at a level that previously required little effort. P.D.H.'s resorting to written reminders is common (3,67,68). The smoothly progressive cognitive impairment over years is consistent with irreversibility since no true irreversible dementia appears abruptly (ie, in a matter of days or weeks) or follows a course other than steady deterioration. Dementia

characterized by an abrupt onset or fluctuating course should not be labeled senile dementia and should be investigated vigorously for a treatable cause.

As P.D.H. becomes aware of his declining cognitive power, affective symptoms appear. At first his anxiety may be adaptive and useful, but it later gives way to irritability and agitation. With more severe memory loss, disorientation, confusion and behavioral problems may become predominant. In the most severe cases, the senile dementia patient suffers from profound defects in memory and orientation which make functioning difficult in all but the most familiar situations. Unable to adapt to changing environmental cues, he may exhibit overactivity, hostility, paranoia and even overt psychosis. The terminal stage, occurring on the average of eight years after onset, is signaled by a profound loss of all higher mental functioning, necessitating continuing nursing care. Characteristic neurological signs develop, such as slouching, wide-based posture, festinating gait, abnormal reflexes and involuntary movements (64–71).

6. In the initial workup, P.D.H.'s cognitive impairment is variously referred to as senility, organic brain syndrome and dementia. Are these terms all correctly applied to P.D.H.?

The term "*senility*" is not a medical diagnosis. It is a catchall term for symptoms ranging from non-pathological senescent forgetfulness to a severely disabling irreversible decline in intellectual functioning, with loss of insight, behavioral disturbances and lack of emotional responsiveness to others. When senility becomes disabling, it is the geriatric equivalent of "failure-to-thrive" in infants and is a signal to investigate further. Mental failure may be the only symptom of a wide range of pathologies, including coronary heart disease, pneumonia, urinary tract infection, thyrotoxicosis and especially drug reactions. It is estimated that between 10 and 30% of older adults presenting with "senility" have an undiagnosed medical problem, and any reversible cause is properly called an *acute organic brain syndrome* (59,69,72).

Dementia describes altered brain function in which memory impairment is the most prominent feature, and may include disordered thinking, judgment and personality changes. Dementia is roughly equivalent to chronic organic brain syndrome except that the latter implies irreversibility, while dementia sometimes is used to describe reversible or partially reversible mental impairment (73). The most common forms of chronic, irreversible organic brain syndrome in older adults are senile dementia, also called Alzheimer's Disease, and multiinfarct dementia, formerly called cerebral arteriosclerosis. These two syndromes account for approximately 80% of the dementias of old age, with senile dementia accounting for two-thirds (69). It is often impossible to differentiate senile dementia from multiinfarct dementia with certainty until autopsy, but certain clinical differences exist. In contrast to senile dementia, the progression of multiinfarct dementia has a downward sawtooth course, with each episode being marked by a sudden progression of symptoms. This is the result of repeated small and widespread microinfarctions. Hypertension, diabetes and definite focal neurological findings are often part of the history, none of which are present in P.D.H. (59,69,72).

Dementia is the correct term to be applied to P.D.H. in view of his history, and in the absence of reversible cause, senile dementia of the Alzheimer's type is the appropriate diagnosis.

7. Comment on how P.D.H. should be studied to rule out any reversible cause of dementia.

The diagnosis of irreversible dementia is a process of elimination. Table 2 summarizes the aggressive workup required (67,74). The most common causes of reversible dementia in the aged are therapeutic drug intoxication, depression and metabolic or infective disorders (69).

8. A final diagnosis of senile dementia is made. What drugs are available to treat P.D.H.'s specific disease process?

Until recently, irreversible dementias of older adults were commonly but incorrectly attributed to cerebrovascular disease and diminished cerebral blood flow and were commonly treated with vasodilators. However, current evidence suggests that arteriosclerotic cerebrovascular disease is not an important etiology of dementia. The diminished cerebral blood flow in senile dementia is now thought to be the consequence of decreased brain mass, due to primary neuronal degeneration. Therefore, although vasodilators can increase cerebral blood flow, they do not modify the basic disease process (71,75–77). Further evi-

Table 2.

RULING OUT REVERSIBLE CAUSES OF DEMENTIA*

	Remedial Cause	Investigation
D	Drug toxicity	history; drug screen
E	Emotional (psychiatric)	EEG; trial of antidepressants
M	Metabolic (endocrine)	blood gasses; electrolytes; blood sugar and glucose tolerances; thyroid, liver and renal function
E	Eyes and ears (sensory)	vision, hearing screens
N	Nutritional state	dietary; alcohol history; B-12 level
T	Tumor and Trauma	EEG; CT scan
I	Infection (pneumonia, CNS, syphilis, etc.)	chest x-ray; serology; lumbar puncture
A	Arteriosclerotic complications (MI, CHF, etc.)	EKG; chest x-ray

*References 67, 74.

dence has been obtained from hyperbaric oxygen treatment, which greatly increases cerebral blood oxygen content without improving cognitive function. Thus, the actions of vasodilating drugs cannot be explained on the basis of increased oxygen supply to the brain (76). Even if cerebral arteriosclerosis were an important etiology of senile dementia, it has been argued that relaxation of smooth muscles would not decrease obstruction due to plaques, and that nonspecific vasodilation of peripheral vessels may actually divert blood from the cerebral circulation (67,75,76).

Some drugs formerly thought to exert their primary effect on smooth muscle may act through other nonspecific mechanisms, and this has led to a differentiation of vasodilator drugs into two classes: the primary vasodilators and the cognitive activators. However, neither class directly affects the underlying biochemical defect, and both should be considered symptomatic treatment at best. Therefore there are no drugs currently approved for use in senile dementia which alter the specific disease process.

9. Evaluate primary vasodilators in the treatment of senile dementia.

The primary vasodilators used in senile dementia are papaverine, cyclandelate, isoxsuprine, and nylidrin. *Papaverine* is a direct smooth muscle relaxant which increases cerebral blood flow (71). In several studies, it has produced statistical improvement over placebo in diverse groups of senile patients (78–81). However, in most controlled, short-term studies, the results have been mixed or negative (71). In a recent review of the literature, papaverine showed practical benefit in only one of nine controlled studies, and in five controlled direct comparisons with dihydrogenated ergot alkaloids (DHE), it was inferior to DHE in all (82). As a result of this unimpressive evidence, the F.D.A. recently concluded that papaverine and its congener ethaverine are ineffective (83). However, two studies suggest that beneficial effects may depend on long-term administration (81,84). In these studies, moderate improvement in overall cognition was observed, and abnormal EEGs, which are pathologically slowed in senile dementia patients, were normalized. This occurred in a significant number of patients after two or more months of papaverine therapy. The known dopamine-blocking effect of papaverine was suggested as a mechanism and implies an effect more like the cognitive activators, but more study is needed.

Cyclandelate is another direct vasodilator with little data to support its effectiveness. A recent review revealed that of 18 total cyclandelate studies performed, 7 were well-controlled, and only 3 of these reported any practical benefit. Four studies showed cyclandelate to be no better than placebo (82). *Isoxsuprine* is a beta-adrenergic stimulant which produces selective vasodilation and which can actually decrease cerebral blood flow when given in parenteral doses (85). Of the five studies of isoxsuprine done since 1958, three were well-controlled and none of these showed isoxsuprine to be of any practical value (82). *Nylidrin* is another beta-adrenergic stimulator which is reportedly useful in the treatment of cognitive impairment, but its use for this disorder has not been widely studied (86).

In conclusion, there is a lack of evidence that primary vasodilator drugs have value in the treatment of senile dementia. In mild cases, vasodilators may induce statistical improvement in some cognitive parameters, but these changes are generally not important clinically.

10. P.D.H.'s physician elects to use the cognitive activator Hydergine, a dihydrogenated ergot derivative, instead of a primary vasodilator. What is the proposed mechanism of Hydergine and is there any evidence of superiority over the primary vasodilators?

Of the cognitive activators, *dihydrogenated ergot alkaloid (DHE)* is the only drug marketed in this country. It is available generically in addition to the trade-named product, Hydergine. Originally marketed as an alpha-blocker and cerebrovasodilator, its mechanism is now known to be much more complex. In addition to its alpha-blocking effects, DHE inhibits phosphodiesterase and exhibits dopaminergic and serotoninergic properties (87–89). DHE possibly improves neuronal intermediary metabolism, and improvement in neuronal metabolism is thought to secondarily cause an increased cerebral blood flow (74,75). DHE also normalizes the pathological EEG changes in senile dementia patients. These improvements begin in three weeks and become statistically significant in 9 to 12 weeks (90). This time course coincides with the drug's usual onset. In a review of 33 studies, 22 were found to be well-controlled and 18 of these reported improvement in cognitive impairment (82). In another study, DHE was found to be superior to papaverine and placebo in institutionalized senile dementia patients (91). Unfortunately there is little standardization of outcome criteria from study to study, and the efficacy issue is still not completely resolved. For example, one review noted that over 60 behavioral scales and psychological tests were in use, making it difficult to cross-compare studies in terms of dementia severity and DHE response (82). Nevertheless, it appears that DHE has the best confirmed efficacy of the drugs commonly used for senile dementia, and is preferable to the primary vasodilators.

11. Given P.D.H.'s history of senile dementia, what response and problems would you anticipate from DHE treatment?

In currently recommended doses, DHE appears to modestly benefit patients in the early stages of senile dementia, although the magnitude of improvement is small and often limited to affective and self-care symptoms. There is little evidence that memory is improved (67). Since P.D.H. has moderate to severe symptoms, it is unlikely that DHE will produce practical benefits. This is true of most patients who have symptoms severe enough to require hospitalization or nursing home care.

The major problems associated with DHE therapy relate to the general lack of pharmacokinetic data and good dose-response relationships in demented geriatric patients. Oral administration of DHE is subject to individual differences in bioavailability due to first pass liver metabolism, but is preferred over sublingual administration. There is better compliance with oral administration because sublingual irritation is avoided. Both tablets and oral liquid are available.

The optimal dose range and necessary duration for DHE are unknown, but on the basis of the literature it appears that doses less than 3 mg/day are suboptimal in most geriatric patients. The data are inadequate to determine whether 3 or even 6 mg is an adequate dose, but the trend in recent studies is to employ doses higher than those currently approved for use (124). Therefore, P.D.H. should be started on the highest approved dose of 1 mg orally three times daily. The trial period should last 8–12 weeks with careful ongoing observation and with a clear understanding that DHE will be discontinued at the end of this period if no benefits are observed.

A perplexing, and as yet unanswered, question is how long DHE should be maintained if a response is obtained. Should P.D.H. continue the drug indefinitely? For one year? Does the physician risk degenerative progression of the disease by stopping the drug? To date, no studies have documented the long-term effects of DHE. Fortunately, at these doses side effects are mild and consist primarily of transient nausea and gastrointestinal disturbance. Rarely, palpitations, sinus bradycardia and headaches have been reported (125,126).

12. P.D.H.'s physician recently read about the experimental use of "precursor loading" therapy to correct the biochemical defect associated with senile dementia. He wonders what it is and how it works. Comment.

The primary neuronal degeneration associated with senile dementia may represent a selective cholinergic abnormality. The hallmark is the formation of pathological senile plaques and neurofibrillary tangles distributed in the neocortex and hippocampus which are associated with declining numbers of cholinergic neurons (50,92–96).

The role of cholinergic fibers in memory processing appears to be established. Animal studies demonstrate that cholinergic drugs facilitate learning and memory retrieval while anticholinergics decrease the speed of learning and worsen retrieval. Large doses of scopolamine in young adult volunteers cause memory defects similar to senile dementia, and these defects are reversed by physostigmine (96–98). Theoretically, the augmentation of central cholinergic activity should improve cognitive function in senile dementia patients.

There also exists preliminary evidence of a selective decline of noradrenergic neurons in senile dementia. In independent post-mortem series, both cholinergic and noradrenergic neuronal markers were reduced in senile dementia but were normal in multiinfarct dementia and depression (99,100). Therefore, although the bulk of biochemical evidence points to a cholinergic deficit, it would be naive to attribute the cognitive decline in senile dementia to a single neurotransmitter or neuronal tract.

If a primary degeneration of the cholinergic neuronal tract emerges as the dominant underlying pathology, it will have important implications for research in the prevention and treatment of senile dementia. It is known that even with severe disease, 25 to 50% of cholinergic neurons survive. Since the enzyme responsible for neuronal synthesis of acetylcholine, choline acetyltransferase, is unsaturated, it would be theoretically possible to boost acetylcholine activity (101). The situation is analogous to Parkinson's disease, where degeneration of the central dopaminergic tracts responds to dopamine precursors; precursor loading therapy with acetylcholine substrates or anticholinesterases may modify senile dementia.

Choline chloride, lecithin and physostigmine have all been studied in senile dementia patients. *Choline* and *lecithin* raise central nervous system acetylcholine levels, enhance memory performance, and possibly exert direct cholinergic actions in normal subjects, but their effects in senile dementia patients are unimpressive. Positive effects are seen only in patients with recent onset of cognitive impairment (101–105). Lecithin, the dietary form of choline, may be preferred because it is an efficient source of choline and lacks the dyspepsia, fishy taste and smell of choline chloride. *Anticholinesterase drugs* show promise but only physostigmine has been investigated, and it must be given parenterally. Both acetylcholine precursors and physostigmine have an extremely narrow therapeutic index, and the future success of cholinergic augmentation therapy will depend on quantifying the dose-response relationship and developing safe, long-acting anticholinesterase drugs (97). Until these problems are resolved, it would be premature to recommend precursor loading therapy for P.D.H.

13. What is the role of neuroleptics in the treatment of behavioral disorders associated with senile dementia?

Phenothiazines and *haloperidol* are among the most commonly used drugs for behavioral disturbances in older adults, particularly those in nursing homes. They are useful for psychotic disturbances commonly associated with moderate to severe senile dementia. For example, the paranoid thought disorder is an indication for neuroleptic use in P.D.H. For nonpsychotic agitation, insomnia or anxiety, neuroleptics are no more effective than antianxiety agents (106). Therefore, neuroleptic drugs should not be used indiscriminately because the risks of Parkinsonism, hypotension, cardiotoxicity and tardive dyskinesia are all concentrated in older adults. In addition, the significant anticholinergic properties of many neuroleptics can aggravate cognitive impairment.

Thioridazine has been singled out for use in geriatric patients, mostly because its promotion has led to the widely held belief that it is a preferred neuroleptic in older adults. It is the only widely used neuroleptic that is specifically approved for use for behavioral disturbances in "geriatric dementia" (107). Thioridazine's superiority over other phenothiazines and haloperidol is not established, and its strong sedative, hypotensive and anticholinergic properties may actually make it a poor choice in certain older adults (71,74).

14. What other drugs have been used in senile dementia? Are there any new drugs on the horizon with potential use in this disorder?

Antianxiety agents and *hypnotics* may aggravate the early stages of senile dementia and are avoided if possible. Anxiety may be a beneficial

adaptive response, and suppression can cloud environmental cues to the extent that confusion is aggravated. In later stages of the disease, these agents may be appropriate for disabling symptoms. Many benzodiazepines can accumulate in elderly patients; thus, the short-acting oxazepam or lorazepam may be preferred in older adults.

Psychostimulants, such as dextroamphetamine, pemoline and methylphenidate theoretically should elevate mood and cognition based on the decreased brain adrenergic activity associated with normal aging. Unfortunately, psychostimulants produce little improvement in learning and memory and in fact have produced temporary paradoxical drowsiness and EEG slowing (108).

Several experimental drugs favorably affect memory and learning in normal adults and will possibly be tried in senile dementia patients in the future. *Piracetam* is a cyclic derivative of gamma-aminobutyric acid which acts specifically on the associative and integrative functions of the brain. It appears to improve memory in both young and old normal adults, and there is some evidence it benefits mild to moderately impaired senile dementia patients (71). *Centrally-acting neuropeptides* have also been shown to improve memory. A peptide fragment of adrenocorticotropin, ACTH 4-10, improves learning in animal models but results in humans are disappointing (71). *Vasopressin*, a posterior pituitary hormone, also appears to improve cognitive skills in normal human volunteers (109,110). The clinical utility of these and other experimental agents in senile dementia awaits further research.

15. P.D.H.'s nurse has recently read about a product called Gerovital-H3 in a health magazine. It is claimed to benefit many symptoms of aging, including "senility." He wants your opinion. Comment.

Gerovital-H3 (G-H3) is a controversial formulation developed in Eastern Europe which has received periodic attention as an anti-aging tonic or rejuvenator. It is approved in Nevada for in-state prescription use. G-H3 is essentially a 2% procaine solution which is administered either orally or intramuscularly. Procaine has a wide range of pharmacological effects, the most germaine of which is its monoamine oxidase inhibiting properties. A few studies suggest that G-H3 may improve depressed geriatric patients (111,

112), but there is no evidence substantiating any favorable cognitive effects in senile dementia. Its antidepressant effects have not been systematically compared to existing tricyclic antidepressants or monoamine oxidase inhibitors.

Pressure Sores

The topic of pressure sores induces boredom in most health professionals; consequently, standards of prevention and treatment are poor. This is probably why one out of five patients in a nursing home develops a pressure sore (113). When pressure sores develop, serious complications such as fever or devastating sepsis often follow (113, 114).

Pressure sores are induced by prolonged obstruction of skin capillary blood flow and lymph drainage which results in ischemia, accumulation of anaerobic metabolic waste products, tissue damage and ulcer formation (113–115). Sores typically develop over pressure points of bony prominances, such as the heel, elbow, ischial or sacral areas. Although commonly referred to as decubitus ulcers or bedsores, the term pressure sore is the best descriptive term.

16. R.K.C. is an 84-year-old nursing home patient with generalized osteoarthritis, diabetes and chronic renal insufficiency. He was institutionalized after recently fracturing his right femur. List the factors that predispose R.K.C. to pressure sores and discuss how pressure sores can be prevented or minimized.

Advanced age, its concomitant multiple chronic disorders, and immobility are major risk factors. R.K.C. is immobilized by osteoarthritis and a fractured femur resulting in a bedridden existence. Diabetes accounts for impaired circulation and poor wound healing. If nursing surveillance is inadequate, R.K.C. is at very high risk for pressure sore problems.

Prevention of pressure sores relies on the identification and minimization of patient risk factors. Immobility is the most important risk factor (116). Other factors are chronic conditions which may impair circulation or retard wound healing, such as diabetes. Mental status is an important risk factor in that impairment interferes with efforts to mobilize the patient.

Surveillance of high risk patients is the next most important factor in the prevention of pressure sores and is a function of good nursing care.

Nurses must follow proper positioning and turning schedules in high risk patients, and close inspection of the skin and skin hygiene are crucial. Clean bedclothes, avoidance of rough, damp or wrinkled bedsheets, and good management of incontinent patients are necessary (115,116).

17. While in the nursing home, R.K.C. develops a 10 cm, Stage 4 pressure sore over the sacral area. Treatment is instituted with pressure redistribution and povidone-iodine soaked gauze applied to the ulcer. It is to be replaced every 4 hours. How is the treatment of pressure sores related to staging?

Once pressure sores occur, they can be staged according to severity; staging is then used to determine appropriate treatment (113,114,116):

Stage 1. Blanching Erythema: skin blanches when pressure is applied; reversible if pressure is eliminated.

Stage 2. Non-blanching Erythema: capillary and dermal tissue have sustained irreversible damage.

Stage 3. Blister and Eschar Formation: well demarcated margins.

Stage 4. Ulcer, Non-infected: tissue enzymes separate eschar and sloughing creates an ulcer.

Stage 5. Ulcer, Infected: same as Stage 4, but infected.

The recommended treatment based on the staging scheme is summarized in Table 3. For all stages, positioning and pressure redistribution are the most important aspects of management. Superficial pressure sores (Stages 1 and 2) comprise 70 to 90% of all sores. They are painful, but usually heal in a few weeks if the patient's condition and mobility can be maintained (117). Stage 1 and 2 pressure sores are conservatively managed with cornstarch or silicone sprays to minimize friction, and cool packs or air to reduce local erythema and edema. Stage 3 pressure sores are treated similarly except that more emphasis is placed on positioning to keep the blister closed and to prevent infection. The deep pressure sore (Stage 4 or 5) exhibited by R.K.C. is painless but far more serious, and may require additional treatment modalities. Topical antiseptics, such as brown soap, povidone-iodine or benzoyl peroxide, are used to cleanse the ulcer. Debriding agents remove the sloughing tissue and facilitate wound granulation. Mechanical debridement with sim-

Table 3.

TREATMENT OF PRESSURE SORES BASED ON STAGING*

Measure	Stage 1 or 2	Stage 3	Stage 4 or 5
topical	cornstarch, silicone spray	not indicated	antiseptic, dextranomer, proteolytic enzyme
thermal	cool packs 5 to 10 min. TID	not indicated	contraindicated
exposure	air (fan)	same	same
positioning	turn every 2 hours; keep pressure off reddened area for 4 hours (Stage 1) or 48 hours (Stage 2)	same; keep pressure off until blister or eschar heals	same; keep pressure off until ulcer heals
ultraviolet light	not indicated	not indicated	may be indicated

*Reference 116.

ple wet-to-dry dressing techniques or chemical debridement with proteolytic enzymes or dextranomer are employed (118,119). If severe, gangrenous ulcers develop or complications such as osteomyelitis appear, and surgical debridement may be necessary (115,119). Once granulation is established, ultraviolet light can be employed for its bacteriocidal and granulation-stimulating properties. Ultraviolet light is avoided in Stages 1 to 3 because it can provoke erythema and edema of intact skin (116).

18. Comment on any potential hazards from R.K.C.'s topical therapy.

Normally, povidone-iodine dressings are an accepted and safe form of topical antiseptic therapy for pressure sores. However, repeated topical applications to large ulcers in patients with renal impairment can have severe consequences. Two case reports describe the development of serious junctional bradycardia and hypotension within three weeks of beginning topical povidone-iodine treatment of pressure sores in patients with renal insufficiency. Iodide retention was blamed when a significant increase in serum iodide concentration was discovered (120). It is assumed that problems with other topical agents are possible when administered under similar conditions.

19. R.K.C.'s nurse recently heard from a colleague at another local nursing home that the topical application of OTC antacid products seems to speed up healing of pressure sores in their patients and requests your opinion about its effectiveness. Comment.

Numerous topical and systemic drugs are claimed to speed the healing of pressure sores, but none has gained universal acceptance. Pressure sore remedies range from sugar and egg white paste, to topical ascorbic acid solutions, to the direct application of Maalox (113,115,121). The fact that no agent has emerged with wide acceptance indicates that none is satisfactory. As one author wrote: "You can put anything you like on a pressure sore except the patient" (122).

Much of the problem stems from the significant placebo response inherent in drug evaluation studies. In one study, a bogus "electromagnetic radiation device" was used by unknowing medical and nursing staff, and resulted in the cure of several "intractable" pressure sores (123). The authors attributed the success to improved care brought on by the study, and stressed that blinded, placebo-controlled design is necessary for the evaluation of any new drug or device used to treat pressure sores. The value of conservative measures with good nursing care was emphasized in another study in which intensive surveillance by a "decubitus ulcer team" resulted in a reduction of pressure sores from an initial prevalence of 69% to 0% in 18 weeks (114). The only topical drug therapy employed was brown soap, benzoyl peroxide and a proteolytic enzyme in Stage 4 and 5 pressure sores. Thus, simple measures and good nursing care are sufficient to treat most pressure sores.

References

1. *A Guide to the 1981 White House Conference on Aging:* U.S. Department of H.H.S., Public. #HHS-393, 1980.

2. Lamy PP: *Prescribing for the Elderly*, 1st ed. PSG Publishing Co., Inc., Littleton, MA, 1980, p 11.

3. Cryer PE: Dementia and the problems of aging. Am J Med. 1979; 67:307.

4. *Recent Developments in Clinical and Research Geriatric Medicine: The NIA Role*, U.S. Department of Health, Education and Welfare, NIH Publication #80-1990, 1980.

5. Campbell WH: Issues and priorities for research in geriatric pharmaceutical care. Drug Intell Clin Pharm. 1981; 15:111.

6. Committee on Ways and Means, U.S. House of Representatives: *Basic Facts of Health Industry*, Washington, D.C., Government Printing Office, 1971.

7. Lamy PP et al: Drug prescribing for the elderly. Hosp Pract. 1976; 11:111.

8. Lamy PP: Drug interactions and the elderly—a new perspective. Drug Intell Clin Pharm. 1980; 14:513.

9. *Handbook for Pharmaceutical Services in Long-Term Care Facilities:* N.A.R.D., 1750 K St. NW, Suite 1200, Washington, D.C., 1979.

10. Lamy PP: *Prescribing for the Elderly*, op. cit., p 94.

11. Hurwitz N: Admission to hospitals due to drugs. Br Med J. 1969; 1:539.

12. Frisk PA et al: Community-hospital pharmacist detection of drug-related problems upon patient admission to small hospitals. Am J Hosp Pharm. 1977; 34:738.

13. Lamy PP: *Prescribing for the Elderly*, op. cit., p 127.

14. Vener AM et al: Drug usage and health characteristics in noninstitutionalized retired persons. J Am Ger Soc. 1979; 27:83.

15. Schwartz D et al: Medication errors made by the elderly chronically ill patient. Am J Pub Health. 1962; 52:2018.

16. Swift CG: Clinical pharmacology in the elderly. Scot Med J. 1979; 24:221.

17. Bender AD: The effect of increasing age on the distribution of peripheral blood flow in man. J Am Ger Soc. 1965; 13:192.

18. Vestal RE et al: Antipyrine metabolism in man: Influence of age, alcohol, caffeine, and smoking. Clin Pharmacol Ther. 1975; 18:425.

19. Shock NW et al: Age differences in the water content of the body as related to basal oxygen consumption in males. J Gerontol. 1963; 18:1.

20. Novak IP: Aging, total body potassium, fat-free mass, and cell mass in males and females between ages 18 and 35 years. J Gerontol. 1972; 27:438.

21. Greenblatt DJ et al: Toxicity of high-dose flurazepam in the elderly. Clin Pharmacol Ther. 1977; 21:355.

22. Greenblatt DJ: Reduced serum albumin concentration in the elderly: A report from the Boston Collaborative Drug Surveillance Program. J Am Ger Soc. 1979; 27:20.

23. Farah F et al: Hepatic drug acetylation and oxidation: Effects of aging in man. Br Med J. 1977; 2:255.

24. O'Malley K et al: Effect of age and sex on human drug metabolism. Br Med J. 1971; 3:607.

25. Thompson EN et al: Effect of age on liver function with particular reference to bromosulphalein excretion. Gut. 1965; 6:266.

26. Triggs EJ et al: Pharmacokinetics in the elderly. Eur J Clin Pharmacol. 1975; 8:55.

27. Crooks J et al: Pharmacokinetics in the elderly. Clin Pharmacokinetics. 1976; 1:280.

28. Hewick DS et al: The effect of age on sensitivity to warfarin sodium. Br J Pharmacol. 1975; 2:189P.

29. Shader RI et al: Absorption and disposition of chlordiazepoxide in young and elderly male volunteers. J Clin Pharmacol. 1977; 17:709.

30. Klotz U et al: Effects of age and liver disease on disposition and elimination of diazepam in adult man. J Clin Invest. 1975; 55:347.

31. Geokas MC et al: The aging gastrointestinal tract. Am J Surg. 1969; 117:881.

32. Nies AS et al: Altered hepatic blood flow and drug disposition. Clin Pharmacokinetics. 1976; 1:125.

33. Richey DP et al: Pharmacokinetic consequences of aging. Ann Rev Pharmacol Toxicol. 1977; 17:49.

34. deWardener HE: Renal function in relation to age. In *The Kidney*, 4th ed., New York, Churchill Livingstone, Division of Longman, 1973, p 100.

35. Rowe JW et al: The effect of age on creatinine clearance in man: A cross sectional and longitudinal study. J Gerontol. 1976; 31:155.

36. Rowe JW et al: The influence of age on renal response to water deprivation in man. Nephron. 1976; 17:270.

37. Epstein M et al: Age as a determinant of renal sodium conservation. J Lab Clin Med. 1976; 87:411.

38. Baylis EM et al: Effects of renal function on plasma digoxin levels in elderly ambulant patients in domiciliary practice. Br Med J. 1972; 1:338.

39. Leikola E et al: On oral penicillin levels in young and geriatric patients. J Gerontol. 1957; 12:48.

40. Bennett WM et al: Drug therapy in renal failure: Dosing guidelines for adults. Ann Intern Med. 1980; 93:62 and 286.

41. Siersback-Nielsen K et al: Rapid evaluation of creatinine clearance (letter). Lancet. 1971; 1:1133.

42. Mølholm-Hansen J et al: Renal excretion of drugs in the elderly. Lancet. 1970; 1:1170.

43. Wollner L et al: Failure of cerebral autoregulation as a cause of brain dysfunction in the elderly. Br Med J. 1979; 1:1117.

44. Schatz IJ: Current management concepts in orthostatic hypotension. Arch Intern Med. 1980; 140:1152.

45. Blumenthal MD et al: Dizziness and falling in elderly outpatients. Am J Psychiatry. 1980; 137:203.

46. Overstall PW et al: Falls in the elderly related to postural imbalance. Br Med J. 1977; 1:261.

47. Anon: Drugs in the elderly. Med Let Drugs Ther. 1979; 21:43.

48. Castleden CM et al: Increased sensitivity to nitrazepam in old age. Br Med J. 1977; 1:10.

49. Smith BH et al: Aging and the nervous system. Geriatrics. 1975; 30:109.

50. Roth M: Senile dementia and its borderlands. Proc Annu Meet Am Psychopathol Assoc. 1980; 69:205.

51. Samorajski T: Age-related changes in brain biogenic amines. In *Aging. Vol. I: Clinical, Morphologic and Neurochemical Aspects in the Aging Central Nervous System*, New York, Raven Press, 1975, pp 199–214.

52. Learoyd BM: Psychotropic drugs and the elderly patient. Med J Austr. 1972; 1:1131.

53. Chung EK: Maintenance digitalization in asymptomatic elderly heart disease patients. JAMA. 1980; 244:2561.

54. Dall JL: Maintenance digoxin in elderly patients. Br Med J. 1970; 2:705.

55. Stewart JE et al: Monitoring drug therapy in skilled nursing facility patients. Drug Intell Clin Phar. 1978; 12:704.

56. Cressman WA et al: Pharmacokinetics of Tolmetin, a new antiinflammatory agent. Clin Pharmacol Ther. 1974; 15:203.

57. Segal JL et al: Drug utilization and prescribing patterns in a skilled nursing facility: The need for a rational approach to therapeutics. J Am Ger Soc. 1979; 27:117.

58. Miller DB et al: Physicians' attitudes toward the ill, aged and nursing homes. J Am Ger Soc. 1976; 24:498.

59. Comfort A: *Practice of Geriatric Psychiatry*, 1st ed., New York, Elsvier, 1980.

60. Miller NE: The measurement of mood in senile brain disease: Examiner ratings and self-reports. Proc Annu Meet Am Psychopathol Assoc. 1980; 69:97.

61. Wells CE: Pseudodementia. Am J Psychiatry. 1979; 136:895.

62. Sripada P: Pseudodementia (letter). JAMA. 1981; 245:235.

63. Marsden CD et al: Outcome of investigation of patients with presenile dementia. Br Med J. 1972; 2:249.

64. Duckworth GS et al: Diagnostic differences in psychogeriatric patients in Toronto, New York, and London. Can Med Assoc J. 1975; 112:84.

65. Nott PN et al: Presenile dementia: The difficulties of early diagnosis. Acta Psychiatr Scand. 1975; 51:210.

66. Fielding S: Tricyclics in elderly patients (letter). Am J Psychiatry. 1979; 136:1100.

67. Hier DB et al: Drugs for senile dementia. Drugs. 1980; 20:74.

68. Ropper AH: A rational approach to dementia. Can Med Assoc J. 1979; 121:1175.

69. Anon: Senility reconsidered: Treatment possibilities for mental impairment in the elderly. JAMA 1980; 244–259.

70. De Boni U et al: Senile dementia and Alzheimer's disease: A current view. Life Sci. 1980; 27:1.

71. Reisberg B et al: Pharmacotherapy of senile dementia. Proc Annu Meet Am Psychopathol Assoc. 1980; 69:233.

72. Charatan FB: Therapeutic supports for the patient with OBS. Geriatrics. 1980; 35:100.

73. Barnes R et al: Strategies for diagnosing and treating agitation in the aging. Geriatrics. 1980; 35:111.

74. Yesavage J: Dementia: Differential diagnosis and treatment. Geriatrics. 1979; 34:51.

75. Anon: Vasodilators in senile dementia (editorial). Br Med J. 1979; 2:511.

76. Yamaguchi F et al: Behavioral activation testing in the dementias. Proceedings of the 9th Salzburg Conference on Cerebral Vascular Disease, *Exerpta Medica*, Amsterdam, 1979.

77. Ingevar DH: Regional cerebral blood flow and psychopathology. Proc Annu Meet Am Psychopathol Assoc. 1980; 69:73.

78. Stern FH: Management of chronic brain syndrome secondary to cerebral arteriosclerosis, with special reference to papaverine HCl. J Am Ger Soc. 1970; 18:507.

79. Ritter RH et al: Effect of papaverine on patients with cerebral arteriosclerosis. Clin Med. 1971; 78:18.

80. Jayne HW et al: The effect of intravenous papaverine HCl on cerebral circulation. J Clin Invest. 1952; 31:111.

81. Branconnier RJ et al: Effects of chronic papaverine administration on mild senile organic brain syndrome. J Am Ger Soc. 1977; 25:458.

82. Yesavage JA et al: Vasodilators in senile dementias—a review of the literature. Arch Gen Psychiatry. 1979; 36:220.

83. Anon: Papaverine and ethaverine studies. FDA Drug Bulletin. 1979; 9:26.

84. McQuillan IM et al: Evaluation of EEG and clinical changes associated with Pavabid therapy in chronic brain syndrome. Curr Ther Res. 1974; 16:49.

85. Anon: Vasodilators in senile dementia (editorial). Br Med J. 1979; 2:866.

86. Goldstein SE et al: Nylidrin HCl in the treatment of symptoms of the aged. J Clin Psych. 1979; 40:520.

87. Emmenegger H et al: The actions of Hydergine on the brain. Pharmacol. 1968; 1:65.

88. Meier-Ruge W et al: Biochemical effects of ergot alkaloids with special reference to the brain. Postgrad Med J. 1976; 52:47.

89. Greengard P et al: Possible role for cyclic nucleotides and phosphorylated membrane proteins in postsynaptic actions of neurotransmitters. Nature. 1976; 260:101.

90. Matejcek M et al: EEG and clinical changes as correlated in geriatric patients treated three months with an ergot alkaloid preparation. J Am Ger Soc. 1979; 27:198.

91. Hughes JR et al: An ergot alkaloid preparation (hydergine) in the treatment of dementia: Critical review of the clinical literature. J Am Ger Soc. 1976; 24:490.

92. Perry EK: The cholinergic system in old age and Alzheimer's disease. Age and Ageing. 1980; 9:1.

93. Perry RH et al: Histochemical observations on cholinesterase activities in the brains of elderly normal and demented (Alzheimer-type) patients. Age and Ageing. 1980; 9:9.

94. Bowen DM et al: Accelerated ageing or selective neuronal loss as an important cause of dementia? Lancet. 1979; 1:11.

95. Kendall MJ: Will drugs help patients with Alzheimer's disease? Age and Ageing. 1979; 8:86.

96. Smith CM et al: Possible biochemical basis of memory disorders in Alzheimer's disease. Age and Ageing. 1979; 8:289.

97. Davis KL et al: Cholinomimetics and memory—the effect of choline chloride. Arch Neurol. 1980; 37:49.

98. Drachman DA: Memory and cognitive function in man: Does the cholinergic system have a specific role? Neurol. 1977; 27:783.

99. Cross AJ et al: Reduced dopamine-beta-hydroxylase activity in Alzheimer's disease. Br Med J. 1981; 282:93.

100. Adolfsson R et al: Changes in the brain catecholamines in patients with dementia of Alzheimer type. Br J Psychiatry. 1979; 135:216.

101. Growdon JL et al: Neurochemical approaches to the treatment of senile dementia. Proc Annu Meet Am Psychopathol Assoc. 1980; 69:281.

102. Boyd WD et al: Clinical effects of choline in Alzheimer senile dementia. Lancet. 1977; 1:711.

103. Signoret JL et al: Influence of choline on amnesia in early Alzheimer's disease. Lancet. 1978; 2:837.

104. Etienne P et al: Alzheimer's disease: Clinical effect of lecithin treatment. In *Choline and Lecithin in Brain Disorders,* New York, Raven Press, 1979, pp 389–396.

105. Smith CM et al: Choline therapy in Alzheimer's disease. Lancet. 1978; 2:318.

106. Cervera AA: Psychoactive drug therapy in the senile patient: Controlled comparison of thioridazine and diazepam. Psychiatry Dig. 1974; 35:15.

107. *Facts and Comparisons,* St. Louis, MO, 1981, p. 266e.

108. Tecce JJ et al: Amphetamine effects in man: Paradoxical drowsiness and lowered electrical brain activity. Science. 1974; 85:451.

109. Legros JJ et al: Influence of vasopressin on learning and memory. Lancet. 1978; 1:41.

110. Oliveros JC et al: Vasopressin in amnesia. Lancet. 1978; 1:42.

111. Sakalis G et al: A trial of Gerovital-H3 in depression during senility. Curr Ther Res. 1974; 16:59.

112. Cohen S et al: Gerovital-H3 in the treatment of the depressed aging patient. Psychosomatics. 1974; 15:15.

113. Isiadinso OO: Decubitus ulcers in geriatric patients; Present status. NY State J Med. 1979; 79:2027.

114. Ameis A et al: Management of pressure sores. Postgrad Med. 1980; 67:127.

115. Mikulic MA: Treatment of pressure ulcers. Am J Nurs. 1980; 80:1125.

116. Tepperman PS et al: Pressure sores: Prevention and step-up management. Postgrad Med. 1977; 62:83.

117. Anon: Treating pressure sores (editorial). Br Med J. 1978; 1:1232.

118. Heel RC et al: Dextranomer: A review of its general properties and therapeutic efficacy. Drugs. 1979; 18:87.

119. Nierman MM: Treatment of dermal and decubitus ulcers. Drugs. 1978; 15:226.

120. Aronoff GR et al: Increased serum iodide concentration from iodide absorption through wounds treated topically with povidone-iodine. Am J Med Sci. 1980; 279:173.

121. Yeats HS: Decubitus ulcer treatment (letter). Am J Nurs. 1980; 80:640.

122. Gutman L: The prevention and treatment of pressure sores. In *Bedsore Biomechanics,* Baltimore, University Park Press, 1976, p 157.

123. Fernie GR et al: The problems of clinical trials with new systems for preventing or healing decubitus. In *Bedsore Biomechanics,* ibid., pp 315–320.

124. Gaitz CM: Ergots in the treatment of mental disorders of old age. Adv Biochem Psychopharmacol. 1980; 23:349.

125. Cayley AC et al: Sinus bradycardia following treatment with Hydergine for cerebrovascular insufficiency. Br Med J. 1975; 2:384.

126. Cohen S: Mental impairment in the aged: Fable and fact. American Psychiatric Association Scientific Exhibit, Chicago, Sandoz, Inc., 1979, p 22.

Chapter 61

Poisonings

Gary M. Oderda and Anthony S. Manoguerra

Both purposeful, for attempted suicide, and accidental ingestions of drugs or chemicals are constituents of the poisoning problem. There were 3900 documented accidental poisoning deaths in the U.S. in 1977, of which 158 occurred in one- to five-year-old children (1). Only a small percentage of poisonings end fatally. More than a quarter million ingestions are recorded annually by the National Clearinghouse for Poison Control Centers and the National Poison Center Network (2,3), but these voluntary reports surely represent only a small fraction of the ingestions that do occur. Most ingestions are accidental and in children four years of age and younger. Internal medications and household products are ingested most commonly. Not all of these substances are potentially toxic.

Potentially Toxic Household Products. Examples of these include:

Drain cleaners are commonly caustic and produce esophageal burns (see Questions 40–42). The most common ingredient of the crystalline products is potassium hydroxide. Some contain strong acids such as sulfuric. The principal ingredient of some of the liquid preparations, 1,1,1-trichloroethane, is not caustic.

Automatic dishwasher detergents. Several different formulations exist. Many are strongly alkaline and may burn the mucous membranes of the mouth, esophagus, and stomach.

Furniture polishes frequently contain petroleum distillates. Products which contain mineral seal oil are the most toxic; when aspirated, they produce a chemical pneumonia which is more severe than that caused by other petroleum distillates (4). (Also see Questions 36–39.)

Insecticide toxicity depends on the individual agent. Many also contain petroleum distillates which add the hazard of aspiration.

Household cleaning agents are generally of low toxicity, with the exception of those which contain hydrocarbons such as pine oil.

Less Toxic Household Products. Many other household products are relatively non-toxic in small amounts:

After shave lotions *(a)*	Body conditioners *(a)*
Airplane glue *(b)*	Bubble bath soaps *(d)*
Ballpoint pen inks	Candles
Battery (dry cell)	Caps for toy pistols
Bleach (sodium hypochlorite 5%) *(c)*	(up to one roll)
	Colognes *(a)*

Crayons marked AP or CP	Porous tip ink markers
Contraceptive pills *(e)*	Play Doh
Cosmetics and skin preparations	Putty
Dehumidifying packets	Roach tablets (1–2)
Deodorizer cakes	Sachets
Fish bowl additives	Shaving creams
Fluoride Tablets (60 tablets)	Silly Putty
Matches (20 wooden or 2 books)	Soaps
Model cement *(b)*	Teething ring fluid
Pencils	Thermometers *(f)*
	Toilet water *(a)*
	Toothpaste

a.   Contains high concentrations of ethyl alcohol: may be toxic in large amounts.
b.   Not harmful unless deliberately inhaled in high concentrations.
c.   Stronger solutions (20%) found in some industrial bleaches are caustic. This concentration (5%) may produce gastrointestinal distress and vomiting.
d.   May produce vomiting or diarrhea.
e.   May produce nausea and, occasionally, vaginal bleeding in young girls.
f.   Metallic mercury is not harmful.

Poison Control Centers. In an attempt to decrease the poisoning problem, the first Poison Control Center was opened in Chicago in 1952 through the efforts of the Illinois chapter of the American Academy of Pediatrics. Since then, over 500 other centers have been established across the country. Most centers are staffed by physicians, pharmacists, and/or nurses and accept calls from the general public as well as medical personnel. Lay callers are told how the ingestion can be treated at home or are referred to a treatment facility if necessary. Recently, a movement to develop large Regional Poison Centers has begun. It is estimated that approximately 60 of these Centers would be necessary to serve the entire country. Each would serve a minimum of one million and perhaps as many as ten million people, and provide a comprehensive list of services.

GENERAL MANAGEMENT

Management of the poisoned patient can be broken down into several distinct categories. In all cases, supportive care holds the highest priority. Beyond that, the initial step is an assessment of the ingestion for potential toxicity. For most oral ingestions, measures aimed at the prevention of absorption are appropriate. Absorption can be prevented by inducing emesis or by performing gastric lavage, administering an adsorbent such as activated charcoal, and by administering a saline cathartic. Enhancement of excretion is possible in some cases, utilizing forced diuresis, alteration of the pH of the urine, hemodialysis, peritoneal dialysis, or hemoperfusion. In a few specific instances, administration of a specific antidote is also possible.

Assessment of Toxicity

Identification of the agent is of primary importance. If the agent is innocuous, other considerations will be irrelevant. Identification of all ingredients is necessary to assess the situation. In situations of ingestion of household products which are not adequately labeled, one can call the manufacturer whose name and address should be on the label.

The amount ingested should be determined if possible. If the original number of tablets in the vial is known, then the amount ingested can be determined by a simple count. In most cases, only an estimate is possible. It is best to overestimate the ingested amount if one cannot be certain of the amount ingested. The amount of substance ingested frequently determines whether or not it is considered a poison. For example, although table salt is not usually considered a poison, death has occurred as a result of salt intoxication (5–11). Most agents commonly considered poisons are toxic in small doses.

The patient's age and weight are useful in evaluating the potential severity of the ingestion and in determining the proper dose of therapeutic agents which might be used.

The patient's symptoms must be ascertained to determine whether or not they correlate with the toxic effects of the ingested agent. If the signs and symptoms are not appropriate, one must consider that the patient may have ingested other agents. Symptomatology is the major determinant of treatment; it is important to "treat the patient, not his poison (12)." Symptomatic and supportive care is the mainstay of therapy.

The time since ingestion, together with knowledge of the agent's bioavailability, onset of action and peak effect, is invaluable in assessing the situation. For example, if a patient is seen shortly after the ingestion, minimal symptoms may not mean that the amounts ingested were subtoxic. This information is also useful in determining whether or not the patient's gastric contents should be emptied by emesis or lavage.

Has any prior treatment been attempted? Some first aid measures, such as the use of salt water as an emetic, can be more toxic than the agent originally ingested.

Once the above information is obtained, one can assess the situation and give instructions for home treatment or refer the patient to an emergency treatment facility. It may also be necessary to support or calm the caller, arrange for transportation, and relay the available information to the treatment center.

Poison Centers are available in most metropolitan areas to help with the interpretation of this information and to assist in evaluating whether there is need for treatment.

Supportive Care

The major principles in providing supportive care to poisoned patients are the same as with others who are acutely ill. Most patients who are provided adequate supportive care will detoxify themselves and survive. The major areas where supportive care is necessary are the respiratory, cardiovascular, and central nervous systems. One must assure that an open airway is present and that respirations are supported if necessary. This may require insertion of an artificial airway and use of a ventilator. Cardiovascular effects may include hypotension, arrhythmias, and hypertension. Hypotension is generally managed first by placing the patient in the Trendelenburg position and administering IV fluids, followed by vasopressors if necessary. Hypertension frequently does not require treatment. Arrhythmias may respond to correction of physiological problems such as acidosis or hypoxia, or may require the use of antiarrhythmics. The major concern with CNS symptoms is the treatment of seizures with anticonvulsants such as diazepam.

Prevention of Absorption

Emetics. Emetics are frequently used to induce vomiting and remove ingested agents from the GI tract prior to absorption. There are several contraindications as well as areas of controversy involving their use.

Unconscious or deeply sedated patients should not be given emetics, because vomiting can be induced only if medullary centers are responsive. Also, if vomiting is produced, these patients are likely to aspirate their gastric contents. Apomorphine may also further depress respiratory and central nervous system function.

Emetics may precipitate or worsen convulsions in patients who are convulsing or have ingested a convulsant. If vomiting occurs, these patients are also at significant risk for aspiration.

Caustics such as strong acids and bases may cause severe esophageal burns. Induction of vomiting in these patients may further traumatize the esophagus through additional exposure to the caustic agent. Also, if the esophagus is badly burned, the trauma of vomiting may produce esophageal perforation.

Ingestion of antiemetic agents such as phenothiazines is theoretically a relative contraindication to the use of emetics, since one would expect that vomiting would not occur. However, two studies suggest that ingestion of these agents does not impair the effectiveness of ipecac (13,14). If an emetic is given and fails to produce vomiting, gastric lavage should be considered.

The use of emetics in petroleum distillate ingestions is controversial. If a small amount has been ingested, emptying the stomach is not necessary, and thus, emetics should not be considered. If a large amount has been taken, or if a potentially dangerous chemical such as a pesticide is dissolved in a petroleum distillate, emptying the stomach is necessary. Traditionally, it was felt that administering an emetic would increase the likelihood of aspiration. Thus, vomiting was not recommended, and gastric lavage was the preferred method of emptying the stomach. In a retrospective study of petroleum distillate ingestions, aspiration pneumonitis occurred less frequently when vomiting was induced than when patients were lavaged or vomited spontaneously (15). Furthermore, radiographic evidence of aspiration is less likely to be observed when petroleum distillate ingestions are treated with ipecac as opposed to lavage. The pneumonitis that did develop was less severe in the ipecac-treated group (16). Thus, administration of syrup of ipecac is the method of choice for emptying the stomach of a petroleum distillate. To reduce the possibility of aspiration, ipecac should only be administered to patients under medical supervision.

Syrup of Ipecac. Syrup of ipecac is the emetic of choice. It can be sold in appropriately labeled one ounce containers without prescription. The fluid extract of ipecac contains approximately 14 times as much active ingredient as the syrup. The fluid extract should never be dispensed, because it is almost impossible to measure accurately and may be easily mistaken for the syrup. Severe toxicity and deaths have resulted when the fluid extract was mistakenly dispensed in place of the syrup (17–19).

Children over one year of age are given one tablespoonful (15 ml) of the syrup as an initial dose. The initial dose in children under one year is 10 ml and in adults is 15–30 ml. Immediately thereafter, the patient should be given approximately 8–12 oz. of a clear liquid, such as water, Kool-Aid, or fruit juice, but not milk. Milk has been shown to delay the onset of vomiting (20). The administration of too much fluid may cause some of the poison to be pushed past the pylorus.

Whether the fluids are given before or after the ipecac (21) or whether the fluids are cold (10°C) or tepid (40°C) (22) does not seem to affect the time of vomiting.

Emesis should occur in 15 to 20 minutes. If it does not, additional fluid may be given, and the initial dose of syrup of ipecac may be repeated once. If vomiting still does not occur, the patient should be gagged. Often this will initiate vomiting. Although it is generally felt that patients who ambulate tend to vomit more quickly than those who do not, a study examining this contention showed that walking on a treadmill had no significant effect on the time to ipecac-induced vomiting in adult volunteers (23).

Frequently encountered side effects following ipecac-induced vomiting include sedation and diarrhea. One ounce of ipecac syrup, the maximum recommended dose in young children, is not toxic even if vomiting does not occur. Slight lethargy and diarrhea are commonly seen. Severe toxicity has been seen in patients given fluid extract of ipecac instead of the syrup or when large amounts of the syrup were given. A 23-month-old child who was given 90 ml of syrup (5 ml every 5 minutes) developed symptoms of ipecac intoxication despite lavage, including lethargy, tachycardia, and EKG changes (24). She was placed on a demand pacemaker, and provided with symptomatic and supportive care. She was discharged without apparent sequelae one day after admission.

Other Emetics. Apomorphine is another agent

that can be used to induce vomiting. It is generally not recommended because of its potential for toxicity and difficulty in administration. Table 1 compares apomorphine and syrup of ipecac.

Other emetics are generally not recommended. Salt is not only unreliable as an emetic but is in fact dangerous. Hysterical parents have been known to give their children large amounts of salt unnecessarily, resulting in death from salt intoxication (5). On one occasion, five infants died when a kitchen employee accidentally substituted salt for sugar in their infant formulas (8). Fatality has also occurred in children lavaged with hypertonic saline solution (6). Ingestion of large amounts of salt may cause gastroenteritis, hypernatremia (serum sodium levels as high as 274 mEq/L have been reported) (8), severe thirst, anorexia, tachypnea, dyspnea, muscular twitching and rigidity, convulsions, and death.

Copper and zinc sulfate have been used as emetics, but their use is no longer recommended.

Table 1.

COMPARISON OF IPECAC AND APOMORPHINE

	Ipecac	Apomorphine
Availability:	OTC	Requires a prescription. Generally available only in a hospital.
Cost:	Low	High. Requires administration under supervision of a physician.
Route:	Oral	Parenteral. (Unsterile.)
Time of onset:	Slow (15–20 minutes)	Fast (3–5 minutes)
Toxicity:	Cardiovascular toxicity in high doses.	May produce protracted vomiting and worsen respiratory and CNS depression. This may not always be reversed with narcotic antagonists (26).
Stability:	Stable in oral solution	Unstable in solution. Must be prepared immediately prior to injection from a hypodermic tablet.
Efficacy:	Excellent	Excellent

Both of these sulfate salts induce emesis by direct gastric irritation. Hopefully, vomiting occurs before significant absorption of the salts occurs. However, only 54–67% of administered copper sulfate is recovered in the vomitus, and significant increases in serum copper levels have occurred following the administration of copper sulfate (27). Copper sulfate administered to a patient with a partial gastrectomy resulted in fatality (28). Since safer, more effective emetics are available, copper or zinc sulfate are not recommended.

An aqueous solution of dry mustard powder is sometimes effective as an emetic; however, prepared table mustard has no emetic properties. Because much better emetics, such as syrup of ipecac, are available for home use, mustard is not recommended.

Gastric Lavage. Gastric lavage is a procedure in which a tube is inserted into the stomach via the esophagus, fluid is instilled, allowed to mix with the gastric contents, and then is removed. This is continued until the returned gastric washings are clear. Lavage is primarily indicated in the comatose or deeply sedated patient. These patients must have their airway protected with a cuffed endotracheal tube to prevent gastric contents from entering their lungs. Patients who are seizing can be lavaged after their seizures are controlled. Lavage can also be used in patients who refuse to take syrup of ipecac. A simpler method in these cases however, is to introduce the ipecac and water into the stomach via a small nasogastric tube.

Early reports comparing ipecac with lavage concluded that ipecac removes more gastric contents than does lavage (29–32). In all of these reports, lavage tubes considerably smaller than the 26-50 French (Fr) (8.7–16.7 mm) orogastric tubes currently recommended were used. Although objective evidence is not available, the larger tubes should empty the stomach much more thoroughly than the smaller tubes. However, the administration of syrup of ipecac is easier and less traumatic than lavage, and until objective evidence is available to demonstrate the superiority of lavage with a large bore tube over ipecac-induced emesis, it is the preferred method for removing gastric contents.

Various fluids have been used for gastric lavage. The advantages and disadvantages of water, normal saline, and sodium bicarbonate are:

Water. In most cases, the composition of the lavage fluid is not as important as the amount of fluid instilled. For this reason, tap water is commonly used. Children have a limited tolerance to electrolyte-free solution; a 5% increase in total body fluid with electrolyte-free solutions is sufficient to produce water intoxication and seizures. In most instances, water is a safe, useful lavage fluid; however, it may be safer to use normal saline or half-normal saline solution in young children.

Normal Saline is the preferred solution for routine use. It is as effective as water and safer. A patient who has taken a large amount of salt as an emetic and has not vomited should be lavaged with water. If silver nitrate is the toxin, normal saline is especially useful, because it precipitates the silver as silver chloride, an insoluble non-corrosive salt.

Sodium bicarbonate should not be used to neutralize an acid ingestion. A 5% solution of sodium bicarbonate or sodium dihydrogen phosphate may be useful for ferrous salt ingestions, since the less corrosive, more insoluble salts, ferrous carbonate and ferrous phosphate, are produced. Whether these fluids produce a significant reduction in GI irritation and iron absorption is difficult to determine from the evidence available.

Lavage or emesis may be useful several hours after ingestion.

In some cases, large numbers of tablets ingested over a short period of time may mass to form a concretion in the stomach. Even soluble drugs may form such a mass. Examples of drugs whose ingestion has caused concretions include glutethimide, barbiturates, aspirin, and meprobamate (33). Since such a mass of tablets dissolves and is absorbed slowly, gastric emptying may be useful even several hours after ingestion. If lavage is to be useful in this situation, a large bore lavage tube must be used. Certain agents, such as methyl salicylate and anticholinergics, delay stomach emptying. This effect delays absorption so that tablets remain in the stomach for a longer period of time. Thus, lavage may be effective long after the ingestion of these agents. The kinetics of absorption for most drugs in the overdose situation have not been studied. One must interpret absorption kinetics data which are based on therapeutic doses with caution when applying them to the overdose situation.

Adsorbents. Adsorbents are used clinically to bind unabsorbed poisons in the gastrointestinal tract. Although other substances have been used, activated charcoal is the most effective. To be effective, it must have a large surface area (usually around 1,000 m^2/gm), be of vegetable origin, and have a low ash content. Charcoal tablets are ineffective because their particle size is too large; thus, their surface area is too small.

Although some feel activated charcoal is an effective local antidote for virtually all organic or inorganic compounds and cite cyanide as the only exception, it is generally felt that it is relatively ineffective in poisonings due to ethanol, methanol, caustic alkalies, and mineral acids (34). A recent presentation suggests, however, that activated charcoal significantly reduces the absorption of ethanol orally administered to dogs (35).

The proper dose of activated charcoal is five to ten times, by weight, the amount of the ingested agent (34). Since the amount of the ingested agent taken is not usually accurately known and activated charcoal is non-toxic, two or more ounces of activated charcoal are mixed with water and administered as a slurry by mouth or via a lavage tube. Some recommend routine doses as high as 100 grams. One ounce of activated charcoal is approximately five or six tablespoonfuls. However, since the density of various activated charcoal preparations is quite different, it is advisable that the desired amount be weighed out ahead of time and prepackaged for use in the emergency room.

Several investigators have attempted to enhance the palatability of activated charcoal. Carboxymethylcellulose has been added as a suspending agent. Various investigators have arrived at differing conclusions as to whether the carboxymethylcellulose impairs adsorption by the charcoal (36). Sweetening agents such as saccharin, sorbitol, and sucrose have been effective at improving palatability without reducing adsorptive capacity (37–39). Two promising developments are medicoal, an effervescent charcoal preparation which is available in Great Britain and experimental high surface area charcoal, Amoco PX21 and PX23 (37,40–42).

The universal antidote has previously been recommended as an adsorbent. The medical formulation for the universal antidote, activated charcoal, tannic acid and magnesium oxide, has been shown to be less effective than activated charcoal alone (43). The home remedy consisting of burnt toast, tea, and milk of magnesia is even more questionable since burnt toast is not an effective adsorbent.

Activated charcoal effectively adsorbs ipecac (44). This renders the ipecac completely ineffective and decreases the adsorptive capacity of the activated charcoal. If activated charcoal and ipecac are to be used together, the charcoal must be given after vomiting has been induced by the ipecac.

Cathartics. Cathartics are recommended to hasten the travel of charcoal-drug complex through the GI tract and prevent further adsorption. The saline cathartics are generally recommended for this purpose. Objective evidence of the effectiveness of cathartics in this instance is not available.

Magnesium sulfate (Epsom Salt) is an effective saline cathartic which is renally excreted. It should not be used if renal function is impaired, because magnesium intoxication may occur. An appropriate dose is 250 mg/kg for children and 15 grams for adults. The dose must be diluted to prevent vomiting. Onset of catharsis is usually within a few hours.

Sodium sulfate (Glauber's Salts), a saline cathartic, is the safest available agent for routine use. Hypernatremia or fluid imbalances may develop secondary to its use, but overall, it is less toxic than magnesium sulfate. The dosage is the same as magnesium sulfate. Alternatively, one-half to one ounce of Fleet's Phospho-Soda (sodium phosphate/sodium biphosphate) may be diluted in a 1:4 solution.

Cathartic oils (such as castor oil) may increase the absorption of fat-soluble agents such as the chlorinated insecticides and therefore should be avoided. In addition, aspiration of the cathartic oil may occur, particularly in patients with CNS depression. Castor oil, one to four ounces, is useful in phenol poisoning because phenol is highly soluble in oil. A saline cathartic may be given after the administration of the castor oil.

Vegetable cathartics, such as cascara and aloes should never be used in poisoning cases, because they are slower in onset and are generally less effective. Sorbitol may be used if saline cathartics are unavailable. Cathartics should not be used in patients who have ingested caustics or in those who have electrolyte imbalances or are hypovolemic.

Enhancement of Excretion

Following absorption, the excretion of some agents can be enhanced by procedures such as forced diuresis, manipulation of urinary pH, hemodialysis, peritoneal dialysis, and hemoperfusion.

Diuresis. Water diuresis is only minimally effective at enhancing renal excretion in most cases. A water load only increases flow through the distal renal tubules and the collecting ducts. However, since passive solute resorption occurs primarily in the proximal tubules, water resorption must be minimized at this site. Osmotic diuretics are far more efficacious, because they increase the excretion rate of many compounds that are passively reabsorbed (eg, salicylates, phenobarbital). The excretion of these agents may be further enhanced by alkalinization of the urine. Mannitol is the most commonly recommended osmotic diuretic. Fluids and osmotic diuretics must be used with caution. Care must be taken not to volume overload the patient and produce pulmonary or cerebral edema.

Following a test dose, adults are usually given mannitol 25 gm IV rapidly to start diuresis. Diuresis is maintained by administering 1.5 gm/kg/day of a 20% solution, up to maximum dose of 100 gm. One aims for an increase in urine output to approximately 3–6 ml/kg/hr.

Urinary pH. Manipulation of urinary pH is sometimes useful as a method of enhancing excretion. Acidification is appropriate for some weak bases and alkalinization for some weak acids.

For tubular reabsorption to occur, the substance must be in the unionized form. If the urinary pH were changed so that more of the compound was in the ionized form, reabsorption would be decreased and excretion would be increased. Using phenobarbital and the Henderson-Hasselbach Equation as an example to describe this effect, approximately 9% of phenobarbital (which has a pK_a of 7.24) is in the unionized, reabsorbable form at pH 6.24:

$$pH = pK_a + \log (A^-)/(HA)$$

$$6.24 = 7.24 + \log (A^-)/(HA)$$

$$(A^-)/(HA) = 0.1$$

However, approximately 90% of the phenobarbital is in the ionized nonreabsorbable form when the urine pH is 8.24, because the ratio of $(A^-)/(HA)$ then becomes 10. Raising the pH to 8.24 is clearly impractical. Generally one aims for a pH of 7–8 for alkalinization, and a pH of 4.5–5.5 for acidification.

This manipulation of urinary pH should increase the excretion significantly. For some agents, particularly salicylates, achievement of an alkaline urine can be quite difficult. In addition one must be concerned about acid-base, fluid and electrolyte problems that may be produced by this procedure.

Dialysis. In dialysis, unwanted plasma solutes diffuse across a semipermeable membrane into a dialysis solution. The dialysis fluid is formulated to allow diffusion of the unwanted agents, nonessential electrolytes, and chemicals. Two basic types of dialysis exist. In peritoneal dialysis, the patient's peritoneum is utilized as the dialysis membrane. In extracorporeal hemodialysis, cellulose serves as the membrane.

Dialysis should not generally be used unless a potentially fatal dose of a dialyzable drug has been ingested by a patient who would not be expected to survive with less heroic measures. Dialysis is also indicated when metabolism of the ingested compound yields a more toxic substance (for example, methanol to formaldehyde; ethylene glycol to oxalic acid) and rapid removal will decrease the amount metabolized.

The main differences between hemodialysis and peritoneal dialysis involve efficiency, availability, and complexity. Peritoneal dialysis is available at most treatment centers and can be performed by health professionals with little special training. Clearance rates for peritoneal dialysis are at best 20% of those achieved by extracorporeal hemodialysis. Although hemodialysis is more efficient, it is generally only available at large referral centers.

Hemoperfusion. Hemoperfusion is a procedure in which blood is passed through adsorbent materials including charcoal and resins. Blood is pumped through a column where it comes in direct contact with the adsorbent material and is then returned to the patient. Charcoal emboli, thrombocytopenia, and leukopenia have been associated with charcoal adsorbents; however, coating the charcoal with various substances has successfully prevented many of these problems. Charcoal hemoperfusion may be three times more efficient than hemodialysis in clearing glutethimide and long acting barbiturates and six times more efficient in clearing short acting barbiturates (45).

Criteria for the use of hemoperfusion remain somewhat controversial. In reviewing reports of the effectiveness of hemoperfusion, one must examine more than clearance values, and look at the amount, or percent, of the total body burden removed, and even more important, the effect on morbidity and mortality. This is particularly true for agents with a high volume of distribution, where one can see high values for clearance but removal of a small percentage of the total body burden.

POISONOUS PLANTS

The ingestion of plants by children is a major cause of poisoning morbidity in the United States today, although death from these ingestions is extremely rare. The most commonly ingested group of plants are those that contain *insoluble oxalates*. The diffenbachias and philodendrons, which are common ornamental house plants, contain insoluble oxalates as well as several other proteinaceous substances. Upon contact with the oral membranes, an intense burning sensation with swelling and erythema is produced. The intense burning is treated by removal of any plant debris from the mouth and by application of cool packs to decrease pain and swelling. If the tongue is involved and begins to swell, the patient should be moved immediately to a medical facility, because extensive swelling of the tongue may produce suffocation. Other plants capable of producing this syndrome include elephant's ear, skunk cabbage, rhubarb leaves, and caladium.

Poisonous plants can be grouped in accordance with the toxic substances that they contain:

Amygdalin-containing plants (50) produce cyanide poisoning. Examples: seeds of peach, pear, apple, apricot, bitter almond.

Anticholinergic-containing plants (51) produce atropine-like anti-cholinergic effects. Examples: Jimson weed, deadly nightshade, potato leaves and sprouts.

Cardiac glycoside-containing plants (52) produce digitalis-like effects on the heart. Examples: foxglove, lily of the valley, oleander.

Colchicine-containing plants (53) produce severe gastrointestinal symptoms with seizures, CNS depression, and bone marrow suppression. Examples: autumn crocus, glory lily.

Nicotine-containing plants (54) produce acute nicotine poisoning. Examples: tobacco, poison hemlock, arnica root, fool's parsley.

Oxalate-containing plants (55): The insoluble oxalate group produces pain, swelling, and erythema of mucous membranes. The soluble oxalate group produces hypocalcemia, gastroenteritis, and oxalate crystalluria. Soluble examples: American ivy, rhubarb leaves, garden sorrel, virginia creeper. Insoluble examples: dieffenbachia, philodendron, caladium, elephant's ear.

Solanine-containing plants (56) produce severe gastroenteritis, bradycardia, fever, muscle weakness, and renal failure. Examples: Jerusalem cherry, black nightshade, jessamine.

Stimulant-containing plants (57) produce CNS excitation with seizures. Examples: water hemlock.

Toxalbumin-containing plants (58) produce severe gastrointestinal burns, shock, hepatic necrosis, and renal failure. Examples: castor bean, jequirity bean, black locust.

SALICYLATES

1. Patient D.B. is a 12 kg, 2-year-old girl who is brought to the emergency room by her parents approximately five hours after being found playing with a half-empty 100-tablet bottle of adult aspirin. Upon arrival at the emergency room she is hyperventilating (respiratory rate of 42 per minute), has a rectal temperature of 101.8°F, a blood pressure of 92/58mm Hg, and a pulse of 125/min. What initial laboratory information should be obtained?

Tests should be ordered to assess the acid-base and fluid and electrolyte status of the patient (arterial blood gasses, pH, bicarbonate, and electrolytes). Determination of BUN and glucose are also important; dehydration is frequently a problem, and hypo- and hyperglycemia may occur.

The presence of salicylate in the urine may be qualitatively determined with either ferric chloride or Phenistix. Either of these tests can be performed quite rapidly in the emergency room; however, they are not always accurate and false positive reactions can occur. A serum salicylate level (Question 6) is much more useful than these qualitative methods and is readily available in most hospitals.

2. How should this patient be treated initially?

Gastric removal may be useful as long as 10 hours after the ingestion of aspirin (even longer for methyl salicylate) (61). Emesis is the treatment of choice unless the patient is deeply sedated or convulsing. If either of these symptoms are present or if syrup of ipecac has been given and emesis has not occurred, the patient should be lavaged with normal saline solution until the returns are clear by the ferric chloride test. Activated charcoal effectively adsorbs aspirin and should be administered after lavage or emesis and followed by a saline cathartic (62).

D.B. was given 15 ml of syrup of ipecac and vomited approximately 20 minutes later. A white powder and large tablet fragments were observed in the vomitus. After emesis, 30 gm of activated charcoal was given as a slurry and followed by 3 gm of magnesium sulfate.

3. What is the cause of this patient's hyperpyrexia and how should it be treated?

Salicylates uncouple oxidative phosphorylation. Although oxidation continues, the formation of ATP is blocked. The energy that normally would go into ATP is released primarily as heat. Temperature elevation can be profound and is most seriously a problem in young children.

Clearly, salicylates should not be given to combat hyperpyrexia. This can be a problem in patients with unrecognized salicylism who are given salicylates to control their fever. Since the hyperpyrexia is not central in origin, other antipyretics, such as acetaminophen, would not be expected to be helpful. Hyperthermia should be treated with sponge bathing or a cooling blanket. Alcohol sponging should be avoided, because it may produce acute alcohol intoxication.

4. The results of D.B.'s initial laboratory work were reported as follows: pH 7.50; pO_2 110 mm Hg; pCO_2 25 mm Hg; bicarbonate 18 mEq/L, potassium 3.2 mEq/L; BUN 30 mg/dl; glucose 85 mg/dl. Explain this patient's acid-base status. Are these acid-base abnormalities typical of those seen in children and adults following an acute salicylate poisoning?

This patient's respiratory alkalosis is consistent with that normally seen in acute salicylate ingestions. Hyperpnea and tachypnea occur as a result of increased CO_2 production and a direct stimulatory effect of salicylate on the respiratory center. This causes the pCO_2 to drop and thus produces a respiratory alkalosis. This effect is commonly seen in both children and adults. In children, and some severely poisoned adults, either a mixed respiratory alkalosis with metabolic acidosis or a metabolic acidosis develop, generally within 12–24 hours after ingestion. The major cause of this acidosis is the accumulation of organic acid ions and a reduction in plasma bicarbonate. Many of these organic acids, such as acetoacetate and β-hydroxybutyrate, are formed or accumulate secondary to metabolic effects of salicylate (uncoupling of oxidative phosphorylation, inhibition of dehydrogenases and aminotransferases).

5. D.B.'s plasma glucose (85 mg/dl) was within normal limits. How do large doses of salicylate affect carbohydrate metabolism? Why should glucose be included in her IV fluids?

In young children and in diabetic adults, one commonly sees hypoglycemia in salicylate poisoning. Although several mechanisms have been proposed, the hypoglycemia is most likely related to an increased rate of tissue glycolysis and a decrease in glucose synthesis from noncarbohydrate precursors (63). Salicylates also increase hepatic glycogenolysis which, in the presence of adequate glycogen stores, normally produces a hyperglycemia. Since infants have lower glycogen stores, hypoglycemia predominates. Other effects that increase plasma glucose include adrenal medullary and cortical stimulation, causing a release of epinephrine and corticosteroids.

Although D.B.'s plasma glucose of 85 mg/dl is within the normal range, it has been clearly shown in mice that high doses of salicylate rapidly decrease brain glucose levels to one-third of control values (64). Because this child may go on to develop hypoglycemia and because her brain glucose level may be low, glucose should be included in all of her IV fluids.

6. A serum salicylate sample obtained 6 hours after D.B.'s ingestion was reported as 90 mg/dl. How can this salicylate level be used to assess the severity of D.B.'s ingestion?

This serum salicylate level can be used to estimate a peak serum salicylate level which is then compared with published categories of severity of ingestion. The peak serum salicylate level (S_0) can be determined from a nomogram developed by Done or can be calculated as follows: $\log S_0 = \log S + 0.015 T$, where S_0 is the hypothetical peak salicylate level at time zero, S is the measured

salicylate level, and T is the time after ingestion that the blood level was drawn. Using this equation, D.B.'s S_0 value is 110; therefore, this is a severe ingestion (59):

S_0	Severity
<50	Not intoxicated
50–80	Mild
80–100	Moderate
>110	Severe
>160	Usually lethal

Levels which are drawn less than 6 hours after ingestion are not useful, since peak absorption has probably not occurred. Although both the above calculation and the nomogram are based on first-order kinetics, a process which is not truly applicable at high salicylate concentrations, the S_0 is clinically useful in the assessment of salicylate ingestions.

7. Eighteen hours after ingestion, D.B. continues to hyperventilate; her respiratory rate is 48/min. She is severely lethargic and has vomited twice in the past 12 hours. Her rectal temperature is 102° F. Laboratory values at this time are: pH 7.30, pO₂ 100 mm Hg, pCO₂ 20 mm Hg, bicarbonate 10 mEq/L, potassium 4.0 mEq/L, BUN 28 mg/dl, glucose 95 mg/dl, and salicylate 85 mg/dl. Why has her serum salicylate not decreased to a greater extent? What should be done?

At high serum concentrations, two of the five salicylate excretion pathways become saturated (see chapter on Rheumatic Diseases), and excretion follows zero-order kinetics. Nevertheless, one would still expect a greater decrease in the serum salicylate level than has occurred in D.B. This may indicate that she is not excreting salicylate at a normal rate, or she may still be absorbing it. Both prevention of further absorption and enhancement of excretion should be attempted. Based on the possibility that an aspirin mass had formed in her gastrointestinal tract, D.B. was relavaged, and activated charcoal was repeated. The enhancement of salicylate excretion is discussed in Question 8.

8. How can the excretion of salicylate be enhanced? What would be appropriate for this patient?

Exchange transfusion, forced diuresis with alkalinization of the urine, hemodialysis, peritoneal dialysis, and hemoperfusion have all been shown to significantly enhance the excretion of salicylate.

Exchange Transfusion. Exchanging 1.7–3.1 blood volumes in dogs given a large intravenous dose of salicylate reduced salicylate levels by 49% and removed 13.3–22.8% of the injected dose (68). Similarly, exchange transfusion of seven salicylate-poisoned children reduced salicylate levels by an average of 48% (69). Exchange transfusion is only practical in infants and has generally been replaced by other methods.

Alkalinization of the Urine. Alkalinization of the urine significantly increases the amount of salicylate excreted. Since salicylate is reabsorbed in the kidney, increasing the urine pH will increase the amount of salicylate in the ionized form, thus inhibiting reabsorption and enhancing excretion. In a group of 18 salicylate-poisoned children, an increase of the mean urine pH from 6.1 to 7.8 with bicarbonate resulted in a nearly three-fold decrease in the interval during which the mean serum salicylate fell 50% (6.1 hours as compared with 17.2 hours in untreated children) (70). The concentration of salicylate in the urine increased three-fold because of the increase in urinary pH (70). A similiar study demonstrated a five-fold increase in the rate of salicylate excretion in the urine when the urinary pH was raised from 5.40–9.90 to 7.65–8.11 (71). It is difficult, if not impossible, to achieve an alkaline urine in patients who are hypokalemic. There is additional concern that forcing fluids in these patients will increase the risk of the development of pulmonary edema as well as further complicate therapy aimed at correcting acid-base and electrolyte problems. The method of choice to alkalinize the urine is intravenous sodium bicarbonate to raise the urine pH to between 7.0 and 8.0. Acetazolamide should be avoided. Even though it will alkalinize the urine, it does so at the expense of worsening acidemia.

Dialysis. Hemodialysis is approximately twice as efficient at removing salicylate as forced diuresis (69). Peritoneal dialysis, particularly if 5% albumin is added to the dialysate, enhances excretion but less so than hemodialysis (68). Hemoperfusion removes salicylate about as efficiently as hemodialysis and more efficiently than alkaline diuresis, although hemoperfusion is less efficient at correcting the metabolic complications of salicylate poisoning than hemodialysis (72). Dialysis or hemoperfusion is generally considered in patients with renal failure or those with severe symptoms and very high blood levels who are not responding to conservative therapy.

Treatment Summary. Dialysis was considered for D.B.; however, since her renal function did not appear to be impaired, it was decided that forced alkaline diuresis would be tried first with IV fluids containing dextrose, potassium, and bicarbonate. Furosemide 12 mg was given and the urine pH and volume were monitored. Urine pH was maintained between 6.8 and 7.4. The salicylate level 24 hours after ingestion was determined to be 60 mg/dl. Administration of sodium bicarbonate also raised the serum pH to 7.41. Forced alkaline diuresis was continued for an additional six hours and then discontinued. D.B. continued to do well throughout her hospital course and was discharged on the fourth hospital day.

9. What other symptoms might be anticipated in a severe salicylate ingestion?

Although rare, pulmonary edema is a significant morbid event. It has been demonstrated that the pulmonary edema is non-cardiac in nature (65) and is related to an increase in pulmonary vascular permeability to protein (66).

Acute renal failure has been reported in acute salicylate intoxication. The presence of azotemia and oliguria may, however, be related to non-renal causes such as dehydration from hyperventilation, sweating, or vomiting. Proteinurea may be caused by increased vascular permeability in the kidneys, a similar effect to that seen in the lungs. Aminoaciduria may be due to the inability of the kidney to reabsorb filtered amino acids; uncoupling of oxidative phosphorylation and the resultant lack of ATP impairs energy-dependent reabsorption. The fluid retention that has been reported in salicylate poisoning may be related to inappropriate ADH secretion (67).

Salicylate-induced hypoprothrombinemia may occur; it is responsive to vitamin K.

In many fatal ingestions, marked CNS depression (manifested by coma and respiratory failure) occurs. Convulsions may occur in some patients. Although the mechanism for the CNS depression has not been elucidated, possible explanations include hypercapnia, hypoglycemia, and alteration of the glutamate/GABA ratio.

10. What is methyl salicylate, and how does it differ from aspirin?

Methyl salicylate (oil of wintergreen) is used in a variety of external products, most commonly liniments. Although it is quite similar toxicologically to aspirin, it is absorbed more slowly. Five ml of methyl salicylate is equivalent to approximately 21.7 adult aspirin tablets, or 7.05 gm of aspirin.

ACETAMINOPHEN

Acetaminophen (N-acetyl-p-aminophenol) is metabolized in the liver by non-cytochrome P450 enzyme systems and excreted. The major pathway involves conjugation to the glucuronide or sulfate (73). A small percentage is metabolized by the hepatic cytochrome P450 mixed function oxidase system to an active intermediate metabolite, perhaps the N-hydroxyl or N-oxime, that is normally conjugated with glutathione and excreted (74). When large doses of acetaminophen are taken, saturation of the sulfate and glucuronide pathways occur, more of the active intermediate is formed, and stores of glutathione are not sufficient to allow for conjugation and excretion. Levels of the intermediate metabolite increase, and this metabolite binds covalently to hepatocytes and produces hepatic necrosis (75).

11. R.J., a 15-year-old, 50 kg female is brought to the emergency room at 1:00 a.m. complaining of nausea and vomiting. These symptoms began approximately two hours earlier. She admits to taking 35 five-grain acetaminophen tablets at approximately 7:00 p.m. the evening prior to admission. The patient appears slightly lethargic, but all vital signs are within normal limits. Is the dose of acetaminophen that was taken by this patient consistent with the production of hepatic necrosis?

Acute ingestions of more than 7.5 gm of acetaminophen in adults or children over 12 are thought to be consistent with the production of hepatic necrosis (76). However, considerable variability exists. This patient weighs 50 kg and by history took 35 five-grain tablets. This is a total dose of 11.3 gm or approximately 227 mg/kg, an amount consistent with the production of hepatic necrosis.

12. A blood sample for serum acetaminophen was drawn one hour after admission (approximately seven hours after the ingestion); the serum level was later reported to be 320 mcg/ml. How should this serum level be interpreted?

Blood levels can be used to predict outcome. Early work suggested that patients with blood levels of 300 mcg/ml or greater at 4 hours postingestion consistently developed hepatic necrosis; those with levels of 120 mcg/ml at 4 hours postingestion consistently did not (77). Prediction of outcome was difficult at levels between 120–300 mcg/ml. Since that time, several nomograms have been developed for evaluation of blood levels at various times after ingestion to predict whether or not toxicity would occur (76,77). This patient's blood level is consistent with the development of hepatic necrosis on each of these nomograms.

13. How should this patient be treated?
Prevention of Absorption. The methods for decreasing absorption discussed earlier in this chapter are appropriate for acetaminophen ingestions. Since significant CNS depression and loss of gag reflex are absent in this patient, there would be no danger in administering syrup of ipecac as an emetic. However, it has been six hours since the ingestion, and acetaminophen, at least with therapeutic doses, appears to be rapidly absorbed. Thus, the likelihood of removing a large amount of acetaminophen from this patient's stomach at this time is small. Activated charcoal effectively binds acetaminophen if given soon after ingestion (79). There is, however, considerable concern that charcoal will adsorb the oral glutathione-like antidotes for acetaminophen poisoning. Two *in vitro* studies have demonstrated significant antidote adsorption by activated charcoal (80,81). However, one *in vivo* study in three adult volunteers seemed to indicate that significant adsorption did not occur (82). Until this issue is resolved, it is generally felt that activated charcoal should not be used.

Antidotes. Since it is the lack of glutathione that prevents metabolism and excretion of the toxic metabolite, administration of glutathione would be expected to decrease the toxicity of large doses of acetaminophen. However, administered glutathione does not enter cells readily and, thus, will not prevent the hepatic necrosis (78). Glutathione precursors, such as *cysteine,* and other nucleophilic sulfhydryl-containing compounds, such as *cysteamine,* have been investigated as potential glutathione substitutes. Intravenously administered cysteamine has been shown to be quite effective in preventing hepatic necrosis from large doses of acetaminophen if given within 10 hours of ingestion (78). Because of the lack of a sterile dosage form, toxicity, and availability of better agents, the use of cysteamine has been abandoned.

Methionine, another glutathione precursor, has been shown to be effective in preventing acetaminophen-induced hepatic necrosis (83–85). It too should be given within 10 hours after the ingestion. Methionine can be given orally. L-methionine is available in powder form and dl-methionine is available commercially in capsules and as a liquid (Pedameth). Since only the l-isomer is effective, a higher dose must be given if the racemic mixture is used. As the use of N-acetylcysteine has increased, methionine use in the United States has fallen into disfavor. N-acetylcystine, another investigational agent, is more readily available since it is routinely stocked in most hospital pharmacies.

N-acetylcysteine is also effective in the treatment of acetaminophen overdose. In mice, which develop acetaminophen-induced hepatic necrosis more quickly than humans, N-acetylcysteine is clearly superior to cysteamine (86). In the first reported human use of N-acetylcysteine, a 32-year-old, 75 kg man who had taken 60 gm of acetaminophen was given N-acetylcysteine 15 hours after ingestion and survived (87). N-acetylcysteine is given orally or by lavage tube in an initial dose of 140 mg/kg and then 70 mg/kg every four hours for 68 hours (88). N-acetylcysteine by this protocol appears to effectively prevent hepatic necrosis in most patients. No deaths were seen in 148 patients with blood levels in the probable or late probable risk categories where treatment was begun within 24 hours of ingestion (89). An IND for this agent has been issued. Contact the Rocky Mountain Poison Center at (800) 525-6115 for further information on this protocol.

Although *BAL* and *d-penicillamine,* two other sulfhydryl-containing compounds, are also available for use in the United States and have been suggested for use in acetaminophen poisoning, their effectiveness in preventing acetaminophen-induced hepatic necrosis has not been demonstrated.

Since this patient had by history taken more than 7.5 grams of acetaminophen, she was given an oral loading dose of 7 grams (140 mg/kg) of N-acetylcysteine at approximately 2:00 a.m. The decision was made to continue therapy with N-acetylcysteine when the acetaminophen level was found to be in the range where one would expect hepatic toxicity to occur.

14. At approximately 2:30 a.m. (30 minutes after the loading dose of N-acetylcysteine), R.J. vomited; the vomitus had the characteristic smell of N-acetylcysteine. What should be done at this time?

Doses of N-acetylcysteine which are vomited within one hour after administration should be repeated. It is thought that chilling the N-acetylcysteine solution reduces GI irritation and prevents vomiting, although objective evidence documenting this effect is not available. If vomiting continues to be a problem, N-acetylcysteine can be administered via duodenal intubation.

R.J. was given a repeat loading dose which was tolerated without further vomiting. Subsequent maintenance doses were also well tolerated.

15. Since oral administration of N-acetylcysteine frequently produces severe vomiting which can limit oral absorption, can it be given intravenously?

In a series of 100 patients treated with intravenous N-acetylcysteine, results were excellent when treatment was begun within 10 hours after acetaminophen ingestion (2% developed severe liver damage). However, more than half of the patients who were treated between 10 and 24 hours after acetaminophen ingestion developed severe liver damage, an incidence comparable with previously reported controls. The dosage was 150 mg/kg over 15 minutes, followed by 50 mg/kg over 4 hours, and then 100 mg/kg over the next 16 hours (90). A pyrogen-tested sterile preparation for intravenous use is not available in the U.S., although the sterile preparation for intrabronchial use has been employed on occasion. Anaphylactoid reactions have been reported (91).

16. Since this patient has a high acetaminophen level, should hemodialysis or hemoperfusion be considered?

Although hemodialysis decreases the acetaminophen excretion half-life (92), there is no evidence that this decreases mortality. This is not unexpected since both the toxic metabolite and damage to the liver are produced quickly; thus, the possibility of removing enough acetaminophen quickly enough to decrease production of the metabolite is unlikely. In addition, since the toxic metabolite is produced intracellularly, it is not removed by dialysis. Likewise, hemoperfusion would not be helpful.

17. Throughout the day, R.J. became progressively more lethargic until approximately 18 hours after admission, when her state of consciousness began to improve. On the second day after admission, the patient was alert, coherent, and well oriented. Pertinent laboratory findings at that time were: SGOT 378 units/ml (nl 5–40), SGPT 606 units/ml (nl 5–35), LDH 119 units/ml (nl 200–450), total bilirubin 1.2 mg/dl (nl 0.3–1.1), and a second acetaminophen level drawn 22 hours after admission was reported to be 6.2 mcg/ml.

Since a second acetaminophen level is available, would calculation of an excretion half-life be useful?

Until recently, it was felt that the excretion half-life of acetaminophen was a better predictor of whether or not toxicity would occur than a single blood level (77). Those patients with a half-life of greater than four hours were expected to develop hepatic toxicity, whereas those with half-lives close to normal (two hours) would not. The use of the half-life has fallen into disfavor. Most feel that the half-life is not a good predictor. This might be expected because acetaminophen metabolism is not first order at high blood levels. In addition, it is difficult in most instances to obtain two blood levels spaced widely enough apart to be useful to make a treatment decision. This is particularly true in this case since the second acetaminophen level was not reported back until the morning of the second day.

CLONIDINE

18. A 3-year-old boy ingested 1.5 mg of clonidine approximately two hours ago. He is semiconscious and has irregular respirations with occasional apneic episodes. Blood pressure is 92/58 mm Hg; heart rate is 65/min. Are these the symptoms that one would expect from a clonidine ingestion?

Clonidine acts on post-synaptic alpha receptors in the medulla, thereby reducing sympathetic tone and decreasing blood pressure. It also may cause a pressor response by direct stimula-

tion of peripheral alpha receptors. In acute overdose, the effects on blood pressure are variable. In a series of 170 acute clonidine overdoses, hypotension occurred in 21% of children and 32% of adults; hypertension occurred in 2% of the children and 11% of the adults; and the remainder were normotensive (93). Central nervous system depression is common and ranges from lethargy to coma. In the above study, respiratory depression occurred in 5% of the adults and 15% of the children (93). Intermittent apneic episodes may occur, as was seen in this patient, although they are not common. Seizures may also occur. Clonidine poisoning has been thoroughly reviewed by Conner and Watanabe (94).

19. What initial treatment should this patient receive?

Provision of supportive care is of primary importance. Because of his respiratory depression, he was intubated. Attempts at decreasing absorption are appropriate; in this case, the patient was lavaged rather than being given syrup of ipecac because he exhibited significant CNS depression. Activated charcoal was administered and followed by a saline cathartic. Although analeptics have been recommended in clonidine overdose, they should be avoided, as in all other ingestions.

20. Two hours later, his blood pressure dropped to 58/44 mm Hg. How are clonidine-induced abnormalities in blood pressure managed? How should this patient be treated?

Hypotension should be treated by placing the patient in the Trendelenburg position and by fluid therapy for volume expansion. If these maneuvers are not successful, dopamine should be considered. Since both hypotension and hypertension appear to be produced by alpha agonist activity, either centrally or peripherally, the use of alpha-blocking agents has been suggested. Tolazoline and phentolamine have been employed for this purpose (93,95) but have not been studied extensively. Therefore, the use of tolazoline and similar drugs is generally reserved for patients who remain unresponsive to fluids, positioning, and dopamine.

Hypertension, if it occurs and is severe enough to require treatment, will generally respond to furosemide and diazoxide (96). Care must be taken in hypertensive patients because they may later become hypotensive (94).

Although forced diuresis has been recommended to enhance excretion (96), it does not appear to be effective (97,98). Data on dialysis are not currently available.

This patient was placed in the Trendelenburg position and given IV fluids; as a result, his blood pressure increased to 84/52 mm Hg. Dopamine was considered initially but judged not to be necessary in this patient. Within 24 hours the patient was alert, breathing normally, and all vital signs were within normal limits.

PROPRANOLOL

21. A previously healthy 20-year-old woman was brought to the emergency room approximately 30 minutes after ingesting fifty 80 mg propranolol tablets (4.0 gm). She was lethargic upon arrival. Her blood pressure was 130/85 mm Hg, and her heart rate was 80/min. Shortly thereafter she had a grand mal seizure and became comatose; blood pressure was unobtainable, and her heart rate was 50/min. Are these symptoms consistent with propranolol overdose?

The predominant effects of propranolol are on the cardiovascular system and are produced by both beta-adrenergic blockade and a direct quinidine-like effect. Negative inotropic and chronotropic effects are produced. AV block as well as disturbances of ventricular function can be seen at high doses (99). Hypotension is common, and congestive heart failure may occur. Increased airway resistance, hypoglycemia, and seizures may also occur (99). GI effects such as nausea, vomiting, and diarrhea may also occur. The severity of the ingestion depends on the medical condition of the patient. Patients with chronic CHF or with preexisting conduction defects are more sensitive to small amounts of propranolol.

22. What treatment is appropriate in propranolol ingestions? How should this patient be treated?

In addition to prevention of absorption, the major goal of treatment is to correct conduction defects, bradycardia, hypotension, hypoglycemia, bronchoconstriction, and seizures. The methods generally used to enhance elimination do not appear to be effective with propranolol. Bradycardia is generally first treated with atropine. If unsuccessful, isoproterenol may be used; because of the beta blockade, larger than usual doses may be needed. Isoproterenol may produce peripheral vasodilation which can further reduce blood pressure; thus, it must be used cautiously. Glucagon has been used successfully in propranolol intoxicated patients and should be considered in patients unresponsive to isoproterenol (104). Glucagon, acting via the adenyl cyclase system, produces positive inotropic and chronotropic effects in the face of beta blockade. A transvenous pacemaker may be necessary in some patients if bradycardia or conduction disturbances cannot be otherwise controlled. Blood pressure is generally restored as other cardiovascular problems are corrected. Hypoglycemia can be corrected with either glucose or glucagon. Bronchoconstriction may require isoproterenol or theophylline. Intravenous diazepam should be used to control seizures.

A total of 1 mg of atropine was given to this patient which resulted in an increase in heart rate to 58 per minute with a slight increase in blood pressure. Three 0.5 mg boluses of epinephrine were given, followed by the institution of an isoproterenol infusion. The dose of isoproterenol was increased to 25 mcg per minute which resulted in a blood pressure of 130/90 mm Hg with a heart rate of 78/min. The isoproterenol infusion was continued for the next 48 hours, at which point she was adequately maintaining her blood pressure.

IRON

23. A 3-year-old boy was brought to the emergency room about 4 hours after ingesting an unknown number of his mother's ferrous sulfate tablets. He was lethargic on arrival, was vomiting spontaneously, and had profuse watery diarrhea. His blood pressure was 80/60 mm Hg; his pulse was 100 beats/min; and respirations were 30/min and regular. Are these symptoms consistent with iron poisoning? What other toxic effects might occur from this ingestion?

This patient's symptoms are typical of those observed in the early hours after iron poisoning. The clinical features of this poisoning are independent of the age of the patient and progress through five distinct phases (105).

Stage one occurs in the first six hours after the ingestion. Diarrhea, vomiting, and melena, caused by the direct irritative effects of iron, dominate this stage. This, along with the vasodilation produced by ferritin which is released from the gastrointestinal mucosa, may lead to shock. A direct depressant effect of iron on the brain or decreased brain perfusion may produce central nervous system depression, lethargy, or coma (106).

Stage two, a period of apparent improvement, occurs 6 to 24 hours after ingestion. The patient may fully recover or may progress to stage three.

Stage three is characterized by numerous metabolic derangements. Profound metabolic acidosis, secondary to interference with metabolism of organic acids, occurs and may be accentuated by loss of large amounts of bicarbonate in diarrheal fluids (107). Fever and leukocytosis result from the extensive gastrointestinal mucosal damage. Alterations in hemodynamics secondary to fluid loss may produce renal failure. Death occurs as a result of this multiplicity of factors. Stage three generally lasts from 12 to 48 hours.

If the patient survives stage three, he may progress to *stage four,* characterized by hepatic necrosis. This stage is seen two to four days after ingestion. Two to four weeks after ingestion, the *fifth phase* is observed and is characterized by scarring of the pylorus and stomach.

24. Approximately how many ferrous sulfate tablets would result in a severe poisoning of this child?

The toxic dose of iron has not been well established, but it is generally accepted that 1–2 gm of elemental iron will produce severe poisoning in a child of two to five years of age (108). Each 325 mg ferrous sulfate tablet contains 65 mg of elemental iron (Table 2); thus, approximately 15 tablets contain 1 gm of elemental iron. Children have been symptomatic after ingesting 300–400 mg of elemental iron, and a fatality has resulted from an ingestion of 65 mg/kg (109,110).

25. What can be done to retard the absorption of iron in this child?

If no contraindication exists, emesis should be induced with syrup of ipecac. As part of the fluids given with ipecac, 2–3 ounces of a 5% solution of either sodium dihydrogen phosphate or sodium bicarbonate should be given (108). The phosphate solution can be prepared by diluting one part of the contents of a Fleet's Enema with four parts of water. The phosphate solution converts the iron

Table 2.

IRON-CONTAINING PRODUCTS

Iron Product	Elemental Iron Content/Tablet
Ferrous sulfate 325 mg	65 mg
Ferrous gluconate 325 mg	39 mg
Ferrous fumarate 325 mg	105 mg
Prenatal vitamins with iron	40–60 mg
Adult multi-vitamins with iron	10–100 mg
Children's multi-vitamins with iron	3–25 mg

salt in the stomach to ferrous phosphate; the bicarbonate solution converts it to ferrous carbonate. Both of these iron salts are relatively insoluble and are poorly absorbed. If contraindications to emesis exist, lavage can be performed with a lavage fluid made by further dilution of the phosphate solution to approximately 2% or with a sodium bicarbonate solution. This fluid should be allowed to remain in the stomach. The phosphate solution also acts as a cathartic which will hasten the movement of any unabsorbed iron through the gastrointestinal tract.

The use of more concentrated phosphate solutions in larger amounts has been associated with hyperphosphatemia and hypocalcemia (111,112).

26. The child was given syrup of ipecac along with 2 ounces of 5% dihydrogen phosphate solution. He vomited forcefully several times, and the vomitus contained many partially disintegrated iron tablets. How can the severity of his iron poisoning be assessed?

Abdominal X-Ray. Iron tablets are radiopaque and will, therefore, visualize on x-ray. An abdominal x-ray should be taken following emesis or lavage to determine the extent of removal. If iron is seen in the small bowel, cathartics should be given. If the tablets appear clumped and stuck in the stomach, surgical removal should be considered (113). Other radiopaque agents include chloral hydrate, heavy metals, and phenothiazines. These radiopaque drugs can more easily be remembered by utilization of the mnemonic CHIP, which represents Chloral hydrate, Heavy metals,

Iron, and Phenothiazines. An x-ray of this child's abdomen showed no remaining iron tablets after emesis.

Serum Iron. If possible, a serum iron and a total iron binding capacity (TIBC) should be performed in all iron poisonings. Since it is the unbound or "free" iron that is toxic, both tests are useful. However, because only a serum iron is available on an emergency basis in most hospitals, guidelines for therapy based on this parameter alone have been established. Patients with levels greater than 300 mcg/dl should be monitored closely. It is highly probable, in these cases, that the TIBC has been exceeded. Patients who have levels greater than 500 mcg/dl or who are in stage three of intoxication should be considered for chelation therapy with deferoxamine. Patients with levels between 300 and 500 mcg/dl may require only fluid replacement therapy (110).

Deferoxamine Chelation Test. For situations where serum iron levels are not available, the provocative deferoxamine chelation test has been proposed as a method for determining whether the TIBC has been exceeded (114). This procedure involves the administration of an intramuscular dose of deferoxamine and then observation of the patient's urine for the vin rose color characteristic of ferrioxamine. The presence of ferrioxamine in the urine indicates that there is free iron in the blood being chelated by the deferoxamine and excreted in the urine. The problem with this test is that the color of ferrioxamine in the urine is pH and concentration dependent (115), and the typical color may not always be seen, even in patients with high iron levels (116).

27. The serum iron level was reported to be 680 mcg/ml, and it was decided to begin chelation therapy with deferoxamine. How much should be given and how should it be administered?

Children and adults are usually given an initial deferoxamine dose of 1 gm followed by 500 mg every four hours for two doses. More may be given, but no more than 6 gm should be given in a 24 hour period. Deferoxamine is generally given intramuscularly unless the patient is in shock. In such cases, it should be given intravenously at a rate not to exceed 15 mg/kg/hr. A vin rose colored urine indicates the presence of the iron-deferox-

amine complex. Although orally administered deferoxamine will bind with iron in the stomach, this complex is absorbable. There is some evidence that the chelate may be toxic, and therefore, the oral use of deferoxamine is no longer suggested (117).

28. Are hemodialysis or peritoneal dialysis useful in the treatment of iron poisoning?

Dialysis is useful only as an adjunct to supportive care, particularly if renal failure is present. It does not remove iron at a rate faster than chelation therapy. Exchange transfusion may be useful (118).

BARBITURATES

29. A 23-year-old woman was brought to the emergency room by a paramedic crew after being found unconscious on the floor of her motel room. Found with her was an empty bottle labeled as pentobarbital 100 mg, 30 capsules, which was dispensed two days previously. Is it likely that this patient has taken a potentially lethal dose?

The lethal dose of a barbiturate depends upon its duration of action. For short and intermediate acting barbiturates (eg, pentobarbital), the lethal dose is estimated to be 3 gm; the estimated lethal dose for long acting barbiturates is about 5 gm. There is tremendous variability of response, however, and individuals who are tolerant to the effects of barbiturates can survive following much higher doses. This factor should also be considered when interpreting blood level information. For non-tolerant individuals, a potentially fatal blood level for short acting barbiturates is 3.5 mg/dl, and for long acting barbiturates it is 8–12 mg/dl (119). This patient's pentobarbital level was subsequently determined to be 3.6 mg/dl.

30. On arrival in the emergency room, she was unconscious with an airway in place and with assisted ventilation. Vital signs were blood pressure 60/? mm Hg, palpable, and pulse 110/min. Her pupils were dilated and sluggishly responsive to light. Neurologic examination showed absence of spinal and corneal reflexes. Pressure sores were present on the patient's forehead, left arm, and left leg. Are these symptoms typical of barbiturate overdose? How should she be treated?

Barbiturates are potent CNS depressants; thus, coma, hypotension, respiratory depression, and hypothermia are consistent with overdose. Blisters or pressure sores, as appeared in this case, are of assistance in the diagnosis of sedative hypnotic overdose. These are seen at areas where skin surfaces are pressured by the unconscious patient's body weight and usually occur within 4 hours of ingestion (120).

The cornerstone of treatment of barbiturate overdose is supportive care. Treatment should be aimed at supporting respirations and blood pressure. Vigorous fluid therapy probably does not alter the outcome of an overdose and is best avoided. Hypothermia should be treated with a heating blanket or by warming IV fluids. Hemodialysis will effectively remove phenobarbital after severe overdose, but it is not effective in removing short acting barbiturates. Hemoperfusion through charcoal or an aberlite resin column may be helpful in severe overdoses of all barbiturates (122).

31. Intravenous fluids and a dopamine drip were started, with a resultant increase in blood pressure to 100/80 mm Hg. Suction was used to remove vomitus from the trachea. The patient was then transferred to the medical intensive care unit where she was treated with supportive care including meticulous pulmonary toilet. Chest x-ray showed a left upper lobe infiltrate, and intravenous penicillin G was started. Her urine was found to be pH 6.5, and an intravenous infusion of sodium bicarbonate was begun in an attempt to increase the urine pH to 8.0.

The patient awoke about 12 hours after admission. About four hours later, she complained of breathing difficulty, and physical examination revealed coarse rales in both lung bases. Chest x-ray showed early pulmonary edema. The sodium bicarbonate infusion was stopped, and intravenous fluids were reduced to maintenance levels. The pulmonary edema resolved, and the patient made an uneventful recovery and was transferred to the psychiatry service after seven days of antibiotic therapy.

Why was the administration of sodium bicarbonate inappropriate for this patient?

Although significant fractions of the longer acting barbiturates are excreted unchanged in the urine, metabolic degradation is the primary means of elimination of the shorter acting barbiturates.

Urinary alkalinization is useful only for phenobarbital, which has one of the lowest pka's of the barbiturates; it is unlikely to be very effective in enhancing pentobarbital excretion.

The major complications of vigorous attempts at urinary alkalinization are hypernatremia, fluid overload, and pulmonary edema. As shown in this case, such treatment may complicate therapy and prolong hospitalization. In one study, pulmonary edema from attempted urinary alkalinization was a frequent complication of barbiturate overdose; aspiration pneumonia was the only complication that occurred more frequently (123).

OPIATES

32. A 28-year-old, 55 kg female was brought into the emergency room after a narcotic overdose. She was apneic, hypotensive, and unconscious. After being given 0.8 mg of naloxone intravenously, she began to breathe on her own and responded to painful stimuli. Five minutes later, an additional 0.4 mg of naloxone was given. At this point she woke up and her respiratory rate increased to 20/minute. Upon awaking the patient admitted to taking her normal daily methadone dose (80 mg) plus two take-home doses, a total of 240 mg orally. After initial stabilization she was moved from the emergency room to an adult medicine ward. Approximately two hours after the last dose of naloxone, a nurse found her apneic and unresponsive. Naloxone 0.8 mg was given again and she awoke and respirations resumed. Explain what happened to this patient.

Intravenously injected naloxone acts within minutes and usually within a few seconds. At best, its duration of action is from one to four hours (127). Clinically, it is often necessary to repeat administration as frequently as every 20–60 minutes to prevent symptoms from recurring (128).

The methadone that this patient had ingested was still present after the naloxone had been eliminated. It is critical that all patients receiving naloxone be carefully monitored and that doses be repeated as needed. (Also see the chapter entitled Drug Abuse.)

33. Did this patient display the characteristic clinical effects of an acute opiate intoxication?

Acute opiate exposure may produce coma and apnea. The degree of central nervous system and respiratory depression depends upon dose and tolerance. Although pinpoint pupils are common, anoxic patients may have dilated pupils. Hypotension, bradycardia, urinary retention, muscle spasm, hyperpyrexia, and leukocytosis may be seen (128). Pulmonary edema has been reported following parenteral or oral ingestions of opioids (129–131).

ANTICHOLINERGIC AND RELATED INGESTIONS

Any drug with anticholinergic effects or side effects can produce anticholinergic toxicity in overdose. Typical examples include antihistamines, antiparkinsonian drugs, antispasmodics, plants that contain belladonna alkaloids, and tricyclic antidepressants.

Tricyclic Antidepressants. In addition to the usual symptoms of anticholinergic toxicity, the tricyclic antidepressants produce a high incidence of cardiac arrhythmias in overdose; these are the usual cause of death in fatal overdoses. These arrhythmias are usually present early in the course of ingestion but may be delayed as long as six days after ingestion (133). Atrial tachycardia, nodal tachycardia, antioventricular block, intraventricular conduction delays, asystole, and other arrhythmias may be observed (113). Late in overdose, severe hypotension and bradycardia may occur. There appears to be a correlation between the duration of the QRS complex and plasma tricyclic antidepressant plasma levels; in one study, patients with high plasma levels had QRS durations of greater than 100 msec (135).

34. A 23-year-old woman was brought to the emergency room after ingesting an unknown amount of amitriptyline. She was comatose with an irregular heart rate of 190 beats/min and a blood pressure of 170/120 mm Hg. An electrocardiogram showed a sinus tachycardia with incomplete right bundle branch block. While the electrocardiogram was being done, she had a grand mal seizure. How should this poisoning be treated?

Physostigmine. This patient has developed several indications for the use of the anticholinesterase drug, physostigmine (136). An initial dose of physostigmine should be given to patients who have central or peripheral signs of anticholinergic toxicity plus one or more of the following: coma, convulsions, severe hallucinations, arrhythmias, and severe hypertension. This initial dose provides diagnostic assistance in that a positive response reinforces the diagnosis. Moreover, patients responding to this initial dose will continue to respond if repeated doses are deemed necessary. Repeated doses should be given to those patients who are experiencing seizures, arrhythmias, or hypertension. Coma and hallucinations are not indications for repeated administration of physostigmine. Coma, in these patients, usually lasts no longer than 24 hours and is not life-threatening. Hallucinations and delirium should be treated with physostigmine only if the patient becomes uncontrollable to the point of threatening injury to himself or others.

Because the antidotal action of physostigmine requires the accumulation of acetylcholine, the maximal effect is not seen until five to ten minutes after administration of the drug. The effect of physostigmine typically lasts from one to three hours; therefore, repeated doses of the drug may be necessary.

Physostigmine is not innocuous; its use carries the risk of inducing seizures and cholinergic crisis. It should not be used routinely.

Arrhythmias. There has been a great deal of debate on the role of physostigmine in the treatment of tricyclic antidepressant-induced cardiac arrhythmias. However, there is good clinical evidence to support its effectiveness in reversing both ventricular arrhythmias and myocardial conduction defects (137). Most clinicians reserve physostigmine for those instances when sodium bicarbonate (see below) fails.

The administration of sodium bicarbonate to increase the systemic blood pH to 7.50 to 7.55 has successfully reversed arrhythmias. The mechanism of this effect is unclear, but it is theorized that alkalinization of the blood increases plasma protein binding, reducing the amount of pharmacologically active free drug (138). Phenytoin has been used with limited success. Theoretically, it should increase A-V conduction while suppressing ventricular arrhythmias (139). Traditional antiarrhythmics such as quinidine and procainamide should be avoided because they add to tricyclic-induced myocardial depression. Lidocaine may be used because it produces less depression of the myocardium. Although propranolol has been advocated, it should be avoided because of its negative inotropic and chronotropic effect on the heart. Propranolol will also worsen the hypotension (137).

35. A decision is made to administer physostigmine; how much should be given, and how should it be administered?

The dose of physostigmine is (132):

Adult. Initial dose: 2 mg IV injected slowly (over at least 2 minutes). Repeat dose: 1–2 mg IV as needed until a desired positive response is achieved or cholinergic signs develop.

Pediatric. Initial dose: 0.5 mg IV injected slowly (over at least 2 minutes). Repeat dose: 0.5 mg is repeated every 5 minutes until the desired positive response is achieved or cholinergic signs develop.

Atropine in a dose one-half the amount of injected physostigmine should be kept on hand and administered if excessive cholinergic symptoms develop.

PETROLEUM DISTILLATES

36. A one-year-old boy is found with a bottle of Old English Furniture Polish; approximately one ounce missing. The child gagged and choked when he first swallowed it but is now asymptomatic except for an occasional cough. What is the hazard with this product? How should this child be managed?

This product contains mineral seal oil which is a petroleum distillate of low viscosity. Mineral seal oil, like many other petroleum distillates, is easily aspirated and can produce a severe chemical pneumonitis. This occurs in 25–40% of children who ingest kerosene and other petroleum distillates (140).

The management of this type of patient is controversial (see Question 39). However, aspiration has occurred in this patient as evidenced by his gagging, choking, and coughing. Therefore, a chest x-ray should be performed, and he should be monitored closely in the hospital.

37. What properties of a petroleum distillate influence its toxicity?

The three properties which influence petroleum distillate toxicity are viscosity, surface tension, and volatility. Agents with low viscosity are more likely to be aspirated into the lungs and penetrate further and more quickly than petroleum distillates with higher viscosity. Those agents with a viscosity of less than 45 SSU are more likely to pose an aspiration hazard (typical examples are naptha, gasoline, and kerosene). More viscous compounds, such as mineral oil and vegetable oil, do not normally pose a significant aspiration hazard. Those agents with low surface tension have a greater tendency to spread in the lung and are thus more toxic. An example of a petroleum distillate with low surface tension is mineral seal oil. Those petroleum distillates with high volatility tend to be more toxic than those with low volatility.

38. Describe the usual clinical course in petroleum distillate ingestion.

There is usually an initial burning sensation in the mouth and throat, followed by gagging and choking. Dyspnea and cyanosis may result if large amounts are aspirated. Continued coughing is common. The child may be lethargic and in respiratory distress with minimal auscultatory findings. Fever may develop within 30 minutes to several hours after ingestion. In severe cases, pulmonary edema, hemoptysis, cyanosis and death occur, usually within 24 hours. In milder cases, symptoms generally plateau at about 24 hours and subside over several days (141). Chest x-ray findings may be apparent after 30 minutes but often take several hours to materialize (142). Approximately 75% of patients ingesting petroleum distillates develop x-ray changes; however, only 25–50% of these develop symptoms (141–144).

39. Under what circumstances should the stomach be emptied in petroleum distillate ingestions?

This is a very controversial issue. What cannot be agreed upon is whether emptying of the stomach provides any therapeutic benefit. There are no well controlled, large population clinical trials that demonstrate whether stomach emptying is a necessary technique. If emptying of the stomach is deemed necessary, emesis is preferred to lavage unless other contraindications exist.

CAUSTICS

40. A 15-month-old child arrived at the emergency room 15 minutes after ingesting an unknown amount of granular drain cleaner (96% potassium hydroxide). He is crying and drooling. Physical examination reveals burns

on the child's lips, tongue, and oropharynx. Upon questioning, the mother states that she found the child with the open drain cleaner can and administered orange juice to the child as instructed on the product label. She then brought the child directly to the hospital. Esophagoscopy, which was performed about 6 hours after the ingestion, showed deep circumferential burns on the esophagus. The child was started on corticosteroids. When corrosive substances are ingested, what is their toxic hazard? How do acids and alkalies differ in their effects?

Alkaline corrosives produce a reaction on the gastrointestinal tract referred to as "liquefaction necrosis." This is a penetrating necrosis that may involve all layers of the gastrointestinal tract, leading to perforation. Upon initial ingestion, intense pain occurs and often makes swallowing and further ingestion difficult. The granular drain cleaner products usually produce severe oral and pharyngeal burns, and in 40–60% of these cases esophageal burns are present (145,146); however, the presence or absence of burns in the mouth is not a reliable indicator of esophageal involvement, and therefore, each patient must be thoroughly evaluated (145–147). About 50% of patients with documented esophageal burns will develop esophageal strictures (145).

The liquid drain cleaners produce a more severe reaction in that the damage often is not limited to the oral, pharyngeal, and esophageal areas but may include the stomach and upper portion of the small bowel (147,148). These products are also more likely to damage adjacent thoracic and abdominal organs (149). Death may occur as a result of hemorrhage, shock, asphyxia due to laryngeal or glottic edema, infection, or damage to thoracic organs (ie, heart and major vessels). Aspiration of the corrosive has been reported, resulting in severe pulmonary necrosis (150).

Acids, such as sulfuric, hydrochloric, nitric, and phosphoric (found in rust removers, toilet bowl cleaners, and similar products) produce an immediate, severe sensation of pain when ingested. They appear to have only a superficial effect on the esophageal mucosa, resulting in burns in only 6–20% of cases (151–153). In such cases the acid produces pylorospasm, trapping the acid in the antrum where it produces its destructive effect. Acids produce a "coagulation necrosis" which differs from "liquefaction necrosis" in that the supporting tissue structures are usually left intact.

Strictures in the pyloric region are late complications which may occur in as many as 80% of cases (154). Death usually occurs from the same complications as with the alkaline corrosives.

41. On the labels of many products containing strong alkalies, the suggested first aid therapy commonly includes the oral administration of dilute vinegar or citric acid solutions. Is this an appropriate first-aid measure?

The combination of an acid (citric or acetic) with an alkali produces an exothermic reaction. The heat produced from this reaction can be severe enough to produce thermal damage to the already damaged esophageal and oral mucosa. The first-aid treatment for this type of ingestion is immediate dilution of the chemical with milk. If milk is unavailable, then water can be used (155). Additionally, it has been shown experimentally that the damage to the mucosa occurs in the first 30–60 seconds after exposure. Therefore, dilution with a weak acid is at best a questionably effective treatment which can produce more severe damage as a result of the exothermic reaction (156,157).

42. How effective are steroids in reducing the complications of corrosive ingestion?

In the 1950's it was shown both experimentally and in clinical trials that steroids, 1–2 mg/kg of prednisone or equivalent, if started within 48 hours of the ingestion of an alkaline agent, decreased the incidence of stricture formation in cases where esophageal burns were demonstrated by esophagoscopy (158,159). Steroids will not stop stricture formation in severe cases but will make the esophagus more pliable and therefore, make dilatation by bougienage easier (160). The use of steroids, however, increases the risk of infection; therefore, patients must be closely monitored for signs of infection and receive appropriate antibiotic therapy when necessary (159).

The effectiveness of steroids in acid corrosive ingestion has not been studied.

SNAKE BITES

In the United States, the pit vipers (rattlesnakes, copperheads, and water moccasins) and the coral snakes are the indigenous snakes which are known to be poisonous. Several other species of snakes, including the Sonoran lyre snake, the

California lyre snake, the Texas lyre snake, the Mexican vine snake, the black striped snake, and the northern annulated snake, should be considered dangerous, because their bites may produce more than a local foreign body reaction (45–47).

Harmless snakes produce a bite characterized by two rows of tiny, shallow teeth wounds, while poisonous snakes produce bites with deep fang punctures connected by a row of very small teeth wounds. Pit vipers have long, retractable fangs that allow the snake to attach to varying shaped surfaces and therefore are very effective at producing envenomation. The coral snakes have short, nonretractable fangs and cannot bite flat surfaces. Most coral snake bites result in no envenomation. The lyre snakes have rear fixed fangs that rarely produce severe or venomous bites (46,47).

Venomous snake bites that show signs of envenomation (rapid swelling, discoloration, and pain) should be treated with the following basic steps: Put the victim at rest; give the victim reassurance; immobilize the affected part; watch for any untoward reactions; and transport to a medical facility as soon as possible (47).

Considerable controversy surrounds the use of incision and suction and the application of cold to the bite. Incision and suction are of no value in coral snake bites (47). In rattle snake bites, if the patient is within 20–30 minutes of medical care, a wide constriction band should be placed immediately proximal to the wound, tight enough to inhibit lymph flow but not blood flow, and the patient should be transported. If the patient is more than 20–30 minutes from medical care, incision and suction may be started. It is of no use if delayed more than 15 minutes after the bite. A 1 cm incision, 3 mm deep should be made through each fangmark, and then suction should be applied. Most snakebites do not happen in areas remote from medical care. In one review of 200 cases, the average time from bite to hospitalization was 34 minutes. Thus, incision and suction will rarely be indicated (47). Surgical excision of the wound area to remove the venom has been used, but this approach is controversial and is not widely accepted.

Administration of antivenin is the single most effective therapy available. The most severe complication of its use is the precipitation of an anaphylactic reaction, because the antivenin is prepared from horse serum. Therefore, the patient must be given a test dose of horse serum prior to administration of the antivenin to determine any sensitivity. This is a conjunctival or skin test. The amount of antivenom required depends upon the seriousness of the envenomation. Severe cases may require more than 20 vials of antivenin. Antivenin should be given intravenously. Administration of antivenin into or around the bite is no longer suggested. Additional therapy aimed at maintenance of a patent airway, control of pain and infection, and local wound care are also necessary (46–49). Serum sickness following antivenin therapy is also seen.

Coral snake bites produce symptoms in a very short period of time, usually 20 minutes. The bite produces minimal pain and usually no local reaction. The venom is a neurotoxin that produces paralysis. Death occurs as a result of respiratory paralysis. Because of the rapid onset of symptoms, local therapy of the bite is not useful. Administration of the specific coral snake antivenin is the only effective treatment (46–49).

ARTHROPOD BITES AND STINGS

Spiders. Of the spiders, only two species, the black widow and the brown recluse, are capable of producing severe toxicity. The black widow venom is neurotoxic, producing ascending paralysis and destruction of peripheral nerve endings. Severe poisonings are characterized by coma, respiratory paralysis, and cardiovascular collapse. Treatment includes supportive care and administration of the specific antivenin in the following patients: victims under 16 years of age or over 60 years of age, victims with hypertension, or those with symptoms of severe envenomation. The patients should be given one ampule of antivenin intravenously (49). Other patients may require only analgesics and muscle relaxants.

The brown recluse spider venom has hemolytic and necrotizing properties. The wound that develops following a bite is ulcerating and does not heal for weeks or months. Treatment is symptomatic and is aimed at treating local infections that may prolong healing (49).

Scorpions. Scorpions are the other group of venomous arthropods that produce significant problems. In the United States only two species are dangerous. All others are relatively harmless. These two species are *Centuroides sculpturatus* and *Vejovis spinigerus,* and they are found only in southwestern Arizona. The venom of *Centuroides sculpturatus* is extremely toxic, with an LD_{50} in mice of 0.096 mg per kilogram of body weight. The adult venom gland contains 0.5 mg of venom. The *Vejovis spinigerus* venom is less toxic but similar in effects. The sting of these scorpions provokes a reaction characterized by erythema and swelling at the site of the sting, flushing, fasciculations, increased parasympathetic activity, hyperirritability, hypertonicity, hypertension, weakness, and paresthesias of the affected extremity. In severe cases, paralysis and respiratory distress can be seen. Treatment involves supportive care and the use of the specific antivenin in the young and very old or those with hypertension. Healthy adult patients may require only muscle relaxants and supportive care.

References

1. Anon: Accident Facts, National Safety Council, 1978.
2. Anon: Natl Clgh Poison Cont Cent Bull. 1981; 25:1.
3. Schultz W: Personal Communication. 1981.
4. Gosselin R et al: *Clinical Toxicology of Commercial Products,* 4th ed, Williams and Wilkins, Baltimore, MD, 1976.
5. Barer J et al: Fatal salt poisoning from salt used as an emetic. Am J Dis Child. 1973; 125:889.
6. Carter RF et al. Fatal salt poisoning due to gastric lavage with hypertonic saline. Med J Aust. 1971; 1:539.
7. DeGenaro F et al: Salt—a dangerous antidote. J Pediatr. 1971; 78:1048.
8. Finberg LF et al: Mass accidental salt poisoning in infancy. JAMA. 1963; 184:187.
9. Laurence BH et al: Hypernatremia following a saline emetic. Med J Aust. 1969; 1:1301.
10. Robertson W: A further warning on the use of salt as an emetic agent. J Pediatr. 1971; 79:877.
11. Ward DJ: Fatal hypernatremia after a saline emetic. Br Med J. 1963; 2:432.
12. Morrelli HF: Rational therapy of drug overdosage, in *Clinical Pharmacology* edited by K Melmon and H Morrelli, MacMillan Co, New York, 1972.
13. Manoguerra AS et al: Rapid emesis from high dose ipecac syrup in adults and children intoxicated with antiemetics or other drugs. Am J Hosp Pharm. 1978; 35:1360.
14. Thoman ME et al: Ipecac syrup in antiemetic ingestion. JAMA. 1966; 196:433.
15. Molinas: Natl Clgh Poison Control Cent Bull (March-April) 1966.
16. Ng RC et al: Emergency treatment of petroleum distillate and turpentine ingestion. Can Med Assoc J. 1974; 111:537.
17. Allport RB: Ipecac not innocuous. Am J Dis Child. 1959; 98:786.
18. Bates T et al: Ipecac poisoning. Am J Dis Child. 1962; 103:169.
19. Speer J et al: Ipecacuanha poisoning—another fatal case. Lancet. 1963; 1:475.
20. Varipapa R et al: Effect of milk on ipecac-induced emesis. N Engl J Med. 1977; 296:112.
21. Bukis OB et al: Results of forcing fluids: pre- versus post-ipecac. Vet and Human Toxicol. 1978; 20:90.
22. Spiegel RW: The effect of temperature on concurrently administered fluid on the onset of ipecac induced emesis. Clin Toxicol. 1979; 14:281.
23. Eisenga BH: Evaluation of the effect of motility on syrup of ipecac-induced emesis. Vet Human Toxicol. 1978; 20:462.
24. MacLeod J: Ipecac intoxication—use of cardiac pacemaker in management. N Engl J Med. 1963; 268:1467.
25. Robertson WO: Syrup of ipecac associated fatality: a case report. Vet and Human Toxicol. 1979; 21:87.
26. Schofferman JA: A clinical comparison of syrup of ipecac and apomorphine: use in adults. J Am Coll Emer Phys. 1976; 5:22.
27. Holtzman NA et al: Evaluation of serum copper following copper sulfate as an emetic. Pediatrics. 1968; 42:189.
28. Stein RS et al: Death after use of cupric sulfate as an emetic. JAMA. 1976; 235:801.
29. Abdallah AH et al: A comparison of the efficacy of emetics and stomach lavage. Am J Dis Child. 1967; 113:571.
30. Arnold FJ et al: Evaluation of the efficacy of lavage and induced emesis in treatment of salicylate poisoning. Pediatrics. 1959; 23:286.
31. Boxer L et al: Comparison of ipecac-induced emesis with gastric lavage in the treatment of acute salicylate ingestion. Pediatric Pharmacol Ther. 1969; 84:800.
32. Goldstein LI: Emesis vs lavage for drug ingestion. JAMA. 1969; 208:2162.
33. Jenis EH et al: Acute meprobamate poisoning. JAMA. 1969; 207:361.
34. Picchioni AL: Activated charcoal—a neglected antidote. Pediatr Clin North Am. 1970; 17:535.
35. Peterson C et al: Methanol poisoning: the influence of activated charcoal on oral ethanol therapy. Presented at the ASHP Midyear Clinical Meeting, San Francisco 1980.
36. Manes M: Easily swallowed formulations of antidote charcoals. Clin Toxicol. 1974; 7:355.
37. Coovey DO: *Activated Charcoal—Antidotal and Other Medicinal Uses,* Marcel Dekker Inc., New York, 1980.
38. Mayersohn M et al: Evaluation of a charcoal-sorbitol mixture as an antidote for oral aspirin overdoses. Clin Toxicol. 1977; 11:561.
39. Schlotz ED et al: Evaluation of five activated charcoal formulations for inhibition of aspirin absorption and palatability in man. Am J Hosp Pharm. 1978; 35:1355.
40. Braithwaite RA: The in vitro and in vivo evaluation of activated charcoal as adsorbent for tricyclic antidepressants. Br J Clin Pharmacol. 1978; 5:369.
41. Coovey DO: A "superactive" charcoal for antidotal use in poisonings. Clin Toxicol. 1977; 11:387.

42. Dowling S et al: Effect of delayed administration of ac-
    tivated charcoal on nortriptyline absorption. Eur J Clin
    Pharmacol. 1978; 14:445.

43. Picchioni AL et al: Activated charcoal versus "univer-
    sal antidote" for poisons. Toxicol Appl Pharmacol. 1966;
    8:447.

44. Coovey DO: In vitro evidence for ipecac inactivation by
    activated charcoal. J Pharm Sci. 1978; 67:426.

45. Vale J et al: Use of charcoal hemoperfusion in the man-
    agement of severely poisoned patients. Br Med J. 1975;
    1:5.

46. Oehme FW et al: Toxins of animal origin, in *Toxicology,
    The Basic Science of Poisons,* edited by L Casarett and
    J Doull, MacMillan Co., New York, 1975.

47. Russell F: *Snake Venom Poisoning.* J B Lippincott Co,
    Philadelphia, 1980, p 45–86, 264, 269, 270, 306–321.

48. Rumack BH: Poisindex management of snake bite. Mi-
    cromedex, Denver, 1981.

49. Russell FE: Venom poisoning. Ration Drug Ther. 1971;
    5:1.

50. Rumack BH: Poisindex management on plants—amyg-
    dalin. Micromedex, Denver, 1981.

51. Rumack BH: Poisindex management on plants—anti-
    cholinergic. Micromedex, Denver, 1981.

52. Rumack BH: Poisindex management on plants—car-
    diac glycoside. Micromedex, Denver, 1981.

53. Rumack BH: Poisindex management on plants—colchi-
    cine. Micromedex, Denver, 1981.

54. Rumack BH: Poisindex management on plants—nico-
    tine. Micromedex, Denver, 1981.

55. Rumack BH: Poisindex management on plants—oxa-
    late. Micromedex, Denver, 1981.

56. Rumack BH: Poisindex management on plants—sola-
    nine. Micromedex, Denver, 1981.

57. Rumack BH: Poisindex management on plants—stim-
    ulants. Micromedex, Denver, 1981.

58. Rumack BH: Poisindex management on plants—toxal-
    bumin. Micromedex, Denver, 1981.

59. Done AK: Salicylate intoxication. Significance of mea-
    suring salicylate in blood. Pediatrics. 1960; 26:800.

60. Ibid.

61. Matthew H: Gastric aspiration and lavage. Clin Toxi-
    col. 1970; 3:179.

62. Decker W et al: Inhibition of aspirin absorption by ac-
    tivated charcoal and apomorphine. Clin Pharmacol
    Therap. 1969; 10:710.

63. Smith MJH: The metabolic basis of the major symp-
    toms in acute salicylate intoxication. Clin Toxicol. 1968;
    1:387.

64. Thurston JH et al: Reduced brain glucose with normal
    plasma glucose in salicylate poisoning. J Clin Invest.
    1970; 49:2139.

65. Hrnicek G et al: Pulmonary edema and salicylate in-
    toxication. JAMA. 1974; 230:866.

66. Hormaecher E et al: Hypovolemia, pulmonary edema
    and protein changes in severe salicylate poisoning. Am
    J Med. 1979; 66:1046.

67. Temple AR et al: Salicylate poisoning complicated by
    fluid retention. Clin Toxicol. 1976; 9:61.

68. James JA et al: Experimental salicylate intoxication.
    1. Comparison of exchange transfusion, intermittent
    peritoneal lavage and hemodialysis as a means for re-
    moving salicylate. Pediatrics. 1962; 29:442.

69. Leikin SL et al: The use of exchange transfusion in
    salicylate intoxication. J Pediatr. 1960; 57:715.

70. Oliver TK et al: The prompt treatment of salicylism
    with sodium bicarbonate. Am J Dis Child. 1960; 99:553.

71. Whitten CF et al: Managing salicylate poisoning in
    children. Am J Dis Child. 1961; 101:178.

72. Winchester JF et al: Extracorporeal treatment of sali-
    cylate or acetaminophen poisoning—is there a role? Arch
    Intern Med. 1981; 141:370.

73. Flower JF et al: Analgesic-antipyretics, anti-inflam-
    matory agents, and drugs employed in the treatment of
    gout, in *The Pharmacological Basis of Therapeutics,* 6th
    ed, edited by AG Gilman and L Goodman, MacMillan
    Co., New York, 1980.

74. Mitchell J et al: Acetaminophen induced hepatic necro-
    sis. I. Role of drug metabolism. J Pharmacol Exper Ther.
    1973; 187:185.

75. Potter W et al: Acetaminophen induced hepatic necro-
    sis. III. Cytochrome p-450 mediated covalent binding in
    vitro. J Pharmacol Exper Ther. 1973; 187:203.

76. Rumack GH et al: Acetaminophen poisoning and tox-
    icity. Pediatrics. 1975; 55:871.

77. Prescott LF et al: Plasma paracetemol half-life and he-
    patic necrosis in patients with paracetamol overdosage.
    Lancet. 1971; 1:519.

78. Prescott LF et al: Successful treatment of severe para-
    cetamol overdosage with cysteamine. Lancet. 1974;
    1:588.

79. Levy G et al: Effect of activated charcoal on acetami-
    nophen absorption. Pediatrics. 1976; 58:432.

80. Chinouth RW et al: N-acetylycysteine adsorption by ac-
    tivated charcoal. Vet Human Toxicol. 1980; 22:392.

81. Klein-Schwartz W et al: Adsorption of antidotes for ace-
    taminophen poisoning (methionine and N-acetylcy-
    steine) by activated charcoal. Clin Toxicol. (In press.)

82. North D et al: The effect of activated charcoal on N-
    acetylcystein serum levels in human subjects. Pre-
    sented at the AAPC-AACT Annual Meeting, Minne-
    apolis, August, 1980.

83. Crome P et al: Oral methionine in the treatment of
    severe paracetamol (Acetaminophen) overdose. Lancet.
    1976; 2:829.

84. Prescot LF et al: Cysteamine, methionine, and pencil-
    lamine in the treatment of paracetamol poisoning. Lan-
    cet. 1976; 2:109.

85. Vale JA et al: Treatment of acetaminophen poisoning -
    the use of oral methionine. Arch Intern Med. 1981;
    141:394.

86. Piperno E et al: Reversal of experimental paracetamol
    toxicosis with N-acetylcysteine. Lancet. 1976; 2:738.

87. Lyons L et al: Treatment of acetaminophen overdose
    with N-acetyl-cysteine. N Engl J Med. 1977; 296:174.

88. Gates TN: *Management of Acetaminophen Over-dose
    With N-Acetylcysteine,* McNeil Consumer Products Co.,
    p 7.

89. Rumack BH et al: Acetaminophen overdose - 662 cases
    with evaluation of oral acetylcysteine therapy. Arch In-
    tern Med. 1981; 141:380.

90. Prescott LF: Treatment of severe acetaminophen poi-
    soning with intravenous acetylcysteine. Arch Intern
    Med. 1981; 141:386.

91. Walton NG et al: Anaphylactoid reaction to N-acetyl-
    cysteine. Lancet. 1979; 2:1298.

92. Farid NR: Haemodialysis in paracetamol self-poisoning. Lancet. 1972; 2:396.

93. Stein B et al: Dixarit overdose: the problem of attractive tablets. Br Med J. 1978; 2:667.

94. Conner CS et al: Clonidine overdose: A review. Am J Hosp Pharm. 1979; 36:906.

95. Amery A et al: Influence of clonidine (Catapressan-ST 155) on the muscle blood flow in the legs of hypertensive patients (Antagonism of Tolazoline). Angiologica. 1970; 7:296.

96. Hunyor SN: Clonidine overdose. Br Med J. 1975; 4:23.

97. Ramsey L: Treatment of clonidine overdose. Br Med J. 1975; 4:283.

98. Wing LMH et al: Clonidine overdose. Br Med J. 1975; 4:408.

99. Buiumsohn A et al: Seizures and intraventricular defect in propranolol poisoning. Ann Intern Med. 1979; 91:860.

100. Wermut W et al: Suicidal attempt with propranolol. Br Med J. 1973; 13:591.

101. Gault R et al: A death involving propranolol (Inderal). Clin Toxicol. 1977; 11:295.

102. Kristinsson J et al: A case of fatal propranolol intoxication. Acta Pharmacol Toxicol. 1977; 41:190.

103. Laegerfelt J et al. Attempted suicide with 5.1 g of propranolol. Acta Med Scand. 1976; 199:517.

104. Kosiaki EJ et al: Glucagon and propranolol (Inderal) toxicity. N Engl J Med. 1971; 285:1325.

105. Jacobs J et al: Acute iron intoxication. N Engl J Med. 1965; 273:1124.

106. Brown RK et al: Mechanism of acute ferrous sulfate poisoning. Can Med Assoc J. 1955; 73:192.

107. Reissman KR et al: Acute intestinal iron intoxication. II. Metabolic, circulatory and respiratory effects of absorbed iron salts. Blood. 1955; 10:46.

108. Greengard J: Iron poisoning in children. Clin Toxicol. 1975; 8:575.

109. Manoguerra AS: Iron poisoning cases treated in a metropolitan general hospital. Presented at the American Association of Poison Control Centers - American Academy of Clinical Toxicology Annual Meeting, Kansas City, Aug. 9, 1975.

110. Rumack BH: Poisindex management on iron. Micromedex, Denver, 1980.

111. Bachrach L et al: Iron poisoning: complications of hypertonic lavage therapy. J Pediatr. 1979; 94:147.

112. Geffner ME et al: Phosphate poisoning complicating treatment for iron ingestion. Am J Dis Child. 1980; 134:509.

113. Peterson C et al: Emergency gastrotomy for acute iron poisoning. Ann Intern Med. 1980; 9:262.

114. Robotham J et al: Acute iron poisoning: A review. Am J Dis Child. 1980; 134:875.

115. Fielding J et al: Estimation of ferrioxamine and deferoxamine in urine. Clin Path. 1964; 17:395.

116. Anon: unpublished case reports. Regional Poison Center. University of California, San Diego, 1979–1980.

117. Whitten C et al: Studies in acute iron poisoning. I: Desferrioxamine in the treatment of acute iron poisonings; clinical observations, experimental studies and theoretical considerations. Pediatrics. 1965; 36:322.

118. Winchester J et al: Dialysis and hemoperfusion of poisons and drugs—update. Trans Am Soc Artif Intern Organs. 1977; 23:762.

119. Schreiner GH: Barbiturate intoxication evaluation of therapy including dialysis in a large series selectively referred because of severity. Arch Intern Med. 1966; 117:224.

120. Matthew H: Barbiturates. Clin Toxicol. 1975; 8:495.

121. Goodman J et al: Barbiturate intoxication. West J Med. 1976; 124:179.

122. Pond S et al: Pharmacokinetics of hemoperfusion for drug overdose. Clin Pharmacokinetics. 1979; 4:329.

123. Goodman JM et al: Barbiturate intoxication. Morbidity and mortality. West J Med. 1976; 124:179–186.

124. Chazan J et al: Clinical spectrum of glutethimide intoxication. JAMA. 1969; 208:837.

125. Hansen AR et al: Glutethimide poisoning. N Engl J Med. 1975; 292:250.

126. Clemesen C et al: Therapeutic trends in the treatment of barbiturate poisoning—the Scandinavian method. Clin Pharmacol Ther. 1961; 2:220.

127. Jaffe JH et al: Opioid analgesics and antagonists, the Pharmacological Basis of Therapeutics, 6th ed, edited by AG Gilman, L Goodman and A Gilman. MacMillan Co., New York, 1980.

128. Rumack BH: Poisindex management of opiates. Micromedex, Denver, 1980.

129. Levine SB: Pulmonary edema and oral ingestion of methadone. JAMA. 1973; 95:330.

130. Malek SK et al: Pulmonary edema and oral ingestion of methadone. JAMA. 1972; 221:915.

131. Tenant F: Complications of propoxyphene abuse. Arch Intern Med. 1973; 132:191.

132. Rumack BH: Anticholinergic poisoning, treatment with physostigmine. Pediatrics. 1973; 52:449.

133. Masters AB: Delayed death in imipramine poisoning. Br Med J. 1967; 3:30.

134. Slovis DG et al: Physostigmine therapy in acute tricyclic antidepressant poisoning. Clin Toxicol. 1971; 4:451.

135. Spiker DG et al: Tricyclic antidepressant overdose; clinical presentation and plasma levels. Clin Pharmacol Ther. 1975; 18:539.

136. Rumack BH: Physostigmine: rational use. J Am Coll Emer Phys. 1976; 5:541.

137. Callahan M: Tricyclic antidepressant overdose. J Am Coll Emer Phys. 1979; 8:413.

138. Hoffman J et al: Bicarbonate therapy for dysrhythmia and hypotension in tricyclic antidepressant overdose. West J Med. 1981; 134:60.

139. Hagerman G et al: Reversal of tricyclic antidepressant-induced cardiac conduction abnormalities by phenytoin. Ann Emerg Med. 1981; 10:82.

140. Eade NR et al: Hydrocarbon pneumonitis. Pediatrics for the Clinician. 1974; 54:351.

141. Foley JC et al: Kerosene poisoning in children. Radiology. 1954; 62:817.

142. Daeschner CW et al: Hydrocarbon pneumonitis. Pediatr Clin North Am. 1957; 4:423.

143. Olstad RB et al: Kerosene intoxication. Am J Dis Child. 1950; 79:623.

144. Press E et al: Co-operative kerosene study; evaluation of gastric lavage and other factors in the treatment of accidental ingestion of petroleum distillate products. Pediatrics. 1962; 29:648.

145. Alford BR et al: Chemical burns of the mouth, pharynx, and esophagus. Ann Otol Rhinol Laryngol. 1959; 68:122.

146. Cardona JC et al: Current management of corrosive esophagitis: an evaluation of results in 239 cases. Ann Otol Rhinol Laryngol. 1971; 80:521.

147. Cello J et al: Liquid caustic ingestion. Arch Intern Med. 1980; 140:501.

148. Ray JF et al: Lye ingestion. JAMA. 1974; 229:765.

149. Hay JF et al: The natural history of liquid lye ingestions. Arch Surg. 1974; 109:436.

150. Danrigal A et al: Necrose totale du poumon par caustique. Med Leg Domm Corpor. 1962; 42:68.

151. Boikan WS: Gastric sequelae of corrosive poisoning. Arch Intern Med. 1930; 46:342.

152. Gray HK et al: Pyloric stenosis caused by ingestion of corrosive substances. Surg Clin North Am. 1948; 28:1041.

153. Penner G: Acid ingestion: toxicology and treatment. Ann Intern Med. 1980; 9:374.

154. Karon AB: The delayed gastric syndrome with pyloric stenosis and achlorhydria following the ingestion of acid—a definite clinical entity. Am J Dig Dis. 1962; 7:1041.

155. Rumack BH: Poisindex management on alkaline corrosives. Micromedex, Denver, 1980.

156. Gago O et al: Aggressive surgical treatment for caustic injury of the esophagus and stomach. Ann Thorac Surg. 1972; 13:243.

157. Leape LL: New liquid drain cleaners. Clin Toxicol. 1974; 7:109.

158. Krey H: On treatment of corrosive lesions in esophagus; experimental study. Acta Otolaryngol. 1952; 102 (suppl):1.

159. Ray ES: Cortisone therapy of lye burns of the esophagus. J Pediatr. 1956; 49:394.

160. Haller JA et al: The comparative effect of current therapy on experimental caustic burns of the esophagus. Pediatrics. 1964; 34:236.

Index

athlete's foot, topical 1193
candida endocarditis 839
candida esophagitis 845
cryptococcal meningitis 847
Midrin 1105
Migraine 1103–1107
clinical presentation
classic 1104
common 1104, 1106
drug-induced
estrogens 1104
oral contraceptives 1261
treatment
abortive 1105–1106
prophylaxis 1106–1107
Milk-alkali syndrome 415–416,
553
also see Antacids, calcium
Milk allergy and intolerance 1494
Milk of magnesia, absorption 108
Miltown. See Meprobamate
Mineral oil 108–109
effects on
prothrombin levels 109
vitamin A absorption 109
interaction with docusate 109
use in hemorrhoids 108
Mineralocorticoids, replacement
therapy 1286
Minimal brain dysfunction. See
Attention deficit disorders
Minimum bactericidal
concentration 728–729
Mini-pills 1242, 1243, 1263–1264
also see Oral contraceptives
Minipres. See Prazosin
Minizide. See Prazosin
Minocycline
use in
acne 1189
gonorrhea, uncomplicated 790
nongonococcal urethritis 787
prophylaxis of meningococcal
meningitis 711
Minoxidil
adverse effects
table of 132
ECG abnormalities 143
heart failure 132, 176
contraindications/precautions
132
use in hypertension 132,
142–143
Miotics
also see specific agents
topical preparations, table 1206
use in glaucoma 1205, 1206,
1208–1210, 1211–1212

Misonidazole
also see Antineoplastic drugs
contraindications/precautions
dehydration 935
hepatic dysfunction 935
renal dysfunction 935
pharmacokinetics 935
Mithramycin
also see Antineoplastic drugs
adverse effects
emesis 917
fever 912
hepatotoxicity 527, 919
myelosuppression 908
nephrotoxicity 914
vesicant reactions 915
contraindications/precautions
renal dysfunction 927, 935
pharmacokinetics 935
use in hypercalcemia 606,
922–923
Mitomycin-C
also see Antineoplastic drugs
adverse effects
bone marrow suppression
906–909
hepatotoxicity 919
pulmonary toxicity 375, 911
vesicant reactions 915
pharmacokinetics 935
Moban. See Molindone
Molindone 992
Molsidomine 257
Monoamine oxidase inhibitors
also see specific agents
adverse effects
hepatotoxicity 527
drug interactions 1026
levodopa 1120
mechanism of action 1026
toxicity 1026
use in
depression 1026
Parkinson's 1121–1122
Monocytes 28
MOPP 904
Morning-after pill 1242, 1244
Morning sickness
also see Nausea; Vomiting;
Antiemetics
associated with pregnancy
92–94
physiological basis 93
treatment
antihistamines 93–34
Bendectin 93–94
cyclizine 93–94
nonpharmacological 92–93

phenothiazines 93
phosphorylated syrups 89, 92
Morphine 51–54
also see Narcotics
abstinence syndrome 1043–1044
addiction in medical setting
1044
administration, intravenous 267,
921
adverse effects
allergic reactions 56
dysphoria 57
hypotension 267
nausea and vomiting 54, 96
respiratory depression 60–61
sedation 53
dosing 51, 52–54, 267
intravenous 54, 921
oral 52–54
drug interactions
dexedrine 53
methylphenidate 53
effectiveness orally 52–53
effect on hemodynamic
parameters 292, 298, 308,
311–312
pharmacokinetics 54–55
preparations, oral 52–53
tolerance 53
use in
cancer pain 52–54, 921
cardiogenic shock 292, 298
migraine 1105
myocardial infarction 58, 267
pulmonary edema 308,
311–312
Motion sickness
also see Nausea; Vomiting
tolerance 92
treatment
amphetamine 92
anticholinergics 87–92
antihistamine 87–92
phenothiazines 87–92
scopolamine 92
sympathomimetics 87–92
Motrin. See Ibuprofen
Moxalactam
also see Cephalosporins
adverse effects 674–675
comparative pharmacology 673
efficacy 674
Moxam. See Moxalactam
MTX. See Methotrexate
Mucolytics, use in cystic fibrosis
370
Mucomyst. See Acetylcysteine
Mumps vaccine 1480–1486